MENDELIAN INHERITANCE IN MAN

MENDELIAN INHERITANCE IN MAN

CATALOGS OF AUTOSOMAL DOMINANT, AUTOSOMAL RECESSIVE, AND X-LINKED PHENOTYPES

THIRD EDITION

Victor A. McKusick, M.D.

The Johns Hopkins Press

Baltimore and London

To my wife, Dr. Anne B. McKusick

The Johns Hopkins Press, Baltimore, Maryland 21218
The Johns Hopkins Press Ltd., London

Library of Congress Catalog Card Number 71-164655
ISBN-0-8018-1296-8

Originally published, 1966
Second edition, 1968
Third edition, 1971

CONTENTS

FOREWORD

These catalogs had their inception in 1960 when, in connection with an inquiry into the genetics of the X chromosome, it seemed advisable to examine the question "What genetic information is carried by the X chromosome of man?" The catalog of X-linked traits in man was first published in 1962 (McKusick, 1962B). Two categories of traits were included—those for which X-linkage was considered proved and those for which the evidence is in various degrees suggestive but not conclusive. All traits, rare and common, were included.

In 1962 a study of genetic disorders in Old Order Amish communities was initiated. The question then arose "What rare recessive disorders might one expect to encounter in inbred groups such as these?" Inbred populations afford an opportunity to detect "new" rare recessive phenotypes in man. A catalog of known recessive phenotypes would obviously be useful in recognizing these. The catalog was confined mainly to rare phenotypes—that is to say, those which in outbred populations have a homozygote frequency of 1 in 1,000 or less.

By 1963 the complexity of the catalog of recessives prompted adoption of computer methods for assembling, revising, and indexing.

In 1964 a catalog of dominant phenotypes was undertaken—with some hesitation because of the magnitude of the undertaking and the questionable status of a large number of traits for which "dominant inheritance with incomplete penetrance" is suggested. Again, the catalog was confined mainly to uncommon traits. "Uncommon" however, was not precisely defined, so that some morphologic traits were included. Furthermore, anomalous hemoglobins, red cell antigenic types, leukocyte types, and serum protein types—co-dominant traits—were included.

As in the original catalog of X-linked traits, two classes of entries have been made in each of the three catalogs. In the case of those marked with an asterisk, the particular mode of inheritance is, in the writer's opinion, quite certain, according to the criteria outlined below. In the case of the others the evidence for the particular mode of inheritance is judged to be incomplete, yet sufficiently strong to warrant inclusion. It is considered important that these less certain items be included so that further families will be studied as they come to attention. In some instances no asterisk is given, not because the mode of inheritance is not established, but because it is not clear that the given phenotype is distinct from that described in another entry.

Each entry consists of three parts: (1) a preferred designation; (2) a brief description of the phenotype, with a resume of genetic information; and (3) key references. An attempt has been made to select references which are up-to-date and/or include particularly useful discussions of the genetics. The catalogs must be considered primarily a bibliographic guide. The discussion of each entry is necessarily brief.

The definitions of *dominant* and *recessive* used in the preparation of these catalogs are those given by Mendel, who introduced the terms: "Those characters which are transmitted entire, or almost unchanged in the hybridization, and therefore in themselves constitute the characters of the hybrid, are termed the dominant, and those which become latent in the process recessive." Following Mendel, care has been taken always to use the terms "dominant" and "recessive" as attributes of a character—that is, a phenotype—and to have a specified phenotype in mind. The question, then, is whether the specific phenotype is observed in the heterozygote or only in the homozygote. Depending on the answer, the specifically defined trait is considered dominant or recessive, respectively.

Many of the phenotypes for which a particular mode of inheritance is indicated as proved might not meet criteria that experimental geneticists would be likely to lay down. A rare phenotype transmitted through several successive generations in a family without consanguinity, affecting both males and females and transmitted by both males and females, with male-to-male transmission, is considered autosomal dominant. When most of the cases are sporadic and few affected persons reproduce because of the gravity of the condition, the possibility that the nonfamilial cases represent the result of a new dominant mutation is supported by the finding of elevated mean paternal age (for example, Apert's syndrome). In the case of a rare phenotype affecting brothers and sisters with normal parents but with instances of parental consanguinity, recessive inheritance has usually been considered very likely. In a "founder population" like the Amish, the ability to trace the ancestry of both parents in all cases back to a single common ancestral couple lends support to the recessive hypothesis. If the phenotype was shown to result from an enzyme deficiency, and especially if both parents showed a partial deficiency, recessive inheritance was considered proved. In the case of oroticaciduria, this judgment was made even when only one homozygote had been observed. Pedigrees showing multiple affected males in two or more sibships connected through females were taken as evidence of X-linked recessive inheritance. Pedigrees revealing a pattern in which all daughters but no sons among the offspring of affected males were affected were taken as evidence of X-linked dominant inheritance. X-linked dominant traits may be mistakenly labeled autosomal dominant, and in early stages, when only a few cases are known, X-linked recessive inheritance may suggest autosomal recessive inheritance. The difficulties of distinguishing X-linked inheritance from male-limited autosomal dominant inheritance (when affected males do not reproduce) are illustrated by disorders such as the testicular feminization syndrome.

Mendelism can be simulated by numerous mechanisms. Multifactorial inheritance is one (Edwards, 1960). Chromosomal aberrations undetectable by present methods are another. Many instances are now known in which, because a parent carries a "balanced" chromosomal rearrangement, two or more offspring suffer from a deficiency or excess of chromosomal material. There is every reason to think that some chromosomal rearrangements are beyond our capacity for detection. SC disease, as well as S-thal and E-thal diseases, is interesting because a characteristic phenotype is present which differs from that resulting from the homozygous state of either gene. In terms of the Mendelian definition of *dominant* and *recessive* these phenotypes cannot be classified as either. There may be some conditions listed in the recessive catalog (because they occur in multiple sibs with normal parents) which when the precise situation is known will be found to be caused by two different mutant alleles at the same locus. This form of disease should not show increased parental consanguinity (Haldane, 1938).

The laboratory, of course, has contributed heavily to the nosology of genetic disease. Studies of fibroblasts have confirmed the distinctness of several mucopolysaccharidoses which had been considered separate on other grounds; for example, co-cultivation of fibroblasts from patients with MPS I (Hurler syndrome) and MPS III (Sanfilippo syndrome) results in mutual correction of the metabolic defects. Although MPS I and MPS V (Scheie syndrome) are also phenotypically distinct, when grown in mixed culture, fibroblasts from patients with these two disorders do not show cross-correction (Wiesmann and Neufeld, 1970). This may indicate that the responsible genes are alleles. The mutation may be in the same codon or in different codons of the particular cistron. I prefer the terms *euallele* and *heteroallele,* respectively, for these two situations (Serra, 1965). Some of the patients with difficult-to-classify disturbances of mucopolysaccharide metabolism may be so-called compounds (heteroallelic homozygotes)— for example, having both the Hurler and the Scheie alleles.

Women with phenylketonuria may have several mentally retarded offspring apparently because of ill-effects of high phenylalanine concentrations on the fetal brain. This is a form of familial and genetic disease based on the genotype of the mother rather than on that of the affected individual. It is to be recalled that before its serologic basis was discovered, erythroblastosis fetalis was thought by some to be a Mendelizing disorder (Macklin, 1937). Congenital infection—for example, toxoplasmosis, listerellosis, rubella, cytomegalic virus disease, and of course syphilis—can affect multiple sibs. The rubella virus acquired *in utero* is known to persist for several years after birth, and at least one instance is known of a rubella-damaged woman giving birth to a rubella-damaged infant (Menser *et al.*, 1968).

The phenotypic simulation of Mendelian disorders by fetal infections is an example of phenocopy. We (McKusick *et al.*, 1966) have observed a recessive syndrome of microcephaly and chorioretinopathy which rather precisely mimics toxoplasmosis. Goldberg and Hardy (1971) studied a family of X-linked cataract in which cytomegalic virus found in the lens of the proband seemed to be the cause of the cataract until a second affected male was born and the mother was found to have sutural cataracts typical of the carrier state. Usher's syndrome (pigmentary retinal degeneration and congenital deafness) is rather closely simulated by rubella infection. In some of their cardiovascular aspects, both the hypercalcemia syndrome and rubella infection closely match the autosomal dominant type of stenotic arterial disease of which supravalvar aortic stenosis is a hallmark.

In dealing with recessives, especially when the parents are known to be related, the problem sometimes arises as to whether two manifestations constitute a syndrome produced by the homozygous state of one mutant gene or occur together in two or more sibs because the parents were both carriers of the separate mutant genes, one for each manifestation. It is possible that some of the rare syndromes which appear as unasterisked entries in the recessive catalog represent the latter phenomenon.

For both applied and scientific reasons I have considered it worthwhile to invest considerable effort in assembling and updating these catalogs. In addition to those already listed, these reasons include the following:

1.   Genetic counseling and the management of hereditary problems demand accurate diagnosis and familiarity with the experience reported in the literature. Genetic heterogeneity—fundamentally distinct hereditary entities that are phenotypically similar—is often not taken into account adequately in connection with genetic counseling.

2.   Genetic disorders give us insight into the normal. These catalogs of hereditary traits are like photographic negatives from which a positive picture of man's genetic constitution can be made. For example, the fact that agammaglobulinemia and classic hemophilia are X-linked disorders tells us that the X chromosome carries loci concerned with the synthesis of gamma globulin and the antihemophilic factor. As complete knowledge as possible of the normal genetic constitution of man is bound to be useful in the long run. Physicians have a unique opportunity to contribute to the knowledge of what Richard Lewontin referred to as "man's mutational repertoire."

Table I presents information on the numerical status of genetic nosology in 1958 and through the successive editions of these catalogs.

TABLE I

| | Verschuer (1958) | These Catalogs | | |
		(1966)	(1968)	(1971)
Autosomal Dominant	285	269 (+568)	344 (+449)	415 (+528)
Autosomal Recessive	89	237 (+294)	280 (+349)	365 (+418)
X-Linked	38	68 (+51)	68 (+55)	86 (+64)
Totals	412	574 (+913)	692 (+853)	866 (+1010)
		1,487	1,545	1,876

The numbers in parentheses relate to nonasterisked entries.

The numbers are of interest from several points of view. The ratio of autosomal dominants to autosomal recessives is of note: 943 dominants to 783 recessives[1]. A few years ago the preponderance of dominants was even greater, but advances in biochemical genetics in the last few years have added many new items to the list of recessives, while fewer new dominants have been added. In experimental species, such as the mouse, recessives predominate.[2] This difference between man and mouse is largely the result of a difference in mating patterns. Most "visible" mutations—that is, those which cause phenotypic changes that are evident to the unaided senses—are recessive. In closely mating mice they are likely to become apparent promptly. In outbred man, however, a recessive mutation can occur and the gene be lost, either by chance or because of a disadvantage in the heterozygote, without ever "meeting up with itself" in a homozygote. Or, if a homozygote occurs, it may, because of the small size of human families, be an isolated case and may not be recognized as representing a distinct genetic entity.

The catalog of X-linked traits represents the largest number of loci that have been identified on one chromosome in any metazoan, excepting *Drosophilia*. Since 86 loci on the X chromosome have been identified, and since the X chromosome represents about 6 percent of the length of the haploid set of chromosomes, one would expect that over 1400 autosomal loci would be known. In fact, less than 800 are confidently known. The main deficiency is undoubtedly in the group of recessives. An X-linked recessive behaves as a dominant in the male. It is, for practical purposes, always expressed if the male has the gene. The number of X-linked dominants is close to what one would expect from the number of autosomal dominants and from the length of the X chromosome relative to that of the autosomal complement.

The total number of loci[3] identified by these catalogs is a very small portion of the total number of genes. Estimates of the number of genes in man have taken two approaches (Vogel, 1964): (1) From the measured amount of DNA, and assuming a triplet code and 150 amino acids per polypeptide chain, one concludes that there is enough DNA to code for about ten milion polypeptide chains. Redundancy, now known to be present in the mammalian genome (DNA-RNA hybridization techniques show that 30 percent or more of the DNA exists in multiple copies), greatly reduces this number. It is certain that much of the DNA must serve some function other than coding for the amino acid sequence of proteins (Markert, 1970). (2) From the relatively extensive information on *E. coli* it is concluded that several thousand genes would be required to code for all the proteins of its cell. Given the greater complexity of any multicellular organism—especially man—the number of genes may be one hundred times as great. The total number of genes in man probably is not less than 100,000. Thus the catalogs reveal perhaps only 1 percent of the whole. The number of entries in the catalogs reflects the degree of genetic variability in man and, even more, man's ingenuity and persistence in detecting this variability.

---

1. These figures refer to all items. The corresponding figures for established (asterisked) items are 415 dominants and 365 recessives. In the X-linkage catalog, 150 items are listed, of which 86 are asterisked.

2. Dr. Margaret C. Green (Bar Harbor, Maine, August, 1967) has estimated that in the house mouse the number of known autosomal dominant mutations is 99, autosomal recessives, 207, and X-linked, 12. In these counts the T locus was counted only once, and loci for protein variants were counted singly, as dominants. Several recessive mutations known to be present at different loci, but having such closely similar phenotypes that they most likely would not be distinguished in man, were counted separately. Alleles producing phenotypes that were sufficiently different for allelism not to be suspected in the absence of genetic tests were also counted separately. The 13 or more histocompatibility loci were not counted.

3. It is likely that some of the phenotypes listed separately here—with the implication that they demonstrate the presence of separate loci—may be determined by mutant genes allelic to the genes for other phenotypes. The opposite error—listing as one locus a phenotype that can be caused by mutation at any one of several different loci—is at least equally likely, however.

3.   Among the uses to which the catalogs may be put is "deletion-mapping" of the chromosomes. Observation of a specific autosomal recessive disorder in a patient with the *cri du chat* syndrome (deletion of the short arm of chromosome no. 5), for example, would provide evidence on the cartography of the particular genetic locus. Although no completely certain chromosomal assignment of a gene locus has yet been made by this approach, deletion mapping is illustrated by the work of Elmore *et al.* (1965).

4.   The mode of inheritance can be a useful guide in the search for the basic defect in genetic disorders. Thanks to the margin of safety with which most enzyme systems are endowed, a gene-determined enzyme deficiency is likely to be reflected in the phenotype only in the homozygote. Contrariwise, when the mutation concerns a nonenzymic protein–for example, a structural protein like collagen–it is plausible to presume that change in the amino acid sequence might alter the physical properties in such a way as to be reflected in the phenotype, even though only about half of the particular protein is of the mutant type. All inborn errors of metabolism (defined in the strict Garrodian sense) are recessives. I believe one would be wasting his time to look for an enzyme defect in the Marfan syndrome, a dominant disorder. Obviously there is much more to biochemical genetics than merely the determination of the amino acid sequence of proteins and the matter of whether these proteins are enzymes or not. Some genes determine enzymes that effect changes in the structure of nonenzymic proteins–for example, hydroxylate proline in collagen. Mutation in such a gene would result in a structural change in a nonenzymic protein and would be expected to behave as a recessive. Speculation here about the existence in man of genetic control mechanisms of the Jacob-Monod type and about the genetic behavior to be expected of mutations therein would be useless. Nonetheless, the generalization stated above is probably true. In recessive disorders an enzyme defect, or a defect in a peptide hormone such as growth hormone (see ateleiotic dwarfism), should be sought. In dominant disorders, abnormality in a nonenzymic protein is more likely. Theoretically, change in the specificity of an enzyme might be the result of mutation, so that it acts on a substrate it ordinarily would not touch. The enzymatic disorder resulting from such a mutation might behave as a dominant (Kirkman, 1970). In bacteria, "noninducible" mutations involve a change in a repressor such that its affinity for an inducer substance is lost and repression is maintained. Again, the enzymic deficiency would be expected to behave as a dominant. This class of mutation has not been proved in man.

In assembling these three catalogs, consideration had constantly to be given to heterogeneity, which is often discovered when a genetic disorder is examined closely; what at first is thought to be one entity is found to be several clinically similar (that is, phenotypically similar) but fundamentally (genotypically) distinct disorders (McKusick, 1969).

The principles of genetics force one to think of mutation as a *specific* etiologic mechanism which results in a *specific* disease entity. In 1930 Knut Faber, professor of medicine in Copenhagen, produced a monograph entitled *Nosography,* in which he traced the development of understanding of the classification of disease. To Gregor Mendel's principles he assigned a leading role in directing thought along lines of specific entities. The one other factor of comparable impact was the advent of the bacteriologic era with its focus on specific etiology and specific entities. One has but to recall that it was only a little more than a century ago that in many circles jaundice, dropsy, anemia, fever, and so on, were thought of as entities to realize the influence of bacteriologic and genetic discoveries on the conceptual base of medicine.

In medical genetics there is little place for expressions such as "spectrum of disease," "disease A is a mild form, or a variant, of disease B," and so on. Disease A and disease B are either the same disease, if they are based on the same mutation, or they are different diseases. Phenotypic overlap is not necessarily grounds for considering them fundamentally the same or even closely related. For example, diagrams purporting to show the interrelationship of neurologic diseases (Myrianthopoulos *et al.,* 1964) are totally meaningless, and useless, except as an indication of phenotypic overlap.

What methods are available for demonstrating the heterogeneity of genetic disease in man? They can be outlined as follows:

I. Genetic Methods
    A. Mode of inheritance—for example, spastic paraplegia
    B. Nonallelism of recessives—for example, deaf-mutism
    C. Linkage relationships—for example, elliptocytosis
II. Analysis of phenotype—for example, the mucopolysaccharidoses
III. Biochemical analysis—for example, the hereditary nonspherocytic hemolytic anemias
IV. Physiological studies—for example, the X-linked hemophilias
V. Studies of cells in culture—for example, the mucopolysaccharidoses

An experience in medical genetics much less frequent than discovery of heterogeneity is demonstration of affinity—that is, the discovery that phenotypes which appeared at first to represent separate entities are in fact the result of one and the same genotype. Wilson's disease can present in young patients as an essentially pure hepatic disorder and in older patients as a predominantly neurologic disorder. Familial Mediterranean fever may present the picture of primary amyloidosis without displaying at any time in its course the picture of episodic fever and polyserositis, and the converse can also occur. In man, final proof of genetic identity depends on demonstrating precisely the same chemical change at the molecular level. (See amaurosis congenita of Leber, type 1, for a possible example of genetic affinity.)

A leading objective of medical genetics is to describe the defect in each disorder in as precise chemical terms as has been possible in many of the hemoglobinopathies. The catalogs provide a listing of all hemoglobin variants together with an indication of the amino acid substitution when known. As similarly detailed information becomes available on the variants of glucose-6-phosphate dehydrogenase, transferrins, and other polymorphic proteins, comprehensive cataloging of these will be undertaken.

Genetics has been defined as the science of variation. Classically, without variation in a character there could be no genetics. Molecular genetics and the development of new techniques in human genetics have to some extent removed the limitation. For example, interspecies cell hybridization permits study of the linkage relationships of gene loci in man, even though no allelic variation at those loci is known. An example is assignment of the thymidine kinase locus to chromosome no. 17. For this reason, thymidine kinase is listed in the catalog. The one cistron—one polypeptide principle[4] leads to the conclusion that any well-characterized, unique polypeptide of man is governed by a specific gene. However, no useful purpose is served by listing such in these catalogs, unless chromosomal or other linkage information is available, as is true of thymidine kinase.

An appreciable homology of genomal organization between man and some of his more closely related fellow animals is demonstrable. The X chromosome has displayed particular stability in evolution, conserving certain loci which it carries in many species, probably because the sex-determining factors scattered through the X chromosome cannot be translocated to autosomes without disruptive effects on reproduction. Attention should be directed constantly to the catalogs of X-linked traits in mice and other nonhuman mammals (Ohno, 1967; Green, 1966), and, although homologous linkage relationships in the autosomes are less likely, mouse linkages, such as albinism with the beta hemoglobin locus and transferrin with one malate dehydrogenase locus, should be kept in mind by students of human linkage. Linkage studies in subhuman primates might be particularly illuminating for human genetics.

---

4. The special case of the immunoglobulins, in which more than one cistron appear to determine a single polypeptide (Edelman, 1970), is an exception that tests the rule.

subhuman primates might be particularly illuminating for human genetics.

Chromosomal aberrations of the relatively gross type demonstrable by means of existing methods are not, of course, within the scope of these catalogs—not even the familial chromosomal aberrations, which are essentially "Mendelizing." Autosomal aberrations were nicely surveyed, with a catalog, by Thompson (1965, 1966).

The terminology related to many genetic disorders presents difficulties, especially when the basic defect is unknown. Personal preference has inevitably played a role in the choice of terms used here. Eponyms (Jablonski, 1969) have been used sparingly; however, some—for example, Marfan, Ehlers-Danlos, Ellis-van Creveld, Pelizaeus-Merzbacher, and Tay-Sachs—are too well established to be avoided, and, in addition, no satisfactory noneponymic designation is available. As a rule, the possessive form of eponyms has *not* been used: for example, Marfan, not Marfan's, syndrome will be found in the catalogs. The reason is that the eponym is merely a "handle"; often the man whose name is thus used was not the first to describe the condition or did not describe the full syndrome as it has subsequently become known. However, agreeing with Emerson that "consistency is the hobgoblin of little minds," I have retained "Wilson's disease" and some others in which the nonpossessive seems awkward to the tongue. Some inconsistency will also be found in the use of designations such as valinemia or hypervalinemia, lysinemia or hyperlysinemia, methylmalonicaciduria or hypermethylmalonicacidemia, and so on. It is hoped that the subject index is sufficiently exhaustive (with a full range of alternative designations indexed) for particular disorders to be found without difficulty, regardless of what designation I have used. Preferred designations have changed some with successive editions, even for conditions of which the defect remains obscure. Usage is the important consideration, as in all language. An example is cystic fibrosis of the pancreas, now generally known simply as *cystic fibrosis,* the designation used here.

When the basic defect underlying a genetic syndrome is known, one might call it a disease—for example, Lesch-Nyhan disease rather than the Lesch-Nyhan syndrome. However, when the basic defect is known one is in a position to devise a specific designation based thereon—for example, HGPRT-deficiency for the Lesch-Nyhan syndrome.

The desideratum in nomenclature is, of course, terminology that is based on the nature of the fundamental defect. Mendelian disorders potentially lend themselves particularly well to precision in nomenclature. In the year 2084, for example, the "compleat" medical geneticist will probably be able to look at the phenotype and at the laboratory data and come up with a diagnostic label that is a statement of the specific abnormality in the genome. It might be something like 14-di-C164-17TA, meaning that on chromosome 14 both alleles of cistron no. 164 have adenine substituted for thymine as base no. 17 (paraphrased from Steinberg, 1971).

It is difficult to master genetic nosology in every branch of medicine and difficult to maintain an overview of all medical literature. Aside from honest differences of opinion regarding the classification of some phenotypes and the interpretation of the evidence on modes of inheritance, errors may have crept in, and important omissions may exist. I have no illusions of either the infallibility or the completeness of these catalogs. I would appreciate suggestions for increasing the usefulness of the catalogs and would like to have errors and omissions called to my attention.

The value of maintaining these catalogs on magnetic tape lies in the ease of revision and republication. I plan to keep them updated on a continuing basis and to republish whenever that is justified by the accumulation of new material. It is hoped that the catalogs will be a *vade mecum* for the clinical geneticist—an inexpensive handbook that will make available the latest information on the nosology and genetics of hereditary diseases.

For the layman the large number of genetic disorders to which man is literally heir may come as an unhappy surprise. I am reminded of the following comment **by** Sir Thomas Browne in his *Religio medici:*

> .....Men that look no further than their outsides, think health an appurtenance unto life, and quarrel with their constitutions for being sick; but I, that have examined the parts of man, and know upon what tender filaments that Fabrick hangs, do wonder that we are not always so; and considering the thousand doors that lead to death, do thank my God that we can die but once.

The Johns Hopkins Hospital   VICTOR A. MCKUSICK, M.D.

REFERENCES

Browne, T. Religio Medici, pt. 1, sec. 44. In *The Works of Sir Thomas Browne,* ed. Geoffrey Keynes. London: Faber & Gwyer, Ltd., 1928. Vol. 1, p. 54.

Edelman, G. M. The Structure and Function of Antibody. Scientific American, August, 1970, pp. 34-42.

Edwards, J. H. The Simulation of Mendelism. Acta Genet. Statist. Med. 10: 63-70, 1960.

Elmore, S. M., Nance, W. E., McGee, B. J., Engel-del Montmollin, M., and Engel, E. Pycnodysostosis, with a Familial Chromosome Anomaly. Amer. J. Med. 40: 273-82, 1966.

Garcia, A. G. P. Congenital Toxoplasmosis in Two Successive Sibs. Arch. Dis. Child. 43: 705-10, 1968.

Goldberg, M. F., and Hardy, J. M. B. X-Linked Cataract. In *Clinical Delineation of Birth Defects,* vol. 8: *The Eye*, ed. D. Bergsma. Baltimore: Williams & Wilkins, 1971.

Green, E. L., ed. *Biology of the Laboratory Mouse.* New York: McGraw-Hill, 1966.

Haldane, J. B. S. A Hitherto Unexpected Complication in the Genetics of Human Recessives. Ann. Eugen. 8: 263-265, 1938.

Jablonski, S. *Illustrated Dictionary of Eponymic Syndromes and Diseases and Their Synonyms.* Philadelphia: W. B. Saunders Co., 1969.

Kirkman, H. N. Dominant Mutations—Biochemical Basis for Phenotype. In *Congenital Malformations,* ed. F. C. Fraser and V. A. McKusick. Amsterdam: Excerpta Medica, 1970.

McKusick, V. A. On Lumpers and Splitters, or the Nosology of Genetic Disease. Perspectives in Biology and Medicine 12: 198-312, 1969.

McKusick, V. A. On the X Chromosome of Man. Quart. Rev. Biol. 37: 69-175, 1962.

McKusick, V. A., Stauffer, M., Knox, D. L., and Clark, D. B. Chorioretinopathy with Hereditary Microcephaly. Arch. Ophthal. 75:597-600, 1966.

Macklin, M. T. Erythroblastosis Foetalis: A Study of Its Mode of Inheritance. Amer. J. Dis. Child. 53: 1245-67, 1937.

Menser, M. A., Slinn, R. F., Dods, L., Herzberg, R., and Harley, J. D. Congenital Rubella in a Mother and Son. Austral. Paed. J. 4: 200-202, 1968.

Myrianthopoulos, N. C., Lane, M. H., Silberberg, D. H., and Vincent, B. L. Nerve Conduction and Other Studies in Families with Charcot-Marie-Tooth Disease. Brain 87:589-608, 1964.

Ohno, S. *Sex Chromosomes and Sex-linked Genes.* Berlin: Springer Verlag, 1967.

Serra, J. A. *Modern Genetics*, Vol. 1, pp. 397-98. London and New York: Academic Press, 1965.

Steinberg, D. The Metabolic Basis of the Refsum Syndrome. In *Clinical Delineation of Birth Defects,* vol. 6: *Nervous System*, ed. D. Bergsma. Baltimore: Williams & Wilkins, 1971.

Thompson, H. Abnormalities of the Autosomal Chromosomes Associated with Human Disease: Selected Topics and Catalogue. Amer. J. Med. Sc. 250: 718-34, 1965, and 251: 706-35, 1966.

Vogel, F. A Preliminary Estimate of the Number of Human Genes. Nature 201:847, 1964.

Wiesmann, V., and Neufeld, E. F. Scheie and Hurler Syndrome: Apparent Identity of the Biochemical Defect. Science 169: 72-74, 1970.

ACKNOWLEDGMENTS

I am indebted to a large number of colleagues in Baltimore and elsewhere for assistance in assembling these catalogs. First, I would mention the research fellows who have worked with me since 1960 when the X-linked catalog was initiated. Second, I have been greatly assisted by the advice of many of my colleagues at The Johns Hopkins University. Colleagues elsewhere who have reviewed the catalogs at one stage or another include Alexander G. Bearn and O. J. Miller of New York City; Dick Hoefnagel of Hanover, N. H.; A. Donald Merritt, W. DeMyer, and Wolfgang Zeman of Indianapolis; J. A. Fraser Roberts of London; Margery W. Shaw, formerly of Ann Arbor, now of Houston; John M. Opitz of Madison; George Fraser, formerly of London, Adelaide, and Seattle, now of Leiden; P. E. Becker of Göttingen; Arno G. Motulsky of Seattle; Herbert A. Lubs, Jr., formerly of New Haven, now of Denver; Mette Warburg of Copenhagen; David J. Weatherall of Liverpool; Robert J. Gorlin of Minneapolis; and many others who will, I hope, forgive my failure to mention them by name. Collaboration with Drs. Margaret O. Dayhoff and Lois T. Hunt of the Biomedical Research Foundation, Silver Spring, Md., was helpful in the cataloging of the protein variants, particularly the hemoglobin variants. A new feature of this edition is a listing of the recognized variants of glucose-6-phosphate dehydrogenase, for which we are endebted to Drs. A. Yoshida and A. G. Motulsky of Seattle and Ernest Beutler of Duarte. None of the errors in these catalogs can be attributed to any of the above, but without their help the catalogs would be much less authoritative and complete.

Computerization was made possible by the sympathetic and ingenious assistance of Drs. Robert P. Rich and Richard H. Shepard of The Johns Hopkins Computing Center and was executed in the Division of Medical Genetics by David R. Bolling and his staff. Mrs. Dixie Palma and Miss Rita Covington deserve special mention for their work, both in computerization and in bibliographic verification. Finally, without the William H. Welch Medical Library this undertaking would have been, quite literally, impossible. Particular thanks are due the library staff for its help.

Some aspects of the process of assembling the catalogs were supported by an NIH Genetics Training Grant (GM 795) and by an NIH Research Grant entitled "Mapping the Chromosomes of Man" (GM 10189). The development of methods for computerization of the material and the processing of the catalogs took place in the Computing Center of The Johns Hopkins University School of Medicine. This facility is supported in part by a grant from the Control Data Corporation.

GENERAL SOURCES

In assembling these catalogs, several general sources, specialized monographs, and textbooks were used.

The older literature was reviewed in the following: R. R. Gates, *Human Heredity*, 2 vols. (New York: Macmillan, 1946); A. Sorsby, ed., *Clinical Genetics* (St. Louis: C. V. Mosby, 1953); and A. Touraine, *L'hérédité en médecine* (Paris: Masson, 1955).

The older literature is also usefully surveyed in *The Treasury of Human Inheritance* (1909-58), a series of reviews of the literature on a variety of genetic disorders: hemophilia, diabetes insipidus, dwarfism, angioneurotic edema, brachydactyly, polydactyly, osteogenesis imperfecta, Leber's optic atrophy, color blindness, retinitis pigmentosa, congenital stationary night blindness, multiple exostoses, cleidocranial dysostosis, Huntington's chorea, peroneal muscular atrophy, hereditary ataxias, spastic paraplegia, pseudohypertrophic muscular dystrophy, myotonic dystrophy, and Laurence-Moon syndrome. *The Treasury* was a publication of the Galton Laboratory, London (Cambridge University Press). Contributors included Julia Bell, Percy Stocks, William Bulloch, and Paul Fildes.

Comparably encyclopedic works of more recent publication include the following: P. E. Becker, ed., *Humangenetik: Ein kürzes Handbuch in fünf Banden*, (Stuttgart: G. Thieme, 1964); and L. Gedda, ed., *De Genetica Medica*, 6 vols. (Rome: G. Mendel Institute, 1961-62).

The medical genetics literature for the six years 1958-63, inclusive, was surveyed by my colleagues and myself in annual reviews published in the *Journal of Chronic Diseases* and collected in the following: V. A. McKusick *et al.*, *Medical Genetics 1958-1960* (St. Louis: C. V. Mosby, 1961); V. A. McKusick *et al.*, *Medical Genetics 1961-1963* (Oxford: Pergamon Press, 1966.)

Exceedingly useful in reviewing those forms of hereditary disease on which biochemical information is fullest was the following:

J. B. Stanbury, J. B. Wyngaarden, and D. S. Fredrickson, eds., *The Metabolic Basis of Inherited Disease*, 2nd ed. (New York: Blakiston Division, McGraw-Hill, 1966).

The following journals were drawn on heavily:

Acta geneticae medicae et gemellologiae; *American Journal of Human Genetics*; *Annals of Human Genetics* (and its predecessor, *Annals of Eugenics*); *Clinical Genetics* (a newcomer); *Human Heredity* (and it spredecessor, *Acta genetica et statistica medica*); *Journal de genetique humaine*; *Journal of Medical Genetics*; and *Social Biology* (and its predecessor, *Eugenics Quarterly*).

The current literature has been surveyed with the assistance of *Current Contents* (a weekly publication of the table of contents of biomedical periodicals) and *Excerpta Medica* (abstracts on human genetics).

In recent years, annual conferences on the nosology of congenital and/or hereditary disorders, entitled "The Clinical Delineation of Birth Defects," have been held in Baltimore. Proceedings of the conferences held in 1968, 1969, and 1970 were published by The National Foundation–March of Dimes, which provided financial support for the conferences, and by Williams & Wilkins Co., Baltimore. Particularly useful in relation to these catalogs were the following volumes in the published proceedings: II, Malformation Syndromes; III, Limb malformations; IV, Skeletal Dysplasias; VI, Nervous System; VII, Muscle; VIII, Eye; IX, Ear; X, Endocrine System; XI, Orofacial Structures; and XII, Skin, Hair and Nails. The 1971 conference is expected to give birth to the following volumes: XIII, Cardiovascular System; XIV, Blood; and XV, Gastrointestinal Tract, Liver and Pancreas.

Specialty monographs used in assembling the catalogs included the following:

I. Eye

Duke-Elder, S. *System of Ophthalmology.* III. *Normal and Abnormal Development.* Part 2. Congenital Deformities. St. Louis: C. V. Mosby, 1963. VIII. *Diseases of the Outer Eye.* Part 1. Conjunctiva. Part 2. Cornea. St. Louis:C. V. Mosby, 1965.

Franceschetti, A., Francois, J., and Babel, J. *Les hérédo–dégénérescences chorio-rétiennes (dégénérescences tapéto-rétiennes).* 2 vols. Paris: Masson, 1963.

Francois, J. *Heredity in Ophthalmology.* St. Louis: C. V. Mosby, 1961.

Francois, J. *Congenital Cataracts.* Springfield, Ill.: Charles C Thomas, 1963.

Fraser, G. R., and Friedman, A. I. *The Causes of Blindness in Childhood:* A Study of 776 Children with Severe Visual Handicaps. Baltimore: The Johns Hopkins Press, 1967.

Waardenburg, P. J., Franceschetti, A., and Klein, D. *Genetics and Ophthalmology,* vols. 1 and 2. Springfield, Ill.: Charles C Thomas, 1961 and 1963.

Walsh, F. B., and Hoyt, W. F. *Clinical Neuro-Ophthalmology,* 3rd ed. Baltimore: Williams & Wilkins, 1969.

II. Skin

Butterworth, R., and Strean, P. *Clinical Genodermatology.* Baltimore: Williams & Wilkins, 1962.

Cockayne, E. A. *Inherited Abnormalities of the Skin and Its Appendages.* London: Oxford University Press, 1933.

Gottron, H. A., and Schnyder, V. W. *Vererbung von Hautkrankheiten.* Berlin: Springer Verlag, 1966 (vol. 7 of *Jadassohn Handbuch).*

III. Nervous System

Allen, N. Developmental and Degenerative Diseases of the Brain. In *Pediatric Neurology,* ed. T. W. Farmer. New York: Hoeber Medical Division, Harper & Row, 1964.

Becker, P. E., ed. *Humangenetik: Ein kürzes Handbuch in fünf Bander,* vol. 5, pt. 1: Krankheiten des Nervensystems. Stuttgart: Georg Thieme Verlag, 1966.

Blackwood, W. *et al. Greenfield's Neuropathology.* Baltimore: Williams & Wilkins, 1963.

Ford, F. R. *Diseases of the Nervous System in Infancy, Childhood, and Adolescence,* 5th ed. Springfield, Ill.: Charles C Thomas, 1966.

Refsum, S. Genetic Aspects of Neurology. In *Clinical Neurology,* ed. A. B. Baker, 2nd ed. New York: Hoeber Medical Division, Harper & Row, 1962.

IV. Muscle

Adams, R. D., Denny-Brown, D., and Pearson, C. M. *Diseases of Muscle,* 2nd ed. New York: Harper & Row, 1962.

V. Hand Malformation

Temtamy, S. Genetic Factors in Hand Malformations. Ph.D. dissertation, The Johns Hopkins University, 1966. (Available through University Microfilms Inc., Ann Arbor, Michigan.)

VI. Genetic Disorders of the Skeleton and of Connective Tissue in General

McKusick, V. A. *Heritable Disorders of Connective Tissue*, 3rd ed. St. Louis: C. V. Mosby, 1966.

Rubin, P. *The Dynamic Classification of Bone Dysplasias*. Chicago: Year Book Medical Publishers, 1963.

VII. Endocrine System

Rimoin, D. L., and Schimke, R. N. *Genetic Disorders of the Endocrine Glands*. St. Louis: C. V. Mosby, 1971.

NOSOLOGIC TABLES

OTHER TABLES

HEREDITARY DEAFNESS

The following classification is that of Dr. Bruce W. Konigsmark (*New Eng. J. Med.* 281: 713-720, 774-778, and 827-832, 1969; *Clinical Delineation of Birth Defects*. IX. *The Ear*. New York: National Foundation–March of Dimes, 1971), with minor modifications and additions. About 70 different varieties of hereditary deafness are recognized.

I.   Hereditary deafness with no associated abnormalities

    A.   Dominant congenital severe deafness

    B.   Dominant progressive nerve deafness (12480)

    C.   Dominant unilateral deafness (12500)

    D.   Dominant low-frequency hearing loss (12490)

    E.   Dominant mid-frequency hearing loss (12470)

    F.   Otosclerosis (16680)

    G.   Recessive congenital severe deafness (22070, 22080)

    H.   Recessive early onset neural deafness (22160)

    I.   Recessive congenital moderate hearing loss (22150)

    J.   Sex-linked deafness with stapes fixation (30450)

    K.   Sex-linked early onset deafness (30440)

    L.   Sex-linked progressive hearing loss (30470)

II.   Hereditary deafness with external ear malformations

    A.   Dominant preauricular pits and neural hearing loss (12510)

    B.   Dominant thickened ears and incudo-stapedial joint abnormality

    C.   Dominant ear malformation and conductive hearing loss

    D.   Dominant facio-cervical abnormalities

    E.   Recessive malformed low set ears and conductive hearing loss.

III.   Hereditary deafness with integumentary system disease

    A.   Waardenburg syndrome (19350)

    B.   Dominant albinism and congenital deafness (10350)

    C.   Leopard syndrome (15110)

    D.   Sex-linked pigmentary abnormality and congenital deafness (30070)

    E.   Recessive atopic dermatitis and neural hearing loss (22110)

    F.   Dominant anhidrosis and progressive hearing loss (12520)

    G.   Recessive ectodermal dysplasia and neurisensory deafness (22480)

    H.   Dominant keratopachydermia, digital constrictions and deafness (12450)

    I.   Recessive pili torti and deafness (26200)

    J.   Dominant knuckle pads, leukonychia, and hearing loss (14920)

    K.   Dominant onychodystrophy, coniform teeth and hearing loss

    L.   Recessive onychodystrophy and deafness (22050)

IV.   Hereditary deafness associated with eye disease

    A.   Dominant saddle nose, myopia, cataract, and hearing loss (12520)

    B.   Dominant myopia, hearing loss, peripheral neuropathy and skeletal abnormalities [Flynn-Aird] (13630)

HAND MALFORMATIONS

IX The system of classification of hand malformations devised by Temtamy[1] has diagnostic usefulness. Three steps are involved in the delineation of specific types:

1. According to the sole or predominant anomaly, the malformation is is placed in one of sevem main categories

I.   Absence deformities
II. Brachydactyly
III. Syndactyly
IV. Polydactyly
V.   Contracture deformities
VI. Symphalangism
VII. Hand malformations with congenital ring constrictions

2. Each main category is divided into two subclasses according to whether or not malformation of other organs is associated.
3. By family studies the groupings achieved in the first two steps can often be extended. Even though categorization is unclear from study of the proband alone, the patterns of familial occurrence (or lack thereof) and—provided affected relatives are identified—the anatomy of malformation in these other affected persons may establish the diagnosis

I. Absence deformities
   A. Absence deformities as isolated malformations
      1. Terminal transverse defects
         a. Ectrodactyly (12980,22530)
         b. Amelia and terminal transverse hemimelia (10440)
         c. Acheiropody (20050)
      2. Radial defects
      3. Ulnar defects
      4. Split-hand/split-foot deformity
         a. Typical split-hand (18360)
         b. Atypical split-hand
   B. Absence deformities as a part of syndromes
      1. The association of absence deformities with orofacial malformations
         a. Terminal transverse defects with orofacial malformations
            (1) Ectrodactyly with orofacial malformations
            (2) Aglossia-adactylia syndrome (10330)
            (3) Ankyloglossum superius syndrome
            (4) Hanhart syndrome:peromelia with micrognathia (26130)
         b. Radial defects with orofacial malformations
            (1) Nager's acrofacial dysostosis (15440)
         c. Ulnar defects with orofacial malformations
            (1) Weyers oligodactyly syndrome (19360)

1. Temtamy, S. and McKusick, V.A.: Synopsis of hand malformations with particular emphasis on genetic factors. In, Bergsma, D. ed.: Clinical Delineation of Birth Defects. III. Limb malformations. New York: National Foundation-March of Dimes, 1969., pp. 125-184.

SKELETAL DISORDERS

The following classification is based on that provided by a conference convened in Paris in November 1969, with Pierre Maroteaux[1] as rapporteur. Standardization of nomenclature was the primary concern of the conference but classification was an inevitable and useful by product.

The classification into dysplasias and dysostoses, as defined below, was sometimes difficult or arbitrary. Certain disorders have features of both. Pycnodysostosis (26580) is such a condition because the mandibular malformation is a dysplasia and the increased density of the skeleton a dysostosis.

A special effort was made to reduce the use of eponyms. Only those were retained which are in almost universal use for conditions which lack another satisfactory designation. Proper names in brackets are formerly used eponyms.

The introduction of new terms was held to a minimum. One of the principle changes was the suggested substitution of *metaphyseal chondrodysplasia* for *metaphyseal dysostosis.* This seems a useful change because the new term more accurately states the nature of the disorder. In the catalogs, however, I have retained the earlier term *metaphyseal dysostosis,* awaiting wider usage of the new term. In some other instances new terms suggested by the Paris conference have not been used in the catalogs, for the same reason.

The conference recognized the tentative nature of the classification.

In adapting the Paris nomenclature/classification to American usage, several changes were made: Hyphens were removed from chondro-ectodermal, spondylo-epiphyseal, chondro-dysplasia, etc., but left in acro-osteolysis, cervico-oculo-acoustic, etc. *Brachydactyly polydactyly;* etc. were used in preference to the forms ending in -ia (e.g., *brachydactylia).* Admittedly, inconsistency was practiced in the retention of *amelia, phocomelia,* etc. Similarly; usage dating from Harvey Cushing's coinage of the term dictated use of *symphalangism* rather than *symphalangy.*

Personal preference has led to the change of some terms from that recommended by the Paris conference–for example; *thrombocytopenia-absent radius(TAR) syndrome* was used rather than*thrombocytopenia-radial aplasia syndrome; Bardet-Biedl syndrome* rather than *Laurence-Moon-Bardet-Biedl syndrome; orofaciodigital syndrome* rather than *oro-digito-facial syndrome; trichorhinophalangeal syndrome* rather than *rhino-tricho-phalangeal syndrome; cockayne syndrome* rather than *Cockayne's syndrome.*

1.   Maroteaux, P.: Nomenclature internationale des maladies osseuses constitutionelles. Ann. Radiol. 13:455-464, 1970.

I. Constitutional Diseases of Bones with Unknown Pathogenesis: Osteochondrodysplasias (abnormalities of cartilage and/or bone growth and development)

A. Defects of growth of tubular bones and/or spine

1. Manifest at birth
   a. Achondroplasia (10080)
   b. Achondrogenesis (20060)
   c. Thanatophoric dwarfism (18770)
   d. Chondrodysplasia punctata (formerly stippled epiphyses or chondrodystrophia calcificans congenita), several forms (21510)
   e. Metatropic dwarfism (25060)
   f. Diastrophic dwarfism (22260)
   g. Chondroectodermal dysplasia [Ellis-van Creveld] (22550)
   h. Asphyxiating thoracic dysplasia [Jeune] (20850)
   i. Spondyloepiphyseal dysplasia, congenital (18390)
   j. Mesomelic dwarfism
      (1) Nievergelt type (16340)
      (2) Langer type (24970)
   k. Cleidocranial dysplasia (formerly cleidocranial dysostosis) (11960)

2. Manifest in later life
   a. Hypochondroplasia (14600)
   b. Dyschondrosteosis (12730)
   c. Metaphyseal chondrodysplasia (formerly metaphyseal dysostosis), Jansen type (15640)
   d. Metaphyseal chondrodysplasia (formerly metaphyseal dysostosis), Schmidt type (15650)
   e. Metaphyseal chondrodysplasia, McKusick type (formerly cartilage-hair hypoplasia) (21230)
   f. Metaphyseal chondrodysplasia with malabsorption and neutropenia (26040)
   g. Metaphyseal chondrodysplasia with thymolymphopenia (20090)
   h. Spondylometaphyseal dysplasis [Kozlowski] (27180)
   i. Multiple epiphyseal dysplasia (several forms) (13240)
   j. Hereditary arthro-ophthalmopathy (10830)
   k. Pseudoachondroplastic dysplasia (formerly pseudo-achondroplastic type of spondyloepiphyseal dysplasia) (18400)
   l. Spondyloepiphyseal dysplasia tarda (31340)
   m. Acrodysplasia
      (1) Trichorhinophalangeal syndrome [Giedion] (12780)
      (2) Epiphyseal type [Thiemann] (16570, 25710, 27370)
      (3) Epiphysometaphyseal type [Brailsford]

B. Disorganized development of cartilage and fibrous components of the skeleton

1. Dysplasia epiphysealis hemimelica (12780)
2. Multiple cartilagenous exostoses (13370)
3. Enchondromatosis [Ollier] (16600)
4. Enchondromatosis with hemangioma [Maffucci] (16600)
5. Fibrous dysplasia [Jaffé-Lichtenstein]

J. Spherophakia-brachymorphia syndrome [Weill-Marchesani] (27760)

K. Marfan syndrome (15470)

V. Constitutional Diseases of Bones with known pathogenesis: Chromosomal aberrations

VI. Constitutional Diseases of Bones with Known Pathogenesis: Primary Metabolic Abnormalities

A. Disorders of Calcium/phosphorus metabolism

1. Hypophosphatemic familial rickets (30780, 19310)

2. Pseudo-deficiency rickets [Royer, Prader] (27-50)

3. Late rickets [McCance]

4. Idiopathic hypercalciuria

5. Hypophosphatasia (several forms) (14630, 24150)

6. Idiopathic hypercalcemia

7. Pseudo-hypoparathyroidism (normo- and hypocalcemic forms) (30080)

B. Mucopolysaccharidoses

1. Mucopolysaccharidosis I [Hurler] (25280)

2. Mucopolysaccharidosis II [Hunter] (30990)

3. Mucopolysaccharidosis III [Sanfilippo] (25290)

4. Mucopolysaccharidosis IV [Morquio] (25300)

5. Mucopolysaccharidosis V [Scheie] (25310)

6. Mucopolysaccharidosis VI [Maroteaux-Lamy] (25320)

C. Mucolipidoses and lipidoses

1. Mucolipidosis I [Spranger-Wiedemann] (25240)

2. Mucolipidosis II [Leroy] (25250)

3. Mucolipidosis III [pseudo-Hurler polydystrophy] (25260)

4. Fucosidosis (23000)

5. Mannosidosis (24850)

6. Generalized Gm1 gangliosidosis (several forms) (23050,23060)

7. Sulfatidosis with mucopolysacchariduria [Austin, Thieffry] (27220)

8. Cerebrosidosis, including Gaucher's disease (23000-23100)

D. Other metabolic extra-osseous disorders

VII. Bone Abnormalities Secondary to Disturbances of Extra-Skeletal Systems

A. Endocrine, e.g., hypothyroidism

B. Hematologic, e.g., thalassemia

C. Neurologic, e.g., sensory neuropathy

D. Renal, e.g., cystinosis

E. Gastrointestinal, e.g., celiac disease

F. Cardiopulmonary, e.g., hypertrophy osteoarthropathy

ENZYMOPATHIES: DISORDERS IN WHICH A DEFICIENT ACTIVITY OF A SPECIFIC ENZYME HAS BEEN DEMONSTRATED IN MAN[a]

	CONDITION	ENZYME WITH DEFICIENT ACTIVITY	CATALOG NO.
1.	Acatalasia	Catalase	20020
2.	Acid phosphatase deficiency	Acid phosphatase	20095
3.	Adrenal hyperplasia I	21-hydroxylase*	20170
4.	Adrenal hyperplasia II	11-beta-hydroxylase*	20180
5.	Adrenal hyperplasia III	3-beta-hydroxysteroid dehydrogenase*	20190
6.	Adrenal hyperplasia V	17-hydroxylase*	20210
7.	Albinism	Tyrosinase	20310
8.	Aldosterone synthesis, defect in	18-hydroxylase	20340
9.	Alkaptonuria	Homogentisic acid oxidase	20350
10.	Angiokeratoma, diffuse [Fabry]	Ceramide trihexosidase	30150
11.	Apnea, drug-induced	Pseudocholinesterase	27240
12.	Argininemia	Arginase	20780
13.	Argininosuccinic	Argininosuccinase	20790
14.	Aspartylglycosaminuria	Specific hydrolase (AADG-ase)	20840
15.	Ataxia, one form	Pyruvate decarboxylase	20880
16.	Carnosinemia	Carnosinase	21220
17.	Cholesterol ester deficiency [Norum's disease]	Lecithin cholesterol acetyltransferase (LCAT)	24590
18.	Citrullinemia	Arginosuccinic acid synthetase	21570
19.	Crigler-Najjar syndrome	Glucuronyl transferase	21880
20.	Cystathioninuria	Cystathionase	21950
21.	Disaccharide intolerance I	Invertase	22290
22.	Diaccharide intolerance II	Invertase, maltase	22300
23.	Disaccharide intolerance III	Lactase	22310
24.	Formininotransferase deficiency	Formininotransferase	22901
25.	Fructose intolerance	Fructose-1-phosphate aldolase	22960
26.	Fructosuria	Hepatic fructokinase	22980
27.	Fucosidosis	Fucosidase	23000

*In some conditions marked in this way (as well as some which are not listed) deficiency of a particular enzyme is suspected but has not been proved by direct study of enzyme activity.

[a]The enzyme defect in many of these conditions is demonstrable in fibroblasts and in amniotic cells, so that antenatal diagnosis is possible.

28.	Galactokinase deficiency	Galactokinase	23020
29.	Galactosemia	Galactose-l-phosphate uridyl	23040
30.	Gangliosidosis, generalized	β -galactosidase	23050
31.	Gaucher's disease	Glucocerebrosidase	23100
32.	G6PD deficiency (favism, etc.)	Glucose-6-phosphate dehydrogenase	30580
33.	Glycogen storage disease I	Glucose-6-phosphatase	23220
34.	Glycogen storage disease II	Alpha-1-4-glucosidase	23220
35.	Glycogen storage disease III	Amylo-1-6-glucosidase	23240
36.	Glycogen storage disease IV	Amylo (1-4 to 1-6)- transglucosidase	23250
37.	Glycogen storage disease V	Muscle phosphorylase	23260
38.	Glycogen storage disease VI	Liver phosphorylase*	23270
39.	Glycogen storage disease VII	Muscle phosphofrucktokinase	23280
40.	Glycogen storage disease VIII	Liver phosphorylase kinase	30600
41.	Gout, primary (one form)	Hypoxanthine guanine phosphoribosyltransferase	30800
42.	Hemolytic anemia	Adenosine triphosphatase	10280
43.	Hemolytic anemia	Adenylate kinase	20160
44.	Hemolytic anemia	Diphosphoglycerate mutase	22280
45.	Hemolytic anemia	Glucose-6-phosphate dehydrogenase	30590
46.	Hemolytic anemia	Glutathione reductase	23180
47.	Hemolytic anemia	Glutathione synthetase	23190
48.	Hemolytic anemia	Hexokinase	23570
49.	Hemolytic anemia	Hexosephosphate isomerase	23575
50.	Hemolytic anemia	Phosphoglycerate kinase	31180
51.	Hemolytic anemia	Pyruvate kinase	26620
52.	Hemolytic anemia	Triosephosphate isomerase	27580
53.	Histidinemia	Histidase	23580
54.	Homocystinuria	Cystathionine synthetase	23620
55.	beta, β -hydroxyisovaleric- aciduria and methyl- crotonylysinuria	β -methylocrotonyl CoA carboxylase*	21020
56.	Hydroxyprolinemia	Hydroxyproline oxidase	23700
57.	Hyperammonemia I	Ornithine transcarbamylase	23720
58.	Hyperammonemia II	Carbamyl phosphate synthetase	23730
59.	Hyperglycinemia, ketotic form	Propionate carboxylase*	23830
60.	Hyperlysinemia	Lysine-ketoglutarate reductase	23870
61.	Hyperoxaluria		14490
	I Glycolic aciduria	2-oxo-glutarate-glyoxylate carboligase	25990

	II Glyceric aciduria	D-glyceric dehydrogenase	26000
62.	Hyperprolinemia I	Proline oxidase deficiency	23950
63.	Hyperprolinemia II	δ-1-pyrroline -5-carboxylate dehydrogenase*	23950
64.	Hypoglycemia and acidosis	Fructose -1-, 6- diphosphatase	22970
65.	Hypophosphatasia	Alkaline phosphatese	14630
66.	Intestinal lactase deficiency (adult)	Lactase	22310
67.	Isovalericacidemia	Isovaleric acid CoA dehydrogenase	24350
68.	Krabbe's disease	A β -galactosidase	24520
69.	Lactosyl ceramidosis	Lactosyl ceramidase	24550
70.	Leigh's necrotizing encephalomyelopathy	Pyruvate carboxylase	25600
71.	Lipase deficiency, congenital	Lipase (pancreatic)	24660
72.	Lysine intolerance	L-lysine: NAD-oxido-reductase	24790
73.	Mannosidosis	α-mannosidase	24850
74.	Maple sugar urine disease	Keto acid decarboxylase	24860
75.	Metachromatic leuko-dystrophy	Arylsulfatase A (sulfatide sulfatase)	25010
76.	Methemoglobinemia	NAD-methemoglobin reductase	25080
77.	Methylmalonic-aciduria I	Methylmalonic CoA mutase	25100
78.	Methylmalonic-aciduria II	Methylmalonic CoA isomerase	25110
79.	Myeloperoxidase deficiency with disseminated candidiasis	Myeloperoxidase	25460
80.	Neonatal jaundice	Glutathione peroxidase	23170
81.	Niemann-Pick disease	Sphingomyelinase	25720
82.	Oroticaciduria	Orotidylic pyrophosphorylase and orotidylic decarboxylase	25890
83.	Phenylketonuria	Phenylalanine hydroxylase	26160
84.	Porphyria, congenital	Uroporphyrinogen III	26370
85.	Propionicacidemia	Mitochondrial propionyl CoA carboxylase	23200
86.	Pulmonary emphysema	d-l-antitrypsin	20740
87.	Pyridoxine-dependent infantile convulsions	Glutamic acid decarboxylase	26610
88.	Pyridoxine-responsive anemia	Delta-aminolevulinic acid synthetase*	30130
89.	Refsum's disease	Phytanic acid oxidase	26650
90.	Sulfite oxidase deficiency	Sulfite oxidase	27230

91.	Tay-Sachs disease	Hexosaminidase A	27280
92.	Testicular feminization	△4-5 α -reductase*	31370
93.	Thyroid hormonogenesis, defect in	Iodotyrosine dehalogenase (deiodinase)	27480
94.	Trypsinogen deficiency	Trypsinogen	27480
95.	Tyrosinemia I	Para-hydroxyphenylpyruvate oxidase	27670
96.	Tyrosinemia II	Tyrosine transaminase	27660
97.	Valinemia	Valine transaminase	27710
98.	Vitamin D resistant rickets	Cholecalciferase*	19310
99.	Wolman's disease	Acid lipase	27800
100.	Xanthinuria	Xanthine oxidase	27830
101.	Xanthurenic aciduria	Kynureninase	27880
102.	Xeroderma pigmentosum	Ultraviolet specific endonuclease	27870
103.	Xylosidase deficiency	Xylosidase	27890

LINKAGES, INCLUDING SPECIFIC AUTOSOMAL ASSIGNMENTS WHERE KNOWN

A. Autosomal linkages 1.

1. Chromosomal assignment

    a. Duffy blood group locus (11070) and locus for a form of cataract (11620)
    b. α-Haptoglobin locus (14010), PGM 3 locus (17210)* and the HL-A locus (or region) (14280)* on chromosome No. 16
    c. Thymidine kinase (18830) on chromosome No. 17

2. Linked loci without chromosomal assignment

    a. ABO blood group locus (11030), adenylate kinase locus (10300) and locus for nail-patella syndrome (16120)
    b. Rhesus blood group locus (11170), 6-phosphogluconate dehydrogenase locus (17220) and locus for one form of elliptocytosis (13050)
    c. Secretor locus (18210), Lutheran blood group locus (11120), and locus for myotonic dystrophy (16090)
    d. Beta hemoglobin locus (14190) and delta hemoglobin locus (14210)
    e. Transferrin locus (19000) and pseudocholinesterase-1 locus (17740)
    f. Albumin locus (10360) and group-specific component (Gc) locus (13920)
    g. Locus for Pelger-Huet anomaly (16940) and locus for unusual form of muscular dystrophy (15900)*
    h. MNSs blood group locus (11130) and sclerotylosis locus (18160)
    i. Locus for Am-2 immunoglobulin type (14700) and locus for Gm immunoglobulin type (14710)
    j. Lactic acid dehydrogenase B (15010) and peptidase B (16990)
    k. ABO blood group locus and locus for xeroderma pigmentosum (11030)*

B. X-borne linkages

    1. Colorblindness loci (30380,30390) and G6PD locus (30590)
    2. Colorblindness loci and hemophilia A (30690)
    3. G6PD locus and hemophilia A locus
    4. Xg blood group locus (31470) and locus for X-linked ichthyosis (30810)
    5. Xg blood group locus and ocular albinism locus (30050)
    6. Xg blood group locus and angiokeratoma locus (30150)
    7. Colorblindness loci and angiokeratoma locus
    8. Xm serum protein locus (31490) and the locus for the Hunter syndrome (30990)*
    9. Hypoxanthine-guanine-phosphoribosyltransferase locus (30800) and Xg locus
    10. Deutan and protan colorblindness loci
    11. Xg blood group locus and locus for X-linked cataract (30220)*
    12. Xg blood group locus and locus for retinoschisis (31270)

*Linkage cannot be considered proven.

PROTEINS IN WHICH GENETICALLY DETERMINED STRUCTURAL VARIATION HAS BEEN DEMONSTRATED IN MAN*[a]

1.	Adenine phosphoribosyltransferase*	10260
2.	Adenosine deaminase*	10270
3.	Adenylate kinase*	20160
4.	Albumin	10360
5.	Alcohol dehydrogenase	10370
6.	Amylase, pancreatic	10470
7.	Amylase, salivary	10470
8.	Antihemophilic globulin	30670
9.	α_1-Antitrypsin (protease inhibitor)*	10740
10.	Carbonic anhydrase	11480
11.	Catalase	11550
12.	Ceruloplasmin	11770
13.	Cholinesterase (E1 locus)*	17740
14.	Cholinesterase (E2 locus)*	17750
15.	Complement component C3	12070
16.	Complement component C4	12080
17.	Esterase (acetylesterase)	13340
18.	Factor IX	26490
19.	Fibrinogen	13480
20.	Galactose-1-phosphate uridyltransferase	23040
21.	α_2-Globulin (PA types)	26010
22.	Glucose-6-phosphate dehydrogenase	30590
23.	Glutamic oxaloacetic transaminase, mitochondrial	13820
24.	Glutathione reductase	13830
25.	Glycoprotein, $\alpha a1$-acid	13860
26.	Group-specific component (Gc)*	13920
27.	Haptoglobin, α chain*	14020
28.	Haptoglobin, β chain	23440
29.	Hemoglobin, α chain	14180
30.	Hemoglobin, β chain	14190
31.	Hemoglobin, γ 136 Gly chain	14200
32.	Hemoglobin, γ 136 Ala chain	14200
33.	Hemoglobin, δ chain	14210
34.	Hemoglobin, $\in$ chain	14220
35.	Hypoxanthine guanine phosphoribosyltransferase	30800
36.	Immunoglobulins, IgA (Am-1)	14690
37.	Immunoglobulins, IgA (Am-2)	14700
38.	Immunoglobulins, IgG, heavy chains (Gm)*	14710
39.	Immunoglobulins, IgG, light chains (InV)*	14720
40.	Inhibitor of C 1-esterase	10610
41.	Lactate dehydrogenase, A chain	15000
42.	Lactate dehydrogenase, B chain	15010
43.	β-Lipoprotein (Ag types)*	15200
44.	β-Lipoprotein (Ld types)	15210
45.	β-Lipoprotein (Lp types)*	15220
46.	α 2-Macroglobulin (Xm)*	31490
47.	Malate dehydrogenase, mitochondrial	15410

48.	Malate dehydrogenase, cytoplasmic	15420
49.	Methemoglobin reductase (NADH diaphorase)	25080
50.	Myoglobin	16000
51.	Pepsinogen	16970
52.	Peptidase A*	16980
53.	Peptidase B*	16990
54.	Peptidase C	17000
55.	Peptidase D	17010
56.	Peptidase E	17020
57.	Phosphatase, acid*	17150
58.	Phosphatase, alkaline	17180
59.	Phosphoglucomutase-1 (PGM-1)*	17190
60.	Phosphoglucomutase-2 (PGM-2)*	17200
61.	Phosphoglucomutase-3 (PGM-3)	17210
62.	6-Phosphogluconate dehydrogenase*	17220
63.	Phosphohexose isomerase	17240
64.	Prothrombin	12790
65.	Pyruvate kinase	26620
66.	Tetrazolium oxidase	18760
67.	Transferrin*	19000

[a]Most are associated with no discernible abnormality of phenotype. Most are demonstrated by electrophoresis, some by immunologic methods, some by immuno-electrophoresis, at least one (HGPRT) by heat stability. The tissue from which the protein was derived was most often serum (or plasma) and next most often red blood cells. White cells, liver, placenta, and saliva have been the source of material in some instances. Multiple alleles have been demonstrated for many of these proteins.

*Proteins marked with an asterisk show variation with gene frequencies in European populations which make them useful in linkage studies (Renwick, Brit. Med. Bull., Jan., 1969, and J. Med. Genet., 1970, with additions). Other markers useful in linkage analysis in European populations include red cell types (ABO, MNSs, P. Rhesus, Lutheran, Kell, Lewis, Duffy, Kidd, Dombrock, Stoltzfus), HL-A white cell types, secretor. In special populations other linkage markers are useful, e.g., G6PD in Mediterranean populations, HbS in African populations and Diego blood group in Oriental populations.

ON THE USE OF THE CATALOGS

In each of the three catalogs the entries are arranged alphabetically according to preferred designation. The entries in the dominant catalog are numbered consecutively beginning with number 10010. The numbers of entries in the recessive catalog begin with 20010. Those in the X-linkage catalog begin with 30010. Beginning with this third edition, a five digit numbering system is used. Numbers 1 through 9 for the terminal digit have been left to accommodate future growth of the catalogs. Some geneticists expressed a desire to use the numbering system of these catalogs as the basis of a diagnostic and bibliographic filing system and were distressed by the change in numbering between the first and second editions.

In the subject index not only the preferred designation but also alternative designations and individual phenotypic features are listed. The author index is provided as an aid in finding a condition whose position in the catalogs is uncertain; the searcher may recall that Dr. So-and-So described a particular unusual syndrome, but he may not know the designation under which it is entered here.

The words "dominant," "recessive," and "X-linked," situated vertically at the margin of each page, are intended to serve as a quick guide for finding the desired section of the book.

An asterisk preceding an entry indicates that the particular mode of inheritance is considered quite certain. In the case of those without an asterisk, suggestions of the particular mode of inheritance are strong enough to warrant inclusion for heuristic purposes.

The computer has certain limitations, but these should not seriously hamper the use of the catalogs. Note that an asterisk is used in place of a colon or semicolon. A question mark (for example, in the title of an article) has been designated ".Q". Special characters from foreign languages such as the German umlaut and the French acute and grave accents could not be reproduced. Greek letters have been written out (for example, γ = gamma, δ = delta, and so on). Genetic notation (particularly superscripts) used in connection with blood groups and serum protein types presented difficulty. As a rule, superscripts and subscripts have been placed in parentheses. For example, Xg^a = XG(A) and Hb M_{Boston} = HB M (BOSTON).

Q.V., an abbreviation used frequently in these catalogs, means *quod vide* "which see."

The nosologic and other tables are a new feature of this edition. They should prove a useful guide to nosology in the three areas covered—hereditary deafness, hand malformations, and skeletal disorders. In future editions other categories of genetic disease will be surveyed in similar tables.

Also included are tables which purport to give an exhaustive listing of identified specific enzyme deficiencies, proved linkages, and structural protein variants. These will be updated on an ongoing basis and will be included in successive editions as an indication of the state of the science.

For other tables see HEMOGLOBIN in the dominant catalog and GLUCOSE-6-PHOSPHATE DEHYDROGENASE VARIANTS in the X-linked catalog.

AUTOSOMAL DOMINANT PHENOTYPES

PRUNE BELLY IS A DESCRIPTIVE TERM FOR THIS SYNDROME, DERIVED FROM THE FACT THAT
THE INTESTINAL PATTERN IS EVIDENT THROUGH THE THIN, LAX, PROTRUDING ABDOMINAL WALL
IN THE INFANT. THE FULL SYNDROME PROBABLY OCCURS ONLY IN MALES (WILLIAMS AND
BURKHOLDER, 1967). MULTIPLE CASES (OF THE FULL SYNDROME) IN FAMILIES HAVE NEVER
BEEN REPORTED. IF THIS IS AN X-LINKED RECESSIVE, MULTIPLE AFFECTED BROTHERS
SHOULD HAVE BEEN OBSERVED. IF THE DISORDER IS DUE TO FRESH DOMINANT MUTATION IN
EACH CASE, THE MALE-LIMITATION WOULD BE UNEXPECTED BUT NOT IMPOSSIBLE. THIS
MALFORMATION SYNDROME IS ONE LIKE POLAND'S SYNDROME (Q.V.) IN BEING RATHER
CONSISTENTLY REPRODUCED IN MANY CASES BUT HAVING NO CLEARLY DEMONSTRABLE MENDELIAN
BASIS. A POSSIBLY RELATED SYNDROME WAS DESCRIBED IN A SINGLE PATIENT BY TEXTER
AND MURPHY (1968). THE TRIAD CONSISTED OF ABSENCE OF THE RIGHT TESTIS, KIDNEY AND
RECTUS ABDOMINIS MUSCLE. A BETTER PROGNOSIS THAN IS USUALLY THOUGHT TO OBTAIN WAS
SUGGESTED BY THE SERIES OF 19 PATIENTS REPORTED BY BURKE ET AL. (1969).

BURKE, E. C., SHIN, M. H. AND KELALIS, P. P.* PRUNE BELLY SYNDROME* CLINICAL
FINDINGS AND SURVIVAL. AM. J. DIS. CHILD. 117* 668-671, 1969.

ROBERTS, P.* CONGENITAL ABSENCE OF THE ABDOMINAL MUSCLES WITH ASSOCIATED
ABNORMALITIES OF THE GENITO-URINARY TRACT. ARCH. DIS. CHILD. 31* 236-239, 1956.

TEXTER, J. H. AND MURPHY, G. P.* THE RIGHT-SIDED SYNDROME* CONGENITAL ABSENCE
OF THE RIGHT TESTIS, KIDNEY AND RECTUS. UROLOGIC DIAGNOSIS AND TREATMENT. JOHNS
HOPKINS MED. J. 122* 224-228, 1968.

WILLIAMS, D. I. AND BURKHOLDER, G. V.* THE PRUNE BELLY SYNDROME. J. UROL. 98*
244-251, 1967.

10020 ABDUCENS PALSY

AFFECTED PERSONS IN TWO OR MORE GENERATIONS HAVE BEEN REPORTED (CHAVASSE, 1938,
1939* FRANCOIS, 1958). NUCLEAR APLASIA HAS BEEN FOUND IN SOME CASES (PHILLIPS ET
AL., 1932). THIS IS A FORM OF HEREDITARY STRABISMUS.

CHAVASSE, F. B.* THE OCULAR PALSIES. TRANS. OPHTHAL. SOC. U.K. 58* 493 AND
497, 1938.

FRANCOIS, J.* HEREDITY IN OPHTHALMOLOGY. ST. LOUIS* C. V. MOSBY CO., 1961. P.
280.

PHILLIPS, W. H., DIRION, J. K. AND GRAVES, G. O.* CONGENITAL BILATERAL PALSY OF
ABDUCENS. ARCH. OPHTHAL. 8* 355-364, 1932.

10030 ABSENCE DEFECT OF LIMBS, SCALP AND SKULL

THE PROBAND DESCRIBED BY ADAMS AND OLIVER (1945) HAD (1) ABSENCE OF THE LOWER
EXTREMITIES BELOW THE MID-CALF REGION AND ABSENCE OF ALL DIGITS AND SOME OF THE
METACARPALS OF THE RIGHT HAND, (2) A DENUDED ULCERATED AREA ON THE VERTEX OF THE
SCALP PRESENT AT BIRTH, AND (3) A BONY DEFECT OF THE SKULL UNDERLYING THE SCALP
DEFECT. THE PROBAND HAD FOUR UNAFFECTED BROTHERS AND A SISTER AND BROTHER WITH
IDENTICAL DEFECTS OF LIMB, SCALP AND SKULL. THE FATHER WAS BORN WITH ABSENCE OF
TOES II-V ON THE LEFT FOOT, WITH SHORT TERMINAL PHALANGES OF ALL FINGERS AND WITH
A SCALP DEFECT. THE FATHER WAS ONE OF 10 CHILDREN OF WHOM THREE OTHERS HAD
DEFECTS OF THE EXTREMITIES. THE FATHER'S FATHER WAS SAID TO HAVE HAD SHORT
FINGERS. THE PROBAND'S PARENTS WERE NOT RELATED. THE SKIN AND SKULL LESIONS ARE
LIKE THOSE OF APLASIA CUTIS CONGENITA (Q.V.).

ADAMS, F. H. AND OLIVER, C. P.* HEREDITARY DEFORMITIES IN MAN DUE TO ARRESTED
DEVELOPMENT. J. HERED. 36* 3-7, 1945.

10040 ABSENCE OF SKIN, BLISTERING, ABNORMALITY OF NAILS

IN 25 PERSONS IN FOUR GENERATIONS DESCENDANT FROM A MAN BORN IN FRANCE, BART
(1970) DESCRIBED CONGENITAL LOCALIZED ABSENCE OF SKIN OF THE LOWER EXTREMITIES (IN
13), BLISTERS OF THE SKIN OR MUCOUS MEMBRANES WHICH HEAL WITHOUT SCARRING (IN 20)
AND ABSENCE OR DEFORMITY OF NAILS (IN 23). FATHER-TO-SON TRANSMISSION WAS NOTED.
THE DISORDER MOST NEARLY RESEMBLES A FORM OF EPIDERMOLYSIS BULLOSA.

BART, B. J.* CONGENITAL LOCALIZED ABSENCE OF SKIN, BLISTERING AND NAIL
ABNORMALITIES. THE CLINICAL DELINEATION OF BIRTH DEFECTS. XII. SKIN, HAIR AND
NAILS. BALTIMORE* WILLIAMS AND WILKINS, 1971.

*10050 ACANTHOCYTOSIS

IN ADDITION TO THE FORM OF ACANTHOCYTOSIS WHICH ACCOMPANIES ABETALIPOPROTEINEMIA
(Q.V.), CRITCHLEY, CLARK AND WIKLER (1967) DESCRIBED AN ADULT FORM OF ACANTHOCYTO-
SIS ASSOCIATED WITH NEUROLOGICAL ABNORMALITIES AND APPARENTLY NORMAL SERUM
LIPOPROTEINS. THE NEUROLOGIC MANIFESTATIONS SUGGESTED THOSE OF THE GILLES DE LA
TOURETTE SYNDROME OR HUNTINGTON'S CHOREA. FIVE OF 10 SIBS HAD NEUROLOGIC
MANIFESTATIONS. A NIECE HAD ACANTHOCYTES AND A NEUROLOGIC DISORDER SUGGESTING

FRIEDREICH'S ATAXIA. THE SAME DISORDER WAS PROBABLY REPORTED BY LEVINE (1964) AND ESTES ET AL.   (1967)   IN A FAMILY IN WHICH 15 PERSONS IN 3 GENERATIONS HAD SOME DEGREE OF NEURONAL IMPAIRMENT AND 9 OF THESE HAD ACANTHOCYTOSIS. LEVINE ET AL. (1968) CONCLUDED THAT THE PREDOMINANT NEUROLOGIC INVOLVEMENT IS NEURONAL.

BETTS, J. J., NICHOLSON, J. T. AND CRITCHLEY, E. M. R.* ACANTHOCYTOSIS WITH NORMOLIPOPROTEINAEMIA* BIOPHYSICAL ASPECTS. POSTGRAD. MED. J. 46* 702-707, 1970.

CRITCHLEY, E. M. R., BETTS, J. J., NICHOLSON, J. T. AND WEATHERALL, D. J.* ACANTHOCYTOSIS, NORMOLIPOPROTEINAEMIA AND MULTIPLE TICS. POSTGRAD. MED. J. 46* 698-701, 1970.

CRITCHLEY, E. M. R., CLARK, D. B. AND WIKLER, A.* AN ADULT FORM OF ACANTHOCYTO-SIS. TRANS. AM. NEUROL. ASS. 92* 132-137, 1967.

ESTES, J. W., MORLEY, T. J., LEVINE, I. M. AND EMERSON, C. P.* A NEW HEREDITARY ACANTHOCYTOSIS SYNDROME. AM. J. MED. 42* 868-881, 1967.

LEVINE, I. M.* AN HEREDITARY NEUROLOGIC DISEASE WITH ACANTHOCYTOSIS. (ABS-TRACT) NEUROLOGY 14* 272 ONLY, 1964.

LEVINE, I. M., ESTES, J. W. AND LOONEY, J. M.* HEREDITARY NEUROLOGICAL DISEASE WITH ACANTHOCYTOSIS. A NEW SYNDROME. ARCH. NEUROL. 19* 403-409, 1968.

10060 ACANTHOSIS NIGRICANS

IN ALL TWENTY-SIX PATIENTS WITH MALIGNANT ACANTHOSIS NIGRICANS - SECONDARY TO VISCERAL CARCINOMA   - CURTH AND ASCHNER (1959) FOUND NO OTHER AFFECTED PERSONS IN THE FAMILY.   ON THE OTHER HAND BENIGN ACANTHOSIS NIGRICANS IS PROBABLY INHERITED AS A MENDELIAN DOMINANT.   JUNG ET AL. (1965) OBSERVED AFFECTED MOTHER AND DAUGHTER.   THE CONDITION CONSISTS OF THICKENING AND HYPERPIGMENTATION OF THE SKIN OF THE ENTIRE BODY BUT ESPECIALLY IN FLEXURAL AREAS.

CURTH, H. O. AND ASCHNER, B. M.* GENETIC STUDIES ON ACANTHOSIS NIGRICANS. ARCH. DERM. 79* 55-66, 1959.

HERMANN, H.* ZUR ERBPATHOLOGIE DER ACANTHOSIS NIGRICANS. Z. MENSCHL. VERERB. KONSTITUTIONSL. 33* 193-202, 1955.

JUNG, H. D., BRUNS, W., WULFERT, P. AND MIELER, W.* EIN BEITRAG ZUM KRANKHEITS-BILD DER ACANTHOSIS NIGRICANS BENIGNA FAMILIARIS. DEUTSCH. MED. WSCHR. 90* 1669-1673, 1965.

10070 ACHARD SYNDROME

ARACHNODACTYLY, RECEDING LOWER JAW AND JOINT LAXITY LIMITED TO THE HANDS AND FEET ARE FEATURES.   PARISH (1960) PICTURED A CASE.   WHEN THURSFIELD (1917-1918) REVIEWED THE LITERATURE ON MARFAN'S SYNDROME, HE REMARKED THAT THE SKELETAL PICTURE IN THE CASES DESCRIBED BY ACHARD (1902) DIFFERED FROM THE OTHERS. THE SKULL IS BROAD AND BRACHYCEPHALIC WITH SMALL MANDIBLE. ALTHOUGH THERE IS ARACHNODACTYLY THE BODY PROPORTIONS ARE NOT ALTERED AND THE PATIENT IS NOT EXCESSIVELY TALL.

ACHARD, C.* ARACHNODACTYLIE. BULL. SOC. MED. HOP. PARIS 19* 834-840, 1902.

PARISH, J. G.* HEREDITABLE DISORDERS OF CONNECTIVE TISSUES WITH ARACHNODACTYLY. PROC. ROY. SOC. MED. 53* 515-518, 1960.

PARISH, J. G.* SKELETAL HAND CHARTS IN INHERITED CONNECTIVE TISSUE DISEASE. J. MED. GENET. 4* 227-238, 1967.

THURSFIELD, H.* ARACHNO-DACTYLY. ST. BART'S HOSP. REP. 53* 35-40, 1917-18.

*10080 ACHONDROPLASIA, CLASSICAL

ALTHOUGH THERE ARE NUMEROUS SIMULATING SKELETAL DISORDERS, TRUE ACHONDROPLASIA IS A WELL-DELINEATED DISTINCT ENTITY WHICH PROBABLY IN ALL INSTANCES OCCURS AS A NEW DOMINANT MUTATION OR BY DOMINANT INHERITANCE. THE CHONDROCRANIUM IS AFFECTED PRODUCING BULGING SKULL, 'SCOOPED OUT' BRIDGE OF THE NOSE, AND SMALL FORAMEN MAGNUM.   TRUE MEGENCEPHALY OCCURS AND APPEARS TO INDICATE EFFECTS OF THE GENE OTHER THAN THOSE ON THE SKELETON ALONE. DISPROPORTION BETWEEN THE BASE OF THE SKULL AND THE BRAIN RESULTS IN INTERNAL HYDROCEPHALUS IN SOME CASES. IN CHILDREN CAUDAD NARROWING OF THE INTERPEDUNCULAR DISTANCE, RATHER THAN THE NORMAL CAUDAD WIDENING, AND NOTCH-LIKE SACRO-ILIAC GROOVE ARE TYPICAL RADIOLOGIC FEATURES. ALSO IN CHILDREN THE EPIPHYSEAL OSSIFICATION CENTER SHOWS A CIRCUMFLEX OR CHEVRON SEAT ON THE METAPHYSIS. ABOUT SEVEN-EIGHTHS OF CASES ARE THE RESULT OF NEW MUTATION, THERE BEING A CONSIDERABLE REDUCTION OF EFFECTIVE REPRODUCTIVE FITNESS. PATERNAL AGE EFFECT ON MUTATION HAS BEEN NOTED (PENROSE, 1955). (IT IS OF HISTORIC INTEREST THAT WEINBERG, OF HARDY-WEINBERG FAME, NOTED (1912) IN THE DATA COLLECTED BY RISCHBIETH AND BARRINGTON THAT SPORADIC CASES WERE MORE OFTEN LAST BORN THAN FIRST BORN.)   THE RADIOLOGIC FEATURES OF TRUE ACHONDROPLASIA AND MUCH CONCERNING THE NATURAL HISTORY OF THE CONDITION WAS PRESENTED BY LANGER ET AL. (1967) ON THE

BASIS OF A STUDY OF 101 CASES. SEE THANATOPHORIC DWARFISM FOR A CONDITION WHICH IS FATAL IN THE FIRST DAYS OF LIFE AND WHICH SIMULATES ACHONDROPLASIA. HOMOZYGOSITY FOR THE ACHONDROPLASIA GENE RESULTS IN A SEVERE DISORDER OF THE SKELETON WITH RADIOLOGIC CHANGES SOMEWHAT DIFFERENT FROM THOSE OF HETEROZYGOUS ACHONDROPLASIA AND WITH EARLY DEATH AS A RESULT OF RESPIRATORY EMBARRASSMENT FROM THE SMALL THORACIC CAGE AND NEUROLOGIC DEFICIT FROM HYDROCEPHALUS (HALL ET AL., 1969). THE CONFUSION OF TRUE ACHONDROPLASIA WITH OTHER ENTITIES IS ILLUSTRATED BY THE TWO FEMALE SIBS REPORTED BY WALLACE ET AL. (1970) AS EXAMPLES OF THIS CONDITION. BOTH DIED IN THE NEONATAL PERIOD AND SHOWED, IN ADDITION TO CHONDRODYSTROPHY, CENTRAL HARELIP, HYPOPLASTIC LUNGS AND HYDROCEPHALUS. WITHOUT RADIOGRAPHIC STUDIES IT IS IMPOSSIBLE TO IDENTIFY THE NATURE OF THIS CONDITION BUT IT IS CERTAINLY NOT TRUE ACHONDROPLASIA. JEUNE'S ASPHYXIATING THORACIC DYSTROPHY, THANATOPHORIC DWARFISM AND ACHONDROGENESIS ARE THREE POSSIBILITIES, BUT WITH THE SECOND AFFECTED SIBS HAVE NOT BEEN DESCRIBED. THE REPORT OF WALLACE ET AL. DEMONSTRATES WHY ESTIMATES OF MUTATION RATE HAVE BEEN FALSELY HIGH.

COHEN, M. E., ROSENTHAL, A. D. AND MATSON, D. D.* NEUROLOGICAL ABNORMALITIES IN ACHONDROPLASTIC CHILDREN. J. PEDIAT. 71* 367-376, 1967.

DENNIS, J. P., ROSENBERG, H. S. AND ALVORD, E. C., JR.* MEGALENCEPHALY, INTERNAL HYDROCEPHALUS AND OTHER NEUROLOGICAL ASPECTS OF ACHONDROPLASIA. BRAIN 84* 427-445, 1961.

HALL, J. G., DORST, J. P., TAYBI, H., SCOTT, C. I., LANGER, L. O., JR. AND MCKUSICK, V. A.* TWO PROBABLE CASES OF HOMOZYGOSITY FOR THE ACHONDROPLASIA GENE. THE CLINICAL DELINEATION OF BIRTH DEFECTS. IV. SKELETAL DYSPLASIAS. NEW YORK* NATIONAL FOUNDATION, 1969. PP. 24-34.

LANGER, L. O., JR., BAUMANN, P. A. AND GORLIN, R. J.* ACHONDROPLASIA. AM. J. ROENTGEN. 100* 12-26, 1967.

MAROTEAUX, P. AND LAMY, P.* ACHONDROPLASIA IN MAN AND ANIMALS. CLIN. ORTHOP. 33* 91-103, 1964.

MORCH, E. T.* CHONDRODYSTROPHIC DWARFS IN DENMARK. OP. EX. DOMO. BIOL. HERED. HUM. U. HAFNIENSIS 3* 1941.

MURDOCH, J. L., WALKER, B. A., HALL, J. G., ABBEY, H., SMITH, K. K. AND MCKUSICK, V. A.* ACHONDROPLASIA - A GENETIC AND STATISTICAL SURVEY. ANN. HUM. GENET. 33* 227-244, 1970.

PENROSE, L. S.* PARENTAL AGE AND MUTATION. LANCET 2* 312-313, 1955.

PENROSE, L. S.* PARENTAL AGE IN ACHONDROPLASIA AND MONGOLISM. AM. J. HUM. GENET. 9* 167-169, 1957.

RIMOIN, D. L., HUGHES, G. N., KAUFMAN, R. L., ROSENTHAL, R. E., MCALISTER, W. H. AND SILBERBERG, R.* ENDOCHONDRAL OSSIFICATION IN ACHONDROPLASTIC DWARFISM. NEW ENG. J. MED. 283* 728-735, 1970.

WALLACE, D. C., EXTON, L. A., PRITCHARD, D. A., LEUNG, Y. AND COOKE, R. A.* SEVERE ACHONDROPLASIA. DEMONSTRATION OF PROBABLE HETEROGENEITY WITHIN THIS CLINICAL SYNDROME. J. MED. GENET. 7* 22-26, 1970.

WEINBERG, W.* ZUR VERERBUNG DES ZWERGWUCHSES. ARCH. RASS. U. GES. BIOL. 9* 710-717, 1912.

*10090 ACHROMATIC REGIONS OF TETRAZOLIUM STAINED STARCH GELS

WHEN STARCH GELS ARE STAINED BY THE PHENAZINE-TETRAZOLIUM TECHNIQUE, IN ADDITION TO THE APPEARANCE OF BLUE BANDS MARKING THE SITE OF ISOZYMES UNDER INVESTIGATION, LIGHT OR ACHROMATIC AREAS APPEAR. THE BANDS ARE THE EFFECTS OF AN OXIDASE WHICH OXIDIZES TETRAZOLIUM DYES IN THE PRESENCE OF PHENAZINE AND LIGHT. BREWER (1967) OBSERVED AN ELECTROPHORETIC VARIANT OF THE OXIDASE IN THREE GENERATIONS OF A FAMILY WITH PRESUMED MALE-TO-MALE TRANSMISSION.

BREWER, G. J.* ACHROMATIC REGIONS OF TETRAZOLIUM STAINED STARCH GELS* INHERITED ELECTROPHORETIC VARIATION. AM. J. HUM. GENET. 19* 674-680, 1967.

*10100 ACOUSTIC NEUROMA, BILATERAL

GARDNER AND FRAZIER (1933) REPORTED A FAMILY OF FIVE GENERATIONS IN WHICH 38 MEMBERS WERE AFFECTED WITH DEAFNESS. OF THESE, 15 LATER BECAME BLIND. THE AVERAGE AGE OF ONSET OF DEAFNESS WAS 20 YEARS. THE AVERAGE AGE AT DEATH OF AFFECTED PERSONS IN THE SECOND GENERATION WAS 72, IN THE THIRD GENERATION 63, IN THE FOURTH 42 AND IN THE FIFTH 28. THERE WAS LITTLE OR NO EVIDENCE OF VON RECKLINGHAUSEN'S DISEASE (Q.V.) IN THE FAMILY, SUGGESTING THAT THIS IS A SEPARATE MUTATION. A FOLLOW-UP OF THE FAMILY WAS PUBLISHED IN 1940. ALTHOUGH ACOUSTIC NEUROMA IS SOMETIMES A FEATURE OF NEUROFIBROMATOSIS (Q.V.) BILATERAL ACOUSTIC NEUROMA IS PROBABLY AN ISOLATED ABNORMALITY WITH DOMINANT INHERITANCE IN SOME CASES. THE MOST CONVINCING FAMILIES ARE THOSE OF GARDNER AND TURNER (1940) AND OF FEILING AND WARD (1920). MOYES (1968) ADDED A WELL-STUDIED, EXTENSIVELY AFFECTED

KINDRED WITH NO EVIDENCE OF VON RECKLINGHAUSEN'S DISEASE. THESE CASES REPRESENT IN ALL PROBABILITY A CENTRAL-NERVOUS SYSTEM FORM OF MULTIPLE NEUROFIBROMATOSIS. ELDRIDGE (1969) FOUND NO EVIDENCE OF VON RECKLINGHAUSEN'S NEUROFIBROMATOSIS OF THE CONVENTIONAL TYPE IN THE FAMILY OF GARDNER WHEN HE RESTUDIED IT EXTENSIVELY. TWO CASES OF THE CNS FORM, ONE OF THEM FAMILIAL, WERE STUDIED AT AUTOPSY BY PEREZ DEMOURA ET AL. (1969), WHO INCORRECTLY REFERRED TO THE CASES OF GARDNER AND FRAZIER (1930) AS REPRESENTING VON RECKLINGHAUSEN'S DISEASE.

ELDRIDGE, R.* BETHESDA, MD.* PERSONAL COMMUNICATION, 1969.

FEILING, A. AND WARD, E.* A FAMILIAL FORM OF ACOUSTIC TUMOUR. BRIT. MED. J. 1* 496-497, 1920.

GARDNER, W. J. AND FRAZIER, C. H.* BILATERAL ACOUSTIC NEUROFIBROMAS. A CLINICAL STUDY AND SURVEY OF A FAMILY OF FIVE GENERATIONS WITH BILATERAL DEAFNESS IN 38 MEMBERS. ARCH. NEUROL. PSYCHIAT. 23* 266-302, 1930. (SEE ALSO J. HERED. 22* 7-8, 1933.)

GARDNER, W. J. AND TURNER, O.* BILATERAL ACOUSTIC NEUROFIBROMAS* FURTHER CLINICAL AND PATHOLOGIC DATA ON HEREDITARY DEAFNESS AND RECKLINGHAUSEN'S DISEASE. ARCH. NEUROL. PSYCHIAT. 44* 76-99, 1940.

MOYES, P. D.* FAMILIAL BILATERAL ACOUSTIC NEUROMA AFFECTING 14 MEMBERS FROM FOUR GENERATIONS. J. NEUROSURG. 29* 78-82, 1968.

PEREZ DEMOURA, L. F., HAYDEN, R. C., JR. AND CONNER, G. H.* BILATERAL ACOUSTIC NEURINOMA AND NEUROFIBROMATOSIS. ARCH. OTOLARYNG. 90* 28-34, 1969.

YOUNG, D. F., ELDRIDGE, R. AND GARDNER, W. J.* BILATERAL ACOUSTIC NEUROMA IN A LARGE KINDRED. J.A.M.A. 214* 347-353, 1970.

10110 ACROCEPHALOPOLYSYNDACTYLY TYPE I (ACPS I, OR NOACK'S SYNDROME)

ACROCEPHALOPOLYSYNDACTYLY DIFFERS FROM APERT'S SYNDROME (ACROCEPHALOSYNDACTYLY) IN THE PRESENCE OF POLYDACTYLY AS AN ADDITIONAL FEATURE. TWO TYPES ARE RECOGNIZED. TYPE I, OR NOACK'S SYNDROME, IS DOMINANT. TYPE II, OR CARPENTER'S SYNDROME, IS RECESSIVE. NOACK (1959) REPORTED A 43 YEAR OLD MAN AND HIS 11 MONTH OLD DAUGHTER, BOTH OF WHOM EXHIBITED ACROCEPHALY AND POLYSYNDACTYLY. ENLARGED THUMBS AND GREAT TOES WITH DUPLICATION OF THE LATTER (PREAXIAL POLYDACTYLY) WERE DESCRIBED, AS WELL AS SYNDACTYLY. INTELLIGENCE WAS APPARENTLY NORMAL. FOLLOW-UP OF NOACK'S KINDRED BY PFEIFFER APPEARS TO INDICATE THAT THEIR DISORDER IS THE SAME AS THAT REFERRED TO ELSEWHERE AS ACROCEPHALOSYNDACTYLY TYPE V (PFEIFFER TYPE).

NOACK, M.* EIN BEITRAG ZUM KRANKHEITSBILD DER AKROZEPHALOSYNDAKTYLIE (APERT). ARCH. KINDERHEILK. 160* 168-171, 1959.

PFEIFFER, R. A.* ASSOCIATED DEFORMITIES OF THE HEAD AND HANDS. THE CLINICAL DELINEATION OF BIRTH DEFECTS. III. LIMB MALFORMATIONS. NEW YORK* NATIONAL FOUNDATION, 1969. PP. 18-34.

*10120 ACROCEPHALOSYNDACTYLY TYPE I (TYPICAL APERT'S SYNDROME)

APERT (1906) DEFINED A SYNDROME CHARACTERIZED BY SKULL MALFORMATION (ACROCEPHALY OF BRACHYSPHENOCEPHALIC TYPE) AND SYNDACTYLY OF THE HANDS AND FEET OF A SPECIAL TYPE (COMPLETE DISTAL FUSION WITH A TENDENCY TO FUSION ALSO OF THE BONY STRUC-TURES). THE HAND WHEN ALL THE FINGERS ARE WEBBED HAS BEEN COMPARED TO A SPOON AND, WHEN THE THUMB IS FREE, TO AN OBSTETRIC HAND. BLANK (1960) IN HIS REVIEW DESIGNATED CASES OF ACS SHOWING THESE MALFORMATIONS AS TYPICAL APERT'S SYNDROME. MOST CASES OF APERT'S SYNDROME ARE SPORADIC, BUT THERE ARE AT LEAST TWO REPORTED INSTANCES OF PARENT-TO-CHILD TRANSMISSION. VAN DEN BOSCH (QUOTED BY BLANK) OBSERVED THE TYPICAL DEFORMITY IN A MOTHER AND HER SON, AND WEECH (1927) REPORTED APERT'S SYNDROME IN A MOTHER AND HER DAUGHTER. BLANK (1960) ASSEMBLED CASE MATERIAL ON 54 PATIENTS BORN IN GREAT BRITIAN. TWO CLINICAL CATEGORIES WERE DISTINGUISHED* (1) 'TYPICAL' ACROCEPHALOSYNDACTYLY, TO WHICH APERT'S NAME IS APPROPRIATELY APPLIED, AND (2) OTHER FORMS LUMPED TOGETHER AS 'ATYPICAL' ACROCE-PHALOSYNDACTYLY. THE FEATURES DISTINGUISHING THE TWO TYPES IS A MIDDIGITAL HAND MASS WITH A SINGLE NAIL COMMON TO DIGITS II - IV, FOUND IN APERT'S SYNDROME AND LACKING IN THE OTHERS. 39 OF THE 54 WERE OF APERT'S TYPE. 6 OF 12 AUTOPSIES SHOWED VISCERAL ANOMALIES BUT IN NO TWO WERE THESE IDENTICAL. A FREQUENCY OF APERT'S SYNDROME OF ONE IN EACH 160,000 BIRTHS WAS ESTIMATED. PATERNAL AGE EFFECT COULD BE DEMONSTRATED. NO PATIENT MARRIED. LOW FREQUENCY OF CONSANGUINITY AND FAILURE TO OBSERVE MULTIPLE SIBS MAKE RECESSIVE INHERITANCE UNLIKELY. NO CHROMOSOMAL ABNORMALITY IS DEMONSTRABLE. THE EVIDENCE STRONGLY SUGGESTS DOMINANT INHERITANCE, PRESUMABLY AUTOSOMAL IN VIEW OF THE EQUAL SEX RATIO. PATERNAL AGE EFFECT IS DEMONSTRABLE. DODSON ET AL. (1970) DESCRIBED DELETION-TRANSLOCATION OF THE SHORT ARM OF A CHROMOSOME 2 TO THE LONG ARM OF A CHROMOSOME 11 OR 12 IN A PATIENT WITH APERT'S SYNDROME. THEY FOUND REPORTS OF CHROMOSOMAL ABNORMALITIES (ALL INVOLVING THE A GROUP) IN THREE OTHER CASES OF APERT'S SYNDROME. WE (ROBERTS AND HALL, 1971) HAVE OBSERVED AFFECTED MOTHER AND DAUGHTER.

APERT, M. E.* DE L'ACROCEPHALOSYNDACTYLIE. BULL. SOC. MED. HOP. PARIS 23* 1310-1330, 1906.

BLANK, C. E.* APERT'S SYNDROME (A TYPE OF ACROCEPHALOSYNDACTYLY). OBSERVATIONS ON A BRITISH SERIES OF THIRTY-NINE CASES. ANN. HUM. GENET. 24* 151-164, 1960.

DODSON, W. E., MUSELES, M., KENNEDY, J. L., JR. AND AL-AISH, M.* ACROCEPHALO-SYNDACTYLIA ASSOCIATED WITH A CHROMOSOMAL TRANSLOCATION* 46,XX,T(2P-*CQ+). AM. J. DIS. CHILD. 120* 360-362, 1970.

HOOVER, G. H., FLATT, A. E. AND WEISS, M. W.* THE HAND AND APERT'S SYNDROME. J. BONE JOINT SURG. 52A* 878-895, 1970.

ROBERTS, K. B. AND HALL, J. G.* APERT'S ACROCEPHALOSYNDACTYLY IN MOTHER AND DAUGHTER, CLEFT PALATE IN THE MOTHER. THE CLINICAL DELINEATION OF BIRTH DEFECTS. XI. OROFACIAL STRUCTURES. BALTIMORE* WILLIAMS AND WILKINS, 1971.

SOLOMON, L. M., FRETZIN, D. AND PRUZANSKY, S.* PILOSEBACEOUS ABNORMALITIES IN APERT'S SYNDROME. ARCH. DERM. 102* 381-385, 1970.

WEECH, A. A.* COMBINED ACROCEPHALY AND SYNDACTYLISM OCCURRING IN MOTHER AND DAUGHTER. A CASE REPORT. BULL. HOPKINS HOSP. 40* 73-76, 1927.

10130 ACROCEPHALOSYNDACTYLY TYPE II (APERT-CROUZON DISEASE, OR VOGT'S CEPHALODACTYLY)

VOGT DESCRIBED CASES PRESENTING THE HAND AND FOOT MALFORMATIONS CHARACTERISTIC OF APERT'S DISEASE, TOGETHER WITH THE FACIAL CHARACTERISTICS OF CROUZON'S DISEASE, CAUSED BY AN EXTREMELY HYPOPLASTIC MAXILLA. IN THE HANDS THE SYNDACTYLY IS LESS SEVERE THAN IN APERT'S DISEASE AND THE THUMBS AND LITTLE FINGERS ARE USUALLY FREE. NAGER AND DE REYNIER (1948) GAVE THIS DEFORMITY THE NAME OF VOGT'S CEPHALODACTYLY, WHILE OTHER AUTHORS CALLED IT APERT-CROUZON DISEASE, INDICATING THE SIMILARITY TO BOTH ABNORMALITIES. THERE ARE NO REPORTED INSTANCES OF HEREDITARY TRANSMISSION* HOWEVER, THIS COULD BE DUE SIMPLY TO LOW REPRODUCTIVE FITNESS. THE ASSOCIATION OF SKULL AND LIMB DEFORMITY COMPRISES A SPECTRUM OF TRAITS WHICH PROBABLY REPRESENTS THE EFFECTS OF MUTATIONS OF VARIOUS GENES OPERATING AT DIFFERENT STAGES OF DIFFERENTIATION AND DEVELOPMENT. IN THIS SPECTRUM THE ASSOCIATION OF ACROCEPHALY WITH SYNDACTYLY IS DISCUSSED. EACH OF THESE TYPES OF ACROCEPHALOSYNDACTYLY (ACS) PROBABLY REPRESENTS A DIFFERENT GENE MUTATION THOUGH THEY ALL SHARE THE PHENOTYPE OF ACROCEPHALY ASSOCIATED WITH SYNDACTYLISM. IN FAVOR OF THE HYPOTHESIS THAT THE DIFFERENT PHENOTYPIC VARIANTS OF ACS REPRESENT EFFECTS OF DIFFERENT GENE MUTATIONS IS THE FACT THAT IN THE TWO CASES OF ACS TYPE I (TYPICAL APERT'S SYNDROME) WHO REPRODUCED, THE CHILDREN HAD THE SAME PHENOTYPE. ON THE OTHER HAND, IN ALL THE PEDIGREES OF AUTOSOMAL DOMINANT TRANSMISSION OF THE OTHER TYPES OF ACS THERE WAS NO TRANSITION FROM ONE TYPE TO THE OTHER IN SPITE OF THE EXISTENCE OF VARIABILITY IN EXPRESSIVITY OF THE TRAIT WITHIN EACH TYPE. PARTICULARLY THERE IS NOT A SINGLE CASE OF TYPICAL APERT'S SYNDROME AMONG THE RELATIVES OF INDIVIDUALS WITH THE OTHER TYPES. SCHAUERTE AND ST-AUBIN (1966) POINTED OUT THAT PROGRESSIVE SYNOSTOSIS OCCURS IN THE FEET, HANDS, CARPUS, TARSUS, CERVICAL VERTEBRAE, AND SKULL AND PROPOSED 'PROGRESSIVE SYNOSTEOSIS WITH SYNDACTYLY' AS A MORE APPROPRIATE DESIGNA-TION.

BLANK, C. E.* APERT'S SYNDROME (A TYPE OF ACROCEPHALOSYNDACTYLY). OBSERVATIONS ON A BRITISH SERIES OF THIRTY-NINE CASES. ANN. HUM. GENET. 24* 151-164, 1960.

NAGER, F. R. AND DE REYNIER, J. P.* DAS GEHORORGAN BEI DEN ANGEBORENEN KOPFMISSBILDUNGEN. PRACT. OTORHINOLARYNG. 10 (SUPPL. 2)* 1-128, 1948.

SCHAUERTE, E. W. AND ST-AUBIN, P. M.* PROGRESSIVE SYNOSTEOSIS IN APERT'S SYNDROME (ACROCEPHALOSYNDACTYLY), WITH A DESCRIPTION OF ROENTGENOGRAPHIC CHANGES IN THE FEET. AM. J. ROENTGEN. 97* 67-73, 1966.

VOGT, A.* DYSKEPHALIE (DYSOSTOSIS CRANIOFACIALIS, MALADIE DE CROUZON 1912) UND EINE NEUARTIGE KOMBINATION DIESER KRANKHEIT MIT SYNDAKTYLIE DER 4 EXTREMITATEN (DYSKEPHALODAKTYLIE). KLIN. MBL. AUGENHEILK. 90* 441-454, 1933.

*10140 ACROCEPHALOSYNDACTYLY TYPE III (ACROCEPHALY, SKULL ASYMMETRY AND MILD SYNDACTY-LY)

IN THE FAMILY DESCRIBED BY SAETHRE (1931), A MOTHER, TWO DAUGHTERS AND PROBABLY OTHER MATERNAL RELATIVES SHOWED MILD ACROCEPHALY, ASYMMETRY OF THE SKULL, AND PARTIAL SOFT TISSUE SYNDACTYLY OF FINGERS II AND III AND TOES III AND IV. CHOTZEN (1932) FOUND IDENTICAL MALFORMATIONS IN A FATHER AND TWO SONS. BARTSOCAS ET AL. (1970) DESCRIBED A LITHUANIAN KINDRED LIVING IN THE UNITED STATES IN WHICH 10 PERSONS IN 3 GENERATIONS WERE AFFECTED, WITH SEVERAL INSTANCES OF MALE-TO-MALE TRANSMISSION.

BARTSOCAS, C. S., WEBER, A. L. AND CRAWFORD, J. D.* ACROCEPHALOSYNDACTYLY TYPE 3* CHOTZEN'S SYNDROME. J. PEDIAT. 77* 267-272, 1970.

CHOTZEN, F.* EINE EIGENARTIGE FAMILIARE ENTWICKLUNGSSTORUNG (AKROCEPHALOSYNDAK-TYLIE, DYSOSTOSIS CRANIOFACIALIS UND HYPERTELORISMUS). MSCHR. KINDERHEILK. 55* 97-122, 1932.

SAETHRE, M.* EIN BEITRAG ZUM TURMSCHADELPROBLEM (PATHOGENESE, ERBLICHKEIT UND SYMPTOMATOLOGIE). DEUTSCH. Z. NERVENHEILK. 119* 533-555, 1931.

*10150 ACROCEPHALOSYNDACTYLY TYPE IV (WAARDENBURG TYPE)

IN 1934 WAARDENBURG DESCRIBED A PEDIGREE COVERING 4 GENERATIONS WITH 8 DEFINITE AND 5 PROBABLE CASES OF ACROCEPHALY, ORBITAL AND FACIAL DEFORMITIES, AND BRACHYDA-CTYLY WITH MILD SOFT TISSUE SYNDACTYLY. IN 1961 HE REPORTED THE FINDINGS IN TWO MORE GENERATIONS OF THE KINDRED. ASYMMETRY OF THE SKULL AND ORBITS (PLAGIOCEPHA-LY), STRABISMUS AND THIN, LONG POINTED NOSE WERE CHANGES IN THE HEAD. SOME AFFECTED PERSONS HAD BIFID TERMINAL PHALANGES OF DIGITS II AND III AND ABSENCE OF THE FIRST METATARSAL. CLEFT PALATE, HYDROPHTHALMOS, CARDIAC MALFORMATION AND CONTRACTURES OF ELBOWS AND KNEES WERE PRESENT IN SOME.

WAARDENBURG, P. J.* EINE MERKWURDIGE KOMBINATION VON ANGEBORENEN MISSBILDUNGEN* DOPPELSEITIGER HYDROPHTHALMUS VERBUNDEN MIT AKROKEPHALOSYNDAKTYLIE, HERZFEHLER, PSEUDOHERMAPHRODITISMUS UND ANDEREN ABWEICHUNGEN. KLIN. MBL. AUGENHEILK. 92* 29-44, 1934.

WAARDENBURG, P. J., FRANCESCHETTI, A. AND KLEIN, D. (EDS.)* IN, GENETICS AND OPHTHALMOLOGY. SPRINGFIELD, ILL.* CHARLES C THOMAS, (PART 1) 1961.

*10160 ACROCEPHALOSYNDACTYLY TYPE V (PFEIFFER TYPE)

PFEIFFER (1964) FOUND 8 AFFECTED IN 3 GENERATIONS, WITH TWO INSTANCES OF MALE-TO-MALE TRANSMISSION. THE STRIKING FEATURE OF THE HAND DEFORMITY WAS BROAD, SHORT THUMBS AND BIG TOES. THE PROXIMAL PHALANX OF THE THUMB WAS EITHER TRIANGULAR OR TRAPEZOID (AND OCCASIONALLY FUSED WITH THE DISTAL PHALANX) SO THAT THE THUMB POINTED OUTWARD (I.E., AWAY FROM THE OTHER DIGITS). MARTSOLF ET AL. (1971) DESCRIBED THE CASE OF AN AFFECTED BOY WHOSE MOTHER AND MATERNAL HALF-BROTHER WERE SAID TO BE AFFECTED ALSO.

MARTSOLF, J. T., CRACCO, J. B., CARPENTER, G. G. AND O'HARA, A. E.* PFEIFFER SYNDROME* AN UNUSUAL TYPE OF ACROCEPHALOSYNDACTYLY WITH BROAD THUMBS AND GREAT TOES. AM. J. DIS. CHILD. 121* 257-262, 1971.

PFEIFFER, R. A.* DOMINANT ERBLICHE AKROCEPHALOSYNDAKTYLIE. Z. KINDERHEILK. 90* 301-320, 1964.

10170 ACROCYANOSIS

THIS MAY BE THE PRESENTING COMPLAINT IN THE EHLERS-DANLOS SYNDROME (Q.V.) AND THIS SYNDROME IS, THEREFORE, AT LEAST ONE BASIS FOR ACROCYANOSIS THAT 'RUNS IN A FAMILY.' (THERE IS NO EVIDENCE OF A SEPARATE GENETIC BASIS FOR ACROCYANOSIS.) FOR EXAMPLE, GILBERT AND COLLEAGUES (1925) DESCRIBED A 22 YEAR OLD MAN WHO HAD HAD CYANOSIS OF THE HANDS, FEET AND EARS FROM BIRTH AND SHOWED OTHER CHARACTERISTIC FEATURES OF E-D. IN HIS FAMILY SEVERAL OTHER PERSONS HAD 'CYANOSED LIMBS AND ULCERATED CHILBLAINS' IN ASSOCIATION WITH E-D.

GILBERT, A., VILLARET, M. AND BOSVIEL, G.* SUR UN CAS D'HYPERELASTICITE CONGENITALE DES LIGAMENTS ARTICULAIRES ET DE LA PEAU. BULL. SOC. MED. HOP. PARIS 49* 303-307, 1925.

10180 ACRODYSOSTOSIS

MAROTEAUX AND MALAMUT (1968) SUGGESTED THAT 'PERIPHERAL DYSOSTOSIS' (Q.V.) IS A HETEROGENEOUS CLASS. THEY DESCRIBED ACRODYSOSTOSIS AS A CONDITION IN WHICH PECULIAR FACIES (SHORT NOSE, OPEN MOUTH AND PROGNATHISM) ARE ASSOCIATED WITH THE SMALL HANDS AND FEET. MENTAL DEFICIENCY IS FREQUENT. INHERITANCE OR PARENTAL CONSANGUINITY IS NOT YET KNOWN. CONE EPIPHYSES OCCUR IN THIS CONDITION. ROBINOW ET AL. (1971) REPORTED NINE CASES AND REVIEWED 11 FROM THE LITERATURE. NONE WERE FAMILIAL.

MAROTEAUX, P. AND MALAMUT, G.* L'ACRODYSOSTOSE. PRESSE MED. 76* 2189-2192, 1968.

ROBINOW, M., PFEIFFER, R. A., GORLIN, R. J., MCKUSICK, V. A., RENUART, A. W., JOHNSON, G. F. AND SUMMITT, R. L.* ACRODYSOSTOSIS* A SYNDROME OF PERIPHERAL DYSOSTOSIS, NASAL HYPOPLASIA, AND MENTAL RETARDATION. AM. J. DIS. CHILD. 121* 195-203, 1971.

*10190 ACROKERATOSIS VERRUCIFORMIS (HOPF)

THE PEDIGREE STUDIED BY NIEDELMAN AND MCKUSICK (1962) CONTAINED INSTANCES OF MALE-TO-MALE TRANSMISSION AS WELL AS UNAFFECTED DAUGHTERS OF AFFECTED MALES. WARTY HYPERKERATOTIC LESIONS ARE FOUND ON THE DORSAL ASPECT OF THE HANDS AND FEET AND ON THE KNEES AND ELBOWS. HERNDON AND WILSON (1966) HAVE EMPHASIZED THE PHENOTYPIC OVERLAP BETWEEN THIS ENTITY AND DARIER-WHITE DISEASE (Q.V.) AND HAVE EVEN PROPOSED THAT THEY MAY NOT BE SEPARATE ENTITIES. IN THE FAMILY THEY STUDIED, 7 PERSONS HAD TYPICAL ACROKERATOSIS VERRUCIFORMIS, ONE OR POSSIBLY TWO HAD DARIER'S DISEASE AND THREE HAD MINOR DISTURBANCES OF KERATINIZATION (WHITE NAILS FROM SUBUNGUAL HYPERKERATOSIS, OR PUNCTATE KERATOSES OF PALMS OR SOLES).

HERNDON, J. H., JR. AND WILSON, J. D.* ACROKERATOSIS VERRUCIFORMIS (HOPF) AND DARIER'S DISEASE. GENETIC EVIDENCE FOR A UNITARY ORIGIN. ARCH. DERM. 93* 305-

NIEDELMAN, M. L. AND MCKUSICK, V. A.* ACROKERATOSIS VERRUCIFORMIS (HOPF). A FOLLOW-UP STUDY. ARCH. DERM. 86* 779-782, 1962.

10200 ACROLEUKOPATHY, SYMMETRIC

SUGAI, SAITO AND HAMADA (1965) DESCRIBED MOTHER AND DAUGHTER WITH SYMMETRIC DEPIGMENTATION OF THE GREAT TOES.

SUGAI, T., SAITO, T. AND HAMADA, T.* SYMMETRIC ACROLEUKOPATHY IN MOTHER AND DAUGHTER. ARCH. DERM. 92* 172-173, 1965.

*10210 ACROMEGALOID CHANGES, CUTIS VERTICIS GYRATA AND CORNEAL LEUKOMA

ROSENTHAL AND KLOEPFER (1962) DESCRIBED A *NEW* SYNDROME WITH THESE THREE FEATURES IN 13 PERSONS OF FOUR GENERATIONS OF A LOUISIANA NEGRO FAMILY. THROUGH THE COURTESY OF KLOEPFER, I SAW AFFECTED MEMBERS OF THIS FAMILY IN 1971. THE CORNEAL LEUKOMA IS AN EPITHELIAL CHANGE. THE HANDS, FEET AND CHIN ARE VERY LARGE AND THE AFFECTED PERSONS UNUSUALLY TALL. ALTHOUGH GROWTH HORMONE ASSAYS HAD NOT BEEN DONE, OTHER ENDOCRINE STUDIES AND X-RAY VIEWS OF THE SELLA TURCICA GIVE NO INDICATION OF PITUITARY DYSFUNCTION. ONE OF THE AFFECTED FEMALES EXAMINED HAD 9 LIVING CHILDREN. THE SKIN OF THE HANDS IS UNUSUALLY SOFT AND HAS AN ABNORMAL DERMAL RIDGE PATTERN, REFERRED TO AS *SPLIT RIDGES,* WHICH PERMITS IDENTIFICATION OF THE DISORDER IN CHILDREN OF PRECLINICAL AGE. A POSSIBLE DIFFERENCE FROM THE USUAL CUTIS VERTICIS GYRATA IS A LONGITUDINAL ORIENTATION OF THE SKIN FOLDS RATHER THAN TRANSVERSE ORIENTATION.

ROSENTHAL, J. W. AND KLOEPFER, H. W.* AN ACROMEGALOID, CUTIS VERTICIS GYRATA, CORNEAL LEUKOMA SYNDROME. ARCH. OPHTHAL. 68* 722-726, 1962.

10220 ACROMEGALY

KOCH AND TIWISINA (1959) REVIEWED 8 EXAMPLES OF AFFECTED PERSONS IN TWO SUCCESSIVE GENERATIONS INCLUDING 4 INSTANCES OF FATHER AND 1 OR MORE SONS AFFECTED. SOME REPORTED INSTANCES OF FAMILIAL ACROMEGALY MAY IN FACT BE PACHYDERMOPERIOSTOSIS, THE ACROMEGALOID-CUTIS GYRATA-LEUKOMA SYNDROME, OR CEREBRAL GIGANTISM. FURTHER- MORE, FAMILIAL ACROMEGALY CAN BE A PARTIAL EXPRESSION OF THE MULTIPLE ENDOCRINE ADENOMATOSIS SYNDROME.

KOCH, G. AND TIWISINA, T.* BEITRAG ZUR ERBLICHKEIT DER AKROMEGALIE UND DER HYPEROSTOSIS GENERALISATA MIT PACHYDERMIE. AERZTL. FORSCH. 13* 489-504, 1959.

KOCH, G.* ERBLICHE HIRNGESCHWULSTE. Z. MENSCHL. VERERB. KONSTITUTIONSL. 29* 400-423, 1949.

10230 ACROMELALGIA, HEREDITARY (*RESTLESS LEGS*)

BECAUSE OF PARESTHESIA WITH FIRST GOING TO BED OR SITTING STILL FOR A TIME, THE AFFECTED PERSON CANNOT RESIST FIDGETING WITH HIS FEET. HUIZINGA (1957) DESCRIBED A FAMILY WITH AFFECTED PERSONS IN FIVE GENERATIONS. THE CONDITION INVOLVING THE FEET WAS RELIEVED BY COLD AND HAD ITS ONSET IN ADOLESCENCE. BORNSTEIN (1961) AND EKBOM (1960) ALSO DESCRIBED FAMILIAL AGGREGATION.

BORNSTEIN, B.* RESTLESS LEGS. PSYCHIAT. NEUROL. 141* 165-201, 1961.

EKBOM, K. A.* RESTLESS LEGS SYNDROME. NEUROLOGY 10* 868-873, 1960.

HUIZINGA, J.* HEREDITARY ACROMELALGIA (OR *RESTLESS LEGS*). ACTA GENET. STATIST. MED. 7* 121-123, 1957.

10240 ACRO-OSTEOLYSIS

LAMY AND MAROTEAUX (1961) DESCRIBED A DOMINANT FORM IN MOTHER AND SON. MEMBERS OF TWO EARLIER GENERATIONS WERE ALSO AFFECTED. NO ABNORMALITY OF SENSATION WAS PRESENT. SCHINZ (1951) DESCRIBED DOMINANT INHERITANCE OF THIS DISORDER WITH ONSET BETWEEN 8 AND 22 YEARS. SLOWLY PROGRESSIVE OSTEOLYSIS OF THE PHALANGES IN THE HANDS AND FEET WAS ASSOCIATED WITH RECURRENT ULCERS OF THE FINGERS AND SOLES OF THE FEET, ELIMINATION OF BONE SEQUESTRA AND HEALING WITH LOSS OF TOES OR FINGERS. MAROTEAUX (1970) FOUND NO BASILAR IMPRESSION, OR OTHER CHANGES IN THE SKULL OR LONG BONES TO SUGGEST THAT THIS WAS CHENEY'S SYNDROME (Q.V.).

HARMS, I.* UBER DIE FAMILIARE AKRO-OSTEOLYSE. FORTSCHR. ROENTGENSTR. 80* 727- 733, 1954.

LAMY, M. AND MAROTEAUX, P.* ACRO-OSTEOLYSE DOMINANTE. ARCH. FRANC. PEDIAT. 18* 693-702, 1961.

MAROTEAUX, P.* PARIS, FRANCE* PERSONAL COMMUNICATION, 1970.

SCHINZ, H. R., BAENSCH, W. E., FRIEDL, E. AND UEHLINGER, E. (EDS.)* ROENTGEN- DIAGNOSTICS. TRANS. IN ENGLISH BY J. T. CASE. NEW YORK* GRUNE AND STRATTON, VOL.

1, 1951. FIG. 969 ON P. 734.

*10250 ACRO-OSTEOLYSIS WITH OSTEOPOROSIS AND CHANGES IN SKULL AND MANDIBLE (CHENEY SYNDROME)

CHENEY (1965) DESCRIBED A FAMILY LIVING IN THE UPPER PENINSULA OF MICHIGAN IN WHICH THE MOTHER AND FOUR CHILDREN HAD ACRO-OSTEOLYSIS, MULTIPLE WORMIAN BONES, HYPOPLASIA OF RAMUS OF MANDIBLE. DIFFERENT FROM PYCNODYSOSTOSIS, A RECESSIVE WITH OSTEOSCLEROSIS, THE CONDITION IN CHENEY'S PATIENTS HAD OSTEOPOROSIS WITH BASILAR IMPRESSION AS A FEATURE. THE MOTHER WAS 57 AND THE AFFECTED CHILDREN (4 OF 6) WERE 35, 26, 21 AND 13. DORST AND MCKUSICK (1969) DESCRIBED A CASE.

CHENEY, W. D.* ACRO-OSTEOLYSIS. AM. J. ROENTGEN. 94* 595-607, 1965.

DORST, J. P. AND MCKUSICK, V. A.* ACRO-OSTEOLYSIS (CHENEY SYNDROME). THE CLINICAL DELINEATION OF BIRTH DEFECTS. III. LIMB MALFORMATIONS. NEW YORK* NATIONAL FOUNDATION, 1969. PP. 215-217.

*10260 ADENINE PHOSPHORIBOSYLTRANSFERASE VARIANT

MUTANT FORMS OF APRT HAVE BEEN DESCRIBED BY KELLEY ET AL. (1968) AND BY HENDERSON ET AL. (1969) WHO FOUND THE INHERITANCE TO BE AUTOSOMAL. THE OTHER PURINE PHOSPHORIBOSYLTRANSFERASE (HGPRT) IS DETERMINED BY AN X-LINKED LOCUS AND IS MUTANT IN THE LESCH-NYHAN SYNDROME (Q.V.). HEAT-STABLE ENZYME ALLELE HAS A FREQUENCY OF ABOUT 15 PERCENT AND THE HEAT-LABILE ENZYME ALLELE OF ABOUT 85 PERCENT. THIS POLYMORPHISM MIGHT BE A USEFUL MARKER FOR LINKAGE STUDIES. NO DISEASE HAS BEEN RELATED TO MUTANT FORMS OF APRT.

HENDERSON, J. F., KELLEY, W. N., ROSENBLOOM, F. M. AND SEEGMILLER, J. E.* INHERITANCE OF PURINE PHOSPHORIBOSYLTRANSFERASES IN MAN. AM. J. HUM. GENET. 21* 61-70, 1969.

KELLEY, W. N., LEVY, R. I., ROSENBLOOM, F. M., HENDERSON, J. F. AND SEEGMILLER, J. E.* ADENINE PHOSPHORIBOSYLTRANSFERASE DEFICIENCY* A PREVIOUSLY UNDESCRIBED GENETIC DEFECT IN MAN. J. CLIN. INVEST. 47* 2281-2289, 1968.

*10270 ADENOSINE DEAMINASE POLYMORPHISM

BY MEANS OF A NEW AND SPECIFIC METHOD, SPENCER ET AL. (1968) DEMONSTRATED ISOZYMES OF ADENOSINE DEAMINASE AND SHOWED THAT THERE ARE 3 GENETICALLY DETERMINED PHENOTYPES* ADA 1, ADA 2-1 AND ADA 2. THE FREQUENCY OF THE ADA(2) ALLELE WAS ESTIMATED AT 0.06 IN EUROPEANS, 0.04 IN NEGROES AND 0.11 IN ASIATIC INDIANS. POLYMORPHISM OF ELECTROPHORETICALLY DEMONSTRATED ADENOSINE DEAMINASE OF RED CELLS WAS STUDIED ALSO BY HOPKINSON ET AL. (1969) AND BY TARIWERDIAN AND RITTER (1969).

COOK, P. J. L., HOPKINSON, D. A. AND ROBSON, E. B.* THE LINKAGE RELATIONSHIPS OF ADENOSINE DEAMINASE. ANN. HUM. GENET. 34* 187-188, 1970.

DETTER, J. C., STAMATOYANNOPOULOS, G., GIBLETT, E. R. AND MOTULSKY, A. G.* ADENOSINE DEAMINASE* RACIAL DISTRIBUTION AND REPORT OF A NEW PHENOTYPE. J. MED. GENET. 7* 356-357, 1970.

DISSING, J. AND KNUDSEN, J. B.* A NEW RED CELL ADENOSINE DEAMINASE PHENOTYPE IN MAN. HUM. HERED. 19* 375-377, 1969.

HOPKINSON, D. A., COOK, P. J. L. AND HARRIS, H.* FURTHER DATA ON THE ADENOSINE DEAMINASE (ADA) POLYMORPHISM AND A REPORT OF A NEW PHENOTYPE. ANN. HUM. GENET. 32* 361-368, 1969.

SPENCER, N., HOPKINSON, D. A. AND HARRIS, H.* ADENOSINE DEAMINASE POLYMORPHISM IN MAN. ANN. HUM. GENET. 32* 9-14, 1968.

TARIWERDIAN, G. AND RITTER, H.* ADENOSINE DEAMINASE POLYMORPHISM (EC 3.5.4.4)* FORMAL GENETICS AND LINKAGE RELATIONS. HUMANGENETIK 7* 176-178, 1969.

10280 ADENOSINE TRIPHOSPHATASE DEFICIENCY, ANEMIA DUE TO

IN TWO KINDREDS HARVALD ET AL. (1964) OBSERVED NONSPHEROCYTIC HEMOLYTIC ANEMIA DUE TO DEFICIENCY OF ATP-ASE. AT LEAST TWO GENERATIONS WERE AFFECTED IN EACH FAMILY AND FATHER-SON TRANSMISSION WAS NOTED.

HARVALD, B., HANEL, K. H., SQUIRES, R. AND TRAP-JENSEN, J.* ADENOSINE-TRIPHOS-PHATASE DEFICIENCY IN PATIENTS WITH NON-SPHEROCYTIC HEMOLYTIC ANEMIA. LANCET 2* 18-19, 1964.

*10290 ADENOSINE TRIPHOSPHATE, ELEVATED, OF ERYTHROCYTES

BREWER (1965) IN THIS COUNTRY AND ZURCHER ET AL. (1965) IN HOLLAND DESCRIBED HIGH ERYTHROCYTE ADENOSINE TRIPHOSPHATE AS A DOMINANTLY INHERITED TRAIT.

BREWER, G. J.* A NEW INHERITED ABNORMALITY OF HUMAN ERYTHROCYTE-ELEVATED ERYTHROCYTE ADENOSINE TRIPHOSPHATE. BIOCHEM. BIOPHYS. RES. COMMUN. 18* 430-434,

LOOS, J. A., PRINS, H. K. AND ZURCHER, C.* ELEVATED ATP LEVELS IN HUMAN
ERYTHROCYTES. IN, BEUTLER, E. (ED.)* HEREDITARY DISORDERS OF ERYTHROCYTE
METABOLISM. NEW YORK* GRUNE AND STRATTON, 1967.

ZURCHER, C., LOOS, J. A. AND PRINS, H. K.* HEREDITARY HIGH ATP CONTENT OF HUMAN
ERYTHROCYTES. FOLIA HAEMAT. 83* 366-376, 1965.

*10300 ADENYLATE KINASE ELECTROPHORETIC VARIANTS

ADENYLATE KINASE, ALSO KNOWN AS MYOKINASE, IS A PHOSPHOTRANSFERASE WHICH CATALYZES
THE REVERSIBLE CONVERSION OF 2 MOLECULES OF ADP TO ONE OF ATP PLUS ONE OF AMP.
THE ENZYME IS PRESENT IN RED CELLS AS WELL. FILDES AND HARRIS (1966) FOUND
ELECTROPHORETIC VARIATION IN RED CELLS AND DEFINIED 3 PHENOTYPES, DESIGNATED AK1,
AK2-1 AND AK2. ALL OF THE 141 CHILDREN OF TWO AK1 PARENTS (62 SUCH MATINGS) WERE
ALSO AK1. AMONG THE 136 CHILDREN OF AK1 BY AK2-1 MATINGS, 72 WERE AK1 AND 64 AK2-
1. AK1 AND AK2 PERSONS ARE THOUGHT TO BE HOMOZYGOTES FOR A TWO ALLELE SYSTEM AND
AK2-1 PERSONS HETEROZYGOTES. THE FREQUENCY OF THE RARER AK(2) ALLELE IS ABOUT
0.05 IN THE ENGLISH AND ABOUT 1 IN 400 PERSONS WOULD BE EXPECTED TO BE HOMOZYGOUS
FOR THIS ALLELE. SURVEY AND FAMILY DATA ARE CONSISTENT. RAPLEY ET AL. (1967)
CONCLUDED THAT THE AK LOCUS IS LINKED TO THE ABO LOCUS WITH A RECOMBINATION VALUE
OF ABOUT 0.20. BOCKELMANN ET AL. (1968) CONCLUDED THAT ADENYLATE KINASE AND
PYRUVATE KINASE ARE ISOZYMES WHICH SHARE A POLYPEPTIDE CHAIN IN COMMON. BECAUSE
OF THEIR SIMILAR FUNCTIONS A COMMON EVOLUTIONARY ORIGIN WOULD BE PLAUSIBLE.

BOCKELMANN, W., WOLF, V. AND RITTER, H.* POLYMORPHISM OF THE PHOSPHOTRANS-
FERASES ADENYLATE KINASE AND PYRUVATE KINASE. EXISTENCE OF A COMMON SUBUNIT.Q
HUMANGENETIK 6* 78-83, 1968.

BOWMAN, J. E., FRISCHER, H., AJMAR, F., CARSON, P. E. AND GOWER, M. K.*
POPULATION, FAMILY AND BIOCHEMICAL INVESTIGATION OF HUMAN ADENYLATE KINASE
POLYMORPHISM. NATURE 214* 1156-1158, 1967.

BROCK, D. J. H.* EVIDENCE AGAINST A COMMON SUBUNIT IN ADENYLATE KINASE AND
PYRUVATE KINASE. HUMANGENETIK 10* 30-34, 1970.

FILDES, R. A. AND HARRIS, H.* GENETICALLY DETERMINED VARIATION OF ADENYLATE
KINASE IN MAN. NATURE 209* 261-262, 1966.

RAPLEY, S., ROBSON, E. B., HARRIS, H. AND SMITH, S. M.* DATA ON THE INCIDENCE,
SEGREGATION AND LINKAGE RELATIONS OF THE ADENYLATE KINASE (AK) POLYMORPHISM. ANN.
HUM. GENET. 31* 237-242, 1967.

SCHLEUTERMANN, D. A., BIAS, W. B., MURDOCH, J. L. AND MCKUSICK, V. A.* LINKAGE
OF THE LOCI FOR THE NAIL-PATELLA SYNDROME AND ADENYLATE KINASE. AM. J. HUM.
GENET. 21* 606-630, 1969.

WEITKAMP, L. R., SING, C. F., SHREFFLER, D. C. AND GUTTORMSEN, S. A.* THE
GENETIC LINKAGE RELATIONS OF ADENYLATE KINASE* FURTHER DATA ON THE ABO-AK LINKAGE
GROUP. AM. J. HUM. GENET. 21* 600-605, 1969.

10310 ADIE SYNDROME

THIS IS A STATIONARY HARMLESS DISORDER CHARACTERIZED BY TONIC, SLUGGISHLY REACTING
PUPIL AND HYPOACTIVE OR ABSENT TENDON REFLEXES. DE RUDOLF (1936) DESCRIBED IT IN
MOTHER AND DAUGHTER, MCKINNEY AND FROCHT (1940) IN FATHER AND SON, AND AFFECTED
SIBS ARE REPORTED (MYLIUS, 1938). THE PUPIL (LATIES AND SCHEIE, 1965) IS
EXCESSIVELY SENSITIVE TO MECHOLYL (METHACHOLINE). IN FAMILIAL DYSAUTONOMIA, A
RECESSIVE (Q.V.), THE PUPIL IS ALSO MECHOLYL-SENSITIVE AND TENDON REFLEXES ARE
ABSENT. IT WOULD BE OF INTEREST TO DETERMINE WHETHER THE REFLEXES RETURN WITH
PARENTERAL ADMINISTRATION OF MECHOLYL AS OCCURS IN DYSAUTONOMIA. AN AUTOPSIED
CASE WAS REPORTED BY HARRIMAN AND GARLAND (1968), WHO FOUND NEURONAL DEGENERATION
IN THE CILIARY GANGLION. SELECTIVE DEGENERATION OF NEURONES IN DORSAL ROOT
GANGLIA MAY HAVE BEEN THE BASIS FOR AREFLEXIA.

ADIE, W. J.* TONIC PUPILS AND ABSENT TENDON REFLEXES* A BENIGN DISORDER SUI
GENERIS* ITS COMPLETE AND INCOMPLETE FORMS. BRAIN 55* 98-113, 1932.

DE RUDOLF, G.* TONIC PUPILS WITH ABSENT TENDON REFLEXES IN MOTHER AND DAUGHTER.
J. NEUROL. PSYCHIAT. 16* 367-368, 1936.

HARRIMAN, D. G. F. AND GARLAND, H.* THE PATHOLOGY OF ADIE'S SYNDROME. BRAIN
91* 401-418, 1968.

LATIES, A. M. AND SCHEIE, H. G.* ADIE'S SYNDROME* DURATION OF METHACHOLINE
SENSITIVITY. ARCH. OPHTHAL. 74* 458-459, 1965.

MCKINNEY, J. M. AND FROCHT, M.* ADIE'S SYNDROME* A NON-LUETIC DISEASE SIMULA-
TING TABES DORSALIS. AM. J. MED. SCI. 199* 546-555, 1940.

MYLIUS, (NI)* UEBER FAMILIARES VORKOMMEN DER PUPILLOTONIE. KLIN. MBL.

10320 ADIPOSIS DOLOROSA (DERCUM'S DISEASE)

LYNCH AND HARLAN (1963) OBSERVED THE DISEASE IN FOUR MEMBERS OF THREE GENERATIONS OF ONE FAMILY AND IN TWO, POSSIBLY FOUR, PERSONS IN TWO GENERATIONS OF A SECOND FAMILY.

LYNCH, H. T. AND HARLAN, W. L.* HEREDITARY FACTORS IN ADIPOSIS DOLOROSA (DERCUM'S DISEASE). AM. J. HUM. GENET. 15* 184-190, 1963.

10330 AGLOSSIA-ADACTYLIA

THE FEATURES ARE INDICATED BY THE NAME ALTHOUGH IT IS TO BE NOTED THAT BOTH THE AGLOSSIA AND THE ADACTYLIA MAY BE ONLY PARTIAL. NO FAMILIAL CASES HAVE BEEN REPORTED (NEVIN ET AL., 1970).

NEVIN, N. C., DODGE, J. A. AND KERNOHAN, D. C.* AGLOSSIA-ADACTYLIA SYNDROME. ORAL SURG. 29* 443-446, 1970.

10340 AINHUM

A NARROW STRIP OF HARDENED SKIN, A CONSTRICTING RING, FORMS ON THE LITTLE TOE AT THE LEVEL OF THE DIGITO-PLANTAR FOLD AND PROGRESSES TO SPONTANEOUS AMPUTATION OF THE DIGIT. FAMILIAL OCCURRENCE HAS BEEN NOTED BY MAASS (1926) AND BY DA SILVA LIMA (1880).

DA SILVA LIMA, J. F.* ON AINHUM. ARCH. DERM. SYPH. 6* 367-376, 1880.

HORWITZ, M. T. AND TUNICK, I.* AINHUM* REPORT OF SIX CASES IN NEW YORK. ARCH. DERM. SYPH. 36* 1058-1063, 1937.

MAASS, E.* BEOBACHTUNGEN UBER AINHUM. ARCH. SCHIFFS- U. TROPENHYGIENE 30* 32-34, 1926.

10350 ALBINISM-DEAFNESS

TIETZ (1963) DESCRIBED 14 AFFECTED PERSONS IN 6 GENERATIONS. THE ALBINISM WAS GENERALIZED BUT DID NOT AFFECT THE EYES. THE IRIDES WERE BLUE. NYSTAGMUS AND OTHER OCULAR ABNORMALITIES WERE ABSENT. THE MEDIAL CANTHI AND NASAL BRIDGE WERE NORMAL. COMPLETE NERVE DEAFNESS WAS PRESENT. THE EYEBROWS WERE ALMOST TOTALLY LACKING, THERE BEING ONLY A FEW ALBINO HAIRS WHERE THE EYEBROWS NORMALLY ARE. THE ALBINISM IN THIS TRAIT IS HYPOPIGMENTATION AND NOT TRUE ALBINISM. THE AFFECTED INDIVIDUALS TAN, FOR EXAMPLE. REED ET AL. (1967) THOUGHT THIS MIGHT HAVE BEEN MERELY A DOMINANT TYPE OF DEAFNESS IN UNUSUALLY BLOND PERSONS.

REED, W. B., STONE, V. M., BODER, E. AND ZIPRKOWSKI, L.* PIGMENTARY DISORDERS IN ASSOCIATION WITH CONGENITAL DEAFNESS. ARCH. DERM. 95* 176-186, 1967.

TIETZ, W.* A SYNDROME OF DEAF-MUTISM ASSOCIATED WITH ALBINISM SHOWING DOMINANT AUTOSOMAL INHERITANCE. AM. J. HUM. GENET. 15* 259-264, 1963.

*10360 ALBUMIN, VARIANTS OF SERUM

BISALBUMINEMIA IS AN ASYMPTOMATIC VARIATION IN SERUM ALBUMIN. HETEROZYGOTES HAVE TWO SPECIES OF ALBUMIN, A NORMAL TYPE AND ONE WHICH MIGRATES ABNORMALLY RAPIDLY OR SLOWLY ON ELECTROPHORESIS. ACROCYANOSIS WAS PRESENT IN TWO AND PROBABLY THREE SUCCESSIVE GENERATIONS OF THE FAMILY REPORTED BY WILLIAMS AND MARTIN (1960) BUT 4 OTHER BISALBUMINEMIC PERSONS DID NOT SHOW ACROCYANOSIS. TARNOKY AND LESTAS (1964) DESCRIBED A NEW TYPE OF BISALBUMINEMIA IN TWO SIBS AND THE SON OF ONE OF THEM. THE USUAL TYPE IS DEMONSTRABLE BY FILTER PAPER ELECTROPHORESIS. THE NEW TYPE WAS DEMONSTRABLE BY ELECTROPHORESIS ON CELLULOSE ACETATE AT PH 8.6, BUT NOT ON FILTER PAPER OR STARCH GEL. A LARGE NUMBER OF ALBUMIN VARIANTS PROBABLY EXIST. 'PARALBUMINEMIA' WAS SUGGESTED BY EARLE ET AL. (1959) AS PREFERABLE TO 'BISALBU-MINEMIA' WHICH IS PERHAPS APPROPRIATE FOR THE HETEROZYGOUS STATE ONLY. ALLOALBU-MINEMIA IS THE TERM SUGGESTED BY BLUMBERG ET AL. (1968) FOR THE VARIANT ALBUMINS. IN THE FAMILY REPORTED BY LAURELL AND NILEHN (1966), A NEW TYPE OF PARALBUMINEMIA WAS ASSOCIATED WITH CONNECTIVE TISSUE DISORDERS* SYSTEMIC LUPUS ERYTHEMATOSUS, RUPTURED KNEE MENISCUS, RECURRENT DISLOCATION OF SHOULDER, BACK PAIN. WEITKAMP ET AL. (1966) CONCLUDED THAT THE ALBUMIN LOCUS INDICATED BY BISALBUMINEMIA IS VERY CLOSELY LINKED WITH THE LOCUS FOR GC TYPE. USING THE NASKAPI VARIANT, KAARSALO ET AL. (1967) FOUND CLOSE LINKAGE OF THE ALBUMIN AND GC LOCI.
MELARTIN AND BLUMBERG (1966) FOUND AN ELECTROPHORETIC VARIANT OF ALBUMIN TO BE FREQUENT IN NASKAPI INDIANS OF QUEBEC AND IN LOWER FREQUENCY IN OTHER NORTH AMERICAN INDIANS. HOMOZYGOTES WERE FOUND.
WIETKAMP ET AL. (1967) COMPARED THE SERUM ALBUMIN VARIANTS OF 19 UNRELATED FAMILIES, USING TWO ELECTROPHORETIC SYSTEMS. FIVE DISTINCT CLASSES WERE FOUND. ONE CLASS OF VARIANTS WAS FOUND ONLY IN NORTH AMERICAN INDIANS. THE OTHERS WERE FOUND ONLY IN PERSONS OF EUROPEAN DESCENT.
FRASER, HARRIS AND ROBSON (1959) FOUND AN ANOMALOUS PLASMA PROTEIN IN 6 PERSONS IN TWO GENERATIONS OF A FAMILY, ON TWO DIMENSIONAL ELECTROPHORESIS (PAPER FIRST, FOLLOWED BY STARCH). THE ELECTROPHORETIC PROPERTIES ON PAPER WERE THE SAME

IN THE ANOMALOUS ALBUMIN AND IN NORMAL ALBUMIN. THIS DISTINGUISHES THE PROTEIN
FROM THAT IN BISALBUMINEMIA AS DOES ALSO THE FACT THAT THE AMOUNT OF THE ANOMALOUS
PROTEIN IS MUCH LESS THAN THAT OF THE NORMAL ALBUMIN IN THE PRESUMABLY HETEROZY-
GOUS PERSONS. THAT THE SAME LOCUS AS THAT WHICH DETERMINES BISALBUMINEMIA IS
INVOLVED HERE IS SUGGESTED BY THE FINDING OF WEITKAMP ET AL. (1967) THAT THE
FRASER ANOMALOUS ALBUMIN IS ALSO LINKED TO THE GC LOCUS. RELATIVELY FREQUENT
DIFFERENT ALLOALBUMINEMIAS OCCUR IN VARIOUS AMERINDIANS (ARENDS ET AL., 1969).
THE ALBUMIN VARIANT FIRST DESCRIBED BY FRASER ET AL. (1959) IN A WELCH FAMILY HAS
BEEN CHARACTERIZED AS A DIMER BY JAMIESON AND GANGULY (1969).

ADAMS, M. S.* GENETIC DIVERSITY IN SERUM ALBUMIN. J. MED. GENET. 3* 198-202,
1966.

ARENDS, T., GALLANGO, M. L., LAYRISSE, M., WILBERT, J. AND HEINEN, H. D.*
ALBUMIN WARAO* NEW TYPE OF HUMAN ALLOALBUMINEMIA. BLOOD 33* 414-420, 1969.

BLUMBERG, B. S., MARTIN, J. R. AND MELARTIN, L.* ALLOALBUMINEMIA. ALBUMIN
NASKAPI IN INDIANS OF THE UNGAVA. J.A.M.A. 203* 180-185, 1968.

EARLE, D. P., HUTT, M. P., SCHMID, K. AND GITLIN, D.* OBSERVATIONS ON DOUBLE
ALBUMIN* A GENETICALLY TRANSMITTED SERUM PROTEIN ANOMALY. J. CLIN. INVEST. 38*
1412-1420, 1959.

EFREMOV, G. AND BRAEND, M.* SERUM ALBUMIN* POLYMORPHISM IN MAN. SCIENCE 146*
1679-1680, 1964.

FRASER, G. R., HARRIS, H. AND ROBSON, E. B.* A NEW GENETICALLY DETERMINED
PLASMA-PROTEIN IN MAN. LANCET 1* 1023-1024, 1959.

JAMIESON, G. A. AND GANGULY, P.* STUDIES ON A GENETICALLY DETERMINED ALBUMIN
DIMER. BIOCHEM. GENET. 3* 403-416, 1969.

KAARSALO, E., MELARTIN, L. AND BLUMBERG, B. S.* AUTOSOMAL LINKAGE BETWEEN THE
ALBUMIN AND GC LOCI IN HUMANS. SCIENCE 158* 123-125, 1967.

KUEPPERS, F., HOLLAND, P. V. AND WEITKAMP, L. R.* ALBUMIN SANTA ANA* A NEW
INHERITED VARIANT. HUM. HERED. 19* 378-384, 1969.

LAURELL, C. B. AND NILEHN, J. E.* A NEW TYPE OF INHERITED SERUM ALBUMIN
ANOMALY. J. CLIN. INVEST. 45* 1935-1945, 1966.

MELARTIN, L. AND BLUMBERG, B. S.* ALBUMIN NASKAPI* A NEW VARIANT OF SERUM
ALBUMIN. SCIENCE 153* 1664-1666, 1966.

MELARTIN, L.* ALBUMIN POLYMORPHISM IN MAN. STUDIES ON ALBUMIN VARIANTS IN
NORTH AMERICAN NATIVE POPULATIONS. ACTA PATH. MICROBIOL. SCAND. 191 (SUPPL.)* 1-
50, 1967.

MELARTIN, L., BLUMBERG, B. S. AND LISKER, R.* ALBUMIN MEXICO, A NEW VARIANT OF
SERUM ALBUMIN. NATURE 215* 1288-1289, 1967.

SARCIONE, E. J. AND AUNGST, C. W.* STUDIES IN BISALBUMINEMIA* BINDING PROPER-
TIES OF THE TWO ALBUMINS. BLOOD 20* 156-164, 1962.

TARNOKY, A. L. AND LESTAS, A. N.* A NEW TYPE OF BISALBUMINAEMIA. CLIN. CHIM.
ACTA 9* 551-558, 1964.

WEITKAMP, L. R. AND CHAGNON, N. A.* ALBUMIN MAKU* A NEW VARIANT OF HUMAN SERUM
ALBUMIN. NATURE 217* 759-760, 1968.

WEITKAMP, L. R., FRANGLEN, G., ROKALA, D. A., POLESKY, H. F., SIMPSON, N. E.,
SUNDERMAN, F. W., JR., BELL, H. E., SAAVE, J., LISKER, R. AND BOHLS, S. W.* AN
ELECTROPHORETIC COMPARISON OF HUMAN SERUM ALBUMIN VARIANTS* EIGHT DISTINGUISHABLE
TYPES. HUM. HERED. 19* 159-169, 1969.

WEITKAMP, L. R., RENWICK, J. H., BERGER, J., SHREFFLER, D. C., DRACHMANN, O.,
WUHRMANN, F., BRAEND, M. AND FRANGLE, G.* ADDITIONAL DATA AND SUMMARY FOR ALBUMIN-
GC LINKAGE IN MAN. HUM. HERED. 20* 1-7, 1970.

WEITKAMP, L. R., ROBSON, E. B., SHREFFLER, D. C. AND CORNEY, G.* AN UNUSUAL
HUMAN SERUM ALBUMIN VARIANT* FURTHER DATA ON GENETIC LINKAGE BETWEEN LOCI FOR
HUMAN SERUM ALBUMIN AND GROUP-SPECIFIC COMPONENT (GC). AM. J. HUM. GENET. 20*
392-397, 1968.

WEITKAMP, L. R., RUCKNAGEL, D. L. AND GERSHOWITZ, H.* GENETIC LINKAGE BETWEEN
STRUCTURAL LOCI FOR ALBUMIN AND GROUP SPECIFIC COMPONENT (GC). AM. J. HUM. GENET.
18* 559-571, 1966.

WEITKAMP, L. R., SHREFFLER, D. C., ROBBINS, J. L., DRACHMANN, O., ADNER, P. L.,
WEIME, R. J., SIMON, N. M., COOKE, K. B., SANDOR, G., WUHRMANN, F., BRAEND, M. AND
TARNOKY, A. L.* AN ELECTROPHORETIC COMPARISON OF SERUM ALBUMIN VARIANTS FROM
NINETEEN UNRELATED FAMILIES. ACTA GENET. STATIST. MED. 17* 399-405, 1967.

WIEME, R. J.* ON THE PRESENCE OF TWO ALBUMINS IN CERTAIN NORMAL HUMAN SERA AND ITS GENETIC DETERMINATION. CLIN. CHIM. ACTA 5* 443-445, 1960.

WILLIAMS, D. I. AND MARTIN, N. H.* BISALBUMINEMIA WITH CURIOUS ACROCYANOTIC SKIN CHANGES (TWO CASES). PROC. ROY. SOC. MED. 53* 566-568, 1960.

10370 ALCOHOL DEHYDROGENASE

POLYMORPHISM WAS INVESTIGATED BY SMITH ET AL. (1971).

SMITH, M., HOPKINSON, D. A. AND HARRIS, H.* DEVELOPMENTAL CHANGES AND POLYMOR-PHISM IN HUMAN ALCOHOL DEHYDROGENASE. ANN. HUM. GENET. 34* 251-272, 1971.

*10380 ALDER ANOMALY

AZUROPHILIC CYTOPLASMIC INCLUSIONS OF THE POLYMORPHONUCLEAR LEUKOCYTES ARE INHERITED AS AN AUTOSOMAL DOMINANT. FRANCOIS, BARBIER AND DE ROUCK (1960) OBSERVED ALDER ANOMALY AND FUCHS' ATROPHIA GYRATA CHORIOIDEAE ET RETINAE IN THE OFFSPRING OF FIRST-COUSIN PARENTS BOTH OF WHOM HAD THE ALDER ANOMALY. THEY SUGGESTED THAT THE EYE DISORDER IS THE HOMOZYGOUS EXPRESSION OF THE ALDER ANOMALY GENE. IT IS POSSIBLE, OF COURSE, THAT THE EYE DISORDER WAS MERELY AN UNRELATED RECESSIVE DISORDER AND INDEED LATER OBSERVATIONS (SEE FUCHS' ATROPHIA GYRATA IN RECESSIVE CATALOG) SUPPORTED THIS VIEW. THIS CHANGE IS PROBABLY MORPHOLOGICALLY INDISTINGUISHABLE FROM THE REILLY GRANULATIONS OBSERVED IN MUCOPOLYSACCHARIDOSES (REILLY, 1941). ALDER (1939) ORIGINALLY DESCRIBED THE CHANGE IN A BROTHER AND SISTER WHO LATER AT PUBERTY DEVELOPED CHANGES IN THEIR HIP JOINTS. THE BROTHER WAS SAID TO BE IN GOOD HEALTH AT AGE 28 (DAVIDSON, 1961). JORDANS (1947) REPORTED A DUTCH FAMILY SHOWING A DOMINANT INHERITANCE PATTERN - 9 AFFECTED PERSONS IN THREE GENERATIONS WITH MALE-TO-MALE TRANSMISSION.

ALDER, A.* UBER KONSTITUTIONELL BEDINGTE GRANULATIONSVERANDERUNGEN DER LEUKOCYTEN. DEUTSCH. ARCH. KLIN. MED. 183* 372-378, 1939.

DAVIDSON, W. M.* INHERITED VARIATIONS IN LEUCOCYTES. BRIT. MED. BULL. 17* 190-195, 1961.

FRANCOIS, J., BARBIER, F. AND DE ROUCK, A.* LES CONDUCTEURS DU GENE DE L'ATROPHIA GYRATA CHORIOIDEAE ET RETINAE DE FUCHS (ANOMALIE D'ALDER). ACTA GENET. MED. GEM. 9* 74-91, 1960.

JORDANS, G. H. W.* HEREDITARY GRANULATION ANOMALY OF THE LEUCOCYTES (ALDER). ACTA MED. SCAND. 129* 348-351, 1947.

REILLY, W. A.* THE GRANULES IN THE LEUKOCYTES IN GARGOYLISM. AM. J. DIS. CHILD. 62* 489-491, 1941.

10390 ALDOSTERONISM, SENSITIVE TO DEXAMETHASONE

SUTHERLAND ET AL. (1966) AND SALTI ET AL. (1969) DESCRIBED A FATHER AND SON WITH HYPERTENSION, LOW PLASMA RENIN ACTIVITY AND INCREASED ALDOSTERONE SECRETION RESPONSIVE TO DEXAMETHASONE. GROWTH AND SEXUAL DEVELOPMENT WERE NORMAL. AT LAPAROTOMY THE FATHER WAS FOUND TO HAVE MULTIPLE ADRENOCORTICAL ADENOMAS. THIS APPEARS TO BE DISTINCT FROM CONN'S SYNDROME (PRIMARY ALDOSTERONISM) WHICH IS NOT SENSITIVE TO DEXAMETHASONE.

SALTI, I. S., STIEFEL, M., RUSE, J. L. AND LAIDLAW, J. C.* NON-TUMOROUS 'PRIMARY ALDOSTERONISM.' CANAD. MED. ASS. J. 101* 1-10, 1969.

SUTHERLAND, D. J., RUSE, J. L. AND LAIDLAW, J. C.* HYPERTENSION, INCREASED ALDOSTERONE SECRETION AND LOW PLASMA RENIN ACTIVITY RELIEVED BY DEXAMETHASONE. CANAD. MED. ASS. J. 95* 1109-1119, 1966.

10400 ALOPECIA AREATA

LUBOWE (1959) DESCRIBED A FAMILY WITH AFFECTED MOTHER AND AFFECTED DAUGHTER AND SON. RECENT EVIDENCE SUGGESTS AN AUTO-IMMUNE MECHANISM IN THIS DISORDER. THEREFORE, A MODEST TENDENCY TO FAMILIAL AGGREGATION AND A FAVORABLE RESPONSE TO ADMINISTRATION OF ADRENOCORTICOSTEROIDS. SEE AUTOIMMUNE DISEASES.

LUBOWE, I. I.* THE CLINICAL ASPECTS OF ALOPECIA AREATA, TOTALIS, AND UNIVERSA-LIS. ANN. N.Y. ACAD. SCI. 83* 458-462, 1959.

10410 ALOPECIA CONGENITA WITH KERATOSIS PALMO-PLANTARIS

STEVANOVIC (1959) DESCRIBED A FAMILY WITH A DOMINANT PATTERN OF INHERITANCE AND HYPERKERATOSIS OF THE PALMS AND SOLES, AND MILD DYSTROPHIC CHANGES OF THE FINGERNAILS.

STEVANOVIC, D. V.* ALOPECIA CONGENITA. THE INCOMPLETE DOMINANT FORM OF INHERITANCE WITH VARYING EXPRESSIVITY. ACTA GENET. STATIST. MED. 9* 127-132, 1959.

PARTIAL SEX LINKAGE (LOCATION OF THE GENE ON PART OF THE X AND Y CHROMOSOMES WHICH ARE HOMOLOGOUS) WAS SUGGESTED ON THE BASIS OF THE LARGE MORMON KINDRED REPORTED BY PERKOFF AND HIS COLLEAGUES (1958). HOWEVER, THIS POSSIBILITY IS EXCLUDED BY OTHER PEDIGREES (E.G., COHEN, CASSADY, HANNA, 1961). AUTOSOMAL DOMINANT INHERITANCE WITH ANOMALOUS SEGREGATION (SHAW, GLOVER, 1961) SEEMS LIKELY. HETEROZYGOUS MOTHERS TRANSMIT THE GENE TO MORE THAN 50 PERCENT OF DAUGHTERS AND PROBABLY ALSO MORE THAN 50 PERCENT OF THEIR SONS. WALKER (1966) HAS STUDIED A FAMILY (N. P., 666088) WITH AFFECTED PERSONS IN FOUR GENERATIONS. ALTHOUGH THE HISTOLOGY IN TWO CASES STUDIED WAS CONSISTENT WITH ALPORT'S SYNDROME INCLUDING THE PRESENCE OF FOAM CELLS, ATYPICAL FEATURES INCLUDED ABSENCE OF DEAFNESS IN ALL AFFECTED PERSONS, UNUSUALLY LONG SURVIVAL OF AFFECTED MALES AND DEATH OF ONE AFFECTED FEMALE IN THE EARLY TWENTIES. THE KINDRED REPORTED BY OHLSSON (1963) DIFFERED FROM OTHERS REPORTED IN THE FACT THAT MYOPIA WAS A CONSPICUOUS FEATURE AND THE IMPAIRMENT OF RENAL FUNCTION IN THE AFFECTED MALES WAS RELATIVELY MILD EVEN IN TWO OVER AGE 30 YEARS. OCULAR ABNORMALITIES HAVE BEEN OBSERVED IN SOME PATIENTS (ARNOTT ET AL., 1966). A POSSIBLY DISTINCT ENTITY IS HEREDITARY NEPHRITIS WITHOUT DEAFNESS REPORTED BY DOCKHORN (1967) AND BY REYERSBACH AND BUTLER (1954). THE CASE OF STANBURY AND CASTLEMAN (1968) HAD HYPOPHOSPHATEMIA AND NEPHROCALCINOSIS. AT LEAST 7 PERSONS IN 3 GENERATIONS WERE AFFECTED, THE PROBAND HAD UNILATERAL DEAFNESS AND FOAM CELLS WERE DEMONSTRATED IN THE KIDNEY. THE FAMILY REPORTED BY ALBERT ET AL. (1969) MAY HAVE SUFFERED FROM A DIFFERENT DISORDER. TWO SISTERS AND A BROTHER WERE AFFECTED. THE FEMALES SHOWED UNUSUALLY SEVERE ABNORMALITY FOR THAT SEX. THE MAJOR MANIFESTATION OF RENAL DISEASE IN ONE SISTER WAS THE NEPHROTIC SYNDROME. NONE HAD DEAFNESS. THE PARENTS WERE NORMAL AND NOT RELATED. TWO OTHERWISE UNAFFECTED BROTHERS HAD CONGENITAL CATARACTS. SEE ALSO NEPHRITIS, FAMILIAL, WITHOUT DEAFNESS OR OCULAR DEFECT. IMMUNOFLUORESCENT STUDIES OF SPEAR ET AL. (1970) WERE INCONCLUSIVE AS FAR AS DECIDING ON A POSSIBLE IMMUNE BASIS OF THE NEPHROPATHY. MILLER ET AL. (1970) SHOWED THAT THE VESTIBULAR NEUROEPITHELIUM IS INVOLVED AS WELL AS THAT OF THE COCHLEA.

ALBERT, M. S., LEEMING, J. M. AND WIGGER, H. J.* FAMILIAL NEPHRITIS ASSOCIATED WITH THE NEPHROTIC SYNDROME. AM. J. DIS. CHILD. 117* 153-155, 1969.

ARNOTT, E. J., CRAWFURD, M. D. AND TOGHILL, P. J.* ANTERIOR LENTICONUS AND ALPORT'S SYNDROME. BRIT. J. OPHTHAL. 50* 390-403, 1966.

COHEN, M. M., CASSADY, G. AND HANNA, B. L.* A GENETIC STUDY OF HEREDITARY RENAL DYSFUNCTION WITH ASSOCIATED NERVE DEAFNESS. AM. J. HUM. GENET. 13* 379-389, 1961.

CRAWFURD, M. D. A. AND TOGHILL, P. J.* ALPORT'S SYNDROME OF HEREDITARY NEPHRITIS AND DEAFNESS. QUART. J. MED. 37* 563-576, 1968.

DOCKHORN, R. J.* HEREDITARY NEPHROPATHY WITHOUT DEAFNESS. AM. J. DIS. CHILD. 114* 135-138, 1967.

GOYER, R. A., REYNOLDS, J., JR., BURKE, J. AND BURKHOLDER, P.* HEREDITARY RENAL DISEASE WITH NEUROSENSORY HEARING LOSS, PROLINURIA AND ICHTHYOSIS. AM. J. MED. SCI. 256* 166-179, 1968.

KRICKSTEIN, H. I., GLOOR, F. J. AND BALOGH, K.* RENAL PATHOLOGY IN HEREDITARY NEPHRITIS WITH NERVE DEAFNESS. ARCH. PATH. 82* 506-517, 1966.

MARIN, O. S. M. AND TYLER, H. R.* HEREDITARY INTERSTITIAL NEPHRITIS ASSOCIATED WITH POLYNEUROPATHY. NEUROLOGY 11* 999-1005, 1961.

MILLER, G. W., JOSEPH, D. J., COZAD, R. L. AND MCCABE, B. F.* ALPORT'S SYNDROME. ARCH. OTOLARYNG. 92* 419-432, 1970.

MULROW, P. J., ARON, A. M., GATHMAN, G. E., YESNER, R. AND LUBS, H. A.* HEREDITARY NEPHRITIS. REPORT OF A KINDRED. AM. J. MED. 35* 737-748, 1963.

OHLSSON, L.* CONGENITAL RENAL DISEASE, DEAFNESS AND MYOPIA IN ONE FAMILY. ACTA MED. SCAND. 174* 77-84, 1963.

PERKOFF, G. T., NUGENT, C. A., JR., DOLOWITZ, D. A., STEPHENS, F. E., CARNES, W. H. AND TYLER, F. H.* A FOLLOW-UP STUDY OF HEREDITARY CHRONIC NEPHRITIS. ARCH. INTERN. MED. 102* 733-746, 1958.

PURRIEL, P., DRETS, M., PASCALE, E., CESTAU, R. S., BORRAS, A., FERREIRA, W. A., DELUCCA, A. AND FERNANDEZ, L.* FAMILIAL HEREDITARY NEPHROPATHY (ALPORT'S SYNDROME). AM. J. MED. 49* 753-773, 1970.

REYERSBACH, G. C. AND BUTLER, A. M.* CONGENITAL HEREDITARY HEMATURIA. NEW ENG. J. MED. 251* 377-380, 1954.

SCHNEIDER, R. G.* CONGENITAL HEREDITARY NEPHRITIS WITH NERVE DEAFNESS. NEW YORK J. MED. 63* 2644-2648, 1963.

SHAW, R. F. AND GLOVER, R. A.* ABNORMAL SEGREGATION IN HEREDITARY RENAL DISEASE WITH DEAFNESS. AM. J. HUM. GENET. 13* 89-97, 1961.

SPEAR, G. S., WHITWORTH, J. M. AND KONIGSMARK, B. W.* HEREDITARY NEPHRITIS WITH NERVE DEAFNESS. IMMUNOFLUORESCENT STUDIES ON THE KIDNEY, WITH A CONSIDERATION OF DISCORDANT IMMUNOGLOBULIN-COMPLEMENT IMMUNOFLUORESCENT REACTIONS. AM. J. MED. 49* 52-63, 1970.

STANBURY, S. W. AND CASTLEMAN, B.* NEPHROCALCINOSIS AND AZOTEMIA IN A YOUNG MAN. NEW ENG. J. MED. 278* 839-846, 1968.

TURNER, J. S., JR.* HEREDITARY HEARING LOSS WITH NEPHROPATHY (ALPORT'S SYNDROME). ACTA OTOLARYNG. 271 (SUPPL.)* 26PP, 1971.

WALKER, W. G.* BALTIMORE, MD.* PERSONAL COMMUNICATION, 1966.

WESTLEY, C. R.* FAMILIAL NEPHRITIS AND ASSOCIATED DEAFNESS IN A SOUTHWESTERN APACHE INDIAN FAMILY. STH. MED. J. 63* 1415-1419, 1970.

WHALEN, R. E., HUANG, S., PESCHEL, E. AND MCINTOSH, H. D.* HEREDITARY NEPHROPA-THY, DEAFNESS AND RENAL FOAM CELLS. AM. J. MED. 31* 171-186, 1961.

WILLIAMSON, D. A. J.* ALPORT'S SYNDROME OF HEREDITARY NEPHRITIS WITH DEAFNESS. LANCET 2* 1321-1323, 1961.

*10430 ALZHEIMER'S DISEASE OF BRAIN

WHEELAN AND RACE (1959) STUDIED A FAMILY IN WHICH THE MOTHER AND FIVE OF TEN CHILDREN HAD ALZHEIMER'S DISEASE. POSSIBLE LINKAGE WITH THE MNS LOCUS WAS SHOWN. CLINICALLY, ALZHEIMER'S DISEASE CANNOT BE DISTINGUISHED FROM PICK'S DISEASE (Q.V.). SCHOTTKY (1932) DESCRIBED PRESENILE DEMENTIA IN FOUR GENERATIONS. THE DIAGNOSIS WAS CONFIRMED AT AUTOPSY IN A PATIENT IN THE FOURTH GENERATION. LOWENBERG AND WAGGONER (1934) REPORTED A FAMILY WITH UNUSUALLY EARLY ONSET. THE FATHER AND FOUR OF FIVE CHILDREN WERE AFFECTED. POSTMORTEM FINDINGS IN ONE CASE WERE DESCRIBED. MCMENEMEY AND COLLEAGUES (1939) DESCRIBED FOUR AFFECTED MALES IN TWO GENERATIONS WITH PATHOLOGIC CONFIRMATION IN ONE. FROM AN EXTENSIVE STUDY IN SWEDEN, SJOGREN, SJOGREN AND LINDGREN (1952) CONCLUDED THAT, ALTHOUGH PICK'S DISEASE MAY BE DOMINANT WITH IMPORTANT MODIFIER GENES, ALZHEIMER'S DISEASE IS PROBABLY MULTIFACTORIAL. HESTON ET AL. (1966) DESCRIBED A FAMILY WITH 19 AFFECTED IN 4 GENERATIONS. DEMENTIA WAS COUPLED WITH CONSPICUOUS PARKINSONISM AND LONG TRACT SIGNS.

HESTON, L. L., LOWTHER, D. L. W. AND LEVENTHAL, C. M.* ALZHEIMER'S DISEASE. A FAMILY STUDY. ARCH. NEUROL. 15* 225-233, 1966.

LOWENBERG, K. AND WAGGONER, R. W.* FAMILIAL ORGANIC PSYCHOSIS (ALZHEIMER'S TYPE). ARCH. NEUROL. PSYCHIAT. 31* 737-754, 1934.

MCMENEMEY, W. H., WORSTER-DROUGHT, C., FLIND, J. AND WILLIAMS, H. G.* FAMILIAL PRESENILE DEMENTIA* REPORT OF A CASE WITH CLINICAL AND PATHOLOGICAL FEATURES OF ALZHEIMER'S DISEASE. J. NEUROL. PSYCHOPATH. 2* 293-302, 1939.

SCHOTTKY, J.* UBER PRASENILE VERBLODUNGEN. ZBL. GES. NEUROL. PSYCHIAT. 140* 333-397, 1932.

SJOGREN, T., SJOGREN, H. AND LINDGREN, A. G. H.* MORBUS ALZHEIMER AND MORBUS PICK. A GENETIC, CLINICAL AND PATHO-ANATOMICAL STUDY. ACTA PSYCHIAT. NEUROL. SCAND. 82 (SUPPL.)* 1-152, 1952.

WHEELAN, L. AND RACE, R. R.* FAMILIAL ALZHEIMER'S DISEASE, NOTE ON THE LINKAGE DATA. ANN. HUM. GENET. 23* 300-310, 1959.

10440 AMELIA AND TERMINAL TRANSVERSE HEMIMELIA

MOST CASES ARE SPORADIC. SOME FAMILIES HAVE AFFECTED RELATIVES SUGGESTING A COMPLEX GENETIC ETIOLOGY.

TEMTAMY, S. A.* GENETIC FACTORS IN HAND MALFORMATIONS. PH. D. THESIS, JOHNS HOPKINS UNIVERSITY, 1966.

*10450 AMELOGENESIS IMPERFECTA, HYPOCALCIFICATION TYPE

THE PRIMARY DEFECT IN AMELOGENESIS IMPERFECTA, HYPOCALCIFICATION TYPE, IS ECTODERMAL ALTHOUGH SECONDARY CHANGES OCCUR IN THE EXPOSED DENTINE. CHAUDHRY AND COLLEAGUES (1959) REPORTED FIVE FAMILIES WITH AN AUTOSOMAL DOMINANT PATTERN OF INHERITANCE. THERE ARE TWO X-LINKED VARIETIES. CLARK AND CLARK (1933) STUDIED TWO KINDREDS LIVING IN MAINE AND ELSEWHERE IN NEW ENGLAND. LEGEND HAD IT THAT THE AFFECTED ANCESTOR OF ONE FAMILY CAME OVER ON THE MAYFLOWER. ALTHOUGH PRESUMED ENAMEL DEFECTS 'RUNNING IN FAMILIES' WERE REPORTED FROM A RELATIVELY EARLY DATE, IT IS OFTEN DIFFICULT TO BE CERTAIN WHETHER A DENTINE DEFECT OR AN ENAMEL DEFECT WAS, IN FACT, INVOLVED IN SPECIFIC INSTANCES. WEINMANN ET AL. (1945) MADE THE USEFUL DIVISION OF ENAMEL DEFECTS INTO TWO CLASSES* (1) HEREDITARY ENAMEL HYPOPLASIA, IN WHICH THE ENAMEL IS DEFICIENT IN QUANTITY BUT HARD IN QUALITY, AND (2) HEREDITARY ENAMEL HYPOCALCIFICATION, IN WHICH THE ENAMEL IS SOFT AND UNDERCAL-CIFIED, ALTHOUGH NORMAL IN QUANTITY AND HISTOLOGY. SEE AMELOGENESIS IMPERFECTA IN

THE X-LINKAGE CATALOG. THIS IS THE MOST FREQUENT TYPE OF ENAMEL DYSPLASIA. BOTH
THE PRIMARY AND THE SECONDARY DENTITIONS ARE AFFECTED. THE ENAMEL IS SOFT AND
FRIABLE. IN OLDER INDIVIDUALS THE ENAMEL MAY BE COMPLETELY WORN AWAY.

17

D
O
M
I
N
A
N
T

CHAUDHRY, A. P., JOHNSON, O. N., MITCHELL, D. F., GORLIN, R. J. AND BARTHOLDI,
W. L.* HEREDITARY ENAMEL DYSPLASIA. J. PEDIAT. 54* 776-785, 1959.

CLARK, F. H. AND CLARK, C. S.* ABSENCE OF TOOTH ENAMEL. A DOMINANT HEREDITARY
ANOMALY IN MAN. J. HERED. 24* 425-429, 1933.

GARDNER, E. J.* A PEDIGREE OF BROWN TEETH. THE INHERITANCE OF BROWN, ENAMEL-
DEFICIENT TEETH IN A UTAH FAMILY. J. HERED. 42* 289-290, 1951.

RUSHTON, M. A.* HEREDITARY ENAMEL DEFECTS. PROC. ROY. SOC. MED. 57* 53-58,
1964.

TSUJII, T. AND OBI, M.* A FAMILY OF HEREDITARY ENAMEL HYPOPLASIA. JAP. J. HUM.
GENET. 6* 118-123, 1961.

WEINMANN, J. P., SVOBODA, J. F. AND WOODS, R. W.* HEREDITARY DISTURBANCES OF
ENAMEL FORMATION AND CALCIFICATION. J. AM. DENT. ASS. 32* 397-418, 1945.

WITKOP, C. J.* GENETICS AND DENTISTRY. EUGEN. QUART. 5* 15-21, 1958.

10460 AMENORRHEA-GALACTORRHEA SYNDROME

THE ASSOCIATION OF SECONDARY AMENORRHEA AND GALACTORRHEA IS GENERALLY THOUGHT TO
OCCUR IN TWO DISTINCT SYNDROMES* THE FORBES-ALBRIGHT SYNDROME, WHERE AMENORRHEA
AND GALACTORRHEA ARE ACCOMPANIED BY A PITUITARY TUMOR, WITH OR WITHOUT PRIOR
PREGNANCY, AND THE CHIARI-FROMMEL SYNDROME, WHERE AMENORRHEA AND GALACTORRHEA
COMMENCE AFTER PREGNANCY, WITHOUT ASSOCIATED PITUITARY TUMOR. THIS DISTINCTION
MAY BE ARTIFICIAL (RIMOIN AND SCHIMKE, 1971), BECAUSE THE PITUITARY ADENOMA MAY BE
TOO SMALL TO IDENTIFY CLINICALLY AND PROGRESSION FROM THE BENIGN TO THE NEOPLASTIC
SYNDROME HAS BEEN DOCUMENTED (YOUNG ET AL., 1967). LINQUETTE ET AL. (1967)
DESCRIBED MOTHER AND DAUGHTER WITH AMENORRHEA-GALACTORRHEA ASSOCIATED WITH
PITUITARY ADENOMA. THE MOTHER FIRST DEVELOPED CLINICAL SIGNS AFTER A PREGNANCY,
WHEREAS THE DAUGHTER WAS NEVER PREGNANT AND AMENORRHEA FOLLOWED EMOTIONAL TRAUMA.
THE SELLA TURCICA WAS ENLARGED IN BOTH AND TUMOR WAS CONFIRMED BY CRANIOTOMY. THE
TUMORS RESEMBLED CHROMOPHOBE ADENOMAS, BUT THERE WAS FIVE EOSINOPHILIC GRANULATION
ON TETRACHROME STAINING, AS SEEN IN PROLACTIN CELLS. SINCE THE AMENORRHEA-
GALACTORRHEA SYNDROME HAS BEEN DESCRIBED AS A PART OF THE MULTIPLE ENDOCRINE
ADENOMATOSIS SYNDROME, IT IS NOT CERTAIN THAT THE AILMENT IN THE MOTHER AND
DAUGHTER REPORTED BY LINQUETTE ET AL. (1967) REPRESENTED A DISTINCT ENTITY.

LINQUETTE, M., HERLANT, M., LAINE, E., FOSSATI, P. AND DUPONT-LECOMPTE, M.*
ADENOME PROLACTIVE CHEZ UNE JEUNE FILLE DONT LA MERE ETAIT PORTEUSE D'UN ADENOME
HYPOPHYSAIRE AVEC AMENORRHEE-GALACTORRHEE. ANN. ENDOCR. 28* 773-780, 1967.

RIMOIN, D. L. AND SCHIMKE, R. N.* GENETIC DISORDERS OF THE ENDOCRINE GLANDS.
ST. LOUIS* C. V. MOSBY CO., 1971.

YOUNG, R. L., BRADLEY, E. M., GOLDZIEHER, J. W., MYERS, P. H. AND LECOCQ, F.
R.* SPECTRUM OF NONPUERPERAL GALACTORRHEA* REPORT OF TWO CASES EVOLVING THROUGH
THE VARIOUS SYNDROMES. J. CLIN. ENDOCR. 27* 461-466, 1967.

*10470 AMYLASE, SERUM (TWO LOCI)

KAMARYT AND LAXOVA (1965, 1966) FOUND TWO AMYLASE ISOENZYMES IN SERUM, ONE
PRODUCED BY THE SALIVARY GLAND AND THE SECOND BY THE PANCREAS. IN 11 OF 120
CHILDREN A DUPLICATION OF PANCREATIC ENZYME BAND WAS FOUND ON STARCH GEL ELECTRO-
PHORESIS AND IN EACH CASE ONE PARENT ALSO SHOWED THE DUPLICATION. IN THE MOUSE
THE SALIVARY AND PANCREATIC AMYLASES ARE DETERMINED BY GENES AT CLOSELY LINKED
LOCI (SICK AND NIELSEN, 1964).

KAMARYT, J. AND LAXOVA, R.* AMYLASE HETEROGENEITY VARIANTS IN MAN. HUMANGENE-
TIK 3* 41-45, 1966.

KAMARYT, J. AND LAXOVA, R.* AMYLASE HETEROGENEITY. SOME GENETIC AND CLINICAL
ASPECTS. HUMANGENETIK 1* 579-586, 1965.

MCGEACHIN, R. L.* MULTIPLE MOLECULAR FORMS OF AMYLASE. ANN. N.Y. ACAD. SCI.
151* 208-212, 1968.

SICK, K. AND NIELSEN, J. T.* GENETICS OF AMYLASE ISOZYMES IN THE MOUSE.
HEREDITAS 51* 291-296, 1964.

*10480 AMYLOIDOSIS I (ANDRADE OR PORTUGUESE TYPE)

AMYLOIDOSIS OCCURS WITH FAMILIAL MEDITERRANEAN FEVER (A RECESSIVE), WITH COLD
HYPERSENSITIVITY (A DOMINANT) AND IN THE SYNDROME OF URTICARIA, DEAFNESS AND
AMYLOIDOSIS (ALSO A DOMINANT). IN ADDITION THREE DOMINANT TYPES OF SYSTEMIC
AMYLOIDOSIS ARE RECOGNIZED. IN THE ANDRADE TYPE, OBSERVED IN MANY PATIENTS IN THE

NORTHERN COASTAL PROVINCES OF PORTUGAL AND IN THEIR BRAZILIAN RELATIVES, NEUROPA-
THIC MANIFESTATIONS BEGIN AND PREDOMINATE IN THE LEGS, LEADING TO THE POPULAR
DESIGNATION OF "FOOT DISEASE." ONSET IS BETWEEN AGE 20 AND 30 AND DEATH OCCURS 7-
10 YEARS LATER. THE DISEASE IS MILDER IN FEMALES. VITREOUS OPACITIES ARE
FREQUENT (KAUFMAN AND THOMAS, 1959). IN BOTH THIS AND AMYLOIDOSIS II THE AMYLOID
IS PERI-COLLAGENOUS. IN FAMILIAL MEDITERRANEAN FEVER IT IS PERI-RETICULAR. THE
ENTIRE TOPIC OF AMYLOIDOSIS WAS EXTENSIVELY REVIEWED BY COHEN (1967). ARAKI ET
AL. (1968) REPORTED A JAPANESE KINDRED WITH MANY MEMBERS AFFECTED WITH THE
PORTUGUESE TYPE OF AMYLOID NEUROPATHY.

ANDRADE, C.* A PECULIAR FORM OF PERIPHERAL NEUROPATHY* FAMILIAL ATYPICAL
GENERALISED AMYLOIDOSIS WITH SPECIAL INVOLVEMENT OF PERIPHERAL NERVES. BRAIN 75*
408-427, 1952.

ANDRADE, C., CANIJO, M., KLEIN, D. AND KAELIN, A.* THE GENETIC ASPECTS OF THE
FAMILIAL AMYLOIDOTIC POLYNEUROPATHY. PORTUGUESE TYPE OF PARAMYLOIDOSIS.
HUMANGENETIK 7* 163-175, 1969.

ARAKI, S., MAWATARI, S., OHTA, M., NAKAJIMA, A. AND KUROIWA, Y.* POLYNEURITIC
AMYLOIDOSIS IN A JAPANESE FAMILY. ARCH. NEUROL. 18* 593-602, 1968.

BECKER, P. E., ANTUNES, L., ROSARIO, M. AND BARROS, F.* PARAMYLOIDOSE DER
PERIPHEREN NERVEN IN PORTUGAL. Z. MENSCHL. VERERB. KONSTITUTIONSL. 37* 329-364,
1963.

COHEN, A. S.* AMYLOIDOSIS. NEW ENG. J. MED. 277* 522-530, 574-583 AND 628-638,
1967.

DA SILVA HORTA, J., FILIPE, I. AND DUARTE, S.* PORTUGUESE POLYNEURITIC FAMILIAL
TYPE OF AMYLOIDOSIS. PATH. MICROBIOL. 27* 809-825, 1964.

HELLER, H., GAFNI, J. AND SOHAR, E.* THE INHERITED SYSTEMIC AMYLOIDOSES. IN,
STANBURY, J. B., WYNGAARDEN, J. B. AND FREDRICKSON, D. S. (EDS.)* THE METABOLIC
BASIS OF INHERITED DISEASE. NEW YORK* MCGRAW-HILL, 1966 (2ND ED.). PP. 995-1014.

HELLER, H., SOHAR, E. AND GAFNI, J.* CLASSIFICATION OF AMYLOIDOSIS WITH SPECIAL
REGARD TO THE GENETIC TYPES. PATH. MICROBIOL. 27* 833-840, 1964.

KAUFMAN, H. E. AND THOMAS, L. B.* VITREOUS OPACITIES DIAGNOSTIC OF FAMILIAL
PRIMARY AMYLOIDOSIS. NEW ENG. J. MED. 261* 1267-1271, 1959.

*10490 AMYLOIDOSIS II (INDIANA OR RUKAVINA TYPE)

THIS TYPE WAS OBSERVED BY RUKAVINA ET AL. (1956) IN MANY MEMBERS OF A RELIGIOUS
SECT OF SWISS ORIGIN LIVING IN INDIANA. WE (MAHLOUDJI ET AL., 1969) HAVE OBSERVED
IT IN AN EQUALLY LARGE NUMBER OF PERSONS OF GERMAN EXTRACTION LIVING IN FREDERICK
AND WASHINGTON COUNTIES OF MARYLAND. NEUROPATHIC MANIFESTATIONS BEGIN AND
PREDOMINATE IN THE UPPER LIMBS. CARPAL TUNNEL SYNDROME (PAIN, NUMBNESS AND
WEAKNESS REFERRABLE TO THE MEDIAN NERVE AND ATROPHY OF THE ABDUCTOR POLLICIS
BREVIS MUSCLE) IS THE CHARACTERISTIC FEATURE AND IS RELIEVED BY DECOMPRESSION OF
THE CARPAL TUNNEL. ONSET IS USUALLY IN THE 40'S AND PROGRESSION TO GENERALIZED
NEUROPATHY IS SLOW SO THAT SURVIVAL FOR 20 YEARS OR MORE AFTER ONSET IS THE RULE.
THE DISEASE IS MILDER IN FEMALES. VITREOUS OPACITIES AND VISCERAL MANIFESTATIONS
ARE LESS CONSPICUOUS THAN IN AMYLOIDOSIS I.

MAHLOUDJI, M., TEASDALL, R. D., ADAMKIEWICZ, J. J., HARTMANN, W. H., LAMBIRD,
P. A. AND MCKUSICK, V. A.* THE GENETIC AMYLOIDOSES WITH PARTICULAR REFERENCE TO
HEREDITARY NEUROPATHIC AMYLOIDOSIS, TYPE II (INDIANA OR RUKAVINA TYPE). MEDICINE
48* 1-37, 1969.

RUKAVINA, J. G., BLOCK, W. D. AND CURTIS, A. C.* FAMILIAL PRIMARY SYSTEMIC
AMYLOIDOSIS* AN EXPERIMENTAL, GENETIC AND CLINICAL STUDY. J. INVEST. DERM. 27*
111-131, 1956.

RUKAVINA, J. G., BLOCK, W. D., JACKSON, C. E., FALLS, H. F., CAREY, J. H. AND
CURTIS, A. C.* PRIMARY SYSTEMIC AMYLOIDOSIS* A REVIEW AND AN EXPERIMENTAL, GENETIC
AND CLINICAL STUDY OF 29 CASES WITH PARTICULAR EMPHASIS ON THE FAMILIAL FORM.
MEDICINE 35* 239-334, 1956.

SCHLESINGER, A. S., DUGGINS, V. A. AND MASUCCI, E. F.* PERIPHERAL NEUROPATHY IN
FAMILIAL PRIMARY AMYLOIDOSIS. BRAIN 85* 357-370, 1962.

10500 AMYLOIDOSIS III (CARDIAC FORM)

FREDERIKSEN AND COLLEAGUES (1962) IN DENMARK DESCRIBED A FAMILY IN WHICH 7 OF 12
SIBS HAD PROGRESSIVE HEART FAILURE DUE TO CARDIAC AMYLOIDOSIS. THE ONSET OF HEART
FAILURE WAS AT ABOUT AGE 40. THE PROCESS PROGRESSED TO DEATH IN 3 TO 6 YEARS.
CARDIAC CATHETERIZATION SHOWED CONSTRICTIVE-TYPE RIGHT-VENTRICULAR PRESSURE
CURVES. THE CHILDREN AND GRANDCHILDREN OF THE AFFECTED PERSONS WERE TOO YOUNG TO
SHOW THE CONDITION. THE FATHER WAS LIVING AND WELL AT AGE 74. THE MOTHER DIED IN
THE INFLUENZA EPIDEMIC OF 1918. SHE WAS SAID TO HAVE BEEN ALWAYS SICKLY AND TO
HAVE SWOLLEN LEGS - BUT DID BEAR 12 OFFSPRING. HARRISON AND DERRICK (1969) IN A

(1955). IN GERMANY HABERLANDT (1961, 1963) CONCLUDED THAT AMYOTROPHIC LATERAL SCLEROSIS (AND ITS EQUIVALENT PROGRESSIVE BULBAR PALSY) IS AN IRREGULAR AUTOSOMAL DOMINANT IN MANY INSTANCES. PROGRESSIVE BULBAR PALSY OF CHILDHOOD (FAZIO-LONDE'S DISEASE) IS MORE LIKELY TO BE RECESSIVE (Q.V.).

ENGEL, W. K., KURLAND, L. T. AND KLATZO, I.* AN INHERITED DISEASE SIMILAR TO AMYOTROPHIC LATERAL SCLEROSIS WITH A PATTERN OF POSTERIOR COLUMN INVOLVEMENT. AN INTERMEDIATE FORM.Q BRAIN 82* 203-220, 1959.

ESPINOSA, R. E., OKIHIRO, M. M., MULDER, D. W. AND SAYRE, G. P.* HEREDITARY AMYOTROPHIC LATERAL SCLEROSIS* A CLINICAL AND PATHOLOGIC REPORT WITH COMMENTS ON CLASSIFICATION. NEUROLOGY 12* 1-7, 1962.

GREEN, J. B.* FAMILIAL AMYOTROPHIC LATERAL SCLEROSIS OCCURRING IN 4 GENERA-TIONS. NEUROLOGY 10* 960-962, 1960.

HABERLANDT, W. F.* ASPECTS GENETIQUES DE LA SCLEROSE LATERALE AMYOTROPHIQUE. WORLD NEUROL. 2* 356-365, 1961.

HABERLANDT, W. F.* ERGEBNISSE EINER NEUROLOGISCH-GENETISCHEN STUDIE IM NORDWEST-DEUTSCHEN RAUM. PROC. SEC. INTERN. CONG. HUM. GENET. (ROME, SEPT. 6-12, 1961) 3* 1645-1651, 1963.

HIRANO, A., KURLAND, L. T. AND SAYRE, G. P.* FAMILIAL AMYOTROPHIC LATERAL SCLEROSIS. A SUBGROUP CHARACTERIZED BY POSTERIOR AND SPINOCEREBELLAR TRACT INVOLVEMENT AND HYALINE INCLUSIONS IN THE ANTERIOR HORN CELLS. ARCH. NEUROL. 16* 232-243, 1967.

KURLAND, L. T. AND MULDER, D. W.* EPIDEMIOLOGIC INVESTIGATIONS OF AMYOTROPHIC LATERAL SCLEROSIS. 2. FAMILIAL AGGREGATIONS INDICATIVE OF DOMINANT INHERITANCE. NEUROLOGY 5* 182 AND 249, 1955.

POSER, C. M., JOHNSON, M. AND BUNCH, L. D.* FAMILIAL AMYOTROPHIC LATERAL SCLEROSIS. DIS. NERV. SYST. 26* 697-702, 1965.

10550 AMYOTROPHIC LATERAL SCLEROSIS-PARKINSONISM DEMENTIA COMPLEX OF GUAM (ALS-PD)

PLATO ET AL. (1969) FOUND ABOUT THE SAME LEVEL OF INBREEDING IN AFFECTED SIBSHIPS AS IN UNAFFECTED SIBSHIPS AND INTERPRETED THIS AS ARGUING AGAINST RECESSIVE INHERITANCE. THEY FOUND THAT AFFECTED SIBSHIPS WERE MORE CLOSELY RELATED TO EACH OTHER THAN TO THE 'GENERAL POPULATION' AND INTERPRETED THIS AS SUGGESTING DOMINANT TRANSMISSION, ALTHOUGH A COMMUNICABLE FACTOR COULD NOT BE EXCLUDED. SEGREGATION ANALYSIS ADJUSTED FOR AGE WAS CONSISTENT WITH THE CONCLUSION THAT THE DISORDER ON GUAM IS AN AUTOSOMAL DOMINANT COMPLETELY PENETRANT IN MALES BUT ONLY ABOUT 50 PERCENT PENETRANT IN FEMALES.

FAGERHOL, M. K. AND LAURELL, C.-B.* THE PI SYSTEM - INHERITED VARIANTS OF SERUM ALPHA(1)-ANTITRYPSIN. IN, STEINBERG, A. G. AND BEARN, A. G. (EDS.)* PROGRESS IN MEDICAL GENETICS, CHAPTER 6 VOL. 7, 1970. PP. 96-111.

PLATO, C. C., CRUZ, M. T. AND KURLAND, L. T.* AMYOTROPHIC LATERAL SCLEROSIS-PARKINSONISM DEMENTIA COMPLEX OF GUAM* FURTHER GENETIC INVESTIGATIONS. AM. J. HUM. GENET. 21* 133-141, 1969.

10560 ANEMIA WITH MULTINUCLEATED ERYTHROBLASTS

WOLFF AND VON HOFE (1951) DESCRIBED IN A MOTHER AND ALL THREE OF HER CHILDREN MILD ANEMIA, MACROCYTOSIS IN THE PERIPHERAL BLOOD, AND GIANT MULTINUCLEAR ERYTHROBLASTS IN THE BONE MARROW. DE LOZZIO ET AL. (1962) STUDIED AN AFFECTED WOMAN WITH TWO AFFECTED SISTERS. THE PARENTS COULD NOT BE EXAMINED. THEY DEMONSTRATED ENDOPOLY-PLOIDY BY CHROMOSOME STUDIES OF BONE MARROW. THE KARYOTYPE OF SKIN CELLS WAS NORMAL. THEY POINTED OUT THAT SEVERAL INSTANCES ARE KNOWN IN PLANTS AND ANIMALS WHERE THE MITOTIC PROCESS IS INFLUENCED BY MUTANT GENES. CROOKSTON ET AL. (1969) OBSERVED 5 PATIENTS (INCLUDING TWO SISTERS) WITH WHAT APPEARS TO BE THE SAME DISORDER* ANEMIA CHARACTERIZED BY MULTIPLE NUCLEI IN ERYTHROBLASTS, INEFFECTIVE ERYTHROPOIESIS AND LYSIS OF RED CELLS BY ACIDIFIED SERUM FROM SOME BUT NOT ALL PERSONS.

CROOKSTON, J. H., CROOKSTON, M. C., BURNIE, K. L., FRANCOMBE, W. H., DACIE, J. V., DAVIS, J. A. AND LEWIS, S. M.* HEREDITARY ERYTHROBLASTIC MULTINUCLEARITY ASSOCIATED WITH A POSITIVE ACIDIFIED-SERUM TEST* A TYPE OF CONGENITAL DYSERYTHRO-POIETIC ANAEMIA. BRIT. J. HAEMAT. 17* 11-26, 1969.

DE LOZZIO, C. B., VALENCIA, J. I. AND ACAME, E.* CHROMOSOMAL STUDY IN ERYTHROB-LASTIC ENDOPOLYPLOIDY. LANCET 1* 1004-1005, 1962.

WOLFF, J. A. AND VON HOFE, F. M.* FAMILIAL ERYTHROID MULTINUCLEARITY. BLOOD 6* 1274-1283, 1951.

*10570 ANEMIA, NON-HEMOLYTIC NORMOCHROMIC

IN NORTHERN SWEDEN BERGSTROM AND JACOBSSON (1962) DISCOVERED A NEW VARIETY OF NON-

DISCUSSION OF ATRIAL STANDSTILL DESCRIBED LATIN-AMERICAN SIBS WITH POSS
CARDIAC AMYLOIDOSIS. BOTH PARENTS AND SISTER HAD DIED SUDDENLY.

FREDERIKSEN, T., GOTZSCHE, H., HARBOE, N., KIAER, W. AND MELLEMGAARD,
FAMILIAL PRIMARY AMYLOIDOSIS WITH SEVERE AMYLOID HEART DISEASE. AM. J. MED.
328-348, 1962.

HARRISON, W. H., JR. AND DERRICK, J. R.* ATRIAL STANDSTILL. A REVIEW,
PRESENTATION OF TWO NEW CASES OF FAMILIAL AND UNUSUAL NATURE WITH REFERENCE
EPICARDIAL PACING IN ONE. ANGIOLOGY 20* 610-617, 1969.

*10510 AMYLOIDOSIS IV (IOWA OR VAN ALLEN TYPE)

IN A FAMILY OF ENGLISH-SCOTTISH-IRISH EXTRACTION VAN ALLEN ET AL. (1968) HAVE B
STUDYING A FORM OF AMYLOIDOSIS APPARENTLY DIFFERENT FROM OTHERS LISTED HE
NEUROPATHY DOMINATES THE CLINICAL PICTURE EARLY IN THE COURSE AND NEUROPATHY, L
IN THE COURSE. ONSET IS AT ABOUT 35 YEARS, ON THE AVERAGE, AND AVERAGE SURVI
AFTER ONSET IS ABOUT 12 YEARS WITH DEATH ASCRIBABLE IN MOST CASES TO RE
AMYLOIDOSIS. SEVERE PEPTIC ULCER DISEASE OCCURRED IN SOME AND HEARING LOSS
ALSO FREQUENT. CATARACTS WERE PRESENT IN SEVERAL BUT VITREOUS OPACITIES WERE N
OBSERVED. THE PEDIGREE WAS TYPICAL OF AUTOSOMAL DOMINANT INHERITANCE.

VAN ALLEN, M. W., FROHLICH, J. A. AND DAVIS, J. R.* INHERITED PREDISPOSITION
GENERALIZED AMYLOIDOSIS* CLINICAL AND PATHOLOGICAL STUDIES OF A FAMILY WI
NEUROPATHY, NEPHROPATHY AND PEPTIC ULCER. NEUROLOGY 19* 10-25, 1968.

*10520 AMYLOIDOSIS, FAMILIAL VISCERAL

IN 1932 AND AGAIN IN 1950, OSTERTAG WROTE ABOUT A FAMILY WITH VISCERAL AMYLOIDO
SIS. A WOMAN, THREE OF HER CHILDREN AND ONE OF HER GRANDCHILDREN WERE AFFECTE
WITH CHRONIC NEPHROPATHY, ARTERIAL HYPERTENSION AND HEPATOSPLENOMEGALY. ALBU
MINURIA, HEMATURIA AND PITTING EDEMA WERE EARLY SIGNS. THE AGE OF ONSET WA
VARIABLE. DEATH OCCURRED ABOUT 10 YEARS AFTER ONSET. THE VISCERAL INVOLVEMENT B
AMYLOID WAS FOUND TO BE EXTENSIVE. MAXWELL AND KIMBELL (1936) DESCRIBED THRE
BROTHERS WHO DIED OF VISCERAL, ESPECIALLY RENAL, AMYLOIDOSIS IN THEIR 40'S.
CHRONIC WEAKNESS, EDEMA, PROTEINURIA AND HEPATOSPLENOMEGALY WERE FEATURES.
ALTHOUGH NEITHER PARENT WAS KNOWN TO BE AFFECTED THIS MAY BE THE SAME DISORDER A
THAT DESCRIBED BY OSTERTAG (1932). I HAVE FOLLOWED UP THE FAMILY REPORTED BY
MAXWELL AND KIMBELL (1936). THE FATHER OF THE THREE AFFECTED BROTHERS DIED AT 72
AFTER AN AUTOMOBILE ACCIDENT AND THEIR MOTHER DIED SUDDENLY AT AGE 87 AFTER BEING
IN APPARENT GOOD HEALTH. A SON OF ONE OF THE BROTHERS HAD FREQUENT BOUTS OF
UNEXPLAINED FEVER IN CHILDHOOD (AS DID HIS FATHER AND TWO UNCLES), ACCOMPANIED AT
TIMES BY NON-SPECIFIC RASH. AT THE AGE OF 35, PROTEINURIA WAS DISCOVERED AND
RENAL AMYLOIDOSIS WAS DIAGNOSED BY RENAL BIOPSY. FOR TWO YEARS THEREAFTER HE
DISPLAYED THE NEPHROTIC SYNDROME FOLLOWED IN THE NEXT TWO YEARS BY UREMIA FROM
WHICH HE DIED AT AGE 39. AUTOPSY REVEALED AMYLOIDOSIS MOST STRIKING IN THE
KIDNEYS BUT ALSO INVOLVING THE ADRENAL GLANDS AND SPLEEN. SOME FEATURES OF THE
FAMILY OF MAXWELL AND KIMBELL (1936) ARE SIMILAR TO THOSE OF URTICARIA, DEAFNESS
AND AMYLOIDOSIS (Q.V.). NO DEAFNESS WAS PRESENT IN THEIR FAMILY, HOWEVER.

MAXWELL, E. S. AND KIMBELL, I.* FAMILIAL AMYLOIDOSIS WITH CASE REPORTS. MED.
BULL. VETERANS ADMIN. 12* 365-369, 1936.

OSTERTAG, B.* DEMONSTRATION EINER EIGENARTIGEN FAMILIAREN PARAMYLOIDOSE. ZBL.
PATH. 56* 253-254, 1932.

OSTERTAG, B.* FAMILIARE AMYLOID-ERKRANKUNG. Z. MENSCHL. VERERB. KONSTITU-
TIONSL. 30* 105-115, 1950.

*10530 AMYOTROPHIC DYSTONIC PARAPLEGIA

GILMAN AND HORENSTEIN (1964) DESCRIBED DYSTONIA, PROGRESSIVE AMYOTROPHY, MENTAL
RETARDATION, NYSTAGMUS, AND INCONTINENCE OF BOWEL AND BLADDER IN ASSOCIATION WITH
SPASTIC PARAPLEGIA. TWELVE MEMBERS OF 3 GENERATIONS WERE INVOLVED TO AN EXTENT
VARYING FROM AN ASYMPTOMATIC CONDITION TO A SEVERELY DISABLING ONE BEGINNING IN
LATE CHILDHOOD.

GILMAN, S. AND HORENSTEIN, S.* FAMILIAL AMYOTROPHIC DYSTONIC PARAPLEGIA. BRAIN
87* 51-66, 1964.

*10540 AMYOTROPHIC LATERAL SCLEROSIS

ESPINOSA ET AL. (1962) CONCLUDED THAT THE FAMILIAL CASES OBSERVED IN THE UNITED
STATES REPRESENT A DIFFERENT DISORDER FROM THAT IN THE CASES ON GUAM AND FROM THAT
IN MANY OF THE SPORADIC CASES. MALES AND FEMALES ARE EQUALLY AFFECTED BY THE
FAMILIAL DISEASE AND THE PROGRESSION IS LESS RAPID THAN IN THE SPORADIC FORM WHICH
AFFECTS MALES TWICE AS OFTEN AS FEMALES.
ENGEL, KURLAND AND KLATZO (1959) DESCRIBED TWO AFFECTED AMERICAN FAMILIES.
IN ONE FAMILY OF PENNSYLVANIA DUTCH STOCK AT LEAST ELEVEN MEMBERS OF FOUR
GENERATIONS WERE AFFECTED BY WHAT WAS LOCALLY AND POPULARLY TERMED *PECKS*
DISEASE.* HISTOPATHOLOGIC STUDIES REVEALED A CONSISTENT PATTERN OF POSTERIOR
COLUMN INVOLVEMENT. THE REPORTS TO 1955 WERE REVIEWED BY KURLAND AND MULDER

HEMOLYTIC, NORMOCHROMIC ANEMIA WITH LOW OR NORMAL RETICULOCYTE COUNT. THEY REFERRED TO IT AS HEREDITARY BENIGN ERYTHRORETICULOSIS. FIFTEEN MEMBERS OF FOUR GENERATIONS WERE AFFECTED. BERGSTROM (1968) STATED THAT NO FURTHER FAMILIES HAD BEEN OBSERVED IN SWEDEN BUT THAT NEW CASES, TO A TOTAL OF ABOUT 20, HAD BEEN DETECTED IN THE REPORTED FAMILY.

BERGSTROM, I. AND JACOBSSON, L.* HEREDITARY BENIGN ERYTHRORETICULOSIS. BLOOD 19* 296-303, 1962.

BERGSTROM, I.* OSTERSUND, SWEDEN* PERSONAL COMMUNICATION, 1968.

10580 ANEURYSM, INTRACRANIAL 'BERRY'

ULLRICH AND SUGAR (1960) REPORTED FOUR FAMILIES IN EACH OF WHICH TWO MEMBERS HAD CEREBRAL ANEURYSMS. WE OBSERVED A 34 YEAR OLD MAN AND HIS 13 YEAR OLD DAUGHTER, BOTH OF WHOM DIED OF INTRACRANIAL BERRY ANEURYSM. IN SOME CASES OF POLYCYSTIC KIDNEYS (Q.V.) BERRY ANEURYSM IS AN ASSOCIATED MALFORMATION. GRAF (1966) REPORTED TWO PAIRS OF AFFECTED SIBS. 'BERRY' ANEURYSM MAY HAVE AN INCREASED FREQUENCY IN PERSONS WITH THE EHLERS-DANLOS SYNDROME AND ALSO OCCURS WITH COARCTATION OF THE AORTA. BEUMONT (1968) DESCRIBED THREE AFFECTED SISTERS.

BANNERMAN, R. M., INGALL, G. B. AND GRAF, C. J.* THE FAMILIAL OCCURRENCE OF INTRACRANIAL ANEURYSMS. NEUROLOGY 20* 283-292, 1970.

BEUMONT, P. J.* THE FAMILIAL OCCURRENCE OF BERRY ANEURYSM. J. NEUROL. NEUROSURG. PSYCHIAT. 31* 399-402, 1968.

CHAKRAVORTY, B. G. AND GLEADHILL, C. A.* FAMILIAL INCIDENCE OF CEREBRAL ANEURYSMS. BRIT. MED. J. 1* 147-148, 1966.

GRAF, C. J.* FAMILIAL INTRACRANIAL ANEURYSMS. REPORT OF FOUR CASES. J. NEUROSURG. 25* 304-308, 1966.

KAK, V. K., GLEADHILL, C. A. AND BAILEY, I. C.* THE FAMILIAL INCIDENCE OF INTRACRANIAL ANEURYSMS. J. NEUROL. NEUROSURG. PSYCHIAT. 33* 29-33, 1970.

ULLRICH, D. P. AND SUGAR, O.* FAMILIAL CEREBRAL ANEURYSMS INCLUDING ONE EXTRACRANIAL INTERNAL CAROTID ANEURYSM. NEUROLOGY 10* 288-294, 1960.

10590 ANGIOLIPOMAS, MULTIPLE

KLEM (1949) DESCRIBED AFFECTED BROTHER AND SISTER WHOSE DECEASED FATHER WAS SAID TO HAVE BEEN SIMILARLY AFFECTED. SEE DESCRIPTION OF HISTOPATHOLOGY AND OTHER FEATURES BY HOWARD AND HELWIG (1960).

HOWARD, W. R. AND HELWIG, E. B.* ANGIOLIPOMA. ARCH. DERM. 82* 924-931, 1960.

KLEM, K. K.* MULTIPLE LIPOMA-ANGIOLIPOMAS. ACTA CHIR. SCAND. 97* 527-532, 1949.

10600 ANGIOMA RACEMOSUM VENOSUM

SEGMENTALLY RELATED VASCULAR ANOMALIES OF THE SPINAL CORD AND SKIN ARE VERY RARE. THERE IS NO EVIDENCE OF A GENETIC BASIS.

FINE, R. D.* ANGIOMA RACEMOSUM VENOSUM OF SPINAL CORD WITH SEGMENTALLY RELATED ANGIOMATOUS LESIONS OF SKIN AND FOREARM. J. NEUROSURG. 18* 546-550, 1961.

*10610 ANGIONEUROTIC EDEMA (TWO TYPES)

A CONSIDERABLE NUMBER OF KINDREDS WITH ANGIONEUROTIC EDEMA TRANSMITTED IN A TYPICAL AUTOSOMAL DOMINANT PATTERN HAVE BEEN DESCRIBED. IN TRIGG'S FAMILY (1961) ABOUT TWICE AS MANY MALES AS FEMALES WERE AFFECTED. THE NATURE OF THE BASIC DEFECT IS NOW KNOWN. TWO TYPES ARE IDENTIFIABLE. SOME FAIL TO SYNTHESIZE THE INHIBITOR OF THE FIRST COMPONENT OF COMPLEMENT, WHEREAS OTHERS SYNTHESIZE AN ABNORMAL, NONFUNCTIONAL PROTEIN. IT IS CURIOUS THAT THIS 'DEFICIENCY' IS EXPRESSED IN THE HETEROZYGOTE. ALL OF THE PARTICULAR PROTEIN IS EITHER ABSENT OR ABNORMAL, NOT APPROXIMATELY HALF AS IN HETEROZYGOTES FOR MOST DISORDERS. SEE COLD HYPERSENSITIVITY FOR RELATED CONDITION. A FAMILY STUDIED BY DONALDSON AND ROSEN (1964) HAD PREVIOUSLY BEEN REPORTED BY HEINER AND BLITZER (1957). COHEN (1961) DESCRIBED A FAMILY WITH MANY CASES IN FIVE GENERATIONS. ALTHOUGH REPORTED AS GIANT URTICARIA, THE SAME FAMILY WAS STUDIED BY ROSEN AND COLLEAGUES (1965) AND SHOWN TO HAVE A DEFECT IN A COMPONENT OF COMPLEMENT. SPAULDING (1960) AND DENNEHY (1970) DESCRIBED APPARENTLY EFFECTIVE PROPHYLAXIS WITH TESTOSTERONE. THE LATTER ALSO CALLED ATTENTION TO THE FACT THAT NATHANIEL HAWTHORNE WAS APPARENTLY FAMILIAR WITH THIS DISORDER FOR IN HIS 'HOUSE OF THE SEVEN GABLES' HE DESCRIBED A FAMILY WITH MEMBERS WHO GURGLED IN THE THROAT AND CHEST WHEN EXCITED AND WHO WOULD SOMETIMES DIE IN THIS WAY, EVER SINCE A CURSE TO CHOKE ON BLOOD HAD BEEN PLACED ON ONE OF THEIR ANCESTORS. DENNEHY (1970) INTERPRETED THE FOLLOWING PASSAGE AS AN INDICATION THAT HAWTHORNE RECOGNIZED THAT A HEREDITARY DISEASE, NOT A CURSE, WAS RESPONSIBLE FOR THE DEATHS* 'THIS MODE OF DEATH HAS BEEN AN IDIOSYNCRASY WITH HIS FAMILY, FOR GENERATIONS PAST. . . . OLD MAULE'S PROPHECY WAS PROBABLY FOUNDED ON A

KNOWLEDGE OF THIS PHYSICAL PREDISPOSITION IN THE PYNCHEON RACE.*

AUSTEN, K. F. AND SHEAFFER, A. L.* DETECTION OF HEREDITARY ANGIONEUROTIC EDEMA BY DEMONSTRATION OF A REDUCTION IN THE SECOND COMPONENT OF HUMAN COMPLEMENT. NEW ENG. J. MED. 272* 649-656, 1965.

COHEN, J. D.* CHRONIC FAMILIAL GIANT URTICARIA. ANN. INTERN. MED. 54* 331-335, 1961.

DENNEHY, J. J.* HEREDITARY ANGIONEUROTIC EDEMA. REPORT OF A LARGE KINDRED WITH DEFECT IN C-PRIME-1 ESTERASE INHIBITOR AND REVIEW OF THE LITERATURE. ANN. INTERN. MED. 73* 55-59, 1970.

PICKERING, R. J., KELLY, J. R., GOOD, R. A. AND GEWURZ, H.* REPLACEMENT THERAPY IN HEREDITARY ANGIOEDEMA. SUCCESSFUL TREATMENT OF TWO PATIENTS WITH FRESH FROZEN PLASMA. LANCET 1* 326-330, 1969.

DONALDSON, V. H. AND EVANS, R. R.* A BIOCHEMICAL ABNORMALITY IN HEREDITARY ANGIONEUROTIC EDEMA. ABSENCE OF SERUM INHIBITOR C*1-ESTERASE. AM. J. MED. 35* 37-44, 1963.

DONALDSON, V. H. AND ROSEN, F. S.* ACTION OF COMPLEMENT IN HEREDITARY AN-GIONEUROTIC EDEMA* THE ROLE OF C-PRIME-1-ESTERASE. J. CLIN. INVEST. 43* 2204-2213, 1964.

HEINER, D. C. AND BLITZER, J. R.* FAMILIAL PAROXYSMAL DYSFUNCTION OF THE AUTONOMIC NERVOUS SYSTEM (A PERIODIC DISEASE), OFTEN PRECIPITATED BY EMOTIONAL STRESS. PEDIATRICS 20* 782-793, 1957.

ROSEN, F. S., CHARACHE, P., PENSKY, J. AND DONALDSON, V.* HEREDITARY AN-GIONEUROTIC EDEMA* TWO GENETIC VARIANTS. SCIENCE 148* 957-958, 1965.

SPAULDING, W. B.* METHYLTESTOSTERONE THERAPY FOR HEREDITARY EPISODIC EDEMA (HEREDITARY ANGIONEUROTIC EDEMA). ANN. INTERN. MED. 53* 739-745, 1960.

TRIGG, J. W.* HEREDITARY ANGIONEUROTIC EDEMA* REPORT OF A CASE WITH GASTROINTE-STINAL MANIFESTATIONS. NEW ENG. J. MED. 264* 761-763, 1961.

*10620 ANIRIDIA

SHAW, FALLS AND NEEL (1960) ASCERTAINED 176 CASES OF ANIRIDIA IN THE LOWER MICHIGAN PENINSULA. FORTY ISOLATED CASES WERE CONSIDERED MUTANTS. THE FREQUENCY IN MICHIGAN WAS ABOUT 1.8 X 10-5 AND THE MUTATION RATE ABOUT 4 X 10-6 PER GAMETE PER GENERATION. AFFECTED PERSONS MAY BE VISUALLY HANDICAPPED BECAUSE OF NYSTAG-MUS, CATARACT OR GLAUCOMA. THE RATIO OF AFFECTED TO NORMAL AMONG THE OFFSPRING OF AN AFFECTED PARENT WAS 38 TO 62, A SIGNIFICANT DIFFERENCE FROM 50 TO 50. UNDOUBTEDLY MORE THAN ONE *CAUSE* OF ANIRIDIA EXISTS. ANIRIDIA IS SOMETIMES ASSOCIATED WITH WILMS* TUMOR (Q.V.) AS A SPORADIC FINDING.

FRAUMENI, J. F.* THE ANIRIDIA-WILMS* TUMOR SYNDROME. THE CLINICAL DELINEATION OF BIRTH DEFECTS. II. MALFORMATION SYNDROMES. NEW YORK* NATIONAL FOUNDATION, 1969. PP. 198-201.

SHAW, M. W., FALLS, H. F. AND NEEL, J. V.* CONGENITAL ANIRIDIA. AM. J. HUM. GENET. 12* 389-415, 1960.

10630 ANKYLOSING SPONDYLITIS

KARTEN AND COLLEAGUES (1962) DEMONSTRATED FAMILIAL AGGREGATION. RHEUMATOID ARTHRITIS AND POSITIVE TESTS FOR RHEUMATOID FACTOR WERE FOUND NO MORE OFTEN IN THE RELATIVES OF SPONDYLITICS THAN IN THOSE OF CONTROLS, SUGGESTING THAT RHEUMATOID ARTHRITIS AND ANKYLOSING SPONDYLITIS ARE DISTINCT ENTITIES. DE BLECOURT, POLMAN AND DE BLECOURT-MEINDERSMA (1961) FOUND SPONDYLITIS 22.6 TIMES MORE FREQUENTLY IN THE RELATIVES OF SPONDYLITIC PATIENTS THAN IN THE RELATIVES OF CONTROLS. THEY SUGGESTED AUTOSOMAL DOMINANT INHERITANCE WITH GREATER PENETRANCE IN MALES THAN IN FEMALES. O*CONNELL (1959) ARRIVED AT THE SAME CONCLUSION. THE FAMILIAL INCIDENCE WAS HIGHER WHEN THE PROBAND WAS FEMALE. KORNSTAD AND KORNSTAD (1960) DESCRIBED TWO FAMILIES IN WHICH ONLY FEMALES WERE AFFECTED. EMERY AND LAWRENCE (1967) PRESENTED DATA WHICH THEY INTERPRETED AS INDICATING MULTIFACTORIAL INHERITANCE.

DE BLECOURT, J. J., POLMAN, A. AND DE BLECOURT-MEINDERSMA, T.* HEREDITARY FACTORS IN RHEUMATOID ARTHRITIS AND ANKYLOSING SPONDYLITIS. ANN. RHEUM. DIS. 20* 215-220, 1961.

EMERY, A. E. H. AND LAWRENCE, J. S.* GENETICS OF ANKYLOSING SPONDYLITIS. J. MED. GENET. 4* 239-244, 1967.

KARTEN, I., DITATA, D., MCEWEN, C. AND TANNER, M.* A FAMILY STUDY OF RHEUMATOID (ANKYLOSING) SPONDYLITIS. ARTHRITIS RHEUM. 5* 131-143* 1962.

KORNSTAD, A. M. G. AND KORNSTAD, L.* ANKYLOSING SPONDYLITIS IN TWO FAMILIES SHOWING INVOLVEMENT OF FEMALE MEMBERS ONLY. WITH A SEARCH FOR LINKAGE TO GENES

O'CONNELL, D.* HEREDITY IN ANKYLOSING SPONDYLITIS. ANN. INTERN. MED. 50* 1115-1121, 1959.

10640 ANKYLOSING VERTEBRAL HYPEROSTOSIS WITH TYLOSIS

BEARDWELL (1969) DESCRIBED A FAMILY OF GREEK CYPRIOT EXTRACTION IN WHICH AT LEAST 8 PERSONS IN 4 SIBSHIPS IN TWO GENERATIONS ARE KNOWN TO HAVE THIS COMBINATION. THE TYLOSIS WAS A PUNCTATE HYPERKERATOSIS OF THE SOLES AND PALMS. IN ADDITION, SIX PERSONS HAD TYLOSIS ALONE.

BEARDWELL, A.* FAMILIAL ANKYLOSING VERTEBRAL HYPEROSTOSIS WITH TYLOSIS. ANN. RHEUM. DIS. 28* 518-523, 1969.

10650 ANNULAR ERYTHEMA

BEARE ET AL. (1966) DESCRIBED AN IRISH FAMILY IN WHICH FOUR PERSONS IN THREE GENERATIONS SUFFERED FROM ANNULAR ERYTHEMA.

BEARE, J. M., FROGGATT, P., JONES, J. H. AND NEILL, D. W.* FAMILIAL ANNULAR ERYTHEMA, AN APPARENTLY NEW DOMINANT MUTATION. BRIT. J. DERM. 78* 59-68, 1966.

*10660 ANODONTIA, PARTIAL

ERWIN AND COCKERN (1949) DESCRIBED ABSENT SECOND BICUSPIDS AND THIRD MOLARS IN NINE MEMBERS OF THREE GENERATIONS.

ERWIN, W. G. AND COCKERN, R. W.* A PEDIGREE OF PARTIAL ANODONTIA. J. HERED. 40* 215-218, 1949.

10670 ANOMALOUS PULMONARY VENOUS RETURN

NEILL AND HER COLLEAGUES (1960) DESCRIBED FATHER AND DAUGHTER WITH HYPOPLASTIC RIGHT LUNG WITH SYSTEMIC ARTERIAL SUPPLY AND VENOUS DRAINAGE. THEY REFERRED TO THE DISORDER AS THE 'SCIMITAR SYNDROME' BECAUSE OF THE RADIOGRAPHIC APPEARANCE CREATED BY THE ANOMALOUS VEIN DRAINING THE RIGHT LOWER LUNG AND CONNECTING WITH THE INFERIOR VENA CAVA. THE FATHER WAS ASYMPTOMATIC BUT HAD BEEN REJECTED FOR MILITARY SERVICE BECAUSE HIS HEART WAS SAID TO BE ON THE RIGHT SIDE. THE DAUGHTER HAD SEVERE PULMONARY HYPERTENSION, FREQUENT RESPIRATORY INFECTIONS AND MARKED HYPOPLASIA OF THE RIGHT LUNG WITH DEXTROPOSITION OF THE HEART. VINH ET AL. (1968) DESCRIBED A BROTHER AND SISTER, OFFSPRING OF NON-CONSANGUINEOUS PARENTS, WITH TOTAL INFRA-DIAPHRAGMATIC PULMONARY VENOUS RETURN. IN TWO BROTHERS AND A MALE PATERNAL FIRST COUSIN COSTELLO (1970) OBSERVED TOTAL ANOMALOUS PULMONARY VENOUS RETURN.

COSTELLO, E.* BUENOS AIRES, VENEZUELA* PERSONAL COMMUNICATION, 1970.

NEILL, C. A., FERENCZ, C., SABISTON, D. C. AND SHELDON, H.* THE FAMILIAL OCCURRENCE OF HYPOPLASTIC RIGHT LUNG WITH SYSTEMIC ARTERIAL SUPPLY AND VENOUS DRAINAGE* 'SCIMITAR SYNDROME.' BULL. HOPKINS HOSP. 107* 1-21, 1960.

VINH, L. T., DUC, T. V., AICARDI, J. AND ST. THIEFFRY, NI* RETOUR VEINEUX PULMONAIRE ANORMAL TOTAL INFRA-DIAPHRAGMATIQUE FAMILIALE. ARCH. FRANC. PEDIAT. 25* 1141-1149, 1968.

10680 ANONYCHIA

IN SOME REPORTED FAMILIES ABSENCE OF SOME OR ALL NAILS APPARENTLY OCCURRED WITHOUT ASSOCIATED MANIFESTATIONS OF THE NAIL-PATELLA SYNDROME (Q.V.) AND WITHOUT ABSENCE OF DIGITS AS IN THE ANONYCHIA-ECTRODACTYLY SYNDROME (Q.V.). WHETHER DIFFERENT FROM 'THUMB NAILS, ABSENCE OF' (Q.V.) IS NOT CERTAIN. RECESSIVE ANONYCHIA HAS ALSO BEEN DESCRIBED.

CHARTERIS, F.* A CASE OF PARTIAL HEREDITARY ANONYCHIA. GLASGOW MED. J. 89* 207-209, 1918.

HOBBS, M. E.* HEREDITARY ONYCHIAL DYSPLASIA. AM. J. MED. SCI. 190* 200-206, 1935.

*10690 ANONYCHIA-ECTRODACTYLY

LEES ET AL. (1957) DESCRIBED A CONDITION OF ABSENCE OF SOME OR ALL FINGER NAILS WITH VARIABLE ABSENCE OF SOME PHALANGES AND METACARPALS. A SUGGESTION OF LINKAGE WITH THE LUTHERAN LOCUS WAS PRESENTED.

LEES, D. H., LAWLER, S. D., RENWICK, J. H. AND THODAY, J. M.* ANONYCHIA WITH ECTRODACTYLY* CLINICAL AND LINKAGE DATA. ANN. HUM. GENET. 22* 69-79, 1957.

10700 ANONYCHIA-ONYCHODYSTROPHY

TIMERMAN ET AL. (1969) DESCRIBED AFFECTED PERSONS IN AT LEAST FOUR GENERATIONS

WITH MALE-TO-MALE TRANSMISSION. SOME DIGITS SHOWED ABSENT NAILS, OTHERS DYSTRO-
PHIC NAILS.

TIMERMAN, I., MUSETEANU, C. AND SIMIONESCU, N. N.* DOMINANT ANONYCHIA AND
ONYCHODYSTROPHY. J. MED. GENET. 6* 105-106, 1969.

VOGEL, F. AND DORN, H.* ANONYCHIA CONGENITA. IN BECKER, P. E. (ED.)* HUMAN-
GENETIC. STUTTGART* GEORG THIEME VERLAG, 1964. 4* 489-490.

10710 ANORECTAL ANOMALIES

VAN GELDER AND KLOEPFER (1961) OBSERVED FOUR SIBS WITH ANORECTAL STENOSIS OR
IMPERFORATE ANUS. ALTHOUGH THE PARENTS WERE UNAFFECTED THE AUTHORS POINTED OUT
THAT FAILURE OF EXPRESSION OF A RECENT DOMINANT MUTATION, CARRIED BY ONE PARENT,
IS A POSSIBILITY. KAIJSER AND MALMSTROM-GROTH (1957) DESCRIBED IMPERFORATE ANUS
WITH RECTOVAGINAL FISTULA IN A MOTHER AND HER TWO DAUGHTERS. FROM THE FINDINGS OF
COZZI AND WILKINSON (1968), ANAL STENOSIS SEEMS PARTICULARLY LIABLE TO FAMILIAL
OCCURRENCE, PROBABLY AS AN IRREGULAR DOMINANT.

COZZI, F. AND WILKINSON, A. W.* FAMILIAL INCIDENCE OF CONGENITAL ANORECTAL
ANOMALIES. SURGERY 64* 669-671, 1968.

KAIJSER, K. AND MALMSTROM-GROTH, A.* ANORECTAL ABNORMALITIES AS A CONGENITAL
FAMILIAL INCIDENCE. ACTA PAEDIAT. 46* 199-200, 1957.

VAN GELDER, D. W. AND KLOEPFER, H. W.* FAMILIAL ANORECTAL ANOMALIES. PEDIA-
TRICS 27* 334-336, 1961.

10720 ANOSMIA, CONGENITAL

PATTERSON AND LAUDER, (1948) DESCRIBED ONE FAMILY WITH ONSET OF ANOSMIA IN MIDDLE
AGE IN MOTHER AND ALL THREE CHILDREN. IN EACH OF TWO FAMILIES, A SINGLE INDIVI-
DUAL COULD NOT SMELL BUTYL MERCAPTAN BUT COULD SMELL OTHER ODORS AND HAD NORMAL
PARENTS. ADMITTING THE MEAGERNESS OF THE MATERIAL, THEY RAISED THE QUESTION OF
RECESSIVE INHERITANCE IN THIS APPARENTLY CONGENITAL FORM OF SMELL-BLINDNESS. IN A
JAPANESE KINDRED YAMAMOTO ET AL. (1966) FOUND TREMOR AND-OR ANOSMIA OR HYPOSMIA IN
14 PERSONS. THEY SUGGESTED THAT THE TWO TRAITS ARE INDEPENDENT DOMINANTS. THEIR
FINDINGS MAY BE EQUALLY CONSISTENT WITH THE PLEIOTROPIC AND VARIABLE EFFECTS OF A
SINGLE GENE. IN THE FAROE ISLANDS LYGONIS (1969) FOUND A LARGE KINDRED IN WHICH 9
MALES AND 19 FEMALES IN 4 GENERATIONS HAD ANOSMIA WITH NO OTHER ABNORMALITY.
MALE-TO-MALE TRANSMISSION WAS OBSERVED SEVERAL TIMES. SINGH ET AL. (1970)
OBSERVED ANOSMIA IN 6 MALES IN THREE GENERATIONS. ONE MALE WHO TRANSMITTED THE
TRAIT HAD ONLY PARTIAL ANOSMIA. DOMINANT INHERITANCE WAS RECORDED BY MAINLAND
(1945) AND JOYNER (1963). SEVERAL INSTANCES OF MALE-TO-MALE TRANSMISSION. SINGH
ET AL. (1970) OBSERVED ANOSMIA OR HYPOSMIA IN 6 MALES IN 3 CONSECUTIVE GENERA-
TIONS. SEE KALLMANN SYNDROME. ONE OF THE PATIENTS OF HOCKADAY (1966) WITH
ANOSMIA-HYPOGONADISM HAD FATHER AND A BROTHER WITH ANOSMIA ALONE.

HOCKADAY, T. D. R.* HYPOGONADISM AND LIFE-LONG ANOSMIA. POSTGRAD. MED. J. 42*
572-574, 1966.

JOYNER, R. E.* OLFACTORY ACUITY IN AN INDUSTRIAL POPULATION. J. OCCUP. MED. 5*
37-42, 1963.

LYGONIS, C. S.* FAMILIAR ABSENCE OF OLFACTION. HEREDITAS 61* 413-415, 1969.

MAINLAND, R. C.* ABSENCE OF OLFACTORY SENSATION. J. HERED. 36* 143-144, 1945.

PATTERSON, P. M. AND LAUDER, B. A.* THE INCIDENCE AND PROBABLE INHERITANCE OF
'SMELL BLINDNESS' TO NORMAL BUTYL MERCAPTAN. J. HERED. 39* 295-297, 1948.

SINGH, N., GREWAL, M. S. AND AUSTIN, J. H.* FAMILIAL ANOSMIA. ARCH. NEUROL.
22* 40-44, 1970.

WENZEL, B. M.* TECHNIQUES IN OLFACTOMETRY* A CRITICAL REVIEW OF THE LAST ONE
HUNDRED YEARS. PSYCHOL. BULL. 45* 231, 1948.

YAMAMOTO, K., ITO, K. AND YAMAGUCHI, M.* A FAMILY SHOWING SMELL DISTURBANCE AND
TREMOR. JAP. J. HUM. GENET. 11* 36-38, 1966.

10730 ANTITHROMBIN DEFICIENCY

EGEBERG (1965) DESCRIBED A PEDIGREE IN WHICH PERSONS IN THREE GENERATIONS HAD
FLORID THROMBOPHLEBITIS AND OTHER THROMBOTIC DISEASE ASSOCIATED WITH LEVELS OF
ANTITHROMBIN III ABOUT HALF NORMAL. HE SUGGESTED THAT ANTITHROMBIN III MAY BE THE
SAME AS HEPARIN COFACTOR. ANTITHROMBIN DEFICIENCY IN INDIVIDUAL PATIENTS WITH
SEVERE VENO-OCCLUSIVE DISEASE AND AN IMPRESSIVE FAMILY HISTORY WAS ALSO REPORTED
BY PENICK (1969) AND BY NESJE AND KORDT (1970).

EGEBERG, O.* INHERITED ANTITHROMBIN DEFICIENCY CAUSING THROMBOPHILIA. THROMB.
DIATH. HAEMORRH. 13* 516-530, 1965.

NESJE, O. A. AND KORDT, K. F.* HYPOANTITHROMBINEMI SOM ARSAK TIL MESENTERIAL-VENETROMBOSE. NORD. MED. 83* 367-368, 1970.

PENICK, G. D.* BLOOD STATES THAT PREDISPOSE TO THROMBOSIS. IN, SHERRY, S., BRINKHOUS, K. M., GENTON, E. AND STENGLE, J. M. (EDS.)* THROMBOSIS. WASHINGTON, D. C.* NATIONAL ACADEMY OF SCIENCES, 1969.

*10740 ANTITRYPSIN, ELECTROPHORETIC VARIANT OF SERUM

ANTITRYPSIN DEFICIENCY IS DISCUSSED IN THE RECESSIVE CATALOG. IN ADDITION, ELECTROPHORETIC VARIANTS OF ALPHA(1)ANTITRYPSIN HAVE BEEN OBSERVED BY AXELSSON AND LAURELL (1965) WHO PROPOSED THAT THE GENE FOR THE ELECTROPHORETIC VARIANT IS ALLELIC WITH THE DEFICIENCY GENE. KUEPPERS AND BEARN (1967) STUDIED AN ITALIAN FAMILY WITH MULTIPLE MEMBERS HETEROZYGOUS FOR AN ELECTROPHORETIC VARIANT WHICH COULD NOT BE DISTINGUISHED FROM THAT WHICH AXELSSON AND LAURELL FOUND IN A SWEDISH FAMILY. THE POLYMORPHISM OF PREALBUMIN DESCRIBED BY FAGERHOL AND BRAEND (1965) WAS SHOWN BY FAGERHOL AND LAURELL (1967) TO BE THE SAME AS THE ALPHA(1)ANTITRYPSIN POLYMORPHISM. FAGERHOL (1968) SUGGESTED THAT THE SYSTEM BE CALLED PI FOR PROTEASE INHIBITOR. A CONSIDERABLE NUMBER OF CODOMINANT ALLELES HAVE BEEN DESCRIBED. THE ALLELES HAVE BEEN GIVEN SYMBOLS ACCORDING TO THE RELATIVE ELECTROPHORETIC MOBILITY OF THE ALLELE PRODUCT. THE DESCRIBED PHENOTYPES INCLUDE FF, FM, FS, FZ, IM, MM, MS, MV, MX, MZ, SS, SZ, XZ AND ZZ. THE LAST PHENOTYPE ZZ IS ASSOCIATED WITH LUNG DISEASE.

AXELSSON, U. AND LAURELL, C.-B.* HEREDITARY VARIANTS OF SERUM ALPHA-1-ANTITRYP-SIN. AM. J. HUM. GENET. 17* 466-472, 1965.

FAGERHOL, M. K. AND BRAEND, M.* SERUM PREALBUMIN* POLYMORPHISM IN MAN. SCIENCE 149* 986-987, 1965.

FAGERHOL, M. K. AND GEDDE-DAHL, T., JR.* GENETICS OF THE PI SERUM TYPES. FAMILY STUDIES OF THE INHERITED VARIANTS OF SERUM ALPHA-1-ANTITRYPSIN. HUM. HERED. 19* 354-359, 1969.

FAGERHOL, M. K. AND HAUGE, H. E.* THE PI PHENOTYPE MP. DISCOVERY OF A NINTH ALLELE BELONGING TO THE SYSTEM OF INHERITED VARIANTS OF SERUM ALPHA-1-ANTITRYPSIN. VOX SANG. 15* 396-400, 1968.

FAGERHOL, M. K. AND LAURELL, C. B.* THE PI SYSTEM-INHERITED VARIANTS OF SERUM ALPHA-1-ANTITRYPSIN. PROG. MED. GENET. 7* 96-111, 1970.

FAGERHOL, M. K. AND LAURELL, C. B.* THE POLYMORPHISM OF *PREALBUMINS* AND ALPHA-1-ANTITRYPSIN IN HUMAN SERA. CLIN. CHIM. ACTA 16* 199-203, 1967.

FAGERHOL, M. K. AND TENFJORD, O. W.* SERUM PI TYPES IN SOME EUROPEAN, AMERICAN, ASIAN AND AFRICAN POPULATIONS. ACTA PATH. MICROBIOL. SCAND. 72* 601-608, 1968.

FAGERHOL, M. K.* THE PI SYSTEM. GENETIC VARIANTS OF SERUM ALPHA-1-ANTITRYPSIN. SERIES HEMAT. 1* 153-161, 1968.

KUEPPERS, F. AND BEARN, A. G.* AN INHERITED ALPHA-1-ANTITRYPSIN VARIANT. HUMANGENETIK 4* 217-220, 1967.

10750 AORTIC ARCH ANOMALY WITH PECULIAR FACIES AND MENTAL RETARDATION

IN A MOTHER AND THREE OF HER CHILDREN, STRONG (1968) FOUND RIGHT AORTIC ARCH, MENTAL SUBNORMALITY AND FACIAL PECULIARITY DIFFICULT TO DESCRIBE. THREE OF THE PATIENTS HAD ESOPHAGEAL INDENTATION DEMONSTRATED BY BARIUM SWALLOW, SUGGESTING LEFT LIGAMENTUM ARTERIOSUM OR ANOMALOUS LEFT SUBCLAVIAN ARTERY. TWO OF THE PATIENTS HAD MICROCEPHALY. A STILLBORN CHILD HAD ANENCEPHALY AND ANOTHER DIED AT 10 MONTHS WITH CONGENITAL HEART DISEASE AND MICROCEPHALY.

STRONG, W. B.* FAMILIAL SYNDROME OF RIGHT-SIDED AORTIC ARCH, MENTAL DEFICIENCY, AND FACIAL DYSMORPHISM. J. PEDIAT. 73* 882-888, 1968.

*10760 APLASIA CUTIS CONGENITA

THE MODE OF INHERITANCE IS NOT CLEAR. PARENT AND CHILD WERE AFFECTED IN AT LEAST THREE FAMILIES AND SIBS AND COUSINS IN OTHERS (HODGMAN ET AL., 1965). A DEFECT IN THE SCALP AND UNDERLYING CALVARIUM CHARACTERIZES THIS CONDITION. PAP (1970) DESCRIBED A DEFECT OF THE SCALP AND SKULL IN FOUR PERSONS IN THREE GENERATIONS. ONLY THE SKIN WAS INVOLVED IN THE AFFECTED PERSONS IN 3 GENERATIONS OF THE FAMILY REPORTED BY TISSERAND-PERRIER (1953). DEEKEN AND CAPLAN (1970) FOUND APLASIA CUTIS CONGENITA OF THE MIDLINE OCCIPITAL SCALP IN A FATHER AND TWO SONS, WHO HAD TWO REPORTEDLY AFFECTED COLLATERAL RELATIVES. THEIR SERIES ALSO CONTAINED TWO PAIRS OF AFFECTED SIBS. CUTLIP ET AL. (1967) DESCRIBED MOTHER AND CHILD.

CUTLIP, B. D., JR., CRYAN, D. M. AND VINEYARD, W. R.* CONGENITAL SCALP DEFECTS IN MOTHER AND CHILD. AM. J. DIS. CHILD. 113* 597-599, 1967.

HODGMAN, J. E., MATHIES, A. W., JR. AND LEVAN, N. E.* CONGENITAL SCALP DEFECTS IN TWIN SISTERS. AM. J. DIS. CHILD. 110* 293-295, 1965.

JOHNSONBAUGH, R. E., LIGHT, I. J. AND SUTHERLAND, J. M.* CONGENITAL SCALP DEFECTS IN FATHER AND SON. AM. J. DIS. CHILD. 110* 297-298, 1965.

LYNCH, P. J. AND KAHN, E. A.* CONGENITAL DEFECTS OF THE SCALP. A SURGICAL APPROACH TO APLASIA CUTIS CONGENITA. J. NEUROSURG. 33* 198-202, 1970.

PAP, G. S.* CONGENITAL DEFECT OF SCALP AND SKULL IN THREE GENERATIONS OF ONE FAMILY* CASE REPORT. PLAST. RECONSTR. SURG. 46* 194-196, 1970.

TISSERAND-PERRIER, M.* TRANSMISSION PENDENT PLUSIEURS GENERATIONS D'UNE APLASIE CUTANEE CIRCONSCRITE DU VERTEX. BULL. SOC. FRANC. DERM. SYPH. 60* 77-78, 1953.

10770 APPENDICITIS, PRONENESS TO

BAKER (1937) AND OTHERS HAVE REPORTED FAMILIES WITH NUMEROUS PERSONS WITH APPENDICITIS IN A PATTERN CONSISTENT WITH DOMINANT INHERITANCE WITH IRREGULAR PENETRANCE.

BAKER, E. G. S.* A FAMILY PEDIGREE FOR APPENDICITIS. J. HERED. 28* 187-191, 1937.

10780 ARCUS CORNEAE (ARCUS SENILIS)

ALTHOUGH ARCUS MAY BE A MANIFESTATION OF A DISORDER OF LIPID METABOLISM, IT IS LIKELY THAT THIS IS BY NO MEANS ALWAYS THE CASE. MACARAEG ET AL. (1968) SHOWED THAT ARCUS CORNEAE OCCURS IN HIGHER FREQUENCY IN NEGROES THAN IN WHITES AND DEVELOPS AT AN EARLIER AGE. THEY COULD NOT RELATE IT TO DIASTOLIC HYPERTENSION, MYOCARDIAL INFARCTION OR CEREBROVASCULAR ACCIDENTS. ARCUS CORNEAE DEVELOPS PRECOCIOUSLY IN TANGIER DISEASE, NORUM'S DISEASE AND IN HOMOZYGOTES FOR TYPE II HYPERLIPOPROTEINEMIA.

AHUJA, Y. R.* L'HEREDITE DE L'ARCUS CORNEAE. J. GENET. HUM. 8* 95-107, 1959.

MACARAEG, P. V. J., JR., LASAGNA, L. AND SNYDER, B.* ARCUS NOT SO SENILIS. ANN. INTERN. MED. 68* 345-354, 1968.

10790 ARMS, MALFORMATION OF

TWELVE CASES OF SHORT, ABSENT OR PARTIALLY FUSED RADIUS AND ULNA AND ABNORMALITIES OF THE DIGITS WERE FOUND IN 3 GENERATIONS BY STILES AND DOUGAN (1940).

STILES, K. A. AND DOUGAN, P.* A PEDIGREE OF MALFORMED UPPER EXTREMITIES SHOWING VARIABLE DOMINANCE. J. HERED. 31* 65-72, 1940.

10800 ARTERIES, ANOMALIES OF

GATES (1946) CITED A FAMILY IN WHICH THE GRANDFATHER SHOWED BILATERALLY A RADIAL ARTERY WHICH PASSED OVER THE SUPINATOR LONGUS MUSCLE 3-4 CM. ABOVE THE WRIST AND RAN OVER THE RADIAL EXTENSORS ABOVE THE STYLOID PROCESS. ALL HIS CHILDREN WERE SAID TO HAVE THE SAME ANOMALY ON THE LEFT SIDE. AMONG HIS GRANDCHILDREN THE ANOMALY WAS FOUND ON BOTH SIDES IN 4, ONE SIDE IN 4 AND NEITHER SIDE IN SEVEN. BARBOSA SUEIRO (1933-34) DESCRIBED THE CASE OF A MAN IN WHOM THE SUPERFICIAL CUBITAL (ULNAR) ARTERY ON THE LEFT ARM RAN ALONG THE MEDIAL BORDER OF THE BICEPS, ARISING BY PRECOCIOUS BIFURCATION OF THE BRANCHIAL ARTERY. THERE WAS ALSO A SUPERFICIAL RIGHT INTEROSSEOUS ARTERY. THE LATTER CONDITION WAS PRESENT ALSO IN THE FATHER AND A BROTHER AND THE FORMER CONDITION IN THE TWO BROTHERS.

BARBOSA SUEIRO, M. B.* OBSERVATION DE QUELQUES ARTERES AVEC SON TRAJET SUPERFICIEL ANORMAL CHEZ QUELQUES MEMBRES D'UNE FAMILLE. ARQ. ANAT. ANTHROP. 16* 163-164, 1933-34.

GATES, R. R.* HUMAN GENETICS. NEW YORK* MACMILLAN, 1946. P. 1304.

10810 ARTHRITIS, SACRO-ILIAC

THERE IS INADEQUATE INFORMATION PROVIDED IN THE REPORT OF STAUFFER AND MERRIHEW (1944) TO BE CERTAIN AS TO THE NATURE OF THE AILMENT REFERRED TO BY THIS DESIGNA-TION. 22 PERSONS IN 4 GENERATIONS WERE SAID TO BE AFFECTED.

STAUFFER, J. AND MERRIHEW, N. H.* A PEDIGREE OF SACRO-ILIAC ARTHRITIS. J. HERED. 35* 112-118, 1944.

10820 ARTHROGRYPOSIS-LIKE HAND ANOMALY AND SENSORI-NEURAL DEAFNESS

STEWART AND BERGSTROM (1971) DESCRIBED A "NEW" SYNDROME OF ARTHROGRYPOSIS-LIKE HAND ANOMALY AND SENSORI-NEURAL DEAFNESS. BOTH FEATURES OF THE SYNDROME VARIED WIDELY IN SEVERITY. TWO MEMBERS OF THE MOST RECENT GENERATION HAD ONLY THE HAND ANOMALY.

STEWART, J. M. AND BERGSTROM, L.* FAMILIAL HAND ABNORMALITY AND SENSORINEURAL DEAFNESS* A NEW SYNDROME. J. PEDIAT. 78* 102-110, 1971.

STICKLER ET AL. (1965) FROM A LONG EXPERIENCE AT THE MAYO CLINIC WITH MULTIPLE
MEMBERS OF A KINDRED DESCRIBED A NEW DOMINANT ENTITY CONSISTING OF PROGRESSIVE
MYOPIA BEGINNING IN THE FIRST DECADE OF LIFE AND RESULTING IN RETINAL DETACHMENT
AND BLINDNESS. AFFECTED PERSONS ALSO EXHIBITED PREMATURE DEGENERATIVE CHANGES IN
VARIOUS JOINTS WITH ABNORMAL EPIPHYSEAL DEVELOPMENT AND SLIGHT HYPERMOBILITY IN
SOME. IN A SECOND PAPER STICKLER AND PUGH (1967) POINTED OUT THAT THE FAMILY
REPORTED BY DAVID (1953) PROBABLY HAD THE SAME CONDITION. CHANGES IN VERTEBRAE
AND HEARING DEFICIT WERE ALSO NOTED.

DAVID, B.* UBER EINEN DOMINANTEN ERBGANG BEI EINER POLYTOPEN ENCHONDRALEN
DYSOSTOSE TYP PFANDLER-HURLER. Z. ORTHOP. 84* 657-660, 1953.

STICKLER, G. B. AND PUGH, D. G.* HEREDITARY PROGRESSIVE ARTHRO-OPHTHALMOPATHY
II. ADDITIONAL OBSERVATIONS ON VERTEBRAL ABNORMALITIES, A HEARING DEFECT, AND A
REPORT OF A SIMILAR CASE. MAYO CLIN. PROC. 42* 495-500, 1967.

STICKLER, G. B., BELAU, P. G., FARRELL, F. J., JONES, J. D., PUGH, D. G.,
STEINBERG, A. G. AND WARD, L. E.* HEREDITARY PROGRESSIVE ARTHRO-OPHTHALMOPATHY.
MAYO CLIN. PROC. 40* 433-455, 1965.

10840 ASPARAGUS, URINARY EXCRETION OF ODORIFEROUS COMPONENT OF

THE ODORIFEROUS COMPONENT SEEMS TO BE METHANETHIOL. FORTY-SIX OF 115 PERSONS WERE
EXCRETORS IN THE EXPERIENCE OF ALLISON AND MCWHIRTER (1956). THEY SUGGESTED,
FURTHERMORE, THAT 'EXCRETOR' IS DOMINANT TO 'NON-EXCRETOR.'

ALLISON, A. C. AND MCWHIRTER, K. G.* TWO UNIFACTORIAL CHARACTERS FOR WHICH MAN
IS POLYMORPHIC. NATURE 178* 748-749, 1956.

*10850 ATAXIA, PERIODIC VESTIBULO-CEREBELLAR

IN 16 MEMBERS OF A WHITE, RURAL NORTH CAROLINA FAMILY, FARMER AND MUSTIAN (1963)
DESCRIBED RECURRENT ATTACKS OF VERTIGO, DIPLOPIA AND ATAXIA BEGINNING IN EARLY
ADULTHOOD. SLOWLY PROGRESSIVE CEREBELLAR ATAXIA OCCURRED IN SOME. HILL AND
SHERMAN (1968) DESCRIBED EPISODIC CEREBELLAR ATAXIA OCCURRING PARTICULARLY IN
CHILDREN, WITH AMELIORATION IN LATER LIFE AND NO PERMANENT OR PROGRESSIVE
CEREBELLAR ABNORMALITIES. A LARGE KINDRED WITH AUTOSOMAL DOMINANT INHERITANCE
PATTERN WAS PRESENTED. THE CONDITION DESCRIBED BY FARMER AND MUSTIAN (1963) WAS
FOLLOWED BY PROGRESSIVE CEREBELLAR DEGENERATION AND MAY BE DIFFERENT. THE SAME
DISORDER MAY HAVE BEEN PRESENT IN THE FAMILIES REPORTED BY HILL AND SHERMAN (1968)
AND BY WHITE (1969).

FARMER, T. W. AND MUSTIAN, V. M.* VESTIBULO-CEREBELLAR ATAXIA. A NEWLY DEFINED
HEREDITARY SYNDROME WITH PERIODIC MANIFESTATIONS. ARCH. NEUROL. 8* 471-480, 1963.

HILL, W. AND SHERMAN, H.* ACUTE INTERMITTENT FAMILIAL CEREBELLAR ATAXIA. ARCH.
NEUROL. 18* 350-357, 1968.

WHITE, J. C.* FAMILIAL PERIODIC NYSTAGMUS, VERTIGO AND ATAXIA. ARCH. NEUROL.
20* 276-280, 1969.

*10860 ATAXIA, SPASTIC

IN AN IRANIAN FAMILY MAHLOUDJI (1963) DESCRIBED A RARE HEREDITARY SYNDROME OF
SPASTIC ATAXIA CLOSELY RESEMBLING DISSEMINATED SCLEROSIS IN 18 PERSONS. THE
PEDIGREE, COVERING FIVE GENERATIONS, STRONGLY SUGGESTS TRANSMISSION AS AN
AUTOSOMAL DOMINANT. IT APPEARS TO BE THE SAME DISORDER AS WAS REPORTED BY
FERGUSON AND CRITCHLEY (1929).

FERGUSON, F. R. AND CRITCHLEY, M.* A CLINICAL STUDY OF AN HEREDO-FAMILIAL
DISEASE RESEMBLING DISSEMINATED SCLEROSIS. BRAIN 52* 203-225, 1929.

MAHLOUDJI, M.* HEREDITARY SPASTIC ATAXIA SIMULATING DISSEMINATED SCLEROSIS. J.
NEUROL. NEUROSURG. PSYCHIAT. 26* 511-513, 1963.

10870 ATAXIA, WITH FASCICULATIONS

SINGH AND SHAM (1964) DESCRIBED AUTOSOMAL DOMINANT INHERITANCE OF PROGRESSIVE
ATAXIA ASSOCIATED WITH PERSISTENT FASCICULATIONS OF THE MUSCLES OF THE LIMBS.
MEMBERS OF FOUR SIBSHIPS IN THREE GENERATIONS WERE AFFECTED.

SINGH, H. AND SHAM, R.* HEREDOFAMILIAL ATAXIA WITH MUSCLE FASCICULATIONS (A
REPORT OF TWO CASES IN BROTHERS). BRIT. J. CLIN. PRACT. 18* 91-92, 1964.

10880 ATRIAL SEPTAL DEFECT

THIS CONGENITAL HEART DEFECT IS ONE WHICH IS ALMOST ALWAYS SPORADIC. YET
OCCASIONAL FAMILIES IN WHICH MULTIPLE PERSONS HAVE ISOLATED ASD SUGGEST THAT A
SINGLE 'MAJOR' GENE MAY SOMETIMES BE RESPONSIBLE. THE FAMILY REPORTED BY
ZUCKERMAN ET AL. (1962) SUGGESTS DOMINANT INHERITANCE. ZETTERQVIST (1960)

REPORTED A FAMILY WITH 8 PROVED AND 5 PROBABLE CASES OF ASD OF SECUNDUM TYPE IN 3 GENERATIONS. JOHANSSON AND SIEVERS (1967) FOUND 6 PROVED AND 1 PROBABLE CASE OF ASD IN 3 GENERATIONS. FURTHERMORE, THEY WERE ABLE TO SHOW THAT ZETTERQVIST'S CASES AND THEIRS TRACED THEIR ANCESTRY TO A COMMON ANCESTRAL COUPLE WHO LIVED IN THE 18TH CENTURY.

JOHANSSON, B. W. AND SIEVERS, J.* INHERITANCE OF ATRIAL SEPTAL DEFECT. (LETTER) LANCET 1* 1224-1225, 1967.

ZETTERQVIST, P.* MULTIPLE OCCURRENCE OF ATRIAL SEPTAL DEFECT IN A FAMILY. ACTA PAEDIAT. 49* 741-747, 1960.

ZUCKERMAN, H. S., ZUCKERMAN, G. H., MAMMEN, R. E. AND WASSERMIL, M.* ATRIAL SEPTAL DEFECT. FAMILIAL OCCURRENCE IN FOUR GENERATIONS OF ONE FAMILY. AM. J. CARDIOL. 9* 515-520, 1962.

*10890 ATRIAL SEPTAL DEFECT WITH ATRIO-VENTRICULAR CONDUCTION DEFECTS

AMARASINGHAM AND FLEMING (1967) AND KAHLER ET AL. (1966) REPORTED A TOTAL OF 3 FAMILIES WITH THIS COMBINATION. BECAUSE OF THE RARITY OF CONDUCTION DEFECTS WITH ATRIAL SEPTAL DEFECTS OF THE SECUNDUM TYPE, THIS MAY BE A SPECIFIC MENDELIZING FORM OF ATRIAL SEPTAL DEFECT. BIZARRO ET AL. (1970) REFERRED TO THE FORM OF ATRIAL SEPTAL DEFECT AS FOSSA OVALIS TYPE (A SYNONYM FOR SECUNDUM TYPE). THEY DEMONSTRATED MALE-TO-MALE TRANSMISSION. THE FAMILY OF WEIL AND ALLENSTEIN (1961) PROBABLY REPRESENTED AN EXAMPLE OF THIS SYNDROME.

AMARASINGHAM, R. AND FLEMING, H. A.* CONGENITAL HEART DISEASE WITH ARRHYTHMIA IN A FAMILY. BRIT. HEART J. 29* 78-82, 1967.

BIZARRO, R. O., CALLAHAN, J. A., FELDT, R. H., KURLAND, L. T., GORDON, H. AND BRANDENBURG, R. O.* FAMILIAL ATRIAL SEPTAL DEFECT WITH PROLONGED ATRIOVENTRICULAR CONDUCTION* A SYNDROME SHOWING THE AUTOSOMAL DOMINANT PATTERN OF INHERITANCE. CIRCULATION 41* 677-684, 1970.

KAHLER, R. L., BRAUNWALD, E., PLAUTH, W. H., JR. AND MORROW, A. G.* FAMILIAL CONGENITAL HEART DISEASE. FAMILIAL OCCURRENCE OF ATRIAL SEPTAL DEFECT WITH A-V CONDUCTION ABNORMALITIES, SUPRAVALVULAR AORTIC AND PULMONIC STENOSIS, AND VENTRICULAR SEPTAL DEFECT. AM. J. MED. 40* 384-399, 1966.

WEIL, M. H. AND ALLENSTEIN, B. J.* A REPORT OF CONGENITAL HEART DISEASE IN FIVE MEMBERS OF ONE FAMILY. NEW ENG. J. MED. 265* 661-667, 1961.

*10900 AURICULO-OSTEODYSPLASIA

BEALS (1967) GAVE THIS DESIGNATION TO A SYNDROME WHICH HE OBSERVED IN MANY MEMBERS OF TWO FAMILIES. MULTIPLE OSSEOUS DYSPLASIA, CHARACTERISTIC EAR SHAPE, AND SOMEWHAT SHORT STATURE WERE FEATURES. DYSPLASIA OF THE RADIOCAPITELLAR JOINT, WITH OR WITHOUT RADIAL-HEAD DISLOCATION, WAS A CONSTANT FINDING. INHERITANCE WAS UNEQUIVOCALLY AUTOSOMAL DOMINANT.

BEALS, R. K.* AURICULO-OSTEODYSPLASIA. A SYNDROME OF MULTIPLE OSSEOUS DYSPLASIA, EAR ANOMALY, AND SHORT STATURE. J. BONE JOINT SURG. 49A* 1541-1550, 1967.

10910 AUTOIMMUNE DISEASES

IN MANY OF THE DISORDERS IN WHICH AUTOIMMUNITY HAS BEEN INCRIMINATED, OR AT LEAST ACCUSED, AS A LEADING ETIOLOGIC FACTOR, FAMILIAL AGGREGATION IS OBSERVED. THE GENETIC SIGNIFICANCE OF THIS IS UNCLEAR. IT IS POSSIBLE THAT IF MATERNAL ANTITHYROID ANTIBODIES ARE RESPONSIBLE FOR ATHYREOTIC CRETINISM, THEN MULTIPLE SIBS MIGHT BE AFFECTED BY THIS CONGENITAL ANOMALY WITHOUT ANY GENETIC BASIS. REPORTS ON THE AGGREGATION OF POSSIBLE ANTOIMMUNE DISORDERS INCLUDE THE FOLLOWING* GREENBERG (1964) DESCRIBED TWO SISTERS WITH MYASTHENIA GRAVIS AND THYROTOXICOSIS AND A THIRD SISTER WITH HASHIMOTO'S STRUMA. SEE THYROID AUTOANTIBODIES. SEE ALOPECIA AREATA. SEE PERNICIOUS ANEMIA. SEE HYPOADRENOCORTICISM WITH HYPOPARA-THYROIDISM AND SUPERFICIAL MONILIASIS. SEE SCHMID'S SYNDROME. PIROFSKY (1968) FOUND THAT 20 PERCENT OF 44 PATIENTS WITH IDIOPATHIC AUTOIMMUNE HEMOLYTIC ANEMIA HAD CLOSE RELATIVES WITH CLINICALLY DETECTABLE AUTOIMMUNE DISEASE.

GREENBERG, J.* MYASTHENIA GRAVIS AND HYPERTHYROIDISM IN TWO SISTERS. ARCH. NEUROL. 11* 219-222, 1964.

PIROFSKY, B.* HEREDITARY ASPECTS OF AUTOIMMUNE HEMOLYTIC ANEMIA* A RETROSPEC-TIVE ANALYSIS. VOX SANG. 14* 334-347, 1968.

*10920 BALDNESS

EARLY BALDNESS OF THE ORDINARY TYPE HAS BEEN THOUGHT TO BE AUTOSOMAL DOMINANT IN MALES AND TO BE AUTOSOMAL RECESSIVE IN FEMALES WHO TRANSMIT THE TRAIT IF HETEROZY-GOUS BUT ARE BALD ONLY IF HOMOZYGOUS (OSBORN, 1916* SNYDER AND YINGLING, 1935). THE TRANSMISSION THROUGH MANY SUCCESSIVE GENERATIONS AS IN THE DESCENDANTS OF PRESIDENT JOHN ADAMS SUGGESTS THE OPERATION OF A SINGLE MAJOR GENE.

OSBORNE, D.* INHERITANCE OF BALDNESS. VARIOUS PATTERNS DUE TO HEREDITY AND SOMETIMES PRESENT AT BIRTH - A SEX-LIMITED CHARACTER-DOMINANT IN MAN - WOMEN NOT BALD UNLESS THEY INHERIT TENDANCY FROM BOTH PARENTS. J. HERED. 7* 347-355, 1916.

SNYDER, L. H. AND YINGLING, H. C.* THE APPLICATION OF THE GENE-FREQUENCY METHOD OF ANALYSIS TO SEX-INFLUENCED FACTORS, WITH SPECIAL REFERENCE TO BALDNESS. HUM. BIOL. 7* 608-615, 1935.

10930 BANKI SYNDROME

BANKI (1965) DESCRIBED A HUNGARIAN FAMILY IN WHICH MEMBERS OF 3 GENERATIONS SHOWED FUSION OF THE LUNATE AND CUNEIFORM BONES OF THE WRIST, CLINODACTYLY, CLINOMETACAR-PY, BRACHYMETACARPY AND LEPTOMETACARPY (THIN DIAPHYSIS). IT APPEARS TO REPRESENT A UNIQUE DOMINANT MUTATION.

BANKI, Z.* KOMBINATION ERBLICHER GELENK- UND KNOCHENANOMALIEN AN DER HAND. ZWEI NEUE RONTGENZEICHEN. FORTSCHR. ROENTGENSTR. 103* 598-604, 1965.

*10940 BASAL CELL NEVUS SYNDROME (MULTIPLE BASAL CELL NEVI, ODONTOGENIC KERATOCYSTS AND SKELETAL ANOMALIES)

GORLIN AND GOLTZ (1960) SUGGESTED AUTOSOMAL DOMINANT INHERITANCE WHICH NOW SEEMS WELL ESTABLISHED. (MEERKOTTER AND SHEAR (1964) FAVORED RECESSIVE INHERITANCE. IN THE FAMILY THEY DESCRIBED BOTH PARENTS WERE NORMAL BUT WERE RELATED AS SECOND COUSINS. OF SIX CHILDREN, ONE (THE PROBAND) WAS TYPICALLY AFFECTED, ONE DIED AT 6 WEEKS FOLLOWING AN EPILEPTIC SEIZURE AND ONE DIED AT TWO YEARS OF MEDULLOBLAS-TOMA.) HERZBERG AND WISKEMANN (1963) DESCRIBED WHAT THEY SUGGESTED MAY BE CONSIDERED THE 'FIFTH PHACOMATOSIS,' BASAL CELL NEVUS WITH MEDULLOBLASTOMA. A FATHER AND SON HAD BASAL CELL NEVUS. THE SON HAD MEDULLOBLASTOMA AND CONGENITAL THORACIC SCOLIOSIS. ONE OF CAWSON AND KERR'S PATIENTS (1964) HAD ASTROCYTOMA WITH SEVERE HYDROCEPHALUS. THE PALMS AND SOLES MAY SHOW PITS. BLOCK AND CLENDENNING (1963) DESCRIBED REDUCED RESPONSIVENESS TO PARATHORMONE. OTHER CLINICAL FEATURES INCLUDE MILD MANDIBULAR PROGNATHISM, LATERAL DISPLACEMENT OF THE INNER CANTHI, FRONTAL AND BIPARIETAL BOSSING, JAW CYSTS, KYPHOSCOLIOSIS, FUSED RIBS, IMPERFECT SEGMENTATION OF CERVICAL VERTEBRAE, CHARACTERISTIC LAMELLAR CALCIFICATION OF THE FALX CEREBRI, OVARIAN FIBROMATA AND LYMPHOMESENTERIC CYSTS WHICH TEND TO CALCIFY, SHORT 4TH AND-OR 5TH METACARPAL. THE BASAL CELL NEVI OCCUR IN ENORMOUS NUMBERS. SOME MAY RESEMBLE SEBORRHEIC KERATOSES. SUICIDE IS RATHER FREQUENT IN THESE UNFORTUNATE PATIENTS. LIP AND-OR PALATAL CLEFTS PROBABLY OCCUR WITH INCREASED FREQUENCY. THE BASAL CELL NEVUS SYNDROME IS ONE OF THE CONDITIONS WHICH IS ACCOMPANIED BY SHORT FOURTH METACARPAL. LILE ET AL. (1968) OBSERVED FOUR CASES IN 3 GENERATIONS. IN TWO OF THESE PATIENTS THE TERMINAL PHALANX OF THE THUMB WAS SHORT. BANG (1970) DESCRIBED AN 18 YEAR OLD PATIENT WITH KERATOCYSTS OF THE JAW, SKELETAL ANOMALIES (BIFID RIBS, BROAD NASAL ROOT, SPINA BIFIDA AT T12, ETC.), UNRESPONSIVENESS TO PARATHYROID HORMONE AND POSSIBLY INCREASED PLASMA CALCITONIN LEVEL. HOWEVER, NO BASAL CELL CARCINOMAS WERE PRESENT. THE MAN AND SEVERAL RELATIVES HAD ICHTHYOSIS. OVARIAN CARCINOMA HAS BEEN OBSERVED (BERLIN ET AL., 1966).

ANDERSON, D. E. AND COOK, W. A.* JAW CYSTS AND BASAL CELL NEVUS SYNDROME. J. ORAL SURG. 24* 15-26, 1966.

ANDERSON, D. E., TAYLOR, W. B., FALLS, H. F. AND DAVIDSON, R. T.* THE NEVOID BASAL CELL CARCINOMA SYNDROME. AM. J. HUM. GENET. 19* 12-22, 1967.

BANG, G.* KERATOCYSTS, SKELETAL ANOMALIES, ICHTHYOSIS, AND DEFECTIVE RESPONSE TO PARATHYROID HORMONE IN A PATIENT WITHOUT BASAL-CELL CARCINOMA. ORAL SURG. 29* 242-248, 1970.

BERLIN, N. I., VAN SCOTT, E. J., CLENDENNING, W. E., ARCHARD, H. O., BLOCK, J. B., WITKOP, C. J. AND HAYNES, H. A.* BASAL CELL NEVUS SYNDROME. ANN. INTERN. MED. 64* 403-421, 1966.

BLOCK, J. B. AND CLENDENNING, W. E.* PARATHYROID HORMONE HYPORESPONSIVENESS IN PATIENTS WITH BASAL-CELL NEVI AND BONE DEFECTS. NEW ENG. J. MED. 268* 1157-1162, 1963.

CAWSON, R. A. AND KERR, G. A.* THE SYNDROME OF JAW CYSTS, BASAL CELL TUMOURS AND SKELETAL ANOMALIES. PROC. ROY. SOC. MED. 57* 799-801, 1964.

GORLIN, R. J. AND GOLTZ, R. W.* MULTIPLE NEVOID BASAL-CELL EPITHELIOMA, JAW CYSTS AND BIFID RIB* A SYNDROME. NEW ENG. J. MED. 262* 908-912, 1960.

GORLIN, R. J. AND PINDBORG, J. J.* MULTIPLE BASAL NEVI, ODONTOGENIC KERATOCYSTS AND SKELETAL ANOMALIES. SYNDROMES OF THE HEAD AND NECK. NEW YORK* BLAKISTON DIVISION, MCGRAW-HILL, 1964. PP. 400-409.

GORLIN, R. J., YUNIS, J. J. AND TUNA, N.* MULTIPLE NEVOID BASAL CELL CARCINOMA, ODONTOGENIC KERATOCYSTS AND SKELETAL ANOMALIES* A SYNDROME. ACTA DERMATOVENER. 43* 39-55, 1963.

HERZBERG, J. J. AND WISKEMANN, A.* DIE FUNFTE PHAKOMATOSE. BASALZELLNAEVUS MIT

FAMILARER BELASTUNG UND MEDULLOBLASTOM. DERMATOLOGICA 126* 106-123, 1963.

HOWELL, J. B. AND MEHREGAN, A. H.* PURSUIT OF THE PITS IN THE NEVOID BASAL CELL CARCINOMA SYNDROME. ARCH. DERM. 102* 586-597, 1970.

LILE, H. A., ROGERS, J. F. AND GERALD, B.* THE BASAL CELL NEVUS SYNDROME. AM. J. ROENTGEN. 103* 214-217, 1968.

MEERKOTTER, V. A. AND SHEAR, M.* MULTIPLE PRIMORDIAL CYSTS ASSOCIATED WITH BIFID RIB AND OCULAR DEFECTS. ORAL SURG. 18* 498-503, 1964.

POLLARD, J. J. AND NEW, P. F. J.* HEREDITARY CUTANEOMANDIBULAR POLYONCOSIS* A SYNDROME OF MYRIAD BASAL-CELL NEVI OF THE SKIN, MANDIBULAR CYSTS, AND INCONSTANT SKELETAL ANOMALIES. RADIOLOGY 82* 840-849, 1964.

RATER, C. J., SELKE, A. C. AND VAN EPPS, E. F.* BASAL CELL NEVUS SYNDROME. AM. J. ROENTGEN. 103* 589-594, 1968.

10950 BASILAR IMPRESSION, PRIMARY

USING A RADIOLOGIC CRITERION BULL, NIXON AND PRATT (1955) FOUND PRIMARY BASILAR IMPRESSION IN 20 SUBJECTS. OF 39 AVAILABLE RELATIVES 11 ALSO SHOWED BASILAR IMPRESSION. ALTHOUGH FIRST COUSIN PARENTS WERE FOUND IN ONE CASE, IT WAS TENTATIVELY CONCLUDED THAT AUTOSOMAL DOMINANT INHERITANCE IS LIKELY. OF THE 20 PROBANDS, 10 WERE ASYMPTOMATIC, 7 HAD A PREVIOUS DIAGNOSIS OF SYRINGOMYELIA AND 3 HAD SYMPTOMS AND SIGNS EXPLICABLE BY A LOCAL LESION AT THE LEVEL OF THE FORAMEN MAGNUM. BROCHER (1955) DESCRIBED AFFECTED MOTHER AND DAUGHTER. SAX (1970) TELLS ME OF A FAMILY IN WHICH AS MANY AS 9 PERSONS IN FOUR GENERATIONS MAY HAVE BEEN AFFECTED, WITH ONE INSTANCE OF MALE-TO-MALE TRANSMISSION. THE PROBAND, A 32 YEAR OLD MAN, PRESENTED WITH WEAKNESS MAINLY IN THE LEFT ARM AND LEG. HE HAD A SHORT NECK, CRANIOFACIAL ASYMMETRY, LEFT HORNER SYNDROME, DEPRESSED REFLEXES IN THE ARMS, EXAGGERATED REFLEXES IN LEGS, BABINSKI SIGN, KYPHOSCOLIOSIS. CERVICAL MYELOGRAM WAS THOUGHT TO DEMONSTRATE HYDROMYELIA.

BROCHER, J. E. W.* DIE OCCIPITO-CERVICAL-GEGEND. STUTTGART* GEORG THIEME VERLAG, 1955.

BULL, J. W. D., NIXON, W. L. B. AND PRATT, R. T. C.* THE RADIOLOGICAL CRITERIA AND FAMILIAL OCCURRENCE OF PRIMARY BASILAR IMPRESSION. BRAIN 78* 229-247, 1955.

SAX, D. S.* BOSTON, MASS.* PERSONAL COMMUNICATION, 1970.

10960 BEETURIA (BETACYANINURIA)

BEETURIA IS THE URINARY EXCRETION OF BEET PIGMENT (BETACYANIN) AFTER ORAL INGESTION OF BEETS. ALLISON AND MCWHIRTER (1956) SUGGESTED THAT THE TRAIT IS UNIFACTORIAL AND POLYMORPHIC. THEY CONCLUDED THAT *NON-EXCRETOR* IS DOMINANT TO *EXCRETOR.* PENROSE (1957) CHALLENGED THIS IDEA. WATSON, LUKE AND INALL (1963) FOUND BEETURIA IN 14 PERCENT OF PERSONS. HOWEVER, 80 PERCENT OF IRON DEFICIENT SUBJECTS HAVE BEETURIA. THEY SUGGESTED THAT IRON AND BETACYANIN MAY COMPETE FOR AN INTESTINAL MUCOSAL ACCEPTOR SUBSTANCE, PERHAPS APOFERRITIN. THUS, IRON DEFICIENCY INTERFERES WITH THE USEFULNESS OF BEETURIA AS A GENETIC TRAIT. PATIENTS WITH IRON DEFICIENCY HAVE BEETURIA (TUNNESSEN ET AL., 1969).

ALLISON, A. C. AND MCWHIRTER, K. G.* TWO UNIFACTORIAL CHARACTERS FOR WHICH MAN IS POLYMORPHIC. NATURE 178* 748-749, 1956.

PENROSE, L. S.* TWO NEW HUMAN GENES. (LETTER) BRIT. MED. J. 1* 282 ONLY, 1957.

TUNNESSEN, W. W., SMITH, C. AND OSKI, F. A.* BEETURIA. AM. J. DIS. CHILD. 117* 424-426, 1969.

WATSON, W. C., LUKE, R. G. AND INALL, J. A.* BEETURIA* ITS INCIDENCE AND A CLUE TO ITS MECHANISM. BRIT. MED. J. 2* 971-973, 1963.

10970 BIEMOND SYNDROME II

THE FEATURES OF THIS SYNDROME, WHICH RESEMBLES LAURENCE-MOON-BIEDL-BARDET (LMBB) SYNDROME, ARE IRIS COLOBOMA, MENTAL RETARDATION, OBESITY, HYPOGENITALISM AND POSTAXIAL POLYDACTYLY. THE 3 BROTHERS DESCRIBED BY BLUMEL AND KNIKER (1959) AS LMBB MAY HAVE HAD THIS CONDITION. HYDROCEPHALUS AND HYPOSPADIAS WERE ALSO PRESENT. IRREGULAR AUTOSOMAL DOMINANT INHERITANCE IS SUGGESTED BY THE SEGREGATION OF IRIS COLOBOMA FOR FOUR GENERATIONS IN THE FAMILY REPORTED BY GREBE (1953) AND THE OCCURRENCE OF POSTAXIAL POLYDACTYLY OF THE TOES IN THE FATHER AND A PATERNAL AUNT OF THE SIBS DESCRIBED BY BLUMEL AND KNIKER.

BIEMOND, A.* HET SYNDROOM VAN LAURENCE-BIEDL EN EEN AANVERWANT, NIEUW SYNDROOM. NEDERL. T. GENEESK. 78* 1801-1814, 1934.

BLUMEL, J. AND KNIKER, W. T.* LAURENCE-MOON-BARDET-BIEDL SYNDROME. REVIEW OF THE LITERATURE AND A REPORT OF FIVE CASES INCLUDING A FAMILY GROUP WITH THREE AFFECTED MALES. TEXAS REP. BIOL. MED. 17* 391-410, 1959.

10980 BLADDER CANCER

FRAUMENI AND THOMAS (1967) OBSERVED AFFECTED FATHER AND 3 SONS. I HAVE ENCOUN-
TERED TWO INSTANCES OF AFFECTED FATHER AND SON.

FRAUMENI, J. F., JR. AND THOMAS, L. B.* MALIGNANT BLADDER TUMORS IN A FAMILY.
J.A.M.A. 201* 507-509, 1967.

*10990 BLEPHAROCHALASIS AND *DOUBLE LIP* (ASCHER*S SYNDROME)

FRANCESCHETTI (1955) DESCRIBED IT IN FATHER AND DAUGHTER. SAGGING EYELIDS AND
DOUBLE UPPER LIP ARE FEATURES. NONTOXIC GOITER IS A VARIABLE FEATURE.

FINDLAY, G. H.* IDIOPATHIC ENLARGEMENTS OF THE LIPS* CHEILITIS GRANULOMATOSA,
ASCHER*S SYNDROME AND DOUBLE LIP. BRIT. J. DERM. 66* 129-138, 1954.

FRANCESCHETTI, A.* CAS OBSERVE* MANIFESTATION DE BLEPHAROCHALASIS CHEZ LE PERE,
ASSOCIE A DES DOUBLES LEVRES APPARAISSANT EGALEMENT CHEZ SA FILETTE AGEE D*UN
MOIS. J. GENET. HUM. 4* 181-182, 1955.

11000 BLEPHAROCHALASIS, SUPERIOR

THE OUTER PORTION OF THE UPPER LID IS LOOSE-SKINNED AND PENDULOUS. SCHULZE (1965)
TRACED THE CONDITION THROUGH 6 GENERATIONS WITH 11 MALES AND 3 FEMALES AFFECTED.
BISMARCK SHOWED THIS CONDITION. IN MINOR FORM, THIS IS SOMETIMES CALLED THE
NORDIC TYPE OF EYE FOLD. PANNETON (1936) FOUND THE TRAIT IN 51 OF 79 MEMBERS OF A
FRENCH-CANADIAN FAMILY.

PANNETON, P.* LA BLEPHARO-CHALAZIS* A PROPOS DE 51 CAS DANS UNE MEME FAMILLE.
ARCH. OPHTAL. 53* 729-755, 1936.

SCHULZE, F.* BEITRAG ZUR HEREDITAREN BLEPHAROCHALASIS. KLIN. MBL. AUGENHEILK.
147* 863-877, 1965.

*11010 BLEPHAROPHIMOSIS, EPICANTHUS INVERSUS AND PTOSIS

VIGNES (1889) PROBABLY FIRST DESCRIBED THIS ENTITY, A DYSPLASIA OF THE EYELIDS.
IN ADDITION TO SMALL PALPEBRAL FISSURES, EPICANTHUS INVERSUS, LOW NASAL BRIDGE,
AND PTOSIS OF THE EYELIDS ARE FEATURES (SACREZ ET AL., 1963* JOHNSON, 1964* SMITH,
1970). THE CONDITION SHOULD BE CONSIDERED DISTINCT FROM CONGENITAL PTOSIS. SMITH
(1970) DESCRIBED AFFECTED MOTHER AND DAUGHTER. OWENS ET AL. (1960) UPDATED THE
PEDIGREE OF A FAMILY WHICH WAS FIRST REPORTED BY DIMITRY (1921) AND WHICH HAD
AFFECTED MEMBERS IN 6 GENERATIONS. THE PATIENTS HAD THE SYNDROME-TRIAD CONSISTING
OF BLEPHAROPHIMOSIS, PTOSIS AND EPICANTHUS INVERSUS (FOLD CURVING IN THE MEDIOLA-
TERAL DIRECTION, INFERIOR TO THE INNER CANTHUS). I GOT A FIRST HAND DESCRIPTION
OF THE DISORDER FROM A PHYSICIAN (RAVIOTTA, 1971) WHO IS AN AFFECTED MEMBER
(NUMBER 38) OF THE PEDIGREE OF OWENS ET AL. (1960).

DIMITRY, T. J.* HEREDITARY PTOSIS. AM. J. OPHTHAL. 4* 655-658, 1921.

JOHNSON, C. C.* SURGICAL REPAIR OF THE SYNDROME OF EPICANTHUS INVERSUS,
BLEPHAROPHIMOSIS AND PTOSIS. ARCH. OPHTHAL. 71* 510-516, 1964.

OWENS, N., HADLEY, R. C. AND KLOEPFER, H. W.* HEREDITARY BLEPHAROPHIMOSIS,
PTOSIS AND EPICANTHUS INVERSUS. J. INTERN. COLL. SURG. 33* 558-574, 1960.

RAVIOTTA, J. J.* NEW ORLEANS, LA.* PERSONAL COMMUNICATION, 1971.

SACREZ, R., FRANCFORT, J., JUIF, J. G. AND DE GROUCHY, J.* LE BLEPHAROPHIMOSIS
COMPLIQUE FAMILIAL. ETUDE DES MEMBRES DE LA FAMILLE BLE. ANN. PEDIAT. 10* 493-
501, 1963.

SMITH, D. W.* RECOGNIZABLE PATTERNS OF HUMAN MALFORMATION. GENETIC, EMBRYOLO-
GIC, AND CLINICAL ASPECTS. PHILADELPHIA* W. B. SANDERS CO., 1970. PP. 114-115.

VIGNES* EPICANTHUS HEREDITAIRE. REV. GEN. OPTHAL. 8* 438, 1889.

11020 BLOOD GROUP (RED CELL ANTIGEN TYPES)

THE BLOOD GROUPS ARE INHERITED AS CO-DOMINANT TRAITS. EXCEPT FOR THE XG SYSTEM,
ALL ARE AUTOSOMAL. (THE SERUM PROTEIN TYPES ARE ALSO BLOOD GROUPS IN THE BROAD
SENSE OF THE TERM BUT ARE DISCUSSED SEPARATELY.) THE STANDARD REFERENCE ON THE
BLOOD GROUPS IS RACE AND SANGER (1962).

RACE, R. R. AND SANGER, R.* BLOOD GROUPS IN MAN. PHILADELPHIA* F. A. DAVIS
CO., 1968 (5TH ED).

THE FOLLOWING ARE THE MAJOR BLOOD GROUPS SYSTEMS. AT LEAST 14 AUTOSOMAL LOCI ARE
IDENTIFIABLE. IN ADDITION, THERE IS A CONSIDERABLE NUMBER OF PRIVATE SYSTEMS

(ANTIGENIC DETERMINANTS OF LOW FREQUENCY IN THE POPULATION) AND PUBLIC SYSTEMS (ANTIGENIC DETERMINANTS OF HIGH FREQUENCY IN THE POPULATION). SOME OF THESE ARE LISTED LATER. HOW MANY OF THEM REPRESENT LOCI SEPARATE FROM THE 14 OTHERS IS NOT KNOWN. IN ADDITION TO THESE, SECRETOR FACTOR (Q.V.) MIGHT BE CONSIDERED AN *HONORARY BLOOD GROUP* AND THE BOMBAY PHENOTYPE (SEE RECESSIVE CATALOG) INVOLVES BLOOD GROUPS.

*11030 BLOOD GROUP-ABO SYSTEM

THIS IS THE FIRST BLOOD GROUP SYSTEM DISCOVERED, BY LANDSTEINER AT THE BEGINNING OF THIS CENTURY. THE OCCURRENCE OF NATURAL ANTIBODY PERMITTED IDENTIFICATION OF RED CELLS TYPES BY AGGLUTINATION OF RED CELLS WHEN MIXED WITH SERUM FROM SOME BUT NOT ALL OTHER PERSONS. AT FIRST THE ALTERNATIVE GENETIC HYPOTHESES WERE MAINLY (1) MULTIPLE ALLELES AT A SINGLE LOCUS AND (2) TWO LOCI EACH WITH TWO ALLELES, ONE LOCUS DETERMINING A AND NON-A AND THE OTHER B AND NON-B. APPLICATION OF THE HARDY-WEINBERG PRINCIPLE TO POPULATION DATA BY BERNSTEIN AND ANALYSIS OF FAMILY DATA EXCLUDED THE SECOND ALTERNATIVE AND ESTABLISHED THE FORMER.

*11040 BLOOD GROUP-AUBERGER SYSTEM

ALTHOUGH THE ALLELES OF THE AUBERGER SYSTEM HAVE A FREQUENCY WHICH WOULD MAKE IT USEFUL IN LINKAGE STUDIES, THE UNAVAILABILITY OF ANTISERUM EXCLUDES IT FROM THE LIST OF LINKAGE MARKERS.

SALMON, C., SALMON, D., LIBERGE, G., ANDRE, R., TIPPETT, P. AND SANGER, R.* UN NOUVEL ANTIGENE DE GROUPE SANGUIN ERYTHROCYTAIRE PRESENT CHEZ 80 PERCENT DES SUJETS DE RACE BLANCHE. NOUV. REV. FRANC. HEMAT. 1* 649-661, 1961.

*11050 BLOOD GROUP-DIEGO SYSTEM

THE DIEGO SYSTEM SHOWS POLYMORPHISM MAINLY IN MONGOLIAN PEOPLES E.G. CHINESE AND AMERICAN INDIANS.

*11060 BLOOD GROUP-DOMBROCK SYSTEM

ANTI-DO(A) ANTIBODY WAS DETECTED IN A TRANSFUSED PATIENT, MRS. DOMBROCK. ABOUT 64 PER CENT OF NORTHERN EUROPEANS ARE DO(A+), MAKING THE SYSTEM A USEFUL MARKER IN LINKAGE STUDY (SWANSON, POLESKY, TIPPETT AND SANGER, 1965).

POLESKY, H. F. AND SWANSON, J. L.* STUDIES ON DISTRIBUTION OF THE BLOOD GROUP ANTIGEN DO(A) (DOMBROCK) AND THE CHARACTERISTICS OF ANTI-DO(A). TRANSFUSION 6* 268-270, 1966.

SWANSON, J. L., POLESKY, H. F., TIPPETT, P. AND SANGER, R.* A *NEW* BLOOD GROUP ANTIGEN, DO(A). NATURE 206* 313 ONLY, 1965.

TIPPETT, P.* GENETICS OF THE DOMBROCK BLOOD SYSTEM. J. MED. GENET. 4* 7-11, 1967.

WILLIAMS, C. H. AND CRAWFORD, M. N.* THE THIRD EXAMPLE OF ANTI-DO. TRANSFUSION 6* 310 ONLY, 1966.

*11070 BLOOD GROUP-DUFFY SYSTEM. SYMBOLIZED FY(A) AND FY(B)

THE DUFFY SYSTEM ENJOYS THE DISTINCTION OF BEING ONE OF THE FIRST WHOSE GENETIC LOCUS WAS ASSIGNED TO A SPECIFIC CHROMOSOME, I.E., NO. 1 (DONAHUE ET AL., 1968).

CRAWFORD, M. N., PUNNETT, H. H. AND CARPENTER, G. G.* DELETION OF THE LONG ARM OF CHROMOSOME 16 AND AN UNEXPECTED DUFFY BLOOD GROUP PHENOTYPE REVEAL A POSSIBLE AUTOSOMAL LINKAGE. NATURE 215* 1075-1076, 1967.

DONAHUE, R. P., BIAS, W. B., RENWICK, J. H. AND MCKUSICK, V. A.* PROBABLE ASSIGNMENT OF THE DUFFY BLOOD GROUP LOCUS TO CHROMOSOME 1 IN MAN. PROC. NAT. ACAD. SCI. 61* 949-955, 1968.

RITTER, H.* ZUR FORMALEN GENETIK DES DUFFY-SYSTEMS. UNTERSUCHUNG VON 247 FAMILIEN. HUMANGENETIK 4* 59-61, 1967.

*11080 BLOOD GROUP-I SYSTEM

TIPPETT ET AL. (1960) DESCRIBED A BALTIMORE NEGRO FAMILY IN WHICH RED CELLS WERE APPARENTLY OF *LITTLE-I* PHENOTYPE AND THEIR SERUM CONTAINED ANTI-*BIG I.* THIS WAS THE FIRST DIRECT EVIDENCE THAT THE *BIG I* ANTIGEN IS UNDER GENETIC CONTROL. ANTI-*BIG I* HAD BEEN FIRST IDENTIFIED BY WIENER ET AL. (1956). ANTI-*LITTLE I* WAS FIRST RECOGNIZED BY MARSH AND JENKINS (1960), LEADING TO THE *RECIPROCAL RELATIONSHIP HYPOTHESIS* OF MARSH (1961). BINGHAM (1970) CONCLUDED, ON THE BASIS OF THE DEVELOPMENTAL PATTERN OF THE *BIG I* AND *LITTLE I* ANTIGENS, THAT THE CORRESPONDING ANTIBODIES MAY DEFINE TWO INDEPENDENT BLOOD GROUP SYSTEMS. THE MATTER CANNOT BE CONSIDERED RESOLVED.

BINGHAM, C. P.* ANTI-I (*BIG I*) AND ANTI-I (*LITTLE I*) DEFINE TWO INDEPENDENT BLOOD GROUP SYSTEMS. TO BE PUBLISHED, 1971.

MARSH, W. L.* ANTI-I* A COLD ANTIBODY DEFINING THE II ("BIG I - LITTLE I")
RELATIONSHIP IN HUMAN RED CELLS. BRIT. J. HAEMAT. 7* 200-209, 1961.

TIPPETT, P., NOADES, J., SANGER, R., RACE, R. R., SAUSAIS, L., HOLMAN, C. A.
AND BUTTIMER, R. J.* FURTHER STUDIES OF THE I ANTIGEN AND ANTIBODY. VOX SANG. 5*
107-121, 1960.

*11090 BLOOD GROUP-KELL-CELLANO SYSTEM. SYMBOLIZED K (CAP) AND K (SMALL)

*11100 BLOOD GROUP-KIDD SYSTEM. SYMBOLIZED JK

*11110 BLOOD GROUP-LEWIS SYSTEM

THE LEWIS SYSTEM INVOLVES GENETICALLY VARIABLE ANTIGENS IN THE BODY FLUIDS AND
ONLY SECONDARILY ARE THE ANTIGENS ADSORBED TO RED CELLS. GROLLMAN ET AL. (1969)
SHOWED THAT LEWIS NEGATIVE WOMEN LACK A SPECIFIC FUCOSYLTRANSFERASE WHICH IS
PRESENT IN THE MILK OF LEWIS POSITIVE WOMEN. THE ENZYME IS APPARENTLY REQUIRED
FOR SYNTHESIS OF THE STRUCTURAL DETERMINANTS OF BOTH LEWIS (A) AND LEWIS (B)
SPECIFICITY. THE SAME ENZYME IS INVOLVED IN THE SYNTHESIS OF MILK OLIGOSAC-
CHARIDES, BECAUSE TWO OLIGOSACCHARIDES CONTAINING THE RELEVANT LINKAGE WERE ABSENT
FROM THE MILK OF LEWIS NEGATIVE WOMEN.

GROLLMAN, E. F., KOBATA, A. AND GINSBURG, V.* AN ENZYMATIC BASIS FOR LEWIS
BLOOD TYPES IN MAN. J. CLIN. INVEST. 48* 1489-1494, 1969.

*11120 BLOOD GROUP-LUTHERAN SYSTEM

LUTHERAN AND SECRETOR (Q.V.) ARE LINKED (REVIEW BY COOK, 1965).

COOK, P. J. L.* THE LUTHERAN-SECRETOR RECOMBINATION FRACTION IN MAN* A POSSIBLE
SEX DIFFERENCE. ANN. HUM. GENET. 28* 393-401, 1965.

*11130 BLOOD GROUP-MNS SYSTEM

ON THE BASIS OF STUDIES IN THE FAMILY OF A CHILD WITH A TRANSLOCATION CHROMOSOME,
GERMAN ET AL. (1968) SUGGESTED THAT THE MN LOCUS IS EITHER IN THE MIDDLE OF
CHROMOSOME NO. 2 OR NEAR THE DISTAL END OF THE LONG ARM OF CHROMOSOME NO. 4.

GERMAN, J., WALKER, M. E., STIEFEL, F. H. AND ALLEN, F. H., JR.* MN BLOOD-GROUP
LOCUS* DATA CONCERNING THE POSSIBLE CHROMOSOMAL LOCATION. SCIENCE 162* 1014-1015,
1968.

*11140 BLOOD GROUP-P SYSTEM

11150 BLOOD GROUP-PRIVATE SYSTEMS (ANTIGENIC DETERMINANTS OF LOW FREQUENCY IN THE
POPULATION)

MANY OF THESE HAVE BEEN FOUND ONLY IN A SINGLE FAMILY. THEY INCLUDE LEVAY,
JOBBINS, BECKER, VEN, CAVALIERE, BERRENS, WRIGHT, BATTY, ROMUNDE, CHR, SWANN,
GOOD, BI, TR, WEBB (WB). THE RELATION IF ANY, OF EACH TO THE MAJOR SYSTEMS LISTED
EARLIER IS NOT KNOWN, MAINLY BECAUSE THE ONE OR FEW FAMILIES IN WHICH THEY HAVE
BEEN FOUND DO NOT CONTRIBUTE ENOUGH INFORMATION.

11160 BLOOD GROUP-PUBLIC SYSTEMS (ANTIGENIC DETERMINANTS OF HIGH FREQUENCY IN THE
POPULATION)

THESE INCLUDE VEL, YT, GERBICH (GE), LAN, SM. THE RELATION IF ANY, TO EACH TO THE
MAJOR SYSTEMS LISTED EARLIER IS NOT KNOWN. THE I ("EYE") BLOOD GROUP SYSTEM MAY
ALSO BE CONSIDERED A PUBLIC SYSTEM.

*11170 BLOOD GROUP-RHESUS SYSTEM (RH)

*11180 BLOOD GROUP-STOLTZFUS SYSTEM

AN ANTIBODY WHICH TESTS FOR AN ANTIGEN IN A SEEMINGLY "NEW" BLOOD GROUP SYSTEM WAS
FOUND IN THE LANCASTER COUNTY AMISH. IT HAS BEEN DESIGNATED STOLTZFUS, SYMBOLIZED
SF.

BIAS, W. B., LIGHT-ORR, J. K., KREVANS, J. R., HUMPHREY, R. L., HAMILL, P. V.
V., COHEN, B. H. AND MCKUSICK, V. A.* THE STOLTZFUS BLOOD GROUP, A NEW POLYMOR-
PHISM IN MAN. AM. J. HUM. GENET. 21* 552-558, 1969.

11190 BLOOD GROUP-SUTTER (PART OF KELL SYSTEM)

THE KELL-CELLANO SYSTEM ILLUSTRATES NICELY THE MANNER IN WHICH THE UNDERSTANDING
OF SEVERAL OF THE BLOOD GROUP SYSTEMS HAVE DEVELOPED. THE KELL TYPE WAS FIRST
IDENTIFIED USING AN ANTIBODY DEVELOPED BY MRS. KELL THROUGH THE MECHANISM OF
MATERNO-FETAL INCOMPATIBILITY. LATER WHEN MRS. CELLANO WAS FOUND TO HAVE AN
ANTIBODY DEVELOPED BY THE SAME MECHANISM IT WAS DEMONSTRATED THAT THESE ANTIBODIES

WERE TESTING FOR ANTIGENS DETERMINED BY ALLELIC GENES.

MORTON, N. E., KRIEGER, H., STEINBERG, A. G. AND ROSENFIELD, R. E.* GENETIC EVIDENCE CONFIRMING THE LOCALIZATION OF SUTTER IN THE KELL BLOOD-GROUP SYSTEM. VOX SANG. 10* 608-613, 1965.

STROUP, M., MACILROY, M., WALKER, R. AND AYDELOTTE, J. V.* EVIDENCE THAT SUTTER BELONGS TO THE KELL BLOOD GROUP SYSTEM. TRANSFUSION 5* 309-314, 1965.

11200 BLOOD GROUP-UL SYSTEM

IN FINLAND FURUHJELM ET AL. (1968) FOUND AN ANTIBODY WHICH TESTS FOR A PREVIOUSLY UNKNOWN ANTIGEN CALLED UL(A). THE ANTIGEN WAS PRESENT IN 2.6 PERCENT OF HELSINKI DONORS. INDEPENDENCE FROM KELL, YT AND DIEGO SYSTEMS WAS NOT YET PROVED BUT IT WAS INDEPENDENT OF OTHER SYSTEMS. THE UL(A) LOCUS MAY BE WITHIN MEASURABLE DISTANCE OF THE ABO AND ADENYLATE KINASE LOCI.

FURUHJELM, U., NEVANLINNA, H. R., NURKKA, R., GAVIN, J., TIPPETT, P., GOOCH, A. AND SANGER, R.* THE BLOOD GROUP ANTIGEN UL(A) (KARHULA). VOX SANG. 15* 118-124, 1968.

11210 BLOOD GROUP-YT SYSTEM

EATON, B. R., MORTON, J. A., PICKLES, M. M. AND WHITE, K. E.* A NEW ANTIBODY ANTI-YT(A), CHARACTERIZING A BLOOD GROUP ANTIGENE OF HIGH INCIDENCE. BRIT. J. HAEMAT. 2* 333-341, 1956.

*11220 BLUE RUBBER BLEB NEVUS

THIS IS A BLADDER-LIKE VARIETY OF HEMANGIOMA FOUND PARTICULARLY ON THE TRUNK AND UPPER ARMS. NOCTURNAL PAIN AND REGIONAL HYPERHIDROSIS ARE FEATURES. BLEEDING HEMANGIOMAS OF THE GASTROINTESTINAL TRACT ARE AN IMPORTANT COMPLICATION. BERLYNE AND BERLYNE (1960) DEMONSTRATED TRANSMISSION THROUGH FIVE GENERATIONS. OTHER CASES HAVE BEEN SPORADIC, PERHAPS NEW DOMINANT MUTATIONS. FRETZIN AND POTTER (1965) DESCRIBED A PARTICULARLY DRAMATIC CASE WITH INVOLVEMENT OF THE SKIN AND GASTROINTESTINAL TRACT AND ANGIOMATOUS GIGANTISM OF THE RIGHT ARM REQUIRING AMPUTATION IN INFANCY. IN A SINGLE CASE IN A JAPANESE WOMAN, SAKURANE ET AL. (1967) DESCRIBED CAVERNOUS HEMANGIOMAS CHARACTERISTIC OF BLUE RUBBER BLEB NEVI OVER THE ENTIRE SURFACE OF THE BODY AND IN THE MUCOSA OF THE OROPHARYNX, ESOPHA- GUS, DISTAL ILEUM AND ANUS. IN ADDITION THE PATIENT HAD MULTIPLE ENCHONDROMATO- SIS. THIS, THEN, HAD MANY OF THE FEATURES OF MAFFUCCI'S SYNDROME (Q.V.). TWO FAMILIES WITH AFFECTED PERSONS IN 3 AND 5 SUCCESSIVE GENERATIONS, SUPPORTING AUTOSOMAL DOMINANT INHERITANCE, WERE REPORTED BY WALSHE ET AL. (1966).

BERLYNE, G. M. AND BERLYNE, N.* ANAEMIA DUE TO *BLUE-RUBBER-BLEB* NAEVUS DISEASE. LANCET 2* 1275-1277, 1960.

FINE, R. M., DERBES, V. J. AND CLARK, W. H.* BLUE RUBBER BLEB NEVUS. ARCH. DERM. 84* 802-805, 1961.

FRETZIN, D. F. AND POTTER, B.* BLUE RUBBER BLEB NEVUS. ARCH. INTERN. MED. 116* 924-929, 1965.

SAKURANE, H. F., SUGAI, T. AND SAITO, T.* THE ASSOCIATION OF BLUE RUBBER BLEB NEVUS AND MAFFUCCI'S SYNDROME. ARCH. DERM. 95* 28-36, 1967.

TALBOT, S. AND WYATT, E. H.* BLUE RUBBER BLEB NAEVI (REPORT OF A FAMILY IN WHICH ONLY MALES WERE AFFECTED). BRIT. J. DERM. 82* 37-39, 1970.

WALSHE, M. M., EVANS, C. D. AND WARIN, R. P.* BLUE RUBBER BLEB NAEVUS. BRIT. MED. J. 2* 931-932, 1966.

*11230 BOOK'S SYNDROME, OR PHC SYNDROME

IN 1950 BOOK REPORTED 25 AFFECTED PERSONS IN 4 GENERATIONS OF A SWEDISH FAMILY. THE FEATURES ARE PREMOLAR APLASIA (P), HYPERHIDROSIS (H) AND CANITIES PREMATURA (C). INHERITANCE IS CLEARLY AUTOSOMAL DOMINANT WITH HIGH PENETRANCE. NO OTHER FAMILY HAS BEEN REPORTED AND THERE IS NO OTHER REPORT OF THIS PARTICULAR SYNDROMAL ASSOCIATION.

BOOK, J. A.* CLINICAL AND GENETICAL STUDIES OF HYPODONTIA. I. PREMOLAR APLASIA, HYPERHIDROSIS, AND CANITIES PREMATURA. A NEW HEREDITARY SYNDROME IN MAN. AM. J. HUM. GENET. 2* 240-263, 1950.

*11240 BRACHYCAMPTODACTYLY

EDWARDS AND GALE (1970) DESCRIBED A FAMILY WITH 28 PERSONS WITH A UNIQUE FORM OF BRACHYDACTYLY DUE TO A COMBINATION OF SHORT METACARPALS AND METATARSALS AND SHORT MIDDLE PHALANGES COMBINED WITH CAMPTODACTYLY. URINARY INCONTINENCE AND LONGITU- DINAL VAGINAL SEPTUM OCCURRED IN MANY AFFECTED PERSONS. THE MARRIAGE OF AFFECTED COUSINS RESULTED IN TWO PRESUMABLY HOMOZYGOUS CHILDREN WITH SEVERE BRACHYDACTYLY, POLYDACTYLY, SYNDACTYLY, DEAFNESS, MENTAL RETARDATION AND, IN THE ONE OF THEM WHO

EDWARDS, J. A. AND GALE, R. P.* A KINDRED WITH AN UNUSUAL HAND AND FOOT ANOMALY* A NEW AUTOSOMAL DOMINANT TRAIT WITH TWO PROBABLE HOMOZYGOTES. (ABSTRACT) AM. J. HUM. GENET. 22* 18A ONLY, 1970.

*11250 BRACHYDACTYLY, TYPE A1 (FARABEE TYPE)

IN THE CLASSIFICATION OF THE BRACHYDACTYLIES, BELL'S (1951) ANALYSIS HAS PROVED MOST USEFUL. THE TYPE A BRACHYDACTYLIES HAVE THE SHORTENING CONFINED MAINLY TO THE MIDDLE PHALANGES. IN THE A1 TYPE THE MIDDLE PHALANGES OF ALL THE DIGITS ARE RUDIMENTARY OR FUSED WITH THE TERMINAL PHALANGES. THE PROXIMAL PHALANGES OF THE THUMBS AND BIG TOES ARE SHORT. THIS TRAIT HAS THE DISTINCTION OF BEING THE FIRST IN MAN TO BE INTERPRETED IN MENDELIAN DOMINANT TERMS (BY FARABEE IN 1903). HAWS AND MCKUSICK (1963) FOLLOWED UP ON FARABEE'S FAMILY. THE SUBJECTS ARE SHORT OF STATURE.

BELL, J.* ON BRACHYDACTYLY AND SYMPHALANGISM. IN, TREASURY OF HUMAN INHERI-TANCE. LONDON* CAMBRIDGE UNIV. PRESS, 5* 1-31, 1951.

HAWS, D. V. AND MCKUSICK, V. A.* FARABEE'S BRACHYDACTYLOUS KINDRED REVISITED. BULL. HOPKINS HOSP. 113* 20-30, 1963.

*11260 BRACHYDACTYLY, TYPE A2 (BRACHYMESOPHALANGY II, MOHR-WRIEDT TYPE)

SHORTENING OF THE MIDDLE PHALANGES IS CONFINED TO THE INDEX FINGER AND THE SECOND TOE, ALL OTHER DIGITS BEING MORE OF LESS NORMAL. BECAUSE OF A RHOMBOID OR TRIANGULAR SHAPE OF THE AFFECTED MIDDLE PHALANX, THE END OF THE SECOND FINGER USUALLY DEVIATES RADIALLY. THIS RARE FORM OF BRACHYDACTYLY HAS BEEN DESCRIBED ONLY 3 TIMES IN THE LITERATURE. TEMTAMY (1966) ADDED A FOURTH FAMILY, THE FIRST CASES IN NEGROES. MOHR AND WRIEDT'S FAMILY (1919) CONTAINED A POSSIBLE HOMOZY-GOTE.

HANHART, E.* DIE ENTSTEHUNG UND AUSBREITUNG VON MUTATIONEN BEIM MENSCHEN. IN, HANDBUCH DER ERBBIOLOGIE DES MENSCHEN. 1* 288-370, 1940.

MOHR, O. L. AND WRIEDT, C.* A NEW TYPE OF HEREDITARY BRACHYPHALANGY I, MAN. WASHINGTON* CARNEG. INST. (PUBL. 295) 1919. PP. 5-64.

TEMTAMY, S. A.* GENETIC FACTORS IN HAND MALFORMATIONS. PH. D. THESIS, JOHNS HOPKINS UNIVERSITY, 1966.

ZIEGNER, H.* KASUISTISCHER BEITRAG ZU DEN SYMMETRISCHEN MISSBILDUNGEN DER EXTREMITATEN. MUNCHEN. MED. WSCHR. 50* 1386-1387, 1903.

*11270 BRACHYDACTYLY, TYPE A3 (BRACHYMESOPHALANGY V, BRACHYDACTYLY-CLINODACTYLY)

SHORTENING IS LIMITED TO THE MIDDLE PHALANX OF THE FIFTH FINGER. BECAUSE OF RHOMBOID OR TRIANGULAR SHAPE OF THE RUDIMENTARY MIDDLE PHALANX, RADIAL CURVATURE (CLINODACTYLY) OF THE FIFTH FINGER RESULTS. DUTTA (1965) DESCRIBED *SIMPLE RADIAL DEVIATION OF THE DISTAL PHALANX* WITHOUT BONEY DEFORMITY OF THE MIDDLE OR DISTAL PHALANX AND WITH NORMAL LENGTH OF THE DIGIT. WHETHER THIS IS A SEPARATE TRAIT IS NOT CERTAIN. TYPE A3 BRACHYDACTYLY IS VARIABLE AND MAY ENCOMPASS THE CASES DESCRIBED BY DUTTA. (SEE ALSO DYSTELEPHALANGY.) BAUER (1907) DESCRIBED THE ANOMALY IN FOUR GENERATIONS. DEFINING SHORTENED FIFTH MEDIAL PHALANGES AS THOSE LESS THAN HALF THE LENGTH OF THE FOURTH MEDIAL PHALANX, HERTZOG (1967) FOUND THE STATE MUCH MORE FREQUENT IN CHINESE THAN IN NEGROES. POPULATION SURVEYS SUGGEST THAT THE TRAIT IS MORE FREQUENT IN MONGOLOIDS AND AMERINDIANS THAN IN WHITES OR NEGROES. THE CONDITION IS MORE FREQUENT IN FEMALES. (NOTE THAT BRACHYMESOPHANGY V AND BRACHYTELOPHALANGY I ARE *NORMAL* FORMS OF BRACHYDACTYLY AND THAT EACH HAS CHARACTERISTIC SEX AND POPULATION DISTRIBUTIONS.) X-RAY CHANGES CONSIST OF CONE-SHAPED EPIPHYSES WITH EARLY UNION.

BAUER, B.* EINE BISHER NICHT BEOBACHTETE KONGENITALE, HEREDITARE ANOMALIE DES FINGERSKELETTES. DEUTSCH. Z. CHIR. 86* 252-259, 1907.

DUTTA, P.* THE INHERITANCE OF THE RADIALLY CURVED LITTLE FINGER. ACTA GENET. STATIST. MED. 15* 70-76, 1965.

HERSH, A. H., DEMARINIS, F. AND STECHER, R. M.* ON THE INHERITANCE AND DEVELOPMENT OF CLINODACTYLY. AM. J. HUM. GENET. 5* 257-268, 1953.

HERTZOG, K. P.* SHORTENED FIFTH MEDIAL PHALANGES. AM. J. PHYS. ANTHROP. 27* 113-118, 1967.

*11280 BRACHYDACTYLY, TYPE A4 (BRACHYMESOPHALANGY II AND V, TEMTAMY TYPE)

TEMTAMY (1966) STUDIED A PEDIGREE WITH AN UNUSUAL TYPE OF BRACHYDACTYLY IN FOUR GENERATIONS. THE MAIN FEATURES WERE BRACHYMESOPHALANGY AFFECTING MAINLY THE 2ND AND 5TH DIGITS. THE 4TH DIGIT WHEN AFFECTED SHOWED AN ABNORMALLY SHAPED MIDDLE PHALANX LEADING TO RADIAL DEVIATION OF THE DISTAL PHALANX. THE FEET ALSO SHOWED ABSENCE OF MIDDLE PHALANGES OF THE LATERAL FOUR TOES. THE PROPOSITUS HAD

CONGENITAL TALIPES CALCANEOVALGUS. A PEDIGREE REPORTED BY JEANSELME (1923) HAD AFFECTED MEMBERS IN FOUR GENERATIONS AND COULD REPRESENT THE SAME TYPE OF BRACHYDACTYLY. IT WAS ONE OF BELL'S UNCLASSIFIED PEDIGREES. THE AFFECTED MEMBERS HAD BRACHYDACTYLY OF THE 2ND AND 5TH FINGERS DUE TO BRACHYMESOPHALANGY, AND ONE AFFECTED MEMBER HAD CLUB FOOT. STILES AND SCHALCK (1945) DESCRIBED A FAMILY IN WHICH MANY MEMBERS OF FOUR GENERATIONS HAD ULNAR CURVATURE OF THE SECOND FINGER. USUALLY THE FIFTH FINGER SHOWED AT LEAST MILD RADIAL CURVATURE AND SOMETIMES ALSO THE FOURTH FINGER. THIS IS REALLY A FORM OF CLINODACTYLY (Q.V.).

JEANSELME, B. AND JOANNON, (NI)* BRACHYDACTYLIE SYMETRIQUE FAMILIALE. REV. ANTHROP. 33* 1-23, 1923.

STILES, K. A. AND SCHALCK, J.* A PEDIGREE OF CURVED FOREFINGERS. J. HERED. 36* 211-216, 1945.

TEMTAMY, S. A.* GENETIC FACTORS IN HAND MALFORMATIONS. PH. D. THESIS, JOHNS HOPKINS UNIVERSITY, 1966.

*11290 BRACHYDACTYLY, TYPE A5 (ABSENT MIDDLE PHALANGES OF DIGITS II-V) WITH NAIL DYSPLASIA

IN 13 PERSONS IN 4 GENERATIONS, WITH MALE-TO-MALE TRANSMISSION, BASS (1968) FOUND ABSENCE OF THE MIDDLE PHALANGES AND NAIL DYSPLASIA. THE TERMINAL PHALANX OF THE THUMB WAS DUPLICATED.

BASS, H. N.* FAMILIAL ABSENCE OF MIDDLE PHALANGES WITH NAIL DYSPLASIA* A NEW SYNDROME. PEDIATRICS 42* 318-323, 1968.

*11300 BRACHYDACTYLY, TYPE B

IN THIS FORM, AS IN THE 4 TYPES A, THE MIDDLE PHALANGES ARE SHORT BUT IN ADDITION THE TERMINAL PHALANGES ARE RUDIMENTARY OR ABSENT. BOTH FINGERS AND TOES ARE AFFECTED. THE THUMBS AND BIG TOES ARE USUALLY DEFORMED. THIS TYPE OF HAND MALFORMATION PRESENTS THE SEVEREST DEFORMITY IN THE BRACHYDACTYLY GROUP. SYMPHALANGISM IS ALSO A FEATURE. THERE IS ALSO MILD SYNDACTYLY BETWEEN THE DIGITS LEADING SOME AUTHORS TO DESCRIBE THIS DEFORMITY AS SYMBRACHYDACTYLY. IN THE FEET THERE IS SYNDACTYLY USUALLY OF THE 2ND AND 3RD TOES. THE FIRST DESCRIPTION OF THIS HAND DEFORMITY WAS IN THE PREMENDELIAN ERA BY MACKINDER (1857) IN SIX GENERATIONS. MACARTHUR AND MCCULLOUGH (1932) DESCRIBED THE SAME DEFORMITY IN THREE GENERATIONS AND PREFERED THE TERM "APICAL DYSTROPHY." (SEE ALSO COLOBOMA OF MACULA WITH TYPE B BRACHYDACTYLY.)

MACARTHUR, J. W. AND MCCULLOUGH, E.* APICAL DYSTROPHY AS INHERITED DEFECT OF HANDS AND FEET. HUM. BIOL. 4* 179-207, 1932.

MACKINDER, D.* DEFICIENCY OF FINGERS TRANSMITTED THROUGH SIX GENERATIONS. BRIT. MED. J. 845-846, 1857.

*11310 BRACHYDACTYLY, TYPE C

HAWS (1963) DESCRIBED AN EXTENSIVELY AFFECTED MORMON KINDRED. THE ANOMALIES OF THE DIGITS ARE OF MANY TYPES* BRACHYDACTYLY OF THE MIDDLE PHALANX OF THE INDEX AND MIDDLE FINGERS, TRIANGULATION OF THE FIFTH MIDDLE PHALANX, BRACHYMETAPODY, HYPERPHALANGY (MORE THAN THREE PHALANGES PER FINGER), SYMPHALANGISM (Q.V.), ETC. ABOUT 600 FAMILY MEMBERS WERE EXAMINED, 86 WERE AFFECTED. THE CHARACTERISTIC CHANGE SHOULD BE CONSIDERED A DEFORMITY OF THE MIDDLE AND PROXIMAL PHALANGES OF THE SECOND AND THIRD FINGERS, SOMETIMES WITH HYPERSEGMENTATION OF THE PROXIMAL PHALANX. THE RING FINGER MAY BE ESSENTIALLY NORMAL AND PROJECT BEYOND THE OTHERS. IN A KINDRED WITH BRACHDACTYLY CONSIDERED BY THE AUTHORS AS TYPE C, ROBINSON ET AL. (1968) FOUND LEGG-PERTHES DISEASE OF THE HIP IN 3 AFFECTED PERSONS, 2 SISTERS AND THEIR MATERNAL UNCLE.

HAWS, D. V.* INHERITED BRACHYDACTYLY AND HYPOPLASIA OF THE BONES OF THE EXTREMITIES. ANN. HUM. GENET. 26* 201-212, 1963.

POL, D.* "BRACHYDACTYLIE," "KLINODAKTYLIE," HYPERPHALANGIE UND IHRE GRUNDLAGEN. VIRCHOW. ARCH. PATH. ANAT. 229* 388-530, 1921.

ROBINSON, G. C., WOOD, B. J., MILLER, J. R. AND BAILLIE, J.* HEREDITARY BRACHYDACTYLY AND HIP DISEASE. UNUSUAL RADIOLOGICAL AND DERMATOGLYPHIC FINDINGS IN A KINDRED. J. PEDIAT. 72* 539-543, 1968.

*11320 BRACHYDACTYLY, TYPE D ("STUB THUMB")

THIS TYPE IS CHARACTERIZED BY SHORT AND BROAD TERMINAL PHALANGES OF THE THUMBS AND BIG TOES. THOMSEN (1928) DESCRIBED THIS ANOMALY. IN A UNILATERAL CASE HE POINTED OUT THAT THE EPIPHYSEAL LINE AT THE BASE OF THE ANOMALOUS PHALANX WAS OBLITERATED BUT WAS STILL DEMONSTRABLE IN THE CORRESPONDING POSITION ON THE NORMAL THUMB. GOODMAN AND COLLEAGUES (1965) HAVE ALSO STUDIED THIS "NORMAL" MORPHOLOGIC TRAIT IN DETAIL. THE TRAIT HAS PICTURESQUE DESIGNATIONS SUCH AS "POTTER'S THUMB" AND "MURDERER'S THUMB." IT OCCURS AS PART OF THE HEART-HAND SYNDROME III (TABATZNIK'S SYNDROME) AND OF RUBINSTEIN'S SYNDROME (Q.V.).

BREITENBECHER, J. K.* HEREDITARY SHORTNESS OF THUMBS. J. HERED. 14* 15-21, 1923.

GOODMAN, R. M., ADAM, A. AND SHEBA, C.* A GENETIC STUDY OF STUB THUMBS AMONG VARIOUS ETHNIC GROUPS IN ISRAEL. J. MED. GENET. 2* 116-121, 1965.

HEFNER, R. A.* INHERITED ABNORMALITIES OF THE FINGERS. II. SHORT THUMBS (BRACHYMEGALODACTYLISM). J. HERED. 15* 433-440, 1924.

SAYLES, L. P. AND JAILER, J. W.* FOUR GENERATIONS OF SHORT THUMBS. J. HERED. 25* 377-378, 1934.

THOMSEN, O.* HEREDITARY GROWTH ANOMALY OF THE THUMB. HEREDITAS 10* 261-273, 1928.

*11330 BRACHYDACTYLY, TYPE E

THE BRACHYDACTYLY IS DUE MAINLY TO SHORTENING OF THE METACARPALS AND METATARSALS. WIDE VARIABILITY IN THE NUMBER OF DIGITS AFFECTED OCCURS FROM PERSON TO PERSON. THE PATIENTS ARE MODERATELY SHORT OF STATURE AND HAVE ROUND FACIES BUT DO NOT HAVE ECTOPIC CALCIFICATION (OR OSSIFICATION), MENTAL RETARDATION OR CATARACT AS IN PSEUDO-PSEUDOHYPOPARATHYROIDISM (Q.V.) WHICH IS AN OTHERWISE SIMILAR ENTITY. MALE-TO-MALE TRANSMISSION OF LOWRY TYPE BRACHYDACTYLY HAS BEEN OBSERVED (MCKUSICK AND MILCH, 1964), WHEREAS THE LATTER CONDITION APPEARS TO BE X-LINKED. THIS PHENOTYPE IS A USEFUL EXAMPLE OF GENETIC HETEROGENEITY, BECAUSE IN ADDITION TO THE AUTOSOMAL DOMINANT ISOLATED TYPE AND THE X-LINKED ALBRIGHT'S HEREDITARY OSTEODYS-TROPHY, IT ALSO OCCURS WITH A CHROMOSOMAL ABERRATION, THE XO TURNER SYNDROME. ALSO SEE BRACHYDACTYLY-NYSTAGMUS-CEREBELLAR ATAXIA (BIEMOND SYNDROME I), A PROBABLE DOMINANT TRAIT. THE OBVIOUSLY AUTOSOMAL DOMINANT PEDIGREE REPORTED BY GOEMINNE (1965) ALSO REPRESENTED THIS ENTITY AND NOT ALBRIGHT'S SYNDROME. HERTZOG (1968) SUGGESTED THAT THERE ARE AT LEAST THREE SUBTYPES* (E1) SHORTENING IS LIMITED TO FOURTH METACARPALS AND-OR METATARSALS (HORTLING, 1960). (E2) VARIABLE COMBINATIONS OF METACARPALS ARE INVOLVED, WITH SHORTENING ALSO OF THE FIRST AND THIRD DISTAL AND THE SECOND AND FIFTH MIDDLE PHALANGES (MCKUSICK AND MILCH, 1964). (E3) A DUBIOUS CATEGORY MAY HAVE A VARIABLE COMBINATION OF SHORT METACARPALS WITHOUT PHALANGEAL INVOLVEMENT. AS PERIPHERAL DYSOSTOSIS, NEWCOMBE AND KEATS (1969) DESCRIBED AN EXTENSIVELY AFFECTED KINDRED WITH A DOMINANT PEDIGREE PATTERN (THEIR PEDIGREE II). THE DESCRIPTION RESEMBLES THAT IN THE FAMILY OF MCKUSICK AND MILCH (1964) EXCEPT FOR CONE EPIPHYSES. THE AUTHORS FELT THAT THE PRESENCE OF CONE EPIPHYSES IN THEIR FAMILY WAS A DISTINGUISHING FEATURE.

GOEMINNE, L.* ALBRIGHT'S HEREDITARY POLY-OSTEOCHONDRODYSTROPHY (PSEUDO-PSEUDO HYPOPARATHYROIDISM WITH DIABETES, HYPERTENSION, ARTERITIS AND POLYARTHROSIS). ACTA GENET. MED. GEM. 14* 226-281, 1965.

HERTZOG, K. P.* BRACHYDACTYLY AND PSEUDO-PSEUDOHYPOPARATHYROIDISM. ACTA GENET. MED. GEM. 17* 428-437, 1968.

HORTLING, H., PUUPPONEN, E. AND KOSKI, K.* SHORT METACARPAL OR METATARSAL BONES* PSEUDO-PSEUDOHYPOPARATHYROIDISM. J. CLIN. ENDOCR. 20* 466-472, 1960.

MCKUSICK, V. A. AND MILCH, R. A.* THE CLINICAL BEHAVIOR OF GENETIC DISEASE* SELECTED ASPECTS. CLIN. ORTHOP. 33* 22-39, 1964.

NEWCOMBE, D. S. AND KEATS, T. E.* ROENTGENOGRAPHIC MANIFESTATIONS OF HEREDITARY PERIPHERAL DYSOSTOSIS. AM. J. ROENTGEN. 106* 178-189, 1969.

11340 BRACHYDACTYLY-NYSTAGMUS-CEREBELLAR ATAXIA

BIEMOND (1934) DESCRIBED A SYNDROME CONSISTING OF BRACHYDACTYLY (DUE TO ONE SHORT METACARPAL AND METATARSAL), NYSTAGMUS AND CEREBELLAR ATAXIA IN FOUR GENERATIONS OF A FAMILY. MENTAL DEFICIENCY AND STRABISMUS WERE ALSO PRESENT. ONLY A FEW MEMBERS OF THE FAMILY HAD THE FULL SYNDROME. ADDITIONAL FAMILIES ARE NEEDED BEFORE THIS COMBINATION CAN BE CONSIDERED A SINGLE GENE SYNDROME.

BIEMOND, A.* BRACHYDACTYLIE, NYSTAGMUS EN CEREBELLAIRE ATAXIE ALS FAMILIAIR SYNDROOM. NEDERL. T. GENEESK. 78* 1423-1431, 1934.

11350 BRACHYRAPHIA

BROWN (1933) DESCRIBED AS MORQUIO'S DISEASE THE CONDITION IN A MOTHER AND TWO DAUGHTERS. LENZ (1964) OBSERVED FATHER AND SON WITH A VERY SHORT SPINE AND DEFORMITY OF THE ANTERIOR CHEST RATHER LIKE THAT IN MORQUIO'S DISEASE. EXCEPT FOR MARKED CHANGES IN THE FEMORAL EPIPHYSES, THE EXTREMITIES WERE NORMAL. THE VERTEBRAL BODIES WERE SMALL, IRREGULAR AND RADIOLUCENT. POSSIBLY THIS IS THE SAME CONDITION AS THAT REFERRED TO ELSEWHERE AS THE DOMINANT TYPE OF SPONDYLOEPIPHYSEAL DYSPLASIA TARDA (Q.V.). PERHAPS THE FAMILY OF LOMUS AND BOYLE (1959) IN WHICH 3 GENERATIONS WERE AFFECTED HAD THE SAME CONDITION.

BROWN, D. O. AND MACDONALD, C.* THREE CASES OF FAMILIAL OSSEOUS DYSTROPHY. AUST. NEW ZEAL. J. SURG. 3* 78-88, 1933.

BROWN, D. O.* MORQUIO'S DISEASE. MED. J. AUST. 1* 598-600, 1933.

LENZ, W.* ANOMALIEN DES WACHSTUMS UND DER KORPERFORM. IN, BECKER, P. E. (ED.)* EIN KURZES HANDBUCH IN FUNF BANDEN. STUTTGART* GEORG THIEME VERLAG, 1964. 2* 88-89, FIG. 30.

LOMAS, J. J. P. AND BOYLE, A. C.* OSTEO-CHONDRODYSTROPHY (MORQUIO'S DISEASE) IN THREE GENERATIONS. LANCET 2* 430-432, 1959.

*11360 BRANCHIAL CLEFT ANOMALIES, INCLUDING BRANCHIAL CYSTS

THE ABNORMALITY MAY BE IN THE FORM OF CYSTS, SINUSES OR FISTULAS, THE LAST TERM BEING RESERVED FOR THOSE INSTANCES IN WHICH THERE IS COMMUNICATION BETWEEN THE SKIN AND THE PHARYNX. THESE ARE CONSIDERED TO BE ANOMALIES OF THE SECOND BRACHIAL CLEFT. ALTHOUGH IN AT LEAST ONE FAMILY, EAR PITS (Q.V.) WERE ALSO PRESENT, THESE ARE LISTED AS SEPARATE MUTATIONS, BECAUSE MOST FAMILIES SHOW EITHER ONE OR THE OTHER. WHEELER, SHAW AND CAWLEY (1958) FOUND BRANCHIAL CYSTS AND SINUSES IN FOUR MEMBERS OF THREE GENERATIONS OF A FAMILY. CYSTS, SINUSES AND SKIN TABS CONTAINING CARTILAGE OCCURRED IN A LINE EXTENDING FROM A POINT ANTERIOR TO THE EAR TO THE ANTERIOR BORDER OF THE STERNOMASTOID MUSCLE AT THE LEVEL OF THE ANGLE OF THE MANDIBLE AND THENCE ALONG THE ANTERIOR BORDER OF THIS MUSCLE TO A POINT NEAR ITS ATTACHMENT TO THE STERNUM.

MUCKLE, T. J.* HEREDITARY BRANCHIAL DEFECTS IN A HAMPSHIRE FAMILY. BRIT. MED. J. 1* 1297-1299, 1961.

WHEELER, C. E., SHAW, R. F. AND CAWLEY, E. P.* BRANCHIAL ANOMALIES IN THREE GENERATIONS OF ONE FAMILY. ARCH. DERM. 77* 715-719, 1958.

11370 BREAST AND NIPPLES, ABSENCE OF

PEDIGREES CONSISTENT WITH DOMINANT INHERITANCE HAVE BEEN REPORTED. FRASER (1956) FOUND ABSENT BREASTS IN 7 MEMBERS OF THREE GENERATIONS. GOLDENRING AND CRELIN (1961) DESCRIBED IT IN MOTHER AND DAUGHTER. RECESSIVE INHERITANCE SEEMED MORE LIKELY IN THE FAMILY OF KOWLESSAR AND ORTI (1968) IN WHICH BROTHER AND SISTER WERE AFFECTED AND THE PARENTS WERE FIRST COUSINS. HYPOPLASIA OR APLASIA OF THE BREASTS AND NIPPLES OCCURS IN ANHIDROTIC ECTODERMAL DYSPLASIA.

FRASER, F. C.* DOMINANT INHERITANCE OF ABSENT NIPPLES AND BREASTS. IN, NOVANT' ANNI DELLE LEGGI MENDELIANE. ROME* ISTITUTO GREGORIO MENDEL, 1956. P. 360.

GOLDENRING, H. AND CRELIN, E. S.* MOTHER AND DAUGHTER WITH BILATERAL CONGENITAL AMASTIA. YALE J. BIOL. MED. 33* 466-467, 1961.

KOWLESSAR, M. AND ORTI, E.* COMPLETE BREAST ABSENCE IN SIBLINGS. AM. J. DIS. CHILD. 115* 91-92, 1968.

*11380 BULLOUS ERYTHRODERMA ICHTHYOSIFORMIS CONGENITA (BROCQ)

HEIMENDINGER AND SCHNYDER (1962) DESCRIBED THIS DISORDER IN A MAN AND TWO OF HIS THREE CHILDREN, A SON AND A DAUGHTER. THE CONDITION IS DISTINCT FROM THE NON-BULLOUS FORM INHERITED AS A RECESSIVE. GASSER (1964) FOUND, AMONG 17 FAMILIES WITH TWO OR MORE AFFECTED PERSONS, ONLY SIBS AFFECTED IN 2, TWO SUCCESSIVE GENERATIONS AFFECTED IN 12, AND THREE GENERATIONS AFFECTED IN 3.

BARKER, L. P. AND SACHS, W.* BULLOUS CONGENITAL ICHTHYOSIFORM ERYTHRODERMIA. ARCH. DERM. 67* 443-455, 1953.

GASSER, V.* ZUR KLINIK, HISTOLOGIE UND GENETIK DER ERYTHRODERMIE CONGENITALE ICHTHYOSIFORME BULLEUSE (BROCQ). ARCH. KLAUS. STIFT. VERERBUNGSFORSCH. 38* 23-59, 1964.

HEIMENDINGER, J. AND SCHNYDER, U. W.* BULLOSE 'ERYTHRODERMIE ICHTHYOSIFORME CONGENITALE' IN ZWEI GENERATIONEN. HELV. PAEDIAT. ACTA 17* 47-55, 1962.

11390 BUNDLE BRANCH BLOCK

COMBRINK, DAVIS AND SNYMAN (1962) DESCRIBED A FAMILY IN WHICH THE MOTHER HAD RIGHT BUNDLE BRANCH BLOCK AND DIED AT AGE 35 YEARS IN A STOKES-ADAMS ATTACK. OF FOUR CHILDREN THREE HAD RIGHT BUNDLE BRANCH BLOCK. THE MOTHER'S PARENTS HAD BOTH DIED SUDDENLY IN THEIR 30'S. ONE OF HER BROTHERS WAS SAID TO HAVE A CARDIAC CONDUCTION DISTURBANCE AND ANOTHER HAD DEXTROCARDIA. THREE OTHER SIBS WERE APPARENTLY NORMAL. SEGALL (1961) DESCRIBED AN INSTANCE OF FATHER, SON AND DAUGHTER (OF FRENCH CANADIAN AND NEGRO INTERMIXTURE) WITH RIGHT BUNDLE BRANCH BLOCK, AND REPEATED STOKES-ADAMS ATTACKS WITH VARIOUS ATRIAL ARRHYTHMIAS AND VENTRICULAR EXTRASYSTOLES. THE FATHER DIED AT 74 YEARS, 14 YEARS AFTER THE FIRST FAINTING EPISODE. TWO ASYMPTOMATIC BROTHERS SHOWED THE ELECTROCARDIOGRAPHIC CHANGES OF WOLFF-PARKINSON-WHITE. DEFOREST (1956) OBSERVED 'BENIGN' LEFT BUNDLE BRANCH BLOCK IN 4 PERSONS IN TWO GENERATIONS.

COMBRINK, J. M., DAVIS, W. H. AND SNYMAN, H. W.* FAMILIAL BUNDLE BRANCH BLOCK. AM. HEART J. 64* 397-400, 1962.

SEGALL, H. N.* CONGENITAL ARRHYTHMIAS AND CONDUCTION ABNORMALITIES IN A FATHER
AND FOUR CHILDREN. CANAD. MED. ASS. J. 84* 1283-1296, 1961.

11400 CAFFEY'S DISEASE (INFANTILE CORTICAL HYPEROSTOSIS)

AUTOSOMAL DOMINANT INHERITANCE IS SUGGESTED BY THE REPORTS OF GERRARD AND
COLLEAGUES (1961), VAN BUSKIRK AND COLLEAGUES (1961), HOLMAN (1962) AND OTHERS.
MULTIPLE SIBS HAVE BEEN AFFECTED, SUGGESTING AUTOSOMAL RECESSIVE INHERITANCE
(E.G., CLEMETT AND WILLIAMS, 1963). HOWEVER, IN AT LEAST TWO FAMILIES (VAN
BUSKIRK, TAMPAS AND PETERSON, 1961* GERRARD, HOLMAN, GORMAN AND MORROW, 1961)
AFFECTED PERSONS OCCURRED IN TWO GENERATIONS. THE CONDITION HAS SOMEWHAT UNUSUAL
FEATURES FOR A HEREDITARY DISORDER. IT RARELY IF EVER APPEARS AFTER 5 MONTHS OF
AGE* IT IS SOMETIMES PRESENT AT BIRTH AND HAS BEEN IDENTIFIED BY X-RAY IN THE
FETUS IN UTERO. THE ACUTE MANIFESTATIONS ARE INFLAMMATORY IN NATURE WITH FEVER
AND HOT, TENDER SWELLING OF INVOLVED BONES (E.G., MANDIBLE, RIBS). DESPITE
STRIKING RADIOLOGIC CHANGES IN THE ACUTE STAGES, PREVIOUSLY AFFECTED BONES ARE
OFTEN COMPLETELY NORMAL ON RESTUDY. INCONTINENTIA PIGMENTI IS ANOTHER FAMILIAL
CONDITION IN WHICH 'ACTIVE' LESIONS AT BIRTH AND EARLY IN LIFE LEAVE LITTLE OR NO
RESIDUA. IN THIS CONDITION AND IN CAFFEY'S DISEASE AN INFECTION COULD PERHAPS BE
THE CAUSE AND NOT A MUTANT GENE. PICKERING AND CUDDIGAN (1969) SUGGESTED THAT
VASCULAR OCCLUSION SECONDARY TO THROMBOCYTOSIS MAY BE INVOLVED IN THE PATHOGENE-
SIS.

CLEMETT, A. R. AND WILLIAMS, J. H.* THE FAMILIAL OCCURRENCE OF INFANTILE
CORTICAL HYPEROSTOSIS. RADIOLOGY 80* 409-416, 1963.

GERRARD, J. W., HOLMAN, G. H., GORMAN, A. A. AND MORROW, I. H.* FAMILIAL
INFANTILE CORTICAL HYPEROSTOSIS. J. PEDIAT. 59* 543-548, 1961.

HOLMAN, G. H.* INFANTILE CORTICAL HYPEROSTOSIS* A REVIEW. QUART. REV. PEDIAT.
17* 24-31, 1962.

PICKERING, D. AND CUDDIGAN, B.* INFANTILE CORTICAL HYPEROSTOSIS ASSOCIATED WITH
THROMBOCYTHAEMIA. LANCET 2* 464-465, 1969.

SHERMAN, M. S. AND HELLYER, D. T.* INFANTILE CORTICAL HYPEROSTOSIS. REVIEW OF
THE LITERATURE AND REPORT OF 5 CASES. AM. J. ROENTGEN. 63* 212-222, 1950.

SIDBURY, J. B.* INFANTILE CORTICAL HYPEROSTOSIS. POSTGRAD. MED. 22* 211-215,
1957.

VAN BUSKIRK, F. W., TAMPAS, J. P. AND PETERSON, O. S.* INFANTILE CORTICAL
HYPEROSTOSIS* AN ENQUIRY INTO ITS FAMILIAL ASPECTS. AM. J. ROENTGEN. 85* 613-632,
1961.

11410 CALCIFICATION OF BASAL GANGLIA AND HYPOCALCEMIA

NICHOLS, HOLDSWORTH AND REINFRANK (1961) REPORTED A FAMILY IN THREE GENERATIONS OF
WHICH MEMBERS HAD A SYNDROME OF CALCIFICATION OF THE BASAL GANGLIA AND HYPOCALCE-
MIA. IT IS NOT CLEAR WHAT RELATION THESE CASES MAY HAVE TO PSEUDOHYPOPARATHYROI-
DISM. ROBERTS (1959) HAD REPORTED A RATHER SIMILAR FAMILY WITH SIX AFFECTED
PERSONS IN TWO GENERATIONS INCLUDING AN INSTANCE OF MALE-TO-MALE TRANSMISSION.
NIGRA (1970) RESTUDIED THE FAMILY OF NICHOLS ET AL. (1961) AND FOUND NO EVIDENCE
OF PARATHORMONE UNRESPONSIVENESS.

NICHOLS, F. L., HOLDSWORTH, D. E. AND REINFRANK, R. F.* FAMILIAL HYPOCALCEMIA,
LATENT TETANY AND CALCIFICATION OF THE BASAL GANGLIA. AM. J. MED. 30* 518-528,
1961.

NIGRA, T. P.* BETHESDA, MD.* PERSONAL COMMUNICATION, 1970.

ROBERTS, P. D.* FAMILIAL CALCIFICATION OF THE CEREBRAL BASAL GANGLIA AND ITS
RELATION TO HYPOPARATHYROIDISM. BRAIN 82* 599-609, 1959.

*11420 CAMPTODACTYLY, CAMPYLODACTYLY

CAMPTODACTYLY IS A HAND MALFORMATION CHARACTERIZED BY A CONTRACTURE DEFORMITY OF
THE PROXIMAL INTERPHALANGEAL JOINTS OF THE FINGERS. THE LITTLE FINGER IS THE MOST
FREQUENTLY AFFECTED THOUGH ANY FINGER MAY BE INVOLVED. THIS DEFORMITY IS
INHERITED AS AN AUTOSOMAL DOMINANT TRAIT WITH VARIABLE PENETRANCE. HEFNER (1929,
1941) REPORTED ITS OCCURRENCE IN FOUR GENERATIONS. CAMPTODACTYLY, THOUGH OFTEN
OCCURRING AS AN ISOLATED ANOMALY, IS OCCASIONALLY A FEATURE OF GENETICALLY
DISTINCT DISORDERS (SEE CRANIOCARPOTARSAL DYSTROPHY). SYMPTOMS INCLUDE STREBLODA-
CTYLY, CONGENITAL CONTRACTURE OF FINGERS, AND CONGENITAL DUPUPTREN'S CONTRACTURE.
PARISH, HORN AND THOMPSON (1963) DESCRIBED FLEXION CONTRACTURES OF THE FINGERS
(STREBLODACTYLY* STREBLOS = GR. TWISTED, CROOKED) AND AMINOACIDURIA IN 10 FEMALES
OF 3 GENERATIONS OF A FAMILY. IN 2 FEMALES THE HANDS WERE NORMAL BUT THE SAME
AMINOACIDURIA WAS PRESENT. 9 MALES WERE NORMAL. SINCE ALL FEMALES IN THE DIRECT
LINE WERE AFFECTED BY ONE OR BOTH OF THE TRAITS MENTIONED, THIS IS BY DEFINITION

HOLOGYNIC. HOWEVER, IT IS NOT, AT LEAST IS NOT NECESSARILY, A SEX-LINKED DOMINANT AS THE AUTHORS PROPOSED. IN MOST PATIENTS FINGERS II TO V WERE AFFECTED. THIS ENTITY MAY NOT BE DIFFERENT FROM CAMPTODACTYLY. NEVIN, HURWITZ AND NEILL (1966) ALSO FOUND TAURINURIA IN ASSOCIATION WITH CAMPTODACTYLY. THE INCREASED EXCRETION OF TAURINE SEEMED TO BE RENAL IN ORIGIN. TAURINE IS NOT AN AMINO ACID BUT A SULFONATED AMINE WHICH ARISES AS AN END PRODUCT OF THE METABOLISM OF SULFUR-CONTAINING AMINO ACIDS. SEVERAL INSTANCES OF MALE-TO-MALE TRANSMISSION WERE NOTED IN THE 4 FAMILIES THEY STUDIED. IN A RURAL AREA OF WESTERN NORTH CAROLINA MURPHY (1926) DESCRIBED CAMPTODACTYLY IN MANY MEMBERS OF 5 GENERATIONS. ELEVEN OF THE AFFECTED PERSONS ALSO HAD KNEE-JOINT SUBLUXATION WHICH WAS USUALLY EASILY REDUCED.

DUTTA, P.* THE INHERITANCE OF THE RADIALLY CURVED LITTLE FINGER. ACTA GENET. STATIST. MED. 15* 70-76, 1965.

HEFNER, R. A.* CROOKED LITTLE FINGER (MINOR STREBLOMICRODACTYLY). J. HERED. 32* 37-38, 1941.

HEFNER, R. A.* INHERITANCE OF CROOKED LITTLE FINGERS (MINOR STREBLOMICRODACTY-LY). J. HERED. 20* 395-398, 1929.

MOORE, W. G. AND MESSINA, P.* CAMPTODACTYLISM AND ITS VARIABLE EXPRESSION. J. HERED. 27* 27-30, 1936.

MURPHY, D. P.* FAMILIAL FINGER CONTRACTURE AND ASSOCIATED FAMILIAL KNEE-JOINT SUBLUXATION. J.A.M.A. 86* 395-397, 1926.

NEVIN, N. C., HURWITZ, L. J. AND NEILL, D. W.* FAMILIAL CAMPTODACTYLY WITH TAURINURIA. J. MED. GENET. 3* 265-268, 1966.

PARISH, J. G., HORN, D. B. AND THOMPSON, M.* FAMILIAL STREBLODACTYLY WITH AMINO-ACIDURIA. BRIT. MED. J. 2* 1247-1250, 1963.

WELCH, J. P. AND TEMTAMY, S. A.* HEREDITARY CONTRACTURES OF THE FINGERS (CAMPTODACTYLY). J. MED. GENET. 3* 104-113, 1966.

11430 CAMPTODACTYLY, CLEFT PALATE, CLUB FOOT

GORDON ET AL. (1969) DESCRIBED AFFECTED PERSONS IN THREE GENERATIONS. NO SIMILAR FAMILY WAS FOUND IN THE LITERATURE. A USEFUL LIST OF CAMPTODACTYLY SYNDROMES WAS PROVIDED.

GORDON, H., DAVIES, D. AND BERMAN, M.* CAMPTODACTYLY, CLEFT PALATE AND CLUB FOOT. SYNDROME SHOWING THE AUTOSOMAL-DOMINANT PATTERN OF INHERITANCE. J. MED. GENET. 6* 266-274, 1969.

11440 CANCER

MALIGNANCY IS OBSERVED WITH VON RECKLINGHAUSEN'S NEUROFIBROMATOSIS, TYLOSIS, THE SEVERAL TYPES OF INTESTINAL POLYPOSIS, VON HIPPEL-LINDAU SYNDROME, AND BASAL CELL NEVUS SYNDROME, ALL CONDITIONS LISTED IN THE DOMINANT CATALOG. XERODERMA PIGMENTOSUM, A RECESSIVE, IS COMPLICATED IN ALL CASES BY SKIN MALIGNANCY. IN ADDITION, NOTABLE INSTANCES OF 'CANCER FAMILIES' ARE ON RECORD. WHETHER THESE REPRESENT MORE THAN CHANCE FAMILIAL AGGREGATION OF COMMON DISORDERS IS UNCLEAR. FOR EXAMPLE, LYNCH ET AL. (1966) REPORTED TWO LARGE 'CANCER FAMILIES.' IN ONE, NINE OF 11 SIBS HAD HISTOLOGICALLY CONFIRMED CANCERS, WITH FOUR OF THESE SHOWING MULTIPLE PRIMARY TUMORS. IN THE SECOND, SEVEN OF 13 SIBS SHOWED HISTOLOGICALLY PROVEN CANCERS, WITH MULTIPLE PRIMARY MALIGNANT NEOPLASM IN FOUR. THE TWO FAMILIES CONTAINED 6 INSTANCES OF THE ORDINARILY RARE COMBINATION OF PRIMARY COLONIC AND ENDOMETRIAL CARCINOMA. THE 'CANCER FAMILY' OF WARTHIN IS ANOTHER NOTABLE EXAMPLE (HAUSER AND WELLER, 1936). A VIROLOGIC BASIS FOR FAMILIAL AGGREGATION, EVEN TRANSMISSION THROUGH SUCCESSIVE GENERATIONS, IS POSSIBLE.

BRISMAN, R., BAKER, R. R., ELKINS, R. AND HARTMANN, W. H.* CARCINOMA OF LUNG IN FOUR SIBLINGS. CANCER 20* 2048-2053, 1967.

HAUSER, I. J. AND WELLER, C. V.* A FURTHER REPORT ON THE CANCER FAMILY OF WARTHIN. AM. J. CANCER 27* 434-449, 1936.

LYNCH, H. T., SHAW, M. W., MAGNUSON, C. W., LARSEN, A. L. AND KRUSH, A. J.* HEREDITARY FACTORS IN CANCER* STUDY OF TWO LARGE MIDWESTERN KINDREDS. ARCH. INTERN. MED. 117* 206-212, 1966.

11450 CANCER OF COLON

CANCER OF THE COLON OCCURRED IN 7 MEMBERS OF 4 SUCCESSIVE GENERATIONS OF THE FAMILY REPORTED BY KLUGE (1964), LEADING HIM TO SUGGEST A SIMPLE GENETIC BASIS FOR COLONIC CANCER INDEPENDENT OF POLYPOSIS.

KLUGE, T.* FAMILIAL CANCER OF THE COLON. ACTA CHIR. SCAND. 127* 392-398, 1964.

*11460 CANINE TEETH, ABSENCE OF UPPER PERMANENT

DOLAMORE (1925) DESCRIBED A CASE OF PERSISTENT DECIDUOUS CANINES WITH ABSENCE OF PERMANENT SUCCESSORS IN FATHER AND SON. GRUNEBERG (1936) DESCRIBED THE SAME IN SEVEN MEMBERS OF THREE GENERATIONS OF A GERMAN JEWISH FAMILY.

DOLAMORE, W. H.* ABSENT CANINES. BRIT. DENT. J. 46* 5-8, 1925.

GRUNEBERG, H.* TWO INDEPENDENT INHERITED TOOTH ANOMALIES IN ONE FAMILY. J. HERED. 27* 225-228, 1936.

11470 CARABELLI'S ANOMALY OF MAXILLARY MOLAR TEETH

KRAUS (1951) WAS OF THE OPINION THAT HOMOZYGOSITY OF A GENE IS RESPONSIBLE FOR A PRONOUNCED TUBERCLE, WHEREAS THE HETEROZYGOTE SHOWS SLIGHT GROOVES, PITS, TUBERCLES OR BULGE. HE PROVIDED GOOD PICTURES OF THE ANOMALY.

DIETZ, V. H.* A COMMON DENTAL MORPHOTROPIC FACTOR* THE CARABELLI CUSP. J. AM. DENT. ASS. 31* 784-789, 1944.

KRAUS, B. S.* CARABELLI'S ANOMALY OF THE MAXILLARY MOLAR TEETH. OBSERVATIONS ON MEXICANS AND PAPAGO INDIANS AND AN INTERPRETATION OF THE INHERITANCE. AM. J. HUM. GENET. 3* 348-355, 1951.

*11480 CARBONIC ANHYDRASE, ERYTHROCYTE, ELECTROPHORETIC VARIANTS OF

BY STARCH GEL ELECTROPHORESIS TASHIAN, PLATO AND SHOWS (1963) DETECTED A GENETI-CALLY DETERMINED VARIANT OF ERYTHROCYTE CARBONIC ANHYDRASE.

TASHIAN, R. E., PLATO, C. C. AND SHOWS, T. B., JR.* INHERITED VARIANT OF ERYTHROCYTE CARBONIC ANHYDRASE IN MICRONESIANS FROM GUAM AND SAIPAN. SCIENCE 140* 53-54, 1963.

11490 CARCINOID, INTESTINAL

ANDERSON (1966) OBSERVED APPENDICEAL CARCINOID IN FATHER AND DAUGHTER. ESCHBACK AND RINALDO (1962) REPORTED FATAL MALIGNANT CARCINOID OF THE ILEUM IN BROTHER AND SISTER. DUODENAL CARCINOID IS DESCRIBED WITH MULTIPLE ENDOCRINE ADENOMATOSIS (Q.V.).

ANDERSON, R. E.* A FAMILIAL INSTANCE OF APPENDICEAL CARCINOID. AM. J. SURG. 111* 738-740, 1966.

ESCHBACH, J. W. AND RINALDO, J. A., JR.* METASTATIC CARCINOID* A FAMILIAL OCCURRENCE. ANN. INTERN. MED. 57* 647-650, 1962.

11500 CARDIAC ARRHYTHMIA (EXTRASYSTOLES)

KUHN, WOLF AND STIELER (1964) DESCRIBED TWO SISTERS WITH POLYMORPHIC AND POLYTOPIC VENTRICULAR EXTRASYSTOLES. ONE HAD SYNCOPAL ATTACKS. A BROTHER DIED SUDDENLY AT AGE 10 AND THE MOTHER AT AGE 40, UNDER CIRCUMSTANCES SUGGESTING THE PRESENCE OF THE SAME DISORDER.

KUHN, E., WOLF, D. AND STIELER, M.* FAMILIAL POLYTOPIC AND POLYMORPHIC EXTRASYSTOLES. JAP. HEART J. 5* 81-84, 1964.

11510 CARDIAC CONDUCTION SYSTEM, DEFECT IN

GREEN ET AL. (1969) DESCRIBED A FAMILY IN WHICH SUDDEN DEATH OCCURRED IN AT LEAST 10 PERSONS IN 3 GENERATIONS AT AN AVERAGE AGE OF 21 YEARS (RANGE 4-44). NO CLINICAL ABNORMALITIES WERE DETECTABLE IN MEMBERS OF THE FAMILY, INCLUDING ONE WHO DIED SUDDENLY. AN ABNORMALITY OF THE CONDUCTION SYSTEM WAS POSTULATED BUT NOT DEFINITELY DEMONSTRATED.

GREEN, J. R., JR., KOROVETZ, M. J., SHANKLIN, D. R., DEVITO, J. J. AND TAYLOR, W. J.* SUDDEN UNEXPECTED DEATH IN THREE GENERATIONS. ARCH. INTERN. MED. 124* 359-363, 1969.

11520 CARDIOMYOPATHY, FAMILIAL IDIOPATHIC

WHITFIELD (1961) DESCRIBED A FAMILY IN WHICH 10 MEMBERS WERE SUFFERING, OR HAD DIED, FROM CARDIOMYOPATHY AND 6 OTHERS WERE PROBABLY AFFECTED. IN THIS, AS IN ALL REPORTED FAMILIES, ALTHOUGH BOTH MALES AND FEMALES ARE AFFECTED, TRANSMISSION SEEMINGLY HAS OCCURRED ONLY THROUGH THE FEMALE. UNAFFECTED WOMEN HAVE NOT BORNE AFFECTED CHILDREN. SCHRADER AND COLLEAGUES (1961) DESCRIBED TWO SISTERS WITH FAMILIAL IDIOPATHIC CARDIOMEGALY. ALMOST CERTAINLY THE MOTHER, WHO DIED AT AGE 34, AND PROBABLY ONE BROTHER, WHO DIED AT 16, HAD THE SAME CONDITION. IN THE FAMILY REPORTED BY BATTERSBY AND GLENNER (1961) AFFECTED PERSONS WERE LIMITED TO ONE SIBSHIP AND DEPOSITS OF A NON-METACHROMATIC, DIASTASE-RESISTANT, PAS-POSITIVE POLYSACCHARIDE WERE DESCRIBED IN THE MYOCARDIUM. ONE AFFECTED MEMBER HAD CHRONIC PERICARDIAL EFFUSION. UNDOUBTEDLY HETEROGENEITY EXISTS IN THE GROUP OF CARDIOMYO-PATHIES. BOYD ET AL. (1965) SUGGESTED THAT THERE MAY BE THREE TYPES* (1) FORM WITH PREDOMINANTLY FIBROSIS, (2) FORM WITH PREDOMINANTLY HYPERTROPHY (SEE VENTRICULAR HYPERTROPHY, HEREDITARY) AND (3) FORM WITH DEPOSITS DESCRIBED ABOVE.

SEE AMYLOIDOSIS, CARDIAC FORM FOR ANOTHER FAMILIAL MYOCARDOPATHY. KARIV AND COLLEAGUES (1966) OBSERVED SIX AFFECTED PERSONS IN 3 GENERATIONS. IN TWO OF THESE PERSONS ADAMS-STOKES ATTACKS REQUIRED AN ARTIFICAL PACEMAKER. THE AFFECTED MALES SHOWED SIGNIFICANT INCREASE IN THE SERUM LEVELS OF MULTIPLE MUSCLE-DERIVED ENZYMES. HETEROGENEITY WAS SUGGESTED BY THE FINDING OF NORMAL SERUM ENZYME LEVELS IN AFFECTED MEMBERS OF A SECOND FAMILY. RYWLIN ET AL. (1969) FAVORED THE VIEW THAT OBSTRUCTIVE AND NON-OBSTRUCTIVE FORMS OF FAMILIAL CARDIOPATHY ARE DIFFERENT EXPRESSIONS OF A SINGLE ENTITY.

BARRY, M. AND HALL, M.* FAMILIAL CARDIOMYOPATHY. BRIT. HEART J. 24* 613-624, 1962.

BATTERSBY, E. J. AND GLENNER, G. G.* FAMILIAL CARDIOMYOPATHY. AM. J. MED. 30* 382-391, 1961.

BIORCK, G. AND ORINIUS, E.* FAMILIAL CARDIOMYOPATHIES. ACTA MED. SCAND. 176* 407-424, 1964.

BISHOP, J. M., CAMPBELL, M. AND JONES, E. W.* CARDIOMYOPATHY IN FOUR MEMBERS OF A FAMILY. BRIT. HEART. J. 24* 715-725, 1962.

BOYD, D. L., MISHKIN, M. E., FEIGENBAUM, H. AND GENOVESE, P. D.* THREE FAMILIES WITH FAMILIAL CARDIOMYOPATHY. ANN. INTERN. MED. 63* 386-401, 1965.

KARIV, I., SZEINBERG, A., FABIAN, I., SHERF, L., KREISLER, B. AND ZELTER, M.* A FAMILY WITH CARDIOMYOPATHY. AM. J. MED. 40* 140-148, 1966.

RYWLIN, A. M., BAROLD, S. S., LINHART, J. W., KRAMER, H. C., MEITUS, M. L. AND SAMET, P.* IDIOPATHIC FAMILIAL CARDIOPATHY. A STUDY OF TWO FAMILIES. J. GENET. HUM. 17* 453-470, 1969.

SCHRADER, W. H., PANKEY, G. A., DAVIS, R. B. AND THEOLOGIDES, A.* FAMILIAL IDIOPATHIC CARDIOMEGALY. CIRCULATION 24* 599-606, 1961.

WHITFIELD, A. G. W.* FAMILIAL CARDIOMYOPATHY. QUART. J. MED. 30* 119-134, 1961.

11530 CAROTINEMIA, FAMILIAL

SHARVILL (1970) DESCRIBED VERY HIGH LEVELS OF BLOOD CAROTINE IN A WOMAN, HER MOTHER, A SIB AND HER SON. LOW LEVELS OF VITAMIN A WERE FOUND AT TIMES. A DEFECT IN CONVERSION OF CAROTINE TO VITAMIN A WAS CONSIDERED ONE POSSIBILITY. MCLAREN AND ZEKIAN (1971) REPORTED A CASE OF VITAMIN A DEFICIENCY IN A LEBANESE ARAB GIRL, THE OFFSPRING OF FIRST-COUSIN-ONCE-REMOVED PARENTS. NIGHT BLINDNESS, HYPERKERATO- SIS FOLLICULARIS, BITOT SPOTS OF THE CONJUNCTIVA AND VERY LOW PLASMA LEVELS OF VITAMIN A. A DEFECT IN ENZYMATIC CONVERSION OF BETA-CAROTENE TO RETINAL IN THE INTESTINE WAS SUGGESTED. RECESSIVE INHERITANCE SEEMS MORE LIKELY THAN DOMINANT.

MCLAREN, D. S. AND ZEKIAN, B.* FAILURE OF ENZYMIC CLEAVAGE OF BETA-CAROTENE. THE CAUSE OF VITAMIN A DEFICIENCY IN A CHILD. AM. J. DIS. CHILD. 121* 278-280, 1971.

SHARVILL, D. E.* FAMILIAL HYPERCAROTINAEMIA AND HYPOVITAMINOSIS A. PROC. ROY. SOC. MED. 63* 605-606, 1970.

11540 CARPAL DISPLACEMENT (CARPAL BOSSING)

ELLSWORTH (1927) FOUND DISPLACEMENT OF THE CARPAL BONE GROUP ON THE RADIUS AND ULNA. THE DISTAL EPIPHYSES OF THESE BONES WERE MISSHAPEN. FIVE FEMALES IN FOUR GENERATIONS WERE AFFECTED IN A PATTERN EQUALLY CONSISTENT WITH EITHER AUTOSOMAL OR X-LINKED INHERITANCE. CARPAL BOSSING APPEARS TO BE THE SAME TRAIT AS ELLSWORTH DESCRIBED. A PROMINENCE IS PRODUCED BY A DOUBLE BEAK BETWEEN THE THIRD METACARPAL AND THE CAPITATE BONE OF THE WRIST. PHOTOGRAPHS AND X-RAYS WERE PRESENTED BY LARSON, LAZCANO AND JANES (1958), WHO ESTIMATED THAT IT IS PRESENT IN ABOUT 26 PERCENT OF ADULTS BUT ONLY ONE OF 50 CHILDREN UNDER 15 YEARS OF AGE. THE GENETICS HAS NOT BEEN WORKED OUT. BOTH GENETIC AND ENVIRONMENTAL (E.G., OCCUPATIONAL) FACTORS MAY BE INVOLVED.

ELLSWORTH, H. A.* INHERITANCE OF CARPAL DISPLACEMENT. J. HERED. 18* 133 ONLY, 1927.

LARSON, R. L., LAZCANO, M. A. AND JANES, J. M.* CARPAL BOSSING, A COMMON CLINICAL ENTITY. MAYO CLIN. PROC. 33* 337-343, 1958.

*11550 CATALASE, ELECTROPHORETIC VARIANTS OF

SEVERAL RARE ELECTROPHORETIC VARIANTS OF RED CELL CATALASE HAVE BEEN IDENTIFIED BY BAUR (1963). NANCE ET AL. (1968) DESCRIBED ELECTROPHORETIC VARIANTS OF CATALASE AND PRESENTED EVIDENCE SUGGESTING LINKAGE OF THE CATALASE LOCUS WITH THE HAPTOGLO- BIN LOCUS. THE RELATIONSHIP OF THE ELECTROPHORETIC VARIANTS TO ACATALASIA (Q.V.) IS UNKNOWN.

NANCE, W. E., EMPSON, J. E., BENNETT, T. W. AND LARSON, L.* HAPTOGLOBIN AND
CATALASE LOCI IN MAN* POSSIBLE GENETIC LINKAGE. SCIENCE 160* 1230-1231, 1968.

*11560 CATARACT, ANTERIOR POLAR

HARMAN (1909) OBSERVED A FAMILY WITH 9 CASES IN 5 GENERATIONS, SHOWING ALSO
MICROPHTHALMIA, NYSTAGMUS AND STRABISMUS. IN THE FAMILY DESCRIBED BY SANDER
(1931) THE FATHER AND THREE DAUGHTERS HAD ASSOCIATED MYOPIA AND MENTAL AND
PHYSICAL RETARDATION.

HARMAN, N. B.* CONGENITAL CATARACT, A PEDIGREE OF FIVE GENERATIONS. TRANS.
OPHTHAL. SOC. U.K. 29* 101-108, 1909.

SANDER, P.* A FAMILY AFFECTED WITH KERATOCONUS AND ANTERIOR POLAR CATARACT.
BRIT. J. OPHTHAL. 15* 23-25, 1931.

*11570 CATARACT, CRYSTALLINE ACULEIFORM OR FROSTED

ALTHOUGH RECESSIVE INHERITANCE IS SUGGESTED BY SOME REPORTS, DOMINANT INHERITANCE
IS CLEAR FROM STUDIES SUCH AS THOSE OF ROMER (1926) AND OF GIFFORD AND PUNTENNEY
(1937).

GIFFORD, S. R. AND PUNTENNEY, I.* CORALLIFORM CATARACT AND A NEW FORM OF
CONGENITAL CATARACT WITH CRYSTALS IN THE LENS. ARCH. OPHTHAL. 17* 885-892, 1937.

ROMER, A.* UNTERSUCHUNG UBER DIE ERBLICHKEIT DER SPIESSKATARAKT (VOGT). ARCH.
KLAUS. STIFT. VERERBUNGSFORSCH. 2* 207-220, 1926.

*11580 CATARACT, CRYSTALLINE CORALLIFORM

BOTH TYPES OF CRYSTALLINE CATARACT (CORALLIFORM AND ACULEIFORM) ARE CHARACTERIZED
BY FINE CRYSTALS IN THE AXIAL REGION OF THE LENS. BOTH ARE USUALLY INHERITED AS
DOMINANTS, ALTHOUGH IN RARE INSTANCES RECESSIVE INHERITANCE IS SUSPECTED.
DOMINANT PEDIGREES OF CORALLIFORM CRYSTALLINE CATARACT WERE REPORTED BY NETTLESHIP
(1909), RIAD (1938) AND JORDAN (1955).

JORDAN, M.* STAMMBAUMUNTERSUCHUNGEN BEI CATARACTA STELLATA CORALLIFORMIS.
KLIN. MBL. AUGENHEILK. 126* 469-475, 1955.

NETTLESHIP, E.* SEVEN NEW PEDIGREES OF HEREDITARY CATARACT. TRANS. OPHTHAL.
SOC. U.K. 29* 188-211, 1909.

RIAD, M.* CONGENITAL FAMILIAL CATARACT WITH CHOLESTERIN DEPOSITS. BRIT. J.
OPHTHAL. 22* 745-749, 1938.

*11590 CATARACT, FLORIFORM

DOGGART (1957) RECORDED ITS TRANSMISSION THROUGH 4 GENERATIONS AND TOSCH (1958)
THROUGH 5 GENERATIONS.

DOGGART, J. H.* CONGENITAL CATARACT. TRANS. OPHTHAL. SOC. U.K. 77* 31-37,
1957.

TOSCH, C.* BEITRAG ZUR STAMMBAUMFORSCHUNG DER CATARACTA FLORIFORMIS. KLIN.
MBL. AUGENHEILK. 133* 60-66, 1958.

*11600 CATARACT, HEREDITARY

KOMAI'S PEDIGREE (REPRODUCED BY FRASER ROBERTS) CONTAINED A PROBABLE HOMOZYGOTE.
IN A LARGE FAMILY FROM SOUTHERN ENGLAND ORIGINALLY REPORTED BY NETTLESHIP (1909),
RENWICK AND LAWLER (1963) FOUND LINKAGE BETWEEN THE LOCUS FOR CONGENITAL ZONULAR
PULVERULENT CATARACT AND THE DUFFY BLOOD GROUP LOCUS. THE FINAL PROBABILITY OF
LINKAGE, AFTER COMBINATION WITH AN A PRIORI PROBABILITY AGAINST LINKAGE, WAS
ASSESSED AS 0.977. THE LARGE CATARACT PEDIGREE REPORTED BY MOHR (1954) SHOWED A
PROBABILITY OF LINKAGE OF ONLY 0.02. HENCE, A DIFFERENT TYPE OF DOMINANTLY
INHERITED CATARACT IS PROBABLY INVOLVED. AMONG THE DOMINANTLY INHERITED DISOR-
DERS, MYOTONIC DYSTROPHY, THE FLYNN-AIRD SYNDROME AND OTHERS HAVE CATARACT AS A
FEATURE.
EXTENSIVE GENETIC HETEROGENEITY OF THIS PARTICULAR PHENOTYPE EXISTS. NOT
ONLY DOES THE PRESENCE OR ABSENCE OF ASSOCIATED FEATURES INDICATE HETEROGENEITY,
BUT ALSO DIFFERENCES IN THE TYPE OF LENS CHANGE IN ISOLATED CATARACT BESPEAK
HETEROGENEITY. OF COURSE, DIFFERENT MODES OF INHERITANCE OF WHAT IS PHENOTYPICAL-
LY ESSENTIALLY IDENTICAL LENS CHANGE ALSO INDICATE HETEROGENEITY. IN CATALOGING
THE FORMS OF CATARACT, HEAVY USE WAS MADE OF FRANCOIS' ENCYCLOPEDIC MONOGRAPH
(1963). ALTHOUGH SEVERAL TYPES OF ISOLATED CATARACT AND OVER 20 CONDITIONS IN
WHICH CATARACT OCCURS AS A FREQUENT OR INVARIABLE FEATURE ARE INCLUDED IN THE
THREE CATALOGS SOME ENTITIES HAVE UNDOUBTEDLY BEEN OVERLOOKED AND SOME INDICATED
AS SEPARATE ENTITIES ARE PROBABLY INSTANCES OF PHENOTYPIC VARIATION IN THE
EXPRESSION OF A SINGLE GENOTYPE. NOSOLOGY IN THIS CATEGORY OF DISEASE IS

COMPLICATED BY THE OCCURRENCE IN THE SAME FAMILY OF CATARACTS OF DIFFERENT MORPHOLOGIC TYPES. EXAMPLES ARE THE FAMILIES OF MARNER (1949), LUTMAN AND NEEL (1945) AND WALSH AND WEGMAN (1937). IN THE LAST FAMILY THE PHENOTYPIC DIFFERENCES PROBABLY ARE EXPLAINED BY X-LINKAGE WITH DIFFERENT MANIFESTATIONS IN HEMIZYGOUS MALE AND HETEROZYGOUS FEMALE.

THE USUAL CLINICAL CLASSIFICATIONS ARE BASED ON EITHER THE LOCALIZATION OF OPACITY (NUCLEAR CATARACT, POLAR CATARACT, ETC.) OR ITS MORPHOLOGY (FLORIFORM, LIFE-BUOY, ETC.). FRANCOIS (1963) FOLLOWED A CLASSIFICATION HE FELT TO BE MORE LOGICAL. THIS DISTINGUISHES CATARACTS WHICH INVOLVE THE CAPSULE AND THOSE AFFECTING ONLY THE LENS FIBERS, AND SUBDIVIDES THE LATTER GROUP INTO THOSE DEVELOPING IN A NORMAL LENS RUDIMENT AND THOSE DEVELOPING IN AN ABNORMAL RUDIMENT. LENTICULAR OPACITIES OCCUR WITH MYOTONIC DYSTROPHY, GALACTOSEMIA, WERNER SYNDROME, ALBRIGHT'S HEREDITARY OSTEODYSTROPHY, PHENYLKETONURIA (RARE), WEIL-MARCHESANI SYNDROME, DIABETES MELLITUS, RETINITIS PIGMENTOSA, ROTHMUND SYNDROME, CHONDRODYS-TROPHIA CALCIFICANS CONGENITA.

I CAPSULAR OR CAPSULO-LENTICULAR CATARACTS

1. ANTERIOR POLAR (D)
2. ANTERIOR CAPSULAR
3. POSTERIOR POLAR (D)
4. POSTERIOR CAPSULAR

II CATARACTS DEVELOPING ON A NORMAL LENS RUDIMENT

1. STELLATE (D)
2. DILACERATED
3. FLORIFORM (D)
4. EMBRYONIC ANTERIOR AXIAL
5. PUNCTATE
6. CENTRAL PULVERULENT
7. NUCLEAR (3D)
8. ZONULAR (D)

III CATARACTS DEVELOPING ON AN ABNORMAL LENS RUDIMENT

1. FUSIFORM
2. DISK-SHAPED OR RING-SHAPED
3. CRYSTALLINE CORALLIFORM (D) OR ACULEIFORM (D)

IV TOTAL (D), MEMBRANOUS (D), OR FIBROUS CATARACTS

V SPECIAL FORMS

FRANCOIS, J.* CONGENITAL CATARACTS. SPRINGFIELD, ILL.* CHARLES C THOMAS, 1963.

LUTMAN, F. C. AND NEEL, J. V.* INHERITED CATARACT IN THE B GENEALOGY. OCCURRENCE OF DIVERSE TYPES OF CATARACTS IN THE DESCENDANTS OF ONE PERSON. ARCH. OPHTHAL. 33* 341-357, 1945.

MARNER, E.* A FAMILY WITH EIGHT GENERATIONS OF HEREDITARY CATARACT. ACTA OPHTHAL. 27* 537-551, 1949.

MOHR, J.* A STUDY OF LINKAGE IN MAN. COPENHAGEN* MUNKSGAARD, 1954.

NETTLESHIP, E.* SEVEN NEW PEDIGREES OF HEREDITARY CATARACT. TRANS. OPHTHAL. SOC. U.K. 29* 188-211, 1909.

RENWICK, J. H. AND LAWLER, S. D.* PROBABLE LINKAGE BETWEEN A CONGENITAL CATARACT LOCUS AND THE DUFFY BLOOD GROUP LOCUS. ANN. HUM. GENET. 27* 67-84, 1963.

ROBERTS, J. A. F.* AN INTRODUCTION TO MEDICAL GENETICS. LONDON* OXFORD U. PRESS, 1959. FIG. 8.

WALSH, F. B. AND WEGMAN, M. E.* A PEDIGREE OF HEREDITARY CATARACT, ILLUSTRATING SEX-LIMITED TYPE. BULL. HOPKINS HOSP. 61* 125-135, 1937.

11610 CATARACT, MEMBRANOUS

GRUBER (1945) DESCRIBED 6 CASES IN 4 GENERATIONS. THIS SHOULD BE CONSIDERED A TOTAL CATARACT WHICH HAS UNDERGONE REGRESSION OR RESORPTION.

GRUBER, M.* UEBER PRIMARE FAMILIARE LINSENDYSPLASIE. OPHTHALMOLOGICA 110* 60-73, 1945.

*11620 CATARACT, NUCLEAR (ALSO KNOWN AS COPPOCK CATARACT, DISCOID CATARACT AND PULVERULENT ZONULAR CATARACT)

NETTLESHIP AND OGILVIE (1906) DESCRIBED 18 CASES IN 4 GENERATIONS. HARMAN (1909) REPORTED 19 CASES IN 5 GENERATIONS, SMITH (1910) 26 IN 4 GENERATIONS, LEE AND

BENEDICT (1950) 63 IN 6 GENERATIONS, ETC. AS NOTED ELSEWHERE, ZONULAR PULVERULENT
CATARACT WAS PRESENT IN THE FAMILY IN WHICH LINKAGE WITH DUFFY BLOOD GROUP WAS
DEMONSTRATED BY RENWICK AND LAWLER (1963).

HARMAN, N. B.* CONGENITAL CATARACT, A PEDIGREE OF FIVE GENERATIONS. TRANS.
OPHTHAL. SOC. U.K. 29* 101-108, 1909.

LEE, J. B. AND BENEDICT, W. L.* HEREDITARY NUCLEAR CATARACT. ARCH. OPHTHAL.
44* 643-650, 1950.

NETTLESHIP, E. AND OGILVIE, F. M.* A PECULIAR FORM OF HEREDITARY CONGENITAL
CATARACT. TRANS. OPHTHAL. SOC. U.K. 26* 191-206, 1906.

SMITH, P.* A PEDIGREE OF DOYNE'S DISCOID CATARACT. TRANS. OPHTHAL. SOC. U.K.
30* 37-42, 1910.

*11630 CATARACT, NUCLEAR DIFFUSE NON-PROGRESSIVE

OPACITY IS LIMITED TO THE FETAL NUCLEUS, RESEMBLES THAT OF SENILE NUCLEAR
SCLEROSIS, AND IS NON-PROGRESSIVE. VOGT (1931) AND WEBER (1940) DOCUMENTED
DOMINANT INHERITANCE.

VOGT, A.* LEHRBUCH UND ATLAS DER SPALTLAMPENMIKROSKOPIE DES LEBENDEN AUGES.
LINSE UND ZONULA. BERLIN* J. SPRINGER, 1931.

WEBER, E.* WEITERE UNTERSUCHUNGEN UBER DEN KONGENITALEN, VERERBTEN KERNSTAR
(CATARACTA NUCLEARIS DIFFUSA CONGENITA HEREDITARIA VOGT). SCHWEIZ. MED. WSCHR.
70* 295-297, 1940.

*11640 CATARACT, NUCLEAR TOTAL

THIS IS ONE OF THE MOST FREQUENT TYPES OF SEVERE CONGENITAL CATARACT WHICH
INTERFERES SERIOUSLY WITH VISION. DOMINANT PEDIGREES WERE REPORTED BY BROWN
(1924), PARROW (1955) AND OTHERS.

BROWN, A. L.* HEREDITARY CATARACT. AM. J. OPHTHAL. 7* 36-38, 1924.

PARROW, R. D.* HEREDITARY CATARACT IN TWO FAMILIES. ACTA PAEDIAT. 44* 460-464,
1955.

11650 CATARACT, OPACITY OF THE SUTURES (STELLATE, CORALLIFORM)

JORDAN (1955) OBSERVED 24 AFFECTED PERSONS IN 3 GENERATIONS.

JORDAN, M.* STAMMBAUMUNTERSUCHUNGEN BEI CATARACTA STELLATA CORALLIFORMIS.
KLIN. MBL. AUGENHEILK. 126* 469-475, 1955.

11660 CATARACT, POSTERIOR POLAR

TULLOH (1955) DESCRIBED 15 AFFECTED IN 5 GENERATIONS. VALK AND BINKHORST (1956)
DESCRIBED ASSOCIATED CHOROIDEREMIA AND MYOPIA IN 2 GENERATIONS. IN NETTLESHIP'S
FAMILY (1909, 1912) CONGENITAL POSTERIOR POLAR OPACITIES WERE PRESENT AND
SCATTERED CORTICAL OPACITIES APPEARED IN CHILDHOOD AND PROGRESSED TO TOTAL
CATARACT.

NETTLESHIP, E.* A PEDIGREE OF PRESENILE OR JUVENILE CATARACT. TRANS. OPHTHAL.
SOC. U.K. 32* 337-352, 1912.

NETTLESHIP, E.* SEVEN NEW PEDIGREES OF HEREDITARY CATARACT. TRANS. OPHTHAL.
SOC. U.K. 29* 188-211, 1909.

TULLOH, C. G.* HEREDITY OF POSTERIOR POLAR CATARACT WITH REPORT OF A PEDIGREE.
BRIT. J. OPHTHAL. 39* 374-379, 1955.

VALK, L. E. M. AND BINKHORST, P. G.* A CASE OF FAMILIAL DWARFISM, WITH
CHOROIDEREMIA, MYOPIA, POSTERIOR POLAR CATARACT AND ZONULAR CATARACT. OPHTHALMO-
LOGICA 132* 299 ONLY, 1956.

11670 CATARACT, TOTAL CONGENITAL

MEISSNER (1933) REPORTED 22 CASES IN 6 GENERATIONS OF ONE FAMILY AND 13 IN FIVE
GENERATIONS IN A SECOND. THREE GENERATIONS WERE AFFECTED IN THE FAMILY REPORTED
BY JAHNS (1938).

JAHNS, H.* ANGEBORENER STAR IN DREI GENERATIONEN. KLIN. MBL. AUGENHEILK. 100*
481-482, 1938.

MEISSNER, M.* AUGENARZTLICHES AUS DEM BLINDENINSTITUT. Z. AUGENHEILK. 80* 48-
58, 1933.

*11680 CATARACT, ZONULAR (PERINUCLEAR OR LAMELLAR)

STRIKING PEDIGREES WERE PRESENTED BY CRIDLAND (1918), HILBERT (1912), JANKIEWICZ AND FREEBERG (1956), KEIZER (1952), KNAPP (1926), AND MARNER (1949), AMONG OTHERS. IN MARNER'S FAMILY, 132 IN 8 GENERATIONS WERE AFFECTED, MAINLY BY ZONULAR CATARACT BUT SOME BY NUCLEAR, ANTERIOR POLAR, OR STELLATE CATARACT. THE OPACITIES WERE PROGRESSIVE AND 'ANTICIPATION' WAS SUGGESTED. IN HARMAN'S FAMILY (1910), MALFORMATION OF THE FINGERS WAS ASSOCIATED.

CRIDLAND, A. B.* THREE CASES OF HEREDITARY CORTICAL CATARACT, WITH A CHART SHOWING THE PEDIGREE OF A FAMILY IN WHICH THEY OCCURRED. TRANS. OPHTHAL. SOC. U.K. 38* 375-376, 1918.

HARMAN, N. B.* CONGENITAL CATARACT. IN, TREASURY OF HUMAN INHERITANCE. LONDON* CAMBRIDGE UNIV. PRESS, 1* (PART 4) 126-169, 1910.

HILBERT, R.* SCHICHTSTARBILDUNG DURCH VIER GENERATIONEN EINER FAMILIE. MUNCHEN. MED. WSCHR. 59* 1272-1273, 1912.

JANKIEWICZ, H. AND FREEBERG, D. D.* A SIX GENERATION PEDIGREE OF CONGENITAL ZONULAR CATARACT. AM. J. OPTOM. 33* 555-557, 1956.

KEIZER, D. P. R.* CONGENITALE CATARACT. NEDERL. T. GENEESK. 96* 763-765, 1952.

KNAPP, F. N.* FAMILIAL CATARACT* A STUDY THROUGH FIVE GENERATIONS. AM. J. OPHTHAL. 9* 683-684, 1926.

MARNER, E.* A FAMILY WITH EIGHT GENERATIONS OF HEREDITARY CATARACT. ACTA OPHTHAL. 27* 537-551, 1949.

11690 CELIAC SPRUE

MCDONALD, DOBBINS AND RUBIN (1965) SUGGESTED THAT THE MECHANISM OF INHERITANCE IS AUTOSOMAL DOMINANT WITH INCOMPLETE PENETRANCE. THE MATTER WAS EXTENSIVELY REVIEWED BY FREZAL AND REY (1970) WHO CONCLUDED THAT MENDELISM IS UNLIKELY. FAMILIAL AGGREGATION IS UNDOUBTED. OF THREE PAIRS OF CAREFULLY STUDIED IDENTICAL TWINS ONLY ONE WAS CONCORDANT. THE AUTHORS THOUGHT THIS MADE A SINGLE-GENE HYPOTHESIS UNLIKELY, ESPECIALLY IN VIEW OF THE INVARIABLE ANATOMIC RELAPSE ON RE-EXPOSURE TO GLUTEN, EVEN WITHOUT CLINICAL OR BIOCHEMICAL SIGNS.

FREZAL, J. AND REY, J.* GENETICS OF DISORDERS OF INTESTINAL DIGESTION AND ABSORPTION. IN, HARRIS, H. AND HIRSCHHORN, K. (EDS.)* ADVANCES IN HUMAN GENETICS 1* 275-336, 1970.

MCDONALD, W. C., DOBBINS, W. O., III AND RUBIN, C. E.* STUDIES OF THE FAMILIAL NATURE OF CELIAC SPRUE USING BIOPSY OF THE SMALL INTESTINE. NEW ENG. J. MED. 272* 448-456, 1965.

*11700 CENTRAL CORE DISEASE OF MUSCLE

THIS DISORDER WAS FIRST DESCRIBED IN 1956 BY SHY AND MAGEE ALTHOUGH THE NAME WAS NOT GIVEN THE ENTITY UNTIL LATER. FIVE PERSONS IN FIVE DIFFERENT SIBSHIPS IN THREE GENERATIONS OF THE ORIGINAL FAMILY WERE AFFECTED. IN THE FAMILY STUDIED BY ENGEL ET AL. (1961) ONLY THE PROBAND HAD CLINICAL MANIFESTATIONS BUT HIS FATHER HAD THE SAME BIOCHEMICAL ABNORMALITY OF MUSCLE, NAMELY, ONE INVOLVING THE LIBERATION OF PHOSPHATE FROM GLUCOSE-6-PHOSPHATE. CENTRAL CORE DISEASE IS ONE OF THE CONDITIONS WHICH PRODUCES THE 'FLOPPY INFANT' (AMYOTONIA CONGENITA OF OPPENHEIM). NEMALINE MYOPATHY (Q.V.) AND CENTRAL CORE DISEASE HAVE BEEN DESCRIBED IN THE SAME FAMILY AND INDEED IN THE SAME PATIENT (AFIFI, SMITH, ZELLWEGER, 1965). IT IS POSSIBLE THAT THE 'CENTRAL CORE' MORPHOLOGIC CHANGE IS NON-SPECIFIC, I.E., MAY OCCUR WITH OTHER TYPES OF MYOPATHY IN ADDITION TO THE SPECIFIC ENTITY TO WHICH THE NAME CAN BE APPLIED. BETHLEM ET AL. (1966) DESCRIBED A NON-PROGRESSIVE MYOPATHY IN 3 FEMALES OF THREE SUCCESSIVE GENERATIONS. THE FATHER OF THE EARLIEST PATIENT MAY HAVE BEEN AFFECTED. HISTOLOGICAL FINDINGS OF CENTRAL CORE DISEASE WERE FOUND. MUSCLE CRAMPS FOLLOWED EXERCISE AND NO HYPOTONIA WAS PRESENT IN INFANCY - FEATURES DIFFERENT FROM PREVIOUSLY REPORTED CASES OF CENTRAL CORE DISEASE. CREATINE EXCRETION IN THE URINE WAS GREATLY INCREASED. CREATINE KINASE AND OXIDATIVE PHOSPHORYLATION IN THE MUSCLES WERE NORMAL. DUBOWITZ AND ROY (1970) DESCRIBED 4 CASES IN 3 GENERATIONS. THE DISORDERS CONSISTED OF SLOWLY PROGRESSIVE WEAKNESS SINCE THE AGE OF 5 YEARS RESEMBLING LIMB GIRDLE MUSCULAR DYSTROPHY. ONLY TYPE 1 MUSCLE FIBERS SHOWED CENTRAL CORES.

AFIFI, A. K., SMITH, J. W. AND ZELLWEGER, H.* CONGENITAL NONPROGRESSIVE MYOPATHY. CENTRAL CORE DISEASE AND NEMALINE MYOPATHY IN ONE FAMILY. NEUROLOGY 15* 371-381, 1965.

BETHLEM, J., VAN GOOL, J., HULSMANN, W. C. AND MEIJER, A. E. F. H.* FAMILIAL NON-PROGRESSIVE MYOPATHY WITH MUSCLE CRAMPS AFTER EXERCISE. A NEW DISEASE ASSOCIATED WITH CORES IN THE MUSCLE FIBRES. BRAIN 89* 569-588, 1966.

DUBOWITZ, V. AND ROY, S.* CENTRAL CORE DISEASE OF MUSCLE* CLINICAL, HISTOCHEMI-CAL AND ELECTRON MICROSCOPIC STUDIES OF AN AFFECTED MOTHER AND CHILD. BRAIN 93* 133-146, 1970.

ENGEL, W. K., FOSTER, J. B., HUGHES, B. P., HUXLEY, H. E. AND MAHLER, R.*
CENTRAL CORE DISEASE - AN INVESTIGATION OF A RARE MUSCLE CELL ABNORMALITY. BRAIN
84* 167-185, 1961.

SHY, G. M. AND MAGEE, K. R.* A NEW CONGENITAL NON-PROGRESSIVE MYOPATHY. BRAIN
79* 610-621, 1956.

SHY, G. M., ENGEL, W. K. AND WANKO, T.* CENTRAL CORE DISEASE* A MYOFIBRILLARY
AND MITOCHONDRIAL ABNORMALITY OF MUSCLE. ANN. INTERN. MED. 56* 511-520, 1962.

*11710 CENTRALOPATHIC EPILEPSY

METRAKOS AND METRAKOS (1961) CONCLUDED THAT THE CENTRENCEPHALIC TYPE OF ELECTROEN-
CEPHALOGRAM (ASSOCIATED WITH 'CENTRALOPATHIC EPILEPSY') IS AN EXPRESSION OF AN
AUTOSOMAL DOMINANT GENE, WITH THE UNUSUAL CHARACTERISTICS OF A VERY LOW PENETRANCE
AT BIRTH, A RAPID RISE TO NEARLY COMPLETE PENETRANCE FOR AGES 4 AND HALF TO 16 AND
HALF YEARS, AND A GRADUAL DECLINE TO ALMOST NO PENETRANCE AFTER THE AGE OF 40 AND
HALF YEARS. IN THIS FORM OF EPILEPSY SEIZURES OF VARYING CLINICAL APPEARANCE ARE
ASSOCIATED WITH PAROXYSMAL, DIFFUSE, BILATERAL SYNCHRONOUS SPIKE-WAVE EEG
ABNORMALITIES. FROM A FAMILY STUDY METRAKOS AND METRAKOS (1961) CONCLUDED THAT
INHERITANCE IS AUTOSOMAL DOMINANT. ALTHOUGH THEIR STUDIES DID NOT LEAD THEM TO A
DEFINITE DOMINANT HYPOTHESIS, BRAY AND WISER (1964, 1965) PRESENTED EVIDENCE FOR A
GENETIC BASIS OF ONE FORM OF TEMPORAL LOBE EPILEPSY.

BRAY, P. F. AND WISER, W. C.* EVIDENCE FOR A GENETIC ETIOLOGY OF TEMPORAL-
CENTRAL ABNORMALITIES IN FOCAL EPILEPSY. NEW ENG. J. MED. 271* 926-933, 1964.

BRAY, P. F. AND WISER, W. C.* HEREDITARY CHARACTERISTICS OF FAMILIAL TEMPORAL-
CENTRAL FOCAL EPILEPSY. PEDIATRICS 36* 207-211, 1965.

METRAKOS, K. AND METRAKOS, J. D.* GENETICS OF CONVULSIVE DISORDERS. II.
GENETIC AND ELECTROENCEPHALOGRAPHIC STUDIES IN CENTRENCEPHALIC EPILEPSY.
NEUROLOGY 11* 474-483, 1961.

11720 CEREBELLAR ATAXIA

THE SPINOCEREBELLAR ATAXIAS REPRESENT A NOSOLOGICALLY CONFUSED CATEGORY.
FRIEDREICH'S ATAXIA IS CLEARLY A RECESSIVE DISORDER. SO-CALLED MARIE'S ATAXIA IS
CHARACTERIZED BY LATE-ONSET AND DOMINANT INHERITANCE. IT PROBABLY IS A HETERO-
GENEOUS CATEGORY ENCOMPASSING SEVERAL OF THE CONDITIONS LISTED HERE AS SEPARATE
DISORDERS UNDER THE GENERAL HEADING OF EITHER OLIVOPONTOCEREBELLAR ATROPHY (Q.V.)
OR CEREBELLAR PARENCHYMAL DISORDER (Q.V.). SEE ALSO SPINO-PONTINE ATROPHY.
NOSOLOGIC AND GENETIC STUDIES OF THE ATAXIAS INCLUDE THOSE OF SJOGREN (1943).
NOSOLOGIC STUDIES BASED ON PATHOLOGIC FINDINGS WERE DONE BY GREENFIELD (1954).
THE MOST EXTENSIVE RECENT NOSOLOGIC STUDIES HAVE BEEN THOSE OF KONIGSMARK AND HIS
COLLEAGUES, WHO HAVE INSISTED ON HISTOPATHOLOGIC STUDIES BEFORE THEY ATTEMPTED TO
CATEGORIZE A GIVEN FAMILY EITHER REPORTED OR IN THEIR OWN EXPERIENCE.

GREENFIELD, J. G.* THE SPINO-CEREBELLAR DEGENERATIONS. OXFORD* BLACKWELL,
1954.

SJOGREN, T.* KLINISCHE UND ERBBIOLOGISCHE UNTERSUCHUNGEN UBER DIE HEREDOATA-
XIEN. ACTA PSYCHIAT. NEUROL. SCAND. 27 (SUPPL.)* 1-200, 1943.

*11730 CEREBELLAR ATAXIA, ACUTE INTERMITTENT FAMILIAL

HILL AND SHERMAN (1968) DESCRIBED ACUTE SELF-LIMITED INTERMITTENT CEREBELLAR
ATAXIA IN AT LEAST 35 MEMBERS IN 5 GENERATIONS OF A NEGRO FAMILY. PRESUMABLY THIS
IS DIFFERENT FROM PERIODIC VESTIBULO-CEREBELLAR ATAXIA (Q.V.) IN WHICH THE ATTACKS
OCCUR MAINLY IN EARLY ADULTHOOD RATHER THAN CHILDHOOD AND SLOWLY PROGRESSIVE,
IRREVERSIBLE SYMPTOMS DEVELOP IN SOME PATIENTS.

HILL, W. AND SHERMAN, H.* ACUTE INTERMITTENT FAMILIAL CEREBELLAR ATAXIA. ARCH.
NEUROL. 18* 350-357, 1968.

11740 CEREBELLO-PARENCHYMAL DISORDER I (CPD I CEREBELLO-OLIVARY ATROPHY)

THE DISORDERS INVOLVING PRIMARILY THE CEREBELLAR PARENCHYMA HAVE BEEN CLASSED INTO
SIX FORMS BY WEINER AND KONIGSMARK (1971). IT IS THEIR CLASSIFICATION WHICH IS
FOLLOWED HERE. CPA I IS CHARACTERIZED BY LATE ONSET (FIFTH OR SIXTH DECADE), WITH
UNSTEADINESS OF GAIT AND SPEECH DIFFICULTIES AND PROGRESSIVE DEMENTIA. PATHOLOGI-
CALLY THERE IS MARKED LOSS OF PURKINJE CELLS, ESPECIALLY IN THE SUPERIOR CEREBEL-
LUM. PRESERVATION OF THE PONTINE NUCLEI AND FIBERS DISTINGUISH IT FROM THE
OLIVOPONTOCEREBELLAR ATROPHIES OF WHICH FIVE TYPES ARE DESCRIBED ELSEWHERE.
AFFECTED FAMILIES HAVE BEEN DESCRIBED BY HALL ET AL. (1941), RICHTER (1950), WEBER
AND GREENFIELD (1942) AND OTHERS.

HALL, B., NOAD, K. B. AND LATHAM, O.* FAMILIAL CORTICAL CEREBELLAR ATROPHY.
BRAIN 64* 178-194, 1941.

RICHTER, R. B.* LATE CORTICAL CEREBELLAR ATROPHY. A FORM OF HEREDITARY
CEREBELLAR ATAXIA. AM. J. HUM. GENET. 2* 1-29, 1950.

WEBER, F. P. AND GREENFIELD, J. G.* CEREBELLO-OLIVARY DEGENERATION* AN EXAMPLE OF HEREDO-FAMILIAL INCIDENCE. BRAIN 65* 220-231, 1942.

WEINER, L. P. AND KONIGSMARK, B. W.* HEREDITARY DISEASE OF THE CEREBELLAR PARENCHYMA. THE CLINICAL DELINEATION OF BIRTH DEFECTS. VI. THE NERVOUS SYSTEM. BALTIMORE* WILLIAMS AND WILKINS, 1970.

11750 CEREBELLO-PARENCHYMAL DISORDER VI (CPA VI* CEREBELLAR GRANULE CELL HYPERTROPHY AND MEGALENCEPHALY)

MENTAL DULLNESS AND IN SOME CASES SIGNS OF INCREASED INTRACRANIAL PRESSURE ARE FEATURES. THE LATTER IS THE RESULT OF HERNIATION OF THE CEREBELLAR TONSILS. FIRST DESCRIBED BY LHERMITTE AND DUCLOS (1920), A TOTAL OF 35 CASES HAVE BEEN REPORTED, ACCORDING TO AMBLER ET AL. (1969), WHO DESCRIBED THE DISORDER IN MOTHER AND SON.

AMBLER, M., POGACAR, S. AND SIDMAN, R.* LHERMITTE-DUCLOS DISEASE (GRANULE CELL HYPERTROPHY OF THE CEREBELLUM)* PATHOLOGICAL ANALYSIS OF THE FIRST FAMILIAL CASES. J. NEUROPATH. EXP. NEUROL. 28* 622-647, 1969.

LHERMITTE, J. AND DUCLOS, P.* SUR UN GANGLIONEUROME DIFFUS DU CORTEX DU CERVELET. BULL. ASSOC. FRANC. CANCER 9* 99, 1920.

*11770 CERULOPLASMIN ELECTROPHORETIC VARIANTS

AT LEAST THREE VARIANTS DETERMINED BY CO-DOMINANT ALLELES HAVE BEEN IDENTIFIED BY STARCH GEL ELECTROPHORESIS (SHREFFLER ET AL., 1967). POLYMORPHISM HAS BEEN FOUND MAINLY IN THE AMERICAN NEGRO.

MCCOMBS, M. L. AND BOWMAN, B. H.* DEMONSTRATION OF INHERITED CERULOPLASMIN VARIANTS IN HUMAN SERUM BY ACRYLAMIDE ELECTROPHORESIS. TEXAS REP. BIOL. MED. 27* 769-772, 1969.

MCCOMBS, M. L., BOWMAN, B. H. AND ALPERIN, J. B.* A NEW CERULOPLASMIN VARIANT, CP GALVESTON. CLIN. GENET. 1* 30-34, 1970.

POULIK, M. D.* HETEROGENEITY AND STRUCTURE OF CERULOPLASMIN. ANN. N.Y. ACAD. SCI. 151* 476-501, 1968.

SHOKEIR, M. H. K. AND SHREFFLER, D. C.* TWO NEW CERULOPLASMIN VARIANTS IN NEGROES - DATA ON THREE POPULATIONS. BIOCHEM. GENET. 4* 517-528, 1970.

SHOKEIR, M. H., SHREFFLER, D. C. AND GALL, J. C., JR.* FURTHER ELECTROPHORETIC VARIATION IN HUMAN CERULOPLASMIN. MEETING, AM. SOC. HUM. GENET., TORONTO, DEC. 1-3, 1967.

SHREFFLER, D. C., BREWER, G. J., GALL, J. C. AND HONEYMAN, M. S.* ELECTROPHORE-TIC VARIATION IN HUMAN SERUM CERULOPLASMIN* A NEW GENETIC POLYMORPHISM. BIOCHEM. GENET. 1* 101-116, 1967.

*11780 CERUMEN, VARIATION IN

IN JAPANESE MATSUNAGA (1962) DESCRIBED A DIMORPHISM OF EAR WAX, THE TWO TYPES BEING WET AND DRY. THIS VARIATION HAS BEEN STUDIED EXTENSIVELY IN JAPAN SINCE AT LEAST 1934. LESS ATTENTION HAS BEEN GIVEN TO THIS VARIATION ELSEWHERE, PROBABLY BECAUSE CAUCASIANS AND NEGROES HAVE ONE TYPE OF CERUMEN, WET. IN 80-85 PERCENT OF JAPANESE THE CERUMEN IS GREY, DRY AND BRITTLE. IT IS REFERRED TO AS *RICE-BRAN EAR WAX* IN JAPANESE. IN THE OTHER JAPANESE THE CERUMEN IS BROWN, STICKY AND WET. THIS IS REFERRED TO AS *HONEY EAR WAX,* *OILY EAR WAX* OR *CAT EAR WAX.* IN ALL EXCEPT ABOUT 0.5 PERCENT OF JAPANESE CLASSIFICATION IS SIMPLE. FAMILY STUDIES INDICATE MONOFACTORIAL INHERITANCE, WITH THE RARER PHENOTYPE, WET WAX, BEING DOMINANT. WET CERUMEN IS OFTEN ASSOCIATED WITH AXILLARY ODOR, WHICH IN JAPAN BECAUSE OF ITS RARITY IS CONSIDERED IN THE LAY MIND A PATHOLOGIC STATE REQUIRING MEDICAL ATTENTION. PETRAKIS ET AL. (1967) FOUND A HIGH FREQUENCY OF DRY CERUMEN IN PURE-BLOODED AMERICAN INDIANS. NO QUALITATIVE DIFFERENCES IN CHEMICAL COMPOSITION HAVE BEEN IDENTIFIED (KATAURA AND KATAURA, 1967).

KATAURA, A. AND KATAURA, K.* THE COMPARISON OF FREE AND BOUND AMINO ACIDS BETWEEN DRY AND WET TYPES OF CERUMEN. TOHOKU J. EXP. MED. 91* 215-225, 1967.

KATAURA, A. AND KATAURA, K.* THE COMPARISON OF LIPIDS BETWEEN DRY AND WET TYPES OF CERUMEN. TOHOKU J. EXP. MED. 91* 227-237, 1967.

MARTIN, L. M. AND JACKSON, J. F.* CERUMEN TYPES IN CHOCTAW INDIANS. SCIENCE 163* 677-678, 1969.

MATSUNAGA, E.* THE DIMORPHISM IN HUMAN NORMAL CERUMEN. ANN. HUM. GENET. 25* 273-286, 1962.

PETRAKIS, N. L., MOLOHAN, K. T. AND TEPPER, D. J.* CERUMEN IN AMERICAN INDIANS* GENETIC IMPLICATIONS OF STICKY AND DRY TYPES. SCIENCE 158* 1192-1193, 1967.

WESTON (1956) FOUND CERVICAL RIBS OR ENLARGED TRANSVERSE PROCESSES IN 14 OF 20 MEMBERS OF A FAMILY. THE ANOMALY WAS PARTICULARLY STRIKING AMONG THE OFFSPRING OF TWO AFFECTED PARENTS, RAISING THE QUESTION OF HOMOZYGOSITY.

WESTON, W. J.* GENETICALLY DETERMINED CERVICAL RIBS* A FAMILY STUDY. BRIT. J. RADIOL. 29* 455-456, 1956.

11800 CERVICAL VERTEBRAL BRIDGE

THE PRESENCE OF A BONY BRIDGE ON THE FIRST CERVICAL VERTEBRA, ROOFING THE GROOVE OCCUPIED BY THE VERTEBRAL ARTERY, BEHAVES AS A DOMINANT TRAIT. THE GENE HAS A FREQUENCY OF ABOUT 0.15.

SELBY, S., GARN, S. M. AND KANAREFF, V.* THE INCIDENCE AND FAMILIAL NATURE OF A BONY BRIDGE ON THE FIRST CERVICAL VERTEBRA. AM. J. PHYS. ANTHROP. 13* 129-141, 1955.

*11810 CERVICAL VERTEBRAL FUSION

C2-C3 FUSION IS THE MOST COMMON FORM OF CONGENITAL FUSED CERVICAL VERTEBRAE AND IS PROBABLY DOMINANT WITH VARIABLE EXPRESSION. THE BEST EVIDENCE FOR DOMINANT INHERITANCE WAS PROVIDED BY GUNDERSON ET AL. (1967).

GUNDERSON, C. H. AND LUBS, H. A.* FAMILIAL C2-3 FUSION. (ABSTRACT) NEUROLOGY 14* 272-273, 1964.

GUNDERSON, C. H., GREENSPAN, R. H., GLASER, G. H. AND LUBS, H. A.* THE KLIPPEL-FEIL SYNDROME* GENETIC AND CLINICAL REEVALUATION OF CERVICAL FUSION. MEDICINE 46* 491-512, 1967.

*11820 CHARCOT-MARIE-TOOTH DISEASE

THIS IS ONE OF THE ENTITIES WHICH, LIKE SPASTIC PARAPLEGIA AND RETINITIS PIGMENTO-SA, DEMONSTRATES AUTOSOMAL DOMINANT INHERITANCE IN SOME FAMILIES, AUTOSOMAL RECESSIVE INHERITANCE IN OTHERS AND X-LINKED RECESSIVE INHERITANCE IN YET OTHERS. NORSTRAND AND MARGULIES (1958) OBSERVED AFFECTED MEMBERS IN THREE GENERATIONS. GASTROINTESTINAL SYMPTOMS IN THE FORM OF CHRONIC DIARRHEA, NAUSEA AND VOMITING WERE STRIKING. AUTOPSY SHOWED DEGENERATION IN THE LATERAL HORN AREA OF THE SPINAL CORD. STARK (1958) DESCRIBED A LARGE AFFECTED KINDRED. WE HAVE OBSERVED ELEVATED CEREBROSPINAL FLUID PROTEIN, HYPERHIDROSIS AND PENETRATING FOOT ULCERS IN A CASE OF THE DOMINANT FORM. THIS DISORDER BEGINS WITH ATROPHY AND WEAKNESS OF THE PERONEAL MUSCLES AND ADVANCES INSIDIOUSLY TO INVOLVE OTHER DISTAL MUSCLES OF THE LEG AND ARM. DEEP TENDON REFLEXES ARE DIMINISHED OR ABSENT AND PES CAVUS IS COMMONLY FOUND. IN THE FAMILY REPORTED FIRST IN THE LAY PRESS BY VERRILL AND FOLLOWED UP BY ENGLAND AND DENNY-BROWN (1952) MEMBERS HAD SENSORY AND TROPHIC CHANGES IN ADDITION TO CLASSIC PERONEAL MUSCULAR ATROPHY. MOST HAVE SOME SENSORY DEFECT AND THIS IS NOT SURPRISING IN VIEW OF THE FACT THAT THIS IS A NEUROPATHY. INDEED, A CASE CAN BE MADE FOR REFERRING TO THE SEVERAL FORMS OF CHARCOT-MARIE-TOOTH DISEASE AS HEREDITARY POLYNEUROPATHIES. CHARCOT'S DESCRIPTION WAS REPRINTED BY BRODY AND WILKINS (1967). THE PHENOMENAL CASE OF A WOMAN WHO WAS A PATIENT IN LA SALPETRIERE, PARIS, FOR 64 YEARS WAS REPORTED BY ALAJOUANINE ET AL. (1967). THE DIAGNOSIS WAS MADE BY CHARCOT IN 1891. SHE DIED AT AGE 80 YEARS. ARGYLL-ROBERTSON PUPILS AND BLINDNESS FROM OPTIC ATROPHY BEGAN 40-50 YEARS AFTER ONSET OF OTHER SIGNS OF DISEASE. WHETHER THIS WAS A SPORADIC CASE OF THE RECESSIVE FORM (WHICH THE AUTHORS FAVORED) OR A NEW MUTANT FOR THE DOMINANT FORM WAS UNCERTAIN. BRADLEY AND AGUAYO (1969) DESCRIBED A FAMILY IN WHICH PERSONS IN 3 GENERATIONS HAD CHRONIC SENSORINEURAL POLYNEUROPATHY.

ALAJOUANINE, T., CASTAIGNE, P., CAMBIER, J. AND ESCOUROLLE, R.* MALADIE DE CHARCOT-MARIE. ETUDE ANATOMO-CLINIQUE D'UNE OBSERVATION SUIVIE PENDANT 65 ANS. PRESSE MED. 75* 2745-2750, 1967.

BRADLEY, W. G. AND AGUAYO, A.* HEREDITARY CHRONIC POLYNEUROPATHY. ELECTROPHY-SIOLOGICAL AND PATHOLOGICAL STUDIES IN AN AFFECTED FAMILY. J. NEUROL. SCI. 9* 131-154, 1969.

BRODY, I. A. AND WILKINS, R. H.* CHARCOT-MARIE-TOOTH DISEASE. ARCH. NEUROL. 17* 552-553, 1967.

DAVIDENKOW, S.* UBER DIE NEUROTISCHE MUSKELATROPHIE CHARCOT-MARIE* KLINISCH-GENETISCHE STUDIEN. ZBL. GES. NEUROL. PSYCHIAT. 107* 259, 1927, AND 108* 344, 1927.

DYCK, P. J.* HISTOLOGIC MEASUREMENTS AND FINE STRUCTURE OF BIOPSIED SURAL NERVE* NORMAL, AND IN PERONEAL MUSCULAR ATROPHY, HYPERTROPHIC NEUROPATHY, AND CONGENITAL SENSORY NEUROPATHY. MAYO CLIN. PROC. 41* 742-774, 1966.

DYCK, P. J., LAMBERT, E. H. AND MULDER, D. W.* CHARCOT-MARIE-TOOTH DISEASE* NERVE CONDUCTION AND CLINICAL STUDIES OF A LARGE KINSHIP. NEUROLOGY 13* 1-11, 1963.

ENGLAND, A. C. AND DENNY-BROWN, D.* SENSORY CHANGES, AND TROPHIC DISORDER, IN PERONEAL MUSCULAR ATROPHY (CHARCOT-MARIE-TOOTH TYPE). ARCH. NEUROL. PSYCHIAT. 67* 1-22, 1952.

LUCAS, G. J. AND FORSTER, F. M.* CHARCOT-MARIE-TOOTH DISEASE WITH ASSOCIATED MYOPATHY* A REPORT OF A FAMILY. NEUROLOGY 12* 629-636, 1962.

MACKLIN, M. T. AND BOWMAN, J. T.* INHERITANCE OF PERONEAL ATROPHY. J.A.M.A. 86* 613-617, 1926.

NORSTRAND, I. F. AND MARGULIES, M. E.* PERIPHERAL NEURONOPATHY (CHARCOT-MARIE-TOOTH DISEASE) IN ASSOCIATION WITH GASTROINTESTINAL SYMPTOMS. NEW YORK J. MED. 58* 863-867, 1958.

STARK, P.* ETUDE CLINIQUE ET GENETIQUE D*UNE FAMILLE ATTEINTE D*ATROPHIE MUSCULAIRE PROGRESSIVE NEURALE (AMYOTROPHIE DE CHARCOT-MARIE). J. GENET. HUM. 7* 1-32, 1958.

11830 CHARCOT-MARIE-TOOTH DISEASE AND NEPHRITIS

LEMIEUX AND NEEMEH (1967) DESCRIBED TWO FAMILIES EACH WITH MULTIPLE CASES OF C-M-T DISEASE. IN TWO OF ONE FAMILY AND ONE OF THE OTHER CHRONIC NEPHRITIS WAS ALSO PRESENT. FOAM CELLS WERE SEEN IN THE INTERSTITIUM IN ONE AND TWO OF THE THREE HAD NERVE DEAFNESS. A NON-SPECIFIC POLYNEUROPATHY, DUE POSSIBLY TO CHRONIC UREMIA, HAS BEEN OBSERVED WITH ALPORT*S SYNDROME. THE NEUROLOGIC DISORDER IN THE CASES OF LEMIEUX AND NEEMEH (1967) WAS FULL-BLOOM C-M-T DISEASE. AMYLOIDOSIS, A CAUSE OF NEPHRITIS AND A CONDITION MIS-DIAGNOSED AS C-M-T DISEASE, WAS APPARENTLY EXCLUDED.

LEMIEUX, G. AND NEEMEH, J. A.* CHARCOT-MARIE-TOOTH DISEASE AND NEPHRITIS. CANAD. MED. ASS. J. 97* 1193-1198, 1967.

*11840 CHERUBISM (FAMILIAL FIBROUS DYSPLASIA OF THE JAWS)

SWELLING OF THE LOWER FACE BEGINS IN THE FIRST YEARS OF LIFE AND PROGRESSES UNTIL THE LATE TEENS. THE ENLARGEMENT IS EXAGGERATED BY ENLARGEMENT OF SUBMANDIBULAR LYMPH NODES. X-RAY REVEALS MULTILOCULAR CYSTIC CHANGES IN THE MANDIBLE AND MAXILLA AND OFTEN IN THE ANTERIOR ENDS OF THE RIBS. THE CONDITION MUST BE DIFFERENTIATED FROM CAFFEY*S DISEASE (Q.V.) IN WHICH THE X-RAY APPEARANCE IS DIFFERENT AND INVOLVEMENT OF THE SKELETON, E.G., THE TIBIA, IS MORE WIDESPREAD. IT IS, LIKE CAFFEY*S DISEASE, A BENIGN SELF-LIMITED CONDITION TREATED BY SIMPLE CURETTAGE. THE CONDITION HAS ALSO BEEN CALLED FAMILIAL BENIGN GIANT-CELL TUMOR OF THE JAW, FAMILIAL MULTILOCULAR CYSTIC DISEASE OF THE JAW, ETC. JONES (1965) POINTED OUT THAT LACK OF SIGNS OR HISTORY IN EITHER PARENT DOES NOT EXCLUDE THE POSSIBILITY OF ONE BEING AFFECTED. IN ONE OF HIS CASES (HE WAS THE FIRST TO DESCRIBE THE ENTITY) THE DISORDER WOULD NOT HAVE BEEN DISCOVERED, OR EVEN SUSPECTED, WERE IT NOT THAT X-RAYS WERE MADE IN CHILDHOOD IN A DELIBERATE SEARCH FOR THE ENTITY BECAUSE OF ITS OCCURRENCE IN OTHER MEMBERS OF THE FAMILY. SEE FIBRO-OSSEOUS DYSPLASIA OF JAWS.

ANDERSON, D. E. AND MCCLENDON, J. L.* CHERUBISM-HEREDITARY FIBROUS DYSPLASIA OF THE JAWS. I. GENETIC CONSIDERATIONS. ORAL SURG. 15* (SUPPL. 2) 5-16, 1962.

BURLAND, J. G.* CHERUBISM* FAMILIAL BILATERAL OSSEOUS DYSPLASIA OF THE JAWS. ORAL SURG. 15 (SUPPL. 2)* 43-68, 1962.

JONES, W. A.* CHERUBISM* A THUMBNAIL SKETCH OF ITS DIAGNOSIS AND A CONSERVATIVE METHOD OF TREATMENT. ORAL SURG. 20* 648-653, 1965.

KHOSLA, V. M. AND KOROBKIN, M.* CHERUBISM. AM. J. DIS. CHILD. 120* 458-461, 1970.

SALZANO, F. M. AND EBLING, H.* CHERUBISM IN A BRAZILIAN KINDRED. ACTA GENET. MED. GEM. 15* 296-301, 1966.

THOMPSON, N.* CHERUBISM* FAMILIAL FIBROUS DYSPLASIA OF THE JAWS. BRIT. J. PLAST. SURG. 12* 89-103, 1959.

11850 CHOLINESTERASE, REDUCTION IN RED CELL

GENETIC VARIATIONS IN SERUM CHOLINESTERASE (*PSEUDOCHOLINESTERASE*) ARE DISCUSSED ELSEWHERE. IN A MAN, HIS MOTHER AND HIS SISTER JOHNS (1962) FOUND RED CELL CHOLINESTERASE REDUCED TO ABOUT ONE-THIRD THE NORMAL VALUE. THE PATIENT WAS PERFECTLY HEALTHY. THE *DEFECT* WOULD NOT HAVE BEEN DETECTED WERE IT NOT FOR THE FACT THAT HE WORKED IN A PLANT MANUFACTURING ORGANOPHOSPHOROUS ANTICHOLINESTERASE COMPOUNDS AND WAS TESTED IN CONNECTION WITH THIS EMPLOYMENT.

JOHNS, R. J.* FAMILIAL REDUCTION IN RED CELL CHOLINESTERASE. NEW ENG. J. MED. 267* 1344-1348, 1962.

11860 CHONDROCALCINOSIS (*CALCIUM GOUT*)

THIS IS A CHRONIC ARTICULAR DISEASE CHARACTERIZED BY ACUTE INTERMITTENT ATTACKS OF

ARTHRITIS, BY THE PRESENCE OF CALCIUM HYPOPHOSPHATE CRYSTALS IN SYNOVAL FLUID, CARTILAGE AND PERIARTICULAR SOFT TISSUE AND BY X-RAY EVIDENCE OF CALCIUM DEPOSITION IN ARTICULAR CARTILAGE. THE CONDITION IS SOMETIMES A FEATURE OF HYPERPARATHYROIDISM. A GENETIC BASIS HAS BEEN POSTULATED IN OTHER CASES. ALSO SEE LIPOCALCIGRANULOMATOSIS. UNDER THE DESIGNATION OF CHONDROCALCINOSIS ARTICULARIS, ASSHOFF ET AL. (1966) DESCRIBED A FAMILY WITH FOUR AFFECTED PERSONS IN TWO GENERATIONS. THE DISORDER WAS MANIFESTED CLINICALLY BY EPISODIC INFLAMMATORY INVOLVEMENT, ACUTE OR SUBACUTE, OF ONE OR MORE JOINTS. CALCIFIED HYALINE AND FIBROUS CARTILAGES ARE DEMONSTRABLE BY X-RAY, PARTICULARLY IN LARGE JOINTS. IN ARTICULAR CARTILAGE A DENSE NARROW BAND FOLLOWS THE CONTOUR OF THE EPIPHYSIS. REGINATO ET AL. (1970) OBSERVED AN UNUSUALLY HIGH FREQUENCY AMONG NATIVES OF THE CHILOE ISLAND GROUP. TWENTY-EIGHT PATIENTS WERE OBSERVED OF WHOM 19 WERE AGGREGATED IN SIX KINDREDS. PARENT-CHILD INVOLVEMENT WITH NO MALE-TO-MALE TRANSMISSION WAS OBSERVED IN 3 OF THE FAMILIES. IN THE OTHER 3 FAMILIES ONE OR BOTH PARENTS WERE NOT SCREENED. SINCE THE CHILOTE GROUP LIVES IN AN ISOLATED AREA AND IS PRESUMABLY INBRED, RECESSIVE INHERITANCE REMAINS A POSSIBILITY. IN THESE CASES INVOLVEMENT WAS POLYARTICULAR. ANKYLOSING OF JOINTS WAS A NEW FEATURE OBSERVED IN THIS STUDY. DEPRESSED ACTIVITY OF SYNONIAL PYROPHOSPHOHYDROLASE WAS SUGGESTED BY THE FINDINGS OF GOOD AND STARKWEATHER (1969).

ASSHOFF, H., BOHM, P., SCHOEN, E. AND SCHURHOLZ, K.* HEREDITARE CHONDROCALCINOSIS ARTICULARIS. UNTERSUCHUNG EINER FAMILIE. HUMANGENETIK 3* 98-103, 1966.

GOOD, A. E. AND STARKWEATHER, W. H.* SYNOVIAL FLUID PYROPHOSPHATE PHOSPHOHYDROLASE (PPPH) IN PSEUDOGOUT, GOUT AND RHEUMATOID ARTHRITIS. (ABSTRACT) ARTHRITIS RHEUM. 12* 298 ONLY, 1969.

MCCARTY, D. J., JR. AND HASKIN, M. E.* THE ROENTGENOGRAPHIC ASPECTS OF PSEUDO GOUT (ARTICULAR CHONDROCALCINOSIS). AN ANALYSIS OF 20 CASES. AM. J. ROENTGEN. 90* 1248-1257, 1963.

MCCARTY, D. J., JR., KOHN, N. N. AND FAIRES, J. S.* THE SIGNIFICANCE OF CALCIUM PHOSPHATE CRYSTALS IN THE SYNOVIAL FLUID OF ARTHRITIC PATIENTS. THE 'PSEUDOGOUT SYNDROME.' I. CLINICAL ASPECTS. ANN. INTERN. MED. 56* 711-737, 1962.

MOSKOWITZ, R. AND KATZ, D.* CHONDROCALCINOSIS (PSEUDOGOUT SYNDROME). A FAMILY STUDY. J.A.M.A. 188* 867-871, 1964.

REGINATO, A., VALENZUELA, F., MARTINEZ, V., PASSANO, G. AND DOZA, S.* POLYARTICULAR AND FAMILIAL CHONDROCALCINOSIS. ARTHRITIS RHEUM. 13* 197-213, 1970.

TWIGG, H. L., ZVAIFLER, N. J. AND NELSON, C. W.* CHONDROCALCINOSIS. RADIOLOGY 82* 655-659, 1964.

VALSIK, J., ZITNAN, D. AND SITAJ, S.* ARTICULAR CHONDROCALCINOSIS. II. GENETIC STUDY. ANN. RHEUM. DIS. 22* 153-157, 1963.

*11865 CHONDRODYSPLASIA PUNCTATA (CHONDRODYSTROPHIA CALCIFICANS CONGENITA)

SPRANGER ET AL. (1971) CONCLUDED THAT THE FORM OF CHONDRODYSPLASIA PUNCTATA TO WHICH THE CONRADI-HUNERMANN EPONYM IS APPROPRIATELY APPLIED HAS PREDOMINANTLY EPIPHYSEAL, FREQUENTLY ASYMMETRIC CALCIFICATIONS AND DYSPLASTIC SKELETAL CHANGES, A RELATIVELY GOOD PROGNOSIS AND AUTOSOMAL DOMINANT INHERITANCE. THEY CONCLUDED THAT CATARACTS OCCUR IN ONLY 17 PERCENT OF CASES AS COMPARED WITH A FREQUENCY OF 72 PERCENT IN THE RHIZOMELIC FORM WHICH IS A RECESSIVE AND USUALLY LETHAL IN THE FIRST YEAR OF LIFE. SKIN CHANGES OCCUR IN ABOUT 28 PERCENT OF CASES OF BOTH FORMS. CONDITIONS CONFUSED WITH CHONDRODYSPLASIA PUNCTATA INCLUDE ZELLWEGER'S CEREBROHEPATORENAL SYNDROME AND MULTICENTRIC EPIPHYSEAL OSSIFICATION IN MULTIPLE EPIPHYSEAL DYSPLASIA.

SPRANGER, J. W., OPITZ, J. M. AND BIDDER, U.* HETEROGENEITY OF CHONDRODYSPLASIA PUNCTATA. HUMANGENETIK 11* 190-212, 1971.

*11870 CHOREA, HEREDITARY BENIGN

PINCUS AND CHUTORIAN (1967) AND HAERER, CURRIER AND JACKSON (1966) DESCRIBED AN EARLY-ONSET, NON-PROGRESSIVE FORM OF CHOREA NOT ASSOCIATED WITH INTELLECTUAL DETERIORATION. THE LATTER REPORT CONCERNED A NEGRO FAMILY. BECAUSE NO MALE-TO-MALE TRANSMISSION WAS NOTED AND BECAUSE THE CONDITION WAS NOT MANIFESTED IN TWO CONDUCTOR FEMALES, X-LINKED DOMINANT INHERITANCE CANNOT BE EXCLUDED.

HAERER, A. F., CURRIER, R. D. AND JACKSON, J. F.* HEREDITARY NONPROGRESSIVE CHOREA OF EARLY ONSET. (ABSTRACT) NEUROLOGY 16* 307 ONLY, 1966.

HAERER, A. F., CURRIER, R. D. AND JACKSON, J. F.* HEREDITARY NONPROGRESSIVE CHOREA OF EARLY ONSET. NEW ENG. J. MED. 276* 1220-1224, 1967.

PINCUS, J. H. AND CHUTORIAN, A.* FAMILIAL BENIGN CHOREA WITH INTENTION TREMOR* A CLINICAL ENTITY. J. PEDIAT. 70* 724-729, 1967.

*11880 CHOREOATHETOSIS, FAMILIAL PAROXYSMAL

MOUNT AND REBACK (1940) DESCRIBED A FAMILY WITH MANY MEMBERS IN FIVE GENERATIONS AFFECTED BY PAROXYSMAL CHOREOATHETOSIS WHICH WAS THOUGHT TO BE SEPARATE AND DISTINCT FROM HUNTINGTON'S CHOREA. THE ATTACKS LASTED ONLY A FEW MINUTES, OCCURRED A FEW TIMES A DAY AND WERE NOT ACCOMPANIED BY UNCONSCIOUSNESS. ALCOHOL, COFFEE, HUNGER, FATIGUE AND TOBACCO WERE PRECIPITATING FACTORS. AFFECTED PERSONS WERE SAID TO BE SCATTERED THOUGHOUT THE SOUTH FROM SOUTH CAROLINA TO OKLAHOMA. WAGNER, MC LEES AND HATCHER (1966) OBSERVED AFFECTED PERSONS IN 3 GENERATIONS. RICHARDS AND BARNETT (1968) SUGGESTED THAT IT BE CALLED PAROXYSMAL DYSTONIC CHOREOATHETOSIS TO DISTINGUISH IT FROM THE MORE FREQUENTLY REPORTED MOVEMENT INDUCED (KINETOGENIC) FAMILIAL (OR NONFAMILIAL) PAROXYSMAL CHOREOATHETOSIS WITH WHICH IT IS OFTEN CONFUSED. THEY ALSO SUGGESTED USE OF THE EPONYM MOUNT-REBACK FOR THE DYSTONIC FORM. SEE DYSTONIA, FAMILIAL PAROXYSMAL.

HUDGINS, R. L. AND CORBIN, K. B.* AN UNCOMMON SEIZURE DISORDER* FAMILIAL PAROXYSMAL CHOREOATHETOSIS. BRAIN 89* 199-204, 1966.

KATO, M. AND ARAKI, S.* PAROXYSMAL KINESIGENIC CHOREOATHETOSIS. ARCH. NEUROL. 20* 508-513, 1969.

MOUNT, L. A. AND REBACK, S.* FAMILIAL PAROXYSMAL CHOREOATHETOSIS* PRELIMINARY REPORT ON A HITHERTO UNDESCRIBED CLINICAL SYNDROME. ARCH. NEUROL. PSYCHIAT. 44* 841-847, 1940.

RICHARDS, R. N. AND BARNETT, H. J.* PAROXYSMAL DYSTONIC CHOREOATHETOSIS. A FAMILY STUDY AND REVIEW OF THE LITERATURE. NEUROLOGY 18* 461-469, 1968.

STEVENS, H.* PAROXYSMAL CHOREO-ATHETOSIS* A FORM OF REFLEX EPILEPSY. ARCH. NEUROL. 14* 415-420, 1966.

WAGNER, G. S., MC LEES, B. D. AND HATCHER, M. A., JR.* FAMILIAL PAROXYSMAL CHOREO-ATHETOSIS. (ABSTRACT) NEUROLOGY 16* 307 ONLY, 1966.

WILLIAMS, J. AND STEVENS, H.* FAMILIAL PAROXYSMAL CHOREA-ATHETOSIS. PEDIATRICS 31* 656-659, 1963.

11890 CIRRHOSIS, FAMILIAL

JOSKE AND LAURENCE (1970) DESCRIBED A FAMILY IN WHICH THE FATHER AND FOUR OF 10 CHILDREN HAD CHRONIC LIVER DISEASE AND RAISED IMMUNOGLOBULIN LEVELS.

JOSKE, R. A. AND LAURENCE, B. H.* FAMILIAL CIRRHOSIS WITH AUTOIMMUNE FEATURES AND RAISED IMMUNOGLOBULIN LEVELS. GASTROENTEROLOGY 59* 546-552, 1970.

*11900 CLEFT CHIN

A BONY PECULIARITY UNDERLIES THE Y-SHAPED FISSURE OF THE CHIN. GUNTHER (1939) FOUND 9 CASES IN 5 GENERATIONS AND MEIROWSKY (1924) 25 CASES IN 4 GENERATIONS.

GUNTHER, H.* ANOMALIEN UND ANOMALIEKOMPLEXE IN DER GEGEND DES ERSTEN SCHLUNDBO-GENS. Z. MENSCHL. VERERB. KONSTITUTIONSL. 23* 43-52, 1939.

LEBOW, M. R. AND SAWIN, P. B.* INHERITANCE OF HUMAN FACIAL FEATURES* A PEDIGREE STUDY INVOLVING LENGTH OF FACE, PROMINANT EARS AND CHIN CLEFT. J. HERED. 32* 127-132, 1941.

MEIROWSKY, VON* KLEINE BEITRAGE ZUR VERERBUNGSWISSENSCHAFT. ARCH. RASS.-U. GES. BIOL. 16* 439-443, 1924.

11910 CLEFT HAND AND ABSENT TIBIA

ROBERTS (1967) DESCRIBED A FAMILY IN WHICH PERSONS IN FOUR GENERATIONS HAD ONE CLEFT HAND WITH A MISSING MIDDLE FINGER AND FLEXED RING FINGER, WHEREAS ONE OTHER HAD IN ADDITION GROSSLY DEFORMED LEGS WITH MISSING TIBIAS REQUIRING AMPUTATION AND A SIB HAD ONLY THE SEVERE LEG DEFORMITY. ANOTHER MEMBER HAD ABSENT FOREARMS WITH THE LEG DEFORMITY.

ROBERTS, J. A. F.* GENETIC PROGNOSIS. AN INTRODUCTION TO MEDICAL GENETICS. LONDON* OXFORD U. PRESS, 1967. (4TH ED.). PP. 253-280.

11920 CLEFT LIP AND-OR PALATE

OVER 30 SYNDROMES INCLUDING A NUMBER WHICH ARE EITHER CHROMOSOMAL OR MENDELIAN IN CAUSATION HAVE CLEFT LIP AND-OR PALATE AS FEATURE(S). AS PRECISE DIAGNOSIS AS POSSIBLE IS NECESSARY BEFORE FALLING BACK ON EMPIRIC RISK FIGURES FOR GENETIC COUNSELLING. IT IS CLEAR FROM FAMILY STUDIES THAT CLEFT PALATE ALONE IS GENETI-CALLY DISTINCT FROM CLEFT LIP WITH OR WITHOUT CLEFT PALATE.

*11930 CLEFT LIP AND-OR PALATE WITH MUCOUS CYSTS OF LOWER LIP

IN 3 GENERATIONS OF A FAMILY LEVY (1962) FOUND MALFORMATIONS OF THE LOWER LIP CONSISTING OF SYMMETRICAL LUMPS. TWO SIBS HAD CLEFT PALATE IN ADDITION TO THE LIP ANOMALY. THE LITERATURE FOR THIS SYNDROME HAS BEEN ANALYZED BY VAN DER WOUDE

(1954) WHERE THE AUTOSOMAL DOMINANT MODE OF INHERITANCE WAS CONFIRMED. IT IS POSSIBLE THAT IN SOME AFFECTED FAMILIES, BECAUSE OF THE VARIABLE EXPRESSIVITY OF THE GENE, THE SYNDROME IS EXPRESSED ONLY AS PITS. BAKER (1964) REPORTED SUCH A PEDIGREE WITH AFFECTED MEMBERS IN THREE GENERATIONS SHOWING PITS AS THE ONLY MALFORMATION. ON THE OTHER HAND, ONLY HARELIP AND-OR CLEFT PALATE WITHOUT PITS COULD SEGREGATE IN FAMILIES AS A DOMINANT TRAIT. TEST AND FALLS (1947) DESCRIBED THE CONDITION TRANSMITTED THROUGH 5 GENERATIONS. THE RULE THAT CLEFT PALATE ALONE AND CLEFT LIP WITH OR WITHOUT CLEFT PALATE BEHAVE DIFFERENTLY DOES NOT HOLD IN THIS DISORDER IN WHICH EITHER TYPE OF CLEFT ALONE OR THE TWO IN COMBINATION MAY OCCUR.

BAKER, B. R.* A FAMILY WITH BILATERAL CONGENITAL PITS OF THE INFERIOR LIP. ORAL SURG. 18* 494-497, 1964.

BOWERS, D. G.* CONGENITAL LOWER LIP SINUSES WITH CLEFT PALATE. PLAST. RECONSTR. SURG. 45* 151-154, 1970.

CERVENKA, J., GORLIN, R. J. AND ANDERSON, V. E.* THE SYNDROME OF PITS OF THE LOWER LIP AND CLEFT LIP AND-OR PALATE. GENETIC CONSIDERATIONS. AM. J. HUM. GENET. 19* 416-432, 1967.

LEVY, J.* ZWILLINGE IN EINER FAMILIE MIT UNTERLIPPEN-MISSBILDUNG. ACTA GENET. STATIST. MED. 12* 33-40, 1962.

TEST, A. R. AND FALLS, H. F.* DOMINANT INHERITANCE OF CLEFT LIP AND PALATE IN FIVE GENERATIONS. J. ORAL SURG. 5* 292-297, 1947.

VAN DER WOUDE, A.* FISTULA LABII INFERIORIS CONGENITA AND ITS ASSOCIATION WITH CLEFT LIP AND PALATE. AM. J. HUM. GENET. 6* 244-256, 1954.

11940 CLEFT LIP-PALATE WITH SPLIT HAND AND FOOT

THE THREE PEDIGREES DESCRIBED BY WALKER AND CLODIUS (1963) SUGGEST IRREGULAR AUTOSOMAL DOMINANT INHERITANCE OF THE COMBINATION OF SPLIT HAND AND-OR FOOT AND CLEFT LIP-PALATE. ATRESIA OF THE LACRIMAL PUNCTA OR OTHER DEFORMITY OF THE LACRIMAL DUCT WAS PRESENT IN SOME. SEE EEC SYNDROME FOR THE ASSOCIATION OF ECTRODACTYLY, ECTODERMAL DYSPLASIA AND CLEFT LIP-PALATE.

WALKER, J. C. AND CLODIUS, L.* THE SYNDROMES OF CLEFT LIP, CLEFT PALATE AND LOBSTER CLAW DEFORMITIES OF HANDS AND FEET. PLAST. RECONSTR. SURG. 32* 627-636, 1963.

*11950 CLEFT LIP-PALATE, MUCOUS CYSTS OF THE LOWER LIP, POPLITEAL PTERYGIUM, DIGITAL AND GENITAL ANOMALIES

ALTHOUGH KLEIN (1962) DESCRIBED A MOTHER AND A DAUGHTER WITH THE FEATURES OF THIS SYNDROME, SUGGESTING DOMINANT INHERITANCE, GORLIN AND PINDBORG (1964) ANALYZING THE LITERATURE FAVORED AN AUTOSOMAL RECESSIVE MODE OF INHERITANCE. CHAMPION AND CREGAN'S REPORT OF THE SYNDROME IN SIBS SUPPORTS THE RECESSIVE HYPOTHESIS. LEWIS (1948) DESCRIBED BROTHER AND SISTER WITH CLEFT PALATE AND WEBBING OF THE LOWER LIMBS WHOSE FATHER HAD HARELIP AND CLEFT PALATE. THE WEBBING EXTENDED FROM THE REGION OF THE ISCHIAL TUBEROSITIES TO THE HEELS. (SURGEONS MUST BE AWARE THAT THE SCIATIC NERVE CAN BE SITUATED IN THE WEB.) THE GIRL WAS SAID TO HAVE *BILATERAL INCOMPLETE HARELIP.* HECHT AND JARVINEN (1967) OBSERVED AFFECTED MOTHER AND TWO SONS IN ONE FAMILY AND AFFECTED MOTHER AND SON AND DAUGHTER IN A SECOND. THE OBSERVATION OF AFFECTED FATHER AND SON BY LEWIS (1948) EXCLUDES X-LINKED INHERITANCE. PTERYGIUM OF THE NECK AND ARMS DOES NOT OCCUR IN THIS SYNDROME. AN INTERCRURAL PTERYGIUM CAUSES DISTORTION OF THE GENITALIA. BIFID SCROTUM AND CRYPTORCHIDISM ARE THE RULE IN MALES AND HYPOPLASIA OF THE LABIA MAJORA IN FEMALES. CONGENITAL ANKYLOBLEPHARON FILIFORME OCCURS IN SOME CASES. THE EPITHELIAL STRANDS CONNECTING THE EYELIDS IN ANKYLOBLEPHARON FILIFORME HAVE THEIR COUNTERPART IN SYMMETRICAL EPITHELIAL STRANDS RUNNING FROM THE MAXILLA, AS PICTURED BY RINTALA ET AL. (1970). PFEIFFER ET AL. (1970) DESCRIBED AFFECTED FATHER AND TWO SONS WITH PREDOMINANTLY UNILATERAL POPLITEAL PTERYGIUM, ANOMALIES OF THE SKIN AROUND THE NAILS, SYNDACTYLY, ABNORMALITY OF THE SCROTUM OR CRYPTORCHIDISM, CLEFT LIP AND PALATE, CONGENITAL FISTULAE OF THE LOWER LIP, CONGENITAL BANDS OF MUCOUS MEMBRANES BETWEEN JAWS, AND ANKYLOBLEPHARON FILIFORME ADNATUM.

CHAMPION, R. AND CREGAN, J. C. F.* CONGENITAL POPLITEAL WEBBING IN SIBLINGS. A REPORT OF TWO CASES. J. BONE JOINT SURG. 41B* 355-357, 1959.

GORLIN, R. J. AND PINDBORG, J. J.* CLEFT LIP-PALATE, POPLITEAL PTERYGIUM DIGITAL AND GENITAL ANOMALY. SYNDROMES OF THE HEAD AND NECK. NEW YORK* BLAKISTON DIVISION, MCGRAW-HILL, 1964. PP. 122-125.

GORLIN, R. J., SEDANO, H. O. AND CERVENKA, J.* POPLITEAL PTERYGIUM SYNDROME* A SYNDROME COMPRISING CLEFT LIP-PALATE, POPLITEAL AND INTERCRURAL PTERYGIA, DIGITAL AND GENITAL ANOMALIES. PEDIATRICS 41* 503-509, 1968.

HECHT, F. AND JARVINEN, J. M.* HERITABLE DYSMORPHIC SYNDROME WITH NORMAL INTELLIGENCE. J. PEDIAT. 70* 927-935, 1967.

KLEIN, D.* UN CURIEUX SYNDROME HEREDITAIRE* CHEILO-PALATOSCHIZIS AVEC FISTULES DE LA LEVRE INFERIEURE ASSOCIE A UNE SYNDACTYLIE, UNE ONYCHODYSPLASIE PARTICU-LIERE, UN PTERYGION POPLITE UNILATERAL ET DES PIEDS VARUS EQUINS. J. GENET. HUM. 11* 65-71, 1962.

LEWIS, E.* CONGENITAL WEBBING OF THE LOWER LIMBS. PROC. ROY. SOC. MED. 41* 864 ONLY, 1948.

PFEIFFER, R. A., TUNTE, W. AND REINKEN, M.* DAS KNIEPTERYGIUM-SYNDROM, EIN AUTOSOMAL-DOMINANT VERERBTES MISSBILDUNGSSYNDROM. Z. KINDERHEILK. 108* 103-116, 1970.

RINTALA, A. E., LALITI, A. Y. AND GYLLING, U. S.* CONGENITAL SINUSES OF THE LOWER LIP IN CONNECTION WITH CLEFT LIP AND PALATE. CLEFT PALATE J. 7* 336-346, 1970.

*11960 CLEIDOCRANIAL DYSOSTOSIS

FEATURES INCLUDE PERSISTENTLY OPEN SKULL SUTURES WITH BULGING CALVARIUM, HYPOPLA-SIA OR APLASIA OF THE CLAVICLES PERMITTING ABNORMAL FACILITY IN APPOSING THE SHOULDERS, WIDE PUBIC SYMPHYSIS, SHORT MIDDLE PHALANX OF THE FIFTH FINGERS, DENTAL ANOMALIES AND OFTEN VERTEBRAL MALFORMATION. THIS DISORDER MUST BE DIFFERENTIATED FROM PYCNODYSOSTOSIS (A RECESSIVE). ACRO-OSTEOLYSIS AND BONE SCLEROSIS WITH TENDENCY TO FRACTURE ARE DIFFERENTIATING FEATURES OF PYCNODYSOSTOSIS. ONE OF THE MOST COLORFUL FAMILIES WAS DESCRIBED BY JACKSON (1951). THE CONDITION OCCURRED IN MANY DESCENDANTS OF A CHINESE NAMED ARNOLD WHO EMBRACED THE MOHAMMEDAN RELIGION AND 7 WIVES. JACKSON WAS ABLE TO TRACE 356 DESCENDANTS OF WHOM 70 WERE AFFECTED BY THE 'ARNOLD HEAD.' FOR TRANSLATION OF ORIGINAL DESCRIPTION BY MARIE AND SAINTON (1898) SEE BICK (1968).

BICK, E. M.* THE CLASSIC* ON HEREDITARY CLEIDO-CRANIAL DYSOSTOSIS. CLIN. ORTHOP. 58* 5-8, 1968.

JACKSON, W. P. U.* OSTEO-DENTAL DYSPLASIA (CLEIDO-CRANIAL DYSOSTOSIS). THE 'ARNOLD HEAD.' ACTA MED. SCAND. 139* 292-307, 1951.

KALLIALA, E. AND TASKINEN, P. J.* CLEIDOCRANIAL DYSOSTOSIS. REPORT OF SIX TYPICAL CASES AND ONE ATYPICAL CASE. ORAL SURG. 15* 808-822, 1962.

LECHELLE, P., THEVENARD, A. AND MIGNOT, H.* DYSOSTOSE CLEIDO-CRANIENNE AVEC MALFORMATIONS VERTEBRALES MULTIPLES ET TROUBLES NERVEUX. CARACTERE FAMILIAL DES MALFORMATIONS. BULL. MEM. SOC. MED. HOP. PARIS 52* 1526-1530, 1936.

LEVIN, E. J. AND SONNENSCHEIN, H.* CLEIDOCRANIAL DYSOSTOSIS. NEW YORK J. MED. 63* 1562-1566, 1963.

MARIE, P. AND SAINTON, P.* THE CLASSIC* ON HEREDITARY CLEIDO-CRANIAL DYSOSTO-SIS. CLIN. ORTHOP. 58* 5-8, 1968.

11970 CLINODACTYLY

CAMPTODACTYLY IS FLEXURE CONTRACTURE OF FINGERS, USUALLY THE FIFTH. CLINODACTYLY, WHICH ALSO INVOLVES THE FIFTH FINGER, IS A RADIAL CURVATURE. IT IS USUALLY DUE TO SHORT, TRIANGULAR MIDDLE PHALANX. CLINODACTYLY ALSO OCCURS IN PERSONS WITH THE MARFAN SYNDROME AND IN 'BIRD-HEADED DWARFS' (SEE RECESSIVE CATALOG), AS WELL AS IN TRISOMY 21 (MONGOLISM).

11980 CLUB FOOT (TALIPES EQUINOVARUS)

ALTHOUGH GENETIC FACTORS ARE CLEARLY IMPORTANT, SIMPLE INHERITANCE HAS NOT BEEN ESTABLISHED. PALMER (1964) SUGGESTED THAT TWO TYPES MAY EXIST* (1) A GROUP WITH NORMAL SEX RATIO, NORMAL MATERNAL AGE CURVE, RECURRENCE RISK OF ABOUT 10 PERCENT AND PROBABLE DOMINANT INHERITANCE WITH ABOUT 40 PERCENT PENETRANCE, AND (2) A GROUP BORN TO YOUNGER MOTHERS WITH PREPONDERANCE OF MALES AND NO CLEAR PATTERN OF INHERITANCE. BOOK (1948) HAD ESTIMATED THAT THE RISK OF RECURRENCE IN SUBSEQUENT-LY BORN CHILDREN IS BETWEEN 3 AND 8 PERCENT IF ONE CHILD IS AFFECTED AND ABOUT 10 PERCENT IF ONE CHILD AND ONE PARENT ARE AFFECTED. CLUB FOOT IS A FEATURE OF DIASTROPHIC DWARFISM (Q.V.).

ALBERMAN, E. D.* THE CAUSES OF CONGENITAL CLUB FOOT. ARCH. DIS. CHILD. 40* 548-554, 1965.

BOOK, J. A.* A CONTRIBUTION TO THE GENETICS OF CONGENITAL CLUBFOOT. HEREDITAS 34* 289-300, 1948.

CHING, G. H. S., CHUNG, C. S. AND NEMECHEK, R. W.* GENETIC AND EPIDEMIOLOGICAL STUDIES OF CLUBFOOT IN HAWAII* ASCERTAINMENT AND INCIDENCE. AM. J. HUM. GENET. 21* 566-580, 1969.

PALMER, R. M.* HEREDITARY CLUBFOOT. CLIN. ORTHOP. 33* 138-146, 1964.

WYNNE-DAVIES, R.* FAMILY STUDIES AND THE CAUSE OF CONGENITAL CLUB FOOT.

11990 CLUBBING OF DIGITS

FAMILIAL CLUBBING MAY BE MORE FREQUENT IN NEGROES THAN IN WHITES. IT IS UNCERTAIN
WHETHER FAMILIAL CLUBBING IS DISTINCT FROM PACHYDERMOPERIOSTOSIS (Q.V.). FISCHER,
SINGER AND FELDMAN (1964) REPORTED NEGRO FAMILIES THAT SHOWED STRONG SEX INF-
LUENCE, WITH MALES ONLY OR PREDOMINANTLY AFFECTED.

CURTH, H. O., FIRSCHEIN, I. L. AND ALPERT, M.* FAMILIAL CLUBBED FINGERS. ARCH.
DERM. 83* 828-836, 1961.

FISCHER, D. S., SINGER, D. H. AND FELDMAN, S. M.* CLUBBING, A REVIEW, WITH
EMPHASIS ON HEREDITARY ACROPACHY. MEDICINE 43* 459-479, 1964.

12000 COARCTATION OF AORTA

GOUGH (1961) DESCRIBED THE ANOMALY IN FATHER AND SON. HE FOUND 6 OTHER REPORTS OF
FAMILIAL COARCTATION.

GOUGH, J. H.* COARCTATION OF THE AORTA IN FATHER AND SON. BRIT. J. RADIOL. 34*
670-674, 1961.

*12010 COLD HYPERSENSITIVITY

AFTER EXPOSURE TO COLD THE PATIENT DEVELOPS URTICARIAL WHEALS, PAIN AND SWELLING
OF JOINTS, CHILLS AND FEVER. AMYLOIDOSIS IS ALSO A FEATURE OF THE SYNDROME OF
URTICARIA, DEAFNESS AND AMYLOIDOSIS (Q.V.), A SEPARATE ALTHOUGH SOMEWHAT SIMILAR
ENTITY. MCKUSICK AND GOODMAN (1962) NOTED THAT SYSTEMIC AMYLOIDOSIS IS A
COMPLICATION OF THIS CONDITION AND THAT AMYLOID NEPHROPATHY IS A FREQUENT CAUSE OF
DEATH.

KILE, R. L. AND RUSK, H. A.* A CASE OF COLD URTICARIA WITH UNUSUAL FAMILY
HISTORY. J.A.M.A. 114* 1067-1068, 1940.

MCKUSICK, V. A. AND GOODMAN, R. M.* PINNAL CALCIFICATION. OBSERVATIONS IN
SYSTEMIC DISEASES NOT ASSOCIATED WITH DISORDERED CALCIUM METABOLISM. J.A.M.A.
179* 230-232, 1962.

TINDALL, J. P., BEEKER, S. K. AND ROSSE, W. F.* FAMILIAL COLD URTICARIA. A
GENERALIZED REACTION INVOLVING LEUKOCYTOSIS. ARCH. INTERN. MED. 124* 129-134,
1969.

WITHERSPOON, F. G., WHITE, C. B., BAZEMORE, J. M. AND HAILEY, H.* FAMILIAL
URTICARIA DUE TO COLD. ARCH. DERM. SYPH. 58* 52-55, 1948.

*12020 COLOBOMA OF IRIS

THE DEFECT IS NOT TYPICALLY LOCATED IN THE LOWER PART OF THE IRIS. NUMEROUS
PEDIGREES SUPPORTING DOMINANT INHERITANCE HAVE BEEN REPORTED. ELDRIDGE (1967)
OBSERVED AN AFFECTED FAMILY WITH DOMINANT PEDIGREE PATTERN. SNELL (1908) OBSERVED
12 CASES IN 5 GENERATIONS.

ELDRIDGE, R.* BETHESDA, MD.* PERSONAL COMMUNICATION, 1967.

FRANCOIS, J.* HEREDITY IN OPHTHALMOLOGY. ST. LOUIS* C. V. MOSBY CO., 1961.
PP. 149-152.

SNELL, S.* CARCINOMA OF ORBIT ORIGINATING IN A MEIBOMIAN GLAND. TRANS.
OPHTHAL. SOC. U.K. 28* 144-147, 1908.

12030 COLOBOMA OF MACULA

CLAUSEN (1921) DESCRIBED AFFECTED BROTHER AND SISTER WHO HAD, RESPECTIVELY, TWO
AFFECTED SONS AND TWO AFFECTED DAUGHTERS. DAVENPORT (1927) DESCRIBED MOTHER AND
SON.

CLAUSEN, (NI)* TYPISCHES, BEIDERSEITIGES HEREDITARES MAKULA-KOLOBOM. KLIN.
MBL. AUGENHEILK. 67* 116 ONLY, 1921.

DAVENPORT, R. C.* BILATERAL 'MACULAR COLOBOMA' IN MOTHER AND SON. PROC. ROY.
SOC. MED. 21* 109-110, 1927.

12040 COLOBOMA OF MACULA WITH TYPE B BRACHYDACTYLY ('APICAL DYSTROPHY')

SORSBY (1935) DESCRIBED A MOTHER AND FIVE CHILDREN WITH BILATERAL PIGMENTED
MACULAR COLOBOMA AND BRACHYDACTYLY. ONE OF THE PATIENTS HAD UNILATERAL ABSENT
KIDNEY. TWO OTHER CHILDREN AND THE FATHER WERE UNAFFECTED. THE SKELETAL DEFECT
WAS OF THE TYPE DESCRIBED BY MACARTHUR AND MCCULLOUGH (1932) AS APICAL DYSTROPHY
AND CLASSIFIED HERE AS BRACHYDACTYLY, TYPE B (Q.V.). ABNORMALITIES ARE CONFINED
TO THE DISTAL TWO PHALANGES. THE DISTAL PHALANX MAY BE COMPLETELY ABSENT. THE

DISTAL PHALANX OF THE THUMB IS USUALLY BROAD OR BIFID.

MACARTHUR, J. W. AND MCCULLOUGH, E.* APICAL DYSTROPHY, AN INHERITED DEFECT OF HANDS AND FEET. HUM. BIOL. 4* 179-207, 1932.

SORSBY, A.* CONGENITAL COLOBOMA OF THE MACULA, TOGETHER WITH AN ACCOUNT OF THE FAMILIAL OCCURRENCE OF BILATERAL MACULAR COLOBOMA IN ASSOCIATION WITH APICAL DYSTROPHY OF HANDS AND FEET. BRIT. J. OPHTHAL. 19* 65-90, 1935.

12050 COMMISSURAL LIP PITS

THESE OCCUR AT THE CORNERS OF THE MOUTH. THEY ARE FREQUENTLY OF PENCIL-LEAD SIZE, FROM 1 TO 4 MM. DEEP AND MAY BE FILLED WITH CELLULAR DEBRIS. PREAURICULAR PITS MAY BE ASSOCIATED. EVERETT AND WESCOTT (1961) FOUND 2 CASES AMONG 1000 SCHOOL CHILDREN OF PORTLAND, ORE. WITKOP (1965) AND THESE AUTHORS FOUND EVIDENCE OF DOMINANT INHERITANCE BUT COULD NOT DISTINGUISH BETWEEN AUTOSOMAL AND X-LINKED DOMINANCE.

EVERETT, F. G. AND WESCOTT, W. B.* COMMISSURAL LIP PITS. ORAL SURG. 14* 202-209, 1961.

WITKOP, C. J.* GENETIC DISEASE OF THE ORAL CAVITY. IN, TIECKE, R. W. (ED.)* ORAL PATHOLOGY. NEW YORK* MCGRAW-HILL, 1965.

*12060 COMPLEMENT COMPONENT-2, VARIANTS OF

BOTH HETEROZYGOTES AND HOMOZYGOTES HAVE BEEN IDENTIFIED. NO GENE PRODUCT IS IDENTIFIABLE IMMUNOLOGICALLY IN THE HOMOZYGOTE (POLLEY, 1968* KLEMPERER, 1969). A STANDARDIZED NOMENCLATURE FOR VARIANTS OF COMPLEMENT COMPONENTS WAS RECOMMENDED BY THE WORLD HEALTH ORGANIZATION (1968). IN ORDER OF THEIR REACTION, THE COMPONENTS OF COMPLEMENT ARE DESIGNATED C1, C2, C3, C4, C5, C6, C7, C8 AND C9.

KLEMPERER, M. R.* HEREDITARY DEFICIENCY OF THE SECOND COMPONENT OF COMPLEMENT IN MAN* AN IMMUNOCHEMICAL STUDY. J. IMMUN. 102* 168-171, 1969.

KLEMPERER, M. R., AUSTEN, K. F. AND ROSEN, F. S.* HEREDITARY DEFICIENCY OF THE SECOND COMPONENT OF COMPLEMENT (C*2) IN MAN* FURTHER OBSERVATIONS ON A SECOND KINDRED. J. IMMUN. 98* 72-78, 1967.

POLLEY, M. J.* INHERITED C-PRIME-2 DEFICIENCY IN MAN* LACK OF IMMUNOCHEMICALLY DETECTABLE C-PRIME-2 PROTEIN IN SERUMS FROM DEFICIENT INDIVIDUALS. SCIENCE 161* 1149-1151, 1968.

RUDDY, S. AND AUSTEN, K. F.* INHERITED ABNORMALITIES OF THE COMPLEMENT SYSTEM IN MAN. PROG. MED. GENET. 7* 69-95, 1970.

WORLD HEALTH ORGANIZATION* BULL. WHO 39* 935-938, 1968.

*12070 COMPLEMENT COMPONENT-3, VARIANT OF

IN GRANDMOTHER, MOTHER, AND TWO SONS, WIEME AND DEMEULENAERE (1967) FOUND A DOUBLE ELECTROPHORETIC BAND CORRESPONDING APPARENTLY TO COMPLEMENT COMPONENT C-PRIME-3. BY MEANS OF HIGH VOLTAGE STARCH GEL ELECTROPHORESIS, AZEN AND SMITHIES (1968) ALSO FOUND ELECTROPHORETIC POLYMORPHISM OF THE THIRD COMPONENT OF COMPLEMENT. THIS COMPONENT HAS MANY IMPORTANT FUNCTIONS IN IMMUNE MECHANISMS. ALPER AND PROPP (1968) INDEPENDENTLY FOUND POLYMORPHISM OF THE THIRD COMPONENT OF COMPLEMENT.

ALPER, C. A. AND PROPP, R. P.* GENETIC POLYMORPHISM OF THE THIRD COMPONENT OF HUMAN COMPLEMENT (C-PRIME-3). J. CLIN. INVEST. 47* 2181-2192, 1968.

ALPER, C. A. AND ROSEN, F. S.* STUDIES OF A HYPOMORPHIC VARIANT OF HUMAN C3. J. CLIN. INVEST. 50* 324-326, 1971.

ALPER, C. A., ABRAMSON, N., JOHNSTON, R. B., JR., JANDL, J. H. AND ROSEN, F. S.* INCREASED SUSCEPTIBILITY TO INFECTION ASSOCIATED WITH ABNORMALITIES OF COMPLEMENT-MEDIATED FUNCTIONS AND OF THE THIRD COMPONENT OF COMPLEMENT (C3). NEW ENG. J. MED. 282* 349-354, 1970.

ALPER, C. A., ABRAMSON, N., JOHNSTON, R. B., JR., JANDL, J. H. AND ROSEN, F. S.* STUDIES IN VIVO AND IN VITRO ON AN ABNORMALITY IN THE METABOLISM OF C3 IN A PATIENT WITH INCREASED SUSCEPTIBILITY TO INFECTION. J. CLIN. INVEST. 49* 1975-1985, 1970.

ALPER, C. A., PROPP, R. P., KLEMPERER, M. R. AND ROSEN, F. S.* INHERITED DEFICIENCY OF THE THIRD COMPONENT OF HUMAN COMPLEMENT (C-PRIME-3). J. CLIN. INVEST. 48* 553-557, 1969.

AZEN, E. A. AND SMITHIES, O.* GENETIC POLYMORPHISM OF C-PRIME-3 (BETA-1C-GLOBULIN) IN HUMAN SERUM. SCIENCE 162* 905-907, 1968.

GOEDDE, H. W., BENKMANN, H.-G. AND HIRTH, L.* GENETIC POLYMORPHISM OF C*3(BETA-1C-GLOBULIN) COMPONENT OF COMPLEMENT IN A GERMAN AND A SPANISH POPULATION.

MULLER-EBERHARD, H. J.* CHEMISTRY AND REACTION MECHANISMS OF COMPLEMENT. ADVANCES IMMUNOLOGY 8* 1-80, 1968.

WIEME, R. J. AND DEMEULENAERE, L.* GENETICALLY DETERMINED ELECTROPHORETIC VARIANT OF THE HUMAN COMPLEMENT COMPONENT C-PRIME-3. NATURE 214* 1042-1043, 1967.

*12080 COMPLEMENT COMPONENT-4, VARIATION IN

BY THE PROCESS OF ANTIGEN-ANTIBODY CROSSED ELECTROPHORESIS, ROSENFELD ET AL. (1969) DEMONSTRATED HETEROGENEITY IN THE FOURTH COMPONENT OF COMPLEMENT. SUBTYPES A AND A(1) SEEM TO BE INHERITED AS CODOMINANT TRAITS INDEPENDENT OF SUBTYPE C. PARTIAL DEFICIENCY OF C4 WAS FOUND IN 3 PERSONS DURING A SCREENING OF 42,000 HEALTHY JAPANESE (TORISU ET AL., 1970). ELLMAN ET AL. (1970) FOUND A DEFICIENCY OF C4 IN THE GUINEA PIG, WHERE TOTAL DEFICIENCY WAS RECESSIVE.

ELLMAN, L., GREEN, I. AND FRANK, M.* GENETICALLY CONTROLLED TOTAL DEFICIENCY OF THE FOURTH COMPONENT OF COMPLEMENT IN THE GUINEA PIG. SCIENCE 170* 74-75, 1970.

ROSENFELD, S. I., RUDDY, S. AND AUSTEN, K. F.* STRUCTURAL POLYMORPHISM OF THE FOURTH COMPONENT OF HUMAN COMPLEMENT. J. CLIN. INVEST. 48* 2283-2292, 1969.

TORISU, M., SONOZAKI, H., INAI, S. AND ARATA, M.* DEFICIENCY OF THE FOURTH COMPONENT OF COMPLEMENT IN MAN. J. IMMUNOL. 104* 728-737, 1970.

*12090 COMPLEMENT COMPONENT-5, DEFICIENCY OF

DYSFUNCTION OF THE FIFTH COMPONENT OF COMPLEMENT (C5) WAS FOUND TO BE THE BASIS FOR THE DEFICIENCY IN PHAGOCYTOSIS - ENHANCING ACTIVITY OF SERUM PRESENT IN THE PROBAND, HER MOTHER AND 15 OTHER RELATIVES (MILLER AND NILSSON, 1970). GENETIC DEFICIENCY OF C5 IN MICE WAS STUDIED ALSO.

MILLER, M. E. AND NILSSON, U. R.* A FAMILIAL DEFICIENCY OF THE PHAGOCYTOSIS-ENHANCING ACTIVITY OF SERUM RELATED TO A DYSFUNCTION OF THE FIFTH COMPONENT OF COMPLEMENT (C5). NEW ENG. J. MED. 282* 354-358, 1970.

12100 CONGENITAL HEART DISEASE

IN THE CASE OF CARDIOVASCULAR MALFORMATIONS AS WELL AS THOSE OF OTHER SYSTEMS, THE OCCASIONAL INSTANCES OF PARENT-CHILD INVOLVEMENT IS TO BE EXPECTED. IT IS OFTEN UNCERTAIN WHETHER THIS IS MORE THAN ONE WOULD EXPECT ON THE BASIS OF THE MODEST FAMILIAL AGGREGATION WHICH OCCURS WITH SUCH MALFORMATIONS. WHEN SUCCESSIVELY AFFECTED GENERATIONS ARE OBSERVED IN THE CASE OF A RARE MALFORMATION SUCH AS SUPRAVALVAR AORTIC STENOSIS OR WHEN THREE, FOUR OR MORE GENERATIONS ARE AFFECTED, ESPECIALLY THROUGH SEVERAL LINES, SIMPLE AUTOSOMAL DOMINANT INHERITANCE IS QUITE LIKELY. SEE THE FAMILIES REPORTED BY KAHLER ET AL. (1966).

CARLETON, R. A., ABELMANN, W. H. AND HANCOCK, E. W.* FAMILIAL OCCURRENCE OF CONGENITAL HEART DISEASE* REPORT OF THREE FAMILIES AND REVIEW OF THE LITERATURE. NEW ENG. J. MED. 259* 1237-1245, 1958.

CHELIUS, C. J., ROWE, G. G. AND CRUMPTON, C. W.* FAMILIAL ASPECTS OF CONGENITAL HEART DISEASE. AM. J. CARDIOL. 9* 508-514, 1962.

KAHLER, R. L., BRAUNWALD, E., PLAUTH, W. H., JR. AND MORROW, A. G.* FAMILIAL CONGENITAL HEART DISEASE. FAMILIAL OCCURRENCE OF ATRIAL SEPTAL DEFECT WITH A-V CONDUCTION ABNORMALITIES, SUPRAVALVULAR AORTIC AND PULMONIC STENOSIS, AND VENTRICULAR SEPTAL DEFECT. AM. J. MED. 40* 384-399, 1966.

NORA, J. J., DODD, P. F., MCNAMARA, D. G., HATTWICK, M. A. W., LEACHMAN, R. D. AND COOLEY, D. A.* RISK TO OFFSPRING OF PARENTS WITH CONGENITAL HEART DEFECTS. J.A.M.A. 209* 2052-2053, 1969.

PITT, D. B.* A FAMILY STUDY OF FALLOT'S TETRAD. AUST. ANN. MED. 11* 179-183, 1962.

12110 CONTRACTURES WITH SCLERODERMA-LIKE CHANGES

PICHLER (1968) DESCRIBED A FATHER, DAUGHTER AND SON WITH FLEXION DEFORMITIES OF FINGERS AND TOES, LIMITED MOTION OF SEVERAL OTHER JOINTS AND THE VERTEBRAL COLUMN, SCLERODERMATOID CHANGES OF THE SKIN AND GENERALIZED INCREASE IN THE CONSISTENCY OF OTHERWISE SLIGHTLY UNDERDEVELOPED MUSCLES. SUSPECTED MYOSCLEROSIS COULD NOT BE CONFIRMED BY BIOPSY. THE APPEARANCE OF THE AFFECTED SON RATHER SUGGESTS THAT OF PSEUDO-HURLER POLYDYSTROPHY (Q.V.) BUT NO CORNEAL CHANGES WERE DESCRIBED AND AUTOSOMAL DOMINANT INHERITANCE SEEMS LIKELY. THIS MAY BE THE SAME ENTITY AS THAT ENTERED ELSEWHERE AS THE STIFF SKIN SYNDROME (18490).

PICHLER, E.* HEREDITARE KONTRAKTUREN MIT SKLERODERMIEARTIGEN HAUTVERANDERUNGEN. Z. KINDERHEILK. 104* 349-361, 1968.

*12120 CONVULSIONS, BENIGN FAMILIAL NEONATAL

FAMILIES HAVE BEEN REPORTED IN WHICH MULTIPLE PERSONS IN AN AUTOSOMAL DOMINANT PATTERN HAD NEONATAL CONVULSIONS WHICH CLEARED SPONTANEOUSLY AFTER A FEW WEEKS AND WERE FOLLOWED BY NORMAL PSYCHOMOTOR DEVELOPMENT (BJERRE AND CORELIUS, 1968* RETT AND TEUBEL, 1964). PYRIDOXINE DEPENDENCY WAS EXCLUDED IN ALL.

BJERRE, I. AND CORELIUS, E.* BENIGN FAMILIAL NEONATAL CONVULSIONS. ACTA PAEDIAT. SCAND. 57* 557-561, 1968.

RETT, A. AND TEUBEL, R.* NEUGEBORENEN KRAMPFE IM RAHMEN EINER EPILEPISCH BELASTETEN FAMILIE. WEIN. KLIN. WSCHR. 76* 609-613, 1964.

*12130 COPROPORPHYRIA

MANY HAVE COMMENTED THAT AFTER THE SWEDISH ACUTE INTERMITTENT AND SOUTH AFRICAN VARIEGATE TYPES OF PORPHYRIA ARE EXCLUDED ONE IS LEFT WITH OVERLAPPING CASES. BARNES AND WHITTAKER (1965) DESCRIBED WHAT MAY BE A DISTINCT ENTITY. FOUR OF 5 SIBS WERE AFFECTED. THE PARENTS WERE NOT TESTED. MARKED ELEVATION OF COPROPOR-PHYRIA IN THE FECES DIFFERENTIATED THE CONDITION FROM THE SWEDISH TYPE IN WHICH STOOL PORPHYRINS ARE USUALLY NORMAL AND FROM VARIEGATE PORPHYRIA, IN WHICH BOTH COPROPORPHYRIN AND PROTOPORPHYRIN FRACTIONS ARE INCREASED IN THE STOOL. THE PROBAND EXPERIENCED TYPICAL ACUTE PORPHYRIA. CONSTIPATION AND ABDOMINAL COLIC WERE STRIKING FEATURES IN THESE PATIENTS. GOLDBERG ET AL. (1967) ADDED 20 NEW CASES. A MASSIVE EXCRETION OF COPROPORPHYRIN III IN THE URINE AND FECES, PREDOMINANTLY THE FECES, WAS DEMONSTRATED. ATTACKS RESEMBLING THOSE OF ACUTE INTERMITTENT PORPHYRIA WERE PRECIPITATED BY DRUGS AND DURING ATTACKS PORPHOBILINO-GEN AND DELTA-AMINOLEVULINIC ACID WERE EXCRETED IN THE URINE IN EXCESS. PHOTOSEN-SITIVITY IS OCCASIONALLY PRESENT AND THE ONLY MANIFESTATIONS MAY BE PSYCHIATRIC. ABOUT HALF OF CASES ARE ASYMPTOMATIC. DOMINANT INHERITANCE SEEMS ADEQUATELY ESTABLISHED. THIS IS A HEPATIC FORM OF PORPHYRIA. HAEGER-ARONSON ET AL. (1968) REPORTED FAMILIAL CASES. CRIPPS AND PETERS (1970) FOUND THAT TRANQUILIZERS INCLUDING MEPROBAMATE AND CHLORPROMAZINE PRECIPITATED TROUBLE. THE FIRST CASE, REPORTED BY BERGER AND GOLDBERG (1955), WAS THE OFFSPRING OF FIRST COUSIN PARENTS, BOTH OF WHOM SHOWED EXCESSIVE EXCRETION OF COPROPORPHYRIN III. THE AUTHORS SUGGESTED THAT THE DISORDER IS AUTOSOMAL DOMINANT AND THAT THEIR PROBAND WAS HOMOZYGOUS. IN THE FAMILY OF HAEGER-ARONSON ET AL. (1968) THIRTEEN PERSONS IN 5 SIBSHIPS OF 2 GENERATIONS SHOWED LATENT COPROPORPHYRIA, IN ADDITION TO THE SYMPTOMATIC PROBAND. KAUFMAN AND MARVER (1970) DEMONSTRATED INCREASED ALA SYNTHETASE ACTIVITY IN COPRPOPORPHYRIA SIMILAR TO THAT IN ACUTE INTERMITTENT PORPHYRIA. INCREASED HEPATIC DELTA-AMINOLEVULINIC ACID SYNTHETASE HAS BEEN DEMONSTRATED IN THREE FORMS OF HEREDITARY PORPHYRIA* ACUTE INTERMITTENT PORPHYRIA, PORPHYRIA VARIEGATA AND COPROPORPHYRIA (MCINTYRE, 1971).

BARNES, H. D. AND WHITTAKER, N.* HEREDITARY COPROPORPHYRIA WITH ACUTE INTERMIT-TENT MANIFESTATIONS. BRIT. MED. J. 2* 1102-1104, 1965.

BERGER, H. AND GOLDBERG, A.* HEREDITARY COPROPORPHYRIA. BRIT. MED. J. 2* 85-88, 1955.

CONNON, J. J. AND TURKINGTON, V.* HEREDITARY COPROPORPHYRIA. LANCET 2* 263-264, 1964.

CRIPPS, D. J. AND PETERS, H. A.* STOOL PORPHYRINS IN ACUTE INTERMITTENT AND HEREDITARY COPROPORPHYRIA. ADVERSE EFFECTS OF TRANQUILIZERS. ARCH. NEUROL. 23* 80-84, 1970.

GOLDBERG, A., RIMINGTON, C. AND LOCHHEAD, A. C.* HEREDITARY COPROPORPHYRIA. LANCET 1* 632-636, 1967.

HAEGER-ARONSON, B., STATHERS, G. AND SWAHN, G.* HEREDITARY COPROPORPHYRIA. STUDY OF A SWEDISH FAMILY. ANN. INTERN. MED. 69* 221-227, 1968.

KAUFMAN, L. AND MARVER, H. S.* BIOCHEMICAL DEFECTS IN TWO TYPES OF HUMAN HEPATIC PORPHYRIA. NEW ENG. J. MED. 283* 954-958, 1970.

LOMHOLT, J. C. AND WITH, T. K.* HEREDITARY COPROPORPHYRIA. A FAMILY WITH UNUSUALLY FEW AND MILD SYMPTOMS. ACTA MED. SCAND. 186* 83-85, 1969.

MCINTYRE, N., PEARSON, A. J. G., ALLAN, D. J., CRASKE, S., WEST, G. M. L., MOORE, M. R., BEATTIE, A. D., PAXTON, J. AND GOLDBERG, A.* HEPATIC DELTA-AMINOLAE-VULINIC ACID SYNTHETASE IN AN ATTACK OF HEREDITARY COPROPORPHYRIA AND DURING REMISSION. LANCET 1* 560-564, 1971.

12140 CORNEA PLANA

LARSEN AND ERIKSEN (1949) DESCRIBED 13 PATIENTS IN 3 GENERATIONS OF EACH OF TWO FAMILIES. RECESSIVE INHERITANCE (Q.V.) SEEMS WELL ESTABLISHED IN MANY OTHER INSTANCES.

LARSEN, V. AND ERIKSEN, A.* CORNEA PLANA. ACTA OPHTHAL. 27* 275-286, 1949.

*12150 CORNEAL DYSTROPHY OF REIS-BUCKLERS

PAUFIQUE AND BONNET (1966) DESCRIBED A FAMILY WITH AFFECTED MEMBERS IN THREE GENERATIONS. MOST OF THE AFFECTED PERSONS ALSO HAD STRABISMUS. THE CORNEA PRESENTED A "DUSTY" OPACITY AND A ROUGH MAP-LIKE SURFACE WITH A PERIPHERAL CONDENSATION RING SEPARATE FROM THE LIMBUS BY A NARROW STRIP OF NORMAL CORNEA. THE LESIONS ARE PRIMARILY IN BOWMAN'S MEMBRANE WITH SECONDARY INVOLVEMENT OF THE EPITHELIUM AND SUPERFICIAL PART OF THE STROMA. RELAPSING CORNEAL EROSIONS OCCUR BETWEEN AGES 8 AND 20 AND AGAIN IN MORE SEVERE FORM AT ABOUT 40 OR 50 YEARS.

PAUFIQUE, L. AND BONNET, M.* LA DYSTROPHIE CORNEENNE HEREDO-FAMILIALE DE REIS-BUCKLERS. ANN. OCULIST. 199* 14-37, 1966.

12160 CORNEAL DYSTROPHY, CONGENITAL

MAUMENEE (1960) OBSERVED 6 KNOWN AFFLICTED PERSONS IN THREE GENERATIONS OF ONE FAMILY. THE CORNEAL DYSTROPHIES CAN, IN THE FIRST INSTANCE, BE CLASSIFIED ACCORDING TO THE SITE OF PREDOMINANT INVOLVEMENT, THE CORNEA HAVING FIVE LAYERS, FROM OUTSIDE INWARD, EPITHELIUM, BOWMAN'S MEMBRANE, STROMA, DESCEMET'S MEMBRANE, AND ENDOTHELIUM. MOST CASES ARE RECESSIVE. IN AN INTERESTING TWICE-REPORTED FAMILY (TURPIN ET AL., 1939* DESVIGNES AND VIGO, 1955) 13 WERE AFFECTED IN 3 CONSECUTIVE GENERATIONS WITH FIVE INSTANCES OF MALE-TO-MALE TRANSMISSION.

DESVIGNES, P. AND VIGO, (NI)* A CASE OF CORNEAL AND PARENCHYMAL DYSTROPHY OF DOMINANT TYPE. BULL. SOC. OPHTAL. FRANC. 4* 220-225, 1955.

FEIGIN, R. D. AND CAPLAN, D. B.* CORNEAL OPACITIES IN INFANCY AND CHILDHOOD. J. PEDIAT. 69* 383-392, 1966.

MAUMENEE, A. E.* CONGENITAL HEREDITARY CORNEAL DYSTROPHY. AM. J. OPHTHAL. 50* 1114-1124, 1960.

TURPIN, R., TISSERAND, M. AND SERANE, J.* OPACITIES CORNEENNES HEREDITARY ET CONGENITALES REPORTIES SUR TROIS GENERATIONS ET ATTEIGNANT DEUX JUMELLES MONCZY-GOTES. ARCH. OPHTAL. 3* 109-111, 1939.

12170 CORNEAL DYSTROPHY, CONGENITAL ENDOTHELIAL

PEARCE ET AL. (1969) DESCRIBED A FAMILY WITH 39 AFFECTED MEMBERS.

PEARCE, W. G., TRIPATHI, R. C. AND MORGAN, G.* CONGENITAL ENDOTHELIAL CORNEAL DYSTROPHY. CLINICAL, PATHOLOGICAL, AND GENETIC STUDY. BRIT. J. OPHTHAL. 53* 577-591, 1969.

*12180 CORNEAL DYSTROPHY, CRYSTALLINE, OF SCHNYDER

THIS DISORDER, BEGINNING EARLY IN LIFE, PRESENTS AS AN OVAL OR ANNULAR CLOUDING OF THE CENTRAL PART OF THE CORNEA WITH THE PERIPHERY REMAINING CLEAR. INVOLVEMENT EXTENDS TOWARD THE LIMBUS BUT USUALLY LEAVES A CLEAR PERIPHERAL AREA. CORNEAL SENSITIVITY IS NORMAL. SLIT LAMP EXAMINATION SHOWS IN THE OPACIFIED AREA MANY SMALL IRIDESCENT NEEDLE-SHAPED SHINY CRYSTALS OF UNKNOWN COMPOSITION. THE OPACITY IS LOCATED IN THE ANTERIOR PORTION OF THE STROMA JUST POSTERIOR TO BOWMAN'S MEMBRANE. THE EPITHELIUM IS NORMAL. GILLESPIE AND COVELLI (1963) REPORTED FATHER-TO-SON TRANSMISSION. THE CORNEA HAS THE APPEARANCE OF CRYSTALLINE DYSTROPHY IN CYSTINOSIS OF WHICH THERE ARE TWO TYPES, BOTH RECESSIVE. MALBRAN ET AL. (1953) DESCRIBED A FAMILY. LUXENBERG (1967) GAVE FURTHER INFORMATION ON MEMBERS OF A FAMILY REPORTED BY FRY AND PICKETT (1950). CLOUDING IS OF EARLY ONSET AND MAY BE CONGENITAL BUT PROGRESSES LITTLE. THE LESIONS ARE BILATERAL, CENTRALLY LOCATED AND IRREGULAR IN OUTLINE. DEPOSITS OCCUR IN THE ANTERIOR STROMA NEAR BOWMAN'S MEMBRANE AND EXTEND IRREGULARLY INTO DEEPER LAYERS. THE DEPOSITS HAVE THE BIOMICROSCOPIC APPEARANCE OF FINE, NEEDLE-SHAPED, COLORED CRYSTALS. THE DISORDER BEGINS IN EARLY YOUTH. INNUMERABLE SMALL NEEDLE-LIKE CRYSTALS ARE SEEN BY SLIT-LAMP IN THE ANTERIOR THIRD OF THE STROMA. DELLEMAN AND WINKELMAN (1968) DESCRIBED TWO FAMILIES. IN THE FIRST 21 PERSONS IN 6 GENERATIONS WERE AFFECTED AND GENU VALGUM WAS RATHER CONSTANTLY ASSOCIATED. THE CRYSTALS ARE THOUGHT TO BE CHOLESTEROL.

DELLEMAN, J. W. AND WINKELMAN, J. E.* DEGENERATIO CORNEAE CRISTALLINEA HEREDITARIA. A CLINICAL, GENETICAL AND HISTOLOGICAL STUDY. OPHTHALMOLOGICA 155* 409-426, 1968.

FRY, W. E. AND PICKETT, W. E.* CRYSTALLINE DYSTROPHY OF CORNEA. TRANS. AM. OPHTHAL. SOC. 48* 220-227, 1950.

GILLESPIE, F. D. AND COVELLI, B.* CRYSTALLINE CORNEAL DYSTROPHY. REPORT OF A CASE. AM. J. OPHTHAL. 56* 465-467, 1963.

LUXENBERG, M.* HEREDITARY CRYSTALLINE DYSTROPHY OF THE CORNEA. AM. J. OPHTHAL. 63* 507-511, 1967.

MALBRAN, J. L., PAUNESSA, J. M. AND VIDAL, F.* HEREDITARY CRYSTALLINE DEGENERA-TION OF CORNEA. OPHTHALMOLOGICA 126* 369-378, 1953.

*12190 CORNEAL DYSTROPHY, GRANULAR TYPE (GROENOUW'S TYPE I)

IN THE MACULAR, GRANULAR AND LATTICE DYSTROPHIES THE CHANGES ARE IN THE CORNEAL STROMA RATHER THAN THE EPITHELIUM. IN THIS AND THE LATTICE TYPE, THE HISTOLOGIC FINDINGS ARE HYALINE DEGENERATION WITH ABSENCE OF ACID MUCOPOLYSACCHARIDE DEPOSITION. SEE RECESSIVE CATALOG FOR MACULAR CORNEAL DYSTROPHY (GROENOUW'S TYPE II). THE OPACITY IN THE GRANULAR TYPE CONSISTS OF GRAYISH WHITE GRANULES WITH SHARP BORDERS MAINLY IN A DISC-SHAPED AREA IN THE CENTER OF THE CORNEA. THE PERIPHERAL CORNEA IS USUALLY CLEAR AND THE CORNEA BETWEEN GRANULES IS CLEAR. HYALINE MATERIAL SEPARATES THE EPITHELIUM FROM BOWMAN'S MEMBRANE. ALTHOUGH THIS TYPE CAN HAVE ITS ONSET IN THE FIRST 10 YEARS, VISUAL ACUITY DURING CHILDHOOD IS USUALLY GOOD.

JONES, S. T. AND ZIMMERMAN, L. E.* HISTOPATHOLOGIC DIFFERENTIATION OF GRANULAR, MACULAR AND LATTICE DYSTROPHIES OF THE CORNEA. AM. J. OPHTHAL. 51* 394-410, 1961.

*12200 CORNEAL DYSTROPHY, HEREDITARY POLYMORPHOUS POSTERIOR

VACUOLES ARE DEMONSTRATED IN THE POSTERIOR PARTS OF THE CORNEA BY SLIT-LAMP EXAMINATION. VISION IS NOT AFFECTED SIGNIFICANTLY IN MOST CASES. HOWEVER, WE HAVE OBSERVED THREE AFFECTED PERSONS IN TWO GENERATIONS OF WHICH ONE IS LEGALLY BLIND. THE AFFECTED PERSONS IN THIS FAMILY ARE OBESE WITH VERY SIMILAR FACIAL FEATURES AND WIDELY SPACED TEETH. THESE CHARACTERISTICS MAY OR MAY NOT BE PRODUCED BY THE GENE RESPONSIBLE FOR THE CORNEAL CHANGE. SCHLICHTING (1941) NOTED DEPRESSIONS, VESICLES AND POLYMORPHOUS OPACITIES IN DESCEMET'S MEMBRANE, WITH OPACITIES IN THE DEEPEST LAYERS OF THE STROMA, IN FATHER AND 4 YEAR OLD DAUGHTER. THEODORE (1939) REPORTED 3 GENERATIONS. RUBINSTEIN AND SILVERMAN (1968) OBSERVED MOTHER AND TWO CHILDREN AFFECTED. THE MOTHER AND ONE CHILD HAD RUPTURE OF DESCEMET'S MEMBRANE AND THE MOTHER HAD GLAUCOMA. MCGEE AND FALLS (1953) REPORTED A FAMILY. THE CONDITION WAS FIRST DESCRIBED BY KOEPPE (1916) UNDER THE NAME OF KERATITIS BULLOSA INTERNA, AN APPROPRIATELY DESCRIPTIVE DESIGNATION. PEARCE ET AL. (1969) REPORTED A FAMILY IN WHICH 39 PERSONS IN FIVE GENERATIONS WERE AFFECTED WITH WHAT THEY TERMED 'CONGENITAL ENDOTHELIAL CORNEAL DYSTROPHY.' A DISTORTION OF SEGREGATION RATIO WAS NOTED IN THE OFFSPRING OF AFFECTED FEMALES - AN INCREASED NUMBER OF AFFECTED FEMALES AND A DEFICIENCY OF AFFECTED MALES. NO BIOLOGIC EXPLANATION COULD BE FOUND AND IT WAS CONCLUDED THAT THE DISTORTED SEX RATIO WAS A CHANCE HAPPENING. THE CLOUDING OF THE CORNEA DEVELOPED IN THE POSTNATAL PERIOD AND WAS USUALLY WELL ESTABLISHED BY EARLY CHILDHOOD. CHANGES IN THE POSTERIOR CORNEA, NAMELY MARKEDLY REDUCED NUMBER OF ENDOTHELIAL CELLS AND THICKENING OF DESCEMET'S MEMBRANE, WAS THOUGHT TO BE PRIMARY.

BERGMAN, G. D.* POSTERIOR POLYMORPHOUS DEGENERATION OF THE CORNEA. AM. J. OPHTHAL. 58* 125-128, 1964.

HOGAN, M. J. AND GIAMBATTISTA, B.* HEREDITARY DEEP DYSTROPHY OF THE CORNEA (POLYMORPHOUS). AM. J. OPHTHAL. 68* 777-788, 1969.

KOEPPE, L.* KLINISCHE BEOBACHTUNGEN MIT DER NERNSTSPALTLAMPE UND DEM HORNHAUT-MIKROSKOP. GRAEFE. ARCH. OPHTHAL. 91* 363-379, 1916.

KWEDAR, E. W.* HEREDITARY NONPROGRESSIVE DEEP CORNEAL DYSTROPHY. ARCH. OPHTHAL. 65* 127-129, 1961.

MCGEE, H. B. AND FALLS, H. F.* HEREDITARY POLYMORPHOUS DEEP DEGENERATION OF THE CORNEA. ARCH. OPHTHAL. 50* 462-467, 1953.

PEARCE, W. G., TRIPATHI, R. C. AND MORGAN, G.* CONGENITAL ENDOTHELIAL CORNEAL DYSTROPHY. CLINICAL, PATHOLOGICAL, AND GENETIC STUDY. BRIT. J. OPHTHAL. 53* 577-591, 1969.

RUBINSTEIN, R. A. AND SILVERMAN, J. J.* HEREDITARY DEEP DYSTROPHY OF THE CORNEA. ASSOCIATED WITH GLAUCOMA AND RUPTURES IN DESCEMET'S MEMBRANE. ARCH. OPHTHAL. 79* 123-126, 1968.

SCHLICHTING, H.* BLASEN- UND DELLENFORMIGE ENDOTHELDYSTROPHIE DER HORNHAUT. KLIN. MBL. AUGENHEILK. 107* 425-435, 1941.

THEODORE, F. H.* CONGENITAL TYPE OF ENDOTHELIAL DYSTROPHY. ARCH. OPHTHAL. 21* 626-638, 1939.

*12210 CORNEAL DYSTROPHY, JUVENILE EPITHELIAL, OF MEESMANN

THE CONDITION USUALLY APPEARS IN THE FIRST YEAR OR TWO OF LIFE, COMMENCING WITH SIGNS OF IRRITATION. THE CORNEAL CHANGES, SEEN ONLY WITH MAGNIFICATION, CONSIST OF MYRIADS OF FINE PUNCTATE OPACITIES IN THE EPITHELIUM AND OCCASIONALLY IN BOWMAN'S MEMBRANE. VISION IS ONLY RARELY IMPAIRED TO A SERIOUS DEGREE. MEESMANN AND WILKE (1939) STUDIED THREE FAMILIES WITH DOMINANT INHERITANCE AND STOCKER AND HOLT (1954, 1955) STUDIED A FAMILY WITH AFFECTED MEMBERS PROBABLY IN 8 GENERATIONS (4 GENERATIONS WERE EXAMINED). BEHNKE AND THIEL (1965) COULD DEMONSTRATE THAT ALL CASES IN SCHLESWIG-HOLSTEIN WERE MEMBERS OF ONE KINDRED TRACED BACK TO 1620. IN THE FOUR LIVING GENERATIONS 120 CASES WERE DEMONSTRATED. PROGRESSION DOES NOT OCCUR. ALKEMADE AND VAN BALEN (1966) OBSERVED 10 AFFECTED PERSONS IN ONE FAMILY. NONE HAD OCULAR COMPLAINTS.

ALKEMADE, P. P. H. AND VAN BALEN, A. T. M.* HEREDITARY EPITHELIAL DYSTROPHY OF THE CORNEA. BRIT. J. OPHTHAL. 50* 603-605, 1966.

BEHNKE, H. AND THIEL, H.-J.* UBER DIE HEREDITARE EPITHELDYSTROPHIE DER HORNHAUT (TYP MEESMAN-WILKE) IN SCHLESWIG-HOLSTEIN. KLIN. MBL. AUGENHEILK. 147* 662-672, 1965.

MEESMANN, A. AND WILKE, F.* KLINISCHE UND ANATOMISCHE UNTERSUCHUNGEN UBER EINE BISHER UNBEKANNTE, DOMINANT VERERBTE EPITHELDYSTROPHIEDER HORNHAUT. KLIN. MBL. AUGENHEILK. 103* 361-391, 1939.

SNYDER, W. B.* HEREDITARY EPITHELIAL CORNEAL DYSTROPHY. AM. J. OPHTHAL. 55* 56-61, 1963.

STOCKER, F. W. AND HOLT, L. B.* A RARE FORM OF HEREDITARY EPITHELIAL DYSTROPHY OF THE CORNEA* A GENETIC, CLINICAL, AND PATHOLOGIC STUDY. TRANS. AM. OPHTHAL. SOC. 52* 133-144, 1954.

STOCKER, F. W. AND HOLT, L. B.* RARE FORM OF HEREDITARY EPITHELIAL DYSTROPHY. ARCH. OPHTHAL. 53* 536-541, 1955.

*12220 CORNEAL DYSTROPHY, LATTICE TYPE

FRAYER AND BLODI (1959) DESCRIBED A FAMILY. GRAYISH LINES LIKE COTTON THREADS ARE MAINLY LIMITED TO A ZONE BETWEEN THE CENTER OF THE CORNEA AND THE PERIPHERY, USUALLY NOT EXTENDING TO THE LIMBUS. ROUNDED DOTS WITH DISTINCT BORDERS ARE SCATTERED EVERYWHERE. THE CORNEA BETWEEN OPACITIES IS RELATIVELY CLEAR. VISUAL ACTIVITY IS USUALLY NORMAL IN CHILDHOOD. IN THIS AND THE GRANULAR TYPE, THE HISTOLOGIC FINDINGS ARE HYALINE DEGENERATION AND ABSENCE OF ACID MUCOPOLYSAC- CHARIDE DEPOSITION. THE CHANGES INVOLVE PARTICULARLY THE CENTRAL PORTION OF THE CORNEA, BECOMING FIRST EVIDENT IN ADOLESCENCE AND CONSISTING OF DELICATE, DOUBLE- CONTOURED, INTERDIGITATING, ELONGATED DEPOSITS WHICH FORM A RETICULAR PATTERN IN THE CORNEAL STROMA. RECURRENT CORNEAL ULCERATION SOMETIMES OCCURS. PROGRESSION TO SEVERE VISUAL IMPAIRMENT BY THE FIFTH OR SIXTH DECADE IS THE RULE. NO SIGNS OF SYSTEMIC ABNORMALITY HAVE BEEN DESCRIBED. KLINTWORTH (1967) PRESENTED EVIDENCE THAT CORNEAL DYSTROFHY OF THE LATTICE TYPE IS A LOCAL VARIETY OF AMYLOIDOSIS.

FRAYER, W. C. AND BLODI, F. C.* THE LATTICE TYPE OF FAMILIAL CORNEAL DEGENERA- TION. A HISTOPATHOLOGIC STUDY. ARCH. OPHTHAL. 61* 712-719, 1959.

KING, R. G., JR. AND GEERAETS, W. J.* LATTICE OR REIS-BUCKLERS CORNEAL DYSTROPHY* A QUESTION OF STROMAL PATHOLOGY. STH. MED. J. 62* 1163-1169, 1969.

KLINTWORTH, G. K.* LATTICE CORNEAL DYSTROPHY* AN INHERITED VARIETY OF AMYLOIDO- SIS RESTRICTED TO THE CORNEA. AM. J. PATH. 50* 371-399, 1967.

RAMSAY, R. M.* FAMILIAL CORNEAL DYSTROPHY-LATTICE TYPE. TRANS. CANAD. OPHTHAL. SOC. 23* 222-229, 1960.

RICE, N. S. C., ASHTON, N., JAY, B. AND BLACH, R. K.* REIS-BUCKLERS' DYSTROPHY* A CLINICO-PATHOLOGICAL STUDY. BRIT. J. OPHTHAL. 52* 577-603, 1968.

*12230 CORNEAL DYSTROPHY, PUNCTATE OR NODULAR

ONSET IS AT ABOUT PUBERTY. BILATERAL NODULAR OPACITIES OF THE CORNEA ARE CHARACTERISTIC. GROENOUW (1933) DEMONSTRATED DOMINANT INHERITANCE.

GROENOUW, A.* KNOTCHENFORMIGE HORNHAUTTRUBUNGEN VERERBT DURCH VIER GENERA- TIONEN. KLIN. MBL. AUGENHEILK. 90* 577-580, 1933.

*12240 CORNEAL EROSIONS, RECURRING HEREDITARY

FRANCESCHETTI (1928) DESCRIBED A FAMILY IN WHICH SIX SUCCESSIVE GENERATIONS WERE AFFECTED. THE DISORDER BECAME MANIFEST BETWEEN 4 AND 6 YEARS. RECURRING ULCERATIONS ARE ALSO SEEN IN MACULAR AND LATTICE TYPES OF CLASSICAL DYSTROPHY. SEE ALSO KERATITIS FUGAX HEREDITARIA. A FOLLOW-UP IN 1958 SHOWED 40 AFFECTED MEMBERS OF THE FAMILY (FRANCESCHETTI AND KLEIN, 1961). VALLE (1967) DESCRIBED A FAMILY WITH SIX AFFECTED PERSONS IN THREE SIBSHIPS IN TWO GENERATIONS. THE PROGENITOR HAD FUCHS' CORNEAL DYSTROPHY. WALES (1956) DESCRIBED AFFECTED PERSONS IN 3 GENERATIONS.

FRANCESCHETTI, A. AND KLEIN, D.* CHAPTER VIII - CORNEA. IN, WAARDENBURG, P. J., FRANCESCHETTI, A. AND KLEIN, D. (EDS.)* GENETICS AND OPHTHALMOLOGY. SPRING- FIELD, ILL.* CHARLES C THOMAS, 1961. PP. 447-543.

FRANCESCHETTI, A.* HEREDITARE REZIVIERENDE EROSION DER HORNHAUT. Z. AUGEN- HEILK. 66* 309-316, 1928.

VALLE, O.* HEREDITARY RECURRING CORNEAL EROSIONS. A FAMILY STUDY, WITH SPECIAL REFERENCE TO FUCH'S DYSTROPHY. ACTA OPHTHAL. 45* 829-836, 1967.

WALES, H. J.* A FAMILY HISTORY OF CORNEAL EROSIONS. TRANS. OPHTHAL. SOC. NEW

12250 CORTICOSTEROID-BINDING GLOBULIN (CBG), DECREASE IN

D
O
M
I
N
A
N
T

DOE ET AL. (1965) FOUND DECREASED LEVELS IN 8 PERSONS IN THREE GENERATIONS OF A FAMILY. IN NO INSTANCE WAS THERE MALE-TO-MALE TRANSMISSION. THE EXTENT OF THE DECREASE WAS THE SAME IN MALES AND FEMALES. CBG, OTHERWISE KNOWN AS TRANSCORTIN, IS AN ALPHA-GLOBULIN. DEMOOR ET AL. (1967) FOUND A BIMODAL DISTRIBUTION OF CBG LEVELS IN MALES BUT NOT IN FEMALES, AND THE FATHERS OF MALES WITH LOW LEVELS SHOWED NORMAL LEVELS. THEY FELT THAT X-LINKED INHERITANCE BEST ACCOUNTS FOR THE FINDINGS. ELEVATED CBG WAS FOUND IN A BROTHER AND SISTER BY LOHRENZ ET AL. (1968). NEITHER SIB HAD CHILDREN AND THE MOTHER, THE ONLY SURVIVING PARENT, HAD NORMAL CBG LEVELS.

DEMOOR, P., MEULEPAS, E., HENDRIKX, A., HEYNS, W. AND VANDENSCHRIECK, H. G.* CORTISOL-BINDING CAPACITY OF PLASMA TRANSCORTIN* A SEX-LINKED TRAIT.Q J. CLIN. ENDOCR. 27* 959-965, 1967.

DOE, R. P., LOHRENZ, F. N. AND SEAL, U. S.* FAMILIAL DECREASE IN CORTICOS-TEROID-BINDING GLOBULIN. METABOLISM 14* 940-943, 1965.

LOHRENZ, F., DOE, R. P. AND SEAL, U. S.* IDIOPATHIC OR GENETIC ELEVATION OF CORTICOSTEROID-BINDING GLOBULIN.Q J. CLIN. ENDOCR. 28* 1073-1075, 1968.

*12260 COSTOVERTEBRAL SEGMENTATION ANOMALIES

WE (RIMOIN ET AL., 1968) HAVE SEEN A FAMILY IN WHICH FATHER AND SON (1122178, 1222180) AND PROBABLY TWO PRECEDING GENERATIONS WERE SHORT OF STATURE (LESS THAN FIVE FEET), THE SHORTENING BEING MAINLY IN THE TRUNK, AND HAD MULTIPLE RIB AND VERTEBRAL ANOMALIES. THE NUMBER OF RIBS WAS REDUCED TO 11 AND SEVERAL RIBS WERE FUSED POSTERIORLY. HEMIVERTEBRA AND VERTEBRAL FUSION WERE NOTED AT MULTIPLE LEVELS IN THE CERVICAL AND THORACIC SPINE. NO NEUROLOGIC MANIFESTATIONS WERE PRESENT. LANGER (1967) HAS SHOWN US ANOTHER FAMILY WITH MULTIPLE AFFECTED GENERATIONS. THE FAMILY REPORTED AS POLYDYSSPONDYLY BY RUTT AND DEGENHARDT (1959) HAD AFFECTED PERSONS IN 4 GENERATIONS. VAN DE SAR (1952) FOUND MULTIPLE HEMIVER-TEBRAE AND RIB ANOMALIES IN A MOTHER AND DAUGHTER. MULTIPLE HEMIVERTEBRAE ALSO OCCUR AS A RECESSIVE. POLYDYSSPONDYLY WAS DESCRIBED BY TURPIN ET AL. (1959) IN ASSOCIATION WITH A TRANSLOCATION INVOLVING GROUP D AND G CHROMOSOMES. DE GROUCHY ET AL. (1963) REPORTED A SIMILAR CONDITION IN MOTHER AND DAUGHTER, BOTH OF WHOM CARRIED A 14-15 TRANSLOCATION.

DE GROUCHY, J., MLYNARSKI, J.-C., MAROTEAUX, P., LAMY, M., DESHAIES, G., BENICHOU, C. AND SALMON, C.* SYNDROME POLYDYSSPONDYLIQUE PAR TRANSLOCATION 14-15 ET DYSCHONDROSTEOSE CHEZ UN MEME SUJET. SEGREGATION FAMILIALE. COMP. REND. ACAD. SCI. 256* 1614-1616, 1963.

LANGER, L. O., JR.* MINNEAPOLIS, MINN.* PERSONAL COMMUNICATION, 1967.

RIMOIN, D. L., FLETCHER, B. D. AND MCKUSICK, V. A.* SPONDYLOCOSTAL DYSPLASIA* A DOMINANTLY INHERITED FORM OF SHORT-TRUNKED DWARFISM. AM. J. MED. 45* 948-953, 1968.

RUTT, A. AND DEGENHARDT, K.-H.* BEITRAG ZUR ATIOLOGIE UND PATHOGENESE VON WIRBELSAULENMISSBILDUNGEN. ARCH. ORTHOP. UNFALLCHIR. 57* 120, 1959. (SEE ALSO, EIN KURZES HANDBUCH IN FUNF BANDEN. BECKER, P. E. (ED.)* STUTTGART* GEORG THIEME VERLAG, 2* 589 ONLY, 1964.).

TURPIN, R., LEJEUNE, J., LAFOURCADE, J. AND GAUTIER, M.* ABERRATIONS CHROMO-SOMIQUES ET MALADIES HUMAINES. LA POLYDYSSPONDYLIE A 45 CHROMOSOMES. COMP. REND. ACAD. SCI. 248* 3636-3638, 1959.

VAN DE SAR, A.* HEREDITARY MULTIPLE HEMIVERTEBRAE. DOC. DE MED. GEOGRAPH. ET TROP. 4* 23-28, 1952.

*12270 COUMARIN RESISTANCE

O'REILLY ET AL. (1964) DESCRIBED RESISTANCE TO THE HYPOPROTHROMBINEMIC EFFECTS OF COUMARIN DRUGS, IN 7 PERSONS IN THREE GENERATIONS OF A FAMILY WITH NO MALE-TO-MALE TRANSMISSION. THEY POSTULATED THAT AN AUTOSOMAL GENE IS RESPONSIBLE FOR THE SYNTHESIS OF A CLOTTING FACTOR DEPENDENT ON VITAMIN K AND THAT IN THIS FAMILY AFFECTED PERSONS HAVE AN ABNORMAL FACTOR WITH DECREASED AFFINITY FOR THE COUMARIN DRUG OR INCREASED AFFINITY FOR VITAMIN K. HEREDITARY RESISTANCE TO WARFARIN IN RATS, WHICH MAY BE A COMPARABLE CONDITION, IS INHERITED AS AN AUTOSOMAL DOMINANT (GREAVES AND AYRES, 1967). O'REILLY (1970) DESCRIBED A SECOND KINDRED OF WHICH 18 MEMBERS WERE SHOWN TO HAVE RELATIVE RESISTANCE TO ORAL ANTICOAGULANT DRUGS. SEVERAL INSTANCES OF MALE-TO-MALE TRANSMISSION WERE OBSERVED. OF THE VARIOUS POSSIBLE MECHANISMS FOR THE RELATIVE RESISTANCE ALL COULD BE EXCLUDED EXCEPT MUTATION IN THE VITAMIN K-ANTICOAGULANT RECEPTOR SITE. POSITIVE EVIDENCE FAVORING THE LATTER INCLUDED THE CORRECTION OF HYPOPROTHROMBINEMIA BY SMALL AMOUNTS OF EXOGENOUS VITAMIN K AND THE FACT THAT THE ANTICOAGULANT DOSE-RESPONSE CURVES FOR THE PROBANDS OF THE TWO FAMILIES STUDIED BY O'REILLY AND NORMAL SUBJECTS ARE PARALLEL. POOL ET AL. (1968) CONCLUDED THAT THE RESISTANCE TO WARFARIN IS DUE TO

GREAVES, J. H. AND AYRES, P.* HERITABLE RESISTANCE TO WARFARIN IN RATS. NATURE
215* 877-878, 1967.

O'REILLY, R. A.* THE SECOND REPORTED KINDRED WITH HEREDITARY RESISTANCE TO ORAL
ANTICOAGULANT DRUGS. NEW ENG. J. MED. 282* 1448-1451, 1970.

O'REILLY, R. A., AGGELER, P. M., HOAG, M. S., LEONG, L. S., AND KROPATKIN, M.
L.* HEREDITARY TRANSMISSION OF EXCEPTIONAL RESISTANCE TO COUMARIN ANTICOAGULANT
DRUGS. THE FIRST REPORTED KINDRED. NEW ENG. J. MED. 271* 809-815, 1964.

POOL, J. G., O'REILLY, R. A., SCHNEIDERMAN, L. J. AND ALEXANDER, M.* WARFARIN
RESISTANCE IN THE RAT. AM. J. PHYSIOL. 215* 627-631, 1968.

12280 CRANIAL DYSOSTOSIS WITH PRONOUNCED DIGITAL IMPRESSIONS (PSEUDO-CROUZON'S
DISEASE)

IN CROUZON'S DISEASE AND PSEUDO-CROUZON'S DISEASE, THE PRONOUNCED DIGITAL
IMPRESSIONS, OR CONVOLUTIONAL MARKINGS, ARE IDENTICAL. THE ESSENTIAL DIFFERENCE
IS IN THE FACE. IN PSEUDO-CROUZON'S DISEASE THERE IS NO PROGNATHISM, THE NOSE IS
NOT CURVED AND DIVERGENT SQUINT IS USUALLY LACKING. PROMINENT FOREHEAD AND SOME
DEGREE OF EXOPHTHALMOS ARE FEATURES. FRANCESCHETTI (1953) FIRST DELINEATED THE
CONDITION. HE (1968) POINTED OUT THAT WALSH (1957) DESCRIBED A CASE AS CROUZON'S
DISEASE. NONE OF FRANCESCHETTI'S CASES WERE FAMILIAL, BUT DOLIVO AND GILLIERON
(1955) DESCRIBED AFFECTED BROTHER AND SISTER. THE MOTHER, GRANDMOTHER AND GREAT-
GRANDMOTHER WERE SAID TO HAVE OXYCEPHALY.

DOLIVO, G. AND GILLIERON, J.-D.* UNE FAMILLE DE PSEUDO-CROUZON. CONFIN.
NEUROL. 15* 114-118, 1955.

FRANCESCHETTI, A.* CRANIAL DYSOSTOSIS WITH PRONOUNCED DIGITAL IMPRESSIONS
(PSEUDO-CROUZON DYSOSTOSIS). IN, CONGENITAL ANOMALIES OF THE EYE. ST. LOUIS* C.
V. MOSBY CO., 1968. PP. 81-84.

FRANCESCHETTI, A.* DYSOSTOSE CRANIENNE AVEC CALOTTE CEREBRIFORME (PSEUDO-
CROUZON). CONFIN. NEUROL. 13* 161-166, 1953.

WALSH, F. B.* CLINICAL NEURO-OPHTHALMOLOGY. BALTIMORE* WILLIAMS AND WILKINS
CO., 1957 (2ND ED.).

12290 CRANIOFACIAL DYSOSTOSIS WITH DIAPHYSEAL HYPERPLASIA

STANESCO ET AL. (1963) DESCRIBED A CURIOUS SYNDROME IN 9 MEMBERS OF A KINDRED WITH
A PATTERN SUGGESTIVE OF AUTOSOMAL DOMINANT INHERITANCE. THE FEATURES INCLUDED A
PECULIAR FORM OF CRANIO-FACIAL DYSOSTOSIS WITH SMALL SKULL, THIN CRANIAL BONE,
DEPRESSIONS OVER THE FRONTO-PARIETAL AND OCCIPITOPARIETAL SUTURES, POORLY
DEVELOPED MANDIBLE, AND EXOPHTHALMOS. THE LIMBS WERE SHORT AND BY X-RAY THE
CORTICES OF THE LONG BONES WERE MASSIVELY THICKENED.

STANESCO, V., MAXIMILIAN, C., POENARU, S., FLOREA, I., STANESCO, R., IONESCO,
V. AND IOANITIU, D.* SYNDROME HEREDITAIRE DOMINANT, REUNISSANT UNE DYSOSTOSE
CRANIO-FACIALE DE TYPE PARTICULIER, UNE INSUFFISANCE DE CROISSANCE D'ASPECT
CHONDRODYSTROPHIQUE ET UN EPAISSISSEMENT MASSIF DE LA CORTICALE DES OS LONGS.
REV. FRANC. ENDOCR. CLIN. 4* 219-231, 1963.

*12300 CRANIOMETAPHYSEAL DYSPLASIA

IN THE FAMILY DESCRIBED BY KOMINS (1954) BROTHER AND SISTER WERE AFFECTED AS WELL
AS THE MOTHER AND A MATERNAL UNCLE. PODLAHA AND KRATOCHVIL (1963) AND LEJEUNE ET
AL. (1966) OBSERVED THAT CRANIOMETAPHYSEAL DYSPLASIA DIFFERS FROM PYLE'S DISEASE
(METAPHYSEAL DYSPLASIA) IN THE PRESENCE OF CONSPICUOUS INVOLVEMENT OF THE
CRANIOFACIAL BONES. WIDENING OF THE BRIDGE OF THE NOSE DEVELOPS AND EVENTUALLY
LEONINE FACIES. PRESSURE ON CRANIAL NERVES IS RESPONSIBLE FOR A CONSIDERABLE PART
OF THE DISABILITY. IT IS LIKELY THAT THE CASES IN THE FAMILY REPORTED BY RIMOIN
ET AL. (1969) AND THOSE REPORTED BY SPRANGER ET AL. (1965) SHOULD BE CONSIDERED
DOMINANT CRANIOMETAPHYSEAL DYSPLASIA RESERVING THE TERM PYLES DISEASE FOR THE
RECESSIVE DISORDER WHICH IS MORE NEARLY A 'PURE' METAPHYSEAL DYSPLASIA WITH LITTLE
OR NO CRANIOFACIAL INVOLVEMENT. SPRANGER (1970) REVIEWED THE SKULL TRAY OF PYLE'S
ORIGINAL CASE AND FAILED TO FIND THE INTENSE INCREASE IN BONE DENSITY CHARACTERIS-
TIC OF CRANIOMETAPHYSEAL DYSPLASIA. FURTHERMORE THE METAPHYSEAL FLARE IS NOTABLY
ABRUPT IN PYLE'S DISEASE, PRODUCING THE 'ERLENMEYER FLASK' DEFORMITY AND MILDER
('CLUB-LIKE') IN CRANIOMETAPHYSEAL DYSPLASIA. PYLE'S DISEASE IS A RECESSIVE,
WHEREAS CRANIOMETAPHYSEAL DYSPLASIA IS A DOMINANT. THE SAME FAMILY WAS REPORTED
BY RIMOIN ET AL. (1969) AND BY GLADNEY AND MONTELEONE (1970).

GLADNEY, J. H. AND MONTELEONE, P. L.* METAPHYSEAL DYSPLASIA. LANCET 2* 44-45,
1970.

HASSLER, R.* FAMILIARE KRANIO-METAPHYSARE DYSPLASIE. FORTSCHR. RONTGENSTR. 90*
704-713, 1959.

HOLT, J. F.* THE EVOLUTION OF CRANIO-METAPHYSEAL DYSPLASIA. ANN. RADIOL. 9* 209-214, 1966.

KOMINS, C.* FAMILIAL METAPHYSEAL DYSPLASIA (PYLE'S DISEASE). BRIT. J. RADIOL. 27* 670-675, 1954.

LEJEUNE, E., ANJOU, A., BOUVIER, M., ROBERT, J., VAUZELLE, J. L. AND JEANNERET, J.* DYSPLASIE CRANIO-METAPHYSAIRE FAMILIALE. REV. RHUM. 33* 714-726, 1966.

MORI, P. A. AND HOLT, J. F.* CRANIAL MANIFESTATIONS OF FAMILIAL METAPHYSEAL DYSPLASIA. RADIOLOGY 66* 335-343, 1956.

PODLAHA, M. AND KRATOCHVIL, L.* FAMILIAL METAPHYSIAL DYSPLASIA* PYLE'S DISEASE. FORTSCHR. ROENTGENSTR. 98* 158-162, 1963.

RIMOIN, D. L., WOODRUFF, S. L. AND HOLMAN, B. L.* CRANIOMETAPHYSEAL DYSPLASIA (PYLE'S DISEASE)* AUTOSOMAL DOMINANT INHERITANCE IN A LARGE KINDRED. THE CLINICAL DELINEATION OF BIRTH DEFECTS. IV. SKELETAL DYSPLASIAS. NEW YORK* NATIONAL FOUNDATION, 1969. PP. 96-104.

SPRANGER, J.* FAMILIAL METAPHYSEAL DYSPLASIA.Q (LETTER) LANCET 2* 475 ONLY, 1970.

SPRANGER, J., PAULSEN, K. AND LEHMANN, W.* DIE KRANIOMETAPHYSARE DYSPLASIE (PYLE). Z. KINDERHEILK. 93* 64-79, 1965.

12310 CRANIOSTENOSIS

GORDON (1959) FOUND MULTIPLE CASES IN FIVE OF NINE SOUTH AFRICAN FAMILIES STUDIED IN DETAIL. IN FOUR MULTIPLE SIBS WERE INVOLVED. IN THE FIFTH THE MOTHER OF AN AFFECTED CHILD WAS ALSO AFFECTED. UNDER THE DESIGNATION "SCAPHOCEPHALY" BELL, CLARE AND WENTWORTH (1961) DESCRIBED THE SAME CONDITION IN TWO FAMILIES. IN ONE FAMILY, 6 PERSONS IN THREE GENERATIONS WERE SAID TO BE AFFECTED WITH MALE-TO-MALE TRANSMISSION AND IN ANOTHER FAMILY TWO CHILDREN OF AN UNAFFECTED WOMAN, EACH BY A DIFFERENT FATHER, WERE AFFECTED. MURPHY (1953) OBSERVED CRANIOSTENOSIS IN FATHER AND SON. NANCE AND ENGEL (1967) DESCRIBED A FAMILY IN WHICH THE MOTHER HAD MARKED DOLICHOCEPHALY AND TWO SONS HAD SEVERE CRANIOSTENOSIS WITH PREMATURE CLOSURE OF SUTURES AND A "BEATEN METAL" APPEARANCE OF THE CALVARIUM BY X-RAY. THE FAMILY WAS OF UNUSUAL INTEREST BECAUSE THE NORMAL FATHER AND THE TWO SONS HAD A DELETION OF THE SHORT ARM OF ONE G CHROMOSOME WHICH HAS BEEN FOUND AS A NORMAL VARIATION IN SOME FAMILIES ("CHRISTCHURCH CHROMOSOME") AND WAS FOUND BY THESE WORKERS IN A PATIENT WITH PYCNODYSOSTOSIS (Q.V.) IN WHICH FAILURE OF CLOSURE OF CRANIAL SUTURES IS A FEATURE. ANDERSON AND GEIGER (1965) OBSERVED AN INFANT WITH LEFT CORONAL SYNOSTOSIS AND FATHER WITH SAGITTAL SYNOSTOSIS. BELL, CLARE AND WENTWORTH (1961) OBSERVED 8 AFFECTED PERSONS IN 3 GENERATIONS OF ONE FAMILY AND IN 2 OFFSPRING OF THE SAME MOTHER BUT DIFFERENT FATHERS. SHELDON (1931) REPORTED FIVE CASES OF OXYCEPHALY IN THREE GENERATIONS. INTELLIGENCE WAS NORMAL. THE MEMBRANE BONES OF THE SKULL SHOWED A "BEATEN COPPER" APPEARANCE BY X-RAY. IN A LARGE EXPERIENCE OF 519 CASES CRANIOSTENOSIS, SHILLITO AND MATSON (1968) ENCOUNTERED 9 FAMILIES IN EACH OF WHICH TWO SIBS WERE AFFECTED. IN ONE THE SIBS WERE IDENTICAL TWINS. FOUR PAIRS HAD SYNOSTOSIS OF ONE OR MORE CORONAL SUTURES. FAMILIAL INVOLVEMENT WAS HIGHEST IN CASES WITH CORONAL SYNOSTOSIS, PARTICULARLY BILATERAL CORONAL INVOLVE-MENT. SUCCESSIVE GENERATIONS WERE ESPECIALLY OFTEN AFFECTED IN CASES OF MULTIPLE OR TOTAL SYNOSTOSIS.

ANDERSON, F. M. AND GEIGER, L.* CRANIOSYNOSTOSIS. A SURVEY OF 204 CASES. J. NEUROSURG. 22* 229-240, 1965.

BELL, H. S., CLARE, F. B. AND WENTWORTH, A. F.* CASE REPORTS AND TECHNICAL NOTES OF FAMILIAL SCAPHOCEPHALY. J. NEUROSURG. 18* 239-241, 1961.

FREEMAN, J. M. AND BERKOWF, S.* CRANIOSTENOSIS* REVIEW OF THE LITERATURE AND REPORT OF THIRTY-FOUR CASES. PEDIATRICS 30* 57-70, 1962.

GORDON, H.* CRANIOSTENOSIS. BRIT. MED. J. 2* 792-795, 1959.

MURPHY, J. W.* FAMILIAL SCAPHOCEPHALY IN FATHER AND SON. U.S. ARMED FORCES MED. J. 4* 1496-1499, 1953.

NANCE, W. E. AND ENGEL, E.* AUTOSOMAL DELETION MAPPING IN MAN. SCIENCE 155* 692-694, 1967.

SHELDON, W.* HEREDITARY AND FAMILIAL OXYCEPHALY. PROC. ROY. SOC. MED. 24* 574-576, 1931.

SHILLITO, J., JR. AND MATSON, D. D.* CRANIOSYNOSTOSIS* A REVIEW OF 519 SURGICAL PATIENTS. PEDIATRICS 41* 829-853, 1968.

12320 CRANIUM BIFIDUM OCCULTUM

TERRAFRANCA AND ZELLIS (1953) DESCRIBED AFFECTED MOTHER AND TWO CHILDREN. IN ONE OF THE CHILDREN A MEDIAL DEFECT IN THE FRONTAL BONE WAS ACCOMPANIED BY SYMMETRICAL

PARIETAL LACUNAE LIKE THOSE DESCRIBED HERE AS PARIETAL FORAMINA (Q.V.), AS WELL AS CERVICAL (C5-C7) AND LUMBOSACRAL (L5-S1) SPINA BIFIDA OCCULTA. THE OTHER OFFSPRING HAD AN IDENTICAL FRONTAL DEFECT BUT LESS CONSPICUOUS PARIETAL FORAMINA AND NO SPINA BIFIDA. THE MOTHER HAD A U-SHAPED FRONTAL DEFECT ASTRIDE THE METOPIC SUTURE.

TERRAFRANCA, R. J. AND ZELLIS, A.* CONGENITAL HEREDITARY CRANIUM BIFIDUM OCCULTUM FRONTALIS. RADIOLOGY 61* 60-66, 1953.

12330 CREATINE KINASE

MULTIPLE FORMS (ISOZYMES) ARE KNOWN. CREATINE KINASE EXISTS AS A DIMER COMPOSED OF TWO SUBUNITS. THE MUSCLE ENZYME (MM) CONSISTS OF TWO IDENTICAL M SUBUNITS. THE BRAIN ENZYME (BB) CONSISTS OF TWO IDENTICAL B SUBUNITS (DAWSON ET AL., 1968). OTHER TISSUES SHOW A THIRD HYBRID MB ENZYME. APPARENTLY POLYMORPHISM OF CREATINE KINASE HAS NOT BEEN IDENTIFIED.

DAWSON, D. M., EPPENBERGER, H. M. AND EPPENBERGER, M. E.* MULTIPLE MOLECULAR FORMS OF CREATINE KINASES. ANN. N.Y. ACAD. SCI. 151* 616-626, 1968.

12340 CREUTZFELDT-JAKOB DISEASE

JACOB ET AL. (1950) AND HIS PREDESCESSORS DESCRIBED THE FIRST REPORTED FAMILY, THE BACKER KINDRED. THREE GENERATIONS MAY HAVE BEEN AFFECTED, WITH MALE-TO-MALE TRANSMISSION. DAVIDSON AND RABINER (1940) DESCRIBED 3 AFFECTED SIBS. SOME QUESTION WHETHER C-J DISEASE SHOULD BE CONSIDERED A DISTINCT ENTITY. FRIEDE AND DEJONG (1964) AND LATER MAY ET AL. (1968) DESCRIBED AFFECTED FATHER AND 3 DAUGHTERS. ONSET WAS BETWEEN 38 AND 45 YEARS. THE ILLNESS LASTED ONLY 10 MONTHS TO TWO YEARS. THE DISORDER BEGAN WITH FORGETFULNESS AND NERVOUSNESS AND PRO-GRESSED WITH JERKY, TREMBLING MOVEMENTS OF THE HANDS, LOSS OF FACIAL EXPRESSION AND UNSTEADY GAIT. PATHOLOGIC FINDINGS INCLUDED SEVERE STATUS SPONGIOSUS, DIFFUSE NERVE CELL DEGENERATION AND SOME GLIAL PROLIFERATION. CREUTZFELDT-JACOB DISEASE IS UNDOUBTEDLY A MIXED CATEGORY. GIBBS ET AL. (1968) REPORTED A TRANSMISSIBLE AGENT WHICH REPRODUCED THE DISEASE IN A CHIMPANZEE INJECTED WITH BRAIN MATERIAL FROM A 59 YEAR OLD ENGLISH MALE.

DAVIDSON, C. AND RABINER, A. M.* SPASTIC PSEUDOSCLEROSIS (DISSEMINATED ENCEPHALOMYELOPATHY* CORTICOPALLIDOSPINAL DEGENERATION). ARCH. NEUROL. PSYCHIAT. 44* 578-598, 1940.

FRIEDE, R. L. AND DEJONG, R. N.* NEURONAL ENZYMIC FAILURE IN CREUTZFELDT-JAKOB DISEASE* A FAMILIAL STUDY. ARCH. NEUROL. 10* 181-195, 1964.

GIBBS, C. J., JR., GAJDUSEK, D. C., ASHER, D. M., ALPERS, M. P., BECK, E., DANIEL, P. M. AND MATTHEWS, W. B.* CREUTZFELDT-JAKOB DISEASE (SPONGIFORM ENCEPHA-LOPATHY)* TRANSMISSION TO THE CHIMPANZEE. SCIENCE 161* 388-389, 1968.

JACOB, H., PYRKOSCH, W. AND STRUBE, H.* HEREDITARY FORM OF CREUTZFELDT-JAKOB DISEASE (BECKER FAMILY). ARCH. PSYCHIAT. 184* 653-674, 1950.

MAY, W. W., ITABASHI, H. AND DEJONG, R. N.* CREUTZFELDT-JAKOB DISEASE. II. CLINICAL, PATHOLOGIC AND GENETIC STUDY OF A FAMILY. ARCH. NEUROL. PSYCHIAT. 19* 137-149, 1968.

*12350 CROUZON'S CRANIOFACIAL DYSOSTOSIS

CROUZON'S DISEASE IS CHARACTERIZED BY CRANIAL SYNOSTOSIS, HYPERTELORISM, EXOPHTHA-LMUS AND EXTERNAL STRABISMUS, PARROT-BEAKED NOSE, SHORT UPPER LIP, HYPOPLASTIC MAXILLA AND A RELATIVE MANDIBULAR PROGNATHISM. THE FAMILIAL OCCURRENCE WAS NOTED BY CROUZON IN 1912 WHEN HE FIRST DESCRIBED THE SYNDROME. SUBSEQUENTLY, SEVERAL INVESTIGATORS HAVE DEMONSTRATED AN AUTOSOMAL DOMINANT MODE OF INHERITANCE. SHILLER (1959) OBSERVED DOMINANT TRANSMISSION IN FOUR GENERATIONS WITH 23 AFFECTED MEMBERS. THERE WAS A MARKED VARIABILITY IN BOTH CRANIAL AND FACIAL MANIFESTATIONS OF THE SYNDROME. ANDERSEN (1943) ALSO TRACED THE CONDITION THROUGH 4 GENERATIONS. DODGE ET AL. (1959) DESCRIBED FIVE PATIENTS, THREE WITH TYPICAL CROUZON'S DISEASE, TWO OF THESE HAD A POSITIVE FAMILY HISTORY AND ONE WAS SPORADIC. THE OTHER TWO CASES, ALSO SPORADIC, HAD SYNDACTYLISM OF BOTH HANDS AND FEET, AN ASSOCIATION WHICH HAS BEEN DESIGNATED AS VOGT'S CEPHALODACTYLY (SEE ACROCEPHALOSYNDACTYLY TYPES). FRANCESCHETTI (1953) DESCRIBED TWO UNRELATED CASES WHICH SIMULATE CROUZON'S DISEASE* HOWEVER THE PATIENTS DO NOT HAVE THE FACIAL MANIFESTATIONS. TO DIFFERENTIATE THESE CASES FROM CROUZON'S DISEASE, FRANCESCHETTI COINED THE TERM 'PSEUDO-CROUZON SYNDROME.' VULLIAMY AND NORMANDALE (1966) IDENTIFIED 14 CASES OF CROUZON'S DISEASE IN 4 GENERATIONS OF A FAMILY WITH SEVERAL INSTANCES OF MALE-TO-MALE TRANSMISSION. SEE PHOSPHATASE, PLACENTAL ALKALINE. SEE CRANIAL DYSOSTOSIS WITH PRONOUNCED DIGITAL IMPRESSIONS (PSEUDO-CROUZON'S DISEASE). THREE GENERATIONS WERE AFFECTED IN THE FAMILY REPORTED BY PALACIOS AND SCHIMKE (1969). FLIPPEN (1950) ALSO TRACED THE MALFORMATION THROUGH FOUR GENERATIONS, AND PINKERTON AND PINKERTON (1952) OBSERVED IT IN A MOTHER AND TWO OF HER THREE DAUGHTERS.

ANDERSEN, P. F.* CRANIOFACIAL DYSOSTOSIS (CROUZON'S DISEASE) AS DOMINANT HEREDITARY DISEASE. NORD. MED. 18* 993-996, 1943.

CROUZON, O.* DYSOSTOSE CRANIO-FACIALE HEREDITAIRE. BULL. SOC. MED. HOP. PARIS 33* 545-555, 1912.

DODGE, H. W., WOOD, M. W. AND KENNEDY, R. L. J.* CRANIOFACIAL DYSOSTOSIS.* CROUZON'S DISEASE. PEDIATRICS 23* 98-106, 1959.

FLIPPEN, J. H., JR.* CRANIO-FACIAL DYSOSTOSIS OF CROUZON. REPORT OF A CASE IN WHICH THE MALFORMATION OCCURRED IN FOUR GENERATIONS. PEDIATRICS 5* 90-96, 1950.

FRANCESCHETTI, A.* DYSOSTOSE CRANIENNE AVEC CALOTTE CEREBRIFORME (PSEUDO-CROUZON). CONFIN. NEUROL. 13* 161-166, 1953.

PALACIOS, E. AND SCHIMKE, R. N.* CRANIOSYNOSTOSIS-SYNDACTYLISM. AM. J. ROENTGEN. 106* 144-155, 1969.

PINKERTON, O. D. AND PINKERTON, F. J.* HEREDITARY CRANIOFACIAL DYSPLASIA. AM. J. OPHTHAL. 35* 500-506, 1952.

SHILLER, J. G.* CRANIOFACIAL DYSOSTOSIS OF CROUZON. A CASE REPORT AND PEDIGREE WITH EMPHASIS ON HEREDITY. PEDIATRICS 23* 107-112, 1959.

VULLIAMY, D. G. AND NORMANDALE, P. A.* CRANIO-FACIAL DYSOSTOSIS IN A DORSET FAMILY. ARCH. DIS. CHILD. 41* 375-382, 1966.

12360 CRYPTORCHIDISM, UNILATERAL

IN 8 MALES IN FOUR GENERATIONS, PERRETT AND O'ROURKE (1969) DESCRIBED IPSILATERAL (RIGHT SIDED) CRYPTORCHIDISM. CORBUS AND O'CONOR (1922) FOUND SEVERAL REPORTS OF FAMILIES WITH MULTIPLE GENERATIONS AFFECTED.

CORBUS, B. C. AND O'CONOR, V. J.* THE FAMILIAL OCCURRENCE OF UNDESCENDED TESTES. REPORT OF SIX BROTHERS WITH TESTICULAR ANOMALIES. SURG. GYNEC. OBSTET. 34* 237-240, 1922.

PERRETT, L. J. AND O'ROURKE, D. A.* HEREDITARY CRYPTORCHIDISM. MED. J. AUST. 1* 1289-1290, 1969.

12370 CUTIS LAXA

IN MOST FAMILIES THE FINDINGS SUGGEST THAT CUTIS LAXA IS INHERITED AS A RECESSIVE (Q.V.). HOWEVER, SESTAK (1962) REPORTED AFFECTED FATHER AND DAUGHTER. SEE ALSO THE EARLIER REPORT OF DOMINANT INHERITANCE BY WIENER (1925). GOLTZ (1966) HAS A FAMILY WITH AFFECTED PERSONS IN SUCCESSIVE GENERATIONS. BALBONI (1963) DESCRIBED A CHILD WITH TYPICAL CUTIS LAXA AND MULTIPLE VASCULAR ANOMALIES INCLUDING COARCTATION OF THE AORTA. THE FATHER AND A PATERNAL UNCLE WERE THOUGHT TO HAVE THE SAME CONDITION.

BALBONI, F. A.* CUTIS LAXA AND MULTIPLE VASCULAR ANOMALIES INCLUDING MULTIPLE COARTATION OF THE AORTA. A CASE REPORT. ST. FRANCIS HOSP. BULL. 19* 26-35, 1963.

GOLTZ, R. W.* DENVER, COL.* PERSONAL COMMUNICATION, 1966.

SESTAK, Z.* EHLERS-DANLOS SYNDROME AND CUTIS LAXA* AN ACCOUNT OF FAMILIES IN THE OXFORD AREA. ANN. HUM. GENET. 25* 313-321, 1962.

WIENER, K.* GUMMIHAUT (CUTIS LAXA) MIT DOMINANTER VERERBUNG. ARCH. DERM. SYPH. 148* 599-601, 1925.

12380 CUTIS LAXA, CORNEAL CLOUDING, MENTAL RETARDATION

DE BARSY ET AL. (1968) DESCRIBED A 22 MONTH OLD GIRL WHO HAD CUTIS LAXA WITH DEFECTIVE DEVELOPMENT OF ELASTIC FIBERS IN THE SKIN. THE CORNEAS WERE CLOUDY DUE TO DEGENERATION IN BOWMAN'S MEMBRANE. PSYCHOMOTOR DEVELOPMENT WAS RETARDED AND SHE WAS GENERALLY HYPOTONIC. THERE WAS NO KNOWN PARENTAL CONSANGUINITY, THE FATHER BEING GREEK AND THE MOTHER FLEMISH. THIS PROBABLY IS A DISTINCT SYNDROME.

DE BARSY, A. M., MOENS, E. AND DIERCKX, L.* DWARFISM, OLIGOPHRENIA AND DEGENERATION OF THE ELASTIC TISSUE IN SKIN AND CORNEA. A NEW SYNDROME.Q HELV. PAEDIAT. ACTA 23* 305-313, 1968.

12390 CYSTS OF THE JAW

SWIFT AND HOROWITZ (1969) OBSERVED MULTIPLE JAW CYSTS AND CALCIFICATION OF THE FALX CEREBRI IN MULTIPLE MEMBERS OF 3 GENERATIONS. THERE WAS NONE OF THE OTHER FEATURES OF BASAL CELL NEVUS SYNDROME (Q.V.) AND CHARCOT-MARIE-TOOTH SYNDROME WAS SEGREGATING IN THE SAME FAMILY. THUS IT IS NOT CERTAIN THAT JAW CYSTS REPRESENTED A DISTINCT ENTITY IN THIS FAMILY.

SWIFT, M. R. AND HOROWITZ, S. L.* FAMILIAL JAW CYSTS IN CHARCOT-MARIE-TOOTH DISEASE. J. MED. GENET. 6* 193-195, 1969.

12400 CYTOCHROME-RELATED DISEASE OF MUSCLE AND NERVOUS SYSTEM

SPIRO ET AL. (1970) DESCRIBED A 46 YEAR OLD MAN AND HIS 16 YEAR OLD SON WITH
PROGRESSIVE ATAXIA, PREDOMINANTLY PROXIMAL MUSCLE WEAKNESS, AREFLEXIA, EXTENSOR
PLANTAR RESPONSES, DEMENTIA, CONCOMITANT NONSPECIFIC MYOPATHIA AND NEUROPATHIC
CHANGES IN MUSCLE. STUDIES OF MUSCLE MITOCHONDRIA SHOWED VERY LOOSE COUPLING OF
OXIDATIVE PHOSPHORYLATION AND MARKED REDUCTION IN CYTOCHROME B CONTENT.

SPIRO, A. J., MOORE, C. L., PRINEAS, J. W., STRASBERG, P. M. AND RAPIN, I.* A
CYTOCHROME-RELATED INHERITED DISORDER OF THE NERVOUS SYSTEM AND MUSCLE. ARCH.
NEUROL. 23* 103-112, 1970.

12410 DANUBIAN ENDEMIC FAMILIAL NEPHROPATHY (DEFN* BALKAN NEPHROPATHY)

THE ENDEMIC NEPHROPATHY, COMMONLY CALLED *BALKAN* IS MORE PROPERLY CALLED
DANUBIAN. IT OCCURS IN A RELATIVELY RESTRICTED RURAL AREA OF ROUMANIA, BULGARIA
AND YUGOSLAVIA NEAR THE DANUBIAN IRON GATES. CLINICAL, EPIDEMIOLOGIC AND
LABORATORY INVESTIGATIONS ARE THOUGHT TO HAVE EXCLUDED SELECTED FORMS (ALTHOUGH
NOT NECESSARILY ALL FORMS) OF INFECTION, PARASITISM, INTOXICATION, AND RADIATION.
*NO GENETIC FACTORS ARE EVIDENT. OF PARAMOUNT IMPORTANCE ARE HOUSEHOLD FACTORS
AND LIVING CONDITIONS* (CRACIUN AND ROSCULESCU, 1970). ON THE OTHER HAND THESE
AUTHORS STATE THAT *THE DISEASE IN A FAMILY MAY DISAPPEAR WITHIN TWO OR THREE
GENERATIONS.* THE HISTOLOGIC END STAGE OF THE KIDNEY LESION IS THOUGHT TO BE A
FORM OF PRIMARY AMYLOIDOSIS.

CRACIUN, E. C. AND ROSCULESCU, I.* ON DANUBIAN ENDEMIC FAMILIAL NEPHROPATHY
(BALKAN NEPHROPATHY). SOME PROBLEMS. AM. J. MED. 49* 774-779, 1970.

*12420 DARIER-WHITE DISEASE (KERATOSIS FOLLICULARIS)

GROSSLY THIS DISORDER IS CHARACTERIZED BY THE FORMATION OF KERATOTIC PAPULES
LOCATED ESPECIALLY IN THE *SEBORRHEIC AREAS.* HISTOLOGICALLY, ONE FINDS (1) MILD
NON-SPECIFIC PERIVASCULAR INFILTRATION IN THE DERMIS, (2) DERMAL VILLI PROTRUDING
INTO THE EPIDERMIS, (3) SUPRA-BASAL DETACHMENT OF THE SPINAL LAYER LEADING TO THE
FORMATION OF LACUNAE CONTAINING ACANTHOLYTIC CELLS, (4) IN THE MORE SUPERFICIAL
EPIDERMIS, DYSKERATOTIC ROUND EPIDERMAL CELLS (*CORPS ROND*), THE MOST DISTINCTIVE
FEATURE, AND (5) IN THE STRATUM CORNEUM, *GRAINS* WHICH RESEMBLE PARAKEROTIC CELLS
EMBEDDED IN A HYPERKERATOTIC HORNY LAYER. A FAMILY WITH AFFECTED MEMBERS IN FIVE
GENERATIONS WAS REPORTED BY HITCH, CALLAWAY AND MOSELEY (1941). SEE ACROKERATOSIS
VERRUCIFORMIS FOR DISCUSSION OF PHENOTYPIC OVERLAP WITH THAT CONDITION. WHEN
BULLOUS LESIONS ARE PRESENT, THE CONDITION IS DIFFICULT TO DISTINGUISH FROM BENIGN
FAMILIAL PEMPHIGUS (Q.V.). NIORDSON AND SYLVEST (1965) ALSO SUGGESTED THAT HAILEY
AND HAILEY'S FAMILIAL BENIGN PEMPHIGUS IS SIMPLY A BULLOUS VARIANT OF DARIER'S
KERATOSIS FOLLICULARIS AND THAT BOTH MAY BE VARIANTS OF ACROKERATOSIS VERRUCIFOR-
MIS. THEY OBSERVED ONE PATIENT WITH CLINICAL AND HISTOPATHOLOGIC FEATURES OF ALL
THREE ENTITIES. THE FATHER, BROTHER, SISTER AND SON HAD ACROKERATOSIS VERRUCIFOR-
MIS.

HITCH, J. M., CALLAWAY, J. L. AND MOSELEY, V.* FAMILIAL DARIER'S DISEASE
(KERATOSIS FOLLICULARIS). STH. MED. J. 34* 578-586, 1941.

MADDEN, J. F.* DARIER'S DISEASE (MOTHER AND FOUR DAUGHTERS). ARCH. DERM. SYPH.
43* 735 ONLY, 1941.

NIORDSON, A. M. AND SYLVEST, B.* BULLOUS DYSKERATOSIS FOLLICULARIS AND
ACROKERATOSIS VERRUCIFORMIS. ARCH. DERM. 92* 166-168, 1965.

WITKOP, C. J. AND GORLIN, R. J.* FOUR HEREDITARY MUCOSAL SYNDROMES. ARCH.
DERM. 84* 762-771, 1961.

12430 DARWINIAN POINT (OF PINNA)

FOR PICTURES, SEE PAGE 292 OF WINCHESTER (1958).

WINCHESTER, A. M.* GENETICS. A SURVEY OF THE PRINCIPLES OF HEREDITY. BOSTON*
HOUGHTON MIFFLIN CO., 1958 (2ND ED.).

12440 DARWINIAN TUBERCLE (OF PINNA)

QUELPRUD (1935) DID AN EXTENSIVE TWIN AND FAMILY STUDY.

QUELPRUD, T.* ZUR ERBLICHKEIT DES DARWINSCHEN HOCKERCHENS. Z. MORPH. ANTHROP.
34* 343-363, 1934. REV. EUGEN. NEWS 20* 3-4, 1935.

*12450 DEAFNESS, CONGENITAL, WITH KERATOPACHYDERMIA AND CONSTRICTIONS OF FINGERS AND
TOES

NOCKEMANN (1961) PRESENTED FOUR GENERATIONS OF A FAMILY IN WHICH FOUR MEMBERS HAD
HYPERKERATOSIS, CONSTRICTIONS ON THE FINGERS AND TOES, AND CONGENITAL DEAFNESS.
THE PROBAND, A 20 YEAR OLD MAN, DEVELOPED HYPERKERATOSIS OF THE PALMS OF HIS HANDS
AND SOLES OF HIS FEET BEGINNING ABOUT TWO YEARS OF AGE, FOLLOWED BY INVOLVEMENT OF
HIS KNEES AND ELBOWS. RUBBING PRODUCED THICKENINGS ELSEWHERE. A FEW YEARS LATER
THERE DEVELOPED RINGSHAPED FURROWS OF THE SKIN IN THE REGION OF THE MIDDLE OF THE
FIVE FINGERS, FOLLOWED BY INVOLVEMENT OF THE TOES. THE PROBAND HAD CONGENITAL

DEAFNESS. THE AUTHOR PRESENTED THREE OTHER FAMILY MEMBERS IN FOUR GENERATIONS WITH SIMILAR FINDINGS. THEY WERE ALL DEAF AND DUMB. DRUMMOND (1939) PRESENTED THE CASE OF A 19 YEAR OLD DEAF MUTE GIRL WITH CONSTRICTING BANDS AROUND THREE FINGERS OF EACH HAND. THE BANDS WERE A QUARTER INCH IN WIDTH COMPLETELY ENCIRC-LING EACH FINGER. MARKED HYPERKERATOSIS OF THE PALMS WAS ALSO PRESENT, TOGETHER WITH EPIDERMAL THICKENING OVER THE KNUCKLES AND KNEES. GIBBS AND FRANK (1966) DESCRIBED AFFECTED FATHER AND DAUGHTER, BUT ARE SURELY MISTAKEN IN CALLING IT A VARIANT OF MAL DE MELEDA, A RECESSIVE. THE PRESENCE OF DIGITAL CONSTRICTIONS AND THE ABSENCE OF LEUKONYCHIA APPEAR TO DISTINGUISH THIS DISORDER FROM THAT LISTED UNDER 'KNUCKLE PADS, LEUKONYCHIA AND SENSINEURAL DEAFNESS' (Q.V.). THE HYPERKERA-TOSIS AND DEAFNESS REPORTED BY MORRIS ET AL. (1969) IS PROBABLY A DISTINCT ENTITY, AS THEY SUGGESTED. THEIR PATIENT WAS AN ISOLATED CASE.

DRUMMOND, M.* A CASE OF UNUSUAL SKIN DISEASE. IRISH J. MED. SCI. 8* 85-86, 1939.

GIBBS, R. C. AND FRANK, S. B.* KERATOMA HEREDITARIA MUTILANS (VOHWINKEL). DIFFERENTIATING FEATURES OF CONDITIONS WITH CONSTRICTION OF DIGITS. ARCH. DERM. 94* 619-625, 1966.

HYDE, J. N. AND MONTGOMERY, F. H.* A PRACTICAL TREATISE OF DISEASES OF THE SKIN. PHILADELPHIA* LEA BROTHERS AND CO., 1901. 6TH ED.

MORRIS, J., ACKERMAN, A. B. AND KOBLENZER, P. T.* GENERALIZED SPINY HYPERKERA-TOSIS, UNIVERSAL ALOPECIA, AND DEAFNESS. A PREVIOUSLY UNDESCRIBED SYNDROME. ARCH. DERM. 100* 692-698, 1969.

NOCKEMANN, P. F.* ERBLICHE HORNHAUTVERDICKUNG MIT SCHNURFURCHEN AN FINGERN UND ZEHEN UND INNENOHRSCHWERHORIGKEIT. MED. WELT. 2* 1894-1900, 1961.

12460 DEAFNESS, ECTODERMAL DYSPLASIA, POLYDACTYLISM AND SYNDACTYLISM

ROBINSON, MILLER, AND BENSIMON (1962) PRESENTED THE PEDIGREE OF 17 PERSONS IN THREE GENERATIONS WITH FIVE AFFECTED. THE PROPOSITUS WAS A 15 YEAR OLD GIRL WITH FISSURED SMALL DYSTROPHIC NAILS, CONIFORM TEETH WITH PARTIAL ANODONTIA, AND SYNDACTYLISM OF THE TOES OF THE RIGHT FOOT WITH UNION OF THE FIRST AND SECOND TOES, AND THE THIRD WITH THE FOURTH TOE. SHE HAD SEVERE SENSORINEURAL HEARING LOSS AND HAD ATTENDED A SCHOOL FOR THE DEAF. ONE BROTHER WAS NORMAL WHILE ANOTHER BROTHER AND A SISTER AND THEIR MOTHER HAD SIMILAR NAIL AND DENTAL DEFECTS. ALL AFFECTED MEMBERS HAD A HIGH FREQUENCY HEARING LOSS TOGETHER WITH A 70 DB LOW FREQUENCY LOSS IN THE PROPOSITUS. THE MATERNAL GRANDMOTHER OF THE PROPOSITUS WAS THOUGHT TO HAVE A SIMILAR SYNDROME BUT WAS NOT AVAILABLE FOR STUDY. THE AUTHORS FOUND ELEVATION OF ELECTROLYTE CONCENTRATIONS IN SWEAT, SUGGESTING THIS WAS A CHARACTERISTIC HIDROTIC FORM OF ECTODERMAL DYSPLASIA WITH DELAYED PRIMARY AND SECONDARY DENTITION, MISSHAPEN AND MISSING TEETH, AND DYSTROPHIC SMALL NAILS. THE PATTERN OF INHERITANCE WAS DOMINANT. FEINMESSER AND ZELIG (1961) DESCRIBED A FAMILY WITH ONYCHODYSTROPHY AND NEURAL DEAFNESS, BUT WITHOUT ABNORMALITIES OF THE TEETH OR DIGITS, AND WITH PROBABLE RECESSIVE INHERITANCE (Q.V.), SUGGESTING THIS IS A SEPARATE DISEASE. THE HIDROTIC NATURE OF THE ECTODERMAL DYSPLASIA DISTIN-GUISHES THIS CONDITION FROM THAT DESCRIBED UNDER 'DEAFNESS WITH ECTODERMAL DYSPLASIA' (Q.V.).

FEINMESSER, M. AND ZELIG, S.* CONGENITAL DEAFNESS ASSOCIATED WITH ONYCHODYSTRO-PHY. ARCH. OTOLARYNG. 74* 507-508, 1961.

ROBINSON, G. C., MILLER, J. R., AND BENSIMON, J. R.* FAMILIAL ECTODERMAL DYSPLASIA WITH SENSORI-NEURAL DEAFNESS AND OTHER ANOMALIES. PEDIATRICS 30* 797-802, 1962.

12470 DEAFNESS, NON-PROGRESSIVE MID-TONE NEURAL

ONSET IS IN CHILDHOOD AND THE RANGE AFFECTED IS 500 TO 4000 CPS. WILLIAMS AND ROBLEE (1962) DESCRIBED AFFECTED MOTHER AND 3 OF HER 6 CHILDREN.

WILLIAMS, F. AND ROBLEE, L. A.* HEREDITARY NERVE DEAFNESS. ARCH. OTOLARYNG. 75* 69-77, 1962.

*12480 DEAFNESS, PROGRESSIVE HIGH-TONE NEURAL

SEVERAL DISTINCT TYPES OF DOMINANTLY INHERITED DEAFNESS ARE IDENTIFIABLE ON THE BASIS OF ASSOCIATED MANIFESTATIONS, AGE OF ONSET, TENDENCY TO PROGRESSION, AND TONAL RANGE INVOLVED. STUDIES OF VESTIBULAR FUNCTION MIGHT PROVIDE FURTHER DIFFERENTIATION. DOMINANT DEAFNESS WITHOUT PIGMENTARY ANOMALY AS IN WAARDENBURG'S SYNDROME (Q.V.) ALMOST CERTAINLY EXISTS (SEE REVIEW BY FRASER, 1964). 8-12 PERCENT OF PROFOUND DEAFNESS OF CHILDHOOD MAY BE DOMINANT (INCLUDING FRESH MUTATIONS). DOLOWITZ AND STEPHENS (1961) DESCRIBED HIGH TONE NEURAL DEAFNESS PRESENT AT ALL AGES BUT MORE SEVERE IN OLDER MEMBERS OF FOUR GENERATIONS OF A MORMON KINDRED. SLOW PROGRESSION OF THE HEARING LOSS OVER A PERIOD OF SEVERAL DECADES WAS WELL DEMONSTRATED. HUIZING ET AL. (1966) STUDIED 5 GENERATIONS OF AN EXTENSIVE KINDRED IN WHICH 67 PERSONS HAD NON-CONGENITAL PROGRESSIVE PERCEPTIVE DEAFNESS. ONSET WAS IN EARLY CHILDHOOD WITH IMPAIRMENT OF HIGH FREQUENCIES. THE LOSS INCREASED RAPIDLY WITH GRADUAL EXTENSION OF THE IMPAIRMENT TO LOWER FREQUEN-

DOLOWITZ, D. A. AND STEPHENS, F. E.* HEREDITARY NERVE DEAFNESS. ANN. OTOL. 70*
851-859, 1961.

FRASER, G. R.* REVIEW ARTICLE* PROFOUND CHILDHOOD DEAFNESS. J. MED. GENET. 1*
118-151, 1964.

HUIZING, E. H., VAN BOLHUIS, A. H. AND ODENTHAL, D. W.* STUDIES ON PROGRESSIVE
HEREDITARY PERCEPTIVE DEAFNESS IN A FAMILY OF 335 MEMBERS. I. GENETICAL AND
GENERAL AUDIOLOGICAL RESULTS. ACTA OTOLARYNG. 61* 35-41, 1966. II. CHARACTERIS-
TIC PATTERNS OF HEARING DETERIORATION. IBID. 61* 161-167, 1966.

PAPARELLA, M. M., SUGIURA, S. AND HOSHINO, T.* FAMILIAL PROGRESSIVE SEN-
SORINEURAL DEAFNESS. ARCH. OTOLARYNG. 90* 44-51, 1969.

*12490 DEAFNESS, PROGRESSIVE LOW-TONE

THE VANDERBILT GROUP (1968) DESCRIBED LOW-FREQUENCY DEAFNESS OF SENSORINEURAL TYPE
IN A LARGE KINDRED. SPEECH DEVELOPMENT, INTELLIGENCE, VESTIBULAR FUNCTION AND
GENERAL PHYSICAL CONDITION WERE NORMAL. AUTOSOMAL DOMINANT INHERITANCE WAS
DEMONSTRATED. ABOVE 2000 CYCLES PER SEC. HEARING WAS NORMAL OR NEAR NORMAL. A
LOCALIZED ABNORMALITY OF THE COCHLEAR APEX WAS SUGGESTED. KONIGSMARK ET AL.
(1971) STUDIED 3 FAMILIES.

KONIGSMARK, B. W., MENGEL, M. AND BERLIN, C. I.* DOMINANT LOW FREQUENCY HEARING
LOSS* REPORT OF THREE FAMILIES. J. OTOL. LARYNG., IN PRESS 1971.

NANCE, W. E. AND SWEENEY, A. J.* DOMINANTLY INHERITED LOW-FREQUENCY HEARING
LOSS. MEETING, AM. SOC. HUM. GENET. (TORONTO, DEC. 1-3), 1967.

VANDERBILT UNIVERSITY HEREDITARY DEAFNESS STUDY GROUP* DOMINANTLY INHERITED
LOW-FREQUENCY HEARING LOSS. ARCH. OTOLARYNG. 88* 242-250, 1968.

12500 DEAFNESS, UNILATERAL

SMITH (1939) DESCRIBED A SIBSHIP OF EIGHT CHILDREN, FOUR OF WHOM HAD TOTAL
DEAFNESS IN ONE OR THE OTHER EAR. THE TYMPANIC MEMBRANES WERE NORMAL. LABYRIN-
THINE TESTING WAS NORMAL. THERE WAS NO HISTORY OF CONSANGUINITY, MUMPS, OR
SYPHILIS. THE MOTHER, HER FATHER, AND HER SISTER ALSO HAD UNILATERAL DEAFNESS
WHILE ANOTHER SISTER BECAME DEAF AND DUMB AFTER MEASLES. THIS LATTER SISTER
MARRIED A DEAF AND DUMB MAN. ONE OF THEIR THREE CHILDREN, A GIRL, HAD UNILATERAL
DEAFNESS. SHE HAD TWO CHILDREN, ONE OF WHOM HAS UNILATERAL DEAFNESS. THUS THERE
WERE NINE PERSONS WITH TOTAL UNILATERAL DEAFNESS IN FOUR GENERATIONS. FOUR WERE
DEAF IN THE RIGHT EAR AND FOUR IN THE LEFT, WHILE THE SIDE WAS UNKNOWN IN ONE
CASE. EVERBERG (1960) STUDIED 122 CHILDREN WITH TOTAL UNILATERAL DEAFNESS IN ONE
EAR AND NORMAL HEARING IN THE OTHER. MORE THAN ONE CASE OF UNILATERAL DEAFNESS IN
THE SAME FAMILY WAS FOUND IN 12 OF THE 122 FAMILIES OF THESE CHILDREN.

EVERBERG, G.* UNILATERAL ANACUSIS. CLINICAL, RADIOLOGICAL AND GENETIC
INVESTIGATIONS. ACTA OTOLARYNG. 158 (SUPPL.)* 366-374, 1960.

SMITH, A. B.* UNILATERAL HEREDITARY DEAFNESS. LANCET 237* 1172-1173, 1939.

*12510 DEAFNESS, WITH EAR PITS (PERHAPS TWO OR MORE TYPES)

FOURMAN AND FOURMAN (1955) DESCRIBED A FAMILY OF 108 IN WHICH 17 MEMBERS HAD
PREAURICULAR PITS. TWELVE WERE DEAF AND ONE WAS NOT. THE OTHERS WERE TOO YOUNG
FOR TESTING. OF THOSE WITHOUT PITS THREE WERE DEAF* ONE OF THESE HAD A BRANCHIAL
PIT. THE DEAFNESS VARIED FROM MILD TO SEVERE. IN SOME IT HAD BEEN RECOGNIZED
FROM CHILDHOOD, OTHERS WERE CERTAIN THEY HAD BEEN ABLE TO HEAR PERFECTLY UNTIL
THEY WERE ABOUT 20 YEARS OLD, WHEN THEIR HEARING BEGAN TO DETERIORATE. AUDIOGRAMS
SHOWED BOTH HIGH AND LOW TONE LOSS, USUALLY HIGH TONES MORE THAN THE LOW. HEARING
TESTING WAS DONE ON TWO OF THE THREE CASES WITH DEAFNESS BUT WITHOUT PITS. THIS
SHOWED THE SAME AUDIOGRAM PATTERN. THERE WAS NO EVIDENCE OF VESTIBULAR DISORDER.
THE AUTHORS SUGGEST EAR-PITS, DEAFNESS, AND BRANCHIAL FISTULAE ARE INDEPENDENT
EFFECTS OF A SINGLE DOMINANT GENE WITH INCOMPLETE PENETRANCE.
WILDERVANCK (1962) REVIEWS 16 MEMBERS OF A FAMILY 14 OF WHOM HAD EITHER
DEFORMED AURICLES, MARGINAL PITS, OR PREAURICULAR APPENDAGES. TWO MEMBERS HAD A
MODERATE CONDUCTIVE DEAFNESS. IN ONE THE DEAFNESS WAS BILATERAL AND IN THE OTHER
IT WAS UNILATERAL. THE MODE OF INHERITANCE IS DOMINANT WITH FULL PENETRATION.
WILDERVANCK SUGGESTS THIS IS A DIFFERENT SYNDROME FROM THAT OF FOURMAN AND
FOURMAN. MCLAURIN ET AL. (1966) REPORTED A KINDRED WITH ABNORMALITIES LIKE THOSE
REPORTED BY WILDERVANCK (1962). SIMILAR BRANCHIAL CLEFT ANOMALIES (Q.V.),
APPARENTLY WITHOUT DEAFNESS, HAVE BEEN REPORTED AND MAY BE GENETICALLY DISTINCT.

FOURMAN, P. AND FOURMAN, J.* HEREDITARY DEAFNESS IN FAMILY WITH EAR-PITS
(FISTULA AURIS CONGENITA). BRIT. MED. J. 2* 1354-1356, 1955.

MCLAURIN, J. W., KLOEPFER, H. W., LAGUAITE, J. K. AND STALLCUP, T. A.*
HEREDITARY BRANCHIAL ANOMALIES AND ASSOCIATED HEARING IMPAIRMENT. LARYNGOSCOPE

76* 1277-1288, 1966.

ROWLEY, P. T.* FAMILIAL HEARING LOSS ASSOCIATED WITH BRANCHIAL FISTULAS. PEDIATRICS 44* 978-985, 1970.

WILDERVANCK, L. S.* HEREDITARY MALFORMATIONS OF THE EAR IN THREE GENERATIONS. ACTA OTOLARYNG. 54* 553-560, 1962.

12520 DEAFNESS, WITH ECTODERMAL DYSPLASIA

HELWEG-LARSEN AND LUDVIGSEN (1946) REPORTED A KINDRED OF 14 WITH ANHIDROTIC ECTODERMAL DYSPLASIA, FOUR OF WHOM HAD DEFECTIVE HEARING WITH ONSET BETWEEN 35 AND 45 YEARS OF AGE. ELLINGSON (1951) FOUND HEARING LOSS IN TWO BROTHERS WITH ECTODERMAL DYSPLASIA. MARSHALL (1958) REPORTED FOUR GENERATIONS OF A FAMILY IN WHICH SEVEN MEMBERS HAD (1) NASAL DEFECT AND FACIES CHARACTERISTIC OF ANHIDROTIC ECTODERMAL DYSPLASIA, (2) CONGENITAL AND JUVENILE CATARACTS, (3) MYOPIA AND FLUID VITREOUS, (4) SPONTANEOUS, SUDDEN MATURATION AND ABSORPTION OF CONGENITAL CATARACT, (5) LUXATION OF CATARACT, (6) CONGENITAL HEARING LOSS. DEFICIENCY IN SWEATING WAS MINIMAL. THE TRANSMISSION WAS DOMINANT. SEE ALSO ECTODERMAL DYSPLASIA, HIDROTIC, WITH NERVE DEAFNESS AND FINGER ANOMALIES. RUPPERT ET AL. (1970) DESCRIBED FATHER AND DAUGHTER WITH FEATURES LIKE THOSE IN MARSHALL'S FAMILY, NAMELY, SADDLE NOSE, MYOPIA, AND DEAFNESS AND IN THE FATHER CATARACTS.

ELLINGSON, R. J.* MAJOR HEREDITARY ECTODERMAL DYSPLASIA. J. PEDIAT. 38* 191-198, 1951.

HELWEG-LARSEN, H. F. AND LUDVIGSEN, K.* CONGENITAL FAMILIAL ANHIDROSIS AND NEUROLABYRINTHITIS. ACTA DERMATOVENER. 26* 489-505, 1946.

MARSHALL, D.* ECTODERMAL DYSPLASIA* REPORT OF KINDRED WITH OCULAR ABNORMALITIES AND HEARING DEFECT. AM. J. OPHTHAL. 45* 143-156, 1958.

RUPPERT, E. S., BUERK, E. AND PFORDRESHER, M. F.* HEREDITARY HEARING LOSS WITH SADDLE-NOSE AND MYOPIA. ARCH. OTOLARYNG. 92* 95-98, 1970.

12530 DENS IN DENTE AND PALATAL INVAGINATIONS

DENS IN DENTE AND DEEP PALATAL INVAGINATIONS (LINGUAL PITS) OF THE SECONDARY MAXILLARY LATERAL INCISORS MAY BE INHERITED AS AN AUTOSOMAL DOMINANT. GRAHNER ET AL. (1959) FOUND IN A STUDY OF 3000 SWEDISH CHILDREN A FREQUENCY OF ABOUT 3 PER CENT. IN 58 FAMILIES STUDIED A SIMILAR DEFECT WAS FOUND IN OVER ONE-THIRD OF PARENTS. IN THE SAME FAMILY SOME HAD DENS IN DENTE AND OTHERS HAD DEEP LINGUAL PITS. LINGUAL PITS OFFER A FAVORABLE SETTING FOR DEVELOPMENT OF CARIES.

GRAHNER, H., LINDAHL, B. AND OMNELL, K. A.* DENS INVAGINATUS. I. A CLINICAL, ROENTGENOLOGICAL AND GENETIC STUDY OF PERMANENT UPPER LATERAL INCISORS. ODONT. REV. 10* 115-137, 1959.

12540 DENTINE DYSPLASIA ('ROOTLESS TEETH,' DENTINE HYPOPLASIA)

BOTH PRIMARY AND SECONDARY DENTITIONS ARE AFFECTED. THE COLOR OF THE TEETH IS USUALLY NORMAL. TEETH ARE OFTEN MALALIGNED IN THE ARCH AND MAY EXFOLIATE WITH MINOR TRAUMA. BY X-RAY, THE DENTAL ROOTS ARE DEMONSTRATED TO BE MARKEDLY DISTORTED AND REDUCED IN SIZE. RUSHTON (1955) DESCRIBED THE HISTOLOGIC CHARAC-TERISTICS. FINN (1962) EXPRESSED THE VIEW THAT THIS IS A SEVERE MANIFESTATION OF DENTINOGENESIS IMPERFECTA AND THAT TRANSITION BETWEEN THE TWO TYPES IS EVIDENT WITHIN FAMILIES. WITKOP (1965) STATES THAT HE 'HAS PERSONALLY EXAMINED OVER 1,000 CASES OF DENTINOGENESIS IMPERFECTA FROM 42 EXTENSIVE KINDREDS AND OVER 50 CASES OF DENTIN HYPOPLASIA FROM 4 KINDREDS AND HAS YET TO FIND ANY CASE REMOTELY RESEMBLING A TRANSITION FROM ONE DISEASE TO THE OTHER. THE CLINICAL, RADIOGRAPHIC AND HISTOLOGIC FINDINGS ARE DISTINCTLY DIFFERENT IN THE TWO CONDITIONS.'

FINN, S. B.* DENTIN AND ENAMEL ANOMALIES. IN, GENETICS AND DENTAL HEALTH. WITKOP, C. J., JR. (ED.)* NEW YORK* MCGRAW-HILL, 1962. PP. 219-245.

LOGAN, J., BECKER, H., SILVERMAN, S., JR. AND PINDBORG, J. J.* DENTINAL DYSPLASIA. ORAL. SURG. 15* 317-333, 1962.

RUSHTON, M. A.* ANOMALIES OF HUMAN DENTINE. ANN. ROY. COLL. SURG. ENG. 16* 94-117, 1955.

WITKOP, C. J.* GENETIC DISEASE OF THE ORAL CAVITY. IN, TIECKE, R. W. (ED.)* NEW YORK* ORAL PATHOLOGY. MCGRAW-HILL, 1965.

*12550 DENTINOGENESIS IMPERFECTA (CAPEDEPONT'S TEETH, OR OPALESCENT DENTINE)

THE PRIMARY DEFECT IS MESODERMAL, INVOLVING DENTINE. AN IDENTICAL DISORDER OCCURS AS PART OF THE OSTEOGENESIS IMPERFECTA SYNDROME. HOWEVER, THERE IS CLEARLY A DISTINCT ENTITY INHERITED AS A DOMINANT AND AFFECTING ONLY THE TEETH. JOHNSON (1959) DESCRIBED THREE FAMILIES CONTAINING AT LEAST SIXTY-TWO AFFECTED PERSONS. THE TEETH VARY IN COLOR FROM OPALESCENT BLUE TO AMBER BROWN. THE ENAMEL SPLITS FROM THE DENTINE READILY WHEN SUBJECTED TO OCCLUSAL STRESS. THE FREQUENCY MAY BE

1 IN 6000 TO 8000 CHILDREN (WITKOP, 1957). STUDY OF A LARGE AFFECTED KINDRED IN A MARYLAND TRIRACIAL ISOLATE SHOWED THE VARIABILITY IN CLINICAL PICTURE (HURSEY ET AL., 1956). THIS CONDITION IS ALSO CALLED HEREDITARY BROWN TEETH.

HURSEY, R. J., WITKOP, C. J., JR., MIKLASHEK, D. AND SACKETT, L. M.* DENTINO-GENESIS IMPERFECTA IN A RACIAL ISOLATE WITH MULTIPLE HEREDITARY DEFECTS. ORAL SURG. 9* 641-658, 1956.

IVANCIE, G. P.* DENTINOGENESIS IMPERFECTA. ORAL SURG. 7* 984-992, 1954.

JOHNSON, O. N., CHAUDHRY, A. P., GORLIN, R. J., MITCHELL, D. F. AND BARTHOLDI, W. L.* HEREDITARY DENTINOGENESIS IMPERFECTA. J. PEDIAT. 54* 786-792, 1959.

ROBERTS, E. AND SCHOUR, I.* HEREDITARY OPALESCENT DENTINE - DENTINOGENESIS IMPERFECTA. AM. J. ORTHODONT. 25* 267-276, 1939.

WALLACE, J. R.* HEREDITARY DENTINOGENESIS IMPERFECTA. J. PEDIAT. 65* 128-130, 1964.

WILSON, G. W. AND STEINBECHER, M.* HEREDITARY HYPOPLASIA OF THE DENTINE. J. AM. DENT. ASS. 16* 866-870, 1929.

WITKOP, C. J.* HEREDITARY DEFECTS IN ENAMEL AND DENTIN. ACTA GENET. STATIST. MED. 7* 236-239, 1957.

12560 DERMATOSIS PAPULOSA NIGRA

ALTHOUGH NOTHING IS CLEARLY ESTABLISHED ABOUT THE GENETICS OF THIS DISORDER, THE OCCURRENCE PREDOMINANTLY IN NEGROES IS CONSISTENT WITH A GENETIC BASIS. AS MANY AS 35 PERCENT OF ADULT NEGROES MAY BE AFFECTED. THE DISORDER IS SOMEWHAT MORE FREQUENT IN FEMALES. THE PAPULES OCCUR MOST TYPICALLY ON THE FACE BELOW THE EYES AND ON THE CHEEKS. CASTELLANI (1925) DESCRIBED AND NAMED THIS DISORDER, WHICH HE FOUND TO BE VERY FREQUENT AMONG THE NEGROES OF JAMAICA AND CENTRAL AMERICA. THE LESIONS ARE BLACK AND DARK-BROWN PAPULES, SOMETIMES CUPOLIFORM OR AT TIMES FLATTENED, SITUATED ON THE FACE, PRINCIPALLY ON BOTH MALAR REGIONS, BEING RARE OR ABSENT ON THE LOWER PARTS OF THE FACE AND CHIN. ONSET IS USUALLY ABOUT THE TIME OF PUBERTY. BUTTERWORTH AND STREAN (1962) EXPRESSED THE OPINION THAT THIS CONDITION IS MERELY A VARIANT OF SEBORRHEIC KERATOSES THAT OCCURS PREDOMINANTLY IN NEGROES.

BUTTERWORTH, T. AND STREAN, L. P.* CLINICAL GENODERMATOLOGY. BALTIMORE* WILLIAMS AND WILKINS. 1962.

CASTELLANI, A.* OBSERVATIONS ON SOME DISEASES OF CENTRAL AMERICA. J. TROP. MED. HYG. 28* 1-14, 1925.

*12570 DIABETES INSIPIDUS, NEUROHYPOPHYSEAL TYPE

NORMALLY THE POSTERIOR PITUITARY HORMONES, ANTIDIURETIC HORMONE AND OXYTOCIN, ARE SYNTHESIZED IN THE SUPRAOPTIC AND PARA-VENTRICULAR NUCLEI OF THE HYPOTHALAMUS AND TRANSPORTED WITHIN AXONS, POSSIBLY IN A BIOLOGICALLY INACTIVE, BOUND FORM, TO THE POSTERIOR LOBE OF THE PITUITARY WHERE THEY ARE STORED. ONE OF THE MOST DRAMATIC EXAMPLES OF FAMILIAL DIABETES INSIPIDUS IS THAT REPORTED BY ADOLPH WEIL (1884) OF HEIDELBERG AND HIS SON ALFRED (1908). SEVEN GENERATIONS WERE AFFECTED. DOLLE (1950-52) REPORTED A FOLLOW-UP ON THIS FAMILY. IT CONTAINED NUMEROUS INSTANCES OF MALE-TO-MALE TRANSMISSION. BRAVERMAN, MANCINI AND MCGOLDRICK (1965) REPORTED THE POSTMORTEM FINDINGS IN A CASE OF PITRESSIN-RESPONSIVE DIABETES INSIPIDUS. AS IN FIVE PREVIOUS REPORTED CASES, A STRIKING DECREASE IN THE NERVE CELLS OF THE SUPRAOPTIC AND PARAVENTICULAR NUCLEI OF THE HYPOTHALAMUS WITH ASSOCIATED MILD GLIOSIS WAS FOUND. IN THIS FAMILY THE FATHER AND PATERNAL GRANDMOTHER WERE THOUGHT TO HAVE HAD DIABETES INSIPIDUS. IN THE SIBSHIP OF THE PROBAND, A MALE, TWO SISTERS HAD DEFINITE DIABETES INSIPIDUS AND A BROTHER MAY HAVE BEEN AFFECTED. ONE CHILD OF EACH OF THREE OF THE SIBS WAS ALSO THOUGHT TO HAVE THE DISORDER. DOMINANT PEDIGREES OF PITRESSIN RESPONSIVE DIABETES INSIPIDUS WERE REPORTED BY PENDER AND FRASER (1953), MOEHLIG AND SCHULTZ (1955) AND MARTIN (1959). ONE WOULD SCARCELY EXPECT A DEFECT IN SYNTHESIS OF ANTIDIURETIC HORMONE TO BEHAVE AS A DOMINANT. ISOLATED DEFICIENCIES OF OTHER PITUITARY HORMONES (E.G., SEXUAL ATELIOSIS) BEHAVE AS RECESSIVES. AN APPARENT DEFECT IN SYNTHESIS OF VASOPRESSIN IN THE RAT RESULTS IN DIABETES INSIPIDUS ONLY IN THE HOMOZYGOTE, ALTHOUGH THE HETEROZYGOTE SHOWS REDUCED VASOPRESSIN. OXYTOCIN SYNTHESIS IS NOT IMPAIRED (VALTIN ET AL., 1965). MORPHOLOGIC FEATURES SUGGEST EXCESSIVE ACTIVITY OF THE HYPOTHALAMO-NEUROHYPOPHYSIAL SYSTEM WHICH CONTROLS SECRETION OF VASOPRESSIN (SOKOL AND VALTIN 1965). BOTH AUTOSOMAL DOMINANT AND X-LINKED INHERITANCE OF BOTH RENAL AND NEUROHYPOPHYSEAL DIABETES INSIPIDUS HAVE BEEN REPORTED. MOST OFTEN, HOWEVER, THE NEUROHYPOPHYSEAL TYPE IS AUTOSOMAL DOMINANT AND THE RENAL TYPE IS X-LINKED. AUTOSOMAL DOMINANT DIABETES INSIPIDUS IS ASSOCIATED WITH OLIGOSYNDACTYLY IN THE MOUSE (FALCONER ET AL., 1964). THE NEUROHYPOPHYSEAL TYPE IS RECESSIVE IN RATS.

BRAVERMAN, L. E., MANCINI, J. P. AND MCGOLDRICK, D. M.* HEREDITARY IDIOPATHIC DIABETES INSIPIDUS. A CASE REPORT WITH AUTOPSY FINDINGS. ANN. INTERN. MED. 63* 503-508, 1965.

DOLLE, W.* EINE WEITERE ERGANZUNG DES WEILSCHEN DIABETES-INSIPIDUS-STAMMBAUMES. Z. MENSCHL. VERERB. KONSTITUTIONSL. 30* 372-374, 1950-52.

FALCONER, D. S., LATSYZEWSKI, M. AND ISAACSON, J. H.* DIABETES INSIPIDUS ASSOCIATED WITH OLIGOSYNDACTYLY IN THE MOUSE. GENET. RES. 5* 473-488, 1964.

MARTIN, F. I. R.* FAMILIAL DIABETES INSIPIDUS. QUART. J. MED. 28* 573-582, 1959.

MOEHLIG, R. C. AND SCHULTZ, R. C.* FAMILIAL DIABETES INSIPIDUS. REPORT OF ONE OF FOURTEEN CASES IN FOUR GENERATIONS. J.A.M.A. 158* 725-727, 1955.

PENDER, C. B. AND FRASER, F. C.* DOMINANT INHERITANCE OF DIABETES INSIPIDUS* A FAMILY STUDY. PEDIATRICS 11* 246-254, 1953.

SOKOL, H. W. AND VALTIN, H.* MORPHOLOGY OF THE NEUROSECRETORY SYSTEM IN RATS HOMOGZYGOUS AND HETEROZYGOUS FOR HYPOTHALAMIC DIABETES INSIPIDUS (BRATTLEBORO STRAIN). ENDOCRINOLOGY 77* 692-700, 1965.

VALTIN, H.* HEREDITARY HYPOTHALAMIC DIABETES INSIPIDUS IN RATS (BRATTLEBORO STRAIN). AM. J. MED. 42* 814-827, 1967

VALTIN, H., SAWYER, W. H. AND SOKOL, H. W.* NEUROHYPOPHYSIAL PRINCIPLES IN RATS HOMOZYGOUS AND HETEROZYGOUS FOR HYPOTHALAMIC DIABETES INSIPIDUS (BRATTLEBORO STRAIN). ENDOCRINOLOGY 77* 701-706, 1965.

WEIL, A.* UEBER DIE HEREDITARE FORM DES DIABETES INSIPIDUS. DEUTSCH. ARCH. KLIN. MED. 93* 180-290, 1908.

WEIL, A.* UEBER DIE HEREDITARE FORM DES DIABETES INSIPIDUS. VIRCHOW. ARCH. PATH. ANAT. 95* 70-95, 1884.

12580 DIABETES INSIPIDUS, RENAL TYPE

CANNON (1955) TRACED A FAMILY BACK TO 1813. THE FAMILY CONTAINED 3 INSTANCES OF MALE-TO-MALE TRANSMISSION. ASSUMING THAT THE INFORMATION WAS ACCURATE AND THAT CONSANGUINITY WAS NOT PRESENT, THIS EXCLUDES X-LINKED INHERITANCE, WHICH IS MORE FREQUENT. CANNON DID NOTE REDUCED PENETRANCE IN FEMALES WITH CONDUCTORS NOT SHOWING THE DISORDER. THIS MAKES ONE SUSPICIOUS THAT THIS WAS IN FACT THE X-LINKED FORM OF DIABETES INSIPIDUS. THE FAMILY SHOULD BE RE-INVESTIGATED. CUTLER ET AL. (1955) PROVED THE RENAL BASIS OF THE PROBLEM IN THIS FAMILY. BODE AND CRAWFORD (1969) SEEM TO HAVE ESTABLISHED THE X-LINKED INHERITANCE OF THE KINDRED REPORTED BY CANNON, BY FINDING A SUGGESTIVE TIE-IN WITH THE VERY LARGE, CLEARLY X-LINKED PEDIGREE DESCENDANT FROM PERSONS WHO CAME TO NORTH AMERICA ON THE SHIP HOPEWELL. TEN BENSEL AND PETERS (1970) RESTUDIED PART OF CANNON'S PEDIGREE AND SHOWED TYPICAL X-LINKED INHERITANCE. WELLER, ELLIOTT AND GUSMAN (1950), AND LEVINGER AND ESCAMILLA (1955), DESCRIBED DOMINANT PEDIGREES. ONE MUST DISTINGUISH RENAL AND NEUROHYPOPHYSEAL TYPES IN THESE REPORTS, HOWEVER.

BODE, H. H. AND CRAWFORD, J. D.* NEPHROGENIC DIABETES INSIPIDUS IN NORTH AMERICA - THE HOPEWELL HYPOTHESIS. NEW ENG. J. MED. 280* 750-754, 1969.

CANNON, J. F.* DIABETES INSIPIDUS* CLINICAL AND EXPERIMENTAL STUDIES WITH CONSIDERATION OF GENETIC RELATIONSHIPS. ARCH. INTERN. MED. 96* 215-272, 1955.

CUTLER, R. E., KLEEMAN, C. R., MAXWELL, M. H. AND DOWLING, J. T.* PHYSIOLOGIC STUDIES IN NEPHROGENIC DIABETES INSIPIDUS. J. CLIN. ENDOCR. 22* 215-272, 1955.

LEVINGER, E. L. AND ESCAMILLA, R. F.* HEREDITARY DIABETES INSIPIDUS* REPORT OF 20 CASES IN SEVEN GENERATIONS. J. CLIN. ENDOCR. 15* 547-552, 1955.

ROBINSON, M. G., AND KAPLAN, S. A.* INHERITANCE OF VASOPRESSIN-RESISTANT ('NEPHROGENIC') DIABETES INSIPIDUS. AM. J. DIS. CHILD. 99* 164-174, 1960.

WELLER, C. G., ELLIOTT, W. AND GUSMAN, A. R.* HEREDITARY DIABETES INSIPIDUS* UNUSUAL URINARY TRACT CHANGES. J. UROL. 64* 716-721, 1950.

*12590 DIASTEMA, DENTAL MEDIAL

A SPACE BETWEEN THE SUPERIOR CENTRAL INCISORS IS PROBABLY INHERITED AS A DOMINANT TRAIT. WENINGER (1933) STUDIED 24 FAMILIES, OBSERVING FOUR GENERATIONS AFFECTED IN SOME. PERSONS WITH THIS TRAIT HAVE, IN THE PAST, BEEN REFERRED TO AS 'GAT-TOOTHED.'

WENINGER, M.* ZUR VERERBUNG DES MEDIANEN OBERKIEFER-TREMAS. Z. MORPH. ANTHROP. 32* 367-393, 1933.

12600 DIBASICAMINOACIDURIA I

WHELAN AND SCRIVER (1968) FOUND EXCESSIVE LYSINE, ORNITHINE AND ARGININE EXCRETION IN 13 MEMBERS OF A FRENCH-CANADIAN KINDRED. PLASMA LEVELS OF THESE AMINO ACIDS WERE NORMAL. THE ENDOGENOUS RENAL CLEARANCE OF THE THREE AMINO ACIDS WAS

INCREASED BUT THAT OF CYSTINE WAS NORMAL. INTESTINAL ABSORPTION L-LYSINE WAS IMPAIRED BUT THAT OF L-CYSTINE WAS NORMAL. THE RELATION TO THE DISORDER DESCRIBED IN FINLAND AND IN JAPAN AND CALLED HERE DIBASICACIDURIA II IS UNCLEAR. THE FRENCH-CANADIAN PATIENTS WERE ASYMPTOMATIC EXCEPT FOR MILD INTESTINAL MALABSORP-TION SYNDROME IN THE PROBAND. THE FINNISH PATIENTS HAD SEVERE PROTEIN INTO-LERANCE.

WHELAN, D. T. AND SCRIVER, C. R.* HYPERDIBASICAMINOACIDURIA* AN INHERITED DISORDER OF AMINO ACID TRANSPORT. PEDIAT. RES. 2* 525-534, 1968.

12610 DIMPLES, FACIAL

CHEEK DIMPLES MAY BE INHERITED AS AN IRREGULAR DOMINANT.

12620 DISSEMINATED SCLEROSIS (MULTIPLE SCLEROSIS)

FAMILIAL AGGREGATION IN THIS DISEASE IS NOT STRONG. HOWEVER, BAS (1964) IN A SERIES OF 91 CASES FOUND 3 INSTANCES OF AFFECTED MOTHER AND DAUGHTER. FROM AN EXTENSIVE REVIEW, MCALPINE (1965) CONCLUDED THAT THE RISK FOR A FIRST DEGREE RELATIVE OF A PATIENT WITH MULTIPLE SCLEROSIS IS AT LEAST 15 TIMES THAT FOR A MEMBER OF THE GENERAL POPULATION BUT THAT NO DEFINITE GENETIC PATTERN IS DISCER-NIBLE. SEE MULTIPLE SCLEROSIS-LIKE DISEASE. SEE ATAXIA, SPASTIC.

BAS, H.* SCLEROSIS MULTIPLEX FAMILIARIS. Z. AERZTL. FORTBILD. 58* 153-155, 1964.

MCALPINE, D.* FAMILIAL INCIDENCE AND ITS SIGNIFICANCE. MULTIPLE SCLEROSIS* A REAPPRAISAL. MCALPINE, D., LUMSDEN, C. E. AND ACHESON, E. D. (EDS.)* BALTIMORE* WILLIAMS AND WILKINS CO., 1965. PP. 61-74.

*12630 DISTICHIASIS (TWO ROWS OF EYELASHES)

FOX (1962) REVIEWED THE HEREDITY OF THIS ANOMALY. DOMINANT PEDIGREES WERE PRESENTED BY ERDMANN (1904) AND BY COCKAYNE (1933). BLATT (1924) TRACED DOUBLE ROWS OF EYELASHES THROUGH THREE GENERATIONS. SEE TRISTICHIASIS. THE TERM *DISTRICHIASIS* AND *TRISTRICHIASIS* REFER TO TWO OR THREE HAIRS PER FOLLICLE. MUCH CONFUSION EXISTS, HOWEVER, AND *DISTICHIASIS* AND *DISTRICHIASIS* ARE OFTEN USED INTERCHANGEABLY TO MEAN *TWO ROWS OF EYELASHES.* IN THREE GENERATIONS OF A FAMILY PICO (1957) FOUND 11 PERSONS WITH CONGENITAL ECTROPION AND OF THESE 8 ALSO HAD DISTICHIASIS. TWO PERSONS HAD DISTICHIASIS ALONE. HISTOLOGIC STUDY IN TWO SHOWED ABSENCE OF MEIBOMIAN GLANDS AND REPLACEMENT OF THE DENSE COLLAGENOUS TISSUE OF THE TARSAL PLATES BY LOOSE AREOLAR TISSUE. SZILY'S OBSERVATION (1923) SUGGESTED RECESSIVE INHERITANCE. SEE LYMPHEDEMA, WITH DISTICHASIS.

BLATT, N.* DISTRICHIASIS CONGENITA VERA. Z. AUGENHEILK. 53* 325-338, 1924.

COCKAYNE, E. A.* INHERITED ABNORMALITIES OF THE SKIN AND ITS APPENDAGES. LONDON* OXFORD U. PRESS, 1933.

ERDMANN, P.* EIN BEITRAG ZUR KENNTNIS DER DISTICHIASIS CONGENITA (HEREDITARIA). Z. AUGENHEILK. 11* 427-444, 1904.

FOX, S. A.* DISTICHIASIS. AM. J. OPHTHAL. 53* 14-18, 1962.

PICO, G.* CONGENITAL ECTROPION AND DISTRICHIASIS. ETIOLOGIC AND HEREDITARY FACTORS* A REPORT OF CASES AND REVIEW OF THE LITERATURE. TRANS. AM. OPHTH. SOC. 55* 663-700, 1957.

SZILY, A. VON* UEBER HAARBILDUNG IN DER MEIBOMSCHEN DRUSE UND UBER BEHAARTE MEIBOM-DRUSEN (SOGENANNTE DISTRICHIASIS CONGENITA VERA). KLIN. MBL. AUGENHEILK. 70* 16-45, 1923.

12640 DOUBLE ATHETOSIS (STATUS MARMORATUS, OR *LITTLE'S DISEASE WITH INVOLUNTARY MOVEMENTS*)

PATZIG (1939) BELIEVED THAT THE GROUP OF INFANTILE CEREBRAL PALSIES CHARACTERIZED BY STATUS MARMORATUS OF THE STRIATUM (VOGT'S DISEASE) IS HEREDITARY. HE DESCRIBED THE DISORDER IN A GIRL, HER FATHER AND HIS UNCLE. ELEVEN MEMBERS OF THE FATHER'S FAMILY EXHIBITED PRONOUNCED INVOLUNTARY MOVEMENTS OF A NON-PROGRESSIVE ATHETOID NATURE.

PATZIG, B.* ERBBIOLOGIE UND ERBPATHOLOGIE DES GEHIRNS. IN, HANDBUCH DER ERBBIOLOGIE DES MENSCHEN. 5* (PART 1) 233-349, 1939.

12650 DOUBLE NAIL FOR FIFTH TOE

TEMTAMY OBSERVED A MOTHER AND SON WITH DOUBLE NAILS ON THE LITTLE TOES - ONE ON TOP OF THE OTHER. THE WOMAN'S GRANDSON (J. A., 988558) THROUGH AN UNAFFECTED DAUGHTER HAD POST-AXIAL POLYDACTYLY (Q.V.).

TEMTAMY, S. A.* GENETIC FACTORS IN HAND MALFORMATIONS. PH. D. THESIS, JOHNS HOPKINS UNIVERSITY, 1966.

12670 DRUSEN OF BRUCH'S MEMBRANE

DEUTMAN AND JANSEN (1970) DESCRIBED A FAMILY IN WHICH 8 PERSONS IN 5 SIBSHIPS HAD CONFIRMED MULTIPLE DRUSEN OF BRUCH'S MEMBRANE. THERE WAS NO INSTANCE OF MALE-TO-MALE TRANSMISSION BUT AN AFFECTED MALE HAD TWO DAUGHTERS WHO WERE NEGATIVE BY EXAMINATION. THEY OBSERVED CONCORDANT MONOZYGOTIC TWINS AND AFFECTED BOYS 12 AND 14 YEARS OLD. THEY CONCLUDED THAT THE FAMILY WITH "CRYSTALLINE RETINAL DEGENERA-TION" REPORTED BY EVANS (1950) HAD THIS CONDITION. THE AUTHORS ALSO CONCLUDED THAT DOYNE'S HONEYCOMB CHOROIDITIS (Q.V.) IS THE SAME CONDITION.

DEUTMAN, A. F. AND JANSEN, L. M. A. A.* DOMINANTLY INHERITED DRUSEN OF BRUCH'S MEMBRANE. BRIT. J. OPHTHAL. 54* 373-382, 1970.

EVANS, P. J.* FIVE CASES OF FAMILIAL RETINAL ABIOTROPHY. TRANS. OPHTHAL. SOC. U.K. 70* 96 ONLY, 1950.

CHARACTERISTICALLY SMALL ROUND WHITE SPOTS INVOLVING THE POSTERIOR POLE OF THE EYE INCLUDING THE AREAS OF THE MACULA AND OPTIC DISC APPEAR IN EARLY ADULT LIFE. PROGRESSION TO FORM A MOSAIC PATTERN WHICH DOYNE (1899) APTLY TERMED "HONEYCOMB" OCCURS THEREAFTER. DOYNE CONSIDERED IT TO REPRESENT "CHOROIDITIS." HOWEVER, TREACHER COLLINS (1913) SHOWED THAT THE CHANGES CONSIST OF SWELLING IN THE INNER PART OF BRUCH'S MEMBRAINE. FAILING VISION USUALLY DEVELOPED CONSIDERABLY LATER THAN THE OPHTHALMOLOGIC CHANGE. DOYNE WAS AN OPHTHALMOLOGIST IN OXFORD, ENGLAND. PEARCE (1967) DID AN EXTENSIVE STUDY OF SIX KINDREDS LIVING NEAR OXFORD. SOME AND POSSIBLY ALL MAY HAVE BEEN DESCENDANTS FROM A COMMON ANCESTOR. DOMINANT INHERI-TANCE WITH COMPLETE MANIFESTATION OF THE TRAIT IN PERSONS SURVIVING BEYOND EARLY ADULT LIFE WAS FOUND. FAMILIES LIVING ELSEWHERE THAN ENGLAND HAVE BEEN REPORTED (SEE REFERENCES GIVEN BY PEARCE, 1968).

COLLINS, E. T.* A PATHOLOGICAL REPORT UPON A CASE OF DOYNE'S CHOROIDITIS. OPHTHALMOSCOPE 11* 537-538, 1913.

DOYNE, R. W.* A PECULIAR CONDITION OF CHOROIDITIS OCCURRING IN SEVERAL MEMBERS OF THE SAME FAMILY. TRANS. OPHTHAL. SOC. U.K. 19* 71 ONLY, 1899.

PEARCE, W. G.* DOYNE'S HONEYCOMB RETINAL DEGENERATION. CLINICAL AND GENETIC FEATURES. BRIT. J. OPHTHAL. 52* 73-78, 1968.

PEARCE, W. G.* GENETIC ASPECTS OF DOYNE'S HONEYCOMB DEGENERATION OF THE RETINA. ANN. HUM. GENET. 31* 173-188, 1967.

*12680 DUANE SYNDROME (RETRACTION SYNDROME)

THE FEATURES OF THE SYNDROME ARE CONGENITAL DEFICIENCY OF OCULAR ABDUCTION, IMPAIRMENT OF ADDUCTION, RETRACTION AND SUPERIOR OR INFERIOR DEVIATION OF THE GLOBE ON ADDUCTION AND NARROWING OF THE PALPEBRAL FISSURE ON ADDUCTION. THE CONDITION IS BILATERAL IN TWENTY PERCENT OF CASES. TRANSMISSION THROUGH 4 GENERATIONS WAS REPORTED BY COOPER (1910) AND THROUGH 3 GENERATIONS BY WAARDENBURG (1923), LAUGHLIN (1937) AND ZENTMAYER (1935). HETEROGENEITY ALMOST CERTAINLY EXISTS. ASSOCIATED DEFORMITY OF THE UPPER EXTREMITY WAS REPORTED BY GIFFORD (1926), CRISP (1918) AND MENNERICH (1923). FERRELL, JONES AND LUCAS (1966) HAVE DESCRIBED THE ASSOCIATION OF A HEART-HAND SYNDROME (PROBABLY TYPE II OF LEWIS Q.V.) IN A DOMINANT PATTERN OF INHERITANCE.

COOPER, H.* A SERIES OF CASES OF CONGENITAL OPHTHALMOPLEGIA EXTERNA (NUCLEAR PARALYSIS) IN THE SAME FAMILY. BRIT. MED. J. 1* 917 ONLY, 1910.

CRISP, W. H.* CONGENITAL PARALYSIS OF THE EXTERNAL RECTUS MUSCLE. AM. J. OPHTHAL. 1* 172-176, 1918.

FERRELL, R. L., JONES, B. AND LUCAS, R. V., JR.* SIMULTANEOUS OCCURRENCE OF THE HOLT-ORAM AND THE DUANE SYNDROMES. J. PEDIAT. 69* 630-634, 1966.

GIFFORD, H.* CONGENITAL DEFECTS OF ABDUCTION AND OTHER OCULAR MOVEMENTS AND THEIR RELATION TO BIRTH INJURIES. AM. J. OPHTHAL. 9* 3-22, 1926.

GOLDFARB, C. AND GANNON, F. L.* FAMILIAL CONGENITAL LATERAL RECTUS PALSY WITH RETRACTION (STILLING-DUANE-TURK SYNDROME). DIS. NERV. SYST. 25* 17-21, 1964.

LAUGHLIN, R. C.* HEREDITARY PARALYSIS OF THE ABDUCENS NERVE. AM. J. OPHTHAL. 20* 396-398, 1937.

MENNERICH, P.* EIN FALL VON RETRAKTIONBEWEGUNGEN DER AUGEN BEI ANGEBORENEN ANOMALIEN DER AUSSEREN AUGENMUSKELN. Z. AUGENHEILK. 50* 173-180, 1923.

WAARDENBURG, P. J.* CONGENITAL DISTURBANCES OF MOTILITY. AM. J. OPHTHAL. 6* 44-45, 1923.

ZENTMAYER, W.* MENGEL'S BILATERAL DEFICIENCY OF ABDUCTION. ARCH. OPHTHAL. 13* 984 ONLY, 1935.

ALTHOUGH THIS CLEARLY RUNS IN FAMILIES AND AUTOSOMAL DOMINANCE WITH VARIABLE PENETRANCE IS LIKELY, THIS MODE OF INHERITANCE CANNOT BE CONSIDERED PROVEN. THERE ARE CERTAIN FUNDAMENTAL SIMILARITIES TO PEYRONIE'S DISEASE (Q.V.) AND THE TWO ARE ASSOCIATED MORE FREQUENTLY THAN CHANCE ALONE WOULD DICTATE. KNUCKLE PADS (Q.V.) ARE ALSO ASSOCIATED FREQUENTLY. MANSON (1931) DESCRIBED AFFECTED FATHER AND THREE SONS.

KOSTIA, J.* A DUPUYTRENS' CONTRACTURE FAMILY. ANN. CHIR. GYNAEC. FENN. 46* 351-358, 1957.

LYGONIS, C.* FAMILIAL DUPUYTREN'S CONTRACTURE. HEREDITAS 56* 142-143, 1966.

MANSON, J. S.* HEREDITY AND DUPUYTREN'S CONTRACTURE. BRIT. MED. J. 2* 11 ONLY, 1931.

MAZA, R. K. AND GOODMAN, R. M.* A FAMILY WITH DUPUYTREN'S CONTRACTURE. J. HERED. 59* 155-156, 1968.

SKOOG, T.* DUPUYTREN'S CONTRACTION WITH SPECIAL REFERENCE TO AETIOLOGY AND IMPROVED SURGICAL TREATMENT* ITS OCCURRENCE IN EPILEPTICS* NOTE ON KNUCKLE-PADS. ACTA CHIR. SCAND. 138 (SUPPL.)* 1-190, 1948.

*12700 DWARFISM, CORTICAL THICKENING OF TUBULAR BONES, AND TRANSIENT HYPOCALCEMIA

KENNY AND LINARELLI (1966) DESCRIBED MOTHER AND SON WHO WERE MARKEDLY DWARFED WITH DENSE TUBULAR BONES AND NARROW MARROW CAVITIES. BOTH HAD SELF-LIMITED BOUTS OF HYPOCALCEMIA AND HYPOPHOSPHATEMIA DOCUMENTED AT AGE 39 YEARS IN THE MOTHER AND AGE 1 TO 15 WEEKS IN THE SON. ASSOCIATED FEATURES WERE DELAYED CLOSURE OF THE FONTANEL, MYOPIA AND LOW BIRTH WEIGHT. MENTATION WAS NORMAL. RADIOLOGIC FEATURES WERE PRESENTED IN DETAIL BY CAFFEY (1967). THE MOTHER WAS 48 INCHES TALL AT AGE 39 YEARS.

CAFFEY, J.* CONGENITAL STENOSIS OF MEDULLARY SPACES IN TUBULAR BONES AND CALVARIA IN TWO PROPORTIONATE DWARFS, MOTHER AND SON, COUPLED WITH TRANSITORY HYPOCALCEMIC TETANY. AM. J. ROENTGEN. 100* 1-11, 1967.

KENNY, F. M. AND LINARELLI, L.* DWARFISM AND CORTICAL THICKENING OF TUBULAR BONES. TRANSIENT HYPOCALCEMIA IN A MOTHER AND SON. AM. J. DIS. CHILD. 111* 201-207, 1966.

12710 DWARFISM, LEVI OR 'SNUB-NOSED' TYPE

IN 1910 LEVI DESCRIBED TWO FAMILIES WITH 'MICROSOMIE ESSENTIALE' DISPLAYING DOMINANT INHERITANCE. BODY PROPORTIONS WERE NORMAL. BLACK (1961) REFERRED TO THESE AS 'SNUB-NOSED DWARFS,' A VARIETY OF LOW BIRTH-WEIGHT DWARFISM, AND SUGGESTED THAT BOTH DOMINANT (ILLUSTRATED BY LEVI'S CASES) AND RECESSIVE FORMS EXIST. THE LOW BIRTH WEIGHT IS, PERHAPS, NOT WELL DOCUMENTED AND THIS CONDITION MAY IN FACT BE SEXUAL ATELIOSIS, A RECESSIVE (Q.V.). THE PHENOTYPES OF THE PRESUMED DOMINANT AND RECESSIVE FORMS SEEM IDENTICAL AND POSSIBLY LEVI'S PEDIGREE WAS AN INSTANCE OF QUASI-DOMINANCE. ON THE OTHER HAND CASES OF PRIMORDIAL DWARFISM IN SUCCESSIVE GENERATIONS ARE CITED BY WARKANY, MONROE AND SUTHERLAND (1961), NOTABLY THE FAMILY STUDIED BY SELLE (1920) IN WHICH 10 PERSONS IN 3 GENERATIONS WERE AFFECTED.

BLACK, J.* LOW BIRTH WEIGHT DWARFISM. ARCH. DIS. CHILD. 36* 633-644, 1961.

LEVI, E.* CONTRIBUTION A LA CONNAISSANCE DE LA MICROSOMIE ESSENTIELLE HEREDO-FAMILIALE* DISTINCTION DE CETTE FORME CLINIQUE D'AVEC LES NANISMES, LES INFANTI-LISMES ET LES FORMES MIXTES DE CES DIFFERENTES DYSTROPHIES. N. ICONOG. SALPET. 23* 552-570, 1910.

SELLE, G.* UBER VERERBUNG DES ECHTEN ZWERGWUCHSES. INAUG. DISSERT., UNIVERSITY OF JENA, 1920.

WARKANY, J., MONROE, B. B. AND SUTHERLAND, B. S.* INTRAUTERINE GROWTH RETARDA-TION. AM. J. DIS. CHILD. 102* 249-279, 1961.

12720 DWARFISM, WITH STIFF-JOINTS AND OCULAR ABNORMALITIES

THE FEATURES (MOORE, FEDERMAN, 1965) ARE DWARFISM WITH DISPROPORTIONATELY SHORT LEGS (HEIGHT 54 TO 57 INCHES), REDUCED JOINT MOBILITY, AND OCULAR ABNORMALITIES (HYPEROPIA, GLAUCOMA, CATARACT, RETINAL DETACHMENT). SEVEN MEMBERS OF THREE GENERATIONS WERE AFFECTED IN THE ONE REPORTED FAMILY, WITH MALE-TO-MALE TRANSMIS-SION. ALTHOUGH SOME FEATURES RESEMBLE THOSE OF LERI'S PLEONOSTEOSIS, THERE IS SUFFICIENT DIFFERENCE TO INDICATE THAT THIS IS A DISTINCT ENTITY. THIS MAY, HOWEVER, BE THE SAME DISORDER AS THAT DESCRIBED UNDER THE DESIGNATION OF ARTHRO-OPHTHALMOPATHY.

MOORE, W. T. AND FEDERMAN, D. D.* FAMILIAL DWARFISM AND 'STIFF JOINTS.' ARCH. INTERN. MED. 115* 398-404, 1965.

THE CHARACTERISTICS ARE TYPICAL DEFORMITY OF THE DISTAL RADIUS AND ULNA AND PROXIMAL CARPAL BONES AND MESOMELIC DWARFISM. THE WRIST DEFORMITY IS OFTEN REFERRED TO AS MADELUNG'S DEFORMITY. LANGER (1965) REPORTED THREE FAMILIES. A STRIKING PREPONDERANCE OF AFFECTED FEMALES MAKES IT IMPORTANT TO OBSERVE MALE-TO-MALE TRANSMISSION BEFORE AUTOSOMAL TRANSMISSION IS COMPLETELY ACCEPTED. IT HAS BEEN MY IMPRESSION THAT FEMALES ARE MORE SEVERELY AFFECTED THAN MALES. HENCE, THE PREPONDERANCE OF AFFECTED FEMALES MAY BE THE RESULT OF BIAS OF ASCERTAINMENT. THE DEFORMITY OF THE FOREARM CONSISTS OF BOWING OF THE RADIUS AND DORSAL DISLOCATION OF THE DISTAL ULNA. MOTION IS LIMITED AT THE ELBOW AND WRIST. LAMY AND BIENEN-FELD (1954) DESCRIBED AFFECTED MOTHER AND SON. THE FIBULA WAS ABSENT IN BOTH. REVIEWING CASES OF MADELUNG DEFORMITY FELMAN AND KIRKPATRICK (1969) CONCLUDED THAT PATIENTS TALLER THAN THE 25TH PERCENTILE FOR HEIGHT PROBABLY DO NOT HAVE DYSCHON-DROSTEOSIS, THAT HEREDITARY ENTITY OF MADELUNG'S DEFORMITY DISTINCT FROM DYSCHON-DROSTEOSIS EXISTS, THAT PATIENTS WITH THE ISOLATED MADELUNG'S DEFORMITY MAY BE SHORT, THAT MARKED SHORTENING OF THE TIBIA RELATIVE TO THE FEMUR SUGGESTS DYSCHONDROSTEOSIS. LANGER (1965) HAD TAKEN THE VIEW THAT MOST OR ALL MADELUNG DEFORMITY IS DYSCHONDROSTEOSIS. THE MOST COMPLETE REVIEW OF THE SUBJECT OF MADELUNG'S DEFORMITY IS THAT BY ANTON ET AL. (1938). RULLIER ET AL. (1968) OBSERVED DYSCHONDROSTEOSIS IN MOTHER AND TWO DAUGHTERS. NASSIF AND HARBOYAN (1970) DESCRIBED TWO BROTHERS WITH LERI'S DYSCHONDROSTEOSIS, WHO ALSO HAD MIDDLE EAR DEFORMITIES AND CONDUCTIVE HEARING LOSS. THREE SISTERS HAD THE SKELETAL DEFORMITY WITH NORMAL HEARING.

ANTON, J. I., REITZ, G. B. AND SPIEGEL, M. B.* MADELUNG'S DEFORMITY. ANN. SURG. 108* 411-439, 1938.

FELMAN, A. H. AND KIRKPATRICK, J. A., JR.* DYSCHONDROSTEOSE. MESOMELIC DWARFISM OF LERI AND WEILL. AM. J. DIS. CHILD. 120* 329-331, 1970.

FELMAN, A. H. AND KIRKPATRICK, J. A., JR.* MADELUNG'S DEFORMITY* OBSERVATIONS IN 17 PATIENTS. RADIOLOGY 93* 1037-1042, 1969.

HERDMAN, R. C., LANGER, L. O. AND GOOD, R. A.* DYSCHONDROSTEOSIS, THE MOST COMMON CAUSE OF MADELUNG'S DEFORMITY. J. PEDIAT. 68* 432-441, 1966.

LAMY, M. AND BIENENFELD, C.* LA DYSCHONDROSTEOSE. DE GENETICA MEDICA. ROME* L. GEDDA (ED.) 1954.

LANGER, L. O., JR.* DYSCHONDROSTEOSIS, A HEREDITABLE BONE DYSPLASIA WITH CHARACTERISTIC ROENTGENOGRAPHIC FEATURES. AM. J. ROENTGEN. 95* 178-188, 1965.

NASSIF, R. AND HARBOYAN, G.* MADELUNG'S DEFORMITY WITH CONDUCTIVE HEARING LOSS. ARCH. OTOLARYNG. 91* 175-178, 1970.

RULLIER, J., LABRAM, C., LAZAROVICI, A. M. AND ROUSSELOT, R.* DYSCHONDROSTEOSE FAMILIALE. ETUDE DE TROIS CAS (MERE ET SIS DEUX FILS). SEM. HOP. PARIS 44* 2474-2479, 1968.

12740 DYSCHROMATOSIS SYMMETRICA HEREDITARIA

THIS DISORDER HAS, LIKE DYSCHROMATOSIS UNIVERSALIS HEREDITARIA, BEEN DESCRIBED ONLY IN JAPANESE. RELATION OF THE TWO CONDITIONS IS NOT CLEAR.

KOMAYA, G.* SYMMETRISCHE PIGMENTANOMALIE DER EXTREMITATEN. ARCH. DERM. SYPH. 147* 389-393, 1924.

12750 DYSCHROMATOSIS UNIVERSALIS HEREDITARIA

THIS ANOMALY HAS BEEN DESCRIBED ONLY IN JAPANESE. IT IS CHARACTERIZED BY PIGMENTED FLECKS AND SPOTS OVER MUCH OF THE BODY. SUENAGA'S FAMILY COULD EQUALLY WELL OR EVEN BETTER, BE RECESSIVE AND ONLY QUASI-DOMINANT, SINCE A CONSANGUINEOUS MARRIAGE OCCURRED IN EACH OF FOUR SUCCESSIVE GENERATIONS. THE APPARENT RESTRIC-TION TO JAPANESE IS MORE CONSISTENT WITH THIS POSSIBILITY.

SUENAGA, M.* GENETICAL STUDIES ON SKIN DISEASES. VII. DYSCHROMATOSIS UNIVERSALIS HEREDITARIA IN FIVE GENERATIONS. TOHOKU J. EXP. MED. 55* 373-376, 1952.

*12760 DYSKERATOSIS, HEREDITARY BENIGN INTRAEPITHELIAL

CHARACTERISTIC HISTOLOGIC CHANGES OF THE PRICKLE CELL LAYER OF THE MUCOSA INCLUDE NUMEROUS ROUND, WAXY-APPEARING, EOSINOPHILIC CELLS WHICH APPEAR TO BE ENGULFED BY NORMAL CELLS GIVING A CELL-WITHIN-CELL APPEARANCE. IN A TRIRACIAL ISOLATE IN NORTH CAROLINA, WITKOP AND COLLEAGUES (1960) FOUND THIS DISORDER IN AT LEAST 83 PERSONS. THE CONJUNCTIVA AND ORAL MUCOUS MEMBRANES ARE AFFECTED. THE ORAL LESION, WHICH GROSSLY RESEMBLES LEUKOPLAKIA, IS NOT PRECANCEROUS. THE EYE LESIONS RESEMBLE PTERYGIA (SEE PTERYGIUM). THE ONLY SYMPTOMS ARE PRODUCED BY INVOLVEMENT OF THE CORNEA WITH BLINDNESS. HISTOLOGICALLY CHARACTERISTIC FINDINGS ARE OBTAINED IN ORAL AND EYE SCRAPING. PENETRANCE IS ABOUT 97 PER CENT AND THERE IS LITTLE EFFECT ON REPRODUCTIVE FITNESS. YANOFF (1968) DESCRIBED THE CONDITION IN MOTHER

AND DAUGHTER. THIS IS THE ONLY REPORT OF THE CONDITION IN PERSONS APPARENTLY UNRELATED TO THE NORTH CAROLINIAN TRI-RACIAL ISOLATE, THE "HALIWA INDIANS," STUDIED BY WITKOP ET AL. (1961).

VON SALLMANN, L. AND PATON, D.* HEREDITARY BENIGN INTRAEPITHELIAL DYSKERATOSIS. I. OCULAR MANIFESTATIONS. ARCH. OPHTHAL. 63* 421-429, 1960.

WITKOP, C. J., JR. AND GORLIN, R. J.* FOUR HEREDITARY MUCOSAL SYNDROMES. ARCH. DERM. 84* 762-771, 1961.

WITKOP, C. J., JR., SHANKLE, C. H., GRAHAM, J. B., MURRAY, M. R., RUCKNAGEL, D. L. AND BYERLY, B. H.* HEREDITARY BENIGN INTRA-EPITHELIAL DYSKERATOSIS. II. ORAL MANIFESTATIONS AND HEREDITARY TRANSMISSION. ARCH. PATH. 70* 696-711, 1960.

YANOFF, M.* HEREDITARY BENIGN INTRAEPITHELIAL DYSKERATOSIS. ARCH. OPHTHAL. 79* 291-293, 1968.

12770 DYSLEXIA, SPECIFIC ("CONGENITAL WORD-BLINDNESS")

HALLGREN (1950) STUDIED 116 FAMILIES. SPEECH DEFECTS WERE ASSOCIATED IN MANY INSTANCES, ESPECIALLY IN MALES, AND WERE PROBABLY DETERMINED BY THE SAME FACTOR AS DYSLEXIA. LEFT-HANDEDNESS AND LEFT-EYEDNESS COULD NOT BE SHOWN TO BE ASSOCIATED. GENETIC ANALYSIS SUGGESTED AUTOSOMAL DOMINANT INHERITANCE.

HALLGREN, B.* SPECIFIC DYSLEXIA ("CONGENITAL WORD-BLINDNESS"). A CLINICAL AND GENETIC STUDY. ACTA PSYCHIAT. NEUROL. SCAND. 65 (SUPPL.)* 1-287, 1950.

12780 DYSPLASIA EPIPHYSEALIS HEMIMELICA

THIS CONDITION IS CHARACTERIZED BY ASYMMETRICAL CARTILAGINOUS OVERGROWTH OF ONE OR MORE EPIPHYSES OF A TARSAL OR CARPAL BONE, AND LESS OFTEN OTHER BONES. MALES ARE AFFECTED ABOUT 3 TIMES MORE OFTEN THAN FEMALES. THE DISORDER APPEARS TO HAVE NO SIMPLE MENDELIAN BASIS. NO FAMILIAL CASE HAS BEEN REPORTED. DONALSON (1953) DESCRIBED A PATIENT WHOSE MONOZYGOTIC CO-TWIN WAS NOT AFFECTED.

DONALSON, J. S., SANKEY, H. H., GIRDANY, B. R. AND DONALSON, W. F.* OSTEOCHON-DROMA OF THE DISTAL FEMORAL EPIPHYSIS. J. PEDIAT. 43* 212-216, 1953.

KETTELKAMP, D. B., CAMPBELL, C. J. AND BONFIGLIO, M.* DYSPLASIA EPIPHYSEALIS HEMIMELICA. A REPORT OF FIFTEEN CASES AND A REVIEW OF THE LITERATURE. J. BONE JOINT SURG. 48A* 746-766, 1966.

SAXTON, H. M. AND WILKINSON, J. A.* HEMIMELIC SKELETAL DYSPLASIA. J. BONE JOINT SURG. 46B* 608-613, 1964.

THEODOROU, S. AND LANITIS, G.* DYSPLASIA EPIPHYSIALIS HEMIMELICA (EPIPHYSEAL OSTEOCHONDROMATA). REPORT OF TWO CASES AND REVIEW OF THE LITERATURE. HELV. PAEDIAT. ACTA 23* 195-204, 1968.

*12790 DYSPROTHROMBINEMIA

IN AN EXTENSIVE KINDRED, SHAPIRO ET AL. (1969) FOUND 11 PERSONS WITH HALF-NORMAL PLASMA CONCENTRATIONS OF BIOLOGICAL PROTHROMBIN ACTIVITY BUT NORMAL IMMUNOREACTIVE PROTHROMBIN. THEY REFERRED TO THE DEFECTIVE MOLECULE AS PROTHROMBIN CARDEZA. THE LOCUS OF THE MUTATION MAY BE THE SAME AS THAT FOR HYPOPROTHROMBINEMIA (Q.V.) IN WHICH NO CROSS-REACTING MATERIAL IS IDENTIFIABLE.

SHAPIRO, S. S., MARTINEZ, J. AND HOLBURN, R. R.* CONGENITAL DYSPROTHROMBINEMIA* AN INHERITED STRUCTURAL DISORDER OF HUMAN PROTHROMBIN. J. CLIN. INVEST. 48* 2251-2259, 1969.

*12800 DYSTELEPHALANGY (KIRNER'S DEFORMITY)

THE TIP OF THE FIFTH FINGER POINTS TOWARD THE THENAR EMINENCE DUE TO BOWING OF THE DISTAL PHALANX. X-RAY SHOWS ANGULATION OF THE METAPHYSIS OF THE PHALANX. THE LESION IS PROBABLY NOT MANIFEST BEFORE THE FIFTH YEAR OF AGE. A GLOBULAR SOFT TISSUE MASS AT THE TIP OF THE FIFTH FINGERS WITHOUT BONE DEFORMITY IS PROBABLY THE MINOR MANIFESTATION. AUTOSOMAL DOMINANT INHERITANCE IS SUPPORTED BY THE FINDINGS OF BLANK AND GIRDANY (1965), BRAILSFORD (1953) AND WILSON (1952).

BLANK, E. AND GIRDANY, B. R.* SYMMETRIC BOWING OF THE TERMINAL PHALANGES OF THE FIFTH FINGERS IN A FAMILY (KIRNER'S DEFORMITY). AM. J. ROENTGEN. 93* 367-373, 1965.

BRAILSFORD, J. F.* RADIOLOGY OF BONES AND JOINTS. BALTIMORE* WILLIAMS AND WILKINS, 1953 (5TH ED.). P. 64.

WILSON, J. N.* DYSTROPHY OF FIFTH FINGER* REPORT OF FOUR CASES. J. BONE JOINT SURG. 34B* 236-239, 1952.

*12810 DYSTONIA MUSCULORUM DEFORMANS

JOHNSON, SCHWARTZ AND BARBEAU (1962) DESCRIBED AN EXTENSIVELY AFFECTED FRENCH-CANADIAN FAMILY. MINOR MANIFESTATIONS INTERPRETED AS FORMES FRUSTES WERE FOUND IN SOME FAMILY MEMBERS. THE NEUROLOGIC PICTURE IN SOME CASES OF WILSON'S DISEASE IS VERY SIMILAR CLINICALLY. ZEMAN ET AL. (1959, 1960) TRACED THE DISORDER THROUGH 4 GENERATIONS AND LARSSON AND SJOGREN (1963) TRACED IT THROUGH 5 GENERATIONS. RATHER THAN A HYPERKINETIC PICTURE, SOME HAD A MYOSTATIC PICTURE, SUCH AS WAS DESCRIBED BY WECHSLER AND BROCK (1922). A RECESSIVE FORM OF THE DISEASE OCCURS WITH INCREASED FREQUENCY AMONG JEWS.

ELDRIDGE, R.* THE TORSION DYSTONIAS* LITERATURE REVIEW AND GENETIC AND CLINICAL STUDIES. NEUROLOGY 20* 1-78, 1970.

JOHNSON, W., SCHWARTZ, G. AND BARBEAU, A.* STUDIES ON DYSTONIA MUSCULORUM DEFORMANS. ARCH. NEUROL. 7* 301-313, 1962.

LARSSON, T. AND SJOGREN, T.* DYSTONIA MUSCULORUM DEFORMANS. A CLINICAL AND GENETIC POPULATION STUDY. PROC. SEC. INTERN. CONG. HUM. GENET. (ROME, SEPT. 6-12, 1961.) 3* 1659-1662, 1963.

WECHSLER, I. S. AND BROCK, S.* DYSTONIA MUSCULORUM DEFORMANS WITH ESPECIAL REFERENCE TO A MYOSTATIC FORM AND THE OCCURRENCE OF DECEREBRATE RIGIDITY PHENOMENA. A STUDY OF SIX CASES. ARCH. NEUROL. PSYCHIAT. 8* 538-552, 1922.

ZEMAN, W. AND DYKEN, P.* DYSTONIA MUSCULORUM DEFORMANS. CLINICAL, GENETIC AND PATHOANATOMICAL STUDIES. PSYCHIAT. NEUROL. NEUROCHIR. 70* 77-121, 1967.

ZEMAN, W., KAELBLING, R. AND PASAMANICK, B.* IDIOPATHIC DYSTONIA MUSCULORUM DEFORMANS. NEUROLOGY 10* 1068-1075, 1960.

ZEMAN, W., KAELBLING, R. AND PASAMANICK, B.* IDIOPATHIC DYSTONIA MUSCULORUM DEFORMANS. I. THE HEREDITARY PATTERN. AM. J. HUM. GENET. 11* 188-202, 1959.

*12820 DYSTONIA, FAMILIAL PAROXYSMAL

PAROXYSMAL DYSTONIA MAY OCCUR IN MULTIPLE SCLEROSIS OR HEPATOLENTICULAR DEGENERATION. IT IS CHARACTERIZED BY ASSUMPTION OF UNILATERAL DYSTONIC POSTURES WITHOUT CLONIC MOVEMENTS OR CHANGE IN CONSCIOUSNESS. IT WAS REPORTED AS A 'PURE ENTITY,' IN MOTHER AND 3 SONS BY WEBER (1967). HE CLAIMED THAT ONLY ONE FAMILY HAD PREVIOUSLY BEEN REPORTED (LANCE, 1963) AND THAT THIS IS DISTINCT FROM FAMILIAL PAROXYSMAL CHOREOATHETOSIS. (POSSIBLY IT IS THE SAME AS THE PERIODIC DYSTONIA REPORTED BY SMITH AND HEERSEMA (1941), ALTHOUGH THEY HAD MULTIPLE AFFECTED SIBS WITH NORMAL PARENTS). KERTESZ (1967) CALLED THE CONDITION PAROXYSMAL KINESIGENIC CHOREOATHETOSIS.

KERTESZ, A.* PAROXYSMAL KINESIGENIC CHOREOATHETOSIS. NEUROLOGY 17* 680-690, 1967.

LANCE, J. W.* SPORADIC AND FAMILIAL VARIETIES OF TONIC SEIZURES. J. NEUROL. NEUROSURG. PSYCHIAT. 26* 51-59, 1963.

SMITH, L. A. AND HEERSEMA, P. H.* PERIODIC DYSTONIA. PROC. MAYO CLIN. 16* 842-846, 1941.

WEBER, M. B.* FAMILIAL PAROXYSMAL DYSTONIA. J. NERV. MENT. DIS. 145* 221-226, 1967.

12830 EAR EXOSTOSES (EXOSTOSES OF EXTERNAL AUDITORY CANAL)

THE TRAIT IS AGE AND SEX DEPENDENT BEING RARE IN YOUNG CHILDREN AND MORE FREQUENT IN MALES. INSTANCES OF INVOLVEMENT IN MULTIPLE GENERATIONS WERE REVIEWED BY HRDLICKA (1935).

HRDLICKA, A.* EAR EXOSTOSES. SMITHSONIAN MISCELLANEOUS COLLECTIONS 93* 1-100, 1935.

12840 EAR FLARE

'NEAR-HEAD,' INTERMEDIATE AND 'FLARE' TYPES CAN BE RECOGNIZED. THE DATA OF KLOEPFER (1946) SUGGESTED COMPLEX GENETICS.

KLOEPFER, H. W.* AN INVESTIGATION OF 171 POSSIBLE LINKAGE RELATIONSHIPS IN MAN. ANN. EUGEN. 13* 35-72, 1946.

12850 EAR FOLDING

VARIOUS UNUSUAL VARIETIES OF FOLDING OF THE HELIX AND OTHER PARTS OF THE EAR ARE DESCRIBED IN FAMILIES USUALLY AS AN AUTOSOMAL DOMINANT 'WITH VARIABLE EXPRESSIVITY AND REDUCED PENETRANCE.'

AHUJA, Y. R. AND GUPTA, M.* INHERITANCE OF AN UNUSUAL EAR TYPE IN MAN. ACTA MED. GENET. GEM. 19* 454-456, 1970.

POTTER (1937) DESCRIBED A BILATERAL CONGENITAL MALFORMATION OF THE PINNA WHICH IS CURLED UP LIKE A CAP OR CUP CONCEALING THE EXTERNAL AUDITORY MEATUS WHEN THE SUBJECT IS IN LATERAL PROFILE. ERICH AND ABU-JAMRA (1965) OBSERVED TRANSMISSION OF THE CONDITION THROUGH FOUR GENERATIONS (IN 17 CASES IN 8 SIBSHIPS) AND REVIEWED SIMILAR REPORTS. PETERSON AND SCHIMKE (1968) OBSERVED CUP-SHAPED EARS IN MEMBERS OF 5 GENERATIONS WITH AT LEAST 4 INSTANCES OF MALE-TO-MALE TRANSMISSION. THEIR PROBAND HAD PIERRE ROBIN SYNDROME (Q.V.). THE EMBRYOLOGY OF THE AURICLE AND A LARGE AMOUNT OF CLINICAL MATERIAL ON VARIOUS ANOMALIES OF THE AURICLE WERE PRESENTED BY ROGERS (1968).

ERICH, J. B. AND ABU-JAMRA, F. N.* CONGENITAL CUP-SHAPED DEFORMITY OF THE EARS TRANSMITTED THROUGH FOUR GENERATIONS. MAYO CLINIC PROC. 40* 597-602, 1965.

PETERSON, D. M. AND SCHIMKE, R. N.* HEREDITARY CUP-SHAPED EARS AND THE PIERRE ROBIN SYNDROME. J. MED. GENET. 5* 52-55, 1968.

POTTER, E. L.* A HEREDITARY EAR MALFORMATION TRANSMITTED THROUGH FIVE GENERA-TIONS. J. HERED. 28* 255-258, 1937.

ROGERS, B. O.* MICROTIC, LOP, CUP AND PROTRUDING EARS* FOUR DIRECTLY INHERI-TABLE DEFORMITIES. PLAST. RECONSTR. SURG. 41* 208-231, 1968.

12870 EAR PITS

ALTHOUGH IN AT LEAST ONE FAMILY (MUCKLE, 1961) BOTH EAR PITS AND LATERAL CERVICAL SINUSES OPENING AT VARIOUS LEVELS ON THE ANTERIOR MARGIN OF THE STERNOMASTOID WERE PRESENT, SOMETIMES IN THE SAME INDIVIDUAL, MOST FAMILIES HAVE SHOWN EITHER EAR-PITS ONLY OR BRANCHIAL CLEFT ANOMALIES (Q.V.) ONLY. HENCE, EAR PITS ARE LISTED AS A SEPARATE MUTATION. THEY OCCUR IN THE UPPER ANTERIOR END OF THE HELIX. EWING (1946) FOUND THEM IN 0.9 PER CENT OF 3500 BRITISH SERVICE MEN. THEY OCCUR MORE FREQUENTLY IN NEGROES. SKIN TAGS CONTAINING CARTILAGE (JENKINS, 1928) OCCUR IN SOME AFFECTED PERSONS (MCKUSICK ET AL., 1964). THESE ARE CONSIDERED ABNORMALITIES OF THE FIRST BRANCHIAL CLEFT. MUCKLE'S FAMILY (1961) SHOWED 'BUCK TEETH' (PROJECTING UPPER FRONT TEETH). GUALANDRI (1969) FOUND 321 CASES AMONG 29,309 MILAN SCHOOL CHILDREN. PEDIGREES WERE PREPARED IN 93 CASES DEMONSTRATING AUTOSOMAL DOMINANT INHERITANCE WITH ABOUT 85 PERCENT PENETRANCE. HIS USE OF THE TERM FISTULA WOULD BE CHALLENGED BY SOME WHO WOULD CALL THE LESION A SINUS OR SIMPLY A PIT.

CANNON, F. E.* INHERITANCE OF EAR PITS IN SIX GENERATIONS OF A FAMILY. J. HERED. 32* 413-414, 1941.

EWING, M. R.* CONGENITAL SINUSES OF EXTERNAL EAR. J. LARYNG. 61* 18-23, 1946.

GUALANDRI, V.* RICERCHE GENETICHE SULLA FISTULA AURIS CONGENITA. ACTA GENET. MED. GEM. 18* 51-68, 1969.

JENKINS, R.* THE OCCURRENCE OF A SKIN PAPILLUS THROUGH FOUR HUMAN GENERATIONS. J. HERED. 19* 174 ONLY, 1928.

MARTINS, A. G.* LATERAL CERVICAL AND PREAURICULAR SINUSES* THEIR TRANSMISSION AS DOMINANT CHARACTERS. BRIT. MED. J. 1* 255-256, 1961.

MCKUSICK, V. A. AND COLLEAGUES* MEDICAL GENETICS 1961-1963. OXFORD* PERGAMON PRESS, 1964. FIG. 12.

MUCKLE, T. J.* HEREDITARY BRANCHIAL DEFECTS IN A HAMPSHIRE FAMILY. BRIT. MED. J. 1* 1297-1299, 1961.

QUELPRUD, T.* EAR PIT AND ITS INHERITANCE. FISTULA AURIS CONGENITA, DESCRIBED IN 1864, STILL A GENETICAL AND EMBRYOLOGICAL PUZZLE. J. HERED. 31* 379-384, 1940.

SIMPKISS, M. AND LOWE, A.* CONGENITAL ABNORMALITIES IN THE AFRICAN NEWBORN. ARCH. DIS. CHILD. 36* 404-406, 1961.

STILES, K. A.* THE INHERITANCE OF PITTED EAR. GENETICS 26* 171 ONLY, 1941. J. HERED. 36* 53-61, 1945.

WHITNEY, D. D.* THREE GENERATIONS OF EAR PITS. J. HERED. 30* 323-324, 1939.

12880 EAR WITHOUT HELIX

WE HAVE OBSERVED MOTHER AND DAUGHTER (L.B., 1110726) WITH THIS PECULIARITY. THE DAUGHTER HAD SPLIT-HAND AND SPLIT-FOOT DEFORMITY. MACCOLLUM (1938) REPORTED A LARGE SERIES BUT GAVE NO GENETIC INFORMATION.

MACCOLLUM, D. W.* THE LOP EAR. J.A.M.A. 110* 1427-1430, 1938.

12890 EARLOBE ATTACHMENT (ATTACHED VS. UNATTACHED)

FREE EARLOBES ARE DOMINANT IN THE VIEW OF SOME. DUTTA AND GANGULY (1965) SUGGESTED POLYGENIC INHERITANCE. THERE IS A VARIETY WHICH IS PERHAPS BETTER CLASSIFIED AS 'LOBELESS' THAN 'ATTACHED.' LAI AND WALSH (1966) CONCLUDED THAT 'A SIMPLE MENDELIAN GENE EFFECT IS UNLIKELY TO BE RESPONSIBLE FOR THE EARLOBE TYPES.'

DUTTA, P. AND GANGULY, P.* FURTHER OBSERVATIONS ON EAR LOBE ATTACHMENT. ACTA GENET. STATIST. MED. 15* 77-86, 1965.

LAI, L. Y. C. AND WALSH, R. J.* OBSERVATIONS ON EAR LOBE TYPES. ACTA GENET. STATIST. MED. 16* 250-257, 1966.

POWELL, E. F. AND WHITNEY, D. D.* EAR LOBE INHERITANCE. AN UNUSUAL THREE-GENERATION PHOTOGRAPHIC PEDIGREE-CHART. J. HERED. 28* 185-186, 1937.

SUZUCHI, A.* GENETIC STUDIES OF THE HUMAN EARLAPPETS. ON THE INHERITANCE OF THE LOBULUS AURICULAE. JAP. J. HUM. GENET. 25* 157 ONLY, 1950.

WIENER, A. S.* COMPLICATIONS IN EAR GENETICS. J. HERED. 28* 425-426, 1937.

12900 EARRING HOLES, NATURAL

EDMONDS AND KEELER (1940) DESCRIBED PITS ON THE EARLOBES AT THE EXACT POINT WHERE LADIES PUNCTURE THEIR EARS FOR EARRINGS. IRREGULAR DOMINANT INHERITANCE WAS SUGGESTED.

EDMONDS, H. W. AND KEELER, C. E.* NATURAL 'EAR-RING' HOLES* INHERITED SINUSES OF EAR LOBE. J. HERED. 31* 507-510, 1940.

12910 EARS, ABILITY TO MOVE

LINDER (1949) FOUND A FREQUENCY OF THE TRAIT AMONG PARENTS AND SIBS OF PROBANDS LEADING TO THE IDEA THAT THE ABILITY IS INHERITED AS A SOMEWHAT IRREGULAR DOMINANT. IN 5 OF 24 CASES BOTH PARENTS LACKED THE TRAIT.

LINDER, L.* THE ABILITY TO MOVE THE EARS. HEREDITAS 35 (SUPPL.)* 620-621, 1949.

12920 ECTODERMAL DYSPLASIA, ABSENT DERMATOGLYPHIC PATTERN, CHANGES IN NAILS AND SIMIAN CREASE

PERSONS OF BOTH SEXES IN 3 GENERATIONS WERE AFFECTED (BASAN, 1965). MALE-TO-MALE TRANSMISSION WAS NOTED.

BASAN, M.* EKTODERMALE DYSPLASIE, FEHLENDES PAPILLARMUSTER. NAGELVERANDERUNGEN UND VIERFINGERFJRCHE. ARCH. KLIN. EXP. DERM. 222* 546-557, 1965.

12930 ECTODERMAL DYSPLASIA, ANHIDROTIC

RICHARDS AND KAPLAN (1969) DESCRIBED A GIRL INFANT WITH NEONATAL PYREXIA DUE TO ANHIDROTIC ECTODERMAL DYSPLASIA. THE MOTHER HAD 'SOMEWHAT SPARCE HAIR AND WRINKLED APPEARANCE OF THE EYELIDS.' TWO OF THE SISTERS AND FOUR OF THE BROTHERS OF THE MOTHER, AS WELL AS HER MOTHER HAD ABSENCE OF UPPER CANINE TEETH, AS DID ALSO THE SON OF A MATERNAL UNCLE. THE AUTHORS SUGGESTED AUTOSOMAL DOMINANT INHERITANCE. EARLIER KERR ET AL. (1966) EXPRESSED THE VIEW THAT DOMINANT INHERITANCE HAD NOT BEEN ADEQUATELY DOCUMENTED. CERTAINLY THE FAMILY OF RICHARDS AND KAPLAN (1969) IS CONSISTENT WITH X-LINKED INHERITANCE WITH PARTIAL EXPRESSION IN HETEROZYGOUS FEMALES.

KERR, C. B., WELLS, R. S. AND COOPER, K. E.* GENE EFFECT IN CARRIERS OF ANHIDROTIC ECTODERMAL DYSPLASIA. J. MED. GENET. 3* 169-176, 1966.

RICHARDS, W. AND KAPLAN, M.* ANHIDROTIC ECTODERMAL DYSPLASIA. AN UNUSUAL CASE OF PYREXIA IN THE NEWBORN. AM. J. DIS. CHILD. 117* 597-598, 1969.

12940 ECTODERMAL DYSPLASIA, ANHIDROTIC, WITH CLEFT LIP AND CLEFT PALATE

RAPP AND HODGKIN (1968) DESCRIBED MOTHER, SON AND DAUGHTER WITH ANHIDROTIC ECTODERMAL DYSPLASIA, CLEFT LIP AND CLEFT PALATE. THE COMBINATION HAD NOT BEEN PREVIOUSLY RECORDED.

RAPP, R. S. AND HODGKIN, W. E.* ANHIDROTIC ECTODERMAL DYSPLASIA* AUTOSOMAL DOMINANT INHERITANCE WITH PALATE AND LIP ANOMALIES. J. MED. GENET. 5* 269-272, 1968.

*12950 ECTODERMAL DYSPLASIA, HIDROTIC

SEVERAL REPORTS HAVE DESCRIBED AN EXTENSIVE KINDRED OF FRENCH EXTRACTION WHICH MIGRATED TO CANADA, SCOTLAND AND NORTHERN UNITED STATES (CLOUSTON, 1929* 1939* JOACHIM, 1936* MACKAY AND DAVIDSON, 1929* WILKEY AND STEVENSON, 1945). IN CONTRAST TO THE X-LINKED FORM, MOST OF THESE PATIENTS HAVE (1) NORMAL SWEAT AND SEBACEOUS GLAND FUNCTION, (2) TOTAL ALOPECIA, (3) SEVERE DYSTROPHY OF THE NAILS, (4) HYPERPIGMENTATION OF THE SKIN, ESPECIALLY OVER THE JOINTS AND (5) NORMAL

TEETH. STRABISMUS, MENTAL DEFICIENCY, CLUBBING OF THE FINGERS AND PALMAR
HYPERKERATOSIS OCCUR IN SOME. SCRIVER ET AL. (1965) SUGGESTED A MOLECULAR
ABNORMALITY OF KERATIN. THE HAIR WAS THIN WITH REDUCED TENSILE STRENGTH,
DISORGANIZED FIBRILLAR STRUCTURE BY LIGHT MICROSCOPY, REDUCED BIREFRINGENCE IN
POLARIZED LIGHT, AND INCREASED AMOUNT OF REACTIVE SH GROUPS.

CLOUSTON, H. R.* A HEREDITARY ECTODERMAL DYSTROPHY. CANAD. MED. ASS. J. 21*
18-31, 1929.

CLOUSTON, H. R.* THE MAJOR FORMS OF HEREDITARY ECTODERMAL DYSPLASIA. CANAD.
MED. ASS. J. 40* 1-7, 1939.

JOACHIM, H.* HEREDITARY DYSTROPHY OF THE HAIR AND NAILS IN SIX GENERATIONS.
ANN. INTERN. MED. 10* 400-402, 1936.

MACKAY, H. AND DAVIDSON, A. M.* CONGENITAL ECTODERMAL DYSPLASIA. BRIT. J.
DERM. 41* 1-5, 1929.

SCRIVER, C. R., SOLOMONS, C. C., DAVIES, E., WILLIAMS, M. AND BOLTON, J.* A
MOLECULAR ABNORMALITY OF KERATIN IN ECTODERMAL DYSPLASIA. (ABSTRACT) J. PEDIAT.
67* 946 ONLY, 1965.

WILKEY, W. D. AND STEVENSON, G. H.* A FAMILY WITH INHERITED ECTODERMAL
DYSTROPHY. CANAD. MED. ASS. J. 53* 226-230, 1945.

WILLIAMS, M. AND FRASER, F. C.* HIDROTIC ECTODERMAL DYSPLASIA - CLOUSTON'S
FAMILY REVISITED. CANAD. MED. ASS. J. 96* 36-38, 1967.

*12960 ECTOPIA LENTIS

USHER (1924) REPORTED SEVEN AFFECTED PERSONS IN THREE SUCCESSIVE GENERATIONS. IN
THESE EARLY REPORTS ONE CANNOT BE CERTAIN THE MARFAN SYNDROME (Q.V.) WAS NOT
PRESENT. FALLS AND COTTERMAN (1943) DESCRIBED A FAMILY WITH A LARGE NUMBER OF
AFFECTED PERSONS IN FIVE GENERATIONS, AND CHACE (1945) OBSERVED THREE GENERATIONS.
I HAVE RESTUDIED THE FAMILY REPORTED BY MCGAVIC (1966) AS HAVING WEILL-MARCHESANI
SYNDROME. THEY PROBABLY SUFFER FROM AN AUTOSOMAL DOMINANT FORM OF 'SIMPLE'
ECTOPIA LENTIS. ELEVEN MEMBERS WERE AFFECTED. ALL MEMBERS WITH OR WITHOUT
ECTOPIA LENTIS WERE SHORT.

CHACE, R. R.* CONGENITAL BILATERAL SUBLUXATION OF THE LENS. ARCH. OPHTHAL. 34*
425-426, 1945.

FALLS, H. F. AND COTTERMAN, C. W.* GENETIC STUDIES ON ECTOPIA LENTIS. A
PEDIGREE OF SIMPLE ECTOPIA OF THE LENS. ARCH. OPHTHAL. 30* 610-620, 1943.

HARSHMAN, J. P.* GLAUCOMA ASSOCIATED WITH SUBLUXATION OF THE LENS IN SEVERAL
MEMBERS OF FAMILY. AM. J. OPHTHAL. 31* 833-836, 1948.

MCGAVIC, J. S.* WEILL-MARCHESANI SYNDROME. BRACHYMORPHISM AND ECTOPIA LENTIS.
AM. J. OPHTHAL. 62* 820-823, 1966.

MEYER, E. T.* FAMILIAL ECTOPIA LENTIS AND ITS COMPLICATIONS. BRIT. J. OPHTHAL.
38* 163-172, 1954.

USHER, C. H.* A PEDIGREE OF CONGENITAL DISLOCATION OF LENSES. BIOMETRIKA 16*
273-282, 1924.

12970 ECTOPIA LENTIS ET PUPILLAE

THIS CONDITION IS ALMOST ALWAYS RECESSIVE (Q.V.). WALLS AND HEATH (1959)
DESCRIBED THREE AFFECTED SIBS AND AN AFFECTED CHILD OF ONE OF THESE. IT SEEMS
MOST LIKELY THAT THIS WAS THE FAMILIAR RECESSIVE DISORDER, THE NORMAL PARENT OF
THE AFFECTED MEMBER IN THE LATER GENERATION BEING A HETEROZYGOTE. FOR DOMINANT
INHERITANCE TO OBTAIN ONE MUST ASSUME GONADAL MOSAICISM OR FAILURE OF EXPRESSION
IN ONE OF THE PARENTS OF THE AFFECTED SIBS. THESE PARENTS, IT SEEMS, WERE NOT
EXAMINED.

WALLS, G. L. AND HEATH, G. G.* DOMINANT ECTOPIA LENTIS ET PUPILLAE. AM. J.
HUM. GENET. 11* 166-168, 1959.

12980 ECTRODACTYLY

ECTRODACTYLY IS DERIVED FROM GREEK EKTROMA (ABORTION) AND DAKTYLOS (FINGER). THE
TERM IS A NON-SPECIFIC ONE APPLIED TO A VARIETY OF MALFORMATIONS. IT IS PROBABLY
BEST RESERVED FOR TRANSVERSE TERMINAL APHALANGIA, ADACTYLIA OR ACHEIRIA. CASES
DEFINED IN THIS WAY ARE USUALLY SPORADIC. ONE HAND IS INVOLVED AND THE FEET ARE
NOT AFFECTED, AS A RULE. CONGENITAL CONSTRICTION RINGS ('AMNIOTIC BANDS') ARE
SOMETIMES ASSOCIATED. MANY CASES DESCRIBED AS EXAMPLES OF AUTOSOMAL DOMINANT
INHERITANCE OF ECTRODACTYLY ARE IN FACT TYPE B BRACHYDACTYLY (Q.V.). THE FAMILY
REPORTED BY KHOSROVANI (1959) MAY BE SUCH AN INSTANCE. THE ANOMALY CALLED HERE
SPLIT-HAND DEFORMITY (Q.V.) AND SOMETIMES CALLED LOBSTER-CLAW DEFORMITY IS ALSO
CALLED ECTRODACTYLY, IMPROPERLY I THINK.

KHOSROVANI, H.* MALFORMATIONS OF THE HANDS AND FEET (ECTRODACTYLIA) THROUGH FIVE SUCCESSIVE GENERATIONS OF A LARGE VAUDOIS FAMILY. J. GENET. HUM. 8* 1-59, 1959.

TEMTAMY, S. A.* GENETIC FACTORS IN HAND MALFORMATIONS. PH. D. THESIS, JOHNS HOPKINS UNIVERSITY, 1966.

12990 EEC SYNDROME (ECTRODACTYLY, ECTODERMAL DYSPLASIA, CLEFT LIP-PALATE)

RUDIGER, HAASE AND PASSARGE (1970) SUGGESTED THE DESIGNATION EEC FOR THE SYNDROME OBSERVED IN A FEMALE CHILD. THE FEATURES WERE ECTRODACTYLY OF BOTH HANDS AND ONE FOOT, ECTODERMAL DYSPLASIA WITH SEVERE KERATITIS AND CLEFT LIP-PALATE. THIS DISORDER IS PROBABLY THE SAME AS THAT REPORTED IN ONE OF THE PATIENTS OF ROSELLI AND GUILIENETTI (1961) AND PROBABLY DIFFERENT FROM THE COMBINATION OF ECTRODACTY-LY, ANODONTIA AND PARTIAL NONCANALIZATION OF THE LACRIMAL DUCT DESCRIBED IN MOTHER AND SON BY TEMTAMY AND MCKUSICK (1969) AND IN A SINGLE PATIENT BY LEVY (1967).

LEVY, W. J.* MESOECTODERMAL DYSPLASIA* A NEW COMBINATION OF ANOMALIES. AM. J. OPHTHAL. 63* 978-982, 1967.

ROSELLI, D. AND GUILIENETTI, R.* ECTODERMAL DYSPLASIA. BRIT. J. PLAST. SURG. 14* 190-204, 1961.

RUDIGER, R. A., HAASE, W. AND PASSARGE, E.* ASSOCIATION OF ECTRODACTYLY, ECTODERMAL DYSPLASIA, AND CLEFT LIP-PALATE. AM. J. DIS. CHILD. 120* 160-163, 1970.

TEMTAMY, S. AND MCKUSICK, V. A.* SYNOPSIS OF HAND MALFORMATIONS WITH PARTICULAR EMPHASIS ON GENETIC FACTORS. THE CLINICAL DELINEATION OF BIRTH DEFECTS. III. LIMB MALFORMATIONS. NEW YORK* NATIONAL FOUNDATION, 1969. PP. 125-184.

*13000 EHLERS-DANLOS SYNDROME

THE MAIN FEATURES ARE LOOSE-JOINTEDNESS AND FRAGILE AND BRUISABLE SKIN WHICH HEALS WITH PECULIAR 'CIGARETTE-PAPER' SCARS. BARABAS (1966) CONCLUDED THAT MOST PERSONS WITH THIS CONDITION ARE BORN PREMATURELY DUE TO PREMATURE RUPTURE OF FETAL MEMBRANES. IN LIGHT OF WHAT IS UNDERSTOOD ABOUT THE NATURE OF THIS CONDITION AND THE FACT THAT THE PLACENTA IS LARGELY FETAL IN ORIGIN (AND GENOTYPE), THE CONCLUSION IS PLAUSIBLE. GRAF (1965) REPORTED BROTHER AND SISTER WITH EHLERS-DANLOS SYNDROME WHO DEVELOPED 'SPONTANEOUS' CAROTID-CAVERNOUS FISTULA. INTERNAL COMPLICATIONS INCLUDE RUPTURE OF LARGE VESSELS, HIATUS HERNIA, SPONTANEOUS RUPTURE OF THE BOWEL, DIVERTICULA OF THE BOWEL. RETINAL DETACHMENT HAS BEEN OBSERVED (PEMBERTON ET AL., 1966). BARABAS (1967) SUGGESTED THE EXISTENCE OF THREE DISTINCT TYPES OF THE EHLERS-DANLOS SYNDROME. IN THE CLASSICAL TYPE THE PATIENTS ARE BORN PREMATURELY BECAUSE OF PREMATURE RUPTURE OF FETAL MEMBRANES, AND HAVE SEVERE SKIN AND JOINT INVOLVEMENT BUT NO VARICOSE VEINS OR ARTERIAL RUPTURES. A SECOND (MILD OR 'VARICOSE') GROUP IS NOT BORN PREMATURELY AND THE SKIN AND JOINT MANIFESTATIONS ARE NOT SEVERE. HOWEVER, VARICOSE VEINS ARE SEVERE. IN A THIRD ('ARTERIAL') GROUP BRUISING IS A PARAMOUNT SIGN, INCLUDING SPONTANEOUS ECCHYMOSES DURING MENSTRUATION. SKIN IS SOFT AND TRANSPARENT BUT LITTLE EXTENSIBLE AND JOINT HYPERMOBILITY IS LIMITED TO THE HANDS. SEVERE AND UNEXPLAINED ABDOMINAL PAIN IS A FEATURE. REPEATED ARTERIAL RUPTURES OCCUR IN THESE PATIENTS. SKIN LIKE THAT OF E-D HAS BEEN OBSERVED WITH A FIBRINOLYTIC DEFECT (Q.V.). NORDSCHOW AND MARSOLAIS (1969) COULD DEMONSTRATE NO ABNORMALITY OF SHRINKAGE TEMPERATURE THERMOGRAMS OF TENDON COLLAGEN FROM A HYPERMOBILE JOINT OF AN E-D PATIENT. THEY SUPPORTED THE SUGGESTION OF WECHSLER AND FISHER (1964) THAT THE DEFECT CONCERNS THE AMOUNT OF COLLAGEN PRODUCED. VARADI AND HALL (1965) CONCLUDED THAT ELASTIN IS NORMAL. SCHOFIELD ET AL. (1970) REPORTED BROTHER AND SISTER IN THEIR 60'S WHO SUFFERED SPONTANEOUS RUPTURE OF THE COLON. THEY HAD JOINT LAXITY, AND BOTH BRUISED EASILY AND SUSTAINED MANY LACERATIONS FROM MINOR TRAUMA. THE FATHER OF THE TWO SIBS AND THE SON OF THE BROTHER MAY HAVE ALSO BEEN AFFECTED.

BARABAS, A. P.* EHLERS-DANLOS SYNDROME ASSOCIATED WITH PREMATURITY AND PREMATURE RUPTURE OF FOETAL MEMBRANES. BRIT. MED. J. 2* 682-684, 1966.

BARABAS, A. P.* HETEROGENEITY OF THE EHLERS-DANLOS SYNDROME* DESCRIPTION OF THREE CLINICAL TYPES AND A HYPOTHESIS TO EXPLAIN THE BASIC DEFECT(S). BRIT. MED. J. 1* 612-613, 1967.

BEIGHTON, P., MURDOCH, J. L. AND VOTTELER, T.* GASTROINTESTINAL COMPLICATIONS OF THE EHLERS-DANLOS SYNDROME. GUT 10* 1004-1008, 1969.

BEIGHTON, P., PRICE, A., LORD, J. AND DICKSON, E.* VARIANTS OF THE EHLERS-DANLOS SYNDROME. CLINICAL, BIOCHEMICAL, HAEMATOLOGICAL, AND CHROMOSOMAL FEATURES OF 100 PATIENTS. ANN. RHEUM. DIS. 28* 228-245, 1969.

BRUNO, M. S. AND NARASIMHAN, P.* THE EHLERS-DANLOS SYNDROME* A REPORT OF FOUR CASES IN TWO GENERATIONS OF A NEGRO FAMILY. NEW ENG. J. MED. 264* 274-277, 1961.

COVENTRY, M. B.* SOME SKELETAL CHANGES IN THE EHLERS-DANLOS SYNDROME. A REPORT OF TWO CASES. J. BONE JOINT SURG. 43A* 855-860, 1961.

DAY, H. J. AND ZARAFONETIS, C. J. D.* COAGULATION STUDIES IN 4 PATIENTS WITH
EHLERS-DANLOS SYNDROME. AM. J. MED. SCI. 242* 565-573, 1961.

GOODMAN, R. M., LEVITSKY, J. M. AND FRIEDMAN, I. A.* THE EHLERS-DANLOS SYNDROME
AND MULTIPLE NEUROFIBROMATOSIS IN A KINDRED OF MIXED DERIVATIONS, WITH SPECIAL
EMPHASIS ON HEMOSTASIS IN THE EHLERS-DANLOS SYNDROME. AM. J. MED. 32* 976-983,
1962.

GRAF, C. J.* SPONTANEOUS CAROTID-CAVERNOUS FISTULA* EHLERS-DANLOS SYNDROME AND
RELATED CONDITIONS. ARCH. NEUROL. 13* 662-672, 1965.

GRAHAME, R. AND BEIGHTON, P.* PHYSICAL PROPERTIES OF THE SKIN IN THE EHLERS-
DANLOS SYNDROME. ANN. RHEUM. DIS. 28* 246-251, 1969.

HEGREBERG, G. A., PADGETT, G. A., OTTO, R. L. AND HENSON, J. B.* A HERITABLE
CONNECTIVE TISSUE DISEASE OF DOGS AND MINK RESEMBLING EHLERS-DANLOS SYNDROME OF
MAN. I. SKIN TENSILE STRENGTH PROPERTIES. J. INVEST. DERM. 54* 377-380, 1970.

IMAHORI, S., BANNERMAN, R. M., GRAF, C. J. AND BRENNAN, J. C.* EHLERS-DANLOS
SYNDROME WITH MULTIPLE ARTERIAL LESIONS. AM. J. MED. 47* 967-977, 1969.

LEES, M. H., MENASHE, V. D., SUNDERLAND, C. O., MORGAN, C. L. AND DAWSON, P.
J.* EHLERS-DANLOS SYNDROME ASSOCIATED WITH MULTIPLE PULMONARY ARTERY STENOSES AND
TORTUOUS SYSTEMIC ARTERIES. J. PEDIAT. 75* 1031-1036, 1969.

MCKUSICK, V. A.* HERITABLE DISORDERS OF CONNECTIVE TISSUE. ST. LOUIS* C. V.
MOSBY CO., 1966 (3RD ED.).

NORDSCHOW, C. D. AND MARSOLAIS, E. B.* EHLERS-DANLOS SYNDROME. SOME RECENT
BIOPHYSICAL OBSERVATIONS. ARCH. PATH. 88* 65-68, 1969.

PEMBERTON, J. W., FREEMAN, H. M. AND SCHEPENS, C. L.* FAMILIAL RETINAL
DETACHMENT AND THE EHLERS-DANLOS SYNDROME. ARCH. OPHTHAL. 76* 817-824, 1966.

SCARPELLI, D. G. AND GOODMAN, R. M.* OBSERVATIONS ON THE FINE STRUCTURE OF THE
FIBROBLAST FROM A CASE OF EHLERS-DANLOS SYNDROME WITH THE MARFAN SYNDROME. J.
INVEST. DERM. 50* 214-219, 1968.

SCHOFIELD, P. F., MACDONALD, N. AND CLEGG, J. F.* FAMILIAL SPONTANEOUS RUPTURE
OF THE COLON* REPORT OF TWO CASES. DIS. COLON RECTUM 13* 394-396, 1970.

SESTAK, Z.* EHLERS-DANLOS SYNDROME AND CUTIS LAXA* AN ACCOUNT OF FAMILIES IN
THE OXFORD AREA. ANN. HUM. GENET. 25* 313-321, 1962.

VARADI, D. P. AND HALL, D. A.* CUTANEOUS ELASTIN IN EHLERS-DANLOS SYNDROME.
NATURE 208* 1224-1225, 1965.

WECHSLER, H. L. AND FISHER, E. R.* EHLERS-DANLOS SYNDROME. PATHOLOGIC,
HISTOCHEMICAL AND ELECTRON MICROSCOPIC OBSERVATIONS. ARCH. PATH. 77* 613-619,
1964.

13010 ELASTOSIS PERFORANS SERGIGINOSA

ALSO KNOWN AS HYPERKERATOSIS FOLLICULARIS ET PARAFOLLICULARIS IN CUTEM PENETRANS,
ELASTOMA INTRAPAPILLARE PERFORANS VERRUCIFORMIS, KYRLE'S DISEASE, MIESCHER'S
ELASTOMA, ETC., THIS CONDITION OCCURS IN THE MARFAN SYNDROME, THE EHLERS-DANLOS
SYNDROME, OSTEOGENESIS IMPERFECTA, PSEUDOXANTHOMA ELASTICUM, AND MONGOLISM. IN
ADDITION IT PROBABLY OCCURS AS AN ISOLATED GENETIC TRAIT OF WHICH THE INHERITANCE
MAY BE DOMINANT.

13020 ELECTROENCEPHALOGRAPHIC PECULIARITY* ('14 AND 6 PER SEC. POSITIVE SPIKE'
PHENOMENON)

THIS PECULIARITY HAS BEEN OBSERVED IN IDENTICAL TWINS (VOGEL, 1965) AND IN PARENTS
AND SIBS OF PROBANDS (RADIN, 1964).

RADIN, E. A.* FAMILIAL OCCURRENCE OF THE 14 AND 6 PER SEC. POSITIVE SPIKE
PHENOMENON. ELECTROENCEPH. CLIN. NEUROPHYSIOL. 17* 566-570, 1964.

VOGEL, F.* '14 AND 6 PER SEC. POSITIVE SPIKES' IN SCHLAF- EEG VON JUGENDLICHEN
EIN- UND ZWEIEIIGEN ZWILLINGEN. HUMANGENETIK 1* 390-391, 1965.

13030 ELECTROENCEPHALOGRAPHIC PECULIARITY* (FRONTO-PRECENTRAL BETA WAVE GROUPS)

VOGEL (1966) SUGGESTED AUTOSOMAL DOMINANT INHERITANCE OF EACH OF TWO TYPES - (1)
FRONTAL BETA-GROUPS WITH HIGH FREQUENCY (25-30 PER SEC.) AND RELATIVELY LOW
VOLTAGE, AND (2) BETA-GROUPS WITH FREQUENCY OF 20-25 PER SEC., HIGHER VOLTAGE AND
PRECENTRAL MAXIMUM.

VOGEL, F.* ZUR GENETISCHEN GRUNDLAGE FRONTO-PRAZENTRALER BETA - WELLENGRUPPEN
IM EEG DES MENSCHEN. HUMANGENETIK 2* 227-237, 1966.

THE ALPHA WAVES ARE REPLACED BY 16-19 PER SEC. BETA WAVES WHICH SHOW AN OCCIPITAL MAXIMUM AND ARE BLOCKED BY OPENING OF THE EYES. FROM FAMILY DATA VOGEL (1966) CONCLUDED THE PATTERN IS INHERITED AS AN AUTOSOMAL DOMINANT. THE FREQUENCY WAS FOUND TO BE ABOUT 0.6 PERCENT AMONG YOUNG MALES.

BERG, K. AND BEARN, A. G.* ANTIBODIES TO INHERITED BETA-LIPOPROTEIN ANTIGENS IN THE SERUM OF MULTIPLY TRANSFUSED PATIENTS. CLIN. GENET. 1* 104-120, 1970.

VOGEL, F.* ZUR GENETISCHEN GRUNDLAGE OCCIPITALER LANGSAMER BETA - WELLEN IM EEG DES MENSCHEN. HUMANGENETIK 2* 238-245, 1966.

*13050 ELLIPTOCYTOSIS, RHESUS-LINKED TYPE

SEE BELOW FOR DESCRIPTION.

*13060 ELLIPTOCYTOSIS, RHESUS-UNLINKED TYPE

TWO GENETICALLY DISTINCT VARIETIES OF ELLIPTOCYTOSIS ARE RECOGNIZED BY THE FACT THAT ONE IS LINKED WITH THE RHESUS LOCUS AND ONE IS NOT. PHENOTYPIC DIFFERENCES MAY BE CORRELATED WITH THE DIFFERENCES IN LINKAGE RELATIONSHIPS. GEERDINK ET AL. (1967) FOUND MORE HEMOLYSIS IN THE *UNLINKED* TYPE THAN IN THE *LINKED* TYPE. PETERS ET AL. (1966) STUDYING ISOLATED RED CELL MEMBRANES DEMONSTRATED AN ABNORMALITY IN ERYTHROCYTE SODIUM TRANSPORT. IN A FAMILY IN WHICH BOTH ELLIPTOCY-TOSIS AND HEREDITARY HEMORRHAGIC TELANGIECTASIA WERE SEGREGATING, ROBERTS (1945) POINTED OUT THAT EVEN VERY SMALL BODIES OF DATA ARE USEFUL FOR EXCLUDING CLOSE LINKAGE. THE EXTENSIVE STUDY OF ELLIPTOCYTOSIS IN ICELAND REPORTED BY JENSSON ET AL. (1967) SHOWS HOW WIDELY THE MANIFESTATIONS MAY VARY. ALL CASES ARE PLAUSIBLY CONSIDERED TO HAVE THE SAME GENE. ADDITIONAL EVIDENCE OF HETEROGENEITY IN ELLIPTOCYTOSIS MAY BE PROVIDED BY THE EFFECTS OF COMBINATION WITH BETA-THALASSE-MIA. AKSOY AND ERDEM (1968) CONCLUDED THAT THE COMBINATION SOMETIMES RESULTS IN MUTUAL ENHANCEMENT, WHEREAS IN OTHER INSTANCES IT DOES NOT. NIELSEN AND STRUNK (1968) DESCRIBED A DUTCH FAMILY IN WHICH, AMONG THE 7 OFFSPRING OF RELATED PARENTS BOTH WITH ELLIPTOCYTOSIS, TWO DIED IN INFANCY OF SEVERE ANEMIA AND A THIRD WHOSE ERYTHROCYTES SHOWED MORE MARKED MORPHOLOGIC CHANGES THAN IN HETEROZYGOTES AND WHOSE SEVERE ANEMIA WAS COMPENSATED BY SPLENECTOMY. ALL THREE WERE PRESUMABLY HOMOZYGOTES. THREE OTHER SIBS WERE HETEROZYGOTES AND ONE WAS STILLBORN. THE ELLIPTOCYTOSIS WAS OF THE RH-LINKED VARIETY.

AKSOY, M. AND ERDEM, S.* COMBINATION OF HEREDITARY ELLIPTOCYTOSIS AND HETEROZY-GOUS BETA-THALASSEMIA* A FAMILY STUDY. J. MED. GENET. 5* 298-301, 1968.

BANNERMAN, R. M. AND RENWICK, J. H.* THE HEREDITARY ELLIPTOCYTOSES* CLINICAL AND LINKAGE DATA. ANN. HUM. GENET. 26* 23-38, 1962.

CLARKE, C. A., DONOHOE, W. T. A., FINN, R., MCCONNELL, R. B., SHEPPARD, P. M. AND NICOL, D. S. H.* DATA ON LINKAGE IN MAN* OVALOCYTOSIS, SICKLING AND THE RHESUS BLOOD GROUP COMPLEX. ANN. HUM. GENET. 24* 283-287, 1960.

GEERDINK, R. A., NIJENHUIS, L. E. AND HUIZINGA, J.* HEREDITARY ELLIPTOCYTOSIS* LINKAGE DATA IN MAN. ANN. HUM. GENET. 30* 363-378, 1967.

JENSSON, O., JONASSON, T. AND OLAFSSON, O.* HEREDITARY ELLIPTOCYTOSIS IN ICELAND. BRIT. J. HAEMAT. 13* 844-854, 1967.

KURODA, S., TAKEUCHI, T. AND NAGAMORI, H.* DATA ON THE LINKAGE BETWEEN ELLIPTOCYTOSIS AND RH BLOOD TYPE. JAP. J. HUM. GENET. 5* 112-118, 1960.

MORTON, N. E.* THE DETECTION AND ESTIMATION OF LINKAGE BETWEEN THE GENES FOR ELLIPTOCYTOSIS AND THE RH BLOOD TYPE. AM. J. HUM. GENET. 8* 80-96, 1956.

NIELSEN, J. A. AND STRUNK, K. W.* HOMOZYGOUS HEREDITARY ELLIPTOCYTOSIS AS THE CAUSE OF HAEMOLYTIC ANEMIA IN INFANCY. SCAND. J. HAEMAT. 5* 486-496, 1968.

PETERS, J. C., ROWLAND, M., ISRAELS, L. G. AND ZIPURSKY, A.* ERYTHROCYTE SODIUM TRANSPORT IN HEREDITARY ELLIPTOCYTOSIS. CANAD. J. PHYSIOL. PHARMACOL. 44* 817-827, 1966.

ROBERTS, J. A. F.* GENETIC LINKAGE IN MAN, WITH PARTICULAR REFERENCE TO THE USEFULNESS OF VERY SMALL BODIES OF DATA. QUART. J. MED. 14* 27-33, 1945.

13070 EMPHYSEMA

LARSON AND BARMAN (1965) DESCRIBED TWO KINDREDS, AND HOLE AND WASSERMAN (1965) REPORTED ONE, WITH MULTIPLE CASES OF CHRONIC OBSTRUCTIVE PULMONARY DISEASE (EMPHYSEMA OR CHRONIC BRONCHITIS OR BOTH). A CORRELATION WITH SMOKING WAS SUGGESTED.

HOLE, B. V. AND WASSERMAN, K.* FAMILIAL EMPHYSEMA. ANN. INTERN. MED. 63* 1009-1017, 1965.

*13080 ENAMEL HYPOPLASIA WITH CURLY HAIR

ROBINSON AND MILLER (1966) DESCRIBED AUTOSOMAL DOMINANT INHERITANCE OF ENAMEL
HYPOPLASIA WITH ASSOCIATED STRIKINGLY CURLY HAIR. WE (LICHTENSTEIN ET AL., 1971)
HAVE TRACED THE SAME CONDITION THROUGH 6 GENERATIONS OF AN IRISH-AMERICAN FAMILY.
IN AFFECTED MEMBERS OF THIS FAMILY, A FEATURE NOT DESCRIBED BY ROBINSON AND MILLER
(1966) IS MILD INCREASE IN BONE DENSITY, PARTICULARLY IN THE SKULL.

LICHTENSTEIN, J. R., WARSON, R. W., JORGENSEN, R. J. AND MCKUSICK, V. A.* THE
TRICHO-DONTO-OSSEOUS SYNDROME. TO BE PUBLISHED, 1971.

ROBINSON, G. C. AND MILLER, J. R.* HEREDITARY ENAMEL HYPOPLASIA* ITS ASSOCIA-
TION WITH CHARACTERISTIC HAIR STRUCTURE. PEDIATRICS 37* 498-502, 1966.

*13090 ENAMEL HYPOPLASIA, HEREDITARY LOCALIZED

THE DISTRIBUTION IS RESTRICTED MAINLY TO THE LABIAL ASPECT OF THE ANTERIOR TEETH
AND MAY AFFECT THE FIRST DENTITION ONLY. PITS AND LINEAR FISSURES ORIENTED
HORIZONTALLY AROUND THE CROWN OF THE TEETH ARE DESCRIBED. WITKOP (1957, 1965)
CONCLUDED THAT THIS IS AN AUTOSOMAL DOMINANT TRAIT WITH INCOMPLETE PENETRANCE AND
VARIABLE EXPRESSIVITY. HE OBSERVED A KINDRED WITH MANY AFFECTED MEMBERS.

DARLING, A. I.* SOME OBSERVATIONS ON AMELOGENESIS IMPERFECTA AND CALCIFICATION
OF THE DENTAL ENAMEL. PROC. ROY. SOC. MED. 49* 759-766, 1956.

WITKOP, C. J.* GENETIC DISEASE OF THE ORAL CAVITY. IN, TIECKE, R. W. (ED.)*
ORAL PATHOLOGY. NEW YORK* MCGRAW-HILL, 1965.

WITKOP, C. J.* HEREDITARY DEFECTS IN ENAMEL AND DENTIN. ACTA GENET. STATIST.
MED. 7* 236-239, 1957.

13100 ENCEPHALO-RETINAL DYSPLASIA (KRAUSE-REESE SYNDROME)

IN REPORTING THE CASE OF A 10 YEAR OLD BOY MATTHES AND STENZEL (1968) DESCRIBED
MINOR CHANGES IN THE MOTHER AND TWO SIBS. KARYOTYPE WAS NORMAL IN THE PROBAND.

KRAUSE, A. C.* CONGENITAL ENCEPHALO-OPHTHALMIC DYSPLASIA. ARCH. OPHTHAL. 36*
387-444, 1946.

MATTHES, A. AND STENZEL, K.* FAMILIARE, ENCEPHALO-RETINALE DYSPLASIE (KRAUSE-
REESE-SYNDROM) MIT MYOKLONISCH-ASTATISCHEN PETIT MAL. Z. KINDERHEILK. 103* 81-89,
1968.

REESE, A. B. AND STRAATSMA, B. R.* RETINAL DYSPLASIA. AM. J. OPHTHAL. 45* 199-
211, 1958.

*13110 ENDOCRINE ADENOMATOSIS, MULTIPLE

UNDERWOOD AND JACOBS (1963) FOUND FATHER, SON AND DAUGHTER AFFECTED. HYPOGLYCEMIA
WAS THE PRESENTING MANIFESTATION IN ALL THREE. IN ADDITION TO ISLET CELL
ADENOMAS, THE FATHER HAD BRONCHIAL CARCINOMA AND HYPERPARATHYROIDISM FROM
PARATHYROID ADENOMAS. THE SON AND DAUGHTER HAD BEEN FOLLOWED FROM CHILDHOOD AS
CASES OF IDIOPATHIC EPILEPSY UNRESPONSIVE TO ANTICONVULSIVE THERAPY. A SOMEWHAT
SIMILAR BUT FUNDAMENTALLY DISTINCT ENTITY IS PHEOCHROMOCYTOMA WITH AMYLOID-
PRODUCING MEDULLARY CARCINOMA OF THE THYROID (Q.V.). FURTHERMORE, THE ZOLLINGER-
ELLISON SYNDROME OF INTRACTABLE PEPTIC ULCER WITH PANCREATIC ISLET ADENOMA IS A
FACET OF MULTIPLE ENDOCRINE ADENOMATOSIS. THIS DISORDER MAY PRESENT PURELY AS
HYPERPARATHYROIDISM. GUIDA ET AL. (1966) DESCRIBED PITUITARY ADENOMA AND DUODENAL
CARCINOID IN PATIENTS WITH THIS CONDITION. BRONCHIAL CARCINOID (WILLIAMS AND
CELESTIN, 1962) OCCURS AS A FEATURE OF ENDOCRINE ADENOMATOSIS (Q.V.). WERMER
FIRST REPORTED *HIS* SYNDROME IN 1954 AND ZOLLINGER AND ELLISON *THEIRS* IN 1955.
RECOGNITION THAT THEY ARE ONE HAS SUBSEQUENTLY OCCURRED (LULU ET AL., 1968).
KIPNIS ET AL. (1969) DESCRIBED A PATIENT WITH MEA WHO SUCCUMBED TO METASTATIC
SCHWANNOMA. ONE MEMBER OF THE FAMILY DESCRIBED AS HEREDITARY HYPERPARATHYROIDISM
BY CUTLER ET AL. (1964) WAS LATER REPORTED TO HAVE A MALIGNANT SCHWANNOMA,
PITUITARY ADENOMAS, MULTIPLE PANCREATIC ISLET CELL ADENOMAS AND MULTIPLE ADRENO-
CORTICAL ADENOMAS.

AACH, R. AND KISSANE, J.* CLINICOPATHOLOGIC CONFERENCE* MULTIPLE ENDOCRINE
ADENOMATOSIS. AM. J. MED. 47* 608-618, 1969.

BALLARD, H. S., FRAME, B. AND HARTSOCK, R. J.* FAMILIAL MULTIPLE ENDOCRINE
ADENOMA-PEPTIC ULCER COMPLEX. MEDICINE 43* 481-516, 1964.

ELLISON, E. H. AND WILSON, S. D.* THE ZOLLINGER-ELLISON SYNDROME UPDATED.
SURG. CLIN. N. AM. 47* 1115-1124, 1967.

ELLISON, E. H. AND WILSON, S. D.* THE ZOLLINGER-ELLISON SYNDROME. RE-APPRAISAL
AND EVALUATION OF 260 REGISTERED CASES. ANN. SURG. 160* 512-530, 1964.

GUIDA, P. M., TODD, J. E., MOORE, S. W. AND BEAL, J. M.* ZOLLINGER-ELLISON SYNDROME WITH INTERESTING VARIATIONS. REPORT OF TWELVE CASES INCLUDING ONE OF CARCINOID OF THE DUODENUM. AM. J. SURG. 112* 807-817, 1966.

JONES, B. S., O'HAGAN, J. J., PHEAR, D. N. AND SHEVILLE, E.* A CASE OF THE ZOLLINGER-ELLISON SYNDROME ASSOCIATED WITH HYPERPLASIA OF SALIVARY AND BRUNNER'S GLANDS. GUT 11* 837-839, 1970.

KIPNIS, D. AND COLLEAGUES* MULTIPLE ENDOCRINE ADENOMATOSIS. (CLINICOPATHOLOGIC CONFERENCE) AM. J. MED. 47* 608-618, 1969.

LULU, D. J., CORCORAN, T. E. AND ANDRE, M.* FAMILIAL ENDOCRINE ADENOMATOSIS WITH ASSOCIATED ZOLLINGER-ELLISON SYNDROME. WERMER'S SYNDROME. AM. J. SURG. 115* 695-701, 1968.

UNDERWOOD, L. E. AND JACOBS, N. M.* FAMILIAL ENDOCRINE ADENOMATOSIS. AM. J. DIS. CHILD. 106* 218-223, 1963.

VANCE, J. E., STOLL, R. W., KITABCHI, A. E., WILLIAMS, R. H. AND WOOD, F. C., JR.* NESIDIOBLASTOSIS IN FAMILIAL ENDOCRINE ADENOMATOSIS. J.A.M.A. 207* 1679-1682, 1969.

WAY, L., GOLDMAN, L. AND DUNPHY, J. E.* ZOLLINGER-ELLISON SYNDROME. AN ANALYSIS OF TWENTY-FIVE CASES. AM. J. SURG. 116* 293-304, 1968.

WERMER, P.* GENETIC ASPECTS OF ADENOMATOSIS OF ENDOCRINE GLANDS. AM. J. MED. 16* 363-371, 1954.

WILLIAMS, E. D. AND CELESTIN, L. R.* THE ASSOCIATION OF BRONCHIAL CARCINOID AND PLURIGLANDULAR ADENOMATOSIS. THORAX 17* 120-127, 1962.

ZOLLINGER, R. M. AND ELLISON, E. H.* PRIMARY PEPTICULCERATIONS OF THE JEJUNUM ASSOCIATED WITH ISLET CELL TUMORS OF THE PANCREAS. ANN. SURG. 142* 709-728, 1955.

13120 ENDOMETRIOSIS

ENDOMETRIOSIS, OFTEN IN THE FORM OF 'CHOCOLATE CYSTS' OF THE OVARY, HAS BEEN REPORTED IN SISTERS RATHER FREQUENTLY AND AT LEAST TWICE IN MOTHER AND DAUGHTER(S).

BARNES, J.* CHOCOLATE CYSTS OF OVARY (OVARIAN ENDOMETRIOSIS) AND PREGNANCY* REPORT OF TWO CASES OCCURRING IN SISTERS. PROC. ROY. SOC. MED. 38* 324-325, 1945.

FREY, G. H.* THE FAMILIAL OCCURRENCE OF ENDOMETRIOSIS. REPORT OF FIVE INSTANCES AND REVIEW OF LITERATURE. AM. J. OBSTET. GYNEC. 73* 418-421, 1957.

GARDNER, G. H., GREENE, R. R. AND RANNEY, B.* HISTOGENESIS OF ENDOMETRIOSIS* RECENT CONTRIBUTIONS. OBSTET. GYNEC. 1* 615-637, 1953.

GOODALL, J. R.* A STUDY OF ENDOMETRIOSIS, ENDOSALPINGIOSIS, ENDOCERVICOSIS, AND PERITONEO-OVARIAN SCLEROSIS* A CLINICAL AND PATHOLOGIC STUDY. PHILADELPHIA* J. B. LIPPINCOTT CO., 1943.

VELDEN, W. H.* FAMILIALE ENDOMETRICOSE EEN ERFELIJKE AANDOENING.Q NEDERL. T. GENEESK. 106* 1276-1281, 1962.

*13130 ENGELMANN'S DISEASE (PROGRESSIVE DIAPHYSEAL DYSPLASIA)

LENNON, SCHECHTER AND HORNABROOK (1961) DESCRIBED A CASE OF ENGELMANN'S DISEASE AND REVIEWED THE LITERATURE. CHARACTERISTIC IS GROSS THICKENING OF THE CORTEX OF BONES, BOTH ON THE PERIOSTEAL SURFACE AND IN THE MEDULLARY CANAL. THE PROCESS USUALLY BEGINS IN THE SHAFT OF THE FEMUR OR TIBIA BUT SPREADS TO INVOLVE ALL BONES. ONSET IS USUALLY BEFORE 30 YEARS, OFTEN BEFORE 10 YEARS OF AGE. ALL RACES AND BOTH SEXES ARE AFFECTED. NINE EXAMPLES OF FAMILIAL OCCURRENCE IN ONE OR TWO GENERATIONS WERE MENTIONED. THE SCLEROTIC BONE DISEASES ARE A CONFUSED GROUP (SEE OSTEOPETROSIS). SEVERAL DIFFERENT AND SEPARATE ENTITIES (INCLUDING VAN BUCHEM'S DISEASE AND RIBBING'S DISEASE) WERE LUMPED TOGETHER BY LENNON ET AL. (1961). TO CONFUSE THE MATTER FURTHER, ENGELMANN'S DISEASE IS CALLED, BY SOME, CAMURATI-ENGELMANN'S DISEASE IN RECOGNITION OF THE EARLIER DESCRIPTION, BUT ON REVIEW IT SEEMS LIKELY THAT CAMURATI DESCRIBED A DIFFERENT ENTITY. THE SKELETAL DISORDER IS OFTEN ASSOCIATED WITH MUSCULAR WEAKNESS, PECULIAR GAIT, PAINS IN THE LEGS, FATIGUABILITY AND APPARENT UNDERNUTRITION. THE MUSCULAR WEAKNESS IS NOT NECESSARILY PROGRESSIVE AND TYPICAL BONE CHANGES MAY BE FOUND IN ASYMPTOMATIC PERSONS. BECAUSE OF THE ASSOCIATED FEATURES MUSCULAR DYSTROPHY OR POLIOMYELITIS IS SOMETIMES DIAGNOSED IN THESE PATIENTS. GIRDANY (1959) DESCRIBED A FAMILY WITH 6 AFFECTED PERSONS IN 3 GENERATIONS (NO MALE-TO-MALE TRANSMISSION). A CASE REPORTED BY SINGLETON ET AL. (1956) HAD STRIKINGLY SIMILAR CLINICAL FEATURES. RESTUDY INDICATE THAT THREE GENERATIONS WERE AFFECTED IN THAT FAMILY ALSO. FATHER AND TWO CHILDREN (SON AND DAUGHTER) WERE AFFECTED IN FAMILY REPORTED BY RAMON AND BUCHNER (1966). THE FATHER WAS MUCH MORE SEVERELY AFFECTED THAN THE OFFSPRING. ALLEN ET AL. (1970) REPORTED IMPROVEMENT WITH CORTICOSTEROIDS. THEY PRESENTED A FAMILY IN WHICH 11 PERSONS IN THREE GENERATIONS WERE KNOWN TO HAVE BEEN AFFECTED. GRAHAM

ALLEN,   D.   T.,   SAUNDERS,   A.   M.,   NORTHWAY,   W. H., JR., WILLIAMS, G. F. AND
SCHAFER,   I. A.* CORTICOSTEROIDS IN THE TREATMENT OF ENGELMANN'S DISEASE* PROGRES-
SIVE DIAPHYSEAL DYSPLASIA. PEDIATRICS 46* 523-531, 1970.

CLAWSON,   D.   K. AND LOOP, J. W.* PROGRESSIVE DIAPHYSEAL DYSPLASIA (ENGELMANN'S
DISEASE). J. BONE JOINT SURG. 46A* 143-150, 1964.

GIRDANY,   B.   R.* ENGELMANN'S DISEASE (PROGRESSIVE DIAPHYSEAL DYSPLASIA) - A
NONPROGRESSIVE FAMILIAL FORM OF MUSCULAR DYSTROPHY WITH CHARACTERISTIC BONE
CHANGES. CLIN. ORTHOP. 14* 102-109, 1959.

GRAHAM, C. B.* SEATTLE, WASH.* PERSONAL COMMUNICATION, 1970.

LENNON,   E.   A.,   SCHECHTER,   M. M. AND HORNABROOK, R. W.* ENGELMANN'S DISEASE.
REPORT OF A CASE WITH REVIEW OF THE LITERATURE. J. BONE JOINT SURG. 43B* 273-284,
1961.

RAMON,   Y.   AND   BUCHNER,   A.* CAMURATI-ENGELMANN'S DISEASE AFFECTING THE JAWS.
ORAL. SURG. 22* 592-599, 1966.

SINGLETON,   E.   B.,   THOMAS, J. R., WORTHINGTON, W. W. AND HILD, J. R.* PROGRES-
SIVE DIAPHYSEAL DYSPLASIA (ENGELMANN'S DISEASE). RADIOLOGY 67* 233-240, 1956.

*13140 EOSINOPHILIA, FAMILIAL

NAIMAN AND COLLEAGUES (1964) OBSERVED EOSINOPHILIA IN THREE GENERATIONS OF A
FAMILY.   NO ALLERGIES WERE RECORDED.   ZENI, NARDI AND FREZZA (1964) OBSERVED
EOSINOPHILIA IN 21 MEMBERS OF 3 GENERATIONS OF A KINDRED. SPARREVOHN (1967)
DESCRIBED   AN   18-MONTH-OLD GIRL WITH RECURRENT ASTHMATIC BRONCHITIS, RECURRENT
PULMONARY INFILTRATES, LEUKOCYTOSIS, PERSISTENT MARKED EOSINOPHILIA WITH 'SHIFT TO
THE LEFT,' INTERMITTENT THROMBOCYTOPENIA, EOSINOPHILIA OF LIVER AND BONE MARROW,
CELLULAR INFILTRATION INCLUDING MAST CELLS AND EOSINOPHILES IN SKIN AND MUSCLE, NO
SIGNS OF ALLERGY BY USUAL SKIN TESTS OR OF PARASITISM AND A CHRONIC BUT BENIGN
COURSE.   THE MOTHER AND A BROTHER HAD TRANSIENT EOSINOPHILIA AND SIMILAR CHANGES
IN SKIN AND MUSCLE BIOPSY. ZUELZER AND APT (1949) DESCRIBED THE ABOVE SYNDROME IN
YOUNG CHILDREN. ONE OF THEIR PATIENTS HAD A SISTER WITH MARKED EOSINOPHILIA.

NAIMAN,   J.   L.,   OSKI,   F. A., ALLEN, F. H. AND DIAMOND, L. K.* HEREDITARY
EOSINOPHILIA.   REPORT OF A FAMILY AND REVIEW OF THE LITERATURE. AM. J. HUM.
GENET. 16* 195-203, 1964.

SPARREVOHN,   S.* DISSEMINATED EOSINOPHILIC COLLAGENOSIS AND FAMILIAL EOSINOPHI-
LIA. ACTA PAEDIAT. SCAND. 56* 307-312, 1967.

STEWART, S. G.* FAMILIAL EOSINOPHILIA. AM. J. MED. SCI. 185* 21-29, 1933.

ZENI,   G., NARDI, F. AND FREZZA, M.* IN TEMA DI IPEREOSINOFILIA CONSTITUZIONALE
FAMILIARE IDIOPATICA. ACTA MED. PATAV. 24* 589-602, 1964.

ZUELZER,   W.   W.   AND APT, L.* DISSEMINATED VISCERAL LESIONS ASSOCIATED WITH
EXTREME EOSINOPHILIA. PATHOLOGICAL AND CLINICAL OBSERVATIONS ON SYNDROME OF YOUNG
CHILDREN. AM. J. DIS. CHILD. 78* 153-181, 1949.

*13150 EPICANTHUS

THIS IS A NORMAL FINDING IN THE FETUS OF ALL RACES. DOMINANT INHERITANCE IS QUITE
CLEAR IN MANY PEDIGREES REVIEWED BY USHER (1935). EPICANTHUS ALSO OCCURS IN
ASSOCIATION WITH HEREDITARY PTOSIS (Q.V.).

USHER, C. H.* PEDIGREES OF HEREDITARY EPICANTHUS. BIOMETRIKA 27* 5-25, 1935.

13160 EPIDERMOID CYSTS

EPIDERMOID CYSTS ARE KERATINOUS CYSTS BUT MAY BE IMPOSSIBLE TO DISTINGUISH
CLINICALLY FROM SEBACEOUS CYSTS (Q.V.).

*13170 EPIDERMOLYSIS BULLOSA DYSTROPHIA

SCARRING OCCURS WITH HEALING OF LESIONS IN THE DYSTROPHIC FORM BUT NOT IN THE
'SIMPLEX' FORM.   IN THE SIMPLEX TYPE THE BLISTERS OCCUR WITHIN THE EPIDERMIS AND
ARE SUBCORNEAL, WHEREAS THE BLISTERS ARE SUBEPIDERMAL IN THE DYSTROPHIC FORM.
DAVISON (1965) HAD SIX FAMILIES WITH THE DYSTROPHIC TYPE OF WHICH FOUR WERE
DOMINANT AND TWO RECESSIVE.

DAVISON, B. C. C.* EPIDERMOLYSIS BULLOSA. J. MED. GENET. 2* 233-242, 1965.

*13180 EPIDERMOLYSIS BULLOSA OF HANDS AND FEET (WEBER-COCKAYNE TYPE)

READETT (1961) DESCRIBED A FAMILY IN WHICH 14 MEMBERS IN 5 GENERATIONS WERE KNOWN

TO HAVE LOCALIZED EPIDERMOLYSIS BULLOSA OF THE HANDS AND FEET. THE PATTERN WAS THAT OF AN AUTOSOMAL DOMINANT. ADRENOSTEROID DEPRESSED BULLA FORMATION BUT RECURRENCE OCCURRED WITH STOPPING THERAPY. THIS DISORDER IS SOMETIMES CALLED WEBER-COCKAYNE SYNDROME. AN ENORMOUS PEDIGREE WITH MANY AFFECTED PERSONS WAS REPORTED FROM WEST VIRGINIA BY CARTLEDGE AND MYERS (1943). THE AFFECTED PERSONS WERE DESCENDANTS OF ONE ZACHARIAH PILES, BORN IN 1762. THE BLISTERING OCCURS ONLY ON THE HANDS AND FEET AND MAINLY IN WARM WEATHER AFTER UNUSUAL WALKING OR LABOR WITH HAND TOOLS.

CARTLEDGE, J. L. AND MYERS, V. W.* INHERITED FOOT BLISTERING IN AN AMERICAN FAMILY. J. HERED. 34* 24 ONLY, 1943.

COCKAYNE, E. A.* RECURRENT BULLOUS ERUPTION OF THE FEET. BRIT. J. DERM. SYPH. 50* 358-362, 1938.

HALDANE, J. B. S. AND POOLE, R.* A NEW PEDIGREE OF RECURRENT BULLOUS ERUPTION OF THE FEET. FOUR GENERATIONS OF FOOT BLISTERS. J. HERED. 33* 17-18, 1942.

READETT, M. D.* LOCALIZED EPIDERMOLYSIS BULLOSA. BRIT. MED. J. 1* 1510-1511, 1961.

*13190 EPIDERMOLYSIS BULLOSA SIMPLEX

DAVISON (1965) LIMITED THE DESIGNATION COCKAYNE TYPE EPIDERMOLYSIS BULLOSA TO THE CONDITION IN WHICH BULLAE ARE CONFINED TO THE FEET. THE TYPE WITH MORE EXTENSIVE INVOLVEMENT WAS REFERRED TO AS EPIDERMOLYSIS BULLOSA SIMPLEX. NINE FAMILIES WERE OF THE SIMPLEX TYPE AND 4 OF THE COCKAYNE TYPE. IT APPEARED THAT IN ANY ONE FAMILY ALL AFFECTED PERSONS WERE OF ONE TYPE OR THE OTHER. PASSARGE (1965) OBSERVED 21 AFFECTED PERSONS IN 4 GENERATIONS OF A FAMILY. ON THE BASIS OF AN EXTENSIVE STUDY IN NORWAY AND REVIEW OF THE LITERATURE, GEDDE-DAHL (1970) ARRIVED AT THE FOLLOWING CLASSIFICATION OF EPIDERMOLYSIS BULLOSA.

I EPIDERMOLYSIS BULLOSA SIMPLEX (AUTOSOMAL DOMINANT)

1. KOEBNER TYPE. GONADAL MOSAICISM (GERMINAL MOSAICISM, I.E., EARLY GERM CELL MUTATION) OCCURRED IN ONE FAMILY.

2. WEBER-COCKAYNE TYPE. BLISTERING LIMITED TO THE FEET OR FEET AND HANDS.

3. OGNA TYPE (FIRST DELINEATED BY GEDDE-DAHL). TRAUMATIC BLISTERING ASSOCIATED WITH CONGENITAL GENERALIZED BRUISING TENDENCY.

II EPIDERMOLYSIS BULLOSA DYSTROPHICA

1. EPIDERMOLYSIS BULLOSA DYSTROPHICA ALBOPAPULOIDEA (PASINI). AUTOSOMAL DOMINANT.

2. EPIDERMOLYSIS BULLOSA DYSTROPHICA (COCKAYNE-TOURAINE). AUTOSOMAL DOMINANT.

3. EPIDERMOLYSIS BULLOSA DYSTROPHICA WITH AUTOSOMAL RECESSIVE INHERI-TANCE.

A. CONGENITAL LOCALIZED NON-LETHAL TYPE

B. CONGENITAL GENERALIZED NON-LETHAL TYPE

C. CONGENITAL GENERALIZED SUB-LETHAL (MUTILATING) TYPE

D. LETHAL TYPE

E. CONGENITAL GENERALIZED INVERSE TYPE

F. NEUROTROPHIC TYPE (SEMITARDIVE LOCALIZED, NON-LETHAL TYPE WITH CONGENITAL DEAFNESS)

GEDDE-DAHL PRESENTED EVIDENCE THAT SOME CLINICAL VARIANTS OF EPIDERMOLYSIS BULLOSA DYSTROPHICA ARE THE RESULT OF THE PRESENCE OF TWO NON-IDENTICAL RECESSIVE ALLELES. THUS, THE GENES RESPONSIBLE FOR SOME OR ALL OF THE SEVERAL FORMS OF RECESSIVE EPIDERMOLYSIS BULLOSA MAY BE AT THE SAME LOCUS.

DAVISON, B. C. C.* EPIDERMOLYSIS BULLOSA. J. MED. GENET. 2* 233-242, 1965.

GEDDE-DAHL, T., JR.* EPIDERMOLYSIS BULLOSA. A CLINICAL, GENETIC AND EPIDERMIO-LOGICAL STUDY. OSLO, 1970.

*13200 EPIDERMOLYSIS BULLOSA WITH CONGENITAL LOCALIZED ABSENCE OF SKIN AND DEFORMITY
OF NAILS

IN THE FAMILY REPORTED BY BART ET AL. (1966), 26 PERSONS WERE AFFECTED. PENE-
TRANCE WAS COMPLETE. THE SYNDROME CONSISTED OF CONGENITAL ABSENCE OF SKIN ON THE
LOWER EXTREMITIES, BLISTERING OF SKIN AND MUCOUS MEMBRANES, AND CONGENITAL ABSENCE
OR DEFORMITY OF NAILS. THE CONDITION SEEMS DISTINCT FROM PREVIOUSLY REPORTED
FORMS OF LOCAL AFLASIA OF SKIN AND FROM VARIOUS OTHER TYPES OF EPIDERMOLYSIS
BULLOSA. CONGENITAL LOCALIZED ABSENCE OF SKIN IS PROBABLY AN OCCASIONAL MANIFES-
TATION OF EPIDERMOLYSIS BULLOSA, THE RESULT OF IN UTERO BLISTERING (BART, 1970).

BART, B. J.* EPIDERMOLYSIS BULLOSA AND CONGENITAL LOCALIZED ABSENCE OF SKIN.
ARCH. DERM. 101* 78-81, 1970.

BART, B. J., GORLIN, R. J., ANDERSON, V. E. AND LYNCH, F. W.* CONGENITAL
LOCALIZED ABSENCE OF SKIN AND ASSOCIATED ABNORMALITIES RESEMBLING EPIDERMOLYSIS
BULLOSA. A NEW SYNDROME. ARCH. DERM. 93* 296-304, 1966.

13210 EPILEPSY, PHOTOGENIC

FRIEDLANDER (1959) DISCUSSED AN HEREDITARY PATTERN OF *CEREBRAL LIGHT SENSITIVI-
TY.* DAVIDSON AND WATSON'S DATA (1956) ON 12 FAMILIES IS CONSISTENT WITH DOMINANT
INHERITANCE WITH REDUCED PENETRANCE. THERE WAS NO INSTANCE OF MALE-TO-MALE
TRANSMISSION.

DAVIDSON, S. AND WATSON, C. W.* HEREDITARY LIGHT SENSITIVE EPILEPSY. NEUROLOGY
6* 231-261, 1956.

FRIEDLANDER, W. J.* EPILEPSY. AM. J. PSYCHOL. 1* 623-628, 1959.

GERKEN, H., DOOSE, H., VOLZKE, E., VOLZ, C. AND HIEN-VOLPEL, K. F.* GENETICS OF
CHILDHOOD EPILEPSY WITH PHOTIC SENSITIVITY. (LETTER) LANCET 1* 1377-1378, 1968.

13220 EPILEPSY, PRIMARY READING

MATTHEWS AND WRIGHT (1967) REPORTED THE CASES OF MOTHER AND DAUGHTER WITH EPILEPSY
AND JAW-JERKING PROVOKED BY READING.

MATTHEWS, W. B. AND WRIGHT, F. K.* HEREDITARY PRIMARY READING EPILEPSY.
NEUROLOGY 17* 919-921, 1967.

13230 EPILEPSY, READING

ROWAN ET AL. (1970) DESCRIBED A GIRL WHO HAD MAJOR AND MINOR SEIZURES WHICH WERE
RELATED TO PATTERN AND PHOTOSENSITIVITY. THE MOTHER ALSO HAD EEG DISCHARGES
DURING READING. THE DAUGHTER'S ATTACKS WERE PRECIPITATED BY TELEVISION-VIEWING.
A YOUNGER SISTER HAD HAD ONE FEBRILE CONVULSION. THE FATHER HAD HAD EPILEPSY
BETWEEN AGES 5 AND 8 YEARS. NO STUDIES OF HIM WERE REPORTED.

ROWAN, A. J., HEATHFIELD, K. W. G. AND SCOTT, D. F.* IS READING EPILEPSY
INHERITED.Q J. NEUROL. NEUROSURG. PSYCHIAT. 33* 476-478, 1970.

*13240 EPIPHYSEAL DYSPLASIA, MULTIPLE

SEVERE OSTEOARTHRITIS OF THE HIPS DEVELOPS IN EARLY ADULTHOOD. THE DIAGNOSIS IN
THE ADULT IS AIDED BY THE CHANGES IN THE DISTAL TIBIA (LEEDS, 1960). A DEFICIENCY
IN THE LATERAL PART OF THE DISTAL TIBIAL OSSIFICATION CENTER SEEN IN CHILDREN
RESULTS IN A SLOPING END OF THE TIBIA IN ADULTHOOD. SHORT STATURE AND BRACHYDAC-
TYLY ARE FEATURES. CONSIDERABLE HETEROGENEITY UNDOUBTEDLY EXISTS WITHIN THIS
CATEGORY. CHONDRODYSTROPHIA CALCIFICANS CONGENITA IS A CONGENITAL FORM OF
MULTIPLE EPIPHYSEAL DYSPLASIA (INHERITED AS A RECESSIVE). BACHMAN AND NORMAN
(1967) DESCRIBED A 47 YEAR OLD WOMAN, HEIGHT 61-AND-ONE-HALF INCHES WITH MARKED
HYPEREXTENSIBILITY OF FINGERS AND PRECOCIOUS OSTEOARTHRITIS OF THE HIPS. A SON
AND A DAUGHTER HAD VERY FLEXIBLE FINGERS AND BY HAND X-RAY DELAY IN CARPAL
OSSIFICATION, PROXIMAL PSEUDO-EPIPHYSES OF METACARPALS II-V, CONE-CUP EPIPHYSES-
METAPHYSES AND WIDENED JOINT SPACES. OTHER JOINTS SHOWED EXTENSIVE CHANGES WITH
WIDENING OF JOINT SPACES AND IRREGULAR EPIPHYSES. THE MOTHER'S MOTHER, AUNT,
UNCLE AND COUSIN HAD HYPEREXTENSIBILITY OF THE FINGERS AND PREMATURE OSTEOARTHRI-
TIS. THESE AUTHORS REFERRED TO THE CONDITION AS PERIPHERAL DYSOSTOSIS BUT IT
SEEMS DIFFERENT FROM THE PERIPHERAL DYSOSTOSIS (Q.V.) DESCRIBED BY SINGLETON ET
AL. (1960), THE TERM *PERIPHERAL* SEEMS INAPPROPRIATE, AND THE DESCRIPTION
SUGGESTS WHAT OTHERS WOULD CALL FAIRBANK'S MULTIPLE EPIPHYSEAL DYSPLASIA. THE
CONDITION DESCRIBED AS ENCHONDRAL DYSOSTOSIS BY ODMAN (1959) IS PROBABLY THE SAME
CONDITION AS IS ALSO ELSBACH'S (1959) MICROEPIPHYSEAL DYSPLASIA. ALMOST CERTAINLY
HETEROGENEITY EXISTS WITHIN THE GROUP OF AUTOSOMAL DOMINANT MULTIPLE EPIPHYSEAL
DYSPLASIA. HOWEVER, NO ONE HAS SUCCEEDED IN SORTING OUT SEPARATE ENTITIES IN A
CONVINCING MANNER. I SUSPECT THAT THE FAMILY WITH FOUR AFFECTED PERSONS IN 3
GENERATIONS REPORTED BY CAMERON AND GARDINER (1963) HAD MULTIPLE EPIPHYSEAL
DYSPLASIA, OR PERHAPS A FORM OF SPONDYLOEPIPHYSEAL DYSPLASIA, INASMUCH AS THE

SPINE WAS INVOLVED. PRECOCIOUS OSTEOARTHRITIS WAS A FEATURE. HULVEY AND KEATS (1969) COMMENTED ON THE VARIABILITY IN THE EXTENT OF SPINAL INVOLVEMENT AND PRESENTED A FAMILY IN WHICH MANY MEMBERS HAD SEVERE PERIPHERAL INVOLVEMENT WITH NO SPINAL INVOLVEMENT. THE DIVIDING LINE BETWEEN MULTIPLE EPIPHYSEAL DYSPLASIA AND SPONDYLOEPIPHYSEAL DYSPLASIA TARDA CAN BE INDISTINCT, WITNESS THE FAMILY REPORTED BY DIAMOND (1970).

BACHMAN, K. AND NORMAN, A. P.* HEREDITARY PERIPHERAL DYSOSTOSIS (3 CASES). PROC. ROY. SOC. MED. 60* 21-22, 1967.

BERG, P. K.* DYSPLASIA EPIPHYSIALIS MULTIPLEX* A CASE REPORT AND REVIEW OF THE LITERATURE. AM. J. ROENTGEN. 97* 31-38, 1966.

CAMERON, J. M. AND GARDINER, T. B.* ATYPICAL FAMILIAL OSTEOCHONDRODYSTROPHY. BRIT. J. RADIOL. 36* 135-139, 1963.

COWAN, D. J.* MULTIPLE EPIPHYSIAL DYSPLASIA. BRIT. MED. J. 2* 1629 ONLY, 1963.

DIAMOND, L. S.* A FAMILY STUDY OF SPONDYLOEPIPHYSEAL DYSPLASIA. J. BONE JOINT SURG. 52A* 1587-1594, 1970.

ELSBACH, L.* BILATERAL HEREDITARY MICRO-EPIPHYSEAL DYSPLASIA OF THE HIPS. J. BONE JOINT SURG. 41B* 514-523, 1959.

HOEFNAGEL, D., SYCAMORE, L. K., RUSSELL, S. W. AND BUCKNALL, W. E.* HEREDITARY MULTIPLE EPIPHYSIAL DYSPLASIA. ANN. HUM. GENET. 30* 201-210, 1967.

HULVEY, J. T. AND KEATS, T.* MULTIPLE EPIPHYSEAL DYSPLASIA. A CONTRIBUTION TO THE PROBLEM OF SPINAL INVOLVEMENT. AM. J. ROENTGEN. 106* 170-177, 1969.

JACOBS, P. A.* DYSPLASIA EPIPHYSIALIS MULTIPLEX. CLIN. ORTHOP. 58* 117-128, 1968.

LEEDS, N. E.* EPIPHYSIAL DYSPLASIA MULTIPLEX. AM. J. ROENTGEN. 84* 506-510, 1960.

MAUDSLEY, R. H.* DYSPLASIA EPIPHYSIALIS MULTIPLEX* A REPORT OF FOURTEEN CASES IN THREE FAMILIES. J. BONE JOINT SURG. 37B* 228-240, 1955.

ODMAN, P.* HEREDITARY ENCHONDRAL DYSOSTOSIS. TWELVE CASES IN THREE GENERATIONS MAINLY WITH PERIPHERAL LOCATION. ACTA RADIOL. 52* 97-113, 1959.

SINGLETON, E. B., DAESCHNER, C. W. AND TENG, C. T.* PERIPHERAL DYSOSTOSIS. AM. J. ROENTGEN. 84* 499-505, 1960.

WATT, J. K.* MULTIPLE EPIPHYSEAL DYSPLASIA* REPORT OF FOUR CASES. BRIT. J. SURG. 39* 533-535, 1952.

13250 EPISTAXIS, HEREDITARY

WHETHER THERE ARE FAMILIES WITH THIS CONDITION TRANSMITTED AS A SIMPLE DOMINANT WITHOUT TELANGIECTASIA IS NOT CLEAR. FINK (1940) DESCRIBED WHAT WAS PRESUMED TO BE SUCH A FAMILY WITH TRANSMISSION THROUGH SIX GENERATIONS.

FINK, H. K.* HEREDITARY EPISTAXIS IN MAN. J. HERED. 31* 319-322, 1940.

13260 EPITHELIOMA CALCIFICANS OF MALHERBE

KAWAMURA AND SEKIMURA (1939) OBSERVED AFFECTED BROTHER AND SISTER. DUPERRAT AND ALBERT (1948) DESCRIBED FIVE AFFECTED PERSONS IN TWO GENERATIONS OF A FAMILY. GEISER (1960) REPORTED AFFECTED FATHER AND DAUGHTER. WE (HARPER, 1971) HAVE OBSERVED TWO AFFECTED SISTERS WHO ALSO HAD TYPICAL MYOTONIC DYSTROPHY A PRESUMABLY UNRELATED TRAIT. NO INFORMATION CONCERNING THEIR PARENTS WAS AVAILABLE. CANTWELL AND REED (1965) REPORTED MULTIPLE CALCIFYING EPITHELIOMA IN ASSOCIATION WITH MYOTONIC DYSTROPHY AND HARPER (1971) REPORTED SIBS WITH THIS COMBINATION AND HAS SEEN AT LEAST 6 OTHER CONFIRMED INSTANCES OF THE ASSOCIATION. PILOMATRIXOMA IS THE TERM FOR THIS TUMOR USED BY JONES AND CAMPBELL (1969). THE LESIONS ARE FIRM, CIRCUMSCRIBED TUMORS, USUALLY IN THE HEAD AND NECK AREA. THEY FEEL LIKE BUTTONS AND ARE ATTACHED TO THE SUBCUTANEOUS TISSUE AND OVERLYING SKIN.

CANTWELL, A. R., JR. AND REED, W. B.* MYOTONIA ATROPHICA AND MULTIPLE CALCIFYING EPITHELIOMA OF MALHERBE. ACTA DERMATOVENER. 45* 387-390, 1965.

DUPERRAT, B. AND ALBERT, (NI)* FORME FAMILIALE DE L'EPITHELIOME DE MALHERBE. BULL. SOC. FRANC. DERM. SYPH. 55* 196, 1948.

GEISER, J. D.* FORME FAMILIALE D'EPITHELIOMA (CALCIFIE) DE MALHERBE. DERMATOLOGICA 120* 361-365, 1960.

HARPER, P. S.* MYOTONIC DYSTROPHY WITH CALCIFYING EPITHELIOMA OF MALHERBE IN SISTERS. THE CLINICAL DELINEATION OF BIRTH DEFECTS. XII. SKIN HAIR AND NAILS. BALTIMORE* WILLIAMS AND WILKINS, 1971.

KAWAMURA, T. AND SEKIMURA, T.* ZWEI FALLE VON BEI BRUDER AND SCHWESTER
VORKOMMENDEM VERKALKTEM EPITHELIOM. JAP. J. DERM. UROL. 45* 41, 1939.

*13270 EPITHELIOMA, HEREDITARY MULTIPLE BENIGN CYSTIC (EPITHELIOMA ADENOIDES CYSTICUM
OF BROOKE)

FLIEGELMAN AND KRUSE (1948) DESCRIBED 10 CASES IN THREE GENERATIONS. THEY
INDICATED THAT DESPITE SOME CLINICAL SIMILARITIES THE DISORDER COULD BE DISTIN-
GUISHED FROM SYRINGOCYSTADENOMA, ADENOMA SEBACEUM AND CYLINDROMA. SOME THINK THAT
THIS AND CYLINDROMA ARE THE SAME ENTITY. GARTLER AND COLLEAGUES (1966), STUDYING
MEMBERS OF A FAMILY WITH AFFECTED MEMBERS IN FOUR GENERATIONS, FOUND THAT FEMALES
HETEROZYGOUS FOR G6PD-DEFICIENCY HAD SHOWN BOTH G6PD-DEFICIENT AND G6PD-NORMAL
CELLS IN THE SAME TUMOR, THUS I DICATING MULTICELLULAR ORIGIN. ZIPRKOWSKI AND
SCHEWACH-MILLET (1966) REPORTED THE DERMATOLOGIC FEATURES IN THE SAME FAMILY. THE
SKIN TUMORS SHOW DIFFERENTIATION IN THE DIRECTION OF HAIR STRUCTURES, HENCE THE
SYNONYM TRICHOEPITHELIOMA. ONE AFFECTED PERSON DEVELOPED BASO-SQUAMOUS CELL
CARCINOMA. WELCH, WELLS AND KERR (1968) PRESENTED FAMILY DATA SUPPORTING THE VIEW
THAT ANCELL-SPIEGLER CYLINDROMAS AND BROOKE-FORDYCE TRICHOEPITHELIOMAS ARE
MANIFESTATIONS OF A SINGLE ENTITY. THE TERM CYLINDROMA WAS ALSO APPLIED BY
BILLROTH (1859) TO A TYPE OF ADENOCARCINOMA ARISING IN SALIVARY GLAND TISSUE
(EVANS ET AL., 1966).

BADEN, H. P.* CYLINDROMATOSIS SIMULATING NEUROFIBROMATOSIS.   NEW ENG. J. MED.
267* 296-297, 1962.

BILLROTH, T.* BEOBACHTUNGEN UBER GESCHWULSTE DER SPEICHELDRUSEN. VIRCHOW.
ARCH. PATH. ANAT. 17* 357-375, 1859.

EVANS, J. C., EFSKIND, J. AND ROBERTS, T. W.* CYLINDROMA.   AM. J. ROENTGEN. 96*
191-196, 1966.

FLIEGELMAN, M. T. AND KRUSE, W. T.* HEREDITARY MULTIPLE BENIGN CYSTIC EPITHE-
LIOMA. J. INVEST. DERM. 11* 189-196, 1948.

GARTLER, S. M., ZIPRKOWSKI, L., KRAKOWSKI, A., EZRA, R., SZEINBERG, A. AND
ADAM, A.* GLUCOSE-6-PHOSPHATE DEHYDROGENASE MOSAICISM AS A TRACER IN THE STUDY OF
HEREDITARY MULTIPLE TRICHOEPITHELIOMA. AM. J. HUM. GENET. 18* 282-287, 1966.

WELCH, J. P., WELLS, R. S. AND KERR, C. B.* ANCELL-SPIEGLER CYLINDROMAS (TURBAN
TUMOURS) AND BROOKE-FORDYCE TRICHOEPITHELIOMAS. EVIDENCE FOR A SINGLE GENETIC
ENTITY. J. MED. GENET. 5* 29-35, 1968.

ZIPRKOWSKI, L. AND SCHEWACH-MILLET, M.* MULTIPLE TRICHOEPITHELIOMA IN A MOTHER
AND TWO CHILDREN. DERMATOLOGICA 132* 248-256, 1966.

*13280 EPITHELIOMA, SELF-HEALING SQUAMOUS (FERGUSON-SMITH TYPE)

THIS IS CONSIDERED TO BE A VARIETY OF MULTIPLE KERATOACANTHOMA. IT GOES UNDER
MANY DIFFERENT NAMES. EREAUX AND SCHOPFLOCHER (1965) OBSERVED AFFECTED BROTHER
AND SISTER. SOMMERVILLE AND MILNE (1950) REPORTED TWO CASES IN EACH OF TWO
SUCCESSIVE GENERATIONS. AFFECTED FATHER AND SON WERE REFERRED TO BY EPSTEIN,
BISKIND AND POLLACK (1957). DEGOS AND COLLEAGUES (1964) DESCRIBED THE CONDITION
IN A WOMAN AND TWO DAUGHTERS. FERGUSON-SMITH, GENETICIST SON OF THE DERMATOLOGIST
WHO ORIGINALLY DESCRIBED THIS CONDITION, AND HIS COLLEAGUES (1971) ASSEMBLED
RELIABLE INFORMATION ON 62 CASES IN THE WEST OF SCOTLAND. IT WAS CONSIDERED
POSSIBLE THAT ALL THE SCOTTISH CASES DERIVED FROM A SINGLE MUTATION WHICH OCCURRED
BEFORE 1790. THE LESIONS WERE FOUND MORE FREQUENTLY ON EXPOSED AREAS OF THE SKIN
AND THEIR DISTRIBUTION CORRESPONDINGLY DIFFERED BETWEEN MALES AND FEMALES.

DEGOS, R., CIVATTE, J., TOURAINE, B. AND GUILAINE, J.* SPONTAN HEILENDE
EPITHELIOME FERGUSON-SMITH UND MULTIPLE FAMILIARE KERATOACANTHOME. HAUTARZT 15*
7-11, 1964.

EPSTEIN, N. N., BISKIND, G. R. AND POLLACK, R. S.* MULTIPLE PRIMARY SELF-
HEALING SQUAMOUS-CELL *EPITHELIOMAS* OF THE SKIN* GENERALIZED KERATOACANTHOMA.
ARCH. DERM. 75* 210-223, 1957.

EREAUX, L. P. AND SCHOPFLOCHER, P.* FAMILIAL PRIMARY SELF-HEALING SQUAMOUS
EPITHELIOMA OF SKIN. ARCH. DERM. 91* 589-594, 1965.

FERGUSON-SMITH, M. A., WALLACE, D. C., JAMES, Z. H. AND RENWICK, J. H.*
MULTIPLE SELF-HEALING SQUAMOUS EPITHELIOMA. THE CLINICAL DELINEATION OF BIRTH
DEFECTS. XII. SKIN, HAIR AND NAILS. BALTIMORE* WILLIAMS AND WILKINS, 1971.

SOMMERVILLE, J. AND MILNE, J. A.* SELF-HEALING SQUAMOUS EPITHELIOMA OF THE
SKIN. BRIT. J. DERM. 62* 485-490, 1950.

13290 ERDHEIM*S CYSTIC MEDIAL NECROSIS OF AORTA

ERDHEIM'S DISEASE WITH DISSECTING ANEURYSM HAS BEEN OBSERVED IN BROTHERS (GRAHAM, MILNE, 1952* VON MEYENBURG, 1939), IN FATHER AND SON (FLEMING, HELWIG, 1941) AND IN MOTHER AND DAUGHTER (GRIFFITHS, HAYHURST, WHITEHEAD, 1951) BUT CLINICAL INFORMATION IN THESE REPORTS IS TOO SCANTY TO PERMIT EXCLUSION OF THE MARFAN SYNDROME (Q.V.). HANLEY AND JONES (1967) REPORTED DISSECTING AORTIC ANEURYSM IN 2 SISTERS AND THE SON OF ONE OF THEM. NO STIGMATA OF MARFAN'S SYNDROME WERE PRESENT.

FLEMING, J. W. AND HELWIG, F. C.* MEDIONECROSIS AORTAE IDIOPATHICA CYSTICA WITH SPONTANEOUS RUPTURE. REPORT OF THREE CASES WITH NECROPSIES. J. MO. MED. ASS. 38* 86-88, 1941.

GRAHAM, J. G. AND MILNE, J. A.* DISSECTING ANEURYSM OF THE AORTA* A REVIEW OF 29 CASES. GLASGOW MED. J. 33* 320-330, 1952.

GRIFFITHS, G. J., HAYHURST, A. P. AND WHITEHEAD, R.* DISSECTING ANEURYSM OF AORTA IN MOTHER AND CHILD. BRIT. HEART J. 13* 364-368, 1951.

HANLEY, W. B. AND JONES, N. B.* FAMILIAL DISSECTING AORTIC ANEURYSM. A REPORT OF THREE CASES WITHIN TWO GENERATIONS. BRIT. HEART J. 29* 852-858, 1967.

VON MEYENBURG, H.* UEBER SPONTANE AORTENRUPTUR BEI ZWEI BRUDERN. SCHWEIZ. MED. WSCHR. 20* 976-979, 1939.

*13300 ERYTHEMA PALMARE HEREDITARIUM

SYMMETRICAL ASYMPTOMATIC REDNESS OF THE PALMS IS SIMILAR TO THAT SEEN WITH HEPATIC CIRRHOSIS. PREGNANCY MAY PRECIPITATE THE APPEARANCE OF HEREDITARY ERYTHEMA. I KNOW OF THE TRAIT IN SUCCESSIVE GENERATIONS. OLIVIER (1956) DESCRIBED AFFECTED FATHER AND 4 (OUT OF 9) AFFECTED CHILDREN.

LANE, J. E.* ERYTHEMA PALMARE HEREDITARIUM. ARCH. DERM. SYPH. 20* 445-448, 1929.

OLIVIER, J.* ERYTHEMA PALMO-PLANTAIRE HEREDITAIRE. MALADIE DE LANE. ARCH. BELG. DERM. SYPH. 12* 202-207, 1956.

13310 ERYTHROCYTOSIS, BENIGN FAMILIAL

THIS DISORDER IS CHARACTERIZED BY AN INCREASE IN RED BLOOD CELL MASS WITH NO INCREASE IN PLATELETS AND LEUKOCYTES, BY A BENIGN COURSE AND FAMILIAL INCIDENCE. THIS IS PROBABLY A CONDITION DISTINCT FROM POLYCYTHEMIA VERA. THE LATTER CONDITION IS MORE FREQUENT IN JEWS THAN NON-JEWS IN THE UNITED STATES (MODAN, 1965) BUT SHOWS NO SIMPLE MENDELIAN PATTERN. A PATIENT REPORTED BY AUERBACH ET AL. (1958) WAS AGAIN REPORTED BY CASSILETH AND HYMAN (1966) WITH FAMILY STUDY. ENGELKING (1920) AND WIELAND (1932) SEPARATELY REPORTED A FAMILY IN WHICH 11 MEMBERS OF 3 GENERATIONS WERE POLYCYTHEMIC. IN SOME THE ABNORMALITY WAS NOTED IN CHILDHOOD. SUCH FAMILIES SHOULD BE STUDIED FOR A HEMOGLOBINOPATHY. POLYCYTHEMIA IS A FEATURE OF SEVERAL VARIANT HEMOGLOBINS* CHESAPEAKE, J (CAPETOWN), YAKIMA, KEMPSEY, RAINIER (WEATHERALL, 1969), YPSILANTI, HIROSHIMA. THE HETEROZYGOTES SHOW POLYCYTHEMIA, HENCE THE PHENOTYPE IS DOMINANT. ALPERIN ET AL. (1967) REPORTED FINDING ELEVATED LEVELS OF ERYTHROPOIETIN IN AFFECTED MEMBERS OF ONE FAMILY. GEARY ET AL. (1967) OBSERVED POLYCYTHEMIA IN 5 PERSONS IN THREE GENERATIONS OF A FAMILY AND SHOWED THAT THE BASIS WAS THALASSEMIA MINOR. THE RED CELL COUNT WAS ELEVATED BUT TOTAL HEMOGLOBIN WAS NORMAL, THUS GIVING HYPOCHROMIA. HEMOGLOBIN A2 WAS ELEVATED. MORE OFTEN THALASSEMIA MINOR PRESENTS AS REFRACTORY HYPOCHROMIC ANEMIA. DAVEY ET AL. (1968) FOUND ERYTHROCYTOSIS IN A BROTHER AND SISTER, OFFSPRING OF A SECOND COUSIN MARRIAGE, AND RAISED THE QUESTION OF RECESSIVE INHERITANCE. THE FATHER HAD SLIGHT BUT PERSISTENT ERYTHROCYTOSIS. APPARENTLY HEMOGLOBIN ELECTROPHORESIS WAS NOT PERFORMED.

ALPERIN, J. B., LEVIN, W. C., ALEXANIAN, R. AND HOUSTON, E. W.* FAMILIAL ERYTHROCYTOSIS* A DISORDER DUE TO INCREASED ERYTHROPOIETIN PRODUCTION. TO BE PUBLISHED.

AUERBACH, M. L., WOLFF, J. A. AND METTIER, S. R.* BENIGN FAMILIAL POLYCYTHEMIA IN CHILDHOOD. PEDIATRICS 21* 54-58, 1958.

CASSILETH, P. A. AND HYMAN, G. A.* BENIGN FAMILIAL ERYTHROCYTOSIS* REPORT OF THREE CASES AND A REVIEW OF THE LITERATURE. AM. J. MED. SCI. 251* 692-697, 1966.

CHARACHE, S.* FAMILIAL POLYCYTHEMIA. MOUNT SINAI J. MED. 37* 418-425, 1970.

DAVEY, M. G., LAWRENCE, J. R., LANDER, H. AND ROBSON, H. N.* FAMILIAL ERYTHRO-CYTOSIS. A REPORT OF TWO CASES, AND A REVIEW. ACTA HAEMAT. 39* 65-74, 1968.

ENGELKING, E.* UEBER FAMILIARE POLYZYTHAEMIE UND DIE DABEI BEOBACHTETEN AUGENVERANDERUNGEN. KLIN. MBL. AUGENHEILK. 64* 645-664, 1920.

GEARY, C. G., AMOS, H. E. AND MACIVER, J. E.* BENIGN FAMILIAL POLYCYTHEMIA. J. CLIN. PATH. 20* 158-160, 1967.

SPODARO, A. AND FORKNER, C. E.* BENIGN FAMILIAL POLYCYTHEMIA. ARCH. INTERN.
MED. 52* 593-602, 1933.

WEATHERALL, D. J.* POLYCYTHEMIA RESULTING FROM ABNORMAL HEMOGLOBINS. NEW ENG.
J. MED. 280* 604-606, 1969.

WIELAND, W.* WEITERE UNTERSUCHUNGEN UBER POLYCYTHAEMIA VERA IM KINDESALTER. Z.
KINDERHEILK. 53* 703-715, 1932.

*13320 ERYTHROKERATODERMIA VARIABILIS

COWAN (1962) PRESENTED CASES OF FATHER AND DAUGHTER WITH ERYTHROKERATODERMIA.
FROM EARLY CHILDHOOD THE FATHER HAD SKIN DISEASE ON THE FACE, HANDS, FOREARMS,
LEGS AND FEET. MARKED HYPERKERATOSIS, HYPERPIGMENTATION AND HYPERTRICHOSIS WERE
SOME OF THE FEATURES AS WELL AS ERYTHEMA WHICH VARIED FROM TIME TO TIME AND VARIED
IN SITE. THE CARDINAL FEATURE IS THE PRESENCE ALMOST FROM BIRTH OF SHARPLY
OUTLINED GEOGRAPHICAL AREAS OF ERYTHROKERATODERMIA. A PARTICULARLY STRIKING
PEDIGREE WAS ASSEMBLED BY NOORDHOECK (1966). THIS WAS PROBABLY THE CONDITION
PRESENT IN THE EXTENSIVELY AFFECTED KINDRED REPORTED BY KELLY AND KOCSARD (1970).

BROWN, J. AND KIERLAND, R. R.* ERYTHROKERATODERMIA VARIABILIS. REPORT OF THREE
CASES AND REVIEW OF THE LITERATURE. ARCH. DERM. 93* 194-201, 1966.

COWAN, M. A.* ERYTHROKERATODERMIA IN FATHER AND DAUGHTER. PROC. ROY. SOC. MED.
55* 875-876, 1962.

KELLY, L. J. AND KOCSARD, E.* CONGENITAL ICHTHYOSIS WITH ERYTHEMA ANULARE
CENTRIFUGUM. A NEW FORM OF ICHTHYOSIS AFFECTING 12 MEMBERS OF A FAMILY OF 31 IN 5
GENERATIONS. DERMATOLOGICA 140* 75-83, 1970.

NOORDHOECK, F. J.* OVER ERYTHRO- ET KERATODERMIA VARIABILIS* ON ERYTHRO- ET
KERATODERMIA VARIABILIS. UTRECHT THESIS, 1950. (CITED BY SCHNYDER, V. W. AND
KLUNKER, W.* ERBLICHE VERHORNUNGSSTORUNGEN DER HAUT. IN GOTTRON, H. A. AND
SCHNYDER, V. W. (EDS.)* VERERBUNG VON HAUTKRANKHEITEN. BERLIN* SPRINGER-VERLAG,
1966. P. 923.)

SCHNYDER, U. W. AND SOMMACAL-SCHOPF, D.* FOURTEEN CASES OF ERYTHRO-KERATODERMIA
FIGURATA VARIABILIS WITHIN ONE FAMILY. ACTA GENET. STATIST. MED. 7* 204-206,
1957.

13330 ESTERASE ES-2, REGULATOR FOR

KLEBE ET AL. (1970) USING MOUSE-HUMAN HYBRID SOMATIC CELLS IN CULTURE, FOUND THAT
ES-2 ESTERASE ACTIVITY WAS DEPRESSED. HUMAN CHROMOSOMES ARE SELECTIVELY LOST FROM
THE HYBRID CELLS. DEPRESSION OF ESTERASE ACTIVITY WAS PRESENT WHEN HUMAN
CHROMOSOME 10 WAS PRESENT AND THE ACTIVITY RETURNED TO NORMAL WHEN CHROMOSOME 10
WAS LOST. THUS, THEY CONCLUDED THAT THE REGULATOR *ELEMENT* IS PROBABLY STRUC-
TURALLY LINKED TO CHROMOSOME 10.

KLEBE, R. J., CHEN, T.-R. AND RUDDLE, F. H.* MAPPING OF A HUMAN GENETIC
REGULATOR ELEMENT BY SOMATIC CELL GENETIC ANALYSIS. PROC. NAT. ACAD. SCI. 66*
1220-1227, 1970.

*13340 ESTERASE OF ERYTHROCYTES, ELECTROPHORETIC VARIANTS OF

TASHIAN AND SHAW (1962) DEMONSTRATED CO-DOMINANT INHERITANCE OF AN ERYTHROCYTE
ACETYLESTERASE VARIANT. THESE ESTERASES CATALYZE THE CLEAVAGE OF CARBOXYL ESTERS.

TASHIAN, R. E. AND SHAW, M. W.* INHERITANCE OF AN ERYTHROCYTE ACETYLESTERASE
VARIANT OF MAN. AM. J. HUM. GENET. 14* 295-300, 1962.

*13350 EXCHONDROSIS OF PINNA, POSTERIOR (*EAR BUMP*)

A CARTILAGINOUS SPUR ON THE POSTERIOR ASPECT OF THE PINNA RATHER CLOSE TO ITS
ATTACHMENT TO THE SIDE OF THE HEAD IS PROBABLY INHERITED AS AN IRREGULAR DOMINANT
(QUELPRUD* SEE GATES, 1947). THE AUTHOR AND SEVERAL MEMBERS OF HIS FAMILY IN 3
GENERATIONS SHOW THIS TRAIT. THERE ARE SEVERAL INSTANCES OF MALE-TO-MALE
TRANSMISSION, A PAIR OF CONCORDANTLY AFFECTED MONOZYGOTIC TWINS AND NO CONSAN-
GUINITY.

GATES, R. R.* HUMAN HEREDITY. NEW YORK* MACMILLAN, 1947. P. 249.

13360 EXOSTOSES OF HEEL

GOULD (1942) DESCRIBED THE CONDITION IN GRANDFATHER, FATHER AND SON, I.E., MALES
OF THREE GENERATIONS. X-RAYS WERE NOT DESCRIBED.

GOULD, E. A.* THREE GENERATIONS OF EXOSTOSES OF THE HEEL. INHERITED FROM
FATHER TO SON. J. HERED. 33* 228 ONLY, 1942.

KROOTH, MACKLIN AND HILBISH (1961) REPORTED ON A STUDY OF THE FAMILIES OF 6 PERSONS WITH DIAPHYSEAL ACLASIS (MULTIPLE EXOSTOSES). THE FAMILIES WERE CHAMOR-ROS, A MICRONESIAN PEOPLE WHO LIVE IN THE MARIANA ISLANDS. THE FREQUENCY OF DIAPHYSEAL ACLASIS IN THE CHAMORROS OF GUAM WAS ESTIMATED AT 1 IN 1000. IN PUBLISHED SERIES THE DISEASE IS MORE FREQUENT IN MALES THAN IN FEMALES AND MORE SEVERE IN AFFECTED MALES THAN IN AFFECTED FEMALES. IN THE 21 GUAM CASES THE TUMORS WERE EVIDENT ON INSPECTION IN ALL MALES BUT IN ONLY HALF THE FEMALES. SCHOLZ AND MURKEN (1963) DID LINKAGE STUDIES WITH NEGATIVE RESULTS. IN A STUDY OF 56 PATIENTS SOLOMON (1963) FOUND A SEX RATIO OF 1 AND REPORTED THAT TWO-THIRDS OF THE PATIENTS HAD AN AFFECTED PARENT. SOLOMON (1964) OBSERVED ONE FAMILY IN WHICH ALL 8 AFFECTED PERSONS IN FOUR SIBSHIPS OF THREE GENERATIONS SHOWED EXOSTOSES ON THE BONES OF THE HANDS AND FINGERS WITH VERY FEW ELSEWHERE. IN NO OTHER PATIENTS OF HIS STUDY DID THE ABNORMALITY TAKE THIS PARTICULAR FORM. OTHER WORKERS HAVE FOUND NO CORRELATION BETWEEN MEMBERS OF THE SAME FAMILY AS TO FORM AND DISTRIBU-TION OF DISEASE. FOR THESE REASONS SOLOMON SUGGESTED THAT THE PARTICULAR FAMILY MAY SUFFER FROM A RARE DISORDER DUE TO A GENE DISTINCT FROM THAT CAUSING MOST CASES. DEFORMITIES OF THE FOREARMS OF THE MADELUNG TYPE OCCUR IN SOME CASES.

KROOTH, R. S., MACKLIN, M. T. AND HILBISH, T. F.* DIAPHYSIAL ACLASIS (MULTIPLE EXOSTOSES) ON GUAM. AM. J. HUM. GENET. 13* 340-347, 1961.

SCHOLZ, W. AND MURKEN, J.-D.* KOPPELUNGSUNTERSUCHUNGEN BEI FAMILIEN MIT MULTIPLEN CARTILAGINAREN EXOSTOSEN. Z. MENSCHL. VERERB. KONSTITUTIONSL. 37* 178-192, 1963.

SOLOMON, L.* HEREDITARY MULTIPLE EXOSTOSIS. AM. J. HUM. GENET. 16* 351-363, 1964.

SOLOMON, L.* HEREDITARY MULTIPLE EXOSTOSIS. J. BONE JOINT SURG. 45B* 292-304, 1963.

13380 EYEBROW, WHORL IN

VIRCHOW (1912) FOUND A WHORL IN THE HAIR OF THE LEFT EYEBROW NEAR THE NOSE IN 8 MEMBERS OF TWO GENERATIONS. THE PROGENITOR IN THE NEXT EARLIER GENERATION MAY HAVE SHOWN IT ALSO.

VIRCHOW, H.* STELLUNG DER HAARE IM BRAUENKOPF. Z. F. ETHNOL. 44* 402-403, 1912.

13390 FACIAL ASYMMETRY, EAR ANOMALY, SIMIAN CREASE

AASE AND SMITH (1970) DESCRIBED A SYNDROME IN FIVE MEMBERS OF THREE GENERATIONS (WITH ONE INSTANCE OF MALE-TO-MALE TRANSMISSION), COMPRISING ASYMMETRY OF THE FACE (HYPOPLASIA OF THE LEFT SIDE), UNUSUALLY SHAPED EAR WITH PROMINENT CRUS, AND SIMIAN CREASE. THEY POINTED OUT SIMILARITIES AND DIFFERENCES FROM WAARDENBURG'S (1961) ASYMMETRY OF THE FACE AND SKULL WITH ABNORMALITIES OF THE DIGITS.

AASE, J. M. AND SMITH, D. W.* FACIAL ASYMMETRY AND ABNORMALITIES OF PALMS AND EARS. A DOMINANTLY INHERITED DEVELOPMENTAL SYNDROME. J. PEDIAT. 76* 928-930, 1970.

WAARDENBURG, P. J., FRANCESCHETTI, A. AND KLEIN, D.* GENETICS AND OPHTHALMOLO-GY, VOL. 1. SPRINGFIELD, ILL.* CHARLES C THOMAS, 1961.

13400 FACIAL HYPERTRICHOSIS

TROTTER AND DANFORTH (1922) ESTIMATED A FREQUENCY OF 27 PERCENT IN WOMEN. OBVIOUSLY THE FREQUENCY IN MAN IS NOT DETERMINABLE. THEY FOUND A CORRELATION OF ABOUT 0.8 BETWEEN MOTHER AND DAUGHTER AND SUGGESTED AUTOSOMAL DOMINANT INHERI-TANCE.

TROTTER, M. AND DANFORTH, C. H.* THE INCIDENCE AND HEREDITY OF FACIAL HYPERTRI-CHOSIS IN WHITE WOMEN. AM. J. PHYS. ANTHROP. 5* 391-397, 1922.

13410 FACIAL PALSY, CONGENITAL UNILATERAL

SKYBERG AND VAN DER HAGEN (1965) OBSERVED THIS IN FOUR GENERATIONS WITH SIXTEEN PROBABLY AFFECTED PERSONS. NO MALE-TO-MALE TRANSMISSION WAS IDENTIFIED BUT ONE AFFECTED MALE HAD AN UNAFFECTED DAUGHTER. THE STAPEDIAL REFLEX WAS ABSENT SUGGESTING INVOLVEMENT OF THE MOTOR NUCLEUS OF THE FACIAL NERVE. CARMENA AND GOMEZ MARCANO (1943) REPORTED FOUR AFFECTED GENERATIONS IN A SPANISH FAMILY. AUTOPSY IN THREE CASES SHOWED PARTIAL AGENESIS OF THE FACIAL MOTOR NUCLEUS. WITTIG, MOREIRA AND FREIRE-MAIA (1967) OBSERVED CONGENITAL FACIAL DIPLEGIA IN THREE GENERATIONS OF A FAMILY. THEY SUGGESTED THAT THE DISORDER IN THIS FAMILY WAS THE SAME AS MOEBIUS' SYNDROME. NUCLEAR APLASIA WAS PRESENT BUT DIFFERENT FROM MOEBIUS' SYNDROME (Q.V.) WHICH IS AN OCULOFACIAL PALSY.

CARMENA, M. AND GOMEZ MARCANO, E.* PARALYSIS FACIAL HEREDITARIA. REV. CLIN. ESP. 8* 266-268, 1943.

WITTIG, E. O., MOREIRA, C. A. AND FREIRE-MAIA, N.* FAMILIAL CONGENITAL
PERIPHERAL FACIAL DIPLEGIA. (LETTER) LANCET 1* 282 ONLY, 1967.

13420 FACIAL PARALYSIS

WE HAVE OBSERVED A MAN (1057218) WHO HAD ONSET OF FACIAL PARALYSIS AT THE AGE OF
ABOUT 56. IT BEGAN AS INABILITY TO CONTROL THE LOWER LIP, WHICH DROOPED.
PROGRESSION OCCURRED SO THAT THE LIP BECAME STRIKINGLY PROTRUBERANT AND EVERTED
WITH EXPOSURE OF THE LOWER GINGIVAL MUCOSA. FIVE YEARS AFTER ONSET HE COULD NOT
WRINKLE HIS FOREHEAD. THERE WAS AN INTERMITTENT TWITCH OF THE RIGHT SIDE OF THE
UPPER LIP. THE EXTRAOCULAR MUSCLES WERE AFFECTED ONLY VERY MINIMALLY AND THERE
WAS NO PTOSIS. A STRIKING FEATURE WAS LAXITY OF THE SKIN RAISING THE QUESTION OF
CUTIS LAXA. SLIT LAMP EXAMINATION SHOWED A LATTICE TYPE OF CORNEAL OPACITY
BILATERALLY. THE MOTHER HAD THE PRECISELY IDENTICAL DISORDER BEGINNING AT ABOUT
THE SAME STAGE OF LIFE AND A SON 20 YEARS THE PROBAND'S JUNIOR WAS SAID TO BE
SHOWING EARLY SIGNS. THE DISORDER MAY REPRESENT A BILATERAL PROGRESSIVE HEREDI-
TARY FACIAL NERVE PALSY. ELECTROMYOGRAMS COULD NOT DISTINGUISH NEURAL AND
MUSCULAR ORIGIN OF THE PARALYSIS. MUSCLE BIOPSY WAS CONSISTENT WITH NEUROGENIC
ATROPHY. I SUSPECT THAT THE DISORDER IN THIS FAMILY IS, IN FACT, MELKERSSON'S
SYNDROME (Q.V.).

13430 FACIAL SPASM

STOCKS (1922-23) MADE A DISTINCTION BETWEEN FACIAL TIC (OR HABIT SPASM), WHICH IS
A MOVEMENT OF A COORDINATED GROUP OF FACIAL MUSCLES NOT ENTIRELY BEYOND THE
CONTROL OF THE WILL AND NOT OCCURRING DURING SLEEP, AND FACIAL SPASM, WHICH IS
USUALLY CONFINED TO THE MUSCLES SUPPLIED BY THE FACIAL NERVE OR ONE BRANCH
THEREOF. THE 18 YEAR OLD PROBAND IN STOCKS' POLISH FAMILY HAD RAPID CLONIC SPASM
OF THE LEVATOR MENTI MUSCLE BETWEEN THE CHIN AND LOWER LIP. THE INVOLVEMENT WAS
SAID TO BE LIMITED TO THAT MUSCLE IN OTHER AFFECTED MEMBERS OF THE FAMILY ALSO.
COLD AND EXCITEMENT AGGRAVATED THE CONDITION. HELLSING'S FAMILY (1930) SHOWED
MORE EXTENSIVE INVOLVEMENT AND ANISOCORIA AND DEPRESSED TENDON REFLEXES WERE
NOTED. CONSIDERABLE CONFUSION EXISTS BETWEEN FACIAL SPASM AND TREMBLING CHIN
(Q.V.). IT SEEMS POSSIBLE THAT THE FAMILIES OF STOCKS AND OF GOLDSMITH ARE ONES
OF TREMBLING CHIN AND HELLSING'S ONE OF FACIAL SPASM.

GOLDSMITH, J. B.* THE INHERITANCE OF 'FACIAL SPASM' AND THE EFFECT OF A
MODIFYING FACTOR ASSOCIATED WITH HIGH TEMPER. J. HERED. 18* 185-187, 1927.

HELLSING, G.* HEREDITARER FACIALISKRAMPF. ACTA MED. SCAND. 73* 526-537, 1930.

STOCKS, P.* FACIAL SPASM INHERITED THROUGH FOUR GENERATIONS. BIOMETRIKA 14*
311-315, 1922-23.

13440 FACTOR V (PROACCELERIN) EXCESS WITH SPONTANEOUS THROMBOSIS

GASTON (1966) REPORTED A FAMILY IN WHICH A 6 YEAR OLD GIRL HAD ILIOFEMORAL
THROMBECTOMY, HER FATHER HAD BILATERAL LEG AMPUTATIONS AT AGE 34 FOR OCCLUSIVE
ARTERIAL DISEASE, A FATHER'S COUSIN HAD RECURRENT THROMBOPHLEBITIS BEGINNING AT
AGE 18 AND A SON OF THE LATTER HAD RECURRENT LEG AND ARM THROMBOPHLEBITIS WITH
PULMONARY EMBOLI. PLASMA FACTOR V WAS FOUND TO BE ELEVATED IN THESE PERSONS.

GASTON, L. W.* STUDIES ON A FAMILY WITH AN ELEVATED PLASMA LEVEL OF FACTOR V
(PROACCELERIN) AND A TENDENCY TO THROMBOSIS. J. PEDIAT. 68* 367-373, 1966.

*13450 FACTOR VIII DEFICIENCY

HENSEN, MATTERN AND LOELIGER (1965) DESCRIBED A FAMILY IN WHICH 8 PERSONS IN FOUR
GENERATIONS IN AN AUTOSOMAL DOMINANT PATTERN HAD FACTOR VIII DEFICIENCY. NORMAL
BLEEDING TIMES AND LACK OF FACTOR VIII ELEVATION AFTER INFUSION OF HEMOPHILIC
PLASMA EXCLUDED VON WILLEBRAND'S DISEASE (Q.V.). VELTKAMP ET AL. (1968) CONFIRMED
THESE FINDINGS. NO RISE OF FACTOR VIII OCCURRED IN A BOY WITH HEMOPHILIA A WHEN
TRANSFUSED PLASMA FROM A GIRL IN HENSEN'S FAMILY. FURTHERMORE, THE GIRL'S PLASMA
TRANSFUSED INTO A WOMAN WITH SEVERE VON WILLEBRAND'S DISEASE HAD NO EFFECT ON HER
FACTOR VIII LEVEL.

HENSEN, A., MATTERN, M. J. AND LOELIGER, E. A.* HAEMOPHILIA A WITH APPARENTLY
AUTOSOMAL DOMINANT INHERITANCE. EVIDENCE FOR A SECOND AUTOSOMAL LOCUS INVOLVED IN
FACTOR VIII PRODUCTION. THROMB. DIATH. HAEMORRH. 14* 341-345, 1965.

VELTKAMP, J. J., TACONIS, W. K. AND LOELIGER, E. A.* AUTOSOMAL FACTOR-VIII
DEFICIENCY. (LETTER) LANCET 2* 1303 ONLY, 1968.

13460 FANCONI RENOTUBULAR SYNDROME

IN THE KINDRED REPORTED BY HUNT ET AL. (1966) 8 PERSONS IN THREE GENERATIONS MAY
HAVE BEEN AFFECTED, ALTHOUGH ONLY A MOTHER AND SON HAD THE FULL-BLOWN PICTURE.
ANOTHER PRESUMABLY DOMINANT PEDIGREE IS THAT OF BEN-ISHAY ET AL. (1961).

BEN-ISHAY, D., DREYFUSS, F. AND ULLMANN, T. D.* FANCONI SYNDROME WITH HYPOURI-CEMIA IN AN ADULT. FAMILY STUDY. AM. J. MED. 31* 793-800, 1961.

HUNT, D. D., STEARNS, G., MCKINLEY, J. B., FRONING, E., HICKS, P. AND BONFIG-LIO, M.* LONG-TERM STUDY OF A FAMILY WITH FANCONI SYNDROME WITHOUT CYSTINOSIS (DETONI-DEBRE-FANCONI SYNDROME). AM. J. MED. 40* 492-510, 1966.

D
O
M
I
N
A
N
T

13470 FAVISM

HEMOLYTIC ANEMIA FOLLOWING INGESTION OF THE BEAN OF VICIA FAVA OR EXPOSURE TO ITS POLLEN IS CONDITIONED PRIMARILY BY A DEFICIENCY OF ERYTHROCYTE GLUCOSE-6-PHOSPHATE DEHYDROGENASE, AN X-LINKED GENETIC TRAIT. VICIA FAVA APPARENTLY PRODUCES A SUBSTANCE WHICH INDUCES HEMOLYSIS OF ENZYME DEFICIENT RED CELLS (MAGER ET AL., 1965). IN AREAS WHERE THE ENZYME DEFICIENCY IS FREQUENT, FAVISM SHOWS FAMILIAL AGGREGATION PROBABLY NOT ACCOUNTED FOR BY THE FAMILIAL OCCURRENCE OF THE ENZYME DEFICIENCY ALONE. STAMATOYANNOPOULOS AND COLLEAGUES (1966) INTERPRETED STUDIES IN GREECE AS INDICATING THE PRESENCE OF AN AUTOSOMAL GENE WHICH IN HETEROZYGOUS STATE ENHANCES THE SUSCEPTIBILITY TO FAVISM OF G6PD-DEFICIENT PERSONS. BEUTLER (1970) SUGGESTED THAT DOPAQUINONE IS THE ACTIVE HEMOLYTIC PRINCIPLE IN FAVA BEANS. (FAVA BEANS ARE THE MAIN COMMERCIAL SOURCE OF L-DOPA.) DIFFERENCES IN SUSCEPTIBILITY TO FAVISM BY G6PD-DEFICIENT PERSONS MAY BE RELATED TO DIFFERENCES IN THE ENZYMATIC SYSTEM WHICH CONVERTS L-DOPA TO DOPAQUINONE. A GENETIC MECHANISM FOR SUSCEPTIBI-LITY TO FAVISM ON THE PART OF G6PD-DEFICIENT PERSONS IS SUGGESTED BY THE FINDINGS OF BOTTINI ET AL. (1971) THAT PERSONS WITH FAVISM ARE MORE OFTEN OF A PARTICULAR RED-CELL ACID PHOSPHATASE TYPE THAN WOULD BE EXPECTED ON THE BASIS OF POPULATION FREQUENCIES.

BEUTLER, E.* L-DOPA AND FAVISM. (EDITORIAL) BLOOD 36* 523-525, 1970.

BOTTINI, E., LUCCERELLI, P., AGOSTINO, R., PALMARINO, R., BUSINCO, L. AND ANTOGNONI, G.* FAVISM* ASSOCIATION WITH ERYTHROCYTE ACID PHOSPHATASE PHENOTYPE. SCIENCE 171* 409-411, 1971.

MAGER, J., GLASER, G., RAZIN, A., IZAK, G., BIEN, S. AND NOAM, M.* METABOLIC EFFECTS OF PYRIMIDINES DERIVED FROM FAVA BEAN GLYCOSIDES ON HUMAN ERYTHROCYTES DEFICIENT IN GLUCOSE-6-PHOSPHATE DEHYDROGENASE. BIOCHEM. BIOPHYS. RES. COMM. 20* 235-240, 1965.

STAMATOYANNOPOULOS, G., FRASER, G. R., MOTULSKY, A. G., FESSAS, P., AKRIVAKIS, A. AND PAPAYANNOPOULOU, T.* ON THE FAMILIAL PREDISPOSITION TO FAVISM. AM. J. HUM. GENET. 18* 253-263, 1966.

*13480 FIBRINOGEN VARIANTS

IN ADDITION TO AFIBRINOGENEMIA (A RECESSIVE), FIBRINOGEN MAY BE FUNCTIONALLY ABNORMAL. EXAMPLES HAVE BEEN REPORTED BY MENACHE (1964), BY IMPERATO AND DETTORI (1958) AND BY JACKSON, BECK AND CHARACHE (1965). THE LAST GROUP (BECK ET AL., 1965), FOLLOWING THE PRACTICE WITH HEMOGLOBINS, REFERRED TO THE ANOMALOUS PROTEIN AS FIBRINOGEN (BALTIMORE). A MOTHER AND THREE DAUGHTERS WERE AFFECTED IN THEIR FAMILY AND A FATHER AND SON IN MENACHE'S FAMILY. BECK, CHARACHE AND JACKSON (1965) DEMONSTRATED AN ANOMALOUS FIBRINOGEN IN A PATIENT WITH INCREASED TENDENCY TO THROMBOSIS AND PARADOXICALLY, A MILD HEMORRHAGIC DIATHESIS. THREE DAUGHTERS BY TWO DIFFERENT HUSBANDS WERE SIMILARLY AFFECTED. MENACHE (1964) DESCRIBED A DIFFERENT FIBRINOGEN VARIANT. IN A FAMILY OF HUNGARIAN EXTRACTION, VON FELTON ET AL. (1966) FOUND PROLONGED PROTHROMBIN TIME WITHOUT HEMORRHAGIC DIATHESIS. CHEMICAL STUDIES SUGGESTED A MOLECULAR ABNORMALITY OF FIBRINOGEN. VON FELTON, DUCKERT AND FRICK (1966) DESCRIBED A CLOTTING DISTURBANCE CHARACTERIZED BY DELAYED AGGREGATION OF FIBRIN MONOMERS, IN FATHER AND SON. FORMAN ET AL. (1968) DESCRIBED A FIBRINOGEN CLEVELAND WHICH IS IMMUNOELECTROPHORETICALLY DISTINCT FROM FIBRINOGEN BALTIMORE. OPERATIVE WOUNDS SHOWED DEHISCENCE IN TWO PERSONS WITH THE ABNORMAL FIBRINOGEN. THE PLASMA IN THEIR 8 RELATED PERSONS OF BOTH SEXES SHOWED ABNORMALLY SLOW COAGULATION WHEN THROMBIN WAS ADDED. THE FIBRINOGEN DESCRIBED BY MAMMEN ET AL. (1969) AND CALLED FIBRINOGEN DETROIT HAD CHARACTERISTICS DIFFERENT FROM FIBRINOGEN BALTIMORE AND FIBRINOGEN CLEVELAND.

BECK, E. A., CHARACHE, P. AND JACKSON, D. P.* A NEW INHERITED COAGULATION DISORDER CAUSED BY AN ABNORMAL FIBRINOGEN (*FIBRINOGEN BALTIMORE*). NATURE 208* 143-145, 1965.

FORMAN, W. B., RATNOFF, O. D. AND BOYER, M. H.* AN INHERITED QUALITATIVE ABNORMALITY IN PLASMA FIBRINOGEN* FIBRINOGEN CLEVELAND. J. LAB. CLIN. MED. 72* 455-472, 1968.

IMPERATO, C. AND DETTORI, A. G.* IPOFIBRINOGENEMIA CONGENITA CON FIBRINOAS-TENIA. HELV. PAEDIAT. ACTA 13* 380-399, 1958.

JACKSON, D. P., BECK, E. A. AND CHARACHE, P.* CONGENITAL DISORDERS OF FIBRINO-GEN. FED. PROC. 24* 816-821, 1965.

MAMMEN, E. F., PRASAD, A. S., BARNHART, M. I. AND AU, C. C.* CONGENITAL DYSFIBRINOGENEMIA* FIBRINOGEN DETROIT. J. CLIN. INVEST. 48* 235-249, 1969.

MENACHE, D.* CONSTITUTIONAL AND FAMILIAL ABNORMAL FIBRINOGEN. THROMB. DIATH. HAEMORRH. 10 (SUPPL. 13)* 173-185, 1964.

VON FELTON, A., DUCKERT, F. AND FRICK, P. G.* FAMILIAL DISTURBANCE OF FIBRIN MONOMER AGGREGATION. BRIT. J. HAEMAT. 12* 667-677, 1966.

13490 FIBRINOLYTIC DEFECT

SELF AND MATTHEWS (1968) DESCRIBED A FAMILY IN WHICH MULTIPLE MEMBERS IN FIVE GENERATIONS SHOWED HYPER-EXTENSIBLE SKIN AND A DEFECT IN FIBRINOLYTIC ACTIVITY AS INDICATED CLINICALLY BY EXCESSIVE BRUISING ON MINOR TRAUMA AND SPONTANEOUS HEMATOMAS. JOINTS WERE NOT EXCESSIVELY MOBILE. THE FIBRINOLYTIC DEFECT WAS DEMONSTRATED BY SHORT EUGLOBULIN CLOT LYSIS TIME AND DECREASED FACTOR XIII ACTIVITY. MALE-TO-MALE TRANSMISSION OCCURRED.

SELF, J. AND MATTHEWS, C.* INHERITED FIBRINOLYTIC HYPERACTIVITY. ARCH. INTERN. MED. 122* 357-358, 1968.

*13500 FIBROCYSTIC PULMONARY DYSPLASIA

KOCH (1965) OBSERVED A FAMILY WITH 3 DEFINITE AND 5 PROBABLE CASES. THE FEATURES WERE PROGRESSIVE DYSPNEA AND CYANOSIS, DIGITAL CLUBBING, PULMONARY HYPERTENSION, POLYCYTHEMIA, DIFFUSE PULMONARY FIBROSIS BY X-RAY. THE DEFINITE CASES INCLUDE AN INSTANCE OF FATHER-SON TRANSMISSION. ONE PATIENT DEVELOPED BRONCHIAL CARCINOMA. THE CONDITION APPEARS TO BE IDENTICAL IN ALL RESPECTS, INCLUDING THE DEVELOPMENT OF CARCINOMA, TO THAT DESCRIBED BY MCKUSICK AND FISHER (1958). REZEK AND TALBERT (1962) REPORTED AFFECTED FATHER AND DAUGHTER. DONOHUE AND COLLEAGUES (1959) DESCRIBED A CANADIAN FAMILY WITH 8 CASES OF PULMONARY FIBROSIS IN FOUR GENERA-TIONS. SWAYE ET AL. (1969) DESCRIBED 8 CASES IN 3 GENERATIONS. IN ONE, THE DIAGNOSIS WAS MADE AT AGE 3.5 YEARS BY LUNG BIOPSY. TWO BROTHERS HAD COEXISTENT PULMONARY FIBROSIS AND BRONCHOGENIC CANCER. IT IS BY NO MEANS CERTAIN THAT THE ENTITY DESCRIBED HERE IS DISTINCT FROM PULMONARY FIBROSIS, IDIOPATHIC (Q.V.).

ADELMAN, A. G., CHERTKOW, G. AND HAYTON, R. C.* FAMILIAL FIBROCYSTIC PULMONARY DYSPLASIA* A DETAILED FAMILY STUDY. CANAD. MED. ASS. J. 95* 603-610, 1966.

DONOHUE, W. L., LASKI, B., UCHIDA, I. AND MUNN, J. D.* FAMILIAL FIBROCYSTIC PULMONARY DYSPLASIA AND ITS RELATION TO THE HAMMAN-RICH SYNDROME. PEDIATRICS 24* 786-813, 1959.

KOCH, B.* FAMILIAL FIBROCYSTIC PULMONARY DYSPLASIA* OBSERVATIONS IN ONE FAMILY. CANAD. MED. ASS. J. 92* 801-808, 1965.

MCKUSICK, V. A. AND FISHER, A. M.* CONGENITAL CYSTIC DISEASE OF THE LUNG WITH PROGRESSIVE PULMONARY FIBROSIS AND CARCINOMATOSIS. ANN. INTERN. MED. 48* 774-790, 1958.

REZEK, P. R. AND TALBERT, W. R., JR.* KONGENITALE (FAMILIARE) ZYSTISCHE FIBROSE DER LUNGE. WIEN. KLIN. WSCHR. 74* 869-873, 1962.

SWAYE, P., VAN ORDSTRAND, H. S., MCCORMICK, L. J. AND WOLPAW, S. E.* FAMILIAL HAMMAN-RICH SYNDROME. DIS. CHEST 55* 7-12, 1969.

YOUNG, W. A.* FAMILIAL FIBROCYSTIC PULMONARY DYSPLASIA* A NEW CASE IN A KNOWN AFFECTED FAMILY. CANAD. MED. ASS. J. 94* 1059-1061, 1966.

*13510 FIBRODYSPLASIA OSSIFICANS PROGRESSIVA

MOST CASES ARE SPORADIC. HOWEVER, SUFFICIENT CASES OF AFFECTED TWINS AND TRIPLETS ARE KNOWN TO SUGGEST A GENETIC BASIS. FURTHERMORE, DOMINANT INHERITANCE IS SUPPORTED BY OBSERVATIONS OF TWO OR THREE SUCCESSIVE GENERATIONS AFFECTED AND THE FINDING OF A PATERNAL AGE EFFECT IN SPORADIC CASES.

MCKUSICK, V. A.* HERITABLE DISORDERS OF CONNECTIVE TISSUE. ST. LOUIS* C. V. MOSBY CO., 1966 (3RD ED.).

TUNTE, W., BECKER, P. E. AND KNORRE, G. V.* ZUR GENETIK DER MYOSITIS OSSIFICANS PROGRESSIVA. HUMANGENETIK 4* 320-351, 1967.

VIPARELLI, V.* LA MIOSITE OSSIFICANTE PROGRESSIVA. ANN. NEUROPSICHIAT. PSICOANAL. 9* 297-324, 1962.

13520 FIBROMATOSIS, CONGENITAL GENERALIZED

THIS DISORDER WAS DESCRIBED BY STOUT (1954) WHO DISTINGUISHED IT FROM OTHER FORMS OF JUVENILE FIBROMATOSIS. THE RADIOLOGIC FINDINGS ARE SIMILAR TO THOSE OF OLLIER'S DISEASE. MULTIPLE CYSTIC LESIONS INVOLVE THE METAPHYSES. MULTIPLE SOFT TISSUE NODULES OCCUR (SHNITKA ET AL., 1958), AS IN MULTIPLE NEUROFIBROMATOSIS, BUT A CUTANEOUS PIGMENTARY ANOMALY IS NOT A FEATURE. THIS IS NO EVIDENCE OF A MENDELIAN BASIS OF THIS DISORDER.

SHNITKA, T. K., ASP, D. M. AND HORNER, R. H.* CONGENITAL GENERALIZED FIBROMATO-

STOUT, A. P.* JUVENILE FIBROMATOSES. CANCER 7* 953-978, 1954.

**D
O
M
I
N
A
N
T**

13530 FIBROMATOSIS, GINGIVAL

IT IS NOT CERTAIN THAT A MUTATION 'GINGIVAL FIBROMATOSIS' EXISTS SEPARATE FROM 'GINGIVAL FIBROMATOSIS WITH HYPERTRICHOSIS.' THE REPORT OF ZACKIN AND WEISBERGER (1961) STATED THAT THERE WAS 'SLIGHT HYPERTRICHOSIS IN ALL MEMBERS OF THE FAMILY' WHICH WAS OF ITALIAN ANCESTRY. WHETHER PERSONS WITHOUT FIBROMATOSIS AS WELL AS THOSE WITH IT WERE HIRSUTE WAS NOT CLEARLY STATED. BECKER ET AL. (1967) DESCRIBED GINGIVAL FIBROMATOSIS WITHOUT OTHER FEATURES IN MOTHER, SON AND DAUGHTER. RAMON ET AL. (1967) DESCRIBED TWO BROTHERS WITH FEATURES OF GINGIVAL FIBROMATOSIS AND OF CHERUBISM. THE PARENTS, SEPHARDIC JEWS, WERE FIRST COUSINS. THEY AND SIX SIBS WERE HEALTHY.

BECKER, W., COLLINGS, C. K., ZIMMERMAN, E. R., DE LA ROSA, M. AND SINGDAHLSEN, D.* HEREDITARY GINGIVAL FIBROMATOSIS. A REPORT ON A FAMILY IN WHICH THREE MEMBERS WERE AFFECTED WITH FIBROMATOSIS OF THE GINGIVA. ORAL SURG. 24* 313-318, 1967.

RAMON, Y., BERMAN, W. AND BUBIS, J. J.* GINGIVAL FIBROMATOSIS COMBINED WITH CHERUBISM. ORAL SURG. 24* 435-448, 1967.

ZACKIN, S. J. AND WEISBERGER, D.* HEREDITARY GINGIVAL FIBROMATOSIS. REPORT OF A FAMILY. ORAL SURG. 14* 828-836, 1961.

*13540 FIBROMATOSIS, GINGIVAL, WITH HYPERTRICHOSIS

EXTREME HIRSUTISM WITH GINGIVAL FIBROMATOSIS FOLLOWS A DOMINANT PATTERN OF INHERITANCE (WESKI, 1920* GARN AND HATCH, 1950). I HAVE SEEN A SPORADIC CASE OF A SEVERELY RETARDED CHILD WHO HAD MUSCULAR HYPOTONIA IN ADDITION TO HYPERTRICHOSIS AND GINGIVAL HYPERPLASIA. THE LAST TWO FEATURES ARE PRODUCED BY DILANTIN - A PHENOCOPY OF THE GENETIC DISORDER. THERE IS NO NECESSARY RELATIONSHIP BETWEEN THE AGE OF DEVELOPMENT OF THE GINGIVAL CHANGES AND THE HYPERTRICHOSIS. THE LATTER MAY BE PRESENT AT BIRTH BUT OFTEN APPEARS AT PUBERTY (ANDERSON ET AL. 1969).

ANDERSON, J., CUNLIFFE, W. J., ROBERTS, D. F. AND CLOSE, H.* HEREDITARY GINGIVAL FIBROMATOSIS. BRIT. MED. J. 3* 218-219, 1969.

FORET, J., DODINVAL, P. AND FORET-KESTLICHER, C.* HYPERPLASIE FIBREUSE IDIOPATHIQUE DES GENCIVES. J. GENET. HUM. 13* 337-350, 1964.

GARN, S. M. AND HATCH, C. E.* HEREDITARY GENERAL GINGIVAL HYPERPLASIA. J. HERED. 41* 41-42, 1950.

WESKI, H.* ELEPHANTIASIS GINGIVAE HEREDITARIA. DEUTSCH. MSCHR. ZAHNHEILK. 38* 557-584, 1920.

*13550 FIBROMATOSIS, GINGIVAL, WITH ABNORMAL FINGERS, FINGERNAILS, NOSE AND EARS AND SPLENOMEGALY

IN TWO ASIATIC INDIAN FAMILIES (ONE LIVING IN THE CARIBBEAN AND ONE IN INDIA) GINGIVAL FIBROMATOSIS OCCURED IN ASSOCIATION WITH 'WHITTLING' OF THE TERMINAL PHALANGES AND ABSENCE OR DYSPLASIA OF THE FINGER NAILS. THE LIVER AND SPLEEN WERE ENLARGED. GORLIN (1967) CALLED MY ATTENTION TO THESE REPORTS. LABAND ET AL. (1964) DESCRIBED THIS DISORDER IN A 38 YEAR OLD TRINIDAD WOMAN AND 5 OF HER SEVEN CHILDREN. THE FAMILY WAS OF EAST-INDIAN ORIGIN. THE MOTHER SHOWED LARGE, SOFT EARS, HYPERTENSION, HYPEREXTENSIBILITY OF METACARPOPHALANGEAL JOINTS AND SPLENOME-GALY. THE FIVE AFFECTED CHILDREN HAD SOFT TISSUE ENLARGMENT OF THE NOSE AND EARS, SPLENOMEGALY, SKELETAL ABNORMALITIES, OBSCURE OR REDUCED SIZE OF TOENAILS AND THUMBNAILS, SHORT TERMINAL PHALANGES AND HYPERMOBILITY OF SEVERAL JOINTS. ALVANDAR (1965) OBSERVED 5 AFFECTED PERSONS IN THREE GENERATIONS WITH ONE INSTANCE OF MALE-TO-MALE TRANSMISSION. ASSOCIATED FEATURES WERE THICKENING OF THE SOFT TISSUES OF THE NOSE AND EAR WITH SOFTNESS OF THE CARTILAGES, HYPEREXTENSIBLE JOINTS, AND HEPATOMEGALY.

ALVANDAR, G.* ELEPHANTIASIS GINGIVAE. REPORT OF AN AFFECTED FAMILY WITH ASSOCIATED HEPATOMEGALY, SOFT TISSUE AND SKELETAL ABNORMALITIES. J. ALL INDIA DENT. ASS. 37* 349-353, 1965.

GORLIN, R. J.* MINNEAPOLIS, MINN.* PERSONAL COMMUNICATION, 1967.

LABAND, P. F., HABIB, G. AND HUMPHREYS, G. S.* HEREDITARY GINGIVAL FIBROMATO-SIS. REPORT OF AN AFFECTED FAMILY WITH ASSOCIATED SPLENOMEGALY AND SKELETAL AND SOFT-TISSUE ABNORMALITIES. ORAL SURG. 17* 339-351, 1964.

13560 FIBRO-OSSEOUS DYSPLASIA OF THE JAWS

CHATTERJEE AND MAZUMDER (1967) DESCRIBED MASSIVE FIBRO-OSSEOUS DYSPLASIA OF THE JAWS IN A MAN AND HIS TWO SONS. THE TUMOROUS INVOLVEMENT REACHED AMAZING PROPORTIONS AS SHOWN IN THE PUBLISHED PHOTOGRAPHS. THE FATHER HAD PROGRESSIVE SWELLING OF THE UPPER JAW FROM CHILDHOOD. INVOLVEMENT OF THE LOWER JAW WAS LATER

CHATTERJEE, S. K. AND MAZUMDER, J. K.* MASSIVE FIBRO-OSSEOUS DYSPLASIA OF THE JAWS IN TWO GENERATIONS. BRIT. J. SURG. 54* 335-340, 1967.

13570 FIBROSIS OF EXTRAOCULAR MUSCLE

HANSEN (1968) DESCRIBED A MOTHER AND A SON AND DAUGHTER WITH FIBROSIS OF THE EXTRAOCULAR MUSCLES. THE DISORDER IS CHARACTERIZED CLINICALLY BY ANCHORING OF THE EYES IN DOWNWARD GAZE, PTOSIS AND BACKWARD TILT OF THE HEAD. LAUGHLIN (1956) OBSERVED THE CONDITION IN AT LEAST FOUR GENERATIONS OF A FAMILY.

HANSEN, E.* CONGENITAL GENERAL FIBROSIS OF THE EXTRAOCULAR MUSCLES. ACTA OPHTHAL. 46* 469-476, 1968.

LAUGHLIN, R. C.* CONGENITAL FIBROSIS OF THE EXTRAOCULAR MUSCLES* A REPORT OF SIX CASES. AM. J. OPHTHAL. 41* 432-438, 1956.

13580 FIBULA, RECURRENT DISLOCATION OF HEAD OF

REEVES (1967) REPORTED TWO FAMILIES, EACH WITH MULTIPLE AFFECTED PERSONS IN THREE GENERATIONS. GENERALIZED JOINT LAXITY WAS NOT PRESENT. ALTHOUGH REEVES FAVORED X-LINKED DOMINANT INHERITANCE, ONE INSTANCE OF MALE-TO-MALE TRANSMISSION WAS DIAGRAMMED.

REEVES, B.* FAMILIAL RECURRENT DISLOCATION OF THE HEAD OF THE FIBULA. PROC. ROY. SOC. MED. 60* 544-545, 1967.

13590 FIFTH FINGER SYNDROME

COFFIN AND SIRIS (1970) DESCRIBED THREE UNRELATED GIRLS WITH MENTAL RETARDATION AND ABSENT NAIL AND TERMINAL PHALANX OF THE FIFTH FINGER. THE NAILS AND DISTAL PHALANGES OF THE LATERAL TOES WERE ABSENT OR HYPOPLASTIC. NO SIMILAR CASES WERE FOUND IN ANY OF THE THREE FAMILIES.

COFFIN, G. S. AND SIRIS, E.* MENTAL RETARDATION WITH ABSENT FIFTH FINGERNAIL AND TERMINAL PHALANX. AM. J. DIS. CHILD. 119* 433-439, 1970.

*13600 FINGERPRINTS, ABSENCE OF

BAIRD (1964) REPORTED A FAMILY IN WHICH 13 PERSONS IN 3 GENERATIONS SHOWED ABSENT DERMAL RIDGES. THE AFFECTED PERSONS ALL SHOWED TRANSIENT CONGENITAL MILIA (SMALL WHITE PAPULES, ESPECIALLY ON THE FACE, REPRESENTING RETENTION CYSTS). SOME AFFECTED MEMBERS ALSO SHOWED BILATERAL PARTIAL FLEXION CONTRACTURES OF THE FINGERS AND TOES AND WEBBING OF THE TOES. SEE ECTODERMAL DYSPLASIA, ABSENT DERMATOGLYPHIC PATTERN, ETC.

BAIRD, H. W., III* KINDRED SHOWING CONGENITAL ABSENCE OF THE DERMAL RIDGES (FINGERPRINTS) AND ASSOCIATED ANOMALIES. J. PEDIAT. 64* 621-631, 1964.

13610 FINGERS, RELATIVE LENGTH OF

THE QUESTION IS WHETHER WHEN THE TIP OF THE RING FINGER IS PLACED ON A LINE, THE INDEX FINGER REACHES THE LINE. SHORT INDEX FINGERS IS SAID TO BE DOMINANT IN MEN, RECESSIVE IN WOMEN. THREE PHENOTYPES WERE NOTED - SECOND LONGER THAN FOURTH, SECOND EQUAL TO FOURTH AND SECOND SHORTER THAN FOURTH. KLOEPFER (1946) STUDIED THE RELATIVE LENGTH OF THE INDEX AND MIDDLE FINGERS.

BLINCOE, H.* SIGNIFICANT HAND TYPES IN WOMEN ACCORDING TO RELATIVE LENGTHS OF FINGERS. AM. J. PHYS. ANTHROP. 20* 45-48, 1962.

KLOEPFER, H. W.* AN INVESTIGATION OF 171 POSSIBLE LINKAGE RELATIONSHIPS IN MAN. ANN. EUGEN. 13* 35-71, 1946.

PHILPS, V. R.* RELATIVE INDEX FINGER LENGTH AS A SEX-INFLUENCED TRAIT IN MAN. AM. J. HUM. GENET. 4* 72-89, 1952.

13620 FLUSHING OF EARS AND SOMNOLENCE

KIM (1969) NOTED A FATHER AND TWO SONS, AGED 7 AND 11 YEARS, WITH INTERMITTENT EPISODES OF FLUSHING OF THE EARS ASSOCIATED WITH SOMNOLENCE. IT HAD ITS ONSET IN ALL THREE AT ABOUT THE SAME TIME. THE MOTHER AND ANOTHER SON WERE UNAFFECTED.

KIM, P. M.* FAMILIAL FLUSHING AND SOMNOLENCE. (LETTER) J.A.M.A. 210* 1289 ONLY, 1969.

*13630 FLYNN-AIRD SYNDROME

IN 10 MEMBERS OF FIVE GENERATIONS OF A FAMILY, FLYNN AND AIRD (1965) OBSERVED A NEUROECTODERMAL SYNDROME WITH SOME SIMILARITIES TO THE SYNDROMES OF WERNER, REFSUM AND COCKAYNE (ALL OF WHICH ARE, HOWEVER, RECESSIVES). MALE-TO-MALE TRANSMISSION OCCURRED IN THREE INSTANCES. FEATURES INCLUDED, IN THE EYE, CATARACTS, ATYPICAL

RETINITIS PIGMENTOSA, MYOPIA* IN THE EAR, BILATERAL NERVE DEAFNESS BEGINNING AS EARLY AS AGE 7* IN THE NERVOUS SYSTEM, ATAXIA, PERIPHERAL NEURITIS, EPILEPSY, ELEVATION OF CEREBROSPINAL FLUID PROTEIN AND DEMENTIA* IN THE ECTODERM, SKIN ATROPHY, CHRONIC ULCERATION, BALDNESS AND STRIKING DENTAL CARIES* IN THE SKELETAL SYSTEM, CYSTIC CHANGES OF BONE AND JOINT STIFFNESS.

FLYNN, P. AND AIRD, R. B.* A NEUROECTODERMAL SYNDROME OF DOMINANT INHERITANCE. J. NEUROL. SCI. 2* 161-182, 1965.

13640 FOCAL EPITHELIAL HYPERPLASIA OF THE ORAL MUCOSA

MOST CASES OF THIS RARE LESION HAVE BEEN NON-FAMILIAL. HOWEVER, SCHOCK (1969) DESCRIBED THE DISORDER IN AN INDIAN WOMAN AND THREE OF HER DAUGHTERS. MOST OF THE CASES HAVE BEEN IN AMERICAN INDIANS, ALL THE WAY FROM THE WARM SPRINGS INDIANS OF OREGON TO THE CHAVANTE INDIANS OF BRAZIL.

SCHOCK, R. K.* FAMILIAL FOCAL EPITHELIAL HYPERPLASIA. REPORT OF A CASE. ORAL SURG. 28* 598-602, 1969.

*13650 FOCAL FACIAL DERMAL DYSPLASIA (HEREDITARY SYMMETRICAL APLASTIC NEVI OF TEMPLES)

BRAUER (1929) DESCRIBED 38 PATIENTS WITH THIS CONDITION AND TRACED IT THROUGH 5 GENERATIONS OF A FAMILY IN WHICH 155 PERSONS WERE SAID TO HAVE BEEN AFFECTED. THE AFFECTED PROGENITOR WAS SAID TO BE ONE JOHANN JOKEB VAN BARGEN, WHO MIGRATED TO GERMANY FROM HOLLAND IN THE 16TH CENTURY. THE RESEMBLANCE TO *FORCEPS MARKS* WAS NOTED. UNILATERAL OCCURRENCE WAS DESCRIBED IN TWO. AFFECTED PERSONS IN 4 GENERATIONS WERE DESCRIBED BY CHURCH (1970). MCGEOCH AND REED (1971) STUDIED AN AUSTRALIAN FAMILY WITH MANY AFFECTED MEMBERS OF MANY GENERATIONS. THEY CALLED IT FOCAL FACIAL DERMAL DYSPLASIA. ALTHOUGH THE MAIN FINDING WAS A WRINKLING OR PUCKERING OF THE SKIN AT THE TEMPLES, SOME PATIENTS SHOWED GUTTATE AREAS ON THE LATERAL ASPECTS OF THE CHIN AND MIDFOREHEAD. FATHER-TO-SON TRANSMISSION HAS BEEN OBSERVED IN EACH OF THE THREE LARGE KINDREDS (GERMAN, ENGLISH, AUSTRALIAN). HISTOLOGICALLY, THE LESION IS A MESODERMAL DYSPLASIA WITH NEAR ABSENCE OF SUBCUTANEOUS FAT AND WITH SKELETAL MUSCLE ALMOST CONTIGUOUS WITH EPIDERMIS. THE PUCKERED SKIN IS WELL ACCOUNTED FOR BY THE HYPOPLASIA OF THE CORIUM AND LACK OF FAT.

BRAUER, A.* HEREDITARER SYMMETRISCHER SYSTEMATISIERTER NAEVUS APLASTICUS BEI 38 PERSONEN. DERM. WSCHR. 89* 1163-1168, 1929.

CHURCH, R. E.* BRIT. ACAD. DERMATOLOGY, SCHEFFIELD, JULY, 1970.

MCGEOCH, A. H. AND REED, W. B.* FAMILIAL FOCAL FACIAL DERMAL DYSPLASIA. THE CLINICAL DELINEATION OF BIRTH DEFECTS. XII. SKIN, HAIR AND NAILS. BALTIMORE* WILLIAMS AND WILKINS, 1971.

13660 FRIEDREICH'S ATAXIA

IT IS LIKELY THAT ALL CASES WHICH LEGITIMATELY DESERVE THIS DESIGNATION HAVE RECESSIVE INHERITANCE. HOWEVER, SYLVESTER (1958) REPORTED WHAT HE TERMED FRIEDREICH'S ATAXIA IN A FATHER AND SIX OF HIS NINE CHILDREN. OPTIC ATROPHY AND NERVE DEAFNESS WERE ASSOCIATED FEATURES. SPILLANE (1940) DESCRIBED A FAMILY IN WHICH 21 PERSONS (12 MALES AND 9 FEMALES) IN 6 GENERATIONS HAD PES CAVUS AND ABSENT DEEP REFLEXES. THIS WAS PROBABLY ROUSSY-LEVY HEREDITARY AREFLEXIC DYSTASIA (Q.V.).

SPILLANE, J. D.* FAMILIAL PES CAVUS AND ABSENT TENDON-JERKS* ITS RELATIONSHIP WITH FRIEDREICH'S DISEASE AND PERONEAL MUSCULAR ATROPHY. BRAIN 63* 275-290, 1940.

SYLVESTER, P. E.* SOME UNUSUAL FINDINGS IN A FAMILY WITH FRIEDREICH'S ATAXIA. ARCH. DIS. CHILD. 33* 217-221, 1958.

13670 FRONTODIGITAL SYNDROME

IN 9 PERSONS IN 5 SIBSHIPS OF 3 GENERATIONS, MARSHALL AND SMITH (1970) DESCRIBED CRANIAL ABNORMALITIES, NAMELY FRONTAL BOSSING AND A SAGITAL RIDGE. IN SIX OF THE NINE THE THUMBS AND-OR TOES WERE BROAD. IN TWO OF THE NINE POLYDACTYLY AND-OR SYNDACTYLY WERE PRESENT.

MARSHALL, R. E. AND SMITH, D. W.* FRONTODIGITAL SYNDROME* A DOMINANTLY INHERITED DISORDER WITH NORMAL INTELLIGENCE. J. PEDIAT. 77* 129-133, 1970.

13680 FUCHS' EPITHELIAL AND ENDOTHELIAL DYSTROPHY OF THE CORNEA

ALTHOUGH EVIDENCE OF A HEREDITARY BASIS IS SCANTY IN THE LITERATURE, FALLS (1968) STATES THAT HIS EXPERIENCE SUGGESTS AUTOSOMAL DOMINANT INHERITANCE WITH GREATER EXPRESSION IN THE FEMALE. CROSS ET AL. (1971) PRESENTED TWO NEW PEDIGREES AND ANALYZED A PREVIOUSLY REPORTED ONE. THEY CONCLUDED THAT THE DISORDER IS PROBABLY AUTOSOMAL DOMINANT. THE FEMALE PREDILECTION WAS AGAIN NOTED. THIS DISORDER HAS AN ADULT-ONSET, PROGRESSIVE CORNEAL DEGENERATION CHARACTERIZED INITIALLY BY CENTRAL GUTTATA AND ENDOTHELIAL EDEMA.

ENDOTHELIAL DYSTROPHY. ARCH. OPHTHAL. 85* 268-272, 1971.

FALLS, H. F.* DETECTION OF THE CARRIER STATE OF GENETICALLY DETERMINED EYE
DISEASES. IN, CONGENITAL ANOMALIES OF THE EYE. ST. LOUIS* C. V. MOSBY CO., 1968.
PP. 34-52.

13690 FUNDUS DYSTROPHY

SORSBY AND MASON (1949) DESCRIBED FIVE FAMILIES WITH A FUNDUS DYSTROPHY WHICH
OCCURRED IN SEVERAL GENERATIONS IN A DOMINANT PEDIGREE PATTERN. IT BECAME
MANIFEST AT ABOUT THE AGE OF 40 YEARS, BEGINNING AS A CENTRAL (MACULAR) LESION
SHOWING EDEMA, HEMORRHAGE AND EXUDATES. IN THE COURSE OF YEARS ATROPHY WITH
PIGMENTATION AND EXTENSION PERIPHERALLY OCCURRED. THE CHOROIDAL VESSELS BECAME
EXPOSED AND APPEARED SOMEWHAT SCLEROTIC. WITHIN ABOUT 35 YEARS AFTER ONSET THE
ENTIRE FUNDUS WAS INVOLVED. THE CHOROIDAL VESSELS DISAPPEARED BY THIS STAGE AND
THE TERMINAL PICTURE WAS ONE OF EXTENSIVE CHOROIDAL ATROPHY WITH PIGMENTATION.
NIGHT-BLINDNESS WAS NOT A FEATURE AT ANY STAGE. THE AUTHORS CONSIDERED THE
PROCESS TO BE PRIMARILY CHOROIDAL. SANDVIG (1955) DESCRIBED 13 CASES OF CENTRAL
CHOROIDAL DEGENERATION IN FOUR GENERATIONS OF A FAMILY.

SANDVIG, K.* FAMILIAL, CENTRAL, AREOLAR, CHOROIDAL ATROPHY OF AUTOSOMAL
DOMINANT INHERITANCE. ACTA OPHTHAL. 33* 71-78, 1955.

SORSBY, A. AND MASON, M. E. J.* A FUNDUS DYSTROPHY WITH UNUSUAL FEATURES (LATE
ONSET AND DOMINANT INHERITANCE OF A CENTRAL RETINAL LESION SHOWING OEDEMA,
HAEMORRHAGE AND EXUDATES DEVELOPING INTO GENERALIZED CHOROIDAL ATROPHY WITH
MASSIVE PIGMENT PROLIFERATION). BRIT. J. OPHTHAL. 33* 67-97, 1949.

13700 FUTCHER'S LINE

FUTCHER'S LINE IS A LINEAR DISCONTINUITY IN INTENSITY OF PIGMENTATION ON THE UPPER
ARM AND DELTOID AREA OF NEGROES. IT IS LOCATED ON THE LATERAL ASPECT OF THE ARM
AND MARKS THE JUNCTION BETWEEN THE DORSAL AND VENTRAL PARTS OF THE EXTREMITY.
FUTCHER (1938, 1940) FOUND IT BILATERALLY IN 17.5 PERCENT OF NEGROES REGARDLESS OF
AGE, SEX AND INTENSITY OF OVER-ALL PIGMENTATION. ANOTHER 2 PERCENT HAD A LINE ON
ONE SIDE ONLY. APPARENTLY NO FAMILY STUDIES HAVE BEEN DONE.

FUTCHER, P. H.* A PECULIARITY OF PIGMENTATION OF THE UPPER ARM OF NEGROES.
SCIENCE 88* 570-571, 1938.

FUTCHER, P. H.* THE DISTRIBUTION OF PIGMENTATION ON THE ARM AND THORAX OF MAN.
BULL. HOPKINS HOSP. 67* 372-373, 1940.

13710 GAMMA-A-GLOBULIN, SELECTIVE DEFICIENCY OF

IN A SWISS KINDRED STOCKER ET AL. (1968) DESCRIBED SELECTIVE COMPLETE DEFICIENCY
OF GAMMA-A-GLOBULIN IN TWO SISTERS, THE SON AND DAUGHTER OF ONE AND THE SON OF THE
OTHER. BOTH PARENTS OF THE TWO SISTERS HAD NORMAL SERUM GLOBULIN. THEY SUGGESTED
AUTOSOMAL DOMINANT INHERITANCE BUT THE EVIDENCE IS MEAGER.

STOCKER, F., AMMANN, P. AND ROSSI, E.* SELECTIVE GAMMA-A-GLOBULIN DEFICIENCY,
WITH DOMINANT AUTOSOMAL INHERITANCE IN A SWISS FAMILY. ARCH. DIS. CHILD. 43* 585-
588, 1968.

13720 GAMSTORP-WOHLFART SYNDROME (MYOKYMIA, MYOTONIA, MUSCLE WASTING, HYPERHIDROSIS)

SOME OF THE FEATURES RESEMBLED CHARCOT-MARIE-TOOTH DISEASE. HOWEVER, MYOKYMIA AND
MYOTONIA ARE NOT FEATURES OF CMT AND HYPERHIDROSIS IS SAID TO BE RARE. THREE
UNRELATED PATIENTS WERE DESCRIBED. IN ONE THE INHERITANCE WAS PROBABLY DOMINANT.
THERE IS LITTLE TO *GO ON* IN THE REPORTS OF THE OTHER TWO. THE MYOTONIA MAY BE
WHAT WAS CALLED NEUROMYOTONIA BY MERTENS AND ZSCHOCKE (1965) BECAUSE THERE IS
CONTINUOUS NERVE ACTIVITY. STIFFNESS IS ALMOST CONTINUAL AND ANTICONVULSANTS GIVE
RELIEF. GRUND (1938) REPORTED AFFECTED BROTHERS.

GAMSTORP, I. AND WOHLFART, G.* A SYNDROME CHARACTERIZED BY MYOKYMIA, MYOTONIA,
MUSCULAR WASTING AND INCREASED PERSPIRATION. ACTA PSYCHIAT. SCAND. 34* 181-194,
1959.

GRUND, G.* UBER GENETISCHE BEZIEHUNGEN ZWISCHEN MYOTONIE, MUSKELKRAMPFEN UND
MYOKYMIE. (ZUGLEICH BEITRAG ZUR PATHOLOGIE DER NEURALEN MUSKELATROPHIE).
DEUTSCH. Z. NERVENHEILK. 146* 3-14, 1938.

MERTENS, H. G. AND ZSCHOCKE, S.* NEUROMYOTONIE. KLIN. WSCHR. 43* 917-925,
1965.

13730 GAUCHER'S DISEASE

HSIA, NAYLOR AND BIGLER (1959) REPORTED GAUCHER'S DISEASE IN FATHER AND SON.
ALTHOUGH IN THE MAJORITY OF INSTANCES GAUCHER'S DISEASE IS AUTOSOMAL RECESSIVE, A
DOMINANT FORM WAS SUGGESTED. THE FATHER IN THEIR CASE WAS GERMAN-JEWISH AND THE
MOTHER SWEDISH-ENGLISH. EVEN HERE, THE MOTHER MAY HAVE BEEN A CARRIER AND THIS

QUASI-DOMINANT MECHANISM IS EVEN MORE LIKELY IN REPORTS OF PRESUMED DOMINANT INHERITANCE IN JEWISH GROUPS WHERE THE FREQUENCY OF THE GAUCHER GENE MAY BE RELATIVELY HIGH.

HSIA, D. Y.-Y., NAYLOR, J. AND BIGLER, J. A.* GAUCHER'S DISEASE* REPORT OF TWO CASES IN FATHER AND SON AND REVIEW OF THE LITERATURE. NEW ENG. J. MED. 261* 164-169, 1959.

13740 GEOGRAPHIC TONGUE AND FISSURED TONGUE

DAWSON AND PIELOU (1967) OBSERVED 18 PERSONS WITH GEOGRAPHIC TONGUE IN 3 GENERA-TIONS WITH PROBABLE AUTOSOMAL DOMINANT PATTERN. SOME HAD FISSURED TONGUE ALSO. TURPIN AND CARATZALI (1936) CONCLUDED THAT ONE AND THE SAME GENE IS RESPONSIBLE FOR BOTH GEOGRAPHIC TONGUE AND FISSURED TONGUE. TOBIAS (1945) REPORTED DOMINANT PEDIGREES.

DAWSON, T. A. J. AND PIELOU, W. D.* GEOGRAPHICAL TONGUE IN THREE GENERATIONS. BRIT. J. DERM. 79* 678-681, 1967.

TOBIAS, N.* SCROTAL TONGUE AND ITS INHERITANCE. ARCH. DERM. SYPH. 52* 266 ONLY, 1945.

TURPIN, R. AND CARATZALI, A.* CONTRIBUTION A L'ETIOLOGIE DE LA GLOSSITE EXFOLIATRICE MARGINEE. PRESSE MED. 44* 1273-1274, 1936.

*13750 GIANT NEUTROPHILE LEUKOCYTES

DAVIDSON, MILNER AND LAWLER (1960) DESCRIBED GIANT NEUTROPHILE LEUKOCYTES IN 7 MEMBERS OF 3 GENERATIONS OF A FAMILY. ONE TO TWO PERCENT OF LEUKOCYTES SHOWED THE CHANGE.

DAVIDSON, W. M., MILNER, R. D. G. AND LAWLER, S. D.* GIANT NEUTROPHILE LEUCOCYTES* AN INHERITED ANOMALY. BRIT. J. HAEMAT. 6* 339-343, 1960.

*13760 GLAUCOMA

USING TOPICAL APPLICATION OF DEXAMETHASONE, ARMALY (1966) CONCLUDED THAT SUBJECTS CAN BE DIVIDED INTO THREE CLASSES ACCORDING TO THE RESPONSE OF INTRA-OCULAR PRESSURE - HIGH, INTERMEDIATE AND LOW. HE INTERPRETED THESE THREE PHENOTYPES TO CORRESPOND TO THE THREE GENOTYPES OF A TWO-ALLELE SYSTEM. CROMBIE AND CULLEN (1964) DESCRIBED JUVENILE OPEN-ANGLE GLAUCOMA IN 11 MEMBERS OF 5 GENERATIONS. HARRIS (1965) OBSERVED 16 CASES IN 3 GENERATIONS. THE AGE OF ONSET IN 8 OF THESE AVERAGED 26 YEARS. THE ANGLES OF THE ANTERIOR CHAMBERS WERE OPEN IN ONE PATIENT ON WHOM GONIOSCOPY WAS PERFORMED EARLY IN THE PROGRESS OF THE DISEASE. IN A SCOTTISH FAMILY SETTLED IN VIRGINIA, COURTNEY AND HILL (1931) DESCRIBED 18 CASES (10 MALES, 8 FEMALES) IN FIVE GENERATIONS WITH TWO INSTANCES OF FAILURE OF PENETRANCE IN THE THIRD GENERATION. ONSET WAS USUALLY IN THE SECOND OR THIRD GENERATION AND THE COURSE WAS RAPID. STUDIES IN FAMILIES WITH AND WITHOUT CASES OF GLAUCOMA LED ARMALY ET AL. (1968) TO THE CONCLUSION THAT INTRAOCULAR PRESSURE AND OUTFLOW FACILITY ARE MULTIFACTORIAL IN DETERMINATION AND THAT OPEN-ANGLE GLAUCOMA IS PROBABLY MULTIFACTORIAL ALSO.

ARMALY, M. F.* THE HERITABLE NATURE OF DEXAMETHASONE INDUCED OCULAR HYPERTEN-SION. ARCH. OPHTHAL. 75* 32-35, 1966.

ARMALY, M. F., MONSTAVICIUS, B. F. AND SAYEGH, R. E.* OCULAR PRESSURE AND AQUEOUS OUTFLOW FACILITY IN SIBLINGS. ARCH. OPHTHAL. 80* 354-360, 1968.

COURTNEY, R. H. AND HILL, E.* HEREDITARY JUVENILE GLAUCOMA SIMPLEX. J.A.M.A. 97* 1602-1609, 1931.

CROMBIE, A. L. AND CULLEN, J. F.* HEREDITARY GLAUCOMA. OCCURRENCE IN FIVE GENERATIONS OF AN EDINBURGH FAMILY. BRIT. J. OPHTHAL. 48* 143-147, 1964.

HARRIS, D.* THE INHERITANCE OF GLAUCOMA. AM. J. OPHTHAL. 60* 91-95, 1965.

*13770 GLAUCOMA, HEREDITARY JUVENILE

TOGETHER BERG (1932) AND JERNDAL (1970) REPORTED OBSERVATIONS ON 11 GENERATIONS OF A FAMILY WITH 25 OUT OF 55 PERSONS EXAMINED BY AN OPHTHALMOLOGIST WERE AFFECTED. ALL AFFECTED MEMBERS SHOWED DYSGENESIS OF THE IRIS AND IRIDO-CORNEAL ANGLE. EVERY MEMBER OF THE KINDRED WITH DYSGENESIS HAD DEVELOPED GLAUCOMA BY AGE 8 YEARS. ELEVATED INTRAOCULAR PRESSURE WAS FOUND IN TWO IN THE NEONATAL PERIOD. THE GONIODYSGENESIS HAD THE SAME APPEARANCE AS THAT IN INFANTILE CONGENITAL GLAUCOMA, WHICH IS, HOWEVER, CLEARLY A DISTINCT DISORDER IN VIEW OF ITS RECESSIVE INHERI-TANCE. IMPRESSIVE 'DOMINANT' PEDIGREES OF JUVENILE GLAUCOMA WERE REPORTED BY COURTNEY AND HILL (1931), BY STOKES (1940), BY ALLEN AND ACKERMAN (1942), AND BY OTHERS. THE FAMILIAL HYPOPLASIA OF THE IRIS WITH GLAUCOMA DESCRIBED BY WEATHERILL AND HART (1969) MAY BE THE SAME BUT DIFFERS IN THE PRESENCE OF GREATER VARIABILITY IN THE GONIODYSGENESIS.

ALLEN, T. D. AND ACKERMAN, W. G.* HEREDITARY GLAUCOMA IN A PEDIGREE OF THREE

BERG, F.* ERBLICHES JUGENDLICHES GLAUKOM. ACTA OPHTHAL. 10* 568-587, 1932.

COURTNEY, R. H. AND HILL, E.* HEREDITARY JUVENILE GLAUCOMA SIMPLEX. J.A.M.A. 97* 1602-1609, 1931.

JERNDAL, T.* GONIODYSGENESIS AND HEREDITARY JUVENILE GLAUCOMA. A CLINICAL STUDY OF A SWEDISH PEDIGREE. ACTA OPHTHAL. (SUPPL. 107)* 1-100, 1970.

STOKES, W. H.* HEREDITARY PRIMARY GLAUCOMA. ARCH. OPHTHAL. 24* 885-909, 1940.

WEATHERILL, J. R. AND HART, C. T.* FAMILIAL HYPOPLASIA OF THE IRIS STROMA ASSOCIATED WITH GLAUCOMA. BRIT. J. OPHTHAL. 53* 433-438, 1969.

13780 GLIOMA OF BRAIN

KING AND EISINGER (1966) DESCRIBED GLIOMA MULTIFORME OF THE FRONTAL LOBES IN FATHER AND DAUGHTER WITH DEVELOPMENT OF SYMPTOMS AT AGE 50 AND 34 YEARS, RESPECTI-VELY. OTHERS HAVE REPORTED MULTIPLE AFFECTED SIBS OR OTHER RELATIVES. ARMSTRONG AND HANSON (1969) DESCRIBED THREE SIBS WHO DIED OF BRAIN GLIOMA IN ADULTHOOD.

ARMSTRONG, R. M. AND HANSON, C. W.* FAMILIAL GLIOMAS. NEUROLOGY 19* 1061-1063, 1969.

KING, A. B. AND EISINGER, G.* MAY GLIOMA MULTIFORME BE HEREDITARY.Q GUTHRIE CLIN. BULL. 35* 169-175, 1966.

KJELLIN, K., MULLER, R. AND ASTROM, K. E.* THE OCCURRENCE OF BRAIN TUMOR IN SEVERAL MEMBERS OF A FAMILY. J. NEUROPATH. EXP. NEUROL. 19* 528-537, 1960.

PARKINSON, D. AND HALL, C. W.* OLIGODENDROGLIOMAS* SIMULTANEOUS APPEARANCE IN FRONTAL LOBES IN SIBLINGS. J. NEUROSURG. 19* 424-426, 1962.

REESE, W., MEREDITH, J. M. AND ZFASS, I. S.* CEREBRAL GLIOMA IN SIBLINGS. STH. MED. J. 37* 424-428, 1944.

13790 GLOBULIN ANOMALY INVOLVING BETA (2A)-GLOBULIN

WYSOCKI AND MACKIEWICZ (1965) DESCRIBED FATHER AND SON WITH ABNORMAL BETA (2A)-GLOBULIN AND A DEFECT IN COAGULATION AND IMMUNOLOGIC RESPONSES. A CIRCULATING ANTICOAGULANT DIRECTED AGAINST FACTOR VIII AND VARIOUS MANIFESTATIONS INTERPRETED AS AUTOIMMUNE WERE DESCRIBED. IN THREE OTHER FAMILY MEMBERS, BETA (2A)-GLOBULIN WAS INCREASED AND IN TWO WAS ASSOCIATED WITH A CLOTTING DEFECT. ANOTHER RELATIVE HAD THE CLOTTING DEFECT WITHOUT THE PROTEIN ABNORMALITY. EXCEPT FOR THE FATHER AND SON THESE PERSONS WERE ALL ASYMPTOMATIC.

WYSOCKI, K. AND MACKIEWICZ, S.* FAMILIAL ANOMALOUS BETA (2A)-GLOBULIN ACCOM-PANIED BY DISORDERS OF BLOOD COAGULATION AND PATHOLOGIC IMMUNE PHENOMENA. ARCH. INTERN. MED. 116* 351-356, 1965.

*13800 GLOMUS TUMORS, MULTIPLE

GORLIN, FUSARO AND BENTON (1960) REPORTED FIVE AFFECTED MEMBERS OF TWO GENERATIONS OF A FAMILY. THE LESIONS TEND TO RESEMBLE CAVERNOUS HEMANGIOMAS. THE DISTINCTIVE FEATURE IS THE PRESENCE OF MULTIPLE LAYERS OF GLOMUS CELLS LINING THE BLOOD-FILLED CAVITIES. THE TUMORS ARE PRESENT AT BIRTH OR APPEAR IN THE FIRST TWO DECADES. ISOLATED GLOMUS TUMOR USUALLY DEVELOPS LATER (AT ABOUT AGE 33 YEARS ON THE AVERAGE), IS MORE FREQUENTLY SUBUNGUAL THAN IS THE CASE WITH MULTIPLE TUMORS, AND HAS NO PARTICULAR FAMILIAL OCCURRENCE. REED (1970) PRESENTED A PEDIGREE OF FOUR PERSONS WITH MULTIPLE GLOMUS TUMORS IN TWO GENERATIONS.

CHASSEUIL, R. AND GAUTARD, J.* TUMEURS GLOMIQUE FAMILIALES* 6 CAS EN 4 GENERATIONS. BULL. SOC. FRANC. DERM. SYPH. 68* 635-636, 1961.

GORLIN, R. J., FUSARO, R. M. AND BENTON, J. W.* MULTIPLE GLOMUS TUMOR OF THE PSEUDOCAVERNOUS HEMANGIOMA TYPE. ARCH. DERM. 82* 776-778, 1960.

KAUFMAN, L. R. AND CLARK, W. T.* GLOMUS TUMORS* REPORT OF 4 CASES IN SAME FAMILY. ANN. SURG. 114* 1102-1105, 1941.

REED, W. B.* GENETISCHE ASPEKTE IN DER DERMATOLOGIE. HAUTARZT 21* 8-16, 1970.

REINHARD, M. AND LUDERS, G.* ZUR PATHOLOGIE UND KLINIK MULTIPLER FAMILIARER GLOMUSTUMOREN. ARCH. KLIN. EXP. DERMAT. 237* 800-810, 1970.

13810 GLUCOGLYCINURIA

RENAL GLYCOSURIA AND HYPERGLYCINURIA WITHOUT INCREASED EXCRETION OF OTHER AMINO ACIDS WERE THE FEATURES OBSERVED BY KASER, COTTIER AND ANTENER (1962). THESE WORKERS FOUND THE COMBINATION IN 14 PERSONS IN 7 SIBSHIPS OF THREE GENERATIONS OF ONE KINDRED WITH PROBABLE AUTOSOMAL DOMINANT INHERITANCE.

KASER, H., COTTIER, P. AND ANTENER, I.* GLUCOGLYCINURIA, A NEW FAMILIAL SYNDROME. J. PEDIAT. 61* 386-394, 1962.

*13820 GLUTAMIC OXALOACETIC TRANSAMINASE OF MITOCHONDRIA, ELECTROPHORETIC VARIANT OF

DAVIDSON ET AL. (1970) DEMONSTRATED POLYMORPHISM OF MITOCHONDRIAL GOT. SOLUBLE GLUTAMIC OXALOACETIC TRANSAMINASE OF RED CELLS, LEUKOCYTES AND FIBROBLASTS WAS NOT ANOMALOUS. IN LOWER ANIMALS AND PLANTS, MANY MITOCHONDRICAL ENZYMES SHOW MATERNAL INHERITANCE, INDICATING THAT A SEPARATE MITOCHONDRIAL GENETIC SYSTEM IS INVOLVED IN THEIR CONTROL. HOWEVER, FAMILY STUDIES SHOWED THAT MITOCHONDRIAL GOT IS UNDER THE CONTROL OF NUCLEAR NOT MITOCHONDRIAL DNA (DAVIDSON ET AL., 1970).

DAVIDSON, R. G., CORTNER, J. A., RATTAZZI, M. C., RUDDLE, F. H. AND LUBS, H. A.* GENETIC POLYMORPHISMS OF HUMAN MITOCHONDRIAL GLUTAMIC OXALOACETIC TRANSA-MINASE. SCIENCE 169* 391-392, 1970.

DELORENZO, R. J. AND RUDDLE, F. H.* GLUTAMATE OXALATE TRANSAMINASE (GOT) GENETICS IN MUS MUSCULUS* LINKAGE, POLYMORPHISM, AND PHENOTYPES OF THE GOT-2 AND GOT-1 LOCI. BIOCHEM. GENET. 4* 259-273, 1970.

*13830 GLUTATHIONE REDUCTASE ELECTROPHORETIC VARIANTS

LONG (1967) FOUND IN A NEGRO A VARIANT RED CELL GLUTATHIONE REDUCTASE, CHARAC-TERIZED BY GREATER ELECTROPHORETIC MOBILITY AND ENZYME ACTIVITY PER UNIT OF HEMOGLOBIN THAN THE NORMAL. INHERITANCE WAS AUTOSOMAL CO-DOMINANT. THREE HOMOZYGOTES WERE IDENTIFIED. THE RELATION TO GOUT IS PROBLEMATICAL. ALSO THE RELATION OF THIS LOCUS TO THAT RESPONSIBLE FOR GLUTATHIONE REDUCTASE DEFICIENCY (Q.V.) IS UNCLEAR.

LONG, W. K.* GLUTATHIONE REDUCTASE IN RED BLOOD CELLS* VARIANT ASSOCIATED WITH GOUT. SCIENCE 155* 712-713, 1967.

13840 GLYCERALDEHYDE-3-PHOSPHATE DEHYDROGENASE VARIANTS

SUCH HAVE BEEN FOUND IN A NUMBER OF PHYLETICALLY DIVERSE ORGANISMS (LEBHERZ AND RUTTER, 1967). THE COMBINATION OF TWO DIFFERENT SUBUNITS (EACH DETERMINED BY A SEPARATE GENE) INTO TETRAMERS WAS SUGGESTED FOR THE EXISTENCE OF 5 SUBUNITS AS IN LACTIC ACID DEHYDROGENASE. NO INFORMATION IS AVAILABLE ON ITS GENETICS IN MAN.

LEBHERZ, H. G. AND RUTTER, W. J.* GLYCERALDEHYDE-3-PHOSPHATE DEHYDROGENASE VARIANTS IN PHYLETICALLY DIVERSE ORGANISMS. SCIENCE 157* 1198-1199, 1967.

13850 GLYCINURIA WITH OR WITHOUT OXALATE UROLITHIASIS

DE VRIES AND COLLEAGUES (1957) FOUND HYPERGLYCINURIA IN A GRANDMOTHER, HER DAUGHTER AND TWO GRANDDAUGHTERS. THE GRANDMOTHER HAD HAD RENAL COLIC AND RENAL OXALATE STONES WERE DEMONSTRATED IN THE TWO GRANDDAUGHTERS OF A ASHKENAZIC JEWISH KINDRED. THIS FAMILY IS APPARENTLY UNIQUE FOR THE ASSOCIATION OF OXALATE STONES. LIETMAN AND COLLEAGUES (1966) DISCOVERED GLYCINURIA IN A NORMAL MALE WHO WAS SERVING AS A 'CONTROL.' THE FATHER AND A MALE SIB ALSO HAD GLYCINURIA. THERE WERE NO RENAL STONES OR OTHER ABNORMALITY. IT WAS PLAUSIBLY SUGGESTED BY SCRIVER (1968) THAT THE GLYCINURIA TRAIT OBSERVED IN THESE FAMILIES WAS THE HETEROZYGOUS STATE OF IMINOGLYCINURIA (Q.V.), A DISORDER WHICH HAS BEEN DESCRIBED SEVERAL TIMES IN ASHKENAZIC FAMILIES.

DE VRIES, A., KOCHWA, S., LAZEBNIK, J., FRANK, M. AND DJALDETTI, M.* GLY-CINURIA, A HEREDITARY DISORDER ASSOCIATED WITH NEPHROLITHIASIS. AM. J. MED. 23* 408-415, 1957.

LIETMAN, P., ROSENBERG, L. E. AND SEEGMILLER, J. E.* REFERRED TO BY WYNGAARDEN IN STANBURY, WYNGAARDEN AND FREDRICKSON, P. 346. TO BE PUBLISHED.

SCRIVER, C. R.* RENAL TUBULAR TRANSPORT OF PROLINE, HYDROXYPROLINE, AND GLYCINE. III. GENETIC BASIS FOR MORE THAN ONE MODE OF TRANSPORT IN HUMAN KIDNEY. J. CLIN. INVEST. 47* 823-835, 1968.

*13860 GLYCOPROTEIN, ALPHA-1-ACID, OF SERUM

VARIANTS OF ALPHA-1-ACID GLYCOPROTEIN HAVE BEEN DEMONSTRATED IN NORMAL CAUCASIAN AND JAPANESE BLOOD (SCHMID ET AL., 1965). FAMILY STUDIES HAVE NOT BEEN REPORTED. JOHNSON ET AL. (1969) PRESENTED TWIN AND FAMILY DATA SUPPORTING THE VIEW THAT THREE PHENOTYPES SS, FF AND FS ARE DETERMINED BY TWO CODOMINANT ALLELES.

JOHNSON, A. M., SCHMID, K. AND ALPER, C. A.* INHERITANCE OF HUMAN ALPHA(1)-ACID GLYCOPROTEIN (OROSOMUCOID) VARIANTS. J. CLIN. INVEST. 48* 2293-2299, 1969.

SCHMID, K., TOKITA, K. AND YOSHIZAKI, H.* THE ALPHA-1-ACID GLYCOPROTEIN VARIANTS OF NORMAL CAUCASIAN AND JAPANESE INDIVIDUALS. J. CLIN. INVEST. 44* 1394-1401, 1965.

13870 GLYCOPROTEIN, CONCENTRATION OF BETA-2-GLYCOPROTEIN I IN SERUM

CLEVE AND RITTNER (1969) FOUND 9 FAMILIES OUT OF 88 IN WHICH ONE PARENT AND ABOUT
HALF THE CHILDREN HAD INTERMEDIATE CONCENTRATIONS OF BETA 2 GLYCOPROTEIN I AND
WERE PRESUMED TO BE HETEROZYGOUS FOR A DEFICIENCY GENE. IRREGULARITIES IN OTHER
FAMILIES LIMIT THE USE OF THE TRAIT IN GENETIC STUDIES.

   CLEVE, H. AND RITTNER, C.* FURTHER FAMILY STUDIES ON THE GENETIC CONTROL OF
BETA 2-GLYCOPROTEIN I CONCENTRATION IN HUMAN SERUM. HUMANGENETIK 7* 93-97, 1969.

   CLEVE, H.* GENETIC STUDIES ON THE DEFICIENCY OF BETA 2-GLYCOPROTEIN I OF HUMAN
SERUM. HUMANGENETIK 5* 294-304, 1968.

13880 GOITER, NON-TOXIC, WITH INTRATHYROIDAL CALCIFICATION

   MURRAY ET AL. (1966) DESCRIBED A FAMILY IN WHICH MEMBERS OF FIVE GENERATIONS HAD
NON-TOXIC GOITER APPEARING IN THE EARLY TEENS. CALCIFICATION AND FIRM, NODULAR
CONSISTENCY WERE UNUSUAL FEATURES. NONE OF THE KNOWN DEFECTS IN THYROID HORMONO-
GENESIS COULD BE DEMONSTRATED. RADIOACTIVE IODINE STUDIES SHOWED INCREASED
THYROID AVIDITY AND RAPID TURNOVER. NO CERTAIN MALE-TO-MALE TRANSMISSION WAS
OBSERVED.

   MURRAY, I. P., THOMSON, J. A., MCGIRR, E. M., MACDONALD, E. M., KENNEDY, J. S.
AND MCLENNAN, I.* UNUSUAL FAMILIAL GOITER ASSOCIATED WITH INTRATHYROIDAL CALCIFI-
CATION. J. CLIN. ENDOCR. 26* 1039-1040, 1966.

13890 GOUT

   GOUT IS A DISORDER IN WHICH, AS IN ESSENTIAL HYPERTENSION, DIABETES MELLITUS AND
HYPERCHOLESTEROLEMIA, THERE IS ROOM FOR DEBATE AS TO WHETHER POLYGENIC OR
MONOMERIC INHERITANCE IS ITS GENETIC BASIS. ALTHOUGH NUMEROUS OTHER FACTORS, SOME
GENETIC, SOME ENVIRONMENTAL, INFLUENCE THE LEVEL OF SERUM URIC ACID AND ALTHOUGH
THE PHENOTYPE GOUT CAN PROBABLY BE PRODUCED BY NON-GENETIC ELEVATIONS OF SERUM
URIC ACID, CLASSIC FAMILIAL GOUT MAY BE A MONOMERIC DOMINANTLY INHERITED DISORDER.
   EVIDENCE FOR BOTH AN INCREASED RATE OF URIC ACID SYNTHESIS AND AN IMPAIRED
NET ELIMINATION OF URIC ACID BY THE KIDNEY HAS BEEN ADVANCED. IN SOME REPORTED
FAMILIES WITH BOTH PARENTS AFFECTED, CHILDREN HAVE BEEN AFFECTED UNUSUALLY EARLY
AND SEVERELY AND MAY REPRESENT HOMOZYGOTES (EMMERSON, 1960). THE NEW VIEW ON THE
POLYGENIC INHERITANCE OF GOUT IS STATED BY NEEL AND COLLEAGUES (1965) AND BY
WYNGAARDEN (1966). HYPERURICEMIA IN FILIPINOS HAS BEEN SHOWN TO RESULT FROM
INTERPLAY OF ENVIRONMENTAL AND GENETIC FACTORS (HEALEY ET AL., 1967).

   EMMERSON, B. T.* HEREDITY IN PRIMARY GOUT. AUST. ANN. MED. 9* 168-175, 1960.

   HEALEY, L. A., SKEITH, M. D., DECKER, J. L. AND BAYANI-SIOSON, P. S.* HYPERURI-
CEMIA IN FILIPINOS* INTERACTION OF HEREDITY AND ENVIRONMENT. AM. J. HUM. GENET.
19* 81-85, 1967.

   NEEL, J. V., RAKIC, M. T., DAVIDSON, R. T., VALKENBURG, H. A. AND MIKKELSON, W.
M.* STUDIES ON HYPERURICEMIA. II. A RECONSIDERATION OF THE DISTRIBUTION OF SERUM
URIC ACID VALUES IN THE FAMILIES OF SMYTH, COTTERMAN, AND FREYBURG. AM. J. HUM.
GENET. 17* 14-22, 1965.

   WYNGAARDEN, J. B.* GOUT. IN STANBURY, J. B., WYNGAARDEN, J. B. AND FREDRICK-
SON, D. S. (EDS.)* THE METABOLIC BASIS OF INHERITED DISEASE. NEW YORK* MCGRAW-
HILL, 1966 (2ND ED.). PP. 667-728.

13900 GRANULOSIS RUBRA NASI

   BINAZZI (1958) DESCRIBED A KINDRED WITH 20 AFFECTED MEMBERS IN A CLEARLY AUTOSOMAL
DOMINANT PEDIGREE PATTERN. HELLIER (1937) DESCRIBED AFFECTED MOTHER AND DAUGHTER.
THIS CONDITION IS CHARACTERIZED BY REDNESS AND MARKED SWEATING CONFINED TO THE
NOSE AND SURROUNDING AREA OF THE FACE, WITH RED PAPULES AND SOMETIMES NUMEROUS
SMALL VESICLES. IT OCCURS MOST COMMONLY IN CHILDREN, CLEARING UP AT PUBERTY, BUT
IN RARE INSTANCES PERSISTS INTO ADULTHOOD.

   BINAZZI, M.* ULTERIORI RELIEVI SU DI UNA OSSERVAZIONE DI GRANULOSIS RUBRA NASI
EREDITARIA. RASS. DERM. SIF. 11* 23-26, 1958.

   HELLIER, F. F.* GRANULOSA RUBRA NASI IN MOTHER AND DAUGHTER. BRIT. MED. J. 2*
1068 ONLY, 1937.

13910 GRAYING OF HAIR, EARLY

   THIS TRAIT IS LIKELY TO HAVE MANY CAUSES. IT IS A FEATURE OF BOTH BOOK'S SYNDROME
AND OF WAARDENBURG'S SYNDROME. PROBABLY A SIMPLE FORM OF PREMATURE GRAYING IS
INHERITED AS A DOMINANT. HARE (1929) DESCRIBED 9 AFFECTED IN FIVE GENERATIONS,
WITH ONE INSTANCE OF MALE-TO-MALE TRANSMISSION. THE HAIR BEGAN TO TURN AT 17 OR
18 YEARS AND WAS WHITE AT 25 OR 26 YEARS. IN SOME PERSONS WITH PREMATURE GRAYING
BLACK PIGMENTATION OF THE EYEBROW PERSISTS.

   HARE, H. J. H.* PREMATURE WHITENING OF HAIR. J. HERED. 20* 31-32, 1929.

*13920 GROUP-SPECIFIC COMPONENT (GC)

BY IMMUNOELECTROPHORESIS HIRSCHFELD (1959) DISCOVERED POLYMORPHISM OF THE SERUM ALPHA-2-GLOBULIN CALLED GC FOR GROUP-SPECIFIC COMPONENT. GC1-1, GC2-2, AND GC2-1 PHENOTYPES CAN BE DISTINGUISHED ALSO BY STARCH OR AGAR ELECTROPHORESIS (BEARN ET AL., 1964). NO EVIDENCE OF LINKAGE OF GC, TRANSFERRINS, ABO, MN, RH, AND HAPTOGLOBINS WAS FOUND IN A STUDY IN FINLAND (SEPPALA ET AL., 1967). SEE ALBUMIN VARIANTS FOR INFORMATION ON LINKAGE.

BEARN, A. G., BOWMAN, B. H. AND KITCHIN, F. D.* GENETIC AND BIOCHEMICAL CONSIDERATION OF THE SERUM GROUP-SPECIFIC COMPONENT. COLD SPRING HARBOR SYMPOSIA QUANT. BIOL. 29* 435-442, 1964.

CLEVE, H., KIRK, R. L., GAJDUSEK, D. C. AND GUIART, J.* ON THE DISTRIBUTION OF THE GC VARIANT GC ABORIGINE IN MELANESIAN POPULATIONS* DETERMINATION OF GC-TYPES IN SERA FROM TONGARIKI ISLAND, NEW HEBRIDES. ACTA GENET. STATIST. MED. 17* 511-517, 1967.

HIRSCHFELD, J.* IMMUNE-ELECTROPHORETIC DEMONSTRATION OF QUALITATIVE DIFFERENCES IN HUMAN SERA AND THEIR RELATION TO THE HAPTOGLOBINS. ACTA PATH. MICROBIOL. SCAND. 47* 160-168, 1959.

RUCKNAGEL, D. L., SHREFFLER, D. C. AND HALSTEAD, S. B.* THE BANGKOK VARIANT OF THE SERUM GROUP-SPECIFIC COMPONENT (GC) AND THE FREQUENCY OF THE GC ALLELES IN THAILAND. AM. J. HUM. GENET. 20* 478-485, 1968.

SEPPALA, M., RUOSLAHTI, E. AND MAKELA, O.* INHERITANCE AND GENETIC LINKAGE OF GC AND TF GROUPS. ACTA GENET. STATIST. MED. 17* 47-54, 1967.

13930 GYNECOMASTIA, HEREDITARY

MALE-LIMITED AUTOSOMAL DOMINANT, AUTOSOMAL RECESSIVE AND X-LINKED MODES OF INHERITANCE HAVE BEEN PROPOSED. WALLACH AND GARCIA (1962) REPORTED A FAMILY IN WHICH TWO BROTHERS, THEIR FATHER AND THEIR PATERNAL UNCLE HAD BILATERAL GYNECOMASTIA BEGINNING AT PUBERTY. THE BREASTS WERE TENDER AT THE TIME OF ENLARGEMENT. THE PATIENTS WERE WELL VIRILIZED AND ALL ENDOCRINE ASSAYS YIELDED NORMAL RESULTS. THE AUTHORS POSTULATED AN INHERITED SENSITIVITY OF THE BREAST TO THE NORMAL HORMONAL MILIEU OF THE MALE.

WALLACH, E. E. AND GARCIA, C.-R.* FAMILIAL GYNECOMASTIA WITHOUT HYPOGONADISM* A REPORT OF THREE CASES IN ONE FAMILY. J. CLIN. ENDOCR. 22* 1201-1206, 1962.

13940 HAIR WHORL ('COW-LICK,' 'CROWN')

WHETHER THE WHORL IN THE SCALP HAIR OF THE OCCIPITAL AREA SHOWS CLOCKWISE OR COUNTER-CLOCKWISE ROTATION IS GENETICALLY DETERMINED. BERNSTEIN (1946) SUGGESTED THAT CLOCKWISE DIRECTION IS DOMINANT TO COUNTER-CLOCKWISE DIRECTION. BREWSTER (1925) REPORTED A FAMILY WITH DOUBLE WHORLS OR DOUBLE CROWN, LAUTERBACK (1927) DESCRIBED THREE CROWNS IN ONE SUBJECT, ONE OF THEM BEING A CONSPICUOUS ONE IN THE FRONTAL AREA.

BERNSTEIN, F.* HEREDITY OF SCALP WHORLS. S. B. AKAD. WISS. WIEN. PHYS.-MATH. KL., PP. 61-62. CITED BY KLOEPFER, H. W.* AN INVESTIGATION OF 171 POSSIBLE LINKAGE RELATIONSHIPS IN MAN. ANN. EUGEN. 13* 35-71, 1946.

BREWSTER, E. T.* THE INHERITANCE OF 'DOUBLE CROWN.' J. HERED. 16* 345-346, 1925.

LAUTERBACK, C. E. AND KNIGHT, J. B.* VARIATION IN WHORL OF THE HEAD HAIR. J. HERED. 18* 107-115, 1927.

13950 HAIRY EARS (HYPERTRICHOSIS PINNAE AURIS)

THE TRAIT CONSISTS OF LONG HAIRS GROWING FROM THE HELIX OF THE PINNA. CONTROVERSY HAS PREVAILED AS TO WHETHER IT IS Y-LINKED OR AUTOSOMAL, OR PERHAPS BOTH (IN DIFFERENT FAMILIES). RAO (1970) PROPOSED THAT HAIRY EARS RESULT FROM THE INTERACTION OF TWO LOCI, ONE ON THE HOMOLOGOUS SEGMENT OF THE X AND Y AND ONE ON THE NON-HOMOLOGOUS SEGMENT OF THE Y.

DRONAMRAJU, K. R.* Y-LINKAGE IN MAN. NATURE 201* 424-425, 1964.

RAO, D. C.* TWO-GENE HYPOTHESIS FOR HAIRY PINNAE OF THE EAR. ACTA GENET. MED. GEM. 19* 448-453, 1970.

STERN, C., CENTERWALL, W. R. AND SARKAR, S. S.* NEW DATA ON THE PROBLEM OF Y-LINKAGE OF HAIRY PINNAE. AM. J. HUM. GENET. 16* 455-471, 1964.

13960 HAIRY ELBOWS

IN AN AMISH KINDRED WE HAVE OBSERVED STRIKING HYPERTRICHOSIS LIMITED MAINLY TO THE ELBOWS (F. K., 1099001). THE CONDITION IS PROBABLY DOMINANT, ALTHOUGH INBREEDING MAKES RECESSIVE INHERITANCE A POSSIBLE EXPLANATION FOR THE FINDINGS.

BEIGHTON, P.* FAMILIAL HYPERTRICHOSIS CUBITI* HAIRY ELBOWS SYNDROME. J. MED.

1397 (HALLERMANN-STREIFF SYNDROME

STEELE AND BASS (1970) EMPHASIZED THE LACK OF MANDIBULAR ANGLE AND HYPOPLASIA OF
THE CLAVICLES AND RIBS. THEY GAVE A USEFUL REVIEW OF 50 PUBLISHED CASES. TWO
PATIENTS HAVE REPRODUCED* AN AFFECTED WOMAN GAVE BIRTH TO TWO NORMAL CHILDREN
(PONTE, 1962) AND AN AFFECTED MAN MARRIED TO A DISTANTLY RELATED WOMAN SIRED AN
AFFECTED DAUGHTER (GUYARD ET AL., 1962). PRESUMEDLY MONOZYGOTIC TWINS OF WHICH
ONLY ONE WAS AFFECTED WERE REPORTED BY SCHONDEL (1943). BOTH OF MONOZYGOTIC TWINS
WERE AFFECTED IN THE REPORT OF VAN BALEN (1961).

PONTE, F.* FURTHER CONTRIBUTIONS TO THE STUDY OF THE SYNDROME OF HALLERMANN AND
STREIFF* (CONGENITAL CATARACT WITH *BIRD'S FACE*). OPHTHALMOLOGICA 143* 399-408,
1962.

SCHONDEL, A.* TWO CASES OF PROGERIA COMPLICATED BY MICROPHTHALMUS. ACTA
PAEDIAT. 30* 286-304, 1943.

VAN BALEN, A. T. M.* DYSCEPHALY WITH MICROPHTHALMOS, CATARACT AND HYPOPLASIA OF
THE MANDIBLE. OPHTHALMOLOGICA 141* 53-63, 1961.

13980 HAND CLASPING PATTERN

FROM TWIN DATA, FREIRE-MAIA (1961) CONCLUDED THAT HAND CLASPING IS GENETIC TO AN
IMPORTANT DEGREE. IF IN CLASPING THE HANDS WITH ENTWINING FINGERS THOSE OF THE
RIGHT HAND ARE POSITIONED ABOVE THE CORRESPONDING FINGERS OF THE LEFT HAND, THE
INDIVIDUAL IS CLASSIFIED AS R WITH THE CONVERSE LABELLED L. THE R FREQUENCY IS
HIGHER IN FEMALES THAN IN MALES. LAI AND WALSH (1965) DOUBTED THAT GENETIC
FACTORS ARE SIGNIFICANT IN DETERMINING THIS TRAIT.

FREIRE-MAIA, A.* TWIN DATA ON HAND CLASPING* A REANALYSIS. ACTA GENET.
STATIST. MED. 10* 207-211, 1961.

LAI, L. Y. AND WALSH, R. J.* THE PATTERNS OF HAND CLASPING IN DIFFERENT ETHNIC
GROUPS. HUM. BIOL. 37* 312-319, 1965.

PONS, J.* HAND CLASPING (SPANISH DATA). ANN. HUM. GENET. 25* 141-144, 1961.

13990 HANDEDNESS

ANNETT (1964) POSTULATED THAT RIGHT HANDEDNESS IS AN INCOMPLETE DOMINANT, OR
INTERMEDIATE, I.E., THAT DOMINANT HOMOZYGOTES ARE ALWAYS RIGHT HANDED WITH *SPEECH
HIGHLY DEVELOPED IN THE LEFT HEMISPHERE.* RECESSIVE HOMOZYGOTES ARE CONSISTENTLY
LEFT HANDED WITH SPEECH IN THE RIGHT HEMISPHERE. HETEROZYGOTES MAY USE EITHER HAND
AND DEVELOP SPEECH IN EITHER HEMISPHERE. FROM TWIN STUDIES RIFE (1940) CONCLUDED
THAT HANDEDNESS IS A MULTIFACTORIAL TRAIT.

ANNETT, M.* A MODEL OF THE INHERITANCE OF HANDEDNESS AND CEREBRAL DOMINANCE.
NATURE 204* 59-60, 1964.

RIFE, D. C.* HANDEDNESS WITH SPECIAL REFERENCE TO TWINS. GENETICS 25* 178-186,
1940.

14000 HAND-FOOT-UTERUS (HFU) SYNDROME

THE CLINICAL FEATURES INCLUDE SMALL FEET WITH UNUSUALLY SHORT GREAT TOES AND
ABNORMAL THUMBS. FEMALES WITH THE DISORDER HAVE DUPLICATION OF THE GENITAL TRACT
(STERN ET AL., 1970). THE RADIOGRAPHIC CHANGES WERE REVIEWED BY POZNANSKI ET AL.
(1970). THESE INCLUDED SHORT FIRST METACARPAL AND METATARSAL, SHORT FIFTH FINGERS
WITH CLINODACTYLY, TRAPEZUIM-SCAPHOID FUSION IN THE WRIST, CUNEIFORM-NAVICULAR
FUSION IN THE FOOT.

POZNANSKI, A. K., STERN, A. M. AND GALL, J. C., JR.* RADIOGRAPHIC FINDINGS IN
THE HAND-FOOT-UTERUS SYNDROME (HFUS). RADIOLOGY 95* 129-134, 1970.

STERN, A. M., GALL, J. C., JR., PERRY, B. L., STIMSON, C. W., WEITKAMP, L. R.
AND POZNANSKI, A. K.* THE HAND-FOOT-UTERUS SYNDROME. A NEW HEREDITARY DISORDER
CHARACTERIZED BY HAND AND FOOT DYSPLASIA, DERMATOGLYPHIC ABNORMALITIES, AND
PARTIAL DUPLICATION OF THE FEMALE GENITAL TRACT. J. PEDIAT. 77* 109-116, 1970.

*14010 HAPTOGLOBIN, ALPHA LOCUS (HP)

THE HAPTOGLOBINS, ALPHA-2-GLOBULINS WHOSE NAME COMES FROM THEIR ABILITY TO BIND
PROTEIN, WERE FOUND TO BE POLYMORPHIC WHEN STUDIED BY SMITHIES USING STARCH GEL
ELECTROPHORESIS. SEVERAL HAPTOGLOBIN VARIANTS HAVE BEEN IDENTIFIED IN ADDITION TO
THE MAIN TYPES AND EVIDENCE OF GENIC EVOLUTION THROUGH DUPLICATION (BY UNEQUAL
CROSSING OVER) AND SUBSEQUENT INDEPENDENT MUTATION HAS BEEN PROVIDED. TWO LOCI
INVOLVED IN HAPTOGLOBIN SYNTHESIS, ONE FOR ALPHA AND ONE FOR BETA CHAINS.
HAPTOGLOBIN VARIANTS WITH CHANGE IN ELECTROPHORETIC MOBILITY OF THE ALPHA
POLYPEPTIDE HAVE BEEN FOUND (GIBLETT, UCHIDA AND BROOKS, 1966), WHEREAS OTHERS,
THE *MARBURG* PHENOTYPES, HAVE ALTERATIONS IN THE BETA POLYPEPTIDE CHAIN (CLEVE

AND DEICHER, 1965). IN MAN AND SOME OTHER MAMMALS FREE HEME IS BOUND NOT BY HAPTOGLOBIN BUT BY ANOTHER PLASMA PROTEIN HEMOPEXIN. POLYMORPHISM OF THIS OTHER PROTEIN HAS BEEN SHOWN IN THE PIG (LUSH, 1966). FROM STUDY OF CASES OF RING CHROMOSOME 13 AND THEIR FAMILIES, BLOOM, GERALD AND REISMAN (1967) CONCLUDE THAT THE HAPTOGLOBIN ALPHA LOCUS MAY BE LOCATED NEAR ONE OR THE OTHER END OF CHROMOSOME 13. BLACK AND DIXON (1968) REPORTED THE AMINO ACID SEQUENCES OF THE ALPHA CHAINS OF HAPTOGLOBIN. THE FINDINGS CONFIRMED THE CONCLUSION THAT THE ALPHA(2) CHAIN AROSE THROUGH PARTIAL GENE DUPLICATION OF THE HP(1) LOCUS. ROBSON ET AL. (1969) PRESENTED EVIDENCE THAT THE ALPHA HAPTOGLOBIN LOCUS IS ON THE LONG ARM OF CHROMOSOME 16. IN A FAMILY WITH 46T(2G-*16G+) AND ONE WITH 46T(1-*16+) HAPTOGLO-BIN TYPE WAS LINKED WITH THE TRANSLOCATION CHROMOSOME. THE ALPHA (1F) AND ALPHA (1S) CHAINS DIFFER BY A SINGLE AMINO ACID* AT POSITION 54, LYSINE AND GLUTAMIC ACID, RESPECTIVELY, ARE PRESENT (BLACK AND DIXON, 1968). THE PRIMARY STRUCTURES OF THE ALPHA CHAIN AND OF LIGHT CHAINS OF GAMMA GLOBULINS BEAR SIMILARITIES AND THERE ARE FUNCTIONAL HOMOLOGIES SINCE BOTH FORM COMPLEXES WITH SPECIFIC PROTEINS. A COMMON EVOLUTIONARY ORIGIN IS POSTULATED.

BIAS, W. B. AND MIGECN, B. R.* HAPTOGLOBIN* A LOCUS ON THE D(1) CHROMOSOME.Q AM. J. HUM. GENET. 19* 393-398, 1967.

BLACK, J. A. AND DIXON, G. H.* AMINO-ACID SEQUENCE OF ALPHA CHAINS OF HUMAN HAPTOGLOBINS. NATURE 218* 736-741, 1968.

BLOOM, G. E., GERALD, P. S. AND REISMAN, L. E.* RING D CHROMOSOME* A SECOND CASE ASSOCIATED WITH ANOMALOUS HAPTOGLOBIN INHERITANCE. SCIENCE 156* 1746-1748, 1967.

CLEVE, H. AND DEICHER, H.* HAPTOGLOBIN *MARBURG* * UNTERSUCHUNGEN UBER EINE SELTENE ERBLICHE HAPTOGLOBIN-VARIANT MIT ZWEI VERSCHIEDENEN PHANOTYPEN INVERHALB EINER FAMILIE. HUMANGENETIK 1* 537-550, 1965.

GIBLETT, E. R., HICKMAN, G. C. AND SMITHIES, O.* VARIANT HAPTOGLOBIN PHENO-TYPES. COLD SPRING HARBOR SYMPOSIA QUANT. BIOL. 29* 321-326, 1964.

GIBLETT, E. R., UCHIDA, I. AND BROOKS, L. E.* TWO RARE HAPTOGLOBIN PHENOTYPES, 1-B AND 2-B, CONTAINING A PREVIOUSLY UNDESCRIBED ALPHA POLYPEPTIDE CHAIN. AM. J. HUM. GENET. 18* 448-453, 1966.

JAVID, J. AND YINGLING, W.* IMMUNOGENETICS OF HUMAN HAPTOGLOBINS. I. THE ANTIGENIC STRUCTURE OF NORMAL HP PHENOTYPES. J. CLIN. INVEST. 47* 2290-2296, 1968.

KIRK, R. L.* THE HAPTOGLOBIN GROUPS IN MAN. (MONOGRAPHS IN HUMAN GENETICS, VOL. 4) BASEL AND NEW YORK* S. KARGER, 1968.

LUSH, I. E.* THE BIOCHEMICAL GENETICS OF VERTEBRATES EXCEPT MAN. PHILADELPHIA* W. B. SAUNDERS, 1966.

MAGENIS, R. E., HECHT, F. AND LOVRIEN, E. W.* HERITABLE FRAGILE SITE ON CHROMOSOME 16* PROBABLE LOCALIZATION OF HAPTOGLOBIN LOCUS IN MAN. SCIENCE 170* 85-87, 1970.

ROBSON, E. B., POLANI, P. E., DART, S. J., JACOBS, P. A. AND RENWICK, J. H.* PROBABLE ASSIGNMENT OF THE ALPHA LOCUS OF HAPTOGLOBIN TO CHROMOSOME 16 IN MAN. NATURE 223* 1163-1165, 1969.

SMITHIES, O., CONNELL, G. E. AND DIXON, G. H.* CHROMOSOMAL REARRANGEMENTS AND THE EVOLUTION OF HAPTOGLOBIN GENES. NATURE 196* 232-236, 1962.

SMITHIES, O., CONNELL, G. E. AND DIXON, G. H.* INHERITANCE OF HAPTOGLOBIN SUBTYPES. AM. J. HUM. GENET. 14* 14-21, 1962.

SUTTON, H. E.* THE HAPTOGLOBINS. IN, STEINBERG, A. G. AND BEARN, A. G. (EDS.)* PROGRESS IN MEDICAL GENETICS, CHAPTER 6, VOL. 7, 1970. PP. 163-216.

SUTTON, H. E.* THE HAPTOGLOBINS. PROG. MED. GENET. 7* 163-216, 1970.

*14020 HAPTOGLOBIN, BETA LOCUS (BP)

JAVID (1967) DESCRIBED A GENETIC VARIANT OF THE HAPTOGLOBIN BETA POLYPEPTIDE CHAIN AND SUGGESTED THAT THE LOCUS BE CALLED BP (*BINDING PEPTIDE* SINCE THE BETA CHAIN BINDS HEMOGLOBIN), THE LONGER KNOWN UNLINKED LOCUS FOR THE ALPHA CHAIN BEING CALLED HP. HAPTOGLOBIN MARBURG IS ALSO A BETA CHAIN VARIANT. CLEVE ET AL. (1969) CONCLUDED THAT HAPTOGLOBIN MARBURG IS THE RESULT OF A MUTATIONAL EVENT OTHER THAN SINGLE BASE SUBSTITUTION. HAPTOGLOBIN P IS ANOTHER BETA VARIANT.

CLEVE, H., BOWMAN, B. H. AND GORDON, S.* BIOCHEMICAL CHARACTERIZATION OF THE BETA-CHAIN VARIANT HAPTOGLOBIN MARBURG. HUMANGENETIK 7* 337-343, 1969.

JAVID, J.* HAPTOGLOBIN 2-1 BELLEVUE, A HAPTOGLOBIN BETA-CHAIN MUTANT. PROC. NAT. ACAD. SCI. 57* 920-924, 1967.

14030 HASHIMOTO'S STRUMA

IN A FAMILY WITH SEVERAL CASES OF HASHIMOTO'S STRUMA, DE GROOT ET AL. (1962)
DEMONSTRATED AN ABNORMAL SMALL IODINATED PROTEIN IN THE SERUM AND SUGGESTED THAT A
DEFECT IN THYROID BASEMENT MEMBRANE MAY ACCOUNT FOR THE APPEARANCE OF THIS PROTEIN
IN THE BLOOD. THREE SIBS, THEIR FATHER AND THEIR PATERNAL AUNT WERE AFFECTED.
THE PATERNAL GRANDPARENTS WERE DEAD. HALL ET AL. (1962) PRESENTED DATA WHICH THEY
FELT SUPPORTED AUTOSOMAL DOMINANT INHERITANCE OF THE TENDENCY TO THYROID AUTOIM-
MUNITY. VOLPE ET AL. (1963) ALSO FOUND AN IMPRESSIVE FAMILIAL AGGREGATION.

DE GROOT, L. J., HALL, R., MCDERMOTT, W. V., JR. AND DAVIS, A. M.* HASHIMOTO'S
THYROIDITIS* A GENETICALLY CONDITIONED DISEASE. NEW ENG. J. MED. 267* 267-273,
1962.

HALL, R., SAXENA, K. M. AND OWEN, S. G.* A STUDY OF THE PARENTS OF PATIENTS
WITH HASHIMOTO'S DISEASE. LANCET 2* 1291-1292, 1962.

VOLPE, R., EZRIN, C., JOHNSTON, M. W. AND STEINER, J. W.* GENETIC FACTORS IN
HASHIMOTO'S STRUMA. CANAD. MED. ASS. J. 88* 915-919, 1963.

*14040 HEART BLOCK

ALTHOUGH MOST REPORTS OF CONGENITAL HEART BLOCK HAVE CONCERNED AFFECTED SIBS, TWO
GENERATIONS HAVE IN A FEW INSTANCES BEEN AFFECTED (FULTON ET AL., 1910* WALLGREN,
WINBLAD, 1937* WENDKOS, STUDY, 1947). IN THE FAMILY REPORTED BY GAZES ET AL.
(1965), CONDUCTION DISTURBANCES OCCURRED IN THREE AND PROBABLY A FOURTH GENERA-
TION. IN MOST OF THE AFFECTED PERSONS THE HEART BLOCK WAS OF SECOND DEGREE WITH
EPISODES OF THIRD DEGREE (COMPLETE) ATRIOVENTRICULAR DISSOCIATION, LEADING TO
ADAMS-STOKES SEIZURES. THE FAMILY OF WENDKOS AND STUDY (1947) CONSISTED OF A
FATHER WITH THE WOLFF-PARKINSON-WHITE SYNDROME AND TWO OFFSPRING WITH CONGENITAL
COMPLETE HEART BLOCK. IN THE FAMILY REPORTED BY FULTON ET AL. (1910) 3 TO 1 BLOCK
WAS THOUGHT TO BE PRESENT IN THE FATHER, COMPLETE BLOCK IN A 22 MONTH OLD SON AND
2 TO 1 BLOCK IN A 20 YEAR OLD DAUGHTER. AMATLLER-TRIAS ET AL. (1966) DESCRIBED
FATHER (AGE 43), SON (AGE 19) AND DAUGHTER (AGE 22) WITH FIRST DEGREE HEART BLOCK
(PROLONGED PR INTERVAL).

AMATLLER-TRIAS, A., PERIZ-SAGUE, A., LORAN-LLEO, J. A., AND OSES, H.* BLOQUEO
AURICULO-VENTRICULAR DE PRIMER GRADO DE TIPO FAMILIAR. MED. CLIN. 46* 27-34,
1966.

FULTON, Z. M. K., JUDSON, C. F. AND NORRIS, G. W.* CONGENITAL HEART BLOCK
OCCURRING IN A FATHER AND TWO CHILDREN, ONE AN INFANT. AM. J. MED. SCI. 140* 339-
348, 1910.

GAZES, P. C., CULLER, R. M., TABER, E. AND KELLY, T. E.* CONGENITAL FAMILIAL
CARDIAC CONDUCTION DEFECTS. CIRCULATION 32* 32-34, 1965.

WALLGREN, A. AND WINBLAD, S.* CONGENITAL HEART-BLOCK. ACTA PAEDIAT. 20* 175-
204, 1937.

WENDKOS, M. H. AND STUDY, R. S.* FAMILIAL CONGENITAL COMPLETE A-V HEART BLOCKS.
AM. HEART J. 34* 138-142, 1947.

14050 HEART, MALFORMATION OF

KOJIMA ET AL. (1969) DESCRIBED HYPOPLASTIC LEFT HEART SYNDROME IN SIBS. SUCH
FAMILIAL AGGREGATION IS TO BE EXPECTED FROM A MULTIFACTORIAL CAUSATION. NORA ET
AL. (1970) CONCLUDED THAT THE FREQUENCY OF CONGENITAL HEART MALFORMATIONS IN FIRST
DEGREE RELATIVES OF PROBANDS IS CLOSE TO THE SQUARE ROOT OF THE POPULATION
FREQUENCY, AS WAS SUGGESTED BY EDWARDS (1960) SHOULD BE THE CASE FOR A MULTIFAC-
TORIAL DISORDER.

EDWARDS, J. H.* SIMUTATION OF MENDELISM. ACTA GENET. 10* 63-70, 1960.

KOJIMA, H., OGIMI, Y., MIZUTANI, K. AND NISHIMURA, Y.* HYPOPLASTIC-LEFT-HEART
SYNDROME IN SIBLINGS. (LETTER) LANCET 2* 701 ONLY, 1969.

NORA, J. J., MCGILL, C. W. AND MCNAMARA, D. G.* EMPIRIC RECURRENCE RISKS IN
COMMON AND UNCOMMON CONGENITAL HEART LESIONS. TERATOLOGY 3* 325-330, 1970.

14060 HEBERDEN'S NODES

THESE ARE BONEY EXCRESCENCES OF THE PHALANGES OF THE DISTAL INTERPHALANGEAL JOINTS
OF THE FINGERS. THEY CAN BE CONSIDERED A VARIETY OF OSTEO-ARTHROSIS, OR DEGENERA-
TIVE ARTHRITIS. STECHER (1955) SUGGESTED THAT THE DISORDER IS SEX-INFLUENCED SO
THAT IT IS DOMINANT IN WOMEN AND RECESSIVE IN MALES. IT IS ALSO AGE-DEPENDENT,
WITH PENETRANCE COMPLETE AFTER 70. IN THE GENERAL POPULATION STECHER ESTIMATED
THAT 27 PERCENT ARE HETEROZYGOTES AND 3 PERCENT HOMOZYGOTES.

STECHER, R. M.* HEBERDEN'S NODES. A CLINICAL DESCRIPTION OF OSTEO-ARTHRITIS OF THE FINGER JOINTS. ANN. RHEUM. DIS. 14* 1-10, 1955.

D
O
M   14070 HEINZ BODY ANEMIA
I
N   THIS IS A FORM OF NON-SPHEROCYTIC HEMOLYTIC ANEMIA OF DACIE'S TYPE I (IN VITRO
A   AUTOHEMOLYSIS IS NOT CORRECTED BY ADDED GLUCOSE). AFTER SPLENECTOMY, WHICH HAS
N   LITTLE BENEFIT, BASOPHILIC INCLUSIONS CALLED HEINZ BODIES ARE DEMONSTRABLE IN THE
T   ERYTHROCYTES. BEFORE SPLENECTOMY DIFFUSE OR PUNCTATE BASOPHILIA MAY BE EVIDENT.
        MOST OR ALL OF THESE CASES ARE PROBABLY INSTANCES OF HEMOGLOBINOPATHY. THE
        HEMOGLOBIN DEMONSTRATES HEAT-LABILITY AND ELECTROPHORETIC HEMOGLOBIN ANOMALY HAS
        BEEN DEMONSTRATED IN SOME, E.G. HB TACOMA (Q.V.).

        DACIE, J. V., GRIMES, A. J., MEISLER, A., STEINGOLD, L., HEMSTED, E. H.,
        BEAVEN, G. H. AND WHITE, J. C.* HEREDITARY HEINZ-BODY ANAEMIA. A REPORT OF
        STUDIES ON FIVE PATIENTS WITH MILD ANAEMIA. BRIT. J. HAEMAT. 10* 388-402, 1964.

14080 HEMANGIOMAS

        NORWOOD AND EVERETT (1964) REPORTED THE REMARKABLE CASE OF A 21 YEAR OLD NEGRO
        FEMALE WHO DURING PREGNANCY DEVELOPED LARGE HEMANGIOMAS AT MANY SITES SUCH AS EAR
        LOBE AND AXILLA AND HEART FAILURE AS A RESULT. AFTER DELIVERY THE HEMANGIOMAS
        RAPIDLY SUBSIDED. THE PATIENT'S MOTHER AND 6 YEAR OLD SON HAD MACULAR HEMANGIOMAS
        OF THE FACE AND TRUNK AND HER BROTHER HAD CLASSICAL KLIPPEL-TRENAUNAY-WEBER
        SYNDROME OF THE RIGHT LOWER EXTREMITY. BEERS AND CLARK (1942) DESCRIBED A FAMILY
        WITH CUTANEOUS HEMANGIOMAS RANGING IN SIZE FROM A MILLIMETER TO MANY CENTIMETERS
        IN DIAMETER, IN 12 PERSONS IN 3 GENERATIONS. METATARSUS ATAVICUS (SECOND TOE
        LONGER THAN THE FIRST TOE) WAS AN INDEPENDENT DOMINANT TRAIT IN THIS FAMILY. (SEE
        TOES, RELATIVE LENGTH OF 1ST AND 2ND.)

        BEERS, C. V. AND CLARK, L. A.* TUMORS AND SHORT-TOE - A DIHYBRID PEDIGREE. A
        FAMILY HISTORY SHOWING THE INHERITANCE OF HEMANGIOMA AND METATARSUS ATAVICUS. J.
        HERED. 33* 366-368, 1942.

        NORWOOD, O. T. AND EVERETT, M. A.* CARDIAC FAILURE DUE TO ENDOCRINE DEPENDENT
        HEMANGIOMAS. ARCH. DERM. 89* 759-760, 1964.

14090 HEMANGIOMAS OF SMALL INTESTINE

        BANDLER (1960) REPORTED A FAMILY IN THREE GENERATIONS OF WHICH THERE WERE 3 PROVED
        AND TWO POSSIBLE INSTANCES OF CAVERNOUS HEMANGIOMA INVOLVING ALMOST THE ENTIRE
        SMALL INTESTINE. ONE PATIENT HAD MUCOCUTANEOUS PIGMENT SPOTS PRECISELY LIKE THOSE
        OF THE PEUTZ-JEGHERS SYNDROME. SEE BLUE RUBBER NEVUS SYNDROME.

        BANDLER, M.* HEMANGIOMAS OF THE SMALL INTESTINE ASSOCIATED WITH MUCOCUTANEOUS
        PIGMENTATION. GASTROENTEROLOGY 38* 641-645, 1960.

14100 HEMANGIOMA-THROMBOCYTOPENIA SYNDROME (KASSABACH-MERRITT SYNDROME)

        WITH GIANT HEMANGIOMAS IN SMALL CHILDREN, THROMBOCYTOPENIA AND RED CELL CHANGES
        COMPATIBLE WITH TRAUMA ('MICROANGIOPATHIC HEMOLYTIC ANEMIA') HAVE BEEN OBSERVED.
        THE MECHANISM OF THE HEMATOLOGIC CHANGES IS OBSCURE. NO EVIDENCE OF A SIMPLE
        GENETIC BASIS HAS BEEN DISCOVERED.

        BRIZEL, H. E. AND RACCUGLIA, G.* GIANT HEMANGIOMA WITH THROMBOCYTOPENIA.
        RADIOISOTOPIC DEMONSTRATION OF PLATELET SEQUESTRATION. BLOOD 26* 751-756, 1965.

        PROPP, R. P. AND SCHARFMAN, W. B.* HEMANGIOMA-THROMBOCYTOPENIA SYNDROME
        ASSOCIATED WITH MICROANGIOPATHIC HEMOLYTIC ANEMIA. BLOOD 28* 623-633, 1966.

        RODRIGUEZ-ERDMANN, F., MURRAY, J. E. AND MOLONEY, W. C.* CONSUMPTION COAGULOPA-
        THY IN KASSABACH-MERRITT SYNDROME. TRANS. ASS. AM. PHYS., 1970.

14110 HEMANGIOMATOSIS, DISSEMINATED

        BURKE ET AL. (1964) DESCRIBED TWO UNRELATED INFANTS WITH A LARGE NUMBER OF SMALL
        HEMANGIOMATA IN MANY AREAS OF THE SKIN AND ALSO IN THE BRAIN. NOTHING IS KNOWN OF
        A POSSIBLE GENETIC BASIS OF THESE.

        BURKE, E. C., WINKELMANN, R. K. AND STRICKLAND, M. K.* DISSEMINATED HEMANGIOMA-
        TOSIS. THE NEWBORN WITH CENTRAL NERVOUS SYSTEM INVOLVEMENT. AM. J. DIS. CHILD.
        108* 418-424, 1964.

14120 HEMATURIA, BENIGN FAMILIAL

        MCCONVILLE, WEST AND MCADAMS (1966) DESCRIBED DOMINANT INHERITANCE OF BENIGN
        FAMILIAL HEMATURIA. A CHEMICAL TEST FOR HEMATURIA (PAPER STRIPS IMPREGNATED AT
        ONE END WITH ORTHOTOLUIDINE WHICH IN THE PRESENCE OF HEMOGLOBIN IS OXIDIZED TO
        YIELD A BLUE COLOR) WAS USED. THE DISORDER IS A NON-PROGRESSIVE CONDITION NOT
        ASSOCIATED WITH OTHER ABNORMALITIES SUCH AS DEAFNESS (SEE ALPORT'S SYNDROME).
        EARLIER REPORTS MAY HAVE INCLUDED SOME PATIENTS OF THIS TYPE (E.G., LIVADITIS AND
        ERICSSON, 1962* AYOUB AND VERNIER, 1965).

AYOUB, E. M. AND VERNIER, R. L.* BENIGN RECURRENT HEMATURIA. AM. J. DIS. CHILD. 109* 217-223, 1965.

LIVADITIS, A. AND ERICSSON, N. O.* ESSENTIAL HEMATURIA IN CHILDREN* PROGNOSTIC ASPECTS. ACTA PAEDIAT. 51* 630-634, 1962.

MCCONVILLE, J. M., WEST, C. D. AND MCADAMS, A. J.* FAMILIAL AND NON-FAMILIAL BENIGN HEMATURIA. J. PEDIAT. 69* 207-214, 1966.

14130 HEMIFACIAL ATROPHY, PROGRESSIVE (PARRY-ROMBERG SYNDROME)

THIS SYNDROME DESCRIBED IN THE LAST CENTURY BY PARRY (1825) AND ROMBERG (1846) CONSISTS OF SLOWLY PROGRESSIVE ATROPHY OF THE SOFT TISSUES OF ESSENTIALLY HALF THE FACE ACCOMPANIED USUALLY BY CONTRALATERAL JACKSONIAN EPILEPSY, TRIGEMINAL NEURALGIA AND CHANGES IN THE EYES AND HAIR (WALSH, 1939* WARTENBERG, 1945). THE NUMBER OF FAMILIAL CASES IS SMALL BUT AUTOSOMAL DOMINANCE WITH REDUCED PENETRANCE IS POSSIBLE.

FRANCESCHETTI, A. AND KOENIG, H.* L'IMPORTANCE DU FACTEUR HEREDO-DEGENERATIF DANS L'HEMIATROPHIE FACIALE PROGRESSIVE (ROMBERG). ETUDE DES COMPLICATIONS OCULAIRES DANS CE SYNDROME. J. GENET. HUM. 1* 27-64, 1952.

KLINGMANN, T.* FACIAL HEMIATROPHY. J.A.M.A. 49* 1888-1891, 1907.

WALSH, F. B.* FACIAL HEMIATROPHY* REPORT OF 2 CASES. AM. J. OPHTHAL. 22* 1-10, 1939.

WARTENBERG, R.* PROGRESSIVE FACIAL HEMIATROPHY. ARCH. NEUROL. PSYCHIAT. 54* 75-96, 1945.

14140 HEMIFACIAL MICROSOMIA

THE LEFT SIDE OF THE FACE IS AFFECTED IN A MAJORITY OF CASES (GORLIN AND PINDBORG, 1964).

GORLIN, R. J. AND PINDBORG, J. J.* SYNDROMES OF THE HEAD AND NECK. NEW YORK* MCGRAW-HILL, 1964. P. 261 FF.

14150 HEMIPLEGIC MIGRAINE, FAMILIAL

ROSENBAUM (1960) DESCRIBED A FAMILY. VASOCONSTRICTION, FOLLOWED BY FOCAL EDEMA, IS THOUGHT TO BE RESPONSIBLE FOR THE NEUROLOGIC MANIFESTATIONS. OHTA ET AL. (1967) DESCRIBED FOUR CASES IN THREE GENERATIONS AND ADDED A 'NEW' FEATURE, PERSISTENT CEREBELLAR MANIFESTATIONS. YOUNG ET AL. (1970) COMMENTED ON THE OCCURRENCE OF HEMIPLEGIC AND ORDINARY MIGRAINE IN THE SAME FAMILY, SUGGESTING THAT THEY ARE BASICALLY THE SAME ENTITY. SEE MIGRAINE.

BLAU, J. N. AND WHITTY, C. W. M.* FAMILIAL HEMIPLEGIC MIGRAINE. LANCET 2* 1115-1116, 1955.

OHTA, M., ARAKI, S. AND KUROIWA, Y.* FAMILIAL OCCURRENCE OF MIGRAINE WITH A HEMIPLEGIC SYNDROME AND CEREBELLAR MANIFESTATIONS. NEUROLOGY 17* 813-817, 1967.

ROSENBAUM, H. E.* FAMILIAL HEMIPLEGIC MIGRAINE. NEUROLOGY 10* 164-170, 1960.

YOUNG, G. F., LEON-BARTH, C. A. AND GREEN, J.* FAMILIAL HEMIPLEGIC MIGRAINE, RETINAL DEGENERATION, DEAFNESS, AND NYSTAGMUS. ARCH. NEUROL. 23* 201-209, 1970.

*14160 HEMOCHROMATOSIS

BOTHWELL AND COLLEAGUES (1959), DEBRE AND COLLEAGUES (1958) AND SEVERAL OTHERS HAVE CONCLUDED THAT ONE FORM OF HEMOCHROMATOSIS IS INHERITED AS AN AUTOSOMAL DOMINANT WITH INCOMPLETE PENETRANCE IN FEMALES BECAUSE OF LOSS OF BLOOD IN MENSTRUATION AND PREGNANCY. FEATURES OF THE DISEASE INCLUDE CIRRHOSIS OF THE LIVER, DIABETES, HYPERMELANOTIC PIGMENTATION OF THE SKIN AND HEART FAILURE. ELEVATED SERUM IRON IS A DIAGNOSTICALLY VALUABLE FINDING WHICH CAN BE SOUGHT IN RELATIVES OF FULL-BLOWN CASES. PROPHYLACTIC VENESECTION IS INDICATED.

BALCERZAK, S. P., WESTERMAN, M. P., LEE, R. E. AND DOYLE, A. P.* IDIOPATHIC HEMOCHROMATOSIS. A STUDY OF THREE FAMILIES. AM. J. MED. 40* 857-873, 1966.

BOTHWELL, T. H., COHEN, I., ABRAHAMS, O. L. AND PEROLD, S. M.* A FAMILIAL STUDY IN IDIOPATHIC HEMOCHROMATOSIS. AM. J. MED. 27* 730-738, 1959.

DEBRE, R., DREYFUS, J.-C., FREZAL, J., LABIE, D., LAMY, M., MAROTEAUX, P., SCHAPIRA, F. AND SCHAPIRA, G.* GENETICS OF HAEMOCHROMATOSIS. ANN. HUM. GENET. 23* 16-30, 1958.

JOHNSON, G. B., JR. AND FREY, W. G., III* FAMILIAL ASPECTS OF IDIOPATHIC HEMOCHROMATOSIS. J.A.M.A. 179* 747-751, 1962.

POLLYCOVE, M.* HEMOCHROMATOSIS. IN, STANBURY, J. B., WYNGAARDEN, J. B. AND

112   FREDRICKSON, D. S. (EDS.)* THE METABOLIC BASIS OF INHERITED DISEASE. NEW YORK*
MCGRAW-HILL, 1966 (2ND ED.). PP. 780-810.

D
O
M
I
N
A
N
T
WILLIAMS, R., SCHEUER, P. J. AND SHERLOCK, S.* THE INHERITANCE OF IDIOPATHIC
HAEMOCHROMATOSIS. QUART. J. MED. 31* 249-265, 1962.

14170 HEMOGLOBIN (5 LOCI - ALPHA, BETA, GAMMA, DELTA, EPSILON)

ACTUALLY EVIDENCE OF TWO SEPARATE GAMMA LOCI HAS BEEN PRESENTED BY SCHROEDER ET
AL. (1968) AND THE FINDINGS ON HEMOGLOBIN PORTLAND-1 (Q.V.) MAY INDICATE THE
PRESENCE OF ANOTHER LOCUS OF THE ALPHA CHAIN TYPE. THE BETA AND DELTA LOCI ARE
CLOSELY LINKED, PERHAPS ADJACENT.   SINCE THE BETA AND GAMMA LOCI ARE CLOSELY
LINKED IN THE MOUSE (GILMAN AND SMITHIES, 1968), THEY MAY BE ALSO IN MAN.

BAGLIONI, C.* CORRELATIONS BETWEEN GENETICS AND CHEMISTRY OF HUMAN HEMOGLOBINS.
IN, J. H. TAYLOR (ED.)* MOLECULAR GENETICS. NEW YORK AND LONDON* ACADEMIC PRESS,
1963. PP. 405-475.

DAYHOFF, M. O. AND ECK, R. V.* ATLAS OF PROTEIN SEQUENCE AND STRUCTURE 1967-68.
SILVER SPRING, MD.* NATIONAL BIOMED. RES. FOUND. (2ND ED.), 1968.

GAMMACK, D. B., HUEHNS, E. R., LEHMANN, H. AND SHOOTER, E. M.* THE ABNORMAL
POLYPEPTIDE CHAINS IN A NUMBER OF HAEMOGLOBIN VARIANTS. ACTA GENET. STATIST. MED.
11* 1-16, 1961.

GILMAN, J. G. AND SMITHIES, O.* FETAL HEMOGLOBIN VARIANTS IN MICE. SCIENCE
160* 885-886, 1968.

HUEHNS, E. R. AND SHOOTER, E. M.* HAEMOGLOBIN. SCI. PROGR. 52* 353-374, 1964.

HUEHNS, E. R. AND SHOOTER, E. M.* HUMAN HAEMOGLOBINS. J. MED. GENET. 2* 48-90,
1965.

HUISMAN, T. H. J.* NORMAL AND ABNORMAL HUMAN HEMOGLOBINS. ADVANCES CLIN. CHEM.
6* 231-261, 1963.

JONXIS, J. H. P. AND DELAFRESNAYE, J. F. (EDS.)* ABNORMAL HAEMOGLOBINS.
OXFORD* BLACKWELL, 1959.

LEHMANN, H. AND BETKE, K. (EDS.)* HAEMOGLOBIN-COLOQUIUM. STUTTGART* GEORG
THIEME VERLAG, 1962.

LEHMANN, H. AND HUNTSMAN, R. G.* MAN*S HEMOGLOBINS. PHILADELPHIA* LIPPINCOTT,
1966.

PERUTZ, M. F. AND LEHMANN, H.* MOLECULAR PATHOLOGY OF HUMAN HAEMOGLOBIN.
NATURE 219* 902-909, 1968.

RANNEY, H. M.* CLINICALLY IMPORTANT VARIANTS OF HUMAN HEMOGLOBIN. NEW ENG. J.
MED. 282* 144-152, 1970.

SCHROEDER, W. A., HUISMAN, T. H. J., SHELTON, J. R., SHELTON, J. B., KLEIHAUER,
E. F., DOZY, A. M. AND ROBBERSON, B.* EVIDENCE FOR MULTIPLE STRUCTURAL GENES FOR
THE GAMMA CHAIN OF HUMAN FETAL HEMOGLOBIN. PROC. NAT. ACAD. SCI. 60* 537-544,
1968.

SCHROEDER, W. A. AND JONES, R. T.* SOME ASPECTS OF THE CHEMISTRY AND FUNCTION
OF HUMAN AND ANIMAL HEMOGLOBINS. FORTSCHR. CHEM. ORGAN. NATURST. 23* 113-194,
1965.

THE FOLLOWING IS THE AMINO ACID SEQUENCE OF THE ALPHA, BETA, GAMMA AND DELTA
CHAINS OF HEMOGLOBIN, STARTING WITH THE -NH2 END OF THE CHAINS. THE ALPHA CHAIN
HAS 141 AMINO ACID RESIDUES AND THE BETA, GAMMA, AND DELTA CHAINS 146. THE
MEANING OF THE THREE LETTER DESIGNATIONS OF THE AMINO ACIDS IS ALSO GIVEN BELOW.
WHEN A STATEMENT SUCH AS *SUBSTITUTION OF VALINE AT BETA 6* APPEARS IN THE
DESCRIPTION OF VARIANT HEMOGLOBINS, THE CHART BELOW WILL INDICATE WHAT AMINO ACID
HAS BEEN REPLACED.

THE ALPHA, BETA, GAMMA AND DELTA CHAINS OF NORMAL HUMAN HEMOGLOBINS

```
         1    2   3   4   5   6   7   8   9  10  11  12  13  14

ALPHA   VAL-   -LEU-SER-PRO-ALA-ASP-LYS-THR-ASN-VAL-LYS-ALA-ALA-TRP-

BETA    VAL-HIS-LEU-THR-PRO-GLU-GLU-LYS-SER-ALA-VAL-THR-ALA-LEU-TRP-
GAMMA   GLY-HIS-PHE-THR-GLU-GLU-ASP-LYS-ALA-THR-ILE-THR-SER-LEU-TRP-
DELTA   VAL-HIS-LEU-THR-PRO-GLU-GLU-LYS-THR-ALA-VAL-ASN-ALA-LEU-TRP-

         1   2   3   4   5   6   7   8   9  10  11  12  13  14  15
```

```
 15   16   17   18   19   20   21   22   23   24   25   26   27   28   29   30   31

GLY-LYS-VAL-GLY-ALA-HIS-ALA-GLY-GLU-TYR-GLY-ALA-GLU-ALA-LEU-GLU-ARG-

GLY-LYS-VAL-ASN-  -   -VAL-ASP-GLU-VAL-GLY-GLY-GLU-ALA-LEU-GLY-ARG-
GLY-LYS-VAL-ASN-  -   -VAL-GLU-ASP-ALA-GLY-GLY-GLU-THR-LEU-GLY-ARG-
GLY-LYS-VAL-ASN-  -   -VAL-ASP-ALA-VAL-GLY-GLY-GLU-ALA-LEU-GLY-ARG-

 16   17   18   19             20   21   22   23   24   25   26   27   28   29   30
```

```
 32   33   34   35   36   37   38   39   40   41   42   43   44   45   46        47

MET-PHE-LEU-SER-PHE-PRO-THR-THR-LYS-THR-TYR-PHE-PRO-HIS-PHE-    -ASP-

LEU-LEU-VAL-VAL-TYR-PRO-TRP-THR-GLN-ARG-PHE-PHE-GLU-SER-PHE-GLY-ASP-
LEU-LEU-VAL-VAL-TYR-PRO-TRP-THR-GLN-ARG-PHE-PHE-ASP-SER-PHE-GLY-ASN-
LEU-LEU-VAL-VAL-TYR-PRO-TRP-THR-GLN-ARG-PHE-PHE-GLU-SER-PHE-GLY-ASP-

 31   32   33   34   35   36   37   38   39   40   41   42   43   44   45   46   47
```

```
 48   49   50   51   52   53                       54   55   56   57   58   59

LEU-SER-HIS-GLY-SER-ALA-   -    -    -    -   -GLN-VAL-LYS-GLY-HIS-GLY-

LEU-SER-THR-PRO-ASP-ALA-VAL-MET-GLY-ASN-PRO-LYS-VAL-LYS-ALA-HIS-GLY-
LEU-SER-SER-ALA-SER-ALA-ILE-MET-GLY-ASN-PRO-LYS-VAL-LYS-ALA-HIS-GLY-
LEU-SER-SER-PRO-ASP-ALA-VAL-MET-GLY-ASN-PRO-LYS-VAL-LYS-ALA-HIS-GLY-

 48   49   50   51   52   53   54   55   56   57   58   59   60   61   62   63   64
```

```
 60   61   62   63   64   65   66   67   68   69   70   71   72   73   74   75   76

LYS-LYS-VAL-ALA-ASP-ALA-LEU-THR-ASN-ALA-VAL-ALA-HIS-VAL-ASP-ASP-MET-

LYS-LYS-VAL-LEU-GLY-ALA-PHE-SER-ASP-GLY-LEU-ALA-HIS-LEU-ASP-ASN-LEU-
LYS-LYS-VAL-LEU-THR-SER-LEU-GLY-ASP-ALA-LLE-LYS-HIS-LEU-ASP-ASP-LEU-
LYS-LYS-VAL-LEU-GLY-ALA-PHE-SER-ASP-GLY-LEU-ALA-HIS-LEU-ASP-ASN-LEU-

 65   66   67   68   69   70   71   72   73   74   75   76   77   78   79   80   81
```

```
 77   78   79   80   81   82   83   84   85   86   87   88   89   90   91   92   93

PRO-ASN-ALA-LEU-SER-ALA-LEU-SER-ASP-LEU-HIS-ALA-HIS-LYS-LEU-ARG-VAL-

LYS-GLY-THR-PHE-ALA-THR-LEU-SER-GLU-LEU-HIS-CYS-ASP-LYS-LEU-HIS-VAL-
LYS-GLY-THR-PHE-ALA-GLN-LEU-SER-GLU-LEU-HIS-CYS-ASP-LYS-LEU-HIS-VAL-
LYS-GLY-THR-PHE-ALA-THR-LEU-SER-GLU-LEU-HIS-CYS-ASP-LYS-LEU-HIS-VAL-

 82   83   84   85   86   87   88   89   90   91   92   93   94   95   96   97   98
```

```
 94   95   96   97   98   99  100  101  102  103  104  105  106  107  108  109  110

ASP-PRO-VAL-ASN-PHE-LYS-LEU-LEU-SER-HIS-CYS-LEU-LEU-VAL-THR-LEU-ALA-

ASP-PRO-GLU-ASN-PHE-ARG-LEU-LEU-GLY-ASN-VAL-LEU-VAL-CYS-VAL-LEU-ALA-
ASP-PRO-GLU-ASN-PHE-LYS-LEU-LEU-GLY-ASN-VAL-LEU-VAL-THR-VAL-LEU-ALA-
ASP-PRO-GLU-ASN-PHE-ARO-LEU-LEU-GLY-ASN-VAL-LEU-VAL-CYS-VAL-LEU-ALA-

 99  100  101  102  103  104  105  106  107  108  109  110  111  112  113  114  115
```

```
111  112  113  114  115  116  117  118  119  120  121  122  123  124  125  126  127

ALA-HIS-LEU-PRO-ALA-GLU-PHE-THR-PRO-ALA-VAL-HIS-ALA-SER-LEU-ASP-LYS-

HIS-HIS-PHE-GLY-LYS-GLU-PHE-THR-PRO-PRO-VAL-GLN-ALA-ALA-TYR-GLN-LYS-
ILE-HIS-PHE-GLY-LYS-GLU-PHE-THR-PRO-GLU-VAL-GLN-ALA-SER-TRP-GLN-LYS-
ARG-ASN-PHE-GLY-LYS-GLU-PHE-THR-PRO-GLN-MET-GLN-ALA-ALA-TYR-GLN-LYS-

116  117  118  119  120  121  122  123  124  125  126  127  128  129  130  131  132
```

```
128  129  130  131  132  133  134  135  136  137  138  139  140  141

PHE-LEU-ALA-SER-VAL-SER-THR-VAL-LEU-THR-SER-LYS-TYR-ARG
```

```
        VAL-VAL-ALA-GLY-VAL-ALA-ASN-ALA-LEU-ALA-HIS-LYS-TYR-HIS
        MET-VAL-THR-GLY-VAL-ALA-SER-ALA-LEU-SER-SER-ARG-TYR-HIS
        VAL-VAL-ALA-GLY-VAL-ALA-ASN-ALA-LEU-ALA-HIS-LYS-TRP-HIS
```

D
O
M
I
N
A
N
T

```
        133 134 135 136 137 138 139 140 141 142 143 144 145 146
```

```
        ALA - ALANINE
        ARG - ARGININE
        ASN - ASPARAGINE
        ASP - ASPARTIC ACID
        CYS - ONE HALF CYSTINE, CYSTEINE
        GLN - GLUTAMINE
        GLU - GLUTAMIC ACID
        GLY - GLYCINE
        HIS - HISTIDINE
        ILE - ISOLEUCINE
        LEU - LEUCINE
        LYS - LYSINE
        MET - METHIONINE
        NIL - AMINO ACID DELETED
        PHE - PHENYLALNINE
        PRO - PROLINE
        SER - SERINE
        THR - THREONINE
        TRP - TRYPTCPHANE
        TYR - TYROSINE
        VAL - VALINE
```

THE BASE SEQUENCES OF THE DNA GENETIC CODE (AS PRESENTLY UNDERSTOOD) IS
GIVEN IN THE FOLLOWING TABLE. FROM IT THE MUTATION RESPONSIBLE FOR EACH
SUBSTITUTION CAN BE DEDUCED.

THE BASE SEQUENCES OF CODING TRIPLETS IN RNA

	U	C	A	G
U	UUU, UUC — PHE UUA, UUG — LEU	UCU, UCC, UCA, UCG — SER	UAU, UAC — TYR UAA ---* UAG ---*	UGU, UGC — CYS UGA ---+ UGG — TRP
C	CUU, CUC, CUA, CUG — LEU	CCU, CCC, CCA, CCG — PRO	CAU, CAC — HIS CAA, CAG — GLN	CGU, CGC, CGA, CGG — ARG
A	AUU, AUC, AUA — ILE AUG — MET	ACU, ACC, ACA, ACG — THR	AAU, AAC — ASN AAA, AAG — LYS	AGU, AGC — SER AGA, AGG — ARG
G	GUU, GUC, GUA, GUG — VAL	GCU, GCC, GCA, GCG — ALA	GAU, GAC — ASP GAA, GAG — GLU	GGU, GGC, GGA, GGG — GLY

* UAA AND UAG ARE OCHRE AND AMBER, RESPECTIVELY. THEY ARE BOTH
NONSENSE AND MAY BE TERMINATION PUNCTUATION. THE CODE IS RE-
VIEWED BY CRICK, SCIENTIFIC, AMERICAN, OCTOBER, 1966.

+ CRICK (NATURE, FEB. 4, 1967) CLAIMS UGA IS NONSENSE. IT MAY
BE A "SPACER" BETWEEN CISTRONS IN A POLYCISTRONIC MESSAGE.

--HEMOGLOBIN A(2) INDONESIA.

ENG, L. I. L., PRIBADI, W., WESTENDORP-BOERMA, F., EFREMOV, G. D., WILSON, J.
B., REYNOLDS, C. A. AND HUISMAN, T. H. J.* HEMOGLOBIN A(2)-INDONESIA OR A(2) B(2)
69(E13)GLY TO ARG(BBA 35755). BIOCHEM. BIOPHYS. ACTA 229* 335-342, 1971.

--HEMOGLOBIN A(2)PRIME, OR B(2).
    SUBSTITUTION OF ARGININE FOR GLYCINE AT DELTA 16.

BALL, E. W., MEYNELL, M. J., BEALE, D., KYNOCH, P., LEHMANN, H. AND STRELTON,
A. O. W.* HAEMOGLOBIN A(2) PRIME* ALPHA 2 GAMMA 2 (16 GLYCINE TO ARGININE).
NATURE 209* 1217-1218, 1966.

HORTON, B., PAYNE, R. A., BRIDGES, M. T. AND HUISMAN, T. H.* STUDIES ON AN
ABNORMAL MINOR HEMOGLOBIN COMPONENT HB-B(2). CLIN. CHIM. ACTA 6* 246-253, 1961.

VELLA, F. AND GRAHAM, B.* A VARIANT OF HEMOGLOBIN A(2) IN ALBERTA INDIANAS.
CLIN. BIOCHEM. 2* 455-460, 1969.

--HEMOGLOBIN AEGINA.
    POSSIBLY ABNORMAL GAMMA CHAIN. FAST HEMOGLOBIN.

FESSAS, P., KARAKLIS, A. AND GNAFAKIS, N.* A FURTHER ABNORMALITY OF FOETAL
HAEMOGLOBIN. ACTA HAEMAT. 25* 62-70, 1961.

--HEMOGLOBIN AGENOGI.
    SUBSTITUTION OF LYSINE FOR GLUTAMIC ACID AT BETA 90.

MIYAJI, T., SUZUKI, H., OHBA, Y. AND SHIBATA, S.* HEMOGLOBIN AGENOGI (ALPHA-2
BETA-2 90 LYS), A SLOW-MOVING HEMOGLOBIN OF A JAPANESE FAMILY RESEMBLING HEMOGLO-
BIN E. CLIN. CHIM. ACTA 14* 624-629, 1966.

--HEMOGLOBIN ALEXANDRA.
    ABNORMAL GAMMA CHAIN.   SEE HEMOGLOBIN F(ALEXANDRA). SUBSTITUTION OF LYSINE FOR
    THREONINE AT GAMMA 12.

FESSAS, P., MASTROKALOS, N. AND FOSTIROPOULOS, G.* NEW VARIANT OF HUMAN FOETAL
HAEMOGLOBIN. NATURE 183* 30-31, 1959.

LOUKOPOULOS, D., KALTSOYA, A. AND FESSAS, P.* ON THE CHEMICAL ABNORMALITY OF HB
'ALEXANDRA,' A FETAL HEMOGLOBIN VARIANT. BLOOD 33* 114-118, 1969.

--HEMOGLOBIN ALLEGRE.
    THIS HEMOGLOBIN MAY HAVE AN OCTOMERIC MOLECULE.

--HEMOGLOBIN ANN ARBOR.
    SUBSTITUTION OF ARGININE FOR LEUCINE AT ALPHA 80.

RUCKNAGEL, D. L.* TO BE PUBLISHED.

--HEMOGLOBIN ATAGO.
    SUBSTITUTION OF TYROSINE FOR ASPARTIC ACID AT ALPHA 85.

FUJIWARO, N.* AN AMINO ACID SUBSTITUTION IN HB ATAGO, AN ABNORMAL HUMAN
HEMOGLOBIN. SEIKAGAKU 42 (NO. 7)* 15-23, 1970.

--HEMOGLOBIN ATWATER ET AL.
    DEFECT UNKNOWN. FAST HEMOGLOBIN.

ATWATER, J., BAGLIONI, C. AND TOCANTINS, L. M.* A VARIETY OF HUMAN HEMOGLOBIN
WITH A 'FAST' COMPONENT, BUT UNALTERED TRYPTIC DIGEST 'FINGERPRINT.' PROC. 9TH
CONGR. INTERN. SOC. HEMATOL., MEXICO CITY, 1962. PP. 115-119.

--HEMOGLOBIN AUGUSTA-1.
    POSSIBLE TETRAMER OF S-BETA CHAIN. FAST HEMOGLOBIN.

HUISMAN, T. H. J.* PROPERTIES AND INHERITANCE OF THE NEW FAST HEMOGLOBIN TYPE
FOUND IN UMBILICAL CORD BLOOD SAMPLES OF NEGRO BABIES. CLIN. CHIM. ACTA 5* 709-
718, 1960.

LABIE, D., SCHROEDER, W. A. AND HUISMAN, T. H. J.* THE AMINO ACID SEQUENCE OF
THE DELTA-BETA CHAINS OF HEMOGLOBIN LEPORE AUGUSTA - LEPORE WASHINGTON. BIOCHIM.
BIOPHYS. ACTA 127* 428-437, 1966.

--HEMOGLOBIN AUGUSTA-2.
    POSSIBLE TETRAMER OF C-BETA CHAIN. FAST HEMOGLOBIN.

HUISMAN, T. H. J.* GENETIC ASPECTS OF TWO DIFFERENT MINOR HAEMOGLOBIN COM-
PONENTS FOUND IN CORD BLOOD SAMPLES OF NEGRO BABIES. NATURE 188* 589-590, 1960.

--HEMOGLOBIN BABINGA.
    SUBSTITUTION OF ASPARTIC ACID FOR GLYCINE AT DELTA 136.

DOMINANT

DE JONG, W. W. W. AND BERNINI, L. F.* HAEMOGLOBIN BABINGA (DELTA 136 GLYCINE-
ASPARTIC ACID)* A NEW DELTA CHAIN VARIANT. NATURE 219* 1360-1362, 1968.

--HEMOGLOBIN BART'S.
TETRAMER OF GAMMA CHAIN. FAST HEMOGLOBIN.

AGER, J. A. M. AND LEHMANN, H.* OBSERVATIONS ON SOME 'FAST' HAEMOGLOBINS* K, J,
N AND BART'S. BRIT. MED. J. 1* 929-931, 1958.

HUNT, J. A. AND LEHMANN, H.* HAEMOGLOBIN BART'S* A FOETAL HAEMOGLOBIN WITHOUT
ALPHA CHAINS. NATURE 184* 872-873, 1959.

--HEMOGLOBIN BEILINSON.
MAY HAVE SUBSTITUTION OF GLYCINE FOR ASPARTIC ACID AT ALPHA 47. THE CHANGE IS IN
TP IV.

DE VRIES, A., JOSHUA, H., LEHMANN, H., HILL, R. L. AND FELLOWS, R. E.* THE
FIRST OBSERVATION OF AN ABNORMAL HAEMOGLOBIN IN A JEWISH FAMILY. HAEMOGLOBIN
BEILINSON. BRIT. J. HAEMAT. 9* 484-486, 1963.

--HEMOGLOBIN BIBBA.
SUBSTITUTION OF PROLINE FOR LEUCINE AT ALPHA 136.

KLEIHAUER, E. F., REYNOLDS, C. A., DOZY, A. M., WILSON, J. B., MOORES, R. R.,
BERENSON, M. P., WRIGHT, C. S. AND HUISMAN, T. H. J.* HEMOGLOBIN BIBBA OR
ALPHA(2)136 PRO BETA(2), AN UNSTABLE ALPHA CHAIN ABNORMAL HEMOGLOBIN. BIOCHEM.
BIOPHYS. ACTA 154* 220-221, 1968.

--HEMOGLOBIN BORAS.
SUBSTITUTION OF ARGININE FOR LEUCINE AT BETA 88.

HOLLENDER, A., LORKIN, P. A., LEHMANN, H. AND SVENSSON, B.* NEW UNSTABLE
HAEMOGLOBIN BORAS* BETA 88 (F4) LEUCINE-ARGININE. NATURE 222* 953-955, 1969.

--HEMOGLOBIN BRISTOL.
SUBSTITUTION OF ASPARATIC ACID FOR VALINE AT BETA 67.

STEADMAN, J. H., YATES, A. AND HUEHNS, E. R.* IDIOPATHIC HEINZ BODY ANAEMIA*
HB-BRISTOL (BETA 67 (E 11) VAL-TO-ASP). BRIT. J. HAEMAT. 18* 435-446, 1970.

--HEMOGLOBIN BRISTOL-SINGAPORE.
POSSIBLY ABNORMAL GAMMA CHAIN. FAST HEMOGLOBIN.

RAPER, A. B., AGER, J. A. M. AND LEHMANN, H.* HAEMOGLOBIN 'SINGAPORE-BRISTOL.'
A 'FAST' HAEMOGLOBIN FOUND IN INFANTS. BRIT. MED. J. 1* 1537-1539, 1960.

--HEMOGLOBIN BROUSSAIS.
SUBSTITUTION OF ASPARAGINE FOR LYSINE AT ALPHA 90.

TRAVERSE, P. M., LEHMANN, H., COQUELET, M. L., BEALE, D. AND ISAACS, W. A.*
ETUDE D'UNE HEMOGLOBINE J-ALPHA NON ENCORE DECRITE, DANS UNE FAMILLE FRANCAISE.
C. R. SEANC. SOC. BIOL. 160* 2270-2272, 1966.

VELLA, F., CHARLESWORTH, D., LORKIN, P. A. AND LEHMANN, H.* HEMOGLOBIN BROUS-
SAIS* ALPHA 90 LYS REPLACED BY ASN. CANAD. J. BIOCHEM. 48* 408-410, 1970.

--HEMOGLOBIN C.
SUBSTITUTION OF LYSINE FOR GLUTAMIC ACID AT BETA 6.

BAGLIONI, C. AND INGRAM, V. M.* FOUR ADULT HAEMOGLOBIN TYPES IN ONE PERSON.
NATURE 189* 465-467, 1961.

HUNT, J. A. AND INGRAM, V. M.* A TERMINAL PEPTIDE SEQUENCE OF HUMAN HAEMOGLO-
BIN.Q NATURE 184* 640-641, 1959.

ITANO, H. A. AND NEEL, J. V.* A NEW INHERITED ABNORMALITY OF HUMAN HEMOGLOBIN.
PROC. NAT. ACAD. SCI. 36* 613-617, 1950.

--HEMOGLOBIN C(GEORGETOWN).
BETA CHAIN ANOMALY. SUBSTITUTION OF LYSINE FOR GLUTAMIC AT BETA 7. SECOND
SUBSTITUTION ALSO PRESENT BUT NOT IDENTIFIED. SICKLES.

PIERCE, L. E., RATH, C. E. AND MCCOY, K.* A NEW HEMOGLOBIN VARIANT WITH
SICKLING PROPERTIES. NEW ENG. J. MED. 268* 862-866, 1963.

--HEMOGLOBIN C(HARLEM).
DOUBLE SUBSTITUTION IN BETA CHAIN (VALINE FOR GLUTAMIC ACID AT BETA 6 AND
ASPARAGINE FOR ASPARTIC ACID AT BETA 73). MAY BE IDENTICAL TO C(GEORGETOWN). SEE
HEMOGLOBIN KORLE-BU.

BOOKCHIN, R. M., DAVIS, R. P. AND RANNEY, H. M.* CLINICAL FEATURES OF HEMOGLO-
BIN C(HARLEM), A NEW SICKLING HEMOGLOBIN VARIANT. ANN. INTERN. MED. 68* 8-18,

BOOKCHIN, R. M., NAGEL, R. L. AND RANNEY, H. M.* THE EFFECT OF BETA 73 ASN ON THE INTERACTIONS OF SICKLING HEMOGLOBINS. BIOCHIM. BIOPHYS. ACTA 221* 373-375, 1970.

BOOKCHIN, R. M., NAGEL, R. L., RANNEY, H. M. AND JACOBS, A. S.* HEMOGLOBIN C(HARLEM)* A SICKLING VARIANT CONTAINING AMINO ACID SUBSTITUTIONS IN TWO RESIDUES OF THE BETA-POLYPEPTIDE CHAIN. BIOCHEM. BIOPHYS. RES. COMM. 23* 122-127, 1966.

--HEMOGLOBIN CASERTA.
BETA CHAIN ANOMALY.

QUATTRIN, N., VENTRUTO, V. AND DE ROSA, L.* HEMOGLOBINOPATHIES IN CAMPANIA WITH PARTICULAR REFERENCE TO THE RARE AND NEW TYPES. BLUT 20* 292-295, 1970.

VENTRUTO, V., BAGLIONI, C., DE ROSA, L., BIANCHI, P., COLOMBO, B. AND QUATTRIN, N.* HAEMOGLOBIN CASERTA* AN ABNORMAL HAEMOGLOBIN OBSERVED IN A SOUTHERN ITALIAN FAMILY. SCAND. J. HAEMAT. 2* 118-125, 1965.

--HEMOGLOBIN CHAD.
SUBSTITUTION OF LYSINE FOR GLUTAMIC ACID AT ALPHA 23.

BOYER, S. H., CROSBY, E. F., FULLER, G. F., ULENURM, L. AND BUCK, A. A.* A SURVEY OF HEMOGLOBINS IN THE REPUBLIC OF CHAD AND CHARACTERIZATION OF HEMOGLOBIN CHAD* ALPHA-2-23GLU-LYS BETA-2. AM. J. HUM. GENET. 20* 570-578, 1968.

--HEMOGLOBIN CHESAPEAKE.
POLYCYTHEMIA IS A CLINICAL FEATURE. LEUCINE IS SUBSTITUTED FOR ARGININE AT ALPHA 92.

CHARACHE, S., WEATHERALL, D. J. AND CLEGG, J. B.* POLYCYTHEMIA ASSOCIATED WITH A HEMOGLOBINOPATHY. J. CLIN. INVEST. 45* 813-822, 1966.

CLEGG, J. B., NAUGHTON, M. A. AND WEATHERALL, D. J.* ABNORMAL HUMAN HAEMOGLO-BINS* SEPARATION AND CHARACTERIZATION OF THE ALPHA AND BETA CHAINS BY CHROMATOGRA-PHY, AND THE DETERMINATION OF TWO NEW VARIANTS, HB CHESAPEAKE AND HB J(BANGKOK). J. MOLEC. BIOL. 19* 91-108, 1966.

--HEMOGLOBIN CHIAPAS.
SUBSTITUTION OF ARGININE FOR PROLINE AT ALPHA 114.

JONES, R. T., BRIMHALL, B. AND LISKER, R.* CHEMICAL CHARACTERIZATION OF HEMOGLOBIN MEXICO AND HEMOGLOBIN CHIAPAS. BIOCHEM. BIOPHYS. ACTA 154* 488-495, 1968.

--HEMOGLOBIN CHRISTCHURCH.
SUBSTITUTION OF SERINE FOR PHENYLALANINE AT BETA 71.

CARRELL, R. W.* CHRISTCHURCH, NEW ZEALAND* PERSONAL COMMUNICATION, 1970.

--HEMOGLOBIN CYPRUS-1.
POSSIBLY ABNORMAL GAMMA CHAIN.

GILLESPIE, J. E. O., WHITE, C. J., ELLIS, M. J., BEAVEN, G. H., GRATZER, W. B., SHOOTER, E. M. AND PARKHOUSE, R. M. E.* HAEMOGLOBIN* A HAEMOGLOBIN WITH UNUSUAL ALKALINE-DENATURATION PROPERTIES IN A TURKISH-CYPRIOT WOMAN. NATURE 184* 1876-1877, 1959.

--HEMOGLOBIN D BETA-BUSHMAN.
SUBSTITUTION OF ARGININE FOR GLYCINE AT BETA 16.

WADE, P. T., JENKINS, T. AND HUEHNS, E. R.* HAEMOGLOBIN VARIANT IN A BUSHMAN* HAEMOGLOBIN D BETA-BUSHMAN (16 GLY TO ARG). NATURE 216* 688-690, 1967.

--HEMOGLOBIN D(CYPRUS).
D(CYPRUS) HAS A SUBSTITION IN THE BETA CHAIN.

BAGLIONI, C.* ABNORMAL HUMAN HAEMOGLOBINS. VII. CHEMICAL STUDIES ON HAEMOGLO-BIN D. BIOCHIM. BIOPHYS. ACTA 59* 437-449, 1962.

GAMMACK, D. B., HUEHNS, E. R., LEHMANN, H. AND SHOOTER, E. M.* THE ABNORMAL POLYPEPTIDE CHAINS IN A NUMBER OF HAEMOGLOBIN VARIANTS. ACTA GENET. STATIST. MED. 11* 1-16, 1961.

--HEMOGLOBIN D(CYPRUS).
SUBSTITUTION IN ALPHA PEPTIDE 23.

BENZER, S., INGRAM, V. M. AND LEHMANN, H.* THREE VARIETIES OF HUMAN HAEMOGLOBIN D. NATURE 182* 852-854, 1958.

--HEMOGLOBIN D(FRANKFURT).

GAMMACK, D. B., HUEHNS, E. R., LEHMANN, H. AND SHOOTER, E. M.* THE ABNORMAL
POLYPEPTIDE CHAINS IN A NUMBER OF HAEMOGLOBIN VARIANTS. ACTA GENET. STATIST. MED.
11* 1-16, 1961.

MARTIN, H., HEUPKE, G., PFLEIDERER, G. AND WOERNER, W.* HAEMOGLOBIN D IN A
FRANKFURT FAMILY. FOLIA HAEMAT. 4* 233-241, 1960.

--HEMOGLOBIN D(IBADAN).
SUBSTITUTION OF LYSINE FOR THREONINE AT BETA 87.

WATSON-WILLIAMS, E. J., BEALE, D., IRVINE, D. AND LEHMANN, H.* A NEW HAEMOGLO-
BIN, D IBADAN (BETA-87 THREONINE TO LYSINE), PRODUCING NO SICKLE-CELL HAEMOGLOBIN
D DISEASE WITH HAEMOGLOBIN S. NATURE 205* 1273-1279, 1965.

--HEMOGLOBIN D(LOS ANGELES).
SAME AS HEMOGLOBIN D(PUNJAB).

SCHNEIDER, R. G., UEDA, S., ALPERIN, J. B., LEVIN, W. C., JONES, R. T. AND
BRIMHALL, B.* HEMOGLOBIN D LOS ANGELES IN TWO CAUCASIAN FAMILIES* HEMOGLOBIN SD
DISEASE AND HEMOGLOBIN D THALASSEMIA. BLOOD 32* 250-259, 1968.

--HEMOGLOBIN D(MICHIGAN I).
PROBABLY SAME AS HEMOGLOBIN KOKURA.

--HEMOGLOBIN D(PUNJAB).
SUBSTITUTION GLUTAMINE FOR GLUTAMIC ACID AT BETA 121.

BENZER, S., INGRAM, V. M. AND LEHMANN, H.* THREE VARIETIES OF HUMAN HAEMOGLOBIN
D. NATURE 182* 852-854, 1958.

BOWMAN, R. AND INGRAM, V. M.* ABNORMAL HUMAN HAEMOGLOBIN. VII. THE COMPARISON
OF NORMAL HUMAN HAEMOGLOBIN AND HAEMOGLOBIN D(CHICAGO). BIOCHIM. BIOPHYS. ACTA
53* 569-573, 1961.

OZSOYLU, S.* HOMOZYGOUS HEMOGLOBIN D PUNJAB. ACTA HAEMAT. 43* 353-359, 1970.

STOUT, C., HOLLAND, C. K. AND BIRD, R. M.* HEMOGLOBIN D IN AN OKLAHOMA FAMILY.
ARCH. INTERN. MED. 114* 296-300, 1964.

--HEMOGLOBIN D(ST. LOUIS).
SUBSTITUTION OF LYSINE FOR ASPARAGINE AT ALPHA 68. SAME AS D(WASHINGTON),
G(PHILADELPHIA), G(BRISTOL), G(AZAKUOLI), KNOXVILLE-1, AND STANLEYVILLE-1.

SCHROEDER, W. A. AND JONES, R. T.* SOME ASPECTS OF THE CHEMISTRY AND FUNCTION
OF HUMAN AND ANIMAL HEMOGLOBINS. FORTSCHR. CHEM. ORGAN. NATURST. 23* 113-194,
1965.

--HEMOGLOBIN DAKAR.
SUBSTITUTION OF GLUTAMINE FOR HISTIDINE AT ALPHA 112.

ROSA, J., MALEKNIA, N., VERGOZ, D. AND DUNET, R.* UNE NOUVELLE HEMOGLOBINE
ANORMALE* L'HEMOGLOBINE JA-PARIS 12 ALA---ASP. NOUV. REV. FRANC. HEMAT. 6* 423-
426, 1966.

--HEMOGLOBIN DELTA CHAIN - TETRAMER.
NOT YET PROVEN TO BE A TETRAMER.

HUEHNS, E. R.* A THIRD HAEMOGLOBIN ABNORMALITY IN TWO INDIVIDUALS WITH HB-H
DISEASE. IN 'HAEMOGLOBIN-COLLOQUIUM.' H. LEHMANN AND K. BETKE (EDS.)* STUTTGART*
GEORG THIEME VERLAG, 1962. PP. 76.

HUEHNS, E. R., DANCE, N., BEAVEN, G. H. AND STEVENS, B. L.* FURTHER INVESTIGA-
TIONS IN HAEMOGLOBIN H DISEASE. PROC. 9TH CONGR. INTERN. SOC. HEMATOL., MEXICO
CITY, 1962. PP. 7-9.

--HEMOGLOBIN DHOFAR.
SUBSTITUTION OF ARGININE FOR PROLINE AT BETA 58.

MARENGO-ROWE, A. J., LORKIN, P. A., GALLO, E. AND LEHMANN, H.* HAEMOGLOBIN DHO-
FAR - A NEW VARIANT FROM SOUTHERN ARABIA. BIOCHEM. BIOPHYS. ACTA 168* 58-63,
1968.

--HEMOGLOBIN DURHAM-I.
BETA CHAIN ANOMALY.

CHERNOFF, A. I. AND PETTIT, N. M.* THE AMINO ACID COMPOSITION OF HEMOGLOBIN.
III. A QUALITATIVE METHOD FOR IDENTIFYING ABNORMALITIES OF THE POLYPEPTIDE CHAINS
OF HEMOGLOBIN. BLOOD 24* 750-756, 1964.

--HEMOGLOBIN E.

BLACKWELL, R. Q., YANG, H. J., LIU, C. S. AND WANG, C. C.* STRUCTURAL IDENTIFI-
CATION OF HAEMOGLOBIN E IN FILIPINOS. TROP. GEOGR. MED. 22* 112-114, 1970.

HUNT, J. A. AND INGRAM, V. M.* ABNORMAL HUMAN HAEMOGLOBINS. VI. THE CHEMICAL
DIFFERENCE BETWEEN HEMOGLOBIN A AND E. BIOCHIM. BIOPHYS. ACTA 49* 520-536, 1961.

SHIBATA, S., IUCHI, I. AND HAMILTON, H. B.* THE FIRST INSTANCE OF HEMOGLOBIN E
IN A JAPANESE FAMILY. PROC. JAP. ACAD. 40* 846-851, 1962.

--HEMOGLOBIN E(SASKATOON).
SUBSTITUTION OF LYSINE FOR GLUTAMIC ACID AT BETA 22.

VELLA, F., LORKIN, P. A., CARRELL, R. W.* A NEW HEMOGLOBIN VARIANT RESEMBLING
HEMOGLOBIN E.   HEMOGLOBIN E(SASKATOON)* BETA-22 GLU REPLACED BY LYS. CANAD. J.
BIOCHEM. 45* 1385-1391, 1967.

--HEMOGLOBIN ETOBICOKE.
SUBSTITUTION OF ARGININE FOR SERINE AT ALPHA 84.

BEALE, D.* 1967, CITED BY DAYHOFF, M. O. AND ECK, R. V., LOC. CIT.

CROOKSTON, J. H., FARQUHARSON, H. A., BEALE, D. AND LEHMANN, H.* HEMOGLOBIN
ETOBICOKE* A 84(F5) SERINE REPLACED BY ARGININE. CANAD. J. BIOCHEM. 47* 143-146,
1969.

--HEMOGLOBIN F.
TWO FORMS OF FETAL HEMOGLOBIN ARE PRESENT IN ALL PERSONS* THAT IN WHICH THE GAMMA
CHAIN HAS GLYCINE AT POSITION 136 AND THAT WHICH HAS ALANINE AT POSITION 136. THE
FINDING IS INTERPRETED AS INDICATING DUPLICATION OF THE GAMMA LOCUS WITH MUTATION
IN ONE LOCUS (SCHROEDER ET AL., 1968).

SCHROEDER, W. A., HUISMAN, T. H. J., SHELTON, J. R., SHELTON, J. B., KLEIHAUER,
E. F., DOZY, A. M. AND ROBBERSON, B.* EVIDENCE FOR MULTIPLE STRUCTURAL GENES FOR
THE GAMMA CHAIN OF HUMAN FETAL HEMOGLOBIN. PROC. NAT. ACAD. SCI. 60* 537-544,
1968.

--HEMOGLOBIN F. HEREDITARY PERSISTENCE OF*
NOT AN ABNORMAL HEMOGLOBIN. THIS STATE WAS FIRST OBSERVED IN NEGROES (CONLEY ET
AL., 1963) AND THEREAFTER IN GREEKS AND SPORADICALLY IN OTHER ETHNIC GROUPS, E.G.,
THAIS (SEE BIBLIOGRAPHY OF WASI ET AL., 1968). TWO TYPES OF HEREDITARY PERSIS-
TENCE OF FETAL HEMOGLOBIN HAVE BEEN FOUND IN NEGROES. SOME HAVE ONLY FETAL
HEMOGLOBIN WITH GLYCINE AT GAMMA 136 AND OTHERS HAVE BOTH GLYCINE 136 AND ALANINE
1 36 FORMS OF FETAL HEMOGLOBIN.   GREEKS STUDIED BY WASI ET AL. (1968) HAD ONLY
FETAL HEMOGLOBIN OF THE ALANINE 136 TYPE. THESE FINDINGS CAN BE INTERPRETED ON
THE BASIS OF VARIOUS DELETIONS INVOLVING A REGION CONTAINING SEVERAL LINKED
HEMOGLOBIN GENES.

CONLEY, C. L., WEATHERALL, D. J., RICHARDSON, S. N., SHEPHARD, M. K. AND
CHARACHE, S.* HEREDITARY PERSISTENCE OF FETAL HEMOGLOBIN. A STUDY OF 79 AFFECTED
PERSONS IN 15 NEGRO FAMILIES IN BALTIMORE. BLOOD 21* 261-281, 1963.

HUISMAN, T. H. J., SCHROEDER, W. A., ADAMS, H. R., SHELTON, J. R., SHELTON, J.
B. AND APELL, G.* A POSSIBLE SUBCLASS OF THE HEREDITARY PERSISTENCE OF FETAL
HEMOGLOBIN. BLOOD 36* 1-9, 1970.

HUISMAN, T. H. J., SCHROEDER, W. A., STAMATOYANNOPOULOS, G., BOUVER, N.,
SHELTON, J. R., SHELTON, J. B. AND APELL, G.* NATURE OF FETAL HEMOGLOBIN IN THE
GREEK TYPE OF HEREDITARY PERSISTENCE OF FETAL HEMOGLOBIN WITH AND WITHOUT
CONCURRENT BETA-THALASSEMIA. J. CLIN. INVEST. 49* 1035-1040, 1970.

SIEGEL, W., COX, R., SCHROEDER, W., HUISMAN, T. H. J., PENNER, O. AND ROWLEY,
P. T.* AN ADULT HOMOZYGOUS FOR PERSISTENT FETAL HEMOGLOBIN. ANN. INTERN. MED. 72*
533-536, 1970.

WASI, P., POOTRAKUL, S. AND NA-NAKORN, S.* HEREDITARY PERSISTENCE OF FOETAL
HAEMOGLOBIN IN A THAI FAMILY* THE FIRST INSTANCE IN THE MONGOL RACE AND IN
ASSOCIATION WITH HAEMOGLOBIN E. BRIT. J. HAEMAT. 14* 501-506, 1968.

WHEELER, J. T. AND KREVANS, J. R.* THE HOMOZYGOUS STATE OF PERSISTENT FETAL
HEMOGLOBIN AND INTERACTION OF PERSISTENT FETAL HEMOGLOBIN WITH THALASSEMIA. BULL.
HOPKINS HOSP. 109* 217-233, 1961.

--HEMOGLOBIN F(ALEXANDRA).
SUBSTITUTION OF LYSINE FOR THREONINE AT GAMMA 12.

LOUKOPOULOS, D., KALTSOYA, A. AND FESSAS, P.* BRIEF REPORT* ON THE CHEMICAL
ABNORMALITY OF HB *ALEXANDRA,* A FETAL HEMOGLOBIN VARIANT. BLOOD 33* 114-118,
1969.

--HEMOGLOBIN F(DICKINSON).

SCHNEIDER, R. G., BRIMHALL, B. AND JONES, R. T.* GALVESTON, TEXAS* PORTLAND, OREGON, PERSONAL COMMUNICATION, 1970.

--HEMOGLOBIN F(FESSAS).

FESSAS, P., KARAKLIS, A. AND GNAFAKIS, N.* A FURTHER ABNORMALITY OF FOETAL HEMOGLOBIN. ACTA HAEMAT. 25* 62-70, 1961.

--HEMOGLOBIN F(HOUSTON).
A GAMMA CHAIN DEFECT. PROBABLY SUBSTITUTION OF ALANINE FOR GLUTAMINE. SIMILAR OR IDENTICAL TO HEMOGLOBIN F(WARREN).

SCHNEIDER, R. G., JONES, R. T. AND SUZUKI, K.* HEMOGLOBIN F-HOUSTON* A FETAL VARIANT. BLOOD 27* 670-676, 1966.

--HEMOGLOBIN F(HULL).
SUBSTITUTION OF LYSINE FOR GLUTAMIC ACID AT GAMMA 121. THE SAME SUBSTITUTION OCCURS AT THE HOMOLOGOUS POSITION IN THE ALPHA CHAIN IN HEMOGLOBIN O(INDONESIA) AND IN THE BETA CHAIN IN HEMOGLOBIN O(ARAB). GLUTAMINE IS SUBSTITUTED FOR GLUTAMIC ACID AT BETA 121 IN HEMOGLOBIN D(PUNJAB).

SACKER, L. S., BEALE, D., BLACK, A. J., HUNTSMAN, R. G., LEHMANN, H. AND LORKIN, P. A.* HAEMOGLOBIN F HULL (GAMMA 121 GLUTAMIC ACID TO LYSINE), HOMOLOGOUS WITH HAEMOGLOBINS O ARAB AND O INDONESIA. BRIT. MED. J. 3* 531-533, 1967.

--HEMOGLOBIN F(JAMAICA).
SUBSTITUTION OF GLUTAMIC ACID FOR LYSINE AT GAMMA 61.

AHERN, E. J., JONES, R. T., BRIMHALL, B. AND GRAY, R. H.* HAEMOGLOBIN F JAMAICA (ALPHA 2-GAMMA-2-61 LYS TO GLU* 136 ALA). BRIT. J. HAEMAT. 18* 369-375, 1970.

--HEMOGLOBIN F(MALTA).
SUBSTITUTION OF ARGININE FOR HISTIDINE AT POSITION 117 IN THE GLYCINE 136 GAMMA CHAIN.

CAUCHI, M. N., CLEGG, J. B. AND WEATHERALL, D. J.* HAEMOGLOBIN F(MALTA)* A NEW FOETAL HAEMOGLOBIN VARIANT WITH A HIGH INCIDENCE IN MALTESE INFANTS. NATURE 223* 311-313, 1969.

--HEMOGLOBIN F(ROMA).
PROBABLE GAMMA CHAIN DEFECT.

SILVESTRONI, E. AND BIANCO, I.* A NEW VARIANT OF HUMAN FETAL HEMOGLOBIN* HB F-ROMA. BLOOD 22* 545-553, 1963.

--HEMOGLOBIN F(TEXAS 1).
SUBSTITUTION OF LYSINE FOR GLUTAMIC ACID AT GAMMA 5.

JENKINS, G. C., BEALE, D., BLACK, A. J., HUNTSMAN, G. R. AND LEHMANN, H.* HAEMOGLOBIN F TEXAS 1(ALPHA-2, GAMMA-2-5 GLU-LYS)* A VARIANT OF HAEMOGLOBIN F. BRIT. J. HAEMAT. 13* 252-255, 1967.

--HEMOGLOBIN F(TEXAS 2).
SUBSTITUTION OF LYSINE FOR GLUTAMIC ACID AT GAMMA 6.

LARKIN, I. L., BAKER, T., LORKIN, P. A., LEHMANN, H., BLACK, A. J. AND HUNTSMAN, R. G.* HAEMOGLOBIN F TEXAS II (ALPHA-2 GAMMA-2 6 GLU-LYS), THE SECOND OF THE HAEMOGLOBIN F TEXAS VARIANTS. BRIT. J. HAEMAT. 14* 233-238, 1968.

SCHNEIDER, R. G. AND JONES, R. T.* HEMOGLOBIN F TEXAS* GAMMA-CHAIN VARIANT. SCIENCE 148* 240-242, 1965.

--HEMOGLOBIN F(WARREN).
A GAMMA CHAIN DEFECT. SIMILAR OR IDENTICAL TO HEMOGLOBIN F(HOUSTON).

HUISMAN, T. H. J., DOZY, A. M., HORTON, B. E. AND WILSON, J. B.* A FETAL HEMOGLOBIN WITH ABNORMAL GAMMA-POLYPEPTIDE CHAINS HEMOGLOBIN (WARREN). BLOOD 26* 668-676, 1965.

--HEMOGLOBIN FESSAS-PAPASPYROU.
SAME AS BART'S.

FESSAS, P. AND PAPASPYROU, A.* NEW *FAST* HEMOGLOBIN ASSOCIATED WITH THALASSE-MIA. SCIENCE 126* 1119 ONLY, 1957.

FESSAS, P.* HAEMOGLOBIN *BART'S.* (LETTER) BRIT. MED. J. 2* 886 ONLY, 1959.

--HEMOGLOBIN FLATBUSH.
SUBSTITUTION OF GLUTAMIC ACID FOR ALANINE AT DELTA 22.

JONES, R. T., BRIMHALL, B. AND HUISMAN, T. H.* STRUCTURAL CHARACTERIZATION OF
TWO DELTA CHAIN VARIANTS. HEMOGLOBIN A-PRIME-2 (B2) AND HEMOGLOBIN FLATBUSH. J.
BIOL. CHEM. 242* 5141-5145, 1967.

D
O
M
I
N
A
N
T

--HEMOGLOBIN FLATBUSH(GEORGIA).
DELTA CHAIN ANOMALY.

LEE, R. C. AND HUISMAN, T. H. J.* A VARIANT OF HEMOGLOBIN A-2 FOUND IN A NEGRO
FAMILY. BLOOD 24* 495-501, 1964.

--HEMOGLOBIN FREIBURG.
DELETION OF VALYL RESIDUE NO. 23 FROM OTHERWISE NORMAL BETA CHAIN PROBABLY
OCCURRED THROUGH TRIPLET DELETION RESULTING FROM UNEQUAL CROSSING-OVER BETWEEN TWO
NORMAL BETA LOCI IN ONE PARENT OF THE PROBAND. TWO OF THREE LIVING CHILDREN OF
THE PROBAND ALSO HAD THE ABNORMAL HEMOGLOBIN WHICH WAS ACCOMPANIED BY SLIGHT
CYANOSIS IN ALL THREE AND BY A HEMOLYTIC PROCESS IN THE PROBAND.

JONES, R. T., BRIMHALL, B., HUISMAN, T. H. J., KLEIHAUER, E. AND BETKE, K.*
HEMOGLOBIN FREIBURG* ABNORMAL HEMOGLOBIN DUE TO DELETION OF A SINGLE AMINO ACID
RESIDUE. SCIENCE 154* 1024-1027, 1966.

--HEMOGLOBIN G TAEGU.
BETA CHAIN DEFECT (PROBABLY IN SEGMENT 18-30).

BLACKWELL, R. Q., HUANG, J. T.-H. AND RO, I. H.* HEMOGLOBIN VARIANTS IN
KOREANS* HEMOGLOBIN G TAEGU. SCIENCE 158* 1056-1057, 1967.

--HEMOGLOBIN G(ACCRA).
SUBSTITUTION OF ASPARAGINE FOR ASPARTIC ACID AT BETA 79. (NO CLINICAL OR
HEMATOLOGIC ABNORMALITY IN THE HOMOZYGOTE.)

EDINGTON, G. M., LEHMANN, H. AND SCHNEIDER, R. G.* CHARACTERIZATION AND
GENETICS OF HAEMOGLOBIN G. NATURE 175* 850-851, 1955.

GAMMACK, D. B., HUEHNS, E. R., LEHMANN, H. AND SHOOTER, E. M.* THE ABNORMAL
POLYPEPTIDE CHAINS IN A NUMBER OF HAEMOGLOBIN VARIANTS. ACTA GENET. STATIST. MED.
11* 1-16, 1961.

LEHMANN, H., BEALE, D. AND BOI-DOKU, F. S.* HAEMOGLOBIN G(ACCRA). NATURE 203*
363-365, 1964.

MILNER, P. F.* HIGH INCIDENCE OF HEMOGLOBIN G(ACCRA) IN A RURAL DISTRICT IN
JAMAICA. J. MED. GENET. 4* 88-90, 1967.

--HEMOGLOBIN G(AUDHALI).
SUBSTITUTION OF VALINE FOR GLUTAMIC ACID AT ALPHA 23.

MARENGO-ROWE, A. J., BEALE, D. AND LEHMANN, H.* NEW HUMAN HEMOGLOBIN VARIANT
FROM SOUTHERN ARABIA* G-AUDHALI (ALPHA-23(B4) GLUTAMIC ACID-VALINE) AND THE
VARIABILITY OF B4 IN HUMAN HAEMOGLOBIN. NATURE 219* 1164-1166, 1968.

--HEMOGLOBIN G(BRISTOL).
SUBSTITUTION OF LYSINE AT ALPHA 68.

ATWATER, J., SCHWARTZ, I. R. AND TOCANTINS, L. M.* A VARIETY OF HUMAN HEMOGLO-
BIN WITH FOUR DISTINCT ELECTROPHORETIC COMPONENTS. BLOOD 15* 901-908, 1960.

BAGLIONI, C. AND INGRAM, V. M.* ABNORMAL HUMAN HEMOGLOBIN. V. CHEMICAL
INVESTIGATION OF HEMOGLOBINS A, G, C, X FROM ONE INDIVIDUAL. BIOCHIM. BIOPHYS.
ACTA 48* 253-265, 1961.

DANCE, N., HUEHNS, E. R. AND SHOOTER, E. M.* THE CHEMICAL INVESTIGATION OF
HAEMOGLOBINS G BRISTOL AND G BRISTOL-C. BIOCHIM. BIOPHYS. ACTA 86* 144-148, 1964.

GAMMACK, D. B., HUEHNS, E. R., LEHMANN, H. AND SHOOTER, E. M.* THE ABNORMAL
POLYPEPTIDE CHAINS IN A NUMBER OF HAEMOGLOBIN VARIANTS. ACTA GENET. STATIST. MED.
11* 1-16, 1961.

HUEHNS, E. R. AND SHOOTER, E. M.* THE POLYPEPTIDE CHAINS OF HAEMOGLOBIN-A2 AND
HAEMOGLOBIN-G2. J. MOLEC. BIOL. 3* 257-262, 1961.

MCCURDY, P. R., PEARSON, H. AND GERALD, P. S.* A NEW HEMOGLOBINOPATHY OF
UNUSUAL GENETIC SIGNIFICANCE. J. LAB. CLIN. MED. 58* 86-94, 1961.

MINNICH, V., CORDONNIER, J. K., WILLIAMS, W. J. AND MOORE, C. V.* ALPHA, BETA
AND GAMMA HEMOGLOBIN POLYPEPTIDE CHAINS DURING THE NEONATAL PERIOD WITH DESCRIP-
TION OF A FETAL FORM OF HEMOGLOBIN D ALPHA-ST. LOUIS. BLOOD 19* 137-167, 1962.

RAPER, A. B., GAMMACK, D. B., HUEHNS, E. R. AND SHOOTER, E. M.* FOUR HAEMOGLO-
BINS IN ONE INDIVIDUAL* A STUDY OF THE GENETIC INTERACTION OF HB-G AND HB-C.
BRIT. MED. J. 2* 1257-1261, 1960.

WEATHERALL, D. J., SIGLER, A. T. AND BAGLIONI, C.* FOUR HEMOGLOBINS IN EACH OF
THREE BROTHERS. GENETIC AND BIOCHEMICAL SIGNIFICANCE. BULL. HOPKINS HOSP. 111*
143-156, 1962.

--HEMOGLOBIN G(CHINESE).
THE ORIGINAL G(CHINESE) WAS FOUND TO HAVE A BETA CHAIN SUBSTITUTION (GAMMACK ET
AL., 1961). SEVERAL HEMOGLOBINS G IN CHINESE PERSONS (HONOLULU, HONG KONG,
SINGAPORE) WERE FOUND BY SWENSON ET AL. (1962) TO HAVE SUBSTITUTION OF GLUTAMINE
FOR GLUTAMIC ACID AT ALPHA 30.

GAMMACK, D. B., HUEHNS, E. R., LEHMANN, H. AND SHOOTER, E. M.* THE ABNORMAL
POLYPEPTIDE CHAINS IN A NUMBER OF HAEMOGLOBIN VARIANTS. ACTA GENET. STATIST. MED.
11* 1-16, 1961.

SWENSON, R. T., HILL, R. L., LEHMANN, H. AND JIM, R. T. S.* A CHEMICAL
ABNORMALITY IN HEMOGLOBIN G FROM CHINESE INDIVIDUALS. J. BIOL. CHEM. 237* 1517-
1520, 1962.

--HEMOGLOBIN G(COPENHAGEN).
SUBSTITUTION OF ASPARAGINE FOR ASPARTIC ACID AT BETA 47.

SICK, K., BEALE, D., IRVINE, D., LEHMANN, H., GOODALL, P. T. AND MACDOUGALL,
S.* HEMOGLOBIN G(COPENHAGEN) AND HEMOGLOBIN J(CAMBRIDGE). TWO NEW BETA-CHAIN
VARIANTS OF HEMOGLOBIN A. BIOCHIM. BIOPHYS. ACTA 140* 231-242, 1967.

--HEMOGLOBIN G(COUSHATTA).
SUBSTITUTION OF ALANINE FOR GLUTAMIC AT BETA 22.

BOWMAN, B. H., BARNETT, D. R. AND HITE, R.* HEMOGLOBIN G(COUSHATTA)* A BETA
VARIANT WITH A DELTA-LIKE SUBSTITUTION. BIOCHEM. BIOPHYS. RES. COMMUN. 26* 466-
470, 1967.

SCHNEIDER, R. G., HAGGARD, M. E., MCNUTT, C. W., JOHNSON, J. E., BOWMAN, B. H.
AND BARNETT, D. R.* HEMOGLOBIN G COUSHATTA* A NEW VARIANT IN AN AMERICAN INDIAN
FAMILY. SCIENCE 143* 697-698, 1964.

--HEMOGLOBIN G(FORT WORTH).
SUBSTITUTION OF GLYCINE FOR GLUTAMIC ACID AT ALPHA 27.

SCHNEIDER, R. G., BRIMHALL, B. AND JONES, R. T.* GALVESTON, TEXAS* PORTLAND,
OREGON, PERSONAL COMMUNICATION, 1970.

--HEMOGLOBIN G(GALVESTON).
SUBSTITUTION OF ALANINE FOR GLUTAMIC AT BETA 43.

BOWMAN, B. H., MORELAND, H. AND SCHNEIDER, R. G.* A NEW HAEMOGLOBIN VARIANT (G-
GALVESTON). NATURE 193* 1298-1300, 1962.

BOWMAN, B. H., OLIVER, C. P., BARNETT, D. R., CUNNINGHAM, J. E. AND SCHNEIDER,
R. G.* CHEMICAL CHARACTERIZATION OF THREE HEMOGLOBINS G. BLOOD 23* 193-199, 1964.

--HEMOGLOBIN G(GEORGIA).
SUBSTITUTION OF LEUCINE FOR PROLINE AT ALPHA 95.

HUISMAN, T. H. J., ADAMS, H. R., WILSON, J. B., EFREMOV, G. D., REYNOLDS, C. A.
AND WRIGHTSTONE, R. N.* HEMOGLOBIN G GEORGIA OR ALPHA 95 LEU (G-2) BETA 2.
BIOCHIM. BIOPHYS. ACTA 200* 578-580, 1970.

--HEMOGLOBIN G(HONAN).
SUBSTITUTION OF LYSINE FOR GLUTAMIC ACID AT BETA 7. SAME AS HB SIRIRAJ.

BLACKWELL, R. Q. AND LIU, C.-S.* HEMOGLOBIN G TAICHUNG* ALPHA 74 ASP TO HIS.
BIOCHIM. BIOPHYS. ACTA 200* 70-75, 1970.

--HEMOGLOBIN G(HONG KONG).
SAME AS HEMOGLOBIN G(HONOLULU).

--HEMOGLOBIN G(HONOLULU).
SAME AS G(HONG KONG) AND G(SINGAPORE). SUBSTITUTION OF GLUTAMINE FOR GLUTAMIC
ACID AT ALPHA 30.

LEHMANN, H.* HAEMOGLOBINS AND HAEMOGLOBINOPATHIES. IN 'HAEMOGLOBIN-COLLO-
QUIUM.' H. LEHMANN AND K. BETKE (EDS.)* STUTTGART* GEORG THIEME VERLAG, 1962.
PP. 1-14.

SWENSON, R. T., HILL, R. L., LEHMANN, H. AND JIM, R. T. S.* A CHEMICAL
ABNORMALITY IN HEMOGLOBIN G FROM CHINESE INDIVIDUALS. J. BIOL. CHEM. 237* 1517-
1520, 1962.

--HEMOGLOBIN G(HSIN-CHU).
SUBSTITUTION OF ALANINE FOR GLUTAMIC ACID AT BETA 22. SAME AS HB G(COUSHATTA) AND
HB G(SASKATOON).

BLACKWELL, R. Q., LIU, C.-S., YANG, H.-J., WANG, C.-C. AND HUANG, J. T.-H.*
HEMOGLOBIN VARIANT COMMON TO CHINESE AND NORTH AMERICAN INDIANS* ALPHA-2 BETA-2
(22 GLU-TO-ALA). SCIENCE 161* 381-382, 1968.

D
O
M
I
N
A
N
T

--HEMOGLOBIN G(IBADAN).
ALPHA CHAIN ANOMALY.

GAMMACK, D. B., HJEHNS, E. R., LEHMANN, H. AND SHOOTER, E. M.* THE ABNORMAL
POLYPEPTIDE CHAINS IN A NUMBER OF HAEMOGLOBIN VARIANTS. ACTA GENET. STATIST. MED.
11* 1-16, 1961.

SHOOTER, E. M., SKINNER, E. R., GARLICK, J. P. AND BARNICOT, N. A.* THE
ELECTROPHORETIC CHARACTERIZATION OF HAEMOGLOBIN G AND A NEW MINOR HAEMOGLOBIN G-2.
BRIT. J. HAEMAT. 6* 140-150, 1960.

--HEMOGLOBIN G(MAKASSAR).
SUBSTITUTION OF ALANINE FOR GLUTAMIC ACID AT BETA 6.

BLACKWELL, R. Q., OEMIJATI, S., PRIBADI, W., WENG, M.-I. AND LIU, C.-S.*
HEMOGLOBIN G(MAKASSAR)* BETA 6 GLU TO ALA. BIOCHIM. BIOPHYS. ACTA 214* 396-401,
1970.

--HEMOGLOBIN G(NORFOLK).
SUBSTITUTION OF ASPARAGINE FOR ASPARTIC ACID AT ALPHA 85.

HUNTSMAN, R. G., LORKIN, P. A. AND LEHMANN, H.* TO BE PUBLISHED.

--HEMOGLOBIN G(PARIS).
ALPHA CHAIN DEFECT. PERHAPS SUBSTITUTION OF LYSINE FOR ASPARTIC ACID AT 64, 74 OR
85. THE PATIENT OF LABIE AND SCHAPIRA (1966) HAD THROMBOCYTOPENIC PURPURA.

LABIE, D. AND SCHAPIRA, G.* NEW VARIANT OF HAEMOGLOBIN G* HAEMOGLOBIN G(PARIS).
NATURE 209* 1033-1034, 1966.

--HEMOGLOBIN G(PHILADELPHIA).
SAME AS D(AZAKOVLI), D(BALTIMORE), D(ST. LOUIS), KNOXVILLE-1, AND G(AZVAKOLI).
SUBSTITUTION OF LYSINE FOR ASPARAGINE AT ALPHA 68.

BAGLIONI, C. AND INGRAM, V. M.* ABNORMAL HUMAN HEMOGLOBIN. V. CHEMICAL
INVESTIGATION OF HEMOGLOBINS A, G, C, X FROM ONE INDIVIDUAL. BIOCHIM. BIOPHYS.
ACTA 48* 253-265, 1961.

--HEMOGLOBIN G(PORT ARTHUR).
SAME AS HB G(GALVESTON) AND HB G(TEXAS), Q.V.

--HEMOGLOBIN G(SAN JOSE).
SUBSTITUTION OF GLYCINE FOR GLUTAMIC ACID AT BETA 7.

HILL, R. L. AND SCHWARTZ, H. C.* A CHEMICAL ABNORMALITY IN HAEMOGLOBIN G.
NATURE 184* 641-642, 1959.

HILL, R. L., SWENSON, R. T. AND SCHWARTZ, H. C.* CHARACTERIZATION OF A CHEMICAL
ABNORMALITY IN HEMOGLOBIN G. J. BIOL. CHEM. 235* 3182-3187, 1960.

SCHWARTZ, H. C., SPAET, T. H., ZUELZER, W. W., NEEL, J. V., ROBINSON, A. R. AND
KAUFMAN, S. F.* COMBINATIONS OF HEMOGLOBIN G, HEMOGLOBIN S AND THALASSEMIA
OCCURRING IN ONE FAMILY. BLOOD 12* 238-250, 1957.

--HEMOGLOBIN G(SASKATOON).
SUBSTITUTION OF LYSINE FOR GLUTAMIC ACID AT BETA 22. SAME AS HEMOGLOBIN G(COU-
SHATTA) AND HEMOGLOBIN G(HSIN-CHU).

VELLA, F., ISAACS, W. A. AND LEHMANN, H.* HEMOGLOBIN G(SASKATOON)* BETA-22-GLU-
ALA. CANAD. J. BIOCHEM. 45* 351-353, 1967.

--HEMOGLOBIN G(SINGAPORE).
SAME AS HEMOGLOBIN G(HONOLULU).

--HEMOGLOBIN G(ST-1).
SUBSTITUTION OF LYSINE FOR ASPARAGINE AT ALPHA 68.

BOWMAN, B. H., BARNETT, D. R., HODGKINSON, K. T. AND SCHNEIDER, R. G.* CHEMICAL
CHARACTERIZATION OF HAEMOGLOBIN G(ST-1). NATURE 211* 1305-1306, 1966.

--HEMOGLOBIN G(SZUHU).
SUBSTITUTION OF LYSINE FOR ASPARAGINE AT BETA 80.

BLACKWELL, R. Q., YANG, H. J. AND WANG, C. C.* HEMOGLOBIN G-SZUHU* BETA 80 ASN
REPLACED BY LYS. BIOCHIM. BIOPHYS. ACTA 188* 59-64, 1969.

--HEMOGLOBIN G(TAEGN).
SAME AS G(COUSHATTA), G(SASKATOON) AND G(HSIN-CHU).

BLACKWELL, R. Q., RO, I.-H., LIU, C.-S., YANG, H.-J., WANG, C.-C. AND HUANG, J. T.-S.* HEMOGLOBIN VARIANT FOUND IN KOREANS, CHINESE, AND NORTH AMERICAN INDIANS* ALPHA2 BETA2(22GLU-TO-ALA). AM. J. PHYS. ANTHROP. 30* 389-391, 1969.

--HEMOGLOBIN G(TAIPEI).
SUBSTITUTION OF GLYCINE FOR GLUTAMIC ACID AT BETA 22.

BLACKWELL, R. Q., YANG, H. J. AND WANG, C. C.* HEMOGLOBIN G-TAIPEI* ALPHA-2-BETA-2-22 GLU REPLACED BY GLY. BIOCHIM. BIOPHYS. ACTA 175* 237-241, 1969.

--HEMOGLOBIN G(TAIWAN-AMI).
SUBSTITUTION OF ARGININE FOR GLYCINE AT BETA 25.

BLACKWELL, R. Q. AND LIU, C.-S.* HEMOGLOBIN G TAIWAN-AMI* ALPHA(2)BETA(2)25GLU-TO-ARG. BIOCHEM. BIOPHYS. RES. COMMUN. 30* 690-696, 1968.

--HEMOGLOBIN G(TEXAS).
SUBSTITUTION OF ALANINE FOR GLUTAMIC ACID AT BETA 43. SAME AS HB G(GALVESTON) AND HB G(PORT ARTHUR).

BOWMAN, B. H., OLIVER, C. P., BARNETT, D. R., CUNNINGHAM, J. E. AND SCHNEIDER, R. G.* CHEMICAL CHARACTERIZATION OF THREE HEMOGLOBINS G. BLOOD 23* 193-199, 1964.

--HEMOGLOBIN GALLIERA GENOVA.
DEFECT UNKNOWN.

SANSONE, G. AND PICK, C.* FAMILIAL HAEMOLYTIC ANAEMIA WITH ERYTHROCYTE INCLUSION BODIES, BILIFUSCINURIA AND ABNORMAL HAEMOGLOBIN (HAEMOGLOBIN GALLIERA GENOVA). BRIT. J. HAEMAT. 11* 511-517, 1965.

--HEMOGLOBIN GENOVA.
SUBSTITUTION OF PROLINE FOR LEUCINE AT BETA 28. UNSTABLE HEMOGLOBIN.

SANSONE, G., CARRELL, R. W. AND LEHMANN, H.* HAEMOGLOBIN GENOVA* BETA 28 (B10) LEUCINE TO PROLINE. NATURE 214* 877-879, 1967.

--HEMOGLOBIN GOWER-1.
POSSIBLE TETRAMER OF EPSILON CHAIN.

--HEMOGLOBIN GOWER-2.
PROBABLY ALPHA-2-EPSILON-2.

HUEHNS, E. R., FLYNN, F. V., BUTLER, E. A. AND BEAVEN, G. H.* TWO NEW HEMOGLO-BIN VARIANTS IN A VERY YOUNG HUMAN EMBRYO. NATURE 189* 496-497, 1961.

--HEMOGLOBIN GUN HILL.
DELETION OF AMINO ACID RESIDUES 93-97 INCLUSIVE OF BETA CHAIN PROBABLY THROUGH UNEQUAL CROSSING OVER. THIS UNSTABLE HEMOGLOBIN ALSO HAS ABSENCE OF HALF OF THE NORMAL COMPLEMENT OF HEME. OTHER UNSTABLE HEMOGLOBINS INCLUDE HB ZURICH, HB KOLN, HB GENOVA, HB SYDNEY, HB HAMMERSMITH AND HB SINAI.

BRADLEY, T. B., JR., WOHL, R. C. AND RIEDER, R. F.* HEMOGLOBIN GUN HILL* DELETION OF FIVE AMINO ACID RESIDUES AND IMPAIRED HEME-GLOBIN BINDING. SCIENCE 157* 1581-1583, 1967.

RIEDER, R. F. AND BRADLEY, T. B., JR.* HEMOGLOBIN GUN HILL* AN UNSTABLE PROTEIN ASSOCIATED WITH CHRONIC HEMOLYSIS. BLOOD 32* 355-369, 1968.

--HEMOGLOBIN H.
TETRAMER OF BETA CHAINS. FAST HEMOGLOBIN. NECHELES ET AL. (1966) PROVIDED FURTHER EVIDENCE THAT HB H DISEASE RESULTS FROM MATING OF A PARENT WITH ALPHA THALASSEMIA AND A PARENT WITH A SILENT H GENE, THAT DOUBLE HETEROZYGOSITY IS NECESSARY FOR HB H DISEASE. THE FINDINGS OF NA-NAKORN ET AL. (1969) LEADS TO ROUGHLY THE SAME CONCLUSION. AMONG THE NEWBORN OFFSPRING OF PERSONS WITH HB H, THEY FOUND SOME WITH 1-2 PERCENT HB BART'S AND OTHERS WITH 5-6 PERCENT. THEY SUGGESTED THAT THESE TWO TYPES OF CHILDREN ARE HETEROZYGOUS FOR TWO DIFFERENT ALPHA-THAL GENES ONE OF WHICH IS NOT DETECTABLE IN THE ADULT HETEROZYGOTE.

JONES, R. T., SCHROEDER, W. A., BALOG, J. E. AND VINOGRAD, J. R.* GROSS STRUCTURE OF HEMOGLOBIN H. J. AM. CHEM. SOC. 81* 3161 ONLY, 1959.

KATTAMIS, C. AND LEHMANN, H.* THE GENETICAL INTERPRETATION OF HAEMOGLOBIN H DISEASE. HUM. HERED. 20* 156-164, 1970.

NA-NAKORN, S., WASI, P., PORNPATKUL, M. AND POOTRAKUL, S.-N.* FURTHER EVIDENCE FOR A GENETIC BASIS OF HAEMOGLOBIN H DISEASE FROM NEWBORN OFFSPRING OF PATIENTS. NATURE 223* 59-60, 1969.

NECHELES, T. F., CATES, M., SHEEHAN, R. G. AND MEYER, H. J.* HEMOGLOBIN H DISEASE. A FAMILY STUDY. BLOOD 28* 501-512, 1966.

RIGAS, D. A., KOLER, R. D. AND OSGOOD, E. E.* NEW HEMOGLOBIN POSSESSING A

HIGHER ELECTROPHORETIC MOBILITY THAN NORMAL ADULT HEMOGLOBIN. SCIENCE 121* 372 ONLY, 1955.

--HEMOGLOBIN HAMMERSMITH.
    SUBSTITUTION OF SERINE FOR PHENYLALANINE AT BETA 42. THE NORMAL PHENYLALANINE AT THIS SITE APPARENTLY *STABILIZES* THE HEME WITH WHICH IT IS IN CONTACT. THE SUBSTITUTION OF SERINE LEADS TO SEVERE HEINZ BODY HEMOLYTIC ANEMIA.

    DACIE, J. V., SHINTON, N. K., GAFFNEY, P. J., JR., CARRELL, R. W. AND LEHMANN, H.* HAEMOGLOBIN HAMMERSMITH (BETA 42 (CD 1) PHE TO SER). NATURE 216* 663-665, 1967.

--HEMOGLOBIN HASHARON.
    SUBSTITUTION OF HISTIDINE FOR ASPARTIC ACID AT ALPHA 47. SAME AS HEMOGLOBIN SINAI.

    CHARACHE, S., MONDZAC, A. M. AND GESSNER, U.* HEMOGLOBIN HASHARON (ALPHA-2 47 HIS(CD5)BETA-2)* A HEMOGLOBIN FOUND IN LOW CONCENTRATION. J. CLIN. INVEST. 48* 834-847, 1969.

    HALBRECHT, I., ISAACS, W. A., LEHMANN, H. AND BEN-PORAT, F.* HEMOGLOBIN HA-SHARON (ALPHA 47 ASPARTIC ACID TO HISTIDINE). ISRAEL J. MED. SCI. 3* 827-831, 1967.

    OSTERTAG, W. AND SMITH, E. W.* HB SINAI, A NEW ALPHA CHAIN MUTANT ALPHA HIS 47. HUMANGENETIK 6* 377-379, 1968.

--HEMOGLOBIN HIJIYAMA.
    SUBSTITUTION OF GLUTAMIC ACID FOR LYSINE AT BETA 120.

    MIYAJI, T., OBA, Y., YAMAMOTO, K., SHIBATA, S., IUCHI, I. AND HAMILTON, H. B.* HEMOGLOBIN HIJIYAMA* A NEW FAST-MOVING HEMOGLOBIN IN A JAPANESE FAMILY. SCIENCE 159* 204-206, 1968.

--HEMOGLOBIN HIKARI.
    SUBSTITUTION OF ASPARAGINE FOR LYSINE AT BETA 61. HETEROZYGOTES HAVE ABOUT 60 PER CENT HEMOGLOBIN HIKARI.

    SHIBATA, S. AND IUCHI, I.* HEMOGLOBIN-HIKARI (ALPHA-2-BETA-2, T-7). A FAST-MOVING HEMOGLOBIN DEMONSTRATED IN TWO FAMILIES OF JAPANESE PEOPLE, WITH A BRIEF NOTE ON THE ABNORMAL HEMOGLOBINS OF JAPAN WHICH ARE LIABLE TO BE CONFUSED WITH IT. PROC. 9TH CONGR. INTERN. SOC. HEMATOL., MEXICO CITY, 1962. PP. 65-70.

    SHIBATA, S., MIYAJI, T., IUCHI, I., UEDA, S. AND TAKEDA, I.* HEMOGLOBIN HIKARI (A(2) A-B(2) 61 ASP NH(2))* A FAST-MOVING HEMOGLOBIN FOUND IN TWO UNRELATED JAPANESE FAMILIES. CLIN. CHIM. ACTA 10* 101-105, 1964.

--HEMOGLOBIN HIROSE.
    SUBSTITUTION OF SERINE FOR TRYPTOPHANE AT BETA 37.

    YANASE, T., HANADA, M., SEITA, M., OHYA, I., OHTA, Y., IMAMURA, T., FUJIMURA, T., KAWASAKI, K. AND YAMAOKA, K.* MOLECULAR BASIS OF MORBIDITY FROM A SERIES OF STUDIES OF HEMOGLOBINOPATHIES IN WESTERN JAPAN. JAP. J. HUM. GENET. 13* 40-53, 1968.

--HEMOGLOBIN HIROSHIMA.
    SUBSTITUTION OF ASPARTIC ACID FOR HISTIDINE AT BETA 143. ASSOCIATED WITH INCREASED OXYGEN AFFINITY, DECREASED BOHR EFFECT AND ERYTHREMIA. SAME AS HB KENWOOD.

    HAMILTON, H. B., IUCHI, I., MIYAJI, T. AND SHIBATA, S.* HEMOGLOBIN HIROSHIMA (BETA 143 HISTIDINE TO ASPARTIC ACID)* A NEWLY IDENTIFIED FAST MOVING BETA CHAIN VARIANT ASSOCIATED WITH INCREASED OXYGEN AFFINITY AND COMPENSATORY ERYTHREMIA. J. CLIN. INVEST. 48* 525-535, 1969.

--HEMOGLOBIN HOFU.
    SUBSTITUTION OF GLUTAMIC ACID FOR VALINE AT BETA 126.

    MIYAJI, T., OHBA, Y., YAMAMOTO, K., SHIBATA, S., IUCHI, I. AND TAKENAKA, M.* JAPANESE HAEMOGLOBIN VARIANT. NATURE 217* 89-90, 1968.

--HEMOGLOBIN HONOLULU.
    DEFECT UNKNOWN.

    SCHNEIDER, R. G. AND JIM, R. T. S.* HAEMOGLOBIN* A NEW HEMOGLOBIN VARIANT (THE *HONOLULU TYPE*) IN A CHINESE. NATURE 190* 454-455, 1961.

--HEMOGLOBIN HOPE.
    SUBSTITUTION OF ASPARTIC FOR GLYCINE AT BETA 136.

    MINNICH, V., HILL, R. J., KHURI, P. D. AND ANDERSON, M. E.* HEMOGLOBIN HOPE* A BETA CHAIN VARIANT. BLOOD 25* 830-838, 1965.

--HEMOGLOBIN HOPKINS-1.
 SUBSTITUTION OF GLUTAMIC ACID FOR LYSINE AT BETA 95. SAME AS HEMOGLOBIN N(BALTI-
 MORE).

 GOTTLIEB, A. J., ROBINSON, E. A. AND ITANO, H. A.* PRIMARY STRUCTURE OF
 HOPKINS-1 HAEMOGLOBIN-A. NATURE 214* 189-190, 1967.

--HEMOGLOBIN HOPKINS-2.
 SUBSTITUTION OF ASPARTIC ACID FOR HISTIDINE AT ALPHA 112. FAST HEMOGLOBIN.

 BRADLEY, T. B., JR., BOYER, S. H. AND ALLEN, F. H., JR.* HOPKINS-2-HEMOGLOBIN*
 A REVISED PEDIGREE WITH DATA ON BLOOD AND SERUM GROUPS. BULL. HOPKINS HOSP. 108*
 75-79, 1961.

 ITANO, H. A. AND ROBINSON, E. A.* GENETIC CONTROL OF THE ALPHA- AND BETA-CHAINS
 OF HEMOGLOBIN. PROC. NAT. ACAD. SCI. 46* 1492-1501, 1960.

 OSTERTAG, W.* BALTIMORE, MD.* PERSONAL COMMUNICATION, 1967.

 SMITH, E. W. AND TORBERT, J. V.* STUDY OF TWO ABNORMAL HEMOGLOBINS WITH
 EVIDENCE FOR A NEW GENETIC LOCUS FOR HEMOGLOBIN FORMATION. BULL. HOPKINS HOSP.
 102* 38-45, 1958.

--HEMOGLOBIN I.
 FAST HEMOGLOBIN. SUBSTITUTION OF ASPARTIC ACID FOR LYSINE AT ALPHA 16 WAS FIRST
 REPORTED BY MURAYAMA (1962). HOWEVER, CRICK POINTED OUT THAT THIS SUBSTITUTION
 COULD NOT BE ACCOMPLISHED BY CHANGE IN ONE BASE. RESTUDY BY BEALE AND LEHMANN
 (1965) AND BY SCHNEIDER ET AL. (1966) SHOWED SUBSTITUTION OF GLUTAMIC ACID FOR
 LYSINE. HEMOGLOBIN I WAS THOUGHT TO SHOW SICKLING BUT THIS HAS BEEN SHOWN TO BE
 DUE TO FAULTY TECHNIQUE (SCHNEIDER ET AL., 1967).

 BEALE, D. AND LEHMANN, H.* ABNORMAL HAEMOGLOBINS AND THE GENETIC CODE. NATURE
 207* 259-261, 1965.

 ITANO, H. A. AND ROBINSON, E. A.* FORMATION OF NORMAL AND DOUBLE ABNORMAL
 HAEMOGLOBINS BY RECOMBINATION OF HAEMOGLOBIN I WITH S AND C. NATURE 183* 1799-
 1800, 1959.

 ITANO, H. A. AND ROBINSON, E. A.* GENETIC CONTROL OF THE ALPHA- AND BETA-CHAINS
 OF HEMOGLOBIN. PROC. NAT. ACAD. SCI. 46* 1492-1501, 1960.

 MURAYAMA, M.* CHEMICAL DIFFERENCE BETWEEN NORMAL HUMAN HAEMOGLOBIN AND
 HAEMOGLOBIN-I. NATURE 196* 276-277, 1962.

 RUCKNAGEL, D. L., PAGE, E. B. AND JENSEN, W. N.* HEMOGLOBIN I* AN INHERITED
 HEMOGLOBIN ANOMALY. BLOOD 10* 999-1009, 1955.

 SCHNEIDER, R. G., ALPERIN, J. B. AND LEHMANN, H.* SICKLING TESTS. PITFALLS IN
 PERFORMANCE AND INTERPRETATION. J.A.M.A. 202* 419-421, 1967.

 SCHNEIDER, R. G., ALPERIN, J. B., BEALE, D. AND LEHMANN, H.* HEMOGLOBIN I IN AN
 AMERICAN NEGRO FAMILY* STRUCTURAL AND HEMATOLOGIC STUDIES. J. LAB. CLIN. MED. 68*
 940-946, 1966.

 SCHWARTZ, I. R., ATWATER, J., REPPLINGER, E. AND TOCANTINS, L. M.* SICKLING OF
 ERYTHROCYTES WITH I-A ELECTROPHORETIC HAEMOGLOBIN PATTERN. FED. PROC. 16* 115
 ONLY, 1957.

 THOMPSON, R. B., RAU, P. J., ODOM, J. AND BELL, W. N.* THE SICKLING PHENOMENON
 IN A WHITE MALE WITHOUT HB-S. ACTA HAEMAT. 34* 347-353, 1965.

--HEMOGLOBIN I(BURLINGTON).
 ALPHA CHAIN DEFECT. SAME AS HEMOGLOBIN I.

 O'BRIEN, C., GREY, M. J. AND JACOBS, A. S.* A SURVEY OF CORD BLOODS FOR
 ABNORMAL HEMOGLOBIN, WITH FURTHER OBSERVATIONS ON HEMOGLOBIN I(BURLINGTON). AM.
 J. OBST. GYNEC. 88* 816-822, 1964.

 RANNEY, H. M., O'BRIEN, C. AND JACOBS, A. S.* AN ABNORMAL HUMAN FOETAL
 HAEMOGLOBIN WITH AN ABNORMAL ALPHA-POLYPEPTIDE CHAIN. NATURE 194* 743-745, 1962.

--HEMOGLOBIN I(HIGH WYCOMBE).
 SUBSTITUTION OF GLUTAMIC ACID FOR LYSINE AT BETA 59.

 BOULTON, F. E., HUNTSMAN, R. G., LEHMANN, H., LORKIN, P. AND ROMERO-HERRERA, A.
 E.* MYOGLOBIN VARIANTS. (ABSTRACT) BIOCHEM. J. 118* 39P ONLY, 1970.

--HEMOGLOBIN I(INTERLAKEN).
 SUBSTITUTION ASPARTIC ACID FOR GLYCINE AT ALPHA 15. SAME AS HEMOGLOBIN J(OXFORD).

 MARTI, H. R., PIK, C. AND MOSIMANN, P.* EINE NEUE HAMOGLOBIN I-VARIANTE* HB
 I(INTERLAKEN). ACTA HAEMAT. 32* 9-16, 1964.

--HEMOGLOBIN I(SKAMANIA).
                SUBSTITUTION OF GLUTAMIC ACID FOR LYSINE AT ALPHA 16. SAME AS HB I(TEXAS), ETC.

BAUR, E. W.* HB ALPHA 2 GLU BETA 2(HB I) IN A CAUCASIAN FAMILY* INDEPENDENT
                MUTATION OR COMMON ORIGIN.Q HUMANGENETIK 6* 368-372, 1968.

      --HEMOGLOBIN I(TEXAS).
                SUBSTITUTION OF GLUTAMIC ACID FOR LYSINE AT ALPHA 16.

                BOWMAN, B. H. AND BARNETT, D. R.* AMINO-ACID SUBSTITUTION IN HAEMOGLOBIN I(TE-
                XAS VARIANT). NATURE 214* 499 ONLY, 1967.

      --HEMOGLOBIN I(TOULOUSE).
                SUBSTITUTION OF GLUTAMIC ACID FOR LYSINE AT BETA 66.

                ROSA, J., LABIE, D., WAJCMAN, H., BOIGNE, J. M., CABANNES, R., BIERME, R.,
                RUFFIE, J.* HEMOGLOBIN I TOULOUSE* BETA 66 (E10) LYS TO GLU* A NEW ABNORMAL
                HEMOGLOBIN WITH A MUTATION LOCALIZED ON THE E10 PORPHYRIN SURROUNDING ZONE.
                NATURE 223* 190-191, 1969.

      --HEMOGLOBIN J(BALTIMORE).
                SUBSTITUTION OF ASPARTIC ACID FOR GLYCINE AT BETA 16. FAST HEMOGLOBIN.

                WEATHERALL, D. J.* HEMOGLOBIN J (BALTIMORE) COEXISTING IN A FAMILY WITH
                HEMOGLOBIN S-I. BULL HOPKINS HOSP. 114* 1-12, 1964.

                WILKINSON, T., KRONENBERG, H., ISAACS, W. A. AND LEHMANN, H.* HAEMOGLOBIN J BA-
                LTIMORE INTERACTING WITH BETA-THALASSAEMIA IN AN AUSTRALIAN FAMILY. MED. J. AUST.
                1* 907-910, 1967.

      --HEMOGLOBIN J(BANGKOK).
                SUBSTITUTION OF ASPARTIC ACID FOR GLYCINE AT BETA 56.

                CLEGG, J. B., NAUGHTON, M. A. AND WEATHERALL, D. J.* ABNORMAL HUMAN HAEMOGLO-
                BINS. SEPARATION AND CHARACTERIZATION OF THE ALPHA AND BETA CHAINS BY CHROMATO-
                GRAPHY, AND THE DETERMINATION OF TWO NEW VARIANTS, HB CHESAPEAK AND HB J(BANGKOK).
                J. MOLEC. BIOL. 17* 91-108, 1966.

                POOTRAKUL, S., WASI, P. AND NAKORN, S.* HAEMOGLOBIN J-BANGKOK* A CLINICAL,
                HAEMATOLOGICAL AND GENETICAL STUDY. BRIT. J. HAEMAT. 13* 303-309, 1967.

      --HEMOGLOBIN J(BROUSSAIS).
                SUBSTITUTION OF ASPARAGINE FOR LYSINE AT ALPHA 90.

                DETRAVERSE, P. M., LEHMANN, H., COQUELET, M. L., BEALE, D. AND ISAACS, W. A.*
                ETUDE D'UNE HEMOGLOBINE J(ALPHA) NON ENCORE DECRITE, DANS UNE FAMILLE FRANCAISE.
                C. R. SOC. BIOL. 160* 2270-2272, 1966.

      --HEMOGLOBIN J(CAMBRIDGE).
                SUBSTITUTION OF ASPARTIC ACID FOR GLYCINE AT BETA 69.

                SICK, K., BEALE, D., IRVINE, D., LEHMANN, H., GOODALL, P. T. AND MACDOUGALL,
                S.* HEMOGLOBIN G(COPENHAGEN) AND HEMOGLOBIN J(CAMBRIDGE). TWO NEW BETA-CHAIN
                VARIANTS OF HEMOGLOBIN A. BIOCHIM. BIOPHYS. ACTA 140* 231-242, 1967.

      --HEMOGLOBIN J(CAPE TOWN).
                GLUTAMINE SUBSTITUTES FOR ARGININE AT ALPHA 92.

                BOTHA, M. C., BEALE, D., ISSACS, W. A. AND LEHMANN, H.* HEMOGLOBIN J CAPE TOWN.
                NATURE 212* 792-794, 1966.

      --HEMOGLOBIN J(GEORGIA).
                BETA CHAIN ANOMALY. FAST HEMOGLOBIN.

                HUISMAN, T. H. J. AND SYDENSTRICKER, V. P.* HAEMATOLOGY* DIFFERENCE IN GROSS
                STRUCTURE OF TWO ELECTROPHORETICALLY IDENTICAL 'MINOR' HEMOGLOBIN COMPONENTS.
                NATURE 193* 489-491, 1962.

                SYDENSTRICKER, V. P., HORTON, B., PAYNE, R. A. AND HUISMAN, T. H. J.* STUDIES
                ON A FAST HEMOGLOBIN VARIANT FOUND IN A NEGRO FAMILY IN ASSOCIATION WITH THALASSE-
                MIA. CLIN. CHIM. ACTA 6* 677-685, 1961.

      --HEMOGLOBIN J(INDIA).
                ALPHA CHAIN ANOMALY.

                LEHMANN, H.* HAEMOGLOBINS AND HAEMOGLOBINOPATHIES. IN 'HAEMOGLOBIN-COLLO-
                QUIUM.' H. LEHMANN AND K. BETKE (EDS.)* STUTTGART* GEORG THIEME VERLAG, 1962.
                PP. 1-14.

                RAPER, A. B.* UNUSUAL HAEMOGLOBIN VARIANT IN A GUJERATI INDIAN. BRIT. MED. J.
                1* 1285-1286, 1957.

    SUBSTITUTION OF ASPARTIC ACID FOR HISTIDINE AT BETA 77.

        GAMMACK, D. B., HUEHNS, E. R., LEHMANN, H. AND SHOOTER, E. M.* THE ABNORMAL   D
    POLYPEPTIDE CHAINS IN A NUMBER OF HAEMOGLOBIN VARIANTS. ACTA GENET. STATIST. MED.   O
    11* 1-16, 1961.   M
                                                                                             I
        RAHBAR, S., BEALE, D., ISAACS, W. A. AND LEHMANN, H.* ABNORMAL HAEMOGLOBINS IN   N
    IRAN. OBSERVATIONS OF A NEW VARIANT - HAEMOGLOBIN J IRAN (ALPHA 2 BETA 2 HIS TO   A
    ASP). BRIT. MED. J. 1* 674-677, 1967.   N
                                                                                             T
--HEMOGLOBIN J(IRELAND).
    SAME AS HEMOGLOBIN J(BALTIMORE).

        WENT, L. N. AND MACIVER, J. E.* SICKLE-CELL HAEMOGLOBIN-J DISEASE. BRIT. MED.
    J. 2* 138-139, 1959.

--HEMOGLOBIN J(JAMAICA).
    BETA CHAIN ANOMALY.

        GAMMACK, D. B., HUEHNS, E. R., LEHMANN, H. AND SHOOTER, E. M.* THE ABNORMAL
    POLYPEPTIDE CHAINS IN A NUMBER OF HAEMOGLOBIN VARIANTS. ACTA GENET. STATIST. MED.
    11* 1-16, 1961.

--HEMOGLOBIN J(KAOHSIUNG).
    SUBSTITUTION OF THREONINE FOR LYSINE AT BETA 59.

        BLACKWELL, R. Q., LIU, C.-S. AND SHIH, T.-B.* HEMOGLOBIN J KAOHSIUNG* BETA 59
    LYS TO THR. BIOCHIM. BIOPHYS. ACTA 229* 343-348, 1971.

--HEMOGLOBIN J(KORAT).
    SUBSTITUTION OF ASPARTIC ACID FOR GLYCINE AT BETA 56.

        BLACKWELL, R. Q. AND LIU, C.-S.* THE IDENTICAL STRUCTURAL ANOMALIES OF
    HEMOGLOBIN J(MEINUNG) AND J(KORAT). BIOCHEM. BIOPHYS. RES. COMMUN. 24* 732-738,
    1966.

--HEMOGLOBIN J(MALAYA).
    ALPHA CHAIN ANOMALY.

        LEHMANN, H.* HAEMOGLOBINS AND HAEMOGLOBINOPATHIES. IN *HAEMOGLOBIN-COLLO-
    QUIUM.* H. LEHMANN AND K. BETKE (EDS.)* STUTTGART* GEORG THIEME VERLAG, 1962.
    PP. 1-14.

--HEMOGLOBIN J(MANADO).
    SUBSTITUTION OF ASPARTIC ACID FOR GLYCINE AT BETA 56. SAME AS HEMOGLOBIN J
    MEINUNG, HEMOGLOBIN J KORAT AND HB J BANGKOK.

        BLACKWELL, R. Q., LIU, C.-S., ENG, L.-I. L. AND PRIBADI, W.* FAST HEMOGLOBIN
    VARIANT IN MINAHASSAN PEOPLE OF SULAWESI, CHINESE AND THAIS* ALPHA(2)BETA(2) 56
    GLY-TO-ASP. AM. J. PHYS. ANTHROP. 32* 147-150, 1970.

--HEMOGLOBIN J(MEDELLIN).
    SUBSTITUTION OF ASPARTIC ACID FOR GLYCINE AT ALPHA 22.

        GOTTLIEB, A. J., RESTREPO, A. AND ITANO, H. A.* HB J(MEDELLIN). CHEMICAL AND
    GENETIC STUDY. FED. PROC. 23* 172 ONLY, 1964.

--HEMOGLOBIN J(MEINUNG).
    SUBSTITUTION OF ASPARTIC ACID FOR GLYCINE AT BETA 56.

        BLACKWELL, R. Q. AND LIU, C.* THE IDENTICAL STRUCTURAL ANOMALIES OF HEMOGLOBIN-
    J(MEINUNG) AND J(KORAT). BIOCHEM. BIOPHYS. RES. COMMUN. 24* 732-738, 1966.

--HEMOGLOBIN J(OXFORD).
    SUBSTITUTION OF ASPARTIC ACID FOR GLYCINE AT ALPHA 15. SAME AS HEMOGLOBIN
    I(INTERLAKEN).

        LIDDELL, J., BROWN, D., BEALE, D., LEHMANN, H. AND HUNTSMAN, R. G.* A NEW
    HAEMOGLOBIN J(ALPHA)-OXFORD, FOUND DURING A SURVEY OF AN ENGLISH POPULATION.
    NATURE 204* 269-270, 1964.

--HEMOGLOBIN J(PARIS-1).
    SUBSTITUTION OF ALANINE FOR ASPARTIC ACID AT ALPHA 12.

        ROSA, J., MALEKNIA, N., VERGOS, D. AND DUNET, R.* UNE NOUVELLE HEMOGLOBINE
    ANORMALE* L*HEMOGLOBINE J(ALPHA-PARIS) 12 ALA A ASP. NOUV. REV. FRANC. HEMAT. 6*
    423-426, 1966.

        TRINCAO, C., DEMELO, J. M., LORKIN, P. A. AND LEHMANN, H.* HAEMOGLOBIN J PARIS
    IN THE SOUTH OF PORTUGAL (ALGARVE). ACTA HAEMAT. 39* 291-298, 1968.

--HEMOGLOBIN J(PARIS-2).
     SUBSTITUTION OF GLUTAMIC ACID FOR GLUTAMINE AT ALPHA 54. IDENTICAL TO HEMOGLOBIN-
     MEXICO.

          LABIE, D. AND ROSA, J.* SUR UNE NOUVELLE HEMOGLOBINE ANORMALE* L*HEMOGLOBINE J
     (ALPHA-54 GLUTAMINE A GLUTAMIQUE). NOUV. REV. FRANC. HEMAT. 6* 426-430, 1966.

--HEMOGLOBIN J(RAMBAM).
     SUBSTITUTION OF ASPARTIC ACID FOR GLYCINE AT BETA 69.

          SALOMON, H., TATARSKI, I., DANCE, N., HUEHNS, E. R. AND SHOOTER, E. M.* A NEW
     HEMOGLOBIN VARIANT FOUND IN A BEDOUIN TRIBE* HEMOGLOBIN *RAMBAM.* (ABSTRACT)
     ISREAL J. MED. SCI. 1* 836-840, 1965. (PUBLISHED SEPARATELY BY GRUNE AND
     STRATTON, N.Y., 1965. G. IZAK AND M. PRYWES (EDS.).

--HEMOGLOBIN J(SARDEGNA).
     SUBSTITUTION OF ASPARTIC ACID FOR HISTIDINE AT ALPHA 50.

          TANGHERONI, W., ZORCOLO, G., GALLO, E. AND LEHMANN, H.* HAEMOGLOBIN J(SARDEG-
     NA)* ALPHA 50(CD8) HISTIDINE - ASPARTIC ACID. NATURE 218* 470-471, 1968.

--HEMOGLOBIN J(TONGARIKI).
     SUBSTITUTION OF ASPARTIC ACID FOR ALANINE AT ALPHA 115. A HOMOZYGOUS INDIVIDUAL
     HAD ONLY ANOMALOUS HEMOGLOBIN SUGGESTING THE EXISTENCE OF ONLY ONE ALPHA LOCUS IN
     MELANESIANS.

          ABRAMSON, R. K., RUCKNAGEL, D. L., SHREFFLER, D. C. AND SAAVE, J. J.* HOMOZY-
     GOUS HB J TONGARIKI* EVIDENCE FOR ONLY ONE ALPHA CHAIN STRUCTURAL LOCUS IN
     MELANESIANS. SCIENCE 169* 194-196, 1970.

          GAJDUSEK, D. C., GUIART, J., KIRK, R. L., CARRELL, R. W., IRVINE, D., KYNOCH,
     P. A. M. AND LEHMANN, H.* HAEMOGLOBIN J TONGARIKI (ALPHA 115 ALANINE TO ASPARTIC
     ACID)* THE FIRST NEW HAEMOGLOBIN VARIANT FOUND IN A PACIFIC (MELANESIAN) POPULA-
     TION. J. MED. GENET. 4* 1-6, 1967.

--HEMOGLOBIN J(TORONTO).
     SUBSTITUTION OF ASPARTIC ACID FOR ALANINE AT ALPHA 5.

          CROOKSTON, J. H., BEALE, D., IRVINE, D. AND LEHMANN, H.* A NEW HAEMOGLOBIN, J
     TORONTO (ALPHA-5 ALANINE TO ASPARTIC ACID). NATURE 208* 1059-1060, 1965.

--HEMOGLOBIN J(TRINIDAD).
     SUBSTITUTION OF GLYCINE FOR ASPARTIC ACID AT BETA 16. SAME AS HEMOGLOBIN J(BALTI-
     MORE).

          GAMMACK, D. B., HUEHNS, E. R., LEHMANN, H. AND SHOOTER, E. M.* THE ABNORMAL
     POLYPEPTIDE CHAINS IN A NUMBER OF HAEMOGLOBIN VARIANTS. ACTA GENET. STATIST. MED.
     11* 1-16, 1961.

--HEMOGLOBIN K.
     BETA CHAIN ANOMALY.

          O*GORMAN, P., LEHMANN, H., ALLSOPP, K. M. AND SUKUMARAN, P. K.* SICKLE CELL
     HAEMOGLOBIN K DISEASE. BRIT. MED. J. 2* 1381-1382, 1963.

--HEMOGLOBIN K(CALCUTTA).
     ALPHA CHAIN ANOMALY. FAST HEMOGLOBIN.

          LEHMANN, H.* HAEMOGLOBINS AND HAEMOGLOBINOPATHIES. IN *HAEMOGLOBIN-COLLO-
     QUIUM.* H. LEHMANN AND K. BETKE (EDS.)* STUTTGART* GEORG THIEME VERLAG, 1962.
     PP. 1-14.

--HEMOGLOBIN K(IBADAN).
     SUBSTITUTION OF GLUTAMIC ACID FOR GLYCINE AT BETA 46. FOR REFERENCE SEE HEMOGLO-
     BIN K(WOOLWICH).

--HEMOGLOBIN K(MADRAS).
     ALPHA CHAIN ANOMALY.

          AGER, J. A. M. AND LEHMANN, H.* HAEMOGLOBIN K IN AN EAST INDIAN AND HIS FAMILY.
     BRIT. MED. J. 1* 1449-1450, 1957.

--HEMOGLOBIN K(WOOLWICH).
     SUBSTITUTION OF GLUTAMINE FOR LYSINE AT BETA 132.

          ALLAN, N., BEALE, D., IRVINE, D. AND LEHMANN, H.* THREE HAEMOGLOBINS K*
     WOOLWICH, AN ABNORMAL, CAMEROON AND IBADAN, TWO UNUSUAL VARIANTS OF HUMAN
     HAEMOGLOBIN A. NATURE 208* 658-661, 1965.

--HEMOGLOBIN KAGOSHIMA.
     SAME AS HEMOGLOBIN NORFOLK.

--HEMOGLOBIN KANSAS.
    ALSO KNOWN AS HEMOGLOBIN REISSMANN (Q.V.). SUBSTITUTION OF THREONINE FOR ASPARTIC
ACID AT BETA 102.

    BONAVENTURA, J. AND RIGGS, A.* HEMOGLOBIN KANSAS, A HUMAN HEMOGLOBIN WITH A
NEUTRAL AMINO ACID SUBSTITUTION AND AN ABNORMAL OXYGEN EQUILIBRIUM. J. BIOL.
CHEM. 243* 980-991, 1968.

--HEMOGLOBIN KARAMOJO.
    ALPHA CHAIN VARIANT.

    ALLBROOK, D., BARNICOT, N. A., DANCE, N., LAWLER, S. D., MARSHALL, R. AND
MUNGAI, J.* BLOOD GROUPS, HAEMOGLOBIN AND SERUM FACTORS OF THE KARAMOJO. HUM.
BIOL. 37* 217-237, 1965.

--HEMOGLOBIN KEMPSEY.
    SUBSTITUTION OF ASPARAGINE FOR ASPARTIC ACID AT BETA 99.

    REED, C. S., HAMPSON, R., GORDON, S., JONES, R. T., NOVY, M. J., BRIMHALL, B.,
EDWARDS, M. J. AND KOLER, R. D.* ERYTHROCYTOSIS SECONDARY TO INCREASED OXYGEN
AFFINITY OF A MUTANT HEMOGLOBIN, HEMOGLOBIN KEMPSEY. BLOOD 31* 623-632, 1968.

--HEMOGLOBIN KENWOOD.
    SUBSTITUTION OF GLUTAMIC ACID FOR LYSINE AT BETA 95. IDENTICAL TO HB N(BALTI-
MORE). THIS WAS PREVIOUSLY REPORTED INCORRECTLY AS HAVING EITHER ASPARTIC ACID OR
GLUTAMIC ACID AT BETA 143. SEE PERSONAL COMMUNICATION FROM HELLER IN HAMILTON ET
AL. (1969).

    HAMILTON, H. B., IUCHI, I., MIYAJI, T. AND SHIBATA, S.* HEMOGLOBIN HIROSHIMA
(BETA-143 HISTIDINE TO ASPARTIC ACID)* A NEWLY IDENTIFIED FAST MOVING BETA CHAIN
VARIANT ASSOCIATED WITH INCREASED OXYGEN AFFINITY AND COMPENSATORY ERYTHREMIA. J.
CLIN. INVEST. 48* 525-535, 1969.

--HEMOGLOBIN KHARTOUM.
    SUBSTITUTION OF ARGININE FOR PROLINE AT BETA 124.

    CLEGG, J. B., WEATHERALL, D. J., BOON, W. H. AND MUSTAFA, D.* TWO NEW HAEMOGLO-
BIN VARIANTS INVOLVING PROLINE SUBSTITUTIONS. NATURE 222* 379-380, 1969.

--HEMOGLOBIN KINGS COUNTY.
    PROBABLY BETA CHAIN DEFECT. OBSERVED IN AN AMERICAN NEGRO FAMILY. AFFECTED
PERSONS HAD NONSPHEROCYTIC HEMOLYTIC HEINZ BODY ANEMIA.

    SATHIAPALAN, R. AND ROBINSON, M. G.* HEREDITARY HAEMOLYTIC ANAEMIA DUE TO AN
ABNORMAL HAEMOGLOBIN (HAEMOGLOBIN KINGS COUNTY).   BRIT. J. HAEMAT. 15* 579-587,
1968.

--HEMOGLOBIN KNOXVILLE-1.
    SAME AS G(PHILADELPHIA).

--HEMOGLOBIN KOELLIKER.
    NOT A GENETIC CHANGE. THE C-TERMINAL AMINO ACID, NO. 141, OF THE ALPHA CHAIN
(ARGININE) IS MISSING, PROBABLY FROM THE ACTION OF A CARBOXYPEPTIDASE PRESENT IN
NORMAL PLASMA. THIS UNUSUAL FAST HEMOGLOBIN IS OBSERVED IN PERSONS WITH HEMOLY-
SIS.

    MARTI, H. R., BEALE, D. AND LEHMANN, H.* HAEMOGLOBIN KOELLIKER* A NEW ACQUIRED
HAEMOGLOBIN APPEARING AFTER SEVERE HAEMOLYSIS* ALPHA-2 (MINUS 141 ARG) BETA-2.
ACTA HAEMAT. 37* 174-180, 1967.

--HEMOGLOBIN KOKURA.
    SUBSTITUTION OF GLYCINE FOR ASPARTIC ACID AT ALPHA 47.

    OOYA, I., KAWAMURA, K., SEITA, M., HANADA, M. AND HITSUMOTO, A.* HEMOGLOBIN
KOKURA WHICH WAS DISCOVERED IN KOKURA. 23RD GEN. MEETING JAPAN. SOC. HEMATOL.
KYOTO, 1961.

    YAMAOKA, K., KAWAMURA, K., HANADA, M., SEITA, M., HITSUMOTO, S. AND OOYA, I.*
STUDIES ON ABNORMAL HAEMOGLOBINS. JAP. J. HUM. GENET. 5* 99-111, 1960.

--HEMOGLOBIN KOLN.
    SUBSTITUTION OF METHIONINE FOR VALINE AT BETA 98.

    CARRELL, R. W., LEHMANN, H. AND HUTCHISON, H. E.* HAEMOGLOBIN KOLN (BETA-98
VALINE TO METHIONINE)* AN UNSTABLE PROTEIN CAUSING INCLUSION BODY ANAEMIA. NATURE
210* 915-917, 1966.

    HUTCHISON, H. E., PINKERTON, P. H., WATERS, P., DOUGLAS, A. S., LEHMANN, H. AND
BEALE, D.* HEREDITARY HEINZ-BODY ANAEMIA, THROMBOCYTOPENIA, AND HAEMOGLOBINOPATHY

(HB KOLN) IN A GLASGOW FAMILY. BRIT. MED. J. 2* 1099-1103, 1964.

D
O
M
I
N
A
N
T

JACKSON, J. M., WAY, B. J. AND WOODLIFF, H. J.* A WEST AUSTRALIAN FAMILY WITH A HAEMOLYTIC DISORDER ASSOCIATED WITH HAEMOGLOBIN KOLN. BRIT. J. HAEMAT. 13* 474-481, 1967.

JONES, R. V., GRIMES, A. J., CARRELL, R. W. AND LEHMANN, H.* KOLN HAEMOGLOBINO-PATHY* FURTHER DATA AND A COMPARISON WITH OTHER HEREDITARY HEINZ BODY ANAEMIAS. BRIT. J. HAEMAT. 13* 394-408, 1967.

PRIBILLA, W.* THALASSEMIE-AHNLICHE ERKRANKUNG MIT NEUEM MINOR-HB (HB KOLN). IN *HAEMOGLOBIN-COLLOQUIUM.* H. LEHMANN AND K. BETKE (EDS.)* STUTTGART* GEORG THIEME VERLAG, 1962. PP. 1-14.

PRIBILLA, W., KLESSE, P., BETKE, K., LEHMANN, H. AND BEALE, D.* HAEMOGLOBIN KOLN DISEASE* FAMILIAL HYPOCHROMIC HEMOLYTIC ANEMIA WITH HEMOGLOBIN ANOMALY. KLIN. WSCHR. 43* 1049-1053, 1965.

--HEMOGLOBIN KORLE-BU.
SUBSTITUTION OF ASPARAGINE FOR ASPARTIC ACID AT BETA 73. SINCE THIS SAME SUBSTITUTION IS PRESENT, WITH THE SICKLE HEMOGLOBIN CHANGE, AS ONE OF THE TWO DEFECTS IN HEMOGLOBIN C(HARLEM), KONOTEY-AHULU ET AL. (1968) SUGGESTED THAT THE LATTER HEMOGLOBIN MAY HAVE ARISEN BY INTRACISTRONIC CROSSING OVER IN AN INDIVIDUAL WITH THE KORLE-BU GENE ON ONE CHROMOSOME AND THE SICKLE GENE ON THE OTHER.

KONOTEY-AHULU, F. I. D., GALLO, E., LEHMANN, H. AND RINGELHANN, B.* HAEMOGLOBIN KORLE-BU (BETA 73 ASPARTIC ACID TO ASPARAGINE) SHOWING ONE OF THE TWO AMINO ACID SUBSTITUTIONS OF HAEMOGLOBIN C HARLEM. J. MED. GENET. 5* 107-111, 1968.

--HEMOGLOBIN KOYA DORA.
EXCESSIVE LENGTH OF ALPHA-LIKE CHAIN (WITH 155 OR 156 AMINO ACIDS RATHER THAN 141).

DE JONG, W. W. W.* LEIDEN, HOLLAND* PERSONAL COMMUNICATION, 1970.

--HEMOGLOBIN L.
BETA CHAIN ANOMALY.

AGER, J. A. M. AND LEHMANN, H.* HAEMOGLOBIN L* A NEW HAEMOGLOBIN FOUND IN A PUNJABI HINDU. BRIT. MED. J. 2* 142-143, 1957.

GAMMACK, D. B., HUEHNS, E. R., LEHMANN, H. AND SHOOTER, E. M.* THE ABNORMAL POLYPEPTIDE CHAINS IN A NUMBER OF HAEMOGLOBIN VARIANTS. ACTA GENET. STATIST. MED. 11* 1-16, 1961.

--HEMOGLOBIN L(BOMBAY).
ALPHA CHAIN ANOMALY.

SUKUMARAN, P. K. AND PIK, C.* SOME OBSERVATIONS ON HAEMOGLOBIN L(BOMBAY). BIOCHIM. BIOPHYS. ACTA 104* 290-292, 1965.

--HEMOGLOBIN L(FERRARA).
SUBSTITUTION OF GLYCINE FOR ASPARTIC ACID AT ALPHA 47. SAME AS HEMOGLOBIN KOKURA. SAME AS HEMOGLOBIN BEILINSON.

NAGEL, R. L., RANNEY, H. M., BRADLEY, T. B., JACOBS, A. AND UDEM, L.* HEMOGLO-BIN L FERRARA IN A JEWISH FAMILY ASSOCIATED WITH A HEMOLYTIC STATE IN THE PROPOSITUS. BLOOD 34* 157-165, 1969.

SILVESTRONI, E., BIANCO, I., LUCCI, R. AND SOFFRITTI, E.* PRESENCE OF HEMOGLO-BIN 'L' IN NATIVES OF FERRARA AND OF HEMOGLOBIN 'D' IN NATIVES OF BOLOGNA. ACTA GENET. MED. GEM. 9* 472-496, 1960.

SILVESTRONI, E., BIANCO, I., LUCCI, R. AND SOFFRITTI, E.* THE HEMATOLOGICAL PICTURE IN CARRIERS OF HB L, LIVING IN FERRARA. ASSOCIATIONS AND RELATIONS TO MICROCYTHENIA. PROGR. MED. 16* 553-561, 1960.

--HEMOGLOBIN L(PERSIAN GULF).
SUBSTITUTION OF ARGININE FOR GLYCINE AT ALPHA 57.

RAHBAR, S., KINDERLERER, J. L. AND LEHMANN, H.* HAEMOGLOBIN L PERSIAN GULF* ALPHA 57 (E6) GLYCINE LEADS TO ARGININE. ACTA HAEMAT. 42* 169-175, 1969.

--HEMOGLOBIN LEIDEN.
DELETION OF GLUTAMIC ACID 6 OR 7 IN THE BETA CHAIN.

DE JONG, W. W. W., WENT, L. N. AND BERNINI, L. F.* ABNORMAL HAEMOGLOBIN - CHEMICAL CHARACTERIZATION OF HEMOGLOBIN LEIDEN. NATURE 220* 788-789, 1968.

--HEMOGLOBIN LEPORE.
BETA-DELTA FUSION.

BAGLIONI, C. AND VENTRUTO, V.* HUMAN ABNORMAL HEMOGLOBINS. II. A CHEMICAL
STUDY OF HEMOGLOBIN LEPORE FROM A HOMOZYGOTE INDIVIDUAL. EUROP. J. BIOCHEM. 5*
29-32, 1968.

GERALD, P. S. AND DIAMOND, L. K.* A NEW HEREDITARY HEMOGLOBINOPATHY (THE LEPORE
TRAIT) AND ITS INTERACTION WITH THALASSEMIA TRAIT. BLOOD 12* 835-844, 1958.

HUISMAN, T. H. K. AND SYDENSTRICKER, V. P.* HAEMOGLOBIN* DIFFERENCE IN GROSS
STRUCTURE OF TWO ELECTROPHORETICALLY IDENTICAL MINOR HAEMOGLOBIN COMPONENTS.
NATURE 193* 489-491, 1962.

--HEMOGLOBIN LEPORE(AUGUSTA).
SAME AS HEMOGLOBIN LEPORE (WASHINGTON).

LABIE, D., SCHROEDER, W. A. AND HUISMAN, T. H. J.* THE AMINO ACID SEQUENCE OF
THE DELTA-BETA CHAINS OF HEMOGLOBIN LEPORE(AUGUSTA) - HEMOGLOBIN LE-
PORE(WASHINGTON). BIOCHIM. BIOPHYS. ACTA 127* 428-437, 1966.

--HEMOGLOBIN LEPORE(BALTIMORE).
BETA-DELTA FUSION.

OSTERTAG, W. AND SMITH, E. W.* HEMOGLOBIN-LEPORE-BALTIMORE, A THIRD TYPE OF A
DELTA, BETA CROSSOVER (DELTA 50, BETA 86). EUROP. J. BIOCHEM. 10* 371-376, 1969.

--HEMOGLOBIN LEPORE(BOSTON).
BETA-DELTA FUSION. SAME AS HEMOGLOBIN PYLOS.

BAGLIONI, C.* THE FUSION OF TWO PEPTIDE CHAINS IN HEMOGLOBIN LEPORE AND ITS
INTERPRETATION AS A GENETIC DELETION. PROC. NAT. ACAD. SCI. 48* 1880-1886, 1962.

--HEMOGLOBIN LEPORE(CYPRUS).
BETA-DELTA FUSION.

BEAVEN, G. H., GRATZER, W. B., STEVENS, B. L., SHOOTER, E. M., ELLIS, M. J.,
WHITE, J. C. AND GILLESPIE, J. E. O.* AN ABNORMAL HAEMOGLOBIN (LEPORE-CYPRUS)
RESEMBLING HAEMOGLOBIN-LEPORE AND ITS INTERACTION WITH THALASSAEMIA. BRIT. J.
HAEMAT. 10* 159-170, 1964.

--HEMOGLOBIN LEPORE(HOLLANDIA).
BETA-DELTA FUSION.

BAGLIONI, C.* THE FUSION OF TWO PEPTIDE CHAINS IN HEMOGLOBIN LEPORE AND ITS
INTERPRETATION AS A GENETIC DELETION. PROC. NAT. ACAD. SCI. 48* 1880-1886, 1962.

BARNABAS, J. AND MULLER, C. J.* HAEMOGLOBIN LEPORE(HOLLANDIA). NATURE 194*
931-932, 1962.

--HEMOGLOBIN LEPORE(THE BRONX).
BETA-DELTA FUSION.

RANNEY, H. M. AND JACOBS, A. S.* SIMULTANEOUS OCCURRENCE OF HAEMOGLOBINS C AND
LEPORE IN AN AFRO-AMERICAN. NATURE 204* 163-166, 1964.

--HEMOGLOBIN M.
AS OUTLINED BELOW, EIGHT OR MORE ABERRANT HEMOGLOBINS ASSOCIATED WITH METHEMOGLO-
BINEMIA HAVE BEEN IDENTIFIED. ALL ARE REFERRED TO AS HEMOGLOBIN M. SOME HAVE
ALPHA CHAIN SUBSTITUTIONS AND SOME HAVE BETA CHAIN SUBSTITUTIONS. IN ALL THE
SUBSTITUTION IS AT A POSITION CRITICAL TO THE GLOBIN-HEME INTERRELATIONSHIP. ALL
MOVE SLOWER THAN HEMOGLOBIN A IN ALKALINE ELECTROPHORESIS.

--HEMOGLOBIN M(AKITA).
SUBSTITUTION OF TYROSINE FOR HISTIDINE AT BETA 92.

SHIBATA, S., MIYAJI, T., IUCHI, I., OHBA, Y. AND YAMAMOTO, K.* AMINO ACID
SUBSTITUTION IN HEMOGLOBIN M(AKITA). J. BIOCHEM. 63* 193-198, 1968.

--HEMOGLOBIN M(BOSTON).
SAME AS M(GOTHENBURG), M(OSAKA) AND PERHAPS M(LEIPZIG-2). SUBSTITUTION OF
TYROSINE FOR HISTIDINE AT ALPHA 58. WITH ONE EXCEPTION THE HEMOGLOBINS M HAVE
SUBSTITUTIONS OF THE HISTIDINE AT ALPHA 53, ALPHA 87, BETA 63 OR BETA 92. THESE
FOUR AMINO ACIDS ARE CRITICAL TO THE BINDING OF THE HEME GROUP. THE EXCEPTION IS
HEMOGLOBIN M(MILWAUKEE-1).

BETKE, K.* HAMOGLOBIN M* TYPEN UND IHRE DIFFERENZIERUNG (UBERSICHT). IN
HAEMOGLOBIN-COLLOQUIUM. H. LEHMANN AND K. BETKE (EDS.)* STUTTGART* GEORG THIEME
VERLAG, 1962. PP. 39-47.

GERALD, P. S. AND EFRON, M. L.* CHEMICAL STUDIES OF SEVERAL VARIETIES OF HB M.
PROC. NAT. ACAD. SCI. 47* 1758-1767, 1961.

GERALD, P. S., COOK, C. D. AND DIAMOND, L. K.* HEMOGLOBIN M. SCIENCE 126* 300-
301, 1957.

HANSEN, H. A., JAGENBURG, O. R. AND JOHANSSON, B. G.* STUDIES ON AN ABNORMAL HEMOGLOBIN CAUSING HEREDITARY CONGENITAL CYANOSIS. ACTA PAEDIAT. 49* 503-511, 1960.

D
O
M
I
N
A
N
T

--HEMOGLOBIN M(CHICAGO).
SAME AS HEMOGLOBIN M(SASKATOON).

HELLER, P.* HEMOGLOBIN M(CHICAGO) AND M(KANKAKEE). IN *HAEMOGLOBIN-COLLO-QUIUM.* H. LEHMANN AND K. BETKE (EDS.)* STUTTGART* GEORG THIEME VERLAG, 1962. PP. 47-49.

JOSEPHSON, A. M., WEINSTEIN, H. G., YAKULIS, V. J., SINGER, L. AND HELLER, P.* A NEW VARIANT OF HEMOGLOBIN M DISEASE. HEMOGLOBIN M(CHICAGO). J. LAB. CLIN. MED. 59* 918-925, 1962.

--HEMOGLOBIN M(FREIBURG).
SEE HEMOGLOBIN FREIBURG.

--HEMOGLOBIN M(HAMBURG).
SAME AS M(SASKATOON).

BETKE, K., KLEIHAUER, E., GEHRING-MULLER, R., BRAUNITZER, G., JACOBI, J. AND SCHMIDT, D.* HB M HAMBURG, EINE BETA-KETTEN-ANOMALIE* ALPHA-2 BETA-2 (63 TYR). KLIN. WSCHR. 44* 961-966, 1966.

--HEMOGLOBIN M(HITA).
SAME AS HEMOGLOBIN M(SASKATOON). HANADA ET AL.* FOR REFERENCE SEE HEMOGLOBIN TAGAWA II.

--HEMOGLOBIN M(HYDE PARK).
SUBSTITUTION OF TYROSINE FOR HISTIDINE AT BETA 92. SAME AS HEMOGLOBIN M(MILWAU-KEE-2).

HELLER, P., COLEMAN, R. D. AND YAKULIS, V.* HEMOGLOBIN M* A NEW VARIANT OF ABNORMAL METHEMOGLOBIN IN A NEGRO. (ABSTRACT) PROC. THIRD INTERN. CONG. HUM. GENET. (CHICAGO, SEPT. 5-10), 1966. (ALSO J. CLIN. INVEST. 45* 1021 ONLY, 1966.)

--HEMOGLOBIN M(IWATE).
SUBSTITUTION OF TYROSINE FOR HISTIDINE AT ALPHA 87.

GERALD, P. S. AND EFRON, M. L.* CHEMICAL STUDIES OF SEVERAL VARIETIES OF HB M. PROC. NAT. ACAD. SCI. 47* 1758-1767, 1961.

MEYERING, C. A., ISRAELS, A. L., SEBENS, T. AND HUISMAN, T. H.* STUDIES ON THE HETEROGENEITY OF HEMOGLOBIN. II. THE HETEROGENEITY OF DIFFERENT HUMAN HEMOGLOBIN TYPES IN CARBOXYMETHYLCELLULOSE AND IN AMBERLITE IRC-50 CHROMATOGRAPHY. QUANTITA-TIVE ASPECTS. CLIN. CHIM. ACTA 5* 208-222, 1960.

MIYAJI, T., UEDA, S., SHIBATA, S., TAMURA, A. AND SASAKI, H.* FURTHER STUDIES ON THE FINGERPRINT OF HB M(IWATE). ACTA HAEMAT. JAP. 25* 169-175, 1962.

SHIBATA, S.* HEREDITARY NIGREMIA (GENETICOBIOCHEMICAL ASPECTS). JAP. J. HUM. GENET. 9* 193-206, 1964.

SHIBATA, S., IUCHI, I., MIYAJI, T. AND UEDA, S.* SPECTROSCOPIC CHARACTERIZATION OF HEMOGLOBIN M(IWATE) AND HEMOGLOBIN M(KURUME), THE TWO VARIANTS OF HEMOGLOBIN M FOUND IN JAPAN. ACTA HAEMAT. JAP. 24* 477-485 AND 486-494, 1961.

SHIBATA, S., TAMURA, A., IUCHI, I. AND TAKAHASHI, H.* HEMOGLOBIN M-1. DEMONS-TRATION OF A NEW ABNORMAL HEMOGLOBIN IN HEREDITARY NIGREMIA. ACTA HAEMAT. JAP. 23* 96-104, 1960.

SHIMIZU, A., TSUGITA, A., HAYASHI, A. AND YAMAMURA, Y.* THE PRIMARY STRUCTURE OF HEMOGLOBIN M(IWATE). BIOCHIM. BIOPHYS. ACTA 107* 270-277, 1965.

TAMURA, A.* BLACK BLOOD DISEASE. JAP. J. HUM. GENET. 9* 183-192, 1964.

--HEMOGLOBIN M(KANKAKEE).
SAME AS HEMOGLOBIN M(IWATE).

HELLER, P.* HEMOGLOBIN M(CHICAGO) AND M(KANKAKEE). IN *HAEMOGLOBIN-COLLO-QUIUM.* H. LEHMANN AND K. BETKE (EDS.)* STUTTGART* GEORG THIEME VERLAG, 1962. PP. 47-49.

HELLER, P., WEINSTEIN, H. G., YAKULIS, V. J. AND ROSENTHAL, I. M.* HEMOGLOBIN M(KANKAKEE), A NEW VARIANT OF HEMOGLOBIN M. BLOOD 20* 287-301, 1962.

--HEMOGLOBIN M(KANSAS).
SUBSTITUTION OF THREONINE FOR ASPARAGINE AT BETA 102.

REISSMAN, K. R., RUTH, W. E. AND NOMURA, T.* A HUMAN HEMOGLOBIN WITH LOWERED OXYGEN AFFINITY AND IMPAIRED HEME-HEME INTERACTIONS. J. CLIN. INVEST. 40* 1826-

--HEMOGLOBIN M(LEIPZIG-1).
    CHAIN ANOMALY UNKNOWN.

    BETKE, K., GROSCHNER, E. AND BOCK, K.* PROPERTIES OF A FURTHER VARIANT OF
HEMOGLOBIN M. NATURE 188* 864-865, 1960.

--HEMOGLOBIN M(MILWAUKEE-1).
    SUBSTITUTION OF GLUTAMIC ACID FOR VALINE AT BETA 67.

    GERALD, P. S. AND EFRON, M. L.* CHEMICAL STUDIES OF SEVERAL VARIETIES OF HB M.
PROC. NAT. ACAD. SCI. 47* 1758-1767, 1961.

    HAYASHI, A., SUZUKI, T., IMAI, K., MORIMOTO, H. AND WATARI, H.* PROPERTIES OF
HEMOGLOBIN M, MILWAUKEE-1 VARIANT AND ITS UNIQUE CHARACTERISTIC. BIOCHIM.
BIOPHYS. ACTA 194* 6-15, 1969.

    PISCIOTTA, A. V., EBRE, S. N. AND HINZ, J. E.* CLINICAL AND LABORATORY FEATURES
OF TWO VARIANTS OF METHEMOGLOBIN-M DISEASE. J. LAB. CLIN. MED. 54* 73-87, 1959.

--HEMOGLOBIN M(MILWAUKEE-2).
    SAME AS HEMOGLOBIN M(HYDE PARK).

    PISCIOTTA, A. V., EBRE, S. N. AND HINZ, J. E.* CLINICAL AND LABORATORY FEATURES
OF TWO VARIANTS OF METHEMOGLOBIN-M DISEASE. J. LAB. CLIN. MED. 54* 73-87, 1959.

--HEMOGLOBIN M(OLDENBURG).
    PROBABLY SUBSTITUTION OF HISTIDINE BY TYROSINE AT ALPHA 87 AND THUS SAME AS
HEMOGLOBIN M(IWATE) AND HEMOGLOBIN M(KANKAKEE).

    PIK, C. AND TONZ, O.* NATURE OF HAEMOGLOBIN M(OLDENBURG). NATURE 210* 1182
ONLY, 1966.

    TONZ, O., SIMON, H. A. AND HASSELFELD, W.* UNTERSUCHUNG EINER GROSSEN HAMOGLO-
BIN-M-SIPPE. ENTDECKUNG EINES NEUEN BLUTFARBSTOFFES* HB M-OLDENBURG. SCHWEIZ.
MED. WSCHR. 92* 1311-1313, 1962.

--HEMOGLOBIN M(OSAKA).
    SUBSTITUTION OF TYROSINE FOR HISTIDINE AT ALPHA 58.

    HAYASHI, A., YAMAMURA, Y., OGITA, S. AND KIKKAWA, H.* HEMOGLOBIN M(OSAKA), A
NEW VARIANT OF HEMOGLOBIN M. JAP. J. HUM. GENET. 9* 87-94, 1964.

    SHIMIZU, A., HAYASHI, A., YAMAMURA, Y., TSUGITA, A. AND KITAYAMA, K.* THE
STRUCTURAL STUDY ON A NEW HEMOGLOBIN VARIANT, HB M(OSAKA). BIOCHIM. BIOPHYS. ACTA
97* 472-482, 1965.

    SUZUKI, T., HAYASHI, A., YAMAMURA, Y., ENOKI, Y. AND TYUMA, I.* FUNCTIONAL
ABNORMALITY OF HEMOGLOBIN M(OSAKA). BIOCHEM. BIOPHYS. RES. COMMUN. 19* 691-695,
1965.

--HEMOGLOBIN M(RADOM).
    SAME AS HEMOGLOBIN M(SASKATOON).

    MURAWSKI, K., CARTA, S., SORCINI, M., TENTORI, L., VIVALDI, G., ANTONINE, E.,
BRUNORI, M., WYMAN, J., BUCCI, E. AND ROSSI-FANELLI, A.* OBSERVATIONS ON THE
STRUCTURE AND BEHAVIOR OF HEMOGLOBIN M(RADOM). ARCH. BIOCHEM. 111* 197-201, 1965.

--HEMOGLOBIN M(RESERVE).
    AN ALPHA CHAIN SUBSTITUTION. REDUCED OXYGEN AFFINITY AND DECREASED REVERSIBLE
OXYGEN BINDING CAPACITY.

    OVERLY, W. L., ROSENBERG, A. AND HARRIS, J. W.* HEMOGLOBIN M(RESERVE)* STUDIES
ON IDENTIFICATION AND CHARACTERIZATION. J. LAB. CLIN. MED. 69* 62-87, 1967.

--HEMOGLOBIN M(SASKATOON).
    SAME AS M(EMORY), M(RADOM) AND POSSIBLY M(KURUME) AND M(H-W). SUBSTITUTION OF
TYROSINE FOR HISTIDINE AT BETA 63.

    GERALD, P. S. AND EFRON, M. L.* CHEMICAL STUDIES OF SEVERAL VARIETIES OF HB M.
PROC. NAT. ACAD. SCI. 47* 1758-1767, 1961.

    GERALD, P. S. AND GEORGE, P.* SECOND SPECTROSCOPICALLY ABNORMAL METHEMOGLOBIN
ASSOCIATED WITH HEREDITARY CYANOSIS. SCIENCE 129* 393-394, 1959.

    HECK, W. AND WOLF, H.* ANGEBORENER HERZFEHLER MIT CYANOSE DURCH PATHOLOGISCHEN
BLUTFARBSTOFF (HB-M). ANN. PAEDIAT. 190* 135-146, 1958.

    HORLEIN, H. AND WEBER, G.* UEBER CHRONISCHE FAMILIARE METHAMOGLOBINS. DEUTSCH.
MED. WSCHR. 73* 476-478, 1948.

SHIBATA, S., IUCHI, I. AND MIYAJI, T.* HEMOGLOBIN M DISEASE IN JAPAN. ISRAEL J. MED. SCI. 1* 766-768, 1965.

SHIBATA, S., IUCHI, I., MIYAJI, T. AND UEDA, S.* SPECTROSCOPIC CHARACTERIZATION OF HEMOGLOBIN M(IWATE) AND HEMOGLOBIN M(KURUME), THE TWO VARIANTS OF HEMOGLOBIN M FOUND IN JAPAN. ACTA HAEMAT. JAP. 24* 477-485, 1961.

SHIBATA, S., MIYAJI, T., IUCHI, I. AND UEDA, S.* A COMPARATIVE STUDY OF HEMOGLOBIN M(IWATE) AND HEMOGLOBIN M(KURUME) BY MEANS OF ELECTROPHORESIS, CHROMATOGRAPHY AND ANALYSIS OF PEPTIDE CHAINS. ACTA HAEMAT. JAP. 24* 486-494, 1961.

--HEMOGLOBIN MAHIDOL.
SUBSTITUTION OF HISTIDINE FOR ASPARTIC ACID AT ALPHA 76.

POOTRAKUL, S. AND DIXON, G. H.* HEMOGLOBIN MAHIDOL* A NEW HEMOGLOBIN ALPHA-CHAIN MUTANT. CANAD. J. BIOCHEM. 48* 1066-1078, 1970.

--HEMOGLOBIN MANITOBA.
SUBSTITUTION OF ARGININE FOR SERINE AT ALPHA 102.

CROOKSTON, J. H., FARQUHARSON, H. A., KINDERLERER, J. L. AND LEHMANN, H.* HEMOGLOBIN MANITOBA* ALPHA 102(G9)SERINE REPLACED BY ARGININE. CANAD. J. BIOCHEM. 48* 911-914, 1970.

--HEMOGLOBIN MALMO.
SUBSTITUTION OF GLUTAMINE FOR HISTIDINE AT BETA 97.

LORKIN, P. A. AND LEHMANN, H.* TWO NEW PATHOLOGICAL HAEMOGLOBINS* OLMSTED BETA 141 (H19) LEU TO ARG AND MALMO BETA 97 (FG4) HIS TO GLU. BIOCHEM. J. 118* 38P ONLY, 1970.

--HEMOGLOBIN MEMPHIS.
SUBSTITUTION OF GLUTAMINE FOR GLUTAMIC ACID AT ALPHA 23. A HB S HOMOZYGOTE WHO ALSO CARRIES THIS ABNORMAL HEMOGLOBIN HAS A MILD FORM OF SICKLE CELL ANEMIA.

KRAUS, A. P., MIYAJI, T., IUCHI, I. AND KRAUS, L. M.* HEMOGLOBIN MEMPHIS, A NEW VARIANT OF SICKLE CELL ANEMIA. TRANS. ASS. AM. PHYSICIANS 80* 297-304, 1968.

KRAUS, A. P., MIYAJI, T., IUCHI, I. AND KRAUS, L. M.* HEMOGLOBIN MEMPHIS, AN ALPHA CHAIN MUTATION - ALPHA 23 GLUTAMINE. (ABSTRACT) PROC. THIRD INTERN. CONG. HUM. GENET. (CHICAGO, SEPT. 5-10), 1966.

--HEMOGLOBIN MEXICO.
SUBSTITUTION OF GLUTAMIC ACID FOR GLUTAMINE AT ALPHA 54. FAST HEMOGLOBIN.

JONES, R. T., BRIMHALL, B. AND LISKER, R.* CHEMICAL CHARACTERIZATION OF HEMOGLOBIN-MEXICO AND HEMOGLOBIN-CHIAPAS. BIOCHIM. BIOPHYS. ACTA 154* 488-495, 1968.

JONES, R. T., KOLER, R. D. AND LISKER, R.* THE CHEMICAL STRUCTURE OF HEMOGLOBIN MEXICO DETERMINED BY AUTOMATIC PEPTIDE CHROMATOGRAPHY AND SUBUNIT HYBRIDIZATION. CLIN. RES. 11* 105 ONLY, 1963.

QUATTRIN, N. AND VENTRUTO, V.* HEMOGLOBIN MEXICO IN A SARDINIAN WOMAN. HELV. MED. ACTA 33* 388-394, 1967.

--HEMOGLOBIN MIYADA.
A BETA-DELTA FUSION VARIANT, I.E., THE COMPLEMENT OF HEMOGLOBIN LEPORE. FOR EXPLANATION SEE HEMOGLOBIN P(CONGO).

YANASE, T., HANADA, M., SEITA, M., OHYA, I., OHTA, Y., IMAMURA, T., FUJIMURA, T., KAWASAKI, K. AND YAMAOKA, K.* MOLECULAR BASIS OF MORBIDITY, FROM A SERIES OF STUDIES OF HEMOGLOBINOPATHIES IN WESTERN JAPAN. JAP. J. HUM. GENET. 13* 40-53, 1968.

--HEMOGLOBIN N.
ALPHA CHAIN ANOMALY.

SILVESTRONI, E., BIANCO, I. AND BRANCATI, C.* HAEMOGLOBINS N AND P IN ITALIAN FAMILIES. NATURE 200* 658-659, 1963.

--HEMOGLOBIN N.
FAST HEMOGLOBIN. SUBSTITUTION OF ASPARTIC ACID FOR LYSINE AT BETA 95.

AGER, J. A. M. AND LEHMANN, H.* OBSERVATIONS ON SOME *FAST* HAEMOGLOBINS* K, J, N AND *BART'S.* BRIT. MED. J. 1* 929-931, 1958.

CHERNOFF, A. I. AND WEICHSELBAUM, T. E.* A MICROHEMOLYZING TECHNIC FOR PREPARING SOLUTIONS OF HEMOGLOBIN FOR PAPER ELECTROPHORETIC ANALYSIS. J. CLIN. PATH. 30* 120-125, 1958.

--HEMOGLOBIN N(BALTIMORE).
GLUTAMIC ACID SUBSTITUTION FOR LYSINE AT BETA 95.

CLEGG, J. B., NAUGHTON, M. A. AND WEATHERALL, D. J.* AN IMPROVED METHOD FOR THE
CHARACTERIZATION OF HUMAN HAEMOGLOBIN MUTANTS* IDENTIFICATION OF ALPHA-2, BETA-2
(95 GLU), HAEMOGLOBIN N(BALTIMORE). NATURE 207* 945-947, 1965.

WEATHERALL, D. J.* HEMOGLOBIN J(BALTIMORE) COEXISTING IN A FAMILY WITH
HEMOGLOBIN S-I. BULL. HOPKINS HOSP. 114* 1-12, 1964.

--HEMOGLOBIN N(JENKINS).
SUBSTITUTION OF GLUTAMIC ACID FOR LYSINE AT BETA 95. SAME AS HEMOGLOBIN N(BALTI-
MORE).

DOBBS, N. B., JR., SIMMONS, J. W., WILSON, J. B. AND HUISMAN, T. H. J.*
HEMOGLOBIN JENKINS OR HEMOGLOBIN-N-BALTIMORE OR ALPHA-2 BETA-2(GLU) 95. BIOCHIM.
BIOPHYS. ACTA 117* 492-494, 1966.

--HEMOGLOBIN N(MEMPHIS).
SUBSTITUTION OF EITHER GLUTAMIC ACID OR GLUTAMINE FOR LYSINE AT BETA 95.

SCHROEDER, W. A. AND JONES, R. T.* SOME ASPECTS OF THE CHEMISTRY AND FUNCTION
OF HUMAN AND ANIMAL HEMOGLOBINS. FORTSCHR. CHEM. ORGAN. NATURST. 23* 113-194,
1965.

--HEMOGLOBIN N(NEW HAVEN-2).
SAME AS HEMOGLOBIN J(BALTIMORE). SUBSTITUTION OF ASPARTIC ACID GLYCINE AT BETA
16.

CHERNOFF, A. I. AND PERILLIE, P. E.* THE AMINO ACID COMPOSITION OF HEMOGLOBIN B
NEW HAVEN-2 OR HGB N(NEW HAVEN). BIOCHEM. BIOPHYS. RES. COMMUN. 16* 368-372,
1964.

--HEMOGLOBIN N(SARDINIA).

SILVESTRONI, E. AND BIANCO, I.* HAEMATOLOGY* ASSOCIATION OF HAEMOGLOBIN N AND
MICROCYTHAEMIA IN A SARDINIAN FAMILY. NATURE 191* 1208-1209, 1961.

--HEMOGLOBIN N(SEATTLE).
SUBSTITUTION OF GLUTAMIC ACID FOR LYSINE AT BETA 61.

JONES, R. T., BRIMHALL, B., HUEHNS, E. R. AND MOTULSKY, A. G.* STRUCTURAL
CHARACTERIZATION OF HEMOGLOBIN N(SEATTLE)* ALPHA(2)BETA(2)61 LYS-TO-GLU. BIOCHIM.
BIOPHYS. ACTA 154* 278-283, 1968.

--HEMOGLOBIN NAGASAKI.
SUBSTITUTION OF LYSINE FOR GLUTAMIC ACID AT BETA 17.

MAEKAWA, M., MAEKAWA, T., FUJIWARA, N., TABARA, K. AND MATSUDA, G.* HEMOGLOBIN
NAGASAKI (ALPHA A2 BETA 17-2 GLU)* A NEW ABNORMAL HUMAN HEMOGLOBIN FOUND IN ONE
FAMILY IN NAGASAKI. INT. J. PROTEIN RES. 2* 147-156, 1970.

--HEMOGLOBIN NEW YORK.
SUBSTITUTION OF GLUTAMIC ACID FOR VALINE AT BETA 113. FOUND IN CHINESE-AMERICAN
FAMILY.

RANNEY, H. M., JACOBS, A. S. AND NAGEL, R. L.* HAEMOGLOBIN NEW YORK. NATURE
213* 876-878, 1967.

--HEMOGLOBIN NICOSIA.
ALPHA CHAIN SUBSTITUTION.

FESSAS, C., KARAKLIS, A., LOUKOPOULOS, D., STAMATOYANNOPOULOS, G. AND FESSAS,
P.* HEMOGLOBIN NICOSIA* AN ALPHA-CHAIN VARIANT AND ITS COMBINATION WITH BETA-
THALASSAEMIA. BRIT. J. HAEMAT. 11* 323-330, 1965.

--HEMOGLOBIN NISHIKI I.
SAME AS HEMOGLOBIN NORFOLK. HANADA ET AL.* FOR REFERENCE SEE HEMOGLOBIN TAGAWA
II.

--HEMOGLOBIN NORFOLK.
SUBSTITUTION OF ASPARTIC ACID FOR GLYCINE AT ALPHA 57. FAST HEMOGLOBIN.

AGER, J. A. M., LEHMANN, H. AND VELLA, F.* HAEMOGLOBIN 'NORFOLK'* A NEW
HAEMOGLOBIN FOUND IN AN ENGLISH FAMILY. BRIT. MED. J. 2* 539-541, 1958.

BAGLIONI, C.* A CHEMICAL STUDY OF HEMOGLOBIN-NORFOLK. J. BIOL. CHEM. 237* 69-

HUNTSMAN, R. G., HALL, M., LEHMANN, H. AND SUKUMARAN, P. K.* A SECOND AND A THIRD ABNORMAL HAEMOGLOBIN IN NORFOLK. HB G-NORFOLK AND HB-D NORFOLK. BRIT. MED. J. 1* 720-722, 1963.

LEHMANN, H. AND CARRELL, R. W.* VARIATIONS IN THE STRUCTURE OF HUMAN HAEMOGLO-BINS* WITH PARTICULAR REFERENCE TO THE UNSTABLE HAEMOGLOBINS. BRIT. MED. BULL. 25* 14-23, 1969.

IMAMURA, T.* HEMOGLOBIN KAGOSHIMA* AN EXAMPLE OF HEMOGLOBIN NORFOLK IN A JAPANESE FAMILY. AM. J. HUM. GENET. 18* 584-593, 1966.

--HEMOGLOBIN NYU.
SUBSTITUTION OF LYSINE FOR ASPARAGINE AT DELTA 12.

RANNEY, H. M., JACOBS, A. S., RAMOT, B. AND BRADLEY, T. B., JR.* HEMOGLOBIN - NYU, A DELTA CHAIN VARIANT, ALPHA 2 DELTA 2(12 LYS). J. CLIN. INVEST. 48* 2057-2062, 1969.

--HEMOGLOBIN O(ARABIA).
SUBSTITUTION OF LYSINE FOR GLUTAMIC ACID AT BETA 121. THIS HEMOGLOBIN HAS BEEN FOUND IN THE AMERICAN NEGROES AND IN BULGARIANS AS WELL AS ARABS (KAMEL ET AL., 1967).

KAMEL, K. A., HOERMAN, K. AND AWNY, A. Y.* HEMOGLOBIN ALPHA(2) BETA(2) 121 LYS CHEMICAL IDENTIFICATION IN AN EGYPTIAN FAMILY. SCIENCE 156* 397-398, 1966.

KAMEL, K. A., HOERMAN, K. AND AWNY, A. Y.* ETHNOLOGICAL SIGNIFICANCE OF HEMOGLOBIN ALPHA 2 BETA 2 (121 LYS). AM. J. PHYS. ANTHROP. 26* 107-108, 1967.

MILNER, P. F., MILLER, C., GREY, R., SEAKINS, M., DEJONG, W. W. AND WENT, L. N.* HEMOGLOBIN O ARAB* INTERACTION WITH HEMOGLOBIN S AND HEMOGLOBIN C. NEW ENG. J. MED. 283* 1417-1424, 1970.

RAMOT, B., FISHER, S., REMEZ, D., SCHNEERSON, R., KAHANE, D., AGER, J. A. M. AND LEHMANN, H.* HAEMOGLOBIN O IN AN ARAB FAMILY* SICKLE-CELL HAEMOGLOBIN O TRAIT. BRIT. MED. J. 2* 1262-1264, 1960.

VELLA, F., BEALE, D. AND LEHMANN, H.* HAEMOGLOBIN O ARAB IN SUDANESE. NATURE 209* 308-309, 1966.

--HEMOGLOBIN O(INDONESIA).
SUBSTITUTION OF LYSINE FOR GLUTAMIC ACID AT ALPHA 116.

BAGLIONI, C. AND LEHMANN, H.* CHEMICAL HETEROGENEITY OF HAEMOGLOBIN O. NATURE 196* 229-231, 1962.

ENG, L.-I. L. AND SADONO, (NI)* HAEMOGLOBIN O (BUGINESE X) IN SULAWESI. BRIT. MED. J. 1* 1461-1462, 1958.

SANSONE, G., CENTA, A., SCIARRATTA, V., GALLO, E. AND LEHMANN, H.* HAEMOGLOBIN-O INDONESIA (ALPHA 116 GLU LEADS TO LYS) IN AN ITALIAN FAMILY. ACTA HAEMAT. 43* 40-47, 1970.

--HEMOGLOBIN OAK RIDGE.
SUBSTITUTION OF ASPARAGINE FOR ASPARTIC ACID AT BETA 94.

LEHMANN, H. AND CARRELL, R. W.* VARIATIONS IN THE STRUCTURE OF HUMAN HAEMOGLO-BINS* WITH PARTICULAR REFERENCE TO THE UNSTABLE HAEMOGLOBINS. BRIT. MED. BULL. 25* 14-23, 1969.

--HEMOGLOBIN OLMSTED.
SUBSTITUTION OF ARGININE FOR LEUCINE AT BETA 141.

FAIRBANKS, V. F., OPFELL, R. W. AND BURGERT, E. O., JR.* THREE FAMILIES WITH UNSTABLE HEMOGLOBINOPATHIES (KOLN, OLMSTED AND SANTA ANA) CAUSING HEMOLYTIC ANEMIA WITH INCLUSION BODIES AND PIGMENTURIA. AM. J. MED. 46* 344-359, 1969.

LORKIN, P. A. AND LEHMANN, H.* TWO NEW PATHOLOGICAL HAEMOGLOBINS* OLMSTED BETA 141 (H19) LEU TO ARG AND MALMO BETA 97 (FG4) HIS TO GLU. BIOCHEM. J. 118* 38P ONLY, 1970.

--HEMOGLOBIN OSU CHRISTIANSBORG.
SUBSTITUTION OF ASPARAGINE FOR ASPARTIC ACID AT BETA 52.

KONOTEY-AHULU, F. I. D., KINDERLERER, J. L., LEHMANN, H. AND RINGELHANN, B.* TO BE PUBLISHED, 1970.

--HEMOGLOBIN P.
SUBSTITUTION OF ARGININE FOR HISTIDINE AT BETA 117.

SILVESTRONI, E., BIANCO, I. AND BRANCATI, C.* HAEMOGLOBIN P IN A FAMILY OF
SOUTHERN ITALIAN EXTRACTION. NATURE 191* 292-294, 1961, AND NATURE 200* 658-659,
1963.

--HEMOGLOBIN P(CONGO).
THIS IS A BETA-DELTA FUSION VARIANT, THE COMPLEMENT OF HEMOGLOBIN LEPORE. UNLIKE
THE DELTA-BETA FUSION PRODUCT OF LEPORE HEMOGLOBIN, THE NON-ALPHA CHAIN RESEMBLES
BETA AT THE NH2-END. FURTHERMORE, HB A2 IS PRESENT IN NORMAL CONCENTRATIONS AND
BOTH HB A AND HB S (OR OTHER BETA VARIANT) CAN BE PRESENT IN THE PATIENT HETEROZY-
GOUS FOR HEMOGLOBIN P(CONGO). THE EXPLANATION FOR THE ORIGIN OF HEMOGLOBIN LEPORE
AND HEMOGLOBIN P(CONGO) (NONHOMOLOGOUS PAIRING AND UNEQUAL CROSSING-OVER) IS
DIAGRAMMED IN FIG. 2.20 (P. 41) OF MCKUSICK (1969).

DHERTE, P., LEHMANN, H. AND VANDEPITTE, J.* HAEMOGLOBIN P IN A FAMILY IN THE
BELGIAN CONGO. NATURE 184* 1133-1135, 1959.

GAMMACK, D. B., HJEHNS, E. R., LEHMANN, H. AND SHOOTER, E. M.* THE ABNORMAL
POLYPEPTIDE CHAINS IN A NUMBER OF HAEMOGLOBIN VARIANTS. ACTA GENET. STATIST. MED.
11* 1-16, 1961.

LAMBOTTE-LEGRAND, J., LAMBOTTE-LEGRAND, C., AGER, J. A. AND LEHMANN, H.*
L'HEMOGLOBINOSE P. A PROPOS D'UN CAS D'ASSOCIATION DES HEMOGLOBINES P ET S. REV.
HEMAT. 15* 10-18, 1960.

LEHMANN, H. AND CHARLESWORTH, D.* OBSERVATIONS ON HAEMOGLOBIN P(CONGO TYPE).
BIOCHEM. J. 118* 12-13P, 1970.

LEHMANN, H., VANDEPITTE, J. AND DHERTE, P.* HAEMOGLOBIN P IN A FAMILY IN THE
BELGIAN CONGO. NATURE 184* 1133-1135, 1959.

MCKUSICK, V. A.* HUMAN GENETICS. ENGLEWOOD CLIFFS, N. J.* PRENTICE-HALL, 1969.

--HEMOGLOBIN P(GALVESTON).
SUBSTITUTION OF ARGININE FOR HISTIDINE AT BETA 117.

SCHNEIDER, R. G., ALPERIN, J. B., BRIMHALL, B. AND JONES, R. T.* HEMOGLOBIN
P(ALPHA 2 BETA 2 117 ARG)* STRUCTURE AND PROPERTIES. J. LAB. CLIN. MED. 73* 616-
622, 1969.

--HEMOGLOBIN PHILLY.
SUBSTITUTION OF PHENYLALANINE FOR TYROSINE AT BETA 35. AN UNSTABLE HEMOGLOBIN
LEADING TO HEMOLYTIC ANEMIA. NO ELECTROPHORETIC ABNORMALITY.

RIEDER, R. F., OSKI, F. A. AND CLEGG, J. B.* HEMOGLOBIN PHILLY (BETA 35
TYROSINE TO PHENYLALANINE)* STUDIES IN THE MOLECULAR PATHOLOGY OF HEMOGLOBIN. J.
CLIN. INVEST. 48* 1627-1642, 1969.

--HEMOGLOBIN PIERCE ET AL.
DEFECT UNKNOWN.

PIERCE, L. E., MCCOY, K. AND RATH, C. E.* A NEW HEMOGLOBIN VARIANT WITH
SICKLING PROPERTIES. NEW ENG. J. MED. 268* 862-866, 1963.

--HEMOGLOBIN PORTLAND-1.
THIS UNIQUE HEMOGLOBIN WAS FOUND IN A NEWBORN INFANT WITH MULTIPLE CONGENITAL
ANOMALIES AND COMPLEX AUTOSOMAL CHROMOSOMAL MOSAICISM. ITS COMPOSITION IS
GAMMA(2) X(2). THE X-CHAIN MAY BE THE EPSILON CHAIN WHOSE SYNTHESIS PERSISTS
UNTIL AFTER BIRTH BECAUSE OF THE CHROMOSOMAL ANOMALY. ON THE OTHER HAND, THE X
POLYPEPTIDE CHAIN MAY BE UNDER THE CONTROL OF A SEPARATE LOCUS.

CAPP, G. I., RIGAS, D. A. AND JONES, R. T.* HEMOGLOBIN PORTLAND 1* A NEW HUMAN
HEMOGLOBIN UNIQUE IN STRUCTURE. SCIENCE 157* 65-66, 1967.

HECHT, F., JONES, R. T. AND KOLER, R. D.* NEWBORN INFANTS WITH HB PORTLAND 1,
AN INDICATOR OF ALPHA-CHAIN DEFICIENCY. ANN. HUM. GENET. 31* 215-218, 1968.

--HEMOGLOBIN PORTO ALEGRE.
SUBSTITUTION OF CYSTINE FOR SERINE AT BETA 9.

BONAVENTURA, J. AND RIGGS, A.* POLYMERIZATION OF HEMOGLOBINS OF MOUSE AND MAN*
STRUCTURAL BASIS. SCIENCE 158* 800-802, 1967.

TONDO, C. V., SALZANO, F. M. AND RUCKNAGEL, D. L.* HEMOGLOBIN PORTO ALEGRE, A
POSSIBLE POLYMER OF NORMAL HEMOGLOBIN IN A CAUCASIAN BRAZILIAN FAMILY. AM. J.
HUM. GENET. 15* 265-279, 1963.

--HEMOGLOBIN PYLOS.
BETA-DELTA CHAIN ANOMALY. SEE LEPORE (BOSTON).

140

FESSAS, P., STAMATOYANNOPOULOS, G. AND KARAKLIS, A.* HEMOGLOBIN *PYLOS** STUDY OF A HEMOGLOBINOPATHY RESEMBLING THALASSEMIA IN THE HETEROZYGOUS, HOMOZYGOUS AND DOUBLE HETEROZYGOUS STATE. BLOOD 19* 1-22, 1962.

D
O
M
I
N
A
N
T

--HEMOGLOBIN Q.
TWO FORMS EXIST, ONE WITH SUBSTITUTION OF HISTIDINE FOR ASPARTIC ACID AT ALPHA 74 AND ONE WITH THE SAME CHANGE AT ALPHA 75.

LORKIN, P. A., CHARLESWORTH, D., LEHMANN, H., RAHBAR, S., TUCHINDA, S. AND ENG, L. I. L.* TWO HAEMOGLOBINS Q, ALPHA 74 (EF3) AND ALPHA 75 (EF4) ASPARTIC ACID TO HISTIDINE. BRIT. J. HAEMAT. 19* 117-125, 1970.

--HEMOGLOBIN Q(CHINESE).
ALPHA CHAIN ANOMALY.

ENG, L.-I. L., PILLAY, R. P. AND THURAISINGHAM, V.* FURTHER CASES OF HAEMOGLO-BIN Q-H DISEASE (HB Q-ALPHA THALASSEMIA). BLOOD 28* 830-839, 1966.

GAMMACK, D. B., HUEHNS, E. R., LEHMANN, H. AND SHOOTER, E. M.* THE ABNORMAL POLYPEPTIDE CHAINS IN A NUMBER OF HAEMOGLOBIN VARIANTS. ACTA GENET. STATIST. MED. 11* 1-16, 1961.

VELLA, F., WELLS, R. H. C., AGER, J. A. M. AND LEHMANN, H.* A HAEMOGLOBINOPATHY INVOLVING HAEMOGLOBIN H AND A NEW (Q) HAEMOGLOBIN. BRIT. MED. J. 1* 752-755, 1958.

--HEMOGLOBIN R.
SAME AS HEMOGLOBIN DURHAM-I.

CHERNOFF, A. I. AND WEICHSELBAUM, T. E.* A MICROHEMOLYZING TECHNIC FOR PREPARING SOLUTIONS OF HEMOGLOBIN FOR PAPER ELECTROPHORETIC ANALYSIS. AM. J. CLIN. PATH. 30* 120-125, 1958.

--HEMOGLOBIN RAINIER.
CAUSES ERYTHROCYTOSIS AND IS ONLY ADULT HEMOGLOBIN THAT IS ALKALI-RESISTANT. SUBSTITUTION OF TYROSINE BY HISTIDINE AT BETA 145.

ADAMSON, J. W., PARER, J. T. AND STAMATOYANNOPOULOS, G.* ERYTHROCYTOSIS ASSOCIATED WITH HEMOGLOBIN RAINIER* OXYGEN EQUILIBRIA AND MARROW REGULATION. J. CLIN. INVEST. 48* 1376-1386, 1969.

STAMATOYANNOPOULOS, G. AND YOSHIDA, A.* SINGLE CHAIN ALKALI RESISTANCE IN HEMOGLOBIN RAINIER* BETA 145 TYROSINE TO HISTIDINE. SCIENCE 166* 1005-1006, 1969.

STAMATOYANNOPOULOS, G., YOSHIDA, A., ADAMSON, J. AND HEINENBERG, S.* HEMOGLOBIN RAINIER (BETA 145 TYROSINE TO HISTIDINE)* ALKALI-RESISTANT HEMOGLOBIN WITH INCREASED OXYGEN AFFINITY. SCIENCE 159* 741-743, 1968.

--HEMOGLOBIN RAJAPPEN.
SUBSTITUTION OF THREONINE FOR LYSINE AT ALPHA 90.

HYDE, R. D., KINDERLERER, J. L., LEHMANN, H. AND HALL, M.* HB RAJAPPEN. TO BE PUBLISHED, 1970.

--HEMOGLOBIN RAMBA.
SUBSTITUTION OF SERINE FOR PROLINE AT ALPHA 95.

DE JONG, W. W. W.* LEIDEN, HOLLAND* PERSONAL COMMUNICATION, 1970.

--HEMOGLOBIN REISSMANN ET AL.
SAME AS HEMOGLOBIN KANSAS. HEMOGLOBIN WITH LOW AFFINITY FOR OXYGEN.

REISSMANN, K. R., RUTH, W. E. AND NORMURA, T.* A HUMAN HEMOGLOBIN WITH LOWERED OXYGEN AFFINITY AND IMPAIRED HEME-HEME INTERACTIONS. J. CLIN. INVEST. 40* 1826-1833, 1961.

--HEMOGLOBIN RICHMOND.
SUBSTITUTION OF LYSINE FOR ASPARAGINE AT BETA 102.

EFREMOV, G. D., HUISMAN, T. H., SMITH, L. L., WILSON, J. B., KITCHENS, J. L., WRIGHTSTONE, R. N. AND ADAMS, H. R.* HEMOGLOBIN RICHMOND, A HUMAN HEMOGLOBIN WHICH FORMS ASYMMETRIC HYBRIDS WITH OTHER HEMOGLOBINS. J. BIOL. CHEM. 244* 6105-6116, 1969.

--HEMOGLOBIN RIVERDALE-BRONX.
SUBSTITUTION OF ARGININE FOR GLYCINE AT BETA 24.

RANNEY, H. M., JACOBS, A. S., UDEM, L. AND ZALUSKY, R.* HEMOGLOBIN RIVERDALE-BRONX* AN UNSTABLE HEMOGLOBIN RESULTING FROM THE SUBSTITUTION OF ARGININE FOR GLYCINE AT HELICAL RESIDUE B6 OF THE B POLYPEPTIDE CHAIN. BIOCHEM. BIOPHYS. RES. COMMUN. 33* 1004-1011, 1968.

--HEMOGLOBIN RUSS.
    SUBSTITUTION OF ARGININE FOR GLYCINE AT ALPHA 51.

        HUISMAN, T. H. AND SYDENSTRICKER, V. P.* DIFFERENCE IN GROSS STRUCTURE OF TWO
    ELECTROPHORETICALLY IDENTICAL 'MINOR' HEMOGLOBIN COMPONENTS. NATURE 193* 489-491,
    1962.

        REYNOLDS, C. A. AND HUISMAN, T. H. J.* HEMOGLOBIN RUSS OR ALPHA-2 (51 ARG)
    BETA-2. BIOCHIM. BIOPHYS. ACTA 130* 541-543, 1966.

--HEMOGLOBIN S.
    SUBSTITUTION OF VALINE FOR GLUTAMIC ACID AT BETA 6. HEMOGLOBIN C(GEORGETOWN) ALSO
    SICKLES.

        INGRAM, V. M.* ABNORMAL HUMAN HAEMOGLOBIN.   III. THE CHEMICAL DIFFERENCE
    BETWEEN NORMAL AND SICKLE CELL HAEMOGLOBINS. BIOCHIM. BIOPHYS. ACTA 36* 402-411,
    1959.

        PAULING, L., ITANO, H. A., SINGER, S. J. AND WELLS, I. C.* SICKLE CELL ANEMIA,
    A MOLECULAR DISEASE. SCIENCE 110* 543-548, 1949.

--HEMOGLOBIN SABINE.
    SUBSTITUTION OF PROLINE FOR LEUCINE AT BETA 91. THE HEMOGLOBIN IS UNSTABLE
    CAUSING HEMOLYTIC ANEMIA IN THE HETEROZYGOTE.

        SCHNEIDER, R. G., UEDA, S., ALPERIN, J. B., BRIMHALL, B. AND JONES, R. T.*
    HEMOGLOBIN SABINE AT BETA 91 (E7) LEU-TO-PRO* AN UNSTABLE VARIANT CAUSING SEVERE
    ANEMIA WITH INCLUSION BODIES. NEW ENG. J. MED. 280* 739-745, 1969.

        SCHNEIDER, R. G., UEDA, S., ALPERIN, J. B., BRIMHALL, B. AND JONES, R. T.*
    HEMOGLOBIN SABINE BETA 91(F7) LEU TO PRO. AN UNSTABLE VARIANT CAUSING SEVERE
    ANEMIA WITH INCLUSION BODIES. NEW ENG. J. MED. 280* 739-745, 1968.

--HEMOGLOBIN SANTA ANA.
    SUBSTITUTION OF PROLINE FOR LEUCINE AT BETA 88.

        OPFELL, R. W., LORKIN, P. A. AND LEHMANN, H.* HEREDITARY NON-SPHEROCYTIC
    HAEMOLYTIC ANAEMIA WITH POST-SPLENECTOMY INCLUSION BODIES AND PIGMENTURIA CAUSED
    BY AN UNSTABLE HAEMOGLOBIN SANTA ANA - BETA 88 (F4) LEUCINE-PROLINE. J. MED.
    GENET. 5* 292-297, 1968.

--HEMOGLOBIN SAVANNAH.
    SUBSTITUTION OF VALINE FOR GLYCINE AT BETA 24.

        HUISMAN, T. H. J., BROWN, A. K., EFREMOV, G. D., WILSON, J. B., REYNOLDS, C.
    A., UY, R. AND SMITH, L. L.* HEMOGLOBIN SAVANNAH (B6 (24) BETA-GLYCINE TO VALINE)*
    AN UNSTABLE VARIANT CAUSING ANEMIA WITH INCLUSION BODIES. J. CLIN. INVEST. 50*
    650-659, 1971.

--HEMOGLOBIN SCOTT ET AL.
    DEFECT UNKNOWN.

        SCOTT, J. L., HAUT, A., CARTWRIGHT, G. E. AND WINTROBE, M. M.* CONGENITAL
    HEMOLYTIC DISEASE ASSOCIATED WITH RED CELL INCLUSION BODIES, ABNORMAL PIGMENT
    METABOLISM AND AN ELECTROPHORETIC HEMOGLOBIN ABNORMALITY. BLOOD 16* 1239-1252,
    1960.

--HEMOGLOBIN SEALY.
    SUBSTITUTION OF HISTIDINE FOR ASPARTIC ACID AT ALPHA 47. (OF INTEREST IS THE FACT
    THAT THE FAMILY IN WHICH THIS WAS FOUND WAS ASHKENAZIC. HEMOGLOBIN BEILINSON WAS
    ALSO FOUND IN AN ASHKENAZIC JEWISH FAMILY AND HAS A SUBSTITUTION OF GLYCINE FOR
    ASPARTIC ACID AT ALPHA 47.)

        SCHNEIDER, R. G., UEDA, S., ALPERIN, J. B., BRIMHALL, B. AND JONES, R. T.*
    HEMOGLOBIN SEALY (ALPHA-47 HIS-2 BETA-2)* A NEW VARIANT IN A JEWISH FAMILY. AM.
    J. HUM. GENET. 20* 151-156, 1968.

--HEMOGLOBIN SEATTLE.
    SUBSTITUTION OF GLUTAMIC ACID FOR ALANINE AT BETA 76.

        HUEHNS, E. R., HECHT, F., YOSHIDA, A., STAMATOYANNOPOULOS, G., HARTMAN, J. AND
    MOTULSKY,   A. G.* HEMOGLOBIN-SEATTLE (ALPHA-2-A-BETA-2-76 GLU)* AN UNSTABLE
    HEMOGLOBIN CAUSING CHRONIC HEMOLYTIC ANEMIA. BLOOD 36* 209-218, 1970.

        STAMATOYANNOPOULOS, G., PARER, J. T. AND FINCH, C. A.* PHYSIOLOGIC IMPLICATIONS
    OF A HEMOGLOBIN WITH DECREASED OXYGEN AFFINITY (HEMOGLOBIN SEATTLE). NEW ENG. J.
    MED. 281* 915-919, 1969.

--HEMOGLOBIN SHEPHERDS BUSH.
    SUBSTITUTION OF ASPARTIC ACID FOR GLYOINE AT BETA 74.

        WHITE, J. M., BRAIN, M. C., LORKIN, P. A., LEHMANN, H. AND SMITH, M.* MILD

'UNSTABLE HAEMOGLOBIN HAEMOLYTIC ANAEMIA' CAUSED BY HAEMOGLOBIN SHEPHERDS BUSH (B74(E18) GLY TO ASP). NATURE 225* 939-941, 1970.

D
O
M   --HEMOGLOBIN SHIMONOSEKI.
I   SUBSTITUTION OF ARGININE FOR GLUTAMINE AT ALPHA 54.
N
A   HANADA, M. AND RUCKNAGEL, D. L.* THE CHARACTERIZATION OF HEMOGLOBIN SHIMONOSE-
N   KI. BLOOD 24* 624-635, 1964.
T
           YAMAOKA, K., KAWAMURA, K., HANADA, M., SEITA, M., HITSUMOTO, S. AND OOYA, I.*
        STUDIES ON ABNORMAL HAEMOGLOBINS. JAP. J. HUM. GENET. 5* 99-111, 1960.

    --HEMOGLOBIN SINAI.
       SUBSTITUTION OF HISTIDINE FOR ASPARTIC ACID AT ALPHA 47. SAME AS HEMOGLOBIN HA-
       SHARON.

           CHARACHE, S.* BALTIMORE, MD.* PERSONAL COMMUNICATION, 1967.

           OSTERTAG, W. AND SMITH, E. W.* HB SINAI, A NEW ALPHA CHAIN MUTANT ALPHA HIS 47.
        HUMANGENETIK 6* 377-379, 1968.

    --HEMOGLOBIN SINGAPORE.
       SUBSTITUTION OF PROLINE FOR ARGININE AT ALPHA 141.

           CLEGG, J. B., WEATHERALL, D. J., BOON, W. H. AND MUSTAFA, D.* TWO NEW HAEMOGLO-
        BIN VARIANTS INVOLVING PROLINE SUBSTITUTIONS. NATURE 222* 379-380, 1969.

    --HEMOGLOBIN SIRIRAJ.
       SUBSTITUTION OF LYSINE FOR GLUTAMIC ACID AT BETA 7.

           TUCHINDA, S., BEALE, D. AND LEHMANN, H.* A NEW HAEMOGLOBIN IN A THAI FAMILY. A
        CASE OF HAEMOGLOBIN SIRIRAJ-BETA THALASSAEMIA. BRIT. MED. J. 1* 1583-1585, 1965.

    --HEMOGLOBIN SOGN.
       SUBSTITUTION OF ARGININE FOR LEUCINE AT BETA 14.

           MONN, E., GAFFNEY, P. J. AND LEHMANN, H.* HAEMOGLOBIN SOGN (B14 ARGININE) - A
        NEW HEMOGLOBIN VARIANT. SCAND. J. HAEMAT. 5* 353-360, 1968.

    --HEMOGLOBIN SPHAKIA.
       SUBSTITUTION OF ARGININE FOR HISTIDINE AT DELTA 2.

           JONES, R. T., BRIMHALL, B., HUEHNS, E. R. AND BARNICOT, N. A.* HEMOGLOBIN
        SPHAKIA* A DELTA-CHAIN VARIANT OF HEMOGLOBIN A2 FROM CRETE. SCIENCE 151* 1406-
        1408, 1966.

    --HEMOGLOBIN ST. MARY'S.
       A POSSIBLE 'CORE' HEMOGLOBIN VARIANT.

           BUCHANAN, A., BARKHAN, P., CROME, P. E., MORRISON, P. L. AND HUEHNS, E. R.*
        1965, UNPUBLISHED.

    --HEMOGLOBIN STANLEYVILLE-1.
       SAME AS G(PHILADELPHIA). CHANGE FROM ASPARAGINE TO LYSINE AT ALPHA 68.

           DHERTE, P., VANDEPITTE, J., AGER, J. A. M. AND LEHMANN, H.* STANLEYVILLE I AND
        II. TWO NEW VARIANTS OF ADULT HEMOGLOBIN. BRIT. MED. J. 2* 282-284, 1959.

    --HEMOGLOBIN STANLEYVILLE-2
       SUBSTITUTION OF LYSINE FOR ASPARAGINE AT ALPHA 78.

           VAN ROS, G., BEALE, D. AND LEHMANN, H.* HEMOGLOBIN STANLEYVILLE-II (ALPHA 78
        ASPARAGINE TO LYSINE). BRIT. MED. J. 4* 92-93, 1968.

    --HEMOGLOBIN SUD-VIETNAM.
       DEFECT UNKNOWN.

           ALBAHARY, C., DREYFUS, J.-C., LABIE, D., SCHAPIRA, G. AND TRAM, L.* HEMOGLO-
        BINES ANORMALES AU SUD-VIETNAM. HEMOGLOBINOSE C HOMOZYGOTE. TRAIT E. HEMOGLOBINE
        NOUVELLE. REV. HEMATOL. 13* 163-170, 1960.

    --HEMOGLOBIN SYDNEY.
       SUBSTITUTION OF ALANINE FOR VALINE AT BETA 67. LIKE HEMOGLOBINS KOLN AND GENOVA,
       THIS HEMOGLOBIN HAS NO ELECTROPHORETIC ABNORMALITY BUT IS UNSTABLE, FORMING
       INTRACELLULAR PRECIPITATES.

           CARRELL, R. W., LEHMANN, H., LORKIN, P. A., RAIK, E. AND HUNTER, E.* HAEMOGLO-
        BIN SYDNEY* BETA 67 (E 11) VALINE TO ALANINE* AN EMERGING PATTERN OF UNSTABLE
        HAEMOGLOBINS. NATURE 215* 626-628, 1967.

    --HEMOGLOBIN TACOMA.
       SUBSTITUTION OF SERINE FOR ARGININE AT BETA 30.

BAUR, E. W. AND MOTULSKY, A. G.* HEMOGLOBIN TACOMA, A BETA-CHAIN VARIANT
ASSOCIATED WITH INCREASED HB A(2). HUMANGENETIK 1* 621-634, 1965.

BRIMHALL, B., JONES, R. T., BAUR, E. W. AND MOTULSKY, A. G.* STRUCTURAL
CHARACTERIZATION OF HEMOGLOBIN TACOMA. BIOCHEMISTRY 8* 2125-2129, 1969.

--HEMOGLOBIN TAGAWA 1.
SUBSTITUTION OF ASPARAGINE FOR LYSINE AT ALPHA 90. SAME AS HB J(BROUSSAIS).

YANASE, T., HANADA, M., SEITA, M., OHYA, I., OHTA, Y., IMAMURA, T., FUJIMURA,
T., KAWASAKI, K. AND YAMAOKA, K.* MOLECULAR BASIS OF MORBIDITY FROM A SERIES OF
STUDIES OF HEMOGLOBINOPATHIES IN WESTERN JAPAN. JAP. J. HUM. GENET. 13* 40-53,
1968.

--HEMOGLOBIN TAGAWA II.
PROBABLY SAME AS HEMOGLOBIN KOKURA.

HANADA, M., OHTA, Y., IMAMURA, T., FEJIMURA, T., KAWASAKI, K., KOSAKA, K.,
YAMAOKA, K. AND SEITA, M.* STUDIES OF ABNORMAL HEMOGLOBINS IN WESTERN JAPAN.
(ABSTRACT) JAP. J. HUM. GENET. 9* 253-254, 1964.

--HEMOGLOBIN TOCHIGI.
DELETION OF RESIDUES 56-59 OF THE BETA CHAIN.

SHIBATA, S., MIYAJI, T., UEDA, S., MATSVOKA, M., IUCHI, I., YAMADA, K. AND
SHINKAI, N.* HEMOGLOBIN TOCHIGI (BETA 56-59 DELETED). A NEW UNSTABLE HEMOGLOBIN
DISCOVERED IN A JAPANESE FAMILY. PROC. JAP. ACAD. 46* 440-445, 1970.

--HEMOGLOBIN TOKUCHI.
SUBSTITUTION OF TYROSINE FOR HISTIDINE AT BETA 2.

SHIBATA, S., IUCHI, I., MAZAGI, T. AND TAKEDA, I.* HEMOGLOBINOPATHY IN JAPAN.
BULL. YAMAGUCHI MED. SCH. 10* 1-9, 1963.

--HEMOGLOBIN TOKYO.
DEFECT UNKNOWN.

FUKUTAKE, K. AND KATO, K.* HEMOLYTIC ANEMIA DUE TO A NEW ABNORMAL HEMOGLOBIN.
PROC. 8TH CONGR. INTERN. SOC. HEMATOL., TOKYO, 1960. 2* 1220-1223, 1961.

--HEMOGLOBIN TORINO.
SUBSTITUTION OF VALINE FOR PHENYLALANINE AT ALPHA 43.

BERETTA, A., PRATO, V., GALLO, E. AND LEHMANN, H.* HAEMOGLOBIN TORINO - ALPHA
43 (CD 1) PHENYLALANINE REPLACED BY VALINE. NATURE 217* 1016-1018, 1968.

PRATO, V., GALLO, E., RICCO, G., MAZZA, U., BIANCO, G. AND LEHMANN, H.*
HAEMOLYTIC ANAEMIA DUE TO HAEMOGLOBIN TORINO. BRIT. J. HAEMAT. 19* 105-115, 1970.

--HEMOGLOBIN TSUKIJI.
BETA CHAIN ANOMALY.

SHIBATA, S. AND IUCHI, I.* HEMOGLOBIN-HIKARI (ALPHA-2-BETA-2,T-7). A FAST-
MOVING HEMOGLOBIN DEMONSTRATED IN TWO FAMILIES OF JAPANESE PEOPLE, WITH A BRIEF
NOTE ON THE ABNORMAL HEMOGLOBINS OF JAPAN WHICH ARE LIABLE TO BE CONFUSED WITH IT.
PROC. 9TH CONGR. INTERN. SOC. HEMATOL., MEXICO CITY, 1962. PP. 65-70.

--HEMOGLOBIN UBE-I.
DEFECT UNKNOWN. POSSIBLY SUBSTITUTION OF CYSTINE AT BETA 93.

SHIBATA, S., IUCHI, I., MIYAJI, T., UEDA, S., YAMASHITA, K. AND SUZUNO, R.* A
CASE OF HEMOLYTIC DISEASE ASSOCIATED WITH THE PRODUCTION OF HEINZ BODIES AND OF AN
ABNORMAL HEMOGLOBIN (HB UBE-1). MED. BIOL. 59* 79-84, 1961.

--HEMOGLOBIN UBE-II.
SUBSTITUTION OF ASPARTIC ACID FOR ASPARAGINE AT ALPHA 68.

MIYAJI, T., IUCHI, I., YAMAMOTO, K., OHBA, Y. AND SHIBATA, S.* AMINO ACID
SUBSTITUTION OF HEMOGLOBIN UBE 2(A2 68ASP B2)* AN EXAMPLE OF SUCCESSFUL APPLICA-
TION OF PARTIAL HYDROLYSIS OF PEPTIDE WITH 5 PERCENT ACETIC ACID. CLIN. CHIM.
ACTA 16* 347-352, 1967.

SHIBATA, S. AND IUCHI, I.* HEMOGLOBIN-HIKARI (ALPHA-2 A-BETA-2,T-7). A
FASTMOVING HEMOGLOBIN DEMONSTRATED IN TWO FAMILIES OF JAPANESE PEOPLE WITH A BRIEF
NOTE ON THE ABNORMAL HEMOGLOBINS OF JAPAN WHICH ARE LIABLE TO BE CONFUSED WITH IT.
PROC. 9TH CONGR. INTERN. SOC. HEMATOL., MEXICO CITY, 1962. PP. 65-70.

--HEMOGLOBIN UMI.
PROBABLY SAME AS HEMOGLOBIN KOKURA. HANADA, ET AL.* FOR REFERENCE SEE HEMOGLOBIN
TAGAWA II.

--HEMOGLOBIN UPPSALA.

BECKMAN, L., CHRISTODOULOU, C., FESSAS, P., LOUKOPOULOS, D., KALTSOYA, A. AND NILSSON, L.-O.* A SWEDISH HAEMOGLOBIN VARIANT. ACTA GENET. STATIST. MED. 16* 362-370, 1966.

FESSAS, P., KALTSOYA, A., LOUKOPOULOS, D. AND NILSSON, L.-O.* ON THE CHEMICAL STRUCTURE OF HAEMOGLOBIN UPPSALA. HUM. HERED. 19* 152-158, 1969.

--HEMOGLOBIN WARREN.
GAMMA CHAIN ANOMALY.

HUISMAN, T. H. J., DOZY, A. M., HORTON, B. E. AND WILSON, J. B.* A FETAL HEMOGLOBIN WITH ABNORMAL GAMMA-POLYPEPTIDE CHAINS* HEMOGLOBIN WARREN. BLOOD 26* 668-676, 1965.

--HEMOGLOBIN WIEN.
SUBSTITUTION OF ASPARTIC ACID FOR TYROSINE AT BETA 130.

PERUTZ, M. F. AND LEHMANN, H.* MOLECULAR PATHOLOGY OF HUMAN HAEMOGLOBIN. NATURE 219* 902-909, 1968.

--HEMOGLOBIN X.
SUBSTITUTIONS IN BOTH ALPHA AND BETA. AT ALPHA 68, CHANGE OF ASPARAGINE TO LYSINE AS IN HEMOGLOBIN G(PHILADELPHIA). AT BETA 6, CHANGE OF GLUTAMIC ACID TO LYSINE AS IN HEMOGLOBIN C.

BAGLIONI, C. AND INGRAM, V. M.* FOUR ADULT HAEMOGLOBIN TYPES IN ONE PERSON. NATURE 189* 465-467, 1961.

--HEMOGLOBIN YAKIMA.
SUBSTITUTION OF HISTIDINE FOR ASPARTIC ACID AT BETA 99. POLYCYTHEMIA OCCURS WITH THIS HEMOGLOBINOPATHY AS WITH HEMOGLOBIN CHESAPEAKE.

JONES, R. T., OSGOOD, E. E., BRIMHALL, B. AND KOLER, R. D.* HEMOGLOBIN YAKINA. I. CLINICAL AND BIOCHEMICAL STUDIES. J. CLIN. INVEST. 46* 1840-1847, 1967.

NOVY, M. J., EDWARDS, M. J. AND METCALFE, J.* HEMOGLOBIN YAKIMA* II. HIGH BLOOD OXYGEN AFFINITY ASSOCIATED WITH COMPENSATORY ERYTHROCYTOSIS AND NORMAL HEMODYNAMICS. J. CLIN. INVEST. 46* 1848-1854, 1967.

NOVY, M. J., EDWARDS, M. J., PETERSON, E. N. AND METCALFE, J.* HEMOGLOBIN YAKI-MA* OXYGEN HEMOGLOBIN EQUILIBRIUM AND CARDIODYNAMIC EFFECTS. (ABSTRACT) CLIN. RES. 15* 133 ONLY, 1967.

OSGOOD, E. E., JONES, R. T., BRIMHALL, B. AND KOLER, R. D.* HEMOGLOBIN YAKIMA* CLINICAL AND BIOCHEMICAL STUDIES. (ABSTRACT) CLIN. RES. 15* 134 ONLY, 1967.

--HEMOGLOBIN YOSHIZUKA.
SUBSTITUTION OF ASPARTIC ACID FOR ASPARAGINE AT BETA 108. REDUCED OXYGEN AFFINITY LIKE HEMOGLOBIN KANSAS.

IMAMURA, T., FUJITA, S., OHTA, Y., HANADA, M. AND YANASE, T.* HEMOGLOBIN YOSHI-ZUKA (G10(108) BETA ASPARAGINE TO ASPARTIC ACID)* A NEW VARIANT WITH A REDUCED OXYGEN AFFINITY FROM A JAPANESE FAMILY. J. CLIN. INVEST. 48* 2341-2348, 1969.

--HEMOGLOBIN YPSI.
SUBSTITUTION IN BETA CHAIN RESULTS IN INCREASED OXYGEN AFFINITY LEADING TO ERYTHREMIA AND ABNORMAL POLYMERIZATION MANIFESTED IN HETEROZYGOTES BY HYBRID HEMOGLOBIN MOLECULES CONTAINING BOTH THE YPSI BETA CHAIN AND THE NORMAL BETA CHAIN.

GLYNN, K. P., PENNER, J. A. AND SMITH, J. R.* FAMILIAL ERYTHROCYTOSIS* A DESCRIPTION OF THREE FAMILIES, ONE WITH HEMOGLOBIN YPSILANTI. ANN. INTERN. MED. 69* 769-776, 1968.

--HEMOGLOBIN YUKUHASHI.
SUBSTITUTION OF ARGININE FOR PROLINE AT BETA 58.

YANASE, T., HANADA, M., SEITA, M., OHYA, I., OHTA, Y., IMAMURA, T., FUJIMURA, T., KAWASAKI, K. AND YAMAOKA, K.* MOLECULAR BASIS OF MORBIDITY FROM A SERIES OF STUDIES OF HEMOGLOBINOPATHIES IN WESTERN JAPAN. JAP. J. HUM. GENET. 13* 40-53, 1968.

--HEMOGLOBIN ZAMBIA.
SUBSTITUTION OF ASPARAGINE FOR LYSINE AT ALPHA 60.

BARCLAY, G. P. T., CHARLESWORTH, D. AND LEHMANN, H.* ABNORMAL HAEMOGLOBINS IN ZAMBIA. A NEW HEMOGLOBIN ZAMBIA ALPHA 60 (E9) LYSINE TO ASPARAGINE. BRIT. MED. J. 2* 595-596, 1969.

--HEMOGLOBIN ZURICH.

FRICK, P. G., HITZIG, W. H. AND BETKE, K.* HEMOGLOBIN ZURICH. I. A NEW HEMOGLOBIN ANOMALY ASSOCIATED WITH ACUTE HEMOLYTIC EPISODES WITH INCLUSION BODIES AFTER SULFONAMIDE THERAPY. BLOOD 20* 261-271, 1962.

HUISMAN, T. H. J., HORTON, B., BRIDGES, M. T., BETKE, K. AND HITZIG, W. H.* A NEW ABNORMAL HUMAN HEMOGLOBIN* HEMOGLOBIN-ZURICH. CLIN. CHEM. ACTA 6* 347-355, 1960.

MULLER, C. J. AND KINGMA, S.* HAEMOGLOBIN ZURICH ALPHA-2 A BETA-2-63 ARG. BIOCHIM. BIOPHYS. ACTA 50* 595 ONLY, 1961.

RIEDER, R. F., ZINKHAM, W. H. AND HOLTZMAN, N. A.* HEMOGLOBIN ZURICH. CLINICAL, CHEMICAL AND KINETIC STUDIES. AM. J. MED. 39* 4-20, 1965.

*14180 HEMOGLOBIN - ALPHA LOCUS

THE ALPHA AND BETA LOCI DETERMINE THE STRUCTURE OF THE TWO TYPES OF POLYPEPTIDE CHAINS IN ADULT HEMOGLOBIN, HB A, ALPHA 2-BETA 2. THE ALPHA LOCUS ALSO DETERMINES ONE POLYPEPTIDE CHAIN, THE ALPHA CHAIN, IN FETAL HEMOGLOBIN (ALPHA 2-GAMMA 2), IN HEMOGLOBIN A2(ALPHA 2-DELTA 2), AND IN EMBRYONIC HEMOGLOBIN (ALPHA 2-EPSILON 2). THE FOLLOWING ARE MUTATIONS AFFECTING THE ALPHA CHAIN, ARRANGED ACCORDING TO LOCATION OF THE AMINO ACID SUBSTITUTION. REFERENCES ARE GIVEN EARLIER UNDER THE NAME OF THE PARTICULAR HEMOGLOBIN VARIANT, IN ALPHABETIC ORDER. IT IS NOTEWORTHY THAT AT LEAST ONE MUTANT SUBSTITUTION IS NOW KNOWN FOR 33 OF THE 141 AMINO ACIDS OF THE ALPHA CHAIN. TWO DIFFERENT MUTANT SUBSTITUTIONS FOR 7 OF THE 33 AMINO ACIDS ARE KNOWN AND IN ONE OTHER THREE SUBSTITUTIONS.

D
O
M
I
N
A
N
T

POSITION	FROM	TO	HEMOGLOBIN
5	ALA	ASP	J(TORONTO)
12	ALA	ASP	J(PARIS-1)
15	GLY	ASP	J(OXFORD)
15	GLY	ASP	I(INTERLAKEN)
16	LYS	GLU	I(BURLINGTON)
16	LYS	GLU	I(SKAMANIA)
22	GLY	ASP	J(MEDELLIN)
23	GLU	GLN	MEMPHIS
23	GLU	LYS	CHAD
23	GLU	VAL	G(AUDHALI)
27	GLU	GLY	G(FORT WORTH)
30	GLU	GLN	G(HONOLULU)
30	GLU	GLN	G(SINGAPORE)
30	GLU	GLN	G(HONGKONG)
43	PHE	VAL	TORINO
47	ASP	HIS	SEALY
47	ASP	HIS	SINAI
47	ASP	HIS	HASHARON
47	ASP	GLY	UMI
47	ASP	GLY	L(FERRARA)
47	ASP	GLY	KOKURA
47	ASP	GLY	TAGAWA II
50	HIS	ASP	J(SARDEGNA)
51	GLY	ARG	RUSS
54	GLN	ARG	SHIMONOSEKI
54	GLN	ARG	HIROSHIMA
54	GLN	GLU	MEXICO
54	GLN	GLU	J(PARIS-2)
54	GLN	GLU	UPPSALA
57	GLY	ASP	NORFOLK
57	GLY	ASP	G(IBADAN)
57	GLY	ASP	NISHIKI I
57	GLY	ASP	KAGOSHIMA
57	GLY	ARG	L(PERSIAN GULF)
58	HIS	TYR	M(BOSTON)
58	HIS	TYR	M(OSAKA)
58	HIS	TYR	M(GOTTENBERG)
58	HIS	TYR	M(LEIPZIG-2)
60	LYS	ASN	ZAMBIA
68	ASN	ASP	UBE II
68	ASN	LYS	G(BRISTOL)
68	ASN	LYS	G(PHILADELPHIA)
68	ASN	LYS	D(ST. LOUIS)
68	ASN	LYS	KNOXVILLE-1
68	ASN	LYS	STANLEYVILLE-1
68	ASN	LYS	G(ST-1)
68	ASN	LYS	X
74	ASP	HIS	G(TAICHUNG)
74	ASP	HIS	Q
75	ASP	HIS	Q
78	ASN	LYS	STANLEYVILLE-2
80	LEU	ARG	ANN ARBOR
84	SER	ARG	ETOBICOKE

85	ASP	ASN	G(NORFOLK)
85	ASP	TYR	ATAGO
87	HIS	TYR	M(KANKAKEE)
87	HIS	TYR	M(IWATE)
90	LYS	THR	RAJAPPEN
90	LYS	ASN	J(BROUSSAIS)
90	LYS	ASN	TAGAWA-I
92	ARG	LEU	CHESAPEAKE
92	ARG	GLN	J(CAPE TOWN)
95	PRO	LEU	G(GEORGIA)
102	SER	ARG	MANITOBA
112	HIS	ASP	HOPKINS-2
112	HIS	GLN	DAKAR
114	PRO	ARG	CHIAPAS
115	ALA	ASP	J(TONGARIKI)
116	GLU	LYS	O(INDONESIA)
136	LEU	PRO	BIBBA
141	ARG	PRO	SINGAPORE
141	ARG	NIL	KOELLIKER

BY DISSOCIATION-RECOMBINATION EXPERIMENTS EACH OF THE FOLLOWING VARIANT HEMOGLOBINS APPEARS TO HAVE A SUBSTITUTION IN THE ALPHA CHAIN BUT ITS NATURE HAS NOT BEEN IDENTIFIED*

HEMOGLOBIN G(IBADAN)
HEMOGLOBIN J(INDIA)
HEMOGLOBIN J(MALAYA)
HEMOGLOBIN K(CALCUTTA)
HEMOGLOBIN K(MADRAS)
HEMOGLOBIN L(BOMBAY)
HEMOGLOBIN M(OLDENBURG)
HEMOGLOBIN Q(CHINESE)
HEMOGLOBIN UBE-2

*14190 HEMOGLOBIN - BETA LOCUS

THE ALPHA AND BETA LOCI DETERMINE THE STRUCTURE OF THE TWO TYPES OF POLYPEPTIDE CHAINS IN ADULT HEMOGLOBIN, HB A. THE FOLLOWING ARE MUTATIONS AFFECTING THE BETA CHAIN, ARRANGED ACCORDING TO LOCATION OF THE AMINO ACID SUBSTITION. REFERENCES ARE GIVEN EARLIER UNDER THE NAME OF THE PARTICULAR HEMOGLOBIN VARIANT, IN ALPHABETIC ORDER. IT IS NOTEWORTHY THAT SINGLE SUBSTITUTION OF 59 OF THE CHAIN HAVE BEEN DETECTED. FOR 9 OF THE 59 AMINO ACIDS, TWO DIFFERENT MUTANT SUBSTITUTIONS HAVE BEEN FOUND AND FOR TWO OTHERS THREE SUBSTITUTIONS ARE KNOWN.

POSITION	FROM	TO	HEMOGLOBIN
2	HIS	TYR	TOKUCHI
6	GLU	VAL	S
6	GLU	LYS	C
6	GLU	LYS	X
6	GLU	ALA	G(MAKASSAR)
6	GLU	VAL	C(HARLEM)
(THE ABOVE HAS A SECOND CHANGE AT BETA 73, Q.V.)			
6	GLU	VAL	C(GEORGETOWN)
(THE ABOVE HAS A SECOND CHANGE IN THE BETA CHAIN.)			
7	GLU	GLY	G(SAN JOSE)
6 OR 7	GLU	NIL	LEIDEN
7	GLU	LYS	SIRIRAJ

D
O
M
I
N
A
N
T

7	GLU	LYS	G(HONAN)
9	SER	CYS	PORTO ALEGRE
14	LEU	ARG	SOGN
16	GLY	ASP	J(BALTIMORE)
16	GLY	ASP	N(NEW HAVEN-2)
16	GLY	ASP	J(TRINIDAD)
16	GLY	ASP	J(IRELAND)
16	GLY	ARG	D(BUSHMAN)
17	LYS	GLU	NAGASAKI
22	GLU	LYS	E(SASKATOON)
22	GLU	ALA	G(HSIN-CHU)
22	GLU	ALA	G(COUSHATTA)
22	GLU	ALA	G(SASKATOON)
22	GLU	GLY	G(TAIPEI)
23	VAL	NIL	FREIBURG
24	GLY	ARG	RIVERDALE-BRONX
24	GLY	VAL	SAVANNAH
25	GLY	ARG	G(TAIWAN-AMI)
26	GLU	LYS	E
28	LEU	PRO	GENOVA
30	ARG	SER	TACOMA
35	TYR	PHE	PHILLY
37	TRP	SER	HIROSE
42	PHE	SER	HAMMERSMITH
43	GLU	ALA	G(GALVESTON)
43	GLU	ALA	G(TEXAS)
43	GLU	ALA	G(PORT ARTHUR)
46	GLY	GLU	K(IBADAN)
47	ASP	ASN	G(COPENHAGEN)
52	ASP	ASN	OSU CHRISTIANSBORG
56	GLY	ASP	J(BANGKOK)
56	GLY	ASP	J(MEINUNG)
56	GLY	ASP	J(KORAT)
56	GLY	ASP	J(MANADO)
58	PRO	ARG	DHOFAR
58	PRO	ARG	YUKUHASHI
59	LYS	GLU	I(HIGH WYCOMBE)
59	LYS	THR	J(KAOHSIUNG)
61	LYS	ASN	HIKARI
61	LYS	GLU	N(SEATTLE)
63	HIS	TYR	M(SASKATOON)
63	HIS	TYR	M(EMORY)
63	HIS	TYR	M(KURUME)
63	HIS	TYR	M(CHICAGO)
63	HIS	TYR	M(HAMBURG)
63	HIS	ARG	ZURICH
66	LYS	GLU	I(TOULOUSE)
67	VAL	GLU	M(MILWAUKEE-1)
67	VAL	ASP	BRISTOL

67	VAL	ALA	SYDNEY
69	GLY	ASP	J(RAMBAM)
69	GLY	ASP	J(CAMBRIDGE)
71	PHE	SER	CHRISTCHURCH
73	ASP	ASN	C(HARLEM)
73	ASP	ASN	KORLE-BU
74	GLY	ASP	SHEPHERDS BUSH
76	ALA	GLU	SEATTLE
77	HIS	ASP	J(IRAN)
79	ASP	ASN	G(ACCRA)
80	ASN	LYS	G(SZUHU)
87	THR	LYS	D(IBADAN)
88	LEU	PRO	SANTA ANA
88	LEU	ARG	BORAS
90	GLU	LYS	AGENOGI
91	LEU	PRO	SABINE
92	HIS	TYR	M(HYDE PARK)
92	HIS	TYR	M(AKITA)
94	ASP	ASN	OAK RIDGE
95	LYS	ASP	N
95	LYS	GLU OR GLN	N(MEMPHIS)
95	LYS	GLU	N(BALTIMORE)
95	LYS	GLU	N(JENKINS)
95	LYS	GLU	HOPKINS-1
97	HIS	GLN	MALMO
98	VAL	MET	KOLN
99	ASP	HIS	YAKIMA
99	ASP	ASN	KEMPSEY
102	ASP	THR	KANSAS
102	ASP	LYS	RICHMOND
108	ASN	ASP	YOSHIZUKA
113	VAL	GLU	NEW YORK
117	HIS	ARG	P(GALVESTON)
120	LYS	GLU	HIJIYAMA
121	GLU	LYS	O(ARABIA)
121	GLU	GLN	D(PUNJAB)
121	GLU	GLN	D(LOS ANGELES)
121	GLU	GLN	D(CYPRUS)
121	GLU	GLN	D(PORTUGAL)
124	PRO	ARG	KHARTOUM
126	VAL	GLU	HOFU
129	ALA	ASP	J(TAICHUNG)
130	TYR	ASP	WIEN
132	LYS	GLN	K(WOOLWICH)
136	GLY	ASP	HOPE
141	LEU	ARG	OLMSTED

DOMINANT

150

		143		HIS		ASP		HIROSHIMA	
		143		HIS		ASP		KENWOOD	

D
O
M
I
N
A
N
T

| | | 145 | | TYR | | HIS | | RAINIER | |

OF THE ABOVE, HEMOGLOBINS C(HARLEM) AND C(GEORGETOWN) HAVE TWO SUBSTITUTIONS IN THE BETA CHAIN, AND HEMOGLOBIN X HAS A SUBSTITUTION IN BOTH THE ALPHA AND THE BETA CHAIN.

BY DISSOCIATION RECOMBINATION EXPERIMENTS, EACH OF THE FOLLOWING VARIANT HEMOGLOBINS APPEARS TO HAVE A SUBSTITUTION IN THE BETA CHAIN BUT ITS NATURE HAS NOT BEEN IDENTIFIED*

HEMOGLOBIN CASERTA
HEMOGLOBIN DURHAM-1
HEMOGLOBIN J(GEORGIA)
HEMOGLOBIN J(JAMAICA)
HEMOGLOBIN J(KORAT)
HEMOGLOBIN J(MEINUNG)
HEMOGLOBIN K
HEMOGLOBIN L
HEMOGLOBIN P
HEMOGLOBIN R(SAME AS DURHAM-1)
HEMOGLOBIN TSUKIJI
HEMOGLOBIN YPSI

```
D
O
M
I
N
A
N
T
```

*14200 HEMOGLOBIN - GAMMA LOCUS (ACTUALLY 2 LOCI)

THE GAMMA LOCUS DETERMINES THE GAMMA, OR NON-ALPHA, CHAIN OF FETAL HEMOGLOBIN
(ALPHA 2-GAMMA 2). SCHROEDER ET AL. (1968) HAVE PROVIDED EVIDENCE FOR THE
EXISTENCE OF TWO TYPES OF GAMMA POLYPEPTIDE CHAINS, DETERMINED PRESUMABLY BY
SEPARATE CISTRONS. ALTHOUGH NOT DISTINGUISHABLE BY MOST OF THE PHYSICAL METHODS
USED, SEQUENCING HAS SHOWN AT LEAST ONE AMINO ACID DIFFERENCE* AT POSITION 136 ONE
TYPE HAS GLYCINE (AS INDICATED IN THE AMINO ACID MAP SHOWN ON A PREVIOUS PAGE) AND
THE SECOND TYPE HAS ALANINE. PRESUMABLY THE TWO LOCI AROSE BY GENE DUPLICATION.
THE FOLLOWING ARE MUTATIONS AFFECTING THE GAMMA CHAIN ARRANGED ACCORDING TO
LOCATION OF THE AMINO ACID SUBSTITUTION. EACH MUTATION OCCURS IN ONLY ONE OF THE
GAMMA CISTRONS, E.G., THE MUTATION OF HB F(MALTA) IS IN THE GLYCINE 136 CISTRON.
REFERENCES ARE GIVEN EARLIER UNDER THE NAME OF THE PARTICULAR HEMOGLOBIN VARIANT,
IN ALPHABETIC ORDER.

SCHROEDER, W. A., HUISMAN, T. H. J., SHELTON, J. R., SHELTON, J. B., KLEIHAUER,
E. F., DOZY, A. M. AND ROBBERSON, B.* EVIDENCE FOR MULTIPLE STRUCTURAL GENES FOR
THE GAMMA CHAIN OF HUMAN FETAL HEMOGLOBIN. PROC. NAT. ACAD. SCI. 60* 537-544,
1968.

POSITION	FROM	TO	HEMOGLOBIN
5	GLU	LYS	F(TEXAS 1)
6	GLU	LYS	F(TEXAS 2)
12	THR	LYS	F(ALEXANDRA)
61	LYS	GLU	F(JAMAICA)
97	HIS	ARG	F(DICKINSON)
117	HIS	ARG	F(MALTA)
121	GLU	LYS	F(HULL)

OTHER VARIANT FETAL HEMOGLOBINS INCLUDE THE FOLLOWING*

HEMOGLOBIN AEGINA
HEMOGLOBIN CYPRUS-1
HEMOGLOBIN BRISTOL-SINGAPORE
HEMOGLOBIN F(ROMA)
HEMOGLOBIN FESSAS-PAPASPYROU

*14210 HEMOGLOBIN - DELTA LOCUS

THE DELTA LOCUS DETERMINES THE DELTA, OR NON-ALPHA, CHAIN OF HEMOGLOBIN A2 (ALPHA
2-DELTA 2). THE FOLLOWING ARE MUTATIONS AFFECTING THE DELTA CHAIN ARRANGED
ACCORDING TO LOCATION OF THE AMINO ACID SUBSTITUTION. REFERENCES ARE GIVEN
EARLIER UNDER THE NAME OF THE PARTICULAR HEMOGLOBIN VARIANT, IN ALPHABETIC ORDER.

POSITION	FROM	TO	HEMOGLOBIN
2	HIS	ARG	SPHAKIA
12	ASN	LYS	NYU
16	GLY	ARG	A(2) PRIME OR B(2)

.	22	.	ALA	.	GLU	.	FLATBUSH		.	
.		.							.	
.	136	.	GLY	.	ASP	.	BABINGA		.	

D
O
M
I
N
A
N
T

*14220 HEMOGLOBIN - EPSILON LOCUS

THE EPSILON LOCUS DETERMINES THE EPSILON, OR NON-ALPHA, CHAIN OF EMBRYONIC HEMOGLOBIN (ORIGINALLY KNOWN AS GOWER-2). NO MUTATIONS AFFECTING THE EPSILON CHAIN HAVE YET BEEN IDENTIFIED.

HUEHNS, E. R., DANCE, N., BEAVEN, G. H., HECHT, F. AND MOTULSKY, A. G.* HUMAN EMBRYONIC HEMOGLOBIN. NATURE 201* 1095-1097, 1964.

THE FOLLOWING VARIANT HEMOGLOBIN REPRESENT UNUSUAL GENETIC AND BIOCHEMICAL CHANGE*

A. TETRAMERS OF A SINGLE TYPE OF POLYPEPTIDE CHAIN
   HEMOGLOBIN AUGUSTA-1. PROBABLY TETRAMER OF S-BETA CHAIN.
   HEMOGLOBIN AUGUSTA-2. PROBABLY TETRAMER OF C-BETA CHAIN.
   HEMOGLOBIN BARTS. TETRAMER OF GAMMA CHAIN.
   HEMOGLOBIN GOWER-1. TETRAMER OF EPSILON CHAIN.
   HEMOGLOBIN H. TETRAMER OF BETA CHAIN.

B. PROBABLE OCTOMER
   HEMOGLOBIN PORTO-ALLEGRE

C. DELTA-BETA FUSION PRODUCTS
   HEMOGLOBIN LEPORE(BOSTON)
   HEMOGLOBIN PYLOS(SAME AS LAST)
   HEMOGLOBIN LEPORE(CYPRUS)
   HEMOGLOBIN LEPORE(HOLLANDIA)
   HEMOGLOBIN LEPORE(THE BRONX)

D. BETA-DELTA FUSION PRODUTS
   HEMOGLOBIN P(CONGO)
   HEMOGLOBIN MIYADA

E. DELETION OF ONE OR MORE AMINO ACIDS
   HEMOGLOBIN FREIBURG
   HEMOGLOBIN GUN HILL
   HEMOGLOBIN LEIDEN
   HEMOGLOBIN TOCHIGI

F. TWO SUBSTITUTIONS IN BETA CHAIN
   HEMOGLOBIN C(HARLEM)
   HEMOGLOBIN C(GEORGETOWN)

G. SUBSTITUTION IN BOTH THE ALPHA AND THE BETA CHAIN
   HEMOGLOBIN X

THE NATURE OF THE FOLLOWING HEMOGLOBINS IS UNKNOWN*

   HEMOGLOBIN ATWATER
   HEMOGLOBIN GALLIERI GENOVA
   HEMOGLOBIN G(PARIS)
   HEMOGLOBIN M(LEIPZIG-1)
   HEMOGLOBIN M(MILWAUKEE-2)
   HEMOGLOBIN N(SARDINIA)
   HEMOGLOBIN PIERCE ET AL.
   HEMOGLOBIN SCOTT
   HEMOGLOBIN ST. MARY*S
   HEMOGLOBIN SUD-VIETNAM
   HEMOGLOBIN TACOMA
   HEMOGLOBIN TOKYO
   HEMOGLOBIN UBE-1

14230 HERNIA, DOUBLE INGUINAL

WEIMER (1949) DESCRIBED A FAMILY IN WHICH AT LEAST ONE MALE IN FOUR SUCCESSIVE GENERATIONS HAD BILATERAL INGUINAL HERNIA. AUTOSOMAL DOMINANCE WITH SEX INFLUENCE WAS SUGGESTED.

WEIMER, B. R.* CONGENITAL INHERITANCE OF INGUINAL HERNIA. J. HERED. 40* 219-220, 1949.

14240 HERNIA, HIATUS

GOODMAN ET AL. (1969) OBSERVED SIX AFFECTED PERSONS IN TWO GENERATIONS. FIVE OF

GOODMAN, R. M., WOOLEY, C. F., RUPPERT, R. D. AND FREIMANIS, A. K.* A POSSIBLE GENETIC ROLE IN ESOPHAGEAL HIATUS HERNIA. J. HERED. 60* 71-74, 1969.

14250 HETEROCHROMIA IRIDIS

ASYMMETRY IN THE PIGMENTATION OF THE IRIDES PROBABLY OCCURS AS AN ISOLATED PHENOMENON INHERITED AS A DOMINANT (CALHOUN, 1919). WE HAVE OBSERVED IT IN AT LEAST THREE CASES OF THE MARFAN SYNDROME. DAMAGE TO THE CERVICAL SYMPATHETICS, AS IN BIRTH INJURY, MAY RESULT IN THIS TRAIT, WHICH REPRESENTS IN SUCH INSTANCES A PHENOCOPY. WHETHER HEREDITARY HETEROCHROMIA IRIDIS EVER EXISTS INDEPENDENT OF HORNER'S SYNDROME (Q.V.), WAARDENBURG'S SYNDROME (Q.V.), OR THE PIEBALD TRAIT (Q.V.) IS NOT CLEAR. THE MELANOCYTES OF THE UVEAL TRAIT CONSTITUTE A BRANCHING PSEUDO-SYNCYTIUM RICHLY INNERVATED BY SYMPATHETIC NERVES. PIGMENTATION OF THE IRIS DOES NOT OCCUR IN THE ABSENCE OF THIS INNERVATION. SYMPATHETIC FIBERS LEAVE THE LATERAL HORN OF THE GRAY MATTER OF THE FIRST AND SECOND THORACIC SEGMENTS, PASS OUT IN THE ANTERIOR ROOTS AND JOIN THE LATERAL SYMPATHETIC CHAIN VIA THE WHITE RAMI COMMUNICANTES. THEY THEN PROCEED TO THE SUPERIOR CERVICAL GANGLION AND ALONG THE DISTRIBUTION OF THE CAROTID ARTERY TO THE HEAD. CONGENITAL HORNER'S SYNDROME WITH ASSOCIATED HETEROCHROMIA IRIDIS CAN BE PRODUCED BY BIRTH INJURY TO THE LOWER ROOTS OF THE BRACHIAL PLEXUS (KLUMPKE PALSY). HETEROCHROMIA IRIDIS IS THE DESIGNATION WHICH THE PURIST RESERVES FOR DIFFERENT PIGMENTATION IN SECTORS OF ONE IRIS, WHEREAS HETEROCHROMIA IRIDUM IS THE TERM USED WHEN THE TWO IRIDES ARE OF DIFFERENT COLOR.

CALHOUN, F. P.* CAUSES OF HETEROCHROMIA IRIDIS WITH SPECIAL REFERENCE TO PARALYSIS OF THE CERVICAL SYMPATHETICS. AM. J. OPHTHAL. 2* 255-269, 1919.

GLADSTONE, R. M.* DEVELOPMENT AND SIGNIFICANCE OF HETEROCHROMIA OF THE IRIS. ARCH. NEUROL. 21* 184-192, 1969.

14260 HEXOKINASE

SCHIMKE AND GROSSBARD (1968) REVIEWED STUDIES OF HEXOKINASE ISOZYMES. POLYMOR- PHISM HAS APPARENTLY NOT BEEN IDENTIFIED IN MAN.

SCHIMKE, R. T. AND GROSSBARD, L.* STUDIES ON ISOZYMES OF HEXOKINASE IN ANIMAL TISSUES. ANN. N.Y. ACAD. SCI. 151* 332-350, 1968.

14270 HIP, DISLOCATION OF, CONGENITAL

THE GENETICS IS CONSIDERED COMPLEX. JOINT LAXITY, NORMALLY GREATER IN FEMALES THAN IN MALES, PROBABLY ACCOUNTS FOR THE PREPONDERANCE OF AFFECTED FEMALES OVER MALES. PERSISTENT LAXITY (Q.V.), OFTEN OF FAMILIAL NATURE, IS PROBABLY A FACTOR ESPECIALLY IN MALES. HIP DYSPLASIA WITH DISLOCATION OCCURS IN HIGH FREQUENCY IN THE GERMAN SHEPHERD DOG. AUTOSOMAL DOMINANT INHERITANCE IS FAVORED BY BORNFORS, PALSSON AND SKUDE (1964). DISLOCATION OF THE HIP IS AN OCCASIONAL FEATURE OF CONDITIONS WITH SIMPLE INHERITANCE, E.G., MARFAN SYNDROME AND EHLERS-DANLOS SYNDROME. RECORD AND EDWARDS (1958) ESTIMATED THE RISK OF RECURRENCE IN SUBSE- QUENTLY BORN SIBS TO BE ABOUT 5 PERCENT.

BORNFORS, S., PALSSON, K. AND SKUDE, G.* HEREDITARY ASPECTS OF HIP DYSPLASIA IN GERMAN SHEPHERD DOGS. J. AM. VET. MED. ASS. 145* 15-20, 1964.

CARTER, C. O. AND WILKINSON, J. A.* GENETIC AND ENVIRONMENTAL FACTORS IN THE ETIOLOGY OF CONGENITAL DISLOCATION OF THE HIP. CLIN. ORTHOP. 33* 119-128, 1964.

CARTER, C. O. AND WILKINSON, J. A.* PERSISTENT JOINT LAXITY AND CONGENITAL DISLOCATION OF THE HIP. J. BONE JOINT SURG. 46B* 40-45, 1964.

RECORD, R. G. AND EDWARDS, J. H.* ENVIRONMENTAL INFLUENCES RELATED TO THE ETIOLOGY OF CONGENITAL DISLOCATION OF THE HIP. BRIT. J. PREV. SOC. MED. 12* 8-22, 1958.

*14280 HL-A HISTOCOMPATIBILITY TYPE

BACH AND AMOS (1967) CONCLUDED THAT A SINGLE LOCUS WITH 15 OR MORE ALLELES CONTROLS REACTIVITY IN MIXED LEUKOCYTE CULTURE TESTS, AND THAT GENES AT THIS LOCUS ALSO CONTROL MOST OF THE SPECIFICITIES MEASURED BY CYTOTOXIC ANTISERUMS TO LEUKOCYTES. THIS MAY BE THE MAJOR HISTOCOMPATIBILITY LOCUS IN MAN. BERNARD (1967) CALLED DISCOVERY OF THE HU-1 (NOW CALLED HL-A) SYSTEM AS IMPORTANT AN EVENT IN BIOLOGY AS DISCOVERY OF THE ABO AND RH SYSTEMS, PERHAPS MORE IMPORTANT. HL-A IN THE NEW NOMENCLATURE MEANS 'HUMAN LEUKOCYTE' AND A REFERS TO THE FACT THAT THIS IS THE FIRST LOCUS DESIGNATED. THE USEFULNESS OF HL-A TYPING FOR SELECTION OF KIDNEY DONORS WAS DEMONSTRATED BY PATEL ET AL. (1968). BY GEL FILTRATION MANN ET AL. (1969) SEPARATED SOLUBLE PREPARATIONS OF HL-A ALLOANTIGENS INTO COMPONENTS HAVING EITHER 'LA' SPECIFICITY OR '4' SPECIFICITY. THIS MAY INDICATE THAT THE HL- A 'LOCUS' IS A REGION WITH SEVERAL DIFFERENT CISTRONS. FURTHERMORE, FAMILY DATA INDICATES THE EXISTENCE OF TWO 'SEGREGANT SERIES.' ANTIGENS 1, 2, 3, 9, 10 AND 11 ARE MUTUALLY EXCLUSIVE MEMBERS OF ONE ALLELIC SERIES WHEREAS A DIFFERENT ARRAY OF ANTIGENS CONSTITUTE A SECOND SERIES (BACH AND BACH, 1970). THE RELATION OF THE

ISOANTIGENIC VARIANTS IDENTIFIED IN HUMAN FIBROBLAST CULTURES TO THE HL-A SYSTEM IS NOT KNOWN. BOTH THE HL-A SYSTEM IN MAN AND THE H-2 SYSTEM IN MICE SEEM TO HAVE HAPLOID EXPRESSION IN SPERM. RECOMBINATION HAS BEEN OBSERVED WITHIN THE LH-A SYSTEM (BODMER ET AL., 1970).

ADMAN, R. AND PIOUS, D. A.* ISOANTIGENIC VARIANTS* ISOLATION FROM HUMAN DIPLOID CELLS IN CULTURE. SCIENCE 168* 370-372, 1970.

BACH, F. H. AND AMOS, D. B.* HU-1 MAJOR HISTOCOMPATIBILITY LOCUS IN MAN. SCIENCE 156* 1506-1508, 1967.

BACH, M. L. AND BACH, F. H.* THE GENETICS OF HISTOCOMPATIBILITY. HOSP. PRACTICE 5 (NO. 8)* 33-44, 1970.

BERNARD, J.* LA DECOUVERTE DU SYSTEME PRINCIPAL D'HISTOCOMPATIBILITE DE L'HOMME. (EDITORIAL) PRESSE MED. 75* 2369 ONLY, 1967.

BODMER, W. F., BODMER, J. G. AND TRIPP, M.* RECOMBINATION BETWEEN THE LA AND 4 LOCI OF THE HL-A SYSTEM. IN, HISTOCOMPATIBILITY TESTING. COPENHAGEN* MUNKSGAARD, 1970. PP. 187-191.

BODMER, W. F., BODMER, J. G., ADLER, S., PAYNE, R. AND BIALEK, J.* GENETICS OF '4' AND 'LA' HUMAN LEUKOCYTE GROUPS. ANN. N. Y. ACAD. SCI. 129* 473-489, 1966.

DAUSSET, J., IVANYI, P., COLOMBANI, J., FEINGOLD, N. AND LEGRAND, L.* LE SYSTEME HU-1. ETUDES GENETIQUES DE POPULATION ET DE FAMILLES. NOUV. REV. FRANC. HEMAT. 7* 897-899, 1967.

ENGELFRIET, C. P. AND BRITTEN, A.* THE CYTOTOXIC TEST FOR LEUCOCYTE ANTIBODIES. A SIMPLE AND RELIABLE TECHNIQUE. VOX. SANG. 10* 660-674, 1965.

FELLOUS, M. AND DAUSSET, J.* PROBABLE HAPLOID EXPRESSION OF HL-A ANTIGENS ON HUMAN SPERMATOZOON. NATURE 225* 191-193, 1970.

KISSMEYER-NIELSEN, F., SVEJGAARD, A. AND HAUGE, M.* GENETICS OF THE HUMAN HL-A TRANSPLANTATION SYSTEM. NATURE 219* 1116-1119, 1968.

KISSMEYER-NIELSEN, F., SVEJGAARD, A., AHRONS, S. AND NIELSEN, L. S.* CROSSING-OVER WITHIN THE HL-A SYSTEM. NATURE 224* 75-76, 1969.

MANN, D. L., ROGENTINE, G. N., JR., FAHEY, J. L. AND NATHENSON, S. G.* MOLECULAR HETEROGENEITY OF HUMAN LYMPHOID (HL-A) ALLOANTIGENS. SCIENCE 163* 1460-1462, 1969.

PATEL, R., MICKEY, M. R. AND TERASAKI, P. I.* SEROTYPING FOR HOMOTRANSPLANTA-TION OF KIDNEYS FROM UNRELATED DONORS. NEW ENG. J. MED. 279* 501-506, 1968.

PAYNE, R., TRIPP, M., WEIGLE, J., BODMER, W. AND BODMER, J.* A NEW LEUKOCYTE ISOANTIGEN SYSTEM IN MAN. COLD SPRING HARBOR SYMPOSIA QUANT. BIOL. 29* 285-295, 1964.

THORSBY, E., SANDBERG, L., LINDHOLM, A. AND KISSMEYER-NIELSEN, F.* THE HL-A SYSTEM. EVIDENCE OF A THIRD SUB-LOCUS. SCAND. J. HAEMAT. 7* 195-200, 1970.

VAN LEEUWEN, A., EERNISSE, J. G. AND VAN ROOD, J. J.* A NEW LEUKOCYTE GROUP WITH TWO ALLELES* LEUCOCYTE GROUP FIVE. VOX SANG. 9* 431-446, 1964.

VAN ROOD, J. J. AND VAN LEEUWEN, A.* LEUKOCYTE GROUPING. A METHOD AND ITS APPLICATION. J. CLIN. INVEST. 42* 1382-1390, 1963.

VAN ROOD, J. J.* LEUCOCYTE GROUPING AND ORGAN TRANSPLANTATION. BRIT. J. HAEMAT. 16* 211-220, 1969.

VAN ROOD, J. J.* TISSUE TYPING AND ORGAN TRANSPLANTATION. LANCET 1* 1142-1146, 1969.

WALFORD, R. L., FINKELSTEIN, S., HANNA, C. AND COLLINS, Z.* THIRD SUBLOCUS IN THE HL-A HUMAN TRANSPLANTATION SYSTEM. NATURE 224* 74-75, 1969.

*14290 HOLT-ORAM SYNDROME (HEART AND HAND SYNDROME)

ALTHOUGH THE ABNORMALITY OF THE UPPER EXTREMITIES IS MORE EXTENSIVE IN SOME CASES, THE CHARACTERISTIC FINDING IS THUMB ANOMALY WITH ATRIAL SEPTAL DEFECT. THE THUMB MAY BE ABSENT OR MAY BE A TRIPHALANGEAL, NON-OPPOSABLE, FINGER-LIKE DIGIT. THE THUMB METACARPAL HAS BOTH A PROXIMAL AND A DISTAL EPIPHYSEAL OSSIFICATION CENTER. MCKUSICK (1961) REPORTED MOTHER AND DAUGHTER WITH ATRIAL SEPTAL DEFECT AND ABSENT OR TRIPHALANGEAL, FINGER-LIKE THUMB. IN 1966 THE DAUGHTER GAVE BIRTH TO A MALE INFANT WITH UPPER EXTREMITY PHOCOMELIA AND VENTRICULAR SEPTAL DEFECT. THE INVOLVEMENT OF THE ARM WAS MORE EXTENSIVE AND THE CARDIOVASCULAR INVOLVEMENT MORE VARIED IN THE FAMILIES DESCRIBED BY LEWIS ET AL. (1965) AND HARRIS ET AL. (1966) THAN IN THAT OF HOLT AND ORAM (1960). HOWEVER IT IS NOT CERTAIN THAT THESE REPRESENT A SEPARATE MUTATION. POZNANSKI ET AL. (1970) POINTED OUT THAT CARPAL

ABNORMALITIES, E.G. EXTRA CARPAL BONES, ARE MORE SPECIFIC FOR THE HOLT-ORAM
SYNDROME THAN CHANGES IN THE THUMB. POSTERIORLY AND LATERALLY PROTRUBERANT MEDIAL
EPICONDYLES OF THE HUMERUS WERE SEEN IN SEVERAL PATIENTS.

EMERIT, I., DE GROUCHY, J., LAVAL-JEANTET, M., CORONE, P. AND VERNANT, P.*
MALFORMATIONS COMPLEXES DES MEMBRES SUPERIEURS ASSOCIEES A UNE CARDIOPATHIE
CONGENITALE. A PROPOS DE SIX OBSERVATIONS. ACTA GENET. MED. GEM. 14* 132-163,
1965.

GALL, J. C., JR., STERN, A. M., COHEN, M. M., ADAMS, M. S. AND DAVIDSON, R. T.*
HOLT-ORAM SYNDROME* CLINICAL AND GENETIC STUDY OF A LARGE FAMILY. AM. J. HUM.
GENET. 18* 187-200, 1966.

HARRIS, L. C. AND OSBORNE, W. P.* CONGENITAL ABSENCE OR HYPOPLASIA OF THE
RADIUS WITH VENTRICULAR SEPTAL DEFECT* VENTRICULO-RADIAL DYSPLASIA. J. PEDIAT.
68* 265-272, 1966.

HOLT, M. AND ORAM, S.* FAMILIAL HEART DISEASE WITH SKELETAL MALFORMATIONS.
BRIT. HEART J. 22* 236-242, 1960.

LEWIS, K. B., BRUCE, R. A., BAUM, D. AND MOTULSKY, A. G.* THE UPPER LIMB-
CARDIOVASCULAR SYNDROME. AN AUTOSOMAL DOMINANT GENETIC EFFECT ON EMBRYOGENESIS.
J.A.M.A. 193* 1080-1086, 1965.

MCKUSICK, V. A. AND COLLEAGUES* MEDICAL GENETICS 1960. J. CHRONIC DIS. 14* 1-
198, 1961 (FIG. 45).

POZNANSKI, A. K., GALL, J. C., JR. AND STERN, A. M.* SKELETAL MANIFESTATIONS OF
THE HOLT-ORAM SYNDROME. RADIOLOGY 94* 45-54, 1970.

ZETTERQVIST, P.* THE SYNDROME OF FAMILIAL ATRIAL SEPTAL DEFECT, HEART ARRHYTH-
MIA AND HAND MALFORMATION (HOLT-ORAM) IN MOTHER AND SON. ACTA PAEDIAT. 52* 115-
122, 1963.

*14300 HORNER SYNDROME

DURHAM (1958) DESCRIBED CONGENITAL HORNER'S SYNDROME IN A BOY AND HIS FATHER,
PATERNAL AUNT AND UNCLE AND A FIRST COUSIN. THE BOY SHOWED PTOSIS AND PUPILLARY
CHANGES ON THE LEFT. THE RIGHT IRIS WAS BROWN, THE LEFT BLUE. THESE FINDINGS
LIKE THOSE OF CALHOUN (1919) ILLUSTRATE THE ROLE OF NORMAL SYMPATHETIC INNERVATION
OF THE IRIS IN ITS PIGMENTATION.

CALHOUN, F. P.* CAUSES OF HETEROCHROMIA IRIDIS WITH SPECIAL REFERENCE TO
PARALYSIS OF CERVICAL SYMPATHETIC. AM. J. OPHTHAL. 2* 256-269, 1919.

DURHAM, D. G.* CONGENITAL HEREDITARY HORNER'S SYNDROME. ARCH. OPHTHAL. 60*
939-940, 1958.

*14310 HUNTINGTON'S CHOREA

CHOREIC MOVEMENTS AND DEMENTIA ARE THE LEADING FEATURES. THE AGE AT ONSET IS
HIGHLY VARIABLE* SOME SHOW SIGNS IN THE FIRST DECADE AND SOME NOT UNTIL OVER 60
YEARS OF AGE. THE MODE IS BETWEEN 30 AND 40 YEARS (CHANDLER AND COLLEAGUES,
1960). REED AND NEEL (1959), IN A STUDY OF 196 KINDREDS, FOUND ONLY EIGHT IN
WHICH BOTH PARENTS OF A SINGLE PATIENT WITH HUNTINGTON'S CHOREA WAS 60 YEARS OF
AGE OR OLDER AND NORMAL. REED AND CHANDLER (1958) ESTIMATED THE FREQUENCY OF
RECOGNIZED HUNTINGTON'S CHOREA IN THE MICHIGAN LOWER PENINSULA TO BE ABOUT 4.12 X
10 (TO THE MINUS 5), AND THE TOTAL FREQUENCY OF HETEROZYGOTES TO BE ABOUT 1.01 X
10 (TO THE MINUS 4). VESSIE (1932) TRACED THE ANCESTRY OF THE FAMILIES STUDIED BY
HUNTINGTON. ABOUT 1000 CASES IN TWELVE GENERATIONS DESCENDANT FROM TWO BROTHERS
IN SUFFOLK, ENGLAND, COULD BE IDENTIFIED. THE INTRAFAMILIAL VARIABILITY IS
ILLUSTRATED BY THE REPORT BY CAMPBELL ET AL. (1961) OF THE JUVENILE RIGID FORM IN
TWO BROTHERS IN A KINDRED IN WHICH FOR THREE PRECEDING GENERATIONS DISEASE OF MORE
CLASSIC TYPE HAD OCCURRED. BARBEAU (1970) POINTED OUT THAT PATIENTS WITH THE
JUVENILE FORM OF HUNTINGTON'S CHOREA SEEM MORE OFTEN TO HAVE INHERITED THEIR
DISORDER FROM THE FATHER THAN FROM THE MOTHER.

BARBEAU, A.* PARENTAL ASCENT IN THE JUVENILE FORM OF HUNTINGTON'S CHOREA.
(LETTER) LANCET 2* 937 ONLY, 1970.

BYERS, R. K. AND DODGE, J. A.* HUNTINGTON'S CHOREA IN CHILDREN* REPORT OF FOUR
CASES. NEUROLOGY 17* 587-596, 1967.

CAMPBELL, A. M. G., CORNER, B. D., NORMAN, R. M. AND URICH, H.* THE RIGID FORM
OF HUNTINGTON'S DISEASE. J. NEUROL. NEUROSURG. PSYCHIAT. 24* 71-77, 1961.

CHANDLER, J. H., REED, T. E. AND DEJONG, R. N.* HUNTINGTON'S CHOREA IN
MICHIGAN. NEUROLOGY 10* 148-153, 1960.

LYON, R. L.* HUNTINGTON'S CHOREA IN THE MORAY FIRTH AREA. BRIT. MED. J. 1*
1301-1306, 1962.

MYRIANTHOPOULOS, N. C.* HUNTINGTON'S CHOREA. J. MED. GENET. 3* 298-314, 1966.

REED, T. E. AND CHANDLER, J. H.* HUNTINGTON'S CHOREA IN MICHIGAN. I.
DEMOGRAPHY AND GENETICS. AM. J. HUM. GENET. 10* 201-225, 1958.

        REED, T. E. AND NEEL, J. V.* HUNTINGTON'S CHOREA IN MICHIGAN. II. SELECTION
AND MUTATION. AM. J. HUM. GENET. 11* 107-136, 1959.

        VESSIE, P. R.* ORIGINAL ARTICLE ON THE TRANSMISSION OF HUNTINGTON'S CHOREA FOR
300 YEARS - THE BURES FAMILY GROUP. J. NERV. MENT. DIS. 76* 553-573, 1932.

*14320 HYALOIDEO-RETINAL DEGENERATION OF WAGNER

        WAGNER (1938) DESCRIBED 13 MEMBERS OF A CANTON ZURICH FAMILY WITH A PECULIAR
LESION OF THE VITREOUS AND RETINA. TEN ADDITIONAL AFFECTED MEMBERS WERE OBSERVED
BY BOHRINGER, DIETERLE AND LANDOLT (1960) AND 5 MORE BY RICCI (1961). IN HOLLAND
JANSEN (1962) DESCRIBED TWO FAMILIES WITH A TOTAL OF 39 AFFECTED PERSONS.
ALEXANDER AND SHEA (1965) REPORTED A DANISH FAMILY. IN THE LAST REPORT, CHARAC-
TERISTIC FACIES (EPICANTHUS, BROAD SUNKEN NASAL BRIDGE, RECEEDING CHIN) WAS NOTED.
GENU VALGUM WAS PRESENT IN ALL. IN ADDITION TO TYPICAL CHANGES IN THE VITREOUS,
RETINAL DETACHMENT OCCURS IN SOME AND CATARACT IS ANOTHER COMPLICATION. SEE
AUTOSOMAL RECESSIVE HYALOIDO-TAPETORETINAL DEGENERATION OF FAVRE. IRREGULAR
AUTOSOMAL DOMINANT INHERITANCE WAS SUGGESTED BY VAN BALEN AND FALGER (1970) ON THE
BASIS OF THREE LARGE PEDIGREES AND THE SYNDROMAL ASSOCIATION OF CLEFT PALATE WAS
EMPHASIZED. THIS DISORDER IS, OF COURSE, A *CAUSE* OF FAMILIAL RETINAL DETACHMENT
(EDMUND, 1961).

        ALEXANDER, R. L. AND SHEA, M.* WAGNER'S DISEASE. ARCH. OPHTHAL. 74* 310-318,
1965.

        BOHRINGER, H. R., DIETERLE, P. AND LANDOLT, E.* ZUR KLINIK UND PATHOLOGIE DER
DEGENERATIO HYALOIDEO-RETINALIS HEREDITARIA (WAGNER). OPHTHALMOLOGICA 139* 330-
338, 1960.

        EDMUND, J.* FAMILIAL RETINAL DETACHMENT. ACTA OPHTHAL. 39* 644-654, 1961.

        FRANDSEN, E.* HEREDITARY HYALOIDEO-RETINAL DEGENERATION (WAGNER) IN A DANISH
FAMILY. ACTA OPHTHAL. 44* 223-232, 1966.

        JANSEN, L. M. A. A.* DEGENERATIO HYALOIDEO-RETINALIS HEREDITARIA. OPHTHALMOLO-
GICA 144* 458-464, 1962.

        RICCI, A.* CLINIQUE ET TRANSMISSION HEREDITAIRE DES DEGENERESCENCES VITREO-
RETINIENNES. BULL. SOC. OPHTAL. FRANC. 61* 618-662, 1961.

        VAN BALEN, A. T. M. AND FALGER, E. L. F.* HEREDITARY HYALOIDEORETINAL DEGENERA-
TION AND PALATOSCHISIS. ARCH. OPHTHAL. 83* 152-162, 1970.

        WAGNER, H.* EIN BISHER UNBEKANNTES ERBLEIDEN DES AUGES (DEGENERATIO HYALOIDEO-
RETINALIS HEREDITARIA), BEOBACHTET IM KANTON ZURICH. KLIN. MBL. AUGENHEILK. 100*
840-858, 1938.

14330 HYALOIDEORETINAL DEGENERATION, CLEFT PALATE, MAXILLARY HYPOPLASIA (CERVENKA'S
        SYNDROME)

        COHEN ET AL. (1971) DESCRIBED A FATHER AND TWO SONS AND TWO DAUGHTERS WITH MYOPIA,
HYALOIDEORETINAL DEGENERATION, RETINAL DETACHMENT, FLAT FACE FROM MAXILLARY
HYPOPLASIA, AND IN THE FATHER AND TWO OF HIS CHILDREN SUBMUCOUS CLEFT PALATE.
FAMILIES WHICH THE AUTHORS FELT HAD THE SAME DISORDER WERE REPORTED BY EDMUND
(1961), DELANEY ET AL. (1963), FRANDSEN (1966), AND VAN BALEN AND FALGER (1970).
PRESUMABLY THIS DISORDER IS DISTINCT FROM HYALOIDEORETINAL DEGENERATION OF WAGNER
(Q.V.) WITHOUT CLEFT PALATE.

        COHEN, M. M., JR., KNOBLOCH, W. H. AND GORLIN, R. J.* A DOMINANTLY INHERITED
SYNDROME OF HYALOIDEORETINAL DEGENERATION, CLEFT PALATE, AND MAXILLARY HYPOPLASIA
(CERVENKA'S SYNDROME). THE CLINICAL DELINEATION OF BIRTH DEFECTS. XI. OROFACIAL
STRUCTURES. BALTIMORE* WILLIAMS AND WILKINS, 1971.

        DELANEY, W. V., PODEDEUORNY, W. AND HAVENER, W. H.* INHERITED RETINAL DETACH-
MENT. ARCH. OPHTHAL. 69* 44-50, 1963.

        EDMUND, J.* FAMILIAL RETINAL DETACHMENT. ACTA OPHTHAL. 39* 644-654, 1961.

        FRANDSEN, E.* HEREDITARY HYALOIDEO-RETINAL DEGENERATION (WAGNER) IN A DANISH
FAMILY. ACTA OPHTHAL. 44* 223-227, 1966.

        VAN BALEN, A. T. M. AND FALGER, E. L. F.* HEREDITARY HYALOIDEORETINAL DEGENERA-
TION AND PALATOSCHISIS. ARCH. OPHTHAL. 83* 152-162, 1970.

14340 HYDRONEPHROSIS

        CANNON (1954) DESCRIBED A CURIOUS FAMILY IN WHICH FIVE MALES IN THREE SUCCESSIVE

GENERATIONS HAD UNILATERAL HYDRONEPHROSIS. MACKAY (1945) OBSERVED CONGENITAL MEGALO-URETERS WITH HYDRONEPHROSIS IN 3 SIBS (BILATERAL IN 2). TWO OTHER SIBS WERE SAID TO HAVE DIED OF CONGENITAL SARCOMA OF THE KIDNEY. THE PATERNAL GRANDFATHER DIED OF PYONEPHROSIS. THE FATHER DIED OF CEREBRAL HEMORRHAGE AT 56. JEWELL AND BUCHERT (1962) OBSERVED FOUR CASES IN THREE GENERATIONS. AARON AND ROBBINS (1948) FOUND HYDRONEPHROSIS WITHOUT HYDROURETERS AND ABERRANT RENAL VESSELS POSSIBLY RESPONSIBLE FOR OBSTRUCTION AT THE URETERO-PELVIC JUNCTION IN SIBS. SIMPSON AND GERMAN (1970) DESCRIBED SEVEN FAMILIES WITH MULTIPLE CASES OF URINARY TRAIT ANOMALIES, MOST OF THEM A FORM OF OBSTRUCTIVE UROPATHY AND REVIEWED THE LITERATURE ON CASES IN SIBS, TWINS AND OTHER RELATIVES.

AARON, G. AND ROBBINS, M. A.* HYDRONEPHROSIS DUE TO ABERRANT VESSELS* REMARKABLE FAMILIAL INCIDENCE WITH REPORT OF CASES. J. UROL. 60* 702-705, 1948.

CANNON, J. F.* HEREDITARY UNILATERAL HYDRONEPHROSIS. ANN. INTERN. MED. 41* 1054-1060, 1954.

JEWELL, J. H. AND BUCHERT, W. I.* UNILATERAL HEREDITARY HYDRONEPHROSIS* A REPORT OF FOUR CASES IN THREE CONSECUTIVE GENERATIONS. J. UROL. 88* 129-136, 1962.

MACKAY, H.* CONGENITAL BILATERAL MEGALO-URETERS WITH HYDRONEPHROSIS. A REMARKABLE FAMILY HISTORY. PROC. ROY. SOC. MED. 38* 567-568, 1945.

SIMPSON, J. L. AND GERMAN, J.* FAMILIAL URINARY TRACT ANOMALIES. (LETTER) J.A.M.A. 212* 2264 ONLY, 1970.

*14350 HYPERBILIRUBINEMIA I (GILBERT'S DISEASE)

IN A SERIES OF 58 PATIENTS, FOULK AND COLLEAGUES (1959) FOUND A FAMILY HISTORY OF JAUNDICE IN 8 AND IN 5 OF THESE JAUNDICE HAD BEEN PRESENT IN SUCCESSIVE GENERATIONS. BILLING, WILLIAMS AND RICHARDS (1964) PRESENTED INDIRECT EVIDENCE OF A DEFECT OF UPTAKE OF BILIRUBIN INTO THE LIVER CELL. THIS DISORDER IS DIFFICULT TO DISTINGUISH FROM PROLONGED POST-HEPATITIC HYPERBILIRUBINEMIA. THE CHARACTERISTICS ARE NORMAL LIVER FUNCTION TESTS OF THE USUAL TYPE, NORMAL LIVER HISTOLOGY, NO EVIDENCE OF HEMOLYSIS AND DELAYED CLEARANCE OF BILIRUBIN FROM THE BLOOD (NIXON AND MONAHAN, 1967). POWELL ET AL. (1967) OBSERVED AFFECTED PERSONS IN SUCCESSIVE GENERATIONS. BLACK AND BILLING (1969) FOUND HEPATIC BILIRUBIN UDP-TRANSFERASE TO BE ABOUT 25 PERCENT OF NORMAL IN 11 PATIENTS WITH GILBERT'S SYNDROME.

BERK, P. D., BLOOMER, J. R., HOWE, R. B. AND BERLIN, N. I.* CONSTITUTIONAL HEPATIC DYSFUNCTION (GILBERT'S SYNDROME). A NEW DEFINITION BASED ON KINETIC STUDIES WITH UNCONJUGATED RADIOBILIRUBIN. AM. J. MED. 49* 296-305, 1970.

BILLING, B. H., WILLIAMS, R. AND RICHARDS, T. G.* DEFECTS IN HEPATIC TRANSPORT OF BILIRUBIN IN CONGENITAL HYPERBILIRUBINAEMIA* AN ANALYSIS OF PLASMA BILIRUBIN DISAPPEARANCE CURVES. CLIN. SCI. 27* 245-257, 1964.

BLACK, M. AND BILLING, B. H.* HEPATIC BILIRUBIN UDP-GLUCORONYL TRANSFERASE ACTIVITY IN LIVER DISEASE AND GILBERT'S SYNDROME. NEW ENG. J. MED. 280* 1266-1271, 1969.

BLACK, M. AND SHERLOCK, S.* TREATMENT OF GILBERT'S SYNDROME WITH PHENOBARBITONE. LANCET 1* 1359-1361, 1970.

FOULK, W. T., BUTT, H. R., OWEN, C. A., JR. WHITCOMB, F. F., JR. AND MASON, H. L.* CONSTITUTIONAL HEPATIC DYSFUNCTION (GILBERT'S DISEASE)* ITS NATURAL HISTORY AND RELATED SYNDROMES. MEDICINE 38* 25-46, 1959.

NIXON, J. C. AND MONAHAN, G. J.* GILBERT'S DISEASE AND THE BILIRUBIN TOLERANCE TEST. CANAD. MED. ASS. J. 96* 370-373, 1967.

POWELL, L. W., HEMINGWAY, E., BILLING, B. H. AND SHERLOCK, S.* IDIOPATHIC UNCONJUGATED HYPERBILIRUBINEMIA (GILBERT'S SYNDROME). A STUDY OF 42 FAMILIES. NEW ENG. J. MED. 277* 1108-1112, 1967.

SCHMID, R.* HYPERBILIRUBINEMIA. IN STANBURY, J. B., WYNGAARDEN, J. B. AND FREDRICKSON, D. S. (EDS.)* THE METABOLIC BASIS OF INHERITED DISEASE. NEW YORK* MCGRAW-HILL, 1966 (2ND ED.). PP. 871-902.

14370 HYPERBILIRUBINEMIA III (ROTOR DISEASE)

LIKE THE DUBIN-JOHNSON SYNDROME THIS IS A FORM OF CONJUGATED HYPERBILIRUBINEMIA. THE TWO DISORDERS ARE NOT CLEARLY DISTINGUISHED. THREE SIBS FROM A FIRST COUSIN MARRIAGE WERE AFFECTED IN THE FAMILY REPORTED BY PEREIRA LIMA, UTZ AND ROISENBERG (1966), SUGGESTING RECESSIVE INHERITANCE. DOLLINGER ET AL. (1967) OBSERVED FATHER AND 3 OF 5 CHILDREN WITH WHAT THEY CONSIDERED TO BE THE ROTOR SYNDROME. HOWEVER, OCCULT HEMOLYSIS WAS ALSO PRESENT.

DOLLINGER, M. R., BRANDBORG, L. L., SARTOR, V. E. AND BERNSTEIN, J. M.* CHRONIC FAMILIAL HYPERBILIRUBINEMIA. HEPATIC DEFECTS ASSOCIATED WITH OCCULT HEMOLYSIS. GASTROENTEROLOGY 52* 875-881, 1967.

PEREIRA LIMA, J. E., UTZ, E. AND ROISENBERG, I.* HEREDITARY NONHEMOLYTIC CONJUGATED HYPERBILIRUBINEMIA WITHOUT ABNORMAL LIVER CELL PIGMENTATION. A FAMILY STUDY. AM. J. MED. 40* 628-633, 1966.

SCHIFF, L., BILLING, B. H. AND OIKAWA, Y.* FAMILIAL NONHEMOLYTIC JAUNDICE WITH CONJUGATED BILIRUBIN IN THE SERUM* A CASE STUDY. NEW ENG. J. MED. 260* 1315-1318, 1959.

*14380 HYPERBILIRUBINEMIA, ARIAS TYPE

ARIAS (1962) DEMONSTRATED GLUCURONYL TRANSFERASE DEFICIENCY IN EIGHT PATIENTS WITH CHRONIC NONHEMOLYTIC JAUNDICE AND SERUM UNCONJUGATED BILIRUBIN LEVELS OF 6.2 TO 18.8 MG. PERCENT. ARIAS ET AL. (1969) CONCLUDED THAT THIS IS A DISORDER DISTINCT FROM CRIGLER-NAJJAR SYNDROME, WHICH ALSO HAS DEFICIENCY OF HEPATIC GLUCURONYL TRANSFERASE ACTIVITY. IN THE CRIGLER-NAJJAR TYPE HYPERBILIRUBINEMIA IS SEVERE AND FREQUENTLY ACCOMPANIED BY KERNICTERUS. THE BILE IS ALMOST COLORLESS AND CONTAINS TRACES OF UNCONJUGATED BILIRUBIN ONLY. TRANSMISSION IS AUTOSOMAL RECESSIVE AND PHENOBARBITAL DOES NOT INFLUENCE THE HYPERBILIRUBINEMIA. IN THE ARIAS TYPE BILIRUBINEMIA IS LESS SEVERE WITHOUT KERNICTERUS. THE BILE IS PIGMENTED AND CONTAINS BILIRUBIN GLUCURONIDE. THE TRANSMISSION IS AUTOSOMAL DOMINANT. PHENOBARBITAL ADMINISTRATION CAUSES PROMPT DISAPPEARANCE OF JAUNDICE. SINCE PATIENTS WITH THE ARIAS TYPE HAVE A DISORDER ALMOST ONLY OF COSMETIC SIGNIFICANCE, LONG-TERM PHENOBARBITAL TREATMENT IS USEFUL. THE RESPONSE TO PHENOBARBITAL, WHICH MAY REPRESENT INDUCTION, AND THE DOMINANT INHERITANCE LEAD ME TO SUSPECT THAT THE DEFECT IN THE ARIAS TYPE IS IN A CONTROLLER GENE AND NOT IN THE STRUCTURAL GENE FOR GLUCURONYL TRANSFERASE. SLEISENGER ET AL. (1967) DESCRIBED AN IRISH KINDRED IN WHICH PERSONS WITH LIFE-LONG JAUNDICE OCCURRED IN 4 GENERATIONS, IN A DOMINANT PEDIGREE PATTERN WITH MALE-TO-MALE TRANSMISSION. HEPATIC GLUCURONYL TRANSFERASE ACTIVITY WAS LOW IN AFFECTED INDIVIDUALS, BY DIRECT OR INDIRECT TEST. THE CONDITION DIFFERS FROM THE CRIGLER-NAJJAR SYNDROME (WHICH HAS DEFICIENCY OF THE SAME ENZYME) IN MODE OF INHERITANCE, LACK OF BRAIN DAMAGE AND FAVORABLE PROGNOSIS. IT IS PROBABLY THE THE SAME CONDITION AS THAT REPORTED BY ARIAS (1962).

ARIAS, I. M.* CHRONIC UNCONJUGATED HYPERBILIRUBINEMIA WITHOUT OVERT SIGNS OF HEMOLYSIS IN ADOLESCENTS AND ADULTS. J. CLIN. INVEST. 41* 2233-2245, 1962.

ARIAS, I. M., GARTNER, L. M., COHEN, M., BEN-EZZER, J. AND LEVI, A. J.* CHRONIC NONHEMOLYTIC UNCONJUGATED HYPERBILIRUBINEMIA WITH GLUCURONYL TRANSFERASE DEFICIEN-CY* CLINICAL, BIOCHEMICAL, PHARMACOLOGIC AND GENETIC EVIDENCE FOR HETEROGENEITY. AM. J. MED. 47* 395-409, 1969.

SLEISENGER, M. H., KAHN, I., BARNIVILLE, H., RUBIN, W., BEN EZZER, J. AND ARIAS, I. M.* NONHEMOLYTIC UNCONJUGATED HYPERBILIRUBINEMIA WITH HEPATIC GLUCURONYL TRANSFERASE DEFICIENCY* A GENETIC STUDY IN FOUR GENERATIONS. TRANS. ASS. AM. PHYSICIANS 80* 259-266, 1967.

14390 HYPERCAROTINEMIA, FAMILIAL

SHARVILL (1970) DESCRIBED VERY HIGH LEVELS OF BLOOD CAROTINE IN A WOMAN, HER MOTHER, A SIB AND HER SON. LOW LEVELS OF VITAMIN A WERE FOUND AT TIMES. A DEFECT IN CONVERSION OF CAROTINE TO VITAMIN A WAS CONSIDERED ONE POSSIBILITY.

SHARVILL, D. E.* FAMILIAL HYPERCAROTINAEMIA AND HYPOVITAMINOSIS A. PROC. ROY. SOC. MED. 63* 605-606, 1970.

14400 HYPERHEPARINEMIA

CONGENITAL HEMORRHAGIC DIATHESIS DUE TO AN EXCESS OF A CLOTTING INHIBITOR HAS NOT BEEN FULLY ESTABLISHED. QUICK (1957) DIAGNOSED CONGENITAL HYPERHEPARINEMIA IN A WOMAN WITH ABNORMAL BLEEDING FROM AGE 3. HENI AND KRAUSS (1956) DESCRIBED A SIMILAR CONDITION IN A FATHER AND DAUGHTER. IN BOTH INSTANCES THE IN VITRO CLOTTING DEFECT WAS REPAIRED BY PROTAMINE SULPHATE AND BY TOLUIDINE BLUE, AND QUICK ACHIEVED CORRECTION OF THE DEFECT IN VIVO AS WELL.

HENI, F. AND KRAUSS, I.* ANGEBORENE FAMILIARE GERINNUNGSSTORUNG DURCH HE-PARINARTIGEN HEMMKORPER. KLIN. WSCHR. 34* 747-749, 1956.

QUICK, A. J.* HEMORRHAGIC DISEASES. PHILADELPHIA* LEA AND FEBIGER, 1957.

14410 HYPERHIDROSIS, GUSTATORY

MAILANDER (1967) DESCRIBED EXCESSIVE SWEATING OF THE FACE WITH EATING IN FIVE PERSONS OF THREE GENERATIONS. THERE WAS NO MALE-TO-MALE TRANSMISSION AND ONE INSTANCE OF 'SKIPPED GENERATION' WAS KNOWN.

MAILANDER, J. C.* HEREDITARY GUSTATORY SWEATING. J.A.M.A. 201* 203-204, 1967.

*14420 HYPERKERATOSIS, LOCALIZED EPIDERMOLYTIC

USUALLY THIS CONDITION HAS NOT BEEN DISTINGUISHED FROM KERATOSIS PALMARIS ET PLANTARIS. THE DISTINGUISHING FEATURE IS THE PRESENCE OF HISTOLOGIC AND KINETIC FINDINGS OF EPIDERMOLYSIS, DESPITE THE SAME CLINICAL PICTURE. KLAUS ET AL. (1970)

KLAUS, S., WEINSTEIN, G. D. AND FROST, P.* LOCALIZED EPIDERMOLYTIC HYPERKERATO-
SIS.   A FORM OF KERATODERMA OF THE PALMS AND SOLES. ARCH. DERM. 101* 272-275,
1970.

14430 HYPERLIPOPROTEINEMIA (TYPE II) AND DEAFNESS

RAPHAEL AND HYDE (1970) DESCRIBED THE ASSOCIATION OF CONGENITAL DEAFNESS WITH TYPE
II HYPERLIPOPROTEINEMIA IN MOTHER AND DAUGHTER.

RAPHAEL, S. S. AND HYDE, T. A.* DEAF-MUTISM AND TYPE-II HYPERLIPOPROTEINAEMIA.
(LETTER) LANCET 1* 892 ONLY, 1970.

*14440 HYPERLIPOPROTEINEMIA II (HYPERBETALIPOPROTEINEMIA, HYPER-LOW-DENSITY-LIPOPRO-
TEINEMIA, ESSENTIAL FAMILIAL HYPERCHOLESTEROLEMIA, FAMILIAL HYPERCHOLESTEROLEMIC
XANTHOMATOSIS, XANTHOMA TUBEROSUM MULTIPLEX, FAMILIAL XANTHOMA)

ON A NORMAL DIET, THE BLOOD SHOWS AN INCREASE IN BETA-LIPOPROTEINS. REFLECTING
THE COMPOSITION OF THESE LIPOPROTEINS, CHOLESTEROL IS INCREASED WHEREAS PHOSPHOLI-
PIDS AND TRIGLYCERIDES REMAIN WITHIN NORMAL LIMITS. THIS IS THE MOST FREQUENT
TYPE OF HYPERLIPIDEMIA. FEATURES ARE XANTHOMA TUBEROSUM AND TENDINOSUM, CORNEAL
ARCUS, AND ATHEROMATOSIS.   THIS IS PROBABLY DOMINANT WITH A WIDE RANGE OF
VARIABILITY OF SEVERITY AS IS COMMONPLACE WITH DOMINANTS.   TERMINOLOGY AND
NOSOLOGY OF THE HYPERLIPOPROTEINEMIAS ARE CONFUSED LARGELY BECAUSE UNDERSTANDING
IS IMPERFECT.   FREDRICKSON AND LEES (1966) MAKE PARTICULAR USE OF PAPER ELECTRO-
PHORESIS IN IDENTIFICATION OF LIPOPROTEIN FACTORS IN THE PLASMA AND CHANGES
THEREIN.   IN A FRENCH CANADIAN KINDRED, HOULD ET AL. (1969) OBSERVED HYPERCHOLES-
TEROLEMIA WITH SEVERE XANTHOMATOSIS IN THREE SIBS AND ONE OF THEIR SECOND COUSINS.
BOTH PARENTS WERE APPARENTLY HETEROZYGOTES. BOTH HAD HYPERCHOLESTEROLEMIA AND
MILD XANTHOMATA, AS DID SOME RELATIVES OF EACH OF THEM. THUS HYPERBETALIPOPRO-
TEINEMIA MIGHT BE LISTED IN EITHER THE DOMINANT OR THE RECESSIVE CATALOG. THIS
PHENOTYPE MAY BE GENETICALLY HETEROGENEOUS.

EPSTEIN, F. H., BLOCK, W. D., HAND, E. A. AND FRANCIS, T., JR.* FAMILIAL
HYPERCHOLESTEROLEMIA, XANTHOMATOSIS AND CORONARY HEART DISEASE. AM. J. MED. 26*
39-53, 1959.

FREDRICKSON, D. S. AND LEES, R. S.* FAMILIAL HYPERLIPOPROTEINEMIA.   IN
STANBURY, J. B., WYNGAARDEN, J. B. AND FREDRICKSON, D. S. (EDS.)* THE METABOLIC
BASIS OF INHERITED DISEASES. NEW YORK* MCGRAW-HILL, 1966 (2ND ED.).   PP. 429-485.

FREDRICKSON, D. S.* PLASMA LIPOPROTEINS* MICELLAR MODELS AND MUTANTS. TRANS.
ASS. AM. PHYS. 82* 68-86, 1969.

FREDRICKSON, D. S., LEVY, R. I. AND LEES, R. S.* FAT TRANSPORT IN LIPOPROTEINS
- AN INTEGRATED APPROACH TO MECHANISMS AND DISORDERS. NEW ENG. J. MED. 276* 215-
225, 1967.

HARLAN, W. R., JR., GRAHAM, J. B. AND ESTES, E. H.* FAMILIAL HYPERCHOLESTEROLE-
MIA* A GENETIC AND METABOLIC STUDY. MEDICINE 45* 77-110, 1966.

HOULD, F., LECLERC, R. AND MARCOUX, J.* ESSENTIAL FAMILIAL HYPERCHOLESTEROLEMIA
WITH XANTHOMATOSIS. PEDIATRICS 43* 455-459, 1969.

KHACHADURIAN, A. K.* THE INHERITANCE OF ESSENTIAL FAMILIAL HYPERCHOLESTEROLE-
MIA. AM. J. MED. 37* 402-407, 1964.

WHEELER, E. O.* THE GENETIC ASPECTS OF ATHEROSCLEROSIS. AM. J. MED. 23* 653-
660, 1957.

14450 HYPERLIPOPROTEINEMIA III (FAMILIAL HYPERBETA AND PREBETALIPOPROTEINEMIA,
FAMILIAL HYPERCHOLESTEROLEMIA WITH HYPERLIPEMIA, HYPERLIPEMIA WITH FAMILIAL
HYPERCHOLESTEROLEMIC XANTHOMATOSIS, CARBOHYDRATE-INDUCED HYPERLIPEMIA)

ON A NORMAL DIET, THE PATIENT SHOWS INCREASED AMOUNTS OF BOTH BETA- AND PRE-BETA-
LIPOPROTEINS. PLASMA CHOLESTEROL AND PHOSPHOLIPIDS ARE ELEVATED AND GLYCERIDES
MAY BE ELEVATED. CARBOHYDRATE INDUCES OR EXACERBATES THE HYPERLIPIDEMIA. OFTEN
TUBEROUS AND PLANAR AND SOMETIMES TENDON XANTHOMAS OCCUR AS WELL AS PRECOCIOUS
ATHEROSCLEROSIS AND ABNORMAL GLUCOSE TOLERANCE. THE RELATION BETWEEN TYPES II
(THE PURE BETA-LIPOPROTEIN DISORDER) AND III IS UNCERTAIN. FURTHERMORE, MATTHEWS
(1968) CONCLUDED THAT TYPES III AND IV ARE CONSEQUENCES OF THE SAME MUTANT
GENE(S).

FREDRICKSON, D. S., LEVY, R. I. AND LEES, R. S.* FAT TRANSPORT IN LIPOPROTEINS
- AN INTEGRATED APPROACH TO MECHANISMS AND DISORDERS. NEW ENG. J. MED. 276* 273-
281, 1967.

MATTHEWS, R. J.* TYPE III AND IV FAMILIAL HYPERLIPOPROTEINEMIA. EVIDENCE THAT
THESE TWO SYNDROMES ARE DIFFERENT PHENOTYPIC EXPRESSIONS OF THE SAME MUTANT
GENE(S). AM. J. MED. 44* 188-199, 1968.

D
O
M
I
N
A
N
T

ON A REGULAR DIET THE PATIENT DEMONSTRATES INCREASED PRE-BETA-LIPOPROTEIN. PLASMA
GLYCERIDES ARE PERSISTENTLY INCREASED. PLASMA CHOLESTROL AND PHOSPHOLIPIDS ARE
USUALLY WITHIN NORMAL LIMITS. PRECOCIOUS SCLEROSIS, ABNORMAL GLUCOSE TOLERANCE
AND ATHERO ERUPTIVE XANTHOMA MAY OCCUR. THE DISORDER IS PROBABLY A DOMINANT BUT
EXPERIENCE IS THUS FAR LIMITED. INDEED, FREDRICKSON AND LEES (1966) HAVE ONLY
RECENTLY SUGGESTED THIS CATEGORY. IN AN OLD AMERICAN FAMILY LIVING IN NEW
ENGLAND, SCHREIBMAN ET AL. (1969) DESCRIBED HYPERPRE-BETA-LIPOPROTEINEMIA BEHAVING
AS AN AUTOSOMAL DOMINANT WITH REDUCED PENETRANCE. ALTHOUGH TRIGLYCERIDE LEVELS AS
HIGH AS 2000 MG. PER 100 ML. WERE OBSERVED IN SOME CHILDREN OF THIS FAMILY,
PRECOCIOUS ATHEROSCLEROSIS WAS NOT OBSERVED. THE ABSENCE OF OBESITY AND GLUCOSE
INTOLERANCE MAY ACCOUNT FOR THE FAVORABLE PROGNOSIS. HETEROGENEITY OF TYPE IV
HYPERLIPOPROTEINEMIA IS SUGGESTED BY THESE OBSERVATIONS.

BLANKENHORN, D. H., CHIN, H. P. AND LAU, F. Y. K.* ISCHEMIC HEART DISEASE IN
YOUNG ADULTS. ANN. INTERN. MED. 69* 21-34, 1968.

FREDRICKSON, D. S. AND LEES, R. S.* FAMILIAL HYPERLIPOPROTEINEMIA. IN
STANBURY, J. B., WYNGAARDEN, J. B. AND FREDRICKSON, D. S. (EDS.)* THE METABOLIC
BASIS OF INHERITED DISEASES. NEW YORK* MCGRAW-HILL, 1966 (2ND ED.). PP. 429-485.

SCHREIBMAN, P. H., WILSON, D. E. AND ARKY, R. A.* FAMILIAL TYPE IV HYPERLIPO-
PROTEINEMIA. NEW ENG. J. MED. 281* 981-985, 1969.

14470 HYPERNEPHROMA (ADENOCARCINOMA OF KIDNEY)

RUSCHE (1953) OBSERVED HYPERNEPHROMA IN TWO BROTHERS. BOTH HAD DISTANT METASTASIS
AS THE FIRST MANIFESTATION AND BOTH WERE IN THEIR EARLY 30'S AT THE TIME OF
DIAGNOSIS. BRINTON (1960) DESCRIBED A FAMILY IN WHICH TWO BROTHERS AND A SISTER
HAD HYPERNEPHROMA. THE FATHER HAD DIED OF KIDNEY TUMOR AND THE MOTHER OF CANCER,
SITE UNSTATED. ONE OF THE PATIENTS HAD POLYCYTHEMIA, A KNOWN ACCOMPANIMENT OF
HYPERNEPHROMA ON OCCASION. IT SHOULD BE NOTED THAT HYPERNEPHROMA AND CEREBELLAR
HEMANGIOBLASTOMA WHICH HISTOLOGICALLY RESEMBLES HYPERNEPHROMA ARE FEATURES OF VON
HIPPEL-LINDAU'S DISEASE. POLYCYTHEMA ALSO OCCURS WITH CEREBELLAR HEMANGIOBLAS-
TOMA.

BRINTON, L. F.* HYPERNEPHROMA - FAMILIAL OCCURRENCE IN ONE FAMILY. J.A.M.A.
173* 888-890, 1960.

RUSCHE, C.* SILENT ADENOCARCINOMA OF THE KIDNEYS WITH SOLITARY METASTASES
OCCURRING IN BROTHERS. J. UROL. 70* 146-151, 1953.

14480 HYPEROSTOSIS FRONTALIS INTERNA (MORGAGNI-STEWART-MOREL SYNDROME)

IN ADDITION TO THICKENING OF THE INNER TABLE OF THE FRONTAL BONE, OBESITY AND
HYPERTRICHOSIS MAY BE PRESENT. THIS CONDITION AFFECTS MAINLY FEMALES. KNIES AND
LE FEVER (1941) REPORTED MOTHER AND THREE CHILDREN AFFECTED. THUS, THE DISORDER
MAY BE DOMINANT, BUT WHETHER AUTOSOMAL OR X-LINKED IS NOT KNOWN. LIEBERMAN (1967)
HAS OBSERVED 5 AFFECTED FEMALES IN THREE GENERATIONS.

KNIES, P. T. AND LE FEVER, H. E.* METABOLIC CRANIOPATHY* HYPEROSTOSIS FRONTALIS
INTERNA. ANN. INTERN MED. 14* 1858-1892, 1941.

LIEBERMAN, B.* OAKLAND, CALIF.* PERSONAL COMMUNICATION, 1967.

MOORE, S.* HYPEROSTOSIS CRANII (STEWART-MOREL SYNDROME, METABOLIC CRANIOPATHY,
MORGAGNI'S SYNDROME, STEWART-MOREL-MOORE SYNDROME (RITVO), LE SYNDROME DE
MORGAGNI-MOREL). SPRINGFIELD, ILL.* CHARLES C THOMAS, 1955.

14490 HYPEROXALURIA

OXALOSIS SEEMS TO BE A RECESSIVE IN MOST INSTANCES. A FEW OBSERVATIONS SUGGEST
DOMINANT INHERITANCE. SHEPARD ET AL. (1960) REPORTED A FAMILY WITH HYPEROXALURIA
IN TWO AND PERHAPS THREE SUCCESSIVE GENERATIONS. OXALATE URINARY STONES OCCUR
COMMONLY THROUGHOUT THE WORLD. MOST PATIENTS WITH OXALATE STONES HAVE NORMAL
URINARY OXALATE EXCRETION. GRAM (1932) DESCRIBED AN EXTENSIVE PEDIGREE OF OXALATE
UROLITHIASIS IN FIVE GENERATIONS. URINARY OXALATE CONCENTRATIONS WERE NOT
REPORTED. SEVERAL PRESUMED CARRIER FEMALES DID NOT HAVE CALCULI. FIFTEEN MALES
(AND NO FEMALES) IN 10 SIBSHIPS WERE AFFECTED. THE SYSTEMATIC GENETIC STUDY OF
CALCIUM OXALATE RENAL CALCULI DONE BY RESNICK ET AL. (1968) LEAD TO THE CONCLUSION
THAT ALTHOUGH FAMILIAL AGGREGATION IS UNDOUBTED, MONOGENIC INHERITANCE CAN BE
EXCLUDED AND THE FINDINGS ARE COMPATIBLE WITH THE HYPOTHESIS THAT THE TENDENCY TO
FORM CALCIUM OXALATE RENAL STONES IS REGULATED BY A POLYGENIC SYSTEM, WITH LESS
RISK FOR FEMALES THAN MALES.

GRAM, H. C.* THE HEREDITY OF OXALIC URINARY CALCULI. ACTA MED. SCAND. 78* 268-
281, 1932.

RESNICK, M., PRIDGEN, D. B. AND GOODMAN, H. O.* GENETIC PREDISPOSITION TO
CALCIUM OXALATE RENAL CALCULI. NEW ENG. J. MED. 278* 1313-1318, 1968.

GENETIC STUDIES IN A FAMILY. PEDIATRICS 25* 869-871, 1960.

14500 HYPERPARATHYROIDISM

FAMILIAL HYPERPARATHYROIDISM IS USUALLY PART OF ENDOCRINE ADENOMATOSIS (Q.V.). PRIMARY CHIEF-CELL HYPERPLASIA IS THE USUAL HISTOLOGIC CHANGE IN THE HYPERPARA-THYROIDISM OF THAT CONDITION AND ALSO IN THE TYPE WHICH OCCURS IN FAMILIES WITHOUT EVIDENCE OF OTHER ENDOCRINE DISEASE. THIS SUGGESTS THAT DISCOVERY OF THIS HISTOLOGIC CHANGE SHOULD PROMPT STUDY FOR OTHER ENDOCRINE DISEASE IN THE PATIENT AND FOR OTHER CASES IN THE FAMILY. CASES OF APPARENTLY ISOLATED FAMILIAL HYPERPARATHYROIDISM HAVE BEEN REPORTED BY CAMERON ET AL. (1966), CUTLER ET AL. (1964), AND PETERS ET AL. (1966), AMONG OTHERS. THE PEDIGREES HAVE USUALLY BEEN CONSISTENT WITH AUTOSOMAL DOMINANT INHERITANCE. FAMILIES WITH MULTIPLE CASES OF PARATHYROID ADENOMA HAVE BEEN DESCRIBED BY CASSIDY AND ANDERSON (1960), JACKSON, TALBERT AND TAYLOR (1960) AND OTHERS. SUCH FAMILIES MAY HAVE MULTIPLE ENDOCRINE ADENOMATOSIS, ALTHOUGH THE POSSIBILITY OF A SEPARATE AND DISTINCT DOMINANTLY INHERITED ENTITY CANNOT BE EXCLUDED (CUTLER, REISS AND ACKERMAN, 1964). CUTLER ET AL. (1964) AMONG OTHERS HAVE EMPHASIZED THAT CHIEF CELL HYPERPLASIA RATHER THAN ADENOMA MAY BE THE CHARACTERISTIC HISTOLOGIC CHANGE IN THE FAMILIAL CASES OF HYPERPARATHYROIDISM. THE TWO TYPES OF CHANGES ARE OFTEN DISTINGUISHED WITH DIFFICULTY. JACKSON AND BOONSTRA (1967) STUDIED 8 FAMILIES EACH WITH MULTIPLE CASES (55 IN ALL) OF PARATHYROID ADENOMA. IN AT LEAST THREE KINDREDS SOME INDIVIDUALS HAD OTHER ENDOCRINE ADENOMATA.

CAMERON, K. M., OGG, C. S. AND HARRISON, A. R.* FAMILIAL HYPERPARATHYROIDISM. LANCET 2* 1006-1007, 1966.

CASSIDY, C. E. AND ANDERSON, A. S.* A FAMILIAL OCCURRENCE OF HYPERPARATHYROI-DISM CAUSED BY MULTIPLE PARATHYROID ADENOMAS. METABOLISM 9* 1152-1158, 1960.

CUTLER, R. E., REISS, E. AND ACKERMAN, L. V.* FAMILIAL HYPERPARATHYROIDISM* A KINDRED INVOLVING ELEVEN CASES, WITH A DISCUSSION OF PRIMARY CHIEF-CELL HYPERPLA-SIA. NEW ENG. J. MED. 270* 859-865, 1964.

GRABER, A. L. AND JACOBS, K.* FAMILIAL HYPERPARATHYROIDISM. MEDICAL AND SURGICAL CONSIDERATIONS. J.A.M.A. 204* 542-544, 1968.

JACKSON, C. E. AND BOONSTRA, C. E.* THE RELATIONSHIP OF HEREDITARY HYPERPARA-THYROIDISM TO ENDOCRINE ADENOMATOSIS. AM. J. MED. 43* 727-734, 1967.

JACKSON, C. E., TALBERT, P. C. AND TAYLOR, H. D.* HEREDITARY HYPERPARATHYROI-DISM. J. INDIANA MED. ASS. 53* 1313-1316, 1960.

PETERS, N., CHALMERS, T. M., RACK, J. H., TRUSCOTT, B. M., AND ADAMS, P. H.* FAMILIAL HYPERPARATHYROIDISM. POSTGRAD. MED. J. 42* 228-233, 1966.

*14510 HYPERPIGMENTATION OF EYELIDS

HUNZIKER (1962) DESCRIBED A FAMILY IN WHICH 10 PERSONS IN THREE GENERATIONS (IN AN AUTOSOMAL DOMINANT PATTERN) SHOWED HYPERPIGMENTATION OF THE EYELIDS. PETERS (1918) TRACED THIS TRAIT THROUGH FIVE GENERATIONS. GOODMAN AND BELCHER (1969) DESCRIBED TWO KINDREDS WITH MANY AFFECTED MEMBERS.

GOODMAN, R. M. AND BELCHER, R. W.* PERIORBITAL HYPERPIGMENTATION. AN OVER-LOOKED GENETIC DISORDER OF PIGMENTATION. ARCH. DERM. 100* 169-174, 1969.

HUNZIKER, N.* A PROPOS DE L'HYPERPIGMENTATION FAMILIALE DES PAUPIERES. J. GENET. HUM. 11* 16-21, 1962.

PETERS, R.* AUFFALLENDE DUNKELFARBUNG DER UNTEREN LIDER ALS ERHEBLICHE ANOMALIE. CENTRBL. PRAKT. AUGENHEILK. 42* 8-11, 1918.

14520 HYPERPIGMENTATION OF FULDAUER AND KUIJPERS

FULDAUER AND KUIJPERS (1964) DESCRIBED A PIGMENTARY ANOMALY IN MANY MEMBERS OF A DUTCH FAMILY. ALTHOUGH THE PAPER WAS ENTITLED 'INCONTINENTIA PIGMENTI,' THE DISTRIBUTION OF THE HYPERPIGMENTATION WAS QUITE DIFFERENT, BEING LOCATED ON THE WRISTS, HANDS, AND NECK AND LESS CONSISTENTLY ON THE AXILLARY FOLDS, DORSA OF THE FEET AND LINES OF THE HANDS. FUTHERMORE INCONTINENTIA PIGMENTI IS PROBABLY AN X-LINKED DOMINANT LETHAL IN MALES. MANY MALES WERE AFFECTED IN THIS FAMILY.

FULDAUER, M. L. AND KUIJPERS, P. B.* AN INHERITED PIGMENTARY ANOMALY (INCON-TINENTIA PIGMENTI.Q). NEDERL. T. GENEESK. 108* 1613-1623, 1964.

14530 HYPER-REFLEXIA, HEREDITARY

SUHREN ET AL. (1966) DESCRIBED A FAMILY IN WHICH 25 PERSONS IN 5 GENERATIONS WITH NUMEROUS INSTANCES OF MALE-TO-MALE TRANSMISSION WERE AFFLICTED WITH TRANSIENT CONGENITAL HYPERTONIA AND HYPOKINESIA IN THE WAKING STATE, LATER IN LIFE GREATLY EXAGGERATED STARTLE REACTION SOMETIMES ASSOCIATED WITH FALLING, MARKEDLY HYPERAC-TIVE BRAIN-STEM REFLEXES (E.G., HEAD RETRACTION, PALMO-MENTAL AND SNOUT REFLEXES)

AND A MOMENTARY GENERALIZED JERKING ON FALLING ASLEEP. THE FINDINGS WERE INTERPRETED AS INDICATING UNINHIBITED NOCICEPTIVE REFLEX PATTERN AS A RESULT OF A DEFECT IN MATURATION. IMPROVEMENT ACCOMPAINED BARBITURATE MEDICATION. THE POSSIBLE RELATIONSHIP TO THE 'JUMPING FRENCHMAN OF MAINE' (Q.V.) WAS MENTIONED. SEE KOK'S DISEASE. (I QUESTION THE ETYMOLOGIC AND ORTHOGRAPHIC PROPRIETY OF 'HYPEREFLEXIA.')

SUHREN, O., BRUYN, G. W. AND TUYNMAN, J. A.* HYPEREFLEXIA. A HEREDITARY STARTLE SYNDROME. J. NEUROL. SCI. 3* 577-605, 1966.

*14540 HYPERTELORISM (GREIG'S SYNDROME)

ALTHOUGH HYPERTELORISM MEANS AN EXCESSIVE DISTANCE BETWEEN ANY PAIRED ORGANS (E.G., THE NIPPLES), THE USE OF THE WORD HAS COME TO BE CONFINED TO OCULAR HYPERTELORISM. PSEUDOHYPERTELORISM OCCURS IN WAARDENBURG'S SYNDROME (Q.V.) IN WHICH LATERAL DISPLACEMENT OF THE INNER CANTHUS GIVES A MISTAKEN IMPRESSION OF EXCESSIVE DISTANCE BETWEEN THE EYES. BOJLEN AND BREMS (1938) TRACED THE ANOMALY THROUGH FIVE GENERATIONS. FRIEDE (1954) DESCRIBED MOTHER AND DAUGHTER. HYPERTE-LORISM IS THOUGHT TO BE THE CONSEQUENCE OF ARREST IN DEVELOPMENT OF THE GREATER WINGS OF THE SPHENOID, MAKING THEM SMALLER THAN THE LESSER WINGS AND THUS FIXING THE ORBITS IN THE WIDELY SEPARATED FETAL POSITION.

ABERNETHY, D. A.* HYPERTELORISM IN SEVERAL GENERATIONS. ARCH. DIS. CHILD. 2* 361-365, 1927.

BOJLEN, K. AND BREMS, T.* HYPERTELORISM (GREIG). ACTA PATH. MICROBIOL. SCAND. 15* 217-258, 1938.

FRIEDE, R.* UBER PHYSIOLOGISCHE EURYOPIE UND PATHOLOGISCHEN HYPERTELORISMUS OCULARIS. GRAEFE ARCH. OPHTHAL. 155* 359-385, 1954.

14550 HYPERTENSION, ESSENTIAL

THE PICKERING SCHOOL HOLDS THAT BLOOD PRESSURE HAS A CONTINUOUS DISTRIBUTION, THAT MULTIPLE GENES AND MULTIPLE ENVIRONMENTAL FACTORS DETERMINE THE LEVEL OF ONE'S BLOOD PRESSURE JUST AS THE DETERMINATION OF STATURE AND INTELLIGENCE IS MULTIFAC-TORIAL, AND THAT 'ESSENTIAL HYPERTENSION' IS MERELY THE UPPER END OF THE DISTRIBU-TION. IN THIS VIEW THE PERSON WITH ESSENTIAL HYPERTENSION IS ONE WHO HAPPENS TO INHERIT AN AGGREGATE OF GENES DETERMINING HYPERTENSION (AND ALSO IS EXPOSED TO EXOGENOUS FACTORS WHICH FAVOR HYPERTENSION). THE PLATT SCHOOL TAKES THE VIEW THAT ESSENTIAL HYPERTENSION IS A SIMPLE MENDELIAN DOMINANT TRAIT. SEE MCKUSICK (1960) FOR REVIEW. I FIND THE PICKERING POINT OF VIEW MORE CONSISTENT WITH THE OBSERVA-TIONS. MCDONOUGH AND COLLEAGUES (1964) DEFENDED THE MONOGENIC IDEA.

ACHESON, R. M. AND FOWLER, G. B.* ON THE INHERITANCE OF STATURE AND BLOOD PRESSURE. J. CHRONIC DIS. 20* 731-746, 1967.

MCDONOUGH, J. R., GARRISON, G. E. AND HAMES, C. G.* BLOOD PRESSURE AND HYPERTENSIVE DISEASE AMONG NEGROES AND WHITES. A STUDY IN EVANS COUNTY, GEORGIA. ANN. INTERN. MED. 61* 208-228, 1964.

MCKUSICK, V. A.* GENETICS AND THE NATURE OF ESSENTIAL HYPERTENSION. (EDI-TORIAL) CIRCULATION 22* 857-863, 1960.

*14560 HYPERTHERMIA OF ANESTHESIA

DENBOROUGH ET AL. (1962) OBSERVED A FAMILY IN WHICH 11 OF 38 PERSONS WHO HAD GENERAL ANESTHESIA DIED. THE 11 INCLUDED FATHER-DAUGHTER AND MOTHER-SON AND DAUGHTER COMBINATIONS. EXPLOSIVE HYPERTHERMIA SEEMS TO OCCUR IN THESE CASES. WILSON ET AL. (1967) SUGGESTED THAT 'UNCOUPLING OF OXIDATION PHOSPHORYLATION' IS THE DEFECT. THUS, THIS CONDITION MAY BE A PHARMACOGENETIC DISORDER. HYPERTONICI-TY OF VOLUNTARY MUSCLES IS OFTEN ASSOCIATED WITH MALIGNANT HYPERPYREXIA. ELEVATION OF CREATINE PHOSPHOKINASE, PHOSPHATE AND POTASSIUM IN THE BLOOD INDICATED SEVERE MUSCLE DAMAGE (DENBOROUGH ET AL. 1970). HIGH LEVELS OF CPK WERE FOUND IN A PATIENT WHO HAD SURVIVED MALIGNANT PYREXIA AND IN HIS FATHER, PATERNAL AUNT AND SISTER. TWO OF THE RELATIVES SHOWED MILD MYOPATHY AFFECTING MAINLY THE LEGS. KALOW (1970) POINTED OUT RIGIDITY AS A FEATURE OF THE SYNDROME AND RAISED THE POSSIBILITY OF TWO DISORDERS ONE WITH AND ONE WITHOUT RIGIDITY. MORTALITY IS HIGHER IN THE CASES WITH RIGIDITY. IN SOME CASES RIGIDITY MAY OCCUR IN THE ABSENCE OF FEVER. KALOW (1970) STATED THAT HIS MOST EXTENSIVELY INVOLVED KINDRED FITS DOMINANT INHERITANCE AND REFERRED TO 11 OTHER INSTANCES OF FAMILIAL OCCUR-RENCE IN HIS SERIES. HE CONCLUDED THAT 'THERE IS NO DOUBT THAT THE CONDITION CAN BE INHERITED AS AN AUTOSOMAL DOMINANT.' THE MALIGNANT HYPERTHERMIA WHICH OCCURS ON THE BASIS OF A GENETIC DEFECT IN LANDRACE PIGS IS NOT ONLY CLINICALLY IDENTICAL WITH THE HUMAN SYNDROME, BUT ALSO IDENTICAL IN MANY OF THE BIOCHEMICAL FEATURES (BRITT AND KALOW, 1970). KALOW ET AL. (1970) SUGGESTED THAT MALIGNANT HYPERTHER-MIA WITH AND WITHOUT RIGIDITY ARE DISTINCT ENTITIES.

ALDRETE, J. A., PADFIELD, A., SOLOMON, C. C. AND RUBRIGHT, M. W.* POSSIBLE PREDICATIVE TESTS FOR MALIGNANT HYPERTHERMIA DURING ANESTHESIA. J.A.M.A. 125* 1465-1469, 1971.

DENBOROUGH, M. A., EBELING, P., KING, J. O. AND ZAPF, P.* MYOPATHY AND
MALIGNANT HYPERPYREXIA. LANCET 1* 1138-1140, 1970.

DENBOROUGH, M. A., FORSTER, J. F. A., HUDSON, M. C., CARTER, N. G. AND ZAPF,
P.* BIOCHEMICAL CHANGES IN MALIGNANT HYPERPYREXIA. LANCET 1* 1137-1138, 1970.

DENBOROUGH, M. A., FORSTER, J. F. A., LOVELL, R. R. H., MAPLESTONE, P. A. AND
VILLIERS, J. D.* ANAESTHETIC DEATH IN A FAMILY. BRIT. J. ANAESTH. 34* 395-396,
1962.

ISAACS, H. AND BARLOW, M. B.* THE GENETIC BACKGROUND TO MALIGNANT HYPERPYREXIA
REVEALED BY SERUM CREATINE PHOSPHOKINASE ESTIMATIONS IN ASYMPTOMATIC RELATIVES.
BRIT. J. ANAESTH. 42* 1077-1084, 1970.

KALOW, W.* RIGIDITY AND MALIGNANT HYPERTHERMIA ASSOCIATED WITH ANAESTHESIA.
HUMANGENETIK 9* 237-239, 1970.

KALOW, W., BRITT, B. A., TERREAU, M. E. AND HAIST, C.* METABOLIC ERROR OF
MUSCLE METABOLISM AFTER RECOVERY FROM MALIGNANT HYPERTHERMIA. LANCET 2* 895-898,
1970.

STEPHENS, C. R.* FULMINANT HYPERTHERMIA DURING ANESTHESIA AND SURGERY.
J.A.M.A. 202* 178-182, 1967.

WILSON, R. D., DENT, T. E., TRABER, D. L., MCCOY, N. R. AND ALLEN, C. R.*
MALIGNANT HYPERPYREXIA WITH ANESTHESIA. J.A.M.A. 202* 183-186, 1967.

*14570 HYPERTRICHOSIS, UNIVERSALIS

WE HAVE OBSERVED A 6 YEAR OLD BOY (JHH, 1251544) WITH EXTREME GENERALIZED
HYPERTRICHOSIS (BEIGHTON, 1970). HE WAS BORN WITH DOUBLE EYEBROWS. THE FATHER,
GRANDFATHER AND GREAT GRANDFATHER HAD EXCESSIVE HAIR OVER THE ENTIRE BODY UNTIL
ABOUT AGE 4. OTHER MALES IN EACH GENERATION ESCAPED THE EXCESSIVE HAIRINESS AND
IT MAY HAVE BEEN TRANSMITTED THROUGH AN UNAFFECTED FEMALE. THERE WAS NO GINGIVAL
FIBROMATOSIS (Q.V.) IN THIS FAMILY. FELGENBAUER (1969) DESCRIBED AFFECTED MOTHER,
SON AND DAUGHTER AND REVIEWED THE LITERATURE EXHAUSTIVELY. DOMINANT INHERITANCE
WAS DEMONSTRATED BY THE FAMILY OF PETER GONZALES WHO WAS BORN IN THE CANARY
ISLANDS IN 1556 AND LATER LIVED IN THE COURT OF KING HENRY II OF FRANCE. HE,
THREE OF HIS CHILDREN AND SOME IN THE NEXT GENERATION WERE AFFECTED (RAVIN AND
HODGE, 1969). AFFECTED MOTHER AND SON ARE DESCRIBED BY DURAND AND DURAND (1957).

BEIGHTON, P.* CONGENITAL HYPERTRICHOSIS LANUGINOSA. ARCH. DERM. 101* 669-672,
1970.

DURAND, J. AND DURAND, A.* PICTORIAL HISTORY OF THE AMERICAN CIRCUS. NEW YORK*
A. S. BARNES, 1957. P. 104.

FELGENBAUER, W. R.* HYPERTRICHOSIS LANUGINOSA UNIVERSALIS. J. GENET. HUM. 17*
1-44, 1969.

RAVIN, J. G. AND HODGE, G. P.* HYPERTRICHOSIS PORTRAYED IN ART. J.A.M.A. 207*
533-535, 1969.

*14580 HYPERTROPHIA MUSCULORUM VERA

THIS CONDITION MUST BE DISTINGUISHED FROM MYOTONIA CONGENITA AND FROM THE DEBRE-
SEMELAIGNE SYNDROME OF CONGENITAL HYPOTHYROIDISM. POCH ET AL. (1971) DESCRIBED A
WELL DOCUMENTED FAMILY WITH MALE-TO-MALE TRANSMISSION. STRIKING HYPERTROPHY OF
THE CALF MUSCLES AND LESS CONSTANTLY OF THE MASSETER MUSCLES WERE FOUND.

POCH, G. F., SICA, E. P., TARATUTO, A. AND WEINSTEIN, I. H.* HYPERTROPHIA
MUSCULORUM VERA. STUDY OF A FAMILY. J. NEUROL. SCI. 12* 53-62, 1971.

*14590 HYPERTROPHIC NEUROPATHY OF DEJERINE-SOTTAS

ANDERMANN AND COLLEAGUES (1962) DESCRIBED DEJERINE-SOTTAS HYPERTROPHIC NEUROPATHY
IN GRANDFATHER, FATHER AND 4 YEAR OLD DAUGHTER. FEATURES WERE NYSTAGMUS, DISTAL
MUSCULAR WEAKNESS, DISTAL SENSORY CHANGE, PES CAVUS AND EXACERBATIONS AND
REMISSIONS. ISAACS (1960) DESCRIBED A FAMILY IN WHICH PARALYSIS OF THE EXTREMI-
TIES WAS PRECIPITATED BY COLD WEATHER. NO SENSORY CHANGES OCCURRED IN THE FAMILY
OF RUSSELL AND GARLAND (1930), RESTUDIED BY CROFT AND WADIA (1957) WITH TRACING OF
THE DISORDER THROUGH FIVE GENERATIONS. ON THE OTHER HAND ANDERMANN ET AL. (1962)
DESCRIBED SENSORY CHANGES. THEY ALSO DEMONSTRATED ADVANCED INVOLVEMENT OF CRANIAL
AND SPINAL NERVES. SPINAL NERVE ROOT ENLARGEMENT WAS DEMONSTRABLE BY MYELOGRAPHY.
AN ABNORMALITY OF PYRUVATE TOLERANCE DESERVES FURTHER STUDY. ELEVATED SPINAL
FLUID PROTEIN IS OFTEN FOUND IN THIS CONDITION AND IN REFSUM'S SYNDROME, A
RECESSIVE (Q.V.). BEDFORD AND JAMES (1956) ALSO OBSERVED A FAMILY WITH AFFECTED
MEMBERS IN FIVE GENERATIONS. THE ONSET IS USUALLY WITH WEAKNESS AND DEFORMITY OF
THE FEET AND LOWER LIMBS. 'ONION BULB' FORMATION MAKES THE HISTOLOGIC DIAGNOSIS.

DESPITE THE APPARENT DOMINANT INHERITANCE AS OUTLINED ABOVE, THE CASES DESCRIBED BY DEJERINE AND SOTTAS (1893) WERE SIBS WITH PRESUMABLY UNAFFECTED PARENTS. ONSET WAS IN INFANCY IN FANNY ROY AND AT AGE 14 IN HENRI ROY. THE PATIENTS SHOWED CLUBFOOT, KYPHOSCOLIOSIS, GENERALIZED WEAKNESS AND MUSCULAR ATROPHY WITH FASCICU-LATIONS BEGINNING FIRST IN THE LEG MUSCLES, DECREASED REACTIVITY TO ELECTRIC STIMULATION, AREFLEXIA, MARKED DISTAL SENSORY LOSS IN ALL FOUR EXTREMITIES, INCOORDINATION IN THE ARMS, ROMBERG'S SIGN, MIOSIS, DECREASED PUPILLARY REACTION TO LIGHT, NYSTAGMUS. FANNY DIED AT 45. AUTOPSY SHOWED THE PERIPHERAL NERVES TO BE INCREASED IN SIZE, FIRM AND GELATINOUS. ONLY RARE NERVE FIBERS CONTAINED MYELIN. DYCK ET AL. (1970) FOUND CHANGES IN NERVES AND LIVER SUGGESTING A SYSTEMIC DEFECT IN THE METABOLISM OF CERAMIDE HEXOSIDES AND CERAMIDE HEXOSIDE SULFATES.

ANDERMANN, F., LLOYD-SMITH, D. L., MAVOR, H. AND MATHIESON, G.* OBSERVATIONS ON HYPERTROPHIC NEUROPATHY OF DEJERINE AND SOTTAS. NEUROLOGY 12* 712-724, 1962.

AUSTIN, J. H.* OBSERVATIONS ON THE SYNDROME OF HYPERTROPHIC NEURITIS (THE HYPERTROPHIC INTERSTITIAL RADICULO-NEUROPATHIES). MEDICINE 35* 187-237, 1956.

BEDFORD, P. D. AND JAMES, F. E.* A FAMILY WITH THE PROGRESSIVE HYPERTROPHIC POLYNEURITIS OF DEJERINE AND SOTTAS. J. NEUROL. NEUROSURG. PSYCHIAT. 19* 46-51, 1956.

CROFT, P. B. AND WADIA, N. H.* FAMILIAL HYPERTROPHIC POLYNEURITIS* REVIEW OF A PREVIOUSLY REPORTED FAMILY. NEUROLOGY 7* 356-366, 1957.

DEJERINE, J. AND SOTTAS, J.* SUR LA NEVRITE INTERSTITIELLE, HYPERTROPHIQUE ET PROGRESSIVE DE L'ENFANCE. C. R. SOC. BIOL. 45* 63-96, 1893.

DELEON, G. A.* PROGRESSIVE VENTRAL SENSORY LOSS IN SENSORY RADICULAR NEUROPATHY AND HYPERTROPHIC NEURITIS. JOHNS HOPKINS MED. J. 125* 53-61, 1969.

DYCK, P. J., ELLEFSON, R. D., LAIS, A. C., SMITH, R. C., TAYLOR, W. F. AND VAN DYKE, R. A.* HISTOLOGIC AND LIPID STUDIES OF SURAL NERVES IN INHERITED HYPERTROPHIC NEUROPATHY* PRELIMINARY REPORT OF A LIPID ABNORMALITY IN NERVE AND LIVER IN DEJERINE-SOTTAS DISEASE. MAYO CLIN. PROC. 45* 286-327, 1970.

ISAACS, H.* FAMILIAL CHRONIC HYPERTROPHIC POLYNEUROPATHY WITH PARALYSIS OF THE EXTREMITIES IN COLD WEATHER. S. AFR. MED. J. 34* 758-761, 1960.

RUSSELL, W. R. AND GARLAND, H. G.* PROGRESSIVE HYPERTROPHIC POLYNEURITIS, WITH CASE REPORTS. BRAIN 53* 376-384, 1930.

*14600 HYPOCHONDROPLASIA

THIS CONDITION RESEMBLING TRUE ACHONDROPLASIA IS PROBABLY NOT RARE AND IT PROBABLY IS A DOMINANT. THE HEAD IS NOT AFFECTED. THE SPINAL CANAL NARROWS IN ITS CAUDAD PORTION AS IN TRUE ACHONDROPLASIA. THE FINGERS ARE SHORT BUT THE HAND IS NOT OF THE TRIDENT TYPE. THIS ENTITY AWAITS FULL DELINEATION CLINICALLY, RADIOLOGICALLY AND GENETICALLY. THE TERM IS LAMY AND MAROTEAUX* (1961). I KNOW OF AFFECTED FATHER AND DAUGHTER. BEALS (1969) DESCRIBED FIVE KINDREDS WITH CLEAR EVIDENCE OF AUTOSOMAL DOMINANT INHERITANCE.

BEALS, R. K.* HYPOCHONDROPLASIA. A REPORT OF FIVE KINDREDS. J. BONE JOINT SURG. 51A* 728-736, 1969.

LAMY, M. AND MAROTEAUX, P.* LES CHONDRODYSTROPHIES GENOTYPIQUES. PARIS* L'EXPANSION* SCIENTIFIQUE FRANCAISE, 1961. P. 26.

14610 HYPOFIBRINOGENEMIA

FAMILIES SEEM TO EXIST IN WHICH HYPOFIBRINOGENEMIA IS SEGREGATING IN A DOMINANT PATTERN AND IN WHICH THE DISORDER ON THE ONE HAND CANNOT BE RELATED TO LIVER DISEASE AND ON THE OTHER HAND IS PROBABLY NOT THE HETEROZYGOUS STATE OF CONGENITAL AFIBRINOGENEMIA (IMPERATO, DETTORI, 1958* REVOL, 1962). SOME OF THESE MAY BE THE SAME ENTITY AS DISCUSSED UNDER FIBRINOGEN VARIANTS (Q.V.).

IMPERATO, C. AND DETTORI, A. G.* IPOFIBRINOGENEMIA CONGENITA CON FIBRINOAS-TENIA. HELV. PAEDIAT. ACTA 13* 380-399, 1958.

REVOL, L.* LES GRANDES HYPOFIBRINEMIES CONSTITUTIONELLES HEMORRHAGIQUES. HEMOSTASE 2* 243-254, 1962.

14620 HYPOPARATHYROIDISM

ACETO ET AL. (1966) REPORTED FETAL AND INFANTILE HYPERPARATHYROIDISM DUE TO MATERNAL HYPOPARATHYROIDISM. THE SECOND AND THIRD OFFSPRING, A GIRL AND A BOY OF THE AFFECTED MOTHER HAD HYPOPARATHYROIDISM. THE FATHERS OF AT LEAST TWO OF THE OFFSPRING WERE DIFFERENT. BENSON AND PARSONS (1964) DESCRIBED HYPOPARATHYROIDISM IN A MOTHER AND TWO OF HER CHILDREN. THEY FOUND NO CIRCULATING ANTIBODIES TO PARATHYROID HORMONE.

ACETO, T., JR., BATT, R. E., BRUCK, E., SCHULTZ, R. B. AND PEREZ, Y. R.*
INTRAUTERINE HYPERPARATHYROIDISM* A COMPLICATION OF UNTREATED MATERNAL HYPOPARA-
THYROIDISM. J. CLIN. ENDOCR. 26* 487-492, 1966.

BENSON, P. F. AND PARSONS, V.* HEREDITARY HYPOPARATHYROIDISM PRESENTING WITH
OEDEMA IN THE NEONATAL PERIOD. QUART. J. MED. 33* 197-208, 1964.

*14630 HYPOPHOSPHATASIA

IN THE FAMILY REPORTED BY SILVERMAN (1962) A FATHER AND 2 SONS HAD HYPOPHOSPHATA-
SIA. THE PATERNAL GRANDMOTHER MAY HAVE BEEN AFFECTED. NO EVIDENCE OF HETEROZYGO-
SITY WAS OBTAINED IN THE PROPOSITUS' WIFE AND TWO UNAFFECTED CHILDREN. CLINICAL
FEATURES WERE EARLY LOSS OF TEETH, BOWED LEGS DIAGNOSED AS RICKETS AND REQUIRING
OSTEOTOMY, AND BEATEN-COPPER APPEARANCE OF SKULL X-RAY. THE PROPOSITUS HAD SERVED
IN THE U.S. AIR FORCE. DANOVITCH ET AL. (1968) ALSO SUGGESTED DOMINANT INHERI-
TANCE AS THE MECHANISM IN THE FAMILY THEY STUDIED. THREE FEMALE COUSINS, THE
DAUGHTERS OF THREE SISTERS, AND THEIR MOTHERS HAD LOW SERUM ALKALINE PHOSPHATASE
AND ELEVATED URINARY PHOSPHOETHANOLAMINE. TWO OF THE COUSINS HAD PREMATURE LOSS
OF PRIMARY TEETH. INTESTINAL ALKALINE PHOSPHATASE WAS NORMAL. JARDON ET AL.
(1970) DESCRIBED A WOMAN WHO WAS ASYMPTOMATIC UNTIL AGE 50 YEARS. SHE SHOWED
PSEUDOFRACTURE OF THE PROXIMAL FEMUR AND CALCIFICATION OF PARASPINOUS LIGAMENTS
LIKE THOSE IN ADULTS WITH HYPOPHOSPHATEMIC RICKETS (Q.V.).

DANOVITCH, S. H., BAER, P. N. AND LASTER, L.* INTESTINAL ALKALINE PHOSPHATASE
ACTIVITY IN FAMILIAL HYPOPHOSPHATASIA. NEW ENG. J. MED. 278* 1253-1260, 1968.

JARDON, O. M., BURNEY, D. W. AND FINK, R. L.* HYPOPHOSPHATASIA IN AN ADULT. J.
BONE JOINT SURG. 52A* 1477-1484, 1970.

SILVERMAN, J. L.* APPARENT DOMINANT INHERITANCE OF HYPOPHOSPHATASIA. ANN.
INTERN. MED. 110* 191-198, 1962.

14640 HYPOPLASIA OF TEETH

BROWN (1944) DESCRIBED A 19 YEAR OLD BOY WITH UNDERDEVELOPED DENTAL ROOTS AND
EARLY EXFOLIATION OF THE TEETH. THE FATHER AND A PATERNAL UNCLE WERE EDENTULOUS.

BROWN, H. C.* HYPOPLASIA OF THE DENTITION. AM. J. ORTH. ORAL SURG. 30* 102-
103, 1944.

14650 HYPOTENSION, ORTHOSTATIC (SHY-DRAGER SYNDROME)

LEWIS (1964) DESCRIBED A FAMILY IN WHICH SEVERAL MEMBERS HAD A NEUROLOGIC DISORDER
MANIFESTED BY ORTHOSTATIC HYPOTENSION, AMYOTROPHY, ATAXIA, RIGIDITY, TREMOR AND
SPHINCTER DISTURBANCE. SIX PERSONS IN THREE GENERATIONS WITH TWO INSTANCES OF
POSSIBLE MALE-TO-MALE TRANSMISSION WERE OBSERVED. ONSET WAS IN MIDDLE LIFE AND
THE DISEASE PROGRESSED SLOWLY WITHOUT IMPAIRMENT OF INTELLECT. VANDERHAEGHEN ET
AL. (1970) SUGGESTED THAT TWO FORMS OF IDIOPATHIC ORTHOSTATIC HYPOTENSION EXIST,
ON THE BASIS OF CLINICO-PATHOLOGIC CORRELATIONS. WALTON (1969) HAS OBSERVED MALE-
TO-MALE TRANSMISSION.

LEWIS, P.* FAMILIAL ORTHOSTATIC HYPOTENSION. BRAIN 87* 719-728, 1964.

SHY, G. M. AND DRAGER, G. A.* A NEUROLOGICAL SYNDROME ASSOCIATED WITH ORTHOSTA-
TIC HYPOTENSION* A CLINICAL-PATHOLOGIC STUDY. ARCH. NEUROL. 2* 511-527, 1960.

VANDERHAEGHEN, J.-J., PERIER, O. AND STERNON, J. E.* PATHOLOGICAL FINDINGS IN
IDIOPATHIC ORTHOSTATIC HYPOTENSION. ARCH. NEUROL. 22* 207-214, 1970.

WALTON, J. N.* NEWCASTLE-UPON-TYNE, ENGLAND* PERSONAL COMMUNICATION, 1969.

*14660 ICHTHYOSIS HYSTRIX GRAVIOR (LAMBERT TYPE ICHTHYOSIS, 'PORCUPINE MAN')

Y-LINKAGE WAS SUGGESTED ON THE BASIS OF THE FAMOUS LAMBERT PEDIGREE. PENROSE AND
STERN (1958) DISPROVED THIS, HOWEVER, AND CONCLUDED THAT AUTOSOMAL DOMINANT
INHERITANCE IS LIKELY.

PENROSE, L. S. AND STERN, C.* RECONSIDERATION OF THE LAMBERT PEDIGREE (ICHTHYO-
SIS HYSTRIX GRAVIOR). ANN. HUM. GENET. 22* 258-283, 1958.

*14670 ICHTHYOSIS VULGARIS (ICHTHYOSIS SIMPLEX)

WELLS AND KERR (1965) SUGGESTED THAT DOMINANT ICHTHYOSIS VULGARIS IS DISTINGUI-
SHABLE CLINICALLY FROM THE X-LINKED VARIETY. IN THE DOMINANT FORM, THE FIRST SKIN
INVOLVEMENT IS USUALLY NOTED AFTER THE FIRST THREE MONTHS OF LIFE AND LESS OF THE
BODY SURFACE IS AFFECTED. LESIONS ARE RARELY OBSERVED IN THE AXILLAE OR ANTICUBI-
TAL AND POPLITEAL FOSSAE BUT THE PALMS AND SOLES OFTEN SHOW INCREASED MARKINGS.
THERE ARE SOME HISTOLOGIC DIFFERENCES ALSO. A CONSIDERABLE PROPORTION OF PATIENTS
WITH DOMINANT ICHTHYOSIS HAVE ASTHMA, ECZEMA OR HAYFEVER. THIS MAY NOT BE A
SEPARATE ENTITY, HOWEVER. FOR A USEFUL CLASSIFICATION AND DISCUSSION OF THE
VARIOUS FORMS OF ICHTHYOSIS, SEE SCHNYDER (1970).

KUOKKANEN, K.* ICHTHYOSIS VULGARIS. A CLINICAL AND HISTOPATHOLOGICAL STUDY OF PATIENTS AND THEIR CLOSE RELATIVES IN THE AUTOSOMAL DOMINANT AND SEX-LINKED FORMS OF THE DISEASE. ACTA DERMATOVENER. 49 (SUPPL. 62)* 1-72, 1969.

SCHNYDER, U. W.* INHERITED ICHTHYOSES. ARCH. DERM. 102* 240-252, 1970.

WELLS, R. S. AND KERR, C. B.* GENETIC CLASSIFICATION OF ICHTHYOSIS. ARCH. DERM. 92* 1-6, 1965.

14680 ICHTHYOSIS, BULLOUS TYPE

SCHNYDER (1970) CONCLUDED THAT THIS REPRESENTS A SEPARATE ENTITY.

SCHNYDER, U. W.* INHERITED ICHTHYOSES. ARCH. DERM. 102* 240-252, 1970.

SIEMENS, H. W.* DICHTUNG UND WAHRHEIT UBER DIE ICHTHYOSIS BULLOSA, MIT BEMERKUNGEN ZUR SYSTEMATIK DER EPIDERMOLYSEN. ARCH. DERM. SYPH. 175* 590-608, 1937.

14690 IMMUNOGLOBULIN TYPES AM(1)

THE GM AND INV TYPES ARE VARIANTS OF IGG, IMMUNOGLOBULIN G. VYAS AND FUDENBERG (1970) DESCRIBED ALLOTYPE OF IGA, USING ISOANTIBODIES FROM A PATIENT WHO DISPLAYED AN ANAPHYLACTOID TRANSFUSION REACTION.

VYAS, G. N. AND FUDENBERG, H. H.* IMMUNOBIOLOGY OF HUMAN ANTI-IGA* A SEROLOGIC AND IMMUNOGENETIC STUDY OF IMMUNIZATION TO IGA IN TRANSFUSION AND PREGNANCY. CLIN. GENET. 1* 44-64, 1970.

14700 IMMUNOGLOBULIN TYPES AM(2)

KUNKEL ET AL. (1969) DEFINED A SYSTEM THEY CALLED AM(2). THE AM(2) AND GM SYSTEMS, INVOLVING IGA AND IGG, RESPECTIVELY, APPEAR TO BE CLOSELY LINKED IN MAN. GAMMA A AND GAMMA G MARKERS ARE CLOSELY LINKED IN THE MOUSE. THE SYSTEM OF VYAS AND FUDENBERG (1969) IS NOT LINKED TO GM. VAN LOGHEM ET AL. (1970) SHOWED THAT THE GM AND AM(2) LOCI ARE CLOSELY LINKED BUT GM AND INV UNLINKED. THE GAMMA 'LOCUS' (SEE BELOW) IS A COMPLEX OF THREE CLOSELY LINKED LOCI* GAMMA-1, GAMMA-2, AND GAMMA-3.

KUNKEL, H. G., SMITH, W. K., JOSLIN, F. G., NATVIG, J. B. AND LITWIN, S. D.* GENETIC MARKER OF THE GAMMA A2 SUBGROUP OF GAMMA A IMMUNOGLOBULINS. NATURE 223* 1247-1248, 1969.

VAN LOGHEM, E., NATVIG, J. B. AND MATSUMOTO, H.* GENETIC MARKERS OF IMMUNOGLO-BULINS IN JAPANESE FAMILIES. INHERITANCE OF ASSOCIATED MARKERS BELONGING TO ONE IGA AND THREE IGG SUBCLASSES. ANN. HUM. GENET. 33* 351-359, 1970.

VYAS, G. N. AND FUDENBERG, H. H.* IMMUNOGENETIC STUDY OF AM(1), THE FIRST ALLOTYPE OF HUMAN IGA. CLIN. RES. 17* 469 ONLY, 1969.

14710 IMMUNOGLOBULIN TYPES GM

AT LEAST TWO SEPARATE AUTOSOMAL LOCI DETERMINING SEROLOGIC TYPE OF GAMMA GLOBULIN HAVE BEEN IDENTIFIED. ONE IS REFERRED TO AS THE GM LOCUS AND THE OTHER AS THE INV LOCUS. THE GENETICS OF THE GAMMA GLOBULINS PROMISES TO BE AS REVEALING OF GENERAL PRINCIPLES AS HAS BEEN THAT OF THE HEMOGLOBINS. THE GM SYSTEM IS ASSOCIATED WITH THE HEAVY CHAINS OF THE IGG MOLECULES AND THE INV SYSTEM WITH THE LIGHT CHAINS. (SEE NATURE 209* 653, 1966, RECOMMENDED NOTATION FOR GM AND INV TYPES.) HOOD AND EIN (1968) PRESENTED EVIDENCE THAT ANTIBODY LIGHT CHAINS ARE AN EXCEPTION TO THE RULE OF 'ONE GENE, ONE POLYPEPTIDE CHAIN.' TWO SEPARATE LOCI (A SPECIFIC REGION LOCUS AND A COMMON REGION LOCUS) APPEAR TO CODE FOR A SINGLE, CONTINUOUS POLYPEP-TIDE CHAIN. ABSENCE OF CERTAIN IMMUNOGLOBULINS IN PATIENTS WITH DELETED CHROMO-SOME 18 SUGGESTS THE LOCALIZATION OF STRUCTURAL AND-OR CONTROLLER GENES TO THAT CHROMOSOME (FINLEY ET AL., 1968).

CEPPELLINI, R., DRAY, S., FABEY, J. L., FRANKLIN, E. C., FUDENBERG, H., GELL, P. G. H., GOODMAN, H. C., GRUBB, R., HARBOE, M., KIRK, R. L., OUDIN, J., ROPARTZ, C., SMITHIES, O., STEINBERG, A. G. AND TRNKA, Z.* NOTATION FOR GENETIC FACTORS IN HUMAN IMMUNOGLOBULINS. GENETICS 53* 235-241, 1966.

FAHEY, J. L.* ANTIBODIES AND IMMUNOGLOBULINS. I. STRUCTURE AND FUNCTION. J.A.M.A. 194* 71-74, 1965.

FINLEY, S. C., FINLEY, W. H., NOTO, T. A., UCHIDA, I. A. AND RODDAM, R. F.* IGA ABSENCE ASSOCIATED WITH A RING-18 CHROMOSOME. (LETTER) LANCET 1* 1095-1096, 1968.

GRUBB, R.* THE GENETIC MARKERS OF HUMAN IMMUNOGLOBINS. NEW YORK* SPRINGER, 1970.

HILL, R. L., DELANEY, R., FELLOWS, R. E., JR. AND LEBOVITZ, H. E.* THE EVOLUTIONARY ORIGINS OF THE IMMUNOGLOBULINS. PROC. NAT. ACAD. SCI. 56* 1762-1769, 1966.

LENNOX, E. S. AND COHN, M.* IMMUNOGLOBULINS. ANN. REV. BIOCHEM. 36* 365-402,
1967.

OUDIN, J.* GENETIC REGULATION OF IMMUNOGLOBULIN SYNTHESIS. J. CELL. PHYSIOL.
67 (SUPPL. 1)* 77-108, 1966.

STEINBERG, A. G. AND BEARN, A. G.* PROGRESS IN MEDICAL GENETICS. NEW YORK*
GRUNE AND STRATTON, 3* 1964.

STEINBERG, A. G.* GAMMAGLOBULIN POLYMORPHISMS IN MAN. ANN. REV. GENET. 3* 25-
32, 1969.

14720 IMMUNOGLOBULIN TYPES INV

INV(-1,3) HOMOZYGOTES HAVE VALINE AT POSITION 191 OF THE KAPPA-TYPE LIGHT
POLYPEPTIDE CHAINS WHEREAS INV(1,3) HETEROZYGOTES HAVE SOME CHAINS WITH LEUCINE
AND SOME WITH VALINE AT THIS POSITION (TERRY ET AL., 1969).

TERRY, W. D., HOOD, L. E. AND STEINBERG, A. G.* GENETICS OF IMMUNOGLOBULIN
KAPPA CHAINS* CHEMICAL ANALYSIS OF NORMAL HUMAN LIGHT CHAINS OF DIFFERING INV
TYPES. PROC. NAT. ACAD. SCI. 63* 71-77, 1969.

14730 INCISORS, LONG UPPER CENTRAL

ALTHOUGH A SINGLE MAJOR GENE MAY BE INVOLVED AND THIS TRAIT BEHAVES AS A SIMPLE
DOMINANT, DATA ACTUALLY PROVING THIS ARE APPARENTLY NOT AVAILABLE.

HRDLICKA, A.* NORMAL VARIATION OF TEETH AND JAWS AND ORTHODONTY. INT. J.
ORTHOD. DENT. CHILD. 21* 1099-1114, 1935.

HYDE, W.* HEREDITY IN RELATION TO SIZE OF THE TEETH. J. AM. DENT. ASS. 25*
1762-1767, 1938.

14740 INCISORS, 'SHOVEL-SHAPED'

THE INCISORS ARE HOLLOWED OUT ON THEIR LINGUAL SURFACE, CREATING A RESEMBLANCE TO
A SHOVEL OR A SUGAR SCOOP. THE LATERAL INCISORS ARE MORE OFTEN OR MORE MARKEDLY
AFFECTED THAN THE MIDDLE INCISORS. THE TRAIT IS PARTICULARLY FREQUENT IN THE
MONGOLOID RACE. FAMILY STUDIES HAVE, APPARENTLY, NOT BEEN PERFORMED.

KOSKI, K. AND HAUTALA, E.* ON THE FREQUENCY OF SHOVEL-SHAPED INCISORS IN THE
FINNS. AM. J. PHYS. ANTHROP. 10* 127-132, 1952.

RIESENFELD, A.* SHOVEL-SHAPED INCISORS AND A FEW OTHER DENTAL FEATURES AMONG
THE NATIVE PEOPLE OF THE PACIFIC. AM. J. PHYS. ANTHROP. 14* 505-521, 1956.

*14750 INHIBITOR OF PROTHROMBIN CONSUMPTION, HEMORRHAGIC DISORDER DUE TO

IN 4 GENERATIONS OF A FAMILY (WITH ONE INSTANCE OF MALE-TO-MALE TRANSMISSION),
ROBINSON ET AL. (1967) DESCRIBED A MILD BLEEDING DISORDER ASSOCIATED WITH
INCREASED CONCENTRATIONS OF A NATURAL INHIBITOR OF PROTHROMBIN CONSUMPTION IN THE
SERUM.

ROBINSON, A. J., AGGELER, P. M., MCNICOL, G. P. AND DOUGLAS, A. S.* AN ATYPICAL
GENETIC HAEMORRHAGIC DISEASE WITH INCREASED CONCENTRATION OF A NATURAL INHIBITOR
OF PROTHROMBIN CONSUMPTION. BRIT. J. HAEMAT. 13* 510-527, 1967.

*14760 IRIS HYPOPLASIA WITH GLAUCOMA

BERG (1932) DESCRIBED 22 AFFECTED IN 6 GENERATIONS. MCCULLOCH (1950) DESCRIBED 18
AFFECTED IN 5 GENERATIONS. WEATHERILL AND HART (1969) OBSERVED IT IN MANY MEMBERS
OF 5 GENERATIONS. NOT ONLY IS THE STROMA OF THE IRIS HYPOPLASTIC BUT THE IRIS IS
ALSO LIGHT IN COLOR, A FEATURE THAT ANTEDATES DEVELOPMENT OF GLAUCOMA AND PERMITS
RECOGNITION OF AFFECTED PERSONS AT BIRTH. SEE RIEGER'S SYNDROME WHICH HAS
SOMEWHAT SIMILAR OCULAR FEATURES.

BERG, F.* ERBLICHES JUGENDLICHES GLAUKOM. ACTA OPHTHAL. 10* 568-587, 1932.

MCCULLOCH, J. C.* IRIDOSCHISIS AS A CAUSE OF GLAUCOMA. AM. J. OPHTHAL. 33*
1398-1400, 1950.

WEATHERILL, J. R. AND HART, C. T.* FAMILIAL HYPOPLASIA OF THE IRIS STROMA
ASSOCIATED WITH GLAUCOMA. BRIT. J. OPHTHAL. 53* 433-438, 1969.

14770 ISOCITRATE DEHYDROGENASE POLYMORPHISM

HENDERSON (1965) DESCRIBED ELECTROPHORETIC POLYMORPHISM OF THIS ENZYME IN MICE BUT
IT HAS NOT TURNED UP IN MAN.

HENDERSON, N. S.* ISOZYMES OF ISOCITRATE DEHYDROGENASE* SUBUNIT STRUCTURE AND INTRACELLULAR LOCATION. J. EXP. ZOOL. 158* 263-273, 1965.

HENDERSON, N. S.* INTRACELLULAR LOCATION AND GENETIC CONTROL OF ISOZYMES OF NADP-DEPENDENT ISOCITRATE DEHYDROGENASE AND MALATE DEHYDROGENASE. ANN. N.Y. ACAD. SCI. 151* 429-440, 1968.

14780 JOINT CONTRACTURES WITH OTHER ABNORMALITIES

AASE AND SMITH (1968) DESCRIBED A SYNDROME IN FATHER AND TWO CHILDREN. THE INFANTS ONE STILLBORN AND ONE WHO SURVIVED ONLY TWO MONTHS HAD VIRTUALLY IDENTICAL FINDINGS* HYDROCEPHALUS, CLEFT PALATE AND SEVERE JOINT CONTRACTURES. THE FATHER HAD JOINT CONTRACTURES FROM BIRTH, DEFORMED EARS AND BILATERAL PTOSIS. ONE OF THE INFANTS WAS MALE. ONE HAD CONGENITAL NEUROBLASTOMA AND THE OTHER HAD MULTIPLE VENTRICULAR SEPTAL DEFECTS AND A SINGLE STERNAL OSSIFICATION CENTER. THE SAME CONDITION MAY HAVE BEEN PRESENT IN THE INFANT REPORTED BY POTTER AND PARRISH (1942). SEE PSEUDO-ARTHROGRYPOSIS.

AASE, J. M. AND SMITH, D. W.* DYSMORPHOGENESIS OF JOINTS, BRAIN AND PALATE* A NEW DOMINANTLY INHERITED SYNDROME. J. PEDIAT. 73* 606-609, 1968.

POTTER, E. L. AND PARRISH, J. M.* NEUROBLASTOMA, GANGLIONEUROMA AND FI-BRONEUROMA IN A STILLBORN FETUS. AM. J. PATH. 18* 141-152, 1942.

*14790 JOINT LAXITY, FAMILIAL

CARTER AND SWEETNAM (1960) NOTED DOMINANT INHERITANCE IN SEVERAL FAMILIES THAT SUFFERED FROM RECURRENT DISLOCATION OF JOINTS, PARTICULARLY THE SHOULDER. RECURRENT DISLOCATION OF THE PATELLA (Q.V.) MAY BE AN INDEPENDENT DOMINANT TRAIT IN SOME FAMILIES. OTHER DOMINANT PEDIGREES ARE REFERRED TO BY MCKUSICK (1966). SEE ALSO RECESSIVE CATALOG.

BEIGHTON, P. H. AND HORAN, F. T.* DOMINANT INHERITANCE IN FAMILIAL GENERALIZED ARTICULAR HYPERMOBILITY. J. BONE JOINT SURG. 52B* 145-147, 1970.

CARTER, C. AND SWEETNAM, R.* RECURRENT DISLOCATION OF THE PATELLA AND OF THE SHOULDER. THEIR ASSOCIATION WITH FAMILIAL JOINT LAXITY. J. BONE JOINT SURG. 42B* 721-727, 1960.

KIRK, J. A., ANSELL, B. M. AND BYWATERS, E. G. L.* THE HYPERMOBILITY SYNDROME. ANN. RHEUM. DIS. 26* 419-425, 1967.

MCKUSICK, V. A.* HERITABLE DISORDERS OF CONNECTIVE TISSUE. ST. LOUIS* C. V. MOSBY CO., 1966 (3RD ED.). P. 215 AND FIGS. 5-10.

14800 KAPOSI'S SARCOMA

ZELIGMAN (1960) OBSERVED THE DISORDER IN FATHER AND SON. ALTHOUGH A CHARACTERIS-TIC ETHNIC OCCURRENCE (ITALIAN AND JEWISH) HAS BEEN NOTED, THIS WAS PERHAPS ONLY THE SECOND INSTANCE OF FAMILIAL INCIDENCE.

ZELIGMAN, I.* KAPOSI'S SARCOMA IN A FATHER AND SON. BULL. HOPKINS HOSP. 107* 208-212, 1960.

14810 KELOIDS

OVER-GROWTH OF CONNECTIVE TISSUE OF THE SKIN OCCURS AFTER TRAUMA. BLOOM (1956) DESCRIBED CASES IN FIVE GENERATIONS. BOHROD (1937) SPECULATED THAT SEXUAL SELECTION FAVORED THE GENOTYPE OF KELOIDS FORMATION. HE PRESENTED EVIDENCE THAT CICATRIZATION WAS PRACTICED AS A PUBERTAL RITE BY AFRICANS AND THAT 'GOOD' SCAR FORMERS MAY HAVE BEEN ON THE AVERAGE MORE FERTILE. COSMAN ET AL. (1961) FOUND A FAMILIAL INCIDENCE OF 3 PERCENT.

BLOOM, D.* HEREDITY OF KELOIDS* REVIEW OF THE LITERATURE AND REPORT OF A FAMILY WITH MULTIPLE KELOIDS IN FIVE GENERATIONS. NEW YORK J. MED. 56* 511-519, 1956.

BOHROD, M. G.* KELOIDS AND SEXUAL SELECTION* A STUDY IN THE RACIAL DISTRIBUTION OF DISEASE. ARCH. DERM. SYPH. 36* 19-25, 1937.

COSMAN, B., CRIKELAIR, G. F., JU, D. M., GAULIN, J. C. AND LATTES, R.* THE SURGICAL TREATMENT OF KELOIDS. PLAST. RECONSTR. SURG. 27* 335-358, 1961.

*14820 KERATITIS FUGAX HEREDITARIA

VALLE (1964) DESCRIBED THIS AS A NEW ENTITY IN 10 MEMBERS OF 4 GENERATIONS. THE DISEASE BEGINS BETWEEN THE AGES OF 4 AND 12 YEARS AND IS CHARACTERIZED BY ACUTE ATTACKS OF KERATITIS OCCURRING 2 TO 8 TIMES A YEAR. NO PERMANENT CORNEAL OPACITIES RESULT. ATTACKS BECOME MILDER AND LESS FREQUENT AFTER AGE 50. ALSO SEE CORNEAL EROSIONS, RECURRING HEREDITARY.

VALLE, O.* KERATITIS FUGAX HEREDITARIA. DUODECIM 80* 659-664, 1964.

IRREGULAR AUTOSOMAL DOMINANT INHERITANCE WAS SUGGESTED BY FALLS AND ALLEN (1969), WHO OBSERVED AFFECTED AUNT AND NEICE. THE MOTHER WHO PRESUMABLY TRANSMITTED THE TRAIT HAD ASTIGMATISM AND OTHER FEATURES THEY INTERPRETED AS FORME FRUSTE OF KERATOCONUS. THEY SITED SEVERAL INSTANCES OF MULTIGENERATION INVOLVEMENT INCLUDING THE FAMILY OF STAHLI (1925) WITH TRANSMISSION THROUGH 3 GENERATIONS.

FALLS, H. F. AND ALLEN, A. W.* DOMINANTLY INHERITED KERATOCONUS. REPORT OF A FAMILY. J. GENET. HUM. 17* 317-324, 1969.

STAHLI, J.* WEITERE MITTEILUNGEN UBER DIE VERERBUNG DES KERATOCONUS. KLIN. MBL. AUGENHEILK. 75* 465-466, 1925.

*14840 KERATOSIS PALMARIS ET PLANTARIS FAMILIARIS (TYLOSIS)

THIS CONDITION IS CHARACTERIZED BY DIFFUSE HYPERKERATOSIS OF THE PALMS AND SOLES. THE CONDITION USUALLY BECOMES FIRST EVIDENT BETWEEN THE AGES OF 3 AND 12 MONTHS. LOW SERUM VITAMIN A HAS BEEN FOUND IN SOME CASES. THE FAMILY OF ANDERSON AND KLINTWORTH (1961) ALSO HAD CLINODACTYLY, PROBABLY AS AN INDEPENDENT TRAIT. IN ADDITION TO THE DIFFUSE TYPE REFERRED TO HERE A PUNCTATE TYPE (SEE KERATOSIS PALMO-PLANTARIS PAPULOSA) AND A LINEAR OR STRIATE FORM (SEE KERATOSIS PALMO-PLANTARIS STRIATA) ARE RECOGNIZED ON MORPHOLOGIC GROUNDS. IT IS QUITE POSSIBLE THAT THESE ARE GENETICALLY DISTINCT FROM THE DIFFUSE TYPE BUT SUCH CANNOT BE CONSIDERED PROVED. SEE HYPERKERATOSIS, LOCALIZED EPIDERMOLYTIC, FOR DESCRIPTION OF A CONDITION GROSSLY INDISTINGUISHABLE BUT HISTOLOGICALLY DIFFERENT. THIS DISORDER IS SOMETIMES REFERRED TO AS KERATOSIS OF GREITHER (1952).

ANDERSON, I. F. AND KLINTWORTH, G. K.* HYPOVITAMINOSIS-A IN A FAMILY WITH TYLOSIS AND CLINODACTYLY. BRIT. MED. J. 1* 1293-1297, 1961.

CHUNG, H.-L.* KERATOMA PALMARE ET PLANTARE HEREDITARIUM, WITH SPECIAL REFERENCE TO ITS MODE OF INHERITANCE AS TRACED IN SIX AND SEVEN GENERATIONS, RESPECTIVELY, IN TWO CHINESE FAMILIES. ARCH. DERM. SYPH. 36* 303-313, 1937.

GREITHER, A.* KERATOSIS EXTREMITATUM HEREDITARIA PROGREDIENS MIT DOMINANTEM ERBGANG. HAUTARZT 3* 198-203, 1952.

KLINTWORTH, G. K. AND ANDERSON, I. F.* TYLOSIS PALMARIS ET PLANTARIS FAMILIARIS ASSOCIATED WITH CLINODACTYLY. S. AFR. MED. J. 35* 170-175, 1961.

*14850 KERATOSIS PALMARIS ET PLANTARIS WITH ESOPHAGEAL CANCER

THE SAME DISORDER AS THAT DESCRIBED ABOVE WAS ASSOCIATED WITH ESOPHAGEAL CANCER IN THE TWO KINDREDS (WHICH PERHAPS ARE RELATED) STUDIED IN LIVERPOOL BY HOWEL-EVANS AND COLLEAGUES (1958). THE DISORDER IS APPARENTLY DISTINCT. WHETHER ALLELIC WITH THE OTHER FORM IS UNKNOWN. FROM OXFORD, SHINE AND ALLISON (1966) DESCRIBED ANOTHER FAMILY IN WHICH MULTIPLE MEMBERS SHOWED THE ASSOCIATION. AFFECTED MEMBERS SHOWED CONGENITAL SLIDING HIATAL HERNIA AND LOWER ESOPHAGUS LINED BY GASTRIC MUCOSA. HARPER ET AL. (1970) GAVE FURTHER INFORMATION ON THE LIVERPOOL FAMILIES AND ADDED TWO FURTHER FAMILIES EACH WITH ONE CASE OF ESOPHAGEAL CANCER WITH TYLOSIS. AGE OF ONSET OF THE TYLOSIS APPEARS TO BE A FEATURE DISTINGUISHING THE CANCER-PRONE FROM THE NONPRONE FORM. TYLOSIS IS LATE IN ONSET IN THE FORM WITH ESOPHAGEAL CANCER.

HARPER, P. S., HARPER, R. M. J. AND HOWEL-EVANS, A. W.* CARCINOMA OF THE OESOPHAGUS WITH TYLOSIS. QUART. J. MED. 39* 317-333, 1970.

HOWEL-EVANS, W., MCCONNELL, R. B., CLARKE, C. A. AND SHEPPARD, P. M.* CARCINOMA OF THE OESOPHAGUS WITH KERATOSIS PALMARIS ET PLANTARIS (TYLOSIS)* A STUDY OF TWO FAMILIES. QUART. J. MED. 27* 413-429, 1958.

SHINE, I. AND ALLISON, P. R.* CARCINOMA OF THE ESOPHAGUS WITH TYLOSIS. LANCET 1* 951-953, 1966.

14860 KERATOSIS PALMO-PLANTARIS PAPULOSA

LATE ONSET COMPLICATES GENETIC STUDY. IN 14 FAMILIES REPORTED BY SCHIRREN AND DINGER (1965) DIRECT TRANSMISSION WAS OBSERVED. FEMALES ARE LESS SEVERELY INVOLVED.

SCHIRREN, V. AND DINGER, R.* UNTERSUCHUNGEN BEI KERATOSIS PALMO-PLANTARIS PAPULOSA. ARCH. KLIN. EXP. DERM. 221* 481-495, 1965.

14870 KERATOSIS PALMO-PLANTARIS STRIATA

THE LESIONS OF THE HANDS CONSIST OF A STREAK OF HYPERKERATOSIS RUNNING THE LENGTH OF EACH FINGER AND ONTO THE PALM. BOLOGNA (1966) REPORTED A CASE IN WHICH INVOLVEMENT OF MALES PREDOMINATED IN A STRIKING MANNER.

BOLOGNA, E. I.* DOMINANT VEREBLICHE DURCH VIER GENERATIONEN GESCHLECHTSGEBUN-DENE KERATOSIS PALMARIS STRIATA (LINEARIA). DERM. WSCHR. 152* 446-457, 1966.

ONLY A FEW DOZEN CASES HAVE BEEN DESCRIBED, ALL SPORADIC. THE HEAD HAS A FLATTENED, TRILOBULAR CONFIGURATION, CAUSED BY HYDROCEPHALUS IN COMBINATION WITH CONGENITAL SYNOSTOSIS OF THE CORONAL AND LAMBDOIDAL SUTURES. IN THE MOST SEVERE FORM THERE IS GROTESQUE EXOPHTHALMOS WITH CORNEAL ULCERATIONS. BONY DEFORMITIES AND ANKYLOSIS AT THE ELBOWS OCCUR IN SOME CASES. NOTHING IS KNOWN OF A POSSIBLE GENETIC BASIS. PATERNAL AGE EFFECT SHOULD BE SOUGHT.

ANGEL, C. R., MCINTRYE, M. S. AND MOORE, R. C.* CLOVERLEAF SKULL* KLEEBLATTS-CHADEL-DEFORMITY SYNDROME. AM. J. DIS. CHILD. 114* 198-202, 1967.

GRUBER, G. B.* UBER EINEN AKROCEPHALEN RELIEFSCHADEL. EIN BIETRAG ZUR FRAGE DER PARTIELLEN CHONDRODYSTROPHIE. BIETR. PATH. ANAT. 97* 9-21, 1936.

HOLTERMUELLER, K. AND WIEDEMANN, H. R.* THE CLOVER-LEAF SKULL SYNDROME. MED. MSCHR. 14* 439-446, 1960.

WELTER, H.* ZUR FRAGE DES HYDROCEPHALUS CHONDRODYSTROPHICUS CONGENITUS. BEITR. PATH. ANAT. 97* 1-8, 1936.

14890 KLIPPEL-FEIL SYNDROME

DOMINANT INHERITANCE WITH REDUCED PENETRANCE AND VARIABLE EXPRESSION IS SUGGESTED BY SEVERAL REPORTS INCLUDING THOSE OF BAUMAN (1932), BIZARRO (1938), CLEMMESEN (1936), ERSKINE (1946) AND JARCHO AND LEVIN (1938). THERE ARE CLEARLY SEVERAL ENTITIES IN THIS GENERAL CATEGORY. ONE OR MORE MAY BE RECESSIVE AND SOME MAY HAVE NO SIMPLE GENETIC BASIS (LUBS, PERSONAL COMMUNICATION). KLIPPEL AND FEIL RECOGNIZED THREE MORPHOLOGIC TYPES OF CERVICAL VERTEBRAL FUSION* I. MASSIVE FUSION OF MANY CERVICAL AND UPPER THORACIC VERTEBRAE INTO BONY BLOCKS. II. FUSION AT ONLY ONE OR TWO INTERSPACES, ALTHOUGH HEMIVERTEBRAE, OCCIPITO-ATLANTAL FUSION, AND OTHER ANOMALIES MIGHT BE ASSOCIATED. III. BOTH CERVICAL FUSION AND LOWER THORACIC OR LUMBAR FUSION. GUNDERSON, GREENSPAN, GLASER AND LUBS (1967) DID FAMILY STUDIES. C2-3 FUSION, A SUBTYPE OF CATEGORY II, MAY BE A SIMPLE DOMINANT.

BAUMAN, G. I.* ABSENCE OF THE CERVICAL SPINE. KLIPPEL-FEIL SYNDROME. J.A.M.A. 98* 129-132, 1932.

BIZARRO, A. H.* BREVICOLLIS. LANCET 2* 828-829, 1938.

CLEMMESEN, V.* CONGENITAL CERVICAL SYNOSTOSIS (KLIPPEL-FEIL'S SYNDROME)* FOUR CASES. ACTA RADIOL. 17* 480-490, 1936.

ERSKINE, C. A.* AN ANALYSIS OF THE KLIPPEL-FEIL SYNDROME. ARCH. PATH. 41* 269-281, 1946.

JARCHO, S. AND LEVIN, P. M.* HEREDITARY MALFORMATION OF THE VERTEBRAL BODIES. BULL. HOPKINS HOSP. 62* 216-226, 1938.

14900 KLIPPEL-TRENAUNAY-WEBER SYNDROME

THE FEATURES ARE LARGE CUTANEOUS HEMANGIOMATA WITH HYPERTROPHY OF THE RELATED BONES AND SOFT TISSUES. IT RESEMBLES, CLINICALLY AND IN ITS LACK OF DEFINITE GENETIC BASIS, STURGE-WEBER SYNDROME AND INDEED THE TWO HAVE BEEN ASSOCIATED IN SOME CASES. SUGGESTIONS OF A GENETIC *CAUSE* ARE MEAGER (WAARDENBURG, 1963). SEE HEMANGIOMAS.

BROOKSALER, F.* THE ANGIOOSTEOHYPERTROPHY SYNDROME (KLIPPEL-TRENAUNAY-WEBER SYNDROME). AM. J. DIS. CHILD. 112* 161-164, 1966.

KOCH, G.* ZUR KLINIK, SYMPTOMATOLOGIE, PATHOGENESE UND ERBPATHOLOGIE DES KLIPPEL-TRENAUNAY-WEBER-SCHEN SYNDROM. ACTA GENET. MED. GEM. 5* 326-370, 1956.

WAARDENBURG, P. J.* HYPERTROPHIC HAEMANGIECTASIA (KLIPPEL-TRENAUNAY-WEBER'S SYNDROME). IN, GENETICS AND OPHTHALMOLOGY. SPRINGFIELD, ILL.* CHARLES C THOMAS, 2* 1381-1386, 1963.

14910 KNUCKLE PADS

THESE ARE SOMETIMES ASSOCIATED WITH DUPUYTREN'S CONTRACTURES (Q.V.) AND IT IS NOT COMPLETELY CERTAIN THAT A DIFFERENT GENE IS INVOLVED. CAMPTODACTYLY (Q.V.) ALSO HAS AN UNCERTAIN RELATIONSHIP.

ALLISON, J. R., JR. AND ALLISON, J. R., SR.* KNUCKLE PADS. ARCH. DERM. 93* 311-316, 1966.

GARROD, A. E.* CONCERNING PADS UPON THE FINGER JOINTS AND THEIR CLINICAL RELATIONSHIP. BRIT. MED. J. 2* 8 ONLY, 1904.

WEBER, F. P.* A NOTE ON DUPUYTREN'S CONTRACTION, CAMPTODACTYLIA AND KNUCKLE-PADS. BRIT. J. DERM. SYPH. 50* 26-31, 1938.

*14920 KNUCKLE PADS, LEUKONYCHIA AND SENSINEURAL DEAFNESS

BART ET AL. (1967) DESCRIBED A KINDRED IN WHICH MANY MEMBERS HAD KNUCKLE PADS, LEUKONYCHIA AND DEAFNESS DUE TO A LESION OF THE COCHLEA. KERATOSIS PALMARIS ET PLANTARIS WAS PRESENT IN SOME.   MALE-TO-MALE TRANSMISSION WAS THOUGHT TO HAVE OCCURRED IN TWO INSTANCES. THE CONDITION DESCRIBED BY SCHWANN (1963) WAS PROBABLY THE SAME.   THE PRESENCE OF LEUKONYCHIA AND THE ABSENCE OF DIGITAL CONSTRICTIONS APPEAR TO DISTINGUISH THIS DISORDER FROM THE ONE LISTED AS 'DEAFNESS, CONGENITAL, WITH KERATOPACHYDERMIA AND CONSTRICTIONS OF FINGERS AND TOES' (Q.V.).

BART, R. S. AND PUMPHREY, R. E.* KNUCKLE PADS, LEUKONYCHIA AND DEAFNESS - A DOMINANTLY INHERITED SYNDROME. NEW ENG. J. MED. 276* 202-207, 1967.

SCHWANN, J.* KERATOSIS PALMARIS ET PLANTARIS CUM SURDITATE CONGENITA ET LEUCONYCHIA TOTALI UNGUIUM. DERMATOLOGICA 126* 335-353, 1963.

*14930 KOILONYCHIA, HEREDITARY

HEIDENSLEBEN (1960) OBSERVED KOILONYCHIA IN FATHER AND CHILD. THE CHILD ALSO HAD CATARACT. BERGESON AND STONE (1967) REPORTED 12 AFFECTED PERSONS IN 4 GENERATIONS WITH SEVERAL INSTANCES OF MALE-TO-MALE TRANSMISSION. HELLIER (1950) REPORTED 16 AFFECTED IN 5 GENERATIONS. SCHLEUTERMANN ET AL. (1970) DESCRIBED EIGHT AFFECTED PERSONS IN 5 GENERATIONS WITH NO MALE-TO-MALE TRANSMISSION AND NO CLEAR EVIDENCE OF CLOSE LINKAGE. LINKAGE WITH THE ABO LOCUS WAS EXCLUDED.

BERGESON, J. R. AND STONE, O. J.* KOILONYCHIA. A REPORT OF FAMILIAL SPOON NAILS. ARCH. DERM. 95* 351-353, 1967.

GRACIANSKY, P. DE AND BOVLLE, S.* ASSOCIATION DE KOILONYCHIE ET DE LEUKONYCHIE TRANSMISES EN DOMINANCE. BULL. SOC. FRANC. DERM. SYPH. 68* 15-17, 1961.

HEIDENSLEBEN, E.* HEREDITARY CONGENITAL KOILONYCHAE ACCOMPANIED BY SYNDERMATO-TIC CATARACT. ACTA OPHTHAL. 38* 1-4, 1960.

HELLIER, F. F.* HEREDITARY KOILONYCHIA. BRIT. J. DERM. 62* 213-214, 1950.

SCHLEUTERMANN, D. A., BIAS, W. B. AND MCKUSICK, V. A.* A KINDRED OF KOILONY-CHIA* LINKAGE DATA. AM. J. HUM. GENET. 22* 390-395, 1970.

*14940 KOK'S DISEASE

KOK AND BRUYN (1962) DESCRIBED A 'NEW' HEREDITARY DISEASE, INHERITED AS AN AUTOSOMAL DOMINANT AND CHARACTERIZED BY ONSET AT BIRTH WITH HYPERTONIA IN FLEXION WHICH DISAPPEARS IN SLEEP, EXAGGERATED STARTLE RESPONSE, STRONG BRAIN-STEM REFLEXES (ESPECIALLY HEAD-RETRACTION REFLEX) AND, IN SOME, EPILEPSY. THERE WERE 29 AFFECTED PERSONS IN SIX GENERATIONS. HYPERTONIA DIMINISHED DURING THE COURSE OF THE FIRST YEAR OF LIFE. THE STARTLE REFLEX WAS SOMETIMES ACCOMPANIED BY ACUTE GENERALIZED HYPERTONIA CAUSING THE PATIENT TO FALL LIKE A LOG TO THE GROUND. THE DESCRIPTION IS SOMEWHAT REMINISCENT OF THE 'JUMPING FRENCHMEN OF MAINE' (STEVENS, 1966). ALSO SEE HYPER-REFLEXIA, HEREDITARY.

KOK, O. AND BRUYN, G. W.* AN UNIDENTIFIED HEREDITARY DISEASE. (LETTER) LANCET 1* 1359 ONLY, 1962.

STEVENS, H.* JUMPING FRENCHMEN OF MAINE. ARCH. NEUROL. 12* 311-314, 1966.

*14950 KYPHOSCOLIOSIS, OSTEOPENIA, CONGENITAL CONTRACTURES

EPSTEIN ET AL. (1968) DESCRIBED FATHER AND SON WITH A CONNECTIVE TISSUE DISORDER WITH SOME FEATURES SUGGESTING THE MARFAN SYNDROME AND SOME SUGGESTING OSTEOGENESIS IMPERFECTA. SEVERE KYPHOSCOLIOSIS, GENERALIZED OSTEOPENIA, FLEXION CONTRACTURES OF THE FINGERS AND ABNORMALLY SHAPED EARS WERE AMONG THE CHARACTERISTICS. BEALS AND HECHT (1971) DESCRIBED FATHER AND TWO SONS AFFECTED IN ONE KINDRED AND FATHER, DAUGHTER AND SON (BY DIFFERENT MOTHERS) AFFECTED IN A SECOND KINDRED. THEY PROPOSED THAT THE DISORDER BE CALLED 'CONTRACTURAL ARACHNODACTYLY' AND FURTHER SUGGESTED THAT MARFAN'S PATIENT (1896) DID NOT HAVE THE MARFAN SYNDROME AS PRESENTLY DELINEATED BUT THIS DISORDER. THEY FOUND SEVERAL OTHER REPORTS APPARENTLY OF THE SAME DISORDER IN THE LITERATURE.

BEALS, R. K. AND HECHT, F.* CONTRACTURAL ARACHNODACTYLY, A HERITABLE DISORDER OF CONNECTIVE TISSUE. J. BONE JOINT SURG., IN PRESS, 1971.

EPSTEIN, C. J., GRAHAM, C. B., HODGKIN, W. E., HECHT, F. AND MOTULSKY, A. G.* HEREDITARY DYSPLASIA OF BONE WITH KYPHOSCOLIOSIS, CONTRACTURES, AND ABNORMALLY SHAPED EARS. J. PEDIAT. 73* 379-386, 1968.

MARFAN, A. B.* UN CAS DE DEFORMATION CONGENITALE DES QUATRE MEMBRES PLUS PRONONCEE AUX EXTREMITIES, CHARACTERISEE PAR L'ALLONGEMENT DES OS AVEC UN CERTAIN DEGRE D'AMINCISSEMENT. BULL. MEM. SOC. MED. HOP. PARIS 13* 220-226, 1896.

D
O
M
I
N
A
N
T

BARBOSA SUEIRO AND PILOTO (1964) REPORTED 5 CASES OCCURRING IN 4 GENERATIONS OF A FAMILY. THE LDH-B LOCUS IS LINKED TO THAT FOR PEPTIDASE B (SILVANA SANTACHIARA ET AL., 1970).

BARBOSA SUEIRO, M. B. AND PILOTO, R.* ADERENCIA INCOMPLETA DOS PEQUENOS LABIOS COM CARACTER FAMILIAR. ARQU. ANAT. ANTROP. 32* 187-192, 1964.

SILVANA SANTACHIARA, A., NABHOLZ, M., MIGGIANO, V., DARLINGTON, A. J. AND BODMER, W.* LINKAGE BETWEEN HUMAN LACTATE DEHYDROGENASE B AND PEPTIDASE B GENES. NATURE 227* 248-251, 1970.

*14970 LACRIMAL DUCT DEFECT

SCHNYDER (1920) DESCRIBED A DEFECT OF THE TEAR DUCTS IN MEMBERS OF THREE GENERA-TIONS OF A FAMILY. IMPERFORATE NASO-LACRIMAL DUCTS WITH OR WITHOUT ABSENCE OF PUNCTA AND CANALICULI HAS BEEN DESCRIBED IN A DOMINANT PEDIGREE PATTERN BY BISCHLER (1957), LUMBROSO (1960), TOWN (1943) AND OTHERS. SEE ALSO ORBITAL MARGIN, HYPOPLASIA OF. SEE ALSO CLEFT LIP-PALATE WITH SPLIT HAND AND FOOT.

BISCHLER, V.* LE FACTEUR HEREDITAIRE DANS OBSTRUCTIONS DES VOIES LACRYMALES ET PLUS PARTICULIEREMENT DANS L*ATRESIE DES POINTS ET CANALICULES LACRYMAUX. MOD. PROB. OPHTHAL. 1* 584-590, 1957.

LUMBROSO, B. D.* ON A CASE OF CONGENITAL ATRESIA OF THE LACRIMAL DUCTS WITH FAMILIAL CHARACTERISTICS. ACTA GENET. MED. GEM. 9* 290-295, 1960.

SCHNYDER, W. F.* UBER FAMILIARES VORKOMMEN RESP. DIE VERERBUNG VON ERKRANKUN-GEN DER TRANENWEGE. Z. AUGENHEILK. 44* 257-261, 1920.

TOWN, A. E.* CONGENITAL ABSENCE OF LACRIMAL PUNCTA IN THREE MEMBERS OF A FAMILY. ARCH. OPHTHAL. 29* 767-771, 1943.

14980 LACTIC ACIDOSIS, CHRONIC ADULT FORM

SUSSMAN ET AL. (1970) DESCRIBED A 28 YEAR OLD WOMAN WITH CHRONICALLY ELEVATED LACTIC ACID, PYRUVIC ACID AND INCREASED LACTATE-TO-PYRUVATE RATIO. ALCOHOL INGESTION AND MODERATE EXERCISE INCREASED LACTATE LEVELS. HYPERURICEMIA WAS PRESENT AS IN GLYCOGEN STORAGE DISEASE AND AS IN THAT CONDITION URIC ACID CLEARANCE WAS APPARENTLY DEPRESSED. THE MOTHER AND THREE OF THE MOTHER*S SIBS ALSO SHOWED ABNORMAL LACTATE RESPONSE TO THE COMBINATION OF ALCOHOL INGESTION AND EXERCISE.

SUSSMAN, K. E., ALFREY, A., KIRSCH, W. M., ZWEIG, P., FELIG, P. AND MESSNER, F.* CHRONIC LACTIC ACIDOSIS IN AN ADULT. A NEW SYNDROME ASSOCIATED WITH AN ALTERED REDOX STATE OF CERTAIN NAD-NADH COUPLED REACTIONS. AM. J. MED. 48* 104-112, 1970.

*14990 LACTIC DEHYDROGENASE VARIANT X OF TESTIS

ZINKHAM ET AL. (1964) HAVE FOUND A DISTINCTIVE LDH ISOZYME IN MATURE TESTIS OF MANY SPECIES INCLUDING MAN. IT IS POLYMORPHIC IN THE PIGEON WHERE ONE CAN INFER THAT A LOCUS SEPARATE FROM THE A AND B LOCI CONTROL IT. THE SAME IS ALMOST CERTAINLY TRUE IN THE HUMAN ALSO. THIS IS A GENE WHICH FUNCTIONS ONLY IN ONE SEX AND ONLY IN ONE TISSUE. THE LOCUS DETERMINING THE TESTICULAR VARIANT X IS CALLED LDH(C). ZINKHAM ET AL. (1969) FOUND THAT THE B AND C LOCI ARE CLOSELY LINKED, POSSIBLY CONTIGUOUS.

BLANCO, A., ZINKHAM, W. H. AND KUPCHYK, L.* GENETIC CONTROL AND ONTOGENY OF LACTATE DEHYDROGENASE IN PIGEON TESTES. J. EXP. ZOOL. 156* 137-152, 1964.

ZINKHAM, W. H., BLANCO, A. AND CLOWRY, L. J., JR.* AN UNUSUAL ISOZYME OF LACTIC DEHYDROGENASE IN MATURE TESTES* LOCALIZATION, ONTOGENY, AND KINETIC PROPERTIES. ANN. N.Y. ACAD. SCI. 121* 571-588, 1964.

ZINKHAM, W. H., BLANCO, A. AND KUPCHYK, L.* LACTATE DEHYDROGENASE IN PIGEON TESTES* GENETIC CONTROL BY THREE LOCI. SCIENCE 144* 1353-1354, 1964.

ZINKHAM, W. H., ISENSEE, H. AND RENWICK, J. H.* LINKAGE OF LACTATE DEHYDRO-GENASE B AND C LOCI IN PIGEONS. SCIENCE 164* 185-187, 1969.

15000 LACTIC DEHYDROGENASE VARIANTS IN SERUM VARIANTS OF SUBUNIT A

BOYER, FAINER AND WATSON-WILLIAMS (1963) DETECTED AN ELECTROPHORETIC VARIANT OF THE B SUBUNIT OF LDH. FAMILY STUDIES COULD NOT BE DONE. THE PATTERN WAS CONSISTENT WITH THE HYPOTHESIS THAT LDH ISOZYMES ARE TETRAMERS OF TWO DIFFERENT SUBUNITS. IN THE HETEROZYGOTE LDH-1, -2, -3, -4 AND -5 OCCUR IN PROPORTIONS 1 * 4 * 6 * 4 * 1, AS IN MARKERT*S DISSOCIATION-REASSOCIATION EXPERIMENTS.
NANCE, CLAFLIN AND SMITHIES (1963) OBSERVED A GENETICALLY DETERMINED VARIANT LDH IN THE RED CELLS OF FOUR MEMBERS OF TWO GENERATIONS OF A BRAZILIAN FAMILY. THE MUTATION INVOLVES THE A SUBUNIT. CLOSE LINKAGE WITH MNS, HAPTOGLOBIN AND GM

LOCI WAS EXCLUDED. THIS IS THE FIRST INSTANCE IN WHICH PRACTICAL CONSIDERATIONS PERMITTED DEMONSTRATION OF THE VARIANT IN MULTIPLE RELATIVES. UNLIKE THE FINDINGS OF SHAW AND BARTO (1963) IN PEROMYSCUS AND OF BOYER, FAINER AND WATSON-WILLIAMS IN MAN, THE FINDINGS IN THE BRAZILIAN FAMILY DID NOT SUGGEST RANDOM ASSOCIATION BETWEEN THE PRODUCTS OF THE MUTANT AND WILD TYPE ALLELES. IN TROUT THE LOCI CODING FOR SUBUNITS A AND B ARE LINKED (MORRISON AND WRIGHT, 1966). STUDIES USING HUMAN-MOUSE SOMATIC CELL HYBRIDS INDICATE THAT THE LDH-A AND LDH-B LOCI ARE NOT LINKED (NABHOLZ ET AL., 1969). LDH VARIANTS, INVOLVING EITHER THE A OR THE B SUBUNIT, SEEM TO BE UNUSUALLY FREQUENT IN INDIA (DAS ET AL., 1970).

BLAKE, N. M., KIRK, R. L., PRYKE, E. AND SINNETT, P.* LACTATE DEHYDROGENASE ELECTROPHORETIC VARIANT IN A NEW GUINEA HIGHLAND POPULATION. SCIENCE 163* 701-702, 1969.

BOYER, S. H., FAINER, D. C. AND WATSON-WILLIAMS, E. J.* LACTATE DEHYDROGENASE VARIANT FROM HUMAN BLOOD* EVIDENCE FOR MOLECULAR SUBUNITS. SCIENCE 141* 642-643, 1963.

DAS, S. R., MUKHERJEE, B. N., DAS, S. K., ANANTHAKRISHNAN, R., BLAKE, N. M. AND KIRK, R. L.* LDH VARIANTS IN INDIA. HUMANGENETIK 9* 107-109, 1970.

DAVIDSON, R. G., FILDES, R. A., GLEN-BOTT, A. M., HARRIS, H., ROBSON, E. B. AND CLEGHORN, T. E.* GENETICAL STUDIES ON A VARIANT OF HUMAN LACTATE DEHYDROGENASE (SUBUNIT A). ANN. HUM. GENET. 29* 5-17, 1965.

MORRISON, W. J. AND WRIGHT, J. E.* GENETIC ANALYSIS OF THREE LACTATE DEHYDRO-GENASE ISOZYME SYSTEMS IN TROUT* EVIDENCE FOR LINKAGE OF GENES CODING SUBUNITS A AND B. J. EXP. ZOOL. 163* 259-270, 1966.

NABHOLZ, M., MIGGIANO, V. AND BODMER, W.* GENETIC ANALYSIS WITH HUMAN-MOUSE SOMATIC CELL HYBRIDS. NATURE 223* 358-363, 1969.

NANCE, W. E., CLAFLIN, A. AND SMITHIES, O.* LACTIC DEHYDROGENASE* GENETIC CONTROL IN MAN. SCIENCE 142* 1075-1077, 1963.

SHAW, C. R. AND BARTO, E.* GENETIC EVIDENCE FOR THE SUBUNIT STRUCTURE OF LACTATE DEHYDROGENASE ISOZYMES. PROC. NAT. ACAD. SCI. 50* 211-214, 1963.

VESELL, E. S.* GENETIC CONTROL OF ISOZYME PATTERNS IN HUMAN TISSUE. PROGRESS IN MEDICAL GENETICS. STEINBERG, A. G. AND BEARN, A. G. (EDS.)* NEW YORK* GRUNE AND STRATTON, 4* 1965.

15010 LACTIC DEHYDROGENASE VARIANTS IN SERUM VARIANTS OF SUBUNIT B

SEE ABOVE.

15020 LAMINA DURA, ABSENCE OF

ORDINARY ABSENCE OF THE LAMINA DURA OF THE TEETH, AS DETECTED BY X-RAY, DIAGNOSIS OF HYPERPARATHYROIDISM. HOWEVER, GRAHAM ET AL. (1965) FOUND SUCH IN A FATHER AND TWO DAUGHTERS WITH NO EVIDENCE OF DERANGED CALCIUM OR PHOSPHORUS METABOLISM. DENTIN WAS ABNORMAL MAKING THIS A PRIMARY DISORDER OF THE TEETH.

GRAHAM, W. L., HARLEY, J. B., ALBERICO, C. AND KELLN, E. E.* ABSENT LAMINA DURA ASSOCIATED WITH A DEVELOPMENTAL DENTIN ABNORMALITY. A FAMILY STUDY. ARCH. INTERN. MED. 116* 837-841, 1965.

15030 LARYNX, CONGENITAL PARTIAL ATRESIA OF

BAKER AND SAVETSKY (1966) DESCRIBED AFFECTED MOTHER AND 2 CHILDREN.

BAKER, D. C., JR. AND SAVETSKY, L.* CONGENITAL PARTIAL ATRESIA OF THE LARYNX. LARYNGOSCOPE 76* 616-620, 1966.

*15040 LATERAL INCISORS, ABSENCE OF

THE UPPER LATERAL INCISORS ARE ABSENT OR HYPOPLASTIC. A POINTED TOOTH IS A PARTIAL EXPRESSION OF THE GENE. THE TRAIT WAS PRESENT IN ONE-THIRD OF A SWISS GROUP STUDIED BY JOHR (1934). FURTHERMORE, ALL AFFECTED MEMBERS OF THE ISOLATE WERE DESCENDANTS OF ONE MAN, BORN IN THE 18TH CENTURY. SCHULTZ (1934) FOUND THE CONDITION IN ONE GORILLA AND ONE GIBBON.

GRAHNEN, H.* HYPODONTIA IN THE PERMANENT DENTITION. ODONT. REV. 7 (SUPPL. 3)* 419-421, 1965.

JOHR, A. C.* REDUKTIONSERSCHEINUNGEN AN DEN OBEREN SEITLICHEN SCHNEIDEZAHNEN. ARCH. KLAUS. STIFT. VERERBUNGSFORSCH. 9* 73-133, 1934.

KEELER, C. E. AND SHORT, R.* HEREDITARY ABSENCE OF UPPER LATERAL INCISORS. J. HERED. 25* 391-392, 1934.

MANDEVILLE, L. C.* CONGENITAL ABSENCE OF PERMANENT MAXILLARY LATERAL INCISOR

TEETH. A PRELIMINARY INVESTIGATION. ANN. EUGEN. 15* 1-10, 1950.

MONTAGU, M. F. A.* THE SIGNIFICANCE OF THE VARIABILITY OF THE UPPER LATERAL INCISOR TEETH IN MAN. HUM. BIOL. 12* 323-358, 1940.

RANTANEN, A. V.* ON THE FREQUENCY OF THE MISSING AND PEG-SHAPED MAXILLARY LATERAL INCISOR AMONG FINNISH STUDENTS. AM. J. PHYS. ANTHROP. 14* 491-496, 1956.

SCHULTZ, A. H.* INHERITED REDUCTIONS IN THE DENTITION OF MAN. HUM. BIOL. 6* 627-631, 1934.

SCHULTZ, A. H.* THE HEREDITARY TENDENCY TO ELIMINATE THE UPPER LATERAL INCISORS. HUM. BIOL. 4* 34-40, 1932.

WITKOP, C. J.* STUDIES OF INTRINSIC DISEASE IN ISOLATES WITH OBSERVATIONS ON PENETRANCE AND EXPRESSIVITY OF CERTAIN ANATOMICAL TRAITS. IN, CONGENITAL ANOMALIES OF THE FACE AND ASSOCIATED STRUCTURES. PRUZANSKY, S. (ED.)* SPRINGFIELD, ILL.* CHARLES C THOMAS, 1961.

15050 LATTICE DEGENERATION OF RETINA LEADING TO RETINAL DETACHMENT

LATTICE DEGENERATION OF THE RETINA WITH LATER DEVELOPMENT OF RETINAL DETACHMENT IN MANY NON-MYOPIC PERSONS WAS OBSERVED BY EVERETT (1968). THE FAMILIAL OCCURRENCE OF LATTICE DEGENERATION IN NON-MYOPES WAS EARLIER REPORTED BY GARTNER (1960).

EVERETT, W. G.* STUDY OF A FAMILY WITH LATTICE DEGENERATION AND RETINAL DETACHMENT. AM. J. OPHTHAL. 65* 229-232, 1968.

GARTNER, J.* ERBBEDINGTE AQUATORIALE DEGENERATIONEN NICHTMYOPER* SOLITARFORMEN UND ORAPARALLELE BANDER. KLIN. MBL. AUGENHEILK. 136* 523-539, 1960.

15060 LEGG-CALVE-PERTHES DISEASE

WAMOSHER AND FARHI (1963) DESCRIBED A JEWISH FAMILY IN WHICH 8 MEMBERS OF 3 GENERATIONS WERE AFFECTED. BOYS PREDOMINATE HEAVILY IN ALL REPORTS OF SPORADIC CASES OF THE DISEASE. IN THE FAMILIES WITH MULTIPLE CASES THE SEX RATIO HAS BEEN CLOSER TO 1. A SIMILAR PHENOMENON HAS BEEN OBSERVED IN ANKYLOSING SPONDYLITIS (Q.V.) AND IN CONGENITAL DISLOCATION OF THE HIP. WHEN FAMILIAL THE DISORDER MAY BE MORE LIKELY TO SHOW BILATERAL INVOLVEMENT. MCNUTT (1962) SUGGESTED THAT A PECULIARITY IN VASCULAR SUPPLY OF THE FEMORAL HEAD AND NECK MAY BE INHERITED AS THE FACTOR PREDISPOSING TO THIS DISORDER. I HAVE SEEN AFFECTED FATHER AND TWO SONS. STEPHENS AND KERBY (1946) OBSERVED MANY AFFECTED PERSONS IN FIVE GENERATIONS. CAFFEY (1968) IS OF THE VIEW THAT COXA PLANA, AS HE TERMS THIS CONDITION, REALLY REPRESENTS AT LEAST IN ITS INITIATION A STRESS FRACTURE AND NOT AVASCULAR NECROSIS.

CAFFEY, J.* THE EARLY ROENTGENOGRAPHIC CHANGES IN ESSENTIAL COXA PLANA* THEIR SIGNIFICANCE IN PATHOGENESIS. AM. J. ROENTGEN. 103* 620-634, 1968.

GOFF, C. W.* LEGG-CALVE-PERTHES SYNDROME (LCPS). AN UP-TO-DATE CRITICAL REVIEW. CLIN. ORTHOP. 22* 93-107, 1962.

MCNUTT, W.* INHERITED VASCULAR PATTERN OF THE FEMORAL HEAD AND NECK AS A PREDISPOSING FACTOR TO LEGG-CALVE-PERTHES DISEASE. TEXAS REP. BIOL. MED. 20* 525-531, 1962.

STEPHENS, F. E. AND KERBY, J. P.* HEREDITARY LEGG-CALVE-PERTHES DISEASE. J. HERED. 37* 153-160, 1946.

WAMOSCHER, Z. AND FARHI, A.* HEREDITARY LEGG-CALVE-PERTHES DISEASE. AM. J. DIS. CHILD. 106* 97-100, 1963.

15070 LEIOMYOMA OF VULVA AND ESOPHAGUS

WAHLEN AND ASTEDT (1965) DESCRIBED THIS COMBINATION IN MOTHER AND DAUGHTER. THE ESOPHAGEAL TUMOR WAS AN OBSTRUCTING LESION IN THE LOWER PORTION. IN BOTH WOMEN THE PRESENTING COMPLAINT WITH REFERENCE TO THE VULVAL LESIONS WAS ENLARGEMENT OF THE CLITORIS DUE TO GROWTH OF THE TUMOR AT ITS BASE. CHROMOSOME AND ENDOCRINOLOGIC STUDIED SHOWED NOTHING ABNORMAL. THE AUTHORS EMPHASIZED THAT LEIOMYOMA OF THE VULVA SHOULD PROMPT X-RAY STUDIES OF THE ESOPHAGUS AND LEIOMYOMA OF THE ESOPHAGUS SHOULD PROMPT SEARCH FOR VULVAL LEIOMYOMA.

WAHLEN, T. AND ASTEDT, B.* FAMILIAL OCCURRENCE OF COEXISTING LEIOMYOMA OF VULVA AND OESOPHAGUS. ACTA OBSTET. GYNEC. SCAND. 44* 197-203, 1965.

*15080 LEIOMYOMATA, HEREDITARY MULTIPLE, OF SKIN

MULTIPLE SMALL TUMORS COMPOSED OF SMOOTH MUSCLE FIBERS DEVELOP IN THE SKIN. MALIGNANT TRANSFORMATION IS RARE. THE TUMORS ARE THOUGHT TO ARISE FROM THE ARRECTOR PILORUM MUSCLES. THE PEDIGREE AS REPORTED BY KLOEPFER ET AL. (1958) WAS MORE SUGGESTIVE OF RECESSIVE INHERITANCE (Q.V.) THAN OF DOMINANT INHERITANCE AS THEY SUGGESTED. HOWEVER, SEVERAL CRITICAL MEMBERS OF THE PEDIGREE WERE NOT

AVAILABLE FOR EXAMINATION. DOMINANT INHERITANCE WITH INCOMPLETE PENETRANCE IS
SUPPORTED BY THE PEDIGREE OF MEZZADRA (1965), WHO DESCRIBED CUTANEOUS LEIOMYOMATA
IN 3 GENERATIONS. UTERINE MYOMATA WERE ASSOCIATED. THIS AND KLOEPFER'S FAMILY
WERE ITALIAN. WEILBAECHER (1967) OBSERVED A SWEDISH FAMILY WITH FIVE AFFECTED IN
THREE GENERATIONS AND MALE-TO-MALE TRANSMISSION.

KLOEPFER, H. W., KRAFCHUK, J., DERBES, V. AND BURKS, J.* HEREDITARY MULTIPLE
LEIOMYOMA OF THE SKIN. AM. J. HUM. GENET. 10* 48-52, 1958.

MEZZADRA, G.* LEIOMIOMA CUTANEO MULTIPLO EREDITARIO. STUDIO DI UN CASO
SISTEMATIZZATO IN SOGGETTO MASCHILE APPARTENENTE A FAMIGLIA PORTATRICE DI
LEIOMIOMATOSI CUTANEA E FIBROMIOMATOSI UTERINA. MINERVA DERM. 40* 388-393, 1965.

WEILBAECHER, R. G.* NEW ORLEANS, LA.* PERSONAL COMMUNICATION, 1967.

15090 LENTIGINES

PIPKIN AND PIPKIN (1950) OBSERVED EIGHT CASES IN THREE GENERATIONS OF A MALTESE-
LEBANESE FAMILY. SIX OF THE AFFECTED HAD NYSTAGMUS.

PIPKIN, A. C. AND PIPKIN, S. B.* A PEDIGREE OF GENERALIZED LENTIGO. J. HERED.
41* 79-82, 1950.

15100 LENTIGINOSIS, CENTROFACIAL NEURO-DYSRAPHIC

TOURAINE (1955), WHO FIRST DESCRIBED THIS CONDITION (1941), STATED THAT IN 17
FAMILIES IN WHICH HE EXAMINED MULTIPLE MEMBERS A TOTAL OF 32 CASES WERE DISCO-
VERED. IN 9 OF THE FAMILIES A PARENT AND ONE OR MORE CHILDREN WERE AFFECTED. IN
5 FAMILIES WITH A TOTAL OF 15 CASES ONLY TWO OR MORE SIBS WERE AFFECTED. HE
QUOTED AN INSTANCE OF AFFECTED MOTHER AND FOUR CHILDREN. MENTAL RETARDATION IS
FREQUENTLY ASSOCIATED.

TOURAINE, A.* L'HEREDITE EN MEDECINE. PARIS* MASSON, 1955.

TOURAINE, A.* UNE NOUVELLE NEURO-ECTODERMOSE CONGENITALE* LA LENTIGINOSE
CENTRO-FACIALE ET SES DYSPLASIES ASSOCIEES. ANN. DERM. SYPH. 8* 453-473, 1941.

*1511(LEOPARD SYNDROME

WALTHER ET AL. (1967) FOUND ASYMPTOMATIC CARDIAC CHANGES IN A MOTHER AND HER SON
AND DAUGHTER, ASSOCIATED WITH GENERALIZED LENTIGO. THE ELECTROCARDIOGRAM IN THE
SON SUGGESTED MYOCARDIAL INFARCTION. THE MOTHER WAS SHOWN BY CARDIAC CATHETERIZA-
TION TO HAVE MILD PULMONARY STENOSIS. WATSON (1967) REPORTED THREE FAMILIES IN
WHICH TWO GENERATIONS CONTAINED PERSONS WITH GENERALIZED LENTIGINES. MANY OF
THESE HAD VALVULAR PULMONARY STENOSIS. IN ALL, 14 PERSONS WERE AFFECTED. WE HAVE
OBSERVED MOTHER AND DAUGHTER WITH STRIKING GENERALIZED LENTIGINES (694841,
693586). BOTH WERE DEAF AND BOTH HAVE A STRIKING HEART MURMUR. THE NATURE OF THE
CARDIAC MALFORMATION HAS NOT BEEN ELUCIDATED. SIMILAR GENERALIZED LENTIGINES WERE
DESCRIBED BY MOYNAHAN (1962) IN THREE UNRELATED PATIENTS (2 FEMALES, 1 MALE).
GROWTH WAS STUNTED. IN ONE GIRL, ONE OVARY WAS ABSENT AND THE OTHER HYPOPLASTIC.
THE BOY HAD HYPOSPADIAS AND UNDESCENDED TESTES. ENDOCARDIAL AND MYOCARDIAL
FIBROELASTOSIS MAY HAVE BEEN PRESENT. INTELLIGENCE WAS NORMAL BUT BEHAVIOR
CHILDISH. MATTHEWS (1968) REPORTED MOTHER AND TWO HALF-SIB CHILDREN WITH
GENERALIZED LENTIGINES, ELECTROCARDIOGRAPHIC CHANGES AND MURMURS. A HISTORY OF
MALE-TO-MALE TRANSMISSION WAS RECORDED. LENTIGINES WERE ALSO PRESENT IN THE
CARDIAC SYNDROME REPORTED BY FORNEY ET AL. (SEE MITRAL REGURGITATION, CONDUCTIVE
DEAFNESS, ETC.). GORLIN ET AL. (1969) PRESENTED EVIDENCE FOR DOMINANT INHERI-
TANCE.

CAPUTE, A. J., RIMOIN, D. L., KONIGSMARK, B. W., ESTERLY, N. B. AND RICHARDSON,
F.* CONGENITAL DEAFNESS AND MULTIPLE LENTIGINES. A REPORT OF CASES IN A MOTHER
AND DAUGHTER. ARCH. DERM. 100* 207-213, 1969.

GORLIN, R. J., ANDERSON, R. C. AND BLAW, M.* MULTIPLE LENTIGINES SYNDROME.
COMPLEX COMPRISING MULTIPLE LENTIGENES, ELECTROCARDIOGRAPHIC CONDUCTION ABNORMALI-
TIES, OCULAR HYPERTELORISM, PULMONARY STENOSIS, ABNORMALITIES OF GENITALIA,
RETARDATION OF GROWTH, SENORINEURAL DEAFNESS, AND AUTOSOMAL DOMINANT HEREDITARY
PATTERN. AM. J. DIS. CHILD. 117* 652-662, 1969.

MATTHEWS, N. L.* LENTIGO AND ELECTROCARDIOGRAPHIC CHANGES. NEW ENG. J. MED.
278* 780-781, 1968.

MOYNAHAN, E. J.* MULTIPLE SYMMETRICAL MOLES, WITH PSYCHIC AND SOMATIC INFANTI-
LISM AND GENITAL HYPOPLASIA* FIRST MALE CASE OF A NEW SYNDROME. PROC. ROY. SOC.
MED. 55* 959-960, 1962.

WALTHER, R. J., POLANSKY, B. AND GROTS, I. A.* ELECTROCARDIOGRAPHIC ABNORMALI-
TIES IN A FAMILY WITH GENERALIZED LENTIGO. MEETING, AM. COLLEGE OF CARDIOL.,
WASHINGTON, D. C., FEB. 17, 1967.

WATSON, G. H.* PULMONARY STENOSIS, CAFE-AU-LAIT SPOTS, AND DULL INTELLIGENCE.
ARCH. DIS. CHILD. 42* 303-307, 1967.

D
O
M
I
N
A
N
T

RUKAVINA AND ASSOCIATES (1959) REPORTED THE DISORDER IN FOUR GENERATIONS OF A FAMILY. THE FEATURES WERE SHORT STATURE, MONGOLOID FACIES, SHORT SPADE-LIKE HANDS, BROAD THUMBS IN VALGUS POSITION, GENU RECURVATUM AND GENERALIZED LIMITATION OF JOINT MOBILITY, THICKENING OF THE PALMAR AND FOREARM FASCIAE, ENLARGEMENT OF THE POSTERIOR NEURAL ARCHES OF THE CERVICAL VERTEBRAE AND SHUFFLING SHORT-STEPPED GAIT.

RUKAVINA, J. G., FALLS, H. F., HOLT, J. F. AND BLOCK, W. D.* LERI'S PLEONOSTEO-SIS* A STUDY OF A FAMILY WITH A REVIEW OF THE LITERATURE. J. BONE JOINT SURG. 41A* 397-408, 1959.

15130 LEUCINE AMINOPEPTIDASE OF PLACENTA

BECKMAN ET AL. (1966) FOUND 3 PLACENTAL LAP TYPES. (LAP ENZYMES IN THE SERUM OF PREGNANT WOMEN PROBABLY ARE NOT DERIVED FROM PLACENTA.) GENETIC STUDIES REMAIN TO BE DONE. BECKMAN ET AL. (1969) IN A LATER PUBLICATION STATED A PREFERENCE FOR THE DESIGNATION AMINO ACID NAPHTHYLAMIDASE.

BECKMAN, L., BECKMAN, G., MI, M. P. AND DE SIMONE, J.* THE HUMAN PLACENTAL AMINO ACID NAPHTHYLAMIDASES* THEIR MOLECULAR INTERRELATIONS AND CORRELATIONS WITH PERINATAL FACTORS. HUM. HERED. 19* 249-257, 1969.

BECKMAN, L., BJORLING, G. AND CHRISTODOULOU, C.* PREGNANCY ENZYMES AND PLACENTAL POLYMORPHISM. II. LEUCINE AMINOPEPTIDASE. ACTA GENET. STATIST. MED. 16* 122-131, 1966.

SCANDALIOS, J. G.* HUMAN SERUM LEUCINE AMINOPEPTIDASE. VARIATION IN PREGNANCY AND IN DISEASE STATES. J. HERED. 58* 153-156, 1967.

15140 LEUKEMIA, CHRONIC LYMPHATIC

CHRONIC LYMPHATIC LEUKEMIA SEEMS ESPECIALLY PRONE TO FAMILIAL OCCURRENCE. FURBETTA AND SOLINAS (1963) REPORTED AFFECTED GRANDFATHER, SON, AND GRANDSON.

FURBETTA, D. AND SOLINAS, P.* HEREDITARY CHRONIC LYMPHATIC LEUKEMIA. PROC. SEC. INTERN. CONG. HUM. GENET. (ROME, SEPT. 6-12, 1961.) 2* 1078-1079, 1963.

MCPHEDRAN, P., HEATH, C. W., JR. AND LEE, J.* PATTERNS OF FAMILIAL LEUKEMIA. TEN CASES OF LEUKEMIA IN TWO INTERRELATED FAMILIES. CANCER 24* 403-407, 1969.

WISNIEWSKI, D. AND WEINREICH, J.* LYMPHATISCHE LEUKAMIE BEI VATER UND SOHN. BLUT 12* 241-244, 1966.

15150 LEUKOCYTE NUCLEAR APPENDAGES, HEREDITARY PREVALENCE OF

SEAMAN (1959) DESCRIBED A FAMILY WITH NUCLEAR PROJECTIONS OF THE NUCLEI OF NEUTROPHILIC LEUKOCYTES SIMULATING THE DRUMSTICKS BUT NOT SEX-SPECIFIC. SUCH WERE PRESENT IN 76 PERCENT OF THE NEUTROPHILES OF THE MALE PROBAND AND IN 25-56 PERCENT OF THOSE OF HIS FATHER, UNCLE, TWO SONS AND A DAUGHTER BUT IN NEITHER OF HIS WIVES.

SEAMAN, G.* SUR UNE ANOMALIE CONSTITUTIONNELLE HEREDITAIRE DU NOYAU DES POLYNUCLEAIRES NEUTROPHILES. REV. HEMAT. 14* 409-412, 1959.

*15160 LEUKONYCHIA TOTALIS

MEDANSKY AND FOX (1960) DESCRIBED WHITE NAILS IN FOURTEEN MEMBERS OF FIVE GENERATIONS OF A FAMILY. KRUSE ET AL. (1951) OBSERVED FATHER-SON TRANSMISSION.

HARRINGTON, J. F.* WHITE FINGERNAILS. ARCH. INTERN. MED. 114* 301-306, 1964.

JUHLIN, L.* HEREDITARY LEUKONYCHIA. ACTA DERM. 43* 136-141, 1963.

KRUSE, W. T., CAWLEY, E. P. AND COTTERMAN, C. W.* HEREDITARY LEUKONYCHIA TOTALIS. J. INVEST. DERM. 17* 135-140, 1951.

MEDANSKY, R. S. AND FOX, J. M.* HEREDITARY LEUKONYCHIA TOTALIS. ARCH. DERM. 82* 412-414, 1960.

15170 LIPOMA OF THE CONJUNCTIVA

SAEBO (1948) DESCRIBED 3 PERSONS IN THREE SUCCESSIVE GENERATIONS* GRANDFATHER, MOTHER AND DAUGHTER. THE TUMOR IS DISTINCTIVE FROM THE DERMO-LIPOMA OF THE GOLDENHAR SYNDROME.

SAEBO, J.* LIPOMA CONJUNCTIVAE IN THREE GENERATIONS. ACTA OPHTHAL. 26* 447-450, 1948.

15180 LIPOMATOSIS, FAMILIAL BENIGN CERVICAL

WE OBSERVED THREE BROTHERS WITH A COLLAR OF FAT AROUND THE NECK IN THE SUBMANDIBU-
LAR AREA AND INVOLVING THE NAPE OF THE NECK. THE AGE OF ONSET WAS SAID TO BE 45,
39 AND 29 YEARS IN THE THREE PATIENTS. THE MOTHER WAS SAID TO BE DEFINITELY
UNAFFECTED, HAVING DIED AT AGE 61, BUT TWO SISTERS AND A MATERNAL AUNT WERE ALSO
AFFECTED. IN ADVANCED STAGES THE PROCESS EXTENDED INTO THE UPPER MEDIASTINUM. IN
THE THREE BROTHERS LIPOMATA OF CONVENTIONAL TYPE WERE PRESENT IN THE EPITROCHLEAR
AREA, BACK, AXILLAE, INTERNAL ASPECT OF FOREARM, ETC. BRODIE (1846) IS SAID TO
HAVE FIRST DESCRIBED DIFFUSE SYMMETRICAL LIPOMATOSIS WITH PREDILECTION FOR THE
NECK. IT WAS CALLED 'FAT NECK' (FETTHALS) BY MADELUNG (1888). MEADORS (1971) HAS
OBSERVATIONS ON A FAMILY WITH MULTIPLE AFFECTED MEMBERS WHO ALSO SHOW HYPERURICE-
MIA AND PYRAMIDAL TRACT DISEASE. IN CRETINISM WE HAVE SEEN NOT ONLY THE SUPRACLA-
VICULAR FOSSA BUT ALSO THE AXILLAE FILLED WITH FAT. WHEN THE CRETINISM IS
FAMILIAL THIS MAY RAISE A SUSPICION OF A SEPARATE RECESSIVELY INHERITED SUPRACLA-
VICULAR LIPOMATOSIS.

BRODIE, B. C.* CLINICAL LECTURES ON SURGERY, DELIVERED AT ST. GEORGE'S
HOSPITAL. PHILADELPHIA* LEA AND BLANCHARD, 1846. PP. 201-202.

MADELUNG, (NI)* UEBER DEN FETTHALS (DIFFUSES LIPOM DES HALSES). ARCH. KLIN.
CHIR. 37* 106-130, 1888.

MCKUSICK, V. A. AND COLLEAGUES* MEDICAL GENETICS 1961. J. CHRONIC DIS. 15*
417-572, 1962 (FIG. 24).

MEADORS, C. K.* BIRMINGHAM, ALA., PERSONAL COMMUNICATION, 1971.

*15190 LIPOMATOSIS, MULTIPLE

STEPHENS AND ISAACSON (1959) OBSERVED SEVENTEEN CASES IN THREE GENERATIONS.
USUALLY THE CONDITION DID NOT BECOME EVIDENT UNTIL THE AGE OF ABOUT 35 YEARS,
ALTHOUGH IN ONE LIPOMAS WERE PRESENT AT AGE 9.

HUMPHREY, A. A. AND KINGSLEY, P. C.* FAMILIAL MULTIPLE LIPOMAS* REPORT OF A
FAMILY. ARCH. DERM. SYPH. 37* 30-34, 1938.

KRABBLE, K. H. AND BARTELS, E. D.* LA LIPOMATOSE CIRCONSCRIPTE MULTIPLE.
COPENHAGEN* MUNKSGAARD, 1944.

KURZWEG, F. T. AND SPENCER, R.* FAMILIAL MULTIPLE LIPOMATOSIS. AM. J. SURG.
82* 762-765, 1951.

SHANKS, J. A., PARANCHYCH, W. AND TUBA, J.* FAMILIAL MULTIPLE LIPOMATOSIS.
CANAD. MED. ASS. J. 77* 881-884, 1957.

STEPHENS, F. E. AND ISAACSON, A.* HEREDITARY MULTIPLE LIPOMATOSIS. J. HERED.
50* 51-53, 1959.

*15200 LIPOPROTEIN TYPES - AG SYSTEM

BLUMBERG ET AL. (1963) DESCRIBED A POLYMORPHIC SYSTEM INCLUDING SERUM BETA
LIPOPROTEIN DISTINCT FROM THAT DISCOVERED BY BERG. THEY DETECTED THIS BY THE
STUDY OF PATIENTS WHO HAD RECEIVED MULTIPLE TRANSFUSIONS. THE FIRST TYPE WAS
CALLED AG-A* THE SECOND WAS CALLED AG-B. BLUMBERG AND COLLEAGUES (1964) PROPOSED
THE SYMBOL LP, FOR LIPOPROTEIN. LOWER CASE LETTERS ARE USED FOR DESIGNATING
DIFFERENT LOCI (I.E., LPA, LPB, LPC, ETC.) AND SUPERSCRIPT NUMBERS FOR ALLELES AT
THE LOCUS (I.E., LPA-1, LPA-2, ETC.). GENE SYMBOLS ARE UNDERLINED IN MANUSCRIPT
OR TYPESCRIPT AND ITALICIZED IN PRINT. RETENTION OF THE AG DESIGNATION MAY BE
ADVISABLE TO AVOID CONFUSION WITH THE BERG TYPE.

ALLISON, A. C. AND BLUMBERG, B. S.* SERUM LIPOPROTEIN ALLOTYPES IN MAN.
PROGRESS IN MEDICAL GENETICS. STEINBERG, A. G. AND BEARN, A. G. (EDS.)* NEW YORK*
GRUNE AND STRATTON, 4* 176-201, 1965.

BLUMBERG, B. S., ALTER, H. J. AND RIDDELL, N. M.* INHERITED ANTIGENIC DIF-
FERENCES IN HUMAN SERUM BETA LIPOPROTEINS. A SECOND ANTISERUM. J. CLIN. INVEST.
42* 867-875, 1963.

BLUMBERG, B. S., ALTER, H. J., RIDDELL, N. M. AND ERLANDSON, M.* MULTIPLE
ANTIGENIC SPECIFICITIES OF SERUM LIPOPROTEINS DETECTED WITH SERA OF TRANSFUSED
PATIENTS. VOX SANG. 9* 128-145, 1964.

BUTLER, R. AND BRUNNER, E.* ON THE GENETICS OF THE LOW DENSITY LIPOPROTEIN
FACTORS AG(C) AND AG(E). HUM. HERED. 19* 174-179, 1969.

BUTLER, R., BRUNNER, E., MORGANTI, G., VIERUCCI, A., SCALOUMBACAS, N. AND
POLITIS, E.* A NEW FACTOR IN THE AG-SYSTEM* AG(G). VOX SANG. 18* 85-89, 1970.

MORGANTI, G., BEOLCHINI, P. E., BUTLER, R., BRUNNER, E. AND VIERUCCI, A.*
CONTRIBUTION TO THE GENETICS OF SERUM BETA-LIPOPROTEINS IN MAN. IV. EVIDENCE FOR
THE EXISTENCE OF THE AG(A1-D) AND AG(C-G) LOCI, CLOSELY LINKED TO THE AG(X-Y)
LOCUS. HUMANGENETIK 10* 244-253, 1970.

D
O
M
I
N
A
N
T

IN THE SERUM OF A MULTIPLY TRANSFUSED BOY, BERG (1965) FOUND AN ISOPRECIPITIN AGAINST A FACTOR IN THE SERUM LOW-DENSITY LIPOPROTEIN OF ABOUT 42 PERCENT OF HEALTHY PERSONS. HE NAMED THE FACTOR LD FOR 'LOW-DENSITY.'

BERG, K.* A NEW SERUM TYPE SYSTEM IN MAN - THE LD SYSTEM. VOX SANG. 10* 513-527, 1965.

*15220 LIPOPROTEIN TYPES - LP SYSTEM

BERG AND MOHR (1963) DISCOVERED A NEW SERUM PROTEIN SYSTEM CALLED LP (FOR LIPOPROTEIN) BY THE INTRAVENOUS INJECTION OF RABBITS WITH ISOLATED HUMAN SERUM BETA-LIPOPROTEIN FROM ONE INDIVIDUAL. THE RESULTING ANTIBODY DISTINGUISHES TWO DISTINCT TYPES OF HUMAN BETA-LIPOPROTEIN. BERG AND MOHR (1963) DEMONSTRATES REGULAR DOMINANT INHERITANCE. THE LP-A ALLELE HAS A FREQUENCY OF 0.19 IN NORWEGIANS. THE AUTHORS CONCLUDED THAT THIS SYSTEM IS INDEPENDENT OF THE AG SYSTEM OF BLUMBERG. BERG AND BEARN (1967) SUGGESTED THAT AT LEAST FOUR LIPOPRO-TEIN SYSTEMS EXIST* AG, LP, LD AND LT.

BERG, K. AND MOHR, J.* GENETICS OF LP SYSTEM. ACTA GENET. STATIST. MED. 13* 349-360, 1963.

BERG, K.* LACK OF LINKAGE BETWEEN THE LP AND AG SERUM SYSTEMS. VOX SANG. 12* 71-74, 1967.

BUTLER, R.* POLYMORPHISM OF THE HUMAN LOW-DENSITY LIPOPROTEINS. VOX SANG. 12* 2-17, 1967.

15230 LIPOPROTEIN TYPES - LT SYSTEM

FOR REFERENCES, SEE ABOVE.

15240 LIPOPROTEIN, VARIANT OF BETA ('DOUBLE BETA-LIPOPROTEIN')

SEEGERS, HIRSCHHORN, BURNETT, ROBSON AND HARRIS (1965) HAVE OBSERVED DOUBLE BETA-LIPOPROTEIN IN 6 FAMILIES. THE RELATION OF THE LOCUS REVEALED BY THIS MUTANT FORM TO THOSE STUDIED BY THE LIPOPROTEIN TYPES OF BERG AND BLUMBERG IS UNKNOWN.

SEEGERS, W., HIRSCHHORN, K., BURNETT, L., ROBSON, E. AND HARRIS, H.* DOUBLE BETA-LIPOPROTEIN* A NEW GENETIC VARIATION IN MAN. SCIENCE 149* 303-304, 1965.

15250 LUDER-SHELDON SYNDROME

LUDER AND SHELDON (1955) AND SHELDON ET AL. (1961) DESCRIBED CASES OF GENERALIZED AMINOACIDURIA WITH LOSS OF GLUCOSE AND PHOSPHATE AS WELL. MILD RICKETS WITH LATE ONSET OR NO BONE DISEASE OCCURRED. THREE GENERATIONS WERE AFFECTED. DOMINANT INHERITANCE IS UNUSUAL FOR A DEFECT OF THIS TYPE. THE AFFECTED PERSONS WERE FEMALE TWINS, THEIR FATHER AND HIS FATHER.

LUDER, J. AND SHELDON, W.* A FAMILIAL TUBULAR ABSORPTION DEFECT OF GLUCOSE AND AMINO-ACIDS. ARCH. DIS. CHILD. 30* 160-164, 1955.

SHELDON, W., LUDER, J. AND WEBB, B.* A FAMILIAL TUBULAR ABSORPTION DEFECT OF GLUCOSE AND AMINO ACIDS. ARCH. DIS. CHILD. 36* 90-95, 1961.

15260 LUNULAE OF FINGERNAILS

SIZE OF THE LUNULAE AND INDEED THEIR PRESENCE OR ABSENCE IS A VARIABLE MATTER PRESUMABLY UNDER GENETIC CONTROL, ALTHOUGH NO SYSTEMIC INVESTIGATION OF THE GENETICS HAS BEEN PERFORMED. THE LUNULAE ARE USUALLY LARGEST ON THE THUMB NAIL AND IF PRESENT AT ALL ARE MOST LIKELY TO BE FOUND ON THE THUMB. AZURE LUNULAE OCCUR IN WILSON'S DISEASE.

15270 LUPUS ERYTHEMATOSUS, SYSTEMIC (SLE)

ALTHOUGH FAMILIAL AGGREGATION OF CLINICAL SLE, OF RELATED DISORDERS SUCH AS DERMATOMYOSITIS, AND OF PROTEIN ABNORMALITIES IS RATHER FREQUENTLY OBSERVED, A SIMPLE MENDELIAN MECHANISM IS NOT ESTABLISHED. LAPPAT AND CAWEIN (1968) SUGGESTED THAT DRUG-INDUCED, SPECIFICALLY PROCAINAMIDE-INDUCED, SYSTEMIC LUPUS ERYTHEMATOSUS IS AN EXPRESSION OF A PHARMACOGENETIC POLYMORPHISM. AMONG CLOSE RELATIVES OF A PROCAINAMIDE SLE PROBAND, THEY FOUND THREE WITH ANTINUCLEAR ANTIBODY IN THE SERUM AND IN ALL FIVE HAD A 'SIGNIFICANT' HISTORY OR LABORATORY FINDINGS SUGGESTING AN IMMUNOLOGIC DISORDER. THREE HAD A COAGULATION ABNORMALITY.

LAPPAT, E. J. AND CAWEIN, M. J.* A FAMILIAL STUDY OF PROCAINAMIDE-INDUCED SYSTEMIC LUPUS ERYTHEMATOSUS. A QUESTION OF PHARMACOGENETIC POLYMORPHISM. AM. J. MED. 45* 846-852, 1968.

LEONHARDT, T.* FAMILY STUDIES IN SYSTEMIC LUPUS ERYTHEMATOSUS. ACTA MED. SCAND. 176 (SUPPL. 416)* 1-156, 1964.

POLLAK, V. E.* ANTINUCLEAR ANTIBODIES IN FAMILIES OF PATIENTS WITH SYSTEMIC
LUPUS ERYTHEMATOSUS. NEW ENG. J. MED. 271* 165-171, 1964.

SIEGEL, M., LEE, S. L., WIDELOCK, D., GWON, N. V. AND KRAVITZ, H.* A COMPARA-
TIVE FAMILY STUDY OF RHEUMATOID ARTHRITIS AND SYSTEMIC LUPUS ERYTHEMATOSUS. NEW
ENG. J. MED. 273* 893-897, 1965.

15280 LYMPHANGIECTASIA, INTESTINAL

UNDER THE DESIGNATION "FAMILIAL IDIOPATHIC DYSPROTEINEMIA" HOMBURGER AND PETERMANN
(1949) DESCRIBED A DISORDER CHARACTERIZED BY EDEMA OF THE LEGS, WITH ULCERS IN THE
MALES AND "FUNCTIONAL VASCULAR CHANGES" IN THE FEMALES, BY DYSPROTEINEMIA OF
VARIABLE TYPE AND SOMETIMES DISCERNABLE ONLY BY ELECTROPHORESIS, BY A NUMBER OF
CONGENITAL MALFORMATIONS AND BY A HIGH INCIDENCE OF STILLBIRTHS. PERSONS IN THREE
GENERATIONS WERE AFFECTED AND MALE-TO-MALE TRANSMISSION OCCURRED. SUBSEQUENTLY
THESE PATIENTS HAVE BEEN FOUND TO HAVE INTESTINAL LOSS OF PROTEIN PRESUMABLY
BECAUSE OF LYMPHANGIECTASIA (WALDMANN ET AL., 1961* WALDMANN AND SCHWAB, 1965).
LYMPHOPENIA DUE TO EXAGGERATED INTESTINAL LOSS IS ALSO A FEATURE. DOUBLE VORTEX
PILORUM ("HAIR WHORL") AND USUALLY PROMINENT "FLOATING RIBS" (RIBS 11 AND 12) WERE
PRESENT. PARFITT (1966) DESCRIBED THREE SIBS (2 FEMALES, ONE MALE) AFFECTED OUT
OF 5. ALL HAD NEONATAL EDEMA. THE SMALL BOWEL SHOWED DILATED LYMPHATIC SPACES
AND PARTIAL VILLOUS ATROPHY. COTTOM, LONDON AND WILSON (1961) REPORTED NEONATAL
HYPOPROTEINEMIA IN TWO SIBS AND OTHER PROBABLE CASES ARE KNOWN. SEE ALSO
LYMPHEDEMA, HEREDITARY I.

COTTOM, D. G., LONDON, D. R. AND WILSON, B. D. R.* NEONATAL OEDEMA DUE TO
EXUDATIVE ENTEROPATHY. LANCET 2* 1009-1012, 1961.

HOMBURGER, F. AND PETERMANN, M. L.* STUDIES ON HYPOPROTEINEMIA. II. FAMILIAL
IDIOPATHIC DYSPROTEINEMIA. BLOOD 4* 1085-1108, 1949.

PARFITT, A. M.* FAMILIAL NEONATAL HYPOPROTEINAEMIA WITH EXUDATIVE ENTEROPATHY
AND INTESTINAL LYMPHANGIECTASIS. ARCH. DIS. CHILD. 41* 54-62, 1966.

WALDMANN, T. A. AND SCHWAB, P. J.* IGG(7S GAMMA GLOBULIN) METABOLISM IN
HYPOGAMMAGLOBULINEMIA* STUDIES IN PATIENTS WITH DEFECTIVE GAMMA GLOBULIN SYNTHE-
SIS, GASTROINTESTINAL PROTEIN LOSS, OR BOTH. J. CLIN. INVEST. 44* 1523-1533,
1965.

WALDMANN, T. A., STEINFELD, J. L., DUTCHER, T. F., DAVIDSON, J. D. AND GORDON,
R. S., JR.* THE ROLE OF THE GASTROINTESTINAL SYSTEM IN "IDIOPATHIC HYPOPROTEINE-
MIA." GASTROENTEROLOGY 41* 197-207, 1961.

15290 LYMPHEDEMA AND CEREBRAL ARTERIOVENOUS ANOMALY

AVASTHEY AND ROY (1968) REPORTED A WOMAN WITH LYMPHEDEMA OF THE FEET BEGINNING IN
HER TEENS AND A CEREBROVASCULAR ANOMALY INDICATED BY A LOUD SYSTOLIC BRUIT OVER
THE TEMPLES AND TRANSMITTED DOWN THE CAROTIDS. A SON, AGED 20 YEARS, LIKEWISE HAD
FOOT LYMPHEDEMA AND A CRANIAL BRUIT AND BY ANGIOGRAM A LARGE EXTRACRANIAL
ARTERIOVENOUS MALFORMATION OVER THE PARIETAL REGION. TWO OTHER SONS HAD LYMPHEDE-
MA, CEREBROVASCULAR MALFORMATION AND PRIMARY PULMONARY HYPERTENSION. ONE SON WAS
NORMAL AND THE ONLY DAUGHTER HAD LYMPHEDEMA OF BOTH FEET AND BILATERAL TEMPORO-
PARIETAL BRUIT.

AVASTHEY, P. AND ROY, S. B.* PRIMARY PULMONARY HYPERTENSION, CEREBROVASCULAR
MALFORMATION, AND LYMPHOEDEMA FEET IN A FAMILY. BRIT. HEART J. 30* 769-775, 1968.

15300 LYMPHEDEMA AND PTOSIS

IN A FAMILY REPORTED BY BLOOM (1941), LYMPHEDEMA OF THE LEGS OCCURRED IN FIVE
GENERATIONS AND SIX AFFECTED PERSONS IN 3 CONSECUTIVE GENERATIONS ALSO HAD PTOSIS.
FALLS AND KERTESZ (1964) MADE BRIEF REFERENCE TO A FAMILY IN WHICH THE MALE
PROBAND HAD PTOSIS AND LYMPHEDEMA AND THE FATHER PTOSIS.

BLOOM, D.* HEREDITARY LYMPHEDEMA (NONNE-MILROY-MEIGE). REPORT OF A FAMILY WITH
HEREDITARY LYMPHEDEMA ASSOCIATED WITH PTOSIS OF THE EYELIDS IN SEVERAL GENERA-
TIONS. NEW YORK J. MED. 41* 856-863, 1941.

FALLS, H. F. AND KERTESZ, E. D.* A NEW SYNDROME COMBINING PTERYGIUM COLLI WITH
DEVELOPMENTAL ANOMALIES OF THE EYELIDS AND LYMPHATICS OF THE LOWER EXTREMITIES.
TRANS. AM. OPHTHAL. SOC. 62* 248-275, 1964.

*15310 LYMPHEDEMA, HEREDITARY I (NONNE-MILROY, OR EARLY-ONSET TYPE)

EDEMA IS PRESENT FROM BIRTH. ROSEN (1962) OBSERVED CONGENITAL CHYLOUS ASCITES IN
AN AFFECTED INFANT. MARKED LOSS OF ALBUMIN INTO THE INTESTINAL TRACT WITH
CONSEQUENT HYPOPROTEINEMIA WAS DEMONSTRATED. THE FATHER HAD RECURRENT SWELLING OF
THE SCROTUM BEGINNING AT THE AGE OF 20 YEARS. HURWITZ AND PINALS (1964) OBSERVED
PERSISTENT BILATERAL PLEURAL EFFUSION IN TWO SUCH PATIENTS. THE PROTEIN CONTENT
OF THE PLEURAL FLUID WAS HIGH. MILROY (1928), A PHYSICIAN IN OMAHA, NEBRASKA,
DESCRIBED THE DISORDER IN A FAMILY IN WHICH MANY OF THE AFFECTED PERSONS WERE
PROMINENT IN PUBLIC AND PROFESSIONAL LIFE.

ESTERLY, J. R.* CONGENITAL HEREDITARY LYMPHOEDEMA. J. MED. GENET. 2* 93-98, 1965.

HURWITZ, P. A. AND PINALS, D. J.* PLEURAL EFFUSION IN CHRONIC HEREDITARY LYMPHEDEMA (NONNE, MILROY, MEIGE'S DISEASE). REPORT OF TWO CASES. RADIOLOGY 82* 246-248, 1964.

MILROY, W. F.* CHRONIC HEREDITARY EDEMA* MILROY'S DISEASE. J.A.M.A. 91* 1172-1175, 1928.

ROSEN, F. S., SMITH, D. H., EARLE, R., JR., JANEWAY, C. A. AND GITLIN, D.* THE ETIOLOGY OF HYPOPROTEINEMIA IN A PATIENT WITH CONGENITAL CHYLOUS ASCITES. PEDIATRICS 30* 696-706, 1962.

15320 LYMPHEDEMA, HEREDITARY II (MEIGE, OR LATE-ONSET TYPE)

EDEMA DEVELOPS ABOUT THE TIME OF PUBERTY (GOODMAN, 1962). MEIGE (1898) DESCRIBED 8 CASES IN FOUR GENERATIONS. NO MALE-TO-MALE TRANSMISSION WAS OBSERVED. GOODMAN (1962) REPORTED THE CONDITION IN TWO SISTERS AND A BROTHER WITH PRESUMED NORMAL PARENTS WHO WERE NOT KNOWN TO BE RELATED.

GOODMAN, R. M.* FAMILIAL LYMPHEDEMA OF THE MEIGE'S TYPE. AM. J. MED. 32* 651-656, 1962.

JUCHEMS, R.* DAS HEREDITARE LYMPHODEM, TYP MEIGE. KLIN. WSCHR. 41* 328-332, 1963.

MEIGE, H.* DYSTROPHIE OEDEMATEUSE HEREDITAIRE. PRESSE MED. 6* 341-343, 1898.

OSTERLAND, G.* BEOBACHTUNGEN ZUM NONNE-MILROY-MEIGE-SYNDROM. Z. MENSCHL. VERERB. KONSTITUTIONSL. 36* 108-117, 1961.

15330 LYMPHEDEMA, WITH ADULT ONSET AND YELLOW NAILS

WELLS (1966) DESCRIBED A FAMILY WITH 8 CASES IN 4 SIBSHIPS OF TWO GENERATIONS. IN THE PROBAND THE ONSET WAS IN THE LEGS AT THE AGE OF 51. AT TIMES EDEMA ALSO AFFECTED THE GENITALIA, HANDS, FACE, AND EVEN THE VOCAL CORDS. LYMPHANGIOGRAMS WERE INTERPRETED AS SHOWING PRIMARY HYPOPLASIA OF LYMPHATICS. THE PROBAND HAD YELLOW NAILS AND GREW POORLY. THE NAIL CHANGES WERE NOTED BEFORE LYMPHEDEMA. ZERFAS AND WALLACE (1966) DESCRIBED A SPORADIC CASE WITH ONSET OF LYMPHEDEMA AT AGE 10. RECURRENT PLEURAL EFFUSION OCCURS IN SOME CASES.

SAMMAN, P. D. AND WHITE, W. F.* THE 'YELLOW NAIL' SYNDROME. BRIT. J. DERM. 76* 153-157, 1964.

WELLS, G. C.* YELLOW NAIL SYNDROME WITH FAMILIAL PRIMARY HYPOPLASIA OF LYMPHATICS, MANIFEST LATE IN LIFE. PROC. ROY. SOC. MED. 59* 447 ONLY, 1966.

ZERFAS, A. J. AND WALLACE, H. J.* YELLOW NAIL SYNDROME WITH BILATERAL BRONCHIE-CTASIS. PROC. ROY. SOC. MED. 59* 448 ONLY, 1966.

*15340 LYMPHEDEMA, WITH DISTICHIASIS

ROBINOW ET AL. (1970) DESCRIBED THE SYNDROME IN A FATHER AND A DAUGHTER AND SON. THE LYMPHEDEMA WAS ALWAYS OF LATE ONSET. SPINAL CHANGES WERE ASYMPTOMATIC. CHYNN (1967) SAW THESE IN COMBINATION WITH SPINAL EXTRADURAL CYST (Q.V.) IN TWO AND PERHAPS THREE NEGRO SIBS. FALLS AND KERTESZ (1964) DESCRIBED (SEE ALSO NEEL AND SCHULL, 1954) A FAMILY WITH DISTICHIASIS AND LYMPHEDEMA. OF A SIBSHIP OF 5, FOUR HAD BILATERAL LYMPHEDEMA OF THE LEGS AND DISTICHIASIS, ONE WAS NORMAL. ONE OF THE FOUR HAD STRIKING WEBBED NECK WHEREAS TWO OF THE OTHERS WERE THOUGHT TO HAVE MILD WEBBING. THE LYMPHEDEMA WAS OF THE TYPE WHICH HAS ONSET AT PUBERTY. SEVERAL OF THE AFFECTED PERSONS COMPLAINED OF PHOTOPHOBIA AND HAD PARTIAL ECTROPION OF THE LATERAL THIRD OF THE LOWER LIDS, GIVING THEM A WIDE-EYED APPEARANCE. THE FATHER AND ONE OF HIS BROTHERS REPORTEDLY HAD LYMPHEDEMA, DISTICHIASIS AND WEBBED NECK. THE PATERNAL GRANDMOTHER HAD LYMPHEDEMA. AN AFFECTED PATERNAL UNCLE DIED OF METASTATIC FIBROSARCOMA ORIGINATING IN AN EDEMATOUS LEG. SEE PTERYGIUM COLLI SYNDROME. HOOVER (1971) HAS STUDIED A FAMILY WITH THE LYMPHEDEMA-DISTICHIASIS SYNDROME IN THREE GENERATIONS. IRRITATION OF THE CORNEA, WITH CORNEAL ULCERATION IN SOME CASES, BRINGS THE PATIENTS TO THE ATTENTION OF OPHTHALMOLOGISTS.

CHYNN, K.-Y.* CONGENITAL SPINAL EXTRADURAL CYST IN TWO SIBLINGS. AM. J. ROENTGEN. 101* 204-215, 1967.

FALLS, H. F. AND KERTESZ, E. D.* A NEW SYNDROME COMBINING PTERYGIUM COLLI WITH DEVELOPMENTAL ANOMALIES OF THE EYELIDS AND LYMPHATICS OF THE LOWER EXTREMITIES. TRANS. AM. OPHTHAL. SOC. 62* 248-275, 1964.

HOOVER, R. E.* BALTIMORE* PERSONAL COMMUNICATION, 1971.

NEEL, J. V. AND SCHULL, W. J.* HUMAN HEREDITY. U. OF CHICAGO PRESS, 1954. PP. 50-51.

1535 (MACROCEPHALY, PSEUDOPAPILLEDEMA AND MULTIPLE HEMANGIOMATA

RILEY AND SMITH (1960) DESCRIBED MOTHER AND TWO CHILDREN OF SEVEN WHO HAD
MACROCEPHALY, PSEUDOPAPILLEDEMA AND MULTIPLE HEMANGIOMATA. TWO OTHER SIBS HAD
MACROCEPHALY AND PSEUDOPAPILLEDEMA. INTELLECT AND VISION WERE UNIMPAIRED.

RILEY, H. D., JR. AND SMITH, W. R.* MACROCEPHALY, PSEUDOPAPILLEDEMA AND
MULTIPLE HEMANGIOMATA* A PREVIOUSLY UNDESCRIBED HEREDOFAMILIAL SYNDROME.
PEDIATRICS 26* 293-300, 1960.

15360 MACROGLOBULINEMIA, WALDENSTROM'S

VANNOTTI (1963) OBSERVED THIS IN MOTHER AND SON AND SELIGMAN, DANON AND FINE
(1963) HAD AN INSTANCE OF MOTHER AND TWO SONS AFFECTED. BROWN ET AL. (1967) FOUND
AN ABNORMAL CHROMOSOME IN SOME LYMPHOCYTES OF 5 MEMBERS OF ONE FAMILY. THREE OF
THE 5 HAD PROTEIN ABNORMALITIES. SEE ALSO ELVES AND BROWN (1968).

BROWN, A. K., ELVES, M. W., GUNSON, H. H. AND PELL-ILDERTON, R.* WALDENSTROM'S
MACROGLOBULINAEMIA. A FAMILY STUDY. ACTA HAEMAT. 38* 184-192, 1967.

ELVES, M. W. AND BROWN, A. K.* CYTOGENETIC STUDIES IN A FAMILY WITH WALDENS-
TROM'S MACROGLOBULINAEMIA. J. MED. GENET. 5* 118-122, 1968.

MASSARI, R., FINE, J. M. AND METAIS, R.* WALDENSTROM'S MACROGLOBULINAEMIA
OBSERVED IN TWO BROTHERS. NATURE 196* 176-178, 1962.

SELIGMAN, M., DANON, F. AND FINE, J. M.* IMMUNOLOGICAL STUDIES IN FAMILIAL
BETA-2-MACROGLOBULINAEMIAS. PROC. SOC. EXP. BIOL. MED. 114* 482-486, 1963.

VANNOTTI, A.* ETUDE CLINIQUE D'UN CAS DE MACROGLOBULINEMIE DE WALDENSTROM A
CARACTERE FAMILIAL, ASSOCIE A DES TROUBLES ENDOCRINIENS. SCHWEIZ. MED. WSCHR. 93*
1744-1746, 1963.

*15370 MACULAR DEGENERATION, POLYMORPHIC

HEREDITARY DEGENERATION OF THE MACULA LUTEA WITHOUT CEREBRAL COMPLICATIONS IS
RARE. AS WILL BE SEEN FROM THE TITLE OF PAPERS REFERENCED BELOW, MANY DIFFERENT
DESIGNATIONS HAVE BEEN EMPLOYED. MORE THAN ONE ENTITY MAY WELL BE REPRESENTED.
YET THE EVIDENCE IS NOT ADEQUATE FOR DELINEATING MORE THAN ONE. DAVIS AND
HOLLENHORST (1955) DESCRIBED A KINDRED CONTAINING AT LEAST 24 AFFECTED PERSONS IN
FIVE GENERATIONS. THE AGE OF ONSET OF MANIFEST VISUAL DISABILITY VARIED FROM VERY
EARLY CHILDHOOD TO ADOLESCENCE. CYSTOID MACULAR DEGENERATION WAS DESCRIBED IN A
DOMINANT PEDIGREE PATTERN BY FALLS (1949) AND SORSBY ET AL. (1956). VAIL AND
SHOCK (1965) FOLLOWED UP ON AN EXTENSIVELY AFFECTED KINDRED AND REPORTED HISTOLO-
GIC FINDINGS IN A PATIENT WHO DIED AT 78 YEARS OF AGE. BEST'S DISEASE IS
SOMETIMES CALLED VITELLINE MACULAR DYSTROPHY. EIGHT PERSONS WERE AFFECTED IN THE
FAMILY REPORTED BY BEST (1905) AND FOLLOW-UP (VOSSIUS, 1921* JUNG, 1936) INCREASED
THE NUMBER TO 22. CHARACTERISTICALLY FUNDUSCOPIC CHANGES ARE IN ADVANCE OF VISUAL
IMPAIRMENT. A YELLOW MASS LIKE THE YOLK OF AN EGG (HENCE THE NAME) IN THE MACULAR
AREA LATER BECOMES DEEPLY AND IRREGULARLY PIGMENTED AND A PROCESS CALLED *SCRAMB-
LING THE EGG* BY BRALEY (1966) TAKES PLACE. THE EGGLIKE LESION IS PROBABLY
PRESENT AT BIRTH. EXAMINATION OF RELATIVES IS ESSENTIAL TO DIAGNOSIS IN ADVANCED
CASES. FRIEDENWALD AND MAUMENEE (1951) OBSERVED AFFECTED MOTHER AND DAUGHTER.

BEST, F.* UEBER EINE HEREDITARE MACULAAFFEKTION. Z. AUGENHEILK. 13* 199-212,
1905.

BRALEY, A. E. AND SPIVEY, B. E.* HEREDITARY VITELLINE MACULAR DEGENERATION. A
CLINICAL AND FUNCTIONAL EVALUATION OF A NEW PEDIGREE WITH VARIABLE EXPRESSIVITY
AND DOMINANT INHERITANCE. ARCH. OPHTHAL. 72* 743-762, 1964.

BRALEY, A. E.* DYSTROPHY OF THE MACULA. AM. J. OPHTHAL. 61* 1-24, 1966.

DAVIS, C. T. AND HOLLENHORST, R. W.* HEREDITARY DEGENERATION OF THE MACULA*
OCCURRING IN FIVE GENERATIONS. AM. J. OPHTHAL. 39* 637-643, 1955.

FALLS, H. F.* HEREDITARY CONGENITAL MACULAR DEGENERATION. AM. J. HUM. GENET.
1* 96-104, 1949.

FRANCOIS, J.* VITELLIFORM DEGENERATION OF THE MACULA. BULL. N.Y. ACAD. MED.
44* 18-27, 1968.

FRIEDENWALD, J. S. AND MAUMENEE, A. E.* PECULIAR MACULAR LESIONS WITH UNACCOUN-
TABLY GOOD VISION. ARCH. OPHTHAL. 45* 567-570, 1951.

JUNG, E. E.* UBER EINE SIPPE MIT ANGEBORENER MACULADEGENERATION. GIESSEN*
SEIBERT, 1936.

KRILL, A. E., MORSE, P. A., POTTS, A. M. AND KLEIN, B. A.* HEREDITARY VITEL-LIRUPTIVE MACULAR DEGENERATION. AM. J. OPHTHAL. 61* 1405-1415, 1966.

SORSBY, A., SAVORY, M., DANEY, J. B. AND FRASER, R. J. L.* MACULAR CYSTS* A DOMINANTLY INHERITED AFFECTION WITH A PROGRESSIVE COURSE. BRIT. J. OPHTHAL. 40* 144-158, 1956.

VAIL, D. AND SHOCK, D.* HEREDITARY DEGENERATION OF THE MACULA. II. FOLLOW-UP REPORT AND HISTOPATHOLOGIC STUDY. TRANS. AM. OPHTHAL. SOC. 63* 51-63, 1965.

VOSSIUS, A.* UBER DIE BESTSCHE FAMILIARE MACULADEGENERATION. ARCH. OPHTAL. 105* 1050-1059, 1921.

15380 MACULAR DEGENERATION, SENILE

STREIFF AND BABEL (1963) DESCRIBED SENILE MACULAR CHANGES IN AN 80 YEAR OLD MOTHER AND HER 50 YEAR OLD DAUGHTER. BECAUSE OF THE LATE ONSET OF THE ABNORMALITY DOMINANT INHERITANCE IS MORE LIKELY. FURTHERMORE BECAUSE OF THE LATE ONSET AFFECTED MEMBERS OF SUCCESSIVE GENERATIONS ARE NOT LIKELY TO BE OBSERVED. BRALEY (1966) STATED THAT SENILE MACULAR DEGENERATION RUNS IN FAMILIES. *NEARLY EVERY PATIENT I HAVE SEEN HAS HAD OTHER MEMBERS OF THE FAMILY SIMILARLY AFFECTED.* VISUAL DISTURBANCE WITHOUT OPHTHALMOSCOPIC FINDINGS MAY BE PRESENT BY AGE 50 AND FUNDUS CHANGES BECOME APPARENT ONLY AFTER AGE 70.

BRALEY, A. E.* DYSTROPHY OF THE MACULA. AM. J. OPHTHAL. 61* 1-24, 1966.

STREIFF, E. B. AND BABEL, J.* LA SENESCENCE DE LA RETINE. PROG. OPHTHAL. 13* 1-75, 1963.

15390 MACULAR DYSTROPHY* BUTTERFLY-SHAPED PIGMENT DYSTROPHY OF FOVEA

DEUTMAN ET AL. (1970) DESCRIBED BUTTERFLY-SHAPED PIGMENT DYSTROPHY OF THE FOVEA IN FOUR OF 5 BROTHERS AND IN THE SON OF ONE OF THE FOUR. THREE HAD NORMAL VISUAL ACUITY AND THE OTHER TWO HAD ONLY SLIGHTLY DIMINISHED VISION. THE ANOMALY APPEARS TO BE DISTINCT FROM ANY PREVIOUSLY DESCRIBED.

DEUTMAN, A. F., VAN BLOMMESTEIN, A., HENKES, H. E., WAARDENBURG, P. J. AND SOLLEVELD VAN DRIEST, E.* BUTTERFLY-SHAPED PIGMENT DYSTROPHY OF THE FOVEA. ARCH. OPHTHAL. 83* 558-569, 1970.

15400 MADELUNG DEFORMITY

PAUS (1942) FOUND 22 AFFECTED (15 MALES, 7 FEMALES) IN 6 GENERATIONS. GATTO (1955) OBSERVED 10 AFFECTED IN 3 GENERATIONS. MADELUNG DEFORMITY OCCURS AS PART OF DYSCHONDROSTEOSIS. THERE MAY BE QUESTION OF WHETHER IT IS EVER AN INDEPENDENT SIMPLY INHERITED ANOMALY. FELMAN AND KIRKPATRICK (1969) DESCRIBED A FAMILY WITH MULTIPLE AFFECTED INDIVIDUALS IN A PATTERN CONSISTENT WITH DOMINANT INHERITANCE. NORMAL STATURE AND LACK OF ABNORMALITY ELSEWHERE SEEMED TO EXCLUDE DYSCHONDROSTEO-SIS (Q.V.).

FELMAN, A. H. AND KIRKPATRICK, J. A., JR.* MADELUNG'S DEFORMITY* OBSERVATIONS IN 17 PATIENTS. RADIOLOGY 93* 1037-1042, 1969.

GATTO, I.* CONTRIBUTO ALLA GENETICA DELLA DEFORMITA DI MADELUNG. ACTA GENET. MED. GEM. 4* 205-216, 1955.

PAUS, B.* MADELUNG'S DEFORMITY. NORSKE VIDENSK. AKAD., 1942. (CITED BY GREBE, H.* MISSBILDUNGEN DER GLIEDMASSEN. IN BECKER, P. E. (ED.)* HUMANGENETIK. STUTTGART* GEORG THIEME VERLAG, 1964. VOL. II, P. 218 ONLY.).

*15410 MALATE DEHYDROGENASE, ELECTROPHORETIC VARIANTS OF MITOCHONDRIAL BOUND

IN LEUKOCYTES AND PLACENTAS DAVIDSON AND CORTNER (1967) FOUND POLYMORPHISM OF THE MALATE DEHYDROGENASE THAT IS BOUND TO MITOCHONDRIA, SO-CALLED M-MDH. THE FACT THAT MITOCHONDRIAL MALATE DEHYDROGENASE WAS INDISTINGUISHABLE FROM NORMAL IN PERSONS WITH VARIATION IN THE SUPERNATANT MDH INDICATES THAT A SEPARATE LOCUS IS INVOLVED IN ITS GENETIC DETERMINATION. MENDELIAN SEGREGATION RATHER THAN MATERNAL INHERITANCE OF M-MDH SUGGESTS THAT NOT ALL MITOCHONDRIAL PROTEINS ARE CODED BY MITOCHONDRIAL DNA. MITOCHONDRIAL GLUTAMIC OXALOACETIC TRANSAMINASE (Q.V.) IS ALSO DETERMINED BY NUCLEAR GENES.

DAVIDSON, R. G. AND CORTNER, J. A.* MITOCHONDRIAL MALATE DEHYDROGENASE* A NEW GENETIC POLYMORPHISM IN MAN. SCIENCE 157* 1569-1571, 1967.

*15420 MALATE DEHYDROGENASE, ELECTROPHORETIC VARIANT OF SOLUBLE CYTOPLASMIC

S-MDH IS THE BRIEF DESIGNATION FOR THE SOLUBLE CYTOPLASMIC ENZYME. DAVIDSON AND CORTNER (1967) OBSERVED AN INHERITED VARIANT OF SUPERNATANT MALATE DEHYDROGENASE OF ERYTHROCYTES. THE VARIANT WAS FOUND IN A NEGRO WOMAN AND HER TWO SONS, UNCOVERED IN A SURVEY OF 1470 NEGROES AND 1440 WHITES. THE ELECTROPHORETIC NATURE OF THE VARIANT SUGGESTED THAT THE MOLECULE IS A DIMER WITH MUTATION IN THE GENE CONTROLLING ONE OF THE ELEMENTS AND THAT THIS GENE IS AUTOSOMAL. SUPERNATANT MDH

IS ALSO POLYMORPHIC IN MICE AND IS APPARENTLY UNDER GENETIC CONTROL INDEPENDENT OF
THAT CONTROLLING MITOCHONDRIAL MDH. FURTHERMORE, IN THE MOUSE THE LOCUS FOR S-MDH
IS IN THE SECOND LINKAGE GROUP (HENDERSON, 1966) WHICH ALSO CONTAINS THE TRANSFER-
RIN LOCUS. LINKAGE OF THESE LOCI SHOULD BE SOUGHT IN MAN. IN MICE SHOWS AND
RUDDLE (1968) FOUND EVIDENCE THAT SUPERNATANT NADP-DEPENDENT MALATE DEHYDROGENASE
HAS A TETRAMERIC STRUCTURE WITH TWO TYPES OF SUBUNITS, DETERMINED PRESUMABLY BY
SEPARATE LOCI.

BLAKE, N. M., KIRK, R. L., SIMONS, M. J. AND ALPERS, M. P.* GENETIC VARIANTS OF
SOLUBLE MALATE DEHYDROGENASE IN NEW GUINEA POPULATIONS. HUMANGENETIK 11* 72-74,
1970.

DAVIDSON, R. G. AND CORTNER, J. A.* GENETIC VARIANT OF HUMAN ERYTHROCYTE MALATE
DEHYDROGENASE. NATURE 215* 761-762, 1967.

HENDERSON, N. S.* ISOZYMES AND GENETIC CONTROL OF NADP-MALATE DEHYDROGENASE IN
MICE. ARCH. BIOCHEM. 117* 28-33, 1966.

SHOWS, T. B. AND RUDDLE, F. H.* MALATE DEHYDROGENASE* EVIDENCE FOR TETRAMERIC
STRUCTURE IN MUS MUSCULUS. SCIENCE 160* 1356-1357, 1968.

15430 MALOCCLUSION DUE TO PROTRUBERANT UPPER FRONT TEETH

STODDARD'S OBSERVATIONS (1947) CONCERNED 19 PERSONS IN 8 SIBSHIPS IN 3 GENERA-
TIONS. NO MALE-TO-MALE TRANSMISSION WAS OBSERVED BUT OF THE 8 DAUGHTERS OF AN
AFFECTED MALE 3 WERE SPARED, MAKING X-LINKED DOMINANCE WITH FULL PENETRANCE
IMPOSSIBLE.

STODDARD, S. E.* INHERITANCE OF MALOCCLUSION. J. HERED. 38* 117-119, 1947.

15440 MANDIBULO-FACIAL DYSOSTOSIS (TREACHER COLLINS TYPE) WITH LIMB ANOMALIES
(NAGER'S ACROFACIAL DYSOSTOSIS)

THE LIMB DEFORMITIES CONSIST OF ABSENCE OF RADIUS, RADIO-ULNAR SYNOSTOSIS AND
HYPOPLASIA OR ABSENCE OF THE THUMBS. ALL REPORTED CASES ARE SPORADIC. HOWEVER,
MARDEN, SMITH AND MCDONALD (1964) DESCRIBED AN INFANT WITH THIS SYNDROME WHOSE
FATHER AND MOTHER WERE 42 AND 41, RESPECTIVELY, AT THE TIME OF HIS BIRTH, THUS
SUGGESTING DOMINANT MUTATION.

MARDEN, P. M., SMITH, D. W. AND MCDONALD, M. J.* CONGENITAL ANOMALIES IN THE
NEWBORN INFANT, INCLUDING MINOR VARIATIONS. A STUDY OF 4,412 BABIES BY SURFACE
EXAMINATION FOR ANOMALIES AND BUCCAL SMEAR FOR SEX CHROMATIN. J. PEDIAT. 64* 357-
371, 1964.

*15450 MANDIBULO-FACIAL DYSOSTOSIS (TREACHER COLLINS-FRANCESCHETTI SYNDROME)

THE FEATURES ARE ANTI-MONGOLOID SLANT OF THE EYES, COLOBOMA OF THE LID, MICROGNA-
THIA, MICROTIA AND OTHER DEFORMITY OF THE EARS, HYPOPLASTIC ZYGOMATIC ARCHES AND
MACROSTOMIA. THE MOUTH IS UNUSUALLY LARGE. IT SHOULD NOT BE CONFUSED WITH
SIMILAR ENTITIES SUCH AS THE OCULO-AURICULO-VERTEBRAL SYNDROME (Q.V.).
ROVIN, DACHI, BORENSTEIN AND COTTER (1964) OBSERVED 14 AFFECTED PERSONS IN 5
GENERATIONS OF A KENTUCKY FAMILY. INTRAFAMILIAL VARIATION WAS WIDE. INTERSIB
VARIATION WAS SMALL. THERE SEEMED TO BE A SIGNIFICANT INCREASE IN AFFECTED
OFFSPRING FROM AFFECTED FEMALES AND A DECREASE IN AFFECTED OFFSPRING FROM AFFECTED
MALES. FAZEN ET AL. (1967) DESCRIBED 10 AFFECTED PERSONS IN 4 GENERATIONS. (THEY
HYPHENATED TREACHER COLLINS, WHICH IS NOT PROPER, TREACHER HAVING BEEN ONE OF DR.
COLLINS' GIVEN NAMES.)

BOOK, J. A. AND FRACCARO, M.* GENETICAL INVESTIGATIONS IN A NORTH-SWEDISH
POPULATION. MANDIBULO-FACIAL DYSOSTOSIS. ACTA GENET. STATIST. MED. 5* 327-333,
1955.

COLLINS, E. TREACHER* CASES WITH SYMMETRICAL CONGENITAL NOTCHES IN THE OUTER
PART OF EACH LOWER LID AND DEFECTIVE DEVELOPMENT OF THE MALAR BONES. TRANS.
OPHTHAL. SOC. U.K. 20* 190-192, 1933.

EDWARDS, W.* CONGENITAL MIDDLE-EAR DEAFNESS WITH ANOMALIES OF THE FACE. J.
LARYNG. 78* 152-170, 1964.

FAZEN, L. E., ELMORE, J. AND NADLER, H. L.* MANDIBULO-FACIAL DYSOSTOSIS.
(TREACHER-COLLINS SYNDROME). AM. J. DIS. CHILD. 113* 405-410, 1967.

FERNANDEZ, A. C. AND RONIS, M. L.* THE TREACHER-COLLINS SYNDROME. ARCH.
OTOLARYNG. 80* 505-520, 1964.

FRANCESCHETTI, A. AND KLEIN, D.* MANDIBULO-FACIAL DYSOSTOSIS* NEW HEREDITARY
SYNDROME. ACTA OPHTHAL. 27* 143-224, 1949.

MONNET, P., BOULEZ, N., NEUMANN, E., MAYNARD, Y. AND HUMBERT, G.* DEUX CAS DE
DYSOSTOSE MANDIBULO-FACIALE OU SYNDROME DE FRANCESCHETTI. PEDIATRIE 15* 537-544,
1960.

ROVIN, S., DACHI, S. F., BORENSTEIN, D. B. AND COTTER, W. B.* MANDIBULOFACIAL DYSOSTOSIS, A FAMILIAL STUDY OF FIVE GENERATIONS. J. PEDIAT. 65* 215-221, 1964.

STOVIN, J. J., LYON, J. A., JR. AND CLEMMENS, R. L.* MANDIBULOFACIAL DYSOSTO-SIS. RADIOLOGY 74* 225-231, 1960.

15460 MARCUS GUNN PHENOMENON ('JAW-WINKING,' OR MAXILLO-PALPEBRAL SYNKINESIS)

ALTHOUGH IT USUALLY PERSISTS INTO ADULT LIFE, THIS PHENOMENON IS SEEN IN ITS MOST MARKED FORMS IN INFANCY WHEN THE RAPID SPASMODIC MOVEMENTS OF THE LID ARE APPARENT DURING SUCKING AND THUS ARE NOTED SOON AFTER BIRTH. IT IS TYPICALLY UNILATERAL AND IS ASSOCIATED WITH PTOSIS. THE PHENOMENON HAS BEEN OBSERVED IN SUCESSIVE GENERATIONS ON SEVERAL OCCASIONS. KIRKHAM (1969) DESCRIBED BROTHER AND SISTER WITH UNILATERAL MARCUS GUNN PHENOMENON.

COOPER, E. L.* THE JAW-WINKING PHENOMENON. REPORT OF A CASE. ARCH. OPHTHAL. 18* 198-203, 1937.

FALLS, H. F., KRUSE, W. T. AND COTTERMAN, C. W.* THREE CASES OF MARCUS GUNN PHENOMENON IN 2 GENERATIONS. AM. J. OPHTHAL. 32* 53-59, 1949.

GRANT, F. C.* THE MARCUS GUNN PHENOMENON* REPORT OF A CASE WITH SUGGESTIONS AS TO RELIEF. ARCH. NEUROL. PSYCHIAT. 35* 487-500, 1936.

KIRKHAM, T. H.* FAMILIAL MARCUS GUNN PHENOMENON. BRIT. J. OPHTHAL. 53* 282-283, 1969.

LERI, A. AND WEILL, J.* PHENOMENE DE MARCUS GUNN (SYNERGIE PALPEBRO-MAXILLAIRE) CONGENITAL ET HEREDITAIRE. BULL. SOC. MED. HOP. PARIS 53* 875-880, 1929.

*15470 MARFAN SYNDROME

CARDINAL FEATURES OCCUR IN THREE AREAS - IN THE EYE, ESPECIALLY SUBLUXATION OF THE LENSES, IN THE SKELETAL SYSTEM, ESPECIALLY EXCESSIVE LENGTH OF THE EXTREMITIES, AND IN THE CARDIOVASCULAR SYSTEM, ESPECIALLY DISSECTING AND-OR DIFFUSE ANEURYSM OF THE ASCENDING AORTA. HOMOCYSTINURIA, A RECESSIVE, ALSO PRODUCES ECTOPIA LENTIS AND VASCULAR LESIONS. FURTHERMORE ECTOPIC LENTIS IS A FEATURE OF SULFO-CYS-TEINURIA AND OF WEILL-MARCHESANI SYNDROME. METACHROMASIA OF FIBROBLASTS WAS REPORTED BY MATALON AND DORFMAN (1968).

MASSUMI, R. A., LOWE, E. W., MISANIK, L. F., JUST, H. AND TAWAKKOI, A.* MULTIPLE AORTIC ANEURYSMS (THORACIC AND ABDOMINAL) IN TWINS WITH MARFAN'S SYNDROME* FATAL RUPTURE DURING PREGNANCY. J. THORAC. CARDIOVASC. SURG. 53* 223-230, 1967.

MATALON, R. AND DORFMAN, A.* THE ACCUMULATION OF HYALURONIC ACID IN CULTURED FIBROBLASTS OF THE MARFAN SYNDROME. BIOCHEM. BIOPHYS. RES. COMMUN. 32* 150-154, 1968.

MCKUSICK, V. A.* HERITABLE DISORDERS OF CONNECTIVE TISSUE. ST. LOUIS* C. V. MOSBY CO., 1966 (3RD ED.).

15480 MAST CELL DISEASE

THE CUTANEOUS MANIFESTATION IS TERMED URTICARIA PIGMENTOSA. GENERALIZED INVOLVE-MENT, WHICH MAY BE FATAL, IS SOMETIMES OBSERVED. BURGOON ET AL. (1968) OBSERVED THE DISORDER IN FATHER AND DAUGHTER.

BURGOON, C. F., JR., GRAHAM, J. H. AND MCCAFFREE, D. L.* MAST CELL DISEASE. A CUTANEOUS VARIANT WITH MULTISYSTEM INVOLVEMENT. ARCH. DERM. 98* 590-605, 1968.

15490 MASTOCYTOSIS

SELMANOWITZ AND ORENTREICH (1970) STATED THAT ABOUT 40 FAMILIAL CASES AND SIX CONCORDANT PAIRS OF MONOZYGOTIC TWINS ARE KNOWN. BOTH DOMINANT AND RECESSIVE INHERITANCE HAS BEEN POSTULATED (SHAW, 1968).

SELMANOWITZ, V. J. AND ORENTREICH, N.* MASTOCYTOSIS* A CLINICAL GENETIC EVALUATION. J. HERED. 61* 91-94, 1970.

SHAW, J. M.* GENETIC ASPECTS OF URTICARIA PIGMENTOSA. ARCH. DERM. 97* 137-138, 1968.

15500 MAXILLOFACIAL DYSOSTOSIS

PETERS AND HOVELS (1960) DESCRIBED THE FAMILIAL NATURE OF THE SYNDROME.

PETERS, A. AND HOVELS, O.* DIE DYSOSTOSIS MAXILLO-FACIALIS, EINE ERBLICHE, TYPISCHE FEHLBILDUNG DES 1. VISCERALBOGENS. Z. MENSCHL. VERERB. KONSTITUTIONSL. 35* 434-444, 1960.

*15510 MAY-HEGGLIN ANOMALY

THE MAY-HEGGLIN ANOMALY CONSISTS OF CYTOPLASMIC RNA-CONTAINING INCLUSIONS OF THE
LEUKOCYTES IN ASSOCIATION WITH GIANT PLATELETS. THE INCLUSIONS ARE THE SO-CALLED
DOHLE BODIES WHICH ARE ALSO SEEN, THOUGH ONLY TRANSIENTLY, WITH ACUTE INFECTIONS.
OSKI AND COLLEAGUES (1962) OBSERVED THE ANOMALY IN A MOTHER AND HER TWO CHILDREN.
OF 24 REPORTED CASES 9 HAD THROMBOCYTOPENIA. ON THE BASIS OF ELECTRON MICROSCOPIC
STUDIES, JENIS ET AL. (1971) SUGGESTED THAT THE INCLUSIONS REPRESENTED PARACRYS-
TALLINE ARRAYS OF DEPOLYMERIZED RIBOSOMES.

JENIS, E. H., TAKEUCHI, A., DILLON, D. E., RUYMANN, F. B. AND RIVKIN, S.* THE
MAY-HEGGLIN ANOMALY* ULTRASTRUCTURE OF THE GRANULOCYTE INCLUSION. AM. J. CLIN.
PATH. 55* 187-196, 1971.

JORDAN, S. W. AND LARSEN, W. E.* ULTRASTRUCTURAL STUDIES OF THE MAY-HEGGLIN
ANOMALY. BLOOD 25* 921-932, 1965.

OSKI, F. A., NAIMAN, J. L., ALLEN, D. M. AND DIAMOND, L. K.* LEUKOCYTIC
INCLUSIONS - DOHLE BODIES - ASSOCIATED WITH PLATELET ABNORMALITY (THE MAY-HEGGLIN
ANOMALY). REPORT OF A FAMILY AND REVIEW OF THE LITERATURE. BLOOD 20* 657-667,
1962.

15520 MEDIOSTERNAL DEPIGMENTATION LINE

KISCH AND NASUHOGLU (1953) DESCRIBED A MEDIOSTERNAL, LONGITUDINALLY DIRECTED
STREAK OF HYPOPIGMENTATION IN FIVE NEGROES. I HAVE OBSERVED THIS, BUT NO
SYSTEMATIC FAMILY STUDIES HAVE BEEN DONE. SEE FUTCHER'S LINE AND RAINDROP
DEPIGMENTATION FOR OTHER PIGMENT PECULIARITIES IN NEGROES.

KISCH, B. AND NASUHOGLU, A.* MEDIOSTERNAL DEPIGMENTATION LINE IN NEGROES. EXP.
MED. SURG. 11* 265-267, 1953.

*15530 MEGADUODENUM AND-OR MEGACYSTIS

LAW AND TEN EYCK (1962) REPORTED THE ASSOCIATION OF MEGADUODENUM AND MEGACYSTIS IN
9 MEMBERS OF A FAMILY OF ITALIAN EXTRACTION. MALE-TO-MALE TRANSMISSION WAS
OBSERVED. WEISS (1938) REPORTED MEGADUODENUM ALONE IN 6 PERSONS IN 3 GENERATIONS
OF A GERMAN FAMILY. NEWTON (1968) TREATED TWO NEGRO MALES WITH MEGADUODENUM. ONE
OF THEM ALSO HAD MAGACYSTIS AND THE FATHER PROBABLY HAD MEGADUODENUM. MARFANOID
HABITUS WAS NOTED. OBERHELMAN, IN DISCUSSING NEWTON'S PAPER REFERRED TO A FAMILY
WITH MULTIPLE CASES OF MEGADUODENUM. TOBENKIN (1964) DESCRIBED MEGACYSTIS WITH
NONOBSTRUCTIVE VESICOURETER REFLUX IN A MOTHER AND HER THREE DAUGHTERS. THE
HISTORY OF UNILATERAL NEPHRECTOMY IN THE MATERNAL GRANDMOTHER SUGGESTED THAT THREE
GENERATIONS MAY HAVE BEEN AFFECTED. NO COMMENT ON ASSOCIATED MEGADUODENUM WAS
MADE.

LAW, D. H. AND TEN EYCK, E. A.* FAMILIAL MEGADUODENUM AND MEGACYSTIS. AM. J.
MED. 33* 911-922, 1962.

NEWTON, W. T.* RADICAL ENTERECTOMY FOR HEREDITARY MEGADUODENUM. ARCH. SURG.
96* 549-553, 1968.

TOBENKIN, M. I.* HEREDITARY VESICOURETERAL REFLUX. STH. MED. J. 57* 139-147,
1964.

WEISS, W.* ZUR ATIOLOGIE DES MEGADUODENUMS. DEUTSCH. Z. CHIR. 251* 317-330,
1938.

15540 MEGALOCORNEA

AUTOSOMAL DOMINANT INHERITANCE IS PROBABLY MUCH RARER THAN X-LINKED RECESSIVE
(Q.V.). MEGALOCORNEA IS AN OCCASIONAL FEATURE OF THE MARFAN SYNDROME.

ALAERTS, L.* FAMILIAL MEGALOCORNEA. BULL. SOC. BELG. OPHTAL. 92* 322-326,
1949.

BONHOMME, F.* UN CAS DE MEGALOCORNEE. BULL. SOC. OPHTAL. FRANC. 49* 184-190,
1937.

GREDIG, C.* EINE NEUE VERERBUNGSART DER MEGALOCORNEA. ARCH. KLAUS STIFT.
VERERBUNGSFORSCH. 2* 79-89, 1926.

KLAR, R.* BEITRAGE ZUR FRAGE DER MEGALOKORNEA AUF GRUND VON UNTERSUCHUNGEN
EINES STAROPERIERTEN PATIENTEN UND SEINER SIPPE. KLIN. MBL. AUGENHEILK. 104* 286-
299, 1940.

15550 MEGALODACTYLY

ONE OR TWO FINGERS ARE GROTESQUELY ENLARGED. BARSKY (1967) AND OTHERS HAVE FOUND
NO REPORT OF FAMILIAL OCCURRENCE.

BARSKY, A. J.* MACRODACTYLY. J. BONE JOINT SURG. 49A* 1255-1266, 1967.

RECHNAGEL, K.* MEGALODACTYLISM. REPORT OF 7 CASES. ACTA ORTHOP. SCAND. 38*

15560 MELANOMA, MALIGNANT

KATZENELLENBOGEN AND SANDBANK (1967) DESCRIBED DIZYGOTIC TWINS EACH WITH MALIGNANT MELANOMA. CAWLEY (1952) OBSERVED THIS MALIGNANCY IN FATHER, SON AND DAUGHTER. SEVERAL WRITERS (E.G. MOSCHELLA, 1961* SCHOCH, 1963* SALOMON ET AL., 1963) COMMENTED ON THE USUAL FAIR COMPLEXION, BLUE EYES AND MULTIPLE EPHELIDES IN THESE PATIENTS. SMITH, HENLY, KNOX AND LANE (1966) DESCRIBED AFFECTED MOTHER AND SON. ANDERSON ET AL. (1967) DESCRIBED MALIGNANT MELANOMA IN AT LEAST 15 MEMBERS OF THREE GENERATIONS OF A SINGLE KINDRED. EARLY AGE OF ONSET AND A TENDENCY FOR MULTIPLE PRIMARY LESIONS WERE FEATURES THEY NOTED. ANDREWS (1968) REPORTED BROTHER AND SISTER. LYNCH AND KRUSH (1968) DESCRIBED TWO FAMILIES WITH MALIGNANT MELANOMA IN TWO GENERATIONS IN ONE AND THREE GENERATIONS IN ANOTHER.

ANDERSON, D. E., SMITH, J. L., JR. AND MCBRIDE, C. M.* HEREDITARY ASPECTS OF MALIGNANT MELANOMA. J.A.M.A. 200* 741-746, 1967.

ANDREWS, J. C.* MALIGNANT MELANOMA IN SIBLINGS. ARCH. DERM. 98* 282-283, 1968.

CAWLEY, E. P.* GENETIC ASPECTS OF MALIGNANT MELANOMA. ARCH. DERM. SYPH. 65* 440-450, 1952.

KATZENELLENBOGEN, I. AND SANDBANK, M.* MALIGNANT MELANOMA IN TWINS. ARCH. DERM. 94* 331-332, 1967.

LYNCH, H. T. AND KRUSH, A. J.* HEREDITY AND MALIGNANT MELANOMA* IMPLICATIONS FOR EARLY CANCER DETECTION. CANAD. MED. ASS. J. 99* 17-21, 1968.

MOSCHELLA, S. L.* A REPORT OF MALIGNANT MELANOMA OF THE SKIN IN SISTERS. ARCH. DERM. 84* 1024-1025, 1961.

SALOMON, T., SCHNYDER, I. W. AND STORCK, H.* A CONTRIBUTION TO THE QUESTION OF HEREDITY IN MALIGNANT MELANOMAS. DERMATOLOGICA 126* 65-75, 1963.

SCHOCH, E. P., JR.* FAMILIAL MALIGNANT MELANOMA. A PEDIGREE AND CYTOGENETIC STUDY. ARCH. DERM. 88* 445-455, 1963.

SMITH, F. E., HENLY, W. S., KNOX, J. M. AND LANE, M.* FAMILIAL MELANOMA. ARCH. INTERN. MED. 117* 820-823, 1966.

15570 MELANOMA, MALIGNANT INTRAOCULAR

BOWEN, BRADY AND JONES (1964) REPORTED MALIGNANT INTRAOCULAR MELANOMA IN A 45 YEAR OLD WHITE FEMALE AND IN HER 26 YEAR OLD DAUGHTER. DAVENPORT (1927) REPORTED THIS MALIGNANCY IN THREE SUCCESSIVE GENERATIONS.

BOWEN, S. F., BRADY, H. AND JONES, V. L.* MALIGNANT MELANOMA OF EYE OCCURRING IN TWO SUCCESSIVE GENERATIONS. ARCH. OPHTHAL. 71* 805-806, 1964.

DAVENPORT, R. C.* FAMILIAL HISTORY OF CHOROIDAL SARCOMA. BRIT. J. OPHTHAL. 11* 443-445, 1927.

*15580 MELANOSIS, UNIVERSAL

SCHEIDT (1926) DESCRIBED 14 AFFECTED IN 4 SUCCESSIVE GENERATIONS. ORTH (1929) DESCRIBED 2 FAMILIES, EACH WITH FOUR AFFECTED GENERATIONS. PEGUM (1955) AND WENDE AND BAUCKUS (1919) DESCRIBED GENERALIZED HYPERPIGMENTATION BEGINNING IN INFANCY IN A PAIR OF SIBS. TVAROH AND KARES (1968) DESCRIBED 5 AFFECTED IN 3 GENERATIONS.

LEBER, R.* UBER EINE FAMILIE MIT ERBLICHEM UNIVERSELLEM MELANISMUS. Z. KINDERHEILK. 58* 142-147, 1936.

ORTH, H.* UBER ZWEI FALLE VON ERBLICHEM MELANISMUS. ARCH. DERM. SYPH. 158* 95-97, 1929.

PEGUM, J. S.* DIFFUSE PIGMENTATION IN BROTHERS. PROC. ROY. SOC. MED. 48* 179-180, 1955.

SCHEIDT, W.* EINIGE ERGEBNISSE BIOLOGISCHER FAMILIENERHEBUNGEN. ARCH. RASS. 17* 135-139, 1926.

TVAROH, F. AND KARES, B.* FAMILIAL OCCURRENCE OF DIFFUSE MELANOSIS. PLZEN. LEK. SBORN. 22 (SUPPL.)* 35-38, 1968.

WENDE, G. W. AND BAUCKUS, H. H.* A HITHERTO UNDESCRIBED GENERALIZED PIGMENTA-TION OF THE SKIN APPEARING IN INFANCY IN BROTHER AND SISTER. J. CUTAN. DIS. 37* 685-701, 1919.

*15590 MELKERSSON'S SYNDROME

THE FEATURES ARE CHRONIC SWELLING OF THE FACE, PERIPHERAL FACIAL PALSY WHICH MAY

BE BILATERAL AND TENDS TO RELAPSE, AND IN SOME CASES LINGUA PLICATA. THE DISEASE OFTEN BEGINS IN CHILDHOOD OR YOUTH. THE SWELLING IS LOCALIZED ESPECIALLY TO THE LIPS. KUNSTADTER (1965) DESCRIBED A CASE WITH ONSET AT 5 AND ONE-HALF YEARS. THE MATERNAL GRANDMOTHER DEVELOPED UNILATERAL BELL'S PALSY WITHOUT FACIAL EDEMA AT AGE 68. A MATERNAL AUNT AT 10 YEARS OF AGE DEVELOPED UNILATERAL BELL'S PALSY WITH QUESTIONABLE EDEMA AND RECOVERED COMPLETELY. CARR (1966) FOUND AT LEAST FOUR OTHER REPORTED FAMILIES IN WHICH TWO GENERATIONS WERE AFFECTED AND ONE INSTANCE OF THREE GENERATIONS AFFECTED.

CARR, R. D.* IS THE MELKERSSON-ROSENTHAL SYNDROME HEREDITARY.Q ARCH. DERM. 93* 426-427, 1966.

KUNSTADTER, R. H.* MELKERSSON'S SYNDROME. A CASE REPORT OF MULTIPLE RECUR-RENCES OF BELL'S PALSY AND EPISODIC FACIAL EDEMA. AM. J. DIS. CHILD. 110* 559-561, 1965.

15600 MENIERE'S DISEASE

ALTHOUGH GENETIC FACTORS PROBABLY ARE INVOLVED TO A SIGNIFICANT EXTENT, IT IS UNUSUAL TO FIND MORE THAN ONE CASE OF EPISODIC VERTIGO AND HEARING LOSS IN THE SAME FAMILY. BERNSTEIN (1965) REPORTED SEVEN SUCH FAMILIES. IN ONE FAMILY IDENTICAL FEMALE TWINS AND THE DAUGHTER OF ONE OF THE TWINS WERE AFFECTED. THREE FAMILIES HAD MIGRAINE ALSO IN CERTAIN MEMBERS. (ALSO SEE ATAXIA, PERIODIC VESTIBULO-CEREBELLAR.)

BERNSTEIN, J. M.* OCCURRENCE OF EPISODIC VERTIGO AND HEARING LOSS IN FAMILIES. ANN. OTOL. 74* 1011-1021, 1965.

15610 MENINGIOMA

ALTHOUGH THE MODE OF INHERITANCE IS NOT CLEAR, A FEW REPORTS HAVE INDICATED FAMILIAL OCCURRENCE OF MENINGIOMA.

GAIST, G. AND PIAZZA, G.* MENINGIOMAS IN TWO MEMBERS OF THE SAME FAMILY (WITH NO EVIDENCE OF NEUROFIBROMATOSIS). J. NEUROSURG. 16* 110-113, 1959.

JOYNT, R. J. AND PERRET, G. E.* MENINGIOMAS IN A MOTHER AND DAUGHTER. CASES WITHOUT EVIDENCE OF NEUROFIBROMATOSIS. NEUROLOGY 11* 164-165, 1961.

SAHAR, A.* FAMILIAL OCCURRENCE OF MENINGIOMAS.* CASE REPORT. J. NEUROSURG. 23* 444-445, 1965.

15620 MENTAL RETARDATION

IN TWO FAMILIES WITH UNDIFFERENTIATED MENTAL RETARDATION OCCURRING IN MEMBERS OF MULTIPLE GENERATIONS, DEKABAN AND KLEIN (1968) CONCLUDED THAT DOMINANT TRANSMIS-SION (I.E., A SINGLE MAJOR GENE) COULD BE RESPONSIBLE.

DEKABAN, A. S. AND KLEIN, D.* FAMILIAL MENTAL RETARDATION. ACTA GENET. STATIST. MED. 18* 206-228, 1968.

15630 METACHROMASIA OF FIBROBLASTS

DANES ET AL. (1970) HAVE DESCRIBED SIX FAMILIES IN WHICH METACHROMASIA CAN BE TRACED THROUGH NORMAL INDIVIDUALS IN AT LEAST THREE GENERATIONS. THE BASIS FOR THE METACHROMASIA IS NOT KNOWN. INCREASED CONCENTRATIONS OF MUCOPOLYSACCHARIDES IS NOT THE EXPLANATION. POSSIBLY THIS CELLULAR CHARACTERISTIC IS AN EXPRESSION OF THE HETEROZYGOUS STATE OF SOME RECESSIVE DISORDERS.

DANES, B. S., SCOTT, J. E. AND BEARN, A. G.* FURTHER STUDIES ON METACHROMASIA IN CULTURED HUMAN FIBROBLASTS. STAINING OF GLYCOSAMINOGLYCANS (MUCOPOLYSAC-CHARIDES) BY ALCIAN BLUE IN SALT SOLUTIONS. J. EXP. MED. 132* 765-774, 1970.

*15640 METAPHYSEAL DYSOSTOSIS, MURK JANSEN TYPE

STOECKENIUS (1966) DESCRIBED AFFECTED MOTHER AND CHILD. THE MOTHER'S CONDITION MAY HAVE BEEN THE RESULT OF NEW DOMINANT MUTATION. HER FATHER WAS 40 YEARS OLD AT HER BIRTH. LENZ (1967) SAW THE SAME FAMILY. THE MOTHER WAS ONLY 102 CM. TALL. THE EXTREME DISORGANIZATION OF THE METAPHYSES OF THE LONG BONES AND OF THE METACARPAL AND METATARSAL BONES IS IN SHARP CONTRAST WITH THE ALMOST NORMAL APPEARANCE OF THE EPIPHYSEAL CENTERS, WHICH ON X-RAY APPEAR WIDELY SEPARATED FROM THE LONG BONES. THE CHIN IS RECEDING. THE FINGERS, ESPECIALLY THE DISTAL PHALANGES, ARE VERY SHORT. THE SPINE, PELVIS AND LOWER LEGS ARE DISTORTED. DE HAAS ET AL. (1969) GAVE A FOLLOW-UP OF THE ORIGINAL CASE OF MURK JANSEN. THE STRIKING FEATURE AT AGE 44 WAS THE DEVELOPMENT OF NEARLY NORMAL BONE STRUCTURE WITH, HOWEVER, MARKED DEFORMITY AND DWARFING. SCLEROSIS IN THE CRANIAL BONES, INCLUDING THE PETROUS BONE LEADING TO DEAFNESS, WAS DEMONSTRATED. HYPERCALCEMIA HAS BEEN NOTED IN CASES IN CHILDHOOD (LENZ, 1969* HOLT AND DENT IN DISCUSSION OF LENZ, 1969). SEE THE FOLLOW-UP BY LENZ (1969).

DE HAAS, W. H. D., DE BOER, W. AND GRIFFIOEN, F.* METAPHYSEAL DYSOSTOSIS. A LATE FOLLOW-UP OF THE FIRST REPORTED CASE. J. BONE JOINT SURG. 51B* 290-299,

LENZ, W.* DIAGNOSIS IN MEDICAL GENETICS. IN CROW, J. F. AND NEEL, J. V. (EDS.)* PROC. 3RD. INTERN. CONG. HUM. GENET., SEPT., 1966. BALTIMORE* JOHNS HOPKINS PRESS, 1967. PP. 29-36.

LENZ, W.* DISCUSSION. THE CLINICAL DELINEATION OF BIRTH DEFECTS. IV. SKELETAL DYSPLASIAS. NEW YORK* NATIONAL FOUNDATION, 1969. PP. 71-72.

OZONOFF, M. B.* METAPHYSEAL DYSOSTOSIS OF JANSEN. RADIOLOGY 93* 1047-1050, 1969.

STOECKENIUS, (NI)* CITED BY LENZ, W.* SYMPOSION UBER GENERALISIERTE ANOMALIEN DES SKELETES. MSCHR. KINDERHEILK. 114* 157-158, 1966.

*15650 METAPHYSEAL DYSOSTOSIS, SCHMIDT TYPE

THIS IS NOT A TRUE DYSOSTOSIS (SINCE IT IS NOT PRIMARILY A DISORDER OF BONE FORMATION), NOR IS THE PRIMARY DEFECT IN THE METAPHYSES. IRREGULARITIES OF THE METAPHYSEAL ENDS OF BONES OF THE EXTREMITIES ARE DEMONSTRATED RADIOLOGICALLY. BOWLEGS AND COXA VARA RESULT. THERE IS A RECESSIVE TYPE OF METAPHYSEAL DYSOSTOSIS (SPAHR TYPE). ROSENBLOOM AND SMITH (1965) DESCRIBED 24 AFFECTED PERSONS IN ONE KINDRED. IN 1943, STEPHENS REPORTED ON A MORMAN KINDRED IN WHICH OVER 40 MEMBERS OF FOUR GENERATIONS WERE AFFECTED WITH WHAT HE CONSIDERED TO BE ACHONDROPLASIA. THE X-RAY FINDINGS AS DEMONSTRATED IN HIS FIGURES AND AS REVIEWED BY CAFFEY (1963) ARE, HOWEVER, THOSE OF METAPHYSEAL DYSOSTOSIS. IN A 3 YEAR OLD CHILD THE INTER-PEDUNCULAR DISTANCES AND GREATER SCIATIC GROOVE WERE QUITE NORMAL AND THE TYPICAL METAPHYSEAL CHANGES WERE DEMONSTRATED. AFFECTED WOMEN WENT THROUGH VAGINAL DELIVERIES SUCCESSFULLY AND WERE USUALLY ACCOMPANIED ONLY BY A MIDWIFE. STEPHENS (1943) SUGGESTED THAT THE ORIGINAL MUTATION COULD BE IDENTIFIED. THE FIRST AFFECTED ANCESTOR, BORN IN 1833, WAS SAID TO HAVE NORMAL PARENTS AND 11 UNAFFECTED SIBS.

CAFFEY, J.* QUOTED BY DR. WILLIAM R. CHRISTENSEN, SALT LAKE CITY, 1963.

DAESCHNER, C. W., SINGLETON, E. B., HILL, L. L. AND DODGE, W. F.* METAPHYSEAL DYSOSTOSIS. J. PEDIAT. 57* 844-854, 1960.

DAVID, J. E. A. AND PALMER, P. E. S.* FAMILIAL METAPHYSIAL DYSPLASIA. J. BONE JOINT SURG. 40B* 86-93, 1958.

DENT, C. E. AND NORMAND, I. C. S.* METAPHYSEAL DYSOSTOSIS, TYPE SCHMID. ARCH. DIS. CHILD. 39* 444-454, 1964.

MILLER, S. M. AND PAUL, L. W.* ROENTGEN OBSERVATIONS IN FAMILIAL METAPHYSEAL DYSOSTOSIS. RADIOLOGY 83* 665-673, 1964.

PETERSON, J. C.* METAPHYSEAL DYSOSTOSIS* QUESTIONABLY A FORM OF VITAMIN D-RESISTANT RICKETS. J. PEDIAT. 60* 656-663, 1962.

ROSENBLOOM, A. L. AND SMITH, D. W.* THE NATURAL HISTORY OF METAPHYSEAL DYSOSTOSIS. J. PEDIAT. 66* 857-868, 1965.

STEPHENS, F. E.* AN ACHONDROPLASTIC MUTATION AND THE NATURE OF ITS INHERITANCE. J. HERED. 34* 229-235, 1943.

STICKLER, G. B., MAHER, F. T., HUNT, J. C., BURKE, E. C. AND ROSEVEAR, J. W.* FAMILIAL BONE DISEASE RESEMBLING RICKETS (HEREDITARY METAPHYSEAL DYSOSTOSIS). PEDIATRICS 29* 996-1004, 1962.

15660 MICROCORIA, CONGENITAL

ARDOUIN ET AL. (1964) DESCRIBED A FAMILY IN WHICH 25 PERSONS HAD SMALL PUPILS DUE APPARENTLY TO HYPOPLASIA OF THE DILATOR MUSCLE OF THE IRIS. MYOPIA WAS PRESENT IN ALL.

ARDOUIN, M., URVOY, M. AND LEFRANC, J.* MICROCORIE CONGENITALE. BULL. SOC. FRANC. OPHTHAL. 64* 356-363, 1964.

15670 MICROCORNEA, GLAUCOMA AND ABSENT FRONTAL SINUSES

GRANDMOTHER, MOTHER, SON AND DAUGHTER SHOWED THIS COMBINATION IN THE FAMILY REPORTED BY HOLMES AND WALTON (1969).

HOLMES, L. B. AND WALTON, D. S.* HEREDITARY MICROCORNEA, GLAUCOMA, AND ABSENT FRONTAL SINUSES* A FAMILY STUDY. J. PEDIAT. 74* 968-972, 1969.

15680 MICRODONTIA, GENERALIZED

IN THE FAMILY REPORTED BY STEINBERG, WARREN AND WARREN (1961) EITHER AUTOSOMAL DOMINANT OR SEX-LINKED DOMINANT INHERITANCE IS POSSIBLE.

STEINBERG, A. G., WARREN, J. F. AND WARREN, L. M.* HEREDITARY GENERALIZED MICRODONTIA. J. DENT. RES. 40* 58-62, 1961.

15690 MICROPHTHALMOS WITH MYOPIA AND CORECTOPIA

USHER (1921) DESCRIBED A FAMILY WITH ELEVEN CASES IN 4 GENERATIONS INCLUDING THREE INSTANCES OF MALE-TO-MALE TRANSMISSION. MYOPIA AND DISPLACED PUPIL WERE ASSO-CIATED WITH MICROPHTHALMOS.

USHER, C. H.* A PEDIGREE OF MICROPHTHALMIA WITH MYOPIA AND CORECTOPIA. BRIT. J. OPHTHAL. 5* 289-299, 1921.

15700 MICROPHTHALMOS, ANTERIOR (MICROCORNEA)

FRIEDMAN AND WRIGHT (1952) REPORTED A PEDIGREE WITH 8 CASES IN 5 GENERATIONS.

FRIEDMAN, M. W. AND WRIGHT, E. S.* HEREDITARY MICROCORNEA AND CATARACT IN FIVE GENERATIONS. AM. J. OPHTHAL. 35* 1017-1021, 1952.

15710 MICROPHTHALMOS, PIGMENTARY RETINOPATHY, GLAUCOMA

HERMANN (1958) REPORTED A FAMILY WITH MICROPHTHALMOS IN 13 MEMBERS OF 4 GENERA-TIONS. SOME ALSO HAD PIGMENTARY RETINOPATHY AND SOME HAD GLAUCOMA.

HERMANN, P.* LE SYNDROME MICROPHTALMIE-RETINITE PIGMENTAIRE-GLAUCOME. ARCH. OPHTHAL. 18* 17-24, 1958.

*15720 MIDPHALANGEAL (MID-DIGITAL) HAIR

THE GENETIC DETERMINATION OF PRESENCE OR ABSENCE OF HAIR ON THE DORSAL ASPECT OF THE MIDDLE PHALANX WAS FIRST SUGGESTED BY DANFORTH (1921). THE PRESENCE OF HAIR IS DOMINANT.

BECKMAN, L. AND BOOK, J. A.* DISTRIBUTION AND INHERITANCE OF MID-DIGITAL HAIR IN SWEDEN. HEREDITAS 45* 215-220, 1959.

BERNSTEIN, M. E.* THE MIDDIGITAL HAIR GENES. THEIR INHERITANCE AND DISTRIBU-TION AMONG THE WHITE RACE. J. HERED. 40* 127-131, 1949.

BERNSTEIN, M. M. AND BURKE, B. S.* THE INCIDENCE AND MENDELIAN TRANSMISSION OF MID-DIGITAL HAIR IN MAN. J. HERED. 33* 45-53, 1942.

DANFORTH, C. H.* DISTRIBUTION OF HAIR ON THE DIGITS IN MAN. AM. J. PHYS. ANTHROP. 4* 189-204, 1921.

SALDANHA, P. H. AND GUINSBURG, S.* DISTRIBUTION AND INHERITANCE OF MIDDLE PHALANGEAL HAIR IN A WHITE POPULATION OF SAO PAULO, BRAZIL. HUM. BIOL. 33* 237-249, 1961.

15730 MIGRAINE

FAMILIAL AGGREGATION FOR MIGRAINE IS UNDOUBTED. ALLAN (1928) FAVORED DOMINANT INHERITANCE. AMONG 500 PATIENTS, AT LEAST ONE PARENT WAS AFFECTED IN 91 PERCENT. AMONG OFFSPRING OF AFFECTED BY AFFECTED MATINGS, 83.3 PERCENT WERE AFFECTED* AFFECTED BY UNAFFECTED, 61 PERCENT* AND UNAFFECTED BY UNAFFECTED, 3.7 PERCENT. GOODELL ET AL. (1953) FOUND VALUES OF 69 PERCENT, 44 PERCENT AND 29 PERCENT IN THE THREE TYPES OF MATINGS AND FAVORED RECESSIVE INHERITANCE WITH ABOUT 70 PERCENT PENETRANCE. REFSUM (1968) GAVE AN EXTENSIVE REVIEW.

ALLAN, W.* INHERITANCE OF MIGRAINE. ARCH. INTERN. MED. 42* 590-599, 1928.

GOODELL, H., LEWONTIN, R. AND WOLFF, H. G.* THE FAMILIAL OCCURRENCE OF MIGRAINE HEADACHE* A STUDY OF HEREDITY. RES. PUBL. ASS. RES. NERV. MENT. DIS. 33* 346-356, 1953.

REFSUM, S.* GENETIC ASPECTS OF MIGRAINE. IN, VINKEN, P. J. AND BRUYN, G. W. (EDS.)* HANDBOOK OF CLINICAL NEUROLOGY. AMSTERDAM* NORTH-HOLLAND PUBLISHING CO. 1968, VOL. 5, CHAPTER 25. PP. 258-269.

*15740 MILIA, MULTIPLE ERUPTIVE

THIES AND SCHWARZ (1961) DESCRIBED THIS CONDITION. HEARD ET AL. (1971) DESCRIBED A SEEMINGLY IDENTICAL SITUATION IN A MAN WHO HAD ONSET OF THE ABNORMALITY IN CHILDHOOD AND WHOSE FATHER HAD THE SAME CONDITION. (THE FATHER DIED AT AGE 72 OF CARCINOMA OF THE COLON.) THE CASE OF THIES AND SCHWARZ WAS UNFAMILIAL AND LATE IN ONSET.

HEARD, M. G., HORTON, W. A. AND HAMBRICK, G. W., JR.* MULTIPLE ERUPTIVE MILIA. THE CLINICAL DELINEATION OF BIRTH DEFECTS. XII. SKIN, HAIR AND NAILS. BALTI-MORE* WILLIAMS AND WILKINS, 1971.

THIES, W. AND SCHWARZ, E.* MULTIPLE ERUPTIVE MILIA - AN ORGANOID FOLLICLE

HAMARTOMA. ARCH. KLIN. EXP. DERMAT. 214* 21-34, 1961.

15750 MILK PROTEINS, VARIANTS OF

POLYMORPHISM IS KNOWN IN THE PROTEINS OF MILK (AS WELL AS IN THOSE OF SEMINAL FLUID) OF CATTLE. SUCH SHOULD BE SOUGHT IN MAN.

BELL, K., HOPPER, K. E., MCKENZIE, H. A., MURPHY, W. H. AND SHAW, D. C.* A COMPARISON OF BOVINE ALPHA-LACTALBIEMIN A AND B OF DROUGHTMASTER. BIOCHIM. BIOPHYS. ACTA 214* 437-444, 1970.

BELL, K., MCKENZIE, H. A., MURPHY, W. H. AND SHAW, D. C.* BETA-LACTOGLOBULIN (DROUGHTMASTER)* A UNIQUE PROTEIN VARIANT. BIOCHIM. BIOPHYS. ACTA 214* 427-436, 1970.

15760 MIRROR MOVEMENTS, HEREDITARY

MIRROR MOVEMENTS PREDOMINANTLY OF THE HAND, NOT ASSOCIATED WITH OTHER NEUROLOGIC ABNORMALITY AND WITH NO ABNORMALITY OF THE CERVICAL VERTEBRAE, IS INHERITED AS A DOMINANT WITH INCOMPLETE PENETRANCE.

REGLI, F., FILIPPA, G. AND WIESENDANGER, M.* HEREDITARY MIRROR MOVEMENTS. ARCH. NEUROL. 16* 620-623, 1967.

*15770 MITRAL REGURGITATION

HUNT AND SLOMAN (1969) DESCRIBED A FAMILY IN WHICH MULTIPLE MEMBERS OF TWO GENERATIONS HAD A SYSTOLIC CLICK FOLLOWED BY A LATE SYSTOLIC MURMUR OR A LATE SYSTOLIC MURMUR ALONE. IN ONE MEMBER THE SYSTOLIC MURMUR BECAME LOUD AND PANSYSTOLIC DURING A FEW YEARS OBSERVATION. SYSTOLIC CLICK AND LATE SYSTOLIC MURMUR HAVE BEEN RELATED TO FLAIL MITRAL VALVE OR FLOPPY MITRAL VALVE. INCOMPE- TENCE OF THE POSTERIOR OR MURAL LEAFLET IS THE USUAL FINDING OF CINEANGIOCARDIO- GRAPHY IN SUCH CASES. THIS ANOMALY OF THE MITRAL VALVE IS FREQUENTLY FOUND IN THE MARFAN SYNDROME BUT CERTAINLY OCCURS AS AN ISOLATED FINDING AND MIGHT BE FAMILIAL. SHELL ET AL. (1969) STUDIED THE FAMILIES OF FOUR PATIENTS WITH THIS SYNDROME AND IN ALL FOUR FOUND A NUMBER OF RELATIVES WITH MID-LATE SYSTOLIC CLICKS, LATE SYSTOLIC MURMURS, PANSYSTOLIC MURMURS, ABNORMAL ELECTROCARDIOGRAMS AND UNEXPLAINED PREMATURE SUDDEN DEATH. SUCCESSIVE GENERATIONS WERE AFFECTED AND MALE-TO-MALE TRANSMISSION OCCURRED. STANNARD ET AL. (1967) OBSERVED FAMILIAL INCIDENCE IN 3 FAMILIES.

HUNT, D. AND SLOMAN, G.* PROLAPSE OF THE POSTERIOR LEAFLET OF THE MITRAL VALVE OCCURRING IN ELEVEN MEMBERS OF A FAMILY. AM. HEART J. 78* 149-153, 1969.

SREENIVASAN, V. V., LIEBMAN, J., LINTON, D. S. AND DOWNS, T. D.* POSTERIOR MITRAL REGURGITATION IN GIRLS POSSIBLY DUE TO POSTERIOR PAPILLARY MUSCLE DYSFUNC- TION. PEDIATRICS 42* 276-290, 1968.

SHELL, W. E., WALTON, J. A., CLIFFORD, M. E. AND WILLIS, P. W., III* THE FAMILIAL OCCURRENCE OF THE SYNDROME OF MID-LATE SYSTOLIC CLICK AND LATE SYSTOLIC MURMUR. CIRCULATION 39* 327-337, 1969.

STANNARD, M. AND RIGO, S. J.* PROLAPSE OF THE POSTERIOR LEAFLET OF THE MITRAL VALVE* CHROMOSOME STUDIES IN THREE SISTERS. AM. HEART J. 75* 282-283, 1968.

STANNARD, M., SLOMAN, J. G., HARE, W. S. C. AND GOBLE, A. J.* PROLAPSE OF THE POSTERIOR LEAFLET OF THE MITRAL VALVE. A CLINICAL, FAMILIAL, AND CINEANGIOGRAPHIC STUDY. BRIT. MED. J. 3* 71-74, 1967.

15780 MITRAL REGURGITATION, CONDUCTIVE DEAFNESS, AND FUSION OF CERVICAL VERTEBRAE AND OF CARPAL AND TARSAL BONES

IN A MOTHER AND TWO DAUGHTERS, FORNEY, ROBINSON AND PASCOE (1966) OBSERVED CONGENITAL MITRAL REGURGITATION, CONGENITAL PERCEPTIVE DEAFNESS DUE TO STAPES FOOTPLATE FIXATION, FUSION OF CERVICAL VERTEBRAE AND OF CARPAL AND TARSAL BONES, STRIKING FRECKLING OF THE FACE AND IRIS, AND SHORT STATURE (MOTHER LESS THAN 5 FEET). THE MATERNAL GRANDFATHER WAS SHORT OF STATURE AND HIS FATHER WAS BOTH SHORT AND DEAF. THUS, THE CONDITION MAY HAVE PASSED THROUGH FOUR GENERATIONS.

FORNEY, W. R., ROBINSON, S. J. AND PASCOE, D. J.* CONGENITAL HEART DISEASE, DEAFNESS, AND SKELETAL MALFORMATIONS* A NEW SYNDROME.Q J. PEDIAT. 68* 14-26, 1966.

*15790 MOEBIUS SYNDROME (CONGENITAL FACIAL DIPLEGIA)

VAN DER WIEL (1957) DESCRIBED THE DISORDER IN 46 PERSONS IN 6 GENERATIONS AND FORTANIER AND SPEIJER (1935) FOUND 15 CASES IN 3 GENERATIONS. CONGENITAL PARALYSIS OF THE SIXTH AND SEVENTH CRANIAL NERVES WAS OBSERVED IN MULTIPLE MEMBERS OF FAMILIES BY WILBRAND AND SAENGER (1921). AFFECTED MEMBERS OF THE FAMILY OF KRUGER AND FRIEDRICH (1963) OCCURRED IN THREE GENERATIONS. SEE FACIAL PALSY, CONGENITAL UNILATERAL. HANISSIAN ET AL. (1970) REPORTED THE MOEBIUS SYNDROME IN BOTH OF PRESUMABLY MONOZYGOTIC, NEGRO, MALE TWINS. THE FACIAL NERVES WERE SMALL

OR ABSENT AT AUTOPSY IN BOTH CASES. SPROFKIN AND HILLMAN (1956) DESCRIBED A PATIENT WITH ARTHROGRYPOSIS AND MOEBIUS SYNDROME WHO HAD A SIB WITH ARTHROGRYPOSIS ONLY.

FORTANIER, A. H. AND SPEIJER, N.* EINE ERBLICHKEITSFORSCHUNG BEI EINER FAMILIE MIT ANGEBORENEN BEWEGLICHKEITSSTORUNGEN DER HIRNNERVEN (INFANTILER KERNSCHWUND VON MOEBIUS). GENETICA 17* 471-486, 1935.

HANISSIAN, A. S., FUSTE, F., HAYES, W. T. AND DUNCAN, J. M.* MOBIUS SYNDROME IN TWINS. AM. J. DIS. CHILD. 120* 472-475, 1970.

KRUGER, K. E. AND FRIEDRICH, D.* FAMILIARE KONGENITALE MOTILITATSSTORUNGEN DER AUGEN. KLIN. MBL. AUGENHEILK. 142* 101-117, 1963.

SPROFKIN, B. E. AND HILLMAN, J. W.* MOEBIUS'S SYNDROME - CONGENITAL OCULOFACIAL PARALYSIS. NEUROLOGY 6* 50-54, 1956.

VAN DER WIEL , H. J.* HEREDITARY CONGENITAL FACIAL PARALYSIS. ACTA GENET. STATIST. MED. 7* 348 ONLY, 1957.

WILBRAND, H. AND SAENGER, A.* DIE NEUROLOGIE DES AUGES. MUNCHEN UND WIESBADEN 8* 179 ONLY, 1921.

*15800 MONILETHRIX

ALOPECIA MAY BE THE PRESENTING MANIFESTATION. THE DEGREE OF ALOPECIA IS VARIABLE FROM PATIENT TO PATIENT AND FROM TIME TO TIME IN THE SAME INDIVIDUAL. PERIFOLLI-CULAR HYPERKERATOSIS IS A CONSISTENT FEATURE. MICROSCOPICALLY THE HAIR IS BEADED.

BAKER, H.* AN INVESTIGATION OF MONILETHRIX. BRIT. J. DERM. 74* 24-30, 1962.

SALAMON, T. AND SCHNYDER, U. W.* UBER DIE MONILETHRIX. ARCH. KLIN. EXP. DERM. 215* 105-136, 1962.

SOLOMON, I. L. AND GREEN, O. C.* MONILETHRIX* ITS OCCURRENCE IN SEVEN GENERA-TIONS, WITH ONE CASE THAT RESPONDED TO ENDOCRINE THERAPY. NEW ENG. J. MED. 269* 1279-1282, 1963.

15810 MONOPHALANGY OF GREAT TOE

MONOPHALANGY OF THE GREAT TOES AS AN ISOLATED HEREDITARY DEFECT WAS DESCRIBED BY FRANKEL (1871).

FRANKEL, B.* UEBER EINEN FALL VON ERBLICHER DIFFORMITAT. KLIN. WSCHR. 8* 418-419, 1871.

15820 MORPHOLOGIC TRAITS (SOMETIMES CALLED ANTHROPOLOGIC TRAITS)

COMMON MORPHOLOGIC TRAITS, LIKE COMMON DISEASES, TEND TO HAVE A COMPLEX GENETIC BACKGROUND. A SINGLE LOCUS IS, HOWEVER, PROBABLY RESPONSIBLE FOR MOST OF THE VARIABILITY IN THE CASE OF MANY OF THESE. MANY HAVE NOT BEEN SUBJECTED TO THOROUGH GENETIC STUDY. MANY OF THESE ARE ILLUSTRATED BY WINCHESTER (1958) AND BY GATES (1947). ALSO WHITNEY (1942) COLLECTED PHOTOGRAPHS ILLUSTRATING THE TRANSMISSION OF A CONSIDERABLE NUMBER OF 'NORMAL' CHARACTERISTICS IN FAMILIES. THEY INCLUDED, IN ADDITION TO MANY OF THOSE LISTED BELOW, HEAVY EYEBROWS, CHARACTERISTIC NOSE SHAPE, LOW FRONTAL HAIR LINE, HIGH FOREHEAD, FULL LOWER LIP, TONGUE CURLING, CHARACTERISTIC EAR CONFIGURATION, ROTATED FINGERS. VARIATIONS IN HAIR, SKIN, EYELASHES AND EYEBROWS, IRIS, NOSE, EARS, TEETH, ETC., ARE DISCUSSED IN A SERIES OF ARTICLES BY DIFFERENT AUTHORS IN VOLUME II OF GEDDA'S ENCYCLOPEDIA (1961).

BECKMAN, L., BOOK, J. A. AND LANDER, E.* AN EVALUATION OF SOME ANTHROPOLOGICAL TRAITS USED IN PATERNITY TESTS. HEREDITAS 46* 543-569, 1960.

GATES, R. R.* HUMAN GENETICS. NEW YORK* MACMILLAN, 1947.

GEDDA, L. (ED.)* DE GENETICA MEDICA. ROME* MENDEL INSTITUTE, 1961.

KLOEPFER, H. W.* AN INVESTIGATION OF 171 POSSIBLE LINKAGE RELATIONSHIPS IN MAN. ANN. EUGEN. 13* 35-71, 1946.

WHITNEY, D. D.* FAMILY TREASURES* A STUDY OF THE INHERITANCE OF NORMAL CHARACTERISTICS IN MAN. LANCASTER, PA.* JAQUES CATTELL PRESS, 1942.

WINCHESTER, A. M.* GENETICS. BOSTON* HOUGHTON MIFFLIN CO., 1958 (2ND ED.).

TRAITS IN THIS CATEGORY WHICH ARE DISCUSSED ELSEWHERE INCLUDE THE FOLLOWING*

        CARABELLI'S ANOMALY OF MAXILLARY MOLAR TEETH
        CERUMEN, VARIATION IN
        CERVICAL RIB
        CERVICAL VERTEBRAL BRIDGE

CLEFT CHIN
DARWINIAN POINT (OF PINNA)
DARWINIAN TUBERCLE
DIMPLES, FACIAL
EAR LOBES, ATTACHED OR UNATTACHED
EAR PITS
EAR FLARE
EAR FOLDING
EXCHONDROSIS OF PINNA ('EAR BUMP')
EYELIDS FOLD, NORDIC TYPE
EPICANTHUS
FACIAL HYPERTRICHOSIS
FINGERS, RELATIVE LENGTH OF
FUTCHER'S LINE
HAIR WHORL
HYPERPIGMENTATION OF EYELIDS
INCISORS, 'SHOVEL-SHAPED'
LUNULAE OF FINGER-NAILS
MIDPHALANGEAL (MID-DIGITAL) HAIR
NAVICULAR BONE, ACCESSORY
NIPPLES, SUPERNUMERARY
NAILBEDS, PIGMENTATION OF
NOSE, ANOMALOUS SHAPE OF
PORT WINE STAIN OF NAPE OF NECK
PERONEUS TERTIUS MUSCLE, ABSENCE OF
RED HAIR
SCAPULA, VERTEBRAL BORDER OF
THUMB, HYPEREXTENSIBLE
TOE, FIFTH, NUMBER OF PHALANGES IN
TOE, ROTATED FOURTH
TOES, RELATIVE LENGTH OF
TONGUE, PIGMENTED FUNGIFORM PAPILLAE OF
VEINS, PATTERN OF, ON ANTERIOR THORAX
WEBBED TOES
WIDOW'S PEAK

D
O
M
I
N
A
N
T

*15830 MOUTH, INABILITY TO OPEN COMPLETELY, AND SHORT FINGER-FLEXOR TENDONS

HECHT AND BEALS (1969) DESCRIBED FATHER AND FOUR CHILDREN (2 SONS, 2 DAUGHTERS) WITH INABILITY TO OPEN THE MOUTH COMPLETELY WITH RESULTING PROBLEMS IN MASTICATION, SHORT FINGER-FLEXOR TENDONS SUCH THAT DORSIFLEXION OF THE WRIST RESULTED IN CAMPTODACTYLY AND SHORT LEG MUSCLES RESULTING IN FOOT DEFORMITY. THE FATHER'S MOTHER WAS PROBABLY ALSO AFFECTED. WILSON ET AL. (1969) DESCRIBED THE SAME SYNDROME IN 9 PERSONS IN 4 GENERATIONS. THEY ASCRIBED THE FINGER PECULIARITY TO SHORTENING OF THE FLEXOR PROFUNDUS MUSCLE-TENDON UNIT.

HECHT, F. AND BEALS, R. K.* INABILITY TO OPEN THE MOUTH FULLY* AN AUTOSOMAL DOMINANT PHENOTYPE WITH FACULTATIVE CAMPYLODACTYLY AND SHORT STATURE. THE CLINICAL DELINEATION OF BIRTH DEFECTS. III. LIMB MALFORMATIONS. NEW YORK* NATIONAL FOUNDATION, 1969. PP. 96-98.

WILSON, R. V., GAINES, D. L., BROOKS, A., CARTER, T. S. AND NANCE, W. E.* AUTOSOMAL DOMINANT INHERITANCE OF SHORTENING OF THE FLEXOR PROFUNDUS MUSCLE-TENDON UNIT WITH LIMITATION OF JAW EXCURSION. THE CLINICAL DELINEATION OF BIRTH DEFECTS. III. LIMB MALFORMATIONS. NEW YORK* NATIONAL FOUNDATION, 1969. PP. 99-102.

15840 MULTIPLE SCLEROSIS-LIKE DISEASE (SEE ATAXIA, SPASTIC)

GAYLE AND WILLIAMS (1933) DESCRIBED 17 CASES IN 4 GENERATIONS OF A DISORDER BEGINNING IN THE SIXTH DECADE WITH STIFFNESS IN THE LEG MUSCLES, FOLLOWED BY STUMBLING, DYSARTHRIA, AND LOSS OF MEMORY. ALTHOUGH PROGRESSION TO SEVERE SPASTIC PARAPLEGIA OCCURRED, THE DISORDER DID NOT SHORTEN LIFE. THESE PATIENTS LIVED IN ACCOMAC AND NORTHAMPTON COUNTIES ON THE EASTERN SHORE OF VIRGINIA.

GAYLE, R. F., JR. AND WILLIAMS, J. P.* A FAMILIAL DISEASE OF THE CENTRAL NERVOUS SYSTEM RESEMBLING MULTIPLE SCLEROSIS. STH. MED. J. 26* 242-246, 1933.

*15850 MUSCULAR ATROPHY, ATAXIA, RETINITIS PIGMENTOSA, DIABETES INSIPIDUS

IN 10 PERSONS IN 4 GENERATIONS, FURUKAWA ET AL. (1968) FOUND MUSCULAR ATROPHY, ATAXIA, RETINITIS PIGMENTOSA AND DIABETES INSIPIDUS. NO REPORTED CASE SEEMED TO BE IDENTICAL.

FURUKAWA, T., TAKAGI, A., NAKAO, K., SUGITA, H., TSUKAGOSHI, H. AND TSUBAKI, T.* HEREDITARY MUSCULAR ATROPHY WITH ATAXIA, RETINITIS PIGMENTOSA, AND DIABETES MELTITUS. A CLINICAL REPORT OF A FAMILY. NEUROLOGY 18* 942-947, 1968.

15860 MUSCULAR ATROPHY, JUVENILE (KUGELBERG-WELANDER SYNDROME)

A DOMINANT FORM OF THIS DISORDER, WHICH IS USUALLY INHERITED AS A RECESSIVE, WAS SUGGESTED BY TSUKAGOSHI ET AL. (1966) AND BY OTHERS. QUASI-DOMINANCE DUE TO CONSANGUINITY IS POSSIBLE, ESPECIALLY IN THE JAPANESE KINDRED. IN THREE GENERA-

TIONS AND 8 SIBSHIPS OF A NEGRO FAMILY, ARMSTRONG, FOGELSON AND SILBERBERG (1966) REPORTED A PROXIMAL MUSCULAR ATROPHY LIKE KUGELBERG-WELANDER DISEASE BUT THE INHERITANCE WAS CLEARLY DOMINANT. SEE SCAPULOPERONEAL AMYOTROPHY IN THIS CATALOG. FENICHEL ET AL. (1967), GARVIE AND WOOLF (1966) AND MAGEE AND DEJONG (1960), AMONG OTHERS, HAVE REPORTED DOMINANT PEDIGREES.

ARMSTRONG, R. M., FOGELSON, M. H. AND SILBERBERG, D. H.* FAMILIAL PROXIMAL SPINAL MUSCULAR ATROPHY. ARCH. NEUROL. 14* 208-212, 1966.

FENICHEL, G. M., EMERY, E. S. AND HUNT, P.* NEUROGENIC ATROPHY SIMULATING FACIOSCAPULOHUMERAL DYSTROPHY. ARCH. NEUROL. 17* 257-260, 1967.

GARVIE, J. M. AND WOOLF, A. L.* KUGELBERG-WELANDER SYNDROME (HEREDITARY PROXIMAL SPINAL MUSCULAR ATROPHY). BRIT. MED. J. 1* 1458-1461, 1966.

MAGEE, K. R. AND DEJONG, R. N.* NEUROGENIC MUSCULAR ATROPHY SIMULATING MUSCULAR DYSTROPHY. ARCH. NEUROL. 2* 677-682, 1960.

TSUKAGOSHI, H., SUGITA, H., FURUKAWA, T., TSUBAKI, T. AND ONO, E.* KUGELBERG-WELANDER SYNDROME WITH DOMINANT INHERITANCE. ARCH. NEUROL. 14* 378-381, 1966.

15870 MUSCULAR ATROPHY, PROGRESSIVE

BROWN (1951, 1960) DESCRIBED TWO NEW ENGLAND FAMILIES, WETHERBEE AND FARR BY NAME, IN WHICH PROGRESSIVE DEGENERATION OF THE ANTERIOR HORN CELLS OF THE SPINAL CORD AND BULBAR PALSY AS A CAUSE OF DEATH BEHAVED AS A DOMINANT TRAIT.

BROWN, M. R.* 'WETHERBEE AIL.' THE INHERITANCE OF PROGRESSIVE MUSCULAR ATROPHY AS A DOMINANT TRAIT IN TWO NEW ENGLAND FAMILIES. NEW ENG. J. MED. 245* 645-647, 1951.

BROWN, M. R.* THE INHERITANCE OF PROGRESSIVE MUSCULAR ATROPHY AS A DOMINANT TRAIT IN TWO NEW ENGLAND FAMILIES. NEW ENG. J. MED. 262* 1280-1282, 1960.

15880 MUSCULAR DYSTROPHY, BARNES TYPE

BARNES (1932) DESCRIBED A FAMILY WITH MUSCULAR DYSTROPHY OF A TYPE WHICH MAY BE DISTINCT FROM ANY OF THE OTHERS PRESENTED IN THESE CATALOGS. THE DISEASE HAD AFFECTED MANY PERSONS IN 6 GENERATIONS OF A FAMILY, WITH MANY INSTANCES OF MALE-TO-MALE TRANSMISSION. THE MYOPATHY WAS EXCEEDINGLY PROTEAN WITH PREDOMINANTLY PSEUDO-HYPERTROPHIC OR DISTAL CHARACTER IN SOME PATIENTS. IN OTHERS IT COULD BE CONFUSED WITH PERONEAL ATROPHY. AT LEAST ONE SHOWED MYOTONIA OF SOME THIGH MUSCLES.

BARNES, S.* MYOPATHIC FAMILY, WITH HYPERTROPHIC, PSEUDOHYPERTROPHIC, ATROPHIC AND TERMINAL (DISTAL IN UPPER EXTREMITIES) STAGES. BRAIN 55* 1-46, 1932.

*15890 MUSCULAR DYSTROPHY, FACIO-SCAPULO-HUMERAL

JUSTIN-BESANCON AND COLLEAGUES (1964) GAVE AUTOPSY FINDINGS IN ONE OF LANDOUZY'S ORIGINAL PATIENTS WHO DIED AT AGE OF 86 YEARS. THREE AFFECTED GENERATIONS WERE ADDED TO THE FOUR DESCRIBED BY LANDOUZY. SOME CASES SHOW CONGENITAL ABSENCE OF PART OR ALL OF CERTAIN MUSCLES SUCH AS A PECTORAL. THE RELATIONSHIP OF THE CONGENITAL DEFECT OF MUSCLE TO THE DYSTROPHY IS UNCLEAR. TYLER AND STEPHENS (1950, 1953) REPORTED 17 FAMILIES. IN ONE KINDRED 150 MEMBERS WERE AFFECTED OVER SIX GENERATIONS. A GIRL, WHOSE FACE ALONE WAS AFFECTED AT AGE 9 WHEN EXAMINED BY LANDOUZY AND DEJERINE (WHOSE NAMES ARE ATTACHED EPONYMOUSLY TO THIS CONDITION), DID NOT DEVELOP WEAKNESS OF THE ARMS UNTIL 60 AND OF THE LEGS UNTIL 70 AND SURVIVED TO AGE 85 YEARS. IN HER FAMILY AFFECTED MEMBERS WERE DISTRIBUTED IN 8 GENERATIONS. MORTON AND CHUNG (1959) ESTIMATED THE FREQUENCY TO BE ABOUT 2 PER MILLION LIVING PERSONS WITH A FREQUENCY IN EACH MILLION BIRTHS, OF ABOUT 4 PERSONS DESTINED TO DEVELOP THE TRAIT. FERTILITY IS LITTLE REDUCED AND THE MUTATION RATE IS NOT MORE THAN 5 PER 10 MILLION GAMETES.

JUSTIN-BESANCON, L., PEQUIGNOT, H., CONTAMIN, F., DELAVIERRE, P. AND ROLLAND, P.* MYOPATHIE DU TYPE LANDOUZY-DEJERINE. RAPPORT D'UNE OBSERVATION HISTORIQUE. SEM. HOSP. PARIS 40* 2990-2999, 1964.

MORTON, N. E. AND CHUNG, C. S.* FORMAL GENETICS OF MUSCULAR DYSTROPHY. AM. J. HUM. GENET. 11* 360-379, 1959.

TYLER, F. H. AND STEVENS, F. E.* STUDIES IN DISORDERS OF MUSCLE. II. CLINICAL MANIFESTATIONS AND INHERITANCE OF FACIOSCAPULOHUMERAL DYSTROPHY IN A LARGE FAMILY. ANN. INTERN. MED. 32* 640-660, 1950.

TYLER, F. H.* THE INHERITANCE OF NEUROMUSCULAR DISORDERS. RES. PUBL. ASS. RES. NERV. MENT. DIS. 33* 283-292, 1953.

15900 MUSCULAR DYSTROPHY, PROXIMAL

SCHNEIDERMAN (1969) DESCRIBED A FAMILY WITH MUSCULAR DYSTROPHY OF GRADUAL ONSET AND SLOW PROGRESSION, AFFECTING MAINLY THE PROXIMAL LIMB MUSCLES AND SPARING THE

FACE. LINKAGE WITH THE PELGER-HUET ANOMALY WAS DEMONSTRATED. THE RECOMBINATION FRACTION WAS ABOUT 0.25.

SCHNEIDERMAN, L. J., SAMPSON, W. I., SCHOENE, W. C. AND HAYDON, G. B.* GENETIC STUDIES OF A FAMILY WITH TWO UNUSUAL AUTOSOMAL DOMINANT CONDITIONS* MUSCULAR DYSTROPHY AND PELGER-HUET ANOMALY. CLINICAL, PATHOLOGIC AND LINKAGE CONSIDERATIONS. AM. J. MED. 46* 380-393, 1969.

15910 MUSCULAR HYPOPLASIA, CONGENITAL UNIVERSAL, OF KRABBE

THE MUSCULAR HYPOPLASIA IS CONGENITAL AND GENERALIZED AND NO OR LITTLE PROGRESSION OF MUSCULAR WEAKNESS OCCURS. THIS CONDITION WAS CALLED MUSCULAR INFANTILISM BY GIBSON (1921) WHO OBSERVED AFFECTED MEMBERS OF FOUR GENERATIONS. SCHREIER AND HUPERZ (1956) DESCRIBED CASES. FORD (1961) DESCRIBED AFFECTED MOTHER AND DAUGHTER WHO HAVE SUBSEQUENTLY BEEN SHOWN TO HAVE NEMALINE MYOPATHY (Q.V.). THIS SUGGESTS THAT A NUMBER OF SEPARATE CONDITIONS WILL BE FOUND TO ANSWER TO THE ABOVE DESCRIPTION. THURMON (1971) HAS SHOWN ME A FATHER AND DAUGHTER WITH UNIVERSAL MUSCULAR HYPOPLASIA IN WHOM NO SPECIFIC MYOPATHY SUCH AS NEMALINE MYOPATHY COULD BE IDENTIFIED BY SPECIAL STUDIES.

FORD, F. R.* DISEASES OF THE NERVOUS SYSTEM IN INFANCY, CHILDHOOD AND ADOLESCENCE. SPRINGFIELD, ILL.* CHARLES C THOMAS, 1961 (4TH ED.). P. 1259.

GIBSON, A.* MUSCULAR INFANTILISM. ARCH. INTERN. MED. 27* 338 ONLY, 1921.

SCHREIER, K. AND HUPERZ, R.* UBER DIE HYPOPLASIA MUSCULORUM GENERALISATA CONGENITA. ANN. PAEDIAT. 186* 241-248, 1956.

THURMON, T. F.* NEW ORLEANS, LA.* PERSONAL COMMUNICATION, 1971.

15920 MUSCULAR SHORTENING AND DYSTROPHY

IN THREE GENERATIONS OF A FRENCH CANADIAN FAMILY, HAUPTMANN AND THANNHAUSER (1941) OBSERVED A DISORDER MANIFESTED BY INABILITY TO FLEX THE NECK AND SLIGHT WEBBING DUE TO SHORTENED MUSCLE AS WELL AS LIMITATION ON SPINAL FLEXION AND ELBOW EXTENSION FROM THE SAME CAUSE. THE LIMB GIRDLE MUSCLES WERE UNDERDEVELOPED AND WEAK. THE CONDITION APPARENTLY WAS NOT PROGRESSIVE.

HAUPTMANN, A. AND THANNHAUSER, S. J.* MUSCULAR SHORTENING AND DYSTROPHY. A HEREDOFAMILIAL DISEASE. ARCH. NEUROL. PSYCHIAT. 46* 654-664, 1941.

15930 MYASTHENIA GRAVIS

NOYES (1930) NOTED MYASTHENIA GRAVIS IN A FATHER AND TWO DAUGHTERS. HERRMANN (1966) REPORTED AFFECTED FATHER AND SON. THE FAMILIAL AGGREGATION, ALTHOUGH DEFINITE AND IMPRESSIVE, DOES NOT CONFORM TO A SIMPLE MENDELIAN PATTERN. JACOB ET AL. (1968) REVIEWED PUBLISHED CASES OF FAMILIAL MYASTHENIA AND REPORTED A STUDY OF THE FAMILIES OF 70 CASES. NO SECONDARY CASES WERE FOUND. THE DISTRIBUTION OF AGE OF ONSET WAS SIGNIFICANTLY DIFFERENT (OLDER) IN THEIR SERIES AND SEVERAL OTHER REPORTED SERIES THAN IN 'FAMILIAL' MYASTHENIA WHICH OFTEN HAD ITS ONSET IN THE FIRST DECADE. IN A SAMPLE OF 70 PATIENTS WITH MYASTHENIA GRAVIS, JACOB ET AL. (1968) FOUND NO INSTANCE OF FAMILIAL OCCURRENCE. THEY PROVIDED A COMPREHENSIVE SURVEY OF THE REPORTED FAMILIAL CASES AND POINTED OUT DIFFERENCES FROM THEIR OWN SERIES, PARTICULARLY EARLIER ONSET IN THE FAMILIAL CASES. NAMBA ET AL. (1971) POINTED OUT, ON THE BASIS OF 85 FAMILIES WITH MULTIPLE CASES (EXCLUDING TRANSIENT NEONATAL MYASTHENIA IN OFFSPRING OF MYASTHENIC MOTHERS), THAT THE FAMILIAL AGGREGATION MOST OFTEN INVOLVES SIBS AND THAT AFFECTED PERSONS IN MORE THAN TWO GENERATIONS HAS NEVER BEEN REPORTED.

HERRMANN, C., JR.* MYASTHENIA GRAVIS OCCURRING IN FAMILIES. NEUROLOGY 16* 75-85, 1966.

JACOB, A., CLACK, E. R. AND EMERY, A. E. H.* GENETIC STUDY OF SAMPLE OF 70 PATIENTS WITH MYASTHENIA GRAVIS. J. MED. GENET. 5* 257-261, 1968.

NAMBA, T., BRUNNER, N. G., BROWN, S. B., MUGURUMA, M. AND GROB, D.* FAMILIAL MYASTHENIA GRAVIS. REPORT OF 27 PATIENTS IN 12 FAMILIES AND REVIEW OF 164 PATIENTS IN 73 FAMILIES. ARCH. NEUROL., IN PRESS, 1971.

NOYES, A. P.* A CASE OF MYASTHENIA GRAVIS WITH CERTAIN UNUSUAL FEATURES. RHODE ISLAND MED. J. 13* 52-59, 1930.

15940 MYASTHENIA, FAMILIAL LIMB-GIRDLE

MCQUILLEN (1966) DESCRIBED LIMB-GIRDLE MYASTHENIA IN 3 OF 3 SIBS AND IN THEIR FATHER. TWO OF THE CHILDREN ALSO HAD DYSTROPHIC CHANGES IN THE WEAK MUSCLES. THE ATROPHY WAS NOT MARKED, HOWEVER, AND NO OCULOBULBAR INVOLVEMENT WAS PRESENT. RESPONSE TO ANTI-CHOLINESTERASE THERAPY WAS STRIKING AND SUSTAINED. ELECTROMYOGRAPHY SUGGESTED A DEFECT OF BOTH MUSCLE AND THE NEUROMYAL JUNCTION.

MCQUILLEN, M. P.* FAMILIAL LIMB-GIRDLE MYASTHENIA. BRAIN 89* 121-132, 1966.

NORMALLY THE OPTIC NERVE FIBERS ARE MYELINATED ONLY AFTER THEIR PASSAGE THROUGH THE LAMINA CRIBOSA. SOMETIMES, HOWEVER, THE MYELIN SHEATH BEGINS SOONER PRODUCING A WHITE AREA NEAR THE DISK. PSEUDOPAPILLEDEMA (Q.V.) IS A DISTINCT CONDITION. FRANCOIS (1961) CITED A FAMILY WITH 10 CASES IN TWO GENERATIONS AND A FEW OTHER INSTANCES SUGGESTING DOMINANT INHERITANCE. IN A FEW DESCRIPTIONS THE ANOMALY WAS LIMITED TO ONE SIBSHIP.

FRANCOIS, J.* HEREDITY IN OPHTHALMOLOGY. ST. LOUIS* C. V. MOSBY CO., 1961. P. 495.

*15960 MYOCLONIC EPILEPSY, HARTUNG TYPE

THIS FORM APPEARS TO BE DISTINCT FROM THE TWO TYPES WHICH ARE INHERITED AS AUTOSOMAL RECESSIVES (Q.V.). FURTHERMORE, UNLIKE THOSE FORMS NO LAFORA BODIES WERE FOUND AT AUTOPSY AND ONLY DIFFUSE ATROPHY WAS PRESENT.

HARTUNG, E.* ZWEI FALLE VON PARAMYOCLONUS MULTIPLEX MIT EPILEPSIE. ZENTHBL. GES. NEUROL. PSYCHIAT. 56* 150-153, 1920.

VOGEL, F., HAFNER, H. AND DIEBOLD, K.* ZUR GENETIK DER PROGRESSIVEN MYOKLONUSE-PILEPSIEN (UNVERRICHT-LUNDBORG). HUMANGENETIK 1* 437-475, 1965.

15970 MYOCLONUS AND ATAXIA

IN 1921, RAMSAY HUNT DESCRIBED THE ASSOCIATION OF GENERALIZED MYOCLONUS AND SIGNS OF CEREBELLAR DYSFUNCTION, ESPECIALLY INTENTION TREMOR, UNDER THE DESIGNATION OF DYSSYNERGIA CEREBELLARIS MYOCLONICA. AUTOPSY IN ONE CASE CONFIRMED HIS IMPRESSION OF A LESION IN THE DENTATE NUCLEUS OF THE CEREBELLUM. HIS CASES WERE NON-FAMILIAL. GILBERT, MCENTEE AND GLASER (1963) DESCRIBED TWO FEMALES AND TWO MALES IN THREE SIBSHIPS OF A FAMILY WITH THE COMBINATION OF MYOCLONUS AND ATAXIA. CEREBROSPINAL FLUID URIC ACID WAS ELEVATED IN TWO. AUTOSOMAL DOMINANT INHERITANCE WITH REDUCED PENETRANCE WAS SUGGESTED.

GILBERT, G. J., MCENTEE, W. J., III AND GLASER, G. H.* FAMILIAL MYOCLONUS AND ATAXIA. PATHOPHYSIOLOGIC IMPLICATIONS. NEUROLOGY 13* 365-372, 1963.

HUNT, J. R.* DYSSYNERGIA CEREBELLARIS MYOCLONICA-PRIMARY ATROPHY OF THE DENTATE SYSTEM* A CONTRIBUTION TO THE PATHOLOGY AND SYMPTOMATOLOGY OF THE CEREBELLUM. BRAIN 44* 490-538, 1921.

15980 MYOCLONUS, CEREBELLAR ATAXIA AND DEAFNESS

MAY AND WHITE (1968) DESCRIBED A NEW SYNDROME OF FAMILIAL MYOCLONUS, CEREBELLAR ATAXIA AND DEAFNESS AND CONCLUDED THAT IT IS AUTOSOMAL DOMINANT. EVIDENCE IS MEAGER, HOWEVER A MOTHER AND SON HAD THE FULL SYNDROME. HEARING LOSS WAS NOTED IN CHILDHOOD OR EARLY ADULTHOOD. MYOCLONIC JERKS AND CEREBELLAR SYMPTOMS BEGAN AT AGE 14 IN THE SON. SEE DEAFMUTISM AND FAMILIAL MYOCLONUS EPILEPSY.

MAY, D. L. AND WHITE, H. H.* FAMILIAL MYOCLONUS, CEREBELLAR ATAXIA, AND DEAFNESS* SPECIFIC GENETICALLY-DETERMINED DISEASE. ARCH. NEUROL. 19* 331-338, 1968.

*15990 MYOCLONUS, HEREDITARY ESSENTIAL

THIS DISORDER CONSISTS OF SUDDEN, BRIEF MUSCULAR CONTRACTIONS AFFECTING MAINLY THE PROXIMAL MUSCLES OF THE EXTREMITIES. THE TWITCHINGS ARE AGGRAVATED BY EXCITEMENT AND DISAPPEAR DURING SLEEP. EPILEPSY AND INTELLECTUAL DETERIORATION DO NOT OCCUR. WE KNOW OF AFFECTED MOTHER AND DAUGHTER AND SON (P7063). IN ANOTHER FAMILY, OF FRENCH-CANADIAN BACKGROUND, A FATHER AND 5 OF HIS 9 CHILDREN SHOW ONSET OF MYOCLONUS IN THE FIRST OR SECOND DECADE AND BENIGN COURSE, WITHOUT SEIZURES, DEMENTIA OR NEUROLOGIC SIGNS OTHER THAN MYOCLONUS (MAHLOUDJI AND PIKIELNY, 1966). BECAUSE OF THE UNCERTAINTY OF THE NATURE OF THE CASE ON THE BASIS OF WHICH FRIEDREICH IN 1881 INTRODUCED THE TERM PARAMYOCLONUS MULTIPLEX, THESE CASES MIGHT BEST BE CALLED HEREDITARY ESSENTIAL MYOCLONUS. DAUBE AND PETERS (1966) REPORTED TWO FAMILIES IN WHICH AFFECTED MEMBERS OCCURRED IN AT LEAST FOUR GENERATIONS OF EACH WITH MALE-TO-MALE TRANSMISSION IN EACH BUT SOME SKIPPED GENERATIONS. SYMONDS (1953) DESCRIBED NOCTURNAL MYOCLONUS IN A MAN AND FIVE OF HIS SIX CHILDREN.

BIEMOND, A.* PARAMYOCLONUS MULTIPLEX (FRIEDREICH). CLINICAL AND GENETIC ASPECTS. PSYCHIAT. NEUROL. NEUROCHIR. 66* 270-276, 1963.

DAUBE, J. R. AND PETERS, H. A.* HEREDITARY ESSENTIAL MYOCLONUS. ARCH. NEUROL. 15* 587-594, 1966.

LINDERMULDER, F. G.* FAMILIAL MYOCLONIA OCCURRING IN THREE SUCCESSIVE GENERA-TIONS. J. NERV. MENT. DIS. 77* 489-491, 1933.

LITTLEJOHN, W. S.* FAMILIAL MYOCLONUS* REPORT OF FOUR CASES WITH ELECTROENCE-PHALOGRAMS. STH. MED. J. 42* 404-410, 1949.

196   MAHLOUDJI, M. AND PIKIELNY, R. T.* HEREDITARY ESSENTIAL MYOCLONUS. BRAIN 90*
        669-674, 1967.

        SYMONDS, C. P.* NOCTURNAL MYOCLONUS. J. NEUROL. NEUROSURG. PSYCHIAT. 16* 166-
        171, 1953.

*16000 MYOGLOBIN MUTANTS

    TWO STRUCTURAL VARIANTS OF MYOGLOBIN WERE DESCRIBED BY BOYER, FAINER AND NAUGHTON
    (1963). BOULTON ET AL. (1969) STUDIED MUSCLE OBTAINED POST MORTEM FROM 2500
    PERSONS. TWO MYOGLOBIN VARIANTS WERE FOUND AND IN ONE OF THESE SUBSTITUTION OF
    LYSINE FOR GLUTAMIC ACID AS THE 53RD RESIDUE WAS DEMONSTRATED. HUMAN MYOGLOBIN
    HAS 152 RESIDUES. LATER BOULTON ET AL. (1970) DESCRIBED A VARIANT MYOGLOBIN WITH
    SUBSTITUTION OF GLUTAMINE FOR ARGININE AS RESIDUE 138.

        BOULTON, F. E. AND HUNTSMAN, R. G.* ABNORMAL HUMAN MYOGLOBIN* 53(D4) GLUTAMIC
    ACID LYSINE. NATURE 223* 832-833, 1969.

        BOULTON, F. E., HUNTSMAN, R. G., LEHMANN, H., LORKIN, P. AND ROMERO-HERRERA, A.
    E.* MYOGLOBIN VARIANTS. (ABSTRACT) BIOCHEM. J. 118* 39P ONLY, 1970.

        BOULTON, F. E., HUNTSMAN, R. G., YAWSON, G. I., ROMERO HERRERA, A. E. AND
    LORKIN, P. A.* THE SECOND VARIANT OF HUMAN MYOGLOBIN* 138(H16) ARGININE TO
    GLUTAMINE. BRIT. J. HAEMAT. 20* 69-74, 1971.

        BOYER, S. H., FAINER, D. C. AND NAUGHTON, M. A.* MYOGLOBIN INHERITED STRUCTURAL
    VARIATION IN MAN. SCIENCE 140* 1228-1231, 1963.

*16010 MYOKYMIA

    SPONTANEOUS MUSCLE TWITCHES OCCUR IN MANY PERSONS AND HAVE NO GRAVE SIGNIFICANCE.
    THEY MAY BE CONFUSED WITH FASCICULATIONS WHICH OCCUR WITH AMYOTROPHIC LATERAL
    SCLEROSIS. I KNOW OF A FAMILY WITH MULTIPLE AFFECTED MEMBERS IN A DOMINANT
    INHERITANCE PATTERN. THE FAMILY DERIVED FROM A TRI-RACIAL (CAUCASOID, NEGRO,
    INDIAN) GROUP IN ROBSON CO., N. C. (H. O., JHH917242). SHEAFF (1952) DESCRIBED
    AFFECTED FATHER AND TWO SONS. WIECZOREK AND GREGER (1962) DESCRIBED A DOMINANT
    PEDIGREE. SHEAFF (1952) OBSERVED MYOKYMIA IN A MAN AND HIS FOUR SONS. IN A
    PORTION OF MUSCLE REMOVED FOR BIOPSY FASCICULATIONS PERSISTED FOR 8 MINUTES.
    AFFECTED PERSONS PROBABLY HAVE AN INCREASED FREQUENCY OF MUSCLE CRAMPS (*NIGHT
    CRAMPS*).

        SHEAFF, H. M.* HEREDITARY MYOKYMIA. SYNDROME OR DISEASE ENTITY ASSOCIATED WITH
    HYPOGLYCEMIA AND DISTURBED THYROID FUNCTION. ARCH. NEUROL. PSYCHIAT. 68* 236-247,
    1952.

        WIECZOREK, V. AND GREGER, J.* UBER EIN FAMILIAR GEHAUFTES VORKOMMEN VON
    MYOKYMIE. PSYCHIAT. NEUROL. MED. PSYCHOL. 14* 452-455, 1962.

16020 MYOPATHY, CONGENITAL, WITH CRYSTALLINE INTRANUCLEAR INCLUSIONS

    JENIS ET AL. (1969) DESCRIBED A WHITE FEMALE FROM UNRELATED PARENTS WHO SHOWED
    EXTREME MUSCULAR WEAKNESS AND HYPOTONIA FROM BIRTH AND DIED OF RESPIRATORY
    INSUFFICIENCY AT 2 MONTHS OF AGE. INTRANUCLEAR AND SARCOPLASMIC INCLUSIONS WERE
    FOUND IN MUSCLE CELLS. THE PARENTS WERE NOT RELATED AND THERE WERE NO SIBS.
    HENCE, THE GENETICS IS COMPLETELY OBSCURE.

        JENIS, E. H., LINDQUIST, R. R. AND LISTER, R. C.* NEW CONGENITAL MYOPATHY WITH
    CRYSTALLINE INTRANUCLEAR INCLUSIONS. ARCH. NEUROL. 20* 281-287, 1969.

*16030 MYOPATHY, DISTAL, WITH ONSET IN INFANCY

    FOOT DROP AND FINGER WEAKNESS ARE LEADING FEATURES. ALTHOUGH ONSET IS IN INFANCY,
    THE AILMENT IS NOT INCAPACITING AND PROGRESSION AFTER ADOLESCENCE DOES NOT OCCUR.
    AUTOSOMAL DOMINANT INHERITANCE SEEMS QUITE CERTAIN.

        MAGEE, K. R. AND DEJONG, R. N.* HEREDITARY DISTAL MYOPATHY WITH ONSET IN
    INFANCY. ARCH. NEUROL. 13* 387-390, 1965.

        WILLEBOIS, A. E. M., BETHLEM, J., MEYER, A. E. F. H. AND SIMONS, A. J. R.*
    DISTAL MYOPATHY WITH ONSET IN EARLY INFANCY. NEUROLOGY 18* 383-390, 1968.

16040 MYOPATHY, DUE TO GLYCOLYTIC ABNORMALITY

    SATOYOSHI AND KOWA (1967) DESCRIBED MYOPATHY STUDIED IN DETAIL IN TWO BROTHERS BUT
    ALSO PRESENT BY HISTORY IN A SISTER, THEIR MOTHER AND A SON OF ONE SISTER. ONSET
    WAS ABOUT AGE 35 YEARS WITH DELAYED MUSCLE PAIN AND STIFFNESS ON EXERTION BUT
    ABSENCE OF CONTRACTURE OR WEAKNESS ON ISCHEMIC EXERCISE. PHOSPHOFRUCTOKINASE
    ACTIVITY WAS ABOUT 40 PERCENT OF NORMAL IN SKELETAL MUSCLE. ORAL INGESTION OF
    FRUCTOSE RELIEVED THE SYMPTOMS. THE POSSIBLE ROLE OF AN INHIBITOR IN THE PROCESS
    WAS PROPOSED. GLYCOGEN STORAGE DISEASE VII (Q.V.), A RECESSIVE, HAS DEFICIENCY OF
    MUSCLE PHOSPHOFRUCTOKINASE.

SATOYOSHI, E. AND KOWA, H.* A MYOPATHY DUE TO GLYCOLYTIC ABNORMALITY. ARCH. NEUROL. 17* 248-256, 1967.

*16050 MYOPATHY, LATE DISTAL HEREDITARY

ON THE BASIS OF 78 PROBANDS AND 171 SECONDARY CASES, WELANDER (1951) DELINEATED DISTAL MYOPATHY AS A DISTINCT ENTITY WITH DOMINANT INHERITANCE. THE 249 AFFECTED PERSONS WERE DISTRIBUTED IN 72 KINDREDS. THE MEAN AGE AT ONSET WAS 47 YEARS (RANGE 20-77). WEAKNESS AND WASTING OF THE SMALL MUSCLES OF HANDS WAS THE FIRST MANIFESTATION IN 89 PERCENT. FASCICULATIONS, MYOTONIA AND SENSORY CHANGES WERE NOTABLY ABSENT. ABOUT 70 PERCENT OF THE PROBANDS WERE AWARE OF THEIR HEREDITARY PREDISPOSITION AT THE TIME OF FIRST EXAMINATION. THE DISORDER WAS VERY SLOWLY PROGRESSIVE AND APPARENTLY DID NOT SHORTEN LIFE. THE FIRST DESCRIPTION OF THIS TYPE IS ATTRIBUTED TO GOWERS. THE RELATIONSHIP TO THE FOUR WITH ONSET IN CHILDHOOD DESCRIBED BY DAHLGAARD (1960) AND THAT WITH ONSET IN INFANCY DESCRIBED BY MAGEE AND DEJONG (1965) IS UNCERTAIN. WELANDER (1957) DESCRIBED THE HOMOZYGOUS STATE. BOTH PARENTS WERE AFFECTED, 7 OF 16 CHILDREN HAD DISTAL MYOPATHY AND 2 OF THESE WERE UNUSUALLY SEVERE WITH EARLY PROXIMAL INVOLVEMENT.

DAHLGAARD, E.* MYOPATHIA DISTALIS TARDA HEREDITARIA. ACTA PSYCHIAT. NEUROL. SCAND. 35* 440-447, 1960.

MAGEE, K. R. AND DEJONG, R. N.* HEREDITARY DISTAL MYOPATHY WITH ONSET IN INFANCY. ARCH. NEUROL. 13* 387-390, 1965.

WALLIS, K., DEUTSCH, V. AND AZIZI, E.* HYPERTENSION IN A CASE OF VON RECKLIN-GHAUSEN'S NEUROFIBROMATOSIS. HELVET. PAEDIAT. ACTA 25* 147-153, 1970.

WELANDER, L.* HOMOZYGOUS APPEARANCE OF DISTAL MYOPATHY. ACTA GENET. STATIST. MED. 7* 321-325, 1957.

WELANDER, L.* MYOPATHIA DISTALIS TARDA HEREDITARIA. ACTA MED. SCAND. 141 (SUPPL. 265)* 1-124, 1951.

16060 MYOPATHY, LIMITED TO FEMALES

HENSON ET AL. (1967) DESCRIBED A SLOWLY PROGRESSIVE LIMB-GIRDLE TYPE OF MUSCULAR DYSTROPHY IN 8 FEMALES IN 4 SIBSHIPS IN 2 GENERATIONS OF A FAMILY. FEMALE-LIMITED AUTOSOMAL DOMINANT INHERITANCE WAS FAVORED.

HENSON, T. E., MULLER, J. AND DEMYER, W. E.* HEREDITARY MYOPATHY LIMITED TO FEMALES. ARCH. NEUROL. 17* 238-247, 1967.

*16070 MYOPIA

MYOPIA OF SEVERE DEGREE WAS TRANSMITTED THROUGH 4 GENERATIONS IN THE FAMILY REPORTED BY FRANCOIS (1961). FRANCESCHETTI (1953) OBSERVED A FAMILY WITH 10 CASES IN 4 GENERATIONS. FOUR SUFFERED DETACHMENT OF THE RETINA. MYOPIA IN A SENSE IS A METRIC CHARACTER. VARIATION IN MANY COMPONENTS OF THE EYE CONTRIBUTES TO ITS REFRACTIVE CAPACITY (SORSBY ET AL., 1962). SOME MYOPIA, PERHAPS MOST, IS MULTIFACTORIAL IN CAUSATION. SOME ENVIRONMENTAL CAUSES OF MYOPIA ARE IDENTI-FIABLE.

FRANCESCHETTI, A.* HAUTE MYOPIE AVEC DECOLLEMENT RETINIEN HEREDITAIRE. J. GENET. HUM. 2* 283-284, 1953.

FRANCOIS, J.* HEREDITY IN OPHTHALMOLOGY. ST. LOUIS* C. V. MOSBY CO., 1961.

SORSBY, A., SHERIDAN, M. AND LEARY, G. A.* REFRACTION AND ITS COMPONENTS IN TWINS. MEDICAL RESEARCH COUNCIL* SPECIAL REPRINT SERIES. LONDON* (NO. 303), 1962.

*16080 MYOTONIA CONGENITA (ALSO SEE PARAMYOTONIA CONGENITA)

THIS IS THE DISORDER DESCRIBED BY THOMSEN (1875) IN HIS OWN FAMILY. ISAACS (1959) STUDIED THE DISORDER IN A MOTHER AND HER SON AND DAUGHTER. QUININE, LOCAL PROCAIN, PROCAIN AMIDE, INSULIN, INJECTIONS OF 50 PERCENT MAGNESIUM SULFATE, CURARIZATION, SODIUM LOADING AND SODIUM DEPLETION HAD NO EFFECT ON THE MOTHER'S MYOTONIA. HOWEVER, MARKED IMPROVEMENT OCCURRED WHEN POTASSIUM DEPLETION WAS ACHIEVED WITH CORTISONE AND CHLOROTHIAZIDE. THE DAUGHTER WAS TREATED WITH CHLOROTHIAZIDE ONLY AND IMPROVED. PASTERNACK AND LINDQVIST (1962) DESCRIBED 6 CASES IN 3 GENERATIONS, AND PERSONALLY EXAMINED FOUR. WITH THE FOLLOW-UP BY THOMASEN (1948), THOMSEN'S FAMILY SHOWED 64 AFFECTED PERSONS IN 7 GENERATIONS WITHOUT SKIPS. THE PEDIGREE OF BIRT (1908), WHO LIKE THOMSEN WAS HIMSELF AFFECTED SHOWED SKIPPED GENERATIONS. POSSIBLE HOMOZYGOTES WERE REPORTED BY TE KAMP (1907). SOMATIC MUTATION IS A POSSIBLE EXPLANATION IN THE CASE OF MONOMELIC MYOTONIA CONGENITA REPORTED BY CELESIA ET AL. (1967).

BIRT, A.* A STUDY OF THOMSEN'S DISEASE (CONGENITAL MYOTONIA) BY A SUFFERER FROM IT. MONTREAL MED. 37* 771-784, 1908.

CELESIA, G. G., ANDERMANN, F., WIGLESWORTH, F. W. AND ROBB, J. P.* MONOMELIC

MYOPATHY. CONGENITAL HYPERTROPHIC MYOTONIC MYOPATHY LIMITED TO ONE EXTREMITY. ARCH. NEUROL. 17* 69-77, 1967.

ISAACS, H.* THE TREATMENT OF MYOTONIA CONGENITA. S. AFR. MED. J. 33* 984-986, 1959.

KATZENSTEIN-SUTRO, E., BOSCH-GWALTER, T. AND ROSENMUND, H.* MYOTONIE CONGENI-TALE DE THOMSEN ET SES CRITERES DIFFERENTIELS AVEC LES AUTRES MALADIES MUSCU-LAIRES* ETUDE D'UNE FAMILLE PRESENTANT UN GROUPEMENT SPECIAL DE SYMPTOMES, EN TENANT SPECIALEMENT COMPTE DE L'ELIMINATION DE RIBOSE DANS L'URINE. J. GENET. HUM. 9* 1-64, 1960.

PASTERNACK, A. AND LINDQVIST, C.* THOMSEN'S DISEASE. OBSERVATIONS ON STRENGTH-DURATION CURVES IN MYOTONIA. ANN. PAEDIAT. FENN. 8* 284-291, 1962.

TE KAMP, (NI)* EIN BIETRAG ZUR KENNTNIS DER MYOTONIA CONGENITA SOG. THOMSENS-CHEN KRANKHEIT. DEUTSCH. MED. WSCHR. 33* 1005 ONLY, 1907.

THOMASEN, E.* MYOTONIA, THOMSEN'S DISEASE. PARAMYOTONIA, AND DYSTROPHIA MYOTONICA. OP. EX. DOMO BIOL. HERED. HUM. U. HAFNIENSIS 17* 11-251, 1948.

THOMSEN, J.* TONISCHE KRAMPFE IN WILLKURLICH BEWEGLICHEN MUSKELN IN FOLGE VON ERERBTER PSYCHISCHER DISPOSITION. ATAXIA MUNULARIS.Q ARCH. PSYCHIAT. NERVENKR. 76* 706, 1875.

*16090 MYOTONIC DYSTROPHY (STEINERT'S DISEASE)

THE FEATURES ARE MYOTONIA, MUSCLE WASTING (E.G., IN THE TEMPORAL MUSCLES AND THOSE OF THE NECK), CATARACT, HYPOGONADISM, FRONTAL BALDING, EKG CHANGES. ANTICIPATION - EARLIER ONSET IN MORE RECENT GENERATIONS - IS DESCRIBED BUT IS PROBABLY AN ARTIFACT OF ASCERTAINMENT (PENROSE, 1948). BOSMA AND BRODIE (1969) DEMONSTRATED BOTH MYOTONIA AND WEAKNESS IN PATIENTS WITH SWALLOWING AND SPEECH DISABILITY. IN THE CYTOPLASM OF CULTURED SKIN FIBROBLASTS SWIFT AND FINEGOLD (1969) FOUND AN ABNORMALLY LARGE AMOUNT OF MATERIAL WITH THE STAINING PROPERTIES OF ACID MUCOPOLY-SACCHARIDES. SCHWINDT ET AL. (1969) CLAIMED THAT 25 TO 50 PERCENT OF PATIENTS HAVE ABDOMINAL SYMPTOMS DUE TO CHOLELITHIASIS. BUNDEY ET AL. (1970) FOUND THAT THE MOST USEFUL METHOD FOR IDENTIFYING SUBCLINICAL CASES IN SLIT-LAMP EXAMINATION (FOR LENS CHANGES), FOLLOWED BY ELECTROMYOGRAPHY (FOR MYOTONIC DISCHARGES), AND IN THIRD POSITION AS TO LEVEL OF SUCCESS, BY MEASUREMENT OF IMMUNOGLOBULINS. THEY ESTIMATED THAT ABOUT A QUARTER OF INDEX CASES ARE THE RESULT OF NEW MUTATION.

BOSMA, J. F. AND BRODIE, D. R.* CINERADIOGRAPHIC DEMONSTRATION OF PHARYNGEAL AREA MYOTONIA IN MYOTONIC DYSTROPHY PATIENTS. RADIOLOGY 92* 104-109, 1969.

BUNDEY, S., CARTER, C. O., SOOTHILL, J. F.* EARLY RECOGNITION OF HETEROZYGOTE FOR THE GENE FOR DYSTROPHIA MYOTONICA. J. NEUROL. NEUROSURG. PSYCHIAT. 33* 279-293, 1970.

CAUGHEY, J. E. AND MYRIANTHOPOULOS, N. C.* DYSTROPHIA MYOTONICA AND RELATED DISORDERS. SPRINGFIELD, ILL.* CHARLES C THOMAS, 1963.

DUMAINE, L. AND LOZERON, P.* CONTRIBUTION A L'ETUDE CLINIQUE ET GENETIQUE DE LA DYSTROPHIE MYOTONIQUE (STEINERT) ET DE LA MYOTONIE CONGENITALE (THOMSEN). J. GENET. HUM. 10* 221-296, 1961.

KLEIN, D.* LA DYSTROPHIE MYOTONIQUE (STEINERT) ET LA MYOTONIE CONGENITALE (THOMSEN) EN SUISSE. GENEVE* EDITION MEDICINE ET HYGIENE, 1957.

LYNAS, M. A.* DYSTROPHIA MYOTONICA WITH SPECIAL REFERENCE TO NORTHERN IRELAND. ANN. HUM. GENET. 21* 318-351, 1957.

PENROSE, L. S.* THE PROELEMS OF ANTICIPATION IN PEDIGREES OF DYSTROPHIA MYOTONICA. ANN. EUGEN. 14* 125-132, 1948.

PRUZANSKI, W.* VARIANTS OF MYOTONIC DYSTROPHY IN PRE-ADOLESCENT LIFE (THE SYNDROME OF MYOTONIC DYSEMBRYOPLASIA). BRAIN 89* 563-568, 1966.

SCHWINDT, W. D., BERNHARDT, L. C. AND PETERS, H. A.* CHOLELITHIASIS AND ASSOCIATED COMPLICATIONS OF MYOTONIA DYSTROPHICA. POSTGRAD. MED. 46* 80-83, 1969.

SWIFT, M. R. AND FINEGOLD, M. J.* MYOTONIC MUSCULAR DYSTROPHY* ABNORMALITIES IN FIBROBLAST CULTURE. SCIENCE 165* 294-296, 1969.

*16100 NAEGELI'S SYNDROME

THIS DISORDER WAS EARLIER CONFUSED WITH INCONTINENTIA PIGMENTI (SEE X-LINKED CATALOG). NAEGELI (1927) DESCRIBED THE SYNDROME IN A FATHER AND TWO DAUGHTERS. FRANCESCHETTI AND JADASSOHN (1954) DOCUMENTED DOMINANT INHERITANCE. DIFFERENCES FROM INCONTINENTIA PIGMENTI INCLUDE (1) EQUAL FREQUENCY IN MALES AND FEMALES, (2) PLANTAR AND PALMAR HYPOHIDROSIS AND HYPERKERATOSIS, AND (3) UNCOMMON BLISTERING AND INFLAMMATORY PHENOMENA. FRANCESCHETTI AND JADASSOHN (1954) MAINTAINED THAT THIS DISORDER IS DISTINCT FROM INCONTINENTIA PIGMENTI (AN X-LINKED TRAIT). THE

CARDINAL FEATURES ARE RETICULAR CUTANEOUS PIGMENTATION, DISCOMFORT PROVOKED BY HEAT WITH DIMINISHED SWEAT GLAND FUNCTION, POOR TEETH AND MODERATE HYPERKERATOSIS OF THE PALMS AND SOLES. MALES AND FEMALES ARE EQUALLY AFFECTED.

BERLIN, C.* CONGENITAL GENERALIZED MELANOLEUCODERMA ASSOCIATED WITH HYPODONTIA, HYPOTRICHOSIS, STUNTED GROWTH AND MENTAL RETARDATION OCCURRING IN TWO BROTHERS AND TWO SISTERS. DERMATOLOGICA. 123* 227-243, 1961.

FRANCESCHETTI, A. AND JADASSOHN, W.* A PROPOS DE L'INCONTINENTIA PIGMENTI, DELIMITATION DE DEUX SYNDROMES DIFFERENTS FIGURANT SOUS LE MEME TERME. DERMATOLOGICA 108* 1-28, 1954.

KITAMURA, K. AND HIRAKO, T.* UBER ZWEI JAPANISCHE FALLE EINER EIGENARTIGEN RETIKULAREN PIGMENTIERUNG* ZUR FRAGE DER DERMATOSE PIGMENTAIRE RETICULEE (FRANCESCHETTI-JADASSOHN). DERMATOLOGICA 110* 97-107, 1955.

NAEGELI, B.* FAMILIARER CHROMATOPHORENNAVUS. SCHWEIZ. MED. WSCHR. 57* 48 ONLY, 1927.

VILANOVA, X. AND AGUADE, J. P.* INCONTINENTIA PIGMENTI. TROUBLES SUDORIPARES FONCTIONNELS DYSPLASTIQUES ET PIGMENTAIRES CHEZ LES ASCENDANTS. ANN. DERM. SYPH. 86* 247-258, 1959.

16110 NAILBEDS, PIGMENTATION OF

PIGMENTED NAILBEDS OCCUR IN A CERTAIN PROPORTION OF NEGROES. THE PIGMENTATION MAY BE CONFUSED WITH CYANOSIS, OR MAY MAKE EVALUATION OF CYANOSIS DIFFICULT.

*16120 NAIL-PATELLA SYNDROME

DYSPLASIA OF THE NAILS AND ABSENT OR HYPOPLASTIC PATELLAE ARE THE CARDINAL FEATURES BUT OTHERS ARE ILIAC HORNS, ABNORMALITY OF THE ELBOWS INTERFERING WITH PRONATION AND SUPINATION, AND IN SOME CASES NEPHROPATHY. THE NAIL-PATELLA LOCUS AND THE ABO BLOOD GROUP LOCUS ARE LINKED. THE RECOMBINATION FRACTION IS ABOUT 10 PERCENT BUT IS HIGHER IN FEMALES THAN IN MALES. NEPHROPATHY WAS AN ASSOCIATED ABNORMALITY IN THE FAMILY OF HAWKINS AND SMITH (1950). THE RENAL CHANGE RESEMBLES GLOMERULONEPHRITIS. IT IS RELATIVELY BENIGN ALTHOUGH FATALITY AT A YOUNG AGE FROM THIS COMPLICATION HAS BEEN DESCRIBED (LEAHY, 1966). THIS CONDITION IS SOMETIMES CALLED TURNER SYNDROME, BUT THIS LEADS TO CONFUSION WITH THE XO SYNDROME. THE RENAL DISORDER IN THE CASE OF SIMILA ET AL. (1970) TOOK THE APPEARANCE OF CONGENITAL NEPHROSIS. IN THE FAMILY EIGHT HAD NAIL-PATELLA SYNDROME OF WHOM FIVE ALSO HAD RENAL DISEASE. THE SEEMING FAMILIAL AGGREGATION OF THE RENAL COMPLICATIONS SUGGESTS TWO SEPARATE GENES, ONE FOR A NEPHROPATHIC FORM AND ONE FOR A NON-NEPHROPATHIC FORM. THEY MIGHT BE ALLELIC SINCE NO HETEROGENEITY HAS BEEN DETECTED IN THE LINKAGE WITH THE ABO LOCUS.

COTTEREILL, C. P. AND JACOBS, P.* HEREDITARY ARTHRO-OSTEO-ONYCHODYSPLASIA ASSOCIATED WITH ILIAC HORNS. BRIT. J. CLIN. PRACT. 15* 933-941, 1961.

DARLINGTON, D. AND HAWKINS, C. F.* NAIL PATELLA SYNDROME WITH ILIAC HORNS AND HEREDITARY NEPHROPATHY. NECROPSY REPORT AND ANATOMICAL DISSECTION. J. BONE JOINT SURG. 49B* 164-174, 1967.

HAWKINS, C. F. AND SMITH, O. E.* RENAL DYSPLASIA IN A FAMILY WITH MULTIPLE HEREDITARY ABNORMALITIES INCLUDING ILIAC HORNS. LANCET 1* 803-808, 1950.

LEAHY, M. S.* THE HEREDITARY NEPHROPATHY OF OSTEO-ONYCHODYSPLASIA NAIL PATELLA SYNDROME AM. J. DIS. CHILD. 112* 237-241, 1966.

PILLAY, V. K.* ONYCHO-OSTEODYSPLASIA (NAIL-PATELLA SYNDROME). STUDY OF A CHINESE FAMILY WITH THIS CONDITION. ANN. HUM. GENET. 28* 301-307, 1965.

RENWICK, J. H. AND LAWLER, S. D.* GENETICAL LINKAGE BETWEEN THE ABO AND NAIL-PATELLA LOCI. ANN. HUM. GENET. 19* 312-331, 1955.

RENWICK, J. H. AND SCHULZE, J.* MALE AND FEMALE RECOMBINATION FRACTIONS FOR THE NAIL PATELLA* ABO LINKAGE IN MAN. ANN. HUM. GENET. 28* 379-392, 1965.

SCHRODER, G.* OSTEO-ONYCHO-DYSPLASIA HEREDITARIA. Z. MENSCHL. VERERB. KONSTITUTIONSL. 36* 42-73, 1961.

SIMILA, S., VESA, L. AND WASZ-HOCKERT, O.* HEREDITARY ONYCHO-OSTEODYSPLASIA (THE NAIL-PATELLA SYNDROME) WITH NEPHROSIS-LIKE RENAL DISEASE IN A NEWBORN BOY. PEDIATRICS 46* 61-65, 1970.

VON KNORRE, G.* UBER DIE HEREDITARE ARTHRO-OSTEO-ONYCHO-DYSPLASIE (TURNER-KIESER-SYNDROM). Z. MENSCHL. VERERB. KONSTITUTIONSL. 36* 118-129, 1961.

ZIMMERMAN, C.* ILIAC HORNS* A PATHOGNOMONIC ROENTGEN SIGN OF FAMILIAL ONYCHO-OSTEODYSPLASIA. AM. J. ROENTGEN. 86* 478-483, 1961.

16130 NANOPHTHALMOS (PURE MICROPHTHALMOS)

THE DEVELOPMENT OF THE GLOBE IS ARRESTED IN ALL DIMENSIONS AFTER THE EMBRYONIC FISSUE HAS CLOSED. HENCE THE EYE IS REDUCED IN VOLUME WITHOUT GROSS CONGENITAL ANOMALIES. BOTH DOMINANT AND RECESSIVE FORMS ARE THOUGHT TO EXIST.

SJOGREN, T. AND LARSSON, T.* MICROPHTHALMOS AND ANOPHTHALMOS WITH OR WITHOUT COINCIDENT OLIGOPHRENIA. ACTA PSYCHIAT. NEUROL. 56 (SUPPL.)* 11-103, 1949.

16140 NARCOLEPSY

IN THREE GENERATIONS OF A FAMILY DALY AND YOSS (1959) FOUND 12 DEFINITE AND 3 POSSIBLE CASES. WHEREAS ABOUT TWO-THIRDS OF ALL CASES OF NARCOLEPSY (SLEEPING ATTACKS) ARE ASSOCIATED WITH CATAPLEXY (PAROXYSMAL ATTACKS OF WEAKNESS OR FRANK PARALYSIS, ASSOCIATED ESPECIALLY WITH STRONG EMOTION), ONLY ONE-THIRD OF THE AFFECTED PERSONS IN THIS FAMILY DISPLAYED CATAPLEXY. FURTHERMORE, IN THESE THE WEAKNESS WAS MILD. NARCOLEPSY IS AS DIFFICULT TO DOCUMENT AND TO STUDY GENETICAL- LY AS IS SCHIZOPHRENIA. THEREFORE, A SIMPLE INHERITED FORM CANNOT BE CONSIDERED FULLY ESTABLISHED. THREE OF THE 12 AFFECTED PERSONS IN THE FAMILY OF DALY AND YOSS (1959) HAD CATAPLECTIC ATTACKS. GELARDI AND BROWN (1967) REPORTED ON A FAMILY IN WHICH 11 PERSONS IN 4 GENERATIONS HAD CATAPLEXY. THREE MAY HAVE HAD NARCOLEPSY. NO INSTANCE OF MALE-TO-MALE TRANSMISSION OCCURRED IN THE PEDIGREE. IN A LATER PUBLICATION, YOSS (1970) REPORTED STUDIES WITH INFRARED PUPILLOGRAPHY IN NARCOLEPSY FAMILIES, LEADING TO THE CONCLUSION THAT NARCOLEPSY IS POLYGENIC, I.E., THAT THE AFFECTED PERSONS ARE AT ONE END OF A SPECTRUM. WHEN A PERSON IS AWAKE AND ALERT IN TOTAL DARKNESS HIS PUPILS ARE LARGE. DURING SLEEP THE PUPILS ARE SMALL. THE PUPILS ARE INTERMEDIATE IN SIZE WHEN THE SUBJECT IS BETWEEN THESE TWO EXTREMES. THIS IS THE BASIS OF INFRARED PUPILLOGRAPHY AS A GUAGE OF WAKEFUL- NESS. THE AUTHOR SUGGESTED THAT IT WOULD BE VERY UNUSUAL FOR TWO PERSONS WITH PHILAGRYPNIA (ABILITY TO STAY ALERT WITH LITTLE SLEEP) TO HAVE AN OFFSPRING WITH NARCOLEPSY.

DALY, D. D. AND YOSS, R. E.* A FAMILY WITH NARCOLEPSY. MAYO CLIN. PROC. 34* 313-320, 1959.

GELARDI, J.-A. M. AND BROWN, J. W.* HEREDITARY CATAPLEXY. J. NEUROL. NEURO- SURG. PSYCHIAT. 30* 455-457, 1967.

YOSS, R. E.* THE INHERITANCE OF DIURNAL SLEEPINESS AS MEASURED BY PUPILLOGRA- PHY. MAYO CLIN. PROC. 45* 426-437, 1970.

*16150 NASAL GROOVE, FAMILIAL TRANSVERSE

THIS IS A RED FURROW WHICH EXTENDS ACROSS THE NOSE JUST PROXIMAL TO THE ALAE NASI. IT IS USUALLY NOTICED EARLY IN CHILDHOOD AND AT THAT STAGE MAY HAVE A ROSE COLOR. ANDERSON OBSERVED TWO RATHER EXTENSIVELY AFFECTED FAMILIES. AN INSTANCE OF MALE- TO-MALE-TRANSMISSION OCCURRED IN ONE.

ANDERSON, P. C.* FAMILIAL TRANSVERSE NASAL GROOVE. ARCH. DERM. 84* 316-317, 1961.

16160 NAVICULAR BONE, ACCESSORY

THIS IS PRESENT IN ABOUT 5 PERCENT OF PERSONS. IT CAUSES AN UNDUE PROMINENCE ON THE MEDIAL SIDE OF THE FOOT. IT IS SOMETIMES REFERRED TO AS AN ACCESSORY OR SECONDARY MEDIAL MALLEOLUS. SOMETIMES IT IS FUSED WITH THE NAVICULAR TO FORM AN ABNORMALLY LARGE TUBEROSITY ON THE LATTER BONE.

MOSELEY, H. F.* STATIC DISORDERS OF THE ANKLE AND FOOT. CIBA CLINICAL SYMPOSIA 9* 83-110, 1957.

16170 NECROBIOSIS LIPOIDICA AND PERIODONTOSIS

IN ONE FAMILY (A. K., 1136340) I HAVE OBSERVED A SKIN LESION RESEMBLING NECROBIO- SIS LIPOIDICA DIABETICORUM IN ASSOCIATION WITH PERIODONTAL DISEASE LEADING TO EARLY LOSS OF TEETH. THE SKIN LESIONS CONSISTED OF SYMMETRICAL PATCHES ON THE FRONT OF THE SHINS, ABOUT FIVE INCHES LONG, COVERED BY PARCHMENT SKIN AND DISCOLORED BY BLOOD PIGMENTS. THE APPEARANCE RESEMBLED THAT IN THE EHLERS-DANLOS SYNDROME. THE KNEES SHOWED SMALL *CIGARETTE-PAPER SCARS* AND EASY BRUISABILITY OF THE SKIN WAS NOTED. LOOSEJOINTEDNESS AND GENERAL BRUISABILITY AND CUTANEOUS FRAGILITY WERE NOT PRESENT. FURTHERMORE, ALTHOUGH THE HISTOLOGY OF THE LESIONS OF THE SKIN SUGGESTED NECROBIOSIS LIPOIDICA DIABETICORUM NO EVIDENCE OF DIABETES WAS UNCOVERED IN ANY MEMBER OF THE FAMILY.

*16180 NEMALINE MYOPATHY

THE MOTHER AND DAUGHTER DESCRIBED BY FORD (1961) AS CASES OF CONGENITAL UNIVERSAL MUSCULAR HYPOPLASIA OF KRABBE WERE SHOWN BY HOPKINS ET AL. (1966) TO HAVE THIS DISORDER. THE ROD-LIKE INCLUSIONS IN MUSCLE MAY BE PRECIPITATED MYOSIN. THE RELATION TO CENTRAL CORE DISEASE (Q.V.) AWAITS CLARIFICATION. THE TWO HAVE BEEN REPORTED IN THE SAME FAMILY. SPIRO AND KENNEDY (1965) ALSO OBSERVED AFFECTED MOTHER AND DAUGHTER. X-LINKED DOMINANT INHERITANCE IS, OF COURSE, ALSO POSSIBLE. THE PATHOLOGIC FIBRILLAR MATERIAL IS SIMILAR TO AND CONTINUOUS WITH THE SUBSTANCE WHICH CONSTITUTES THE Z-BANDS (PRICE ET AL., 1965) AND MAY BE TROPOMYOSIN B.

CONVENTIONAL HISTOPATHOLOGICAL PREPARATIONS MAY BE NORMAL OR NEARLY NORMAL. THE
CONDITION DESCRIBED BY GIBSON (1921) WAS PRESENT IN THREE GENERATIONS AND MAY BE
THIS DISORDER. THE DOMINANT INHERITANCE AND THE ANOMALOUS MATERIAL OF Z BAND
ORIGIN SUGGEST THAT A SIMPLE AMINO ACID SUBSTITUTION MAY BE DEMONSTRATED EVENTUAL-
LY IN THIS DISORDER. THIS IS A NON-PROGRESSIVE FORM OF CONGENITAL MYOPATHY WITH
ABNORMAL THREADLIKE STRUCTURES IN MUSCLE CELLS ON HISTOLOGIC EXAMINATION. IN THE
FAMILY OF SHY ET AL. (1963) BOTH PARENTS OF TWO AFFECTED SIBS SHOWED MINOR
ABNORMALITIES WHICH MIGHT BE INTERPRETED AS HETEROZYGOUS EFFECTS. THE CLINICAL
PICTURE IS THAT OF THE "FLOPPY INFANT" (SEE MYOTONIA CONGENITA). AN OLDER CASE
STUDIED BY ENGEL ET AL. (1964) SUGGESTED SLOW PROGRESSION OF THE DISEASE THROUGH
LATE CHILDHOOD. PEARSON ET AL. (1967) DESCRIBED 3 AFFECTED SIBS OUT OF 8. THE
MOTHER, ALTHOUGH CLINICALLY NORMAL, HAD MINOR HISTOLOGIC ALTERATIONS OF SKELETAL
MUSCLE. NARROW, HIGHLY ARCHED PALATE IS A FEATURE OF ALL THESE CASES, AS IT
SOMETIMES IS IN MYOTONIC DYSTROPHY WITH CHILDHOOD ONSET OF MANIFESTATIONS.

ENGEL, W. K., WANKO, T. AND FENI HEL, G. M.* NEMALINE MYOPATHY. A SECOND CASE.
ARCH. NEUROL. 11* 22-39, 1964.

FORD, F. R.* DISEASES OF THE NERVOUS SYSTEM IN INFANCY, CHILDHOOD AND ADOLES-
CENCE. SPRINGFIELD, ILL.* CHARLES C THOMAS, 1961. (4TH ED.) PP. 1259-1260.

GIBSON, A.* MUSCULAR INFANTILISM. ARCH. INTERN. MED. 27* 333 ONLY, 1921.

GONATAS, N. K., SHY, G. M. AND GODFREY, E. H.* NEMALINE MYOPATHY. THE ORIGIN
OF NEMALINE STRUCTURES. NEW ENG. J. MED. 274* 535-539, 1966.

HOPKINS, I. J., LINDSEY, J. R. AND FORD, F. R.* NEMALINE MYOPATHY. A LONG-TERM
CLINICOPATHOLOGIC STUDY OF AFFECTED MOTHER AND DAUGHTER. BRAIN 89* 299-310, 1966.

PEARSON, C. M., COLEMAN, R. F., FOWLER, W. M., JR., MOMMAERTS, W. F. H. M.,
MUNSAT, T. L. AND PETER, J. B.* SKELETAL MUSCLE. BASIC AND CLINICAL ASPECTS AND
ILLUSTRATIVE NEW DISEASES. ANN. INTERN. MED. 67* 614-650, 1967.

PRICE, H. M., GORDON, G. B., PEARSON, C. M., MUNSAT, T. L. AND BLUMBERG, J. M.*
NEW EVIDENCE FOR EXCESSIVE ACCUMULATION OF Z-BAND MATERIAL IN NEMALINE MYOPATHY.
PROC. NAT. ACAD. SCI. 54* 1398-1406, 1965.

SHY, G. M.* CENTRAL CORE DISEASE AND NEMALINE MYOPATHY. IN STANBURY, J. B.,
WYNGAARDEN, J. B. AND FREDRICKSON, D. S. (EDS.)* THE METABOLIC BASIS OF INHERITED
DISEASE. NEW YORK* MCGRAW-HILL, 1966 (2ND ED.). PP. 952-962.

SHY, G. M., ENGEL, W. K., SOMERS, J. E. AND WANKO, T.* NEMALINE MYOPATHY. A
NEW CONGENITAL MYOPATHY. BRAIN 86* 793-810, 1963.

SPIRO, A. J. AND KENNEDY, C.* HEREDITARY OCCURRENCE OF NEMALINE MYOPATHY.
ARCH. NEUROL. 13* 155-159, 1965.

16190 NEPHRITIS, FAMILIAL, WITHOUT DEAFNESS OR OCULAR DEFECT

BEN-ISHAY, BIRAN AND ULLMAN (1967) DESCRIBED A JEWISH-KURDISH FAMILY WITH MANY
CASES OF NEPHRITIS IN FOUR GENERATIONS. DIFFERENCES FROM ALPORT'S SYNDROME
INCLUDED RARITY OF GROSS HEMATURIA, PROTEINURIA BEING THE PRESENTING MANIFESTA-
TION, AND ABSENCE OF DEAFNESS. THE FAMILY OF GOLDMAN AND HABERFELDE (1959) MAY BE
OF THE SAME TYPE. PERKOFF (1967) GAVE A GENERAL REVIEW OF HEREDITARY RENAL
DISEASE.

BEN-ISHAY, D., BIRAN, S. AND ULLMANN, T. D.* FAMILIAL NEPHRITIS. ISRAEL J.
MED. SCI. 3* 106-112, 1967.

GOLDMAN, R. AND HABERFELDE, G. C.* HEREDITARY NEPHRITIS* REPORT OF A KINDRED.
NEW ENG. J. MED. 261* 734-738, 1959.

PERKOFF, G. T.* THE HEREDITARY RENAL DISEASES. NEW ENG. J. MED. 277* 79-85,
AND 129-138, 1967.

16200 NEPHROPATHY, FAMILIAL, WITH GOUT

ROSENBLOOM ET AL. (1967) DESCRIBED A FAMILY IN WHICH MULTIPLE MALES IN THREE
GENERATIONS DIED FROM RENAL FAILURE AT A RELATIVELY EARLY AGE. ALL HAD HYPERURI-
CEMIA EARLY IN THE COURSE AND GOUT. NO DISTINCTIVE HISTOLOGIC FINDINGS WERE
YIELDED BY RENAL BIOPSY. TRANSMISSION FROM FATHER TO SON EXCLUDED X-LINKED
INHERITANCE.

ROSENBLOOM, F. M., KELLEY, W. N., CARR, A. A. AND SEEGMILLER, J. E.* FAMILIAL
NEPHROPATHY AND GOUT IN A KINDRED. (ABSTRACT) CLIN. RES. 15* 270 ONLY, 1967.

*16210 NEURITIS WITH BRACHIAL PREDILECTION

THE DISORDER DESCRIBED BY JACOB, ANDERMANN AND ROBB (1961) IS MANIFESTED BY
RECURRING BRACHIAL NEURITIS OR MONONEURITIS MULTIPLEX. THE LEGS ARE INVOLVED ONLY
IN INSTANCES OF SEVERE ARM INVOLVEMENT. THEY OBSERVED 14 SIMILAR EPISODES IN 7
PATIENTS IN TWO UNRELATED FAMILIES. ATTACKS WERE FEATURED BY INCAPACITATING PAIN,

WEAKNESS, WASTING, DEPRESSION OF REFLEXES, AND SENSORY LOSS. NARROW FACE WITH CLOSE-SET EYES WAS A FEATURE. TAYLOR (1960) STUDIED A FAMILY IN WHICH FIVE GENERATIONS WERE AFFECTED BY SINGLE OR RECURRENT ATTACKS OF MONONEURITIS WITH A PARTICULAR PREDILECTION FOR PROXIMAL BRACHIAL LOCALIZATION. THE TRAIT BEHAVED AS AN AUTOSOMAL DOMINANT ONE WITH HIGH PENETRANCE. CLINICALLY, THE PICTURE CLOSELY RESEMBLED SERUM NEURITIS, SUGGESTING THAT THE FUNDAMENTAL DEFECT MIGHT BE A GENETIC SUSCEPTIBILITY TO 'HYPERERGIC REACTIONS.'

JACOB, J. C., ANDERMANN, F. AND ROBB, J. P.* HEREDOFAMILIAL NEURITIS WITH BRACHIAL PREDILECTION. NEUROLOGY 11* 1025-1033, 1961.

TAYLOR, R. A.* HEREDOFAMILIAL MONONEURITIS MULTIPLEX WITH BRACHIAL PREDILEC-TION. BRAIN 83* 113-137, 1960.

*16220 NEUROFIBROMATOSIS

THE ONLY CONSISTENT FEATURES ARE CAFE-AU-LAIT SPOTS AND FIBROMATOUS SKIN TUMORS. TUMORS OF NERVE TRUNKS ARE LIKELY TO BE PALPABLE. OTHER OCCASIONAL FEATURES INCLUDED PENDULOUS TUMORS, SCOLIOSIS, PSEUDOARTHROSIS OF THE TIBIA, PHEOCHROMOCY-TOMA, MENINGIOMA, GLIOMA, ACOUSTIC NEUROMA, OPTIC NEUROMA, MENTAL RETARDATION, HYPERTENSION, HYPOGLYCEMIA. HAYES AND COLLEAGUES (1961) REPORTED HYPOGLYCEMIA ASSOCIATED WITH MASSIVE INTRAPERITONEAL TUMOR OF MESODERMAL ORIGIN IN A PATIENT WITH TYPICAL CUTANEOUS LESIONS. GASTROINTESTINAL BLEEDING IS ANOTHER MANIFESTA-TION. FIBROMAS MAY OCCUR IN THE IRIS AND GLAUCOMA OCCURS IN RARE INSTANCES (GRANT AND WALTON, 1968). UNUSUAL CLINICAL MANIFESTATIONS WERE DESCRIBED BY DIEKMANN ET AL. (1967)* HYPERTENSION DUE TO RENAL ARTERY STENOSIS, HYPERTROPHY OF THE CLITORIS. BENEDICT ET AL. (1968) STUDIED THE PIGMENTARY ANOMALY OF NEUROFIBROMA-TOSIS IN RELATION TO THAT OF ALBRIGHT'S POLYOSTOTIC FIBROUS DYSPLASIA. GROSS APPEARANCE OF THE PIGMENTED AREAS WAS NOT ALWAYS RELIABLE. HOWEVER SPECIAL MICROSCOPIC STUDIES SHOWED GIANT PIGMENT GRANULES IN MALPIGHIAN CELLS OR MELANO-CYTE OF NORMAL SKIN AND OF NEUROFIBROMATOSIS SPOTS BUT RARELY IN ALBRIGHT'S SYNDROME. NICOLLS (1969) DESCRIBED TWO CASES OF SECTORIAL NEUROFIBROMATOSIS WHICH HE PLAUSIBLY INTERPRETED AS REPRESENTING SOMATIC MUTATION. ONE HAD A MEDIASTINAL NEUROFIBROMA AND IN THE SKIN ARE / CORRESPONDING SEGMENTALLY TO THE SITE OF THE INTERNAL LESION FIVE SMALL NEUROFIBROMAS. INVOLVEMENT OF THE HEART IN NEUROFI-BROMATOSIS WAS DESCRIBED AND REVIEWED BY ROSENQUIST ET AL. (1970) WHO ALSO REVIEWED INVOLVEMENT OF RENAL AND OTHER ARTERIES, ABDOMINAL AORTA AND CAROTID ARTERY. CROWE ET AL. (1956) SUGGESTED THAT THE PRESENCE OF SIX SPOTS EACH MORE THAN 1.5 CM. IN DIAMETER IS NECESSARY FOR THE DIAGNOSIS. CROWE (1964) SUGGESTED AXILLARY FRECKLING AS AN ESPECIALLY USEFUL DIAGNOSTIC CLUE. SEE ACOUSTIC NEUROMA FOR A DISCUSSION OF 'CENTRAL NEUROFIBROMATOSIS,' A PROBABLY SEPARATE ENTITY. THE PATIENTS DESCRIBED BY HASHEMIAN (1953) APPARENTLY HAD RECKLINGHAUSEN'S NEUROFI-BROMATOSIS (Q.V.), ALTHOUGH THE SKIN CHANGES WERE NOT AS STRIKING AS IN SOME PATIENTS. WE HAVE OBSERVED VERY SIMILAR INTESTINAL TUMORS IN A PATIENT (G. R., 368525) WITH STRIKING SKIN CHANGES OF NEUROFIBROMATOSIS. JOHNSON AND CHARNECO (1970) SUGGESTED THAT THE CAFE-AU-LAIT SPOT OF NEUROFIBROMATOSIS CAN BE DISTIN-GUISHED FROM THE INNOCENT SPOT WHICH OCCURS IN NORMAL PERSONS AND FROM THE PIGMENTED AREAS OF ALBRIGHT'S DISEASE BY THE PRESENCE OF A LARGE NUMBER OF DOPA-POSITIVE MELANOCYTES WHICH HAVE GIANT PIGMENT GRANULES IN THE CYTOPLASM. FIALKOW ET AL. (1971) CONCLUDED FROM ANALYSIS OF NEUROFIBROMAS FROM G6PD A-B HETEROZYGOTES WITH VON RECKLINGHAUSEN'S DISEASE THAT EACH TUMOR MUST ORIGINATE IN MANY CELLS, PERHAPS AT LEAST 150.

BENEDICT, P. H., SZABO, G., FITZPATRICK, T. B. AND SINESI, S. J.* MELANOTIC MACULES IN ALBRIGHT'S SYNDROME AND IN NEUROFIBROMATOSIS. J.A.M.A. 205* 618-626, 1968.

BOUDIN, G., PEPIN, B. AND VERNANT, C.* LES TUMEURS MULTIPLES DU SYSTEME NERVEUX AU COURS DE LA MALADIE DE RECKLINGHAUSEN. A PROPOS D'UNE OBSERVATION ANATOMO-CLINIQUE AVEC ADENOME CHROMOPHOBE DE L'HYPOPHYSE. PRESSE MED. 78* 1427-1430, 1970.

BUNTIN, P. T. AND FITZGERALD, J. F.* GASTROINTESTINAL NEUROFIBROMATOSIS* A RARE CAUSE OF CHRONIC ANEMIA. AM. J. DIS. CHILD. 119* 521-523, 1970.

CHARRON, J. W. AND GARIEPY, G.* NEUROFIBROMATOSIS OF BLADDER* CASE REPORT AND REVIEW OF THE LITERATURE. CANAD. J. SURG. 13* 303-306, 1970.

CROWE, F. W., SCHULL, W. J. AND NEEL, J. V.* A CLINICAL, PATHOLOGICAL AND GENETIC STUDY OF MULTIPLE NEUROFIBROMATOSIS. SPRINGFIELD, ILL.* CHARLES C THOMAS, 1956.

CROWE, F. W.* AXILLARY FRECKLING AS A DIAGNOSTIC AID IN NEUROFIBROMATOSIS. ANN. INTERN. MED. 61* 1142-1143, 1964.

DIEKMANN, L., HUTHER, W. AND PFEIFFER, R. A.* UNGEWOHNLICHE ERSCHEINUNGSFORMEN DER NEUROFIBROMATOSE (VON RECKLINGHAUSENSCHE KRANKHEIT) IM KINDESALTER. Z. KINDERHEILK. 101* 191-222, 1967.

FIALKOW, P. J., SAGEBIEL, R. W., GARTTER, S. M. AND RIMOIN, D. L.* MULTIPLE CELL ORIGIN OF HEREDITARY NEUROFIBROMAS. NEW ENG. J. MED. 284* 298-300, 1971.

FIENMAN, N. L. AND YAKOVAC, W. C.* NEUROFIBROMATOSIS IN CHILDHOOD. J. PEDIAT. 76* 339-346, 1970.

GRANT, W. M. AND WALTON, D. S.* DISTINCTIVE GONIOSCOPIC FINDINGS IN GLAUCOMA DUE TO NEUROFIBROMATOSIS. ARCH. OPHTHAL. 79* 127-134, 1968.

HASHEMIAN, H.* FAMILIAL FIBROMATOSIS OF SMALL INTESTINE. BRIT. J. SURG. 40* 346-350, 1953.

HAYES, D. M., SPURR, C. L., FELTS, J. H. AND MILLER, E. C., JR.* VON RECKLIN-GHAUSEN'S DISEASE WITH MASSIVE INTRA-ABDOMINAL TUMOR AND SPONTANEOUS HYPOGLYCEMIA* METABOLIC STUDIES BEFORE AND AFTER PERFUSION OF ABDOMINAL CAVITY WITH NITROGEN MUSTARD. METABOLISM 10* 183-199, 1961.

JOHNSON, B. L. AND CHARNECO, D. R.* CAFE AU LAIT SPOT IN NEUROFIBROMATOSIS AND IN NORMAL INDIVIDUALS. ARCH. DERM. 102* 442-446, 1970.

MILES, J., PENNYBACKER, J. AND SHELDON, P.* INTRATHORACIC MENINGOCELE. ITS DEVELOPMENT AND ASSOCIATION WITH NEUROFIBROMATOSIS. J. NEUROL. NEUROSURG. PSYCHIAT. 32* 99-110, 1969.

NAGER, G. T.* ASSOCIATION OF BILATERAL VIIITH NERVE TUMORS WITH MENINGIOMAS IN VON RECKLINGHAUSEN'S DISEASE. LARYNGOSCOPE 74* 1220-1261, 1964.

NICOLLS, E. M.* SOMATIC VARIATION AND MULTIPLE NEUROFIBROMATOSIS. HUM. HERED. 19* 473-479, 1969.

PHILIPPART, M.* NEUROFIBROMATOSE HEREDITAIRE A LARGE SPECTRE PHENOTYPIQUE (FAMILLE SN). J. GENET. HUM. 10* 338-346, 1961.

ROSENQUIST, G. C., KROVETZ, L. J., HALLER, J. A., JR., SIMON, A. L. AND BANNAYAN, G. A.* ACQUIRED RIGHT VENTRICULAR OUTFLOW OBSTRUCTION IN A CHILD WITH NEUROFIBROMATOSIS. AM. HEART J. 79* 103-108, 1970.

SMITH, C. J., HATCH, F. E., JOHNSON, J. G. AND KELLY, B. J.* RENAL ARTERY DYSPLASIA AS A CAUSE OF HYPERTENSION IN NEUROFIBROMATOSIS. ARCH. INTERN. MED. 125* 1022-1026, 1970.

TAYLOR, P. E.* ENCAPSULATED GLIOMA OF THE SYLVIAN FISSURE ASSOCIATED WITH NEUROFIBROMATOSIS. REPORT OF A CASE WITH HISTOPATHOLOGICAL COMPARISON OF SURGICAL LESION AND AUTOPSY SPECIMEN FOLLOWING RECURRENCE. J. NEUROPATH. EXP. NEUROL. 21* 566-578, 1962.

*16230 NEUROMATA, MUCOSAL, WITH ENDOCRINE TUMORS

WILLIAMS AND POLLOCK (1966) DESCRIBED TWO UNRELATED PATIENTS WITH MULTIPLE TRUE NEUROMAS, PHEOCHROMOCYTOMA AND THYROID CARCINOMA. THE THYROID CANCER WAS OF THE MEDULLARY TYPE AS IN THE PTC SYNDROME (Q.V.). INDEED THE RELATIONSHIP OF THESE IS UNCLEAR. ALTHOUGH THE ASSOCIATION OF PHEOCHROMOCYTOMA WITH NEUROFIBROMATOSIS IS WELL KNOWN, THE NERVOUS TUMOR IS A TRUE NEUROMA, I.E., CONSISTS MAINLY OF NERVE CELLS, IN THIS CONDITION. THEY ARE NOT ASSOCIATED WITH CAFE-AU-LAIT SPOTS. THEY OCCUR AS PEDUNCULATED NODULES ON THE EYELID MARGINS, LIPS AND TONGUE. THE LIPS ARE DIFFUSELY HYPERTROPHIED WITH A 'NEGROID' APPEARANCE. NEUROMAS OCCUR ALSO IN THE TONGUE. THE FATHER OF ONE OF WILLIAMS AND POLLOCK'S CASES HAD VERY THICK LIPS AND EYELID AND TONGUE LESIONS LIKE HIS DAUGHTERS. HE HAD A MEDULLARY THYROID CANCER AND HAD DIED AT AGE 38 AFTER AN ABDOMINAL OPERATION, HAVING HAD SYMPTOMS SUGGESTIVE OF PHEOCHROMOCYTOMA. SCHIMKE ET AL. (1968) REPORTED CASES ALSO. CUNLIFFE ET AL. (1968) DEMONSTRATED CALCITONIN-SECRETION IN A MEDULLARY CARCINOMA OF THE THYROID. THE PATIENT WAS A 19 YEAR OLD GIRL WITH ACNE, FEATURES OF MARFAN SYNDROME, NEUROMAS OF TONGUE AND EYELID, PROMINENT LIPS, NODULAR GOITER, PIGMENTA-TION OF HANDS, FEET AND CIRCUMORAL AREA, PROXIMAL MYOPATHY, LOOSE MOTIONS, AND FLUSHING ATTACKS. (THE FIRST PATIENT WITH THIS SYNDROME I SAW WAS REFERRED TO ME AS POSSIBLE MARFAN SYNDROME.) THE FEATURES SUGGESTING MARFAN SYNDROME WERE HIGH ARCHED PALATE, PECTUS EXCAVATUM, BILATERAL PES CAVUS, HIGH PATELLA AND SCOLIOSIS. MARFANOID HABITUS AND PES CAVUS ARE STRIKING FEATURES IN MOST. MEGACOLON OR COLONIC DIVERTICULA ALSO OCCUR. MUCOSAL NEUROMAS INVOLVE THE LIPS, ANTERIOR TONGUE, CONJUNCTIVA AND NASAL AND LARYNGEAL MUCOSA. MEDULLATED NERVE FIBERS TRAVERSE THE CORNEA. BARTLETT ET AL. (1968) DESCRIBED AFFECTED PERSONS IN 6 GENERATIONS.

BARTLETT, R. C., BEAN, L. R. AND MANDELSTAM, P.* HEREDITARY STUDY OF NEUROENDO-CRINE DYSPLASIA IN SIX GENERATIONS. INT. ASS. DENT. RES. (SAN FRANCISCO, MARCH 21-24), 1968. P. 36.

BAYLIN, S. B., BEAVEN, M. O. ENGELMAN, K. AND SJOERDSMA, A.* ELEVATED HISTA-MINASE ACTIVITY IN MEDULLARY CARCINOMA OF THE THYROID GLAND. NEW ENG. J. MED. 283* 1239-1244, 1970.

BRALEY, A. E.* MEDULLATED CORNEAL NERVES AND PLEXIFORM NEUROMA ASSOCIATED WITH PHEOCHROMOCYTOMA. TRANS. AM. OPHTHAL. SOC. 52* 189-197, 1954.

CUNLIFFE, W. J., BLACK, M. M., HALL, R., JOHNSTON, I. D. A., HUDGSON, P.,

SHUSTER, S., GUDMUNDSSON, T. V., JOPLIN, G. F., WILLIAMS, E. D., WOODHOUSE, N. J. Y., GALANTE, L. AND MACINTYRE, I.* A CALCITONIN-SECRETING THYROID CARCINOMA. LANCET 2* 63-66, 1968.

GORLIN, R. J., SEDANO, H. O., VICKERS, R. A. AND CERVENKA, J.* MULTIPLE MUCOSAL NEUROMAS, PHEOCHROMOCYTOMA AND MEDULLARY CARCINOMA OF THE THYROID - A SYNDROME. CANCER 22* 293-299, 1968.

SCHIMKE, R. N., HARTMANN, W. H., PROUT, T. E. AND RIMOIN, D. L.* PHEOCHROMOCY-TOMA, MEDULLARY THYROID CARCINOMA AND MULTIPLE NEUROMAS. NEW ENG. J. MED. 279* 1-7, 1968.

WILLIAMS, E. D. AND POLLOCK, D. J.* MULTIPLE MUCOSAL NEUROMATA WITH ENDOCRINE TUMOURS* A SYNDROME ALLIED TO VON RECKLINGHAUSEN'S DISEASE. J. PATH. BACT. 91* 71-80, 1966.

*16240 NEUROPATHY, HEREDITARY SENSORY RADICULAR

MANDELL AND SMITH (1960) DESCRIBED A CASE. THE MANIFESTATIONS WERE CHARCOT-TYPE ARTHROPATHY, RECURRENT ULCERATION OF THE LOWER EXTREMITIES AND SIGNS OF RADICULAR SENSORY DEFICIENCY IN BOTH THE UPPER AND THE LOWER EXTREMITIES, WITHOUT ANY MOTOR DYSFUNCTION.

HICKS (1922) DESCRIBED A FAMILY IN WHICH TEN MEMBERS SUFFERED FROM PERFORA-TING ULCERS OF THE FEET AND SHOOTING PAINS ABOUT THE BODY, AND DEAFNESS. THE FIRST SYMPTOMS APPEARED BETWEEN 15 TO 36 YEARS OF AGE. FIRST TO APPEAR WAS A CORN ON A BIG TOE, FOLLOWED BY A PAINLESS ULCER WITH BONY DEBRIS. OTHER TOES THEN BECAME INVOLVED. SHOOTING PAINS THEN APPEARED, SIMILAR TO THE LIGHTNING PAINS OF TABES DORSALIS. AT ABOUT THE SAME TIME THE PATIENT BEGINS TO SUFFER FROM BILATERAL DEAFNESS, PROGRESSING TO TOTAL DEAFNESS OVER SEVERAL YEARS. NEUROLOGI-CAL EXAMINATION SHOWS DISAPPEARANCE OF ANKLE, THEN KNEE JERKS. CRANIAL NERVES ARE NORMAL WITH THE EXCEPTION OF THE AUDITORY NERVE. AN EXTENSOR PLANTAR RESPONSE IS NEVER OBTAINED, THE PUPILS REACT NORMALLY, AND THERE IS NO NYSTAGMUS. SENSATION OF THE ARMS IS NORMAL. THERE IS LOSS OF PAIN, TOUCH, HEAT AND COLD OVER THE FEET. THE PATHOLOGY IS COMPLETELY UNKNOWN. THOUGH OTHERS HAVE REPORTED HEREDITARY PERFORATING ULCERS OF THE FEET (Q.V.) THERE IS NO MENTION OF DEAFNESS OR SHOOTING PAINS.

DENNY-BROWN (1951) REPORTED THE CLINICAL AND AUTOPSY FINDINGS OF A 53-YEAR-OLD WOMAN, A MEMBER OF THE FAMILY REPORTED BY HICKS (1922). AT THE AGE OF 22 AN ULCER FORMED ON HER RIGHT GREAT TOE REQUIRING A YEAR TO HEAL. SINCE THEN SHE SUFFERED FROM RECURRENT ULCERATION, EACH LASTING SIX TO NINE MONTHS, SOMETIMES EXTENDING TO BONE. IN HER EARLY TWENTIES SHE FIRST NOTICED SHOOTING PAINS IN HER LEGS, SOMETIMES IN HER ARMS. DEAFNESS BEGAN AT THE AGE OF 40 YEARS AND PROGRESSED TO ALMOST TOTAL DEAFNESS BY 53 YEARS OF AGE. NEUROLOGICAL EXAMINATION 53 YEARS OF AGE SHOWED LOSS OF ALL SENSATION IN THE LOWER LEGS WITH LOSS OF PAIN AND TEMPERA-TURE SENSATION IN THE THIGHS AND HANDS. AUTOPSY SHOWED A SMALL BRAIN. THE MOST SEVERE CHANGES WERE A MARKED LOSS OF GANGLION CELLS IN THE SACRAL AND LUMBAR DORSAL ROOT GANGLIA. THERE WERE LESS SEVERE CHANGES IN C-8 AND T-1 GANGLIA. THE REMAINING GANGLION CELLS SHOWED GREAT PROLIFERATION OF SUBCAPSULAR DENDRITES. CLEAR HYALIN BODIES WERE SEEN IN THE INVOLVED GANGLIA REPRESENTING POSSIBLY AN AMYLOID MASS AROUND CAPILLARIES. NO MENTION WAS MADE OF THE TEMPORAL BONES.

HELLER AND ROBB (1955) DESCRIBED A FRENCH-CANADIAN FAMILY IN WHICH FIVE HAD FULL-BLOWN DISEASE AND THREE HAD AN INCOMPLETE FORM. ALTHOUGH DOMINANT INHERITANCE WAS PROPOSED FOR THIS FAMILY ALSO, RECESSIVE INHERITANCE SEEMS EQUALLY OR MORE LIKELY. NO AMYLOID WAS FOUND ON DORSAL ROOT GANGLION BIOPSY. THESE AUTHORS SUGGESTED THAT MORVAN'S DISEASE WAS THE SAME AS THIS. MOST OF MORVAN'S CASES (1883-1889) CAME FROM BRITTANY. MANY OF THE FEATURES SUGGEST ACRO-OSTEOLYSIS (RECESSIVE CATALOG). MANDELL AND SMITH (1960) OBSERVED SENSORY RADICULAR NEUROPATHY IN GRANDFATHER, FATHER AND MALE PROBAND.

DYCK, KENNEL, MAGAL AND KRAYBILL (1965) DESCRIBED A FAMILY IN WHICH THE PRESENCE OF PERONEAL MUSCULAR ATROPHY AND PES CAVUS SUGGESTED CHARCOT-MARIE-TOOTH DISEASE. BIOPSY OF THE SKIN FROM THE PAD OF THE GREAT TOE OF AFFECTED PERSONS USING THE CHOLINESTERASE TECHNIQUE SHOWED NORMAL NUMBERS OF MEISSNER CORPUSCLES IN A 14 YEAR OLD BOY WITH EARLY SIGNS SUGGESTIVE OF THE DISORDER BUT NO CORPUSCLES IN A 37 YEAR OLD MAN AND A 28 YEAR OLD WOMAN WITH WELL-DEVELOPED DISEASE. THE AUTHORS COMMENTED ON THE SIMILARITIES BETWEEN FOUR ENTITIES - THIS ONE AND THOSE WHICH CARRY THE EPONYMS CHARCOT-MARIE-TOOTH, ROUSSY-LEVY AND DEJERINE-SOTTAS.

CAMPBELL AND HOFFMAN (1964) REPORTED TWO FAMILIES. DELEON (1969) DESCRIBED A CASE WHICH LIKE THEIRS HAD AMYOTROPHY. THIS MAY, THEREFORE, BE A SEPARATE ENTITY. CONGENITAL SENSORY NEUROPATHY RESULTING IN INSENSITIVITY TO PAIN SEEMED TO BE DOMINANT IN THE FAMILY REPORTED BY ERVIN AND STERNBACH (1960) AND THAT OF SILVERMAN AND GILDEN (1959). WALLACE (1968) STUDIED AN EXTENSIVELY AFFECTED AUSTRALIAN KINDRED.

CAMPBELL, A. M. G. AND HOFFMAN, H. L.* SENSORY RADICULAR NEUROPATHY ASSOCIATED WITH MUSCLE WASTING IN TWO CASES. BRAIN 87* 67-74, 1964.

CLARKE, J. M. AND GROVES, E. W. H.* REMARKS ON SYRINGOMYELIA (SACRO-LUMBAR TYPE) OCCURRING IN A BROTHER AND SISTER. BRIT. MED. J. 2* 737-740, 1909.

DELEON, G. A.* PROGRESSIVE VENTRAL SENSORY LOSS IN SENSORY RADICULAR NEUROPATHY AND HYPERTROPHIC NEURITIS. JOHNS HOPKINS MED. J. 125* 53-61, 1969.

DENNY-BROWN, D.* HEREDITARY SENSORY RADICULAR NEUROPATHY. J. NEUROL. NEURO-SURG. PSYCHIAT. 14* 237-252, 1951.

DYCK, P. J., KENNEL, A. J., MAGAL, I. V. AND KRAYBILL, E. N.* A VIRGINIA KINSHIP WITH HEREDITARY SENSORY NEUROPATHY* PERONEAL MUSCULAR ATROPHY AND PES CAVUS. MAYO CLIN. PROC. 40* 685-694, 1965.

ERVIN, F. R. AND STERNBACH, R. A.* HEREDITARY INSENSITIVITY TO PAIN. TRANS. AM. NEUROL. ASS. 86* 70-74, 1960.

HELLER, I. H. AND ROBB, P.* HEREDITARY SENSORY NEUROPATHY. NEUROLOGY 5* 15-29, 1955.

HICKS, E. P. AND CAMP, M. B.* HEREDITARY PERFORATING ULCER OF THE FOOT. LANCET 1* 319-321, 1922.

MANDELL, A. J. AND SMITH, C. K.* HEREDITARY SENSORY RADICULAR NEUROPATHY. NEUROLOGY 10* 627-630, 1960.

OGRYZLO, M. A.* A FAMILIAL PERIPHERAL NEUROPATHY OF UNKNOWN ETIOLOGY RESEMBLING MORVAN'S DISEASE. CANAD. MED. ASS. J. 54* 547-553, 1946.

SCHULTZE, F.* FAMILIAR AUFTRETENDES MALUM PERFORANS DER FUSSE (FAMILIARE LUMBALE SYRINGOMYELIE). DEUTSCH. MED. WSCHR. 43* 545-547, 1917.

SILVERMAN, F. N. AND GILDEN, J. J.* CONGENITAL INSENSITIVITY TO PAIN, A NEUROLOGIC SYNDROME WITH BIZARRE SKELETAL LESIONS. RADIOLOGY 72* 176-190, 1959.

SMITH, E. M.* FAMILIAL NEUROTROPHIC OSSEOUS ATROPHY. A FAMILIAL NEUROTROPHIC CONDITION OF THE FEET WITH ANESTHESIA AND LOSS OF BONE. J.A.M.A. 102* 593-595, 1934.

TOCANTINS, L. M., AND REIMANN, H. A.* PERFORATING ULCERS OF FEET, WITH OSSEOUS ATROPHY IN FAMILY WITH OTHER EVIDENCES OF DYSGENESIS (HARE LIP, CLEFT PALATE)* AN INSTANCE OF PROBABLE MYELODYSPLASIA. J.A.M.A. 112* 2251-2255, 1939.

WALLACE, D. C.* A STUDY OF AN HEREDITARY NEUROPATHY. U. OF SYDNEY M.D. THESIS, 1968.

*16250 NEUROPATHY, HEREDITARY, WITH LIABILITY TO PRESSURE PALSIES

THIS DISORDER SEEMS TO BE DISTINCT FROM NEURITIS WITH BRACHIAL PREDILECTION (Q.V.). FAMILIES WERE REPORTED BY DAVIES (1954) AND BY EARL AND COLLEAGUES (1964). THE LATTER GROUP FOUND THAT MOTOR NERVE CONDUCTION VELOCITY WAS REDUCED IN SOME CLINICALLY NORMAL FAMILY MEMBERS. STAAL, DE WEERDT, AND WENT (1965) STUDIED A FAMILY IN WHICH MEMBERS IN 4 GENERATIONS SHOWED TRANSIENT UNILATERAL PERONEAL PALSIES. THE NEUROPATHY MANIFESTED ITSELF ESPECIALLY AFTER PROLONGED WORK IN A KNEELING POSITION. THE FAMILY, LIVING IN HOLLAND, KNEW THE DISEASE AS 'BULB DIGGERS' PALSY. OTHER NERVE PALSIES, SUCH AS ULNA, OCCUR AS WELL (DAVIES, 1954). FEMALES ARE LESS SEVERELY AFFECTED. THE RELATIONSHIP TO NEURITIS WITH BRACHIAL PREDILECTION IS UNCLEAR.

DAVIES, D. M.* RECURRENT PERIPHERAL-NERVE PALSIES IN A FAMILY. LANCET 2* 266-268, 1954.

EARL, C. J., FULLERTON, P. M., WAKEFIELD, G. S. AND SCHRETTA, H. S.* HEREDITARY NEUROPATHY, WITH LIABILITY TO PRESSURE PALSIES* A CLINICAL AND ELECTROPHYSIOLOGI-CAL STUDY OF FOUR FAMILIES. QUART. J. MED. 33* 481-498, 1964.

STAAL, A., DE WEERDT, C. J. AND WENT, L. N.* HEREDITARY COMPRESSION SYNDROME OF PERIPHERAL NERVES. NEUROLOGY 15* 1008-1017, 1965.

16260 NEUROPATHY, WITH PARAPROTEIN IN SERUM, CEREBROSPINAL FLUID AND URINE

GIBBERD AND GAVRILESCU (1966) DESCRIBED A FAMILY IN WHICH FOUR PERSONS IN THREE GENERATIONS HAD A PROGRESSIVE HYPERTROPHIC POLYNEURITIS ASSOCIATED WITH AN ABNORMAL PROTEIN IN SERUM, CEREBROSPINAL FLUID AND URINE. MOTOR AND SENSORY CHANGES BEGAN AT ABOUT AGE 50 YEARS. NERVE CONDUCTION VELOCITY WAS DELAYED. SURAL NERVE ON BIOPSY SHOWED MARKED DEMYELINATION WITH SCHWANN CELL PROLIFERATION. THE TOTAL SPINAL FLUID PROTEIN WAS ONLY SLIGHTLY INCREASED.

GIBBERD, F. B. AND GAVRILESCU, K.* A FAMILIAL NEUROPATHY ASSOCIATED WITH A PARAPROTEIN IN THE SERUM, CEREBROSPINAL FLUID AND URINE. NEUROLOGY 16* 130-134, 1966.

*16270 NEUTROPENIA, CHRONIC FAMILIAL

LEVINE (1959) DESCRIBED AN AFFECTED 14 AND ONE HALF YEAR OLD BOY WHO ALSO SHOWED HYPERPLASTIC GINGIVITIS. THE FATHER AND TWO SIBS ALSO HAD CHRONIC NEUTROPENIA. CLUBBING OF THE FINGERS AND HYPERGLOBULINEMIA WERE OTHER FEATURES. ALTHOUGH RECESSIVE FORMS OF CONGENITAL NEUTROPENIA HAVE BEEN MORE FREQUENTLY DESCRIBED, THE FAMILY DESCRIBED BY HITZIG (1959) SUGGESTS DOMINANT INHERITANCE OF ONE FORM. THE

FATHER, AGE 36, A SON AGE 8 AND A DAUGHTER AGE 4 WERE AFFECTED. THE BLOOD AND MARROW FINDINGS WERE SIMILAR TO THOSE IN THE RECESSIVE FORM DESCRIBED BY KOSTER-MANN. HOWEVER, SEVERE INFECTIONS WERE NOT A FEATURE. CUTTING AND LANG (1964) OBSERVED 9 CASES OF BENIGN CHRONIC NEUTROPENIA IN 3 GENERATIONS OF A FAMILY. THE NEUTROPENIA WAS CONSTANT.

CUTTING, H. O. AND LANG, J. E., JR.* FAMILIAL BENIGN CHRONIC NEUTROPENIA. ANN. INTERN. MED. 61* 876-887, 1964.

HITZIG, W. H.* FAMILIARE NEUTROPENIE MIT DOMINANTEM ERBGANG UND HYPERGAMMAGLO-BULINAMIE. HELV. MED. ACTA 26* 779-784, 1959.

LEVINE, S.* CHRONIC FAMILIAL NEUTROPENIA, WITH MARKED PERIODONTAL LESIONS. REPORT OF A CASE. ORAL SURG. 12* 310-314, 1959.

16280 NEUTROPENIA, CYCLIC

HAHNEMAN AND ALT (1958) DESCRIBED A 29 YEAR OLD MAN WHO FROM AN EARLY AGE HAD NEUTROPENIA RECURRING EVERY 21 DAYS AND ACCOMPANIED BY INFECTION. COMPLETE REMISSION OCCURRED AT AGE 18 YEARS. THE MAN'S DAUGHTER WAS SEEN AT THE AGE OF 2 YEARS WITH SIMILAR PERIODIC DISEASE RECURRING EACH 14 DAYS. TORRIOLI-RIGGIO (1958) ALSO REPORTED CASES. MORLEY ET AL. (1967) DESCRIBED 20 CASES IN 5 FAMILIES. CLINICAL MANIFESTATIONS USUALLY BEGAN IN CHILDHOOD AND IMPROVED THEREAFTER. THE COMMONEST ARE FEVER, ORAL ULCERATIONS AND SKIN INFECTIONS. NEUTROPENIA OCCURS AT INTERVALS OF 15-35 DAYS. IT IS OFTEN ACCOMPANIED BY MONOCYTOSIS AND SOMETIMES BY ANEMIA, EOSINOPHILIA OR THROMBOCYTOPENIA. MALE-TO-MALE TRANSMISSION OCCURRED. CYCLIC NEUTROPENIA IN THE COLLIE DOG IS ACCOMPANIED BY GRAY FUR, LEADS TO EARLY DEATH FROM PYOGENIC INFECTIONS AND IS AN AUTOSOMAL RECESSIVE (DALE ET AL., 1970).

DALE, D. C., KIMBALL, H. R. AND WOLFF, S. M.* STUDIES OF CYCLIC NEUTROPENIA IN GRAY COLLIE DOGS. (ABSTRACT) CLIN. RES. 18* 402 ONLY, 1970.

HAHNEMAN, B. M. AND ALT, H. L.* CYCLIC NEUTROPENIA IN A FATHER AND DAUGHTER. J.A.M.A. 168* 270-272, 1958.

MORLEY, A. A., CAREW, J. P. AND BAIKIE, A. G.* FAMILIAL CYCLICAL NEUTROPENIA. BRIT. J. HAEMAT. 13* 719-738, 1967.

TORRIOLI-RIGGIO, G.* CONSIDERAZIONI SU UNA FAMIGLIA DI GRANULOPENICI. ACTA GENET. MED. GEM. 7* 237-248, 1958.

*16290 NEVI (PIGMENTED MOLES)

ALTHOUGH IT IS A COMMON OBSERVATION THAT NEVI OCCUR IN FAMILIES, PROBABLY WITH DOMINANT TRANSMISSION, THE STUDY BY DENARO (1944) IS ONE OF THE FEW WHICH HAS EXAMINED THE MATTER SPECIFICALLY. MULTIPLE PIGMENTED MOLES ARE A FEATURE OF ONE CHROMOSOMAL ABERRATION, THE TURNER SYNDROME, AS POINTED OUT BY SHARPEY-SCHAFER (1941). ESTABROOK (1928) REPORTED AFFECTED PERSONS IN 5 GENERATIONS OF A FAMILY. (HIS TERM NEVUS SPILUS COMES FROM THE GREEK 'SPILOS' FOR 'SPOT.').

DENARO, S. J.* THE INHERITANCE OF NEVI. J. HERED. 35* 215-218, 1944.

ESTABROOK, A. H.* A FAMILY WITH BIRTHMARKS (NEVUS SPILUS) FOR FIVE GENERATIONS. (ABSTRACT) EUGEN. NEWS 13* 90-92, 1928.

MEIROWSKI, E.* MOLES AND MALFORMATIONS OF THE SKIN IN THEIR RELATIONSHIP TO INHERITANCE AND PHYLOGENESIS (NEW AND OLD INVESTIGATIONS). BRIT. J. DERM. 54* 99-121, 1942.

SHARPEY-SCHAFER, E. P.* CASE OF PTERYGO-NUCHAL INFANTILISM (TURNER'S SYNDROME), WITH POST-MORTEM FINDINGS. LANCET 2* 559-560, 1941.

*16300 NEVI FLAMMEI, FAMILIAL MULTIPLE

SHELLEY AND LIVINGOOD (1949) DESCRIBED 12 CASES IN 7 SIBSHIPS IN 4 GENERATIONS OF A FAMILY, WITH FIVE INSTANCES OF MALE-TO-MALE TRANSMISSION. TWO GENERATIONS WERE SKIPPED IN ONE BRANCH OF THE FAMILY. REFERRED TO AS BIRTHMARKS, THESE CONSIST OF DARK RED, NONELEVATED, SHARPLY CIRCUMSCRIBED PATCHES WHICH BLANCH ON PRESSURE WITH A GLASS, LEAVING A RESIDUAL BROWN HYPERPIGMENTATION.

SHELLEY, W. B. AND LIVINGOOD, C. S.* FAMILIAL MULTIPLE NEVI FLAMMEI. ARCH. DERM. SYPH. 59* 343-345, 1949.

*16310 NEVUS FLAMMEUS OF THE NAPE OF THE NECK

NEVUS FLAMMEUS NUCHAE OCCURS IN ABOUT 5 PERCENT OF PERSONS. SOMETIMES CALLED PORT WINE STAINS, THESE CONSIST OF A FAINT NON-ELEVATED RED AREA OF VARIABLE SIZE AND IRREGULAR OUTLINE ON THE NAPE OF THE NECK. AN EXCEEDINGLY EXTENSIVE PEDIGREE DEMONSTRATING DOMINANT INHERITANCE WAS PUBLISHED BY ZUMKELLER (1957). SKLARZ (1955) QUESTIONED THE SIGNIFICANCE OF GENETIC FACTORS. HOWEVER, SHAFAR AND DOIG (1955), LIKE ZUMKELLER (1957) AND OTHERS, INSISTED ON A GENETIC BASIS.

CORSON, E. F.* NEVUS FLAMMEUS NUCHAE, ITS OCCURRENCE AND ABNORMALITIES. AM. J. MED. SCI. 187* 121-124, 1934.

OSTER, J. AND NIELSEN, A.* NUCHAL NAEVI AND INTERSCAPULAR TELANGIECTASES. INCIDENCE IN DANISH SCHOOL CHILDREN. ACTA PAEDIAT. SCAND. 59* 416-423, 1970.

SHAFAR, J. AND DOIG, A.* THE 'NAPE NAEVUS.' BRIT. MED. J. 1* 913 ONLY, 1955.

SKLARZ, E.* TELANGIECTATIC ('NAPE') NAEVI. BRIT. MED. J. 1* 1221 ONLY, 1955.

ZUMKELLER, R.* A PROPOS DE LA FREQUENCE ET DE L'HEREDITE DU NAEVUS VASCULOSUS NUCHAE (UNNA). INCIDENCE AND HEREDITY OF NEVUS VASCULOSUS NUCHAE UNNA. J. GENET. HUM. 6* 1-12, 1957.

16320 NEVUS SEBACEUS OF JADASSOHN

CONVULSIVE DISORDERS AND MULTIPLE DEVELOPMENTAL ABNORMALITIES AS WELL AS MENTAL RETARDATION ARE OFTEN ASSOCIATED. MEHREGAN AND PINKUS (1965) POINTED OUT CHARACTERISTICS OF THE NATURAL HISTORY. IN THE FIRST STAGE THERE IS ALOPECIA WITH ABSENT OR PRIMITIVE HAIR FOLLICES AND NUMEROUS SMALL HYPOPLASTIC SEBACEOUS GLANDS. AT PUBERTY THE LESIONS BECOME VERRUCOUS WITH HYPERPLASTIC SEBACEOUS GLANDS. IN LATE STAGES BENIGN OR MALIGNANT TUMORS DEVELOP. APPARENTLY NO FAMILIAL CASES HAVE BEEN OBSERVED. THE SYNDROME IS INCLUDED HERE FOR HEURISTIC PURPOSES ONLY.

LANTIS, S., LEYDEN, J., THEW, M. AND HEATON, C.* NEVUS SEBACEUS OF JADASSOHN. ARCH. DERM. 98* 117-123, 1968.

MEHREGAN, A. H. AND PINKUS, H.* LIFE HISTORY OF ORGANOID NEVI. ARCH. DERM. 91* 574-588, 1965.

16330 NEVUS SEBACEUS, LINEAR, WITH CONVULSIONS AND MENTAL RETARDATION

FEUERSTEIN AND MIMS (1962) DESCRIBED 2 UNRELATED PATIENTS WITH LINEAR NEVUS SEBACEUS OF THE MIDLINE OF THE FACE ASSOCIATED WITH EPILEPSY, FOCAL EEG ABNORMALI-TIES AND MENTAL RETARDATION. NOTHING IS KNOWN ABOUT A POSSIBLE GENETIC BASIS.

FEUERSTEIN, R. C. AND MIMS, L. C.* LINEAR NEVUS SEBACEUS WITH CONVULSIONS AND MENTAL RETARDATION. AM. J. DIS. CHILD. 104* 675-679, 1962.

*16340 NIEVERGELT SYNDROME

COMPLEX DIGITAL MALFORMATIONS (BRACHYDACTYLY, SYNDACTYLY, ETC.) ARE ASSOCIATED WITH HYPOPLASIA OF TIBIA, FIBULA, ULNA, AND RADIUS. NIEVERGELT (1944) REPORTED AN AFFECTED MAN WHO TRANSMITTED THE SYNDROME TO THREE SONS, EACH BY A DIFFERENT WIFE. IN A SECOND FAMILY 9 PERSONS (2 MALES AND 7 FEMALES) IN 3 GENERATIONS WERE AFFECTED. A CHARACTERISTIC RHOMBOIDAL SHAPE OF THE TIBIA AND FIBULA HELP DIFFERENTIATE THIS CONDITION FROM ACHONDROGENESIS (Q.V.) AND FROM RECESSIVE MICROMELIC DWARFISM (Q.V.) WITH HYPOPLASTIC ULNA AND FIBULA BUT NO HAND MALFORMA-TION. THE X-RAY CHANGES, COMPLETELY SPECIFIC, ARE WELL DEMONSTRATED IN THE SPORADIC CASE REPORTED BY SOLONEN AND SULAMAA (1958). THE CASES CALLED NIEVER-GELT'S SYNDROME BY BLOCKEY AND LAWRIE (1963) WERE IN FACT INSTANCES OF MESOMELIC DWARFISM, A RECESSIVE (Q.V.).

DUBOIS, H. J.* NIEVERGELT-PEARLMAN SYNDROME* SYNOSTOSIS IN FEET AND HANDS WITH DYSPLASIA OF ELBOWS. REPORT OF A CASE. J. BONE JOINT SURG. 52B* 325-329, 1970.

NIEVERGELT, K.* POSITIVER VATERSCHAFTSNACHWEIS AUF GRUND ERBLICHER MISSBILDUN-GEN DER EXTREMITATEN. ARCH. KLAUS. STIFT. VERERBUNGSFORSCH. 19* 157 ONLY, 1944.

SOLONEN, K. A. AND SULAMAA, M.* NIEVERGELT SYNDROME AND ITS TREATMENT. A CASE REPORT. ANN. CHIR. GYNAEC. FENN. 47* 142-147, 1958.

*16350 NIGHT BLINDNESS, CONGENITAL STATIONARY (HEMERALOPIA)

THE MOST FAMOUS AFFECTED FAMILY IS THAT DESCENDANT FOR SOME 11 GENERATIONS FROM JEAN NOUGARET, A BUTCHER FROM PROVENCE WHO SETTLED IN A SMALL VILLAGE NEAR MONTPELLIER IN THE SOUTH OF FRANCE. FLORENT CUNIER, THE BELGIAN OPHTHALMOLOGIST WHO FOUNDED ANNALES D'OCULISTIQUE, HEARD OF THE FAMILY, EXAMINED SOME AFFECTED MEMBERS AND STIMULATED M. CHAUVET, A LOCAL ANTIQUARIAN, TO ASSEMBLE THE FAMILY GENEALOGY. IT WAS CHAUVET WHO SHOWED THAT NOUGARET WAS THE COMMON ANCESTOR OF ALL PERSONS IN THE DISTRICT WITH NIGHT BLINDNESS. HIS GENEALOGY LISTED 629 PERSONS OF WHOM 86 WERE NIGHT BLIND. CUNIER PUBLISHED THE FINDINGS IN 1838. NETTLESHIP FOLLOWED UP ON THE FAMILY IN 1907. BY THIS TIME 135 NIGHT-BLIND PERSONS WERE KNOWN. VISION WAS UNIMPAIRED IN DAYLIGHT, THE FUNDI WERE NORMAL AND GENERAL HEALTH WAS EXCELLENT. THE EXCESS OF NORMAL OVER AFFECTED OBSERVED IN THIS FAMILY AMONG OFFSPRING OF AFFECTED PERSONS MAY BE A MATTER OF INCOMPLETE PENETRANCE OR INCOMPLETE RECORDING OF MILD CASES - A VIEW SUBSCRIBED TO BY THE GENETICIST WILLIAM BATESON WHO DISCUSSED THE PAPER. ATTEMPTS AT FURTHER FOLLOW UP IN 1949 BY DEJEAN ET AL. INDICATED THAT THE VILLAGE INHABITED BY NOUGARET'S DESCENDANTS WAS NO LONGER AN ISOLATE. FRANCOIS, VERRIEST AND DE ROUCK (1965) OBSERVED A FAMILY WITH AT LEAST FOUR AFFECTED IN THREE GENERATIONS. ALL WERE FEMALES. SEE EDITORIAL (1970) FOR AN INTERESTING BIOGRAPHY OF NETTLESHIP.

CARROLL, F. AND HAIG, C.* CONGENITAL STATIONARY NIGHT BLINDNESS WITHOUT OPHTHALMOSCOPIC OR OTHER ABNORMALITIES. ARCH. OPHTHAL. 50* 35-44, 1953.

CUNIER, F.* ANN. OCUL. 1* 32, 1838.

CUNIER, F.* ANNALES DE LA SOCIETE DE MEDICIN DE GAND 4* 385-395, 1838.

DEJEAN, C. AND GASSENC, R.* NOTE SUR LA GENEALOGIE DE LA FAMILLE NOUGARET, DE VENDEMIAN. BULL. SOC. OPHTAL. FRANC. 96* 96-100, 1949.

EDITORIAL* EDWARD NETTLESHIP (1845-1913)* VETERINARIAN-DERMATOLOGIST-OPHTHALMO-LOGIST-GENETICIST. J.A.M.A. 214* 751-752, 1970.

FRANCOIS, J., VERRIEST, G. AND DE ROUCK, A.* A NEW PEDIGREE OF IDIOPATHIC CONGENITAL NIGHT-BLINDNESS* TRANSMITTED AS A DOMINANT HEREDITARY TRAIT. AM. J. OPHTHAL. 59* 621-625, 1965.

NETTLESHIP, E.* A HISTORY OF CONGENITAL STATIONARY NIGHT-BLINDNESS IN NINE CONSECUTIVE GENERATIONS. TRANS. OPHTHAL. SOC. U.K. 27* 269-293, 1907.

SNYDER, C.* JEAN NOUGARET, THE BUTCHER FROM PROVENCE, AND HIS FAMILY. ARCH. OPHTHAL. 69* 676-678, 1963.

*16360 NIPPLES INVERTED (MAMMILLAE INVERTITA)

ROMANUS (1948) DESCRIBED 7 CASES IN 5 SIBSHIPS IN 4 GENERATIONS.

ROMANUS, T.* A PEDIGREE SHOWING THE INCIDENCE OF MALFORMATION OF THE NIPPLES. ACTA GENET. STATIST. MED. 1* 168-173, 1948.

16370 NIPPLES, SUPERNUMERARY

RATHER EXTENSIVE LITERATURE SUPPORTING DOMINANT INHERITANCE WAS REVIEWED BY GATES (1947). IN THE GUINEA PIG THIS TRAIT BEHAVES AS AN AUTOSOMAL DOMINANT. KLINKER-FUSS (1924) FOUND POLYMASTIA IN 5 FEMALES IN 4 GENERATIONS. THE EXTRA BREAST CONSISTED OF A MASS IN ONE OR BOTH AXILLAE WHICH ENLARGED IN PREGNANCY AND LACTATION. IN SOME BUT NOT ALL A NIPPLE WAS ASSOCIATED WITH THE ADVENTITIOUS BREAST TISSUE. IT MAY HAVE COMMUNICATED WITH THE MAIN BREAST TISSUE BECAUSE IT SWELLED BEFORE NURSING AND SHRUNK WITH NURSING. PIERRE MARIE (1893) ALSO OBSERVED SUPERNUMERARY BREASTS IN FOUR GENERATIONS AND NOTED AN ASSOCIATION WITH TWINNING.

FERNET, C.* BULL. SOC. MED. HOP. PARIS 10* 457-484, 1893.

GATES, R. R.* HUMAN GENETICS. NEW YORK* MACMILLAN, 1947. 2* 843 FF.

GOERTZEN, B. L. AND IBSEN, H. L.* SUPERNUMERARY MAMMAE IN GUINEA PIGS. J. HERED. 42* 307-311, 1951.

KLINKERFUSS, G. H.* FOUR GENERATIONS OF POLYMASTIA. J.A.M.A. 82* 1247-1248, 1924.

*16380 NODAL RHYTHM

BACOS, EAGAN AND ORGAIN (1960) PRESENTED A FAMILY IN WHICH 9 MEMBERS OF 3 GENERATIONS EXHIBITED NODAL RHYTHM WITH BRADYCARDIA AND TENDED TO DEVELOP PAROXYSMS OF ATRIAL FIBRILLATION IN THE FOURTH DECADE OF LIFE.

BACOS, J. M., EAGAN, J. T. AND ORGAIN, E. S.* CONGENITAL FAMILIAL NODAL RHYTHM. CIRCULATION 22* 887-895, 1960.

16390 NON-HEME PROTEIN OF ERYTHROCYTE

HEWITT (1963) FOUND IN THE RED CELLS OF CYNOMOLGUS AND RHESUS MONKEYS A NON-HEME PROTEIN WHICH MIGRATES TOWARD THE CATHODE ON ELECTROPHORESIS IN STARCH GEL AT PH 8.5. TWO VARIANT FORMS, Y AND Z, EXISTED, WITH YY, YZ AND ZZ ANIMALS IN PROPOR-TIONS CONSISTENT WITH SIMPLE INHERITANCE. POLYMORPHISM OF THE PROTEIN HAS NOT BEEN RECOGNIZED IN MAN.

HEWITT, L. F.* PROTEINS IN THE ERYTHROCYTE OF MONKEYS. PROC. ROY. SOC. BIOL. 159* 536-543, 1963.

16400 NOSE, ANOMALOUS SHAPE OF ('POTATO NOSE')

BENJAMINS AND STIBBE (1926) DESCRIBED A DUTCH FAMILY IN WHICH 6 MALES AND 8 FEMALES IN TWO GENERATIONS SHOWED A 'POTATO NOSE.'

BENJAMINS, C. E. AND STIBBE, F. H.* EEN MERKWAARDIG GEVAL VAN AANGEBOREN AFWIJKING VAN DEN UITWENDIGEN NEUS. (BIGDRAGE TOT DE KENNIS DER ERFELIJKHEID VAN DERGELIJDE AFIVIJKINGEN). NEDERL. T. GENEESK. 70* 2543-2549, 1926.

*16410 NYSTAGMUS, CONGENITAL

ALLEN (1942) DESCRIBED A FAMILY WITH MANY AFFECTED MEMBERS. WE HAVE OBSERVED THIS AS A PROBABLY DOMINANT TRAIT AMONG THE OLD ORDER AMISH OF HOLMES CO., OHIO.

ALLEN, M.* THREE PEDIGREES OF EYE DEFECTS* PRIMARY HEREDITARY NYSTAGMUS. CASE STUDY WITH GENEALOGY. J. HERED. 33* 454-456, 1942.

DICHGANS, J. AND KORNHUBER, H. H.* EINE SELTENE ART DES HEREDITAREN NYSTAGMUS MIT AUTOSOMAL-DOMINANTEM ERBGANG UND BESONDEREM ERSCHEINUNGSBILD* VERTIKALE NYSTAGMUSKOMPONENTE UND STORUNG DES VERTIKALEN UND HORIZONTALEN OPTOKINETISCHEN NYSTAGMUS. ACTA GENET. STATIST. MED. 14* 240-250, 1964.

JAYALAKSHMI, P., SCOTT, T. F. M., RUCKER, S. H. AND SCHAFFER, D. B.* INFANTILE NYSTAGMUS* A PROSPECTIVE STUDY OF SPASMUS NUTANS, CONGENITAL NYSTAGMUS, AND UNCLASSIFIED NYSTAGMUS OF INFANCY. J. PEDIAT. 77* 177-187, 1970.

16420 OCULODENTODIGITAL DYSPLASIA (ODD SYNDROME) OCULO-DENTO-OSSEOUS SYNDROME

GILLESPIE (1964) DESCRIBED BROTHER AND SISTER WITH BILATERAL MICROPHTHALMOS, ABNORMALLY SMALL NOSE, HYPOTRICHOSIS, DENTAL ANOMALIES, FIFTH FINGER CAMPTODACTY-LY, SYNDACTYLY OF THE FOURTH AND FIFTH FINGERS AND MISSING TOE PHALANGES. THE CONDITION REPORTED AS ACROCEPHALOSYNDACTYLY BY MOHR (1939) AND CHARACTERIZED BY BILATERAL SYNDACTYLY OF THE 4TH AND 5TH FINGERS IS PROBABLY THE SAME CONDITION. THE FATHER AND FIVE OF HIS CHILDREN (INCLUDING THREE SONS) PRESENTED CRANIOFACIAL DEFORMITY AND COMPLETE SYNDACTYLY OF THE 4TH AND 5TH FINGERS OF THE HAND. THIS TYPE OF SYNDACTYLY, DESIGNATED AS TYPE III SYNDACTYLY (Q.V.), ALSO OCCURS AS AN ISOLATED MALFORMATION. IN TWO UNPUBLISHED PEDIGREES RENWICK (1967) FOUND THAT A CONSTANT AND CHARACTERISTIC FEATURE OF THE SYNDROME IS THE ABSENCE OF THE MIDDLE PHALANX OF THOSE TOES (2ND THROUGH 5TH) THAT NORMALLY HAVE THREE PHALANGES. LIGHTWOOD AND LEWIS (1963) REPORTED FATHER AND SON. EIDELMAN ET AL. (1967) OBSERVED AFFECTED BROTHER AND SISTER. RAJIC AND DE VEBER (1966) REPORTED A FAMILY WITH MANY AFFECTED MEMBERS IN 3 GENERATIONS BUT NO MALE-TO-MALE TRANSMISSION. EYE FEATURES INCLUDE MICROPHTHALMOS, MICROCORNEA AND GLAUCOMA. THE TEETH WERE SMALL WITH WHAT WAS TERMED ENAMELOGENESIS IMPERFECTA. THE PHALANGES AND METACARPALS WERE WIDENED AND SYNDACTYLY OF FINGERS 4 AND 5 WAS PRESENT. THESE AUTHORS USED THE DESIGNATION 'OCULODENTOOSSEOUS DYSPLASIA.' O'ROURK AND BRAVOS (1969) HAVE OBSERVED THE SPORADIC CASE OF A BOY WITH AN OCULODENTODIGITAL DYSPLASIA PROBABLY DISTINCT FROM THAT DESCRIBED ABOVE AND THEREFORE TENTATIVELY DESIGNATED ODD SYNDROME II. RATHER THAN SYNDACTYLY OF FINGERS 4 AND 5 THE PATIENT SHOWED UNILATERAL PRE-AXIAL POLYDACTYLY OF THE HAND, LATERALLY CURVED FIFTH FINGER ON RIGHT AND FIFTH FINGER CAMPTODACTYLY ON THE LEFT, ABSENT PHALANGES OF RIGHT FINGERS II AND V. O'ROURK AND BRAVOS (1969) DESCRIBED A SINGLE CASE WITH OCULAR, DENTAL AND DIGITAL ANOMALIES, WHICH DO NOT CORRESPOND PRECISELY, HOWEVER, DO SYNDROME. THEY PROPOSED TO CALL IT ODD SYNDROME II. THE MAIN POINT OF DISTINC-TION WAS THE ABSENCE OF SYNDACTYLY OF FINGERS IV AND V CHARACTERISTIC OF THE USUAL ODD SYNDROME.

EIDELMAN, E., CHOSACK, A. AND WAGNER, M. L.* ORODIGITOFACIAL DYSOSTOSIS AND OCULODENTODIGITAL DYSPLASIA. ORAL SURG. 23* 311-319, 1967.

GILLESPIE, F. D.* A HEREDITARY SYNDROME* 'DYSPLASIA OCULODENTODIGITALIS.' ARCH. OPHTHAL. 71* 187-192, 1964.

GORLIN, R. J., MESKIN, L. H. AND GEME, J. W.* OCULODENTODIGITAL DYSPLASIA. J. PEDIAT. 63* 69-75, 1963.

LIGHTWOOD, J. M. AND LEWIS, G. M.* THE HOLMES-ADIE SYNDROME IN A BOY WITH ACUTE JUVENILE RHEUMATISM AND BILATERAL SYNDACTYLY. ARCH. DIS. CHILD. 38* 86-88, 1963.

MOHR, O. L.* DOMINANT ACROCEPHALOSYNDACTYLY. HEREDITAS 25* 193-203, 1939.

O'ROURK, T. R., JR. AND BRAVOS, A.* AN OCULO-DENTO-DIGITAL DYSPLASIA. THE CLINICAL DELINEATION OF BIRTH DEFECTS. II. MALFORMATION SYNDROMES. NEW YORK* NATIONAL FOUNDATION, 1969. PP. 226-227.

RAJIC, D. S. AND DE VEBER, L. L.* HEREDITARY OCULODENTOOSSEOUS DYSPLASIA. ANN. RADIOL. 9* 224-231, 1966.

RENWICK, J. H.* GLASGOW, SCOTLAND* PERSONAL COMMUNICATION, 1967.

SUGAR, H. S., THOMPSON, J. P. AND DAVIS, J. D.* THE OCULO-DENTO-DIGITAL DYSPLASIA SYNDROME. AM. J. OPHTHAL. 61* 1448-1451, 1966.

*16430 OCULOPHARYNGEAL MUSCULAR DYSTROPHY

VICTOR, HAYES AND ADAMS (1962) DESCRIBED A FAMILY WITH OCULOPHARYNGEAL MUSCULAR DYSTROPHY, AN AUTOSOMAL DOMINANT DISORDER COMING ON IN LATE LIFE AND CHARACTERIZED BY DYSPHAGIA AND PROGRESSIVE PTOSIS OF THE EYELIDS. NINE MEMBERS OF THREE GENERATIONS WERE KNOWN TO BE AFFECTED. ONE AFFECTED MEMBER ALSO HAD TOTAL EXTERNAL OPHTHALMOPLEGIA AND WEAKNESS OF THE LIMB-GIRDLE MUSCLES. THE COMBINATION OF PTOSIS AND PHARYNGEAL PALSY WAS FIRST NOTED IN 1915 BY TAYLOR WHO ALSO COMMENTED ON THE FAMILIAL NATURE OF THE SYNDROME. HAYES AND COLLEAGUES (1963) SUCCEEDED IN LOCATING TAYLOR'S ORIGINAL FAMILY AND FOUND THAT MEMBERS OF TWO

SUBSEQUENT GENERATIONS HAD DEVELOPED THE DISORDER. IN A FAMILY WITH THIS DISORDER OBSERVED IN THE JOHNS HOPKINS HOSPITAL THE ANAL AND VESICAL SPHINCTERS WERE ALSO INVOLVED (TEASDALL, SCHUSTER, WALSH, 1964). MANY CASES HAVE BEEN OF FRENCH CANADIAN DESCENT. THE FAMILY REPORTED BY SCHOTLAND AND ROWLAND (1964) MAY HAVE HAD THIS DISORDER. TEN MEMBERS HAD PTOSIS, OPHTHALMOPARESIS, DYSPHAGIA, AND WEAKNESS AND WASTING OF FACE, NECK AND DISTAL LIMB MUSCLES. BARBEAU (1966) SHOWED THAT ALL OF THE NUMEROUS REPORTED FRENCH-CANADIAN CASES COULD BE TRACED BACK TO A SINGLE ANCESTOR WHO IMMIGRATED FROM FRANCE IN THE 1600'S.

BARBEAU, A.* THE SYNDROME OF HEREDITARY LATE ONSET PTOSIS AND DYSPHAGIA IN FRENCH-CANADA. IN KUHN, E. (ED.)* SYMPOSIUM UBER PROGRESSIVE MUSKELDYSTROPHIE, MYOTONIE, MYASTHENIE. BERLIN* SPRINGER-VERLAG, 1966. PP. 102-109.

BRAY, G. M., KAARSOO, M. AND ROSS, R. T.* OCULAR MYOPATHY WITH DYSPHAGIA. NEUROLOGY 15* 678-684, 1965.

HAYES, R., LONDON, W., SEIDMAN, J. AND EMBREE, L.* OCULOPHARYNGEAL MUSCULAR DYSTROPHY. (LETTER) NEW ENG. J. MED. 268* 163 ONLY, 1963.

MURPHY, S. F. AND DRACHMAN, D. B.* THE OCULOPHARYNGEAL SYNDROME. J.A.M.A. 203* 1003-1008, 1968.

SCHOTLAND, D. L. AND ROWLAND, L. P.* MUSCULAR DYSTROPHY. FEATURES OCULAR MYOPATHY, DISTAL MYOPATHY, AND MYOTONIC DYSTROPHY. ARCH. NEUROL. 10* 433-445, 1964.

TAYLOR, E. W.* PROGRESSIVE VAGUS-GLOSSOPHARYNGEAL PARALYSIS WITH PTOSIS. CONTRIBUTION TO GROUP OF FAMILY DISEASES. J. NERV. MENT. DIS. 42* 129-139, 1915.

TEASDALL, R. D., SCHUSTER, M. M. AND WALSH, F. B.* SPHINCTER INVOLVEMENT IN OCULAR MYOPATHY. ARCH. NEUROL. 10* 446-448, 1964.

VICTOR, M., HAYES, R. AND ADAMS, R. D.* OCULOPHARYNGEAL MUSCULAR DYSTROPHY. A FAMILIAL DISEASE OF LATE LIFE CHARACTERIZED BY DYSPHAGIA AND PROGRESSIVE PTOSIS OF THE EYELIDS. NEW ENG. J. MED. 267* 1267-1272, 1962.

16440 OLIVOPONTOCEREBELLAR ATROPHY I (OPCA I MENZEL TYPE)

SYMPTOMS USUALLY BEGIN IN THE THIRD OR FOURTH DECADES OF LIFE USUALLY ABOUT 30. IN ADDITION TO CEREBELLAR SIGNS, THERE ARE UPPER MOTOR NEURONE SIGNS AND EXTENSOR PLANTAR RESPONSES. INVOLUNTARY CHOREIFORM MOVEMENTS MAY OCCUR. CHARACTERISTIC FAMILIES WERE REPORTED BY MENZEL (1890) AND BY WAGGONER ET AL. (1938), DESTUNIS (1944). THE NOSOLOGY OF THE OLIVOPONTOCEREBELLAR ATROPHIES FOLLOWED HERE IS THAT OF KONIGSMARK AND WEINER (1970) WHO IDENTIFY FIVE TYPES. IN ADDITION SOME REPORTED FAMILIES DEFY PRECISE CLASSIFICATION INTO ONE OF THE FIVE TYPES. SEE ALSO CEREBELLO-PARENCHYMAL DISORDER, OF WHICH SIX TYPES ARE RECOGNIZED.

CRITCHLEY, M. AND GREENFIELD, J. G.* OLIVO-PONTO-CEREBELLAR ATROPHY. BRAIN 71* 343-364, 1948.

DESTUNIS, G.* DIE OLIVO-PONTOCEREBELLARE HEREDOATAXIE. ZBL. GES. NEUROL. PSYCHIAT. 177* 683, 1944.

GEARY, J. R., JR., EARLE, K. M. AND ROSE, A. S.* CASE REPORT* OLIVOPONTOCERE-BELLAR ATROPHY. NEUROLOGY 6* 218-224, 1956.

KONIGSMARK, B. W. AND WEINER, L. P.* THE OLIVOPONTOCEREBELLAR ATROPHIES* A REVIEW. MEDICINE 49* 227-242, 1970.

MENZEL, P.* BEITRAG ZUR KENNTNISS DER HEREDITAREN ATAXIE UND KLEINHIRNATROPHIE. ARCH. PSYCHIAT. NERVENKR. 22* 160-190, 1890.

WAGGONER, R. W., LOWENBERG, K. AND SPEICHER, K. G.* HEREDITARY CEREBELLAR ATAXIA. REPORT OF A CASE AND GENETIC STUDY. ARCH. NEUROL. PSYCHIAT. 39* 570-586, 1938.

16450 OLIVOPONTOCEREBELLAR ATROPHY III (OPCA III WITH RETINAL DEGENERATION)

WEINER ET AL. (1967) FOUND 27 AFFECTED PERSONS IN 5 GENERATIONS. THEY SUGGESTED THAT THE FAMILIES OF WOODWORTH ET AL. (1959) AND OF CARPENTER AND SCHUMACHER (1966) MAY HAVE SUFFERED FROM THE SAME ENTITY. FROMENT, BONNET AND COLRAT (1937) DESCRIBED FOUR AFFECTED PERSONS IN THREE SUCCESSIVE GENERATIONS. THEY REFERRED TO THE NEUROLOGIC LESION AS SPINOCEREBELLAR DEGENERATION. THE CHARACTER OF THE RETINOPATHY WAS VARIABLE BEING PERIPHERAL IN THE FIRST GENERATION, MACULAR IN THE SECOND AND MACULAR AND CIRCUMPAPILLARY IN THE THIRD. RETINAL DEGENERATION WITH CEREBELLAR ATAXIA IN A DOMINANT PEDIGREE PATTERN WAS ALSO REPORTED BY BJORK, LINDBLOM AND WADENSTEN (1956) AND OTHERS. HAVENER (1951) DESCRIBED MACULAR DEGENERATION WITH CEREBELLAR ATAXIA IN A 28 YEAR OLD NEGRO. CEREBELLAR INVOLVE-MENT WAS MUCH LESS SEVERE THAN IN A DAUGHTER WHO DIED AT 3 YEARS WITH PROFOUND INVOLVEMENT. SEE ALSO SPINOCEREBELLAR ATAXIA WITH EXTERNAL OPHTHALMOPLEGIA AND RETINAL DEGENERATION. FOSTER AND INGRAM (1962) DESCRIBED A FAMILY WITH AT LEAST 7 AFFECTED MEMBERS OF 3 GENERATIONS. SEVERITY VARIED WIDELY WITH INFANT DEATH IN AT

LEAST ONE CASE AND SURVIVAL TO MIDDLE AGE IN OTHER AFFECTED PERSONS. HALSEY ET
AL. (1967) FOUND DEGENERATIVE CHANGES IN THE RETINA AND CEREBELLUM OF 11 PERSONS
IN THREE GENERATIONS OF A NORTH CAROLINA NEGRO FAMILY. BLINDNESS AND ATAXIA WERE
THE CLINICAL FEATURES. FUNDUS CHANGES WERE MAINLY MACULAR. ONSET WAS USUALLY IN
MIDDLE AGE ALTHOUGH 3 HAD ONSET IN ADOLESCENCE. CONSANGUINITY AND SKIPPED
GENERATIONS SUGGEST RECESSIVE INHERITANCE. HOWEVER, A HIGH ILLEGITIMACY RATE IN
THIS POPULATION COULD ACCOUNT FOR THE PEDIGREE PATTERN BY ACCOUNTING FOR APPARENT-
LY 'SKIPPED' GENERATIONS WITH A DOMINANT TRAIT. JAMPEL, OKAZAKI AND BERNSTEIN
(1961) REPORTED SPINOCEREBELLAR ATAXIA WITH EXTERNAL OPHTHALMOPLEGIA AND RETINAL
DEGENERATION IN 8 MEMBERS OF A NEGRO FAMILY (IN 4 SIBSHIPS OF 3 GENERATIONS).
OPHTHALMOPLEGIA WAS PROGRESSIVE AND APPEARED TO HAVE A SUPRANUCLEAR BASIS. PTOSIS
NEVER OCCURRED. RETINAL DEGENERATION BEGAN IN THE MACULAR AREA AND PROGRESSED TO
THE PERIPHERY. REPORTS OF THE SAME SYNDROME WERE FOUND IN THE LITERATURE, E.G.,
ALFANO AND BERGER (1957). IN OTHER REPORTS ONLY EXTERNAL OPHTHALMOPLEGIA OR ONLY
RETINAL DEGENERATION WAS ASSOCIATED WITH ATAXIA.

ALFANO, J. E. AND BERGER, J. P.* RETINITIS PIGMENTOSA, OPHTHALMOPLEGIA, AND
SPASTIC QUADRIPLEGIA. AM. J. OPHTHAL. 43* 231-240, 1957.

BJORK, A., LINDBLOM, U. AND WADENSTEN, L.* RETINAL DEGENERATION IN HEREDITARY
ATAXIA. J. NEUROL. NEUROSURG. PSYCHIAT. 19* 186-193, 1956.

CARPENTER, S. AND SCHUMACHER, G. A.* FAMILIAL INFANTILE CEREBELLAR ATROPHY
ASSOCIATED WITH RETINAL DEGENERATION. ARCH. NEUROL. 14* 82-94, 1966.

FOSTER, J. B. AND INGRAM, T. T. S.* FAMILIAL CEREBRO-MACULAR DEGENERATION AND
ATAXIA. J. NEUROL. NEUROSURG. PSYCHIAT. 25* 63-68, 1962.

FROMENT, J., BONNET, P. AND COLRAT, A.* HEREDO-DEGENERATIONS RETINIENNE ET
SPINO CEREBELLEUSE. VARIANTES OPHTALMOSCOPIQUES ET NEUROLOGIQUES PRESENTEES PAR
TROIS GENERATIONS SUCCESSIVES. J. MED. LYON, NO VOL* 153-163, 1937.

HALSEY, J. H., JR., SCOTT, T. R. AND FARMER, T. W.* ADULT HEREDITARY CEREBEL-
LORETINAL DEGENERATION. NEUROLOGY 17* 87-90, 1967.

HAVENER, W. H.* CEREBELLAR-MACULAR ABIOTROPHY. ARCH. OPHTHAL. 45* 40-43, 1951.

JAMPEL, R. S., OKAZAKI, H. AND BERNSTEIN, H.* OPHTHALMOPLEGIA AND RETINAL
DEGENERATION ASSOCIATED WITH SPINOCEREBELLAR ATAXIA. ARCH. OPHTHAL. 66* 247-259,
1961.

WEINER, L. P., KONIGSMARK, B. W., STOLL, J., JR. AND MAGLADERY, J. W.*
HEREDITARY OLIVOPONTOCEREBELLAR ATROPHY WITH RETINAL DEGENERATION. REPORT OF A
FAMILY THROUGH SIX GENERATIONS. ARCH. NEUROL. 16* 364-376, 1967.

WOODWORTH, J. A., BECKETT, R. S. AND NETSKY, M. G.* A COMPOSITE OF HEREDITARY
ATAXIAS. A FAMILIAL DISORDER WITH FEATURES OF OLIVOPONTOCEREBELLAR ATROPHY,
LEBER'S OPTIC ATROPHY AND FRIEDREICH'S ATAXIA. ARCH. INTERN. MED. 104* 594-606,
1959.

16460 OLIVOPONTOCEREBELLAR ATROPHY IV (OPCA IV SCHUT-HAYMAKER TYPE)

BOTH THE CLINICAL AND THE PATHOLOGIC PICTURES IN THE DISORDER DESCRIBED IN A LARGE
KINDRED BY SCHUT (1950) AND BY SCHUT AND HAYMAKER (1951) WERE VARIABLE. SYMPTOMS
VARIED FROM THOSE OF SPINOCEREBELLAR ATAXIA TO SPASTIC PARAPLEGIA. IDENTIFICATION
AS A FORM OF OPCA IS BASED ON THE PRESENCE OF THE MAJOR PATHOLOGY IN THE INFERIOR
OLIVARY NUCLEUS AND CEREBELLUM WITH VARIABLE POSITIVE INVOLVEMENT. THE SPINAL
CORD SHOWED VARIABLE LOSS OF ANTERIOR MOTOR HORN CELLS AND CHANGES IN THE
SPINOCEREBELLAR TRACTS AND POSTERIOR FUNICULUS. INVOLVEMENT OF CRANIAL NERVES IX,
X AND XII WAS ANOTHER DISTINGUISHING FEATURE.

SCHUT, J. W. AND HAYMAKER, W.* HEREDITARY ATAXIA* PATHOLOGIC STUDY OF 5 CASES
OF COMMON ANCESTRY. J. NEUROPATH. CLIN. NEUROL. 1* 183-213, 1951.

SCHUT, J. W.* HEREDITARY ATAXIA* CLINICAL STUDY THROUGH SIX GENERATIONS. ARCH.
NEUROL. PSYCHIAT. 63* 535-568, 1950.

16470 OLIVOPONTOCEREBELLAR ATROPHY V (OPCA V WITH DEMENTIA AND EXTRAPYRAMIDAL SIGNS)

AFFECTED KINDREDS WERE REPORTED BY CARTER AND SUKAVAJANA (1956), KONIGSMARK AND
LIPTON (1970) AND CHANDLER AND BEBIN (1956). IN ADDITION TO CEREBELLAR SIGNS,
RIGIDITY AND MENTAL DETERIORATION WERE CONSISTENT FEATURES. NEURONAL LOSS WAS
OBSERVED IN THE BASAL GANGLIA IN ALL CASES. CORTICAL CHANGES CORRELATED WITH
DEMENTIA. CARTER AND SUKAVAJANA (1956) DESCRIBED A FATHER AND FIVE SONS AND A
DAUGHTER (OUT OF A SIBSHIP OF 19) WITH A FAMILIAL FORM OF CEREBELLO-OLIVARY
DEGENERATION WITH LATE DEVELOPMENT OF RIGIDITY AND DEMENTIA. POST-MORTEM SHOWED
PROFOUND CEREBELLAR ATROPHY WITH DEGENERATION IN THE OLIVARY NUCLEI AND SUBSTANTIA
NIGRA.

CARTER, H. R. AND SUKAVAJANA, C.* FAMILIAL CEREBELLO-OLIVARY DEGENERATION WITH
LATE DEVELOPMENT OF RIGIDITY AND DEMENTIA. NEUROLOGY 6* 876-884, 1956.

CHANDLER, J. H. AND BEBIN, J.* HEREDITARY CEREBELLAR ATAXIA* OLIVOPONTOCEREBEL-
LAR TYPE. NEUROLOGY 6* 187-195, 1956.

KONIGSMARK, B. W. AND LIPTON, H. L.* DOMINANT OLIVOPONTOCEREBELLAR ATROPHY WITH
DEMENTIA AND EXTRAPYRAMIDAL SIGNS. THE CLINICAL DELINEATION OF BIRTH DEFECTS.
VI. THE NERVOUS SYSTEM. BALTIMORE* WILLIAMS AND WILKINS, 1970.

KONIGSMARK, B. W. AND WEINER, L. P.* THE OLIVOPONTOCEREBELLAR ATROPHIES* A
REVIEW. MEDICINE 49* 227-242, 1970.

16480 ONYCHOLYSIS, PARTIAL, WITH SCLERONYCHIA

SCHULZE (1966) DESCRIBED MOTHER AND TWO CHILDREN WITH ONYCHOLYSIS OF THE DISTAL
PART OF THE FINGERNAILS, WHICH WERE THICKENED. THE DISEASE WAS THOUGHT TO HAVE
OCCURRED IN FIVE GENERATIONS.

SCHULZE, H. D.* HEREDITARE ONYCHOLYSIS PARTIALIS MIT SKLERONYCHIE. DERM.
WSCHR. 152* 766-775, 1966.

*16490 OPHTHALMO-MANDIBULO-MELIC DYSPLASIA

THE ABOVE DESIGNATION WAS GIVEN BY PILLAY (1964) TO A SYNDROME HE OBSERVED IN A
FATHER AND TWO SONS. CHANGES WERE FOUND IN THE EYE (CORNEAL CLOUDING), IN THE
MANDIBLE (TEMPORO-MANDIBULAR FUSION, ABSENT CORONOID PROCESS, OBTUSE MANDIBULAR
ANGLE) AND LIMBS (RADIO-HUMERAL AND RADIO-ULNAR DISLOCATIONS, APLASIA OF THE
LATERAL HUMERAL CONDYLE, RADIAL HEAD AND DISTAL ULNA, ETC.). CHROMOSOME STUDIES
WERE NEGATIVE.

PILLAY, V. K.* OPHTHALMO-MANDIBULO-MELIC DYSPLASIA, AN HEREDITARY SYNDROME. J.
BONE JOINT SURG. 46A* 858-862, 1964.

*16500 OPHTHALMOPLEGIA, FAMILIAL STATIC

LEES (1960) DESCRIBED CONGENITAL STATIC FAMILIAL OPHTHALMOPLEGIA. PTOSIS, ALMOST
COMPLETELY FIXED EYES, NYSTAGMOID MOVEMENTS AND UNEQUAL PUPILS WERE FEATURES.
MALES IN THREE SUCCESSIVE GENERATIONS AND 7 PERSONS IN ALL WERE AFFECTED. LEES
THOUGHT THE LESION TO BE IN THE POSTERIOR LONGITUDINAL BUNDLE AND ITS CONNECTIONS
WITH THE OCULOMOTOR NUCLEI. TRANSMISSION THROUGH SEVERAL GENERATIONS WITH MALE-
TO-MALE TRANSMISSION HAS BEEN NOTED BY BRADBURNE (1912) AND MANY OTHERS. THE
PALSY IS THOUGHT TO BE OF NUCLEAR ORIGIN. PTOSIS, IMMOBILITY OF THE EYEBALL AND
PARALYSIS OF THE PUPIL TO ACCOMMODATION ARE FEATURES. HOLMES (1955) DESCRIBED 9
AFFECTED IN FOUR GENERATIONS OF A FAMILY, WITH CONGENITAL ONSET.

BRADBURNE, A. A.* HEREDITARY OPHTHALMOPLEGIA IN FIVE GENERATIONS. TRANS.
OPHTHAL. SOC. U.K. 32* 142-153, 1912.

HOLMES, W. J.* HEREDITARY CONGENITAL OPHTHALMOPLEGIA. TRANS. AM. OPHTHAL. SOC.
53* 245-253, 1955.

LEES, F.* CONGENITAL STATIC FAMILIAL OPHTHALMOPLEGIA. J. NEUROL. NEUROSURG.
PSYCHIAT. 23* 46-51, 1960.

16510 OPHTHALMOPLEGIA, PIGMENTARY DEGENERATION OF RETINA AND CARDIOMYOPATHY

KEARNS (1965) REPORTED 9 UNRELATED PATIENTS WITH OPHTHALMOPLEGIA, PIGMENTARY
DEGENERATION OF THE RETINA AND CARDIOMYOPATHY AS LEADING FEATURES. LESS CONSIS-
TENT FEATURES WERE WEAKNESS OF FACIAL, PHARYNGEAL, TRUNK AND EXTREMITY MUSCLES,
DEAFNESS, SMALL STATURE, ELECTROENCEPHALOGRAPHIC CHANGES AND MARKEDLY INCREASED
CEREBROSPINAL FLUID PROTEIN. IN NONE OF THE 9 WAS A POSITIVE FAMILY HISTORY
PRESENT. REFSUM'S DISEASE (Q.V.) SHOULD BE CONSIDERED.

KEARNS, T. P.* EXTERNAL OPHTHALMOPLEGIA, PIGMENTARY DEGENERATION OF THE RETINA,
AND CARDIOMYOPATHY* A NEWLY RECOGNIZED SYNDROME. TRANS. OPHTHAL. SOC. U.K. 63*
559-625, 1965.

16520 OPTIC ATROPHY WITH DEMYELINATING DISEASE OF CNS

LEES, MACDONALD AND TURNER (1964) DESCRIBED A KINDRED IN 5 GENERATIONS OF WHICH 12
MALES AND 3 FEMALES WERE AFFECTED WITH OPTIC NEURITIS ACCOMPANIED IN SOME BY
NEUROLOGIC MANIFESTATIONS RESEMBLING DISSEMINATED SCLEROSIS. ONE HAD ATAXIA,
RIGHT LEG WEAKNESS AND DYSARTHRIA. ANOTHER DEVELOPED LEFT HEMIPARESIS DURING A
TWO WEEK PERIOD AND THEN RECOVERED PARTIALLY.

LEES, F., MACDONALD, A. M. E. AND TURNER, J. W. A.* LEBER'S DISEASE WITH
SYMPTOMS RESEMBLING DISSEMINATED SCLEROSIS. J. NEUROL. NEUROSURG. PSYCHIAT. 27*
415-421, 1964.

16530 OPTIC ATROPHY, CATARACT AND NEUROLOGIC DISORDER

GARCIN ET AL. (1961) DESCRIBED OPTIC ATROPHY, CATARACT, AND NEUROLOGIC DISORDER IN
14 PERSONS IN 7 SIBSHIPS OF FOUR GENERATIONS WITH SEVERAL INSTANCES OF MALE-TO-
MALE TRANSMISSION. CONSIDERABLE VARIABILITY WAS OBSERVED. CATARACT WAS USUALLY

RECOGNIZED IN THE FIRST DECADE. THE AUTHORS DISCUSSED THE RELATION OF THIS DISORDER TO SYNDROME OF BEHR, OF MARINESCO AND SJOGREN AND OF FRIEDREICH. SINCE ALL OF THESE THREE ARE RECESSIVES THERE CAN BE NO DOUBT THAT THE ENTITY THEY REPORTED WAS DISTINCT.

GARCIN, R., RAVERDY, P., DELTHIL, S., MAN, H. X. AND CHIMENES, H.* SUR UNE AFFECTION HEREDO-FAMILIALE ASSOCIANT CATARACTE, ATROPHIE OPTIQUE, SIGNES EXTRA-PYRAMIDAUX ET CERTAINS STIGMATES DE LA MALADIE DE FRIEDREICH. (SA POSITION NOSOLOGIQUE PAR RAPPORT AU SYNDROME DE BEHR, AU SYNDROME DE MARINESCO-SJOGREN ET A LA MALADIE DE FRIEDREICH AVEC SIGNES OCULAIRES). REV. NEUROL. 104* 373-379, 1961.

*16540 OPTIC ATROPHY, CONGENITAL

IVERSON (1958) REPORTED CONGENITAL OPTIC ATROPHY IN THREE GENERATIONS. THE CLEAR AUTOSOMAL DOMINANT PATTERN OF INHERITANCE AND CONGENITAL NATURE DISTINGUISH IT FROM LEBER'S OPTIC ATROPHY.

IVERSON, H. A.* HEREDITARY OPTIC ATROPHY. ARCH. OPHTHAL. 59* 850-853, 1958.

KJER, P.* INFANTILE OPTIC ATROPHY WITH DOMINANT MODE OF INHERITANCE. OP. EX. DOMO BIOL. HERED. HUM. U. HAFNIENSIS 42* 146 ONLY, 1959.

*16550 OPTIC ATROPHY, JUVENILE

CALDWELL ET AL. (1971) DESCRIBED TWO FAMILIES WITH INSIDIOUS ONSET OF OPTIC ATROPHY IN CHILDHOOD. THERE WERE NO NEUROLOGIC, CONGENITAL OR DEVELOPMENTAL ABNORMALITIES. THEY CLASSIFIED THE FAMILIAL OPTIC ATROPHIES INTO SIX GROUPS* CONGENITAL DOMINANT, CONGENITAL RECESSIVE, JUVENILE DOMINANT, JUVENILE RECESSIVE, LEBER'S (PERHAPS X-LINKED), AND BEHR'S (RECESSIVE). THE FEATURES OF THE SIX WERE USEFULLY COMPARED.

CALDWELL, J. B. H., HOWARD, R. O. AND RIGGS, L. A.* DOMINANT JUVENILE OPTIC ATROPHY. A STUDY OF TWO FAMILIES AND REVIEW OF HEREDITARY DISEASE IN CHILDHOOD. ARCH. OPHTHAL. 85* 133-147, 1971.

16560 ORBITAL MARGIN, HYPOPLASIA OF

URRETS-ZAVALIA (1955) OBSERVED TWO FAMILIES WITH A SYNDROME CONSISTING OF AGENESIS OF THE ORBITAL MARGIN, HYPOPLASIA OF THE PALPEBRAL SKIN AND TARSAL PLATES AND VARIABLE DEFECTS OF THE LACRIMAL PASSAGES INCLUDING ECTOPIA AND ELONGATION OF THE LOWER PUNCTUM, SHORTENING OR ABSENCE OF THE INFERIOR CANALICULI, SUPERNUMERARY CANALICULI, OR ATRESIA OF THE NASO-LACRIMAL DUCT. IN SOME A SMALL COLOBOMA OF THE INNER PART OF THE LOWER LIDS AND CONGENITAL ANOMALIES OF THE EXTRA-OCULAR MUSCLES WERE PRESENT.

URRETS-ZAVALIA, A., JR.* FAMILIAL PRIMARY HYPOPLASIA OF THE ORBITAL MARGIN. TRANS. AM. ACAD. OPHTH. OTOLARYNG. 59* 42-59, 1955.

*16570 OSTEOARTHROPATHY OF FINGERS, FAMILIAL

ALLISON AND BLUMBERG (1958) DESCRIBED THE TYPE OF AVASCULAR NECROSIS OF THE PHALANGEAL EPIPHYSES TO WHICH THE NAME OF THIEMANN IS SOMETIMES ATTACHED. PAINLESS DEFORMITY AT THE PROXIMAL INTERPHALANGEAL JOINTS BEGAN IN CHILDHOOD OR ADOLESCENCE. A CONSANGUINEOUS MATING OF TWO AFFECTED PERSONS RESULTED IN PARTICULARLY SEVERE DEFORMITY IN TWO OF SIX OFFSPRING. THESE TWO MAY HAVE BEEN HOMOZYGOTES.

ALLISON, A. C. AND BLUMBERG, B. S.* FAMILIAL OSTEOARTHROPATHY OF THE FINGERS. J. BONE JOINT SURG. 40B* 538-545, 1958.

16580 OSTEOCHONDRITIS DISSECANS (ASEPTIC NECROSIS)

EACH OF THE LARGE NUMBER OF POSSIBLE LOCALIZATIONS HAS AN EPONYM, E.G., OF PHALANGEAL EPIPHYSES (THIEMANN'S, Q.V.), OF TIBIAL TUBERCLE (OSGOOD-SCHLATTER'S), OF HEAD OF FEMUR (LEGG-CALVE-PERTHES'), OF SPINE (SCHEUERMANN'S), OF TARSAL SCAPHOID (KOHLER'S), OF SEMILUNAR BONE OF THE WRIST (KIENBOCK'S), OF THE HEAD OF THE SECOND METATARSAL (FRIEBERG'S), OF THE CAPITELLUM OF THE HUMERUS (PANNER'S), OF THE PATELLA (LARSEN-JOHANSSEN'S). DOMINANT INHERITANCE HAS BEEN SUGGESTED IN RELATION TO SEVERAL OF THESE. GARDINER (1955) REPORTED OSTEOCHONDRITIS DISSECANS OF THE KNEES IN A SISTER AND TWO BROTHERS. THE TERM 'DISSECANS' COMES FROM 'DIS' MEANING 'FROM' AND 'SECARE' MEANING 'CUT OFF,' AND IS NOT TO BE CONFUSED WITH 'DESICCANS' DERIVED FROM 'DESICCARE' MEANING TO 'DRY UP.' DISSECANS REFERS TO THE APPEARANCE OF PART OF THE BONE HAVING BEEN CUT AWAY.

GARDINER, T. B.* OSTEOCHONDRITIS DISSECANS IN THREE MEMBERS OF ONE FAMILY. J. BONE JOINT SURG. 37E* 139-141, 1955.

HARBIN, M. AND ZOLLINGER, R.* OSTEOCHONDRITIS OF GROWTH CENTERS. SURG. GYNEC. OBSTET. 51* 145-161, 1930.

SMITH, A. D.* OSTEOCHONDRITIS OF THE KNEE JOINT* A REPORT OF THREE CASES IN ONE FAMILY AND A DISCUSSION OF THE ETIOLOGY AND TREATMENT. J. BONE JOINT SURG. 42A*

16590 OSTEOCHONDRITIS DISSECANS OF MULTIPLE SITES

D
O
M
I
N
A
N
T

STOUGAARD (1961) OBSERVED OSTEOCHONDRITIS DISSECANS OF THE KNEES AND-OR ELBOWS IN 9 PERSONS IN THREE GENERATIONS. A PAIR OF TWINS THOUGHT TO BE IDENTICAL WERE AFFECTED. WE HAVE OBSERVED OSTEOCHONDRITIS DISSECANS IN THE FEMUR AT THE KNEE AND IN THE CAPITELLUM OF THE HUMERUS IN TWO BROTHERS WHO ALSO SHOW HYPERTELORISM, FINGER CONTRACTURES, PECULIARLY SHAPED EARS, STERNAL DEFORMITY AND CRYPTORCHIDISM. THIS MAY BE A SYNDROME. (IT IS ALSO LISTED IN THE RECESSIVE CATALOG BECAUSE OF THE UNCERTAINTY IN THE MODE OF INHERITANCE.) BOTH PARENTS SEEM NORMAL. ZELLWEGER AND EBNOTHER (1951) REPORTED A FAMILY IN WHICH THE FOUR AFFECTED MEMBERS WERE ALSO DWARFED. IN THE FAMILY REPORTED BY PICK (1955) THE AFFECTED MOTHER AND 3 AFFECTED DAUGHTERS WERE SHORT. ON THE OTHER HAND SOME AUTHORS HAVE COMMENTED ON A TALL, SLENDER HABITUS. TOBIN (1957) DESCRIBED FATHER AND 2 SONS WITH THE COMBINATION OF OSTEOCHONDRITIS DISSECANS AND TIBIA VARA (Q.V.). A DAUGHTER HAD ONLY OSTEOCHON-DRITIS DISSECANS.

HANLEY, W. B., MCKUSICK, V. A. AND BARRANCO, F. T.* OSTEOCHONDRITIS DISSECANS AND ASSOCIATED MALFORMATIONS IN BROTHERS. A REVIEW OF FAMILIAL ASPECTS. J. BONE JOINT SURG. 49A* 925-937, 1967.

MULLER, W. AND HETZAR, W.* FAMILIARE GENERALISIERTE OSTEOCHONDRITIS DISSECANS ZAHLREICHER GELENKE UND DER WIRBELSAULE. DEUTSCH. Z. CHIR. 241* 795-804, 1933.

PICK, M. P.* FAMILIAL OSTEOCHONDRITIS DISSECANS. J. BONE JOINT SURG. 37B* 142-145, 1955.

STOUGAARD, J.* THE HEREDITARY FACTOR IN OSTEOCHONDRITIS DISSECANS. J. BONE JOINT SURG. 43B* 256-258, 1961.

TOBIN, W. J.* FAMILIAL OSTEOCHONDRITIS DISSECANS WITH ASSOCIATED TIBIA VARA. J. BONE JOINT SURG. 39A* 1091-1105, 1957.

ZELLWEGER, H. AND EBNOTHER, M.* UBER EINE FAMILIARE SKELETTSTORUNG MIT MULTILOCULAREN, ASEPTISCHEN KNOCHENNEKROSEN, INSBESONDERE MIT OSTEOCHONDRITIS DISSECANS. HELV. PAEDIAT. ACTA 6* 95-111, 1951.

16600 OSTEOCHONDROMATOSIS (ENCHONDROMATOSIS, DYSCHONDROPLASIA)

OLLIER'S DISEASE IS THE EPONYMOUS DESIGNATION. WHEN HEMANGIOMATA ARE ASSOCIATED, THE CONDITION IS KNOWN AS MAFFUCCI'S SYNDROME. NEITHER CONDITION SEEMS TO BE GENETICALLY DETERMINED IN A SIMPLE MENDELIAN MANNER. THERE ARE A FEW INSTANCES OF FAMILIAL OCCURRENCE OF OLLIER'S DISEASE, HOWEVER. STEUDEL (1891-2) DESCRIBED TWO AFFECTED BROTHERS AND ROSSBERG (1959) REPORTED AFFECTED BROTHER AND SISTER WHOSE PATERNAL GRANDFATHER WAS ALSO AFFECTED. LAMY ET AL. (1954) OBSERVED 3 AFFECTED SIBS AND CARBONELL AND VINETA (1962) REPORTED AFFECTED BROTHER AND SISTER. DOMINANT INHERITANCE WITH REDUCED PENETRANCE IS POSSIBLE.

ANDERSON, I. F.* MAFFUCCI'S SYNDROME* REPORT OF A CASE WITH A REVIEW OF THE LITERATURE. S. AFR. MED. J. 39* 1066-1070, 1965.

ANDREN, L., DYMLING, J.-F., ELNER, A. AND HOGEMAN, K. E.* MAFFUCCI'S SYNDROME* REPORT OF FOUR CASES. ACTA CHIR. SCAND. 126* 397-405, 1963.

CARBONELL JUANICO, M. AND VINETA TEIXIDO, J.* OTRO CASO DE DISCONDROTEOSIS GENERALIZADA CONGENITA, TIPO OLLIER. REV. ESP. PEDIAT. 18* 91-99, 1962.

CAUBLE, W. G. AND BOWMAN, H. S.* DYSCHONDROPLASIA AND HEMANGIOMAS (MAFFUCCI'S SYNDROME)* PRESENTATION OF A CASE. ARCH. SURG. 97* 678-681, 1968.

LAMY, M., AUSSANNAIRE, M., JAMMET, M. L. AND NEZELOF, C.* TROIS CAS DE MALADIE D'OLLIER DANS UNE FRATRIE. BULL. SOC. MED. HOP. PARIS 70* 62-70, 1954.

ROSSBERG, A.* ZUR ERBLICHKEIT DER KNOCHENCHONDROMATOSE. FORTSCHR. RONTGENSTR. 90(1)* 138-139, 1959.

STEUDEL, (NI)* MULTIPLE ENCHONDROME DER KNOCHEN IN VERBINDUNG MIT VENOSEN ANGIOMEN DER WEICHTEILE. BRUNS BEIR. KLIN. CHIR. 8* 503-521, 1891-2.

*16610 OSTEODYSPLASTY OF MELNICK AND NEEDLES

MELNICK AND NEEDLES (1966) DESCRIBED FAMILIES WHICH CONTAINED MULTIPLE CASES IN MULTIPLE GENERATIONS OF A SEVERE CONGENITAL BONE DISORDER CHARACTERIZED BY TYPICAL FACIES (EXOPHTHALMOS, FULL CHEEKS, MICROGNATHIA AND MALALIGNMENT OF TEETH), FLARING OF THE METAPHYSES OF LONG BONES, S-LIKE CURVATURE OF BONES OF LEGS, IRREGULAR CONSTRICTIONS IN THE RIBS, SCLEROSIS OF BASE OF SKULL. MALE-TO-MALE TRANSMISSION WAS NOTED IN ONE CASE. 'OSTEODYSPLASTY' WAS THE TERM SUGGESTED BY COSTE ET AL. (1968) WHO DESCRIBED AN AFFECTED 58 YEAR OLD WOMAN. BONE DISEASE WAS RECOGNIZED IN INFANCY WHEN SHE BEGAN TO WALK. NORMAL CHILDBIRTH WAS IMPOSSIBLE BECAUSE OF CONTRACTED PELVIS. OSTEOARTHRITIS OF THE LUMBAR SPINE AND HIPS GAVE MUCH PAIN. HER HEIGHT WAS NORMAL. STRIKING FACIES COMPRISED EXOPHTHALMOS, HIGH

COSTE, F., MAROTEAUX, P. AND CHOURAKI, L.* OSTEODYSPLASTY (MELNICK AND NEEDLES' SYNDROME). REPORT OF A CASE. ANN. RHEUM. DIS. 27* 360-366, 1968.

MELNICK, J. C. AND NEEDLES, C. F.* AN UNDIAGNOSED BONE DYSPLASIA. A TWO FAMILY STUDY OF 4 GENERATIONS AND 3 GENERATIONS. AM. J. ROENTGEN. 97* 39-48, 1966.

*16620 OSTEOGENESIS IMPERFECTA

ALTHOUGH IT NOW SEEMS CLEAR THAT SOME CASES OF OSTEOGENESIS IMPERFECTA CONGENITA ARE RECESSIVE, OSTEOGENESIS IMPERFECTA IS USUALLY DOMINANT. IN ADDITION TO FREQUENT FRACTURES, LOOSE JOINTEDNESS, BLUE SCLERAE, AND PROGRESSIVE DEAFNESS ARE FEATURES. AORTIC REGURGITATION HAS BEEN REPORTED IN OI, E.G., BY JORNOD ET AL. (1968). SOLOMONS AND STYNER (1969) REPORTED THAT BONE COLLAGEN OF OI INHIBITS CALCIFICATION IN VITRO. TREATMENT OF THE COLLAGEN WITH PYROPHOSPHATASE IN THE PRESENCE OF MAGNESIUM ION REMOVED THE INHIBITION. ELEVATED SERUM AND URINARY PYROPHOSPHATE IN PATIENTS DECLINED WITH ADMINISTRATION OF MAGNESIUM SULFATE.

FREDA, V. J., VOSBURGH, G. J. AND DI LIBERTI, C.* OSTEOGENESIS IMPERFECTA CONGENITA* A PRESENTATION OF 16 CASES AND REVIEW OF THE LITERATURE. OBSTET. GYNEC. 18* 535-547, 1961.

HECKMAN, B. A. AND STEINBERG, I.* CONGENITAL HEART DISEASE (MITRAL REGURGITATION) IN OSTEOGENESIS IMPERFECTA. AM. J. ROENTGEN. 103* 601-607, 1968.

JORNOD, J., ROTHLIN, M. AND UEHLINGER, E.* ANOMALIES CARDIOVASCULAIRES DE LA MALADIE DE LOBSTEIN. SCHWEIZ. MED. WSCHR. 98* 795-798, 1968.

MCKUSICK, V. A.* HERITABLE DISORDERS OF CONNECTIVE TISSUE. ST. LOUIS* C. V. MOSBY CO., 1966 (3RD ED).

SCOTT, P. P., MCKUSICK, V. A. AND MCKUSICK, A. B.* THE NATURE OF OSTEOGENESIS IMPERFECTA IN CATS. EVIDENCE THAT THE DISORDER IS PRIMARILY NUTRITIONAL, NOT GENETIC, AND THEREFORE NOT ANALOGOUS TO THE DISEASE IN MAN. J. BONE JOINT SURG. 45A* 125-134, 1963.

SMARS, G.* OSTEOGENESIS IMPERFECTA IN SWEDEN* CLINICAL GENETIC, EPIDEMIOLOGICAL AND SOCIO-MEDICAL ASPECTS. STOCKHOLM* SVENSKA BOKFORLAGET, 1961.

SMARS, G., BECKMAN, L. AND BOOK, J. A.* OSTEOGENESIS IMPERFECTA AND BLOOD GROUPS. ACTA GENET. STATIST. MED. 11* 133-136, 1961.

SOLOMONS, C. C. AND STYNER, J.* OSTEOGENESIS IMPERFECTA* EFFECT OF MAGNESIUM ADMINISTRATION ON PYROPHOSPHATE METABOLISM. CALC. TISS. RES. 3* 318-326, 1969.

*16630 OSTEOLYSIS, HEREDITARY, OF CARPAL BONES WITH NEPHROPATHY

SHURTLEFF AND COLLEAGUES (1964) OBSERVED A FAMILY WITH 11 AFFECTED PERSONS IN THREE GENERATIONS. OSTEOLYSIS OF THE CARPAL BONES LEADS TO DISAPPEARANCE OF THESE IN OLDER CASES. DEFORMITY OF THE HANDS SUGGESTING ARTHRITIS ALSO OCCURRED IN SEVERE CASES. HYPERTENSION AND RENAL FAILURE WERE INTERNAL COMPLICATIONS. ARTERIOLAR THICKENING WAS THE BASIS OF THESE CHANGES. CAFFEY (1961) DESCRIBED FATHER AND SON. THE FATHER DIED OF UREMIA (PERSONAL OBSERVATION). TORG ET AL. (1969) SUGGESTED THAT SPORADIC CASES SUCH AS THAT OF LAGIER AND RUTISHAUER (1965) AND THAT OF TORG AND STEEL (1968) REPRESENT A SEPARATE DISORDER. IT SEEMS THAT THEY ARE INDISTINGUISHABLE (EXCEPT QUANTITATIVELY IN TERMS OF SEVERITY OF RENAL DISEASE) FROM THE INHERITED CASES AND PROBABLY REPRESENT NEW DOMINANT MUTATIONS.

CAFFEY, J.* IDIOPATHIC FAMILIAL MULTIPLE CARPAL NECROSIS. PEDIATRIC X-RAY DIAGNOSIS. CHICAGO* YEARBOOK MEDICAL PUBLISHERS, (4TH ED.) 1961. P. 984.

LAGIER, R. AND RUTISHAUER, E.* OSTEOARTICULAR CHANGES IN A CASE OF ESSENTIAL OSTEOLYSIS. J. BONE JOINT SURG. 47B* 339-353, 1965.

SHURTLEFF, D. B., SPARKES, R. S., CLAWSON, D. K., GUNTHEROTH, W. G. AND MOTTET, N. K.* HEREDITARY OSTEOLYSIS WITH HYPERTENSION AND NEPHROPATHY. J.A.M.A. 188* 363-368, 1964.

THIEFFRY, S. AND SORREL-DEJERINE, J.* FORME SPECIALE D'OSTEOLYSE ESSENTIALLE HEREDITAIRE ET FAMILIALE A STABILISATION SPONTANEE, SURVENANT DANS L'ENFANCE. PRESSE MED. 66* 1858-1861, 1958.

TORG, J. S. AND STEEL, H. H.* ESSENTIAL OSTEOLYSIS WITH NEPHROPATHY* A REVIEW OF THE LITERATURE AND CASE REPORT OF AN UNUSUAL SYNDROME. J. BONE JOINT SURG. 50A* 1629-1638, 1968.

TORG, J. S., DIGEORGE, A. M., KIRKPATRICK, J. A., JR. AND TRUJILLO, M. M.* HEREDITARY MULTICENTRIC OSTEOLYSIS WITH RECESSIVE TRANSMISSION* A NEW SYNDROME. J. PEDIAT. 75* 243-252, 1969.

MULTIPLE SMOOTHLY OUTLINED GLOBOID OSTEOMAS OCCUR ON THE JAW IN GARDNER'S SYNDROME (SEE POLYPOSIS III). WHETHER THIS TUMOR EVER OCCURS AS AN INHERITED TRAIT INDEPENDENT OF INTESTINAL POLYPS AND OTHER BONY AND SOFT-TISSUE TUMORS IS NOT CLEAR. FRANGENHEIM (1914) DESCRIBED THIS TYPE OF TUMOR IN A FATHER AND 3 OF HIS CHILDREN BUT INTESTINAL POLYPS WERE NOT EXCLUDED.

FRANGENHEIM, P.* FAMILIARE HYPEROSTOSEN DER KIEFER. BEITR. KLIN. CHIR. 90* 139-152, 1914.

16650 OSTEOPATHIA STRIATA

THE NAME OF THE CONDITION REFERS TO A FEATURE OF RELATIVELY LITTLE PRACTICAL IMPORTANCE, LONGITUDINAL STRIATIONS OF OSTEOSCLEROSIS IN THE LONG BONES. OSTEOSCLEROSIS IN THE CRANIAL AND FACIAL BONES LEADS TO DISFIGUREMENT AND TO DISABILITY DUE TO PRESSURE ON CRANIAL NERVES. WALKER (1969) AND JONES AND MULCAHY (1968) DESCRIBED TYPICAL CASES. RUCKER AND ALFIDI (1964) DESCRIBED A PATIENT WITH SCLEROTIC BONE DISEASE WHICH HAD THE ADDITIONAL FEATURE OF STRIATIONS. THE FATHER AND GRANDFATHER WERE SAID TO HAVE THE SAME DISORDER. THE FATHER DIED OF SEVERE AORTIC STENOSIS. ONLY ONE EARLIER CASE WAS FOUND, THAT REPORTED BY FAIRBANK (1951).

FAIRBANK, T.* AN ATLAS OF GENERAL AFFECTIONS OF THE SKELETON. BALTIMORE* WILLIAMS AND WILKINS, 1951.

JONES, M. D. AND MULCAHY, N. D.* OSTEOPATHIA STRIATA, OSTEOPETROSIS, AND IMPAIRED HEARING. A CASE REPORT. ARCH. OTOLARYNG. 87* 116-118, 1968.

RUCKER, T. N. AND ALFIDI, R. J.* A RARE FAMILIAL SYSTEMIC AFFECTION OF THE SKELETON, FAIRBANK'S DISEASE. RADIOLOGY 82* 63-66, 1964.

WALKER, B. A.* OSTEOPATHIA STRIATA WITH CATARACTS AND DEAFNESS. THE CLINICAL DELINEATION OF BIRTH DEFECTS. IV. SKELETAL DYSPLASIAS. NEW YORK* NATIONAL FOUNDATION, 1969. PP. 295-297.

*16660 OSTEOPETROSIS ('MARBLE BONES,' OSTEOSCLEROSIS FRAGILIS GENERALISATA, ALBERS-SCHONBERG'S DISEASE)

SALZANO (1961) ESTIMATED THE FREQUENCY OF THE DOMINANT FORM OF OSTEOPETROSIS IN BRAZIL TO BE ABOUT 1 IN 100,000. FRAGILITY OF BONES AND DENTAL ABSCESS ARE LEADING COMPLICATIONS. A MORE MALIGNANT FORM, INHERITED AS A RECESSIVE, CAUSES ANEMIA AND EARLY DEATH FROM INTERFERENCE WITH THE BONE MARROW. WELFORD (1959) DESCRIBED 14 AFFECTED MALE MEMBERS OF FIVE GENERATIONS OF A FAMILY. ALL AFFECTED PERSONS HAD FACIAL PARALYSIS BEGINNING USUALLY AT ABOUT THE AGE OF 12 YEARS. MAIN CLINICAL FEATURES ARE FRACTURES AND OSTEOMYELITIS, ESPECIALLY OF THE MANDIBLE. BY X-RAY THE VERTEBRAL BODIES HAVE A CHARACTERISTIC 'SANDWICH' APPEARANCE RESULTING FROM SCLEROSIS OF THE UPPER AND LOWER PLATES WITH INTERVENING LESS DENSE AREA. LONG BONES OF THE EXTREMITIES MAY SHOW A 'BONE-WITHIN-BONE' APPEARANCE. OSTEOSC- LEROSIS SOMETIMES TERMED OSTEOPETROSIS IS A FEATURE OF PYCNODYSOSTOSIS. FOLLOW-UP ON THE FAMILY REPORTED BY GHORMLEY (1922) WAS PROVIDED BY MCKUSICK (1961). JOHNSTON ET AL. (1968) STUDIED TWO FAMILIES. IN ONE PEDIGREE, THE DISORDER WAS TWICE NONPENETRANT. ELEVATED ACID PHOSPHATASE WAS A FEATURE IN ALL BUT ONE OF THE AFFECTED PERSONS.

GHORMLEY, R. K.* A CASE OF CONGENITAL OSTEOSCLEROSIS. BULL. HOPKINS HOSP. 33* 444-446, 1922.

ILHA, D. O. AND SALZANO, F. M.* A ROENTGENOLOGIC AND GENETIC STUDY OF A RARE OSSEOUS DYSTROPHY. ACTA GENET. MED. GEM. 10* 340-352, 1961.

JOHNSTON, C. C., JR., LAVY, N., LORD, T., VELLIOS, F., MERRITT, A. D. AND DEISS, W. P., JR.* OSTEOPETROSIS. A CLINICAL, GENETIC, METABOLIC, AND MORPHOLOGIC STUDY OF THE DOMINANTLY INHERITED, BENIGN FORM. MEDICINE 47* 149-167, 1968.

MCKUSICK, V. A. AND COLLEAGUES* MEDICAL GENETICS 1960. J. CHRONIC DIS. 14* 1-198, 1961 (FIG. 67).

SALZANO, F. M.* OSTEOPETROSIS* REVIEW OF DOMINANT CASES AND FREQUENCY IN A BRAZILIAN STATE. ACTA GENET. MED. GEM. 10* 353-358, 1961.

WELFORD, N. T.* FACIAL PARALYSIS ASSOCIATED WITH OSTEOPETROSIS (MARBLE BONES). J. PEDIAT. 55* 67-72, 1959.

*16670 OSTEOPOIKILOSIS

THE TERM MEANS LITERALLY 'SPOTTED BONES.' CIRCUMSCRIBED SCLEROTIC AREAS OCCUR NEAR THE ENDS OF MANY BONES. IT IS OF NO PATHOLOGIC CONSEQUENCE. SPOTTY SKIN LESIONS ALSO ARE FOUND IN MANY CASES. THESE ARE CONNECTIVE TISSUE NEVI. BERLIN ET AL. (1967) SHOWED THAT EITHER THE SKIN OR THE BONE LESIONS CAN BE ABSENT IN FAMILIES IN WHICH SOME MEMBERS HAVE BOTH. STRIKING PEDIGREES SUPPORTING AUTOSOMAL DOMINANT INHERITANCE WERE PUBLISHED BY MELNICK (1959), JONASCH (1955) AND BUSCH

FATHER AND SON. RAQUE AND WOOD (1970) FOUND DERMATO-OSTEOPOIKILOSIS IN A BROTHER
AND SISTER AND IN A SON OF THE BROTHER.

BERLIN, R., HEDENSIO, B., LILJA, B. AND LINDER, L.* OSTEOPOIKILOSIS - A
CLINICAL AND GENETIC STUDY. ACTA MED. SCAND. 181* 305-314, 1967.

BUSCH, K. F. B.* FAMILIAL DISSEMINATED OSTEOSCLEROSIS. ACTA RADIOL. 18* 693-
714, 1937.

DANIELSEN, L., MIDTGAARD, K. AND CHRISTENSEN, H. E.* OSTEOPOIKILOSIS ASSOCIATED
WITH DERMATOFIBROSIS LENTICULARIS DISSEMINATA. ARCH. DERM. 100* 465-470, 1969.

GREEN, A. E., ELLSWOOD, W. H. AND COLLINS, J. R.* MELORHEOSTOSIS AND OSTEOPOI-
KILOSIS* WITH A REVIEW OF THE LITERATURE. AM. J. ROENTGEN. 87* 1096-1111, 1962.

JONASCH, E.* 12 FALLE VON OSTEOPOIKILIE. FORTSCHR. ROENTGENSTR. 82* 344-353,
1955.

LANDBERG, T. AND AKESSON, H. O.* A STUDY OF OSTEOPOIKILOSIS. ACTA GENET. MED.
GEM. 12* 256-268, 1963.

LUZSA, G.* OSTEOPOIKILIA FAMILIARIS. ORV. HETIL. 103* 1267-1269, 1962.

MELNICK, J. C.* OSTEOPATHIA CONDENSANS DISSEMINATA (OSTEOPOIKILOSIS). STUDY OF
A FAMILY OF 4 GENERATIONS. AM. J. ROENTGEN. 82* 229-238, 1959.

RAQUE, C. J. AND WOOD, M. G.* CONNECTIVE-TISSUE NEVUS. DERMATOFIBROSIS
LENTICULARIS DISSEMINATA WITH OSTEOPOIKILOSIS. ARCH. DERM. 102* 390-396, 1970.

SMITH, A. D. AND WAISMAN, M.* CONNECTIVE TISSUE NEVI* FAMILIAL OCCURRENCE AND
ASSOCIATION WITH OSTEOPOIKILOSIS. ARCH. DERM. 81* 249-252, 1960.

16680 OTOSCLEROSIS

LARSSON (1960) REVIEWED ALL CASES SEEN IN THE UNIVERSITY OF GOTEBORG HOSPITAL FROM
1949 TO 1957. IN ABOUT 80 PERCENT IT WAS POSSIBLE TO VERIFY A POSITIVE FAMILY
HISTORY AFTER EXAMINING SIBS AND PARENTS. HE CONCLUDED THAT AUTOSOMAL DOMINANT
INHERITANCE WITH PENETRANCE BETWEEN 25 AND 40 PERCENT ACCOUNTS FOR THE FINDINGS.
DEAFNESS INTERPRETED AS OTOSCLEROSIS AND BEGINNING AS EARLY AS AGE FIVE IN SOME
CASES WAS DESCRIBED BY KABAT (1943) IN NINETEEN MEMBERS OF FOUR GENERATIONS OF A
FAMILY. OTOSCLEROSIS IS SAID TO BE RARE IN JAPAN (SHIMIZU, 1965). MORRISON
(1967) PRESENTED A SURVEY OF 150 ENGLISH CASES AND THEIR FAMILIES. HE CONCLUDED
THAT OTOSCLEROSIS IS DOMINANT WITH LESS THAN 50 PERCENT PENETRANCE. THE RISK TO A
CHILD OF AN AFFECTED PERSON IS OF THE ORDER OF 25 PERCENT.

AMIDON, E. W.* HEREDITY AND ENVIRONMENT IN OTOSCLEROSIS. J. HERED. 39* 223-
227, 1948.

CHUMLEA, B. J.* A PEDIGREE OF OTOSCLEROSIS. J. HERED. 33* 93-99, 1942.

KABAT, C.* A FAMILY HISTORY OF DEAFNESS. J. HERED. 34* 377-378, 1943.

LARSSON, A.* OTOSCLEROSIS, A GENETIC AND CLINICAL STUDY. ACTA OTOLARYNG. 154
(SUPPL.)* 1-86, 1960.

MACGREGOR, A. G. AND HARRISON, R.* CONGENITAL TOTAL COLOR BLINDNESS ASSOCIATED
WITH OTOSCLEROSIS. ANN. EUGEN. 15* 219-233, 1950.

MORRISON, A. W.* GENETIC FACTORS IN OTOSCLEROSIS. ANN. ROY. COLL. SURG. ENG.
41* 202-237, 1967.

SHIMIZU, H.* BALTIMORE, MD.* PERSONAL COMMUNICATION, 1965.

16690 OVALOCYTOSIS, HEREDITARY HEMOLYTIC

CUTTING ET AL. (1965) REPORTED SEVEN AFFECTED MEMBERS IN THREE GENERATIONS OF A
CAUCASIAN FAMILY WITH THREE INSTANCES OF MALE-TO-MALE TRANSMISSION. ALL 7 HAD
FULL OVALOCYTES AND 6 HAD UNCOMPENSATED HEMOLYTIC ANEMIA WHICH UNDERWENT
REMISSION WITH SPLENECTOMY. THESE WRITERS SUGGESTED THAT THERE ARE TWO TYPES OF
NON-LINKED ELLIPTOCYTOSIS OF WHICH ONE TYPE IS HEMOLYTIC WITH PREDOMINANT
OVALOCYTES. THEY SUGGESTED THIS SHOULD BE CALLED OVALOCYTOSIS AND *ELLIPTOCYTO-
SIS* RESERVED FOR THE OTHER CONDITIONS. SEE ELLIPTOCYTOSIS.

CUTTING, H. O., MCHUGH, W. J., CONRAD, F. G. AND MARLOW, A. A.* AUTOSOMAL
DOMINANT HEMOLYTIC ANEMIA CHARACTERIZED BY OVALOCYTOSIS. A FAMILY STUDY OF SEVEN
INVOLVED MEMBERS. AM. J. MED. 39* 21-34, 1965.

16700 OVARIAN TUMOR

JACKSON (1967) REPORTED A JAMAICAN FAMILY IN WHICH GRANDMOTHER, MOTHER AND
DAUGHTER (I.E., MEMBERS OF 3 GENERATIONS) DEVELOPED OVARIAN TUMORS WHICH IN TWO

WERE KNOWN TO HAVE BEEN DYSGERMINOMAS. SEE PEUTZ-JEGHERS SYNDROME FOR DESCRIPTION
OF OVARIAN TUMORS WITH THAT CONDITION.   LEWIS AND DAVISON (1969) DESCRIBED A
FAMILY IN WHICH 5 SISTERS (OUT OF 6) AND THEIR MOTHER HAD OVARIAN CANCER. ONE OF
THE FIVE HAD A MALIGNANT OVARIAN CYST BUT SUBSEQUENTLY DIED OF COLONIC CANCER.
PROPHYLACTIC OOPORECTOMY WAS PERFORMED IN THE SIXTH SISTER AND IN 5 FEMALES OF THE
FOLLOWING GENERATION. LIBER (1950) DESCRIBED A FAMILY WITH HISTOLOGICALLY PROVEN
PAPILLARY ADENOCARCINOMA OF THE OVARY IN 5 SISTERS AND THEIR MOTHER. LI ET AL.
(1970) REPORTED A FAMILY IN WHICH 7 WOMEN (FOUR OF THEM SISTERS) WERE PROVED TO
HAVE OVARIAN CARCINOMA AND THIS FORM OF MALIGNANCY WAS SUSPECTED IN 3 OTHERS.
OVARIAN TUMORS ALSC OCCUR IN THE PEUTZ-JEGHERS' SYNDROME (Q.V.), GONADAL DYSGENE-
SIS IN WHICH XY CELLS ARE PRESENT AND IN THE BASAL CELL NEVUS SYNDROME (Q.V.).

JACKSON, S. M.* OVARIAN DYSGERMINOMA IN THREE GENERATIONS.Q J. MED. GENET. 4*
112-113, 1967.

LEWIS, A. C. W. AND DAVISON, B. C. C.* FAMILIAL OVARIAN CANCER. LANCET 2* 235-
237, 1969.

LI, F. P., RAPOPORT, A. H., FAUMENI, J. F., JR. AND JENSEN, R. D.* FAMILIAL
OVARIAN CARCINOMA. J.A.M.A. 214* 1559-1561, 1970.

LIBER, A. F.* OVARIAN CANCER IN MOTHER AND FIVE DAUGHTERS. ARCH. PATH. 49*
280-290, 1950.

16710 PACHYDERMOPERIOSTOSIS (PRIMARY OR IDIOPATHIC HYPERTROPHIC OSTEOARTHROPATHY)

THE MANIFESTATIONS INCLUDE CLUBBING OF THE FINGERS, THICKENING OF THE SKIN AND
PERIOSTEUM OF THE DISTAL PART OF THE EXTREMITIES, THICKENING AND SEBORRHEA OF THE
SKIN OF THE FACE AND FOREHEAD AND HYPERHIDROSIS (VOGL AND GOLDFISCHER, 1962).
SIMPLE DIGITAL CLUBBING (Q.V.) MAY BE A SEPARATE GENETIC DEFECT. RIMOIN (1965)
OBSERVED AFFECTED PERSONS IN SUCCESSIVE GENERATIONS.   FEMALES WERE MUCH MORE
MILDLY AFFECTED THAN MALES. EITHER HETEROGENEITY IN THIS CONDITION OR RECESSIVE
INHERITANCE IS SUGGESTED BY THE CONSIDERABLE NUMBER OF INSTANCES OF AFFECTED SIBS
WITH APPARENTLY NORMAL PARENTS AND THE SEVERAL EXAMPLES OF CONSANGUINEOUS PARENTS
(LEVA, 1915* SIMONS, 1918* SHEN AND YAMANOUCHI, 1934).

HAMBRICK, G. W., JR. AND CARTER, D. M.* PACHYDERMOPERIOSTOSIS. TOURAINE-
SOLENTE-GOLE SYNDROME. ARCH. DERM. 94* 594-608, 1966.

LEVA, J.* UEBER FAMILIARE AKROMEGALIE. MED. KLIN. 11* 1266-1268, 1915.

RIMOIN, D. L.* PACHYDERMOPERIOSTOSIS (IDIOPATHIC CLUBBING AND PERIOSTOSIS).
GENETIC AND PHYSIOLOGIC CONSIDERATIONS. NEW ENG. J. MED. 272* 923-931, 1965.

SHEN, R. AND YAMANOUCHI, N.* UBER CUTIS GYRATA UND CUTIS VERITIS GYRATA LATENS.
DERM. WSCHR. 98* 254 ONLY, 1934.

SIMONS, A.* FAMILIARE TROMMELSCHLAGELBILDUNG UND KNOCHENKYPERTROPHIE. DEUTSCH.
NERVENHEILK. 59* 301-321, 1918.

VOGL, A. AND GOLDFISCHER, S.* PACHYDERMOPERIOSTOSIS* PRIMARY OR IDIOPATHIC
OSTEOARTHROPATHY. AM. J. MED. 33* 166-187, 1962.

*16720 PACHYONYCHIA CONGENITA

THIS DOMINANTLY INHERITED DISORDER IS CHARACTERIZED BY ONYCHOGRYPOSIS, HYPERKERA-
TOSIS OF THE PALMS, SOLES, KNEES AND ELBOWS, TINY CUTANEOUS HORNS IN MANY AREAS,
AND LEUKOPLAKIA OF THE ORAL MUCOUS MEMBRANES. HYPERHIDROSIS OF THE HANDS AND FEET
IS USUALLY PRESENT. JACKSON AND LAWLER (1951-52) REPORTED 6 AFFECTED MEMBERS OF 3
GENERATIONS. MURRAY (1921) FOUND 7 AFFECTED IN 3 GENERATIONS. KUMER AND LOOS
(1935) FOUND 24 AFFECTED IN 5 GENERATIONS. THE SYNDROME MAY BE MORE FREQUENT IN
JEWS THAN IN NON-JEWS.   AT BIRTH SOME TEETH ARE USUALLY ALREADY ERUPTED. IN A
JEWISH KINDRED WE HAVE OBSERVED AN APPARENT NEW MUTATION WITH TRANSMISSION TO A
SON OF THE MALE PROBAND.

AKESSON, H. O.* PACHYONYCHIA CONGENITA IN SIX GENERATIONS. HEREDITAS 58* 103-
110, 1967.

JACKSON, A. D. M. AND LAWLER, S. D.* PACHYONYCHIA CONGENITA. A REPORT OF SIX
CASES IN ONE FAMILY, WITH A NOTE ON LINKAGE DATA. ANN. EUGEN. 16* 142-146, 1951-
52.

JOSEPH, H. L.* PACHYONYCHIA CONGENITA. ARCH. DERM. 90* 594-603, 1964.

KUMER, L. AND LOOS, H. O.* UBER PACHYONYCHIA CONGENITA (TYPUS RIEHL). WIEN.
KLIN. WSCHR. 48* 174-178, 1935.

MURRAY, F. A.* CONGENITAL ANOMALIES OF THE NAILS. FOUR CASES OF HEREDITARY
HYPERTROPHY OF THE NAIL BED ASSOCIATED WITH A HISTORY OF ERUPTED TEETH AT BIRTH.
BRIT. J. DERM. 33* 409-412, 1921.

SODERQUIST, N. A. AND REED, W. B.* PACHYONYCHIA CONGENITA WITH EPIDERMAL CYSTS

WITKOP, C. J., JR. AND GORLIN, R. J.* FOUR HEREDITARY MUCOSAL SYNDROMES. ARCH. DERM. 84* 762-771, 1961.

16730 PAGET'S DISEASE OF BONE

REPORTS OF FAMILIAL AGGREGATION ARE RATHER NUMEROUS, INCLUDING OCCURRENCE IN SUCCESSIVE GENERATIONS. MONTAGU (1949) REVIEWED THE REPORTED FAMILIES WITH MULTIPLE INSTANCES OF PAGET'S DISEASE OF BONE AND CONCLUDED THAT 'WHEN INHERITED, IT IS TRANSMITTED AS AN INCOMPLETELY DOMINANT GENE CARRIED ON AN X-CHROMOSOME.' MCKUSICK (1960) REVIEWED 35 PEDIGREES REPORTED TO 1956 AND ADDED TWO OTHERS. IN ONLY ONE FAMILY, THAT OF VAN BOGAERT (1933), WAS THERE MALE-TO-MALE TRANSMISSION. ALL THE PERSONS AFFECTED BY THE BONE DISEASE AND SOME MEMBERS OF THE FAMILY NOT SO AFFECTED ALSO HAD RETINITIS PIGMENTOSA, WHICH MAY HAVE BEEN AN INDEPENDENT, I.E., COINCIDENTAL, GENETIC DISORDER. JONES AND REED (1967) OBSERVED 6 CASES IN 3 GENERATIONS OF A FAMILY. EVENS AND BARTTER (1968) DESCRIBED 7 DEFINITE AND TWO PROBABLE CASES IN ONE KINDRED.

EVENS, R. G. AND BARTTER, F. C.* THE HEREDITARY ASPECTS OF PAGET'S DISEASE (OSTEITIS DEFORMANS). J.A.M.A. 205* 900-902, 1968.

JONES, J. V. AND REED, M. F.* PAGET'S DISEASE* A FAMILY WITH SIX CASES. BRIT. MED. J. 2* 90-91, 1967.

MCKUSICK, V. A.* PAGET'S DISEASE OF THE BONE. HERITABLE DISORDERS OF CONNEC-TIVE TISSUE. ST. LOUIS* C. V. MOSBY CO., 1960 (2ND ED.). PP. 304-309.

MONTAGU, M. F. A.* PAGET'S DISEASE (OSTEITIS DEFORMANS) AND HEREDITY. AM. J. HUM. GENET. 1* 94-95, 1949.

VAN BOGAERT, L.* UBER EINE HEREDITARE UND FAMILIARE FORM DER PAGETSCHEN OSTITIS DEFORMANS MIT CHORIORETINITIS PIGMENTOSA. ZBL. GES. NEUROL. PSYCHIAT. 147* 327-345, 1933.

16740 PAIN, SUBMANDIBULAR, OCULAR AND RECTAL, WITH FLUSHING

HAYDEN AND GROSSMAN (1959) DESCRIBED A SYNDROME CONSISTING OF VERY BRIEF, EXCRUCIATING PAIN OF THE SUBMANDIBULAR, OCULAR AND RECTAL AREAS WITH FLUSHING OF THE SURROUNDING SKIN. AUTOSOMAL DOMINANT INHERITANCE WITH VARIABLE PENETRANCE OF THE COMPONENTS WAS SUGGESTED. SUBMANDIBULAR AND OCULAR PAIN IS A MORE CONSISTENT FEATURE THAN RECTAL PAIN. THEY CONSIDERED THE CONDITION A 'DYSAUTONOMIA.'

HAYDEN, R. AND GROSSMAN, M.* RECTAL, OCULAR AND SUBMAXILLARY PAIN. A FAMILIAL AUTONOMIC DISORDER RELATED TO PROCTALGIA FUGAX. REPORT OF A FAMILY. AM. J. DIS. CHILD. 97* 479-482, 1959.

16750 PALATOPHARYNGEAL INCOMPETENCE

CONGENITAL PALATOPHARYNGEAL INCOMPETENCE IS CHARACTERIZED BY CLEFT PALATE SPEECH (RHINOLALIA APERTA) IN THE ABSENCE OF OVERT CLEFT PALATE. ABOUT A FOURTH OF CASES ARE 'UNMASKED' BY ADENOIDECTOMY. ABNORMALITIES OF THE UVULA, SOFT PALATE AND HARD PALATE MAY BE VISIBLE. OCCASIONALLY DOMINANT INHERITANCE MAY OBTAIN, WITH GREAT VARIABILITY.

PRUZANSKY, S. AND MASON, R.* FAMILY STUDIES OF CONGENITAL PALATOPHARYNGEAL INCOMPETENCE. (ABSTRACT) PROC. THIRD INTERN. CONG. HUM. GENET. (CHICAGO, SEPT. 5-10, 1966.).

16760 PALMARIS LONGUS MUSCLE, ABSENCE OF

AT THE WRIST THE TENDON OF THE PALMARIS LONGUS MUSCLE IS LOCATED IN THE MIDDLE OF THE VENTRAL SURFACE. IT IS FLANKED BY THE TENDONS OF THE FLEXOR CARPI ULNARIS AND FLEXOR CARPI RADIALIS. SCHAEFFER (1953) RECORDED THAT THE MUSCLE WAS ABSENT FROM 12.6 PERCENT OF THE 310 LIMBS OF 155 SUBJECTS AND WAS BILATERALLY ABSENT IN 7.7 PERCENT OF SUBJECTS. THE MUSCLE IS SAID TO BE ABSENT MORE OFTEN IN FEMALES AND ON THE LEFT SIDE. FOR EXAMPLE, THOMPSON, MCBATTS AND DANFORTH (1921) FOUND THE MUSCLE MISSING IN ABOUT 16 PERCENT OF MALES AND 24 PERCENT OF FEMALES, THESE FIGURES BEING BASED ON STUDIES OF CADAVERS. ABSENCE WAS THOUGHT TO BE A DOMINANT TRAIT, WITH INCOMPLETE PENETRANCE AND LATERAL VARIABILITY. THOMPSON, MCBATTS AND DANFORTH (1921) CONCLUDED THAT ABSENCE IS DOMINANT. THEIR STUDY INVOLVED 81 FAMILIES WITH A TOTAL OF 188 CHILDREN.

SCHAEFFER, J. P.* IN, HUMAN ANATOMY. MORRIS (ED.) NEW YORK* BLAKISTON CO., 1953 (11TH ED.) PP. 482-483.

THOMPSON, J. W., MCBATTS, J. AND DANFORTH, C. H.* HEREDITARY AND RACIAL VARIATIONS IN THE MUSCULUS PALMARIS LONGUS. AM. J. PHYS. ANTHROP. 4* 205-218, 1921.

16770 PALMO-MENTAL REFLEX

D
O
M
I
N
A
N
T

THE PALMO-MENTAL REFLEX IS AN IPSILATERAL OR BILATERAL CONTRACTION OF THE MENTALIS MUSCLE ELICITED BY A SCRATCH APPLIED TO THE THENAR EMINENCE. IN JAPANESE, ABE (1965) FOUND IT IN ONE-THIRD OF 3 YEAR OLD CHILDREN AND ONE-SIXTH OF THE MOTHERS, SUGGESTING THAT ABOUT HALF THE POSITIVE CHILDREN BECOME NEGATIVE BY ADULTHOOD. THE REFLEX WAS MUCH MORE OFTEN POSITIVE IN MOTHERS OF CHILDREN WITH THE REFLEX THAN IN MOTHERS OF 'NEGATIVE' CHILDREN. FURTHER ANALYSIS OF THE DATA SUGGESTED DOMINANT INHERITANCE. THE DESIGN OF THIS STUDY DID NOT PERMIT EXCLUSION OF X-LINKED DOMINANCE. A MARKED, SLOWLY SUBSIDING REFLEX IN AN ADULT MAY INDICATE CEREBRAL DISEASE.

ABE, K.* GENETIC ASPECTS OF THE PALMO-MENTAL REFLEX. ACTA GENET. STATIST. MED. 15* 327-336, 1965.

*16780 PANCREATITIS, HEREDITARY

GROSS, GAMBILL AND ULRICH (1962) DESCRIBED A KINDRED WITH AFFECTED PERSONS IN FOUR GENERATIONS. FOUR OTHER FAMILIES HAVE BEEN REPORTED FROM THE MAYO CLINIC. A PUZZLING FEATURE IS THE URINARY EXCRETION OF LYSINE AND CYSTINE BY ABOUT HALF THE MEMBERS OF AFFECTED KINDREDS (WITH OR WITHOUT PANCREATITIS). CYSTINE URINARY STONES HAVE NOT BEEN OBSERVED. SINGER AND COHEN (1966) REPORTED ONSET AT ABOUT AGE 20 IN A MAN WHOSE YOUNGER SISTER AND A COUSIN WERE SIMILARLY AFFECTED. THE ATTACKS WERE CHARACTERIZED BY SEVERE ABDOMINAL PAINS, FEVER AND MARKED ELEVATION OF SERUM AMYLASE. EXCEPT FOR THE LAST, DIFFERENTIATION FROM FAMILIAL MEDITER-RANEAN FEVER (Q.V.), ALSO CALLED 'FAMILIAL PAROXYSMAL PERITONITIS.' MIGHT BE DIFFICULT. THE AMINOACIDURIA WAS ALMOST CERTAINLY AN INCIDENTAL FINDING SINCE FAMILY MEMBERS WITHOUT PANCREATITIS SHOWED IT AND BECAUSE OTHER FAMILIES WITH PANCREATITIS HAVE NOT HAD THIS FEATURE (DAVIDSON ET AL., 1968). ROBECHEK (1967) OBSERVED A FAMILY WITH 5 AFFECTED PERSONS. HE SUGGESTED THAT HYPERTROPHY OF THE SPHINCTER OF ODDI TOGETHER WITH A COMMON AMPULLA OF THE BILIARY AND PANCREATIC DUCTS MAY BE THE INHERITED FACTOR. MANN AND RUBIN (1969) DESCRIBED A 17 MONTH OLD BOY WITH STEATORRHEA WHOSE 26 YEAR OLD BROTHER AND MOTHER HAD STEATORRHEA AND PANCREATIC CALCIFICATION. HEREDITARY PANCREATITIS OCCURS WITH HYPERPARATHYROIDISM IN THE MULTIPLE ENDOCRINE ADENOMATOSIS SYNDROME (Q.V.).

CAREY, M. C. AND FITZGERALD, O.* HYPERPARATHYROIDISM ASSOCIATED WITH CHRONIC PANCREATITIS IN A FAMILY. GUT 9* 700-703, 1968.

DAVIDSON, P., COSTANZA, D., SWIECONEK, J. A. AND HARRIS, J. B.* HEREDITARY PANCREATITIS* A KINDRED WITHOUT GROSS AMINOACIDURIA. ANN. INTERN. MED. 68* 88-96, 1968.

GROSS, J. B., GAMBILL, E. E. AND ULRICH, J. A.* HEREDITARY PANCREATITIS. DESCRIPTION OF A FIFTH KINDRED AND SUMMARY OF CLINICAL FEATURES. AM. J. MED. 33* 358-364, 1962.

GROSS, J. B., ULRICH, J. A. AND JONES, J. D.* URINARY EXCRETION OF AMINOACIDS IN A KINDRED WITH HEREDITARY PANCREATITIS AND AMINOACIDURIA. GASTROENTEROLOGY 47* 41-48, 1964.

MANN, T. P. AND RUBIN, J.* FAMILIAL PANCREATIC EXOCRINE DYSFUNCTION WITH PANCREATIC CALCIFICATION. PROC. ROY. SOC. MED. 62* 326 ONLY, 1969.

ROBECHEK, P. J.* HEREDITARY CHRONIC RELAPSING PANCREATITIS. A CLUE TO PANCREATITIS IN GENERAL.Q AM. J. SURG. 113* 819-824, 1967.

SINGER, M. AND COHEN, F. B.* HEREDITARY CHRONIC RELAPSING PANCREATITIS. J. NEWARK BETH ISRAEL HOSP. 21* 121-126, 1966.

16790 PAPILLOMATOSIS, FAMILIAL CUTANEOUS

BADEN (1965) DESCRIBED A CONFLUENT, RETICULAR TYPE OF PAPILLOMATOSIS IN TWO SISTERS AND THE DAUGHTER OF ONE.

BADEN, H. P.* FAMILIAL CUTANEOUS PAPILLOMATOSIS. ARCH. DERM. 92* 394-395, 1965.

*16800 PARAGANGLIOMATA

KROLL AND COLLEAGUES (1964) FOUND CAROTID BODY TUMORS IN 12 MEMBERS OF A FAMILY IN AN AUTOSOMAL DOMINANT PATTERN OF INHERITANCE. CAROTID BODY TUMORS AND GLOMUS JUGULARE TUMORS ARE CONSIDERED TO BE CHEMODECTOMAS, THIS BEING A TERM FOR TUMORS ARISING IN CHEMORECEPTOR STRUCTURES. SOME WOULD QUESTION THE APPROPRIATENESS OF CALLING THESE PARAGANGLIOMAS. RESLER ET AL. (1966) DESCRIBED A PATIENT WITH BILATRAL CAROTID BODY TUMORS AND A GLOMUS JUGULARE TUMOR. THEY COMMENTED THAT FAMILIAL CAROTID BODY TUMORS TEND TO BE MULTIPLE. FAMILIAL GLOMUS JUGULARE TUMORS ARE PROBABLY RARE. THE ONLY REPORTED FAMILY MAY BE THAT WITH THREE AFFECTED SISTERS DESCRIBED IN 1937 BY GOEKOOP (CITED BY ROSEN, 1952). BARTELS (1949) FOUND CAROTID BODY TUMOR IN MEMBERS OF 3 SUCCESSIVE GENERATIONS. WILSON (1970) REVIEWED THE FAMILIAL REPORTS AND DESCRIBED A FAMILY WITH MALE-TO-MALE TRANSMISSION AND A 'SKIPPED GENERATION.'

BARTELS, J.* DE TUMOREN VAN HET GLOMUS JUGULARE. THESIS. GRONINGEN, 1949.

KROLL, A. J., ALEXANDER, B., COCHIOS, F. AND PECHET, L.* HEREDITARY DEFICIEN-
CIES OF CLOTTING FACTORS VII AND X ASSOCIATED WITH CAROTID-BODY TUMORS. NEW ENG.
J. MED. 270* 6-13, 1964.

RESLER, D. R., SNOW, J. B. AND WILLIAMS, G. R.* MULTIPLICITY AND FAMILIAL
INCIDENCE OF CAROTID BODY AND GLOMUS JUGULARE TUMORS. ANN. OTOL. 75* 114-122,
1966.

ROSEN, S.* GLOMUS JUGULARE TUMOR OF THE MIDDLE EAR WITH NORMAL DRUM, IMPROVED
BIOPSY TECHNIQUE. ANN. OTOL. 61* 448-451, 1952.

WILSON, H.* CAROTID BODY TUMORS* FAMILIAL AND BILATERAL. ANN. SURG. 171* 843-
848, 1970.

16810 PARALYSIS AGITANS, JUVENILE, OF HUNT

RAMSEY HUNT (1917) DESCRIBED A DISORDER WITH TYPICAL PARKINSONISM BEGINNING IN THE
TEENS OR EARLIER WITH TREMOR, MASK-LIKE FACIES, BRADYKINESIA, DYSARTHRIA AND
RIGIDITY. PROGRESSION IS VERY SLOW. DAVID B. CLARK HAS SEEN THE DISORDER IN
FATHER AND DAUGHTER (FORD, 1961). THE SUBSTANTIA NIGRA IS NORMAL BUT DEGENERATION
AND LOSS OF LARGE CELLS OF THE LENTICULAR NUCLEI OCCUR. HUNT'S SECOND CASE WAS
THE OFFSPRING OF FIRST COUSINS. SHE DIED AT THE AGE OF 65 YEARS. AUTOPSY SHOWED
PALLIDO-PYRAMIDAL DISEASE WHICH IS LISTED IN THE RECESSIVE CATALOG (Q.V.).

FORD, F. R.* HYPERTROPHIC INTERSTITIAL POLY-NEURITIS. DISEASES OF THE NERVOUS
SYSTEM IN INFANCY, CHILDHOOD AND ADOLESCENCE. SPRINGFIELD, ILL.* CHARLES C
THOMAS, 1961 (4TH ED.). PP. 369-399.

HUNT, J. R.* PROGRESSIVE ATROPHY OF THE GLOBUS PALLIDUS (PRIMARY ATROPHY OF THE
PALLIDAL SYSTEM). BRAIN 40* 58-148, 1917.

MJONES, H.* PARALYSIS AGITANS* A CLINICAL AND GENETIC STUDY. COPENHAGEN* E.
MUNKSGAARD, 1949.

16820 PARAMOLAR TUBERCLE OF BOLK

THIS IS AN EXTRA SMALL CUSP LOCATED ON THE BUCCAL SIDE OF THE PERMANENT MOLAR
TEETH. ITS SIGNIFICANCE IS UNKNOWN.

DAHLBERG, A. A.* PARAMOLAR TUBERCLE (BOLK). AM. J. PHYS. ANTHROP. 3* 97-103,
1945.

*16830 PARAMYOTONIA CONGENITA OF EULENBURG

LAJOIE (1961) DESCRIBED A FAMILY WITH MANY AFFECTED MEMBERS. THE CONDITION IS
MANIFESTED MAINLY BY PARALYSIS OF MUSCLES EXPOSED TO COLD, IS ALREADY EVIDENT IN
INFANCY, IS NOT PROGRESSIVE, DOES NOT INTERFERE WITH A REASONABLY NORMAL SOCIAL
AND ECONOMIC LIFE, AND DOES NOT AFFECT LONGEVITY. HUDSON'S FAMILY (1963) SHOWED
17 AFFECTED IN 5 GENERATIONS. DRAGER, HAMMILL AND SHY (1958) FOUND THIRTY
AFFECTED MEMBERS IN SIX GENERATIONS OF A FAMILY. THE CHARACTERISTICS OF THIS
DISEASE DESCRIBED BY EULENBURG ARE (1) INHERITANCE AS A DOMINANT WITH HIGH
PENETRANCE, (2) MYOTONIA, INCREASED BY EXPOSURE TO COLD, (3) INTERMITTENT FLACCID
PARESIS, NOT NECESSARILY DEPENDENT ON COLD OR MYOTONIA, (4) LABILITY OF SERUM
POTASSIUM, (5) NON-PROGRESSIVE NATURE AND (6) LACK OF ATROPHY OR HYPERTROPHY OF
MUSCLES. HUDSON (1963) COMMENTED ON THE PHENOTYPIC OVERLAP OF THIS CONDITION WITH
HYPOKALEMIC, EUKALEMIC AND HYPERKALEMIC PERIODIC PARALYSIS, WITH MYOTONIA
CONGENITA AND WITH MYOTONIC DYSTROPHY. SIX AND POSSIBLY 9 GENERATIONS HAD
AFFECTED MEMBERS IN THE FRENCH CANADIAN FAMILY REPORTED BY SAMAHA (1964). EATING
ICE-CREAM OR SWIMMING IN COLD WATER WAS DANGEROUS TO AFFECTED MEMBERS. SERUM
POTASSIUM LEVELS WERE MODERATELY INCREASED AND THE PATIENTS WERE SENSITIVE TO
ADMINISTERED POTASSIUM. CHLOROTHIAZIDE WAS REMARKABLY BENEFICIAL. BECKER (1970)
GAVE AN EXTENSIVE REVIEW OF THE SUBJECT AND DESCRIBED STUDIES IN 18 KINDREDS.

BECKER, P. E.* PARAMYOTONIA CONGENITA (EULENBERG). FORTSCHRITTE DER ALLGE-
MEINEN UND KLINISCHEN. HUMANGENETIK 3* 134, 1970.

DRAGER, G. A., HAMMILL, J. F. AND SHY, G. M.* PARAMYOTONIA CONGENITA. ARCH.
NEUROL. PSYCHIAT. 80* 1-9, 1958.

HUDSON, A. J.* PROGRESSIVE NEUROLOGICAL DISORDER AND MYOTONIA CONGENITA
ASSOCIATED WITH PARAMYOTONIA. BRAIN 86* 811-826, 1963.

LAJOIE, W. J.* PARAMYOTONIA CONGENITA, CLINICAL FEATURES AND ELECTROMYOGRAPHIC
FINDINGS. ARCH. PHYS. MED. 42* 507-512, 1961.

MAGEE, K. R.* PARAMYOTONIA CONGENITA* ASSOCIATED WITH CUTANEOUS COLD SENSITIVI-
TY AND DESCRIPTION OF PECULIAR SUSTAINED POSTURES AFTER MUSCLE CONTRACTION. ARCH.
NEUROL. 14* 590-594, 1966.

SAMAHA, F. J.* VON EULENBERG'S PARAMYOTONIA. TRANS. AM. NEUROL. ASS. 89* 87-
91, 1964.

THOMASEN, E.* MYOTONIA. THOMSEN'S DISEASE (MYOTONIA CONGENITA). PARAMYOTONIA AND DYSTROPHIA MYOTONICA. A CLINICAL AND HEREDOBIOLOGIC INVESTIGATION. AARHUS* UNIVERSITETSFORLAGET. 1948.

D
O
M
I
N
A
N
T

16840 PARASTREMMATIC DWARFISM

LANGER ET AL. (1970) DESCRIBED 3 PATIENTS WITH A FORM OF DWARFISM IN WHICH DEFORMITIES ARE RECOGNIZED IN THE FIRST 6 TO 12 MONTHS OF LIFE. THEY NAMED THE DISORDER PARASTREMATIC FROM THE GREEK TERM FOR TWISTED. CLINICALLY THE FULL SYNDROME IS MANIFESTED BY 10 YEARS. ADULT HEIGHT IS 90 TO 110 CM. THERE ARE BIZZARE AND SYMMETRIC DEFORMITIES OF THE LEGS WITH SEVERE GENU VALGUM, BOWING OF THE LONG BONES, TWISTED THIGHS AND SHANKS ALONG THE LONG AXIS, SHORT NECK, KYPHOSCOLIOSIS, MULTIPLE CONTRACTURES OF MAJOR JOINTS, CLEAR CORNEA AND NORMAL CARDIOVASCULAR SYSTEM. INTELLIGENCE IS ALSO NORMAL AND THERE IS NO ABNORMAL MUCOPOLYSACCHARIDURIA. RADIOGRAPHS SHOW VERY COARSE TRABECULATIONS WITH AREAS OF IRREGULAR, DENSE STIPPLING AND STREAKING PRODUCING A 'FLOCKY OR WOOLY' APPEARANCE. IN THE PELVIS THIS IS SEEN AS A LACE LIKE BORDER OF THE ILIAC CRESTS. THE METAPHYSES ARE CLEAR AND CONTAIN 'FLOCKY' BONE* SEVERELY DEFORMED AND RADIOLUCENT EPIPHYSES ARE PRESENT. THE EVIDENCE FOR DOMINANT INHERITANCE COMES FROM THE REPORT OF FATHER AND DAUGHTER BY RASK (1963). SINCE THE DAUGHTER WAS AS SEVERELY AFFECTED AS THE FATHER, THE CAUSATIVE GENE IS PROBABLY AUTOSOMAL.

LANGER, L. O., PETERSEN, D. AND SPRANGER, J.* AN UNUSUAL BONE DYSPLASIA* PARASTREMMATIC DWARFISM. AM. J. ROENTGEN. 110* 550-560, 1970.

RASK, M. R.* MORQUIO-BRAILSFORD OSTEOCHONDRODYSTROPHY AND OSTEOGENESIS IMPERFECTA* REPORT OF A PATIENT WITH BOTH CONDITIONS. J. BONE JOINT SURG. 45A* 561-570, 1963.

*16850 PARIETAL FORAMINA, SYMMETRICAL (FORAMINA PARIETALIA PERMAGNA)

PARIETAL FORAMINA ARE SYMMETRICAL, OVAL DEFECTS IN THE PARIETAL BONE SITUATED ON EACH SIDE OF THE SAGGITAL SUTURE AND SEPARATED FROM EACH OTHER BY A NARROW BRIDGE OF BONE. GOLDSMITH (1922) CALLED THIS CONDITION CATLIN MARKS BECAUSE HE OBSERVED 16 INSTANCES IN 5 GENERATIONS OF THE CATLIN FAMILY. THIS, LIKE HARTNUP DISEASE, IS ONE OF THE FEW EXAMPLES OF HEREDITARY TRAITS NAMED FOR THE FAMILY IN WHICH IT WAS FIRST OBSERVED. LOTHER (1959) DESCRIBED FIVE CASES IN TWO GENERATIONS. MANY OF THE AFFECTED PERSONS IN GOLDSMITH'S FAMILY HAD CIRCUMSCRIBED APLASIA OF THE SCALP AND THE SAME WAS TRUE OF LOTHER'S FAMILY. KITE (1961) OBSERVED ASSOCIATION WITH SEIZURES. THE POSSIBILITY OF CONFUSION WITH ABORIGINAL TREPINATION WAS POINTED OUT BY POWELL (1970).

GOLDSMITH, W. M.* 'THE CATLIN MARK'* THE INHERITANCE OF AN UNUSUAL OPENING IN THE PARIETAL BONES. J. HERED. 13* 69-71, 1922.

KITE, W. C., JR.* SEIZURES ASSOCIATED WITH THE CATLIN MARK. NEUROLOGY 11* 345-348, 1961.

LOTHER, K.* FAMILIARES VORKOMMEN VON FORAMINA PARIETALIA PERMAGNA. ARCH. KINDERHEILK. 160* 156-168, 1959.

MURPHY, J. AND GOODING, C. A.* EVOLUTION OF PERSISTENTLY ENLARGED PARIETAL FORAMINA. RADIOLOGY 97* 391-392, 1970.

POWELL, B. W.* ABORIGINAL TREPINATION* CASE FROM SOUTHERN NEW ENGLAND.Q SCIENCE 170* 732-734, 1970.

*16860 PARKINSONISM

SPELLMAN (1962) DESCRIBED A FAMILY IN WHICH MULTIPLE MEMBERS IN FOUR GENERATIONS HAD PARKINSONISM BEGINNING IN THE 30'S AND PROGRESSING RAPIDLY TO DEATH IN 2-12 YEARS. BELL AND CLARK (1926) REVIEWED PUBLISHED PEDIGREES AND PUBLISHED AN ADDITIONAL ONE. ALLAN (1937) REPORTED IMPRESSIVE PEDIGREES FROM NORTH CAROLINA.

ALLAN, W.* INHERITANCE OF SHAKING PALSY. ARCH. INTERN. MED. 60* 424-436, 1937.

BELL, J. AND CLARK, A. J.* A PEDIGREE OF PARALYSIS AGITANS. ANN. EUGEN. 1* 455-462, 1926.

SPELLMAN, G. G.* REPORT OF FAMILIAL CASES OF PARKINSONISM* EVIDENCE OF A DOMINANT TRAIT IN A PATIENT'S FAMILY. J.A.M.A. 179* 372-374, 1962.

16870 PARKINSONISM-DEMENTIA

IT IS NOT CERTAIN THAT THIS DISORDER, ENDEMIC AMONG THE NATIVES OF GUAM, IS GENETIC OR, IF GENETIC, IS DOMINANT.

HIRANO, A., KURLAND, L. T., KROOTH, R. S. AND LESSELL, S.* PARKINSONISM-DEMENTIA COMPLEX, AN ENDEMIC DISEASE ON THE ISLAND OF GUAM. BRAIN 84* 642-661, 1961.

16880 PAROTIDOMEGALY, HEREDITARY BILATERAL

MARIE ET AL. (1968) DESCRIBED SIX CASES IN 3 GENERATIONS.

MARIE, R., MARIE, M., GRELLET, M., GOUYGOU, C., CARIOU, P., GAUTHEY, J. C. AND REVERSE, C.* PAROTIDOMEGALIE BILATERALE D'ALLURE HEREDITAIRE. DYSPLASIE MICROKYS-TIQUE DE LA PAROTIDE* ETUDE CLINIQUE, SIALOGROPHIQUE ET ANATOMO-PATHOLOGIQUE. REV. STOMAT. 68* 578-585, 1967.

*16890 PATELLA, CHONDROMALACIA OF

THIS DISORDER IS CHARACTERIZED BY WELL-LOCALIZED PAIN WHEN THE PATELLA IS GRATED AGAINST THE FEMORAL CONDYLES OR WHEN THE KNEE IS ACTIVELY EXTENDED WITH THE PATELLA MANUALLY DISPLACED DISTALLY. RUBACKY (1963) DESCRIBED FIVE FAMILIES WITH MULTIPLE AFFECTED PERSONS IN MULTIPLE GENERATIONS AND MALE-TO-MALE TRANSMISSION. THE ASSOCIATION OF PATELLAR CHONDROMALACIA WITH RECURRENT DISLOCATION OF THE PATELLA (Q.V.) IS WELL KNOWN AND THE FORMER IS USUALLY ATTRIBUTED TO THE LATTER. HOWEVER, RUBACKY (1963) SUGGESTED THAT THE CAUSE AND EFFECT RELATION MAY BE THE OTHER WAY AROUND, IN SOME CASES. THIS CONDITION IS PROBABLY NOT A FORM OF OSTEODRONDRITIS DISSECANS (Q.V.), WHICH CAN AFFECT THE PATELLA.

RUBACKY, G. E.* INHERITABLE CHONDROMALACIA OF THE PATELLA. J. BONE JOINT SURG. 45A* 1685-1688, 1963.

16900 PATELLA, FAMILIAL RECURRENT DISLOCATION OF

CARTER AND SWEETNAN (1960) SUGGESTED THAT THIS IS A DOMINANT TRAIT INDEPENDENT OF FAMILIAL JOINT LAXITY (Q.V.).

CARTER, C. AND SWEETNAN, R.* RECURRENT DISLOCATION OF THE PATELLA AND OF THE SHOULDER. THEIR ASSOCIATION WITH FAMILIAL JOINT LAXITY. J. BONE JOINT SURG. 42B* 721-727, 1960.

16910 PATENT DUCTUS ARTERIOSUS (PDA)

OCCASIONALLY PATENT DUCTUS ARTERIOSUS OCCURS IN SO MANY MEMBERS OF MULTIPLE GENERATIONS OF A FAMILY THAT SIMPLE AUTOSOMAL DOMINANT INHERITANCE SEEMS LIKELY. FOR EXAMPLE, BURMAN (1961) DESCRIBED PDA IN A GIRL, HER FATHER AND TWO PATERNAL AUNTS WITH THE PATERNAL GRANDFATHER AND SOME OTHER MEMBERS OF THE FAMILY POSSIBLY ALSO AFFECTED. GOODYEAR (1961) OBSERVED A FAMILY IN WHICH THE MOTHER HAD PATENT DUCTUS ARTERIOSUS AND TWO OF HER THREE CHILDREN HAD PERSISTENT TRUNCUS ARTERIOSUS. AN ESTABLISHED EXOGENOUS CAUSE OF PDA IS MATERNAL RUBELLA.

BURMAN, D.* FAMILIAL PATENT DUCTUS ARTERIOSUS. BRIT. HEART J. 23* 603-604, 1961.

GOODYEAR, J. E.* PERSISTENT TRUNCUS ARTERIOSUS IN TWO SIBLINGS. BRIT. HEART J. 23* 194-196, 1961.

LYNCH, H. T., GRISSOM, R. L., MAGNUSON, C. R. AND KRUSH, A.* PATENT DUCTUS ARTERIOSUS* STUDY OF TWO FAMILIES. J.A.M.A. 194* 135-138, 1965.

16920 PECHET FACTOR DEFICIENCY

PECHET (1964, 1966) DESCRIBED A *NEW* CLOTTING DEFECT IN A 15 YEAR OLD BOY, HIS MOTHER, ONE BROTHER AND ONE SISTER. THE PROBAND HAD FREQUENT TRAUMATIC HEMORR-HAGES. THE RELATIVES WITH LABORATORY ABNORMALITIES WERE ASYMPTOMATIC. THE MATERNAL GRANDFATHER ALSO SHOWED A DEFECT OF CLOTTING. THE AUTHORS SUGGESTED THAT THESE PERSONS LACK A CLOTTING FACTOR WHICH PLAYS A ROLE IN THE FIRST PHASE OF COAGULATION, FOLLOWING THE ACTIVATION OF FACTOR IX BUT BEFORE THE ACTIVATION OF FACTOR X.

PECHET, L., GOLDSTEIN, C. AND DEYKIN, D.* A HITHERTO UNDESCRIBED HEREDOFAMILIAL CLOTTING DEFECT. BLOOD 24* 854-855, 1964.

PECHET, L., GOLDSTEIN, C., COCHIOS, F. AND DEYKIN, D.* A PREVIOUSLY UNDESCRIBED HEREDITARY CLOTTING ABNORMALITY. THROMB. DIATH. HAEMORRH. 20 (SUPPL.)* 269-274, 1966.

16930 PECTUS EXCAVATUM

STODDARD (1939) REPORTED AN EXTENSIVELY AFFECTED FAMILY WITH A PATTERN CONSISTENT WITH AUTOSOMAL DOMINANT INHERITANCE. THIS DEFORMITY ALSO OCCURS IN THE MARFAN SYNDROME AND SOME OTHER HEREDITARY DISORDERS. NOWAK (1936) TRACED PECTUS EXCAVATUM IN 2-4 GENERATIONS IN 12 FAMILIES. A GENERATION WAS SKIPPED IN 5 FAMILIES.

NOWAK, H.* DIE ERBLICHE TRICHTERBRUST. DEUTSCH. MED. WSCHR. 62* 2003-2004, 1936.

PEIPER, A.* UBER DIE ERBLICHKEIT DER TRICHTERBRUST. KLIN. WSCHR. 1* 1647 ONLY, 1922.

SAINSBURY, H. S. K.* CONGENITAL FUNNEL CHEST. LANCET 2* 615-616, 1947.

224   SNYDER, L. H. AND CURTIS, G. M.* AN INHERITED 'HOLLOW CHEST,' KOILOSTERNIA, A
NEW CHARACTER DEPENDENT UPON A DOMINANT AUTOSOMAL GENE. J. HERED. 25* 445-447,
1934.

D
O   STODDARD, S. E.* THE INHERITANCE OF 'HOLLOW CHEST' 'COBBLER'S CHEST' DUE TO
M   HEREDITY-NOT AN OCCUPATIONAL DEFORMITY. J. HERED. 30* 139-141, 1939.
I
N   *16940 PELGER-HUET ANOMALY
A
N   THE NUCLEUS OF THE GRANULOCYTES IS HYPOSEGMENTED, BEING ROD-LIKE, DUMBBELL,
T   PEANUT-SHAPED OR SPECTACLE-LIKE. IN SPOKANE, WASH., LUDDEN AND HARVEY (1962)
FOUND 4 CASES AMONG 43,000 PERSONS. AFFECTED PERSONS WERE OF GERMAN OR DUTCH
DESCENT. IN CLEVELAND, SKENDZEL AND HOFFMAN (1962) FOUND A FREQUENCY OF 1 IN 4785
ROUTINE SMEARS. ALL FIGURES IN THIS COUNTRY AND ALSO THAT OF DAVIDSON IN ENGLAND
(1 IN 6000) ARE LOWER THAN THAT OF NACHTSHEIM (1 IN 1020). THIS ANOMALY ALSO IS
FOUND IN THE RABBIT. THE HOMOZYGOTE IN THE RABBIT HAS CHONDRODYSTROPHY (NACHT-
SHEIM, 1950). SKELETAL ABNORMALITY APPARENTLY DOES NOT OCCUR IN THE HUMAN
HOMOZYGOTE (STOBBE AND JORKE, 1965). SEE MUSCULAR DYSTROPHY, PROXIMAL, FOR
INFORMATION ON LINKAGE. RIOUX ET AL. (1968) REPORTED AN EXTENSIVELY AFFECTED
FRENCH CANADIAN KINDRED. THE NUCLEI OF LEUKOCYTES HAD A PINCE-NEZ APPEARANCE.

LUDDEN, T. E. AND HARVEY, M.* PELGER-HUET ANOMALY OF LEUKOCYTES. REPORT OF A
CASE AND SURVEY OF INCIDENCE. AM. J. CLIN. PATH. 37* 302-304, 1962.

NACHTSHEIM, H.* THE PELGER-ANOMALY IN MAN AND RABBIT* MENDELIAN CHARACTER OF
THE NUCLEI OF THE LEUCOCYTES. J. HERED. 41* 131-137, 1950.

RIOUX, E., ST.-ARNEAULT, G. AND BROSSEAU, C.* THE PELGER-HUET ANOMALY OF
LEUKOCYTES* DESCRIPTION OF A QUEBEC KINDRED. CANAD. MED. ASS. J. 99* 621-624,
1968.

ROSSE, W. F. AND GURNEY, C. W.* THE PELGER-HUET ANOMALY IN THREE FAMILIES AND
ITS USES IN DETERMINING THE DISAPPEARANCE OF TRANSFUSED NEUTROPHILS FROM THE
PERIPHERAL BLOOD. BLOOD 14* 170-186, 1959.

SKENDZEL, L. P. AND HOFFMAN, G. C.* THE PELGER ANOMALY OF LEUKOCYTES* FORTY-ONE
CASES IN SEVEN FAMILIES. AM. J. CLIN. PATH. 37* 294-301, 1962.

STOBBE, H. AND JORKE, D.* BEFUNDE AN HOMOZYGOTEN PELGER-MERKMALSTRAGERN.
SCHWEIZ. MED. WSCHR. 95* 1524-1529, 1965.

*16950 PELIZAEUS-MERZBACHER DISEASE (LATE FORM)

ZERBIN-RUDIN AND PEIFFER (1964) DESCRIBED A LATE FORM OF THIS CONDITION WHICH
SHOWED AUTOSOMAL DOMINANT INHERITANCE RATHER THAN X-LINKED INHERITANCE TYPICAL OF
THE FORM WITH EARLY ONSET. THE DISEASE SIMULATED DISSEMINATED SCLEROSIS IN SOME
RESPECTS. IT MAY BE THE SAME DISORDER AS THAT REPORTED BY CAMP AND LOWENBERG
(1941).

CAMP, C. D. AND LOWENBERG, K.* AN AMERICAN FAMILY WITH PELIZAEUS-MERZBACHER
DISEASE. ARCH. NEUROL. PSYCHIAT. 45* 261-264, 1941.

ZERBIN-RUDIN, E. AND PEIFFER, J.* EIN GENETISCHER BEITRAG ZUR FRAGE DER
SPATFORM DER PELIZAEUS-MERZBACHERSCHEN KRANKHEIT. HUMANGENETIK 1* 107-122, 1964.

*16960 PEMPHIGUS, BENIGN FAMILIAL (HAILEY-HAILEY DISEASE)

RECURRENT ERUPTION OF VESICLES AND BULLAE INVOLVING PREDOMINANTLY THE NECK, GROIN
AND AXILLARY REGIONS IS CHARACTERISTIC. HISTOLOGICAL EXAMINATION SHOWS NUMEROUS
ACANTHOLYTIC CELLS AND THE SUPRA-BASAL TYPE OF BLISTER FORMATION, STRIKINGLY
RESEMBLING THOSE IN PEMPHIGUS VULGARIS MALIGNUS. LOEWENTHAL (1959) THOUGHT THAT
PYOGENIC BACTERIA ACT AS A PRECIPITATING FACTOR. THIS POSSIBILITY IS SUPPORTED BY
THE BENEFICIAL EFFECTS OF ANTIBIOTICS, USE OF WHICH HAS CONVERTED THIS CONDITION
INTO A RELATIVELY INSIGNIFICANT DISORDER. IN FOUR CASES OF ONE FAMILY, BURNS ET
AL. (1967) WILSON ET AL. (1968) FOUND CANDIDA ALBICANS IN THE LESIONS AND FOUND
THAT THE FUNGUS WOULD INDUCE LESIONS IN PREVIOUSLY UNINVOLVED SKIN.

BURNS, R. A., REED, W. B., SWATEK, F. E. AND OMIECZYNSKI, D. T.* FAMILIAL
BENIGN CHRONIC PEMPHIGUS. INDUCTION OF LESIONS BY CANDIDA ALBICANS. ARCH. DERM.
96* 254-258, 1967.

ELLIS, F. A.* VESICULAR DARIER'S DISEASE (SO-CALLED BENIGN FAMILIAL PEMPHIGUS).
ARCH. DERM. SYPH. 61* 715-736, 1950.

HAILEY, H. AND HAILEY, H.* FAMILIAL BENIGN CHRONIC PEMPHIGUS. REPORT OF 13
CASES IN 4 GENERATIONS OF A FAMILY AND REPORT OF 9 ADDITIONAL CASES IN 4 GENERA-
TIONS OF A FAMILY. ARCH. DERM. SYPH. 39* 679-685, 1939.

LOEWENTHAL, L. J. A.* FAMILIAL BENIGN CHRONIC PEMPHIGUS. THE ROLE OF PYOGENIC
BACTERIA. ARCH. DERM. 80* 318-326, 1959.

POLANO, M. K.* PEMPHIGUS BENIGNUS FAMILIARIS (WITH SPECIAL REFERENCE TO THE

WILSON, J. W., BURNS, R. A., REED, W. B. AND HAGERMAN, R. D.* PENFIGO FAMILIAR BENIGNO CRONICO. LESIONES INDUCIDAS POR 'CANDIDA ALBICANS.' MEDICINA CUTANEA 3* 275-280, 1968.

WINER, L. H. AND LEEB, A. J.* BENIGN FAMILIAL PEMPHIGUS. ARCH. DERM. 67* 77-83, 1953.

16970 PEPSINOGEN

SAMLOFF AND TOWNES (1970) SHOWED THAT THE PEPSINOGEN 5 DERIVED FROM THE STOMACH AND EXCRETED IN THE URINE IS ABSENT IN SOME PERSONS. FAMILY AND POPULATION DATA SUPPORTED THE VIEW THAT ABSENCE OF PEPSINOGEN 5 IS RECESSIVE, I.E., PERSONS WITH THE PEPSINOGEN 5 BAND ON ELECTROPHORESIS ARE EITHER HOMOZYGOUS OR HETEROZYGOUS FOR A PARTICULAR ALLELE.

SAMLOFF, I. M. AND TOWNES, P. L.* PEPSINOGENS* GENETIC POLYMORPHISM IN MAN. SCIENCE 168* 144-145, 1970.

*16980 PEPTIDASE A

LEWIS ET AL. (1968) HAVE IDENTIFIED GENETICALLY VARIABLE PEPTIDASES DETERMINED BY ALLELES AT TWO SEPARATE AND NOT CLOSELY LINKED STRUCTURAL LOCI (PEP A AND PEP B). THE PEPTIDASES STUDIED ARE PRESENT IN RED CELLS AND ARE CAPABLE OF HYDROLYZING DI-AND TRI-PEPTIDES. FIVE DISTINCT ENZYMES A, B, C, D AND E HAVE BEEN IDENTIFIED. LEWIS AND HARRIS (1969) STATED THAT PEPTIDASES A, B, C AND D ARE PRODUCTS OF SEPARATE GENE LOCI AND THAT E PROBABLY IS ALSO.

LEWIS, W. H. P. AND HARRIS, H.* HUMAN RED CELL PEPTIDASES. NATURE 215* 351-355, 1967.

LEWIS, W. H. P. AND HARRIS, H.* MOLECULAR SIZE ESTIMATES OF HUMAN PEPTIDASES DETERMINED BY SEPARATE GENE LOCI. ANN. HUM. GENET. 33* 89-92, 1969.

LEWIS, W. H. P., CORNEY, G. AND HARRIS, H.* PEP A5-1 AND PEP A6-1* TWO NEW VARIANTS OF PEPTIDASE A WITH FEATURES OF SPECIAL INTEREST. ANN. HUM. GENET. 32* 35-42, 1968.

*16990 PEPTIDASE B

SEE PEPTIDASE A. THE PEPTIDASE B LOCUS IS LINKED TO THE LDH-B LOCUS (RUDDLE ET AL., 1970).

BLAKE, N. M., KIRK, R. L., LEWIS, W. H. P. AND HARRIS, H.* SOME FURTHER PEPTIDASE B PHENOTYPES. ANN. HUM. GENET. 33* 301-305, 1970.

RUDDLE, F. H., CHAPMAN, V. M., CHEN, T. R. AND KLEBE, R. J.* LINKAGE BETWEEN HUMAN LACTATE DEHYDROGENASE A AND B AND PEPTIDASE B. NATURE 227* 251-257, 1970.

*17000 PEPTIDASE C

SEE PEPTIDASE A. AMONG THE BABINGA PYGMIES BENERECETTI (1970) FOUND POLYMORPHISM OF PEPTIDASE C AND PROVIDED THE FIRST EVIDENCE ON THE GENETICS OF THIS RED CELL ENZYME. THREE ALLELES WERE POSTULATED, ONE OF WHICH IS SILENT AND HAS A FREQUENCY OF 0.208 IN THE POPULATION STUDIED. NO ABNORMALITY WAS DETECTED IN PERSONS WITH DEFICIENCY OF THE ENZYME.

BENERECETTI, S. A. S.* STUDIES OF AFRICAN PYGMIES. III. PEPTIDASE C POLYMOR-PHISM IN BABINGA PYGMIES* A FREQUENT ERYTHROCYTIC ENZYME DEFICIENCY. AM. J. HUM. GENET. 22* 228-231, 1970.

*17010 PEPTIDASE D

LEWIS AND HARRIS (1969) IDENTIFIED A NUMBER OF ELECTROPHORETIC VARIANTS OF PEPTIDASE D OF RED CELLS.

LEWIS, W. H. P. AND HARRIS, H.* PEPTIDASE D (PROLIDASE) VARIANTS IN MAN. ANN. HUM. GENET. 32* 317-322, 1969.

*17020 PEPTIDASE E

SEE PEPTIDASE A.

*17030 PERIODIC FEVER

BOURONCLE AND DOAN (1957) DESCRIBED 12 CASES OF PERIODIC FEVER IN 6 SIBSHIPS IN 5 GENERATIONS OF A FAMILY. NO ABNORMALITY WAS DETECTED BY CLINICAL EXAMINATIONS DURING AND BETWEEN ATTACKS OR BY MANY LABORATORY STUDIES. IN TWO BROTHERS WITH PERIODIC FEVER, DRIESSEN ET AL. (1968) FOUND THAT THE NON-ESTERIFIED ETIOCHOLANO-LONE LEVEL OF THE BLOOD WAS RAISED NOT ONLY DURING FEBRILE ATTACKS BUT ALSO IN FEVER-FREE PERIODS. A SISTER HAD ATTACKS OF FEVER OF UNEXPLAINED ORIGIN ACCOM-

PANIED BY ABDOMINAL PAIN AND RASH BUT HAD NO SYMPTOMS AFTER MENARCHE.

BOURONCLE, B. A. AND DOAN, C. A.* 'PERIODIC FEVER.' OCCURRENCE IN FIVE GENERATIONS. AM. J. MED. 23* 502-506, 1957.

DRIESSEN, O., VOUTE, P. A., JR. AND VERMEULEN, A.* A DESCRIPTION OF TWO BROTHERS WITH PERMANENTLY RAISED NON-ESTERIFIED AETIOCHOLANOLONE BLOOD LEVEL. ACTA ENDOCR. 57* 177-186, 1968.

*17040 PERIODIC PARALYSIS I (HYPOKALEMIC TYPE)

THE CLASSIC PICTURE IS EPISODIC WEAKNESS ACCOMPANIED BY LOW SERUM POTASSIUM LEVELS. THE ATTACKS ARE ABORTED BY ADMINISTRATION OF POTASSIUM OR BY EXERCISE AND ARE PRECIPITATED BY INSULIN OR GLUCOSE ADMINSTRATION.

CUSINS, P. J. AND VAN ROOYEN, R. J.* FAMILIAL PERIODIC PARALYSIS. SEVEN CASES IN A DURBAN FAMILY. S. AFR. MED. J. 37* 1180-1183, 1963.

STREETEN, D. H. P.* PERIODIC PARALYSIS. IN STANBURY, J. B., WYNGAARDEN, J. B. AND FREDRICKSON, D. S. (EDS.)* THE METABOLIC BASIS OF INHERITED DISEASE. NEW YORK* MCGRAW-HILL, 1966 (2ND ED.). PP. 905-938.

TALBOTT, J. H.* PERIODIC PARALYSIS* A CLINICAL SYNDROME. MEDICINE 20* 85-143, 1941.

*17050 PERIODIC PARALYSIS II (HYPERKALEMIC TYPE)

MYOTONIC SYMPTOMS IN PERIODIC PARALYSIS CAN BE A CLUE THAT THE DISORDER IS OF THE HYPERKALEMIC TYPE. OCULAR MUSCLE MYOTONIA IS INDICATED BY SLOW OPENING OF THE LIDS AFTER FORCED ACTIVE CLOSURE OF THE EYES. POTASSIUM PRECIPITATES WEAKNESS. GAMSTORP (1956, 1963) WHO FIRST DESCRIBED HYPERKALEMIC PERIODIC PARALYSIS (CALLING IT ADYNAMIA EPISODICA HEREDITARIA) DID NOT FIND MYOTONIA IN HER CASES. WHETHER TWO DISTINCT ENTITIES ARE REPRESENTED IS NOT CLEAR. MYOTONIA WAS PRESENT IN SAMAHA'S FAMILY (1965). KRULL ET AL. (1966) CLAIMED TO HAVE DEMONSTRATED A HUMORAL SUBSTANCE, NOT POTASSIUM, ORIGINATING FROM THE CONTRACTING MUSCLES OF THE FOREARM AND PRODUCING STRIKING GENERALIZED MYOTONIA. VAN'T HOFF (1962) FOUND NINE AFFECTED PERSONS IN FOUR GENERATIONS. ALL SUFFERED FROM PERIODIC ATTACKS OF WEAKNESS WHICH COULD BE INDUCED BY ADMINISTERING POTASSIUM AND ALLEVIATED BY ADMINISTERING OF CALCIUM. BOTH BETWEEN AND DURING ATTACKS, AFFECTED PERSONS HAD MYOTONIC LID LAG LASTING 15-20 SECONDS AFTER ELEVATION OF THE EYES. THE FAMILY OF SAUNDERS ET AL. (1968) SHOWED MYOTONIC PERIODIC PARALYSIS WITH MUSCLE WASTING.

ARMSTRONG, F. S.* HYPERKALEMIC FAMILIAL PERIODIC PARALYSIS (ADYNAMIA EPISODICA HEREDITARIA). ANN. INTERN. MED. 57* 455-461, 1962.

GAMSTORP, I.* ADYNAMIA EPISODICA HEREDITARIA AND MYOTONIA. ACTA NEUROL. SCAND. 39* 41-58, 1963.

GAMSTORP, I.* ADYNAMIA EPISODICA HEREDITARIA. ACTA PAEDIAT. 45 (SUPPL. 108)* 1-126, 1956.

HERMAN, R. H. AND MCDOWELL, M. K.* HYPERKALEMIC PARALYSIS (ADYNAMIA EPISODICA HEREDITARIA). REPORT OF 4 CASES AND CLINICAL STUDIES. AM. J. MED. 35* 749-767, 1963.

KRULL, G. H., LEIJNSE, B., DE VLIEGER, M., VIETOR, W. P. J., TER BRAAK, J. W. G. AND GERBRANDY, J.* MYOTONIA PRODUCED BY AN UNKNOWN HUMORAL SUBSTANCE. LANCET 2* 668-672, 1966.

LAYZER, R. B., LOVELACE, R. E. AND ROWLAND, L. P.* HYPERKALEMIC PERIODIC PARALYSIS. ARCH. NEUROL. 16* 455-472, 1967.

SAMAHA, F. J.* HYPERKALEMIC PERIODIC PARALYSIS. A GENETIC STUDY, CLINICAL OBSERVATIONS, AND REPORT OF A NEW METHOD OF THERAPY. ARCH. NEUROL. 12* 145-154, 1965.

SAUNDERS, M., ASHWORTH, B., EMERY, A. E. H. AND BENEDIKZ, J. E. G.* FAMILIAL MYOTONIC PERIODIC PARALYSIS WITH MUSCLE WASTING. BRAIN 91* 295-304, 1968.

VAN'T HOFF, W.* FAMILIAL MYOTONIC PERIODIC PARALYSIS. QUART. J. MED. 31* 385-402, 1962.

*17060 PERIODIC PARALYSIS III (NORMOKALEMIC TYPE)

IN THE FAMILY REPORTED BY POSKANZER AND KERR (1961) 21 MEMBERS WERE AFFECTED. IN ADDITION TO NORMOKALEMIA, FAVORABLE RESPONSE TO SODIUM CHLORIDE WAS AN UNUSUAL FEATURE.

POSKANZER, D. C. AND KERR, D. N. S.* A THIRD TYPE OF PERIODIC PARALYSIS, WITH NORMOKALEMIA AND FAVORABLE RESPONSE TO SODIUM CHLORIDE. AM. J. MED. 31* 328-342, 1961.

SINGLETON, DAESCHNER AND TENG (1960) REPORTED A FORM OF DYSOSTOSIS LIMITED ESSENTIALLY TO THE TUBULAR BONES OF THE HANDS AND FEET. THE EPIPHYSES IN THE FINGERS ARE CONICAL IN SHAPE WITH THEIR APEX SET INTO THE METAPHYSEAL ENDS OF THE PHALANGES (WHICH LOOK LIKE THE BOTTOM OF WINE-BOTTLES). THE CONE-SHAPED EPIPHYSES IN THE PHALANGES WITH A PAUCITY OF SIGNS AND SYMPTOMS ELSEWHERE IS CHARACTERISTIC. BACHMAN AND NORMAN (1967) REPORTED AFFECTED MOTHER AND HER SON AND DAUGHTER, THE MOTHER, AGE 47, WAS 61.5 INCHES TALL, HAD SHORT FINGERS AND SUFFERED FROM SEVERE OSTEOARTHRITIS OF THE HIPS. THIS IS PROBABLY A HETEROGENEOUS CATEGORY IN WHICH ONE ENTITY IS THE CONDITION TERMED ACRODYSOSTOSIS (Q.V.), IN WHICH PUG NOSE, OPEN MOUTH AND PROGNATHISM, TOGETHER WITH MENTAL DEFICIENCY ARE ADDITIONAL FEATURES. CHANGES WERE ALMOST LIMITED TO THE HANDS AND FEET IN THE PATIENT REPORTED BY COHEN AND VAN CREVELD (1963). THE FACIES WERE CHARACTERIZED BY PUG NOSE AND SUNKEN BRIDGE BUT THE SKULL DID NOT SUGGEST ACHONDROPLASIA. INTELLIGENCE WAS CONSIDERED NORMAL.

BACHMAN, R. K. AND NORMAN, A. P.* HEREDITARY PERIPHERAL DYSOSTOSIS (THREE CASES). PROC. ROY. SOC. MED. 60* 21 ONLY, 1967.

COHEN, P. AND VAN CREVELD, S.* PERIPHERAL DYSOSTOSIS. BRIT. J. RADIOL. 36* 761-765, 1963.

NEWCOMBE, D. S. AND KEATS, T. E.* ROENTGENOGRAPHIC MANIFESTATIONS OF HEREDITARY PERIPHERAL DYSOSTOSIS. AM. J. ROENTGEN. 106* 178-189, 1969.

SINGLETON, E. B., DAESCHNER, C. W. AND TENG, C. T.* PERIPHERAL DYSOSTOSIS. AM. J. ROENTGEN. 84* 499-505, 1960.

17080 PERIPHERAL DYSOSTOSIS AND MENTAL RETARDATION

THE PATIENT REPORTED BY ARKLESS AND GRAHAM (1967) RESEMBLES A CASE WITH THIS COMBINATION I HAVE OBSERVED (C.M., 381867). NO GENETICALLY RELEVANT INFORMATION IS AVAILABLE. ROBINOW ET AL. (1971) REPORTED 9 CASES. NO FAMILIAL INCIDENCE OR PARENTAL CONSANGUINITY WAS OBSERVED.

ARKLESS, R. AND GRAHAM, C. B.* AN UNUSUAL CASE OF BRACHYDACTYLY. AM. J. ROENTGEN. 99* 724-735, 1967.

ROBINOW, M., PFEIFFER, R. A., GORLIN, R. J., MCKUSICK, V. A., RENUART, A. W., JOHNSON, G. F. AND SUMMITT, R. L.* ACRODYSOSTOSIS. A SYNDROME OF PERIPHERAL DYSOSTOSIS, NASAL HYPOPLASIA, AND MENTAL RETARDATION. AM. J. DIS. CHILD. 121* 195-203, 1971.

17090 PERNICIOUS ANEMIA

IN THE RELATIVES OF THIRTY-FOUR PERNICIOUS ANEMIA PROBANDS, MCINTYRE AND HER ASSOCIATES (1959) TESTED THE ABILITY TO ABSORB ORALLY GIVEN DOSES OF COBALT-60 LABELLED VITAMIN B12 (SCHILLING TEST). THE RELATIVES OF PERNICIOUS ANEMIA PATIENTS SHOWED A NEGATIVE CORRELATION WITH AGE* CONTROL SUBJECTS DID NOT. THE RELATIVES SHOWED A TENDENCY TO BIMODALITY. 48 PERCENT OF SIBS AND 32 PERCENT OF OFFSPRING HAD ABNORMAL ABSORPTION. THE AUTHORS SUGGESTED AUTOSOMAL DOMINANT INHERITANCE. WANGEL ET AL. (1968) SUGGESTED THAT THE TENDENCY TO FORM AUTOANTIBO- DIES AGAINST GASTRIC PARIETAL CELLS MAY BE INHERITED AS A DOMINANT WITH INCOMPLETE PENETRANCE. LATER STUDIES (MCINTYRE, 1968) YIELDED RESULTS WHICH MAKE A SIMPLE GENETIC HYPOTHESIS DIFFICULT TO SUPPORT.

MCINTYRE, P. A.* GENETIC AND AUTO-IMMUNE FEATURES OF PERNICIOUS ANEMIA. I. UNRELIABILITY OF THE SCHILLING TEST IN DETECTING GENETIC PREDISPOSITION TO THE DISEASE. JOHNS HOPKINS MED. J. 122* 181-183, 1968.

MCINTYRE, P. A., HAHN, R., CONLEY, C. L. AND GLASS, B.* GENETIC FACTORS IN PREDISPOSITION TO PERNICIOUS ANEMIA. BULL. HOPKINS HOSP. 104* 309-342, 1959.

WANGEL, A. G., CALLENDER, S. T., SPRAY, G. H. AND WRIGHT, R.* A FAMILY STUDY OF PERNICIOUS ANAEMIA. I. AUTOANTIBODIES, ACHLORHYDRIA, SERUM PEPSINOGEN AND VITAMIN B12. BRIT. J. HAEMAT. 14* 161-181, 1968. II. INTRINSIC FACTOR SECRE- TION, VITAMIN B12 ABSORPTION AND GENETIC ASPECTS OF GASTRIC AUTOIMMUNITY. BRIT. J. HAEMAT. 14* 183-204, 1968.

17100 PEYRONIE'S DISEASE

THIS CONDITION, A FIBROUS CONTRACTURE OF THE PENIS, BEARS CERTAIN FUNDAMENTAL SIMILARITIES TO DUPUYTREN'S CONTRACTURE OF THE HAND AND THE TWO OCCUR RATHER FREQUENTLY IN THE SAME SUBJECT.

MURLEY, R. S.* PEYRONIE'S DISEASE. BRIT. MED. J. 1* 908 ONLY, 1964.

SCHOURUP, K.* PLASTIC INDURATION OF THE PENIS. ACTA RADIOL. 26* 313-323, 1945.

17110 PHAGOCYTOSIS, PLASMA-RELATED DEFECT IN

MILLER ET AL. (1968) DESCRIBED A FAMILIAL DISORDER OF PHAGOCYTOSIS DUE TO A PLASMA-ASSOCIATED DEFECT RATHER THAN A PRIMARY DEFECT OF POLYMORPHONUCLEAR LEUKOCYTE FUNCTION. LEUKOCYTES FROM THE PROBAND, INCUBATED IN HER OWN PLASMA, SHOWED GREATLY DIMINISHED ABILITY TO INGEST YEAST, RICE-STARCH, OR STAPHYLOCOCCUS AUREUS, BUT INGESTED THE SAME PARTICLES NORMALLY IN THE PRESENCE OF HETEROZYGOTES PLASMA. NORMAL LEUKOCYTES SHOWED IMPAIRED PHAGOCYTOSIS WHEN INCUBATED IN PLASMA FROM THE PATIENT. THE MOTHER AND MANY RELATIVES HAD PLASMA WHICH GAVE THE SAME RESULT. THE FATHER AND TWO SIBS WERE 'NEGATIVE.' BOTH MATERNAL GRANDPARENTS AND SIBS OF BOTH OF THEM WERE 'POSITIVE.' CONSANGUINITY OF THESE GRANDPARENTS WAS CONSIDERED POSSIBLE BUT NOT PROVED. INFUSION OF FRESH PLASMA CORRECTED THE DEFICIENCY OF OPSONIZATION AND WAS REGULARLY FOLLOWED BY CLINICAL IMPROVEMENT. THE POSSIBILITY OF NON-PATERNITY WAS APPARENTLY NOT INVESTIGATED. A PRIORI, RECESSIVE INHERITANCE WOULD SEEM MORE LIKELY, THE PROBAND BEING HOMOZYGOUS.

MILLER, M. E., SEALS, J., KAYE, R. AND LEVITSKY, L.* A FAMILIAL, PLASMA-ASSOCIATED DEFECT OF PHAGOCYTOSIS. A NEW CAUSE OF RECURRENT BACTERIAL INFECTIONS. LANCET 2* 60-63, 1968.

*17120 PHENYLTHIOCARBAMIDE (PTC) TASTING

SUPPLEMENTATION OF THE STANDARD TEST USING QUININE IN THE INTERMEDIATE CASES WAS SUGGESTED BY KALMUS (1958). ABILITY TO TASTE IS DOMINANT.

HARRIS, H. AND KALMUS, H.* THE MEASUREMENT OF TASTE SENSITIVITY TO PHENYL-THIOUREA (PTC). ANN. EUGEN. 15* 24-31, 1949.

KALMUS, H.* IMPROVEMENTS IN THE CLASSIFICATION OF THE TASTER GENOTYPES. ANN. HUM. GENET. 22* 222-230, 1958.

17130 PHEOCHROMOCYTOMA

ADRENAL MEDULLARY TUMORS OCCUR SOMETIMES WITH VON HIPPEL-LINDAU SYNDROME (Q.V.), WITH NEUROFIBROMATOSIS (Q.V.), AND WITH FAMILIAL ENDOCRINE ADENOMATOSIS. (SEE NEUROMATA, MUCOSAL, WITH ENDOCRINE TUMORS AND SEE PHEOCHROMOCYTOMA WITH AMYLOID-PRODUCING MEDULLARY THYROID CARCINOMA, AS EXAMPLES OF TWO OTHER SYNDROMES WITH PHEOCHROMOCYTOMA AS A FEATURE.) OCCURRING AS AN ISOLATED DEFECT IT PROBABLY IS ALSO INHERITED AS A SIMPLE DOMINANT IN SOME FAMILIES. THE RELATION OF THE CONDITION IN THE FAMILY REPORTED BY HADORN (1963) IS UNCERTAIN. THREE SIBS HAD ADRENAL TUMORS. A BROTHER AND SISTER SUFFERED FROM TACHYCARDIA, SWEATING, HYPERTENSION AND ALBUMINURIA. THE SISTER HAD ADVANCED HYPERTENSIVE RETINOPATHY AND THE BROTHER HAD CONGESTIVE HEART FAILURE. AT AUTOPSY THE SISTER SHOWED CEREBRAL HEMORRHAGE AND BILATERAL ADRENOCORTICAL TUMORS. A SURVIVING SIB DEVELOPED SIMILAR SYMPTOMS. PHEOCHROMOCYTOMA WAS TENTATIVELY DIAGNOSED. THE REGITINE TEST WAS STRONGLY POSITIVE, THE URINE CONTAINED LARGE AMOUNTS OF NOREPINEPHRINE AND PNEUMOPERITONEUM DEMONSTRATED AN ENLARGED RIGHT ADRENAL. AT OPERATION A MIXED TUMOR CONTAINING HYPERNEPHROMATOUS AND PARAGANGLION TISSUE WAS FOUND. THE VERY LARGE KINDRED STUDIED BY TISHERMAN ET AL. (1962) HAD AT LEAST 7 PATIENTS WITH PHEOCHROMOCYTOMA. ONE OR MORE CAFE-AU-LAIT SPOTS (IN 22 PERSONS), EXTENSIVE HEMANGIOMAS (IN 2 PERSONS) AND ANGIOMATOSIS RETINAE (IN 2 PERSONS) WERE DISCOVERED IN MEMBERS OF THE FAMILY. PHEOCHROMOCYTOMA WAS ASSOCIATED WITH CONGENITAL CATARACTS IN ONE PATIENT AND WITH RENAL ARTERY STENOSIS IN ANOTHER.

CARMAN, C. T. AND BRASHEAR, R. E.* PHEOCHROMOCYTOMA AS AN INHERITED ABNORMALI-TY* REPORT OF THE TENTH AFFECTED KINDRED AND REVIEW OF THE LITERATURE. NEW ENG. J. MED. 263* 419-423, 1960.

COOK, J. E., ULRICH, R. W., SAMPLE, H. G., JR. AND FAWCETT, N. W.* PECULIAR FAMILIAL AND MALIGNANT PHEOCHROMOCYTOMAS OF THE ORGANS OF ZUCKERKANDL. ANN. INTERN. MED. 52* 126-133, 1960.

HADORN, W.* MALIGNE HYPERNEPHROIDE UND PARAGANGLIONARE MISCHGESCHWULSTE DER NEBENNIERE BEI DREI GESCHWISTERN. HELV. MED. ACTA 30* 291-296, 1963.

TISHERMAN, S. E., GREGG, F. J. AND DANOWSKI, T. S.* FAMILIAL PHEOCHROMOCYTOMA. J.A.M.A. 182* 152-156, 1962.

TRADEC, E., MARATKA, Z. AND PALECROVA, M.* LE PHEOCHROMOCYTOME AVEC CARACTERE FAMILIAL. J. CHIR. 81* 479, 1961.

VON DOEPP, C. E.* DAS PHAOCHROMOCYTOM ALS DOMINANT VERERBBARE DYSGENETISCHE GESCHWULST. VIRCHOW. ARCH. PATH. ANAT. 335* 231-239, 1962.

*17140 PHEOCHROMOCYTOMA AND AMYLOID-PRODUCING MEDULLARY THYROID CARCINOMA (PTC SYNDROME)

SCHIMKE AND HARTMANN (1965) DESCRIBED A SYNDROME OF PHEOCHROMOCYTOMA AND MEDULLARY THYROID CARCINOMA WITH ABUNDANT AMYLOID STROMA. A SIMILAR ALTHOUGH PERHAPS DISTINCT CONDITION IS DESCRIBED UNDER 'NEUROMATA, MUCOSAL, WITH ENDOCRINE TUMORS.' STEINER ET AL. (1967) DESCRIBED A FAMILY WITH 11 CASES IN SUCCESSIVE GENERATIONS. THE PHEOCHROMOCYTOMAS WERE BILATERAL. PARATHYROID ADENOMA WAS PRESENT IN SEVERAL. ONE PATIENT HAD CUSHING'S SYNDROME. URBANSKI (1967) ALSO FOUND PARATHYROID ADENOMA TO BE PART OF THE SYNDROME. MEYER AND ABDEL-BARI (1968) PRESENTED

OBSERVATIONS CONSISTENT WITH THE VIEW THAT MEDULLARY CARCINOMA IS A THYROCALCI-TONIN-PRODUCING NEOPLASM OF PARAFOLLICULAR CELLS OF THE THYROID. PARATHYROID HYPERPLASIA OR ADENOMAS IN SOME OF THESE PATIENTS MAY BE SECONDARY TO HYPOCALCEMIC EFFECTS OF THYROCALCITONIN. JOHNSTON ET AL. (1970), AS WELL AS OTHERS, HAVE SHOWN CALCITONIN-SECRETION BY MEDULLARY THYROID CARCINOMA. STEINER ET AL. (1967) REFERRED TO THIS DISORDER AS "MULTIPLE ENDOCRINE NEOPLASIA, TYPE 2" TO DISTINGUISH IT FROM THE MULTIPLE ENDOCRINE ADENOMATOSIS DESCRIBED BY WERMER (Q.V.), CALLED TYPE I BY STEINER ET AL. (1967). KAPLAN ET AL. (1970) SHOWED THAT THE ADRENAL MEDULLA PRODUCES A CALCITONIN-LIKE MATERIAL INDISTINGUISHABLE FROM THAT OF THE THYROID BY BIO- AND RADIOIMMUNOASSAY. THEY SUGGEST THAT THE PARAFOLLICULAR CELLS OF THE THYROID ARE OF NEURAL CREST ORIGIN. THE FINDING THAT MEDULLARY CARCINOMA OF THE THYROID ARISES FROM PARAFOLLICULAR CELLS AND THAT LIKE THE CELL OF ORIGIN IT SOMETIMES PRODUCES THYROCALCITONIN MAY ACCOUNT FOR THE ASSOCIATION OF PARA-THYROID HYPERPLASIA AND PERHAPS PARATHYROID ADENOMA. PALOYAN ET AL. (1970) WAS IMPRESSED WITH THE HISTOLOGIC SIMILARITY BETWEEN THE MEDULLARY THYROID CANCER AND PHEOCHROMOCYTOMA METASTASES.

BLOCK, M. A., HORN, R. C., JR., MILLER, J. M., BARRETT, J. L. AND BRUSH, B. E.* FAMILIAL MEDULLARY CARCINOMA OF THE THYROID. ANN. SURG. 166* 403-412, 1967.

CUSHMAN, P., JR.* FAMILIAL ENDOCRINE TUMORS. REPORT OF TWO UNRELATED KINDRED AFFECTED WITH PHEOCHROMOCYTOMAS, ONE ALSO WITH MULTIPLE THYROID CARCINOMAS. AM. J. MED. 32* 352-360, 1962.

JOHNSTON, C. I., MARTIN, T. J. AND RIDDELL, J.* MEDULLARY THYROID CARCINOMA* A FUNCTIONAL PEPTIDE SECRETING TUMOR. AUST. ANN. MED. 19* 50-53, 1970.

KAPLAN, E. L., ARNAUD, C. D., HILL, B. J. AND PESKIN, G. W.* ADRENAL MEDULLARY CALCITONIN-LIKE FACTOR* A KEY TO MULTIPLE ENDOCRINE NEOPLASIA, TYPE 2.Q SURGERY 68* 146-149, 1970.

MEYER, J. S. AND ABDEL-BARI, W.* GRANULES AND THYROCALCITONIN-LIKE ACTIVITY IN MEDULLARY CARCINOMA OF THE THYROID GLAND. NEW ENG. J. MED. 278* 523-529, 1968.

POLOYAN, E., SCANU, A., STRAUS, F. H., PICKLEMAN, J. R. AND PALOYAN, D.* FAMILIAL PHEOCHROMOCYTOMA, MEDULLARY THYROID CARCINOMA, AND PARATHYROID ADENOMAS. J.A.M.A. 214* 1443-1447, 1970.

SAROSI, G. AND DOE, R. P.* FAMILIAL OCCURRENCE OF PARATHYROID ADENOMAS, PHEOCHROMOCYTOMA, AND MEDULLARY CARCINOMA OF THE THYROID WITH AMYLOID STROMA (SIPPLE'S SYNDROME). ANN. INTERN. MED. 68* 1305-1309, 1968.

SCHIMKE, R. N. AND HARTMANN, W. H.* FAMILIAL AMYLOID-PRODUCING MEDULLARY THYROID CARCINOMA AND PHEOCHROMOCYTOMA, A DISTINCT GENETIC ENTITY. ANN. INTERN. MED. 63* 1027-1039, 1965.

SIPPLE, J. H.* THE ASSOCIATION OF PHEOCHROMOCYTOMA WITH CARCINOMA OF THE THYROID GLAND. AM. J. MED. 31* 163-166, 1961.

STEINER, A. L., GOODMAN, A. D. AND POWERS, S. R., JR.* STUDY OF A KINDRED WITH PHEOCHROMOCYTOMA, MEDULLARY THYROID CARCINOMA, HYPERPARATHYROIDISM AND CUSHING'S DISEASE* MULTIPLE ENDOCRINE NEOPLASIA, TYPE 2. MEDICINE 47* 371-409, 1968.

TASHJIAN, A. H., JR. AND MELVIN, K. E. W.* MEDULLARY CARCINOMA OF THE THYROID* THYROCALCITONIN IN PLASMA AND TUMOR. NEW ENG. J. MED. 279* 279-283, 1968.

URBANSKI, F. X.* MEDULLARY THYROID CARCINOMA, PARATHYROID ADENOMA, AND BILATERAL PHEOCHROMOCYTOMA. AN UNUSUAL TRIAD OF ENDOCRINE TUMORS. J. CHRONIC DIS. 20* 627-636, 1967.

*17150 PHOSPHATASE, ACID, OF ERYTHROCYTE

HOPKINSON, SPENCER AND HARRIS, (1963) DESCRIBED A NEW HUMAN POLYMORPHISM INVOLVING ERYTHROCYTE ACID PHOSPHATASE AS DEMONSTRATED IN STARCH-GEL ELECTROPHORESIS. THREE ALLELES, P-(A), P-(B) AND P-(C) ARE THOUGHT TO BE INVOLVED, THEIR FREQUENCY BEING ESTIMATED TO BE ABOUT 0.35, 0.60 AND 0.05, RESPECTIVELY. ANOTHER RARE ALLELE, P(R), WAS DESCRIBED BY GIBLETT AND SCOTT (1965).

FUHRMANN, W. AND LICHTE, K.-H.* HUMAN RED CELL ACID PHOSPHATASE POLYMORPHISM. A STUDY ON GENE FREQUENCY AND FORENSIC USE OF THE SYSTEM IN CASES OF DISPUTED PATERNITY. HUMANGENETIK 3* 121-126, 1966.

GIBLETT, E. R. AND SCOTT, N. M.* RED CELL ACID PHOSPHATASE* RACIAL DISTRIBUTION AND REPORT OF A NEW PHENOTYPE. AM. J. HUM. GENET. 17* 425-432, 1965.

HERBICH, J., FISHER, R. A. AND HOPKINSON, D. A.* ATYPICAL SEGREGATION OF HUMAN RED CELL ACID PHOSPHATASE PHENOTYPES* EVIDENCE FOR A RARE "SILENT" ALLELE P(O). ANN. HUM. GENET. 34* 145-152, 1970.

HOPKINSON, D. A., SPENCER, N. AND HARRIS, H.* RED CELL ACID PHOSPHATASE VARIANTS* A NEW HUMAN POLYMORPHISM. NATURE 199* 969-971, 1963.

KARP, G. W., JR. AND SUTTON, H. E.* SOME NEW PHENOTYPES OF HUMAN RED CELL ACID PHOSPHATASE. AM. J. HUM. GENET. 19* 54-62, 1967.

17160 PHOSPHATASE, ACID, OF PLACENTA AND LEUKOCYTES

BECKMAN ET AL. (1970) STUDIED A RARE VARIANT OF PLACENTAL AND LEUKOCYTE ACID PHOSPHATASE PRESUMABLY UNDER THE CONTROL OF A LOCUS SEPARATE FROM THAT DETERMINING THE RED CELL ACID PHOSPHATASE POLYMORPHISM.

BECKMAN, G., BECKMAN, L. AND TARNVIK, A.* A RARE SUBUNIT VARIANT SHARED BY FIVE ACID PHOSPHATASE ISOZYMES FROM HUMAN LEUKOCYTES AND PLACENTAE. HUM. HERED. 20* 81-85, 1970.

17170 PHOSPHATASE, ALKALINE, BLOOD-GROUP-ASSOCIATED

BOTH THE ABO AND THE SECRETOR LOCI INFLUENCE THE APPEARANCE OF ALKALINE PHOSPHATASE IN THE SERUM. MANY UNCERTAINTIES ABOUT THE GENETIC CONTROL OF ALKALINE PHOSPHATASE EXIST.

BECKMAN, L., BJORLING, G. AND HEIKEN, A.* HUMAN ALKALINE PHOSPHATASES AND THE FACTORS CONTROLLING THEIR APPEARANCE IN SERUM. ACTA GENET. STATIST. MED. 16* 305-312, 1966.

SHREFFLER, D. C.* GENETIC STUDIES OF BLOOD GROUP - ASSOCIATED VARIATIONS IN HUMAN SERUM ALKALINE PHOSPHATASE. AM. J. HUM. GENET. 17* 71-86, 1965.

*17180 PHOSPHATASE, PLACENTAL ALKALINE

BOYER (1961, 1963) DESCRIBED AN ELECTROPHORETIC VARIANT OF ALKALINE PHOSPHATASE WHICH APPEARS IN THE SERUM DURING PREGNANCY IN SOME BUT NOT ALL WOMEN AND DEMONSTRATED ITS ORIGIN IN THE PLACENTA. SINCE THE HUMAN PLACENTA IS LARGELY FETAL IN ORIGIN, THE POLYMORPHISM MAY BE A CHARACTERISTIC DETERMINED BY THE FETAL GENOTYPE. ROBSON AND HARRIS (1965) STUDIED THE GENETICS. BECKMAN ET AL. (1967) FOUND A RARE PHENOTYPE, ABSENCE OF PLACENTAL ALKALINE PHOSPHATASE, IN TWINS AND SUGGESTED THAT THESE TWINS MIGHT BE HOMOZYGOUS FOR A *SILENT ALLELE.* THE TWINS WERE ALSO CONCORDANT FOR CROUZON'S CRANIOFACIAL DYSOSTOSIS, RAISING THE QUESTION OF A CASUAL RELATIONSHIP.

BECKMAN, L., BECKMAN, G., CHRISTODOULOU, C. AND IFEKWUNIGWE, A.* VARIATIONS IN HUMAN PLACENTAL ALKALINE PHOSPHATASE. ACTA GENET. STATIST. MED. 17* 406-412, 1967.

BECKMAN, L., BJORLING, G. AND CHRISTODOULOU, C.* PREGNANCY ENZYMES AND PLACENTAL POLYMORPHISM. I. ALKALINE PHOSPHATASE. ACTA GENET. STATIST. MED. 16* 59-73, 1966.

BOYER, S. H.* ALKALINE PHOSPHATASE IN HUMAN SERA AND PLACENTA. SCIENCE 134* 1002-1004, 1961.

BOYER, S. H.* HUMAN ORGAN ALKALINE PHOSPHATASES* DISCRIMINATION BY SEVERAL MEANS INCLUDING STARCH GEL ELECTROPHORESIS OF ANTIENZYME-ENZYME SUPERNATANT FLUIDS. ANN. N.Y. ACAD. SCI. 103* 938-950, 1963.

ROBINSON, J. C. AND GOLDSMITH, L. A.* GENETICALLY DETERMINED VARIANTS OF SERUM ALKALINE PHOSPHATASE* A REVIEW. VOX SANG. 13* 289-307, 1967.

ROBSON, E. B. AND HARRIS, H.* GENETICS OF THE ALKALINE PHOSPHATASE POLYMORPHISM OF THE HUMAN PLACENTA. NATURE 207* 1257-1259, 1965.

17190 PHOSPHOGLUCOMUTASE POLYMORPHISM PGM(1)

BY STARCH GEL ELECTROPHORESIS, SPENCER, HOPKINSON AND HARRIS (1964) DEMONSTRATED POLYMORPHISM OF PHOSPHOGLUCOMUTASE, THE ENZYME WHICH CATALYZES THE TRANSFER OF A PHOSPHATE GROUP BETWEEN THE 1- AND 6- POSITIONS OF GLUCOSE. HOPKINSON AND HARRIS (1965) PRESENTED EVIDENCE FOR THE EXISTENCE OF TWO STRUCTURAL LOCI PGM(1) AND PGM(2). LOCUS PGM(1) IS THOUGHT TO BE RESPONSIBLE FOR ELECTROPHORETICALLY SLOW-MOVING COMPONENTS AND AT LEAST 5 ALLELES HAVE BEEN IDENTIFIED. LOCUS PGM(2) DETERMINES THE ELECTROPHORETICALLY FAST-MOVING COMPONENTS AND AT LEAST 3 ALLELES MAY EXIST AT THIS LOCUS. EVIDENCE OF A THIRD STRUCTURAL LOCUS CONTROLLING PHOSPHOGLUCOMUTASE WAS PRESENTED BY HOPKINSON (1966). THE PHOSPHOGLUCOMUTASES ARE MONOMERS. THE EXISTENCE OF THREE GENETIC FORMS MUST MEAN THAT THREE SEPARATE ENZYMES HAVE PGM SPECIFICITY. THIS IS NOT A SITUATION IN WHICH POLYPEPTIDE CHAINS OF DIFFERENT GENETIC ORIGIN COMBINE IN A SINGLE PROTEIN, AS IS THE CASE WITH LACTATE DEHYDROGENASE AND HEMOGLOBIN. PARRINGTON ET AL. (1968) FOUND THAT THE THREE PGM LOCI ARE NOT CLOSELY LINKED WITH EACH OTHER.

GEDDE-DAHL, T., JR. AND MONN, E.* LINKAGE RELATIONS OF THE PHOSPHOGLUCOMUTASE PGM(1) LOCUS IN MAN. PROBABLE LINKAGE TO PHENYLTHIOCARBAMID (PTC) TASTER LOCUS. ACTA GENET. STATIST. MED. 17* 482-494, 1967.

HOPKINSON, D. A. AND HARRIS, H.* EVIDENCE FOR A SECOND *STRUCTURAL* LOCUS DETERMINING HUMAN PHOSPHOGLUCOMUTASE. NATURE 208* 410-412, 1965.

ISHIMOTO, G.* PLACENTAL PHOSPHOGLUCOMUTASE IN JAPANESE. JAP. J. HUM. GENET.
14* 183-188, 1969.

MCALPINE, P. J., HOPKINSON, D. A. AND HARRIS, H.* THERMOSTABILITY STUDIES ON
THE ISOENZYMES OF HUMAN PHOSPHOGLUCOMUTASE. ANN. HUM. GENET. 34* 61-71, 1970.

MONN, E.* A NEW RED CELL PHOSPHOGLUCOMUTASE PHENOTYPE IN MAN. ACTA GENET.
STATIST. MED. 18* 123-127, 1967.

PARRINGTON, J. M., CRUICKSHANK, G., HOPKINSON, D. A., ROBSON, E. B. AND HARRIS,
H.* LINKAGE RELATIONSHIPS BETWEEN THE THREE PHOSPHOGLUCOMUTASE LOCI PGM(1), PGM(2)
AND PGM(3). ANN. HUM. GENET. 32* 27-34, 1968.

SHINODA, T. AND MATSUNAGA, E.* POLYMORPHISM OF RED CELL PHOSPHOGLUCOMUTASE
AMONG JAPANESE. JAP. J. HUM. GENET. 14* 316, 1970.

SPENCER, N., HOPKINSON, D. A. AND HARRIS, H.* PHOSPHOGLUCOMUTASE POLYMORPHISM
IN MAN. NATURE 204* 742-745, 1964.

17200 PHOSPHOGLUCOMUTASE POLYMORPHISM PGM(2)

SEE ABOVE DESCRIPTION.

17210 PHOSPHOGLUCOMUTASE POLYMORPHISM PGM(3)

SEE ABOVE DESCRIPTION. PGM(1) AND PGM(3) ARE NOT CLOSELY LINKED (HOPKINSON AND
HARRIS, 1968). THE PGM-3 LOCUS AND THE HL-A LOCUS ARE LINKED (LAMM ET AL., 1970*
KISSMEYER-NIELSEN, 1970). WHEREAS PGM-1 AND PGM-2 POLYMORPHISM IS DETERMINED IN
RED CELLS, PGM-3 IS DETECTED IN WHITE CELLS.

HOPKINSON, D. A. AND HARRIS, H.* A THIRD PHOSPHOGLUCOMUTASE LOCUS IN MAN. ANN.
HUM. GENET. 31* 359-368, 1968.

KISSMEYER-NIELSEN, F.* ARHUS, DENMARK* PERSONAL COMMUNICATION, 1970.

LAMM, L. U., KISSMEYER-NIELSEN, F. AND HENNINGSEN, K.* LINKAGE AND ASSOCIATION
STUDIES OF TWO PHOSPHOGLUCOMUTASE LOCI (PGM-1 AND PGM-3) TO EIGHTEEN OTHER
MARKERS. HUM. HERED. 20* 305-318, 1970.

*17220 6-PHOSPHOGLUCONATE DEHYDROGENASE, VARIANTS OF, IN ERYTHROCYTE

BREWER AND DERN (1964) REPORTED DEFICIENCY OF 6-PGD IN 10 MEMBERS OF 4 GENERATIONS
OF AN AMERICAN NEGRO FAMILY. THEY CONCLUDED THAT THE INHERITANCE IS AUTOSOMAL
DOMINANT, ALL 6-PGD-DEFICIENT PERSONS OBSERVED BEING HETEROZYGOTES. HOWEVER, NO
MALE-TO-MALE TRANSMISSION WAS OBSERVED* INDEED, NO OFFSPRING OF AFFECTED MALES
WERE TESTED. AGAINST X-LINKAGE IS THE FACT THAT THE AVERAGE ENZYME LEVEL IN THREE
6-PGD-DEFICIENT MALES WAS SOMEWHAT HIGHER THAN THAT IN SEVEN 6-PGD-DEFICIENT
FEMALES. THE OPPOSITE WOULD BE EXPECTED OF AN X-LINKED TRAIT. THE AUTHORS
COMMENTED ON THE AUTOSOMAL CONTROL OF AN ENZYME WHICH IS CLOSELY RELATED METABOLI-
CALLY TO G6PD, AN ENZYME CONTROLLED BY AN X-LINKED GENE. IN A SURVEY OF UNRELATED
PERSONS, DERN, BREWER, TASHIAN AND SHOWS (1966) FOUND IN 3 OF 873 AMERICAN NEGROES
AND 2 OF 275 CAUCASIANS A REDUCTION IN ERYTHROCYTE 6-PHOSPHOGLUCONATE DEHYDRO-
GENASE (6-PGD) TO THE RANGE OF 42 TO 65 PERCENT OF NORMAL. LEUKOCYTE ENZYME WAS
ALSO REDUCED. NO CORRELATION WAS FOUND BETWEEN ELECTROPHORETIC PHENOTYPE AND THE
QUANTITATIVE VARIATION. THE INHERITANCE WAS CLEARLY AUTOSOMAL DOMINANT.
USING STARCH-GEL ELECTROPHORESIS, FILDES AND PARR DETECTED TWO DISTINCT TYPES
OF HUMAN RED CELL 6-PHOSPHOGLUCONATE DEHYDROGENASE (6-PGD). TEN OF 150 RANDOM
BLOOD SAMPLES SHOWED TWO BROAD, LESS DISTINCT BANDS IN CONTRAST TO THE SINGLE
NARROW, SHARP BAND IN THE REMAINDER. INHERITANCE APPEARS TO BE AUTOSOMAL, A POINT
OF PARTICULAR NOTE. SINCE THE G6PD LOCUS IS X-LINKED, THESE TWO FUNCTIONALLY
RELATED GENES DO NOT SHOW CLUSTERING. HETEROZYGOTES AND HOMOZYGOTES SHOWED NO
QUANTITATIVE DIFFERENCE IN RED BLOOD CELL 6-PGD ACTIVITY. DEFICIENCY OF THIS
ENZYME, BOTH WITH AND WITHOUT ELECTROPHORETIC ABNORMALITY, HAS BEEN OBSERVED
(PARR, 1966). A POSSIBILITY OF LINKAGE BETWEEN THE RHESUS AND 6-PGD LOCI WAS
FOUND BY WEITKAMP ET AL. (1970).

BLAKE, N. M. AND KIRK, R. L.* NEW GENETIC VARIANT OF 6-PHOSPHOGLUCONATE
DEHYDROGENASE IN AUSTRALIAN ABORIGINES. NATURE 221* 278 ONLY, 1969.

BOWMAN, J. E., CARSON, P. E., FRISCHER, H. AND DE GARAY, A. L.* GENETICS OF
STARCH-GEL ELECTROPHORETIC VARIANTS OF HUMAN 6-PHOSPHOGLUCONIC DEHYDROGENASE*
POPULATION AND FAMILY STUDIES IN THE UNITED STATES AND IN MEXICO. NATURE 210*
811-812, 1966.

BREWER, G. J. AND DERN, R. J.* A NEW INHERITED ENZYMATIC DEFICIENCY OF HUMAN
ERYTHROCYTES* 6-PHOSPHOGLUCONATE DEHYDROGENASE DEFICIENCY. AM. J. HUM. GENET. 16*
472-476, 1964.

DAVIDSON, R. G.* ELECTROPHORETIC VARIANTS OF HUMAN 6-PHOSPHOGLUCONATE DEHYDRO-

GENASE* POPULATION AND FAMILY STUDIES AND DESCRIPTION OF A NEW VARIANT. ANN. HUM. GENET. 30* 355-362, 1967.

DERN, R. J., BREWER, G. J., TASHIAN, R. E. AND SHOWS, T. B.* HEREDITARY VARIATION OF ERYTHROCYTIC 6-PHOSPHOGLUCONATE DEHYDROGENASE. J. LAB. CLIN. MED. 67* 255-264, 1966.

FILDES, R. A. AND PARR, C. W.* HUMAN RED-CELL PHOSPHOGLUCONATE DEHYDROGENASES. NATURE 200* 890-891, 1963.

PARR, C. W. AND FITCH, L. I.* INHERITED QUANTITATIVE VARIATIONS OF HUMAN PHOSPHOGLUCONATE DEHYDROGENASE. ANN. HUM. GENET. 30* 339-353, 1967.

PARR, C. W.* ERYTHROCYTE PHOSPHOGLUCONATE DEHYDROGENASE POLYMORPHISM. NATURE 210* 487-489, 1966.

PARR, C. W.* STRUCTURAL ALLELES AT THE SAME LOCUS DETERMINING BOTH ELECTRO-PHORETIC VARIATION AND PARTIAL DEFICIENCY OF ERYTHROCYTE PHOSPHOGLUCONATE DEHYDROGENASE IN THE HUMAN. (ABSTRACT) PROC. THIRD INTERN. CONG. HUM. GENET., (CHICAGO, SEPT. 5-10), 1966. PP. 75-76.

TARIVERDIAN, G., ROPERS, H., OP*T HOF, J. AND RITTER, H.* ZUR GENETIK DER 6-PHOSPHOGLUCONATDEHYDROGENASE (EC* 1.1.1.44)* EINE NEUE VARIANTE F (FREIBURG). HUMANGENETIK 10* 355-357, 1970.

WEITKAMP, L. R., GUTTORMSEN, S. A., SHREFFLER, D. C., SING, C. F. AND NAPIER, J. A.* GENETIC LINKAGE RELATIONS OF THE LOCI FOR 6-PHOSPHOGLUCONATE DEHYDROGENASE AND ADENOSINE DEAMINASE IN MAN. AM. J. HUM. GENET. 22* 216-220, 1970.

17230 PHOSPHOHEXOKINASE

FROM QUANTITATIVE STUDIES OF RED CELL ENZYMES IN CASES OF TRISOMY 21, PANTELAKIS ET AL. (1970) FOUND SUGGESTIVE EVIDENCE THAT THE LOCUS FOR PHOSPHOHEXOKINASE IS SITUATED ON CHROMOSOME 21.

PANTELAKIS, S. N., KARAKLIS, A. G., ALEXIOU, D., VARDAS, E. AND VALAES, T.* RED CELL ENZYMES IN TRISOMY 21. AM. J. HUM. GENET. 22* 184-193, 1970.

*17240 PHOSPHOHEXOSE ISOMERASE, VARIANTS OF

PHOSPHOHEXOSE ISOMERASE IS ALSO KNOWN AS GLUCOSEPHOSPHATE, ISOMERASE AND PHOSPHOG-LUCOSE ISOMERASE. BAUGHAN ET AL. (1968) FOUND DEFICIENCY OF ERYTHROCYTE GLUCOSE-PHOSPHATE ISOMERASE (GPI), WHICH CATALYZES THE INTERCONVERSION OF GLUCOSE-6-PHOSPHATE AND FRUCTOSE-6-PHOSPHATE IN AN ADOLESCENT BOY WITH LIFE-LONG NONSPHERO-CYTIC HEMOLYTIC ANEMIA. THE AUTOHEMOLYSIS PATTERN CONFORMED TO DACIE*S TYPE I. BOTH PARENTS, A SIB AND FIVE OTHER RELATIVES SHOWED INTERMEDIATE ENZYME LEVELS. THE PROBAND SHOWED LOW ENZYME IN LEUKOCYTES AND NO DETECTABLE ENZYME IN PLASMA. GLUCOSEPHOSPHATE ISOMERASE IS THE CATALYST SPECIFIC TO THE SECOND STEP OF THE EMBDEN-MEYERHOF GLYCOLYTIC PATHWAY. THE DEFICIENCY OCCURS IN LEUKOCYTES AND PLASMA AS WELL AS ERYTHROCYTES BUT THE ONLY CLINICAL MANIFESTATION IS HEMOLYTIC ANEMIA. DETTER ET AL. (1968) FOUND THAT THE PARENTS OF A PATIENT WITH HEMOLYTIC ANEMIA HAD DIFFERENT ELECTROPHORETIC VARIANTS OF PHI, EACH ASSOCIATED WITH REDUCED ENZYME ACTIVITY. THE DEFINITION OF *RECESSIVE* IS STRAINED, THIS BECOMING A SITUATION LIKE THAT IN THE HB SC PERSON. IN THE MOUSE THE HEMOGLOBIN BETA CHAIN LOCUS IS LOOSELY LINKED TO THAT FOR GLUCOSEPHOSPHATE ISOMERASE (RECOMBINATION FRACTION, 32 PERCENT). EVEN IF HOMOLOGY EXISTS IN MAN, A LINKAGE THIS LOOSE WOULD BE HARD TO ESTABLISH.

BAUGHAN, M. A., VALENTINE, W. N., PAGLIA, M. D., WAYS, P. O., SIMON, E. R. AND DEMARSH, Q. B.* HEREDITARY HEMOLYTIC ANEMIA ASSOCIATED WITH GLUCOSEPHOSPHATE ISOMERASE (GPI) DEFICIENCY - A NEW ENZYME DEFECT OF HUMAN ERYTHROCYTES. BLOOD 32* 236-249, 1968.

DETTER, J. C., WAYS, P. O., GIBLETT, E. R., BAUGHAN, D. A., HOPKINSON, D. A., POVEY, S. AND HARRIS, H.* INHERITED VARIATIONS IN HUMAN PHOSPHOHEXOSE ISOMERASE. ANN. HUM. GENET. 31* 329-338, 1968.

HUTTON, J. J.* LINKAGE ANALYSIS USING BIOCHEMICAL VARIANTS IN MICE. I. LINKAGE OF THE HEMOGLOBIN BETA-CHAIN AND GLUCOSEPHOSPHATE ISOMERASE LOCI. BIOCHEM. GENET. 3* 507-515, 1969.

KRONE, W., SCHNEIDER, G., SCHULZ, D., ARNOLD, H. AND BLUME, K. G.* DETECTION OF PHOSPHOHEXOSE ISOMERASE* DEFICIENCY IN HUMAN FIBROBLAST CULTURES. HUMANGENETIK 10* 224-230, 1970.

PAGLIA, D. E., HOLLAND, P., BAUGHAN, M. A. AND VALENTINE, W. N.* OCCURRENCE OF DEFECTIVE HEXOSEPHOSPHATE ISOMERIZATION IN HUMAN ERYTHROCYTES AND LEUKOCYTES. NEW ENG. J. MED. 280* 66-71, 1969.

TARIVERDIAN, G., ARNOLD, H., BLUME, K. G., LENKEIT, U. AND LOHR, G. W.* ZUR FORMALGENETIK DER PHOSPHOGLUCOSEISOMERASE (EC* 5.3.1.9). UNTERSUCHUNG EINER SIPPE MIT PGI-DEFIZIENZ. HUMANGENETIK 10* 218-223, 1970.

HERRMANN, AGUILAR, AND SACKS (1964) REPORTED 14 MEMBERS IN FIVE GENERATIONS OF A
FAMILY WITH DIABETES MELLITUS, NEPHROPATHY, EPILEPSY, AND DEAFNESS. THE PROBAND,
A 43 YEAR OLD WOMAN, HAD PHOTOMYOCLONIC SEIZURES FOR 20 YEARS AND PROGRESSIVE
NERVE DEAFNESS FOR SEVEN YEARS. HER TERMINAL ILLNESS BEGAN SIX MONTHS BEFORE
DEATH WITH MILD PERSONALITY CHANGE, SLOWING AND SLURRING OF SPEECH, FOLLOWED BY
DEPRESSION, MILD DIABETES, FOCAL MOTOR SEIZURES AFFECTING EITHER SIDE OF THE FACE,
EMACIATION, AND CONFUSION. TERMINALLY A COARSE HORIZONTAL NYSTAGMUS AND GROSS
ATAXIA OF THE TRUNK AND LIMBS APPEARED. SERIAL AUDIOGRAMS FROM PRECEDING YEARS
WERE CONSISTENT WITH PROGRESSIVE COCHLEAR DEGENERATION. THE KIDNEYS AT AUTOPSY
SHOWED SMALL FOCI OF INTERSTITIAL CHRONIC INFLAMMATION. THE RENAL TUBULES SHOWED
VACUOLATION AND PAS-POSITIVE CYTOPLASMIC GRANULES. THE BRAIN SHOWED DIFFUSE
NEURONAL DEGENERATION AND ASTROCYTOSIS. CEREBELLAR GRANULE CELLS WERE DECREASED.
NEURONS IN THE DENTATE AND INFERIOR OLIVARY NUCLEUS WERE DECREASED. REMAINING
NEURONS WERE BALLOONED BY A PAS-POSITIVE, NEUTRAL FAT POSITIVE MATERIAL. OTHER
NUCLEAR GROUPS WERE INVOLVED TO A LESSER DEGREE. A FEMALE COUSIN OF THE PROBAND
HAD A SIMILAR ILLNESS WITH PHOTOMYOCLONIC SEIZURES, AND PROGRESSIVE NERVE DEAFNESS
IN EARLY ADULT LIFE. PROGRESSIVE DEMENTIA BEGAN AT AGE 40. RENAL TESTS WERE
NORMAL. DIABETES AND PHOTIC SENSITIVITY WERE FOUND IN THE TWO SIBS OF THE
PROBAND, THE MOTHER OF THE PROBAND, AND HER SIBS, THE MATERNAL GRANDMOTHER AND
SCATTERED OTHER MEMBERS OF THE KINDRED. 'BRIGHT'S DISEASE' OCCURRED IN THREE
FEMALE RELATIVES. SEVEN MEMBERS IN THE FAMILY OF THE MATERNAL GRANDFATHER, ALL
MALE, SUCCUMBED IN CHILDHOOD OR ADOLESCENCE TO A RAPID NEUROLOGICAL DETERIORATION
AND DEMENTIA. THE AUTHORS SUGGESTED THE FEATURES OF PHOTOMYOCLONUS, COCHLEAR
DEGENERATION, DIABETES, AND NEPHROPATHY ARE INHERITED TOGETHER AS AN AUTOSOMAL
DOMINANT OF VARIABLE PENETRANCE. NO INSTANCE OF MALE-TO-MALE TRANSMISSION WAS
OBSERVED.

HERRMANN, C., JR., AGUILAR, M. J. AND SACKS, O. W.* HEREDITARY PHOTOMYOCLONUS
ASSOCIATED WITH DIABETES MELLITUS, DEAFNESS, NEPHROPATHY, AND CEREBRAL DYSFUNC-
TION. NEUROLOGY 14* 212-221, 1964.

17260 PHYSIOLOGIC TRAITS

THE 'NORMAL' PHYSIOLOGIC TRAITS THAT SHOW VARIATION WHICH MAY BE UNIFACTORIAL
INCLUDE THE FOLLOWING*
    ASPARAGUS, URINARY EXCRETION OF ODORIFEROUS COMPONENT OF
    BEETURIA
    BETA-AMINOISOBUTYRIC (BAIB), URINARY EXCRETION OF
    EARS, ABILITY TO MOVE
    HANDEDNESS
    PHENYLTHIOCARBAMIDE (PTC) TASTING
    PITCH DISCRIMINATION
    SECRETOR FACTOR
    SMELL BLINDNESS
    TONGUE CURLING, ROLLING, FOLDING
    TUNE DEAFNESS

*17270 PICK'S DISEASE OF BRAIN (LOBAR ATROPHY)

SCHENK (1959) FOLLOWED UP ON A FAMILY WITH PICK'S DISEASE (LOBAR ATROPHY)
ORIGINALLY STUDIED IN 1938, AT WHICH TIME TEN CASES WERE IDENTIFIED IN THE FAMILY.
TEN FURTHER CASES WERE FOUND IN A DOMINANT PATTERN OF INHERITANCE. SEE ALZHEI-
MER'S DISEASE.

SCHENK, V. W. D.* RE-EXAMINATION OF A FAMILY WITH PICK'S DISEASE. ANN. HUM.
GENET. 23* 325-333, 1959.

*17280 PIEBALD TRAIT

KEELER (1934) DESCRIBED A LOUISIANA NEGRO FAMILY IN WHICH THE DISORDER COULD BE
TRACED BACK TO A WOMAN BORN IN 1853. SUNDFOR (1939) DESCRIBED A FAMILY IN WHICH
MANY PERSONS HAD A WHITE FORELOCK OFTEN WITH UNPIGMENTED PATCHES ON THE FOREHEAD,
LIMBS, BODY, ETC. THE FEATURES ARE LIKE THOSE OF WAARDENBURG'S SYNDROME (Q.V.)
EXCEPT FOR ABSENCE OF DEAFNESS AND DISPLACED INNER CANTHUS. SPECIFICALLY THE
FEATURES ARE WHITE FORELOCK AND ABSENCE OF PIGMENTATION OF THE MEDIAL PORTION OF
THE FOREHEAD, EYEBROWS AND CHIN AND OF THE VENTRAL CHEST, ABDOMEN AND EXTREMITIES.
THE BORDERS OF UNPIGMENTED AREAS ARE HYPERPIGMENTED. HETEROCHROMIA IRIDIS OCCURS
IN SOME. A DEFECT IN MIGRATION OR DIFFERENTIATION OF MELANOBLASTS IN HYPOPIG-
MENTED AREAS WAS SUGGESTED BY COMINGS AND ODLAND (1965). LOEWENTHAL (1959)
ASSIGNED THE NAME ALBINOIDISM TO A DOMINANTLY INHERITED CONDITION CHARACTERIZED BY
A WHITE 'BLAZE' IN THE SCALP HAIR, USUALLY THE FORELOCK AND-OR PATCHES OF
LEUKODERMA. EPITHELIOMAS OCCURRED WITH INCREASED FREQUENCY. THE DESIGNATION
ALBINOIDISM IS BETTER RESERVED FOR THE RECESSIVE CONDITION SIMULATING TRUE
ALBINISM. WHITE FORELOCK AND PATCHES OF LEUKODERMA OCCUR ALSO IN WAARDENBURG'S
SYNDROME (Q.V.) AND IN FANCONI'S ANEMIA (A RECESSIVE). IN MICE AGANGLIONIC
MEGACOLON IS ASSOCIATED WITH THE PIEBALD TRAIT (BIELSCHOWSKY AND SCHOFIELD, 1962),
INHERITED PROBABLY AS AN AUTOSOMAL RECESSIVE. COMINGS AND ODLAND (1966) FOUND THE
TRAIT IN 6 GENERATIONS. A GENETIC DEFECT IN MELANOBLAST DIFFERENTIATION WAS
POSTULATED. GEORGE CATLIN (1796-1872), PAINTER OF THE AMERICAN INDIANS, PAINTED

AN AFFECTED MANDAN INDIAN. MULTIPLE MEMBERS OF THE GROUP WERE SAID TO HAVE BEEN AFFECTED.

BIELSCHOWSKY, M. AND SCHOFIELD, G. C.* STUDIES ON MEGACOLON IN PIEBALD MICE. AUST. J. EXP. BIOL. MED. SCI. 40* 395-403, 1962.

COMINGS, D. E. AND ODLAND, G. F.* ELECTRON MICROSCOPE STUDY OF PARTIAL ALBINISM. (ABSTRACT) CLIN. RES. 13* 265 ONLY, 1965.

COMINGS, D. E. AND ODLAND, G. F.* PARTIAL ALBINISM. J.A.M.A. 195* 510-523, 1966.

CROMWELL, A. M.* INHERITANCE OF WHITE FORELOCK IN A MULATTO FAMILY. J. HERED. 31* 94-96, 1940.

FITCH, L.* INHERITANCE OF A WHITE FORELOCK* THROUGH FIVE SUCCESSIVE GENERATIONS IN THE LOGSDON FAMILY. J. HERED. 28* 413-414, 1937.

FROGGATT, P.* AN OUTLINE WITH BIBLIOGRAPHY OF HUMAN PIE-BALDISM AND WHITE FORELOCK. IRISH J. MED. SCI. 398* 86-94, 1951.

JAHR, H. M. AND MCINTYRE, M. S.* PIEBALDNESS, OF FAMILIAL WHITE SKIN SPOTTING (PARTIAL ALBINISM). AM. J. DIS. CHILD. 88* 481-484, 1954.

KEELER, C. E.* THE HEREDITY OF A CONGENITAL WHITE SPOTTING IN NEGROES. J.A.M.A. 103* 179-180, 1934.

LOEWENTHAL, L. J. A.* ALBINOIDISM WITH EPITHELIOMATOSIS. BRIT. J. DERM. 71* 37-38, 1959.

SUNDFOR, H.* A PEDIGREE OF SKIN-SPOTTING IN MAN* 42 PIEBALDS IN A NORWEGIAN FAMILY. J. HERED. 30* 67-77, 1939.

*17290 PIGMENTED PURPURIC ERUPTION

GOULD AND FARBER (1966) DESCRIBED A FAMILY IN WHICH 6 PERSONS IN 3 GENERATIONS (WITH ONE INSTANCE OF MALE-TO-MALE TRANSMISSION) SHOWED A BILATERALLY SYMMETRICAL PIGMENTED AND PURPURIC ERUPTION BEGINNING EARLY IN LIFE. THE CONDITION MAY BE THE SAME AS SCHAMBERG'S DISEASE (1901) WHICH BADEN (1964) OBSERVED IN FATHER AND SON.

BADEN, H. P.* FAMILIAL SCHAMBERG'S DISEASE. ARCH. DERM. 90* 400 ONLY, 1964.

GOULD, W. M. AND FARBER, E. M.* A FAMILIAL PIGMENTED PURPURIC ERUPTION. DERMATOLOGICA 132* 400-408, 1966.

SCHAMBERG, J. G.* A PECULIAR PIGMENTARY DISEASE OF THE SKIN. BRIT. J. DERM. 13* 1-5, 1901.

17300 PILONIDAL SINUS

HOLMES AND TURNER (1969) OBSERVED 9 AFFECTED MEMBERS IN A FAMILY IN A PATTERN CONSISTENT WITH AUTOSOMAL DOMINANT INHERITANCE, ALTHOUGH NO MALE-TO-MALE TRANSMISSION WAS OBSERVED. HOWEVER, FATHER-SON TRANSMISSION WAS NOTED BY STONE (1924).

HOLMES, L. B. AND TURNER, E. A., JR.* HEREDITARY PILONIDAL SINUS. J.A.M.A. 209* 1525-1526, 1969.

STONE, H. B.* PILONIDAL SINUS (COCCYGEAL FISTULA). ANN. SURG. 79* 410-414, 1924.

*17310 PITUITARY DWARFISM

WHETHER SEXUAL ATELEIOSIS (PRESUMED OR PROVED ISOLATED GROWTH HORMONE DEFICIENCY) IS EVER INHERITED AS A DOMINANT IS NOT KNOWN. PERSONS WHO APPEAR TO HAVE THIS CONDITION HAVE BEEN OBSERVED IN SUCCESSIVE GENERATIONS. FURTHERMORE, DOMINANT INHERITANCE IS A POSSIBLE EXPLANATION FOR THE FINDINGS IN A FAMILY IN WHICH TWO MIDGET PARENTS WITH DEMONSTRATED ISOLATED GROWTH HOROMONE DEFICIENCY HAVE THREE OFFSPRING, TWO DWARFED AND ONE OF NORMAL STATURE (RIMOIN ET AL., 1966). ONE EXPLANATION IS THAT AT LEAST ONE OF THE PARENTS HAS DIFFERENT ALLELES EACH OF WHICH DETERMINES AN INEFFECTIVE GROWTH HORMONE MOLECULE AND THAT THROUGH INTRACIS- TRONIC CROSSING OVER A WILD-TYPE GENE WAS RECONSTITUTED. ANOTHER POSSIBILITY IS THAT THE FATHER'S CONDITION IS THE RESULT OF NEW DOMINANT MUTATION AND THAT HE TRANSMITTED THE CONDITION TO THE TWO AFFECTED OFFSPRING. DOMINANT INHERITANCE SEEMS POSSIBLE IN THE CASE OF THOSE PATIENTS WHO HAVE ISOLATED GROWTH HORMONE DEFICIENCY BUT DO NOT HAVE INSULINOPENIA AS IS FOUND IN MOST SUCH CASES. SELLE (1920) IS SAID (WARKANY ET AL., 1961) TO HAVE DESCRIBED A KINDRED IN WHICH 'PRIMORDIAL DWARFISM' WAS TRANSMITTED THROUGH 3 GENERATIONS, 10 PERSONS BEING AFFECTED. MULTIGENERATION KINDREDS WERE INCLUDED IN THE REVIEW OF RISCHBIETH AND BARRINGTON (1912). WHETHER THESE WERE INSTANCES OF GROWTH HORMONE DEFICIENCY IS, OF COURSE, UNKNOWN. WE (MERIMEE ET AL., 1969 TYSON, 1971) HAVE OBSERVED A FAMILY WITH AFFECTED PERSONS IN FOUR GENERATIONS. UNLIKE TYPE I ISOLATED GROWTH HORMONE DEFICIENCY, A RECESSIVE, INSULIN RESPONSES TO GLUCOSE AND TO ARGININE ARE USUALLY

MERIMEE, T. J., HALL, J. G., RIMOIN, D. L. AND MCKUSICK, V. A.* A METABOLIC AND
HORMONAL BASIS FOR CLASSIFYING ATELIOTIC DWARFS. LANCET 1* 963-965, 1969.

RIMOIN, D. L., MERIMEE, T. J. AND MCKUSICK, V. A.* GROWTH HORMONE DEFICIENCY IN
MAN* AN ISOLATED RECESSIVELY INHERITED DEFECT. SCIENCE 152* 1635-1637, 1966.

RISCHBIETH, H. AND BARRINGTON, A.* DWARFISM. IN, TREASURY OF HUMAN INHERI-
TANCE. PEARSON, K. (ED.)* LONDON* DULAU AND CO., 1912, VOL. 1, PT. 7, SEC. 15A,
P. 355.

SELLE, G.* UBER VERERBUNG, DES ECHTEN ZWERGWUCHSES. INAUG. DISSERT., U. OF
JENA, 1920.

TYSON, J. E. A.* ISOLATED GROWTH HORMONE DEFICIENCY, TYPE II (SEXUAL ATELEIO-
SIS, TYPE II). THE CLINICAL DELINEATION OF BIRTH DEFECTS. X. ENDOCRINE SYSTEM.
BALTIMORE* WILLIAMS AND WILKINS, 1971.

WARKANY, J., MONROE, B. B. AND SUTHERLAND, B. S.* INTRAUTERINE GROWTH RETARDA-
TION. AM. J. DIS. CHILD. 102* 249-279, 1961.

*17320 PITYRIASIS RUBRA PILARIS

THE LESIONS WERE DESCRIBED AS *CONSISTING OF ACUMINATE FOLLICULAR PLUGGING ABOUT
THE DORSAL ASPECTS OF THE HANDS AND FEET, AND LARGE PLAQUELIKE, SCALING PSORIASI-
FORM LESIONS OF THE EXTENSOR SURFACES OF THE ARMS, LEGS AND THIGHS AS WELL AS THE
NECK AND CALVES.* THIS DISORDER IS *CHARACTERIZED BY SCALY AND HORNY PRODUCTIONS
SITUATED CHIEFLY IN THE SEBACEOUS FOLLICLES AND BY A MORE OR LESS GENERALIZED
HYPEREMIA* TO USE THE WORDS OF DEVERGIE WHO FIRST DESCRIBED IT (ZEISLER, 1923).
HE OBSERVED IT IN A MAN AND HIS SON AND TWO DAUGHTERS. WEINER AND LEVIN (1943)
FOUND 39 CASES IN THREE GENERATIONS.

PARISH, L. C. AND WOO, T. H.* PITYRIASIS RUBRA PILARIS IN KOREA. TREATMENT
WITH METHOTREXATE. DERMATOLOGICA 139* 399-403, 1969.

WEINER, A. L. AND LEVIN, A. A.* PITYRIASIS RUBRA PILARIS OF FAMILIAL TYPE*
EXPERIENCE IN THE THERAPY WITH CAROTENE AND VITAMIN A. ARCH. DERM. SYPH. 48* 288-
296, 1943.

ZEISLER, E. P.* PITYRIASIS RUBRA PILARIS - FAMILIAL TYPE. ARCH. DERM. SYPH. 7*
195-208, 1923.

17330 PLACENTAL ENZYMES

NUMEROUS POLYMORPHISMS INVOLVING PLACENTAL ENZYMES AND OTHER CONSTITUENTS ARE
LIKELY TO BE UNCOVERED IN THE NEXT FEW YEARS. SOME OF THESE MAY BE UNDER THE
CONTROL OF LOCI SEPARATE FROM THOSE DETERMINING PROTEINS WITH COMPARABLE FUNCTION
IN EXTRA-UTERINE LIFE. THE FIRST POLYMORPHISM INVOLVING A PLACENTAL PROTEIN, THAT
OF PLACENTAL ALKALINE PHOSPHATASE (Q.V.), WAS DISCOVERED BY BOYER (1961).

BOYER, S. H.* ALKALINE PHOSPHATASE IN HUMAN SERA AND PLACENTA. SCIENCE 134*
1002-1004, 1961.

17340 PLATELET ABNORMALITIES, QUALITATIVE

QUALITATIVE GENETIC DISORDERS OF THE BLOOD PLATELET ARE IN AN UNSATISFACTORY
NOSOLOGIC STATE (MARCUS AND ZUCKER, 1965* ULUTIN, 1961). SEE THROMBASTHENIC
THROMBOPATHY.

MARCUS, A. J. AND ZUCKER, M. B.* THE PHYSIOLOGY OF BLOOD PLATELETS. RECENT
BIOCHEMICAL, MORPHOLOGIC, AND CLINICAL RESEARCH. NEW YORK* GRUNE AND STRATTON,
1965.

ULUTIN, O. N.* THE QUALITATIVE PLATELET DISEASES. IN, HENRY FORD HOSPITAL
INTERNATIONAL SYMPOSIUM. S. A. JOHNSON, R. W. MONTO, J. W. REBUCK AND R. C. HORN,
JR. (EDS.)* BOSTON* LITTLE BROWN AND CO., 1961.

*17350 PLATELET GROUPS

IN A LONG REVIEW DAUSSET AND TANGUN (1965) DISCUSSED ANTIGENS COMMON TO RED CELLS,
LEUKOCYTES AND PLATELETS, THOSE LIMITED TO ONE OF THESE AND THOSE SHARED BY
PLATELETS AND LEUKOCYTES. KO AND ZW (VAN DER WEERDT ET AL., 1963) ARE TWO OF THE
PLATELET SYSTEMS.

DAUSSET, J. AND TANGUN, Y.* LEUCOCYTE AND PLATELET GROUPS AND THEIR PRACTICAL
SIGNIFICANCE. (EDITORIAL) VOX SANG. 10* 641-659, 1965.

VAN DER WEERDT, C. M., VEENHOVEN-VON RIESZ, L. E., NIJENHUIS, L. E. AND
VAN LOGHEM, J. L.* THE ZW BLOOD GROUP SYSTEM IN PLATELETS. VOX SANG. 8* 513-530,
1963.

THIS IS A COMPLICATION OF CERTAIN HERITABLE DISORDERS OF CONNECTIVE TISSUE, PARTICULARLY THE MARFAN SYNDROME AND EHLERS-DANLOS SYNDROME, BUT MAY OCCUR AS AN ISOLATED FAMILIAL DISORDER WITHOUT OTHER STIGMATA OF CONNECTIVE TISSUE DISEASE (BOYD, 1957). BROCK (1948) FAVORED THE PRESENCE OF HEREDITARY LUNG CYSTS AS THE ANATOMIC SUBSTRATE.

BERLIN, R.* FAMILIAL OCCURRENCE OF PNEUMOTHORAX SIMPLEX. ACTA MED. SCAND. 137* 268-275, 1950.

BOYD, D. H. A.* FAMILIAL SPONTANEOUS PNEUMOTHORAX. SCOT. MED. J. 2* 220-221, 1957.

BROCK, R. C.* RECURRENT AND CHRONIC SPONTANEOUS PNEUMOTHORAX. THORAX 3* 88-111, 1948.

17370 POIKILODERMA, HEREDITARY SCLEROSING

WEARY ET AL. (1969) REPORTED AN APPARENTLY NEW DISORDER CHARACTERIZED BY GENERA-LIZED POIKILODERMA ACCENTUATED IN FLEXURAL AREAS AND ON EXTENSOR SURFACES, SCLEROSIS OF THE PALMS AND SOLES, AND IN ONE PATIENT LATE DEVELOPMENT OF SUBCU-TANEOUS CALCIFICATION. CLUBBING OF THE FINGERS MAY BE A FEATURE. ALL SEVEN PATIENTS WERE NEGRO. SIX WERE FROM ONE FAMILY (MOTHER AND FIVE AFFECTED CHILDREN OUT OF 10, BY THREE DIFFERENT HUSBANDS).

WEARY, P. E., HSU, Y. T., RICHARDSON, D. R., CARAVATI, C. M. AND WOOD, B. T.* HEREDITARY SCLEROSING POIKILODERMA. REPORT OF TWO FAMILIES WITH AN UNUSUAL AND DISTINCTIVE GENODERMATOSIS. ARCH. DERM. 100* 413-422, 1969.

17380 POLAND SYNDROME (OR POLAND'S SYNDACTYLY)

THIS CONDITION CONSISTS OF UNILATERAL SYMBRACHYDACTYLY AND IPSILATERAL APLASIA OF THE STERNAL HEAD OF THE PECTORALIS MAJOR MUSCLE. ALL REPORTED CASES SEEM TO HAVE BEEN SPORADIC. THERE IS NO EVIDENCE FOR A SIMPLE GENETIC MECHANISM IN THE CASE OF THIS SYNDROME.

BROWN, J. B. AND MCDOWELL, F.* SYNDACTYLISM WITH ABSENCE OF THE PECTORALIS MAJOR. SURGERY 7* 599-601, 1940.

CLARKSON, P.* POLAND'S SYNDACTYLY. GUY HOSP. REP. 111* 335-346, 1962.

*17390 POLYCYSTIC KIDNEYS

DITLEFSEN AND TONJUM (1960) DESCRIBED A FAMILY IN WHICH THERE WERE 15 VERIFIED AND 2 SUSPECTED CASES. SIX OF THE PATIENTS SUFFERED FROM CEREBRAL HEMORRHAGE. IN ONE OF THE SIX, ANEURYSM OF THE MIDDLE CEREBRAL ARTERY WAS VERIFIED. INTRACRANIAL 'BERRY' ANEURYSM IS A RATHER FREQUENT ASSOCIATED MALFORMATION. DALGAARD (1963) FOUND LIVER CYSTS IN 43 PERCENT OF 173 AUTOPSIED CASES IN DENMARK. IN A REVIEW OF CASES, LARGELY FROM THE LITERATURE, POINSO ET AL. (1954) FOUND THAT POLYCYSTIC KIDNEYS OCCURRED IN 53 PERCENT OF 224 CASES OF POLYCYSTIC LIVERS. DALGAARD (1963) SAID HE HAS FOUND A REGULAR TRANSITION FROM POLYCYSTIC LIVER DEGENERATION TO THE SOLITARY LIVER CYST IN ASSOCIATION WITH POLYCYSTIC KIDNEY. ELLIS AND PUTSCHAR (1968) PRESENTED THE CASE OF A 42 YEAR OLD WOMAN WITH POLYCYSTIC KIDNEYS AND PORTAL HYPERTENSION FOR WHICH SPLENORENAL SHUNT WAS PERFORMED. LIVER BIOPSY SHOWED 'DISSEMINATED MICROCYSTIC BILIARY HAMATOMAS, WITH CONGENITAL FIBROSIS.' THE MOTHER DIED WITH HYPERTENSION, RENAL DISEASE AND STROKE AT AGE 64. TWO OF HER SISTERS DIED OF RENAL DISEASE. TWO SISTERS OF THE PROBAND WERE SAID TO HAVE POLYCYSTIC KIDNEY DISEASE.

DALGAARD, O. Z.* BILATERAL POLYCYSTIC DISEASE OF THE KIDNEYS. A FOLLOW-UP OF TWO-HUNDRED AND EIGHTY-FOUR PATIENTS AND THEIR FAMILIES. COPENHAGEN* E. MUNKS-GAARD, 1957. (ALSO ACTA. MED. SCAND. 328 (SUPPL.)* 1957).

DALGAARD, O. Z.* BILATERAL POLYCYSTIC DISEASE OF THE KIDNEYS. IN STRAUSS, M. B. AND WELT, L. G. (EDS.)* DISEASES OF THE KIDNEY. BOSTON* LITTLE, BROWN AND CO., 1963. PP. 907-910.

DITLEFSEN, E. M. L. AND TONJUM, A. M.* INTRACRANIAL ANEURYSMS AND POLYCYSTIC KIDNEYS. ACTA MED. SCAND. 168* 51-54, 1960.

ELLIS, D. S. AND PUTSCHAR, W. G. J.* PERSISTENT FATIGUE, HEPATOSPLENOMEGALY AND PORTAL HYPERTENSION. NEW ENG. J. MED. 278* 899-904, 1968.

OSATHANONDH, V. AND POTTER, E. L.* PATHOGENESIS OF POLYCYSTIC KIDNEYS. ARCH. PATH. 77* 459-465, 1964.

POINSO, R., MONGES, H. AND PAYAN, H.* LA MALADIE KYSTIQUE DU FOIE. EXPANSION SCIENTIFIQUE FRANCAISE, 1954.

*17400 POLYCYSTIC KIDNEYS, MEDULLARY TYPE

GOLDMAN AND COLLEAGUES (1966) DESCRIBED 17 AFFECTED MEMBERS IN FIVE GENERATIONS OF
A FAMILY. FIFTEEN HAD DIED IN THE SECOND DECADE OF LIFE WITH RAPID CLINICAL
DETERIORATION AFTER THE ONSET OF SYMPTOMS. THE KIDNEYS SHOWED THIN CORTICES,
PROMINENT GLOMERULAR HYALINIZATION, NUMEROUS CORTICOMEDULLARY AND INTRAMEDULLARY
CYSTS LINED BY LOW CUBOIDAL EPITHELIUM, AND INCREASE IN MEDULLARY CONNECTIVE
TISSUE. THESE ARE THE FINDINGS ALSO REPORTED IN SPORADIC CASES OF MEDULLARY
CYSTIC DISEASE. DIFFERENCES FROM THE USUAL TYPE OF POLYCYSTIC KIDNEY INCLUDE
USUAL ABSENCE OF FLANK PAIN, HYPERTENSION AND HEMATURIA AND SMALL KIDNEYS BY X-
RAY. IN TWO EXTENSIVELY AFFECTED SIBSHIPS ON WHICH GARDNER (1971) PROVIDED
FOLLOW-UP INFORMATION, THE AVERAGE AGE OF ONSET OF SYMPTOMS WAS 23 YEARS IN ONE
AND 35 YEARS IN A SECOND. THE AVERAGE DURATION OF ILLNESS WAS ONLY 2.2 YEARS.

ABESHOUSE, B. S. AND ABESHOUSE, G. A.* SPONGY KIDNEY* A REVIEW OF THE LITERA-
TURE AND A REPORT OF FIVE CASES. J. UROL. 84* 252-267, 1960.

COPPING, G. A.* MEDULLARY SPONGE KIDNEYS* ITS OCCURRENCE IN A FATHER AND
DAUGHTER. CANAD. M. ASS. J. 96* 608-611, 1967.

DALGAARD, O. Z.* BILATERAL POLYCYSTIC DISEASE OF THE KIDNEYS. IN, DISEASES OF
THE KIDNEY. STRAUSS, M. B. AND WELT, L. G. (EDS.)* BOSTON* LITTLE, BROWN AND CO.,
1963. PP. 907-910.

GARDNER, K. D., JR.* EVOLUTION OF CLINICAL SIGNS IN ADULT-ONSET CYSTIC DISEASE
OF THE RENAL MEDULLA. ANN. INTERN. MED. 74* 47-54, 1971.

GOLDMAN, S. H., WALKER, S. R., MERIGAN, T. C., JR., GARDNER, K. D., JR. AND
BULL, J. M. C.* HEREDITARY OCCURRENCE OF CYSTIC DISEASE OF THE RENAL MEDULLA. NEW
ENG. J. MED. 274* 984-992, 1966.

17410 POLYDACTYLY, IMPERFORATE ANUS, VERTEBRAL ANOMALIES

SAY AND GERALD (1968) FOUND, AMONG 186 CASES OF POLYDACTYLY, 10 WHO ALSO HAD
IMPERFORATE ANUS. OF THE 10, 8 HAD SEVERE SKELETAL ANOMALIES, PREDOMINANTLY
VERTEBRAL. NONE OF THE CASES WERE FAMILIAL. MUTATIONS IN MICE THAT PRODUCE THIS
TRIAD WERE NOTED.

SAY, B. AND GERALD, P. S.* A NEW POLYDACTYLY - IMPERFORATE-ANUS - VERTEBRAL-
ANOMALIES SYNDROME.Q (LETTER) LANCET 2* 688 ONLY, 1968.

*17420 POLYDACTYLY, POSTAXIAL (PROBABLY AT LEAST TWO TYPES)

THIS FORM OF POLYDACTYLY IS ABOUT TEN TIMES MORE FREQUENT IN THE NEGRO THAN IN
CAUCASIANS (FRAZIER, 1960). FROM THE STUDY OF VARIOUS PEDIGREES OF POSTAXIAL
POLYDACTYLY IT IS SUGGESTED THAT TWO PHENOTYPIC AND POSSIBLY GENETICALLY DIFFERENT
VARIETIES EXIST. IN ONE OF THEM, POSTAXIAL POLYDACTYLY TYPE A, THE EXTRA DIGIT IS
RATHER WELL FORMED AND ARTICULATES WITH THE FIFTH OR AN EXTRA METACARPAL. THIS
TYPE IS INHERITED AS A DOMINANT TRAIT WITH MARKED PENETRANCE. IN POSTAXIAL
POLYDACTYLY (TYPE B OR PEDUNCULATED POSTMINIMI) THE EXTRA DIGIT IS NOT WELL FORMED
AND IS FREQUENTLY IN THE FORM OF A SKIN TAG. THE GENETICS OF THIS TYPE IS MORE
COMPLICATED. WALKER (1961) STUDIED A PEDIGREE WITH THIS TRAIT AND OWING TO LACK
OF PENETRANCE, SUGGESTED THAT THE PRESENCE OF TWO DOMINANT GENES WOULD BEST
EXPLAIN THE FINDING. THE LARGEST PEDIGREE OF POSTAXIAL POLYDACTYLY IS THAT
DESCRIBED BY ODIORNE (1943). SVERDRUP (1922) STUDIED A LARGE KINDRED AND NOTED
THE OCCURRENCE OF BOTH TYPES A AND B IN THE SAME PEDIGREE AND DISCUSSED THE
POSSIBILITY OF A GENETIC DIFFERENCE.

FRAZIER, T. M.* A NOTE ON RACE-SPECIFIC CONGENITAL MALFORMATION RATES. AM. J.
OBST. GYNEC. 80* 184-185, 1960.

MOHAN, J.* POSTAXIAL POLYDACTYLY IN THREE INDIAN FAMILIES. J. MED. GENET. 6*
196-200, 1969.

ODIORNE, J. M.* POLYDACTYLISM IN RELATED NEW ENGLAND FAMILIES. J. HERED. 34*
45-56, 1943.

SVERDRUP, A.* POSTAXIAL POLYDACTYLISM IN SIX GENERATIONS OF A NORWEGIAN FAMILY.
J. GENET. 12* 217-240, 1922.

WALKER, J. T.* A PEDIGREE OF EXTRA-DIGIT-V POLYDACTYLY IN A BATUTSI FAMILY.
ANN. HUM. GENET. 25* 65-68, 1961.

17430 POLYDACTYLY, POSTAXIAL, WITH MEDIAN CLEFT OF UPPER LIP

RISCHBIETH (1910) PICTURED A HINDU PATIENT WITH THIS COMBINATION. HIS BROTHER WAS
IDENTICALLY AFFECTED. THURSTON HAD EARLIER (1909) REPORTED THESE BROTHERS.
RISCHBIETH CITED THE FAMILY OF ROUX (1847) IN WHICH THE FATHER HAD UNILATERAL
HARELIP AND SIX DIGITS OF ALL FOUR LIMBS, WHEREAS THE SON HAD DOUBLE HARELIP AND
THE SAME DEFORMITY OF HANDS AND FEET.

RISCHBIETH, H.* HARE-LIP AND CLEFT PALATE. IN, TREASURY OF HUMAN INHERITANCE.
LONDON* CAMBRIDGE UNIV. PRESS, 1910. VOL. I, PART IV, PLATE J.

ROUX, (NI)* BEC-DE-LIEVRE UNILATERAL. GAZ. HOP., P. 274, 1847.

THURSTON, E. O.* A CASE OF MEDIAN HARE-LIP ASSOCIATED WITH OTHER MALFORMATIONS. LANCET 2* 996-997, 1909.

17440 POLYDACTYLY, PREAXIAL I ('THUMB POLYDACTYLY')

PREAXIAL POLYDACTYLY, I.E. POLYDACTYLY ON THE RADIAL SIDE OF THE HAND, IS A HETEROGENEOUS CATEGORY. FOUR TYPES ARE (1) THUMB POLYDACTYLY, (2) POLYDACTYLY OF TRIPHALANGEAL THUMB, (3) POLYDACTYLY OF INDEX FINGER, AND (4) POLYSYNDACTYLY. PREAXIAL POLYDACTYLY I, 'THUMB POLYDACTYLY,' INVOLVES DUPLICATION OF ONE OR MORE OF THE SKELETAL COMPONENTS OF A BIPHALANGEAL THUMB. SEVERITY VARIES FROM MERELY BROADENING OF THE DISTAL PHALANX WITH SLIGHT BIFURCATION AT THE TIP TO FULL DUPLICATION OF THE THUMB INCLUDING THE METACARPALS. THIS TYPE IS THE MOST FREQUENT FORM OF POLYDACTYLY IN MANY POPULATIONS (HANDFORTH, 1950). THE GENETICS IS NOT COMPLETELY CLEAR. DIGBY (1645) REPORTED PREAXIAL POLYDACTYLY, PRESUMABLY OF THIS TYPE, IN FEMALES IN 5 GENERATIONS. POTT (1884) OBSERVED 10 AFFECTED (6 FEMALES AND 4 MALES) IN 3 GENERATIONS. SINHA (1918) FOUND IRREGULAR SEGREGATION IN A FAMILY WITH AFFECTED PERSONS IN 3 GENERATIONS. IN ONE GENERATION, ONLY 1 OF 13 PERSONS AT RISK WERE AFFECTED. DE MARINIS AND SOBBOTA (1957) OBSERVED A GIRL WITH BILATERAL THUMB POLYDACTYLY WHOSE MOTHER HAD RADIAL DEVIATION OF THE TERMINAL PHALANX (A FEATURE WHICH POTT ALSO CONSIDERED A MANIFESTATION OF THE SAME TRAIT). NO MALE-TO-MALE TRANSMISSION SEEMS TO HAVE BEEN DOCUMENTED.

DE MARMINIS, F. AND SOBBOTA, A.* ON THE INHERITANCE AND DEVELOPMENT OF PREAXIAL AND POSTAXIAL TYPES OF POLYDACTYLISM. ACTA. GENET. MED. GEM. 6* 85-93, 1957.

DIGBY, SIR KENELM* THE IMMORTALITY OF REASONABLE SOULS. LONDON* JOHN WILLIAMS, 1645.

HANDFORTH, J. R.* POLYDACTYLISM OF HAND IN SOUTHERN CHINESE. ANAT. REC. 106* 119-125, 1950.

POTT, R.* EIN BEITRAG ZU DEN SYMMETRISCHEN MISSBILDUNGEN DER FINGER UND ZEHEN. JAHRB. KINDERHEILK. 21* 392-407, 1884.

SINHA, S.* POLYDACTYLISM AND TOOTH COLOR. J. HERED. 9* 96 ONLY, 1918.

*17450 POLYDACTYLY, PREAXIAL II (POLYDACTYLY OF TRIPHALANGEAL THUMB)

THE THUMB IN THIS MALFORMATION IS OPPOSABLE AND POSSESSES A NORMAL METACARPAL. POLYDACTYLY CONSISTS OF DUPLICATION OF THE DISTAL PHALANX GIVING A 'DUCK-BILL' APPEARANCE. REPORTED FAMILIES INCLUDE THE SECOND IN THE PAPER BY HAAS (1939), AND THOSE DESCRIBED BY ATWOOD AND POND (1917), HEFNER (1940) AND ECKE (1962).

ATWOOD, E. S. AND POND, C. P.* A POLYDACTYLOUS FAMILY. J. HERED. 8* 96 ONLY, 1917.

ECKE, H.* BEITRAG ZU DEN DOPPELMISSBILDUNGEN IN BEREICH DER FINGER. BRUNS' BEITR. KLIN. CHIR. 205* 463-468, 1962.

HAAS, S. L.* THREE-PHALANGEAL THUMBS. AM. J. ROENTGEN. 42* 677-682, 1939.

HEFNER, R. A.* HEREDITARY POLYDACTYLY* ASSOCIATED WITH EXTRA PHALANGES IN THE THUMB. J. HERED. 31* 25-27, 1940.

*17460 POLYDACTYLY, PREAXIAL III ('INDEX FINGER POLYDACTYLY')

AN HISTORICALLY NOTABLE EXAMPLE IS THE SCIPION FAMILY IN WHICH THE MALFORMATION WAS TRANSMITTED FOR OVER TWO THOUSAND YEARS (MANOILOFF, 1931). THE THUMB IS REPLACED BY ONE OR TWO TRIPHALANGEAL DIGITS, WHICH MAY OR MAY NOT BE OPPOSABLE (SWANSON AND BROWN, 1962). THE FEET, IN SOME CASES, SHOW PREAXIAL POLYDACTYLY OF THE 1ST OR 2ND TOES (MANOILOFF, 1931* JAMES AND LAMB, 1963). A CONSTANT RADIOLO-GIC FINDING IS DISTAL EPIPHYSIS FOR THE METACARPAL OF THE ACCESSORY DIGITS (SWANSON AND BROWN, 1962).

JAMES, J. I. R. AND LAMB, D. W.* CONGENITAL ABNORMALITIES OF THE LIMBS. PRACTITIONER 191* 159-172, 1963.

MANOILOFF, E. O.* A RARE CASE OF HEREDITARY HEXADACTYLISM. AM. J. PHYS. ANTHROP. 15* 503-508, 1931.

SWANSON, A. B. AND BROWN, K. S.* HEREDITARY TRIPHALANGEAL THUMB. J. HERED. 53* 259-265, 1962.

*17470 POLYDACTYLY, PREAXIAL IV (POLYSYNDACTYLY)

ALTHOUGH BOTH PREAXIAL POLYDACTYLY AND SYNDACTYLY ARE CARDINAL FEATURES OF THIS MALFORMATION, IT IS CLASSIFIED AS A FORM OF POLYDACTYLY BECAUSE SYNDACTYLY DOES NOT OCCUR IN THE ABSENCE OF POLYDACTYLY (MCCLINTIC, 1935), THE OPPOSITE NOT BEING TRUE. ON THE OTHER HAND, SYNPOLYDACTYLY (Q.V.) IS HERE CLASSIFIED AS A TYPE OF SYNDACTYLY BECAUSE POLYDACTYLY (OF THE 3RD OR 4TH FINGERS AND 5TH TOES) DOES NOT

OCCUR IN THE ABSENCE OF SYNDACTYLY. IN THE HAND THE THUMB SHOWS ONLY THE MILDEST DEGREE OF DUPLICATION AND SYNDACTYLY OF VARIOUS DEGREES AFFECTS FINGERS 3 AND 4. THE FOOT MALFORMATION IS MORE CONSTANT AND CONSISTS OF DUPLICATION OF PART OR ALL OF THE FIRST OR SECOND TOES AND SYNDACTYLY AFFECTS ALL OF THE TOES, ESPECIALLY THE SECOND AND THIRD. THOMSEN (1927) DESCRIBED 10 AFFECTED FEMALES AND 5 AFFECTED MALES IN 5 GENERATIONS. MCCLINTIC (1935) OBSERVED 15 AFFECTED IN 5 GENERATIONS AND GOODMAN (1965), 5 AFFECTED IN 3 GENERATIONS.

GOODMAN, R. M.* A FAMILY WITH POLYSYNDACTYLY AND OTHER ANOMALIES. J. HERED. 56* 37-38, 1965.

MCCLINTIC, B. S.* FIVE GENERATIONS OF POLYDACTYLISM. J. HERED. 26* 141-144, 1935.

THOMSEN, O.* EINIGE EIGENTHUMLICHKEITEN DER ERBLICHEN POLY- UND SYNDAKTYLIE BEI MENSCHEN. ACTA MED. SCAND. 65* 609-644, 1927.

17480 POLYOSTOTIC FIBROUS DYSPLASIA

THIS DISORDER IS ALSO CALLED ALBRIGHT'S SYNDROME BUT SHOULD NOT BE CONFUSED WITH ALBRIGHT'S HEREDITARY OSTEODYSTROPHY, OR PSEUDOHYPOPARATHYROIDISM (Q.V.). THERE IS LITTLE EVIDENCE OF AN HEREDITARY BASIS. HIBBS AND RUSH (1952) REPORTED THE CASE OF A 50 YEAR OLD WOMAN WITH TYPICAL SKIN PIGMENTATION AND INVOLVEMENT OF MULTIPLE BONES. THE DAUGHTER HAD NO SKIN PIGMENTATION (WHICH IS ABSENT IN SOME CASES) BUT HAD A PATHOLOGIC FRACTURE OF THE LEFT RADIUS AND RADIOLOGIC AND HISTOLOGIC CHANGES INTERPRETED AS THOSE OF FIBROUS DYSPLASIA. FIRAT AND STUTZMAN (1968) DESCRIBED HYPERTHYROIDISM IN ONE PATIENT WHO ALSO HAD PITUITARY GIGANTISM AND HYPERPARATHYROIDISM IN TWO OTHERS. THE LAST TWO CASES WERE MOTHER AND DAUGHTER. THE FIBROUS DYSPLASIA WAS LIMITED TO THE JAW. HYPERTHYROIDISM WAS NOTED BY LICHTENSTEIN AND JAFFE (1942) AS WELL AS OTHER AUTHORS AND WAS PRESENT IN A PATIENT SEEN AT THIS HOSPITAL.

ALBRIGHT, F., BUTLER, A. M., HAMPTON, A. O. AND SMITH, P.* SYNDROME CHARAC-TERIZED BY OSTEITIS FIBROSA DISSEMINATA, AREAS OF PIGMENTATION AND ENDOCRINE DYSFUNCTION, WITH PRECOCIOUS PUBERTY IN FEMALES. REPORT OF FIVE CASES. NEW ENG. J. MED. 216* 727-746, 1937.

ALBRIGHT, F., SCOVILLE, B. AND SULKOWITCH, H. W.* SYNDROME CHARACTERIZED BY OSTEITIS FIBROSA DISSEMINATA, AREAS OF PIGMENTATION, AND A GONADAL DYSFUNCTION. FURTHER OBSERVATIONS INCLUDING THE REPORT. ENDOCRINOLOGY 22* 411-421, 1938.

FIRAT, D. AND STUTZMAN, L.* FIBROUS DYSPLASIA OF THE BONE. REVIEW OF TWENTY-FOUR CASES. AM. J. MED. 44* 421-429, 1968.

HIBBS, R. E. AND RUSH, H. P.* ALBRIGHT'S SYNDROME. ANN. INTERN. MED. 37* 587-593, 1952.

LICHTENSTEIN, L. AND JAFFE, H. L.* FIBROUS DYSPLASIA OF THE BONE. A CONDITION AFFECTING ONE, SEVERAL OR MANY BONES, THE GRAVER CASES OF WHICH MAY PRESENT ABNORMAL PIGMENTATION OF SKIN, PREMATURE SEXUAL DEVELOPMENT, HYPERTHYROIDISM OR STILL OTHER EXTRASKELETAL ABNORMALITIES. ARCH. PATH. 33* 777-816, 1942.

*17490 POLYPOSIS COLI, JUVENILE TYPE

VEALE ET APER SE L. (1966) INVESTIGATED THE FAMILIES OF 11 PATIENTS. JUVENILE POLYPS MAY BE ISOLATED OR MULTIPLE, EVEN VERY NUMEROUS. THE HISTOLOGY AND NATURAL HISTORY OF THESE POLYPS SUGGESTS THEY ARE HAMARTOMAS. THEY PROBABLY ARE NOT PRECANCEROUS. IN FOUR FAMILIES MULTIPLE POLYPOSIS AND-OR COLONIC CARCINOMA OCCURRED IN RELATIVES. FOR EXAMPLE, THE FATHER OF AN AFFECTED BROTHER AND SISTER HAD COLONIC CANCER. IN TWO INSTANCES A PARENT OF A CASE OF JUVENILE POLYPOSIS HAD COLONIC CANCER AND MULTIPLE POLYPOSIS. SMILOW ET AL. (1966) DESCRIBED A 7 YEAR OLD BOY WITH JUVENILE POLYPOSIS, HIS MOTHER WHO AT 10 YEARS OF AGE HAD NOTED A PROLAPSED POLYP DURING DEFECATION AND HIS MATERNAL GRANDFATHER WHO AT AGE 60 HAD SURGERY FOR ADENOCARCINOMA OF THE COLON. VARIOUS POLYPS WERE PRESENT IN THE LATTER PERSON, SOME RESEMBLING ADENOMATOUS POLYPS AND OTHERS RESEMBLING THE JUVENILE POLYPS FOUND IN THE PROBAND AND HIS MOTHER. IN THE PROBAND'S MOTHER THE LESIONS WERE SO NUMEROUS THAT TOTAL COLECTOMY AND ILEOSTOMY WERE PERFORMED. VEALE (1966) DESCRIBED JUVENILE POLYPS IN TWO SISTERS AND THEIR MOTHER. HAGGITT AND PITCOCK (1970) DESCRIBED A GIRL WHO HAD ONSET OF INTERMITTENT BRIGHT RED RECTAL BLEEDING AT AGE 3 YEARS. HER FATHER, AN AUNT AND AN UNCLE HAD 'WELL-DIFFEREN-TIATED ADENOCARCINOMA WITH INVASIN OF THE SUBMUCOSA.' THE GRANDFATHER DIED AT 42 OF COLONIC CANCER.

HAGGITT, R. C. AND PITCOCK, J. A.* FAMILIAL JUVENILE POLYPOSIS OF THE COLON. CANCER 26* 1232-1238, 1970.

SMILOW, P. C., PRYOR, C. A., JR. AND SWINTON, N. W.* JUVENILE POLYPOSIS COLI* A REPORT OF THREE PATIENTS IN THREE GENERATIONS OF ONE FAMILY. DIS. COLON RECTUM 9* 248-254, 1966.

VEALE, A. M. O., MCCOLL, I., BUSSEY, H. J. R. AND MORSON, B. C.* JUVENILE POLYPOSIS COLI. J. MED. GENET. 3* 5-16, 1966.

D
O
M
I
N
A
N
T

YONEMOTO ET AL. (1969) DESCRIBED A FAMILY WITH MULTIPLE CASES CONSISTENT WITH DOMINANT INHERITANCE. ONE PATIENT HAD A DESMOID TUMOR OF THE ABDOMINAL WALL. WHETHER DISTINCT FROM GARDNER'S SYNDROME OR FAMILIAL POLYPOSIS OF THE COLON IS UNCLEAR. EARLY DEVELOPMENT OF SYMPTOMS IS TYPICAL. RAVITCH (1948) DESCRIBED A CASE.

RAVITCH, M. M.* POLYPOID ADENOMATOSIS OF ENTIRE GASTRO-INTESTINAL TRACT. ANN. SURG. 128* 283-298, 1948.

YONEMOTO, R. H., SLAYBACK, J. B., BYRON, R. L., JR. AND ROSEN, R. B.* FAMILIAL POLYPOSIS OF THE ENTIRE GASTROINTESTINAL TRACT. ARCH. SURG. 99* 427-434, 1969.

*17510 POLYPOSIS, INTESTINAL I (FAMILIAL POLYPOSIS OF THE COLON)

NO EXTRA-INTESTINAL MANIFESTATIONS ARE ASSOCIATED WITH THIS FORM AND THE POLYPS ARE PROBABLY ALWAYS LIMITED TO THE COLON. IN EXTREME CASES THE COLON BECOMES CARPETED WITH MYRIADS OF POLYPS. THIS IS A VICIOUSLY PREMALIGNANT CONDITION. CARCINOMA MAY ARISE IN THE TEENS OR BE POSTPONED UNTIL THE SEVENTH DECADE. BLOODY DIARRHEA AND INANITION MAY LEAD TO THE DIAGNOSIS OF ENTERITIS AS THE CAUSE OF DEATH. PIERCE (1968) REPORTED THE FINDINGS IN A PARTICULARLY EXTENSIVELY AFFECTED KINDRED.

ASMAN, H. B. AND PIERCE, E. R.* FAMILIAL MULTIPLE POLYPOSIS. A STATISTICAL STUDY OF A LARGE KENTUCKY KINDRED. CANCER 25* 972-981, 1970.

DUHAMEL, J., BERTHON, G. AND DUBARRY, J. J.* ETUDE MATHEMATIQUE DE L'HEREDITE DE LA POLYPOSE RECTO-COLIQUE. J. GENET. HUM. 9* 65-77, 1960.

MCKUSICK, V. A.* GENETIC FACTORS IN INTESTINAL POLYPOSIS. J.A.M.A. 182* 271-277, 1962.

PIERCE, E. R.* SOME GENETIC ASPECTS OF FAMILIAL POLYPOSIS OF THE COLON IN A KINDRED OF 1,422 MEMBERS. DIS. COLON RECTUM 11* 321-329, 1968.

VEALE, A. M.* CLINICAL AND GENETIC PROBLEMS IN FAMILIAL INTESTINAL POLYPOSIS. GUT 1* 285-290, 1960.

VEALE, A. M.* INTESTINAL POLYPOSIS. EUGENICS LABORATORY MEMOIRS, XL. LONDON* CAMBRIDGE UNIV. PRESS, 1965.

*17520 POLYPOSIS, INTESTINAL II (PEUTZ-JEGHERS SYNDROME)

POLYPS MAY OCCUR IN ANY PART OF THE GASTROINTESTINAL TRACT BUT JEJUNAL POLYPS ARE A CONSISTENT FEATURE. INTUSSUSCEPTION AND BLEEDING ARE THE USUAL SYMPTOMS. MELANIN SPOTS OF THE LIPS, BUCCAL MUCOSA AND DIGITS REPRESENT THE SECOND PART OF THE SYNDROME. MALIGNANT DEGENERATION OF THE INTESTINAL POLYPS IS RARE. THE FEMALES ARE PRONE TO DEVELOP OVARIAN TUMOR, ESPECIALLY GRANULOSA CELL TUMOR (CHRISTIAN ET AL., 1964). METASTASES IN A MALIGNANT POLYP IN PEUTZ-JEGHERS SYNDROME WAS REPORTED BY WILLIAMS AND KNUDSEN (1965). IN THE FAMILY REPORTED BY FARMER ET AL. (1963) THE FATHER HAD ONLY POLYPS, THE SON APPARENTLY ONLY PIGMENTA-TION AND THE DAUGHTER BOTH POLYPS AND PIGMENTATION. A DISSOCIATION OF SIGNS WAS ALSO NOTED BY KIESELSTEIN ET AL. (1969), WHO ALSO FOUND POLYCYSTIC KIDNEY DISEASE IN THE SAME FAMILY. SOMMERHAUG AND MASON (1970) ADDED THE URETER TO THE SITE OF POLYPS DESCRIBED IN THE PEUTZ-JEGHERS SYNDROME. PREVIOUSLY DESCRIBED EXTRA-INTESTINAL SITES INCLUDE ESOPHAGUS, BLADDER, RENAL PELVIS, BRONCHUS AND NOSE.

ANDRE, R., DUHAMEL, G., BRUAIRE, M. AND TIOLLAIS, P.* SYNDROME DE PEUTZ-JEGHERS AVEC POLYPOSE OESOPHAGIENNE. BULL. SOC. MED. HOP. PARIS 117* 505-510, 1966.

BARTHOLOMEW, L. G., MOORE, C., DAHLIN, D. C. AND WAUGH, J. M.* INTESTINAL POLYPOSIS ASSOCIATED WITH MUCOCUTANEOUS PIGMENTATION. SURG. GYNEC. OBSTET. 115* 1-11, 1962.

CHRISTIAN, C. D., MCLOUGHLIN, T. G., CATHCART, E. S. AND EISENBERG, M. M.* PEUTZ-JEGHERS SYNDROME ASSOCIATED WITH FUNCTIONING OVARIAN TUMOR. J.A.M.A. 190* 935-938, 1964.

FARMER, R. G., HAWKS, W. A. AND TURNBULL, R. B.* THE SPECTRUM OF THE PEUTZ-JEGHERS SYNDROME. REPORT OF 3 CASES. AM. J. DIG. DIS. 8* 953-961, 1963.

KEEN, G. AND MURRAY, M. A.* PEUTZ-JEGHERS SYNDROME* A FURTHER FAMILY HISTORY. BRIT. MED. J. 1* 923-924, 1962.

KIESELSTEIN, M., HERMAN, G., WAHRMAN, J., VOSS, R., GITELSON, S., FEUCHTWANGER, M. AND KADAR, S.* MUCOCUTANEOUS PIGMENTATION AND INTESTINAL POLYPOSIS (PEUTZ-JEGHERS SYNDROME) IN A FAMILY OF IRAQI JEWS WITH POLYCYSTIC KIDNEY DISEASE, WITH A CHROMOSOME STUDY. ISRAEL J. MED. SCI., IN PRESS, 1969.

MCALLISTER, A. J., HICKEN, N. F., LATIMER, R. G. AND CONDON, V. R.* SEVENTEEN PATIENTS WITH PEUTZ-JEGHERS SYNDROME IN FOUR GENERATIONS. AM. J. SURG. 114* 839-

MICHALANY, J. AND FERRAZ, M. D.* PEUTZ SYNDROME IN A MULATTO FAMILY. WITH SPECIAL REFERENCE TO THE HISTOLOGICAL STRUCTURE OF THE INTESTINAL POLYPS. GASTROENTEROLOGIA 97* 119-129, 1962.

SCULLY, R. E.* SEX CORD TUMORS WITH ANNULAR TUBULES - A DISTINCTIVE OVARIAN TUMOR OF THE PEUTZ-JEGHERS SYNDROME. CANCER 25* 1107-1121, 1970.

SHEWARD, J. D.* PEUTZ-JEGHERS SYNDROME IN CHILDHOOD* UNUSUAL RADIOLOGICAL FEATURES. BRIT. MED. J. 1* 921-923, 1962.

SOMMERHAUG, R. G. AND MASON, T.* PEUTZ-JEGHERS SYNDROME AND URETERAL POLYPOSIS. J.A.M.A. 211* 120-122, 1970.

WILLIAMS, J. P. AND KNUDSEN, A.* PEUTZ-JEGHERS SYNDROME WITH METASTASIZING DUODENAL CARCINOMA. GUT 6* 179-184, 1965.

*17530 POLYPOSIS, INTESTINAL III (GARDNER'S SYNDROME)

POLYPS OF THE COLON AND SOMETIMES OF THE STOMACH AND SMALL INTESTINE ARE ASSO-CIATED WITH OSSEOUS AND SOFT TISSUE TUMORS. GLOBOID OSTEOMATA OF THE MANDIBLE WITH OVERLYING FIBROMATA ARE CHARACTERISTIC. OSTEOMATOUS CHANGES IN THE CALVARIUM WITH ASSOCIATED FIBROMAS (OF THE FOREHEAD, FOR EXAMPLE) ARE ALSO OBSERVED. SEBACEOUS OR EPIDERMOID CYSTS OCCUR ON THE BACK. MESENTERIC FIBROMATOSIS MAY DEVELOP, ESPECIALLY AFTER SURGERY (SIMPSON ET AL., 1964). THE COLONIC POLYPS FREQUENTLY UNDERGO MALIGNANT DEGENERATION. OLDFIELD'S FAMILY (1954) HAD ONLY SEBACEOUS CYSTS WITH COLONIC POLYPOSIS. WHETHER THIS IS THE SAME MUTATION AS THAT OF THE GARDNER SYNDROME IS UNCLEAR. THE FAMILY REPORTED BY OLDFIELD (1954) WERE SPECIFICALLY STATED TO HAVE MULTIPLE SEBACEOUS CYSTS, OR SEBOCYSTOMATOSIS. IN FACT THE SAME FAMILY HAD BEEN PREVIOUSLY REPORTED BY INGRAM AND OLDFIELD (1937) IN CONNECTION WITH THE SKIN TUMORS ALONE. DRAMATIC PICTURES WERE PUBLISHED. IN THE PAPER BY INGRAM AND OLDFIELD (1937) THE QUESTION OF ORIGIN - RETENTION VS. NEW FORMATION - WAS DISCUSSED AND THE REVIEW OF BENECKE (1931) WAS CITED TOGETHER WITH HIS VIEW THAT MOST SO-CALLED SEBACEOUS CYSTS ARE MORE PROPERLY TERMED EPIDERMOID CYSTS. IN THE FAMILY REPORTED BY KENNY AND O'NEILL (1958) THE CYSTS WERE DESCRIBED AS EPIDERMOID. THE PATHOLOGIST DESCRIBED 'AN OVAL CYST 5 X TWO AND ONE HALF X TWO AND ONE HALF CMS. CONTAINING CHEESY MATERIAL. MICROSCOPICALLY, THE LESION IS AN EPIDERMOID CYST, SIMILAR TO THAT REMOVED FROM THE PATIENT'S BROTHER.' FRAUMENI ET AL. (1968) DESCRIBED A FAMILY IN WHICH THE FATHER AND A DAUGHTER HAD A MALIGNANT MESENCHYMAL TUMOR, A SON HAD POLYPOSIS COLI, AND ANOTHER SON HAD BOTH POLYPOSIS COLI AND MALIGNANT MESENCHYMAL TUMOR. (FATAL METASTIC CARCINOMA OF THE COLON OCCURRED IN AN 11 YEAR OLD BOY, PROBABLY THE YOUNGEST REPORTED.) THE RELATION OF THIS FAMILY'S DISORDER TO GARDNER'S SYNDROME WAS DISCUSSED. MARSHALL ET AL. (1967) REPORTED A PATIENT WITH GARDNER'S SYNDROME (PRESENT ALSO IN MULTIPLE RELATIVES) WHO DEVELOPED ADRENAL CARCINOMA WITH CUSHING'S SYNDROME. CAMIEL ET AL. (1968) DESCRIBED THYROID CARCINOMA IN TWO SISTERS WHO ALSO HAD GARDNER'S SYNDROME WHICH WAS PROBABLY PRESENT IN AT LEAST 3 GENERATIONS OF THE FAMILY. SMITH (1968) ALSO DESCRIBED PATIENTS WITH THE ASSOCIATION OF COLONIC POLYPS AND PAPILLARY CARCINOMA OF THE THYROID. FURTHERMORE, SMITH (1968) QUESTIONED THAT GARDNER'S SYNDROME IS DISTINCT FROM FAMILIAL MULTIPLE POLYPOSIS. THE BEST EVIDENCE OF DISTINCTNESS IS PROVIDED BY LARGE KINDRED SUCH AS THAT OF ASMAN AND PIERCE (1970) IN WHICH NO EXTRA-INTESTINAL FEATURES WERE FOUND AND THAT OF GARDNER (1962) IN WHICH ASSOCIATION OF EXTRA-BOWEL FEATURES WAS CONSISTENTLY FOUND. FURTHERMORE, RESTUDY OF AN EARLIER REPORTED KINDRED (KELLY AND MCKINNON, 1961) SHOWS THAT THE DISORDER IS IN FACT GARDNER'S SYNDROME WITH ABOUT 60 AFFECTED PERSONS PIERCE ET AL. (1970). HOFFMANN AND BROOKE (1970) DESCRIBED A FAMILY IN WHICH 6 PERSONS IN 3 GENERATIONS HAD POLYPOSIS COLI AND A MOTHER AND SON HAD SARCOMA OF BONE LEADING TO DEATH FROM METACTASES AT 28 AND 13 YEARS OF AGE, RESPECTIVELY. NO EVIDENCE OF POLYPOSIS WAS FOUND IN EITHER BUT SPECIAL STUDIES INCLUDING AUTOPSIES WERE NOT DONE.

ASMAN, H. B. AND PIERCE, E. R.* FAMILIAL MULTIPLE POLYPOSIS* A STATISTICAL STUDY OF A LARGE KENTUCKY KINDRED. CANCER 25* 972-981, 1970.

BENECKE, E.* UBER EPITHELIOME AUF ATHEROMEN (EPIDERMOIDE) UND DERMOIDCYSTEN DER HAUT. FRANKFURT. Z. PATH. 42* 502-515, 1931.

CAMIEL, M. R., MULE, J. E., ALEXANDER, L. L. AND BENNINGHOFF, D. L.* ASSOCIA-TION OF THYROID CARCINOMA WITH GARDNER'S SYNDROME IN SIBLINGS. NEW ENG. J. MED. 278* 1056-1058, 1968.

CHANG, C. H., PLATT, E. D., THOMAS, K. E. AND WATNE, A. L.* BONE ABNORMALITIES IN GARDNER'S SYNDROME. AM. J. ROENTGEN. 103* 645-652, 1968.

FADER, M., KLINE, S. N., SPATZ, S. S. AND ZUBROW, H. J.* GARDNER'S SYNDROME (INTESTINAL POLYPOSIS, OSTEOMAS, SEBACEOUS CYSTS) AND A NEW DENTAL DISCOVERY. ORAL SURG. 15* 153-172, 1962.

FRAUMENI, J. F., JR., VOGEL, C. L. AND EASTON, J. M.* SARCOMAS AND MULTIPLE POLYPOSIS IN A KINDRED. A GENETIC VARIETY OF HEREDITARY POLYPOSIS.Q ARCH. INTERN. MED. 121* 57-61, 1968.

GARDNER, E. J.* FOLLOW-UP STUDY OF A FAMILY GROUP EXHIBITING DOMINANT INHERI-
TANCE FOR A SYNDROME INCLUDING INTESTINAL POLYPS, OSTEOMAS, FIBROMAS AND EPIDERMAL
CYSTS. AM. J. HUM. GENET. 14* 376-390, 1962.

GORLIN, R. J. AND CHAUDHRY, A. P.* MULTIPLE OSTEOMATOSIS, FIBROMAS, LIPOMAS AND
FIBROSARCOMAS OF THE SKIN AND MESENTERY, EPIDERMOID INCLUSION CYSTS OF THE SKIN,
LEIOMYOMAS AND MULTIPLE INTESTINAL POLYPOSIS* AN HERITABLE DISORDER OF CONNECTIVE
TISSUE. NEW ENG. J. MED. 263* 1151-1158, 1960.

HAGGITT, R. C. AND BOOTH, J. L.* BILATERAL FIBROMATOSIS OF THE BREAST IN
GARDNER'S SYNDROME. CANCER 25* 161-166, 1970.

HOFFMANN, D. C. AND BROOKE, B. N.* FAMILIAL SARCOMA OF BONE IN A POLYPOSIS COLI
FAMILY. DIS. COLON RECTUM 13* 119-120, 1970.

INGRAM, J. T. AND OLDFIELD, M. C.* HEREDITARY SEBACEOUS CYSTS. BRIT. MED. J.
1* 960-963, 1937.

KELLY, P. B. AND MCKINNON, D. A.* FAMILIAL MULTIPLE POLYPOSIS OF THE COLON*
REVIEW AND DESCRIPTION OF A LARGE KINDRED. MCGILL MED. J. 30* 67-85, 1961.

KENNY, P. J. AND O'NEILL, J.* FAMILIAL INTESTINAL POLYPOSIS ASSOCIATED WITH
FURTHER ABNORMALITIES OF GROWTH. AUST. NEW ZEAL. J. SURG. 28* 145-150, 1958.

LEWIS, R. J. AND MITCHELL, J. C.* BASAL CELL CARCINOMA IN GARDNER'S SYNDROME.
ACTA DERMATOVENER. 51* 67-68, 1970.

MACDONALD, J. M., DAVIS, W. C., CRAGO, H. R. AND BERK, A. D.* GARDNER'S
SYNDROME AND PERIAMPULLARY MALIGNANCY. AM. J. SURG. 113* 425-430, 1967.

MARSHALL, W. H., MARTIN, F. I. R. AND MACKAY, I. R.* GARDNER'S SYNDROME WITH
ADRENAL CARCINOMA. AUST. ANN. MED. 16* 242-244, 1967.

MCKUSICK, V. A.* GENETIC FACTORS IN INTESTINAL POLYPOSIS. J.A.M.A. 182* 271-
277, 1962.

OLDFIELD, M. C.* THE ASSOCIATION OF FAMILIAL POLYPOSIS OF THE COLON WITH
MULTIPLE SEBACEOUS CYSTS. BRIT. J. SURG. 41* 534-541, 1954.

PIERCE, E. R., WEISBORD, T. AND MCKUSICK, V. A.* GARDNER'S SYNDROME* FORMAL
GENETICS AND STATISTICAL ANALYSIS OF A LARGE CANADIAN KINDRED. CLIN. GENET. 1*
65-80, 1970.

SAVAGE, P. T.* POLYPOSIS COLI ASSOCIATED WITH MULTIPLE TUMOURS IN OTHER PARTS
OF THE BODY (GARDNER'S SYNDROME). PROC. ROY. SOC. MED. 57* 402-403, 1964.

SIMPSON, R. D., HARRISON, E. G., JR. AND MAYO, C. W.* MESENTERIC FIBROMATOSIS
IN FAMILIAL POLYPOSIS* A VARIANT OF GARDNER'S SYNDROME. CANCER 17* 526-534, 1964.

SMITH, W. G.* FAMILIAL MULTIPLE POLYPOSIS* RESEARCH TOOL FOR INVESTIGATING THE
ETIOLOGY OF CARCINOMA OF THE COLON.Q DIS. COLON RECTUM 11* 17-31, 1968.

VANHOUTTE, J. J.* POLYPOID LYMPHOID HYPERPLASIA OF THE TERMINAL ILEUM IN
PATIENTS WITH FAMILIAL POLYPOSIS COLI AND WITH GARDNER'S SYNDROME. AM. J.
ROENTGEN. 110* 340-342, 1970.

17540 POLYPOSIS, INTESTINAL IV (SCATTERED, DISCRETE POLYPS)

WOOLF, RICHARDS AND GARDNER (1955) SUGGESTED THAT SOME FAMILIES HAVE SCATTERED
POLYPS AS A DOMINANT TRAIT DISTINCT FROM MULTIPLE POLYPOSIS OF THE COLON. STUDIES
OF POLYPOSIS I FAMILIES SHOW, HOWEVER, SUCH WIDE VARIABILITY IN THE NUMBER OF
POLYPS THAT IT IS DIFFICULT TO ACCEPT THE IDEA THAT A SEPARATE MUTATION EXISTS.
THE EVIDENCE IS, TO SAY THE LEAST, INCONCLUSIVE.

WOOLF, C. M., RICHARDS, R. C. AND GARDNER, E. J.* OCCASIONAL DISCRETE POLYPS OF
THE COLON AND RECTUM SHOWING INHERITED TENDENCY IN A KINDRED. CANCER 8* 403-408,
1955.

17550 POLYPOSIS, SKIN PIGMENTATION, ALOPECIA AND FINGERNAIL CHANGES (CRONKITE-CANADA
SYNDROME)

THIS SYNDROME WAS FIRST DESCRIBED BY CRONKITE AND CANADA (1955) AND LATER BY
JARNUM AND JENSEN (1966). MANOUSOS AND WEBSTER (1966) REPORTED THE FOURTH
PATIENT. ALL CASES HAVE BEEN SPORADIC. NO EVIDENCE OF A GENETIC BASIS IS
AVAILABLE. ALL HAVE BEEN ADULT. THE PROGNOSIS IS POOR. THE CRONKITE-CANADA
SYNDROME IS GENERALIZED INTESTINAL POLYPOSIS WITH MUCOCUTANEOUS PIGMENTATION,
ATROPHY OF FINGER NAILS AND ALOPECIA (CRONKITE AND CANADA, 1955* DACRUZ, 1967).
THE ETIOLOGY IS UNKNOWN BUT IT APPEARS TO BE NON-GENETIC.

CRONKITE, L. W., JR. AND CANADA, W. J.* GENERALIZED GASTROINTESTINAL POLYPOSIS*
AN UNUSUAL SYNDROME OF POLYPOSIS, PIGMENTATION, ALOPECIA AND ONYCHOTROPHIA. NEW
ENG. J. MED. 252* 1011-1015, 1955.

DACRUZ, G. M. G.* GENERALIZED GASTROINTESTINAL POLYPOSIS. AN UNUSUAL SYNDROME OF ADENOMATOUS POLYPOSIS, ALOPECIA, ONYCHOROTROPHIA. AM. J. GASTROENT. 47* 504-510, 1967.

JARNUM, S. AND JENSEN, H.* DIFFUSE GASTROINTESTINAL POLYPOSIS WITH ECTODERMAL CHANGES. A CASE WITH SEVERE MALABSORPTION AND ENTERIC LOSS OF PLASMA PROTEINS AND ELECTROLYTES. GASTROENTEROLOGY 50* 107-118, 1966.

MANOUSOS, O. AND WEBSTER, C. V.* DIFFUSE GASTROINTESTINAL POLYPOSIS WITH ECTODERMAL CHANGES. GUT 7* 375-378, 1966.

*17560 POLYSYNDACTYLY

BOTH PREAXIAL POLYDACTYLY AND SYNDACTYLY ARE FEATURES. TEMTAMY (1966) CLASSIFIED POLYSYNDACTYLY AMONG THE POLYDACTYLIES BECAUSE SYNDACTYLY DID NOT OCCUR WITHOUT POLYDACTYLY. (SYNPOLYDACTYLY, OR SYNDACTYLY TYPE II, WAS CLASSIFIED AS A FORM OF SYNDACTYLY BECAUSE POLYDACTYLY, WHICH AFFECTS THE THIRD OR FOURTH FINGERS AND THE FIFTH TOES, DOES NOT OCCUR IN THE ABSENCE OF SYNDACTYLY.) THE THUMB SHOWS MINOR DUPLICATION IN THE FORM OF A BROAD BIFID OR RADIALLY DEVIATED TERMINAL PHALANX. SYNDACTYLY OF VARIOUS DEGREES AFFECTS THE 3RD AND 4TH FINGERS. WHILE HAND INVOLVEMENT IS MILD AND VARIABLE, FOOT INVOLVEMENT IS NEARLY UNIFORM. PREAXIAL POLYDACTYLY IN THE FOOT TAKES THE FORM OF DUPLICATION OF ALL OR PART OF TOES I OR II. OCCASIONALLY THE FIRST METATARSAL IS SHORT AND TIBIALLY DEVIATED, PRODUCING HALLUX VARUS. SYNDACTYLY AFFECTS ALL TOES, BUT MAXIMALLY THE SECOND AND THIRD.

GOODMAN, R. M.* A FAMILY WITH POLYSYNDACTYLY AND OTHER ANOMALIES. J. HERED. 56* 37-38, 1965.

MCCLINTIC, B. S.* FIVE GENERATIONS OF POLYDACTYLISM. J. HERED. 26* 141-144, 1935.

TEMTAMY, S. A.* GENETIC FACTORS IN HAND MALFORMATIONS. PH. D. THESIS, JOHNS HOPKINS UNIVERSITY, 1966.

THOMSEN, O.* EINIGE EIGENTUMLICHKEITEN DER ERBLICHEN POLY- UND SYNDAKTYLIE BEI MENSCHEN. ACTA MED. SCAND. 65* 609-644, 1927.

*17570 POLYSYNDACTYLY WITH PECULIAR SKULL SHAPE

GREIG (1928) DESCRIBED DIGITAL MALFORMATIONS AND PECULIAR SKULL SHAPE IN MOTHER AND DAUGHTER. THE MOTHER HAD SYNDACTYLY OF BOTH HANDS. THE DAUGHTER HAD POLYSYNDACTYLY AND A PECULIAR SKULL SHAPE IN THE FORM OF EXPANDED CRANIAL VAULT LEADING TO HIGH FOREHEAD AND BREGMA, WITH NO EVIDENCE OF PRECOCIOUS CLOSURE OF CRANIAL SUTURES. THE DAUGHTER WAS OF ABOVE AVERAGE INTELLIGENCE. THE THUMBS AND GREAT TOES HAD BIFID TERMINAL PHALANGES. TEMTAMY (1966) STUDIED A PARTICULARLY INSTRUCTIVE FAMILY IN WHICH 10 MEMBERS OF 4 GENERATIONS IN 6 SIBSHIPS WERE AFFECTED IN THE PATTERN OF A FULLY PENETRANT AUTOSOMAL DOMINANT TRAIT.

GREIG, D. M.* OXYCEPHALY. EDINB. MED. J. 33* 189-218, 1928.

TEMTAMY, S. A.* GENETIC FACTORS IN HAND MALFORMATIONS. PH. D. THESIS, JOHNS HOPKINS UNIVERSITY, 1966.

*17580 POROKERATOSIS OF MIBELLI

THIS IS A RARE HEREDITARY KERATOATROPHODERMA CHARACTERIZED BY CENTRIFUGALLY SPREADING PATCHES SURROUNDED BY NARROW HORNY RIDGES AND WITH CENTRAL ATROPHY. THE LESIONS ARE CRATER-LIKE. MORE CASES HAVE BEEN DESCRIBED IN ITALIANS THAN IN OTHER NATIONALITIES, ACCORDING TO SOME, ALTHOUGH BLOOM AND ABRAMOWITZ (1943) WERE IMPRESSED WITH THE WIDE ETHNIC DISTRIBUTION OF CASES INCLUDING NEGROES. THEY DESCRIBED THE DISORDER IN AN ITALIAN MAN AND HIS TWO SONS. THE GRANDFATHER WAS SAID TO BE AFFECTED. AUTOSOMAL DOMINANT INHERITANCE, PROBABLY WITH SOME REDUCTION IN PENETRANCE IN FEMALES, SEEMS QUITE CERTAIN. THE PREFIX PORO- COMES FROM THE GREEK FOR CALLUS. MIBELLI (1860-1910), WHO DESCRIBED THIS CONDITION, WAS AN ITALIAN DERMATOLOGIST.

BLOOM, D. AND ABRAMOWITZ, E. W.* POROKERATOSIS MIBELLI* REPORT OF THREE CASES IN ONE FAMILY* HISTOLOGIC STUDIES. ARCH. DERM. SYPH. 47* 1-15, 1943.

REED, R. J. AND LEONE, P.* POROKERATOSIS - A MUTANT CLONAL KERATOSIS OF THE EPIDERMIS. I. HISTOGENESIS. ARCH. DERM. 101* 340-347, 1970.

SAUNDERS, T. S.* POROKERATOSIS. A DISEASE OF EPIDERMAL ECCRINE-SWEAT-DUCT UNITS. ARCH. DERM. 84* 980-988, 1961.

*17590 POROKERATOSIS, DISSEMINATED SUPERFICIAL ACTINIC (DSAP)

LESIONS OCCUR ALMOST ONLY IN SUN-EXPOSED AREAS OF THE SKIN. LESIONS DEVELOP AFTER AGE 16 AND PENETRANCE BECOMES ALMOST COMPLETE BY AGE 30 OR 40. DSAP IS MUCH MORE FREQUENT THAN POROKERATOSIS OF MIBELLI FROM WHICH IT MUST BE DISTINGUISHED.

ANDERSON, D. E. AND CHERNOSKY, M. E.* DISSEMINATED SUPERFICIAL ACTINIC

POROKERATOSIS. GENETIC ASPECTS. ARCH. DERM. 99* 408-412, 1969.

    CHERNOSKY, M. E. AND ANDERSON, D. E.* DISSEMINATED SUPERFICIAL ACTINIC POROKERATOSIS. CLINICAL STUDIES AND EXPERIMENTAL PRODUCTION OF LESIONS. ARCH. DERM. 99* 401-407, 1969.

*17600 PORPHYRIA, ACUTE INTERMITTENT (SWEDISH TYPE OF PORPHYRIA)

    SKIN LESIONS DO NOT OCCUR IN THIS DISORDER. PORPHOBILINOGEN IS PRESENT IN THE URINE AT ALL TIMES. ACUTE NEUROPATHIC ATTACKS MAY BE PRECIPITATED BY BARBI- TURATES. WALDENSTROM AND HAEGER-ARONSEN (1963) ESTIMATED THAT THERE MAY BE AS MANY AS 600 SUCH CASES IN SWEDEN. WITH (1969) CONCLUDED THAT 'GENE PENETRATION' AND DRUG SENSITIVITY DIFFER FROM FAMILY TO FAMILY. 'EVERY PORPHYRIC FAMILY HAS ITS OWN CHARACTERISTIC DISEASE.'

    DEAN, G.* THE PORPHYRIAS. A STORY OF INHERITANCE AND ENVIRONMENT. PHILADEL- PHIA* J. B. LIPPINCOTT CO., 1963.

    DRABKIN, D. L.* SOME HISTORICAL HIGHLIGHTS IN KNOWLEDGE OF PORPHYRINS AND PORPHYRIAS. ANN. N.Y. ACAD. SCI. 104* 658-665, 1963.

    GOLDBERG, A. AND RIMINGTON, C.* DISEASE OF PORPHYRIN METABOLISM. SPRINGFIELD, ILL.* CHARLES C THOMAS, 1963.

    LABBE, R. F.* METABOLIC ABNORMALITY IN PORPHYRIA. THE RESULT OF IMPAIRED BIOLOGICAL OXIDATION.Q LANCET 1* 1361-1364, 1967.

    MACALPINE, I., HUNTER, R., RIMINGTON, C., BROOKE, J. AND GOLDBERG, A.* PORPHYRIA - A RARE ROYAL MALADY. LONDON* BRIT. MED. ASS., 1968.

    STEIN, J. A. AND TSCHUDY, D. P.* ACUTE INTERMITTENT PORPHYRIA. A CLINICAL AND BIOCHEMICAL STUDY OF 46 PATIENTS. MEDICINE 49* 1-16, 1970.

    STRAND, L. J., FELSHER, B. F., REDEKER, A. G. AND MARVER, H. S.* HEME BIOSYN- THESIS IN INTERMITTENT ACUTE PORPHYRIA* DECREASED HEPATIC CONVERSION OF PORPHOBI- LINOGEN TO PORPHYRINS AND INCREASED DELTA AMINOLEVULINIC ACID SYNTHETASE ACTIVITY. PROC. NAT. ACAD. SCI. 67* 1315-1320, 1970.

    SWEENEY, V. P., PATHALS, M. A. AND ASBURY, A. K.* ACUTE INTERMITTENT PORPHYRIA. INCREASED ALA-SYNTHETASE ACTIVITY DURING AN ACUTE ATTACK. BRAIN 93* 369-380, 1970.

    TSCHUDY, D. P.* BIOCHEMICAL LESIONS IN PORPHYRIA. J.A.M.A. 191* 718-730, 1965.

    WALDENSTROM, J. AND HAEGER-ARONSEN, B.* DIFFERENT PATTERNS OF HUMAN PORPHYRIA. BRIT. MED. J. 2* 272-276, 1963.

    WALDENSTROM, J.* STUDIES ON THE INCIDENCE AND HEREDITY OF ACUTE PORPHYRIA IN SWEDEN. ACTA GENET. STATIST. MED. 6* 122-131, 1956.

    WITH, T. K.* HEREDITARY HEPATIC PORPHYRIAS. GENE PENETRATION, DRUG SENSITIVITY AND SUBDIVISION IN THE LIGHT OF SYSTEMATIC FAMILY STUDIES. ACTA MED. SCAND. 186* 117-124, 1969.

17610 PORPHYRIA, HEPATIC-CUTANEOUS TYPE (PORPHYRIA CUTANEA TARDA)

    THIS TYPE OCCURS PARTICULARLY IN ALCOHOLICS, PRODUCING SOME OF THE SAME NEUROLOGIC AND CUTANEOUS MANIFESTATIONS AS ARE SEEN IN OTHER FORMS OF PORPHYRIA. GENETICALLY DETERMINED IDIOSYNCRASY IS SUSPECTED. FEATURES INCLUDE HYPERPIGMENTATION AND SCLERODERMA-LIKE CHANGES. WATSON (1965) HAS OBSERVED AFFECTED BROTHERS. ZIPRKOWSKI (1966) OBSERVED PORPHYRIA CUTANEA TARDA IN THREE SUCCESSIVE GENERA- TIONS. VENOSECTION, ORIGINALLY PERFORMED BECAUSE OF CONFUSION WITH HEMOCHROMATO- SIS, SEEMS TO BE BENEFICIAL. PHLEBOTOMY WAS SYMPTOMATICALLY AND BIOCHEMICALLY BENEFICIAL (EPSTEIN AND REDEKER, 1968).

    EPSTEIN, J. H. AND REDEKER, A. G.* PORPHYRIA CUTANEA TARDA* A STUDY OF THE EFFECT OF PHLEBOTOMY. NEW ENG. J. MED. 279* 1301-1304, 1968.

    WATSON, C. J.* MINNEAPOLIS, MINN.* PERSONAL COMMUNICATION, 1965.

    ZIPRKOWSKI, L., KRAKOWSKI, A., CRISPIN, M. AND SZEINBERG, A.* PORPHYRIA CUTANEA TARDA HEREDITARIA. ISRAEL J. MED. SCI. 2* 338-343, 1966.

*17620 PORPHYRIA, VARIEGATA (SOUTH AFRICAN TYPE OF PORPHYRIA)

    DEAN (1963) HAS DESCRIBED IN AN ENGAGING MANNER HIS STUDIES OF PORPHYRIA IN SOUTH AFRICA AND COMPARATIVE STUDIES IN SWEDEN, HOLLAND, TURKEY AND ELSEWHERE. THE HIGH FREQUENCY OF THE GENE FOR PORPHYRIA VARIEGATA IN SOUTH AFRICA IS A CARDINAL EXAMPLE OF FOUNDER EFFECT. DEAN ESTIMATES THAT ABOUT 8,000 PERSONS IN SOUTH AFRICA NOW SUFFER FROM PORPHYRIA INHERITED FROM EITHER GERRIT JANSZ, A DUTCH SETTLER IN THE CAPE, OR HIS WIFE, ARIAANTJE JACOBS, WHO WAS ONE OF EIGHT SENT FROM AN ORPHANAGE IN ROTTERDAM TO PROVIDE WIVES FOR DUTCH SETTLERS IN THE CAPE. HE

ESTIMATES, FURTHERMORE, THAT ONE MILLION OF THREE MILLION WHITES ARE DESCENDANTS OF 40 ORIGINAL SETTLERS AND THEIR WIVES, A 12,000-FOLD INCREASE. AFFECTED PERSONS SHOW INCREASED FECAL EXCRETION OF PROTOPORPHYRIN AND COPROPORPHYRIN AT ALL TIMES. PORPHYRIA VARIEGATA WAS OBSERVED IN THREE FAMILIES IN SWEDEN BY HAMNSTROM ET AL. (1967). NO GENERALOGIC CONNECTION WITH ANY OF THE 600 KNOWN CASES OF ACUTE INTERMITTENT PORPHYRIA COULD BE SHOWN. MACALPINE ET AL. (1968) SUGGESTED THAT GEORGE III SUFFERED FROM PORPHYRIA AND THAT THE DISEASE CAN BE TRACED BACK TO MARY QUEEN OF SCOTS. IDENTIFICATION OF PORPHYRIA IN TWO LIVING PERSONS IN THE KINDRED SUPPORTED THEIR SUGGESTION. PRESUMABLY IF BARBITURATES HAD BEEN PART OF THE PHARMACEUTICAL ARMANENTARIUM 2 OR 3 CENTURIES AGO THE COURSE OF WORLD HISTORY WOULD HAVE BEEN QUITE DIFFERENT. ALTHOUGH THE MALADY OF GEORGE III WAS INDISTIN-GUISHABLE RETROSPECTIVELY FROM ACUTE INTERMITTENT PORPHYRIA, THE DERMATOLOGIC MANIFESTATIONS AND FECAL FINDINGS IN TWO LIVING MEMBERS OF THE FAMILY SUPPORT THE POSITION THAT THE ROYAL PORPHYRIA WAS THE VARIEGATE TYPE. COCHRANE AND GOLDBERG (1968) REPORTED STUDIES OF AN EXTENSIVE KINDRED OF WHICH THE FIRST AUTHOR IS A MEMBER.

COCHRANE, A. L. AND GOLDBERG, A.* A STUDY OF FAECAL PORPHYRIN LEVELS IN A LARGE FAMILY. ANN. HUM. GENET. 32* 195-208, 1968.

DEAN, G.* THE PORPHYRIAS. A STORY OF INHERITANCE AND ENVIRONMENT. PHILADEL-PHIA* J. B. LIPPINCOTT, CO., 1963.

HAMNSTROM, B., HAEGER-ARONSEN, B., WALDENSTROM, J., HYSING, B. AND MOLANDER, J.* THREE SWEDISH FAMILIES WITH PORPHYRIA VARIEGATA. BRIT. MED. J. 2* 449-453, 1967.

MACALPINE, I., HUNTER, R. AND RIMINGTON, C.* PORPHYRIA IN THE ROYAL HOUSES OF STUART, HANOVER AND PRUSSIA* A FOLLOW-UP STUDY OF GEORGE III'S ILLNESS. BRIT. MED. J. 1* 7-17, 1968.

17630 PREALBUMIN, POLYMORPHISM OF SERUM

FAGERHOL AND BRAEND (1965) DEMONSTRATED POLYMORPHISM BY STARCH GEL ELECTROPHORESIS AND PRESENTED FAMILY DATA SUPPORTING GENETIC CONTROL BY THREE CODOMINANT ALLELES. POLYMORPHISM OF PREALBUMIN IS KNOWN IN THE MOUSE AND PIG (REVIEWED BY LUSH, 1966). THE PREALBUMINS, SERUM PROTEINS WHICH MIGRATE FASTER THAN ALBUMIN IN ACIDIC STARCH GELS, INCLUDE ALPHA(1)-ANTITRYPSIN, THYROXINE BINDING PREALBUMIN AND OROSOMUCOID, AN ALPHA(1)-ACID GLYCOPROTEIN (Q.V.). POLYMORPHISM OF THE FIRST AND LAST ARE KNOWN. THE POLYMORPHISM OF PREALBUMIN WHICH FAGERHOL AND BRAEND (1965, 1966) DESCRIBED WAS SHOWN BY FAGERHOL AND LAURELL (1967) TO BE IDENTICAL TO ALPHA(1)-ANTITRYPSIN.

FAGERHOL, M. K. AND BRAEND, M.* CLASSIFICATION OF HUMAN SERUM PREALBUMIN AFTER STARCH GEL ELECTROPHORESIS. ACTA PATH. MICROBIOL. SCAND. 68* 434-438, 1966.

FAGERHOL, M. K. AND BRAEND, M.* SERUM PREALBUMIN* POLYMORPHISM IN MAN. SCIENCE 149* 986-987, 1965.

FAGERHOL, M. K. AND LAURELL, C.-B.* THE POLYMORPHISM OF *PREALBUMINS* AND ALPHA(1)-ANTITRYPSIN IN HUMAN SERA. CLIN. CHIM. ACTA. 16* 199-203, 1967.

LUSH, I. E.* THE BIOCHEMICAL GENETICS OF VERTEBRATES EXCEPT MAN. PHILADELPHIA* W. B. SAUNDERS, 1966.

*17640 PRECOCIOUS PUBERTY

THESE CASES ARE OFTEN MIS-DIAGNOSED ADRENOGENITAL SYNDROME. PUBERTY MAY OCCUR BEFORE 3 YEARS OF AGE. MALE-TO-MALE TRANSMISSION HAS BEEN OBSERVED. NO PECU-LIARITY HAS BEEN NOTED IN FEMALES, WHO CAN TRANSMIT THE TRAIT. ADULT HEIGHT IS REDUCED. RUSH ET AL. (1937) AND JACOBSEN AND MACKLIN (1952) REPORTED A FAMILY IN WHICH 27 MALES (BUT NO FEMALES) IN 4 GENERATIONS SHOWED SEXUAL PRECOCITY. WILKINS (1965) STATED THAT 'AMONG GIRLS WE ALSO HAVE SEEN A FAMILIAL TENDENCY TO SEXUAL PRECOCITY AND HAVE HAD ONE FAMILY IN WHICH BOTH SEXES WERE AFFECTED.' FERRIER ET AL. (1961) OBSERVED AFFECTED BROTHER AND SISTER. HAMPSON AND MONEY (1955) SUGGESTED THAT FEMALE SEXUAL PRECOCITY MAY BE TRANSMITTED THROUGH THE MALE. JUNGCK ET AL. (1957) OBSERVED TRANSMISSION OF MALE PRECOCITY THROUGH FEMALES. THE FAMILY OF BEAS ET AL. (1962) CONTAINED AN AFFECTED BROTHER AND SISTER. THIS IS SO-CALLED ISOSEXUAL PRECOCIOUS PUBERTY. A USUAL DEFINITION IS ONSET OF MENARCHE IN THE FEMALE BEFORE AGE 10 OR PUBERTAL CHANGES IN THE MALE BEFORE AGE EIGHT AND ONE HALF YEARS. IT IS A MORE FREQUENT OCCURRENCE IN FEMALES THAN IN MALES, BUT FAMILIAL OCCURRENCE SEEMS RARER IN FEMALES.

BEAS, F., ZURBRUGG, R. P., LEIBOW, S. G., PATTON, R. G. AND GARDNER, L. I.* FAMILIAL MALE SEXUAL PRECOCITY* REPORT OF THE ELEVENTH KINDRED FOUND, WITH OBSERVATIONS ON BLOOD GROUP LINKAGE AND URINARY C-19-STEROID EXCRETION. J. CLIN. ENDOCR. 22* 1095-1102, 1962.

FERRIER, P., SHEPARD, T. H. AND SMITH, E. K.* GROWTH DISTURBANCES AND VALUES FOR HORMONE EXCRETION IN VARIOUS FORMS OF PRECOCIOUS SEXUAL DEVELOPMENT. PEDIATRICS 28* 258-275, 1961.

HAMPSON, J. G. AND MONEY, J.* IDIOPATHIC SEXUAL PRECOCITY IN THE FEMALE. REPORT OF THREE CASES. PSYCHOSOM. MED. 17* 16-35, 1955.

JACOBSEN, A. W. AND MACKLIN, M. T.* HEREDITARY SEXUAL PRECOCITY* REPORT OF A FAMILY WITH 27 AFFECTED MEMBERS. PEDIATRICS 9* 682-694, 1952.

JUNGCK, E. C., THRASH, A. M., OHLMACHER, A. P., KNIGHT, A. M., JR. AND DYRENFORTH, L. Y.* SEXUAL PRECOCITY DUE TO INTERSTITIAL-CELL TUMOR OF THE TESTIS* REPORT OF 2 CASES. J. CLIN. ENDOCR. 17* 291-295, 1957.

MORTIMER, E. A.* FAMILIAL CONSTITUTIONAL PRECOCIOUS PUBERTY IN A BOY THREE YEARS OF AGE. REPORT OF A CASE. PEDIATRICS 13* 174-177, 1954.

NOVAK, E.* CONSTITUTIONAL TYPE OF FEMALE PRECOCIOUS PUBERTY WITH A REPORT OF 9 CASES. AM. J. OBSTET. GYNEC. 47* 20-42, 1944.

RUSH, H. P., BILDERBACK, J. B., SLOCUM, D. AND ROGERS, A.* PUBERTAS PRAECOX (MACROGENITOSOMIA). ENDOCRINOLOGY 21* 404-411, 1937.

WILKINS, L.* DIAGNOSIS AND TREATMENT OF ENDOCRINE DISORDERS IN CHILDHOOD AND ADOLESCENCE. SPRINGFIELD, ILL.* CHARLES C THOMAS, 1965 (3RD ED.).

17650 PRESENILE DEMENTIA WITH SPASTIC PARALYSIS

WORSTER-DROUGHT AND COLLEAGUES (1933, 1940) DESCRIBED 9 AFFECTED PERSONS IN THREE GENERATIONS. ONSET OCCURRED BETWEEN 40 AND 60 YEARS WITH EARLY ONSET OF SPASTICI-TY (INCREASED DTR AND TONE). MUSCULAR RIGIDITY OF EXTRAPYRAMIDAL TYPE WAS PRESENT. NO TREMORS, SPONTANEOUS MOVEMENTS OR SENSORY CHANGES WERE OBSERVED. MENTAL DETERIORATION WAS PROGRESSIVE, WITH SURVIVAL AS LONG AS 13 YEARS AFTER ONSET. PARESIS OF PYRAMIDAL AND EXTRAPYRAMIDAL TYPE IS RARE IN PICK'S DISEASE AND OCCURS LATE. NO MALE-TO-MALE TRANSMISSION WAS NOTED BY WORSTER-DROUGHT ET AL. (1940), ALTHOUGH 12 PERSONS IN 3 GENERATIONS WERE AFFECTED.

WORSTER-DROUGHT, C., GREENFIELD, J. G. AND MCMENEMEY, W. H.* A FORM OF FAMILIAL PRESENILE DEMENTIA WITH SPASTIC PARALYSIS (INCLUDING PATHOLOGICAL EXAMINATION OF A CASE). BRAIN 63* 237-254, 1940.

WORSTER-DROUGHT, C., HILL, T. R. AND MCMENEMEY, W. H.* FAMILIAL PRESENILE DEMENTIA WITH SPASTIC PARALYSIS. J. NEUROL. PSYCHOPATH. 14* 27-34, 1933.

17660 PRESENILE DEMENTIA, KRAEPELIA TYPE

A NONSPECIFIC TYPE OF FAMILIAL PRESENILE DEMENTIA APPARENTLY DISTINCT FROM BOTH ALZHEIMER'S DISEASE AND PICK'S DISEASE (Q.V.) WAS DESCRIBED BY SCHAUMBURG AND SUZUKI (1968) IN 6 PERSONS IN 3 GENERATIONS WITH MALE-TO-MALE TRANSMISSION. THE HISTOLOGIC CHANGES CORRESPONDED TO THOSE DESCRIBED FOR KRAEPELIN'S DISEASE. ONSET WAS BETWEEN AGES 28 AND 34 YEARS IN 4 OF THE PATIENTS.

SCHAUMBURG, H. H. AND SUZUKI, K.* NON-SPECIFIC FAMILIAL PRESENILE DEMENTIA. J. NEUROL. NEUROSURG. PSYCHIAT. 31* 479-486, 1968.

*17670 PROGNATHISM, MANDIBULAR

MANDIBULAR PROGNATHISM WAS TRANSMITTED THROUGH MANY GENERATIONS OF THE HABSBURG LINE AS A SIMPLE DOMINANT (RUBBRECHT, 1930* STROHMAYER, 1937). WE HAVE OBSERVED A DOMINANT INHERITANCE PATTERN IN A NEGRO FAMILY. INVOLVEMENT IN FOUR GENERATIONS WAS DESCRIBED BY STILES AND LUKE (1953). AN APPARENT CONDUCTOR DID NOT SHOW THE CONDITION. MANDIBULAR PROGNATHISM IS A FEATURE OF THE XXY, XXXY, AND XXXXY SYNDROMES AND OF INTEREST IS THE PROGRESSIVE INCREASE OF THIS FEATURE AS THE NUMBER OF X CHROMOSOMES INCREASED (GORLIN ET AL., 1965). ALTHOUGH THE X CHROMO-SOME HAS A ROLE, THE MENDELIAN TRAIT IS NOT X-LINKED.

GORLIN, R. J., REDMAN, R. S. AND SHAPIRO, B. L.* EFFECT OF X-CHROMOSOME ANENPLOIDY ON JAW GROWTH. J. DENTAL RES. 44* 269-282, 1965.

GRABB, W. C., HODGE, G. P., DINGMAN, R. O. AND ONEAL, R. M.* THE HABSBURG JAW. PLAST. RECONSTR. SURG. 42* 442-445, 1968.

HAECKER, V.* DER FAMILIENTYPUS DER HABSBURGER. Z. ABST. VERERB. 6* 61-89, 1911.

RUBBRECHT, O.* DER UNTERKIEFERPROGNATHISMUS UND DESSEN VEREBUNG NACH DEM MENDELSCHEN. GESETZ. PROVINCE DENTAIRE, P. 322, 1930.

RUBBRECHT, O.* L'ORIGIN DU TYPE FAMILIAL DE LA MAISON DE HABSBOURG. BRUXELLES* G. VAN OEST ET CIE, 1910.

RUBBRECHT, O.* STUDY OF THE HEREDITY OF THE ANOMALIES OF THE JAWS. AM. J. ORTHODONT. 25* 751-779, 1939.

STILES, K. A. AND LUKE, J. E.* THE INHERITANCE OF MALOCCLUSION DUE TO MANDIBU-LAR PROGNATHISM. J. HERED. 44* 241-245, 1953.

17680 PRONATION-SUPINATION OF THE FOREARM, IMPAIRMENT OF

THOMPSON ET AL. (1968) DESCRIBED A FAMILY IN WHICH MALES IN THREE SUCCESSIVE
GENERATIONS HAD LIMITATION IN PRONATION AND SUPINATION OF THE FOREARMS. RADIO-
ULNAR SYNOSTOSIS (Q.V.) WAS NOT PRESENT.

THOMPSON, J. S., MCLAUGHLIN, P. R. AND HESLIN, D. J.* IMPAIRED PRONATION-
SUPINATION OF THE FOREARM* AN INHERITED CONDITION. J. MED. GENET. 5* 48-51, 1968.

17690 PROTEOLYTIC CAPACITY OF PLASMA

JACOBSEN (1968) CONCLUDED THAT LOW PROTEOLYTIC CAPACITY IS INHERITED AS AN
AUTOSOMAL DOMINANT. INCREASED TENDENCY TO THROMBOSIS DID NOT OCCUR IN THESE
PERSONS.

JACOBSEN, C. D.* PROTEOLYTIC CAPACITY IN HUMAN PLASMA. GENETICS AND CLINICAL
STUDY. SCAND. J. CLIN. LAB. INVEST. 21* 227-237, 1968.

*17700 PROTOPORPHYRIA, ERYTHROPOIETIC

HAEGER-ARONSEN (1963) FOUND FIVE CASES IN THREE GENERATIONS OF A SWEDISH FAMILY.
IT SEEMS POSSIBLE, HOWEVER, THAT TWO OF THE CASES ARE IN FACT HETEROZYGOTES AND A
FATHER AND HIS TWO DAUGHTERS ARE HOMOZYGOUS. THE MOTHER OF THESE DAUGHTERS (A
HETEROZYGOTE BY THIS LINE OF THOUGHT) WAS APPARENTLY NOT TESTED. FIRST DESCRIBED
BY MAGNUS ET AL. (1961), THE CONDITION IS CHARACTERIZED BY THE SUDDEN ONSET IN
CHILDHOOD OF ITCHING, ERYTHEMA AND EDEMA FOLLOWING EXPOSURE TO ULTRAVIOLET LIGHT.
VESICLES NEVER DEVELOP. THE MOST CONSPICUOUS BIOCHEMICAL CHANGE IS A MARKED
INCREASE IN THE PROTOPORPHYRIN AND COPROPORPHYRIN CONTENT OF RED BLOOD CELLS. THE
URINARY EXCRETION OF PORPHYRINS AND THEIR PRECURSORS IS NORMAL. FECAL EXCRETION
OF COPROPORPHYRIN AND PROTOPORPHYRIN MAY BE INCREASED. IT IS OF NOTE THAT BOTH OF
THE BRITISH PATIENTS OF MAGNUS ET AL. AND ONE OF HAEGER-ARONSEN'S PATIENTS WERE
OPERATED ON FOR GALLSTONES AT A RELATIVELY YOUNG AGE. THREE GENERATIONS WERE
AFFECTED IN THE FAMILY STUDIED BY LYNCH AND MIEDLER (1965). CRIPPS (1966) CLAIMED
THAT PATIENTS WITH THIS CONDITION HAVE BEEN INCORRECTLY REPORTED AS EXAMPLES OF
LIPOID PROTEINOSIS. RATHER NUMEROUS INSTANCES OF PARENT-OFFSPRING INVOLVEMENT
HAVE BEEN OBSERVED. BETA-CAROTENE IS AN EFFECTIVE PHOTOPROTECTIVE AGENT (MAT-
THEWS-ROTH ET AL., 1970). BECAUSE OF EVIDENCE THEY ADDUCED FOR FORMATION OF
PROTOPORPHYRIN IN AT LEAST THE TWO TISSUES, SCHOLNICK ET AL. (1971) PROPOSED THAT
THE DISORDER BE RENAMED ERYTHROHEPATIC PROTOPORPHYRIA.

CRIPPS, D. J.* ERYTHROPOIETIC PROTOPORPHYRIA (ANTEA LIPOID PROTEINOSIS) IN
SISTERS. ARCH. DERM. 94* 682-686, 1966.

DONALDSON, E. M., DONALDSON, A. D. AND RIMINGTON, C.* ERYTHROPOIETIC PROTOPOR-
PHYRIA* A FAMILY STUDY. BRIT. MED. J. 1* 659-663, 1967.

HAEGER-ARONSEN, B. AND KROOK, G.* ERYTHROPOIETIC PROTOPORPHYRIA. A STUDY OF
KNOWN CASES IN SWEDEN. ACTA MED. SCAND. 445 (SUPPL.)* 48-55, 1966.

HAEGER-ARONSEN, B.* ERYTHROPOIETIC PROTOPORPHYRIA. A NEW TYPE OF INBORN ERROR
OF METABOLISM. AM. J. MED. 35* 450-454, 1963.

LYNCH, P. J. AND MIEDLER, L. J.* ERYTHROPOIETIC PROTOPORPHYRIA. REPORT OF A
FAMILY AND A CLINICAL REVIEW. ARCH. DERM. 92* 351-356, 1965.

MAGNUS, I. A., JARRETT, A., PRANKERD, T. A. AND RIMINGTON, C.* ERYTHROPOIETIC
PORPHYRIA. A NEW PROTOPORPHYRIA SYNDROME WITH SOLAR URTICARIA DUE TO PROTOPOR-
PHYRINAEMIA. LANCET 2* 448-451, 1961.

MATTHEWS-ROTH, M. M., PATHAK, M. A., FITZPATRICK, T. B., HARBER, L. C. AND
KASS, E. H.* BETA-CAROTENE AS A PHOTOPROTECTIVE AGENT IN ERYTHROPOIETIC PROTOPOR-
PHYRIA. NEW ENG. J. MED. 282* 1231-1234, 1970.

PETERKA, E. S., FUSARO, R. M., RUNGE, W. J., JAFFE, M. O. AND WATSON, C. J.*
ERYTHROPOIETIC PROTOPORPHYRIA. I. CLINICAL AND LABORATORY FEATURES IN SEVEN NEW
CASES. J.A.M.A. 193* 1036-1042, 1965.

REED, W. B., WUEPPER, K. D., EPSTEIN, J. H., REDEKER, A., SIMONSON, R. J. AND
MCKUSICK, V. A.* ERYTHROPOIETIC PROTOPORPHYRIA. J.A.M.A. 214* 1060-1066, 1970.

SCHOLNICK, P., MARVER, H. S. AND SCHMID, R.* ERYTHROPOIETIC PROTOPORPHYRIA*
EVIDENCE FOR MULTIPLE SITES OF EXCESS PROTOPORPHYRIN FORMATION. J. CLIN. INVEST.
50* 203-207, 1971.

17710 PRURITUS, HEREDITARY LOCALIZED

COMINGS AND COMINGS (1965) DESCRIBED THE ENTITY IN 8 MEMBERS OF THREE SIBSHIPS IN
TWO GENERATIONS IN A PATTERN CONSISTENT WITH EITHER AUTOSOMAL OR X-LINKED DOMINANT
INHERITANCE. ONSET WAS IN THE THIRD DECADE AND THE ITCHING WAS LOCATED IN AN AREA

COMINGS, D. E. AND COMINGS, S. N.* HEREDITARY LOCALIZED PRURITUS. ARCH. DERM. 92* 236-237, 1965.

17720 PSEUDO-ALDOSTERONISM (LIDDLE SYNDROME)

LIDDLE ET AL. (1963) DESCRIBED HYPERTENSION ASSOCIATED WITH HYPOKALEMIC ALKALOSIS NOT DUE TO HYPERALDOSTERONISM BUT RATHER TO A RENAL TUBULAR PECULIARITY. THREE GENERATIONS HAD BEEN AFFECTED WITH NO KNOWN MALE-TO-MALE TRANSMISSION. SEE POTASSIUM AND MAGNESIUM DEPLETION IN THE RECESSIVE CATALOG. LIDDLE'S SYNDROME IS CHARACTERIZED BY HYPOALDOSTERONISM, HYPOKALEMIA, DECREASED RENIN AND ANGIOTENSIN. GARDNER ET AL. (1970) PRESENTED EVIDENCE FOR A PRIMARY DEFECT IN MEMBRANE TRANSPORT.

GARDNER, J., LAPEY, A., SIMOPOULOS, A. AND BRAVO, E.* EVIDENCE FOR A PRIMARY DISTURBANCE OF MEMBRANE TRANSPORT IN BARTTER'S SYNDROME AND LIDDLE'S SYNDROME. (ABSTRACT) J. CLIN. INVEST. 49* 32A ONLY, 1970.

LIDDLE, G. W., BLEDSOE, T. AND COPPAGE, W. S., JR.* A FAMILIAL RENAL DISORDER SIMULATING PRIMARY ALDOSTERONISM BUT WITH NEGLIGIBLE ALDOSTERONE SECRETION. TRANS. ASS. AM. PHYSICIANS 76* 199-213, 1963.

17730 PSEUDO-ARTHROGRYPOSIS (HEREDITARY CONGENITAL RIGIDITY OF ELBOWS AND KNEES)

PASMA AND WILDERVANCK (1956) DESCRIBED A GRANDMOTHER, HER DAUGHTER AND THREE GRANDDAUGHTERS WITH RIGIDITY OF THE ELBOWS AND KNEES. THE GRANDMOTHER SHOWED BONY ANKYLOSIS AT THE ELBOW AND PROXIMAL FUSION OF THE TIBIA AND FIBULA. THEY POINTED OUT A SIMILARITY TO THE CASES IN FEMALES IN THREE GENERATIONS DESCRIBED BY SIWON (1928). IN THE LATTER FAMILY THE RIGIDITY APPEARS TO HAVE BEEN CONFINED TO THE ELBOWS. ONE PATIENT WAS SHOWN TO HAVE BILATERAL FUSION OF THE HUMERUS, RADIUS AND ULNA AS IN ONE OF THE PATIENTS OF PASMA AND WILDERVANCK. SEE ALSO PRONATION-SUPINATION OF FOREARM, IMPAIRMENT OF. SEE RADIO-ULNAR SYNOSTOSIS. SEE KUSKOKWIN SYNDROME.

PASMA, A. AND WILDERVANCK, L. S.* HEREDITARY OCCURRENCE OF CONGENITAL RIGIDITY OF THE ELBOWS AND KNEES (CONGENITAL MULTIPLE 'PSEUDOARTHROGRYPOSIS'). ARCH. CHIR. NEERL. 8* 43-56, 1956.

SIWON, P.* KONGENITALE, HEREDITARE, DOPPELSEITIGE ANKYLOSEN DER ELLENBOGENGE-LENKE. DUETSCH. Z. CHIR. 209* 338-349, 1928.

*17740 PSEUDOCHOLINESTERASE TYPES, E(1) VARIANTS

ALTHOUGH SUCCINYLCHOLINE SENSITIVITY (PSEUDOCHOLINESTERASE DEFICIENCY) IS A RECESSIVE, METHODS FOR DEMONSTRATING THE HETEROZYGOTE AND SEVERAL DIFFERENT RARE HETEROZYGOUS PHENOTYPES ARE KNOWN, HENCE INCLUSION HERE. FOUR ALLELIC FORMS OF THE GENE RESPONSIBLE FOR SERUM PSEUDOCHOLINESTERASE ARE RECOGNIZED. IN ADDITION TO THAT DETERMINING THE TYPICAL PSEUDOCHOLINESTERASE, THESE ARE (1) GENE FOR ATYPICAL FORM OF ENZYME LESS INHIBITED BY DIBUCAINE THAN THE NORMAL, (2) GENE FOR FORM WITH NORMAL DIBUCAINE INHIBITION BUT LESS INHIBITION BY FLUORIDE THAN THE NORMAL, AND (3) GENE DETERMINING COMPLETE ABSENCE OF CHOLINESTERASE ACTIVITY ('SILENT GENE'). IN ADDITION TO THE ABOVE ALLELES AT THE E(1) LOCUS, A SECOND SEPARATE LOCUS CALLED E(2) WAS DESCRIBED BY HARRIS ET AL. (1963). MOTULSKY AND MORROW (1968), USING A RAPID SCREENING TEST, DEMONSTRATED A LOW FREQUENCY OF HETEROZYGOTES AMONG CONGOLESE AFRICANS, JAPANESE, TAIWANESE, FILIPINOS AND ESKIMOS. U.S. CAUCASIANS, GREEKS, YUGOSLAVS AND EAST INDIANS HAD A RELATIVELY HIGH FREQUENCY (2.8 TO 3.3 PERCENT). THEY PREDICTED A LOW FREQUENCY OF SUXAME-THONIUM APNEA IN THE LOW FREQUENCY GROUPS. SEE TRANSFERRINS FOR REFERENCE TO LINKAGE BETWEEN TRANSFERRIN LOCUS AND PSEUDOCHOLINESTERASE LOCUS. THE CYNTHIANA VARIANT IS ASSOCIATED WITH INCREASED ENZYME ACTIVITY (YOSHIDA AND MOTULSKY, 1969). WHETHER IT IS DETERMINED BY THE (E1) OR (E2) LOCUS IS NOT KNOWN.

ALTLAND, K. AND GOEDDE, H. W.* HETEROGENEITY IN THE SILENT GENE PHENOTYPE OF PSEUDOCHOLINESTERASE OF HUMAN SERUM. BIOCHEM. GENET. 4* 321-338, 1970.

DIETZ, A. A., LUBRANO, T. AND RUBINSTEIN, H. M.* FOUR FAMILIES SEGREGATING FOR THE SILENT GENE FOR SERUM CHOLINESTERASE. ACTA GENET. STATIST. MED. 15* 208-217, 1965.

GOEDDE, H. W. AND BAITSCH, H.* ON NOMENCLATURE OF PSEUDOCHOLINESTERASE POLYMORPHISM. ACTA GENET. STATIST. MED. 14* 366-369, 1964.

HARRIS, H., HOPKINSON, D. A., ROBSON, E. B. AND WHITTAKER, M.* GENETICAL STUDIES ON A NEW VARIANT OF SERUM CHOLINESTERASE DETECTED BY ELECTROPHORESIS. ANN. HUM. GENET. 26* 359-382, 1963.

MOTULSKY, A. G. AND MORROW, A.* ATYPICAL CHOLINESTERASE GENE E(1)(A)* RARITY IN NEGROES AND MOST ORIENTALS. SCIENCE 159* 202-203, 1968.

WHITTAKER, M.* PSEUDOCHOLINESTERASE VARIANTS* A STUDY OF FOURTEEN FAMILIES SELECTED VIA THE FLUORIDE RESISTANT PHENOTYPE. ACTA GENET. STATIST. MED. 17* 1-

YOSHIDA, A. AND MOTULSKY, A. G.* A PSEUDOCHOLINESTERASE VARIANT (E CYNTHIANA)
ASSOCIATED WITH ELEVATED PLASMA ENZYME ACTIVITY. AM. J. HUM. GENET. 21* 486-498,
1969.

*17750 PSEUDOCHOLINESTERASE TYPES, E(2) VARIANTS

SEE ABOVE.

17760 PSEUDOCHOLINESTERASE, INCREASE IN PLASMA LEVEL OF

NEITLICH (1966) DESCRIBED A KINDRED WITH INCREASED PLASMA CHOLINESTERASE ACTIVITY
AND DECREASED RESPONSIVENESS TO SUCCINYLCHOLINESTERASE. SEE CHOLINESTERASE,
REDUCTION IN RED CELL.

NEITLICH, H. W.* INCREASED PLASMA CHOLINESTERASE ACTIVITY AND SUCCINYLCHOLINE
RESISTANCE* A GENETIC VARIANT. J. CLIN. INVEST. 45* 380-387, 1966.

17770 PSEUDOGLAUCOMA

THIS TERM APPLIES TO A CONDITION CHARACTERIZED BY NORMAL INTRAOCULAR TENSION WITH
CUPPING OF THE OPTIC DISC AND GLAUCOMATOUS VISUAL FIELD DEFECTS. SANDVIG (1961)
DESCRIBED NORWEGIAN FAMILIES WITH A DOMINANT INHERITANCE PATTERN.

SANDVIG, K.* PSEUDOGLAUCOMA OF AUTOSOMAL DOMINANT INHERITANCE. ACTA OPHTHAL.
39* 33-43, 1961.

17780 PSEUDOPAPILLEDEMA

HOYT AND PONT (1962) DESCRIBED 28 PATIENTS WHO WERE FIRST THOUGHT TO HAVE BRAIN
TUMORS. IDENTICAL TWINS WERE BOTH AFFECTED. WE HAVE OBSERVED AFFECTED FATHER AND
DAUGHTER. 'BURIED DRUSEN' WERE THOUGHT TO BE THE CAUSE. JACQUEMIN (1964)
REPORTED MOTHER AND TWO DAUGHTERS. THERE MAY BE MORE THAN ONE TYPE OF PSEUDOPA-
PILLEDEMA. FITE AND LEWIS (1966) DESCRIBED FATHER AND TWO SONS WITH A TYPE DUE
APPARENTLY TO 'HYPEREMIA.'

CHAMBERS, J. W. AND WALSH, F. B.* HYALINE BODIES IN THE OPTIC DISCS* REPORT OF
10 CASES EXEMPLIFYING IMPORTANCE IN NEUROLOGICAL DIAGNOSIS. BRAIN 74* 95-108,
1951.

FITE, J. D. AND LEWIS, A. D.* FAMILIAL ANOMALY SIMULATING PAPILLEDEMA* A CASE
REPORT. J. PEDIAT. 68* 927-931, 1966.

HOYT, W. F. AND PONT, M. E.* PSEUDOPAPILLEDEMA* ANOMALOUS ELEVATION OF OPTIC
DISK. PITFALLS IN DIAGNOSIS AND MANAGEMENT. J.A.M.A. 181* 191-196, 1962.

JACQUEMIN, P. J.* OEDEME PAPILLAIRE FAMILIAL ET HEREDITAIRE. ANN. OCULIST.
197* 449-460, 1964.

LORENTZEN, S. E.* DRUSEN OF OPTIC DISK, IRREGULARLY DOMINANT HEREDITARY
AFFECTION. ACTA OPHTHAL. 39* 626-643, 1961.

LORENTZEN, S. E.* DRUSEN OF THE OPTIC DISK. A CLINICAL AND GENETIC STUDY.
ACTA OPHTHAL. 90 (SUPPL.)* 1-181, 1966.

*17790 PSORIASIS

A VERY LARGE FAMILY TREE HAS BEEN ASSEMBLED IN NORTH CAROLINA (ABELE ET AL.,
1963). THE AUTHORS CONCLUDED THAT PENETRANCE WAS REDUCED TO ABOUT 60 PERCENT.
THE PREVALENCE OF ARTHRITIS WAS NOT INCREASED IN THE PSORIATIC MEMBERS OF THE
KINDRED. LOMHOLT (1965) DID A COMPREHENSIVE STUDY IN THE FAROE ISLANDS. HE FOUND
THAT 91 PERCENT OF PATIENTS HAD AFFECTED RELATIVES. TRANSMISSION THROUGH MANY
GENERATIONS OF MANY LINES OF THE LARGE KINDRED REPORTED BY ABELE ET AL. (1963)
SUPPORTS DOMINANT INHERITANCE, THE MODE OF INHERITANCE ESPOUSED BY ROMANUS (1945).
STEINBERG ET AL. (1951) SUGGESTED THAT HOMOZYGOSITY AT TWO SEPARATE LOCI WOULD
BEST EXPLAIN THEIR FAMILY DATA.

ABELE, D. C., DOBSON, R. L. AND GRAHAM, J. B.* HEREDITY AND PSORIASIS. STUDY
OF A LARGE FAMILY. ARCH. DERM. 88* 38-47, 1963.

LOMHOLT, G.* PSORIASIS* PREVALENCE, SPONTANEOUS COURSE, AND GENETICS. A CENSUS
STUDY ON THE PREVALENCE OF SKIN DISEASE ON THE FAROE ISLANDS. COPENHAGEN* G. E.
C. GAD, 1963.

LOMHOLT, G.* PSORIASIS-PRAVALENZ, SPONTANER VERLAUF UND VERERBUNG. EINE
ZENSUSUNTERSUCHUNG VON DEN FARINSELN. Z. HAUT GESCHLECHTSKR. 38* 223-238, 1965.

ROMANUS, T.* PSORIASIS FROM A PROGNOSTIC AND HEREDITARY POINT OF VIEW.
DISSERTATION, UPPSALA, 1945.

STEINBERG, A. G., BECKER, S. W., FITZPATRICK, T. B. AND KIERLAND, R. R.* A

GENETIC AND STATISTICAL STUDY OF PSORIASIS. AM. J. HUM. GENET. 3* 267-281, 1951. (A FURTHER NOTE ON THE GENETICS OF PSORIASIS. AM. J. HUM. GENET. 4* 373-375, 1952.)

WARD, J. H. AND STEPHENS, F. E.* INHERITANCE OF PSORIASIS IN A UTAH KINDRED. ARCH. DERM. 84* 589-592, 1961.

17800 PTERYGIUM

WHEN THIS TERM IS USED WITHOUT FURTHER QUALIFICATION IT REFERS TO A WING-SHAPED THICKENING IN THE CONJUNCTIVA IN THE INTERPALPEBRAL FISSURE AREA. (PTERYGIUM COLLI IS WEBBED NECK. WEBBING IN THE POPLITEAL (Q.V.) OR ANTECUBITAL AREA IS ALSO REFERRED TO AS PTERYGIUM.) HILGERS (1960) AND SCHWARTZ (1960) CONCLUDED THAT PTERYGIUM IS IN MANY INSTANCES A DOMINANT TRAIT. ENVIRONMENTAL FACTORS MAY INFLUENCE PENETRANCE. THE DISORDER IS MORE FREQUENT IN PERSONS WHO WORK OUT-OF-DOORS. ITS FREQUENCY IS PROBABLY THE SAME IN MEN AND WOMEN WORKING INDOORS. ALTHOUGH PTERYGIUM DEVELOPS SOMETIME FAIRLY LATE IN LIFE IN MOST CASES, IT IS ALREADY EVIDENT AT BIRTH IN RARE INSTANCES (SCHWARTZ, 1960). MURKEN AND DANNHEIM (1965) CONCLUDED THAT THE RARE CONGENITAL TYPE OF PTERYGIUM IS INHERITED AS A DOMINANT WITH 70 PERCENT PENETRANCE. JACKLIN (1964) REPORTED 6 AFFECTED PERSONS (4 FEMALES, 2 MALES) IN 3 GENERATIONS OF A FAMILY.

HILGERS, J. H. C.* PTERYGIUM, ITS INCIDENCE, HEREDITY AND ETIOLOGY. AM. J. OPHTHAL. 50* 635-644, 1960.

JACKLIN, H. N.* FAMILIAL PREDISPOSITION TO PTERYGIUM FORMATION. REPORT OF A FAMILY. AM. J. OPHTHAL. 57* 481-482, 1964.

MURKEN, J. D. AND DANNHEIM, R.* ZUR GENETIK DES PTERYGIUM CORNEAE. KLIN. MBL. ANGENHEILK. 147* 574-579, 1965.

SCHWARTZ, V. J.* CONGENITAL PTERYGIUM. J.A.M.A. 174* 2078-2079, 1960.

17810 PTERYGIUM COLLI SYNDROME

SOME FEMALES HAVE WEBBED NECK (PTERYGIUM COLLI), SHORT STATURE AND LYMPHEDEMA - FEATURES SUGGESTING THE XO TURNER SYNDROME - BUT HAVE NORMAL SEXUAL DEVELOPMENT. PULMONIC STENOSIS IS FREQUENT IN THESE CASES. THE ETIOLOGY AND PATHOGENESIS ARE OBSCURE. CHROMOSOMAL MOSAICISM SEEMS TO HAVE BEEN ADEQUATELY EXCLUDED IN MANY CASES AND FAMILIAL INCIDENCE IS NOT STRIKING. WE SOMETIMES REFER TO THIS CONDITION AS THE FEMALE PSEUDO-TURNER SYNDROME. WHEN THE SAME SITUATION OCCURS IN MALES, IT IS SOMETIMES REFERRED TO AS THE MALE TURNER SYNDROME. MOLDENHAUER (1964) DESCRIBED A CONDITION HE CALLED NIELSON'S SYNDROME IN 4 FEMALES OF THREE GENERATIONS OF A FAMILY. THE FEATURES WERE SHORT STATURE, PTOSIS, CLEFT PALATE, CAMPTODACTYLY, PTERYGIUM COLLI AND VERTEBRAL ANOMALIES. FERTILITY WAS NORMAL. THE DIFFERENCE FROM THE KLIPPEL-FEIL SYNDROME AND FROM THE BONNEVIE-ULLRICH SYNDROME IS NOT CLEAR. EITHER X-LINKED OR AUTOSOMAL DOMINANT INHERITANCE COULD ACCOUNT FOR THE FINDINGS. DORNSTEIN (1966) DESCRIBED TWO UNRELATED MALES WITH WHAT HE TERMED PTERYGOLYMPHANGIECTASIA. IN ADDITION TO PTERYGIUM COLLI, PERI-PHERAL EDEMA PERSISTED TO THE THIRD DECADE. THE FAMILY HISTORY WAS UNREMARKABLE. IN BOTH, THE GENITALIA WERE FULLY DEVELOPED AND SPERM PRODUCTION WAS NORMAL. CHROMOSOME STUDY IN ONE YIELDED NORMAL FINDINGS. TO DATE ONLY FEMALES HAVE TRANSMITTED THIS DISORDER (NORA AND SINHA, 1967* POLANI ET AL., 1967). MATOLCSY (1936) DESCRIBED A BROTHER AND SISTER WITH SEVERE WEBBING OF THE NECK, AXILLAE, POPLITEAL FOSSAE AND FINGERS. THE BOY, AGE 13, HAD CRYPTORCHIDISM. ALSEV AND REINWEIN (1958) DESCRIBED BROTHERS AGED 16 AND 19 WHO HAD WEBBING OF THE NECK, CONGENITAL HEART DISEASE, LYMPHEDEMA OF LATE ONSET (MEIGE TYPE) AND CRYPTORCHI-DISM. GOLDEN AND LAKIM (1959) REPORTED AS EXAMPLES OF THE MARFAN SYNDROME TWO BROTHERS WITH WEB NECK, FIXED FLEXION OF THE KNEES AND DISTAL INTRAPHALANGEAL JOINTS, KYPHOSCOLIOSIS, PECTUS EXCAVATUM AND ATRIAL SEPTAL DEFECT WHICH IN ONE BOY WAS CONFIRMED BY AUTOPSY. THE FATHER HAD PECTUS EXCAVATUM AND HEART DISEASE. MIGEON AND WHITEHOUSE (1967) DESCRIBED TWO FAMILIES EACH WITH TWO SIBS WITH SOMATIC FEATURES OF THE TURNER SYNDROME. IN ONE TWO BROTHERS HAD WEBBING OF THE NECK, COARCTATION OF THE AORTA AND CRYPTORCHIDISM. IN THE SECOND, A BROTHER AND SISTER WERE AFFECTED. SIMPSON ET AL. (1969) REPORTED EXPERIENCES WHICH SUGGEST THAT RUBELLA EMBRYOPATHY MAY RESULT IN THE TURNER PHENOTYPE THEREBY ACCOUNTING FOR EITHER THE MALE TURNER SYNDROME OR THE FEMALE PSEUDO-TURNER SYNDROME. KIND (1970) DESCRIBED AFFECTED MOTHER AND DAUGHTER. IN ADDITION TO BILATERAL POPLITEAL PTERYGIUM, APLASIA OF THE LABIA MAJORA, ANKYLOBLEPHARON FILIFORME, FILIFORM BANDS BETWEEN THE JAWS, LIP PITS AND CLEFT PALATE WERE PRESENT. SEE TURNER PHENOTYPE.

ALSLEV, J. AND REINWEIN, H.* UBER DAS FAMILIARE VORKOMMEN DES SOGENANNTENULL-RICH-TURNER-SYNDROMES UN DAS VORHANDENSEIN EINES PTERYGIUM COLLI, EINES KRYPTOR-CHISMUS UND DES MEIGE-SYNDROMES BEI ZWEIBRUDERN MIT KONGENITALEN VITIEN. DEUTSCH. MED. WSCHR. 83* 601-604, 1958.

DORNSTEIN, P.* PTERYGOLYMPHANGIECTASIA. J. ALBERT EINSTEIN MED. CENT. 14* 149-156, 1966.

GOLDEN, R. L. AND LAKIM, H.* THE FORME FRUSTE IN MARFAN'S SYNDROME. NEW ENG. J. MED. 260* 797-801, 1959.

KOPITS, E.* DIEALS 'FLUGHAUT' BEZEICHNETEN MISSBILDUNGEN UND DEREN OPERATIVE BEHANDLUNG (MUSCULO-DYSPLASIA CONGENITA). LANGENBECK. ARCH. KLIN. CHIR. 37* 539-549, 1937.

MATOLCSY, T.* UBER DIE CHIRURGISCHE BEHANDLUNG DER ANGEBORENEN FLUGHAUT. LANGENBECK. ARCH. KLIN. CHIR. 185* 675-681, 1936.

MIGEON, B. R. AND WHITEHOUSE, D.* FAMILIAL OCCURRENCE OF THE SOMATIC PHENOTYPE OF TURNER'S SYNDROME. JOHNS HOPKINS MED. J. 120* 78-80, 1967.

MOLDENHAUER, E.* ZUR KLINIK DES NIELSON-SYNDROMES. DERM. WSCHR. 150* 594-601, 1964.

NORA, J. J. AND SINHA, A. K.* HEREDITARY TURNER PHENOTYPES. (LETTER) LANCET 2* 256 ONLY, 1967.

POLANI, P. E., ANGELL, R. AND POLANI, N.* ULLRICH'S SYNDROME. (LETTER) LANCET 2* 421 ONLY, 1967.

ROSSI, E. AND CAFLISCH, A.* LE SYNDROME DU PTERYGIUM STATUS BONNEVIE-ULLRICH, DYSTROPHIA BREVICOLLI CONGENITA, SYNDROME DE TURNER ET ARTHROMYODYSPLASIA CONGENITA. HELV. PAEDIAT. ACTA 6* 119-148, 1951.

ROSSI, E. AND HOWALD, E.* UBER DIE ERBLICHKEIT DES STATUS BONNEVIE-ULLRICH. HELV. PAEDIAT. ACTA 2* 98-102, 1947.

SIMPSON, J. W., NORA, J. J., SINGER, D. B. AND MCNAMARA, D. G.* MULTIPLE VALVULAR SCLEROSIS IN TURNER PHENOTYPES AND RUBELLA SYNDROME. AM. J. CARDIOL. 23* 94-97, 1969.

17820 PTERYGIUM, ANTECUBITAL

SHUN-SHIN (1954) DESCRIBED 8 AFFECTED INDIVIDUALS IN 3 GENERATIONS OF A MAURITIAN FAMILY. THERE WAS ONE INSTANCE OF A 'SKIPPED GENERATION.' THE WEB EXTENDED ACROSS THE CUBITAL FOSSA FROM THE DISTAL ONE-THIRD OF THE UPPER ARM TO THE PROXIMAL ONE-THIRD OF THE FOREARM. ELBOW EXTENSION WAS LIMITED TO 90 DEGREES, ALTHOUGH FLEXION WAS UNIMPEDED. RADIOLOGICALLY, POSTERIOR SUBLUXATION OF THE RADIAL HEAD (Q.V.) AND MALDEVELOPMENT OF THE RADIO-ULNAR JOINT WERE DEMONSTRATED.

SHUN-SHIN, M.* CONGENITAL WEB FORMATION. J. BONE JOINT SURG. 36B* 268-271, 1954.

*17830 PTOSIS, HEREDITARY

RODIN AND BARKAN (1935) RECOGNIZED FOUR TYPES* (1) HEREDITARY CONGENITAL PTOSIS, (2) HEREDITARY PTOSIS WITH EXTERNAL OPHTHALMOPLEGIA, (3) HEREDITARY NON-CONGENITAL PTOSIS, AND (4) HEREDITARY PTOSIS WITH EPICANTHUS. THE SECOND TYPE IS SAID TO BE MOST FREQUENT. ON THE OTHER HAND, DUKE-ELDER (1963) STATED THAT AT LEAST 8 TYPES OF CONGENITAL PTOSIS ARE RECOGNIZABLE OF WHICH 7 SHOW A GENETIC BASIS* (1) SIMPLE PTOSIS, DUE TO FAILURE OF PERIPHERAL DIFFERENTIATION OF MUSCLES, TRANSMITTED AS A DOMINANT. THE RECTUS SUPERIOR MUSCLE MAY BE INVOLVED ALSO. (2) PTOSIS WITH BLEPHAROPHIMOSIS, ALSO DUE TO FAULTY PERIPHERAL DIFFERENTIATION AND TRANSMITTED AS A DOMINANT. (3) PTOSIS DUE TO OPHTHALMOPLEGIA (Q.V.) USUALLY OF CENTRAL ORIGIN. (4) PTOSIS ASSOCIATED WITH MYASTHENIA GRAVIS AND MYOTONIA, BOTH RARE AS CONGENITAL DISORDERS. (5) PTOSIS DUE TO CONGENITAL SYMPATHETIC PALSY. (6) SYNKINETIC PTOSIS (SEE MARCUS GUNN PHENOMENON). (7) INTERMITTENT PSEUDO-PTOSIS ASSOCIATED WITH THE RETRACTION SYNDROME. THE EXTENSIVE METCALF KINDRED IN LAFAYETTE, TENN., HAS HEREDITARY CONGENITAL PTOSIS (BRIGGS, 1919). THE GEORGIA MOUNTAIN FAMILY REPORTED BY STUCKEY (1916) MAY HAVE BEEN RELATED. THE SAME CONDITION WAS DESCRIBED BY USHER (1925) AS 'EPICANTHUS AND PTOSIS.' I DOUBT THAT THE EXCESS SKIN AT THE INNER CANTHUS IN THESE 'SLIT-EYED PEOPLE' SHOULD BE CALLED EPICANTHUS. BLEPHARO-PHIMOSIS IS PRESENT. SEE PURPURA SIMPLEX. FAMILIES WITH LATE ONSET PTOSIS SUCH AS THAT OF FAULKNER (1939) MAY HAVE REPRESENTED OCULOPHARYNGEAL MUSCULAR DYSTROPHY (Q.V.). CONGENITAL PTOSIS MAY BE ONLY UNILATERAL. EPICANTHUS MAY BE ASSOCIATED (RANK, THOMPSON, 1959).

BRIGGS, H. H.* HEREDITARY CONGENITAL PTOSIS WITH REPORT OF 64 CASES CONFORMING TO THE MENDELIAN RULE OF DOMINANCE. AM. J. OPHTHAL. 2* 408-417, 1919.

DUKE-ELDER, S.* CONGENITAL DEFORMITIES. SYSTEM OF OPHTHALMOLOGY NORMAL AND ABNORMAL DEVELOPMENT. ST. LOUIS* C. V. MOSBY CO., 3* (PART 2) 1963.

FAULKNER, S. H.* FAMILIAL PTOSIS WITH OPHTHALMOPLEGIA EXTERNA STARTING LATE IN LIFE. BRIT. MED. J. 1* 854 ONLY, 1939.

RANK, B. K. AND THOMSON, J. A.* THE GENETIC APPROACH TO HEREDITARY CONGENITAL PTOSIS. AUST. NEW ZEAL. J. SURG. 28* 274-279, 1959.

RODIN, F. H. AND BARKAN, H.* HEREDITARY CONGENITAL PTOSIS. REPORT OF A PEDIGREE AND REVIEW OF LITERATURE. AM. J. OPHTHAL. 18* 213-225, 1935.

STUCKEY, H. P.* THE SLIT-EYED PEOPLE* CONSTRICTED EYELIDS FOUND IN FOUR GENERATIONS OF A GEORGIA FAMILY. J. HERED. 7* 147 ONLY, 1916.

USHER, C. H.* A PEDIGREE OF EPICANTHUS AND PTOSIS. ANN. EUGEN. 1* 128-138, 1925.

17840 PULMONARY EDEMA OF MOUNTAINEERS

FRED AND COLLEAGUES (1962) DESCRIBED ACUTE PULMONARY EDEMA PRECIPITATED IN SOME PERSONS AT HIGH ALTITUDE. THEIR TWO PATIENTS WERE BOTH PHYSICIANS WHO ON ONE OR MORE OCCASIONS WERE NEAR DEATH FROM PULMONARY EDEMA DEVELOPING WHEN SKIING AT ALTITUDES OF 6000 TO 10,000 FEET. THE FATHER OF ONE OF THESE, PREVIOUSLY IN GOOD HEALTH, DIED AT AGE 43, WHILE MOUNTAIN CLIMBING AND ACUTE PULMONARY EDEMA WAS THOUGHT TO BE THE CAUSE. HULTGREN AND COLLEAGUES (1961) ALSO NOTED FAMILIAL OCCURRENCE. CARDIAC CATHETERIZATION DURING THE ACUTE EPISODE SHOWED NORMAL LEFT ATRIAL AND PULMONARY VEIN PRESSURES BUT ELEVATION OF PULMONARY ARTERY PRESSURE. PULMONARY EDEMA, IT WAS PROPOSED, RESULTS FROM INCREASED VASOMOTOR ACTIVITY OF THE PULMONARY VENOUS CAPILLARIES OR VENULES.

FRED, H. L., SCHMIDT, A. M., BATES, T. AND HECHT, H. H.* ACUTE PULMONARY EDEMA OF ALTITUDE. CLINICAL AND PHYSIOLOGIC OBSERVATIONS. CIRCULATION 25* 929-937, 1962.

HULTGREN, H. N., SPICKARD, W. B., HELLRIEGEL, K. AND HOUSTON, C. S.* HIGH ALTITUDE PULMONARY EDEMA. MEDICINE 40* 289-313, 1961.

17850 PULMONARY FIBROSIS, IDIOPATHIC (SEE FIBROCYSTIC PULMONARY DYSPLASIA)

JACOX, FRYMOYER AND BONANNI (1964) DESCRIBED A FAMILY IN WHICH IDIOPATHIC PULMONARY FIBROSIS HAD BEEN OBSERVED IN 8 DEFINITE AND 3 PROBABLE INSTANCES IN A DOMINANT PEDIGREE PATTERN. APPARENT MALE-TO-MALE TRANSMISSION HAD OCCURRED IN ONE INSTANCE. INCREASE OF A GAMMA GLOBULIN FRACTION WAS THOUGHT TO BE A POSSIBLE INTEGRAL PART OF THE SYNDROME. HUGHES (1964) DESCRIBED THE DISORDER IN A MOTHER AND TWO DAUGHTERS. DANIES AND POTTS (1964) OBSERVED AFFECTED BROTHERS IN WHOM CLUBBING OF THE FINGERS WAS PRESENT FOR MANY YEARS BEFORE THE DEVELOPMENT OF RESPIRATORY SYMPTOMS. IT IS BY NO MEANS CERTAIN THAT THE CONDITION IN THESE REPORTS IS AN ENTITY SEPARATE FROM THAT REFERRED TO ELSEWHERE AS FIBROCYSTIC PULMONARY DYSPLASIA (Q.V.).

BONANNI, P. P., FRYMOYER, J. W. AND JACOX, R. F.* A FAMILY STUDY OF IDIOPATHIC PULMONARY FIBROSIS, A POSSIBLE DYSPROTEINEMIC AND GENETICALLY DETERMINED DISEASE. AM. J. MED. 39* 411-421, 1965.

DANIES, G. M. AND POTTS, M. W.* CHRONIC DIFFUSE INTERSTITIAL PULMONARY FIBROSIS IN BROTHERS. GUY. HOSP. REP. 113* 36-44, 1964.

HUGHES, E. W.* FAMILIAL INTERSTITIAL PULMONARY FIBROSIS. THORAX 19* 515-525, 1964.

JACOX, R. F., FRYMOYER, J. W. AND BONANNI, P. P.* A FAMILY STUDY OF IDIOPATHIC PULMONARY FIBROSIS* A POSSIBLE DYSPROTEINEMIC AND GENETICALLY DETERMINED DISEASE. TRANS. ASS. AM. PHYSICIANS 77* 232-238, 1964.

SWAYE, P., VAN ORDSTRAND, H. S., MCCORMACK, L. J. AND WOLPAW, S. E.* FAMILIAL HAMMAN-RICH SYNDROME* REPORT OF EIGHT CASES. DIS. CHEST 55* 7-12, 1969.

*17860 PULMONARY HYPERTENSION, PRIMARY

MELMON AND BRAUNWALD (1963) OBSERVED TWO PROVED CASES AND 3 PRESUMPTIVE CASES IN THREE GENERATIONS OF A FAMILY. THE FAMILY REPORTED BY KUHN, SCHAAF AND WAGNER (1963) MAY IN FACT BE AN EXAMPLE OF THE LEWIS TYPE OF HEART-HAND SYNDROME (Q.V.). PARRY AND VEREL (1966) DESCRIBED THE DISORDER IN A MOTHER AND HER TWO DAUGHTERS AND REFERRED TO AT LEAST TWO OTHER REPORTS OF TWO GENERATIONS BEING AFFECTED. X-LINKED DOMINANCE WOULD ACCOUNT NICELY FOR THE PREPONDERANCE OF FEMALE CASES. KINGDON ET AL. (1966) DESCRIBED THE CONDITION IN BROTHER AND SISTER AND THEIR FATHER, THUS EXCLUDING, IN THIS FAMILY AT LEAST, X-LINKAGE.

KINGDON, H. S., COHEN, L. S., ROBERTS, W. C. AND BRAUNWALD, E.* FAMILIAL OCCURRENCE OF PRIMARY PULMONARY HYPERTENSION. ARCH. INTERN. MED. 118* 422-426, 1966.

KUHN, E., SCHAAF, J. AND WAGNER, A.* PRIMARY PULMONARY HYPERTENSION, CONGENITAL HEART DISEASE AND SKELETAL ANOMALIES IN THREE GENERATIONS. JAP. HEART J. 4* 205-223, 1963.

MELMON, K. L. AND BRAUNWALD, E.* FAMILIAL PULMONARY HYPERTENSION. NEW ENG. J. MED. 269* 770-775, 1963.

PARRY, W. R. AND VEREL, D.* FAMILIAL PRIMARY PULMONARY HYPERTENSION. BRIT. HEART J. 28* 193-198, 1966.

ROGGE, J. D., MISHKIN, M. E. AND GENOVESE, P. D.* THE FAMILIAL OCCURRENCE OF

THOMPSON, P. AND MCRAE, C.* FAMILIAL PULMONARY HYPERTENSION. EVIDENCE OF AUTOSOMAL DOMINANT INHERITANCE. BRIT. HEART J. 32* 758-760, 1970.

17870 PULMONARY VALVULAR DYSPLASIA

KORETZKY ET AL. (1969) DESCRIBED AN UNUSUAL TYPE OF PULMONARY VALVULAR DYSPLASIA WHICH SHOWED A FAMILIAL TENDENCY WITH EITHER AFFECTED PARENT AND OFFSPRING OR AFFECTED SIBS. ALTHOUGH SOME RELATIVES HAD PULMONARY VALVULAR STENOSIS OF THE STANDARD DOME-SHAPED VARIETY, THE VALVULAR DYSPLASIA IN OTHERS WAS CHARACTERIZED BY THE PRESENCE OF THREE DISTINCT CUSPS AND NO COMMISSURAL FUSION. THE OBSTRUC-TIVE MECHANISM WAS RELATED TO MARKEDLY THICKENED, IMMOBILE CUSPS, WITH DISOR-GANIZED MYXOMATOUS TISSUE. OTHER FEATURES WERE RETARDED GROWTH, ABNORMAL FACIES (TRIANGULAR FACE, HYPERTELORISM, LOW-SET EARS AND PTOSIS OF THE EYELIDS), ABSENCE OF EJECTION CLICK AND UNUSUALLY MARKED RIGHT AXIS DEVIATION BY ELECTROCARDIOGRAM.

KORETZKY, E. D., MOLLER, J. H., KORNS, M. E., SCHWARTZ, C. J. AND EDWARDS, J. E.* CONGENITAL PULMONARY STENOSIS RESULTING FROM DYSPLASIA OF VALVE. CIRCULATION 40* 43-53, 1969.

17880 PUPIL, EGG-SHAPED

WHITE AND FULTON (1937) DESCRIBED OVOID PUPILS WHICH WERE LARGE AND REACTED POORLY TO CONSTRICTING STIMULI IN A WOMAN OF RUSSIAN-JEWISH EXTRACTION AND BOTH HER IDENTICAL TWIN DAUGHTERS.

WHITE, B. V., JR. AND FULTON, M. N.* A RARE PUPILLARY DEFECT INHERITED BY IDENTICAL TWINS. J. HERED. 28* 177-179, 1937.

*17890 PUPILLARY MEMBRANE, PERSISTENCE OF

REMNANTS OF THE PUPILLARY MEMBRANE PERSIST AS STRANDS AND OTHER IRREGULAR TISSUE IN THE REGION OF THE PUPIL. CASSADY AND LIGHT (1957) DESCRIBED A FAMILY IN WHICH 11 PERSONS IN 4 GENERATIONS SHOWED REMNANTS OF THE PUPILLARY MEMBRANE. FOUR OF THESE ALSO HAD CONGENITAL CATARACT AND 3 HAD INCREASED CORNEAL DIAMETER.

CASSADY, J. R. AND LIGHT, A.* FAMILIAL PERSISTENT PUPILLARY MEMBRANES. ARCH. OPHTHAL. 58* 438-448, 1957.

17900 PURPURA SIMPLEX

PURPURA OF THE EXTREMITIES, EPISTAXIS, ECCHYMOSES ON SLIGHT TRAUMA AND MENORRHAGIA ARE FEATURES. TOURNIQUET TEST IS POSITIVE BUT ALL OTHER TESTS OF CLOTTING ARE NORMAL. IN THE FAMILY REPORTED BY FISHER ET AL. (1954) PURPURA AND PTOSIS OCCURRED TOGETHER WITH MALE-TO-MALE TRANSMISSION IN AT LEAST THREE GENERATIONS. AMONG DAVIS' 27 FAMILIES, 9 HAD 2 OR MORE GENERATIONS AFFECTED. WOMEN WERE MORE OFTEN AFFECTED AND HE APPARENTLY HAD NO INSTANCE OF MALE-TO-MALE TRANSMISSION.

DAVIS, E.* HEREDITARY FAMILIAL PURPURA SIMPLEX* REVIEW OF 27 FAMILIES. LANCET 1* 145-146, 1941.

FISHER, B., ZUCKERMAN, G. H. AND DOUGLASS, R. C.* COMBINED INHERITANCE OF PURPURA SIMPLEX AND PTOSIS IN FOUR GENERATIONS OF ONE FAMILY. BLOOD 9* 1199-1204, 1954.

17910 RADIAL DEFECTS (DEFICIENCY OF RADIAL RAYS AND RADIUS AND PHOCOMELIA)

MANY OF THESE CASES ARE SPORADIC AND IN MOST OF THE REPORTED FAMILIAL INSTANCES IT IS IMPOSSIBLE TO EXCLUDE THE HEART-HAND SYNDROME I AND II, FANCONI'S PANMYELOPH-THISIS, RADIUS-PLATELET HYPOPLASIA AND OTHER SYNDROMES WITH RADIAL DEFECTS AS A FEATURE. IN ITS GROSSER FORM THE DISORDER CONSISTS OF PHOCOMELIA DUE TO LACK OF THE RADIUS AND ULNA AND HYPOPLASIA OF THE HUMERUS WITH CARPALS AND DIGITS ARTICULATING WITH IT, WHILE MILDER CASES SHOW ONLY UNDERDEVELOPMENT OF THE THUMB OR THE FIRST METACARPAL.

REEDY, J. J. AND BODNER, L. M.* DOMINANT INHERITANCE OF RADIAL HEMIMELIA. J. HERED. 44* 254-256, 1953.

TEMTAMY, S. A.* GENETIC FACTORS IN HAND MALFORMATIONS. PH. D. THESIS, JOHNS HOPKINS UNIVERSITY, 1966.

17920 RADIAL HEADS, POSTERIOR DISLOCATION OF

COCKSHOTT AND OMOLOLU (1958) DESCRIBED MULTIPLE CASES OF CONGENITAL POSTERIOR DISLOCATION OF THE RADIAL HEAD IN A FAMILY. ABBOTT (1892) OBSERVED SEVEN CASES IN ONE FAMILY. SHUN-SHIN (1954) OBSERVED THIS DISORDER ASSOCIATED WITH ANTECUBITAL WEBBING OR PTERYGIUM (Q.V.) IN MEMBERS OF THREE GENERATIONS OF A FAMILY. GUNN AND PILLAY (1964) DESCRIBED CONGENITAL POSTERIOR DISLOCATION OF THE HEAD OF THE RADIUS IN A MOTHER AND DAUGHTER IN MALAYA. THE MOTHER'S PARENTS WERE CONSANGUINEOUS AND SHE HAD MARRIED WITHIN A RESTRICTED GROUP. A THIRD UNRELATED PATIENT CAME FROM FIRST COUSIN PARENTS WHO WERE STATED TO BE NORMAL. THE AUTHORS FAVORED RECESSIVE

ABBOTT, F. C.* CONGENITAL DISLOCATIONS OF RADIUS. LANCET 1* 800 ONLY, 1892.

COCKSHOTT, W. P. AND OMOLOLU, A.* FAMILIAL CONGENITAL POSTERIOR DISLOCATION OF BOTH RADIAL HEADS. J. BONE JOINT SURG. 40B* 483-486, 1958.

GUNN, D. R. AND PILLAY, V. K.* CONGENITAL POSTERIOR DISLOCATION OF THE HEAD OF THE RADIUS. CLIN. ORTHOP. 34* 108-113, 1964.

SHUN-SHIN, M.* CONGENITAL WEB FORMATION. J. BONE JOINT SURG. 36B* 268-271, 1954.

*17930 RADIO-ULNAR SYNOSTOSIS

DOMINANT INHERITANCE THROUGH SEVERAL LINES IN SEVERAL GENERATIONS WAS DEMONSTRATED BY A FAMILY REPORTED BY DAVENPORT, TAYLOR AND NELSON (1924). RADIO-ULNAR SYNOSTOSIS IS A FEATURE OF CERTAIN CHROMOSOME ABNORMALITIES, NOTABLY THE TRIPLE X-Y SYNDROME (XXXY). SEE PRONATION-SUPINATION OF THE FOREARM, IMPAIRMENT OF. HANSEN AND ANDERSEN (1970) FOUND A POSITIVE FAMILY HISTORY IN 5 OF 37 CASES.

DAVENPORT, C. B., TAYLOR, H. L. AND NELSON, L. A.* RADIO-ULNAR SYNOSTOSIS. ARCH. SURG. 8* 705-762, 1924.

FERGUSON-SMITH, M. A., JOHNSON, A. W. AND HANDMAKER, S. D.* PRIMARY AMENTIA AND MICRO-ORCHIDISM ASSOCIATED WITH THE XXXY CHROMOSOME CONSTITUTION. LANCET 2* 184-187, 1960.

HANSEN, O. H. AND ANDERSEN, N. O.* CONGENITAL RADIO-ULNAR SYNOSTOSIS. REPORT OF 37 CASES. ACTA ORTHOP. SCAND. 41* 225-230, 1970.

17940 RADIUS, APLASIA OF, WITH CLEFT LIP-PALATE

AT LEAST 18 CASES HAVE BEEN REPORTED (IMMEYER, 1967). NO INFORMATION ON ITS GENETICS IS AVAILABLE.

IMMEYER, F.* LIPPEN-KIEFER-GAUMENSPALTEN BEI THALIDOMIDGESCHADIGTEN KINDERN. ACTA GENET. MED. GEM. 16* 244-274, 1967.

17950 RAINDROP HYPOPIGMENTATION

WEARY AND BEHLEN (1965) DESCRIBED A DISTINCTIVE BILATERAL, SYMMETRICAL, SHARPLY LOCALIZED HYPOPIGMENTATION OF THE UPPER CHEST IN A NEGRO WOMAN AND HER FOUR CHILDREN. A SINGLE SPOT OF DEPIGMENTATION, WITH A SHAPE SUGGESTING A RAINDROP, WAS PRESENT BELOW THE MID-CLAVICLE ON EACH SIDE. EITHER X-LINKED OR AUTOSOMAL DOMINANT INHERITANCE IS POSSIBLE.

WEARY, P. E. AND BEHLEN, C. H.* UNUSUAL FAMILIAL HYPOPIGMENTARY ANOMALY. ARCH. DERM. 92* 54-55, 1965.

*17960 RAYNAUD'S DISEASE ('HEREDITARY COLD FINGERS')

LEWIS AND PICKERING (1933) DESCRIBED TWO WORKING CLASS BRITISH FAMILIES WITH MULTIPLE PERSONS SUFFERING FROM INTERMITTENT ATTACKS OF NUMB AND WHITE FINGERS. ONE FAMILY HAD 9 CASES IN TWO GENERATIONS, THE SECOND 14 CASES IN 3 GENERATIONS. MALES AND FEMALES WERE EQUALLY AFFECTED AND SEVERAL INSTANCES OF MALE-TO-MALE TRANSMISSION WERE NOTED.

LEWIS, T. AND PICKERING, G. W.* OBSERVATIONS UPON MALADIES IN WHICH THE BLOOD SUPPLY TO DIGITS CEASES INTERMITTENTLY OR PERMANENTLY, AND UPON BILATERAL GANGRENE OF DIGITS, OBSERVATIONS RELEVANT TO SO-CALLED 'RAYNAUD'S DISEASE.' CLIN. SCI. 1* 327-366, 1933.

*17970 RED CELL PHOSPHOLIPID DEFECT WITH HEMOLYSIS

IN 8 MEMBERS OF A FAMILY FROM THE DOMINICAN REPUBLIC, JAFFE AND GOTTFRIED (1968) FOUND A HEMOLYTIC DISORDER WITH MILD HYPERBILIRUBINEMIA AND RETICULOCYTOSIS OF 6 TO 15 PERCENT BUT WITH LITTLE OR NO ANEMIA, AND WAS ABLE TO SHOW AN INCREASE IN LECITHIN. THE PEDIGREE SUGGESTED REGULAR AUTOSOMAL DOMINANT INHERITANCE. IN A POLISH-BORN JEWISH FAMILY, DANON ET AL. (1962) DESCRIBED AN ELECTRON MICROSCOPIC ABNORMALITY OF THE RED-CELL MEMBRANE WHICH PROBABLY WAS RESPONSIBLE FOR SUSCEPTI-BILITY TO HEMOLYSIS ON EXPOSURE TO DRUGS AND POSSIBLY VIRUSES. TWO SISTERS HAD SIMILAR FINDINGS. QUESTIONABLE ANOMALY WAS FOUND IN THE PROBAND'S SON.

DANON, D., DE VRIES, A., DJALDETTI, M. AND KIRSCHMANN, C.* EPISODES OF ACUTE HAEMOLYTIC ANAEMIA IN A PATIENT WITH FAMILIAL ULTRASTRUCTURAL ABNORMALITY OF THE RED-CELL MEMBRANE. BRIT. J. HAEMAT. 8* 274-282, 1962.

JAFFE, E. R. AND GOTTFRIED, E. L.* HEREDITARY NONSPHEROCYTIC HEMOLYTIC DISEASE ASSOCIATED WITH AN ALTERED PHOSPHOLIPID COMPOSITION OF THE ERYTHROCYTES. J. CLIN. INVEST. 47* 1375-1388, 1968.

RANDALL AND TARGGART (1961) OBSERVED RENAL TUBULAR ACIDOSIS IN MEMBERS OF SEVERAL SUCCESSIVE GENERATIONS. ALL AFFECTED MEMBERS SHOWED BOTH ACIDOSIS AND NEPHROCAL- CINOSIS. SEEDAT (1964) PRESENTED A FAMILY WITH 8 AFFECTED IN 4 GENERATIONS. THE PROBAND WAS BORN OF FIRST COUSIN PARENTS. IN ANOTHER FIRST COUSIN MARRIAGE, 4 OF HIS HALF-SIBS WERE AFFECTED. RANDALL (1967) PROVIDED FOLLOW-UP OF THE FAMILY REPORTED BY TARGGART AND HIM. THE PEDIGREE INCLUDED FOUR INSTANCES OF MALE-TO- MALE TRANSMISSION. THE FEATURES ARE NEPHROCALCINOSIS, FIXED URINARY SPECIFIC GRAVITY, FIXED URINARY PH OF ABOUT 5.0, HIGH SERUM CHLORIDE, LOW SERUM BICAR- BONATE, OSTEOMALACIA, HYPOCALCEMIA. ALKALINIZATION IS EFFECTIVE THERAPY. KOLB (1967) SHOWED ME A PEDIGREE WITH THREE GENERATIONS AFFECTED AND INSTANCES OF MALE- TO-MALE TRANSMISSION. SEEDAT (1968) OBSERVED 18 AFFECTED PERSONS IN THREE GENERATIONS. IN THE WELL-STUDIED FAMILY REPORTED BY GYORY ET AL. (1968), 10 PERSONS WERE AFFECTED BY TEST, 3 OTHERS WERE (BY GENEALOGIC CONNECTIONS) PRESUMAB- LY AFFECTED AND TWO OTHERS WERE REPORTEDLY AFFECTED. MALE-TO-MALE TRANSMISSION OCCURRED. KUHLENCORDT ET AL. (1967) OBSERVED AFFECTED MZ TWINS WHOSE PARENTS WERE FIRST COUSINS AND SUGGESTED THAT A FORM OF THIS DISORDER IS RECESSIVE. THUS, THERE MAY BE MORE THAN ONE FORM OF THIS DISORDER. SEE RTA II AND RTA III IN THE RECESSIVE CATALOG. RENAL TUBULAR ACIDOSIS WITH PERCEPTIVE DEAFNESS (Q.V.) IS A DISTINCT ENTITY. MORRIS (1970) SUGGESTED THAT AT LEAST THREE TYPES OF RENAL TUBULAR ACIDOSIS CAN BE RECOGNIZED. IN THE CLASSIC TYPE (RTA I) THE BICARBONATE THRESHOLD IS NORMAL, THE DEFECT IS PRIMARILY IN THE DISTAL TUBULE AND INHERITANCE IS DOMINANT. IN RTA II THE DEFECT IS IN THE PROXIMAL TUBULE, THE BICARBONATE THRESHOLD IS LOW AND INHERITANCE IS RECESSIVE. A THIRD TYPE OF RTA IS CALLED 'DISLOCATION' TYPE AND MAY ALSO BE RECESSIVELY INHERITED.

A PHENOCOPY OF THE GENETIC DISORDER IS PRODUCED BY AMPHOTERICIN B (MCCURDY ET AL., 1968).

BUCKALEW, V. M., JR.* FAMILIAL RENAL TUBULAR ACIDOSIS. ANN. INTERN. MED. 68* 1367-1368, 1968.

GYORY, A. Z. AND EDWARDS, K. D. G.* RENAL TUBULAR ACIDOSIS. A FAMILY WITH AN AUTOSOMAL DOMINANT GENETIC DEFECT IN RENAL HYDROGEN ION TRANSPORT, WITH PROXIMAL TUBULAR AND COLLECTING DUCT DYSFUNCTION AND INCREASED METABOLISM OF CITRATE AND AMMONIA. AM. J. MED. 45* 43-62, 1968.

KOLB, F. O.* SAN FRANCISCO, CALIF.* PERSONAL COMMUNICATION, 1967.

KUHLENCORDT, F., LENZ, W., SEEMAN, N. AND ZUKSCHWERDT, L.* RENAL TUBULAR ACIDOSIS AND BILATERAL NEPHROCALCINOSIS IN UNIOVULAR TWINS. GERMAN MED. MONTHLY 12* 565-570, 1967.

MCCURDY, D. K., FREDERIC, M. AND ELKINTON, J. R.* RENAL TUBULAR ACIDOSIS DUE TO AMPHOTERICIN B. NEW ENG. J. MED. 278* 124-131, 1968.

MORRIS, R. C.* RENAL TUBULAR ACIDOSIS. MECHANISMS, CLASSIFICATION AND IMPLICATIONS. NEW ENG. J. MED. 281* 1405-1413, 1970.

RANDALL, R. E., JR. AND TARGGART, W. H.* FAMILIAL RENAL TUBULAR ACIDOSIS. ANN. INTERN. MED. 54* 1108-1116, 1961.

RANDALL, R. E., JR.* FAMILIAL RENAL TUBULAR ACIDOSIS REVISITED. (LETTER) ANN. INTERN. MED. 66* 1024-1025, 1967.

SEEDAT, Y. K.* FAMILIAL RENAL TUBULAR ACIDOSIS. (LETTER) ANN. INTERN. MED. 69* 1329 ONLY, 1968.

SEEDAT, Y. K.* SOME OBSERVATIONS OF RENAL TUBULAR ACIDOSIS - A FAMILY STUDY. S. AFR. MED. J. 38* 606-610, 1964.

SELDIN, D. W. AND WILSON, J. D.* RENAL TUBULAR ACIDOSIS. IN STANBURY, J. B., WYNGAARDEN, J. B. AND FREDRICKSON, D. S. (EDS.)* THE METABOLIC BASIS OF INHERITED DISEASE. NEW YORK* MCGRAW-HILL, 1966 (2ND ED.). PP. 1230-1246.

*17990 RETINAL APLASIA

SORSBY AND WILLIAMS (1960) OBSERVED A FAMILY WITH MULTIPLE CASES OF RETINAL APLASIA IN WHICH INHERITANCE WAS AUTOSOMAL DOMINANT. 'RETINAL APLASIA' IS THE BRITISH TERM FOR WHAT IS CALLED 'CONGENITAL AMAUROSIS' ON THE CONTINENT. MUCH GENETIC HETEROGENEITY UNDOUBTEDLY EXISTS, WITNESS THE DEMONSTRATION OF BOTH AUTOSOMAL DOMINANT AND AUTOSOMAL RECESSIVE FORMS.

SORSBY, A. AND WILLIAMS, C. E.* RETINAL APLASIA AS A CLINICAL ENTITY. BRIT. MED. J. 1* 293-297, 1960.

*18000 RETINAL ARTERIES, TORTUOSITY OF

BEYER (1958) DESCRIBED TORTUOUS RETINAL ARTERIES WITH FOVEAL HEMORRHAGE IN A 43 YEAR OLD MAN AND HIS 17 YEAR OLD SON. A 12 YEAR OLD SON SHOWED EARLY CHANGES. POLYCYTHEMIA WAS PRESENT IN THE 17 YEAR OLD. WERNER AND GAFNER (1961) DESCRIBED TORTUOUS ARTERIES IN A 47 YEAR OLD MAN AND HIS SON AND 2 DAUGHTERS. CAGIANUT AND

WERNER (1968) OBSERVED FOUR PERSONS IN ONE FAMILY WITH RETINAL ARTERIOLAR TORTUOSITY AND RECURRENT HEMORRHAGES. POLLACK AND GOLDBERG (1970) OBSERVED RETINAL VASCULAR TORTUOSITY AND RETINAL HEMORRHAGE IN 10 PERSONS IN 4 SIBSHIPS OF A FAMILY, INCLUDING A FATHER AND TWO SONS. ONE OF THE 10 HAD RETINAL HEMORRHAGES WITHOUT TORTUOSITY.

BEYER, E.* FAMILIARE TORTUOSITAS DER KLEINEN NETZHAUTARTERIEN MIT MAKULABLU-TUNG. (FAMILIAL TORTUOSITY OF THE SMALL RETINAL ARTERIES WITH MACULAR HEMORR-HAGE). KLIN. MBL. AUGENHEILK. 132* 532-539, 1958.

CAGIANUT, B. AND WERNER, H.* ZUM KRANKHEITSBILD DER FAMILIAREN TORTUOSITAS DER KLEINEN NETZHAUTARTERIEN MIT MACULABLUTUNG. KLIN. MBL. AUGENHEILK. 153* 533-542, 1968.

CAGIANUT, B.* ZUM KRANKHEITSBILD DER FAMILIAREN TORTUOSITAS DER KLEINEN NETZHAUTGEFASSE. OPHTHALMOLOGICA 156* 322-324, 1968.

POLLACK, I. AND GOLDBERG, M. F.* BALTIMORE, MD.* PERSONAL COMMUNICATION, 1970.

WERNER, H. AND GAFNER, F.* BEITRAG ZUR FAMILIAREN TORTUOSITAS DER KLEINEN NETZHAUTARTERIEN. OPHTHALMOLOGICA 141* 350-356, 1961.

*18010 RETINITIS PIGMENTOSA (RP)

THIS IS ONE OF THE SIMPLY INHERITED TRAITS WHICH APPEARS IN ALL THREE CATALOGS. ATYPICAL RP OCCURS IN THE FLYNN-AIRD SYNDROME (Q.V.). DOMINANT INHERITANCE IS NOTED IN 3 OR 4 PERCENT OF CASES. AYRES (1886) REPORTED 4 GENERATIONS, ALLAN AND HERNDON (1944) - 5 GENERATIONS, BORDLEY (1908) - 5 GENERATIONS, HEUSCHER-ISLER ET AL. (1949) - 11 CASES IN 3 GENERATIONS, REHSTEINER (1949) - 16 CASES IN 4 GENERATIONS, AND SO ON. CONSTRICTION OF THE VISUAL FIELDS AND NIGHT BLINDNESS ARE TYPICAL AS WELL AS THE CHARACTERISTIC FUNDUS CHANGES INCLUDING 'BONE CORPUSCLE' LUMPS OF PIGMENT. THE MOST EXTENSIVELY AFFECTED FAMILY REPORTED IS PROBABLY THAT STUDIED BY BECKERSHAUS (1925). THE PATHOPHYSIOLOGY OF RETINITIS PIGMENTOSA WAS DISCUSSED BY DOWLING (1966), WHO PRESENTED EXPERIMENTS SUGGESTING THAT EXPOSURE TO BRIGHT LIGHT MAY ACCELERATE THE DEGENERATIVE PROCESS. SUNGA AND SLOAN (1967) DESCRIBED A FAMILY WITH 13 AFFECTED IN 3 GENERATIONS, INCLUDING 2 INSTANCES OF MALE-TO-MALE TRANSMISSION. THEY REMARKED ON THE WIDE VARIABILITY IN THE RATE OF VISUAL DETERIORATION AMONG INDIVIDUALS OF THE SAME FAMILY.

ALLAN, W. AND HERNDON, C. N.* RETINITIS PIGMENTOSA AND APPARENTLY SEX-LINKED IDIOCY IN A SINGLE SIBSHIP. J. HERED. 35* 40-43, 1944.

AMMANN, F., KLEIN, D. AND BOHRINGER, H. R.* RESULTATS PRELIMINAIRES D'UNE ENQUET SUR LA FREQUENCE ET LA DISTRIBUTION GEOGRAPHIQUE DES DEGENERESCENCES TAPETC-RETINIENNES EN SUISSE (ETUDE DE CINQ CANTONS). J. GENET. HUM. 10* 99-127, 1961.

AYRES, S. C.* RETINITIS PIGMENTOSA. AM. J. OPHTHAL. 3* 81-90, 1886.

BECKERSHAUS, F.* DOMINANTE VERERBUNG DER RETINITIS PIGMENTOSA. KLIN. MBL. AUGENHEILK. 75* 96-109, 1925.

BORDLEY, J.* A FAMILY OF HEMERALOPES. BULL. HOPKINS HOSP. 19* 278-281, 1908.

DOWLING, J. E.* NIGHT BLINDNESS. SCI. AM. 215 (NO. 4)* 78-84, 1966.

HEUSCHER-ISLER, R., GYSIN, W. AND HEGNER, H.* BEITRAG ZUR KASUISTIK DER DOMINANTEN VERERBUNG DER RETINITIS PIGMENTOSA. OPHTHALMOLOGICA 118* 858-865, 1949.

REHSTEINER, K.* EIN WEITERER SCHWEIZERISCHER STAMMBAUM VON DOMINANT VERERBTER RETINITIS PIGMENTOSA. OPHTHALMOLOGICA 117* 51-59, 1949.

SUNGA, R. N. AND SLOAN, L. L.* PIGMENTARY DEGENERATION OF THE RETINA* EARLY DIAGNOSIS AND NATURAL HISTORY. INVEST. OPHTHAL. 6* 309-325, 1967.

*18020 RETINOBLASTOMA

SMITH AND SORSBY (1958) CONCLUDED THAT BILATERAL CASES ARE MOST OFTEN FAMILIAL. MANY UNILATERAL CASES MAY BE SPORADIC WITH A LOW RISK (ABOUT 4 PERCENT) TO SUBSEQUENT CHILDREN OR TO OFFSPRING OF THE PROBAND. IN THEIR OPINION ESTIMATES OF MUTATION RATE OF 2.3 X 10 (TO THE MINUS 5) AS GIVEN BY FALLS AND NEEL (1951) ARE TOO HIGH. MACKLIN (1959) DEMONSTRATED IRREGULARITIES IN THE INHERITANCE SUGGES-TING INCOMPLETE PENETRANCE. IN 10.5 PERCENT OF CASES, AFFECTED PERSONS WERE IDENTIFIED IN COLLATERAL LINES. EXAMPLES INCLUDED (1) A BILATERAL CASE, HIS UNILATERALLY AFFECTED BROTHER AND A BILATERALLY AFFECTED DAUGHTER OF THE LATTER PERSON, (2) SIX BILATERALLY AFFECTED OFFSPRING OF A WOMAN WHO HAD ONE MICROPHTHAL-MIC EYE BUT REFUSED EXAMINATION, (3) SEVERAL INSTANCES OF TWO OR MORE AFFECTED SIBS WITH NORMAL PARENTS. THE GENETIC NATURE OF RETINOBLASTOMA AND ITS DOMINANT INHERITANCE CAME TO LIGHT EARLY BECAUSE EARLY RECOGNITION AND TREATMENT OF INDIVIDUAL CASES PERMITTED SURVIVAL. THE GENETIC BASIS OF OTHER EMBRYONIC TUMORS, SUCH AS WILMS' TUMOR, NEUROBLASTOMA AND MEDULLOBLASTOMA, IS BEGINNING TO BE

APPRECIATED.   IN ALL   OF   THESE TUMORS SPONTANEOUS REGRESSION ("CURE") OCCURS IN
SOME CASES.

FALLS, H. F. AND NEEL, J. V.* GENETICS OF RETINOBLASTOMA. ARCH. OPHTHAL. 46*
367-389, 1951.

FRANCOIS, J.* HEREDITARY MALIGNANT TUMOR OF THE EYE. CONGENITAL ANOMALIES OF
THE EYE. (CHAPTER 9), ST. LOUIS* C. V. MOSBY CO., 1968. PP. 205-246.

MACKLIN, M. T.* INHERITANCE OF RETINOBLASTOMA IN OHIO. ARCH. OPHTHAL. 62* 842-
851, 1959.

MANCHESTER, P. T., JR.* RETINOBLASTOMA AMONG OFFSPRING OF ADULT SURVIVORS.
ARCH. OPHTHAL. 65* 546-549, 1961.

NIRANKARI, M. S., GULATI, G. C. AND CHADDAH, M. R.* RETINOBLASTOMA* GENETICS
AND REPORT OF A FAMILY. AM. J. OPHTHAL. 53* 523-532, 1962.

SCHAPPERT-KIMMIJSER, (NI)., HEMMES, G. D. AND NIJLAND, R.* THE HEREDITY OF
RETINOBLASTOMA. OPHTHALMOLOGICA 151* 197-213, 1966.

SMITH, S. M. AND SORSBY, A.* RETINOBLASTOMA* SOME GENETIC ASPECTS. ANN. HUM.
GENET. 23* 50-58, 1958.

VOGEL, F.* GENETICS OF RETINOBLASTOMA. MODERN TRENDS IN OPHTHALMOLOGY, 1968.

VOGEL, F.* GENETICS OF RETINOBLASTOMA. IN, GENETIC COUNSELING. HEIDELBERG
UNIVERSITY, SCIENCE LIBRARY. TRANS. BY SABINE KURTH. NEW YORK* SPRINGER VERLAG,
1969.

18030 RHEUMATOID ARTHRITIS

OCCASIONAL FAMILIES SHOW A CONSIDERABLE NUMBER OF CASES OF THIS COMMON DISORDER.
A SIMPLE MENDELIAN MECHANISM CANNOT BE PROVED, HOWEVER. INDEED, SOME (BURCH,
O'BRIEN AND BUNIM, 1964) CANNOT DEMONSTRATE SIGNIFICANT FAMILIAL AGGREGATION.

BURCH, T. A., O'BRIEN, W. M. AND BUNIM, J. J.* FAMILY AND GENETIC STUDIES OF
RHEUMATOID ARTHRITIS AND RHEUMATOID FACTOR IN BLACKFEET INDIANS. AM. J. PUBLIC
HEALTH 54* 1184-1190, 1964.

GOWANS, J. D. C., EVANGELISTA, I. AND O'SULLIVAN, M. A.* FAMILIAL FACTORS IN
RHEUMATOID ARTHRITIS. ARCH. INTERN. MED. 113* 744-747, 1964.

18040 RIBBING'S DISEASE (HEREDITARY MULTIPLE DIAPHYSEAL SCLEROSIS)

RIBBING (1949) DESCRIBED A FAMILY IN WHICH FOUR OF SIX SIBS WERE AFFECTED. THE
DIAPHYSEAL OSTEOSCLEROSIS AND HYPEROSTOSIS WERE LIMITED TO ONE OR MORE (UP TO
FOUR) OF THE LONG BONES, THE TIBIA BEING AFFECTED IN ALL. THE FATHER, WHO WAS
DEAD, HAD COMPLAINED FOR MANY YEARS OF PAINS IN THE LEGS. THUS, THE CONDITION MAY
BE DOMINANT* NO X-RAY STUDIES OF THE FATHER WERE AVAILABLE AND RIBBING NOTED THAT
THE BODY HAD BEEN CREMATED. PAUL (1953) REPORTED THE SAME ENTITY IN 2 OF 4 SIBS,
ONE OF WHOM ALSO HAD OTOSCLEROSIS, WHICH WAS PRESENT IN SEVERAL OTHER MEMBERS OF
THE KINDRED.   IN AN ADDENDUM, PAUL NOTED THAT THE INFANT SON OF ONE OF HIS
PATIENTS HAD DIFFICULTY WALKING AND WAS FOUND TO HAVE MULTIPLE SCLEROSING LESIONS
OF LONG BONES. AGAIN DOMINANT INHERITANCE IS SUGGESTED.

PAUL, L. W.* HEREDITARY MULTIPLE DIAPHYSEAL SCLEROSIS (RIBBING). RADIOLOGY 60*
412-416, 1953.

RIBBING, S.* HEREDITARY, MULTIPLE, DIAPHYSEAL SCLEROSIS. ACTA RADIOL. 31* 522-
536, 1949.

*18050 RIEGER'S SYNDROME (HYPODONTIA, MESOECTODERMAL DYSGENESIS OF IRIS AND CORNEA,
AND MYOTONIC DYSTROPHY)

HYPODONTIA (PARTIAL ANODONTIA) WITH MALFORMATION OF THE ANTERIOR CHAMBER OF THE
EYE WAS RECOGNIZED AS A DOMINANTLY INHERITED DISORDER BY RIEGER (1935, 1941). THE
OCULAR FEATURES ARE MICROCORNEA WITH OPACITY, HYPOPLASIA OF THE IRIS AND ANTERIOR
SYNECHIAE.   IN FIVE GENERATIONS OF A FAMILY BUSCH AND COLLEAGUES (1960) FOUND
MYOTONIC DYSTROPHY AS A CONSISTENTLY ASSOCIATED FEATURE. PEARCE AND KERR (1965)
STUDIED A LARGE KINDRED WITH MANY AFFECTED MEMBERS AND EMPHASIZED THE VARIABILITY
IN EXPRESSION OF THE SYNDROME. A LESS WELL-KNOWN COMPONENT OF THIS SYNDROME IS
ANAL STENOSIS (CRAWFORD, 1967* BRAILEY, 1890). IT IS INTERESTING TO NOTE THAT
SCHACHENMANN ET AL. (1965) DESCRIBED A FAMILY IN WHICH THE COMBINATION OF COLOBOMA
OF THE IRIS, ANAL STENOSIS AND RENAL MALFORMATION WAS INHERITED IN A DOMINANT
MANNER AND ASSOCIATED WITH A SPECIFIC CHROMOSOME ABERRATION. ALKEMADE (1969)
AMPLY CONFIRMED AUTOSOMAL DOMINANT INHERITANCE. HE POINTED OUT CHARACTERISTIC
FACIES CONSISTING OF BROAD NASAL ROOT WITH TELECANTHUS AND MAXILLARY HYPOPLASIA
WITH PROTRUDING LOWER LIP. A MOTHER AND 2 OF HER 3 CHILDREN HAD SEVERE DEVELOP-
MENTAL ANOMALIES OF THE IRIS, ASSOCIATED WITH MALDEVELOPMENT OF THE EAR AND
MAXILLA, UMBILICAL HERNIA AND ANAL STENOSIS. GLAUCOMA OCCURRED IN ALL 3 PATIENTS.
IT IS DOUBTFUL THAT AXENFELD ANOMALY SHOULD BE CONSIDERED A SEPARATE ENTITY. IT

IS ONE FEATURE OF RIEGER'S SYNDROME.

ALKEMADE, P. P. H.* DYSGENESIS MESODERMALIS OF THE IRIS AND THE CORNEA. A STUDY OF RIEGER'S SYNDROME AND PETER'S ANOMALY. (ROTTERDAM THESIS) VAN GORCUM, 1969.

BRAILEY, W. A.* DOUBLE MICROPHTHALMOS WITH DEFECTIVE DEVELOPMENT OF IRIS, TEETH AND ANUS. GLAUCOMA AT AN EARLY AGE. TRANS. OPHTHAL. SOC. U.K. 10* 139 ONLY, 1890.

BUSCH, G., WEISKOPF, J. AND BUSCH, K.-T.* DYSGENESIS MESODERMALIS ET ECTODERMA-LIS RIEGER ODER RIEGER'S CHE KRANKHEIT. KLIN. MBL. AUGENHEILK. 36* 512-523, 1960.

CRAWFORD, R. A.* IRIS DYSGENESIS WITH OTHER ANOMALIES. BRIT. J. OPHTHAL. 51* 438-440, 1967.

PEARCE, W. G. AND KERR, C. B.* INHERITED VARIATION IN RIEGER'S MALFORMATION. BRIT. J. OPHTHAL. 49* 530-537, 1965.

RIEGER, H.* BEITRAGE ZUR KENNTNIS SELTENER MISSBILDUNGEN DER IRIS* UBER HYPOPLASIE DES IRISVORDERBLATTES MIT VERLAGERUNG UND ENTRUNDUNG DER PUPILLE. GRAEFE ARCH. OPHTHAL. 133* 602-635, 1935.

RIEGER, H.* ERBFRAGEN IN DER AUGENHEILKUNDE. GRAEFE ARCH. OPHTHAL. 143* 277-299, 1941.

SCHACHENMANN, G., SCHMID, W., FRACCARO, M., MANNINI, A., TIEPOLO, L., PERONA, G. P. AND SARTORI, E.* CHROMOSOMES IN COLOBOMA AND ANAL ATRESIA. LANCET 2* 290 ONLY, 1965.

*18060 RINGED HAIR (PILI ANNULATI)

ON CLOSE INSPECTION WITH THE UNAIDED EYE ALTERNATING LIGHT AND DARK BANDS ARE VISIBLE ON THE HAIR. THE LIGHT AREAS ARE DUE TO INCLUSION OF AIR IN THE CORTEX. THE HAIR TENDS TO BREAK OFF AT THESE POINTS. SEE PEDIGREE OF ASHLEY AND JACQUES (1950) WITH SIX AFFECTED IN FOUR GENERATIONS.

ASHLEY, L. M. AND JACQUES, R. S.* FOUR GENERATIONS OF RINGED HAIR. J. HERED. 41* 82-84, 1950.

JUON, M.* EINE BEOBACHTUNG FAMILIAREN AUFTRETENS VON PILI ANULATI. DERMATOLO-GIA 86* 117-122, 1942.

18070 ROBINOW DWARFISM

ROBINOW ET AL. (1969) DESCRIBED A DWARF SYNDROME IN SIX GENERATIONS OF A FAMILY BUT WITH NO INSTANCE OF MALE-TO-MALE TRANSMISSIONS. NORMAL VAGINAL DELIVERY OF AFFECTED FEMALES WAS POSSIBLE. INTERORBITAL DISTANCE WAS INCREASED AND THE TEETH WERE MALALIGNED. BECAUSE OF BULGING FOREHEAD, DEPRESSED NASAL BRIDGE AND SHORT LIMBS ACHONDROPLASIA IS SUGGESTED BUT THE SPINE AND PELVIC RADIOLOGIC FINDINGS ARE NEARLY NORMAL.

ROBINOW, M., SILVERMAN, F. N. AND SMITH, H. D.* A NEWLY RECOGNIZED DWARFING SYNDROME. AM. J. DIS. CHILD. 117* 645-651, 1969.

*18080 ROUSSY-LEVY HEREDITARY AREFLEXIC DYSTASIA

THIS DISORDER USUALLY BEGINS IN CHILDHOOD BUT CAUSES LITTLE DISABILITY. THE CONDITION WAS DESCRIBED INDEPENDENTLY IN 1926 BY ROUSSY AND LEVY, BY SYMONDS AND SHAW (WHO CALLED IT 'FAMILIAL CLAW-FOOT WITH ABSENT TENDON JERKS') AND BY ROMBOLD AND RILEY (WHO CALLED IT AN 'ABORTIVE TYPE OF FRIEDREICH'S DISEASE'). THIS CONDITION RESEMBLES CHARCOT-MARIE-TOOTH DISEASE IN ITS DOMINANT INHERITANCE, CLAWFOOT, WEAKNESS AND ATROPHY OF DISTAL LIMB MUSCLES ESPECIALLY THE PERONEI, DECREASED EXCITABILITY OF MUSCLES TO GALVANIC AND FARADIC STIMULATION, AND SOME DISTAL SENSORY LOSS. THE SYNDROME DIFFERS IN THAT IT INCLUDES STATIC TREMOR OF THE HANDS. ROUSSY AND LEVY (1926, 1934) STRESSED THE ABSENCE OF CEREBELLAR SIGNS, SPEECH DISTURBANCES, BABINSKI SIGN AND NYSTAGMUS. LOW CONDUCTION VELOCITY OF PERIPHERAL NERVES WAS A STRIKING FEATURE OF THE CASES REPORTED BY YUDELL ET AL. (1965). ROZANSKI (1951) DESCRIBED A FAMILY WITH AFFECTED MEMBERS IN FOUR GENERATIONS AND WITH SEVERAL INSTANCES OF MALE-TO-MALE TRANSMISSION. LAPRESLE (1956) GAVE FOLLOW-UP INFORMATION ON THE FAMILY OF ROUSSY AND LEVY.

LAPRESLE, J.* CONTRIBUTION A L'ETUDE DE LA DYSTASIE AREFLEXIQUE HEREDITAIRE. ETAT ACTUEL DE QUATRE DES SEPT CAS PRINCEPS DE ROUSSY ET MLLE. LEVY, TRENTE ANS APRES LA PREMIERE PUBLICATION DE CES AUTEURS. SEM. HOP. PARIS 32* 2473-2482, 1956.

ROMBOLD, C. R. AND RILEY, H. A.* THE ABORTIVE TYPE OF FRIEDREICH'S DISEASE. ARCH. NEUROL. PSYCHIAT. 16* 301-312, 1926.

ROUSSY, G. AND LEVY, G.* A PROPOS DE LA DYSTASIE AREFLEXIQUE HEREDITAIRE. REV. NEUROL. 62* 763-773, 1934.

ROUSSY, G. AND LEVY, G.* SEPT CAS D'UNE MALADIE FAMILIALE PARTICULAIERE. REV.
NEUROL. 45* 427-450, 1926.

ROZANSKI, J.* HEREDITARY AREFLEXIC DYSTASIA* REPORT ON A FAMILY WITH ROUSSY-
LEVY DISEASE IN ISRAEL. MSCHR. PSYCHIAT. NEUROL. 122* 141-156, 1951.

SYMONDS, C. P. AND SHAW, M. E.* FAMILIAL CLAW-FOOT WITH ABSENT TENDON JERKS.
BRAIN 49* 387-403, 1926.

YUDELL, A., DYCK, P. J. AND LAMBERT, E. H.* A KINSHIP WITH THE ROUSSY-LEVY
SYNDROME. ARCH. NEUROL. 13* 432-440, 1965.

D
O
M
I
N
A
N
T

*18090 RUTHERFURD'S SYNDROME

HOUSTON AND SHOTTS (1966) RESTUDIED THE FAMILY REPORTED BY RUTHERFURD IN 1931. IN
FIVE GENERATIONS AFFECTED PERSONS SHOWED CORNEAL DYSTROPHY, HYPERTROPHY OF GUMS
AND FAILURE OF TOOTH ERUPTION. SEVEN PERSONS IN 4 GENERATIONS WERE AFFECTED WITH
THREE INSTANCES OF MALE-TO-MALE TRANSMISSION.

HOUSTON, I. B. AND SHOTTS, N.* RUTHERFURD'S SYNDROME. A FAMILIAL OCULO-DENTAL
DISORDER. A CLINICAL AND ELECTROPHYSIOLOGIC STUDY. ACTA PAEDIAT. SCAND. 55* 233-
238, 1966.

RUTHERFURD, M. E.* THREE GENERATIONS OF INHERITED DENTAL DEFECT. BRIT. MED. J.
2* 9-11, 1931.

18100 SARCOIDOSIS

FAMILIAL AGGREGATION WAS STUDIED BY BUCK AND MCKUSICK (1961) AND BY ALLISON
(1964), AMONG OTHERS. THE FAMILIAL AGGREGATION IN THIS DISEASE OF UNKNOWN
ETIOLOGY MAY HAVE A NON-GENETIC BASIS. THE MUCH GREATER FREQUENCY IN U.S. NEGROES
THAN IN U.S. WHITES SUGGESTS A GENETIC CONTRIBUTION TO ETIOLOGY. THE FAMILY
PATTERN DOES NOT CONFORM TO A SIMPLE MENDELIAN MODE OF INHERITANCE. IN ALLISON'S
FAMILY AFFECTED PERSONS WERE TWO BROTHERS OUT OF 4 SIBS AND TWO OF THE 4 CHILDREN
OF ONE OF THESE.

ALLISON, J. R., JR.* SARCOIDOSIS. I. FAMILIAL OCCURRENCE. II. PSEUDOTUMOR
CEREBRI AND UNUSUAL SKIN LESIONS. STH. MED. J. 57* 27-32, 1964.

BUCK, A. A. AND MCKUSICK, V. A.* EPIDEMIOLOGIC INVESTIGATIONS OF SARCOIDOSIS.
III. SERUM PROTEINS, SYPHILIS, ASSOCIATION WITH TUBERCULOSIS* FAMILIAL AGGREGA-
TION. AM. J. HYG. 74* 174-188, 1961.

18110 SATELLITE ASSOCIATION RESULTING IN FAMILIAL CHROMOSOMAL MOSAICISM

ZELLWEGER AND ABBO (1965) DESCRIBED MOSAICISM IN THREE SUCCESSIVE GENERATIONS.
CLONES WITH NORMAL KARYOTYPE, D-G AND D-D TRANSLOCATIONS, PARTIAL TRISOMY 21 AND
MONOSOMY X WERE FOUND. BECAUSE OF AN UNUSUAL FREQUENCY OF SATELLITE ASSOCIATION
THEY POSTULATED THE EXISTENCE OF A 'DOMINANT GENE' WHICH LEADS TO MOSAICISM OF
SOMATIC ORIGIN. THE FAMILY WAS DESCRIBED IN FULL BY ABBO, ZELLWEGER AND CUANY
(1966), WHO IN THIS PUBLICATION CONCLUDED THAT INHERITANCE OF A POSTULATED GENE
FOR INCREASED SATELLITE ASSOCIATION FROM BOTH PARENTS MIGHT LEAD TO MOSAICISM.

ABBO, G. N., ZELLWEGER, H. V. AND CUANY, R.* SATELLITE ASSOCIATION (SA) IN
FAMILIAL MOSAICISM. HELV. PAEDIAT. ACTA 21* 293-299, 1966.

ZELLWEGER, H. V. AND ABBO, G. N.* ABOUT A NEW GENE AS A CAUSE OF INCREASED
SATELLITE ASSOCIATION. (ABSTRACT) J. PEDIAT. 67* 935 ONLY, 1965.

ZELLWEGER, H. V., ABBO, G. N. AND CUANY, R.* SATELLITE ASSOCIATION AND
TRANSLOCATION MONGOLISM. J. MED. GENET. 3* 186-189, 1966.

18120 SC(1) TRAIT OF SALIVA

SC(1) IS A COMPONENT OF SALIVA DEMONSTRATED IMMUNO-ELECTROPHORETICALLY. THE
PRECISE MECHANISM OF GENETIC CONTROL HAS NOT BEEN DETERMINED ALTHOUGH THE
IMPORTANCE OF GENETIC FACTORS HAS BEEN DEMONSTRATED (NISWANDER ET AL., 1964) BY
FAMILY DATA AND TWIN STUDIES. ENVIRONMENTAL INFLUENCES SEEM RATHER STRONG. THE
COMPONENT IS LACKING FROM SERUM.

NISWANDER, J. D., SHREFFLER, D. C. AND NEEL, J. V.* GENETIC STUDIES OF
QUANTITATIVE VARIATION IN A COMPONENT OF HUMAN SALIVA. ANN. HUM. GENET. 27* 319-
328, 1964.

18130 SCAPULA, CONTOUR OF VERTEBRAL BORDER OF

GRAVES (1921) FOUND THAT ABOUT 54 PERCENT OF PERSONS HAVE A CONVEX VERTEBRAL
BORDER, ABOUT 26 PERCENT HAVE A STRAIGHT VERTEBRAL BORDER AND ABOUT 20 PERCENT
HAVE A CONCAVE BORDER.

GRAVES, W. W.* METHOD OF RECOGNIZING SCAPULAR TYPES IN LIVING. ARCH. INTERN.
MED. 36* 51-61, 1925.

GRAVES, W. W.* OBSERVATIONS ON AGE CHANGES IN THE SCAPULA* A PRIMARY NOTE. AM. J. PHYS. ANTHROP. 5* 21-33, 1922.

GRAVES, W. W.* THE RELATIONS OF THE SCAPULAR TYPES TO PROBLEMS OF HUMAN HEREDITY, LONGEVITY, MORBIDITY AND ADAPTABILITY IN GENERAL. ARCH. INTERN. MED. 34* 1-26, 1924.

GRAVES, W. W.* THE TYPES OF SCAPULAE. A COMPARATIVE STUDY OF SOME CORRELATED CHARACTERS IN HUMAN SCAPULAE. AM. J. PHYS. ANTHROP. 4* 111-128, 1921.

18140 SCAPULOPERONEAL AMYOTROPHY

PERONEAL ATROPHY IS ACCOMPANIED BY BILATERAL FOOT DROP AND TALIPES EQUINOVARUS. FOLLOWING ATROPHY OF THE LOWER LEGS, THE SHOULDER GIRDLE IS INVOLVED. BULBAR INVOLVEMENT IS LATE. AUTOPSY SHOWS MUSCULAR ATROPHY AND INVOLVEMENT OF CAUDAL CRANIAL NUCLEI. PALMER (1932) DESCRIBED A FAMILY WITH 8 PERSONS AFFECTED, THE EARLIEST HAVING ONSET ABOUT 1800. PALMER'S CASE LOOKS LIKE CHARCOT-MARIE-TOOTH DISEASE. DAVIDENKOV (1939) SUGGESTED THAT CASES REPORTED BY WOHLFART WERE THE SAME AS THOSE HE DESIGNATED SCAPULOPERONEAL AMYOTROPHY. THUS, SCAPULOPERONEAL MYOPATHY MIGHT BE VIEWED AS A DOMINANT TYPE OF WOHLFART-KUGELBERG-WELANDER JUVENILE MUSCULAR ATROPHY. SEE MUSCULAR ATROPHY, JUVENILE, IN THIS CATALOG.

DAVIDENKOV, S.* SCAPULOPERONEAL AMYOTROPHY. ARCH. NEUROL. PSYCHIAT. 41* 694-701, 1939.

KAESER, H. E.* DIE FAMILIARE SCAPULOPERONEALE MUSKELATROPHIE. DEUTSCH. Z. NERVENHEILK. 186* 379-394, 1964.

PALMER, H. D.* FAMILIAL SCAPULOPERONEAL AMYOTROPHY. ARCH. NEUROL. PSYCHIAT. 28* 473-477, 1932.

18150 SCHIZOPHRENIA

THIS MAY NOT BE A SINGLE ENTITY. ALTHOUGH THE IMPORTANCE OF GENETIC FACTORS AND THE DISTINCTNESS FROM MANIAC-DEPRESSIVE PSYCHOSIS ARE INDICATED BY TWIN STUDIES, THE MODE OF INHERITANCE IS UNCLEAR. SOME (E.G., GARRONE, 1962) SUGGEST RECESSIVE INHERITANCE. OTHERS (E.G., BOOK, 1953 AND SLATER, 1958) FAVOR IRREGULAR DOMINANT INHERITANCE. A PRIORI, POLYGENIC INHERITANCE SEEMS MOST LIKELY, ACCORDING TO THE RULE THAT RELATIVELY FREQUENT DISORDERS SUCH AS THIS DO NOT HAVE SIMPLE MONOMERIC GENETIC DETERMINATION. WITHIN THE LARGER GROUP THERE MAY BE ENTITIES WHICH BEHAVE IN A SIMPLE MENDELIAN MANNER. HESTON (1970) REVIEWED THE EVIDENCE AND CONCLUDED THAT IT SUPPORTS THE AUTOSOMAL DOMINANT HYPOTHESIS. HE POINTS OUT THAT THE DEFINITION OF SCHIZOPHRENIA USED BY RECENT RESEARCHERS IS A BROAD ONE ENCOMPASSING THE SCHIZOID STATE, THE "SCHIZOPHRENIC SPECTRUM." SCHIZOIDS AND SCHIZOPHRENICS OCCUR WITH ABOUT EQUAL FREQUENCY AMONG THE COTWINS OF SCHIZOPHRENIC MONOZYGOTIC TWIN PROBANDS, BRINGING THE CONCORDANCE RATE CLOSE TO 100 PERCENT. ABOUT 45 PERCENT OF SIBS, PARENTS AND OFFSPRING OF SCHIZOPHRENICS ARE SCHIZOID OR SCHIZOPH-RENIC, AS ARE ABOUT 66 PERCENT OF THE CHILDREN OF TWO SCHIZOPHRENIC PARENTS. ABOUT 4 PERCENT OF THE GENERAL POPULATION IS AFFECTED WITH SCHIZOID-SCHIZOPHRENIC DISEASE. SEE REVIEW (ANON., LANCET, 1970).

ANNOTATION* GENETICS OF SCHIZOPHRENIA. (EDITORIAL) LANCET 1* 26 ONLY, 1970.

BOOK, J. A.* SCHIZOPHRENIA AS A GENE MUTATION. ACTA GENET. STATIST. MED. 4* 133-139, 1953.

GARRONE, G.* ETUDE STATISTIQUE ET GENETIQUE DE LA SCHIZOPHRENIE A GENEVE DE 1901 A 1950. J. GENET. HUM. 11* 91-219, 1962.

HESTON, L. L.* THE GENETICS OF SCHIZOPHRENIC AND SCHIZOID DISEASE. SCIENCE 167* 249-256, 1970.

KARLSSON, J. L.* A DOUBLE DOMINANT GENETIC MECHANISM FOR SCHIZOPHRENIA. HEREDITAS 65* 261-268, 1970.

MORAN, P. A. P.* CLASS MIGRATION AND THE SCHIZOPHRENIC POLYMORPHISM. ANN. HUM. GENET. 28* 261-268, 1965.

SLATER, E.* THE MONOGENIC THEORY OF SCHIZOPHRENIA. ACTA GENET. STATIST. MED. 8* 50-56, 1958.

*18160 SCLERO-ATROPHIC AND KERATOTIC DERMATOSIS OF LIMBS

HURIEZ ET AL. (1968) DESCRIBED A "NEW" GENO-DERMATOSIS IN 44 MEMBERS OF THREE FRENCH KINDREDS. THE CHARACTERISTICS WERE ATROPHIC FIBROSIS OF THE SKIN OF THE LIMBS, HYPOPLASIA OF NAILS, AND KERATODERMIA OF THE PALMS AND SOLES. SKIN CANCER AND BOWEL CANCER WERE FREQUENT. LINKAGE WITH THE MNS BLOOD GROUP LOCUS HAS BEEN ESTABLISHED (MENNECIER, 1967).

HURIEZ, C., DEMINATTI, M., AGACHE, P. AND MENNECIER, M.* A PROPOS DE 28 CAS D'EPIDERMOLYSE BULLEUSE DANS 11 FAMILIES DONT UNE FAMILE ETUDIEE DU POINT DE UNE GENETIQUE, SANS MISE EN EVIDENCE DE LINKAGE. BULL. SOC. FRANC. DERM. SYPH. 75*

HURIEZ, C., DEMINATTI, M., AGACHE, P. AND MENNECIER, M.* UNE GENODYSPLASIE NON
ENCORE INDIVIDUALISEE* LA GENODERMATOSE SCLERO-ATROPHIANTE ET KERATODERMIQUE DES
EXTREMITES FREQUEMMENT DEGENERATIVE. SEM. HOP. PARIS 44* 481-488, 1968.

MENNECIER, M.* INDIVIDUALISATION D'UNE NOUVELLE ENTITE* LA GENODERMATOSE
SCLERO-ATROPHIANTE ET KERATODERMIQUE DES EXTREMITES FREQUEMMENT DEGENERATIVE.
ETUDE CLINIQUE ET GENETIQUE (POSSIBILITE DE LINKAGE AVEC LE SYSTEME MNSS). M.D.
THESIS, U. DE LILLE, 1967.

18170 SCLEROCORNEA

IN THIS CONGENITAL MALFORMATION OF THE CORNEA, THE LIMITS OF THE CORNEA AND SCLERA
ARE INDISTINCT. A SEVERE FORM IS INHERITED AS A RECESSIVE (Q.V.). SCLEROCORNEA
IS ALSO A FEATURE OF CORNEA PLANA (Q.V.).

18180 SCOLIOSIS, IDIOPATHIC

DEGEORGE AND FISHER (1967) COULD NOT FIND EVIDENCE FOR OPERATION OF SIMPLE GENETIC
FACTORS. HIGH CONCORDANCE IN BOTH MONOZYGOTIC AND DIZYGOTIC TWINS AND AN EXCESS
OF PROPOSITI BORN TO OLDER MOTHERS SUGGESTED TO THESE WORKERS THAT MATERNAL
FACTORS PREDOMINATE. WYNNE-DAVIES (1968) FAVORED EITHER DOMINANT OR MULTIFAC-
TORIAL INHERITANCE. DOMINANT INHERITANCE WAS SUGGESTED BY FABER (1936), GARLAND
(1934) WHO OBSERVED THE CONDITION IN 5 GENERATIONS, AND GILLY ET AL. (1963).
MALE-TO-MALE TRANSMISSION IS APPARENTLY RARE AND WAS SPECIFICALLY ABSENT IN 17
FAMILIES STUDIED BY COWELL (1971), WHO SUGGESTED X-LINKED DOMINANT INHERITANCE.
THE 8 TO 1 RATIO OF FEMALES TO MALES SUPPORTS THIS CONCLUSION. SCOLIOSIS OCCURS
SECONDARY TO OTHER HEREDITARY DISORDERS SUCH AS MARFAN SYNDROME, DYSAUTONOMIA,
NEUROFIBROMATOSIS, FRIEDREICH'S ATAXIA, MUSCULAR DYSTROPHIES, ETC.

COWELL, H. R.* GENETIC ASPECTS OF IDIOPATHIC SCOLIOSIS. J. BONE JOINT SURG.,
IN PRESS, 1971.

DEGEORGE, F. V. AND FISHER, R. L.* IDIOPATHIC SCOLIOSIS* GENETIC AND ENVIRON-
MENTAL ASPECTS. J. MED. GENET. 4* 251-257, 1967.

FABER, A.* UNTERSUCHUNGEN UBER DIE ERBLICHKEIT DER SKOLIOSE. ARCH. ORTHOP.
UNFALLCHIR. 36* 217-296, 1936.

GARLAND, H. G.* HEREDITARY SCOLIOSIS. BRIT. MED. J. 1* 328 ONLY, 1934.

GILLY, R., STAGNARA, P., FREDERICH, A., DALLOZ, C., ROBERT, J. M. AND GOLDB-
LATT, B.* MEDICAL ASPECTS OF ESSENTIAL STRUCTURAL SCOLIOSIS IN CHILDREN. LYON
MED. 95* 79-95, 1963.

WYNNE-DAVIES, R.* FAMILIAL IDIOPATHIC SCOLIOSIS. A FAMILY SURVEY. J. BONE
JOINT SURG. 50A* 24-30, 1968.

*18190 SCROTAL TONGUE (LINGUA PLICATA)

THE TONGUE IS FURROWED AND GROOVED. TOBIAS (1945) REPORTED TWO FAMILIES, ONE WITH
TWO GENERATIONS AND THE OTHER WITH FOUR AFFECTED. GEOGRAPHIC TONGUE WAS AN
ASSOCIATED FEATURE IN THE PROBAND OF ONE FAMILY. SEILER (1936) ASSEMBLED THE MOST
EXTENSIVE PEDIGREE DATA SUPPORTING AUTOSOMAL DOMINANT INHERITANCE.

ROLLERI, F.* UBER DAS VORKOMMEN DER LINGUA PLICATA (FALTENZUNGE). Z. MENSCHL.
VERERB. KONSTITUTIONSL. 23* 587-593, 1939.

SEILER, A.* ZUR VERBREITUNG UND VERERBUNG DER FALTENZUNGE (LINGUA PLICATA).
ARCH. KLAUS STIFT. VERERBUNGSFORSCH. 11* 541-569, 1936.

TOBIAS, N.* SCROTAL TONGUE AND ITS INHERITANCE. ARCH. DERM. SYPH. 52* 266
ONLY, 1945.

18200 SEBORRHEIC KERATOSES

BUTTERWORTH AND STREAN (1962) DESCRIBED MOTHER AND DAUGHTER AND STATED THAT
INHERITANCE IS AUTOSOMAL DOMINANT. RIECHES (1952) DESCRIBED 7 FAMILIES IN WHICH
SEBORRHEIC KERATOSIS WAS TRANSMITTED THROUGH TWO OR THREE GENERATIONS. THE SKIN
LESIONS OF THE BASAL CELL NEVUS SYNDROME SOMETIMES RESEMBLE SEBORRHEIC KERATOSES.

BUTTERWORTH, T. AND STREAN, L. P.* CLINICAL GENODERMATOLOGY. BALTIMORE*
WILLIAMS AND WILKINS, 1962.

RIECHES, A. J.* SEBORRHEIC KERATOSES. ARE THEY DELAYED HEREDITARY NEVI.Q
ARCH. DERM. SYPH. 65* 596-600, 1952.

*18210 SECRETOR FACTOR

THIS MIGHT BE CONSIDERED EITHER A PHYSIOLOGIC TRAIT OR AN HONORARY BLOOD GROUP.
THE SO-CALLED SECRETOR HAS DEMONSTRABLE ABH BLOOD GROUP ANTIGEN IN THE SALIVA AND

OTHER BODY FLUIDS. THE NON-SECRETOR DOES NOT. SECRETOR IS DOMINANT. THE SECRETOR LOCUS IS LINKED TO THE LUTHERAN BLOOD GROUP LOCUS.

RACE, R. R. AND SANGER, R.* BLOOD GROUPS IN MAN. PHILADELPHIA* F. A. DAVIS CO., 1968 (5TH ED.).

18220 SELLA TURCICA, BRIDGED

IN A MOTHER AND THREE CHILDREN CAREY ET AL. (1968) OBSERVED OSSEOUS BRIDGING BETWEEN THE ANTERIOR AND POSTERIOR CLINOIDS.

CAREY, M. C., FITZGERALD, O. AND MCKIERNAN, E.* OSTEOGENESIS IMPERFECTA IN TWENTY-THREE MEMBERS OF A KINDRED WITH HERITABLE FEATURES CONTRIBUTED BY A NON-SPECIFIC SKELETAL DISORDER. QUART. J. MED. 37* 437-449, 1968.

18230 SERUM PROTEIN TYPES

THOSE FOR WHICH GENETIC VARIATION IS KNOWN INCLUDE PREALBUMIN, ALBUMIN, GROUP SPECIFIC COMPONENT (GC TYPES), HAPTOGLOBINS, TRANSFERRINS, LIPOPROTEINS, GAMMA GLOBULINS, COMPLEMENT COMPONENTS, ANTITRYPSIN. THE XM TYPE IS X-LINKED. SEE ALSO BISALBUMINEMIA, ANGIONEUROTIC EDEMA AND ENZYMES, ELECTROPHORETIC VARIANTS OF.

BEARN, A. G. AND CLEVE, H.* GENETIC VARIATIONS IN THE SERUM PROTEINS. IN STANBURY, J. B., WYNGAARDEN, J. B. AND FREDRICKSON, D. S. (EDS.)* THE METABOLIC BASIS OF INHERITED DISEASE. NEW YORK* MCGRAW-HILL, 1966 (2ND ED.). PP. 1321-1342.

BECKMAN, L.* ISOZYME VARIATIONS IN MAN. MONOGRAPHS IN HUMAN GENETICS. NEW YORK* S. KARGER, 1966.

18240 SILVER-RUSSELL DWARFISM

NO MENDELIAN OR CHROMOSOMAL BASIS FOR THIS CONDITION HAS BEEN ESTABLISHED. NEW DOMINANT MUTATION IS A POSSIBILITY. THE TWO MAIN FEATURES ARE HEMIHYPERTROPHY (OR BETTER, LATERAL ASYMMETRY) AND LOW BIRTH WEIGHT DWARFISM. TANNER AND HAM (1969) SUGGESTED THE DESIGNATION OF SILVER DWARF BE RESERVED FOR CHILDREN OF SHORT STATURE (WITHOUT MICROCEPHALY OR OTHER SPECIAL FEATURES) WHO HAVE LOW BIRTH WEIGHT FOR THE LENGTH OF GESTATION, ASYMMETRY OF ARMS, LEGS, BODY OR HEAD AND INCURVED 5TH FINGERS. THEY SUGGESTED THAT THE DESIGNATION OF RUSSELL DWARF BE RESERVED FOR THE SIMILAR SITUATION WHEN ASYMMETRY IS LACKING. RIMOIN (1969) DESCRIBED MONOZYGOTIC MALE TWINS CONCORDANT FOR SILVER DWARFISM.

MOSELEY, J. E., MOLOSHOK, R. E. AND FREIBERGER, R. H.* THE SILVER SYNDROME* CONGENITAL ASYMMETRY, SHORT STATURE AND VARIATIONS IN SEXUAL DEVELOPMENT. AM. J. ROENTGEN. 97* 74-81, 1966.

RIMOIN, D. L.* THE SILVER SYNDROME IN TWINS. THE CLINICAL DELINEATION OF BIRTH DEFECTS. II. MALFORMATION SYNDROMES. NEW YORK* NATIONAL FOUNDATION, 1969. PP. 183-187.

SILVER, H. K.* ASYMMETRY, SHORT STATURE, AND VARIATIONS IN SEXUAL DEVELOPMENT* A SYNDROME OF CONGENITAL MALFORMATIONS. AM. J. DIS. CHILD. 107* 495-515, 1964.

TANNER, J. M. AND HAM, T. J.* LOW BIRTHWEIGHT DWARFISM WITH ASYMMETRY (SILVER'S SYNDROME)* TREATMENT WITH HUMAN GROWTH HORMONE. ARCH. DIS. CHILD. 44* 231-243, 1969.

18250 SORBITOL DEHYDROGENASE VARIANTS

OP'T HOF (1969) STATED THAT 'PRELIMINARY STUDIES WITH HUMAN POST MORTEM LIVER SPECIMENS SUGGEST THAT A POLYMORPHISM FOR SDH ISOENZYMES EXIST ALSO IN MAN.

OP'T HOF, J.* ISOENZYMES AND POPULATION GENETICS OF SORBIT DEHYDROGENASE (EC* 1.1. 1.14) IN SWINE (SUS SCROFA). HUMANGENETIK 7* 258-259, 1969.

*18260 SPASTIC PARAPLEGIA

PROBABLY IN LARGE PART BECAUSE OF THEIR EXCEPTIONAL LENGTH, THE PYRAMIDAL TRACTS ARE UNUSUALLY VULNERABLE TO BOTH ACQUIRED AND GENETIC DERANGEMENT. AUTOSOMAL DOMINANT, AUTOSOMAL RECESSIVE AND X-LINKED RECESSIVE VARIETIES OF SPASTIC PARAPLEGIA HAVE BEEN RECOGNIZED AND MORE THAN ONE RECESSIVE FORM EXISTS. IN THE AMISH OF LANCASTER COUNTY, PA., A KINDRED WITH AFFECTED MEMBERS IN THREE GENERA-TIONS WAS OBSERVED. IN THIS CLOSED COMMUNITY THE ORIGIN OF THE DE NOVO MUTATION COULD BE IDENTIFIED WITH CONSIDERABLE CERTAINTY. THE DISEASE WAS EARLY IN ONSET BUT VERY SLOWLY PROGRESSIVE OR EVEN STATIC. THIS SAME TYPE OF CONGENITAL STATIONARY FAMILIAL PARAPLEGIA WAS DESCRIBED IN 7 MEMBERS OF TWO GENERATIONS BY HOHMANN (1957). SCHWARZ (1956) REPORTED SEVERAL FAMILIES INCLUDING ONE ORIGINALLY REPORTED BY BAYLEY (1897) AND NOW CONTAINING 22 AFFECTED PERSONS IN 6 GENERATIONS. IN CONTRAST TO THE EARLY ONSET, STATIC FORM OF DISEASE IN THE AMISH FAMILY, A FAMILY WITH MANY AFFECTED MEMBERS I HAVE STUDIED ON DEER ISLE, MAINE, HAS ONSET IN THE SECOND OR THIRD DECADE AND STEADY PROGRESSION OF NEUROLOGIC DEFECT.
AAGENAES (1959) DESCRIBED A FAMILY WITH THIRTY-ONE CASES IN FOUR GENERATIONS.

PROGNOSIS FOR LIFE WAS GOOD. HISTOPATHOLOGIC CHANGES WERE FOUND BILATERALLY IN THE LATERAL CORTICOSPINAL TRACTS IN THE THORACIC CORD AND IN THE FASCICULUS GRACILIS. ALTHOUGH A MAJORITY OF REPORTED FAMILIES HAVE DISPLAYED RECESSIVE INHERITANCE, 10-30 PERCENT OF FAMILIES HAVE A DOMINANT PATTERN. THE CONFUSION OF THE SPINOCEREBELLAR DEGENERATIONS IS ILLUSTRATED BY THE FACT THAT SOME MEMBERS OF AAGENAES' FAMILY HAD ATAXIA IN ADDITION TO SPASTIC PARAPLEGIA.

AAGENAES, O.* HEREDITARY SPASTIC PARAPLEGIA. ACTA PSYCHIAT. NEUROL. SCAND. 34* 489-494, 1959.

BAYLEY, W. D.* HEREDITARY SPASTIC PARAPLEGIA. J. NERV. MENT. DIS. 24* 697-701, 1897.

GARLAND, H. G. AND ASTLEY, C. E.* HEREDITARY SPASTIC PARAPLEGIA WITH AMYOTROPHY AND PES CAVUS. J. NEUROL. NEUROSURG. PSYCHIAT. 13* 130-133, 1950.

HARIGA, J. AND MATTHYS, E.* DE LA PARAPLEGIE SPASMODIQUE DE STRUMPELL-LORRAIN A L'AMYOTROPHIE DE CHARCOT-MARIE-TOOTH* (ETUDE D'UNE FAMILLE). J. GENET. HUM. 10* 326-337, 1961.

HOHMANN, H.* DIE DIPLEGIA SPASTICA INFANTILIS HEREDITARIA UND IHRE BEZIEHUNGEN ZUR FAMILIAREN SPASTISCHEN SPINALPARALYSE. NERVENARZT 28* 323-325, 1957.

SCHWARZ, G. A. AND LIU, C.-N.* HEREDITARY FAMILIAL SPASTIC PARAPLEGIA. FURTHER CLINICAL AND PATHOLOGIC OBSERVATIONS. ARCH. NEUROL. PSYCHIAT. 75* 144-162, 1956.

VAN BOGAERT, L.* ETUDE GENETIQUE SUR LES PARAPLEGIES SPASMODIQUES FAMILIALES. J. GENET. HUM. 1* 6-23, 1952.

18270 SPASTIC PARAPLEGIA WITH AMYOTROPHY OF HANDS

SILVER (1966) DESCRIBED TWO UNRELATED ENGLISH FAMILIES WITH THIS COMBINATION WHICH, HE SUGGESTED, MAY REPRESENT A DISTINCT TYPE OF SPASTIC PARAPLEGIA. WASTING OF THE HAND MUSCLES WAS THE FIRST AND MOST MARKED MANIFESTATION. SEE ALSO AMYOTROPHIC DYSTONIC PARAPLEGIA.

SILVER, J. R.* FAMILIAL SPASTIC PARAPLEGIA WITH AMYOTROPHY OF THE HANDS. ANN. HUM. GENET. 30* 69-75, 1966.

18280 SPASTIC PARAPLEGIA WITH ASSOCIATED EXTRAPYRAMIDAL SIGNS

DICK AND STEVENSON (1953) OBSERVED 7 CASES OF SPASTIC PARAPLEGIA IN 3 GENERATIONS, WITH TWO INSTANCES OF MALE-TO-MALE TRANSMISSION. FOUR OF THE AFFECTED HAD ASSOCIATED EXTRAPYRAMIDAL SIGNS.

DICK, A. P. AND STEVENSON, C. J.* HEREDITARY SPASTIC PARAPLEGIA* REPORT OF A FAMILY WITH ASSOCIATED EXTRAPYRAMIDAL SIGNS. LANCET 1* 921-923, 1953.

*18290 SPHEROCYTOSIS, HEREDITARY

MACKINNEY AND COLLEAGUES (1962) AND MORTON AND COLLEAGUES (1962) STUDIED 26 FAMILIES. THEY CONCLUDED THAT AFTER THE INITIAL CASE IN A FAMILY HAS BEEN IDENTIFIED, FOUR TESTS SUFFICE FOR THE DIAGNOSIS IN OTHER FAMILY MEMBERS - SMEAR, RETICULOCYTE COUNT, HEMOGLOBIN, BILIRUBIN. THE FRAGILITY TEST (INCREASED OSMOTIC FRAGILITY CHARACTERIZES THE DISEASE) IS UNNECESSARY AFTER THE DIAGNOSIS HAS BEEN MADE IN THE PROBAND. TYPICAL OF OTHER RARE DOMINANT TRAITS IN MAN, HEREDITARY SPHEROCYTOSIS SHOWS PHENOCOPIES, INCOMPLETE PENETRANCE AND INCOMPLETE ASCERTAIN-MENT AND MAY BE GENETICALLY HETEROGENEOUS. IT WAS ESTIMATED THAT PREVALENCE IS 2.2 PER 10,000, THAT MUTATION RATE IS 0.000022 (2.2 X 10 *TO THE MINUS 5*) AND THAT ABOUT ONE-FOURTH OF CASES ARE SPORADIC. NO EVIDENCE OF REPRODUCTIVE COMPENSATION OR OF INCREASED PRENATAL AND INFANT MORTALITY WAS FOUND.
NO ENZYME DEFECT HAS BEEN IDENTIFIED (MIWA, TANAKA, VALENTINE, 1962) AND INDEED WOULD NOT BE EXPECTED, IN VIEW OF THE DOMINANT INHERITANCE. JACOB AND JANDL (1964) ARE OF THE VIEW THAT THE PRIMARY DEFECT IS IN THE RED CELL MEMBRANE, WHICH IS ABNORMALLY PERMEABLE TO SODIUM. A MORPHOLOGICALLY COMPARABLE DISORDER IN THE DEER MOUSE PEROMYSCUS IS INHERITED AS A RECESSIVE (ANDERSON, HUESTIS, MOTULSKY, 1960). SEVERAL OBSERVATIONS SUGGEST THAT MORE THAN ONE TYPE OF HEREDITARY SPHEROCYTOSIS EXISTS IN MAN (REVIEW BY ZAIL ET AL., 1967). BARRY ET AL. (1968) POINTED OUT THAT HEMOCHROMATOSIS IS A SERIOUS COMPLICATION OF UNTREATED SPHEROCYTOSIS. IN A FAMILY WITH 6 PERSONS AFFECTED IN 3 GENERATIONS, WILEY AND FIRKIN (1970) FOUND A FORM OF HEREDITARY SPHEROCYTOSIS WITH UNUSUAL FEATURES* OTHER REPORTS OF ATYPICAL DISEASE WERE REVIEWED. CHANMUGAM ET AL. (1971) FOUND CONCORDANT FOR POLYCYSTIC DISEASE AND HEREDITARY SPHEROCYTOSIS IN A FATHER AND THREE CHILDREN. THREE OTHER CHILDREN AND FOUR SIBS OF THE FATHER WERE THOUGHT TO BE FREE OF BOTH DISEASES. OF THE SEVERAL POSSIBLE EXPLANATIONS, LINKAGE IS A PARTICULAR INTRIGUING ONE. SEE ELLIPTOCYTOSIS FOR AN EXAMPLE OF EXCLUSION OF LINKAGE WITH HEREDITARY HEMORRHAGIC TELANGIECTASIA ON THE BASIS OF A SMALL BODY OF DATA.

ANDERSON, R., HUESTIS, R. R. AND MOTULSKY, A. G.* HEREDITARY SPHEROCYTOSIS IN THE DEER MOUSE. ITS SIMILARITY TO THE HUMAN DISEASE. BLOOD 15* 491-504, 1960.

BARRY, M., SCHEUER, P. J., SHERLOCK, S., ROSS, C. F. AND WILLIAMS, R.* HEREDITARY SPHEROCYTOSIS WITH SECONDARY HAEMOCHROMATOSIS. LANCET 2* 481-485, 1968.

CHANMUGAM, D., ROSARETNAM, R. AND KARUNARATNE, K. E. S.* HEREDITARY SPHEROCYTOSIS AND POLYCYSTIC DISEASE OF THE KIDNEYS IN FOUR MEMBERS OF A FAMILY. AM. J. HUM. GENET. 23* 66 ONLY, 1971.

JACOB, H. S. AND JANDL, J. H.* INCREASED CELL MEMBRANE PERMEABILITY IN THE PATHOGENESIS OF HEREDITARY SPHEROCYTOSIS. J. CLIN. INVEST. 43* 1704-1720, 1964.

JACOB, H. S.* ABNORMALITIES IN THE PHYSIOLOGY OF THE ERYTHROCYTE MEMBRANE IN HEREDITARY SPHEROCYTOSIS. AM. J. MED. 41* 734-741, 1966.

JACOB, H. S.* DYSFUNCTION OF THE RED BLOOD CELL MEMBRANE IN HEREDITARY SPHEROCYTOSIS. BRIT. J. HAEMAT. 14* 99-104, 1968.

JACOB, H. S.* HEREDITARY SPHEROCYTOSIS* A DISEASE OF THE RED CELL MEMBRANE. SEMINARS IN HEMAT. 2* 139-166, 1965.

JANDL, J. H.* HEREDITARY SPHEROCYTOSIS. IN STANBURY, J. B., WYNGAARDEN, J. B. AND FREDRICKSON, D. S. (EDS.)* THE METABOLIC BASIS OF INHERITED DISEASE. NEW YORK* MCGRAW-HILL, 1966 (2ND ED.). PP. 1035-1050.

MACKINNEY, A. A.* HEREDITARY SPHEROCYTOSIS. CLINICAL FAMILY STUDIES. ARCH. INTERN. MED. 116* 257-265, 1965.

MACKINNEY, A. A., MORTON, N. E., KOSOWER, N. S. AND SCHILLING, R. F.* ASCERTAINING GENETIC CARRIERS OF HEREDITARY SPHEROCYTOSIS BY STATISTICAL ANALYSIS OF MULTIPLE LABORATORY TESTS. J. CLIN. INVEST. 41* 554-567, 1962.

MACPHERSON, A. I. S., RICHMOND, J., DONALDSON, G. W. K. AND MUIR, A. R.* THE ROLE OF THE SPLEEN IN CONGENITAL SPHEROCYTOSIS. AM. J. MED. 50* 35-41, 1971.

MIWA, S., TANAKA, K. R. AND VALENTINE, W. N.* ENOLASE ACTIVITY OF ERYTHROCYTES IN HEREDITARY SPHEROCYTOSIS. NATURE 195* 613-614, 1962.

MORTON, N. E., MACKINNEY, A. A., KOSOWER, N., SCHILLING, R. F. AND GRAY, M. P.* GENETICS OF SPHEROCYTOSIS. AM. J. HUM. GENET. 14* 170-184, 1962.

MOTULSKY, A. G., ANDERSON, R., SPARKES, R. S. AND HUESTIS, R. H.* MARROW TRANSPLANTATION IN NEWBORN MICE WITH HEREDITARY SPHEROCYTOSIS. A MODEL SYSTEM. TRANS. ASS. AM. PHYSICIANS 75* 64-72, 1962.

WILEY, J. S. AND FIRKIN, B. G.* AN UNUSUAL VARIANT OF HEREDITARY SPHEROCYTOSIS. AM. J. MED. 48* 63-71, 1970.

ZAIL, S. S., KRAWITZ, E., VILJOEN, E., KRAMER, S. AND METZ, J.* ATYPICAL HEREDITARY SPHEROCYTOSIS* BIOCHEMICAL STUDIES AND SITES OF ERYTHROCYTE DESTRUCTION. BRIT. J. HAEMAT. 13* 323-334, 1967.

*18300 SPINOCEREBELLAR ATAXIA AND PLAQUE-LIKE DEPOSITS

SEITELBERGER (1962) DESCRIBED A KINDRED WITH A UNIQUE NEUROLOGIC DISORDER TRACED THROUGH 5 GENERATIONS. PLAQUE-LIKE DEPOSITS WERE FOUND IN THE CEREBRAL CORTEX, BASAL GANGLIA AND (MOST EXTREMELY) ALL LAYERS OF THE CEREBELLUM. CLINICALLY AND PATHOLOGICALLY THE DISORDER MOST CLOSELY RESEMBLED KURU. HOWEVER, IN KURU THE POSTERIOR WHITE COLUMNS ARE SPARED AND PLAQUE-FORMATION IN THE CEREBRAL CORTEX IS MORE INTENSE.

SEITELBERGER, F.* EIGENARTIGE FAMILIAR-HEREDITARE KRANKHEIT DES ZENTRALNERVENSYSTEMS IN EINER NIEDEROSTERREICHISCHER SIPPE (ZUGLEICH EIN BEITRAG ZUR VERGLEICHENDEN NEUROPATHOLOGIE DES KURU). WIEN. KLIN. WSCHR. 74* 687-691, 1962.

18310 SPINOCEREBELLAR ATROPHY WITH PUPILLARY PARALYSIS

IN A 37 YEAR OLD WOMAN AND HER 14 YEAR OLD SON AND 6 YEAR OLD DAUGHTER SUTHERLAND, TYRER AND EADIE (1963) DESCRIBED SPINOCEREBELLAR ATROPHY WITH ABSENCE OF PUPILLARY REACTION TO LIGHT OR CONVERGENCE, BUT PRESERVATION OF ACCOMMODATION REFLEXES.

INDEMINI, M. AND AMMANN, F.* HEREDO-DEGENERESCENCE SPINO-CEREBELLEUSE (HDSC) ASSOCIEE AU SYNDROME DE KLINEFELTER. J. GENET. HUM. 10* 297-325, 1961.

SUTHERLAND, J. M., TYRER, J. H. AND EADIE, M. J.* ATROPHIE SPINO-CEREBELLEUSE FAMILIALE AVEC MYDRIASE FIXE. REV. NEUROL. 108* 439-442, 1963.

*18320 SPINO-PONTINE ATROPHY

BOLLER AND SEGARRA (1969) OBSERVED 24 PERSONS WITH LATE ONSET ATAXIA IN FOUR GENERATIONS OF AN ANGLO-SAXON FAMILY. TANIGUCHI AND KONIGSMARK (1971) DESCRIBED 16 AFFECTED PERSONS IN THREE GENERATIONS OF A NEGRO FAMILY. THE PATHOLOGIC FINDINGS WERE SIMILAR IN THE TWO FAMILIES. THE CEREBELLUM WAS RELATIVELY SPARED

AND THE INFERIOR OLIVES WERE NORMAL. THE SPINAL CORD SHOWED LOSS OF MYELINATED
FIBERS IN THE SPINOCEREBELLAR TRACTS AND POSTERIOR FUNICULI. THERE WAS ALSO
MARKED LOSS OF NUCLEI BASIS PONTI.

BOLLER, F. AND SEGARRA, J. M.* SPINO-PONTINE DEGENERATION. EUROPEAN NEUROL. 2*
356-373, 1969.

TANIGUCHI, R. AND KONIGSMARK, B. W.* DOMINANT SPINO-PONTINE ATROPHY. REPORT OF
A FAMILY THROUGH THREE GENERATIONS. BRAIN, IN PRESS, 1971.

18330 SPLENO-GONADAL FUSION WITH LIMB DEFECTS AND MICROGNATHIA

AN EXCEEDINGLY BIZARRE SYNDROME IS THAT OF FUSION OF SPLEEN AND GONAD WITH
ECTROMELIA. HIVES AND EGGUM (1961) REPORTED A NINTH CASE. SEVEN WERE STILLBORN
OR DIED IN INFANCY. THE EIGHTH DIED AT AGE 10. THEIR PATIENT WAS 15 YEARS OLD.
THIS MAY BE A LETHAL DOMINANT.

HIVES, J. R. AND EGGUM, P. R.* SPLENIC-GONADAL FUSION CAUSING BOWEL OBSTRUC-
TION. ARCH. SURG. 83* 887-889, 1961.

18340 SPLIT LOWER LIP

HERBST (1936) DESCRIBED A KINDRED IN WHICH 18 PERSONS IN FOUR GENERATIONS HAD A
MEDIAN GROOVE OR SPLIT IN THE LOWER LIP. THE UPPER LIP WAS FLESHY AND MODERATELY
EVERTED BUT ONLY ONE OF THE EXAMINED PERSONS HAD A MEDIAN CLEFT OF THE UPPER LIP.
THE MAXILLA WAS NARROW AND THE TEETH CROWDED AND IRREGULARLY ALLIGNED. GORLIN
(1968) THINKS THIS MAY HAVE BEEN AN EXAMPLE OF LOWER LIP PITS.

GORLIN, R. J.* MINNEAPOLIS, MINN.* PERSONAL COMMUNICATION, 1968.

HERBST, E.* ERBLICHE SPALTBILDUNGEN DER UNTERLIPPE MIT SCHWEREN KIEFERDEFORMA-
TIONEN UND INTELLIGENZSTORUNGEN. VOLK. RASSE. 11* 276-280, 1936.

18350 SPLIT-HAND AND FOOT WITH HYPODONTIA

TEMTAMY AND MCKUSICK (1971) DESCRIBED MOTHER AND SON.

TEMTAMY, S. AND MCKUSICK, V. A.* THE GENETICS OF HAND ANOMALIES. BALTIMORE*
JOHNS HOPKINS PRESS, 1971.

*18360 SPLIT-HAND DEFORMITY

TYPICAL AND ATYPICAL FORMS ARE RECOGNIZED. ATYPICAL CASES ARE USUALLY SPORADIC.
TYPICAL CASES MAY BE OF THE LOBSTER-CLAW VARIETY (ABSENCE OF CENTRAL RAYS) OR
MONODACTYLY TYPE (DEFICIENCY OF RADIAL RAYS WITH NO CLEFT). GRADATIONS BETWEEN
THESE TYPES OCCUR AND CASES OF EACH TYPE SOMETIMES ARE FOUND IN THE SAME FAMILY.
FEATURES OF GENETIC INTEREST IN REPORTED FAMILIES INCLUDE REGULAR DOMINANT
INHERITANCE IN THREE OR MORE GENERATIONS, LACK OF PENETRANCE WITH SKIPPED
GENERATIONS, MARKEDLY IRREGULAR 'DOMINANT' INHERITANCE, TWO OR MORE AFFECTED
OFFSPRING OF NORMAL PARENTS, AND ANOMALOUS SEGREGATION RATIOS IN OFFSPRING OF
AFFECTED MALES. VOGEL (1958) SUGGESTED THAT TWO VARIETIES OF SPLIT-HAND DEFORMITY
EXIST* (1) TYPE WITH CONSTANT INVOLVEMENT OF THE FEET AND REGULAR AUTOSOMAL
DOMINANT INHERITANCE, (2) TYPE WITH INCONSISTENT INVOLVEMENT OF THE FEET AND
IRREGULAR INHERITANCE. BIRCH-JENSEN (1949) RECOGNIZED TWO ANATOMICAL TYPES* (1)
TYPICAL LOBSTER CLAW, AND (2) MONODACTYLY. THE ANATOMICAL CLASSIFICATION HAS NO
GENETIC SIGNIFICANCE BECAUSE EITHER TYPE MAY OCCUR IN THE SAME FAMILY OR ON
DIFFERENT LIMBS OF THE SAME PERSON (TEMTAMY, 1966). ABSENCE OF THE CENTRAL RAYS
CHARACTERIZED THE FIRST ANATOMICAL TYPE. THE HAND IS DIVIDED INTO TWO PARTS BY A
CONE-SHAPED CLEFT TAPERING PROXIMALLY. THE TWO PARTS OF THE HAND CAN BE APPOSED
LIKE A LOBSTER CLAW. A COMPARABLE DEFORMITY OF THE FEET MAY BE PRESENT. IN THE
SECOND ANATOMICAL TYPE, OR MONODACTYLY, THE RADIAL RAYS ARE ABSENT WITH ONLY THE
FIFTH DIGIT REMAINING, AS A RULE. IN DENMARK BIRCH-JENSEN (1949) ESTIMATED THE
FREQUENCY AT BIRTH TO BE ABOUT 1 IN 90,000. ABOUT 70 PEDIGREES WERE REPORTED
PRIOR TO 1965 (TEMTAMY, 1966). REGULAR AUTOSOMAL DOMINANT INHERITANCE THROUGH
THREE OR MORE GENERATIONS WAS DEMONSTRATED BY ABOUT 27 OF THE 70 PEDIGREES.
SKIPPING OF A GENERATION WAS NOTED BY AT LEAST 4 AUTHORS. TWO OR MORE AFFECTED
SIBS WITH BOTH PARENTS NORMAL WERE NOTED BY SEVERAL AUTHORS (MACKENZIE, PENROSE,
1951* GRAHAM, BADGLEY, 1955* NEUGEBAUER, 1962* AND OTHERS). GONADAL MOSAICISM WAS
SUGGESTED BY AUERBACH (1956) AS A POSSIBLE EXPLANATION. IN THOSE PEDIGREES WITH
INCONSTANT INVOLVEMENT OF THE FEET THE GENETICS IS LESS CLEAR. A DISTURBED
SEGREGATION RATIO WAS FOUND IN THE FAMILY FIRST REPORTED BY MCMULLAN AND PEARSON
(1913) AND BROUGHT UP TO DATE BY STEVENSON AND JENNINGS (1960). A MARKED
PREPONDERANCE OF AFFECTED SONS OF AFFECTED FATHERS SUGGESTED GERMINAL SELECTION TO
THE LATTER WORKERS. FORD (1963) RAISED THE QUESTION OF CHROMOSOMAL ABERRATION BUT
COULD DEMONSTRATE NONE BY THE AVAILABLE METHODS. ANOMALOUS SEGREGATION HAS ALSO
BEEN OBSERVED WITH ANIRIDIA (Q.V.) AND WITH ALPORT'S SYNDROME (Q.V.). RAY (1970)
DESCRIBED TWO CASES AMONG THE CHILDREN OF FIRST-COUSIN, UNAFFECTED PARENTS.

AUERBACH, C.* A POSSIBLE CASE OF DELAYED MUTATION IN MAN. ANN. HUM. GENET. 20*
266-269, 1956.

BIRCH-JENSEN, A.* CONGENITAL DEFORMITIES OF THE UPPER EXTREMITIES. COPENHAGEN*

FORD, C. E.* AUTOSOMAL ABNORMALITIES. SEC. INTERN. CONF. ON CONG. MALFORMA-
TIONS, NEW YORK* NATIONAL FOUNDATION, 1963. P. 25.

GRAHAM, J. B. AND BADGLEY, C. E.* SPLIT-HAND WITH UNUSUAL COMPLICATIONS. AM.
J. HUM. GENET. 7* 44-50, 1955.

MACKENZIE, H. J. AND PENROSE, L. S.* TWO PEDIGREES OF ECTRODACTYLY. ANN.
EUGEN. 16* 88-96, 1951.

MCMULLEN, G. AND PEARSON, K.* ON THE INHERITANCE OF THE DEFORMITY KNOWN AS
SPLIT FOOT OR LOBSTER CLAW. BIOMETRIKA 9* 381-390, 1913.

NEUGEBAUER, H.* SPALTHAND UND -FUSS MIT FAMILIARER BESONDERHEIT. Z. ORTHOP.
95* 500-506, 1962.

RAY, A. K.* ANOTHER CASE OF SPLIT-FOOT MUTATION IN TWO SIBS. J. HERED. 61*
169-170, 1970.

STEVENSON, A. C. AND JENNINGS, L. M.* ECTRODACTYLY - EVIDENCE IN FAVOUR OF A
DISTURBED SEGREGATION IN THE OFFSPRING OF AFFECTED MALES. ANN. HUM. GENET. 24*
89-96, 1960.

TEMTAMY, S. A.* GENETIC FACTORS IN HAND MALFORMATIONS. PH. D. THESIS. JOHNS
HOPKINS UNIVERSITY, 1966.

VOGEL, F.* VERZOGERTE MUTATION BEIM MENSCHEN* EINIGE KRITISCHE BEMERKUNGEN ZU
CH. AUERBACHS ARBEIT (1956). ANN. HUM. GENET. 22* 132-137, 1958.

18370 SPLIT-HAND DEFORMITY WITH MANDIBULOFACIAL DYSOSTOSIS

PATTERSON AND STEVENSON (1964) STUDIED A FATHER WITH THE FULL SYNDROME AND HIS SON
WHO HAD ONLY THE SPLIT-FOOT DEFORMITY. SEE MANDIBULOFACIAL DYSOSTOSIS WITH LIMB
ANOMALIES (NAGER'S ACROFACIAL DYSOSTOSIS).

PATTERSON, T. J. S. AND STEVENSON, A. C.* CRANIOFACIAL DYSOSTOSIS AND MALFORMA-
TIONS OF THE FEET. J. MED. GENET. 1* 112-114, 1964.

18380 SPLIT-HAND WITH CONGENITAL NYSTAGMUS, FUNDAL CHANGES, CATARACTS

IN A FATHER AND DAUGHTER WITH SPLIT-HAND SPLIT-FOOT DEFORMITY, KARSCH (1936) FOUND
HORIZONTAL UNDULATORY NYSTAGMUS, SQUINT, FUNDAL CHANGES AND CATARACT, WHICH IN THE
FATHER APPEARED AT A LATE AGE AND IN THE DAUGHTER APPEARED EARLIER. NEUGEBAUER
(1962) DESCRIBED AFFECTED HALF SIBS, A BROTHER AND SISTER AGES 7 MONTHS AND 42
MONTHS, RESPECTIVELY. THE MOTHER OF THE TWO CHILDREN (BY DIFFERENT HUSBANDS) WAS
NORMAL. CATARACT WAS NOT PRESENT.

KARSCH, J.* ERBLICHE AUGENMISSBILDUNG IN VERBINDUNG MIT SPALTHAND UND -FUSS.
Z. AUGENHEILK. 89* 274-279, 1936.

NEUGEBAUER, H.* SPALTHAND UND -FUSS MIT FAMILIARER BESONDERHEIT. Z. ORTHOP.
95* 500-506, 1962.

*18390 SPONDYLOEPIPHYSEAL DYSPLASIA, CONGENITAL TYPE

SPRANGER AND WIEDEMANN (1966) SUGGESTED THIS DESIGNATION FOR A DISORDER AFFECTING
PARTICULARLY THE VERTEBRAE AND JUXTA-TRUNCAL EPIPHYSES. FOUR OF 6 PATIENTS HAD
PROGRESSIVE MYOPIA. THREE PERSONS (MOTHER AND 2 SONS) WERE AFFECTED IN ONE
FAMILY. THEY COLLECTED 14 CASES FROM THE LITERATURE. BACH ET AL. (1967) REPORTED
AN ISOLATED CASE. PLATYSPONDYLY, SHORT LIMBS AND CLEFT PALATE WERE EVIDENT AT
BIRTH. OTHER MALFORMATIONS INCLUDED MYOPIA, HYPOPLASIA OF ABDOMINAL MUSCULATURE,
ABDOMINAL AND INGUINAL HERNIAS AND MENTAL RETARDATION. DETACHMENT OF THE RETINA
OCCURS IN SOME PATIENTS EVEN WITHOUT SIGNIFICANT MYOPIA. ROAF ET AL. (1967)
REPORTED 4 SPORADIC CASES. POSSIBLY THE PATIENT DESCRIBED BY MCKUSICK (1966) HAD
THIS CONDITION. FRASER (1968) OBSERVED DOMINANT INHERITANCE (HIS CASE M 13).
SEVERE MYOPIA IN PARTICULAR WAS A SERIOUS PROBLEM IN THE CASES REPORTED BY FRASER
ET AL. (1969). MOTHER AND TWO CHILDREN WERE AFFECTED IN ONE OF THEIR FAMILIES.
SPRANGER AND LANGER (1970) REPORTED 20 CASES. IN THE AFFECTED NEWBORN INFANT X-
RAYS SHOW LACK OF OSSIFICATION OF THE OS PUBIS, DISTAL FEMORAL AND PROXIMAL TIBIAL
EPIPHYSES, TALUS AND CALCANEUS AND FLATTENING OF VERTEBRAL BODIES (SPRANGER AND
LANGER, 1970).

BACH, C., MAROTEAUX, P., SCHAEFFER, P., BITAN, A. AND CRUMIERE, C.* DYSPLASIA
SPONDYLO-EPIPHYSAIRE CONGENITALE AVEC ANOMALIES MULTIPLES. ARCH. FRANC. PEDIAT.
24* 23-34, 1967.

FRASER, G. R., FRIEDMANN, A. I., MAROTEAUX, P., GLEN-BOTT, A. M. AND MITTWOCH,
V.* DYSPLASIA SPONDYLOEPIPHYSARIA CONGENITA AND RELATED GENERALIZED SKELETAL
DYSPLASIAS AMONG CHILDREN WITH SEVERE VISUAL HANDICAPS. ARCH. DIS. CHILD. 44*
490-498, 1969.

D
O
M
I
N
A
N
T

BALTIMORE* JOHNS HOPKINS PRESS, 1968.

MCKUSICK, V. A.* HERITABLE DISORDERS OF CONNECTIVE TISSUE.   ST. LOUIS* C. V.
MOSBY CO., 1966. (3RD ED.).   P. 467.

ROAF, R., LONGMORE, J. B. AND FORRESTER, R. M.* A CHILDHOOD SYNDROME OF BONE
DYSPLASIA, RETINAL DETACHMENT AND DEAFNESS. DEVELOP. MED. CHILD. NEUROL. 9* 464-
473, 1967.

SPRANGER, J. AND LANGER, L. O., JR.* SPONDYLOEPIPHYSEAL DYSPLASIA CONGENITA.
RADIOLOGY 94* 313-322, 1970.

SPRANGER, J. AND WIEDEMANN, H.-R.* DYSPLASIA SPONDYLOEPIPHYSARIA CONGENITA.
(LETTER) LANCET 2* 642 ONLY, 1966.

SPRANGER, J. AND WIEDEMANN, H.-R.* DYSPLASIA SPONDYLOEPIPHYSARIA CONGENITA.
HELV. PAEDIAT. ACTA 21* 598-611, 1966.

*18400 SPONDYLOEPIPHYSEAL DYSPLASIA, PSEUDO-ACHONDROPLASTIC TYPES

DWARFISM IS DELAYED IN ONSET AND THE HEAD AND FACE ARE NOT INVOLVED. THE
RADIOLOGIC CHANGES ARE QUITE DIFFERENT FROM THOSE OF TRUE ACHONDROPLASIA. HALL
AND DORST (1969) SUGGESTED THAT THERE ARE FOUR TYPES OF PSEUDOACHONDROPLASIA SED*
DOMINANT AND RECESSIVE KOZLOWSKI TYPES* DOMINANT AND RECESSIVE MAROTEAUX-LAMY
TYPES. ALTHOUGH THE DOMINANT AND RECESSIVE TYPES ARE CLEARLY SEPARATE, THE
RELATIONSHIP OF THE TWO DOMINANT AND TWO RECESSIVE TYPES TO EACH OTHER IS UNCLEAR.
THEY MIGHT, FOR EXAMPLE, BE ALLELIC.

FORD, N., SILVERMAN, F. N. AND KOZLOWSKI, K.* SPONDYLO-EPIPHYSEAL DYSPLASIA
(PSEUDO-ACHONDROPLASTIC TYPE). AM. J. ROENTGEN. 86* 462-472, 1961.

HALL, J. G. AND DORST, J. P.* PSEUDOACHONDROPLASTIC SED.   THE CLINICAL
DELINEATION OF BIRTH DEFECTS.   IV.   SKELETAL DYSPLASIAS. NEW YORK* NATIONAL
FOUNDATION, 1969. PP. 254-259.

MAROTEAUX, P. AND LAMY, M.* LES FORMES PSEUDO-ACHONDROPLASIQUES DES DYSPLASIES
SPONDYLO-EPIPHYSAIRES. PRESSE MED. 67* 383-386, 1959.

MCKUSICK, V. A.* HERITABLE DISORDERS OF CONNECTIVE TISSUE.   ST. LOUIS* C. V.
MOSBY CO., 1966 (3RD ED.).

18410 SPONDYLOEPIPHYSEAL DYSPLASIA, TARDA TYPE

A LATE FORM OF SED PRODUCING MARKED DWARFISM WAS OBSERVED IN MOTHER AND SON
(1215027, 1215026). THE RADIOGRAPHIC CHANGES WERE DIFFERENT FROM THOSE OF THE X-
LINKED SED. THE DWARFING WAS MARKED, THE MOTHER BEING ONLY ABOUT 4 FEET TALL.
THIS CONDITION IS DISTINGUISHED FROM BRACHYRAPHIA (Q.V.) BY THE FACT THAT THE ARMS
ARE SHORTENED TO A DEGREE ABOUT PROPORTIONATE TO THE DEGREE OF SHORTENING IN THE
TRUNK. FELMAN (1969) DESCRIBED A NEGRO FATHER AND HIS SON AND DAUGHTER WITH
EPIPHYSEAL AND VERTEBRAL DYSPLASIA PRODUCING SEVERE SCOLIOSIS AND TRUNCAL
SHORTENING AS WELL AS COMPLETE DESTRUCTION OF THE FEMORAL CAPITAL EPIPHYSES AND
NECKS. THE HANDS AND FEET WERE SHORT AND STUBBY. CLINICALLY AND RADIOLOGICALLY
THE PATIENTS WERE NORMAL AT BIRTH. RUBIN (1964) PRESENTED (FIGS. 7.10-7.14) AN
INSTRUCTIVE FAMILY IN WHICH PLATYSPONDYLY ACCOMPANIED CHANGES IN THE EPIPHYSES IN
THE LIMBS.

FELMAN, A. H.* MULTIPLE EPIPHYSEAL D'SPLASIA.   THREE CASES WITH UNUSUAL
VERTEBRAL ABNORMALITIES. RADIOLOGY 93* 119-125, 1969.

RUBIN, P.* DYNAMIC CLASSIFICATION OF BONE DYSPLASIAS. CHICAGO* YEAR BOOK
MEDICAL PUBLISHERS, 1964.

18420 SPONDYLOLISTHESIS AND SPINA BIFIDA OCCULTA

AMUSO AND MANKIN (1967) REPORTED ON A FAMILY IN WHICH FIVE MEMBERS IN THREE
GENERATIONS HAD SPONDYLOLISTHESIS OF THE FIFTH LUMBAR VERTEBRA ON THE FIRST SACRAL
IN ASSOCIATION WITH DEFECTS IN THE POSTERIOR SPINOUS PROCESSES OF THE FIFTH LUMBAR
VERTEBRA AND SACRUM. TRANSMISSION FROM FATHER TO SON OCCURRED ONCE. SHAHRIAREE
AND HARKESS (1970) FOUND SPONDYLOLISTHESIS IN A FATHER AND THREE SONS. THE DEFECT
WAS THOUGHT TO CONCERN THE PARS INTERARTICULARIS.

AMUSO, S. J. AND MANKIN, H. J.* HEREDITARY SPONDYLOLISTHESIS AND SPINA BIFIDA.
REPORT OF A FAMILY IN WHICH THE LESION IS TRANSMITTED AS AN AUTOSOMAL DOMINANT
THROUGH THREE GENERATIONS. J. BONE JOINT SURG. 49A* 507-513, 1967.

SHAHRIAREE, H. AND HARKESS, J. W.* A FAMILY WITH SPONDYLOLISTHESIS. RADIOLOGY
94* 631-633, 1970.

18430 SPONDYLOSIS, CERVICAL

BULL ET AL. (1969) FROM AN X-RAY STUDY OF THE CERVICAL SPINE IN TWINS CONCLUDED

THAT GENETIC FACTORS ARE SIGNIFICANT IN DEGENERATIVE CHANGES IN THE CERVICAL SPINE.

BULL, J., EL GAMMAL, T. AND POPHAM, M.* A POSSIBLE GENETIC FACTOR IN CERVICAL SPONDYLOSIS. BRIT. J. RADIOL. 42* 9-16, 1969.

18440 SPRENGEL'S DEFORMITY ('HIGH SCAPULA')

CONGENITAL UPWARD DISPLACEMENT OF THE SCAPULA ALMOST ALWAYS OCCURS SPORADICALLY. HOWEVER, GOTTESLEBEN (1927) OBSERVED 9 CASES IN 6 SIBSHIPS OF 3 GENERATIONS OF A FAMILY WITH MALE-TO-MALE TRANSMISSION. SCHWARZWELLER (1937) FOUND TWO AFFECTED SIBS IN TWO OUT OF 9 FAMILIES. IN ONE OF THESE THE FATHER HAD MILD ABNORMALITY. AUBERT AND ARROYO (1967) OBSERVED THE DISORDER IN FATHER AND DAUGHTER.

AUBERT, L. AND ARROYO, H.* MALADIE DE SPRENGEL FAMILIALE. MARSEILLE MED. 104* 287-290, 1967.

GOTTESLEBEN, A.* UBER DEN DOPPELSEITIGEN UND EINSEITIGEN SCHULTERBLATTHOCHSTAND. ARCH. KLIN. CHIR. 144* 723-731, 1927.

SCHWARZWELLER, F.* DER ANGEBORENE SCHULTERBLATTHOCHSTAND DEN WIRBELSAULE. (EINE ERBBIOLOGISCHE UNTERSUCHUNG UBER DIE ENTSTEHUNG DES ENTSTEHUNG DES ANGEBORENE SCHULTERBLATTHOCHSTANDES). Z. MENSCHL. VERERB. KONSTITUTIONSL. 20* 341-349, 1937.

*18450 STEATOCYSTOMA MULTIPLEX (SEBACEOUS CYSTS, MULTIPLE)

NOOJIN AND REYNOLDS (1948) OBSERVED TWELVE CASES IN THREE GENERATIONS. IN TYPICAL CASES THE PATIENT MAY EXHIBIT 100 TO 2000 ROUND OR OVAL CYSTIC TUMORS WIDELY DISTRIBUTED ON THE BACK, ANTERIOR TRUNK, ARMS, SCROTUM AND THIGHS. SEBACEOUS CYSTS PRESENTING MAINLY AS WENS OF THE SCALP WERE REPORTED BY STEPHENS (1959) IN A VERY LARGE NUMBER OF INDIVIDUALS IN FIVE GENERATIONS IN A DOMINANT PEDIGREE PATTERN. SEBACEOUS AND OTHER SOFT TISSUE TUMORS OCCUR AS PART OF GARDNER'S SYNDROME (SEE POLYPOSIS III). ACTUALLY THE SO-CALLED SEBACEOUS CYSTS OF GARDNER'S SYNDROME ARE USUALLY EPIDERMOID CYSTS.

NOOJIN, R. O. AND REYNOLDS, J. P.* FAMILIAL STEATOCYSTOMA MULTIPLEX. TWELVE CASES IN THREE GENERATIONS. ARCH. DERM. SYPH. 57* 1013-1018, 1948.

STEPHENS, F. E.* HEREDITARY MULTIPLE SEBACEOUS CYSTS. J. HERED. 50* 299-301, 1959.

*18460 STEATOCYSTOMA MULTIPLEX WITH PACHYONYCHIA CONGENITA

IN FOUR GENERATIONS OF A FAMILY, VINEYARD AND SCOTT (1961) OBSERVED STEATOCYSTOMA ASSOCIATED WITH PACHYONYCHIA CONGENITA (Q.V.).

VINEYARD, W. R. AND SCOTT, R. A.* STEATOCYSTOMA MULTIPLEX WITH PACHYONYCHIA CONGENITA. EIGHT CASES IN FOUR GENERATIONS. ARCH. DERM. 84* 824-827, 1961.

18470 STEIN-LEVENTHAL SYNDROME

THE FATHERS TEND TO BE ABNORMALLY HAIRY, FEMALE SIBS ARE HIRSUTE AND MOTHERS AND SISTERS OFTEN HAVE OLIGOMENORRHEA. CULDOSCOPY HAS OFTEN SHOWN SIGNS OF S-L, E.G., 8 OF 12 SISTERS OF CASES SHOWED OVARIAN CHANGES CONSISTENT WITH THAT DIAGNOSIS (COOPER ET AL., 1968). URINARY STEROID DETERMINATIONS ALSO SUGGEST A GENETIC BASIS.

COOPER, H. E., SPELLACY, W. N., PREM, K. A. AND COHEN, W. D.* HEREDITARY FACTORS IN THE STEIN-LEVENTHAL SYNDROME. AM. J. OBSTET. GYNEC. 100* 371-387, 1968.

18480 STERNUM, PREMATURE OBLITERATION OF SUTURES OF

CURRARINO AND SILVERMAN (1958) REPORTED CASES IN WHICH THE STERNAL SUTURES WERE HYPOPLASTIC OR CLOSED PREMATURELY LEADING TO A CHARACTERISTIC DEFORMITY OF THE STERNUM WHICH WAS ABNORMALLY SHORT WITH AN ACUTE ANGULATION IN THE NORMAL POSITION OF THE ANGLE OF LOUIS AND DEPRESSED IN ITS LOWER PART. ASSOCIATED MANIFESTATIONS IN SOME CASES INCLUDED MICROGNATHIA, CRYPTORCHIDISM, CONGENITAL HEART MALFORMATION. DORST (1966) OBSERVED THE STERNAL ANOMALY IN MOTHER AND DAUGHTER WHO WERE OTHERWISE NORMAL. THE STERNAL DEFORMITY IS SEEN IN THE MALE TURNER SYNDROME, PTERYGIUM COLLI SYNDROME. IT WAS ALSO SEEN IN BROTHERS WITH MULTIPLE OSTEOCHONDRITIS DISSECANS (Q.V.).

CURRARINO, G. AND SILVERMAN, F. N.* PREMATURE OBLITERATION OF THE STERNAL SUTURES AND PIGEON-BREAST DEFORMITY. RADIOLOGY 70* 532-540, 1958.

DORST, J. P.* BALTIMORE, MD.* PERSONAL COMMUNICATION, 1966.

18490 STIFF SKIN SYNDROME

ESTERLY AND MCKUSICK (1971) DESCRIBED A DISORDER CHARACTERIZED BY THICKENED AND

INDURATED SKIN OF THE ENTIRE BODY AND LIMITATION OF JOINT MOBILITY WITH FLEXION CONTRACTURES. ONE PATIENT THEY REPORTED WAS A SPORADIC CASE BUT THE OTHER HAD AN AFFECTED SISTER AND MOTHER. THIS MAY BE THE SAME DISORDER AS THAT ENTERED ELSEWHERE AS CONTRACTURES WITH SCLERODERMA-LIKE CHANGES (12110).

ESTERLY, N. B. AND MCKUSICK, V. A.* STIFF SKIN SYNDROME. PEDIATRICS 47* 360-369, 1971.

18500 STOMATOCYTOSIS

LOCK, SMITH AND HARDISTY (1961) DESCRIBED A *NEW* HEREDITARY RED CELL ANOMALY ASSOCIATED WITH HEMOLYTIC ANEMIA. THEY REFERRED TO IT AS STOMATOCYTOSIS BECAUSED OF A PALE-STAINING BAND IN THE ERYTHROCYTES. ERYTHROCYTES SHOWED SHORTENED SURVIVAL AND INCREASED OSMOTIC FRAGILITY.

LOCK, S. P., SMITH, R. AND HARDISTY, R. M.* STOMATOCYTOSIS* A HEREDITARY RED CELL ANOMALY ASSOCIATED WITH HAEMOLYTIC ANAEMIA. BRIT. J. HAEMAT. 7* 303-314, 1961.

18510 STRABISMUS

ALTHOUGH THE FAMILIAL NATURE OF STRABISMUS HAS BEEN RECOGNIZED IN THE MEDICAL LITERATURE SINCE HIPPOCRATES (SEE CANTOLINO AND VON NOORDEN, 1969), NO SIMPLE MENDELIAN INHERITANCE IS ESTABLISHED (RICHTER, 1967). CANTOLINO AND VON NOORDEN (1969) ARRIVED AT THE SAME CONCLUSION FROM A FAMILY STUDY OF MICROTROPIA, THE MINOR FORM OF STRABISMUS. RICHTER (1967) FOUND LOWER RISK IN FIRST DEGREE RELATIVES WITH DIVERGENT STRABISMUS THAN WITH CONVERGENT STRABISMUS. WHEN TWO FIRST DEGREE RELATIVES (E.G., TWO PARENTS, ONE PARENT AND A CHILD, OR TWO CHILDREN) ARE AFFECTED THE RISK IS ABOUT 1 IN 4 AND 1 IN 2 FOR THE TWO FORMS, RESPECTIVELY.

CANTOLINO, S. J. AND VON NOORDEN, G. K.* HEREDITY IN MICROTROPIA. ARCH. OPHTHAL. 81* 753-759, 1969.

RICHTER, S.* UNTERSUCHUNGEN UBER DIE HEREDITAT DES STRABISMUS CONCOMITANS. HUMANGENETIK. 3* 235-243, 1967.

*18520 STRIAE DISTENSAE

I HAVE OBSERVED TRANSVERSE STRIAE OF THE LUMBAR AREA IN FATHER AND TWO SONS. THE STRIAE APPEARED IN THEIR TEENS AND FADED AS THEY GREW OLDER. CARR AND HAMILTON (1969) NOTED THAT SUCH STRIAE ARE MORE COMMON IN MALES. F. PARKES WEBER (1935) CALLED THEM IDIOPATHIC STRIAE ATROPHICAE OF PUBERTY. STRIAE DISTENSAE OCCUR, ESPECIALLY IN THE DELTOID, PECTORAL, HIP AND THIGH AREAS, IN THE MARFAN SYNDROME.

CARR, R. D. AND HAMILTON, J. F.* TRANSVERSE STRIAE OF THE BACK. ARCH. DERM. 99* 26-30, 1969.

WEBER, F. P.* *IDIOPATHIC* STRIAE ATROPHICAE OF PUBERTY. LANCET 2* 885-886, AND 1347 ONLY, 1935.

18530 STURGE-WEBER SYNDROME

THIS CONDITION, SOMETIMES CALLED THE FOURTH PHACOMATOSIS, IS CHARACTERIZED BY NEVUS FLAMMEUS OF THE FACE AND ANGIOMA OF THE MENINGES. UNLIKE THE OTHER PHACOMATOSES (TUBEROUS SCLEROSIS, NEUROFIBROMATOSIS AND VON HIPPEL-LINDAU'S DISEASE), NO CLEAR EVIDENCE OF HEREDITY HAS BEEN DISCOVERED. SOMETIMES (SEE BONSE, 1951, AND NONNENMACHER, 1955) THE KLIPPEL-TRENAUNAY-WEBER SYNDROME (Q.V.), WHICH ALSO DOES NOT SEEM TO MENDELIZE, IS ASSOCIATED. SEE KLIPPEL-TRENAUNAY-WEBER SYNDROME.

BONSE, G.* RONTGENBEFUNDE BEI EINER PHAKOMATOSE (STURGE-WEBER KOMBINIERT MIT KLIPPEL-TRENAUNAY). FORTSCHR. RONTGENSTR. 74* 727, 1951.

FURUKAWA, T., IGATA, A., TOYOKURA, Y. AND IKEDA, S.* STURGE-WEBER AND KLIPPEL-TRENAUNAY SYNDROME WITH NEVUS OF OTA AND ITO. ARCH. DERM. 102* 640-645, 1970.

NONNENMACHER, H.* AUGENARZTLICHE BETRACHTUNGEN ZUM SYMPTOMENKOMPLEX MORBUS STURGE-WEBER, KLIPPEL-TRENAUNAY UND PARKES-WEBER. KLIN. MBL. AUGENHEILK. 126* 154-164, 1955.

18540 SUBGLOTTIC BAR

HOWIE, LADEFOGED AND STARK (1961) DESCRIBED SUBGLOTTIC BAR IN A GRANDFATHER, MOTHER AND TWO DAUGHTERS (4 PERSONS IN THREE GENERATIONS). SEVERE DYSPNEA WITH RESPIRATORY INFECTION IN A 6-YEAR-OLD BROUGHT THE CONDITION TO ATTENTION. ALL FOUR HAD A HARSH, QUIVERING, HIGH-PITCHED, WEAK VOICE AND THREE HAD SUFFERED FROM RESPIRATORY DISTRESS WITH INSPIRATORY STRIDOR. IMPERFECT ADDUCTION OF THE VOCAL CORDS WAS AN ASSOCIATED FINDING.

HOWIE, T. O., LADEFOGED, P. AND STARK, R. E.* CONGENITAL SUBGLOTTIC BARS FOUND IN 3 GENERATIONS OF ONE FAMILY. FOLIA PHONIAT. 13* 56-61, 1961.

EISENBERG AND COLLEAGUES (1964) REPORTED 22 CASES INVOLVING 3 GENERATIONS OF EACH OF TWO FAMILIES. SOME HAD ASSOCIATED PULMONARY VALVULAR OR PERIPHERAL ARTERIAL STENOSIS. NONE HAD UNUSUAL FACIES. A SIMILAR CONDITION WHICH MAY BE THE RESULT OF FETAL HYPERCALCEMIA IS CHARACTERIZED BY ELFIN FACIES (ANTEVERTED NOSTRILS AND PATULOUS LIPS) AND MENTAL RETARDATION WITH SUPRAVALVAR AORTIC STENOSIS. IT IS APPARENTLY NON-FAMILIAL AND A PHENOCOPY OF FAMILIAL SUPRAVALVAR AORTIC STENOSIS. PULMONARY ARTERY STENOSIS WAS NOTED IN MOTHER AND SON BY GYLLENSWARD ET AL. (1957). LEWIS ET AL. (1969) DESCRIBED A SIBSHIP IN WHICH 5 OF 9 SIBS HAD SUPRAVALVAR AORTIC STENOSIS WITH PECULIAR FACIES BUT NORMAL INTELLIGENCE. ANTIA ET AL. (1967) COMMENTED ON THE LACK OF CLEAR DISTINCTION BETWEEN THE FAMILIAL SUPRAVALVAR AORTIC STENOSIS WITH NORMAL FACIES AND MENTALITY AND THE NON-FAMILIAL TYPE WITH ABNORMAL FACIES AND MENTAL RETARDATION. MCDONALD ET AL. (1969) DESCRIBED AN ARTERIOPATHY, WITH MULTIPLE PULMONARY AND SYSTEMIC ARTERIAL STENOSES, IN A MOTHER AND THREE DAUGHTERS. TWO HAD SUPRAVALVAR AORTIC STENOSIS. THE FAMILIAL OCCURRENCE OF PULMONARY ARTERIAL STENOSES IS DOCUMENTED (MCCUE ET AL., 1965) AND THEIR OCCURRENCE AFTER MATERNAL RUBELLA IS WELL ESTABLISHED (ROWE, 1963). IT CAN BE ARGUED THAT SUPRAVALVAR AORTIC STENOSIS IS AN INADEQUATE OR INAPPROPRIATE DESIGNATION. STRONG ET AL. (1970) OBSERVED SUDDEN DEATH FOLLOWING PREMEDICATION FOR CARDIAC CATHETERIZATION IN AN 11 MONTH OLD MALE. POSTMORTEM SHOWED SEVERE FIBROMUSCULAR DYSPLASIA OF BOTH SYSTEMIC AND PULMONARY ARTERIES. A SISTER HAD SIGNS OF MILD PULMONARY ARTERY AND SUPRAVALVULAR AORTIC STENOSIS. THE MOTHER HAD SIGNS OF MILD AORTIC STENOSIS.

ANTIA, A. U., WILTSE, H. E., ROWE, R. D., PITT, E. L., LEVIN, S., OTTESEN, O. E. AND COOKE, R. E.* PATHOGENESIS OF THE SUPRAVALVULAR AORTIC STENOSIS SYNDROME. J. PEDIAT. 71* 431-441, 1967.

EISENBERG, R., YOUNG, D., JACOBSON, B. AND BOITO, A.* FAMILIAL SUPRAVALVAR AORTIC STENOSIS. AM. J. DIS. CHILD. 108* 341-347, 1964.

GARCIA, R. E., FRIEDMAN, W. F., KABACK, M. M. AND ROWE, R. D.* IDIOPATHIC HYPERCALCEMIA AND SUPRAVALVULAR AORTIC STENOSIS* DOCUMENTATION OF A NEW SYNDROME. NEW ENG. J. MED. 271* 117-120, 1964.

GYLLENSWARD, A., LODIN, H., LUNDBERG, A. AND MOLLER, T.* CONGENITAL, MULTIPLE PERIPHERAL STENOSIS OF THE PULMONARY ARTERY. PEDIATRICS 19* 399-410, 1957.

JORGENSEN, G. AND BEUREN, A. J.* GENETISCHE UNTERSUCHUNGEN BEI SUPRAVALVULAREN AORTENSTENOSEN. HUMANGENETIK 1* 497-515, 1965.

LEWIS, A. J., ONGLEY, P. A., KINCAID, O. W. AND RITTER, D. G.* SUPRAVALVULAR AORTIC STENOSIS. REPORT OF A FAMILY WITH PECULIAR SOMATIC FEATURES AND NORMAL INTELLIGENCE. DIS. CHEST 55* 372-379, 1969.

LOGAN, W. F., JONES, E. W., WALKER, E., COULSHED, II. AND EPSTEIN, E. J.* FAMILIAL SUPRAVALVAR AORTIC STENOSIS. BRIT. HEART J. 27* 547-559, 1965.

MCCUE, C. M., ROBERTSON, L. W., LESTER, R. G. AND MAUCK, H. P., JR.* PULMONARY ARTERY COARCTATIONS. A REPORT OF 20 CASES WITH REVIEW OF 319 CASES FROM THE LITERATURE. J. PEDIAT. 67* 222-238, 1965.

MCCUE, C. M., SPICUZZA, T. J., ROBERTSON, L. W. AND MAUCK, H. P., JR.* FAMILIAL SUPRAVALVULAR AORTIC STENOSIS. J. PEDIAT. 73* 889-895, 1968.

MCDONALD, A. H., GERLIS, L. M. AND SOMERVILLE, J.* FAMILIAL ARTERIOPATHY WITH ASSOCIATED PULMONARY AND SYSTEMIC ARTERIAL STENOSIS. BRIT. HEART J. 31* 375-385, 1969.

MORRISON, R. C. AND MCNALLEY, M. C.* THE SPECTRUM OF ABNORMALITIES IN SUPRAVAL-VULAR AORTIC STENOSIS. (ABSTRACT) AM. J. CARDIOL. 19* 143 ONLY, 1967.

PAGE, H. L., JR., VOGEL, J. H. K., PRYOR, R. AND BLOUNT, S. G., JR.* SUPRAVAL-VULAR AORTIC STENOSIS. UNUSUAL OBSERVATIONS IN THREE PATIENTS. AM. J. CARDIOL. 23* 270-277, 1969.

ROWE, R. D.* MATERNAL RUBELLA AND PULMONARY ARTERY STENOSES. REPORT OF ELEVEN CASES. PEDIATRICS 32* 180-185, 1963.

STRONG, W. B., PERRIN, E., LIEBMAN, J. AND SILBERT, D. R.* SYSTEMIC AND PULMONARY ARTERY DYSPLASIA ASSOCIATED WITH UNEXPECTED DEATH IN INFANCY. J. PEDIAT. 77* 233-238, 1970.

WILLIAMS, J. C., BARRATT-BOYES, B. G. AND LOWE, J. B.* SUPRAVALVULAR AORTIC STENOSIS. CIRCULATION 24* 1311-1318, 1961.

18560 SYMPHALANGISM OF TOES

GARN ET AL. (1965) DESCRIBED FUSION ACROSS THE INTERPHALANGEAL JOINTS OF THE TOES AS AN ISOLATED INHERITED ANATOMICAL VARIANT, OFTEN SECONDARY TO ABSENCE OF SECONDARY OSSIFICATION CENTERS OF THE FEET. THE HANDS ARE NOT COMPARABLY

GARN, S. M., ROHMANN, C. G. AND SILVERMAN, F. N.* MISSING SECONDARY OSSIFICA-
TION CENTERS OF THE FOOT. INHERITANCE AND DEVELOPMENTAL MEANING. ANN. RADIOL. 8*
629-644, 1965.

*18570 SYMPHALANGISM, DISTAL

A SEPARATE DOMINANT MUTATION PRODUCES ANKYLOSIS OF THE DISTAL INTERPHALANGEAL
JOINTS.   SEE RECESSIVE CATALOG FOR THE SYMPHALANGISM-DWARFISM SYNDROME. PROXIMAL
SYMPHALANGISM OCCURS WITH THE RECESSIVE DISORDER DIASTROPHIC DWARFISM (Q.V.).
SYMPHALANGISM ALSO OCCURS AMONG THE MULTIPLE DIGITAL ANOMALIES OF BRACHYDACTYLY,
TYPE C (Q.V.).

STEINBERG, A. G. AND REYNOLDS, E. L.* FURTHER DATA ON SYMPHALANGISM. J. HERED.
39* 23-27, 1948.

*18580 SYMPHALANGISM, PROXIMAL (HEREDITARY ABSENCE OF THE PROXIMAL INTERPHALANGEAL
JOINTS)

CUSHING (1916) DESCRIBED A LARGE AMERICAN FAMILY WITH MANY AFFECTED MEMBERS AND
ASSIGNED THE DESIGNATION SYMPHALANGISM. FUSION OF CARPAL AND TARSAL BONES IS ALSO
A FEATURE. (SEE CALCANEO-NAVICULAR COALITION.) THIS TRAIT WAS THOUGHT TO ENJOY
THE DISTINCTION OF BEING TRACED THROUGH MORE GENERATIONS THAN ALMOST ANY OTHER,
HAVING BEEN IDENTIFIED IN THE FIRST EARL OF SHREWSBURY WHO LIVED IN THE 15TH
CENTURY (DRINKWATER, 1917).   AFTER A RE-EXAMINATION OF THE EVIDENCE, HOWEVER,
ELKINGTON AND HUNTSMAN (1967) CONCLUDED THAT THE EARL PROBABLY DID NOT HAVE
SYMPHALANGISM AND THE MUTATION IS OF MORE RECENT ORIGIN IN THAT KINDRED. IN THE
FAMILY REPORTED BY VESELL (1960) MOTHER AND DAUGHTER HAD CONDUCTIVE DEAFNESS. THE
MOTHER WAS APPARENTLY THE NEW MUTATION.   STRASBURGER AND COLLEAGUES (1965)
FOLLOWED UP ON CUSHING'S FAMILY. CONDUCTIVE DEAFNESS WITH EARLY ONSET OCCURRED
SUFFICIENTLY OFTEN IN AFFECTED MEMBERS OF THIS LARGE KINDRED TO SUGGEST THAT IT IS
AN EFFECT OF THE SAME GENE. WILDERVANCK ET AL. (1967) OBSERVED TWO ACCESSORY
BONES IN THE FEET OF MULTIPLE AFFECTED PERSONS IN ONE FAMILY.

CUSHING, H.* HEREDITARY ANCHYLOSIS OF PROXIMAL PHALANGEAL JOINTS (SYMPHALAN-
GISM). GENETICS 1* 90-106, 1916.

DRINKWATER, H.* PHALANGEAL ANARTHROSIS (SYNOSTOSIS, ANKYLOSIS) TRANSMITTED
THROUGH 14 GENERATIONS. PROC. ROY. SOC. MED. 10* 60-68, 1917.

ELKINGTON, S. G. AND HUNTSMAN, R. G.* THE TALBOT FINGERS* A STUDY IN SYMPHALAN-
GISM. BRIT. MED. J. 1* 407-411, 1967.

GORLIN, R. J., KIETZER, G. AND WOLFSON, J.* STAPES FIXATION AND PROXIMAL
SYMPHALANGISM. Z. KINDERHEILK. 108* 12-16, 1970.

STRASBURGER, A. K., HAWKINS, M. R., ELDRIDGE, R., HARGRAVE, R. L. AND MCKUSICK,
V. A.* SYMPHALANGISM* GENETIC AND CLINICAL ASPECTS. BULL. HOPKINS HOSP. 117* 108-
127, 1965.

VESELL, E. S.* SYMPHALANGISM, STRABISMUS AND HEARING LOSS IN MOTHER AND
DAUGHTER. NEW ENG. J. MED. 263* 839-842, 1960.

WILDERVANCK, L. S., GOEDHARD, G. AND MEIJER, S.* PROXIMAL SYMPHALANGISM OF
FINGERS ASSOCIATED WITH FUSION OF OS NAVICULARE AND TALUS AND OCCURRENCE OF TWO
ACCESSORY BONES IN THE FEET (OS PARANAVICULARE AND OS TIBIALE EXTERNUM) IN A
EUROPEAN-INDONESIAN-CHINESE FAMILY. ACTA GENET. STATIST. MED. 17* 166-177, 1967.

*18590 SYNDACTYLY, TYPE I (ZYGODACTYLY)

FROM THE MEDICAL LITERATURE AND FROM OUR OWN EXPERIENCE WE CONCLUDED THAT THERE
ARE AT LEAST 5 PHENOTYPICALLY DIFFERENT TYPES OF SYNDACTYLY INVOLVING THE HANDS
WITH OR WITHOUT FOOT INVOLVEMENT. ALL ARE INHERITED AS AUTOSOMAL DOMINANT TRAITS
AND WITHIN ANY PEDIGREE THERE IS UNIFORMITY OF TYPE OF SYNDACTYLY, ALLOWING FOR
THE VARIATION CHARACTERISTIC FOR DOMINANT TRAITS.   THESE GENETIC TYPES OF
SYNDACTYLY HAVE TO BE DIFFERENTIATED FROM SYNDACTYLY ASSOCIATED WITH CONGENITAL
BANDS FOR WHICH THERE IS NO EVIDENCE OF A GENETIC BASIS. IN THIS COMMON TYPE OF
SYNDACTYLY, SOMETIMES CALLED ZYGODACTYLY, THERE IS USUALLY WEBBING BETWEEN THE 3RD
AND 4TH FINGERS, EITHER COMPLETE OR PARTIAL AND OCCASIONALLY ASSOCIATED WITH
FUSION OF THE DISTAL PHALANGES OF THESE FINGERS. OTHER FINGERS ARE SOMETIMES ALSO
INVOLVED BUT THE 3RD AND 4TH FINGERS ARE THE MOST COMMONLY AFFECTED. IN THE FEET,
THERE IS USUALLY WEBBING BETWEEN THE 2ND AND 3RD TOES, EITHER COMPLETE OR PARTIAL.
SOMETIMES THE HANDS ARE ONLY AFFECTED AND SOMETIMES ONLY THE FEET. LUEKEN (1938)
REPORTED THIS TYPE OF SYNDACTYLY IN 18 MALES AND 29 FEMALES OF 5 GENERATIONS
ILLUSTRATING THE VARIOUS DEGREES OF EXPRESSIVITY OF THE SAME GENE. SOME DEGREE OF
WEBBING BETWEEN THE SECOND AND THIRD TOES IS FREQUENT. SCHOFIELD (1921) PRESENTED
A PEDIGREE WHICH SUGGESTED HOLANDRIC INHERITANCE TO CASTLE (1922). STERN (1957)
WAS UNABLE, HOWEVER, TO OBTAIN FURTHER EVIDENCE OF SAME AND SUGGESTED THAT
INHERITANCE IS AUTOSOMAL DOMINANT. STRAUS (1926) SUPPORTED THIS MODE OF INHERI-
TANCE. HSU (1965) DESCRIBED BILATERAL SYNDACTYLY IN 6 GENERATIONS OF A CHINESE
FAMILY. OF THE 31 DESCENDANTS OF ONE SYNDACTYLOUS WOMAN, 22 WERE AFFECTED. SKIN

AND BONEY FUSION OF THE DISTAL PHALANGES OF THE THIRD, FOURTH AND FIFTH FINGERS WERE PRESENT. AT LEAST ONE PERSON ALSO SHOWED UNION OF THE THIRD, FOURTH AND FIFTH TOES.

CASTLE, W. E.* THE Y-CHROMOSOME TYPE OF SEX-LINKED INHERITANCE IN MAN. SCIENCE 55* 703-704, 1922.

HSU, C.-K.* HEREDITARY SYNDACTYLIA IN A CHINESE FAMILY. CHIN. MED. J. 84* 482-485, 1965.

LUEKEN, K. G.* UBER EINE FAMILIE MIT SYNDACKTYLIE. Z. MENSCHL. VERERB. KONSTITUTIONSL. 22* 152-159, 1938.

SCHOFIELD, R.* INHERITANCE CF WEBBED TOES. J. HERED. 12* 400-401, 1921.

STERN, C.* THE PROBLEM OF COMPLETE Y-LINKAGE IN MAN. AM. J. HUM. GENET. 9* 147-166, 1957.

STRAUS, W. L., JR.* THE NATURE AND INHERITANCE OF WEBBED TOES IN MAN. J. MORPH. 41* 427-439, 1926.

*18600 SYNDACTYLY, TYPE II (SYNPOLYDACTYLY)

IN THE HANDS THERE IS USUALLY SYNDACTYLY OF THE 3RD AND 4TH FINGERS ASSOCIATED WITH POLYDACTYLY OF ALL COMPONENTS OR OF PART OF THE 4TH FINGER IN THE WEB. IN THE FEET THERE IS POLYDACTYLY OF THE 5TH TOE INCLUDED IN A WEB OF SYNDACTYLY OF THE 4TH AND 5TH TOES. THE MOST EXTENSIVE PEDIGREE IS THAT DESCRIBED BY THOMSEN (1927) SHOWING 31 AFFECTED MALES AND 11 AFFECTED FEMALES IN 7 GENERATIONS. OTHER KINDREDS WERE REPORTED BY ALVORD (1947), AND PIPKIN AND PIPKIN (1946) AMONG OTHERS. CROSS ET AL. (1968) OBSERVED A KINDRED WITH 27 AFFECTED PERSONS. TWO PERSONS TRANSMITTED THE GENE WITHOUT SHOWING ANY EFFECTS THEMSELVES. ALL PERSONS WITH CLINICALLY EVIDENT MALFORMATION IN THE HAND SHOWED ANOMALOUS PALMAR DERMATOG-LYPHICS. NO LINKAGE WITH ANY OF 12 LOCI WAS DEMONSTRABLE. AN EXCESS OF AFFECTED MALES HAS BEEN A CONSISTENT FEATURE. CROSS ET AL. (1968) FOUND, IN THE LITERATURE AND IN THEIR KINDRED, 133 FEMALES AND 174 MALES AFFECTED.

ALVORD, R. M.* ZYGODACTYLY AND ASSOCIATED VARIATIONS IN A UTAH FAMILY. J. HERED. 38* 49-53, 1947.

CROSS, H. E., LERBERG, D. B. AND MCKUSICK, V. A.* TYPE II SYNDACTYLY. J. MED. GENET. 20* 368-380, 1968.

PIPKIN, S. B. AND PIPKIN, A. C.* TWO NEW PEDIGREES OF ZYGODACTYLY. VARIATION OF EXPRESSION OF POLYDACTYLY. J. HERED. 37* 93-96, 1946.

THOMSEN, O.* EINIGE EIGENTUMLICHKEITEN DER ERBLICHEN POLY- UND SYNDAKTYLIE BEI MENSCHEN. ACTA MED. SCAND. 65* 609-644, 1927.

*18610 SYNDACTYLY, TYPE III (RING AND LITTLE FINGER SYNDACTYLY)

IN THIS TYPE THERE IS SYNDACTYLY BETWEEN THE 4TH AND 5TH FINGERS, USUALLY COMPLETE AND BILATERAL. USUALLY IT IS SOFT TISSUE SYNDACTYLY BUT OCCASIONALLY THE DISTAL PHALANGES ARE FUSED. IN THIS TYPE THE 5TH FINGER IS SHORT WITH ABSENT OR RUDIMENTARY MIDDLE PHALANX. THE FEET ARE NOT AFFECTED IN THIS TYPE. THE LARGEST PEDIGREE IS THAT DESCRIBED BY JOHNSTON AND KIRBY (1955) OF SEVEN AFFECTED MALES AND SEVEN AFFECTED FEMALES IN FIVE GENERATIONS.

JOHNSTON, O. AND KIRBY, V. V.* SYNDACTYLY OF THE RING AND LITTLE FINGER. AM. J. HUM. GENET. 7* 80-82, 1955.

18620 SYNDACTYLY, TYPE IV (HASS TYPE)

THIS TYPE OF SYNDACTYLY HAS BEEN REPORTED ONLY BY HAAS, OCCURRING IN A MOTHER AND HER TWO CHILDREN. THE SYNDACTYLY IS COMPLETE, AFFECTING THE FINGERS OF BOTH HANDS WITH SIX METACARPALS AND SIX DIGITS, AND IS ASSOCIATED WITH FLEXION OF THE FINGERS, GIVING THE HANDS A CUP-SHAPED FORM. IN CONTRADISTINCTION TO THE TYPE OF SYNDACTYLY IN APERT'S SYNDROME THERE WAS NO BONE FUSION. THERE WAS NO MENTION OF THE CONDITION OF THE FEET AND THERE WERE NO ASSOCIATED MALFORMATIONS.

HAAS, S. L.* BILATERAL COMPLETE SYNDACTYLISM OF ALL FINGERS. AM. J. SURG. 50* 363-366, 1940.

*18630 SYNDACTYLY, TYPE V (SYNDACTYLY WITH METACARPAL AND METATARSAL FUSION)

THE CHARACTERISTIC FINDING IN THIS RARE TYPE OF SYNDACTYLY IS THE PRESENCE OF AN ASSOCIATED METACARPAL AND METATARSAL FUSION. THE METACARPALS AND METATARSALS MOST COMMONLY FUSED ARE THE 4TH AND 5TH OR THE 3RD AND 4TH. SOFT TISSUE SYNDACTYLY USUALLY AFFECTS THE 3RD AND 4TH FINGERS AND THE 2ND AND 3RD TOES. SYNDACTYLY IS USUALLY MORE EXTENSIVE AND COMPLETE. KEMP AND RAVN (1932) DESCRIBED THIS ANOMALY IN FIVE GENERATIONS.

KEMP, T. AND RAVN, J.* UBER ERBLICHE HAND- UND FUSSDEFORMITATEN IN EINEM 140-

KOPFIGEN GESCHLECHT, NEBST EINIGEN BEMERKUNGEN UBER POLY- UND SYNDAKTYLIE BEIM MENSCHEN. ACTA PSYCHIAT. NEUROL. 7* 275-296, 1932.

18640 SYNOSTOSES (TARSAL, CARPAL AND DIGITAL)

PEARLMAN, EDKIN AND WARREN (1964) DESCRIBED MOTHER AND DAUGHTER WITH MULTIPLE CARPAL AND TARSAL SYNOSTOSES (CARPAL AND TARSAL COALITION) AS WELL AS RADIAL-HEAD SUBLUXATION, APLASIA OR HYPOPLASIA OF THE MIDDLE PHALANGES AND METACARPOPHALANGEAL SYNOSTOSES. THE LATTER SYNOSTOSES SEEM COMPARABLE TO THOSE WHICH OCCUR IN THE TWO MORE DISTAL JOINTS IN THE TWO FORMS OF SYMPHALANGISM (Q.V.). ALTHOUGH THE AUTHORS FELT THIS TO BE THE DISORDER DESCRIBED BY NIEVERGELT (SEE NIEVERGELT'S SYNDROME), THIS IS ALMOST CERTAINLY NOT THE CASE BUT A DISTINCT ENTITY IS INVOLVED. BERSANI AND SAMILSON (1957) DESCRIBED A MOTHER AND HER DAUGHTER AND SON WITH MASSIVE SYNOSTOSIS OF TARSAL BONES. NO SPECIFIC STATEMENT WAS MADE ABOUT THE STATE OF THE CARPAL BONES. WRAY AND HERNDON (1963) OBSERVED CALCANEO-NAVICULAR COALITION IN THREE GENERATIONS. FUSION OF CARPAL AND TARSAL BONES OCCURS IN SYMPHALANGISM (Q.V.).

BERSANI, F. A. AND SAMILSON, R. L.* MASSIVE FAMILIAL TARSAL SYNOSTOSIS. J. BONE JOINT SURG. 39A* 1187-1190, 1957.

PEARLMAN, H. S., EDKIN, R. E. AND WARREN, R. F.* FAMILIAL TARSAL AND CARPAL SYNOSTOSIS WITH RADIAL-HEAD SUBLUXATION (NIEVERGELT'S SYNDROME). J. BONE JOINT SURG. 46A* 585-592, 1964.

WRAY, J. B. AND HERNDON, C. N.* HEREDITARY TRANSMISSION OF CONGENITAL COALITION OF THE CALCANEUS TO THE NAVICULAR. J. BONE JOINT SURG. 45A* 365-372, 1963.

18650 SYNOSTOSES, MULTIPLE, WITH BRACHYDACTYLY

FUHRMANN ET AL. (1966) DESCRIBED MOTHER AND SON WITH BILATERAL DYSPLASIA AND SYNOSTOSIS OF THE ELBOW JOINT, SYNOSTOSES IN THE FINGERS, WRIST AND FOOT, AND SHORT MIDDLE PHALANGES AND METACARPALS. THE COMBINATION WAS DESCRIBED IN FATHER AND DAUGHTER AND FATHER AND SON BY EARLIER AUTHORS.

FUHRMANN, W. G., STEFFENS, C. AND ROMPE, U.* DOMINANT ERBLICHE DOPPELSEITIGE DYSPLASIE UND SYNOSTOSE DES ELLENBOGENGELENKS. MIT SYMMETRISCHER BRACHYMESOPHA-LANGIE UND BRACHYMETAKARPIE SOWIE SYNOSTOSEN IM FINGER-, HAND- UND FUSSWURZEL-BEREICH. HUMANGENETIK 3* 64-75, 1966.

18660 SYRINGOMAS, MULTIPLE

MULTIPLE SYRINGOMAS OR SWEAT GLAND TUMORS OCCUR PARTICULARLY ON THE FACE AND AROUND THE EYES. THEY ARE NOT TO BE CONFUSED WITH MILIA, WHICH ARE INTRAEPITHE-LIAL CYSTS. FAMILIAL OCCURRENCE IS, IT SEEMS, A COMMONPLACE OBSERVATION OF DERMATOLOGISTS AND AUTOSOMAL DOMINANT INHERITANCE IS LIKELY (REED, 1967). REED (1970) DESCRIBED A FAMILY IN WHICH 7 FEMALES AND 1 MALE IN 4 GENERATIONS WERE AFFECTED.

REED, W. B.* BURBANK, CALIF.* PERSONAL COMMUNICATION, 1967.

REED, W. B.* GENETISCHE ASPEKTE IN DER DERMATOLOGIE. HAUTARZT 21* 8-16, 1970.

18670 SYRINGOMYELIA, LUMBOSACRAL

GREENFIELD (1954) STATED THAT THIS IS PROBABLY THE SAME AS DENNY BROWN'S *HEREDI-TARY SENSORY RADICULAR NEUROPATHY* (Q.V.). OSTERTAG (1930) FOUND DOMINANT INHERITANCE OF SYRINGOMYELIA IN RABBITS. CURTIUS (1939) SUGGESTED THAT THE SAME MODE OF INHERITANCE OCCURS IN MAN. MULVEY AND RIELY (1942) DESCRIBED A FAMILY WITH AFFECTED PERSONS IN 3 GENERATIONS. THEY RECOGNIZED THAT THIS WAS PROBABLY NOT TRUE SYRINGOMYELIA.

BARRAQUER, L. U. AND DE GISPERT, I.* DIE SYRINGOMYELIE, EINE FAMILIARE UND HEREDITARE KRANKHEIT (13 FALLE IN 2 GENERATIONEN DERSELBEN FAMILIE). DEUTSCH. Z. NERVENHEILK. 141* 146-157, 1936.

CURTIUS, F.* STATUS DYSRAPHICUS UND MYELODYSPLASIE. FORTSCHR. ERBPATHOL. 3* 199-258, 1939.

GOLDBLADT, A.* SYRINGOMYELIE BEI MUTTER UND TOCHTER* ZUGLEICH EIN BEITRAG ZUR PATHOLOGIE DES SYMPATHICUS. DEUTSCH. MED. WSCHR. 36* 1523-1526, 1910.

GREENFIELD, J. G.* THE SPINO-CEREBELLAR DEGENERATIONS. OXFORD* BLACKWELL, 1954.

KARPLUS, J. P.* SYRINGOMYELIE BEI VATER UND SOHN. MED. KLIN. 11* 1344-1347, 1915.

KINO, F.* UEBER HEREDO-FAMILIARE SYRINGOMYELIE (ZUGLEICH EIN BIETRAG ZUR TOPISCHEN GLIEDERUNG IM QUERSCHNITT DES VORDENHORNS). Z. GES. NEUROL. PSYCHIAT. 107* 1-15, 1927.

MULVEY, B. E. AND RIELY, L. A.* FAMILIAL SYRINGOMYELIA AND STATUS DYSRAPHICUS. ANN. INTERN. MED. 16* 966-994, 1942.

OSTERTAG, B.* DIE SYRINGOMYELIE ALS ERBBIOLOGISCHES PROBLEM. VERH. DEUTSCH. GES. PATH. 25* 166-174, 1930.

TENNER, J.* SYRINGOMYELIE BEI VATER UND TOCHTER. DEUTSCH. Z. NERVENHEILK. 106* 13-25, 1928.

VAN EPPS, C. AND KERR, H. D.* FAMILIAL LUMBOSACRAL SYRINGOMYELIA. RADIOLOGY 35* 160-173, 1940.

18680 TABATZNIK HEART-HAND SYNDROME

THE FEATURES ARE CARDIAC ARRHYTHMIA AND MALFORMATION OF THE UPPER EXTREMITIES, PARTICULARLY 'STUB THUMB' (BRACHYDACTYLY, TYPE D).

TABATZNIK, B.* BALTIMORE, MD.* PERSONAL COMMUNICATION.

18690 TEETH, GENETIC VARIATION AND DISORDER OF

THE DOMINANT OR PROBABLY DOMINANT MUTATIONS AFFECTING THE TEETH INCLUDE DENTINO-GENESIS IMPERFECTA, OSTEOGENESIS IMPERFECTA, ENAMEL DYSPLASIA, 'SHOVEL-SHAPED' INCISORS, LONG INCISORS, ABSENT LATERAL INCISORS, CARABELLI TUBERCLES, ABSENCE OF UPPER PERMANENT CANINES, ANODONTIA, ENAMEL HYPOPLASIA, DENTINE HYPOPLASIA, PIGMENTED HYPOMATURATION OF TEETH, HYPOPLASIA OF TEETH, PARAMOLAR TUBERCLE OF BOLK, DIASTEMA, MICRODONTIA. ALSO SEE DEAFNESS WITH ECTODERMAL DYSPLASIA.

KROGMAN, W. M.* ORAL STRUCTURES GENETICALLY AND ANTHROPOLOGICALLY CONSIDERED. ANN. N.Y. ACAD. SCI. 85* 17-41, 1960.

LASKER, G. W.* GENETIC ANALYSIS OF RACIAL TRAITS OF THE TEETH. COLD SPRING HARBOR SYMPOSIA QUANT. BIOL. 15* 191-202, 1950.

*18700 TEETH, ODD SHAPES OF

ROBBINS AND KEENE (1964) PRESENTED A 19 YEAR OLD BOY WHOSE TEETH SHOWED PARTIAL PEGGING, DEEP LINGUAL PITS, EXAGGERATION OF MIDDLE LABIAL LOBES OF THE CANINES, AND REDUCED PREMOLAR SIZE. ONE SIB WAS NORMAL. IN 5 GENERATIONS, 10 PERSONS SHOWED ODD SHAPED TEETH, 16 WERE NORMAL AND 8 WERE UNKNOWN.

ROBBINS, I. M. AND KEENE, H. J.* MULTIPLE MORPHOLOGIC DENTAL ANOMALIES. REPORT OF A CASE. ORAL SURG. 17* 683-690, 1964.

18710 TEETH, SUPERNUMERARY

FINN (1967) PRESENTED A PEDIGREE IN WHICH ALL FEMALES (NUMBERING 14) WERE AFFECTED AND ALL MALES (NUMBERING 3) WERE UNAFFECTED, IN FIVE SIBSHIPS IN THREE GENERA-TIONS. THE AUTHOR SUGGESTED X-LINKED DOMINANT INHERITANCE WITH FEMALE LIMITATION, OR FEMALE-LIMITED AUTOSOMAL DOMINANT INHERITANCE. IN SOME OF THE AFFECTED FEMALES THE SUPERNUMERARY TEETH OCCURRED IN THE MIDLINE OF THE MAXILLA, SO-CALLED MESIODENS.

FINN, S. B.* CLINICAL PEDODONTICS. PHILADELPHIA* W. B. SAUNDERS CO., 1967.

18720 TELANGIECTASES OF BRAIN

MICHAEL AND LEVIN (1936) DESCRIBED A SWEDISH FAMILY IN WHICH A MOTHER, HER TWO BROTHERS AND THREE DAUGHTERS HAD MULTIPLE TELANGIECTASES OF THE BRAIN. CONVUL-SIONS AND MIGRAINE ATTACKS WERE OBSERVED. AUTOPSY IN ONE CASE DEMONSTRATED CALCIFICATION IN THE VASCULAR LESIONS OF THE BRAIN.

MICHAEL, J. C. AND LEVIN, P. M.* MULTIPLE TELANGIECTASES OF BRAIN* DISCUSSION OF HEREDITARY FACTORS IN THEIR DEVELOPMENT. ARCH. NEUROL. PSYCHIAT. 36* 514-529, 1936.

*18730 TELANGIECTASIA, HEREDITARY HEMORRHAGIC, OF RENDU, OSLER AND WEBER

THE TIP OF THE TONGUE AND MUCOSAL SURFACE OF THE LIPS ARE FREQUENT SITES OF TELANGIECTASES WHICH ALSO OCCUR ON THE FACE, CONJUNCTIVA, EARS, FINGERS, AND MUCOSA OF THE NASOPHARYNX, GASTROINTESTINAL TRACT AND BLADDER. BLEEDING FROM ALL THESE SITES IS A MAJOR PROBLEM. CIRRHOSIS OF THE LIVER OCCURS IN SOME CASES. PULMONARY ARTERIOVENOUS FISTULA WITH POLYCYTHEMIA AND CLUBBING OCCUR IN SOME CASES. OVER HALF THE CASES OF PULMONARY ARTERIOVENOUS FISTULA ARE ON THE BASIS OF THIS DISORDER. SNYDER AND DOAN (1944) REPORTED A POSSIBLE INSTANCE OF HOMOZYGOSI-TY, A STILLBORN OFFSPRING OF TWO AFFECTED PARENTS HAD EXTENSIVE ANGIOMATOUS MALFORMATION OF THE VISCERA. AN IMPORTANT PHENOCOPY IS THE CRST SYNDROME (CALCINOSIS, RAYNAUD'S SYNDROME, SCLERODACTYLY, TELANGIECTASIA), A PROBABLE 'COLLAGEN VASCULAR DISEASE.' THE MUCOSAL AND CUTANEOUS TELANGIECTASES ARE INDISTINGUISHABLE FROM THOSE OF THE HEREDITARY DISORDER (WINTERBAUER, 1964). TUNTE (1964) STUDIED 18 FAMILIES. LIVER DISEASE WAS TWICE AS FREQUENT IN AFFECTED MEMBERS AS IN UNAFFECTED ONES. THE FREQUENCY OF THE CONDITION WAS ESTIMATED TO BE

1 OR 2 IN 100,000. THE MUTATION RATE WAS ESTIMATED TO BE 2 X 10-6 TO 3 X 10-6. REPORTED INSTANCES OF FAMILIAL EPISTAXIS (E.G., LANE, 1916) PROBABLY REPRESENT THIS DISORDER. BY ANGIOGRAPHIC METHODS VARIOUS TYPES OF VISCERAL ANGIODYSPLASIAS HAVE BEEN DEMONSTRATED (HALPERN ET AL., 1968). THESE INCLUDE ARTERIAL ANEURYSM, ARTERIOVENOUS COMMUNICATION INCLUDING DISCRETE A-V FISTULA, CONGLOMERATE MASSES OF ANGIECTASIA, PHLEBECTASIA AND ANGIOMA. MICHAELI ET AL. (1968) DESCRIBED A 47 YEAR OLD WOMAN WITH O-R-W DISEASE AND HEPATIC PORTOCAVAL SHUNTS OF SUFFICIENT MAGNITUDE TO CAUSE REPEATED EPISODES OF ENCEPHALOPATHY. THE LIVER WAS NOT SCARRED.

BERGQVIST, N., HESSEN, I. AND HEY, M.* ARTERIOVENOUS PULMONARY ANEURYSMS IN OSLER'S DISEASE. ACTA MED. SCAND. 171* 301-309, 1962.

HALPERN, M., TURNER, A. F. AND CITRON, B. P.* HEREDITARY HEMORRHAGIC TELANGIEC-TASIA. A VISCERAL ANGIODYSPLASIAS ASSOCIATED WITH GASTROINTESTINAL HEMORRHAGE. RADIOLOGY 90* 1143-1149, 1968.

HARRISON, D. F. N.* HEREDITARY HAEMORRHAGIC TELANGIECTASIA AND ORAL CONTRACEP-TIVES. (LETTER) LANCET 1* 721 ONLY, 1970.

HODGSON, C. H., BURCHELL, H. B., GOOD, C. A. AND CLAGETT, O. T.* HEREDITARY HEMORRHAGIC TELANGIECTASIA AND PULMONARY ARTERIOVENOUS FISTULA* SURVEY OF A LARGE FAMILY. NEW ENG. J. MED. 261* 625-636, 1959.

LANE, W. C.* HEREDITARY NOSE-BLEED. J. HERED. 7* 132-134, 1916.

MICHAELI, D., BEN-BASSAT, I., MILLER, H. I. AND DEUTSCH, V.* HEPATIC TELANGIEC-TASES AND PORTOSYSTEMIC ENCEPHALOPATHY IN OSLER-WEBER-RENDU DISEASE. GASTROEN-TEROLOGY 54* 929-932, 1968.

ROWLEY, P. T., KURNICK, J. AND CHEVILLE, R.* HEREDITARY HAEMORRHAGIC TELANGIEC-TASIA* AGGRAVATION BY ORAL CONTRACEPTIVE.Q (LETTER) LANCET 1* 474-475, 1970.

SNYDER, L. H. AND DOAN, C. A.* CLINICAL AND EXPERIMENTAL STUDIES IN HUMAN INHERITANCE* IS THE HOMOZYGOUS FORM OF MULTIPLE TELANGIECTASIA LETHAL.Q J. LAB. CLIN. MED. 29* 1211-1216, 1944.

TUNTE, W.* KLINIK UND GENETIK DER OSLERSCHEN KRANKHEIT. Z. MENSCHL. VERERB. KONSTITUTIONSL. 37* 221-250, 1964.

WINTERBAUER, R. H.* MULTIPLE TELANGIECTASIA, RAYNAUD'S PHENOMENON, SCLERODACTY-LY AND SUBCUTANEOUS CALCINOSIS. A SYNDROME MIMICKING HEREDITARY HEMORRHAGIC TELANGIECTASIA. BULL. HOPKINS HOSP. 114* 361-383, 1964.

18740 TESTICULAR TORSION

CUNNINGHAM (1960) OBSERVED TESTICULAR TORSION IN THREE BROTHERS, AGES 14, 15 AND 21. THE FATHER AND TWO OTHER BROTHERS HAD HYPERMOBILITY OF THE TESTICLE BUT HAD NOT SUFFERED ACUTE TORSION. THE ANATOMIC PECULIARITY IS PRESUMABLY INHERITED AND IS EITHER AUTOSOMAL DOMINANT (OBVIOUSLY MALE-LIMITED), OR Y-LINKED.

CUNNINGHAM, R. F.* FAMILIAL OCCURRENCE OF TESTICULAR TORSION. J.A.M.A. 174* 1330-1331, 1960.

18750 TETRALOGY OF FALLOT

PITT (1962) DESCRIBED A FAMILY IN WHICH 11 PERSONS HAD EITHER TETRALOGY OF FALLOT OR ONE OF ITS COMPONENTS. THE DIAGNOSIS WAS CONFIRMED AT OPERATION OR AUTOPSY IN FIVE OF THE 11.

PITT, D. B.* A FAMILY STUDY OF FALLOT'S TETRAD. AUST. ANN. MED. 11* 179-183, 1962.

18760 TETRAZOLIUM OXIDASE VARIANTS

BREWER (1967) DEMONSTRATED TETRAZOLIUM OXIDASE IN SEVERAL HUMAN TISSUES AND CLASSIFIED THE ENZYME AS AN INDOPHENOL OXIDASE. THE PHYSIOLOGIC FUNCTION OF THE ENZYME IS NOT KNOWN. IN THE DOG THERE IS A GENETIC POLYMORPHISM OF RED CELL TETRAZOLIUM OXIDASE (BAUR AND SCHORR, 1969). IN MAN GENETIC VARIATION IS RARE. BAUR (CITED BY BAUR AND SCHORR, 1969) HAS OBSERVED AN ELECTROPHORETIC VARIANT OF TETRAZOLIUM OXIDASE IN A CAUCASIAN MOTHER AND ONE OF HER TWO CHILDREN.

BAUR, E. W. AND SCHORR, R. T.* GENETIC POLYMORPHISM OF TETRAZOLIUM OXIDASE IN DOGS. SCIENCE 166* 1524-1525, 1969.

BREWER, G. J.* ACHROMATIC REGIONS OF TETRAZOLIUM STAINED STARCH GELS* INHERITED ELECTROPHORETIC VARIATION. AM. J. HUM. GENET. 19* 674-680, 1967.

18770 THANATOPHORIC DWARFISM

MAROTEAUX, LAMY AND ROBERT (1967) GIVE THIS NAME TO THE CONDITION IN CERTAIN MICROMELIC DWARFS WHO DIE IN THE FIRST HOURS OF LIFE. THE RIBS AND BONES OF THE EXTREMITIES ARE VERY SHORT. VERTEBRAL BODIES ARE GREATLY REDUCED IN HEIGHT WITH

WIDE INTERVERTEBRAL SPACES BUT CAUDAD NARROWING OF THE SPINAL CANAL IS NOT PRESENT. THEY FOUND CASES IN THE LITERATURE WHICH ANSWERED THIS DESCRIPTION, THE EARLIEST BEING ONE REPORTED BY MAYGRIER IN 1898. THEY CONCLUDED THAT DOMINANT MUTATION IS THE MOST LIKELY BASIS BUT THAT RECESSIVE INHERITANCE CANNOT BE EXCLUDED. ASPHYXIATING THORACIC DYSTROPHY (Q.V.) IS TO BE DIFFERENTIATED. MAROTEAUX ET AL. (1967) REFERRED TO YET ANOTHER RARE TYPE OF MICROMELIC CHONDRODY-STROPHY WITH EARLY DEATH. GIEDION (1968) DESCRIBED A SWISS CASE WHICH DIFFERED FROM OTHER CASES IN THE PRESENCE OF RADIOULNAR SYNOSTOSIS AND SURVIVAL FOR 96 HOURS. IN UTERO DIAGNOSIS WAS DEMONSTRATED BY KEATS ET AL. (1970).

GIEDION, A.* THANATOPHORIC DWARFISM. HELV. PAEDIAT. ACTA 23* 175-183, 1968.

KEATS, T. E., RIDDERVOLD, H. O. AND MICHAELIS, L. L.* THANATOPHORIC DWARFISM. AM. J. ROENTGEN. 108* 473-480, 1970.

KAUFMAN, R. L., RIMOIN, D. L., MCALISTER, W. H. AND KISSANE, J. M.* THANATO-PHORIC DWARFISM. AM. J. DIS. CHILD. 120* 53-57, 1970.

KOZLOWSKI, K., PROKOP, E. AND ZYBACZYNSKI, J.* THANATOPHORIC DWARFISM. BRIT. J. RADIOL. 43* 565-568, 1970.

MAROTEAUX, P. AND LAMY, M.* LE DIAGNOSTIC DES NANISMES CHONDRO-DYSTROPHIQUES CHEZ LES NOUVEAU-NES. ARCH. FRANC. PEDIAT. 25* 241-262, 1968.

MAROTEAUX, P., LAMY, M. AND ROBERT, J.-M.* LE NANISME THANATOPHORE. PRESSE MED. 75* 2519-2524, 1967.

MAYGRIER, C.* FOETUS ACHONDROPLASIQUE* PRESENTATION DE PHOTOGRAPHIES, DU MOULAGE, D'UNE RADIOGRAPHIE ET DU SQUELETTE. BULL. SOC. OBSTET. GYNEC. 1* 248-255, 1898.

*18780 THROMBASTHENIA OF GLANZMANN AND NAEGELI

IN ONE FAMILY STUDIED BY GROSS AND COLLEAGUES (1960) THREE GENERATIONS HAD AFFECTED MEMBERS. CLINICALLY PETECHIAE, BLEEDING FROM MUCOUS MEMBRANE, PROLONGED BLEEDING AFTER INJURY, AND SEVERE ANEMIA WERE FEATURES. STUDIES REVEALED PROLONGED BLEEDING TIME, ABNORMAL CAPILLARY FRAGILITY, NORMAL OR INCREASED NUMBER OF PLATELETS, WITH GIANT PLATELETS. ALTERATION IN THE CONCENTRATION OF SEVERAL PLATELET ENZYMES WERE FOUND. OF 13 FAMILIES STUDIED BY CAEN ET AL. (1966), ONLY ONE SEEMED TO HAVE DOMINANT INHERITANCE WITH PROBABLE TRANSMISSION THROUGH FOUR GENERATIONS WITH MALE-TO-MALE TRANSMISSION.

CAEN, J. P., CASTALDI, P. A., LECLERC, J. C., INCEMAN, S., LARRIERE, M. J., PROBST, M. AND BERNARD, J.* CONGENITAL BLEEDING DISORDERS WITH LONG BLEEDING TIME AND NORMAL PLATELET COUNT. I. GLANZMANN'S THROMBASTHENIA (REPORT OF FIFTEEN PATIENTS). AM. J. MED. 41* 11-26, 1966.

GROSS, R., GEROK, W., LOHR, G. W., VOGELL, W., WALKER, H. D. AND THEOPOLD, W.* UBER DIE NATUR DER THROMBASTHENIE* THROMBOPATHIE GLANZMANN NAEGELI. KLIN. WSCHR. 38* 193-206, 1960.

18790 THROMBASTHENIA-THROMBOCYTOPENIA, HEREDITARY

QUICK AND HUSSEY (1962) DIFFERENTIATED THIS DISORDER FROM VON WILLEBRAND'S DISEASE BY A NEGATIVE TOURNIQUET TEST AND POOR PROTHROMBIN CONSUMPTION. BLEEDING TIME IS PROLONGED. ONSET IS IN INFANCY WITH A HEMOPHILIA-LIKE PICTURE. PLATELETS ARE NORMAL IN NUMBERS. THE DISORDER IS NOT INFLUENCED BY SPLENECTOMY. SEIP (1964) OBSERVED AUTOSOMAL DOMINANT TRANSMISSION IN TWO FAMILIES. MARROW PREPARATIONS SHOWED NORMAL OR INCREASED MEGAKARYOCYTES WITH LITTLE OR NO SIGNS OF ACTIVE THROMBOPOIESIS. NO RESPONSE TO ADRENAL STEROIDS OR SPLENECTOMY WAS NOTED. MOST INSTANCES SEEM TO BE RECESSIVE (Q.V.) MAKING IT UNCLEAR WHAT CONDITION WAS PRESENT IN THE FAMILY DESCRIBED ABOVE. SEIP AND KJAERHEIM (1965) STUDIED A MOTHER AND HER ONLY SON. SYMPTOMS AND SIGNS WERE PRESENT FROM BIRTH. BLEEDING TIME EXCEEDED 30 MINUTES. PLATELET COUNTS VARIED FROM 60,000 TO 120,000. ELECTRON MICROSCOPY SHOWED LIKED VACUOLES IN THE PLATELETS AND SOME HAD ABNORMAL GRANULES.

KURSTJENS, R., BOLT, C., VOSSEN, M. AND HAANEN, C.* FAMILIAL THROMBOPATHIC THROMBOCYTOPENIA. BRIT. J. HAEMAT. 15* 305-317, 1968.

QUICK, A. J. AND HUSSEY, C. V.* HEREDITARY THROMBASTHENIA-THROMBOCYTOPENIA. J. LAB. CLIN. MED. 60* 1006 ONLY, 1962.

SEIP, M. AND KJAERHEIM, A.* A FAMILIAL PLATELET DISEASE - HEREDITARY THROMBAS-THENIC-THROMBOPATHIC THROMBOCYTOPENIA. SCAND. J. CLIN. LAB. INVEST. 17 (SUPPL. 84)* 159-169, 1965.

SEIP, M. F.* HEREDITARY HYPOPLASTIC THROMBOCYTOPENIA. SANGRE 9* 382-384, 1964.

*18800 THROMBOCYTOPENIA

SEIP (1963) DESCRIBED A MOTHER AND HER TWO SONS WITH THROMBOCYTOPENIA. PLATELET ANTIBODIES WERE NOT DEMONSTRATED. ONE SON HAD BILATERAL APLASIA OF THE 12TH RIB

AND MILD RIGHT HYDRONEPHROSIS. THE OTHER SON HAD FREQUENT EPISODES OF HEMATURIA AND RECURRENT HYDRONEPHROSIS. ATA, FISHER AND HOLMAN (1965) FOUND UNDUE BLEEDING IN 10 MEMBERS OF 6 SIBSHIPS IN 5 GENERATIONS OF A FAMILY. INHERITANCE WAS THOUGHT TO BE AUTOSOMAL DOMINANT WITH INCOMPLETE PENETRANCE IN FEMALES. SPLENECTOMY PERFORMED IN 3 AFFECTED PERSONS CORRECTED THROMBOCYTOPENIA. THE ONLY AFFECTED WOMAN RECOVERED SPONTANEOUSLY. HARMS AND SACHS (1965) DESCRIBED 3 SISTERS, THEIR MOTHER AND THEIR MATERNAL GRANDMOTHER WITH CHRONIC IDIOPATHIC THROMBOCYTOPENIA AND PLATELET AUTO-ANTIBODIES ASSOCIATED WITH A DIMINUTION OF CLOTTING FACTOR IX. A PARTICULARLY CONVINCING PEDIGREE STUDIED BY BITHELL ET AL. (1965) HAD 8 PROVEN CASES OF THROMBOCYTOPENIA IN THREE GENERATIONS. IN ADDITION, A HISTORY OF HEMORRHAGIC DIATHESIS WAS GIVEN BY 7 OTHER PERSONS SO THAT THE INVOLVED SPANNED AT LEAST 4 GENERATIONS, INVOLVING AT LEAST 11 SIBSHIPS. MURPHY ET AL. (1969) DESCRIBED A FAMILY WITH FIVE CASES OF THROMBOCYTOPENIA IN THREE GENERATIONS, WITH NO EXAMPLE OF MALE-TO-MALE TRANSMISSION. SHORTENED PLATELET LIFESPAN WAS DEMONSTRATED AND WAS SHOWN TO BE AN INTRINSIC PROPERTY OF THE PLATELET. MORPHOLO-GIC AND BIOCHEMICAL STUDIES FAILED TO ELUSIDATE THE NATURE OF THE DEFECT. OTHER APPARENTLY DOMINANT PEDIGREES WERE REPORTED BY BETHARD AND BOYER (1964) AND WOOLEY (1956).

ATA, M., FISHER, O. D. AND HOLMAN, C. A.* INHERITED THROMBOCYTOPENIA. LANCET 1* 119-123, 1965.

BETHARD, W. F. AND BOYER, J. L.* FAMILIAL THROMBOCYTOPENIA. (ABSTRACT) J. LAB. CLIN. MED. 64* 842 ONLY, 1964.

BITHELL, T. C., DIDISHEIM, P., CARTWRIGHT, G. E. AND WINTROBE, M. M.* THROMBO-CYTOPENIA INHERITED AS AN AUTOSOMAL DOMINANT TRAIT. BLOOD 25* 231-240, 1965.

GROTTUM, K. A. AND SOLUM, N. O.* CONGENITAL THROMBOCYTOPENIA WITH GIANT PLATELETS* A DEFECT IN THE PLATELET MEMBRANE. BRIT. J. HAEMAT. 16* 277-290, 1969.

HARMS, D. AND SACHS, V.* FAMILIAL CHRONIC THROMBOCYTOPENIA WITH PLATELET AUTOANTIBODIES. ACTA HAEMAT. 34* 30-35, 1965.

KURSTJENS, R., BOLT, C. AND HAANEN, C. A.* FAMILIALE THROMBOCYTOPENIA. NEDERL. T. GENEESK. 111* 1897-1898, 1967.

MURPHY, S., OSKI, F. A. AND GARDNER, F. H.* HEREDITARY THROMBOCYTOPENIA WITH AN INTRINSIC PLATELET DEFECT. NEW ENG. J. MED. 281* 857-862, 1969.

MYLLYLA, G., PELKONEN, R., IKKALA, E. AND APAJALAHTI, J.* HEREDITARY THROMBOCY-TOPENIA* REPORT OF THREE FAMILIES. SCAND. J. HAEMAT. 4* 441-452, 1967.

QUICK, A. J. AND HUSSEY, C. V.* HEREDITARY THROMBOPATHIC THROMBOCYTOPENIA. AM. J. MED. SCI. 245* 643-653, 1963.

SEIP, M.* HEREDITARY HYPOPLASTIC THROMBOCYTOPENIA. ACTA PAEDIAT. 52* 370-376, 1963.

WOOLEY, E. S. J.* FAMILIAL IDIOPATHIC THROMBOCYTOPENIC PURPURA. BRIT. MED. J. 1* 440 ONLY, 1956.

18810 THUMB DEFORMITY

BILBREY (1966) DESCRIBED THUMB DEFORMITY OF THE TYPE SEEN WITH THE HEART-HAND SYNDROME. THE THUMB WAS EITHER ABSENT OR HYPOPLASTIC. THE PUBLISHED X-RAYS DO NOT DEMONSTRATE WHETHER THE METACARPAL OF THE THUMB WHEN PRESENT HAD AN EPIPHYSEAL OSSIFICATION CENTER AT EACH END. NO CARDIAC ANOMALY WAS DETECTED IN ANY OF THE 13 AFFECTED PERSONS IN 3 GENERATIONS. THE PEDIGREE CONTAINED NO EVIDENCE OF MALE-TO-MALE TRANSMISSION.

BILBREY, G. L.* ISOLATED CONGENITAL FAMILIAL THUMB DEFORMITIES. REPORT OF A FAMILY. NEW ENG. J. MED. 274* 1057-1060, 1966.

18820 THUMBNAILS, ABSENT

STRANDSKOV (1939) OBSERVED ABSENT THUMBNAILS IN A WOMAN, TWO OF HER THREE DAUGHTERS AND IN A SON OF ONE OF THE DAUGHTERS. THUS THE FINDINGS WERE EQUALLY CONSISTENT WITH AUTOSOMAL AND X-LINKED DOMINANCE. HE WAS OF THE OPINION THAT THE MUTATION IS SEPARATE AND DISTINCT FROM THE NAIL-PATELLA MUTATION. NO SKELETAL ABNORMALITIES WERE DETECTED IN HIS FAMILY, BUT NO X-RAY INFORMATION WAS AVAILABLE, IT SEEMS. ABSENT THUMBNAILS IN FEMALE MEMBERS OF THREE GENERATIONS OF A FAMILY (V. D., 845898) PROVED ON FURTHER STUDY TO BE THE NAIL-PATELLA SYNDROME (SCHLEU-TERMANN, 1968).

SCHLEUTERMANN, D. A.* BALTIMORE, MD.* PERSONAL COMMUNICATION, 1968.

STRANDSKOV, H. H.* INHERITANCE OF ABSENCE OF THUMB NAILS. J. HERED. 30* 53-54, 1939.

*18830 THYMIDINE KINASE

GENETIC VARIATION IN THIS ENZYME HAS NOT BEEN IDENTIFIED IN MAN. HOWEVER, LOCALIZATION OF THE GENE HAS BEEN ACHIEVED BY HYBRIDIZATION EXPERIMENTS. WEISS AND GREEN (1967) FOUND THAT FUSION OF MOUSE CELLS LACKING THIS ENZYME WITH NORMAL HUMAN CELLS COULD BE ACHIEVED, THAT PROGRESSIVE LOSS OF HUMAN CHROMOSOMES FROM THE HYBRID OCCURRED WITH PASSAGE OF TIME AND THAT AT A STAGE WHEN ONLY ONE HUMAN CHROMOSOME REMAINED THE CELL STILL HAD THE CAPACITY TO SYNTHESIZE THYMIDINE KINASE. THE ASUMPTION WAS THAT THE REMAINING CHROMOSOME PRESENTLY TENTATIVELY IDENTIFIED AS CHROMOSOME 17 CARRIES THE THYMIDINE KINASE LOCUS.

MIGEON, B. R. AND MILLER, C. S.* HUMAN-MOUSE SOMATIC CELL HYBRIDS WITH SINGLE HUMAN CHROMOSOME (GROUP E)* LINK WITH THYMIDINE KINASE ACTIVITY. SCIENCE 162* 1005-1006, 1968.

WEISS, M. AND GREEN, H.* HUMAN-MOUSE HYBRID CELL LINES CONTAINING PARTIAL COMPLEMENTS OF HUMAN CHROMOSOMES AND FUNCTIONING HUMAN GENES. PROC. NAT. ACAD. SCI. 58* 1104-1111, 1967.

18840 THYMUS AND PARATHYROIDS, ABSENCE OF (DIGEORGE SYNDROME)

THIS IS A CONGENITAL ANOMALY IN DEVELOPMENT OF DERIVATIVES OF THE 3RD AND 4TH PHARYNGEAL POUCHES. IT IS PROBABLY NOT GENETIC TO A SIGNIFICANT EXTENT. DEFORMITIES OF THE EAR, NOSE, MOUTH AND AORTIC ARCH ARE OFTEN ASSOCIATED. TRANSPLANTATION OF FETAL THYMUS HAS BEEN SUCCESSFULLY ACCOMPLISHED, WITH DRAMATIC RECONSTRUCTION OF THE IMMUNE MECHANISM. THE POSSIBILITY OF NEW AUTOSOMAL DOMINANT MUTATION SHOULD BE INVESTIGATED BY DETERMINATION OF MEAN PATERNAL AGE.

CLEVELAND, W. W., FOGEL, B. J., BROWN, W. T. AND KAY, H. E. M.* FOETAL THYMIC TRANSPLANT IN A CASE OF DIGEORGE'S SYNDROME. LANCET 2* 1211-1214, 1968.

DIGEORGE, A. M.* CONGENITAL ABSENCE OF THE THYMUS AND ITS IMMUNOLOGIC CONSEQUENCES* CONCURRENCE WITH CONGENITAL HYPOPARATHYROIDISM. IN GOOD, R. A. (ED.).* IMMUNOLOGIC DEFICIENCY DISEASES. NEW YORK* NATIONAL FOUNDATION, 1968. PP. 116-123.

18850 THYROID AUTOANTIBODIES

HALL, OWEN AND SMART (1964) STUDIED SIX FAMILIES IN WHICH THE FATHER HAD THYROID AUTOANTIBODY AND THE MOTHER DID NOT. IN EACH CASE FEMALE CHILDREN HAD THYROID AUTOANTIBODIES. TRANSPLACENTAL TRANSMISSION WAS THUS RULED OUT AND GENETIC TRANSMISSION WAS SUGGESTED.

HALL, R., OWEN, S. G. AND SMART, G. A.* PATERNAL TRANSMISSION OF THYROID AUTOIMMUNITY. LANCET 2* 115 ONLY, 1964.

*18860 THYROXINE-BINDING GLOBULIN (TBG) OF SERUM, VARIANTS OF

IN ADDITION TO THE USUAL X-LINKED FORM OF DECREASED OR INCREASED TBG, AN AUTOSOMAL DOMINANT FORM APPEARS TO EXIST. PERSONS WITH THE AUTOSOMAL FORM SHOW AN INCREASE IN TBG LEVEL WITH ADMINISTRATION OF ESTROGEN, SUGGESTING THAT THE MUTATION MAY CONCERN A REGULATOR GENE RATHER THAN A STRUCTURAL GENE. FOR REVIEW, SEE RIVAS ET AL. (1971). ELECTROPHORETIC VARIANTS OF TBG WERE DESCRIBED BY THORSON ET AL. (1966) AND THERE MAY BE BOTH AUTOSOMAL AND X-LINKED VARIETIES. EVIDENCE FOR AUTOSOMAL DOMINANT TRANSMISSION OF TBG DEFICIENCY WAS PRESENTED BY NICOLOFF ET AL. (1964) AND BY KRAEMER AND WISWELL (1968). IN THE LAST REPORT THREE BROTHERS HAD ABSENT TBG, AND THEIR FATHER, PATERNAL UNCLE AND PATERNAL GRANDMOTHER HAD LOW VALUES WHEREAS THE MOTHER AND SEVERAL OTHER RELATIVES ON HER SIDE HAD NORMAL VALUES.

KRAEMER, E. AND WISWELL, J. G.* FAMILIAL THYROXINE-BINDING GLOBULIN DEFICIENCY. METABOLISM 17* 260-262, 1968.

NICOLOFF, J. T., DOWLING, J. T. AND PATTON, D. D.* INHERITANCE OF DECREASED THYROXINE-BINDING BY THE THYROXINE-BINDING GLOBULIN. J. CLIN. ENDOCR. 24* 294-298, 1964.

RIVAS, M.* INDIANAPOLIS, IND.* PERSONAL COMMUNICATION, 1968.

RIVAS, M., MERRITT, A. D. AND OLIVER, L.* GENETIC VARIANTS OF THYROXINE BINDING GLOBULIN (TBG). THE CLINICAL DELINEATION OF BIRTH DEFECTS. X. THE ENDOCRINE SYSTEM. BALTIMORE* WILLIAMS AND WILKINS, 1971.

THORSON, S. C., TAUXE, W. N. AND TASWELL, H. F.* EVIDENCE FOR THE EXISTENCE OF TWO THYROXINE-BINDING GLOBULIN MOIETIES* CORRELATION BETWEEN PAPER AND STARCH-GEL ELECTROPHORETIC PATTERNS UTILIZING THYROXINE-BINDING GLOBULIN-DEFICIENT SERA. J. CLIN. ENDOCR. 26* 181-188, 1966.

TORKINGTON, P., HARRISON, R. J., MACLAGAN, N. F. AND BURSTON, D.* FAMILIAL THYROXINE-BINDING GLOBULIN DEFICIENCY. BRIT. MED. J. 3* 27-29, 1970.

18870 TIBIA VARA (BLOUNT'S DISEASE, OR OSTEOCHONDROSIS DEFORMANS TIBIAE)

LITTLE IS KNOWN ABOUT THIS CONDITION WHICH BEARS SOME SIMILARITY TO OSTEOCHONDRI-

SUGGESTED THE EXISTENCE OF AN INFANTILE TYPE WITH ONSET IN THE FIRST YEAR OR TWO
OF LIFE AND AN ADOLESCENT TYPE DEVELOPING JUST BEFORE PUBERTY. TOBIN'S DESCRIP-
TION (1957) OF TIBIA VARA BEGINNING AT PUBERTY WITH OSTEOCHONDRITIS DISSECANS OF
THE KNEES IN FATHER AND TWO SONS STRENGTHENS THE VIEW THAT THE TWO DISORDERS ARE
FUNDAMENTALLY IDENTICAL.

BLOUNT, W. P.* TIBIA VARA* OSTEOCHONDROSIS DEFORMANS TIBIAE. J. BONE JOINT
SURG. 19A* 1-29, 1937.

TOBIN, W. J.* FAMILIAL OSTEOCHONDRITIS DISSECANS WITH ASSOCIATED TIBIA VARA.
J. BONE JOINT SURG. 39A* 1091-1105, 1957.

18880 TIBIAL TORSION, BILATERAL MEDIAL

BLUMEL ET AL. (1957) REPORTED A FAMILY WITH 8 AFFECTED PERSONS IN FOUR GENERA-
TIONS. NO MALE-TO-MALE TRANSMISSION WAS OBSERVED. BOWLEGS ARE THE MAIN CLINICAL
FEATURE.

BLUMEL, J., EGGERS, G. W. AND EVANS, E. B.* EIGHT CASES OF HEREDITARY BILATERAL
TIBIAL TORSION IN FOUR GENERATIONS. J. BONE JOINT SURG. 39A* 1198-1202, 1957.

18890 TOE, FIFTH ROTATED

I HAVE OBSERVED TWO KINDREDS IN WHICH ROTATION OF THE FIFTH TOES ON THEIR LONG
AXIS, WITH LATTERALLY FACING NAIL, WAS TRANSMITTED AS AN AUTOSOMAL DOMINANT.

18900 TOE, FIFTH, NUMBER OF PHALANGES IN

THE FIFTH TOE MAY SHOW EITHER TWO OR THREE PHALANGES (VENNING, 1954). SIB PAIRS
SHOWED A CORRELATION COEFFICIENT OF 0.28.

VENNING, P.* SIB CORRELATIONS WITH RESPECT TO THE NUMBER OF PHALANGES ON THE
FIFTH TOE. ANN. EUGEN. 18* 232-254, 1953-1954.

18910 TOE, MISSHAPEN

GARBER (1950) REPORTED FIVE PERSONS IN THREE GENERATIONS WITH TOES PECULIARLY
POSITIONED IN RELATION TO EACH OTHER. THERE WAS MALE-TO-MALE TRANSMISSION.

GARBER, M. J.* MISSHAPEN TOES IN THREE GENERATIONS OF THE G FAMILY. J. HERED.
41* 215-216, 1950.

LARSON, C. A.* GARBER'S TOE DEFORMITY. REPORT OF A KINDRED. ACTA GENET.
STATIST. MED. 4* 414-416, 1953.

18920 TOES, RELATIVE LENGTH OF 1ST AND 2ND

KAPLAN (1964) CLAIMS THE RELATIVE LENGTH OF THE HALLUX AND SECOND TOE IS SIMPLY
INHERITED, LONG HALLUX BEING RECESSIVE. IN CLEVELAND CAUCASOIDS THE FREQUENCY OF
THE DOMINANT AND RECESSIVE PHENOTYPES WAS 24 PERCENT AND 76 PERCENT RESPECTIVELY.
USUALLY THE FIRST TOE IS LONGEST, ALTHOUGH IN THE AINU THE SECOND TOE IS SAID TO
BE LONGEST IN 90 PERCENT OF PERSONS. IN SWEDEN ROMANUS (1949) FOUND THE SECOND
TOE LONGEST IN 2.95 PERCENT OF 8,141 MEN. ROMANUS THOUGHT THAT LONG SECOND TOE IS
DOMINANT WITH REDUCED PENETRANCE. BEERS AND CLARK (1942) DESCRIBED A FAMILY IN
WHICH LONG SECOND TOE OCCURRED IN 10 PERSONS IN 3 GENERATIONS.

BEERS, C. V. AND CLARK, L. A.* TUMORS AND SHORT-TOE - A DIHYBRID PEDIGREE* A
FAMILY HISTORY SHOWING THE INHERITANCE OF HEMANGIOMA AND METATARSUS ACTIVITUS. J.
HERED. 33* 366-368, 1942.

KAPLAN, A. R.* GENETICS OF RELATIVE TOE LENGTHS. ACTA GENET. MED. GEM. 13*
295-304, 1964.

ROMANUS, T.* HEREDITY OF A LONG SECOND TOE. HEREDITAS 35* 651-652, 1949.

18930 TONGUE CURLING, FOLDING, OR ROLLING

STURTEVANT (1940) DESCRIBED TWO CLASSES, *ROLLER* AND *NON-ROLLER,* THE ROLLER
PHENOTYPE BEING DOMINANT. HOWEVER, STURTEVANT (1965) CITED MATLOCK AS FINDING A
HIGH FREQUENCY OF DISCORDANCE IN MONOZYGOTIC TWINS, SUGGESTING LITTLE GENETIC
BASIS FOR THE TRAIT. HSU (1948) DESCRIBED THE ABILITY TO FOLD UP THE TIP OF THE
TONGUE AS A RECESSIVE. LIU AND HSU (1949) AND LEE (1955) DEMONSTRATED INDEPEN-
DENCE OF THE TWO TRAITS. THE CLOVER-LEAF TONGUE (ABILITY TO FOLD THE TONGUE IN A
PARTICULAR CONFIGURATION) MAY BE YET ANOTHER DISTINCT TRAIT (WHITNEY, 1950),
INHERITED PROBABLY AS A DOMINANT. HIRSCHHORN (1970) EMPHASIZED THAT AMPLE TIME
FOR LEARNING MUST BE ALLOWED IN DOING FAMILY STUDIES OF TONGUE GYMNASTIC ABILITY.

GAHRES, E. E.* TONGUE ROLLING AND TONGUE FOLDING AND OTHER HEREDITARY MOVEMENTS
OF THE TONGUE. J. HERED. 43* 221-225, 1952.

HIRSCHHORN, H. H.* TRANSMISSION AND LEARNING OF TONGUE GYMNASTIC ABILITY. AM.

J. PHYS. ANTHROP. 32* 451-454, 1970.

HSU, T. C.* TONGUE UPFOLDING* A NEWLY REPORTED HERITABLE CHARACTER IN MAN.   J. HERED. 39* 187-188, 1948.

KOMAI, T.* NOTES ON LINGUAL GYMNASTICS.   FREQUENCY OF TONGUE ROLLERS AND PEDIGREES OF TIED TONGUES IN JAPAN.   J. HERED. 42* 293-297, 1951.

LEE, J. W.* TONGUE-FOLDING AND TONGUE-ROLLING IN AN AMERICAN NEGRO POPULATION SAMPLE.   J. HERED. 46* 289-291, 1955.

LIU, T. T. AND HSU, T.* TONGUE-FOLDING AND TONGUE-ROLLING IN A SAMPLE OF THE CHINESE POPULATION.   J. HERED. 40* 19-21, 1949.

MATLOCK, P.* IDENTICAL TWINS DISCORDANT IN TONGUE-ROLLING.   J. HERED. 43* 24 ONLY, 1952.

STURTEVANT, A. H.* A HISTORY OF GENETICS.   NEW YORK* HARPER, ROW, 1965.   P. 127.

STURTEVANT, A. H.* A NEW INHERITED CHARACTER IN MAN.   PROC. NAT. ACAD. SCI. 26* 100-102, 1940.

URBANOWSKI, A. AND WILSON, J.* TONGUE CURLING.   J. HERED. 38* 365-366, 1947.

VOGEL, F.* UEBER DIE FAHIGKEIT, DIE ZUNGE UM DIE LANGSACHSE ZU ROLLEN.   ACTA GENET. MED. GEM. 6* 225-230, 1957.

WHITNEY, D. D.* CLOVER-LEAF TONGUES.   J. HERED. 41* 176 ONLY, 1950.

18940 TONGUE, PIGMENTED FUNGIFORM PAPILLAE OF

NEGROES IN PARTICULAR MAY SHOW SPOTTED PIGMENTATION OF THE TIP OF THE TONGUE. THE MELANIN IS LOCATED ON THE SUMMIT OF THE FUNGIFORM PAPILLAE. NO SYSTEMATIC FAMILY STUDY HAS, IT SEEMS, BEEN DONE.   DAVIS (1968) COMMENTED ON THE OCCURRENCE OF PIGMENTED SPOTS AND PATCHES OF THE TONGUE, A POSSIBLY DIFFERENT PHENOTYPE. RAO (1970) COLLECTED DATA ON 132 FAMILIES FROM WEST BURGAL AND CONCLUDED THAT THE TRAIT SEGREGATES, THE *NORMAL* ALLELE BEING DOMINANT OVER THE *PIGMENTED* ALLELE, I.E., PIGMENT SPOTS (OR PATCHES) BEING A RECESSIVE TRAIT.

DAVIS, T. A.* BIOLOGY IN THE TROPICS. IN, DRONAMRAJU, K. (ED.)* HALDANE AND MODERN BIOLOGY. BALTIMORE* JOHNS HOPKINS PRESS, 1968. PP. 327-333.

KOPLON, B. S. AND HURLEY, H. J.* PROMINENT PIGMENTED PAPILLAE OF THE TONGUE. ARCH. DERM. 95* 394-396, 1967.

MONASH, S.* NORMAL PIGMENTATION OF THE ORAL MUCOSA. ARCH. DERM. SYPH. 26* 139-147, 1932.

RAO, D. C.* TONGUE PIGMENTATION IN MAN. HUM. HERED. 20* 8-12, 1970.

18950 TOOTH-AND-NAIL SYNDROME (DYSPLASIA OF NAILS WITH HYPODONTIA)

CHANGES ARE LIMITED LARGELY TO TEETH (SOME OF WHICH ARE MISSING) AND NAILS (WHICH ARE POORLY FORMED EARLY IN LIFE, ESPECIALLY TOENAILS). THIS CONDITION IS DISTINGUISHED FROM ANHIDROTIC ECTODERMAL DYSPLASIA BY AUTOSOMAL DOMINANT INHERI-TANCE AND LITTLE INVOLVEMENT OF HAIR AND SWEAT GLANDS. THE TEETH ARE NOT AS SEVERELY AFFECTED. WITKOP (1965) STATED THAT THE CONDITION IS FREQUENT AMONG DUTCH MENNONITES IN CANADA. HE PRESENTED A PEDIGREE SUPPORTING AUTOSOMAL DOMINANT INHERITANCE. THE TEETH ARE NOT AFFECTED IN THE AUTOSOMAL DOMINANT HIDROTIC ECTODERMAL DYSPLASIA.

WITKOP, C. J.* GENETIC DISEASE OF THE ORAL CAVITY. ORAL PATHOLOGY. TIECKE, R. W. (ED.)* NEW YORK* MCGRAW-HILL, 1965.

18960 TORTICOLLIS

MALE-TO-MALE TRANSMISSION (ISIGKEIT, 1931* GARCEAU, 1962) AND TRANSMISSION THROUGH 3 OR MORE GENERATIONS (ARMSTRONG ET AL., 1965) HAS BEEN REPORTED. FACIAL ASYMMETRY MAY BE A PARTIAL MANIFESTATION.

ARMSTRONG, D., PICKRELL, K., FETTER, B. AND PITTS, W.* TORTICOLLIS* AN ANALYSIS OF 271 CASES. PLAST. RECONSTR. SURG. 35* 14-25, 1965.

GARCEAU, G. J.* CONGENITAL MUSCULAR TORTICOLLIS (HEMATOMA, FACT OR MYTH). RHODE ISLAND MED. J. 45* 401-404, 1962.

ISIGKEIT, E.* UNTERSUCHUNGEN UBER HEREDITAT ORTHOPADISCHER LEIDEN* DER ANGEBORENE SCHIEFHALS. ARCH. ORTHOP. UNFALLCHIR. 30* 459-494, 1931.

*18970 TORUS PALATINUS AND TORUS MANDIBULARIS

THE STUDY OF SUZUKI AND SAKAI (1960) SUGGESTS THAT THE TWO ANOMALIES ARE EQUIVA-
LENT, I.E., DUE TO THE SAME GENE, AND THAT THE INHERITANCE IS AUTOSOMAL DOMINANT
WITH REDUCED PENETRANCE. A STUDY BY JOHNSON, GORLIN AND ANDERSON (1965) SUPPORTED
DOMINANT INHERITANCE OF TORUS MANDIBULARIS. THEY FOUND THAT 85.7 AND 89.7
PERCENT, RESPECTIVELY, OF CHILDREN WITH TORUS PALATINUS OR TORUS MANDIBULARIS HAD
AT LEAST ONE PARENT WITH ONE OR THE OTHER ANOMALY. A SEX PREDILECTION WAS NOTED,
MALES HAVING TORUS ONLY 70 PERCENT AS OFTEN AS FEMALES.

JOHNSON, C. C., GORLIN, R. J. AND ANDERSON, V. E.* TORUS MANDIBULARIS* A
GENETIC STUDY. AM. J. HUM. GENET. 17* 433-439, 1965.

SUZUKI, M. AND SAKAI, T.* A FAMILIAL STUDY OF TORUS PALATINUS AND TORUS
MANDIBULARIS. AM. J. PHYS. ANTHROP. 18* 263-272, 1960.

18980 TOXEMIA OF PREGNANCY

HUMPHRIES (1960) MADE THE FIRST SYSTEMATIC STUDY OF HYPERTENSIVE TOXEMIA OF
PREGNANCY IN MOTHER-DAUGHTER PAIRS DELIVERED AT THE JOHNS HOPKINS HOSPITAL.
TOXEMIA OCCURRED IN 28 PERCENT OF DAUGHTERS OF WOMEN WHO HAD TOXEMIA IN THE
PREGNANCY IN WHICH THEY WERE DELIVERED AS COMPARED WITH 13 PERCENT IN A COMPARISON
GROUP. CHESLEY ET AL. (1968) DID A SIMILAR STUDY WITH VERY SIMILAR RESULTS. IN
CASES IN WHICH 2 OR MORE DAUGHTERS OF AN ECLAMPTIC WOMAN HAVE BEEN TESTED BY
PREGNANCY, TOXEMIA DEVELOPED IN THE FIRST PREGNANCY OF AT LEAST 1 DAUGHTER IN 53
PERCENT OF THE FAMILIES.

CHESLEY, L. C., ANNITTO, J. E. AND COSGROVE, R. A.* THE FAMILIAL FACTOR IN
TOXEMIA OF PREGNANCY. OBSTET. GYNEC. 32* 303-311, 1968.

HUMPHRIES, J. O.* OCCURRENCE OF HYPERTENSIVE TOXEMIA OF PREGNANCY IN MOTHER-
DAUGHTER PAIRS. BULL. JOHNS HOPKINS HOSP. 107* 271-277, 1960.

18990 TRACHEOESOPHAGEAL FISTULA WITH ESOPHAGEAL ATRESIA

ENGEL ET AL. (1970) DESCRIBED AFFECTED MOTHER AND DAUGHTER.

ENGEL, M. A., VOS, L. J. M., DE VRIES, J. A. AND KUIJJER, P. J.* ESOPHAGEAL
ATRESIA WITH TRACHEOESOPHAGEAL FISTULA IN MOTHER AND CHILD. J. PEDIAT. SURG. 5*
564-565, 1970.

*19000 TRANSFERRINS

TRANSFERRIN, THE IRON-BINDING PROTEIN OF SERUM, IS A BETA-GLOBULIN. POLYMORPHISM
WAS FIRST DEMONSTRATED BY SMITHIES USING STARCH GEL ELECTROPHORESIS. EIGHTEEN OR
MORE TYPES HAVE BEEN IDENTIFIED. ROBSON ET AL. (1966) PRESENTED EVIDENCE OF
LINKAGE BETWEEN THE TRANSFERRIN LOCUS AND THE SERUM CHOLINESTERASE LOCUS (E1).

PARKER, W. C. AND BEARN, A. G.* ADDITIONAL GENETIC VARIATION OF HUMAN SERUM
TRANSFERRIN. SCIENCE 137* 854-856, 1962.

ROBSON, E. B., SUTHERLAND, I. AND HARRIS, H.* EVIDENCE FOR LINKAGE BETWEEN THE
TRANSFERRIN LOCUS (TF) AND THE SERUM CHOLINESTERASE LOCUS (E1) IN MAN. ANN. HUM.
GENET. 29* 325-336, 1966.

WANG, A.-C. AND SUTTON, H. E.* HUMAN TRANSFERRINS C AND D(1)* CHEMICAL
DIFFERENCE IN A PEPTIDE. SCIENCE 149* 435-437, 1965.

WANG, A.-C., SUTTON, H. E. AND HOWARD, P. N.* HUMAN TRANSFERRINS C AND D(CHI)*
AN IMINO-ACID DIFFERENCE. BIOCHEM. GENET. 1* 55-60, 1967.

WANG, A.-C., SUTTON, H. E. AND RIGGS, A.* A CHEMICAL DIFFERENCE BETWEEN HUMAN
TRANSFERRINS B2 AND C. AM. J. HUM. GENET. 18* 454-458, 1966.

*19010 TREMBLING CHIN

WADLINGTON (1958) FOUND THE CONDITION IN EIGHT MEMBERS OF THREE GENERATIONS, WITH
NO ASSOCIATED NEUROLOGIC OR OTHER ABNORMALITIES. ANXIETY OR EMOTIONAL UPSET WAS A
TRIGGER MECHANISM AND TRANQUILIZING AND ANTICONVULSANT AGENTS REDUCED THE ATTACKS.
ATTACKS WERE OBSERVED AS EARLY AS TWO MONTHS OF AGE. THERE WAS NO INSTANCE OF
MALE-TO-MALE TRANSMISSION AND ALL THREE DAUGHTERS OF THE ONE MALE WITH CHILDREN
WERE AFFECTED. TREMBLING OF THE CHIN OCCURS AS PART OF THE ORAL-FACIAL-DIGITAL
SYNDROME (Q.V.). OTHER FAMILIES OF TREMBLING CHIN WERE REPORTED BY GROSSMAN
(1957), FREY (1930) AND GANNER (1938), AND THOSE REPORTED BY STOCKS (1922-23) AND
BY GOLDSMITH (1927) AS FACIAL SPASM (Q.V.) WERE PROBABLY TREMBLING CHIN. MALE-TO-
MALE TRANSMISSION OCCURRED IN SOME OF THESE FAMILIES. THE CONDITION WAS PROBABLY
FIRST REPORTED BY MASSARO (1894), WHO DESCRIBED 26 CASES IN 5 GENERATIONS.
LAURANCE ET AL. (1968) DESCRIBED TWO FAMILIES. THE CONDITION AMELIORATES WITH
AGE. ALSO SEE FACIAL TIC.

FREY, E.* EIN STRENG DOMINANT ERBLICHES KINNMUSKELZITTERN (BIETRAG ZUR
ENFORSCHUNG DER MENSCHLICHEN AFFEKTAUSSERUNGEN). DEUTSCH. Z. NERVENHEILK. 115* 9-
26, 1930.

GANNER, H.* ERBLICHES KINNZITTERN IN EINER TIROLER TALSCHAFT. Z. GES. NEUROL. PSYCHIAT. 161* 259-266, 1938.

GOLDSMITH, J. B.* INHERITANCE OF 'FACIAL SPASM,' AND EFFECT OF MODIFYING FACTOR ASSOCIATED WITH HIGH TEMPERATURE. J. HERED. 18* 185-187, 1927.

GROSSMAN, B.* TREMBLING OF THE CHIN - AN INHERITABLE DOMINANT CHARACTER. PEDIATRICS 19* 453-455, 1957.

LAURANCE, B. M., MATTHEWS, W. B. AND DIGGLE, J. H.* HEREDITARY QUIVERING OF THE CHIN. ARCH. DIS. CHILD. 43* 249-251, 1968.

STOCKS, P.* FACIAL SPASM INHERITED THROUGH FOUR GENERATIONS. BIOMETRIKA 14* 311-315, 1922-23.

WADLINGTON, W. B.* FAMILIAL TREMBLING OF THE CHIN. J. PEDIAT. 53* 316-321, 1958.

19020 TREMOR OF INTENTION, ATAXIA AND LIPOFUSCINOSIS

FELDMAN ET AL. (1969) DESCRIBED THREE PERSONS IN THREE SUCCESSIVE GENERATIONS WITH THIS COMBINATION. AUTOPSY AT AGE 80 IN ONE CASE SHOWED INTRACYTOPLASMIC LIPOFUS-CIN GRANULES IN THE INFERIOR OLIVARY NUCLEI AND HEPATOCYTES. THE AFFECTED PERSONS HAD PREMATURE GRAYING.

FELDMAN, R. G., ISERI, O. A., GOTTLIEB, L. S. AND GREENBERG, J. P.* FAMILIAL INTENTION TREMOR, ATAXIA, AND LIPOFUSCINOSIS. LIVER BIOPSY STUDIES. NEUROLOGY 19* 503-509, 1969.

*19030 TREMOR, HEREDITARY ESSENTIAL

LARSSON AND SJOGREN (1960) DID A THOROUGH STUDY OF HEREDITARY ESSENTIAL TREMOR IN A PARISH OF SWEDEN. IN ALL, 210 CASES WERE ASCERTAINED. THE AGE OF ONSET WAS ON THE AVERAGE ABOUT 50 YEARS AND SOMEWHAT LATER IN WOMEN THAN IN MEN. THE AGE OF ONSET SHOWED HIGH INTRAFAMILIAL CORRELATION. 'ANTICIPATION' WAS NOT OBSERVED. FINE RAPID TREMOR OF THE HANDS WAS USUALLY THE FIRST SYMPTOM. TREMOR OF THE ARMS, TONGUE (WITH DYSARTHRIA), HEAD, LEGS AND TRUNK DEVELOPED LATER, USUALLY IN THE ORDER LISTED. MILD EXTRAPYRAMIDAL SYMPTOMS IN THE FORM OF RIGIDITY AND STIFFNESS OF GAIT OCCURRED FREQUENTLY, BUT THE CLINICAL PICTURE WAS EASILY DISTINGUISHABLE FROM PARKINSONISM. MENTAL DETERIORATION WAS NOT A FEATURE. WITH TWO EXCEPTIONS, ALL 210 CASES COULD BE TRACED BACK TO FOUR ANCESTRAL COUPLES. THE INHERITANCE WAS AUTOSOMAL DOMINANT. FROM OBSERVATION OF ABOUT 15 PRESUMED HOMOZYGOUS INDIVIDUALS, IT WAS CONCLUDED THAT THERE IS NO DIFFERENCE FROM THE DISEASE IN HETEROZYGOTES. IT WAS ESTIMATED THAT MORE THAN 9 PERCENT OF THE MALES AND 6 TO 6.5 PERCENT OF FEMALES OF THE PARISH CARRY THE GENE FOR ESSENTIAL TREMOR. THE AUTHORS COULD FIND NO REASON TO SUSPECT SELECTIVE FERTILITY, SELECTIVE MORTALITY, OR ASSORTATIVE MATING AS FACTORS IN THE HIGH GENE FREQUENCY OBSERVED. RATHER, CHANCE VARIATIONS THAT OCCURRED WHEN THE POPULATION WAS SMALL - ABOUT 150 PERSONS IN THE LATE 1700'S - SEEM TO HAVE BEEN RESPONSIBLE. KEHRER (1965) DESCRIBED A FAMILY IN WHICH MEMBERS OF 3 SUCCESSIVE GENERATIONS HAD TREMOR OF THE HANDS AND FACE AND IN TWO PATIENTS STUDIED IN DETAIL, CEREBRAL ATROPHY DEMONSTRABLE BY PNUEMOENCEPHALOGRA-PHY. HE SUGGESTED THAT THIS REPRESENTS A DISTINCT ENTITY.

KEHRER, H. E.* UBER HEREDITAREN ESSENTIELLEN TREMOR MIT HIRNATROPHIE. ARCH. PSYCHIAT. NERVENKR. 207* 6-22, 1965.

LARSSON, T. AND SJOGREN, T.* ESSENTIAL TREMOR. A CLINICAL AND GENETIC POPULATION STUDY. ACTA PSYCHIAT. NEUROL. SCAND. 36 (SUPPL. 144)* 1-176, 1960.

SCHADE, H.* VERERBUNGSFRAGEN BEI EINER FAMILIE MIT ESSENTIELLEM HEREDITAREN TREMOR. Z. MENSCHL. VERERB. KONSTITUTIONSL. 33* 355-364, 1966.

19040 TRIGEMINAL NEURALGIA (TIC DOULOUREUX)

AULD AND BUERMANN (1965) OBSERVED SIX AFFECTED SIBS. ONLY ONE SIB WAS UNAFFECTED. NO COMMENT ON PARENTAL CONSANGUINITY WAS MADE. HARRIS (1936) OBSERVED 9 CASES IN 3 GENERATIONS. ALLAN (1938) DESCRIBED THE CONDITION IN A 32 YEAR OLD MAN, HIS MATERNAL UNCLE AND HIS MATERNAL GRANDMOTHER.

ALLAN, W.* FAMILIAL OCCURRENCE OF TIC DOULOUREUX. ARCH. NEUROL. PSYCHIAT. 40* 1019-1020, 1938.

AULD, A. W. AND BUERMANN, A.* TRIGEMINAL NEURALGIA IN SIX MEMBERS OF ONE GENERATION. ARCH. NEUROL. 13* 194 ONLY, 1965.

HARRIS, W.* BILATERAL TRIGEMINAL TIC* ITS ASSOCIATION WITH HEREDITY AND DISSEMINATED SCLEROSIS. ANN. SURG. 103* 161-172, 1936.

19050 TRIPHALANGEAL THUMB WITH DOUBLE PHALANGES

ECKE (1962) DESCRIBED TRIPHALANGY OF THE THUMB WITH DOUBLING OF THE TWO DISTAL PHALANGES IN A GRANDFATHER, SON AND GRANDSON.

*19060 TRIPHALANGEAL THUMB, NON-OPPOSABLE

SWANSON AND BROWN (1962) DESCRIBED A FAMILY IN WHICH 30 PERSONS IN 5 GENERATIONS
HAD FIVE DIGITS OF EACH HAND TRIPHALANGEAL AND APPARENTLY LACKED A TRUE THUMB.
THE 'THUMB' COULD NOT BE OPPOSED. NO ASSOCIATED INTERNAL MALFORMATIONS WERE
DETECTED. TRIPHALANGEAL THUMB OF THIS TYPE OCCURS IN SOME CASES OF THE HOLT-ORAM
SYNDROME (Q.V.), ALTHOUGH THE THUMB WHEN PRESENT WAS OPPOSABLE IN THE FAMILY I
REPORTED. WHEREAS IN THE CASES OF SWANSON AND BROWN THE METACARPAL OF THE
TRIPHALANGEAL THUMB HAD ONLY A DISTAL EPIPHYSIS AS IS NORMAL FOR METACARPALS II-V,
THE METACARPAL I IN THE HOLT-ORAM SYNDROME SHOWS BOTH A PROXIMAL AND A DISTAL
EPIPHYSIS. IN THREE OF THE AFFECTED PERSONS SWANSON AND BROWN (1962) FOUND
POLYDACTYLISM (SEE NEXT ITEM).

SWANSON, A. B. AND BROWN, K. S.* HEREDITARY TRIPHALANGEAL THUMB. J. HERED. 53*
259-265, 1962.

*19070 TRIPHALANGEAL THUMB, OPPOSABLE, WITH POLYDACTYLY

PREAXIAL POLYDACTYLY IS OFTEN ASSOCIATED (ATWOOD AND POND, 1917* HEFNER, 1940).
FOR EXAMPLE, THE PROBAND OF A FAMILY STUDIED BY TEMTAMY (1966) HAD OPPOSABLE
TRIPHALANGEAL THUMBS, ALL THREE PHALANGES BEING WELL DEVELOPED, AND IN BOTH FEET
HAD DUPLICATION OF THE GREAT TOES. THE TRAIT HAD PASSED THROUGH AT LEAST 6
GENERATIONS.

ATWOOD, E. S. AND POND, C. P.* A POLYDACTYLOUS FAMILY. J. HERED. 8* 96-98,
1917.

HEFNER, R. A.* HEREDITARY POLYDACTYLY ASSOCIATED WITH EXTRA PHALANGES IN THE
THUMBS. J. HERED. 31* 25-27, 1940.

TEMTAMY, S. A.* THE GENETICS OF HAND MALFORMATIONS. PH.D. THESIS, JOHNS
HOPKINS UNIVERSITY, 1966.

19080 TRISTICHIASIS (THREE ROWS OF EYELASHES)

A DOMINANT PEDIGREE PATTERN WAS REFERRED TO BY DANFORTH (1925) AND BY LOEFFLER
(1940). SEE DISTRICHIASIS.

DANFORTH, C. H.* STUDIES ON HAIR, WITH SPECIAL REFERENCE TO HYPERTRICHOSIS.
ARCH. DERM. SYPH. 11* 494-508, 1925.

LOEFFLER, L.* ERBBIOLOGIE DES MENSCHLICHEN HAUTORGANS. IN, HANDBUCH DER
ERBBIOLOGIE DES MENSCHEN. BERLIN* SPRINGER VERLAG, 1940. PP. 391-406.

19090 TRITANOPIA

KALMUS (1955) CONCLUDED THAT TRITANOPIA IS AUTOSOMAL DOMINANT WITH INCOMPLETE
MANIFESTATION. THE MINIMUM FREQUENCY IN GREAT BRITAIN WAS ESTIMATED AS 1 IN
13,000 AND ACCORDING TO KALMUS IS PROBABLY HIGHER. DEFECTIVE BLUE VISION IS
CHARACTERISTIC. AN X-LINKED FORM ALSO IS KNOWN.

KALMUS, H.* THE FAMILIAL DISTRIBUTION OF CONGENITAL TRITANOPIA WITH SOME
REMARKS ON SOME SIMILAR CONDITIONS. ANN. HUM. GENET. 20* 39-56, 1955.

19100 TROCHLEA OF THE HUMERUS, APLASIA OF

MEAD AND MARTIN (1963) DESCRIBED A NEGRO FAMILY IN WHICH A MOTHER AND FOUR
CHILDREN HAD APLASIA OF THE TROCHLEA OF THE HUMERUS (THAT PART WHICH ARTICULATES
WITH THE ULNA). THREE OF THE CHILDREN WERE BY ONE FATHER AND ONE BY ANOTHER. HE
COULD FIND NO IDENTICAL CASE IN THE LITERATURE. THE DEFORMITY WAS BILATERALLY
SYMMETRICAL. THE PATIENT HELD THE ELBOWS IN FLEXION AND THE FOREARMS IN PRONA-
TION. THE HUMERUS WAS SHORTENED. A WEB OF SOFT TISSUE STRETCHED ACROSS THE
ANTECUBITAL SPACE. THE ELBOWS COULD NOT BE EXTENDED BEYOND A RIGHT ANGLE BUT
COULD BE FLEXED TO ABOUT 30-0. PRONATION WAS MODERATELY LIMITED* SUPINATION WAS
NORMAL. THE BICEPS BRACHII APPEARED TO BE EITHER HYPOPLASTIC OR ABSENT. ONE OF
THE AFFECTED CHILDREN HAD A CLEFT PALATE. WHEREAS THE LATERAL PART OF THE DISTAL
HUMERUS INCLUDING THE CAPITELLUM WAS ESSENTIALLY NORMAL, THE MEDIAL PART HAD NO
TROCHLEA OR MEDIAL EPICONDYLE. THE ULNA WAS DISPLACED AND DID NOT ARTICULATE WITH
THE HUMERUS. THE AUTHORS SUGGESTED THAT THIS IS A 'NEW' MUTATION BOTH IN THE
SENSE OF HAVING OCCURRED FIRST IN THE MOTHER AND THAT OF NOT HAVING BEEN DESCRIBED
PREVIOUSLY. BECAUSE OF THE HIGH ILLEGITIMACY RATE IN NEGROES NEW MUTATION IS
DIFFICULT TO DEFEND. IT IS ALSO RASH TO SUGGEST THE DISORDER HAS NEVER BEEN
REPORTED. CERTAINLY THIS MUST BE A VERY RARE ANOMALY.

MEAD, C. A. AND MARTIN, M.* APLASIA OF THE TROCHLEA - AN ORIGINAL MUTATION. J.
BONE JOINT SURG. 45A* 379-383, 1963.

*19110 TUBEROUS (OR TUBEROSE) SCLEROSIS

THE PREFERRED DESIGNATION FOR THIS SYNDROME REFERS TO THE CHANGES OBSERVED IN THE BRAIN. ADENOMA SEBACEUM AND EPILOIA ARE SYNONYMS WHICH REFER TO THE CUTANEOUS FEATURES. RHABDOMYOMA OF THE MYOCARDIUM AND MIXED TUMOR OF THE KIDNEY ALSO OCCUR. FITZPATRICK ET AL. (1968) POINTED OUT THE DIAGNOSTIC USEFULNESS OF WHITE MACULES SHAPED LIKE THE LEAF OF A MOUNTAIN ASH IN PATIENTS WITH TUBEROUS SCLEROSIS. THE WHITE MACULE IS PROBABLY PRESENT AT BIRTH IN MOST CASES, THUS PERMITTING EARLY DIAGNOSIS. THEY MAY BE EVIDENT ONLY UNDER WOOD'S LIGHT. KIDNEY LESIONS ARE IN THE FORM OF ANGIOMYOLIPOMA (ANDERSON AND TANNEN, 1969). TEPLICK (1969) STATED THAT ADENOMA SEBACEUM IS ABSENT IN HALF THE CASES-SURELY TOO HIGH AN ESTIMATE. HE DESCRIBED A 53 YEAR OLD WOMAN OF NORMAL INTELLIGENCE WITH BONE AND PULMONARY LESIONS MISINTERPRETED AS THOSE OF SARCOID.

ANDERSON, D. AND TANNEN, R. L.* TUBEROUS SCLEROSIS AND CHRONIC RENAL FAILURE. POTENTIAL CONFUSION WITH POLYCYSTIC KIDNEY DISEASE. AM. J. MED. 47* 163-168, 1969.

BJORNBERG, A.* ADENOMA SEBACEUM. REVIEW, CASE REPORTS AND DISCUSSION OF EUGENIC ASPECTS. ACTA DERMATOVENER. 41* 213-223, 1961.

BORBERG, A.* CLINICAL AND GENETIC INVESTIGATIONS INTO TUBEROUS SCLEROSIS AND RECKLINGHAUSEN'S NEUROFIBROMATOSIS. COPENHAGEN* MUNKSGAARD, 1951.

DE LA CRUZ, F. F. AND LAVECK, G. D.* TUBEROUS SCLEROSIS* A REVIEW AND REPORT OF EIGHT CASES. AM. J. MENT. DEFIC. 67* 369-380, 1962.

FITZPATRICK, T. B., SZABO, G., HORI, Y., SIMONE, A. A., REED, W. B. AND GREENBERG, M. H.* WHITE LEAF-SHAPED MACULES. ARCH. DERM. 98* 1-6, 1968.

HUDOLIN, V.* LA SCLEROSE TUBEREUSE (COMPTE RENDU DES CAS YOUGOSLAVES). J. GENET. HUM. 10* 128-155, 1961.

LAGOS, J. C. AND GOMEZ, M. R.* TUBEROUS SCLEROSIS* REAPPRAISAL OF A CLINICAL ENTITY. MAYO CLIN. PROC. 42* 26-49, 1967.

MILLEDGE, R. D., GERALD, B. E. AND CARTER, W. J.* PULMONARY MANIFESTATIONS OF TUBEROUS SCLEROSIS. AM. J. ROENTGEN. 98* 734-738, 1966.

NEVIN, N. C. AND PEARCE, W. G.* DIAGNOSTIC AND GENETICAL ASPECTS OF TUBEROUS SCLEROSIS. J. MED. GENET. 5* 273-280, 1968.

NICKEL, W. R. AND REED, W. B.* TUBEROUS SCLEROSIS. SPECIAL REFERENCE TO THE MICROSCOPIC ALTERATIONS IN THE CUTANEOUS HAMARTOMAS. ARCH. DERM. 85* 209-226, 1962.

SCHEIG, R. L. AND BORNSTEIN, P.* TUBEROUS SCLEROSIS IN THE ADULT. AN UNUSUAL CASE WITHOUT MENTAL DEFICIENCY OR EPILEPSY. ARCH. INTERN. MED. 108* 789-795, 1961.

SCHULL, W. J. AND CROWE, F. W.* NEUROCUTANEOUS SYNDROMES IN A KINDRED* A CASE OF SIMULTANEOUS OCCURRENCE OF TUBEROUS SCLEROSIS AND NEUROFIBROMATOSIS. NEUROLOGY 3* 904-909, 1953.

STEVENSON, A. C. AND FISHER, O. D.* FREQUENCY OF EPILOIA IN NORTHERN IRELAND. BRIT. J. PREV. SOC. MED. 10* 134-135, 1956.

TEPLICK, J. G.* TUBEROUS SCLEROSIS. EXTENSIVE ROENTGEN FINDINGS WITHOUT USUAL CLINICAL PICTURE* A CASE REPORT. RADIOLOGY 93* 53-55, 1969.

19120 TUNE DEAFNESS

SEASHORE (1940) REVIEWED THE COMPLEXITY OF THE PROBLEM OF THE INHERITANCE OF MUSICAL ABILITY. KALMUS (1949) STUDIED TUNE DEAFNESS IN A GROUP OF CONTINENTAL AND BRITISH STUDENTS AT UNIVERSITY COLLEGE IN LONDON. HE FOUND A BIMODAL DISTRIBUTION IN POPULATION INVESTIGATIONS, WITH FREQUENT SEGREGATION IN FAMILIES AND SIB PAIRS. HE SUGGESTED THIS MIGHT BE CAUSED BY A UNIT GENE SUBSTITUTION, POSSIBLY A DOMINANT.

KALMUS, H.* TUNE DEAFNESS AND ITS INHERITANCE. HEREDITAS 35* 605 ONLY, 1949.

SEASHORE, C. E.* MUSICAL INHERITANCE. SCIENTIFIC MONTHLY 50* 351-356, 1940.

19130 TURNER PHENOTYPE

AMONG 95 MALE PATIENTS WITH PULMONARY STENOSIS, CELERMAJER ET AL. (1968) FOUND THE TURNER PHENOTYPE IN 8. IN 5 OF THESE, KARYOTYPING WAS PERFORMED. IN 4 THE CHROMOSOMES WERE NORMAL. IN ONE AN EXTRA ACROCENTRIC CHROMOSOME WAS PRESENT. NOONAN (1968) REPORTED 19 CASES OF WHOM 17 HAD PULMONARY STENOSIS AND 2 HAD PATENT DUCTUS ARTERIOSUS. TWELVE WERE MALES AND 7 WERE FEMALES. DEFORMITY OF THE STERNUM WITH PRECOCIOUS CLOSURE OF SUTURES WAS A FREQUENT FEATURE. KAPLAN ET AL. (1968) DESCRIBED TWO BROTHERS WITH ELEVATED ALKALINE PHOSPHATASE LEVELS AND IN ONE OF THEM MALIGNANT SCHWANNOMA OF THE FOREARM. IN 3 FAMILIES NORA AND SINHA (1968) OBSERVED MOTHER-TO-OFFSPRING TRANSMISSION, THROUGH 3 GENERATIONS IN ONE FAMILY.

THEY SUGGESTED X-LINKED DOMINANT INHERITANCE EITHER OF A SINGLE MUTANT GENE OR A
SUBMICROSCOPIC DELETION. SEE PTERYGIUM COLLI SYNDROME.

CELERMAJER, J. M., BOWDLER, J. D. AND COHEN, D. H.* PULMONARY STENOSIS IN
PATIENTS WITH THE TURNER PHENOTYPE IN THE MALE. AM. J. DIS. CHILD. 116* 351-358,
1968.

KAPLAN, M. S., OPITZ, J. M. AND GOSSET, F. R.* NOONAN*S SYNDROME. A CASE WITH
ELEVATED SERUM ALKALINE PHOSPHATASE LEVELS AND MALIGNANT SCHWANNOMA OF THE LEFT
FOREARM. AM. J. DIS. CHILD. 116* 359-366, 1968.

LEVY, E. P., PASHAYAN, H., FRASER, F. C. AND PINSKY, L.* XX AND XY TURNER
PHENOTYPES IN A FAMILY. AM. J. DIS. CHILD. 120* 36-43, 1970.

NOONAN, J. A.* HYPERTELORISM WITH TURNER PHENOTYPE. A NEW SYNDROME WITH
ASSOCIATED CONGENITAL HEART DISEASE. AM. J. DIS. CHILD. 116* 373-380, 1968.

NORA, J. J. AND SINHA, A. K.* DIRECT FAMILIAL TRANSMISSION OF THE TURNER
PHENOTYPE. AM. J. DIS. CHILD. 116* 343-350, 1968.

*19140 ULNA AND FIBULA, HYPOPLASIA OF

PFEIFFER (1966) AND REINHARDT AND PFEIFFER (1967) STUDIED A KINDRED WITH 14
PERSONS AFFECTED BY HYPOPLASIA OF ULNA AND FIBULA IN THE PATTERN OF A REGULAR
AUTOSOMAL DOMINANT. SEE MESOMELIC DWARFISM OF HYPOPLASTIC ULNA, FIBULA AND
MANDIBLE TYPE. ALSO SEE NIEVERGELT SYNDROME.

REINHARDT, K. AND PFEIFFER, R. A.* ULNO-FIBULARE DYSPLASIE. EINE AUTOSOMAL-
DOMINANT VERERBTE MIKROMESOMELIE AHNLICH DEM NIEVERGELTSYNDROM. FORTSCHR.
RONTGENSTR. 107* 379-391, 1967.

PFEIFFER, R. A.* BEITRAG ZUR ERBLICHEN VERKURZUNG VON ULNA UND FIBULA. IN,
WIEDEMANN, H.-R. (ED.)* DYSOSTOSEN. STUTTGART* GUSTAV FISHER VERLAG, 1966.

*19150 UNDRITZ ANOMALY (HYPERSEGMENTATION OF THE NUCLEI OF THE POLYMORPHONUCLEAR
LEUKOCYTES)

HYPERSEGMENTATION OF THE NUCLEI OF NEUTROPHILES WAS KNOWN IN RABBITS AS A GENETIC
TRAIT BEFORE THE DESCRIPTION IN MAN BY UNDRITZ. UNDRITZ (1958) OBSERVED A
POSSIBLE INSTANCE OF HOMOZYGOSITY IN AN OFFSPRING OF TWO AFFECTED PARENTS.
HYPERSEGMENTATION WAS EXTREME. BARBIER (1958) OBSERVED THE ANOMALY IN THREE
GENERATIONS OF A FAMILY. ONE PATIENT DEVELOPED HYPERSEGMENTATION OF THE NUCLEI OF
LYMPHOCYTES, MONOCYTES AND PLASMA CELLS DURING A BOUT OF HENOCH-SCHOENLEIN
PURPURA. UNDRITZ (1954) ALSO DESCRIBED HYPERSEGMENTATION OF THE EOSINOPHILES, A
GENETIC TRAIT POSSIBLY DISTINCT FROM HYPERSEGMENTATION OF THE NEUTROPHILES. HE
OBSERVED THE TRAIT IN OTHERWISE NORMAL MOTHER AND DAUGHTER. INHERITED VARIATIONS
IN LEUKOCYTES WERE USEFULLY REVIEWED BY DAVIDSON (1961).

BARBIER, F.* UN CAS PARTICULIER D*HYPERSEGMENTATION CONSTITUTIONNELLE DES
NOYAUX DES NEUTROPHILES CHEZ L*HOMME. ACTA HAEMAT. 19* 121-125, 1958.

DAVIDSON, W. M.* INHERITED VARIATIONS IN LEUCOCYTES. BRIT. MED. BULL. 17* 190-
195, 1961.

UNDRITZ, E.* EINE NEUE SIPPE MIT ERBLICH-KONSTITUTIONELLER HOCHSEGMENTIERUNG
DER NEUTROPHILENKERNE. SCHWEIZ. MED. WSCHR. 88* 1000-1001, 1958.

UNDRITZ, E.* LES MALFORMATIONS HEREDITAIRES DES ELEMENTS FIGURES DU SANG. SANG
25* 296-324, 1954.

19160 URETER, CANCER OF

BURKLAND AND JUZEK (1966) REPORTED CANCER OF THE RIGHT URETER IN MOTHER AND SON.

BURKLAND, C. E. AND JUZEK, R. H.* FAMILIAL OCCURRENCE OF CARCINOMA OF THE
URETER. J. UROL. 96* 697-701, 1966.

19170 URIC ACID UROLITHIASIS

DE VRIES, FRANK AND ATSMON (1962) PRESENTED EVIDENCE, BASED ON THREE EXTENSIVELY
STUDIED FAMILIES, THAT URIC ACID UROLITHIASIS CAN BE INHERITED AS AN AUTOSOMAL
DOMINANT TRAIT INDEPENDENT OF GOUT. IN THESE FAMILIES NO GOUT AND HYPERURICEMIA
WERE FOUND. CASES OF THIS TYPE HAVE RATHER LONG BEEN RECOGNIZED AND HAVE BEEN
REFERRED TO BY HENNEMAN AS *IDIOPATHIC URIC ACID STONE FORMERS.* THE FAMILIAL
NATURE HAS APPARENTLY NOT BEEN PREVIOUSLY RECOGNIZED. RECOGNITION OF THE DISORDER
AS FAMILIAL IS IMPORTANT TO ITS PREVENTION. ORAL ALKALINIZATION AND HIGH FLUID
INTAKE WILL OFTEN DISSOLVE STONES ALREADY FORMED AND CAN BE DEPENDED ON TO PREVENT
STONE FORMATION. HENNEMAN ET AL. (1962) SUGGESTED THAT ELDERLY ITALIAN OR JEWISH
PATIENTS ARE MOST LIKELY TO GET INTO TROUBLE WITH URIC ACID STONES DESPITE NORMAL
SERUM AND URINE CONCENTRATIONS OF URIC ACID. CONSTANT ACIDITY OF THE URINE AND
LOW AMMONIUM EXCRETION MAY BE INVOLVED IN PATHOGENESIS.

DE VRIES, A., FRANK, M. AND ATSMON, A.* INHERITED URIC ACID LITHIASIS. AM. J. MED. 33* 880-892, 1962.

HENNEMAN, P. H., WALLACH, S. AND DEMPSEY, E. F.* THE METABOLIC DEFECT RESPONSIBLE FOR URIC ACID STONE FORMATION. J. CLIN. INVEST. 41* 537-542, 1962.

19180 URINARY BLADDER, ATONY OF

GUNDRUM (1922) DESCRIBED 9 (8 MALE, 1 FEMALE) CASES IN THREE GENERATIONS. MOST PERFORMED CATHETERIZATION DAILY ON THEMSELVES.

GUNDRUM, F. F.* FAMILIAL BLADDER ATONY. J.A.M.A. 78* 411-412, 1922.

*19190 URTICARIA, DEAFNESS AND AMYLOIDOSIS

MUCKLE AND WELLS (1962) DESCRIBED A FAMILY IN WHICH URTICARIA, PROGRESSIVE PERCEPTIVE DEAFNESS AND AMYLOIDOSIS WERE COMBINED IN A DOMINANTLY INHERITED SYNDROME. FIVE GENERATIONS WERE AFFECTED. AUTOPSY IN TWO PATIENTS SHOWED ABSENT ORGAN OF CORTI, ATROPHY OF THE COCHLEAR NERVE AND AMYLOID INFILTRATION OF THE KIDNEYS. AMYLOIDOSIS IS A COMPLICATION OF URTICARIA DUE TO COLD SENSITIVITY (Q.V.). BLACK (1969) DESCRIBED AFFECTED PERSONS IN THREE GENERATIONS OF A FAMILY AND EMPHASIZED LIMB PAINS AS A FEATURE.

BLACK, J. T.* AMYLOIDOSIS DEAFNESS, URTICARIA AND LIMB PAINS* A HEREDITARY SYNDROME. ANN. INTERN. MED. 70* 989-994, 1969.

MUCKLE, T. J. AND WELLS, M.* URTICARIA, DEAFNESS AND AMYLOIDOSIS* A NEW HEREDO-FAMILIAL SYNDROME. QUART. J. MED. 31* 235-248, 1962.

19200 UTERINE ANOMALIES

HOLMES (1956) REPORTED A MOTHER WITH UTERUS ARCUATUS WHO DELIVERED A STILLBORN FEMALE IN WHOM UTERUS BICORNIS UNICOLLIS WAS DEMONSTRATED AT AUTOPSY. SIMILAR UTERINE ANOMALIES WERE DESCRIBED IN MOTHER AND DAUGHTER BY STEVENSON ET AL. (1959) AND IN SISTERS BY DRESCHER (1966) AND NYKIFORUK (1938).

DRESCHER, H.* ZUR FRAGE GEHAUFTEN FAMILIAREN VORKOMMENS VON UTERUSMISSBILDUN-GEN. ZBL. GYNAEK. 88* 1673-1675, 1966.

HOLMES, J. A.* CONGENITAL ABNORMALITIES OF THE UTERUS AND PREGNANCY. BRIT. MED. J. 1* 1144-1147, 1956.

NYKIFORUK, N. E.* UTERUS DIDELPHYS. CANAD. MED. ASS. J. 38* 175 ONLY, 1938.

STEVENSON, A. C., DUDGEON, M. Y. AND MCCLURE, H. I.* PREGNANCIES IN WOMEN RESIDENT IN BELFAST. II. ABORTIONS, HYDATIFORM MOLES AND ECTOPIC PREGNANCIES. ANN. HUM. GENET. 23* 395-411, 1959.

19210 UVULA, BIFID (SPLIT UVULA, CLEFT UVULA)

THE UVULA IS SPLIT INTO TWO LOBES BY A CENTRAL FISSURE. ABOUT 1 PERCENT OF CAUCASIANS AND 10 PERCENT OF AMERICAN INDIANS AND JAPANESE SHOW IT IN SOME DEGREE. THE FREQUENCY IN SIBS AND PARENTS OF AFFECTED PERSONS IS SAID TO BE ABOUT 18 PERCENT.

MESKIN, L. H., GORLIN, R. J. AND ISAACSON, R. J.* ABNORMAL MORPHOLOGY OF THE SOFT PALATE. II. THE GENETICS OF CLEFT UVULA. CLEFT PALATE J. 2* 40-45, 1965.

19220 VARICOSE VEINS

DOMINANT INHERITANCE WITH REDUCED PENETRANCE WAS SUGGESTED BY ARNOLDI (1958). HE THOUGHT THAT LATE MENARCHE IS RELATED TO VARICOSITY. VARICOSE VEINS WERE ABOUT TWICE AS FREQUENT IN FEMALES AS IN MALES AND NO MALE-TO-MALE TRANSMISSION WAS INDICATED IN HIS ILLUSTRATIVE PEDIGREE. POSSIBLE X-LINKED DOMINANCE SHOULD BE CONSIDERED. VARICOSE VEINS ARE FREQUENT IN SOME GENETIC DISORDERS SUCH AS THE MARFAN SYNDROME. HAUGE AND GUNDERSEN (1969) PRESENTED A FAMILY STUDY OF 249 PROBANDS, WITH THE CONCLUSION THAT MULTIFACTORIAL INHERITANCE SEEMS 'VERY PROBABLE.'

ARNOLDI, C. C.* THE HEREDITY OF VENOUS INSUFFICIENCY. DANISH MED. BULL. 5* 169-176, 1958.

HAUGE, M. AND GUNDERSEN, J.* GENETICS OF VARICOSE VEINS OF THE LOWER EXTREMI-TIES. HUM. HERED. 19* 573-580, 1969.

19230 VASCULAR HELIX OF UMBILICAL CORD

MALPAS AND SYMONDS (1966) FOUND IN LIVERPOOL, ENG., THAT OF 652 CORDS THE HELIX WAS RIGHT-HANDED IN 133 AND LEFT-HANDED IN 519. ALTHOUGH A GENETIC BASIS FOR THE DIFFERENCE WAS SUGGESTED, FAMILY DATA ARE YET TO BE COLLECTED.

MALPAS, P. AND SYMONDS, E. M.* THE DIRECTION OF THE HELIX OF THE HUMAN

19240 VEINS, PATTERN OF, ON ANTERIOR THORAX

SPUHLER (1950) FOUND TWO ALTERNATIVE PATTERNS. (1) IN THE TRANSVERSE TYPE, THE SUPERFICIAL VEINS RADIATE LATERALLY FROM THE PECTORAL VENOUS PLEXUS TOWARD THE AXILLARY REGION. (2) IN THE LONGITUDINAL TYPE THE VEINS RADIATE IN A FAN-LIKE PATTERN DOWNWARD AND LATERALLY FROM THE POINT WHERE THE ANTERIOR JUGULAR VEIN TURNS BENEATH THE STERNOCLEIDOMASTOID MUSCLE. IN A STUDY IN THE NAVAJO INDIANS, THE TRANSVERSE PATTERN APPEARED TO BEHAVE AS A DOMINANT.

SPUHLER, J. N.* GENETICS OF THREE NORMAL MORPHOLOGICAL VARIATIONS* PATTERN OF SUPERFICIAL VEINS OF THE ANTERIOR THORAX, PERONEUS TERTIUS MUSCLE, AND NUMBER OF VALLATE PAPILLAE. COLD SPRING HARBOR SYMPOSIA QUANT. BIOL. 15* 175-188, 1950.

*19250 VENTRICULAR FIBRILLATION WITH PROLONGED Q-T INTERVAL

WARD (1964) OBSERVED SYNCOPE DUE TO VENTRICULAR FIBRILLATION IN A BROTHER AND SISTER WHOSE RESTING ELECTROCARDIOGRAM SHOWED ABNORMAL PROLONGATION OF THE QT INTERVAL. THE MOTHER, ALTHOUGH ASYMPTOMATIC HAD A PROLONGED QT INTERVAL ALSO. HER SISTER HAD ATTACKS OF SYNCOPE AND DIED IN ONE OF THESE AT THE AGE OF 30 YEARS. THIS DISORDER APPEARS TO BE DISTINCT FROM THE RECESSIVELY INHERITED SYNDROME DESCRIBED BY JERVELL AND LANGE-NIELSEN (SEE DEAFMUTISM III). DEAFNESS IS NOT A FEATURE. SIMILAR FAMILIES WERE REPORTED BY ROMANO ET AL. (1963) AND BY BARLOW ET AL. (1964). TRANSMISSION THROUGH THREE GENERATIONS WAS DESCRIBED BY GARZA ET AL. (1970). PROPRANOLOL EFFECTIVELY PREVENTED VENTRICULAR ARRHYTHMIA. MULTIPLE GENERATION INVOLVEMENT WAS REPORTED ALSO BY BARLOW ET AL. (1964) AND BY ROMANO (1965). MALE-TO-MALE TRANSMISSION HAS, IT SEEMS, NOT BEEN ADEQUATELY DOCUMENTED. GAMSTORP ET AL. (1964) REPORTED A FAMILY WITH PROLONGED Q-T INTERVAL AND CARDIAC ARRHYTHMIAS WITHOUT DEAFNESS BUT UNLIKE THE FAMILIES MENTIONED ABOVE HYPOKALEMIA AND BENEFICIAL EFFECTS OF ADMINISTRATION OF POTASSIUM WERE NOTED. GALE ET AL. (1970) ALSO SUGGESTED THAT ADRENERGIC BETA-BLOCKADE IS THE BEST METHOD OF TREATMENT.

BARLOW, J. B., BOSMAN, C. K. AND COCHRANE, J. W. C.* CONGENITAL CARDIAC ARRHYTHMIA. LANCET 2* 531 ONLY, 1964.

GALE, G. E., BOSMAN, C. K., TUCKER, R. B. K. AND BARLOW, J. B.* HEREDITARY PROLONGATION OF QT INTERVAL. STUDY OF TWO FAMILIES. BRIT. HEART J. 32* 505-509, 1970.

GAMSTORP, I., NILSEN, R., WESTLING, H.* CONGENITAL CARDIAC ARRHYTHMIA. (LETTER) LANCET 2* 965 ONLY, 1964.

GARZA, L. A., VICK, R. L., NORA, J. J. AND MCNAMARA, D. G.* HERITABLE Q-T PROLONGATION WITHOUT DEAFNESS. CIRCULATION 41* 39-48, 1970.

ROMANO, C.* CONGENITAL CARDIAC ARRHYTHMIA. (LETTER) LANCET 1* 658-659, 1965.

ROMANO, C., GEMME, G. AND PONGIGLIONE, R.* ARITMIE CARDIACHE RARE DELL' ETA PEDIATRICA. II. ACCESSI SINCOPALI PER FIBRILLAZIONE VENTRICOLARE PAROSSISTICA. (PRESENTAZIONE DEL PRIMO CASO DELLA LETTERATURA PEDIATRICA ITALIANA). CLIN. PEDIAT. 45* 656-683, 1963.

WARD, O. C.* A NEW FAMILIAL CARDIAC SYNDROME IN CHILDREN. J. IRISH MED. ASS. 54* 103-106, 1964.

*19260 VENTRICULAR HYPERTROPHY, HEREDITARY

THIS CONDITION HAS BEEN CALLED MUSCULAR SUBAORTIC STENOSIS BUT MORE GENERALIZED VENTRICULAR HYPERTROPHY IS OFTEN AN EARLIER AND MORE IMPRESSIVE FEATURE AND OBSTRUCTION TO OUTFLOW FROM THE RIGHT VENTRICLE CAN ALSO OCCUR. STUDY OF THE FAMILIES OF PROBANDS WITH THE FULL-BLOWN CONDITION SHOWS THAT AN ATRIAL HEART SOUND ('PRESYSTOLIC GALLOP') AND EKG CHANGES OF VENTRICULAR HYPERTROPHY ARE THE EARLIEST SIGNS. SUDDEN DEATH OCCURS IN SOME CASES. BRAUNWALD AND COLLEAGUES (1964) REPORTED IN DETAIL ON 64 PATIENTS. MULTIPLE CASES WERE OBSERVED IN 11 FAMILIES, WHICH CONTAINED IN ALL AT LEAST 41 DEFINITE OR PROBABLE CASES. IN THE FAMILY REPORTED BY HORLICK ET AL. (1966), 10 PERSONS IN FOUR GENERATIONS WERE THOUGHT TO HAVE BEEN AFFECTED. PARE AND COLLEAGUES (1961) DESCRIBED THIS DISORDER IN 30 OUT OF 87 MEMBERS OF A FRENCH-CANADIAN KINDRED. THE GENEALOGIC SURVEY WAS CARRIED BACK TO THE ORIGINAL IMMIGRANT FROM FRANCE IN THE 1600'S. THE PATTERN OF OCCURRENCE OVER FIVE GENERATIONS AND 160 YEARS SINCE THE DEATH OF THE MAN BELIEVED TO BE THE FIRST INSTANCE OF THE HEART DISEASE INDICATES AUTOSOMAL DOMINANT INHERITANCE. AS POINTED OUT BY NASSER ET AL. (1967) AMONG OTHERS, OUTFLOW OBSTRUCTION MAY BE ABSENT IN SOME AFFECTED MEMBERS OF FAMILIES IN WHICH OTHERS DO HAVE OUTFLOW OBSTRUCTION. ELEVATED PATERNAL AGE OF SPORADIC (POSSIBLE FRESH MUTATION) CASES WAS OBSERVED BY JORGENSEN (1968).

BRAUNWALD, E., LAMBREW, C. T., ROCKOFF, S. D., ROSS, J., JR. AND MORROW, A. G.* IDIOPATHIC HYPERTROPHIC SUBAORTIC STENOSIS. I. A DESCRIPTION OF THE DISEASE BASED ON AN ANALYSIS OF 64 PATIENTS. CIRCULATION 30 (SUPPL. 4)* 3-119, 1964.

CRILEY, J., LEWIS, K. B., WHITE, R. I., JR. AND ROSS, R. S.* PRESSURE GRADIENTS WITHOUT OBSTRUCTION* A NEW CONCEPT OF *HYPERTROPHIC SUBAORTIC STENOSIS.* CIRCULATION 32* 881-887, 1965.

HORLICK, L., PETKOVICH, N. J. AND BOLTON, C. F.* IDIOPATHIC HYPERTROPHIC SUBVALVULAR STENOSIS. A STUDY OF A FAMILY INVOLVING FOUR GENERATIONS. CLINICAL, HEMODYNAMIC AND PATHOLOGIC OBSERVATIONS. AM. J. CARDIOL. 17* 411-418, 1966.

JORGENSEN, G.* GENETISCHE UNTERSUCHUNGEN BEI FUNKTIONELL-OBSTRUKTIVER SUBVALVU-LARER AORTENSTENOSE (IRREGULAR HYPERTROPHISCHER KARDIOMYOPATHIE). HUMANGENETIK 6* 13-28, 1968.

MANCHESTER, G. H.* MUSCULAR SUBAORTIC STENOSIS. NEW ENG. J. MED. 269* 300-306, 1963.

NASSER, W. K., WILLIAMS, J. F., MISHKIN, M. E., CHILDRESS, R. H., HELMEN, C., MERRITT, A. D. AND GENOVESE, P. D.* FAMILIAL MYOCARDIAL DISEASE WITH AND WITHOUT OBSTRUCTION TO LEFT VENTRICULAR OUTFLOW* CLINICAL, HEMODYNAMIC AND ANGIOGRAPHIC FINDINGS. CIRCULATION 35* 638-652, 1967.

PARE, J. A. P., FRASER, R. G., PIROZYNSKI, W. J., SHANKS, J. A. AND STUBINGTON, D.* HEREDITARY CARDIOVASCULAR DYSPLASIA. A FORM OF FAMILIAL CARDIOMYOPATHY. AM. J. MED. 31* 37-62, 1961.

WOOD, R. S., TAYLOR, W. J., WHEAT, M. W. AND SCHIEBLER, G. L.* MUSCULAR SUBAORTIC STENOSIS IN CHILDHOOD. REPORT OF OCCURRENCE IN THREE SIBLINGS. PEDIATRICS 30* 749-758, 1962.

19270 VENULAR INSUFFICIENCY, SYSTEMIC

SEIJFFERS, GROEN AND DAVIS (1964) DESCRIBED WHAT THEY TERMED SYSTEMIC VENULAR INSUFFICIENCY IN A 40 YEAR OLD ASHKENAZI JEW. MARKED CYANOSIS AND SWELLING OF THE HEAD AND NECK FOLLOWED BENDING OVER AND THE HANDS AND FEET WERE SIMILARLY AFFECTED WHEN IN THE DEPENDENT POSITION. SMALL VEINS AND VENULES IN CONJUNCTIVA SHOWED MARKED DILATION. ERECTION DID NOT OCCUR BUT COULD BE INDUCED BY MANUAL COMPRES-SION OF THE ROOT OF THE PENIS. THE AUTHORS SUGGESTED A VENOUS DEFECT, EITHER ABSENCE OF VALVES OR ABSENCE OF SMOOTH MUSCLE IN THE WALLS OF SMALL VEINS. THE PARENTS WERE FIRST COUSINS AND THE FATHER MAY HAVE HAD THE SAME DISORDER IN MILDER FORM. THUS, THE POSSIBILITY OF EITHER RECESSIVE OR DOMINANT INHERITANCE COULD BE ENTERTAINED.

SEIJFFERS, M. J., GROEN, J. J. AND DAVIS, E.* SYSTEMIC VENULAR INSUFFICIENCY. AM. J. MED. 36* 158-166, 1964.

19280 VERTEBRAL FUSION, POSTERIOR LUMBOSACRAL, WITH BLEPHAROPTOSIS

FAULK ET AL. (1970) DESCRIBED A MOTHER AND TWO DAUGHTERS WITH CONGENITAL PTOSIS AND POSTERIOR FUSION OF LUMBOSACRAL VERTEBRAE. THE MOTHER'S MOTHER HAD PTOSIS AND *HAD NEVER BEEN ABLE TO PLACE HER FEET FLAT ON THE FLOOR* BECAUSE OF *TIGHTNESS OF THE HEEL CORDS.* SERUM LACTIC DEHYDROGENASE ACTIVITY WAS ELEVATED IN THE MOTHER AND ONE DAUGHTER STUDIED.

FAULK, W. P., EPSTEIN, C. J. AND JONES, M. D.* FAMILIAL POSTERIOR LUMBOSACRAL VERTEBRAL FUSION AND EYELID PTOSIS. AM. J. DIS. CHILD. 119* 510-512, 1970.

19290 VERTEBRAL HYPOPLASIA WITH LUMBAR KYPHOSIS

BEALS (1969) OBSERVED MULTIPLE CASES OF VERTEBRAL HYPOPLASIA LEADING TO KYPHOSIS IN THE UPPER LUMBAR AREA, IN MULTIPLE GENERATIONS OF A FAMILY, WITH MALE-TO-MALE TRANSMISSION. THE FAMILIAL CASES REPORTED BY VAN ASSEN (1930) AND BY BAUER (1933) MAY HAVE BEEN THE SAME CONDITION.

BAUER, H.* UBER ANGEBORENE WIRBELSAULENMISSBILDUNGEN, INSBESONDERE ANGEBORENE KYPHOSEN. ZTSCHR. ORTHOP. CHIR. 58* 354-381, 1933.

BEALS, R. K.* FAMILIAL VERTEBRAL HYPOPLASIA AND KYPHOSIS. J. BONE JOINT SURG. 51* 190-196, 1969.

VAN ASSEN, J.* ANGEBORENE KYPHOSE. ACTA CHIR. SCAND. 67* 14-33, 1930.

19300 VESICOURETERAL REFLUX

MULCAHY ET AL. (1970) DESCRIBED A HIGH FAMILIAL INCIDENCE. THE DISORDER IS RARE IN NEGROES.

MULCAHY, J. J., KELALIS, P. P., STICKLER, G. B. AND BURKE, E. C.* FAMILIAL VESICOURETERAL REFLUX. J. UROL. 104* 762-764, 1970.

*19310 VITAMIN-D-RESISTANT RICKETS

AUTOSOMAL DOMINANT INHERITANCE IN SOME FAMILIES WAS SUGGESTED BY PRADER ET AL. (1961). HOWEVER, LATER OBSERVATIONS LED PRADER TO CONCLUDE THAT HIS *HEREDITARE

PSEUDO-MANGELRACHITIS* IS AN AUTOSOMAL RECESSIVE (SEE PSEUDO-VITAMIN D DEFICIENCY RICKETS). HARRISON ET AL. (1966) MENTIONED AFFECTED BROTHER AND TWO SISTERS, WHOSE FATHER HAD HYPOPHOSPHATEMIA, SEVERE OSTEOMALACIA AND STUNTING OF GROWTH AND WHOSE MOTHER WAS NORMAL (ALSO SEE BIANCHINE ET AL., 1971). THEY EMPHASIZED THAT SERUM PHOSPHORUS IS LIKELY TO BE AT A NORMAL LEVEL AT BIRTH AND DURING EARLY LIFE. WILSON ET AL. (1965) REPORTED A FAMILY STUDY INITIATED FROM A FEMALE PROBAND WITH TYPICAL VITAMIN-D-RESISTANT RICKETS. ONLY THE PROBAND WAS CLINICALLY AFFECTED, BUT, ALTHOUGH THE PARENTS HAD NORMAL BLOOD PHOSPHORUS, MANY MORE REMOTE RELATIVES HAD HYPOPHOSPHATEMIA. FATHER-TO-SON TRANSMISSION OF HYPOPHOSPHATEMIA WAS OBSERVED. ALTHOUGH THE NORMAL PARENTS AND THEIR RELATIONSHIP AS SECOND COUSINS SUGGESTED AUTOSOMAL RECESSIVE INHERITANCE, THE AUTHORS FAVORED AUTOSOMAL DOMINANCE WITH REDUCED PENETRANCE. IT IS CERTAINLY POSSIBLE FOR MORE THAN ONE GENETIC VARIETY OF VITAMIN-D-RESISTANT RICKETS TO EXIST. ALTHOUGH THE X-LINKED VARIETY MAY HAVE A DEFECT IN THE CONVERSION OF VITAMIN D3 TO 25-HYDROXYCHOLECALCIFEROL (25-HCC) IN THE LIVER, ALTERNATIVE POSSIBLE MECHANISMS INCLUDE MUTATION IN A GENE CONCERNED WITH THE CALCIUM-BINDING PROTEIN IN INTESTINAL MUCOSA WHICH IS ACTIVATED BY 25-HCC.

BIANCHINE, J. W., STAMBLER, A. A. AND HARRISON, H. E.* FAMILIAL HYPOPHOSPHATE-MIC RICKETS SHOWING AUTOSOMAL DOMINANT INHERITANCE. THE CLINICAL DELINEATION OF BIRTH DEFECTS. X. THE ENDOCRINE SYSTEM. BALTIMORE* WILLIAMS AND WILKINS, 1971.

DELUCA, H. F.* VITAMIN D. NEW ENG. J. MED. 281* 1103-1104, 1969.

HARRISON, H. E., HARRISON, H. C., LIFSHITZ, F. AND JOHNSON, A. D.* GROWTH DISTURBANCE IN HEREDITARY HYPOPHOSPHATEMIA. AM. J. DIS. CHILD. 112* 290-297, 1966.

MATSUDA, I., SUGAI, M. AND OHSAWA, T.* LABORATORY FINDINGS IN A CHILD WITH PSEUDO-VITAMIN D DEFICIENCY RICKETS. HELVET. PAEDIAT. ACTA 24* 329-336, 1969.

PRADER, A., ILLIG, R. AND HEIERLI, E.* EINE BESONDERE FORM DER PRIMAREN VITAMIN-D-RESISTENTEN RACHITIS MIT HYPOCALCAMIE UND AUTOSOMAL-DOMINANTEM ERBGANG* DIE HEREDITARE PSEUDO-MANGELRACHITIS. HELV. PAEDIAT. ACTA 16* 452-468, 1961.

WILSON, D. R., YORK, S. E., JAWORSKI, Z. F. AND YENDT, E. R.* STUDIES IN HYPOPHOSPHATEMIC VITAMIN D-REFRACTORY OSTEOMALACIA IN ADULTS. ORAL PHOSPHATE SUPPLEMENTS AS AN ADJUNCT TO THERAPY. MEDICINE 44* 99-134, 1965.

19320 VITILIGO

VITILIGO DIFFERS FROM PIEBALD TRAIT (Q.V.) IN ONSET AFTER BIRTH, ABSENCE OF PREDILECTION FOR VENTRAL SKIN AND TENDENCY TO PROGRESS OR REGRESS. FEW PEDIGREES HAVE BEEN REPORTED, BUT LERNER (1959) SUGGESTED AUTOSOMAL DOMINANT INHERITANCE.

LERNER, A. B.* VITILIGO. J. INVEST. DERM. 32* 285-310, 1959.

*19330 VON HIPPEL-LINDAU SYNDROME

THE CARDINAL FEATURES ARE ANGIOMATA OF THE RETINA AND HEMANGIOBLASTOMA OF THE CEREBELLUM. HEMANGIOMA OF THE SPINAL CORD HAS ALSO BEEN OBSERVED. PHEOCHROMOCY-TOMA OCCURS IN SOME PATIENTS. THE COMBINATION OF HYPERTENSION WITH ANGIOMA MAY LEAD TO SUBARACHNOID HEMORRHAGE. HYPERNEPHROMA-LIKE RENAL TUMORS OCCUR IN SOME PATIENTS. POLYCYTHEMIA MAY BE DUE TO EITHER THE HEMANGIOBLASTOMA OF THE CEREBEL-LUM OR THE HYPERNEPHROMA. HEMANGIOMAS OF THE ADRENALS, LUNGS AND LIVER AND MULTIPLE CYSTS OF THE PANCREAS AND KIDNEYS HAVE BEEN OBSERVED IN SOME INSTANCES. THE CONDITION OF ARTERIOVENOUS ANEURYSM OF RETINA AND MID-BRAIN WITH FACIAL NEVUS, DESCRIBED BY BONNET AND OTHERS (1938) AND BY WYBURN-MASON (1943) IS OF UNCERTAIN RELATIONSHIP TO THIS CONDITION. METASTATIC RENAL CANCER OCCURS IN SOME INSTANCES (KRANES AND BALOGH, 1966). GOLDBERG AND DUKE (1968) EXAMINED THE EYES OF AN AFFECTED 51 YEAR OLD NEGRO MALE WHOSE MOTHER DIED OF CEREBELLAR TUMOR AT AGE 26 YEARS. THE SAME CASE WAS DESCRIBED BY MCKUSICK ET AL. (1961). IN ADDITION TO THE ASSOCIATION OF TUMORS OF THE BRAIN AND ADRENAL MEDULLA WHICH OCCUR IN NEUROFI-BROMATOSIS AND IN VON HIPPEL-LINDAU'S DISEASE, CEREBELLAR TUMORS SOMETIMES PRODUCE PAROXYSMAL HYPERTENSION LIKE THAT OF PHEOCHROMOCYTOMA. URINARY CATECHOLAMINES ARE NORMAL IN SUCH CASES (CAMERON, DOIG, 1970).

BONNET, P., DECHAUME, J. AND BLANC, E.* L'ANEVRISME CIRSOIDE DE LA RETINE L'ANEVRISME RACEMEUX, SES RELATIONS AVEC L'ANEVRISME CIRSOIDE DE LA FACE ET L'ANEVRISME CIRSOID DU CERVEAU. BULL. SOC. FRANC. OPHTAL. 51* 521-524, 1938.

CAMERON, S. J. AND DOIG, A.* CEREBELLAR TUMORS PRESENTED WITH CLINICAL FEATURES OF PHAEOCHROMOCYTOMA. LANCET 1* 492-494, 1970.

CHAPMAN, R. C. AND DIAZ-PEREZ, R.* PHEOCHROMOCYTOMA ASSOCIATED WITH CEREBELLAR HEMANGIOBLASTOMA. J.A.M.A. 182* 1014-1017, 1962.

CHRISTOFERSON, L. A., GUSTAFSON, M. B. AND PETERSEN, A. G.* VON HIPPEL-LINDAU'S DISEASE. J.A.M.A. 178* 280-282, 1961.

GOLDBERG, M. F. AND DUKE, J. R.* VON HIPPEL-LINDAU DISEASE* HISTOPATHOLOGIC FINDINGS IN A TREATED AND UNTREATED EYE. AM. J. OPHTHAL. 66* 693-705, 1968.

HENNESSY, T. G., STERN, W. E. AND HERRICK, S. E.* CEREBELLAR HEMANGIOBLASTOMA* ERYTHROPOIETIC ACTIVITY BY RADIOIRON ASSAY. J. NUCLEAR MED. 8* 601-606, 1967.

KAPLAN, C., SAYRE, G. P. AND GREENE, L. F.* BILATERAL NEPHROGENIC CARCINOMAS IN LINDAU-VONHIPPEL DISEASE. J. UROL. 86* 36-42, 1961.

KRANES, A. AND BALOGH, K., JR.* LIVER DISEASE IN A PATIENT WITH VON HIPPEL-LINDAU DISEASE. NEW ENG. J. MED. 275* 950-959, 1966.

MCKUSICK, V. A. AND COLLEAGUES* MEDICAL GENETICS 1960. J. CHRONIC DIS. 14* 1-198, 1961. FIG. 71.

NIBBELINK, D. W., PETERS, B. H. AND MCCORMICK, W. F.* ON THE ASSOCIATION OF PHEOCHROMOCYTOMA AND CEREBELLAR HEMANGIOBLASTOMA. NEUROLOGY 19* 455-460, 1969.

OTENASEK, F. J. AND SILVER, M. L.* SPINAL HEMANGIOMA (HEMANGIOBLASTOMA) IN LINDAU'S DISEASE. REPORT OF SIX CASES IN A SINGLE FAMILY. J. NEUROSURG. 18* 295-300, 1961.

RHO, Y. M.* VON HIPPEL-LINDAU'S DISEASE* A REPORT OF 5 CASES. CANAD. MED. ASS. J. 101* 135-142, 1969.

SCHECHTERMAN, L.* LINDAU'S DISEASE* REPORT OF AN UNUSUAL CASE AND TWO ADDITIONAL CASES IN A NEGRO FAMILY. MED. ANN. D.C. 30* 64-76, 1961.

SILVER, M. L.* HEREDITARY VASCULAR TUMORS OF THE NERVOUS SYSTEM. J.A.M.A. 156* 1053-1056, 1954.

THOMAS, M. AND BURNSIDE, R. M.* VON HIPPEL-LINDAU DISEASE. AM. J. OPHTHAL. 51* 140-146, 1961.

WISE, K. S. AND GIBSON, J. A.* VON HIPPEL-LINDAU'S DISEASE AND PHAEOCHROMOCYTOMA. BRIT. MED. J. 1* 441 ONLY, 1971.

WYBURN-MASON, R.* ARTERIOVENOUS ANEURYSM OF MID-BRAIN AND RETINA, FACIAL NAEVI AND MENTAL CHANGES. BRAIN 66* 163-203, 1943.

*19340 VON WILLEBRAND'S DISEASE

VON WILLEBRAND (1931) DISCOVERED A HEMORRHAGIC CONDITION IN PERSONS LIVING ON THE ALAND ISLANDS IN THE SEA OF BOTHNIA BETWEEN SWEDEN AND FINLAND AND CALLED IT *PSEUDOHEMOPHILIA.* THE MAIN DIFFERENCES FROM CLASSIC HEMOPHILIA WAS PROLONGED BLEEDING TIME. MAIN PROBLEMS WERE GASTROINTESTINAL, URINARY AND UTERINE BLEEDING. HEMARTHROSES WERE RARE. THE CONDITION AMELIORATED WITH AGE. LATER JERGENS (1937) WORKING WITH WILLEBRAND AND USING THE CAPILLARY THROMBOMETER SUGGESTED THE DESIGNATION, *CONSTITUTIONAL THROMBOPATHY.* IN 1953, ALEXANDER AND GOLDSTEIN DISCOVERED LOW ANTI-HEMOPHILIC GLOBULIN (FACTOR VIII) IN THIS DISORDER. THEREAFTER THE CONDITION BECAME KNOWN AS *VASCULAR HEMOPHILIA.* IN RECENT YEARS THE MAIN DEVELOPMENTS HAVE BEEN THE DEMONSTRATIONS (1) THAT THE PLATELET IS INTRINSICALLY NORMAL BUT HAS REDUCED ADHESIVENESS BECAUSE OF THE FACTOR VIII DEFICIENCY AND (2) THAT PLASMA FROM PERSONS WITH CLASSICAL HEMOPHILIA WILL CORRECT BOTH THE VASCULAR DEFECT AND THE FACTOR VIII DEFICIENCY. IN A FAMILY WHICH APPEARED TO CONTAIN BOTH HOMOZYGOTES AND HETEROZYGOTES FOR THE VON WILLEBRAND GENE, BARROW ET AL. (1965) FOUND THAT HEMOPHILIC PLASMA RESULTED IN ABOUT 8 TIMES AS GREAT SYNTHESIS OF AHG IN HETEROZYGOTES AS IN HOMOZYGOTES. THEY INTERPRETED THIS AS SUGGESTING THE PRESENCE OF TWO SUBUNITS OF AHG WHICH ARE UNDER SEPARATE GENETIC CONTROL. SEVERAL OBSERVATIONS (CORNU, ET AL., 1963* BIGGS AND MATTHEWS, 1963) ARE PERTINENT TO THE NATURE OF THE AHG DEFECT IN VON WILLEBRAND'S DISEASE. (1) BLOOD FROM A PATIENT WITH HEMOPHILIA A WILL CORRECT THE CLOTTING DEFECT IN VON WILLEBRAND'S DISEASE. (2) THE CONVERSE IS NOT TRUE. BLOOD FROM A PATIENT WITH VON WILLEBRAND'S DISEASE WILL NOT CORRECT THE CLOTTING DEFECT IN HEMOPHILIA A. (3) THE BLEEDING TENDENCY IN VON WILLEBRAND'S DISEASE IS CORRECTED PROMPTLY BY NORMAL BLOOD. (4) AFTER ADMINISTRATION OF HEMOPHILIA A BLOOD TO VON WILLEBRAND PATIENTS THERE IS A DELAY OF SEVERAL HOURS BEFORE THE LEVEL OF AHG REACHES NORMAL. THESE OBSERVATIONS ARE CONSISTENT WITH THE FOLLOWING SCHEMA* AT LEAST TWO BIOCHEMICAL STEPS ARE INVOLVED IN THE SYNTHESIS OF AHG. THE FIRST STEP UNDER CONTROL OF AN AUTOSOMAL LOCUS PRODUCES THE WILLEBRAND FACTOR WHICH IS CONCERNED WITH PLATELET ADHESIVENESS AND THEREFORE WITH VASCULAR INTEGRITY. THE WILLEBRAND FACTOR IS ALSO THE SUBSTRATE FOR THE SECOND STEP WHICH IS UNDER X-CHROMOSOME CONTROL AND WHICH RESULTS IN AHG. THE ABOVE SCHEMA CONCEIVES, THEREFORE, A CHAIN OF BIOCHEMICAL PROCESSES, EACH UNDER SEPARATE GENETIC CONTROL - THE TYPE OF SYSTEM OF WHICH MANY INSTANCES HAVE NOW BEEN DEMONSTRATED. TELANGIECTASIA AND VON WILLEBRAND'S DISEASE OCCURRED IN A MOTHER AND DAUGHTER REPORTED BY QUICK (1967). THE DIFFICULT TOPIC OF DIAGNOSTIC CRITERIA WAS REVIEWED BY WEISS (1968). A PHENOCOPY OF VON WILLEBRAND'S DISEASE IN A PATIENT WITH SYSTEMIC LUPUS ERYTHEMATOSUS WAS REPORTED BY SIMONE ET AL. (1968).

ALEXANDER, B. AND GOLDSTEIN, R.* DUAL HEMOSTATIC DEFECT IN PSEUDOHEMOPHILIA. (ABSTRACT) J. CLIN. INVEST. 32* 551 ONLY, 1953.

BARROW, E. M., HEINDEL, C. C., ROBERTS, H. R. AND GRAHAM, J. B.* HETEROZYGOSITY AND HOMOZYGOSITY IN VON WILLEBRAND'S DISEASE. PROC. SOC. EXP. BIOL. MED. 118* 684-687, 1965.

D
O
M
I
N
A
N
T

BIGGS, R. AND MATTHEWS, J. M.* THE TREATMENT OF HAEMORRHAGE IN VON WILLEBRAND'S DISEASE AND THE BLOOD LEVEL OF FACTOR VIII (AHG). BRIT. J. HAEMAT. 9* 203-214, 1963.

BLOMBACK, M., JORPES, J. E. AND NILSSON, I. M.* VON WILLEBRAND'S DISEASE. AM. J. MED. 34* 236-241, 1963.

CORNU, P., LARRIEU, M. J., CAEN, J. AND BERNARD, J.* TRANSFUSION STUDIES IN VON WILLEBRAND'S DISEASE* EFFECT ON BLEEDING TIME AND FACTOR VIII. BRIT. J. HAEMAT. 9* 189-202, 1963.

DODDS, W. J.* CANINE VON WILLEBRAND'S DISEASE. J. LAB. CLIN. MED. 76* 713-721, 1970.

NEVANLINNA, H. R., IKKALA, E. AND VUOPIO, P.* VON WILLEBRAND'S DISEASE. ACTA HAEMAT. 27* 65-77, 1962.

QUICK, A. J.* TELANGIECTASIA* ITS RELATIONSHIP TO THE MINOT-VON WILLEBRAND SYNDROME. AM. J. MED. SCI. 254* 585-601, 1967.

RACCUGLIA, G. AND NEEL, J. V.* CONGENITAL VASCULAR DEFECT ASSOCIATED WITH PLATELET ABNORMALITY AND ANTIHEMOPHILIC FACTOR DEFICIENCY. BLOOD 15* 807-829, 1960.

SIMONE, J. V., CORNET, J. A. AND ABILDGAARD, C. F.* ACQUIRED VON WILLEBRAND'S SYNDROME IN SYSTEMIC LUPUS ERYTHEMATOSUS. BLOOD 31* 806-812, 1968.

STRAUSS, H. S. AND BLOOM, G. E.* VON WILLEBRAND'S DISEASE* USE OF A PLATELET-ADHESIVENESS TEST IN DIAGNOSIS AND FAMILY INVESTIGATION. NEW ENG. J. MED. 273* 171-181, 1965.

VON WILLEBRAND, E. A.* UBER HEREDITARE PSEUDOHAMOPHILIE. ACTA MED. SCAND. 76* 521-550, 1931.

WEISS, H. J.* VON WILLEBRAND'S DISEASE - DIAGNOSTIC CRITERIA. BLOOD 32* 668-679, 1968.

*19350 WAARDENBURG'S SYNDROME

THE FEATURES ARE WIDE BRIDGE OF THE NOSE OWING TO LATERAL DISPLACEMENT OF THE INNER CANTHUS OF EACH EYE, PIGMENTARY DISTURBANCE (FRONTAL WHITE BLAZE OF HAIR, HETEROCHROMIA IRIDIS, WHITE EYE LASHES, LEUKODERMA), AND COCHLEAR DEAFNESS. THE SEVERITY VARIES WIDELY AND SOME AFFECTED PERSONS ESCAPE DEAFNESS. LATERAL DISPLACEMENT OF THE INNER CANTHI IS SEEN ALSO IN THE ORODIGITOFACIAL SYNDROME (X-LINKED). THE DISORDER HAS BEEN DESCRIBED IN THE AMERICAN NEGRO (HANSEN, ACKAOUY AND CRUMP, 1965) AND THE MAORI (HOUGHTON, 1964) AS WELL AS IN EUROPEANS. CLEFT PALATE AND-OR LIP OCCURS IN SOME CASES. PREMATURE GRAYING OF THE HAIR IS AN EFFECT OF THE GENE. THE FUNDUS MAY BE ALBINOTIC COMPLETELY OR PARTIALLY AND DEPIGMENTED AREAS LIKE PIEBALD TRAIT (Q.V.) MAY BE PRESENT ELSEWHERE. IN THE STATE OF SOUTH AUSTRALIA, THE WAARDENBURG SYNDROME IS A LEADING CAUSE OF DEAFNESS AND 'ENJOYS' A POSITION COMPARABLE TO PORPHYRIA IN SOUTH AFRICA HAVING BEEN INTRODUCED BY EARLY SETTLERS WHO HAVE MANY DESCENDANTS (FRASER, 1967). THE WHITE FORELOCK MAY BE PRESENT AT BIRTH AND LATER DISAPPEAR (FEINGOLD ET AL., 1967). AN AFFECTED CHINESE FAMILY WAS REPORTED BY CHEW ET AL. (1968). THE WORK OF BOSHER AND HALLPIKE (1966) ON AN ANIMAL ANALOG MIGHT HAVE IMPORTANT IMPLICATIONS FOR PREVENTION OF DEAFNESS. THEIR WORK WITH DEAF WHITE CATS SUGGESTED THAT DESTRUC-TION OF THE INNER EAR MECHANISM OCCURS IN THE FIRST DAYS OF EXTRA-UTERINE LIFE AND WAS CORRELATED WITH AN INABILITY TO REGULATE PROPERLY THE CONSTITUTION OF THE ENDOLYMPHATIC FLUID. THE CAT, LIKE MAN, MAY ESCAPE DEAFNESS IN ONE OR BOTH EARS. IF WE KNEW MORE OF THE FACTORS THAT LEAD TO RETENTION OF HEARING WE MIGHT BE ABLE TO PREVENT DEAFNESS. SKIPPED GENERATIONS AND THE OCCURRENCE OF BILATERAL CLEFT LIP WERE DOCUMENTED BY GIACOIA AND KLEIN (1969). LAESTADIUS ET AL. (1969) PROVIDED NORMAL STANDARDS FOR THE MEASUREMENT OF INNER CANTHAL AND OUTER CANTHAL DISTANCE. STANDARDS WERE ALSO PRESENTED BY CHRISTIAN ET AL. (1969). KLEIN'S NAME IS SOMETIMES COMBINED WITH WAARDENBURG'S IN THE EPINYMIC DESIGNATION OF THIS DISORDER, ON THE BASIS OF A PATIENT WHICH KLEIN (1949) DESCRIBED WITH 'PARTIAL ALBINISM,' BLUE EYES, DEAFMUTISM, UNDEVELOPED MUSCLES AND FUSED JOINTS IN THE ARMS, SKELETAL DYSPLASIA ETC. THIS WAS RATHER CLEARLY A SEPARATE DISORDER.

BOSHER, S. K. AND HALLPIKE, C. S.* OBSERVATIONS ON THE HISTOGENESIS OF THE INNER EAR DEGENERATION OF THE DEAF WHITE CAT AND ITS POSSIBLE RELATIONSHIP TO THE AETIOLOGY OF CERTAIN UNEXPLAINED VARIETIES OF HUMAN CONGENITAL DEAFNESS. J. LARYNG. 80* 222-235, 1966.

CHEW, K. L., CHEN, A. J. AND TAN, K. H.* A CHINESE FAMILY WITH WAARDENBURG'S SYNDROME. AM. J. OPHTHAL. 65* 174-182, 1968.

CHRISTIAN, J. C., BIXLER, D., BLYTHE, S. C. AND MERRITT, A. D.* FAMILIAL TELECANTHUS WITH ASSOCIATED CONGENITAL ANOMALIES. THE CLINICAL DELINEATION OF BIRTH DEFECTS. II. MALFORMATION SYNDROMES. NEW YORK* NATIONAL FOUNDATION, 1969. PP. 82-85.

FEINGOLD, M., ROBINSON, M. J. AND GELLIS, S. S.* WAARDENBURG'S SYNDROME DURING THE FIRST YEAR OF LIFE. J. PEDIAT. 71* 874-876, 1967.

FRASER, G. R.* ADELAIDE, AUSTRALIA* PERSONAL COMMUNICATION, 1967.

GIACOIA, J. P. AND KLEIN, S. W.* WAARDENBURG'S SYNDROME WITH BILATERAL CLEFT LIP. AM. J. DIS. CHILD. 117* 344-348, 1969.

GOLDBERG, M. F.* WAARDENBURG'S SYNDROME WITH FUNDUS AND OTHER ANOMALIES. ARCH. OPHTHAL. 76* 797-810, 1966.

HANSEN, A. C., ACKAOUY, G. AND CRUMP, E. P.* WAARDENBURG'S SYNDROME* REPORT OF A PEDIGREE. J. NAT. MED. ASS. 57* 8-12, 1965.

HOUGHTON, N. I.* WAARDENBURG'S SYNDROME WITH DEAFNESS AS THE PRESENTING SYMPTOM. REPORT OF TWO CASES. NEW ZEALAND J. MED. 63* 83-89, 1964.

KLEIN, D.* ALBINISME PARTIEL (LEUCISME) AVEC SURDI-MUTITE, BLEPHAROPHIMOSIS ET DYSPLASIE MYO-OSTEO-ARTICULAIRE. HELVET. PAEDIAT. ACTA 5* 38-58, 1950.

LAESTADIUS, N. D., AASE, J. M. AND SMITH, D. W.* NORMAL INNER CANTHAL AND OUTER ORBITAL DIMENSIONS. J. PEDIAT. 74* 465-468, 1969.

SETTELMAYER, J. R. AND HOGAN, M.* WAARDENBURG'S SYNDROME - REPORT OF A CASE IN A NON-DUTCH FAMILY. NEW ENG. J. MED. 264* 500-501, 1961.

19360 WEYERS' OLIGODACTYLY SYNDROME

THIS SYNDROME IS CHARACTERIZED BY THE ASSOCIATION OF DEFICIENCY OF ULNA AND ULNAR RAYS, ANTECUBITAL PTERYGIA, REDUCED STERNAL SEGMENTS, AND MALFORMATION OF THE KIDNEY AND SPLEEN WITH CLEFT LIP, CLEFT PALATE. THE TWO REPORTED CASES WERE SPORADIC.

WEYERS, H.* DAS OLIGODACTYLIE-SYNDROM DES MENSCHEN UND SEINE PARALLELMUTATION BEI DER HAUSMANS. ANN. PAEDIAT. 189* 351-370, 1957.

19370 WHISTLING FACE-WINDMILL VANE HAND SYNDROME (CRANIOCARPOTARSAL DYSTROPHY FREEMAN-SHELDON SYNDROME)

IN CRANIOCARPOTARSAL DYSTROPHY, A SYNDROME FIRST DESCRIBED BY FREEMAN AND SHELDON (1938), CERTAIN SKELETAL MALFORMATIONS ARE ASSOCIATED WITH FACIAL CHARACTERISTICS. THE SKELETAL MALFORMATIONS ARE MAINLY, IN THE HANDS, CAMPTODACTYLY WITH ULNAR DEVIATION, IN THE FEET, TALIPES EQUINOVARUS, AND IN THE SKULL, AN ABNORMAL X-RAY APPEARANCE OF THE FLOOR OF THE ANTERIOR CRANIAL FOSSA. THE FACIAL CHARACTERISTICS ARE DEEP SUNKEN EYES WITH HYPERTELORISM, INCREASED PHILTRUM LENGTH, SMALL NOSE AND NOSTRILS AND A SMALL MOUTH. RINTALA (1968) DESCRIBED A CASE. HE ACCEPTED ONLY FREEMAN AND SHELDON'S AND OTTO'S AS 'GENUINE.' STEEP ANTERIOR CEREBRAL FOSSA WAS STRIKING IN HIS PATIENT. HE ALSO POINTED OUT IN HIS AND THE OTHER PATIENTS VERTICAL 'FOLDS OF SKIN IN THE JAW.' IN A STUDY OF GENETIC FACTORS IN HAND MALFORMATIONS TEMTAMY (1966) NOTED THE OCCURRENCE OF THIS SYNDROME IN TWO GENERATIONS OF THREE DIFFERENT FAMILIES. JACQUEMAIN (1966) DESCRIBED CONGENITAL WINDMILL VANE POSITION OF THE HAND* BILATERAL ULNAR DEVIATION AND CONTRACTURE OF FINGERS II-V AT THE METACARPOPHALANGEAL JOINTS WITH ADDUCTION OF THUMBS. THE DEFORMITY RESEMBLED THAT OF RHEUMATOID ARTHRITIS. CLUBFOOT WAS ALSO PRESENT. THEY FOUND THAT 7 WERE AFFECTED IN FOUR GENERATIONS. 14 OF 23 CASES IN THE LITERATURE WERE FAMILIAL AND CASES OCCURRED IN SUCCESSIVE GENERATIONS, WITH FATHER-TO-SON TRANSMISSION. THE DEFECT WAS THOUGHT TO CONCERN THE PALMAR FASCIA. THIS TYPE OF DEFORMITY, ESPECIALLY WHEN COMBINED WITH CLUBFOOT, MIGHT MISTAKENLY BE CALLED ARTHROGRYPOSIS MULTIPLEX CONGENITA. WEINSTEIN AND GORLIN (1969) GAVE A FULL CLINICAL DESCRIPTION AND REFERRED TO OBSERVATION OF AFFECTED FATHER AND DAUGHTER BY FRASER (PERSONAL COMMUNICATION). THEY ALSO SUGGESTED 'DYSPLASIA' AS MORE APPROPRIATE THAN 'DYSTROPHY.' CERVENKA, FIGALOVA AND GORLIN (1969) PROVIDED NORMAL STANDARDS FOR THE MEASUREMENT OF ORAL INTERCOMMISSURAL DISTANCE IN CHILDREN. FRASER ET AL. (1970) REPORTED THE SYNDROME IN FATHER AND SON. DRAMATIC PICTURES OF FRASER AND PASHAYAN'S EXAMPLE OF AFFECTED FATHER AND SON HAVE BEEN PUBLISHED (GELLIS AND FEINGOLD, 1970).

BURIAN, F.* THE 'WHISTLING FACE' CHARACTERISTIC IN A COMPOUND CRANIO-FACIO-CORPORAL SYNDROME. BRIT. J. PLAST. SURG. 16* 140-143, 1963.

CERVENKA, J., FIGALOVA, P. AND GORLIN, R. J.* CRANIO-CARPO-TARSAL DYSPLASIA OR THE WHISTLING FACE SYNDROME. II. ORAL INTERCOMMISSURAL DISTANCE IN CHILDREN. AM. J. DIS. CHILD. 117* 434-435, 1969.

CERVENKA, J., GORLIN, R. J., FIGALOVA, P. AND FARKASOVA, J.* CRANIOCARPOTARSAL DYSPLASIA OR WHISTLING FACE SYNDROME. ARCH. OTOLARYNG. 91* 183-187, 1970.

FRASER, F. C., PASHAYAN, H. AND KADISH, M. E.* CRANIO-CARPO-TARSAL DYSPLASIA. REPORT OF A CASE IN FATHER AND SON. J.A.M.A. 211* 1374-1376, 1970.

FREEMAN, E. A. AND SHELDON, J. H.* CRANIO-CARPOTARSAL DYSTROPHY* UNDESCRIBED CONGENITAL MALFORMATION. ARCH. DIS. CHILD. 13* 277-283, 1938.

GELLIS, S. S. FEINGOLD, M. AND GORLIN, R.* PICTURE OF THE MONTH. ORAL-FACIAL-
DIGITAL SYNDROME. AM. J. DIS. CHILD. 120* 241-242, 1970.

JACQUEMAIN, B.* DIE ANGEBORENE WINDMUHLENFLUGELSTELLUNG AL ERBLICHE KOMBINA-
TION-SMISSBILDUNG. Z. ORTHOP. 102* 146-154, 1966.

LUNDBLOM, A.* ON CONGENITAL ULNAR DEVIATION OF THE FINGERS OF FAMILIAL
OCCURRENCE (*DEVIATION DES DOIGTS EN COUP DE VENT*). ACTA ORTHOP. SCAND. 3* 393-
404, 1932.

OTTO, F. M.* DIE CRANIO-CARPO-TARSAL DYSTROPHIE (FREEMAN AND SHELDON) EIN
RASUISTISCHER BEITRAG. Z. KINDERHEILK. 73* 240-250, 1953.

RINTALA, A. E.* FREEMAN-SHELDON'S SYNDROME, CRANIO-CARPO-TARSAL DYSTROPHY.
ACTA PAEDIAT. SCAND. 57* 553-556, 1968.

SHARMA, R. N. AND TANDON, S. N.* *WHISTLING FACE* DEFORMITY IN COMPOUND CRANIO-
FACIO-CORPORAL SYNDROME. BRIT. MED. J. 4* 33 ONLY, 1970.

TEMTAMY, S. A.* GENETIC FACTORS IN HAND MALFORMATIONS. PH. D. THESIS, JOHNS
HOPKINS UNIVERSITY, 1966.

WEINSTEIN, S. AND GORLIN, R. J.* CRANIO-CARPO-TARSAL DYSPLASIA OR THE WHISTLING
FACE SYNDROME. I. CLINICAL CONSIDERATIONS. AM. J. DIS. CHILD. 117* 427-433,
1969.

*19380 WHITE HAIR, PREMATURE

HARE (1929) DESCRIBED 9 CASES IN 5 GENERATIONS WITH MALE-TO-MALE TRANSMISSION.
ONSET OF WHITENING WAS IN THE TEENS.

HARE, H. J. H.* PREMATURE WHITENING OF THE HAIR. J. HERED. 20* 31-32, 1929.

*19390 WHITE SPONGE NEVUS OF CANNON

THIS DISORDER IS MANIFESTED BY THICKENED SPONGY FOLD MUCOSA IN THE MOUTH WITH A
WHITE OPALESCENT TINT. IT MAY BE THE SAME AS THE CONDITION REFERRED TO BY
ZEGARELLI, EVERETT AND KUTSCHER (1961) AS WHITE FOLDED HYPERPLASIA OF THE MUCOUS
MEMBRANES. IT IS DIFFERENTIATED FROM BENIGN INTRAEPITHELIAL DYSKERATOSIS (Q.V.)
BY THE PRESENCE OF VAGINAL AND ANAL LESIONS AND THE ABSENCE OF CONJUNCTIVAL
INVOLVEMENT AND THE CHARACTERISTIC CELL-WITHIN-CELL HISTOLOGIC CHANGE. SCOTT
(1966) FOUND THREE GENERATIONS AFFECTED. HAYE AND WHITEHEAD (1968) REPORTED ON 7
CASES IN 3 GENERATIONS WITH MALE-TO-MALE TRANSMISSION. VERMA (1967) DESCRIBED THE
DISORDER IN ASIATIC INDIANS.

BROWNE, W. G., IZATT, M. M. AND RENWICK, J. H.* WHITE SPONGE NAEVUS OF THE
MUCOSA* CLINICAL AND LINKAGE DATA. ANN. HUM. GENET. 32* 271-282, 1969.

HAYE, K. R. AND WHITEHEAD, F. I. H.* HEREDITARY LEUKOKERATOSIS OF THE MUCOUS
MEMBRANES. BRIT. J. DERM. 80* 529-533, 1968.

SCOTT, C. R.* HEREDITARY LEUKOKERATOSIS, WHITE MOUTH. J. PEDIAT. 68* 768-772,
1966.

VERMA, B. S.* HEREDITARY MUCOSAL KERATOSIS. INDIAN J. MED. SCI. 21* 310-313,
1967.

WITKOP, C. J. AND GORLIN, R. J.* FOUR HEREDITARY MUCOSAL SYNDROMES. ARCH.
DERM. 84* 762-771, 1961.

ZEGARELLI, E. V., EVERETT, F. G. AND KUTSCHER, A. H.* FAMILIAL WHITE FOLDED
DYSPLASIA OF THE MUCOUS MEMBRANES. AN ATLAS OF ORAL LESIONS. ORAL SURG. 14*
1436-1443, 1961.

19400 WIDOW'S PEAK

A POINTED FRONTAL HAIRLINE MAY BE INHERITED AS A DOMINANT. FOR PICTURE SEE P. 359
OF WINCHESTER.

WINCHESTER, A. M.* GENETICS. BOSTON* HOUGHTON MIFFLIN CO., 1958 (2ND ED.).

19410 WISDOM TEETH, ABSENCE OF

GRUNEBERG (1936) DESCRIBED A FAMILY IN WHICH A MOTHER AND FOUR OF FIVE CHILDREN
LACKED SOME OR ALL WISDOM TEETH. THE EVIDENCE FOR SIMPLE DOMINANT INHERITANCE IS
MEAGER.

GRUNEBERG, H.* TWO INDEPENDENT INHERITED TOOTH ANOMALIES IN ONE FAMILY. J.
HERED. 27* 225-228, 1936.

19420 WOLFF-PARKINSON-WHITE SYNDROME

THE FEATURES OF THIS ELECTROCARDIOGRAPHIC SYNDROME ARE SHORT PR INTERVAL AND PROLONGED QRS, SPECIFICALLY WITH A SLURRED-UP STROKE OF THE R WAVE CALLED A DELTA WAVE. THE PATIENTS ARE PRONE TO PAROXYSMAL SUPRA-VENTRICULAR TACHYCARDIA. THE FAMILIAL OCCURRENCE OF THE WOLFF-PARKINSON-WHITE SYNDROME HAS BEEN REPORTED MANY TIMES (HARNISCHFEGER, 1959). IN AT LEAST TWO REPORTED FAMILIES IT HAS BEEN ASSOCIATED WITH FAMILIAL CARDIOMYOPATHY (MASSUMI, 1967). SCHNEIDER (1969) OBSERVED AFFECTED MOTHER AND SON.

HARNISCHFEGER, W. W.* HEREDITARY OCCURRENCE OF THE PRE-EXCITATION (WOLFF-PARKINSON-WHITE) SYNDROME WITH RE-ENTRY MECHANISM AND CONCEALED CONDUCTION. CIRCULATION 19* 28-40, 1959.

MASSUMI, R. A.* FAMILIAL WOLFF-PARKINSON-WHITE SYNDROME WITH CARDIOMYOPATHY. AM. J. MED. 43* 951-955, 1967.

SCHNEIDER, R. G.* FAMILIAL OCCURRENCE OF WOLFF-PARKINSON-WHITE SYNDROME. AM. HEART J. 78* 34-36, 1969.

*19430 WOOLLY HAIR

THE HAIR IS SHORT, TIGHTLY CURLED AND WOOLLY, RESEMBLING THAT OF A NEGRO. MOHR (1932) CONSIDERED NEGRO ADMIXTURE VERY UNLIKELY IN THE NORWEGIAN KINDRED WITH MANY PERSONS AFFECTED. ANDERSON (1936) AND SCHOKKING (1934) ALSO REPORTED CAUCASIAN FAMILIES WITH MANY AFFECTED. ANDERSON (1936), WHO HAD CLOSE FAMILIARITY WITH NEGRO HAIR, FELT THAT THE WOOLLY HAIR WAS DIFFERENT.

ANDERSON, E.* AN AMERICAN PEDIGREE FOR WOOLLY HAIR. J. HERED. 27* 444 ONLY, 1936.

MOHR, O. L.* WOOLLY HAIR, A DOMINANT MUTANT CHARACTER IN MAN. J. HERED. 23* 345-352, 1932.

SANDERS, J.* EINE FAMILIE MIT KRAUSHAAR. GENETICA 18* 97-104, 1936.

SCHOKKING, C. P.* ANOTHER WOOLLY HAIR MUTATION IN MAN. J. HERED. 25* 337-340, 1934.

19440 XERODERMA PIGMENTOSUM

IN ADDITION TO THE USUAL SEVERE, RECESSIVELY INHERITED XERODERMA PIGMENTOSUM, THE EXISTENCE OF A MILDER FORM BEHAVING AS A DOMINANT HAS BEEN CLAIMED BY ANDERSON AND BEGG (1950) WHO DESCRIBED 11 AFFECTED PERSONS IN 5 SIBSHIPS OF FOUR GENERATIONS OF A SCOTTISH FAMILY BY THE NAME OF MACPHERSON. THE PATIENTS SHOWED FRECKLING AND MULTIPLE SKIN CANCERS AS IN THE RECESSIVE FORM BUT DID NOT GET TROUBLE AS EARLY IN LIFE AND SURVIVED LONGER. INDEED, ANDERSON AND BEGG EXAMINED ONE AFFECTED MEMBER OF THE FAMILY WHO WAS 74 YEARS OF AGE. THE FAMILY OF ANDERSON AND BEGG (1950) WAS FROM SCOTLAND AND HAD THE NAME MACPHERSON. INDEED, FULL NAMES WERE GIVEN OF OTHER AFFECTED MEMBERS OF THE FAMILY, WHICH SHOULD FACILITATE FOLLOW-UP IN THE FUTURE. NO AFFECTED MEMBER WAS SAID TO HAVE DIED OF THE DISEASE.

ANDERSON, T. E. AND BEGG, M.* XERODERMA PIGMENTOSUM OF MILD TYPE. BRIT. J. DERM. 62* 402-407, 1950.

AUTOSOMAL RECESSIVE PHENOTYPES

FEATURES ARE CELIAC SYNDROME, PIGMENTARY DEGENERATION OF THE RETINA, PROGRESSIVE ATAXIC NEUROPATHY, AND A PECULIAR "BURR-CELL" MALFORMATION OF THE RED CELLS CALLED ACANTHOCYTOSIS (SOMETIMES INCORRECTLY WRITTEN "ACANTHROCYTOSIS"). INTESTINAL ABSORPTION OF LIPIDS IS DEFECTIVE, SERUM CHOLESTEROL VERY LOW AND SERUM BETA LIPOPROTEIN ABSENT. FEW CASES HAVE TO DATE BEEN DISCOVERED AND ALMOST ALL HAVE BEEN JEWS. AUTOPSY (SOBREVILLA ET AL., 1964) AND BIOPSY OF PERIPHERAL NERVES SHOW EXTENSIVE CENTRAL AND PERIPHERAL DEMYELINATION. LEES (1967) DEMONSTRATED THAT THE LIPID-FREE APOPROTEIN OF BETA-LIPOPROTEIN IS PRESENT IN ABETALIPOPROTEINEMIA. THE DEFECT MUST CONCERN FORMATION OF THE COMPLETE MACROMOLECULE. SEE LIPID TRANSPORT DEFECT OF INTESTINE FOR A DISORDER WITH SOME OF THE SAME FEATURES AS ABETALIPOPRO-TEINEMIA.

DISCHE, M. R. AND PORRO, R. S.* THE CARDIAC LESIONS IN BASSEN-KORNZWEIG SYNDROME. REPORT OF A CASE, WITH AUTOPSY FINDINGS. AM. J. MED. 49* 568-571, 1970.

DODGE, J. T., COHEN, G., KAYDEN, H. J. AND PHILLIPS, G. B.* PEROXIDATIVE HEMOLYSIS OF RED BLOOD CELLS FROM PATIENTS WITH ABETALIPOPROTEINEMIA (ACANTHOCYTO-SIS). J. CLIN. INVEST. 46* 357-368, 1967.

FARQUHAR, J. W. AND WAYS, P.* ABETALIPOPROTEINEMIA. IN, STANBURY, J. B., WYNGAARDEN, J. B. AND FREDRICKSON, D. S. (EDS.)* THE METABOLIC BASIS OF INHERITED DISEASE. NEW YORK* MCGRAW-HILL, 1966 (2ND ED.). PP. 509-522.

ISSELBACHER, K. J., SCHEIG, R., PLOTKIN, G. R. AND CAULFIELD, J. B.* CONGENITAL BETA-LIPOPROTEIN DEFICIENCY* AN HEREDITARY DISORDER INVOLVING A DEFECT IN THE ABSORPTION AND TRANSPORT OF LIPIDS. MEDICINE 43* 347-361, 1964.

LEES, R. S.* IMMUNOLOGICAL EVIDENCE FOR THE PRESENCE OF B PROTEIN (APOPROTEIN OF BETA-LIPOPROTEIN) IN NORMAL AND ABETALIPOPROTEINEMIA PLASMA. J. LIPID. RES. 8* 396-405, 1967.

MIER, M., SCHWARTZ, S. O. AND BOSHES, B.* ACANTHOCYTOSIS, PIGMENTARY DEGENERA-TION OF THE RETINA AND ATAXIC NEUROPATHY* A GENETICALLY DETERMINED SYNDROME WITH ASSOCIATED METABOLIC DISORDER. BLOOD 16* 1586-1608, 1960.

SALT, H. B., WOLFF, O. H., LLOYD, J. K., FOSBROOKE, A. S., CAMERON, A. H. AND HUBBLE, D. V.* ON HAVING NO BETA-LIPOPROTEIN. A SYNDROME COMPRISING A-BETA-LIPOPROTEINAEMIA, ACANTHOCYTOSIS AND STEATORRHOEA. LANCET 2* 325-329, 1960.

SCHWARTZ, J. F., ROWLAND, L. P., EDER, H., MARKS, P. A., OSSERMAN, E. F., HIRSCHBERG, E. AND ANDERSON, H.* BASSEN-KORNZWEIG SYNDROME. DEFICIENCY OF SERUM BETA-LIPOPROTEIN. ARCH. NEUROL. 8* 438-454, 1963.

SOBREVILLA, L. A., GOODMAN, M. L. AND KANE, C. A.* DEMYELINATING CENTRAL NERVOUS SYSTEM DISEASE, MACULAR ATROPHY AND ACANTHOCYTOSIS (BASSEN-KORNZWEIG SYNDROME). AM. J. MED. 37* 821-832, 1964.

*20020 ACATALASEMIA (TWO OR MORE TYPES)

ACATALASIA WAS FIRST DISCOVERED IN JAPAN BY TAKAHARA, AN OTOLARYNGOLOGIST, WHO, IN CASES OF PROGRESSIVE ORAL GANGRENE, FOUND THAT PEROXIDE APPLIED TO THE ULCERATED AREAS DID NOT FROTH IN THE USUAL MANNER. HETEROZYGOTES HAVE AN INTERMEDIATE LEVEL OF CATALASE IN THE BLOOD. THE FREQUENCY OF THE GENE, ALTHOUGH RELATIVELY HIGH IN JAPAN, IS VARIABLE. THE FREQUENCY OF HETEROZYGOTES IS 0.09 PERCENT IN HIROSHIMA AND NAGASAKI BUT IS OF THE ORDER OF 1.4 PERCENT IN OTHER PARTS OF JAPAN (HAMILTON ET AL., 1961). ACATALASIA HAS BEEN DETECTED IN SWITZERLAND (AEBI ET AL., 1962), AND IN ISRAEL (SZEINBERG ET AL., 1963). IN BOTH OF THE LATTER SITUATIONS THE HOMOZYGOTES SHOWED SOME RESIDUAL CATALASE ACTIVITY SUGGESTING THAT THIS MAY BE A DIFFERENT MUTATION THAN THAT RESPONSIBLE FOR THE JAPANESE DISEASE IN WHICH CATALASE ACTIVITY IS ZERO AND NO CROSS-REACTING MATERIAL HAS BEEN IDENTIFIED. HAMILTON AND NEEL (1963) PRESENTED EVIDENCE THAT AT LEAST TWO FORMS OF ACATALASIA EXIST IN JAPAN. IN AN EXTENSIVE KINDRED WITH ACATALASIA IN TWO SIBSHIPS, HETEROZYGOTES SHOWED CATALASE VALUES OVERLAPPING WITH THE NORMAL. HYPOCATALASIA HAS ALSO BEEN FOUND IN THE GUINEA PIG, DOG AND DOMESTIC FOWL (SEE REVIEW BY LUSH, 1966). ELECTROPHORETIC VARIANTS OF RED CELL CATALASE HAVE BEEN DESCRIBED (SEE DOMINANT CATALOG). THESE MAY BE DETERMINED BY GENES ALLELIC WITH THAT FOR ACATALASEMIA.

AEBI, H., BAGGIOLINI, M., DEWALD, B., LAUBER, E., SUTTER, H., MICHELI, A. AND FREI, J.* OBERVATIONS IN TWO SWISS FAMILIES WITH ACATALASIA. ENZYM. BIOL. CLIN. 4* 121-151, 1964.

AEBI, H., JEUNET, F., RICHTERICH, R., SUTER, H., BUTLER, R., FREI, J. AND MARTI, H. R.* OBSERVATIONS IN TWO SWISS FAMILIES WITH ACATALASIA. ENZYM. BIOL. CLIN. 2* 1-22, 1962.

BAUR, E. W.* CATALASE ABNORMALITY IN A CAUCASIAN FAMILY IN THE UNITED STATES. SCIENCE 140* 816-817, 1963.

FEINSTEIN, R. N., HOWARD, J. B., BRAUN, J. T. AND SEAHOLM, J. E.* ACATALASEMIC AND HYPOCATALASEMIC MOUSE MUTANTS. GENETICS 53* 923-933, 1966.

HAMILTON, H. B. AND NEEL, J. V.* GENETIC HETEROGENEITY IN HUMAN ACATALASIA. AM. J. HUM. GENET. 15* 408-419, 1963.

HAMILTON, H. B., NEEL, J. V., KOBARA, T. Y. AND OZAKI, K.* THE FREQUENCY IN JAPAN OF CARRIERS OF THE RARE *RECESSIVE* GENE CAUSING ACATALASEMIA. J. CLIN. INVEST. 40* 2199-2208, 1961.

LUSH, I. E.* THE BIOCHEMICAL GENETICS OF VERTEBRATES EXCEPT MAN. PHILADELPHIA* W. B. SAUNDERS, 1966.

MATSUBARA, S., SUTER, H. AND AEBI, H.* FRACTIONATION OF ERYTHROCYTE CATALASE FROM NORMAL, HYPOCATALATIC AND ACATALATIC HUMANS. HUMANGENETIK 4* 29-41, 1967.

SZEINBERG, A., DE VRIES, A., PINKHAS, J., DJALDETTI, M. AND EZRA, R.* A DUAL HEREDITARY RED BLOOD CELL DEFECT IN ONE FAMILY* HYPOCATALASEMIA AND GLUCOSE-6-PHOSPHATE DEHYDROGENASE DEFICIENCY. ACTA GENET. MED. GEM. 12* 247-255, 1963.

WYNGAARDEN, J. B. AND HOWELL, R. R.* ACATALASIA. IN, STANBURY, J. B., WYNGAARDEN, J. B. AND FREDRICKSON, D. S. (EDS.)* THE METABOLIC BASIS OF INHERITED DISEASE. NEW YORK* MCGRAW-HILL, 1966 (2ND ED.). PP. 1343-1369.

*20030 ACETOPHENETIDIN SENSITIVITY

SHAHIDI (1967) DESCRIBED A 17 YEAR OLD GIRL WITH SEVERE METHEMOGLOBINEMIA AND HEMOLYSIS FOLLOWING INGESTION OF ACETOPHENETIDIN. THE ACTIVITY OF G6PD, 6PGD, DIAPHORASE, AND GLUTATHIONE REDUCTASE WAS NORMAL, AS WAS ALSO THE CONCENTRATION OF REDUCED GLUTATHIONE. HEMOGLOBIN WAS PHYSICALLY NORMAL. PREVIOUSLY UNKNOWN METABOLITES OF ACETOPHENETIDIN WERE FOUND IN THE URINE. A 38 YEAR OLD SISTER SHOWED THE SAME ABNORMALITY. INADEQUATE DEETHYLATION WAS SUGGESTED WITH INCREASED HYDROXYLATION OF ACETOPHENETIDIN TO HYDROXYPHENETIDIN WHICH WAS THOUGHT TO BE RESPONSIBLE FOR METHEMOGLOBIN PRODUCTION. PHENOBARBITAL ADMINISTRATION HAD ADVERSE EFFECTS POSSIBLY BY STIMULATION OF THE HYDROXYLATION PROCESS. THE PARENTS WERE NOT RELATED. THE FAMILY WAS OF GERMAN EXTRACTION (SHAHIDI, 1967).

SHAHIDI, N. T.* ACETOPHENETIDIN SENSITIVITY. AM. J. DIS. CHILD. 113* 81-82, 1967.

SHAHIDI, N. T.* MILWAUKEE, WIS.* PERSONAL COMMUNICATION, 1967.

20040 ACHALASIA, FAMILIAL ESOPHAGEAL

THIBERT ET AL. (1965) DESCRIBED TWO FAMILIES EACH WITH TWO AFFECTED SIBS UNDER 16 YEARS OF AGE. CLOUD ET AL. (1966) OBSERVED THE DISORDER IN 4 FULL-BLOODED APACHE INDIAN SIBS LESS THAN 6 YEARS OLD. POLONSKY AND GUTH (1970) REPORTED THE CONDITION IN TWO SIBS, AND POSSIBLY A THIRD, ALL LESS THAN 5 YEARS OLD.

CLOUD, D. T., JR., WHITE, R. F., LINKNER, L. M. AND TAYLOR, L. C.* SURGICAL TREATMENT OF ESOPHAGEAL ACHALASIA IN CHILDREN. J. PEDIAT. SURG. 1* 137-144, 1966.

POLONSKY, L. AND GUTH, P. H.* FAMILIAL ACHALASIA. AM. J. DIGEST. DIS. 15* 291-295, 1970.

THIBERT, F., CHICOINE, R., CHARTIER-RATELLE, G.* FORME FAMILIALE DE L*ACHALASIE DE L*OESOPHAGE CHEZ L*ENFANT. UN. MED. CANADA 94* 1293-1300, 1965.

*20050 ACHEIROPODY (BRAZILIAN TYPE)

ABSENCE OF HANDS AND FEET HAS PROBABLY BEEN OBSERVED ONLY IN MULTIPLE MEMBERS OF AN INBRED BRAZILIAN KINDRED OF PORTUGUESE ANCESTRY.

BOHOMOLETZ, M.* FURTHER LIGHT ON THE HANDLESS AND FOOTLESS FAMILY OF BRAZIL. EUGEN. NEWS 15* 143-145, 1930.

KOEHLER, O.* DIE HAND- UND FUSSLOSEN BRASILIANISCHEN GESCHWISTER. EIN BEITRAG ZUR FRAGE DER ERBBEDINGHEIT ANGEBORENER MISSBILDUNGEN. Z. MENSCHL. VERERB. KONSTITUTIONSL. 19* 670-690, 1936.

QUELCE-SALGADO, A., FREIRE-MAIA, N. AND KOEHLER, R. A.* MARILIA AND CURITIBA, BRAZIL* PERSONAL COMMUNICATION, 1966.

TOLEDO, S. P. A. AND SALDANHA, P. H.* A RADIOLOGICAL AND GENETIC INVESTIGATION OF ACHEIROPODY IN A KINDRED INCLUDING SIX CASES. J. GENET. HUM. 17* 81-94, 1969.

*20060 ACHONDROGENESIS, TYPE I (PARENTI-FRACCARO OR LETHAL TYPE)

TWO QUITE DISTINCT DISORDERS HAVE BEEN GIVEN THE NAME ACHONDROGENESIS. THAT DESCRIBED BY PARENTI (1936) AND BY FRACCARO (1952) IS A SEVERE CHONDRODYSTROPHY CHARACTERIZED RADIOGRAPHICALLY BY DEFICIENT OSSIFICATION IN THE LUMBAR VERTEBRAE AND ABSENT OSSIFICATION IN THE SACRAL, PUBIC AND ISCHIAL BONES AND CLINICALLY BY

STILLBIRTH OR EARLY DEATH (MAROTEAUX AND LAMY, 1968* LANGER ET AL., 1969). SALDINO (1970) OBSERVED A GYPSY FAMILY IN WHICH THE PARENTS WERE SECOND COUSINS AND TWO OFFSPRING HAD WELL DOCUMENTED ACHONDROGENESIS AND TWO OTHER OFFSPRING MAY HAVE BEEN AFFECTED. SILVERMAN (1970) ALSO HAS INFORMATION ON A FAMILY WITH MULTIPLE AFFECTED SIBS. HOUSTON (1970) HAS OBSERVED 4 SIBS WITH ACHONDROGENESIS OUT OF A FAMILY OF 9.

FRACCARO, M.* CONTRIBUTO ALLO STUDIO DELLE MALATTIE DEL MESENCHIMA OSTEOPOIETI-CO. L'ACONDROGENESI. FOLIA HERED. PATH. 1* 190-208, 1952.

HOUSTON, C. S.* SASKATOON, SASKATCHEWAN, CANADA* PERSONAL COMMUNICATION, 1970.

LANGER, L. O., JR., SPRANGER, J. W., GREINACHER, I. AND HERDMAN, R. C.* THANATOPHORIC DWARFISM. A CONDITION CONFUSED WITH ACHONDROPLASIA IN THE NEONATE, WITH BRIEF COMMENTS ON ACHONDROGENESIS AND HOMOZYGOUS ACHONDROPLASIA. RADIOLOGY 92* 285-294, 1969.

MAROTEAUX, P. AND LAMY, M.* LE DIAGNOSTIC DES NANISMES CHONDRO-DYSTROPHIQUES CHEZ LES NOUVEAU-NES. ARCH. FRANC. PEDIAT. 25* 241-262, 1968.

PARENTI, G. C.* LA ANOSTEOGENESI* (UNA VARIETA DELLA OSTEOGENESI IMPERFETTA). PATHOLOGICA 28* 447-462, 1936.

SALDINO, R. M.* SAN FRANCISCO, CALIF.* PERSONAL COMMUNICATION, 1970.

SILVERMAN, F.* CINCINNATI, OHIO* PERSONAL COMMUNICATION, 1970.

*20070 ACHONDROGENESIS, TYPE II (GREBE OR BRAZILIAN TYPE)

GREBE (1952, 1955) DESCRIBED THE DISORDER IN 7 AND 11 YEAR OLD SISTERS, OFFSPRING OF A CONSANGUINEOUS MATING. THE SAME DISORDER WAS FOUND IN BRAZIL BY QUELCE-SALGADO (1964). IN THESE CASES ALL FOUR LIMBS ARE MARKEDLY SHORTENED AND END IN TINY DIGITS. THE TRUNK AND HEAD ARE NORMAL. A CASE WITH CHILDHOOD AND ADULT RADIOGRAPHIC STUDIES WAS PRESENTED BY SCOTT (1969).

GREBE, H.* CHONDRODYSPLASIE. ROME* INST. GREG. MENDEL, 1955. PP. 300-303.

GREBE, H.* DIE ACHONDROGENESIS* EIN EINFACH REZESSIVES ERBMERKMAL. FOLIA HERED. PATH. 2* 23-28, 1952.

QUELCE-SALGADO, A.* A NEW TYPE OF DWARFISM WITH VARIOUS BONE APLASIAS AND HYPOPLASIAS OF THE EXTREMITIES. ACTA GENET. STATIST. MED. 14* 63-66, 1964.

SCOTT, C. I.* DISCUSSION. THE CLINICAL DELINEATION OF BIRTH DEFECTS. IV. SKELETAL DYSPLASIAS. NEW YORK* NATIONAL FOUNDATION, 1969. PP. 14-16.

R
E
C
E
S
S
I
V
E

20080 ACHONDROPLASIA

WHETHER ACHONDROPLASIA COMPLETELY INDISTINGUISHABLE FROM THE ACHONDROPLASIA WHICH IS DEMONSTRABLY DOMINANT IS EVER INHERITED AS A RECESSIVE IS A MOOTED MATTER. DOCUMENTATION OF THE DIAGNOSIS IS INADEQUATE IN MOST REPORTS OF POSSIBLE RECESSIVE INHERITANCE. COHN AND WEINBERG (1956) REPORTED AFFECTED TWINS WITH AN AFFECTED SIB. CHIARI (1913) REPORTED AFFECTED HALF-SIBS. THE FATHER WAS THE SAME. I HAVE OBSERVED TWO COUSINS WITH UNDOUBTED ACHONDROPLASIA, A MALE AND FEMALE. THE MOTHERS ARE SISTERS. (THIS MAY HAVE BEEN ACHONDROGENESIS, Q.V.) MOST DOMINANTS SHOW SUFFICIENT VARIABILITY TO ACCOUNT FOR OBSERVATIONS SUCH AS THESE ON THE BASIS OF REDUCED PENETRANCE BUT SUCH IS NOT THE CASE WITH ACHONDROPLASIA. GONADAL MOSAICISM (OR SPERMATOGONIAL MUTATION) IS A POSSIBLE EXPLANATION FOR AFFECTED SIBS FROM NORMAL PARENTS. AFFECTED COUSINS COULD BE COINCIDENCE OF TWO NEW MUTATIONS. DURR (1968) DESCRIBED AN ACHONDROPLASIA-LIKE DISORDER IN TWO SIBS. RETARDATION OF GROWTH, MICROMELIA AND SQUARE ILIAC WINGS RESEMBLED ACHONDROPLASIA. SPINE AND OTHER PELVIC CHANGES OF ACHONDROPLASIA WERE MISSING.

CHIARI, H.* UEBER FAMILIARE CHONDRODYSTROPHIA FOETALIS. MUNCHEN. MED. WSCHR. 60* 248-249, 1913.

COHN, S. AND WEINBERG, A.* IDENTICAL HYDROCEPHALIC ACHONDROPLASTIC TWINS. SUBSEQUENT DELIVERY OF SINGLE SIBLING WITH SAME ABNORMALITY. AM. J. OBSTET. GYNEC. 72* 1346-1348, 1956.

DURR, D. K.* EINE NEUE DYSOSTOSEFORM MIT MIKROMELIE BEI ZWEI GESCHWISTERN. HELV. PAEDIAT. ACTA 23* 184-194, 1968.

*20090 'ACHONDROPLASIA' AND SWISS-TYPE AGAMMAGLOBULINEMIA

DAVIS (1967) STATES THAT AT LEAST FIVE CASES ARE KNOWN TO HIM. THE CASE HE PERSONALLY DESCRIBED WAS A FEMALE INFANT WHOSE PARENTS WERE JEWISH BUT NOT KNOWN TO BE RELATED. THE CHILD DIED AT 2 MONTHS OF AGE. GATTI ET AL. (1969) DESCRIBED AFFECTED BROTHER AND SISTER. THEY SUGGESTED THAT OTHER CASES HAD BEEN REPORTED BY MCKUSICK AND CROSS (1966), DAVIS (1966), FULGINITI ET AL. (1967), ALEXANDER AND DUNBAR (1968).

ALEXANDER, W. J. AND DUNBAR, J. S.* UNUSUAL BONE CHANGES IN THYMIC ALYMPHOPLA-SIA. ANN. RADIOL. 11* 389-394, 1968.

DAVIS, J. A.* A CASE OF SWISS-TYPE AGAMMAGLOBULINAEMIA AND ACHONDROPLASIA. BRIT. J. MED. 2* 1371-1374, 1966.

DAVIS, J. A.* SWISS-TYPE AGAMMAGLOBULINAEMIA AND ACHONDROPLASIA. (LETTER) BRIT. MED. J. 3* 110 ONLY, 1967.

FULGINITI, V. A., HATHAWAY, W. E., PEARLMAN, D. S. AND KEMPE, C. H.* AGAMMAGLO-BULINAEMIA AND ACHONDROPLASIA. (LETTER) BRIT. MED. J. 2* 242 ONLY, 1967.

GATTI, R. A., PLATT, N., POMERANCE, H. H., HONG, R., LANGER, L. O., KAY, H. E. M. AND GOOD, R. A.* HEREDITARY LYMPHOPENIC AGAMMAGLOBULINEMIA ASSOCIATED WITH A DISTINCTIVE FORM OF SHORT-LIMBED DWARFISM AND ECTODERMAL DYSPLASIA. J. PEDIAT. 75* 675-684, 1969.

MCKUSICK, V. A. AND CROSS, H. E.* ATAXIA-TELANGIECTASIA AND SWISS-TYPE AGAMMAGLOBULINEMIA. TWO GENETIC DISORDERS OF THE IMMUNE MECHANISM IN RELATED AMISH SIBSHIPS. J.A.M.A. 195* 739-745, 1966.

*20095 ACID PHOSPHATASE DEFICIENCY

NADLER AND EGAN (1970) DISCOVERED THIS DISORDER. THE CLINICAL FEATURES ARE INTERMITTENT VOMITING, HYPOTONIA, LETHARGY, OPISTHOTONOS, TERMINAL BLEEDING AND DEATH IN EARLY INFANCY. THE LYSOSOMAL ENZYME ACID PHOSPHATASE IS DEFICIENT IN CULTURED FIBROBLASTS AND MULTIPLE TISSUES. PRENATAL DIAGNOSIS WAS POSSIBLE. THE PARENTS WERE FIRST COUSINS. AFTER TREATMENT WITH PHYTOHEMAGGLUTININ, LYMPHOCYTES FROM HETEROZYGOTES AND CONTROLS COULD BE DISTINGUISHED.

NADLER, H. L. AND EGAN, T. J.* DEFICIENCY OF LYSOSOMAL ACID PHOSPHATASE* A NEW FAMILIAL METABOLIC DISORDER. NEW ENG. J. MED. 282* 303-307, 1970.

*20100 ACROCEPHALOPOLYSYNDACTYLY TYPE II (ACPS II, CARPENTER'S SYNDROME)

R
E
C
E
S
S
I
V
E

CARPENTER (1909) DESCRIBED TWO SISTERS AND A BROTHER WITH ACROCEPHALY, PECULIAR FACIES, BRACHYDACTYLY, AND SYNDACTYLY IN THE HANDS, AND PREAXIAL POLYDACTYLY AND SYNDACTYLY OF THE TOES. TEMTAMY (1966) COULD FIND 9 OTHER REPORTED CASES AND ADDED ONE. IN OLDER PATIENTS OBESITY, MENTAL RETARDATION AND HYPOGONADISM HAVE BEEN NOTED. IN ALL CASES THE PARENTS HAVE BEEN NORMAL. PARENTAL CONSANGUINITY WAS SUSPECTED IN ONE CASE. IN THE DOMINANT CATALOG, SEE ACPS I AND SEE POLYSYNDA-CTYLY WITH PECULIAR SKULL SHAPE. THE CASE OF ACROCEPHALOSYNDACTYLY WITH FOOT POLYDACTYLY REPORTED BY OWEN (1952) PROBABLY REPRESENTED THIS ENTITY, AS DO ALSO THE SIBS REPORTED BY SCHONENBERG AND SCHEIDHAUER (1966). ONE PATIENT THOUGHT TO HAVE THIS CONDITION BY PALACIOS AND SCHIMKE (1969) WAS 49 YEARS OLD.

CARPENTER, G.* CASE OF ACROCEPHALY WITH OTHER CONGENITAL MALFORMATIONS. PROC. ROY. SOC. MED. 2* 45-53, 199-201, 1909.

OWEN, R. H.* ACROCEPHALOSYNDACTYLY* A CASE WITH CONGENITAL CARDIAC ABNORMALI-TIES. BRIT. J. RADIOL. 25* 103-106, 1952.

PALACIOS, E. AND SCHIMKE, R. N.* CRANIOSYNOSTOSIS - SYNDACTYLISM. AM. J. ROENTGEN. 106* 144-155, 1969.

SCHONENBERG, H. AND SCHEIDHAUER, E.* UBER ZWEI UNGEWOHNLICHE DYSCRANIO-DYSPHALANGIEN BEI GESCHWISTERN (ATYPISCHE AKROCEPHALOSYNDAKTYLIE UND FRAGLICHE DYSENCEPHALIA SPLANCHNOCYSTICA). MSCHR. KINDERHEILK. 114* 322-327, 1966.

TEMTAMY, S. A.* CARPENTER'S SYNDROME* ACROCEPHALOPOLYSYNDACTYLY. AN AUTOSOMAL RECESSIVE SYNDROME. J. PEDIAT. 69* 111-120, 1966.

*20110 ACRODERMATITIS ENTEROPATHICA

THE DISORDER IS CHARACTERIZED BY INTERMITTENT SIMULTANEOUS OCCURRENCE OF DIARRHEA AND DERMATITIS WITH FAILURE TO THRIVE. ALOPECIA OF THE SCALP, EYEBROWS AND EYELASHES IS A USUAL FEATURE. THE SKIN LESIONS ARE BULLOUS. NOTEWORTHY IS THE CURE BY DIODOQUIN, OR DIIODOHYDROXYQUINOLINE (DILLAHA AND COLLEAGUES, 1953, BLOOM AND SOBEL, 1955). MOYNAHAN ET AL. (1963) FOUND A DEFICIENCY OF SUCCINIC DEHYDRO-GENASE IN INTESTINAL MUCOSAL CELLS BY HISTOCHEMICAL METHODS. ONE OF TWO CASES SHOWED ELECTRON MICROSCOPIC ABNORMALITY. CASH AND BERGER (1969) FOUND DEFECTIVE INTERCONVERSION OF UNSATURATED FATTY ACIDS, IN PARTICULAR, IN THE SYNTHESIS OF ESSENTIAL FATTY ACIDS. RODIN AND GOLDMAN (1969) DESCRIBED AUTOPSY FINDINGS, INCLUDING PANCREATIC ISLET HYPERPLASIA, ABSENCE OF THE THYMUS AND OF GERMINAL CENTERS AND PLASMOCYTOSIS OF LYMPH NODES AND SPLEEN.

BLOOM, D. AND SOBEL, N.* ACRODERMATITIS ENTEROPATHICA SUCCESSFULLY TREATED WITH DIODOQUIN. J. INVEST. DERM. 24* 167-177, 1955.

CASH, R. AND BERGER, C. K.* ACRODERMATITIS ENTEROPATHICA* DEFECTIVE METABOLISM OF UNSATURATED FATTY ACIDS. J. PEDIAT. 74* 717-729, 1969.

DILLAHA, C. J., LORINCZ, A. L. AND AAVIK, O. R.* ACRODERMATITIS ENTEROPATHICA. REVIEW OF THE LITERATURE AND REPORT OF A CASE SUCCESSFULLY TREATED WITH DIODOQUIN. J.A.M.A. 152* 509-512, 1953.

LINDSTROM, B.* FAMILIAL ACRODERMATITIS ENTEROPATHICA IN AN ADULT. ACTA DERMATOVENER. 43* 522-527, 1963.

MARGILETH, A. M.* ACRODERMATITIS ENTEROPATHICA. CASE REPORT AND REVIEW OF LITERATURE. AM. J. DIS. CHILD. 105* 285-291, 1963.

MOYNAHAN, E. J., JOHNSON, F. R. AND MCMINN, R. M. H.* ACRODERMATITIS ENTEROPA-THICA* DEMONSTRATION OF POSSIBLE INTESTINAL ENZYME DEFECT. PROC. ROY. SOC. MED. 56* 300-301, 1963.

RODIN, A. E. AND GOLDMAN, A. S.* AUTOPSY FINDINGS IN ACRODERMATITIS ENTEROPA-THICA. AM. J. CLIN. PATH. 51* 315-322, 1969.

STEVENSON, J. R., FIDONE, G. S. AND LELAND, L. S.* ACRODERMATITIS ENTEROPATHI-CA. ARCH. DERM. 89* 224-228, 1964.

20120 ACROGERIA

GOTTRON (1940) REPORTED A BROTHER AND SISTER, 16 AND 19 YEARS OLD, WHOSE HANDS AND FEET HAD APPEARED OLD SINCE INFANCY BECAUSE OF THIN SKIN. GENERAL PHYSICAL AND MENTAL DEVELOPMENT WERE NORMAL. LESS SEVERE SKIN ATROPHY WAS PRESENT ELSEWHERE. HUTTOVA ET AL. (1967) ALSO DESCRIBED AFFECTED SIBS. THE EHLERS-DANLOS SYNDROME IS OFTEN MIS-DIAGNOSED.

CALVERT, H. T.* ACROGERIA (GOTTRON TYPE). BRIT. J. DERM. 69* 69 ONLY, 1957.

GOTTRON, H.* FAMILIARE AKROGERIE. ARCH. DERM. SYPH. 181* 571-583, 1940.

HUTTOVA, M., RUSNAK, M. AND LYSA, G.* AKROGERIA. CESK. PEDIAT. 22* 233-237, 1967.

20130 ACRO-OSTEOLYSIS, NEUROGENIC

GIACCAI (1952) FOUND FOUR CASES AMONG THE CHILDREN OF AN ARAB MAN WHO MARRIED TWO FIRST COUSINS. BY THE FIRST, ONE OF THE CHILDREN WAS AFFECTED AND BY THE SECOND, THREE OUT OF FIVE WERE AFFECTED. THE SPINAL CORD WAS NORMAL AT AUTOPSY. HE CONCLUDED THAT THE ABNORMALITY RESIDES IN PERIPHERAL SENSORY NERVES. SEE INSENSITIVITY TO PAIN.

GIACCAI, L.* FAMILIAL AND SPORADIC NEUROGENIC ACRO-OSTEOLYSIS. ACTA RADIOL. 38* 17-29, 1952.

HOZAY, J.* SUR UNE DYSTROPHIE FAMILIALE PARTICULIERE (INHIBITION PRECOE DE LA CROISSANCE ET OSTEOLYSE NON MUTILANTE ACRALES AVEC DYSMORPHIE FACIALE). REV. NEUROL. 89* 245-258, 1953.

VAN BOGAERT, L.* FAMILIAL ULCERS, MUTILATING LESIONS OF THE EXTREMITIES AND ACRO-OSTEOLYSIS. BRIT. MED. J. 2* 367-371, 1957.

20140 ACTH DEFICIENCY

HUNG AND MIGEON (1968) DESCRIBED A 34 MONTH OLD NEGRO BOY WITH APPARENT ISOLATED ACTH DEFICIENCY. THE ADRENAL MEDULLA WAS UNRESPONSIVE TO INSULIN-INDUCED HYPOGLYCEMIA. TREATMENT OF THE ADRENOCORTICAL INSUFFICIENCY RESTORED RESPONSI-VENESS. THE ENZYME PHENYLETHANOLAMINE-N-METHYL TRANSFERASE (PNMT) IS LOCALIZED TO THE ADRENAL MEDULLA AND CATALYZES THE N-METHYLATION OF NOREPINEPHRINE TO EPINEPH-RINE. THE ACTIVITY OF THIS ENZYME IS CONTROLLED BY GLUCOCORTICOIDS. NO FAMILIAL CASES HAVE, IT SEEMS, BEEN REPORTED.

HUNG, W. AND MIGEON, C. J.* HYPOGLYCEMIA IN A TWO-YEAR-OLD BOY WITH ADRENOCOR-TICOTROPIC HORMONE (ACTH) DEFICIENCY (PROBABLY ISOLATED) AND ADRENAL MEDULLARY UNRESPONSIVENESS TO INSULIN-INDUCED HYPOGLYCEMIA. J. CLIN. ENDOCR. 28* 146-152, 1968.

ODELL, W. D., GREEN, G. M. AND WILLIAMS, R. H.* HYPOADRENOTROPISM* THE ISOLATED DEFICIENCY OF ADRENOTROPIC HORMONE. J. CLIN. ENDOCR. 20* 1017-1028, 1960.

20150 ADDISON'S DISEASE AND SPASTIC PARAPLEGIA

HARRIS-JONES AND NIXON (1955) DESCRIBED TWO BROTHERS IN WHOM ADDISON'S DISEASE WAS FIRST RECOGNIZED AT 39 AND 40 AND WHO SUBSEQUENTLY DEVELOPED SPASTIC PARAPLEGIA. NO AUTOPSY WAS PERFORMED. A SIMILAR CASE WAS REPORTED BY PENMAN (1960) IN A 28 YEAR OLD WOMAN. THE LATE ONSET AND THE OCCURRENCE IN A FEMALE PATIENT PROBABLY INDICATES THAT THIS IS A DISORDER DISTINCT FROM ADDISON'S DISEASE AND CEREBRAL SCLEROSIS, A WELL-ESTABLISHED X-LINKED RECESSIVE.

HARRIS-JONES, J. N. AND NIXON, P. G. F.* FAMILIAL ADDISON'S DISEASE WITH SPASTIC PARAPLEGIA. J. CLIN. ENDOCR. 15* 739-744, 1955.

PENMAN, R. W. B.* ADDISON'S DISEASE IN ASSOCIATION WITH SPASTIC PARAPLEGIA. BRIT. MED. J. 1* 402 ONLY, 1960.

*20160 ADENYLATE KINASE DEFICIENCY, ANEMIA DUE TO

IN TWO OFFSPRING OF SECOND COUSIN ARAB PARENTS SZEINBERG ET AL. (1969) FOUND MARKED AK DEFICIENCY WITH INTERMEDIATE LEVELS IN THE PRESUMED HETEROZYGOTES. SEVERE ANEMIA WAS PRESENT IN BOTH.

BOIVIN, P., GALAND, C., HAKIM, J., SIMONY, D. AND SELIGMAN, M.* DEFICIT CONGENITAL EN ADENYLATE-KINASE ERYTHROCYTAIRE. (LETTER) PRESSE MED. 78* 1443 ONLY, 1970.

SZEINBERG, A., GAVENDO, S. AND CAHANE, D.* ERYTHROCYTE ADENYLATE-KINASE DEFICIENCY. (LETTER) LANCET 1* 315-316, 1969.

SZEINBERG, A., KAHANA, D., GAVENDO, S., ZAIDMAN, J. AND BEN-EZZER, J.* HEREDITARY DEFICIENCY OF ADENYLATE KINASE IN RED BLOOD CELLS. ACTA HAEMAT. 42* 111-126, 1969.

*20170 ADRENAL HYPERPLASIA I (WITH DEFECT IN 21-HYDROXYLASE)

ALL FORMS OF ADRENAL HYPERPLASIA SHOW SIGNS OF EXCESSIVE SECRETION OF ADRENAL ANDROGENS IN THE FORM OF VIRILIZATION AND RAPID SOMATIC ADVANCE. IN SOME CASES VOMITING AND DEHYDRATION RESEMBLING ADDISONIAN CRISIS DEVELOP WITHIN A FEW WEEKS AFTER BIRTH AND LEAD TO RAPID DETERIORATION AND DEATH. HYPOGLYCEMIA SOMETIMES OCCURS. RECURRENT FEVER ALSO MAY OCCUR AND MAY BE RELATED TO ETIOCHOLANOLONE, ALTHOUGH THIS REMAINS TO BE CLARIFIED. HYPERTENSION OCCURS IN THIS FORM IN ADDITION TO THE OTHER FEATURES. EVEN AFTER BEING PRESENT FOR SEVERAL YEARS IT IS RELIEVED BY STEROID THERAPY. ALL TYPES OF ADRENAL HYPERPLASIA WERE REVIEWED EXHAUSTIVELY BY BONGIOVANNI AND ROOT (1963). PRADER AND COLLEAGUES (1962) REPORTED AN ENORMOUS INTERLOCKING SWISS KINDRED. TWO TYPES OF 21-HYDROXYLASE DEFECT APPEAR TO OCCUR, ONE MILD AND ONE SEVERE. IN THE SEVERE FORM, ALDOSTERONE PRODUCTION IS CURTAILED AND ALDOSTERONE ANTAGONISTS ACCUMULATE LEADING TO SEVERE SALT WASTING AND ADDISONIAN CRISIS. IN FEMALES VIRILIZATION IS USUALLY EVIDENT AT BIRTH. INDEED SOME AFFECTED FEMALES ARE REARED AS MALES. IN THE MALE THE CONDITION IS OFTEN NOT RECOGNIZED UNTIL LATE INFANCY OR CHILDHOOD. OTHER FEATURES OF THE ADRENOGENITAL SYNDROME ARE SALT AND WATER LOSS, HYPERTENSION, POSSIBLY FEVER, AND ADDISONIAN CRISIS. THE COMMON DENOMINATOR OF THE SEVERAL FORMS, IN BOTH MALES AND FEMALES, IS EXCESSIVE SECRETION OF ADRENAL ANDROGENS. (SEE PRECOCIOUS PUBERTY OF MALE IN DOMINANT CATALOG FOR SIMULATING CONDITION.) IN THE CANTON OF ZURICH, SWITZERLAND, PRADER (1958) ESTIMATED THE FREQUENCY TO BE 1 IN 5041 LIVE BIRTHS, GIVING A FREQUENCY OF CARRIERS OF 1 IN 35. CHILDS, GRUMBACH AND VAN WYK (1956) HAD ESTIMATED THE FREQUENCY IN MARYLAND TO BE 1 IN 67,000 BIRTHS. A REMARKABLE AND POSSIBLY SIGNIFICANT FEATURE FROM THE POINT OF VIEW OF SELECTION AND GENE FREQUENCY IS THE FINDING OF LEWIS ET AL. (1968) THAT INTELLIGENCE IS INCREASED IN THE ADRENOGENITAL SYNDROME. MERKATZ ET AL. (1969) COULD NOT DIAGNOSE THE DISORDER EARLY IN PREGNANCY BY AMNIOCENTESIS AND HORMONE ASSAY OF THE AMNIOTIC FLUID. GALAL ET AL. (1969) CONCLUDED THAT THE TWO CLINICAL FORMS OF 21-HYDROXY-LASE DEFICIENCY (WITH AND WITHOUT SALT-LOSING) CORRELATE WITH THE EXTENT OF THE DEFECT IN THE CORTISOL PATHWAY.

R
E
C
E
S
S
I
V
E

BONGIOVANNI, A. M. AND ROOT, A. W.* THE ADRENOGENITAL SYNDROME. NEW ENG. J. MED. 268* 1283-1289, 1342-1351, AND 1391-1399, 1963.

CHILDS, B., GRUMBACH, M. M. AND VAN WYK, J. J.* VIRILIZING ADRENAL HYPERPLASIA* GENETIC AND HORMONAL STUDIES. J. CLIN. INVEST. 35* 213-222, 1956.

GALAL, O. M., RUDD, B. T. AND DRAYER, N. M.* EVALUATION OF DEFICIENCY OF 21-HYDROXYLATION IN PATIENTS WITH CONGENITAL ADRENAL HYPERPLASIA. ARCH. DIS. CHILD. 43* 410-414, 1969.

LEWIS, V. G., MONEY, J. AND EPSTEIN, R.* CONCORDANCE OF VERBAL AND NONVERBAL ABILITY IN THE ADRENOGENITAL SYNDROME. JOHNS HOPKINS MED. J. 122* 192-195, 1968.

MERKATZ, I. R., NEW, M. I., PETERSON, R. E. AND SEAMAN, M. P.* PRENATAL DIAGNOSIS OF ADRENOGENITAL SYNDROME BY AMNIOCENTESIS. J. PEDIAT. 75* 977-982, 1969.

PRADER, A.* DIE HAUFIGKEIT DES KONGENITALEN ADRENOGENITALEN SYNDROMS. HELV. PAEDIAT. ACTA 13* 426-431, 1958.

PRADER, A., ANDERS, G. J. P. A. AND HABICH, H.* ZUR GENETIK DES KONGENITALEN ADRENOGENITALEN SYNDROMS (VIRILISIERENDE NEBENNIERENHYPERPLASIA). HELV. PAEDIAT. ACTA 17* 271-284, 1962.

STEMPFEL, R. S., JR. AND TOMKINS, G. M.* CONGENITAL VIRILIZING ADRENOCORTICAL HYPERPLASIA (THE ADRENOGENITAL SYNDROME). IN, STANBURY, J. B., WYNGAARDEN, J. B. AND FREDRICKSON, D. S. (EDS.)* THE METABOLIC BASIS OF INHERITED DISEASE. NEW YORK* MCGRAW-HILL, 1966 (2ND ED.). PP. 635-664.

*20180 ADRENAL HYPERPLASIA II (WITH DEFECT IN 11-BETA-HYDROXYLASE)

WHEN THE DEFECT INVOLVES THE ENZYME SYSTEM CONCERNED IN HYDROXYLATION OF C11, 11-
DEOXYCORTICOSTERONE, A POTENT SALT-RETAINER, ACCUMULATES, LEADING TO ARTERIAL
HYPERTENSION.

VISSER, H. K. A.* INHERITED VARIATION IN THE BIOSYNTHESIS OF ADRENAL CORTICOS-
TEROIDS IN MAN. IN, ENDOCRINE GENETICS. SPICKETT, S. G. (ED.)* MEM. SOC.
ENDOCRINOLOGY, 1967. PP. 145-178.

*20190 ADRENAL HYPERPLASIA III (WITH DEFECT IN 3-BETA-HYDROXYSTEROID DEHYDROGENASE)

VIRILIZATION IS MUCH LESS MARKED OR DOES NOT OCCUR IN THIS TYPE, SUGGESTING THAT
THE GENE-DETERMINED DEFECT INVOLVES THE TESTIS AS WELL AS THE ADRENAL. MALES WITH
THE DEFECT HAVE HYPOSPADIAS. SALT LOSS IS FREQUENT CAUSE OF DEATH. FOR ANOTHER
GENETIC DISORDER OF THE ADRENAL WITH SALT LOSS, SEE ALDOSTERONE SYNTHESIS, DEFECT
IN.

BONGIOVANNI, A. M.* THE ADRENOGENITAL SYNDROME WITH DEFICIENCY OF 3-BETA-
HYDROXYSTEROID DEHYDROGENASE. J. CLIN. INVEST. 41* 2086-2092, 1962.

HAMILTON, W. AND BRUSH, M. G.* FOUR CLINICAL VARIANTS OF CONGENITAL ADRENAL
HYPERPLASIA. ARCH. DIS. CHILD. 39* 66-72, 1964.

20200 ADRENAL HYPERPLASIA IV (WITH DEFECT IN ENZYME PRIOR TO DELTA 5-PREGNENOLONE)
LIPOID HYPERPLASIA OF ADRENAL CORTEX WITH MALE PSEUDOHERMAPHRODITISM

THIS FORM OF THE SYNDROME IS CHARACTERIZED IN THE MALE BY VARIOUS DEGREES OF
HYPOSPADIAS OR EVEN ALMOST COMPLETE FAILURE OF THE EXTERNAL GENITALIA TO UNDERGO
MASCULINE DEVELOPMENT. IT IS BELIEVED THAT THE GENETIC DEFECT INVOLVES AN ENZYME
NECESSARY FOR THE SYNTHESIS OF BOTH TESTICULAR AND ADRENOCORTICAL HORMONES.
PROBABLY THE TESTES ARE UNABLE TO SECRETE THE FETAL MALE 'INDUCTOR' HORMONE WHICH
RESULTS IN NORMAL MASCULINE GENITAL ORGANOGENESIS. THE NATURE OF THE DEFECT WAS
STATED TO BE UNKNOWN BY BONGIOVANNI AND ROOT (1963). THE FIRST CLUE TO THE
GENETIC BASIS OF THIS SYNDROME WAS THE OBSERVATION OF CONSANGUINITY IN THE PARENTS
OF CASES (PRADER AND SIEBENMANN, 1957). IT IS NOT COMPLETELY CERTAIN THAT THIS
CONDITION DESCRIBED BY PRADER IS DISTINCT FROM TYPE III, ABOVE.

BONGIOVANNI, A. M. AND ROOT, A. W.* THE ADRENOGENITAL SYNDROME. NEW ENG. J.
MED. 268* 1283-1289, 1342-1351, AND 1391-1399, 1963.

CAMACHO, A. M., KOWARSKI, A., MIGEON, C. J. AND BROUGH, A. J.* CONGENITAL
ADRENAL HYPERPLASIA DUE TO A DEFICIENCY OF ONE OF THE ENZYMES INVOLVED IN THE
BIOSYNTHESIS OF PREGNENOLONE. J. CLIN. ENDOCR. 28* 153-161, 1968.

PRADER, A. AND ANDERS, G. J. P. A.* ZUR GENETIK DER KONGENITALEN LIPOIDHYPERP-
LASIE DER NEBENNIEREN. HELV. PAEDIAT. ACTA 17* 285-289, 1962.

PRADER, A. AND SIEBENMANN, R. E.* NEBENNIERENINSUFFIZIENZ BEI KONGENITALER
LIPOIDHYPERPLASIE DER NEBENNIEREN. HELV. PAEDIAT. ACTA 12* 569-595, 1957.

RECESSIVE

20210 ADRENAL HYPERPLASIA V (WITH DEFECT IN 17-HYDROXYLASE)

NEW AND PETERSON (1967) DESCRIBED WHAT THEY SUGGESTED IS A NEW FORM OF ADRENAL
HYPERPLASIA IN A 12 YEAR OLD BOY. FEATURES INCLUDED (1) CLASSIC SIGNS OF PRIMARY
HYPERALDOSTERONISM (MILD HYPERTENSION, HYPOKALEMIC ALKALOSIS, LOW PLASMA RENIN,
HYPERVOLEMIA AND FIXED HYPERALDOSTERONE LEVELS IN BLOOD UNINFLUENCED BY SODIUM
RESTRICTION OR EXCESS), (2) LOW NORMAL PLASMA CORTISOL AND CORTICOSTERONE, (3)
ELEVATED PLASMA ACTH, (4) FALL IN ALDOSTERONE PRODUCTION AND IN BLOOD PRESSURE
DURING TREATMENT WITH GLUCOCORTICOIDS, (5) NORMAL RISE OF PLASMA TESTOSTERONE TO
CHORIONIC GONADOTROPIN. THE FATHER AND TWO NORMOTENSIVE SIBS SHOWED NO ABNORMALI-
TY ON MULTIPLE TESTING BUT THE HYPERTENSIVE MOTHER HAD ABNORMAL ALDOSTERONE
REGULATION. THUS X-LINKED RECESSIVE INHERITANCE IS POSSIBLE. A 17-HYDROXYLASE
DEFECT IN THE KIDNEY BUT NOT THE TESTIS WAS POSTULATED. A DEFICIENCY OF ADRENAL
17-HYDROXYLATION ACTIVITY WAS DEMONSTRATED IN A SINGLE PATIENT BY BIGLIERI ET AL.
(1966). A SIMILAR DEFECT IN THE GONAD WAS SUGGESTED. PRODUCTION OF EXCESSIVE
CORTICOSTERONE AND DEOXYCORTICOSTERONE RESULTED IN HYPERTENSION AND HYPOKALEMIC
ALKALOSIS. ALDOSTERONE SYNTHESIS WAS ALMOST TOTALLY ABSENT. AMENORRHEA WAS
PRESENT. STATURE WAS NORMAL. ALTHOUGH THERE WERE NO OTHER CASES IN THE FAMILY
AND PARENTAL CONSANGUINITY WAS NOT NOTED, RECESSIVE INHERITANCE IS POSSIBLE,
INDEED LIKELY. GOLDSMITH ET AL. (1967) REPORTED A SECOND CASE IN WHOM THE DEFECT
IN 17-ALPHA-HYDROXYLATION MAY HAVE BEEN LESS COMPLETE THAN IN THE FIRST CASE.
AGAIN A SINGLE PERSON WAS AFFECTED - A 26 YEAR OLD WOMAN WITH HYPERTENSION,
PRIMARY AMENORRHEA AND LACK OF SECONDARY SEXUAL CHARACTERISTICS. MALLIN (1969)
DESCRIBED AFFECTED SISTERS. 17-HYDROXYLASE IS NECESSARY FOR BOTH CORTISOL AND
ESTROGEN SYNTHESIS. BECAUSE OF LACK OF THESE HORMONES INCREASE IN ACTH AND FSH
OCCURS. EXCESSIVE SYNTHESIS OF DEOXYCORTICOSTERONE AND CORTICOSTERONE PRODUCE
HYPERTENSION. ESTROGEN LACK RESULTS IN PRIMARY AMENORRHEA AND ABSENT SEXUAL
MATURATION. OVARIAN ENLARGEMENT AND INFARCTION FROM TWISTING ALSO OCCUR. THERAPY
WITH DEXAMETHASONE AND ESTROGEN LOWERS BLOOD PRESSURE AND PRODUCE FEMINIZATION.
NEW (1970) REPORTED THE FIRST AFFECTED MALE. THE CLINICAL FEATURES WERE PSEUDO-
HERMAPHRODITISM WITH AMBIGUOUS EXTERNAL GENITALIA AND PROMINENT BREAST DEVELOPMENT
AT PUBERTY. UNLIKE THE PREVIOUSLY REPORTED FEMALE CASES THIS MALE PATIENT DID NOT
DEMONSTRATE SEVERE HYPERTENSION OR HYPOKALEMIA.

BIGLIERI, E. G., HERRON, M. A. AND BRUST, N.* 17-HYDROXYLATION DEFICIENCY IN MAN. J. CLIN. INVEST. 45* 1946-1954, 1966.

GOLDSMITH, O., SOLOMON, D. H. AND HORTON, R.* HYPOGONADISM AND MINERALOCORTI-COID EXCESS* 17-HYDROXYLASE DEFICIENCY. NEW ENG. J. MED. 277* 673-677, 1967.

MALLIN, S. R.* CONGENITAL ADRENAL HYPERPLASIA SECONDARY TO 17-HYDROXYLASE DEFICIENCY. ANN. INTERN. MED. 70* 69-76, 1969.

NEW, M. I. AND PETERSON, R. E.* A NEW FORM OF CONGENITAL ADRENAL HYPERPLASIA. J. CLIN. ENDOCR. 27* 300-305, 1967.

NEW, M. I.* MALE PSEUDOHERMAPHRODITISM DUE TO 17 ALPHA-HYDROXYLASE DEFICIENCY. J. CLIN. INVEST. 49* 1930-1941, 1970.

*20220 ADRENAL UNRESPONSIVENESS TO ACTH

MIGEON AND COLLEAGUES (1968) HAVE DESCRIBED AN ENTITY OF ADRENAL UNRESPONSIVENESS TO ACTH. FEATURES ARE HYPOGLYCEMIA, HYPERPIGMENTATION, FEEDING PROBLEMS IN INFANCY, LOW URINARY 17-OHCS, NORMAL TOLERANCE TO SALT DEPRIVATION, AND NO ELEVATION OF 17-OHCS EXCRETION OR PLASMA CORTISOL CONCENTRATION WITH ADMINISTRA-TION OF ACTH. TWO OF THEIR PATIENTS WERE BROTHERS. SIBS OF TWO OTHER PATIENTS WERE PROBABLY AFFECTED. AFFECTED MALE AND FEMALE SIBS HAVE BEEN REPORTED (SHEPARD, LANDING, MASON, 1959). FRANKS AND NANCE (1970) OBSERVED THE CONDITION IN TWO SISTERS AND A BROTHER, OFFSPRING OF FIRST COUSIN PARENTS, AND REVIEWED 8 OTHER FAMILIAL CASES. AN EXCESS OF MALES AND A DEFICIENCY OF CONSANGUINITY SUGGESTED THE EXISTENCE OF BOTH AUTOSOMAL AND X-LINKED RECESSIVE FORMS. PLASMA ACTH LEVELS WERE GREATLY ELEVATED.

FRANKS, R. C. AND NANCE, W. E.* HEREDITARY ADRENOCORTICAL UNRESPONSIVENESS TO ACTH. PEDIATRICS 45* 43-48, 1970.

MIGEON, C. J., KENNY, E. M., KOWARSKI, A., SNIPES, C. A., SPAULDING, J. S., FINKELSTEIN, J. W. AND BLIZZARD, R. M.* THE SYNDROME OF CONGENITAL ADRENOCORTICAL UNRESPONSIVENESS TO ACTH. REPORT OF SIX CASES. PEDIAT. RES. 2* 501-513, 1968.

SHEPARD, T. H., LANDING, B. H. AND MASON, D. G.* FAMILIAL ADDISON'S DISEASE. CASE REPORTS OF TWO SISTERS WITH CORTICOID DEFICIENCY UNASSOCIATED WITH HYPOALDOS-TERONISM. AM. J. DIS. CHILD. 97* 154-162, 1959.

STEMPFEL, R. S., JR. AND ENGEL, F. L.* A CONGENITAL, FAMILIAL SYNDROME OF ADRENOCORTICAL INSUFFICIENCY WITHOUT HYPOALDOSTERONISM. J. PEDIAT. 57* 443-451, 1960.

20230 ADRENOCORTICAL CARCINOMA

FRAUMENI AND MILLER (1967) MENTIONED AFFECTED SIBS. MAHLOUDJI ET AL. (1970) OBSERVED AFFECTED BROTHER AND SISTER WHO WERE PRODUCTS OF A CONSANGUINEOUS UNION. NICHOLS (1968) ALSO DESCRIBED AFFECTED BROTHER AND SISTER.

FRAUMENI, J. F., JR. AND MILLER, R. W.* ADRENOCORTICAL NEOPLASMS WITH HEMIHY-PERTROPHY, BRAIN TUMORS, AND OTHER DISORDERS. J. PEDIAT. 70* 129-138, 1967.

MAHLOUDJI, M., RONAGHI, H. AND DUTZ, W.* FAMILIAL ADRENAL CORTICAL CARCINOMA. TO BE PUBLISHED, 1970.

NICHOLS, J.* ADRENAL CORTEX. IN, BLOODWORTH, J. M. B. (ED.)* BALTIMORE* WILLIAMS AND WILLIAMS CO., 1968.

*20240 AFIBRINOGENEMIA, CONGENITAL

RELATIVELY FEW CASES HAVE BEEN REPORTED. HOWEVER, THE HIGH PROPORTION WITH CONSANGUINEOUS PARENTS AND-OR AFFECTED SIBS MAKES RECESSIVE INHERITANCE VERY LIKELY. THE BLOOD IS COMPLETELY INCOAGULABLE, YET SOME OF THE AFFECTED PERSONS HAVE REMARKABLY LITTLE TROUBLE WITH BLEEDING. IN SOME CASES THE DISORDER WAS DETECTED AT BIRTH BECAUSE OF EXCESS BLEEDING FROM THE UMBILICAL STUMP. A PARTIAL DEFICIENCY OF FIBRINOGEN HAS BEEN OBSERVED IN PARENTS AND OTHER HETEROZYGOTES. IN TWO BROTHERS REPORTED BY LEMOINE ET AL. (1963) CONGENITAL AFIBRINOGENEMIA WAS ASSOCIATED WITH OSSEOUS AND HEPATIC LESIONS, THOUGHT TO BE OF HEMORRHAGIC ORIGIN.

BOMMER, W., KUNZER, W. AND SCHROER, H.* KONGENITALE AFIBRINOGENAMIE. ANN. PAEDIAT. 200* 46-59, 1963.

BRONNIMANN, R.* KONGENITALE AFIBRINOGENAMIE. ACTA HAEMAT. 11* 40-51, 1954.

LAWSON, H. A.* CONGENITAL AFIBRINOGENEMIA* REPORT OF A CASE. NEW ENG. J. MED. 248* 552-554, 1953.

LEMOINE, P., HAROUSSEAU, H., GUIMBRETIERE, J., LENNE, Y. AND ANGEBAUD, Y.* AFIBRINEMIE CONGENITALE CHEZ DEUX FRERES AVEC LESIONS OSSEUSES ET HEPATIQUES. ARCH. FRANC. PEDIAT. 20* 463-483, 1963.

R
E
C
E
S
S
I
V
E

PRICHARD, R. W. AND VANN, R. L.* CONGENITAL AFIBRINOGENAEMIA* REPORT ON A CHILD WITHOUT FIBRINOGEN AND REVIEW OF THE LITERATURE. AM. J. DIS. CHILD. 88* 703-710, 1954.

WERDER, E.* KONGENITALE AFIBRINOGENAMIE. HELV. PAEDIAT. ACTA 18* 208-229, 1963.

*20250 AGAMMAGLOBULINEMIA, SWISS OR ALYMPHOCYTOTIC TYPE

IN ADDITION TO THE MORE FREQUENT X-LINKED VARIETY, A PRESUMED AUTOSOMAL RECESSIVE FORM HAS BEEN DESCRIBED BY SEVERAL AUTHORS. GOOD (1963) REFERRED TO THE LATTER AS THE SWISS TYPE OF AGAMMAGLOBULINEMIA. UNLIKE THE X-LINKED VARIETY, THE PATIENT IS UNUSUALLY SUSCEPTIBLE TO FUNGAL AND VIRAL AS WELL AS PYOGENIC PATHOGENS AND LACKS DELAYED HYPERSENSITIVITY AS WELL AS SHOWING FAILURE OF ANTIBODY PRODUCTION. FURTHERMORE, THE THYMUS IS VERY SMALL AND SHOWS LACK OF LYMPHOID CELLS AND HASSALL'S CORPUSCLES, WHEREAS IT MAY BE QUITE NORMAL IN THE X-LINKED FORM. COOPER, PETERSON AND GOOD (1965) HAVE SUGGESTED THAT BOTH THE THYMUS SYSTEM RESPONSIBLE FOR CELLULAR IMMUNITY AND THE TONSILLAR SYSTEM RESPONSIBLE FOR IMMUNOGLOBULIN PRODUCTION ARE ABSENT IN THIS DISORDER WHEREAS ONLY THE LATTER IS AFFECTED IN BRUTON TYPE AGAMMAGLOBULINEMIA (X-LINKED FORM). ONLY THE THYMUS SYSTEM MAY BE DEFECTIVE IN THE DISORDER DESCRIBED UNDER IMMUNE DEFECT DUE TO ABSENCE OF THYMUS (Q.V.). SEE ATAXIA-TELANGIECTASIA FOR POSSIBLE RELATIONSHIP TO THAT DISORDER. THIS DISORDER IS RELATIVELY FREQUENT AMONG MENNONITES LIVING IN SOUTHERN MANITOBA (HAWORTH ET AL., 1967). HETEROGENEITY IN THE AUTOSOMAL RECESSIVE IMMUNE DISORDERS IS INDICATED BY THE REPORT OF LIPSEY ET AL. (1967) OF THREE FAMILIES WITH MULTIPLE SIBS WITH AN IMMUNE DISORDER WHICH DEFIES CLASSIFICA- TION. THE THREE PROBANDS DIED IN THE FIRST THREE YEARS OF LIFE OF PNEUMONIA.

COMINGS, D. E.* A THIRD GAMMA-GLOBJLIN CHAIN.Q (LETTER) LANCET 2* 786, 1963.

COOPER, M. D., PETERSON, R. D. AND GOOD, R. A.* *NEW* CONCEPT OF THE CELLULAR BASIS OF IMMUNITY. (ABSTRACT) J. PEDIAT. 67* 907-908, 1965.

GREENWOOD, R. D., TRAISMAN, H. S., RICE, H. M. AND OH-PAIK, S. G.* SWISS TYPE AGAMMAGLOBULINEMIA IN THE UNITED STATES. AM. J. DIS. CHILD. 121* 30-34, 1971.

GITLIN, D., JANEWAY, C. A., APT, C. AND CRAIG, J. M.* AGAMMAGLOBULINEMIA. IN, LAURENCE, H. S. (ED.)* CELLULAR AND HUMORAL ASPECTS OF HYPERSENSITIVE STATES. NEW YORK* HOEBER-HARPER, 1959.

GITLIN, D., ROSEN, F. S. AND JANEWAY, C. A.* UNDUE SUSCEPTIBILITY TO INFECTION. PEDIAT. CLIN. N. AM. 9* 405-423, 1962.

GOOD, R. A.* IMMUNOLOGIC COMPETENCE - ITS DEVELOPMENT AND RELATION TO THYMUS FUNCTION. SEC. INTERN. CONF. ON CONG. MALFORMATIONS, 1963.

GOOD, R. A., KELLEY, W. D., ROTSTEIN, J. AND VARCO, R. L.* AGAMMAGLOBULINEMIA, HYPOGAMMAGLOBULINEMIA, HODGKIN'S DISEASE AND SARCOIDOSIS. PROGR. ALLERG. 6* 187- 319, 1962.

HAWORTH, J. C., HOOGSTRATEN, J. AND TAYLOR, H.* THYMIC ALYMPHOPLASIA. ARCH. DIS. CHILD. 42* 40-54, 1967.

HITZIG, W. H. AND WILLI, H.* HEREDITARE LYMPHO-PLASMOCYTARE DYSGENESIE ('ALYMPHOCYTOSE MIT AGAMMAGLOBULINAMIE'). SCHWEIZ. MED. WSCHR. 91* 1625-1633, 1961.

HITZIG, W. H.* THE SWISS TYPE OF AGAMMAGLOBULINEMIA. IN, GOOD, R. A. (ED.)* IMMUNOLOGIC DEFICIENCY DISEASES. NEW YORK* NATIONAL FOUNDATION, 1968. PP. 82-90.

LIPSEY, A. I., KAHN, M. J. AND BOLANDE, R. P.* PATHOLOGIC VARIANTS OF CONGENI- TAL HYPOGAMMAGLOBULINEMIA* AN ANALYSIS OF 3 PATIENTS DYING OF MEASLES. PEDIATRICS 39* 659-674, 1967.

ROSEN, F. S., GITLIN, D. AND JANEWAY, C. A.* ALYMPHOCYTOSIS, AGAMMAGLOBULINAE- MIA, HOMOGRAFTS, AND DELAYED HYPERSENSITIVITY* REPORT OF A CASE. LANCET 2* 380- 381, 1962.

TOBLER, R. AND COTTIER, H.* FAMILIARE LYMPHOPENIE MIT AGAMMAGLOBULINAEMIE UND SCHWERER MONILIASIS. HELV. PAEDIAT. ACTA 13* 313-338, 1958.

20260 AGENESIS OF CEREBRAL WHITE MATTER

WAGGONER ET AL. (1942) DESCRIBED SIX SISTERS IN A SIBSHIP OF 11 WITH AGENESIS OF THE WHITE MATTER AND IDIOCY, SURVIVING TO ADULTHOOD. THE FAMILY WAS OF FINNISH EXTRACTION. NO PARENTAL CONSANGUINITY WAS KNOWN.

WAGGONER, R. W., LOWENBERG-SCHARENBERG, K. AND SCHILLING, M. E.* AGENESIS OF WHITE MATTER WITH IDIOCY. AM. J. MENT. DEFIC. 47* 20-24, 1942.

*20270 AGRANULOCYTOSIS, INFANTILE GENETIC, OF KOSTMANN

R
E
C
E
S
S
I
V
E

IN ADDITION TO KOSTMANN'S AGRANULOCYTOSIS, RECESSIVELY INHERITED NEUTROPENIC SYNDROMES INCLUDE (1) NEUTROPENIA, CONGENITAL, WITH EOSINOPHILIA. (2) CHEDIAK-HIGASHI SYNDROME, AND (3) FANCONI PANCYTOPENIC SYNDROME. HEDENBERG (1959) FOUND THAT ADDITION OF SULFUR-CONTAINING AMINO ACIDS TO TISSUE CULTURES LED TO MATURATION OF WHITE CELLS.

ANDREWS, J. P., MCCLELLAN, J. T. AND SCOTT, C. H.* LETHAL CONGENITAL NEUTROPENIA WITH EOSINOPHILIA OCCURRING IN TWO SIBLINGS. AM. J. MED. 29* 358-362, 1960.

HEDENBERG, F.* INFANTILE AGRANULOCYTOSIS OF PROBABLY CONGENITAL ORIGIN. ACTA PAEDIAT. 48* 77-84, 1959.

KOSTMANN, R.* INFANTILE GENETIC AGRANULOCYTOSIS (AGRANULOCYTOSIS INFANTILIS HEREDITARIA)* A NEW RECESSIVE LETHAL DISEASE IN MAN. UPPSALA* ALMUVIST AND WIKSELLS BOKTRYCKERI, 1956.

20280 ALACRIMIA CONGENITA

KRUGER (1954) DESCRIBED BROTHER AND SISTER WITH PTOSIS, DISTICHIASIS, CONJUNCTIVITIS, KERATITIS, AND ALACRIMIA CONGENITA. THE FATHER AND ANOTHER BROTHER WERE SAID TO HAVE DEFECTIVE LACRIMATION. A NUCLEAR DEFECT WAS POSTULATED.

KRUGER, K. E.* ANGEBORENES FEHLEN DER TRANENSEKRETION IN EINER FAMILIE. KLIN. MBL. AUGENHEILK. 124* 711-713, 1954.

20290 ALANINURIA WITH MICROCEPHALY, DWARFISM, ENAMEL HYPOPLASIA, DIABETES MELLITUS

STIMMLER ET AL. (1970) DESCRIBED TWO SISTERS BORN IN 1963 AND 1964 WITH MICROCEPHALY AT BIRTH, LOW BIRTH WEIGHT, SEVERE MENTAL RETARDATION AND DWARFISM, SMALL TEETH, AND DIABETES MELLITUS. EXCESSIVE QUANTITIES OF ALANINE WERE FOUND IN THE URINE. ALANINE, PYRUVATE AND LACTATE WERE ELEVATED IN THE BLOOD. PYRUVATE WAS THOUGHT TO BE A SOURCE OF THE ALANINE. THE AUTHORS CONTRASTED THE FINDINGS WITH THOSE IN THE CONDITION DESCRIBED BY HAWORTH ET AL. (1967) AND IN LEIGH'S SUBACUTE NECROTIZING ENCEPHALOPATHY WITH LACTIC ACIDOSIS (WORSLEY ET AL., 1965). THE MAIN DIFFERENCES WERE ELEVATED PLASMA CHLORIDE AND LACK OF HYPERALANINEMIA IN THE OTHER TWO CONDITIONS.

HAWORTH, J. C., FORD, J. D. AND YOUNOSZAI, M. K.* FAMILIAL CHRONIC ACIDOSIS DUE TO AN ERROR IN LACTATE AND PYRUVATE METABOLISM. CANAD. MED. ASS. J. 97* 773-779, 1967.

STIMMLER, L., JENSEN, N. AND TOSELAND, P.* ALANINURIA, ASSOCIATED WITH MICROCEPHALY, DWARFISM, ENAMEL HYPOPLASIA, AND DIABETES MELLITUS IN TWO SISTERS. ARCH. DIS. CHILD. 45* 682-685, 1970.

WORSLEY, H. E., BROOKFIELD, R. W., ELWOOD, J. S., NOBLE, R. L. AND TAYLOR, W. H.* LACTIC ACIDOSIS WITH NECROTIZING ENCEPHALOPATHY IN TWO SIBS. ARCH. DIS. CHILD. 40* 492-501, 1965.

20300 ALAR-NASAL CARTILAGES, COLOBOMA OF, WITH TELECANTHUS

RIMOIN (1969) DESCRIBED TWO SISTERS WITH AN IDENTICAL MALFORMATION OF THE NOSE CONSISTING MAINLY OF HYPOPLASIA AND COLOBOMA OF THE ALAR CARTILAGES. BOTH ALSO SHOWED TELECANTHUS. THE PARENTS AND OTHER RELATIVES WERE UNAFFECTED AND NO PARENTAL CONSANGUINITY WAS REPORTED.

RIMOIN, D. L.* HYPOPLASIA AND COLOBOMA OF THE ALAR-NASAL CARTILAGES WITH PSEUDOHYPERTELORISM IN SIBS. THE CLINICAL DELINEATION OF BIRTH DEFECTS. II. MALFORMATION SYNDROMES. NEW YORK* NATIONAL FOUNDATION, 1969. PP. 224-225.

*20310 ALBINISM I

AMELANIC MELANOCYTES ARE PRESENT IN THE SKIN OF ALBINOS. THESE CONTAIN GRANULES SIMILAR TO THE PREMELANOSOMES OF NORMAL MELANOCYTES. THE NATURE OF THE BASIC DEFECT IS UNKNOWN. IN MICE THE NON-ALPHA HEMOGLOBIN LOCUS IS LINKED TO THE ALBINISM LOCUS. THEREFORE, THE FAMILY WITH BOTH ALBINISM AND SICKLEMIA, REPORTED BY MASSIE AND HARTMANN (1957), IS OF INTEREST. FROGGATT (1960) ESTIMATED A PHENOTYPE FREQUENCY OF 1 IN 10,000 IN NORTHERN IRELAND. FIRST COUSIN MARRIAGES OCCURRED IN 4.5 PERCENT OF THE PARENTS. AN EXCESS OF MALES WAS ALMOST EXCLUSIVELY IN THE PROBANDS AND THE SEX RATIO OF SECONDARY CASES WAS ABOUT 1* THEREFORE, BIAS OF ASCERTAINMENT PROBABLY ACCOUNTED FOR THE EXCESS OF MALES. THE MUTATION RATE WAS ESTIMATED TO BE BETWEEN 3.3 AND 7 X 10-5 PER GENE PER GENERATION. ABNORMAL IRIS TRANSLUCENCY, OCCURRING IN 70 PERCENT OF THE PARENTS AND CHILDREN OF ALBINOS, WAS INTERPRETED AS A HETEROZYGOUS MANIFESTATION. KEELER (1953) IN DESCRIBING ALBINISM IN THE CARIBE CUNA INDIANS COMMENTED ON THE ABUNDANT STRAIGHT WHITE DOWN CONSISTING OF HAIRS UP TO TWO AND ONE HALF CM IN LENGTH WHICH DEVELOPS ON THE BODY AND EXTREMITIES. IT IS NOT CLEAR THAT THIS INDICATES GENETIC DISTINCTNESS BUT MAY SOMEHOW BE RELATED TO THE EXPOSURE OF THE SUBJECTS. PARTIAL ALBINISM IN ASSOCIATION WITH DEAFMUTISM OCCURS AS A DOMINANT TRAIT IN WAARDENBURG SYNDROME (Q.V.). PIPKIN AND PIPKIN (1942) CLAIMED DOMINANT INHERITANCE FOR TOTAL ALBINISM WITHOUT OTHER FEATURES IN ONE FAMILY, BUT A QUASIDOMINANT PEDIGREE PATTERN OF THE USUAL RECESSIVE FORMS SEEMS QUITE LIKELY. WORKING WITH ALBINO MELANOMAS AND TYROSINASE

R
E
C
E
S
S
I
V
E

INHIBITOR IN ANIMALS, CHIAN AND WILGRAM (1967) FOUND THAT THE INHIBITOR IS EFFECTIVE AGAINST SOLUBLE TYROSINASE BUT NOT AGAINST TYROSINASE AGGREGATED INTO MELANOSOMES. IN ONE TYPE OF ALBINO MUTATION, TYROSINASE APPARENTLY COULD NOT AGGREGATE BECAUSE OF GENETIC ALTERATION IN ITS PROTEIN CARRIER AND THEREFORE WAS VULNERABLE TO THE EFFECTS OF THE INHIBITOR. THESE WORKERS SUGGESTED THAT A SIMILAR SITUATION MAY OBTAIN IN SOME TYPE OF ALBINISM OF MAN.

CHIAN, L. T. Y. AND WILGRAM, G. F.* TYROSINASE INHIBITION* ITS ROLE IN SUNTANNING AND IN ALBINISM. SCIENCE 155* 198-200, 1967.

FITZPATRICK, T. B. AND QUEVEDO, W. C., JR.* ALBINISM. IN, STANBURY, J. B., WYNGAARDEN, J. B. AND FREDRICKSON, D. S. (EDS.)* THE METABOLIC BASIS OF INHERITED DISEASE. NEW YORK* MCGRAW-HILL, 1966 (2ND ED.). PP. 324-340.

FROGGATT, P.* ALBINISM IN NORTHERN IRELAND. ANN. HUM. GENET. 24* 213-238, 1960.

HANHART, E.* UBER 18 LEBENDE UND 13 VERSTORBENE ALBINOS IN EINEM DORF DES PIEMONT NEBST WEITEREN BEITRAGEN ZUR POPULATIONSGENETIK DES ALBINISMUS UNIVERSALIS. ARCH. KLAUS STIFT. VERERBUNGSFORSCH. 27* 178-188, 1952.

KEELER, C. E.* THE CARIBE CUNA MOON-CHILD AND ITS HEREDITY. J. HERED. 44* 163-171, 1953.

MASSIE, R. W. AND HARTMANN, R. C.* ALBINISM AND SICKLEMIA IN A NEGRO FAMILY. AM. J. HUM. GENET. 9* 127-132, 1957.

PIPKIN, A. C. AND PIPKIN, S. B.* ALBINISM IN NEGROES. J. HERED. 33* 419-427, 1942.

*20320 ALBINISM II

THE EVIDENCE FOR A SECOND NON-ALLELIC FORM OF RECESSIVE ALBINISM IS DERIVED MAINLY FROM THE FAMILY REPORTED BY TREVOR-ROPER (1952, 1963). TWO ALBINO PARENTS HAD FOUR NORMALLY PIGMENTED CHILDREN. ASSUMING PATERNITY (AND BLOOD GROUPS PROVIDED NO REASON TO QUESTION IT), IT IS POSSIBLE THAT THE FATHER HAD X-LINKED OCULAR ALBINISM AND A LIGHT COMPLEXION. HOWEVER, IF SUCH WERE THE CASE, HIS DAUGHTERS, NECESSARILY HETEROZYGOUS FOR THE X-LINKED GENE, SHOULD HAVE HAD THE MOSAIC PIGMENTARY PATTERN CHARACTERISTIC OF THE FUNDUS OCULI IN THE HETEROZYGOTE. SUCH WAS NOT FOUND. THE EXISTENCE OF MORE THAN ONE LOCUS MAY ALSO BE SUPPORTED BY THE FACT THAT THE RATE OF PARENTAL CONSANGUINITY IS HIGHER THAN WOULD BE EXPECTED IF ONLY ONE LOCUS WERE INVOLVED. FINALLY, APPLYING THE CHEMICAL METHOD OF KUGELMAN AND VAN SCOTT (1961), WITKOP (1962) FOUND SUGGESTIVE EVIDENCE OF SEPARATE FORMS OF ALBINISM. WITKOP (1966) EXAMINED TREVOR-ROPER'S FAMILY AND FOUND THAT WHEREAS THE MOTHER DID NOT SHOW PIGMENTATION IN THE KUGELMAN-VAN SCOTT TEST, THE FATHER DID SHOW PIGMENT.

RECESSIVE

IT SEEMS CLEAR THAT THERE IS A SEPARATE RECESSIVELY INHERITED CONDITION CALLED ALBINOIDISM CHARACTERIZED BY OCULAR ALBINISM, NYSTAGMUS, MYOPIA AND REDUCED PIGMENTATION GENERALLY. THE DEFICIENCY IN PIGMENTATION IS STRIKING EARLY IN LIFE, BUT AS THE AFFECTED PERSON GROWS OLDER THE HAIR AND SKIN DARKEN. HETEROZYGOTES DO NOT SHOW THE MOSAIC PIGMENTARY PATTERN OF THE FUNDUS AS DO THE CARRIERS FOR X-LINKED OCULAR ALBINISM. PROBABLY IN THE FAMILY REPORTED BY TREVOR-ROPER THE MOTHER HAD TRUE ALBINISM AND THE FATHER HAD ALBINOIDISM. KLEIN (1961) REFERRED TO ALBINOIDISM AS UNIVERSAL INCOMPLETE ALBINISM. NANCE ET AL. (1970) DESCRIBED A DISTINCTIVE FORM OF RECESSIVE ALBINISM IN AN AMISH ISOLATE. AFFECTED PERSONS SHOWED PROFOUND GENERALIZED ALBINISM AT BIRTH BUT DEVELOPED NORMAL SKIN PIGMENTATION AND YELLOW HAIR BY AGE TWO, ALTHOUGH PERSISTENT OCULAR ALBINISM AND NYSTAGMUS PERMITTED DIAGNOSIS IN THE ADULT. RESULTS OF HAIR-BULB INCUBATION STUDIES WERE CONSIDERED TO BE INTERMEDIATE BETWEEN THOSE OF TYROSINASE-POSITIVE AND TYROSINASE-NEGATIVE ALBINISM.

KLEIN, D.* LES DIVERSES FORMES HEREDITAIRES DE L'ALBINISME. BULL. ACAD. SERBE. SCI. (BULL. SCHWEIZ. AKAD. MED. WISS.) 17* 351-364, 1961.

KUGELMAN, T. P. AND VAN SCOTT, E.* TYROSINASE ACTIVITY IN MELANOCYTES OF HUMAN ALBINOS. J. INVEST. DERM. 37* 73-76, 1961.

MCKUSICK, V. A. AND COLLEAGUES* MEDICAL GENETICS 1963. J. CHRONIC DIS. 17* 1077-1215, 1964.

NANCE, W. E., JACKSON, C. E. AND WITKOP, C. J., JR.* AMISH ALBINISM* A DISTINCTIVE AUTOSOMAL RECESSIVE PHENOTYPE. AM. J. HUM. GENET. 22* 579-586, 1970.

NANCE, W. E., WITKOP, C. J. AND RAWLS, R. F.* GENETIC AND BIOCHEMICAL EVIDENCE FOR TWO FORMS OF OCULOCUTANEOUS ALBINISM IN MAN. THE CLINICAL DELINEATION OF BIRTH DEFECTS. VIII. EYE. BALTIMORE* WILLIAMS AND WILKINS, 1970.

TREVOR-ROPER, P. D.* MARRIAGE OF TWO COMPLETE ALBINOS WITH NORMALLY PIGMENTED OFFSPRING. BRIT. J. OPHTHAL. 36* 107-110, 1952, AND PROC. ROY. SOC. MED. 56* 21-24, 1963.

WAARDENBURG, P. J.* GENETICS AND OPHTHALMOLOGY. SPRINGFIELD, ILL.* CHARLES C

WITKOP, C. J., JR.* BETHESDA, MD.* PERSONAL COMMUNICATION, 1966.

WITKOP, C. J., JR.* DENTAL PROBLEMS OF AN HEREDITARY NATURE. IN, WITKOP, C. J. (ED.)* GENETICS AND DENTAL HEALTH. NEW YORK* MCGRAW-HILL, 1962.

WITKOP, C. J., JR., VAN SCOTT, E. J. AND JACOBY, G. A.* EVIDENCE FOR TWO FORMS OF AUTOSOMAL RECESSIVE ALBINISM IN MAN. PROC. SEC. INTERN. CONG. HUM. GENET. (ROME, SEPT. 6-12, 1961.) 2* 1064-1065, 1963.

*20330 ALBINISM WITH HEMORRHAGIC DIATHESIS AND PIGMENTED RETICULOENDOTHELIAL CELLS

HERMANSKY AND PUDLAK (1959) DESCRIBED TWO UNRELATED ALBINOS WITH LIFELONG BLEEDING TENDENCY AND PECULIAR PIGMENTED RETICULAR CELLS IN THE BONE MARROW AS WELL AS IN LYMPH NODE AND LIVER BIOPSIES. ONE WAS MALE AND ONE FEMALE* BOTH WERE 33 YEARS OLD. THE FEMALE HAS SINCE DIED AND WAS FOUND TO HAVE LARGE AMOUNTS OF THE PIGMENT IN RETICULOENDOTHELIAL CELLS EVERYWHERE AND IN THE WALLS OF SMALL BLOOD VESSELS (HERMANSKY, 1963). TWO FAMILIES, EACH WITH TWO SIBS AFFECTED WITH THIS SYNDROME, HAVE COME TO HERMANSKY'S ATTENTION (1963). THIS SYNDROME IS CLEARLY DIFFERENT FROM THE CHEDIAK-HIGASHI SYNDROME (Q.V.) BECAUSE NO QUALITATIVE CHANGES OF LEUKOCYTES ARE FOUND IN HERMANSKY'S SYNDROME AND NO PIGMENTED MACROPHAGES ARE FOUND IN THE CHEDIAK-HIGASHI SYNDROME. REPORT OF A FAMILY BY VERLOOP ET AL. (1964) SUPPORTS THIS CONCLUSION.

HERMANSKY, F. AND PUDLAK, P.* ALBINISM ASSOCIATED WITH HEMORRHAGIC DIATHESIS AND UNUSUAL PIGMENTED RETICULAR CELLS IN THE BONE MARROW* REPORT OF TWO CASES WITH HISTOCHEMICAL STUDIES. BLOOD 14* 162-169, 1959.

HERMANSKY, F.* PRAGUE, CZECHOSLOVAKIA* PERSONAL COMMUNICATION, 1963.

VERLOOP, M. C., VON WIERINGEN, A., VUYLSTEKE, J., HART, H. C. AND HUIZINGA, J.* ALBINISMUS, HEMORRHAGISCHE DIATHESE UND ANOMALE PIGMENTZELLEN IM KNOCKENMARK. MED. KLIN. 59* 408-412, 1964.

*20340 ALDOSTERONE DEFICIENCY, DUE TO, DEFECT IN 18-HYDROXYLASE OR 18-DEHYDROGENASE

R
E
C
E
S
S
I
V
E

VISSER AND COST (1964) DESCRIBED THREE INFANTS WITH A TYPICAL CLINICAL PICTURE CONSISTING OF DEHYDRATION, OCCASIONAL VOMITING, POOR FEEDING, FAILURE TO GAIN WEIGHT, INTERMITTENT FEVER, HYPERNATREMIA, AND HYPOKALEMIA. DOCA WAS SUCCESSFUL IN THE TREATMENT OF THESE CASES. ALL SIX PARENTS OF THE THREE PATIENTS SHARED A GREAT-GRANDPARENTAL ANCESTRAL COUPLE IN COMMON. THE TOTAL URINARY EXCRETION OF 17-KETOSTEROIDS, 17 KETOGENIC STEROIDS AND 17-HYDROXYCORTICOSTEROIDS WAS NORMAL. NO ALDOSTERONE WAS DETECTED. AUTOPSY IN ONE INFANT SHOWED THE ADRENALS TO BE GROSSLY NORMAL, BUT ON MICROSCOPIC EXAMINATION THE ZONA GLOMERULOSA SHOWED TUBULAR AND EMPTY AREAS. THE FINDINGS SUGGESTED A DEFECT IN 18-OXIDATION, WHICH WOULD BE EXPECTED TO AFFECT BIOSYNTHESIS OF ALDOSTERONE AT THE STEP BETWEEN CORTICOSTERONE AND ALDOSTERONE. DAVID ET AL. (1968) CONCLUDED THAT THE ENZYMATIC DEFECT IS IN THE DEHYDROGENATION OF 18-HYDROXYCORTICOSTERONE TO ALDOSTERONE. THE CLINICAL MANIFESTATIONS MAY BE SUBTLE. GROWTH RETARDATION WAS THE LEADING FEATURE IN TWO INFANT PUERTO RICAN SIBS REPORTED BY DAVID ET AL. (1968). ABNORMALITY IN SERUM ELECTROLYTES WAS TRANSIENT IN ONE. RAPPAPORT ET AL. (1968) OBSERVED TWO BROTHERS WITH A SALT-LOSING SYNDROME DUE TO 18-OH-DEHYDROGENASE DEFICIENCY. SPONTANEOUS IMPROVEMENT OCCURRED.

DAVID, R., GOLAN, S. AND DRUCKER, W.* FAMILIAL ALDOSTERONE DEFICIENCY* ENZYME DEFECT, DIAGNOSIS AND CLINICAL COURSE. PEDIATRICS 41* 403-412, 1968.

RAPPAPORT, R., DRAY, F., LEGRAND, J. C. AND ROYER, P.* HYPOALDOSTERONISME CONGENITAL FAMILIAL PAR DEFAUT DE LA 18-OH-DEHYDROGENASE. PEDIAT. RES. 2* 456-463, 1968.

ULICK, S., GAUTIER, E., VETTER, K. K., MARKELLO, J. R., YAFFE, S. AND LOWE, C. U.* AN ALDOSTERONE BIOSYNTHETIC DEFECT IN A SALT-LOSING DISORDER. J. CLIN. ENDOCR. 24* 669-672, 1964.

VISSER, H. K. A. AND COST, W. S.* A NEW HEREDITARY DEFECT IN THE BIOSYNTHESIS OF ALDOSTERONE* URINARY C(21)-CORTICOSTEROID PATTERN IN THREE RELATED PATIENTS WITH A SALT-LOSING SYNDROME, SUGGESTING AN 18-OXIDATION DEFECT. ACTA ENDOCR. 47* 589-612, 1964.

*20350 ALKAPTONURIA

ALKAPTONURIA ENJOYS THE HISTORIC DISTINCTION OF BEING ONE OF THE FIRST CONDITIONS IN WHICH MENDELIAN RECESSIVE INHERITANCE WAS PROPOSED (BY GARROD, 1902, ON THE SUGGESTION OF BATESON) AND OF BEING ONE OF THE FOUR CONDITIONS IN THE CHARTER GROUP OF INBORN ERRORS OF METABOLISM. THE MANIFESTATIONS ARE URINE THAT TURNS DARK ON STANDING AND ALKALINIZATION, BLACK OCHRONOTIC PIGMENTATION OF CARTILAGE AND COLLAGENOUS TISSUES AND ARTHRITIS, ESPECIALLY CHARACTERISTIC IN THE SPINE. SANDLER ET AL. (1970) RAISED THE QUESTION OF WHETHER PARKINSONISM OCCURS IN INCREASED FREQUENCY WITH ALKAPTONURIA, EITHER AS A COMPLICATION OR AS A DISTINCT SYNDROMAL ENTITY SEPARATE FROM ORDINARY ALKAPTONURIA. LUSTBERG ET AL. (1970)

PRESENTED EVIDENCE THAT ASCORBIC ACID IN HIGH DOSES DECREASES BINDING OF C(14)-HOMOGENTISIC ACID IN CONNECTIVE TISSUES OF RATS WITH EXPERIMENTAL ALKAPTONURIA. LONG-TERM THERAPY IN YOUNG PATIENTS WITH ALKAPTONURIA IS INDICATED.

ABE, Y., OSHIMA, N., HATANAKA, R., AMAKO, T. AND HIROHATA, R.* THIRTEEN CASES OF ALKAPTONURIA FROM ONE FAMILY TREE WITH SPECIAL REFERENCE TO OSTEO-ARTHROSIS ALKAPTONURICA. J. BONE JOINT SURG. 42A* 817-831, 1960.

GARROD, A. E.* THE INCIDENCE OF ALKAPTONURIA* A STUDY IN CHEMICAL INDIVIDUALITY. LANCET 2* 1616-1620, 1902.

KNOX, A. E.* SIR ARCHIBALD GARROD'S 'INBORN ERRORS OF METABOLISM.' II. ALKAPTONURIA. AM. J. HUM. GENET. 10* 95-124, 1958.

LA DU, B. N.* ALCAPTONURIA. IN, STANBURY, J. B., WYNGAARDEN, J. B. AND FREDRICKSON, D. S. (EDS.)* THE METABOLIC BASIS OF INHERITED DISEASE. NEW YORK* MCGRAW-HILL, 1966 (2ND ED.). PP. 303-323.

LUSTBERG, T. J., SCHULMAN, J. D. AND SEEGMILLER, J. E.* DECREASED BINDING OF (14)C-HOMOGENTISIC ACID INDUCED BY ASCORBIC ACID IN CONNECTIVE TISSUES OF RATS WITH EXPERIMENTAL ALKAPTONURIA. NATURE 228* 770-771, 1970.

SANDLER, M., KAROUM, F. AND RUTHVEN, C. R. J.* PARKINSONISM WITH ALKAPTONURIA* A NEW SYNDROME.Q (LETTER) LANCET 2* 770 ONLY, 1970.

20360   ALOPECIA-EPILEPSY-OLIGOPHRENIA SYNDROME OF MOYNAHAN (FAMILIAL CONGENITAL ALOPECIA, EPILEPSY, MENTAL RETARDATION AND UNUSUAL EEG)

IN THE FAMILY REPORTED BY MOYNAHAN (1962) TWO BROTHERS WERE AFFECTED. THE ALOPECIA CONSISTED OF A DELAY IN THE GROWTH OF HAIR. THE FATHER OF THE BOYS HAD BEEN BALD UNTIL AGE 2 AND A MATERNAL AUNT UNTIL AGE 4.

MOYNAHAN, E. J.* FAMILIAL CONGENITAL ALOPECIA, EPILEPSY, MENTAL RETARDATION WITH UNUSUAL ELECTROENCEPHALOGRAMS. PROC. ROY. SOC. MED. 55* 411-412, 1962.

*20370 ALPERS' DIFFUSE DEGENERATION OF CEREBRAL GRAY MATTER (POLIODYSTROPHIA CEREBRI PROGRESSIVA) WITH HEPATIC CIRRHOSIS

THE ILLNESS USUALLY BEGINS IN EARLY LIFE WITH CONVULSIONS. A PROGRESSIVE NEUROLOGIC DISORDER CHARACTERIZED BY SPASTICITY, MYOCLONUS AND DEMENTIA ENSUES. STATUS EPILEPTICUS IS OFTEN THE TERMINATING DEVELOPMENT. THE CASES, IN BROTHER AND SISTER, REPORTED BY FORD ET AL. (1951) ARE THOUGHT TO BE IN THIS CATEGORY. (SEE MYOCLONIC EPILEPSY FOR REFERENCE TO SAME CASES REPORTED BY MORSE.) FAMILIAL CASES WERE ALSO REPORTED BY PALINSKY ET AL. (1954), BY CHRISTENSEN AND HOJGAARD (1964) AND BY BLACKWOOD ET AL. (1963).
IT IS NOW REALIZED THAT PROGRESSIVE NEURONAL DEGENERATION CAN FOLLOW CONVULSIONS AND ANOXIC EPISODES FROM OTHER CAUSES. CARDIORESPIRATORY ARREST, HYPOTENSION, CYANOSIS AND THE VASCULAR CHANGES OBSERVED IN THE EXPOSED BRAIN BY NEUROSURGICAL INVESTIGATORS OF EPILEPSY ARE LIKELY TO LEAD TO BRAIN DAMAGE IN WHICH THE CEREBELLUM PARTICIPATES AS WELL AS THE CEREBRUM. (CEREBELLAR DAMAGE DUE TO CONVULSIONS MUST BE DISTINGUISHED FROM THAT DUE TO DILANTIN USED IN THEIR TREATMENT.) ALPERS' DISEASE MAY BE A NON-SPECIFIC ENTITY, ONLY SOME CASES OF WHICH HAVE A SPECIFIC GENETIC BASIS. IN THE FAMILY REPORTED BY ALBERCA-SERRANO ET AL. (1965) FOUR OF 6 SIBS WERE AFFECTED. THE PARENTS WERE UNRELATED. SEVERAL RELATIVES OF THE FATHER MAY HAVE HAD THE SAME DISORDER, WHICH HAD THE PICTURE OF ENCEPHALITIS PROGRESSING TO INFANTILE SPASTIC DIPLEGIA. POST-MORTEM STUDY IN ONE SHOWED 'DIFFUSE ANOXIC ENCEPHALOPATHY.' ALL THE CASES HAD REACTED TO INFECTIONS WITH VIOLENT CONVULSIONS. THE AUTHORS SUGGESTED THAT THIS REPRESENTS A FAMILIAL SUSCEPTIBILITY AND THAT THE CEREBRAL DAMAGE WAS SECONDARY TO ANOXIA. WEFRING AND LAMVIK (1967) DESCRIBED BROTHER AND SISTER WHO DEVELOPED CONVULSIONS AT AGES 11 AND 14 MONTHS, FOLLOWED BY PROGRESSIVE HYPOTONIA, DEMENTIA AND JAUNDICE 4 AND 2 WEEKS BEFORE DEATH AT THE AGE OF 15 AND 20 MONTHS. IN ADDITION TO THE TYPICAL FINDINGS OF ALPERS' DISEASE, THE LIVER SHOWED EXTENSIVE ATROPHY WITH FIBROSIS, INFLAMMATION AND BILE DUCT PROLIFERATION. BLACKWOOD ET AL. (1963) ALSO DESCRIBED SIBS WITH THIS COMBINATION, WHICH MAY REPRESENT A SEPARATE ENTITY.

ALBERCA-SERRANO, R., FABIANI, F., DENEVE, V. AND MACKEN, J.* FAMILIAL SPASTIC DIPLEGIA DUE TO ANOXIC ENCEPHALOPATHY (ALPERS). A CONTRIBUTION TO THE STUDY OF VASCULAR FRAGILITIES OF THE NERVOUS SYSTEM OF GENETIC TYPE. J. NEUROL. SCI. 2* 419-433, 1965.

ALPERS, B. J.* DIFFUSE PROGRESSIVE DEGENERATION OF GRAY MATTER OF CEREBRUM. ARCH. NEUROL. PSYCHIAT. 25* 469-505, 1931.

BLACKWOOD, W., BUXTON, P. H., CUMINGS, J. N., ROBERTSON, D. J. AND TUCKER, S. M.* DIFFUSE CEREBRAL DEGENERATION IN INFANCY (ALPERS' DISEASE). ARCH. DIS. CHILD. 38* 193-204, 1963.

CHRISTENSEN, E. AND HOJGAARD, K.* POLIODYSTROPHIA CEREBRI PROGRESSIVA INFANTILIS. ACTA NEUROL. SCAND. 40* 21-40, 1964.

FORD, F. R., LIVINGSTON, S. AND PRYLES, C. V.* FAMILIAL DEGENERATION OF THE

CEREBRAL GRAY MATTER IN CHILDHOOD WITH CONVULSIONS, MYOCLONUS, SPASTICITY, CEREBRAL ATAXIA, CHOREOATHETOSIS, DEMENTIA, AND DEATH IN STATUS EPILEPTICUS. DIFFERENTIATION OF INFANTILE AND JUVENILE TYPES. J. PEDIAT. 39* 33-43, 1951.

PALINSKY, M., KOZINN, P. J. AND ZAHTZ, H.* ACUTE FAMILIAL INFANTILE HEREDODE-GENERATIVE DISORDER OF THE CENTRAL NERVOUS SYSTEM. J. PEDIAT. 45* 538-545, 1954.

WEFRING, K. W. AND LAMVIK, J. O.* FAMILIAL PROGRESSIVE POLIODYSTROPHY WITH CIRRHOSIS OF THE LIVER. ACTA PAEDIAT. SCAND. 56* 295-300, 1967.

20380 ALSTROM SYNDROME

ALTHOUGH THIS RECESSIVE DISORDER BEARS MANY SIMILARITIES TO THE LAURENCE-MOON-BIEDL SYNDROME (Q.V.), ALSTROM ET AL. (1959) CLAIMS IT IS A DISTINCT ENTITY BECAUSE THERE IS NO MENTAL DEFECT, POLYDACTYLY OR HYPOGONADISM. THE PRESENCE OF RETINITIS PIGMENTOSA, DEAFNESS, OBESITY AND DIABETES MELLITUS ARE ELEMENTS OF SIMILARITY. THE RETINAL LESICN CAUSES NYSTAGMUS AND EARLY LOSS OF CENTRAL VISION IN CONTRAST TO LOSS OF PERIPHERAL VISION FIRST, IN OTHER PIGMENTARY RETINOPATHIES. WEINSTEIN ET AL. (1969) DESCRIBED THE CONDITION OF TWO BROTHERS WITH A DISORDER WHICH THEY SUGGESTED 'RESEMBLES THAT DESCRIBED BY ALSTROM AND HIS CO-WORKERS.' IN SPITE OF THE PRESENCE OF SMALL TESTES AND ELEVATED URINARY GONADOTROPIN LEVELS, SECONDARY SEXUAL CHARACTERISTICS WERE NORMAL. ASSOCIATED FINDINGS WERE BLINDNESS, DEAFNESS, OBESITY, AND SEVERAL METABOLIC ABNORMALITIES INCLUDING HYPERURICEMIA AND ELEVATED SERUM TRIGLYCERIDE AND PRE-BETA-LIPOPROTEIN. AUTOSOMAL RECESSIVE AND X-LINKED RECESSIVE INHERITANCE CANNOT BE DISTINGUISHED AND EVEN MALE-LIMITED AUTOSOMAL DOMINANT INHERITANCE IS POSSIBLE. HOWEVER, THE PEDIGREE DATA OF AHLSTROM MAKE BOTH X-LINKED RECESSIVE AND AUTOSOMAL DOMINANT INHERITANCE UNLIKELY.

ALSTROM, C. H., HALLGREN, B., NILSSON, L. B. AND ASANDER, H.* RETINAL DEGENERA-TION COMBINED WITH OBESITY, DIABETES MELLITUS AND NEUROGENOUS DEAFNESS. A SPECIFIC SYNDROME (NOT HITHERTO DESCRIBED) DISTINCT FROM THE LAURENCE-MOON-BIEDL SYNDROME. A CLINICAL ENDOCRINOLOGICAL AND GENETIC EXAMINATION BASED ON A LARGE PEDIGREE. ACTA PSYCHIAT. NEUROL. SCAND. 34 (SUPPL. 129)* 1-35, 1959.

WEINSTEIN, R. L., KLIMAN, B. AND SCULLY, R. E.* FAMILIAL SYNDROME OF PRIMARY TESTICULAR INSUFFICIENCY WITH NORMAL VIRILIZATION, BLINDNESS, DEAFNESS AND METABOLIC ABNORMALITIES. NEW ENG. J. MED. 281* 969-977, 1969.

*20390 ALYMPHOCYTOSIS, PURE (THYMIC DYSPLASIA WITH NORMAL IMMUNOGLOBINS AND IMMUNOLO-GIC DEFICIENCY)

NEZELOF (1968) LISTS THE CHARACTERISTICS OF THIS DISORDER AS SEVERE LYMPHOPENIA, TISSUE ALYMPHOCYTOSIS, THYMIC HYPOPLASIA, FATAL COURSE, NORMAL OR SUBNORMAL SERUM IMMUNOGLOBULINS AND PRESENCE OF PLASMA CELLS. HE PRESENTED A PEDIGREE STRONGLY SUGGESTIVE OF AUTOSOMAL RECESSIVE INHERITANCE. FIREMAN ET AL. (1966) REPORTED A CASE. WHEREAS BOTH CELLULAR AND HUMORAL IMMUNE MECHANISMS ARE AFFECTED IN THE SWISS TYPE AGAMMAGLOBULINEMIA AND ONLY THE HUMORAL MECHANISM IN THE BRUTON (X-LINKED) TYPE, ONLY THE CELLULAR MECHANISM IS AFFECTED IN THIS CONDITION.

FIREMAN, P., JOHNSON, H. A. AND GITLIN, D.* PRESENCE OF PLASMA CELLS AND GAMMA-1-M-GLOBULIN SYNTHESIS IN A PATIENT WITH THYMIC ALYMPHOPLASIA. PEDIATRICS 37* 485-492, 1966.

NEZELOF, C.* THYMIC DYSPLASIA WITH NORMAL IMMUNOGLOBULINS AND IMMUNOLOGIC DEFICIENCY* PURE ALYMPHOCYTOSIS. IN, GOOD, R. A. (ED.)* IMMUNOLOGIC DEFICIENCY DISEASES. NEW YORK* NATIONAL FOUNDATION, 1968. PP. 104-115.

*20400 AMAUROSIS CONGENITA OF LEBER I

ALSTROM (1957) FOUND THAT A SINGLE DISORDER INHERITED AS AN AUTOSOMAL RECESSIVE WAS RESPONSIBLE FOR 10 PERCENT OF BLINDNESS IN SWEDEN. TOTAL BLINDNESS OR GREATLY IMPAIRED VISION WITH LOSS OF CENTRAL VISION WAS PRESENT. EARLY IN LIFE FUNDUS CHANGES WERE LACKING, BUT BY AGE 50 YEARS WIDESPREAD ATROPHY EXPOSED WHITE AREAS OF SCLERA. CATARACT AND KERATOCONUS WERE ASSOCIATED. KERATOCONUS WAS OF DIAGNOSTIC USEFULNESS. NO MANIFESTATIONS EXCEPT IN THE EYE WERE DISCOVERED. 'IT WAS NOT UNTIL COMBINED GENEALOGIC AND GENETICO-STATISTICAL STUDIES HAD BEEN MADE, AND CLINICAL DATA COLLECTED OVER A LONG PERIOD THAT THE CONGENITAL DEVELOPMENT AND AFFINITY OF THESE APPARENTLY HETEROGENEOUS CASES COULD BE ESTABLISHED WITH SOME DEGREE OF PROBABILITY' (ALSTROM, 1957). STRIKING PEDIGREES WERE PRESENTED. IN HOLLAND, SCHAPPERT-KIMMIJSER, HENKES AND VAN DEN BOSCH (1959) STUDIED 227 CASES AND ALSO PRESENTED PEDIGREES TYPICAL OF AUTOSOMAL RECESSIVE INHERITANCE. AMONG THE CAUSES OF PROFOUND VISUAL IMPAIRMENT OF CHILDHOOD, AMAUROSIS CONGENITA IS COMPARABLE TO RECESSIVE CONGENITAL DEAFNESS AS THE CAUSE OF PROFOUND DEAFNESS OF CHILDHOOD. UNDOUBTEDLY GREAT HETEROGENEITY EXISTS. PROBABLY A MINIMUM OF 6 DIFFERENT LOCI AND POSSIBLY MANY MORE EXIST, HOMOZYGOSITY AT ANY ONE OF WHICH CAN RESULT IN THE SAME PHENOTYPE. SEPARATE ENTITIES ARE BEGINNING TO BE SEPARATED ON THE BASIS OF ASSOCIATED ABNORMALITIES ESPECIALLY NEUROLOGIC. SEE RENAL DYSPLASIA AND RETINAL APLASIA.
CONGENITAL NYSTAGMUS AND CEREBRAL (OR CORTICAL) BLINDNESS WERE TERMS OFTEN ASSIGNED TO THESE CASES IN THE PAST BEFORE THE CHORIORETINAL SITE OF ABNORMALITY WAS APPRECIATED. SOMETIMES IT IS CONFUSED WITH RETINITIS PIGMENTOSA. RETINAL APLASIA IS THE TERM MOST FREQUENTLY USED IN ENGLAND. CONGENITAL ABSENCE OF THE

R
E
C
E
S
S
I
V
E

RODS AND CONES IS A DESIGNATION OFTEN USED IN THE U.S.A. PHOTOPHOBIA IS FREQUENT-
LY PRESENT AND IN YOUNG CHILDREN MAY BE ASSOCIATED WITH FORCEFUL DIGGING OF THE
FINGERS AND FISTS INTO THE ORBITS. THIS MAY BE RESPONSIBLE FOR THE KERATOCONUS.
IN A FAMILY REPORTED BY RAHN ET AL. (1968) THERE WERE CIGARETTE-PAPER SCARS AND
SKETCHABLE SKIN SUGGESTING EHLERS-DANLOS SYNDROME.

ALSTROM, C. H.* HEREDO-RETINOPATHIA CONGENITALIS MONOHYBRIDA RECESSIVA
AUTOSOMALIS. HEREDITAS 43* 1-178, 1957.

GILLESPIE, F. D.* CONGENITAL AMAUROSIS OF LEBER. AM. J. OPHTHAL. 61* 874-880,
1966.

RAHN, E. K., MEADOW, E., FALLS, H. F., KNAGGS, J. C. AND PROUX, D. J.* LEBER'S
CONGENITAL AMAUROSIS WITH EHLERS-DANLOS-LIKE SYNDROME. STUDY OF AN AMERICAN
FAMILY. ARCH. OPHTHAL. 79* 135-141, 1968.

SCHAPPERT-KIMMIJSER, J., HENKES, H. E. AND VAN DEN BOSCH, J.* AMAUROSIS
CONGENITA (LEBER). ARCH. OPHTHAL. 61* 211-218, 1959.

*20410 AMAUROSIS CONGENITA OF LEBER II

ONE REASON FOR SUSPECTING THE EXISTENCE OF TWO FORMS OF THE DISEASE IS A PEDIGREE
PUBLISHED BY WAARDENBURG (1963) WHICH SHOWS ALL NORMAL CHILDREN FROM TWO AFFECTED
PARENTS. THE MOTHER HAD TWO AFFECTED SISTERS AND THE FATHER WAS THE PRODUCT OF A
FIRST COUSIN MARRIAGE (WAARDENBURG AND SCHAPPERT-KIMMIJSER, 1963). KERATOCONUS
(OR KERATOGLOBUS), A FREQUENT FEATURE OF THIS CONDITION, WAS NOT PRESENT IN EITHER
PARENT BUT WAS FOUND IN ONE OF THE MOTHER'S AFFECTED SISTERS. THIS CONDITION, IS,
OF COURSE, NOT TO BE CONFUSED WITH LEBER'S OPTIC ATROPHY.

WAARDENBURG, P. J. AND SCHAPPERT-KIMMIJSER, J.* IN, GENETICS AND OPHTHALMOLOGY,
WAARDENBURG, P. J., FRANCESCHETTI, A. AND KLEIN, D. (EDS.)* SPRINGFIELD, ILL.*
CHARLES C THOMAS, 2* 1579 ONLY, 1963.

WAARDENBURG, P. J. AND SCHAPPERT-KIMMIJSER, J.* ON VARIOUS RECESSIVE BIOTYPES
OF LEBER'S CONGENITAL AMAUROSIS. ACTA OPHTHAL. 41* 317-320, 1963.

*20420 AMAUROTIC FAMILY IDIOCY, JUVENILE TYPE (BATTEN'S DISEASE IN ENGLAND, VOGT-
SPIELMEYER'S DISEASE ON THE CONTINENT)

THE FIRST MANIFESTATION IS OFTEN RAPID DETERIORATION OF VISION AND A SLOWER BUT
PROGRESSIVE DETERIORATION OF INTELLECT. SEIZURES AND PSYCHOTIC BEHAVIOR DEVELOPED
LATER. THE FUNDI SHOW PIGMENTARY DEGENERATION. KYPHOSCOLIOSIS MAY DEVELOP.
ONSET IS AT AGE 5-10 YEARS. BRAIN BIOPSY AND RECTAL BIOPSY USUALLY MAKE THE
DIAGNOSIS BY DEMONSTRATION OF NERVE CELLS HEAVILY LADEN WITH LIPID. THE RELATIVE-
LY HIGH FREQUENCY IN NON-JEWISH NORTHERN EUROPEANS (E.G., SWEDES) EMPHASIZES THE
FACT THAT THIS FORM IS DISTINCT FROM TAY-SACHS DISEASE, WHICH, OF COURSE, IT
DIFFERS FROM GREATLY IN CLINICAL BEHAVIOR. VACUOLATION OF THE LYMPHOCYTES IS A
WELL ESTABLISHED FEATURE OF THE HOMOZYGOTE (MCKUSICK ET AL., 1963). WHAT IS NOT
SO CERTAIN IS VACUOLATION IN HETEROZYGOTES. RAYNER (1963) CLAIMS THAT ABOUT 1
PERCENT OF LYMPHOCYTES ARE VACUOLATED IN HETEROZYGOTES. BESSMAN AND BALDWIN
(1962) FOUND IMIDAZOLE AMINOACIDURIA IN FIVE PATIENTS AND SOME OF THEIR IMMEDIATE
RELATIVES IN THREE UNRELATED FAMILIES. POTENTIALLY THE METHOD MIGHT BE USEFUL FOR
DETECTION OF HETEROZYGOTES AND FOR IDENTIFYING HETEROGENEITY IN THIS CATEGORY OF
DISEASE. STROUTH, ZEMAN AND MERRITT (1966) FOUND AZUROPHILIC CYTOPLASMIC GRANULES
IN THE PERIPHERAL LEUKOCYTES IN 12 OUT OF 16 PATIENTS. FURTHERMORE, BOTH PARENTS
AND TWO-THIRDS OF NORMAL SIBS SHOWED THESE GRANULATIONS WHICH RESEMBLE THOSE OF
THE ALDER ANOMALY (Q.V.). THE CASES WITH ABSENT LEUKOCYTE GRANULATIONS MAY
REPRESENT A DIFFERENT ENTITY. ANATOMIC FEATURES ARE (1) SEVERE WIDESPREAD
NEURONAL DEGENERATION RESULTING IN SIMPLE RETINAL ATROPHY AND IN MASSIVE LOSS OF
BRAIN SUBSTANCE, THE AVERAGE BRAIN WEIGHT BEING ABOUT 600 GM, AND (2) ACCUMULATION
OF LIPOFUSCIN IN NEURONAL PERIKARYON. THE LIPOFUSCIN ACCUMULATION HAS BEEN
DEMONSTRATED BY ELECTRON MICROSCOPY (ZEMAN AND DONAHUE, 1963* GONATAS AND TERRY ET
AL., 1963). ALTHOUGH THE SIMILAR NAME ASSIGNED BECAUSE OF SOME HISTOLOGIC
SIMILARITY TO TAY-SACHS DISEASE MIGHT SUGGEST BIOCHEMICAL RELATEDNESS, THERE IS NO
EVIDENCE THAT BATTEN'S DISEASE IS A GANGLIOSIDE LIPIDOSIS AS IS TAY-SACHS DISEASE.
DANES AND BEARN (1968) SHOWED THAT BOTH HOMOZYGOTES AND HETEROZYGOTES CAN BE
IDENTIFIED ON THE BASIS OF METACHROMASIA IN SKIN FIBROBLASTS IN CELL CULTURE.
SEITELBERGER ET AL. (1967) CALLED THE CONDITION 'MYOCLONIC VARIANT OF CEREBRAL
LIPIDOSIS.' DAYAN AND TRICKEY (1970) FOUND LARGE AMOUNTS OF LIPOFUSCIN IN THE
THYROID.

BESSMAN, S. P. AND BALDWIN, R.* IMIDAZOLE AMINOACIDURIA IN CEREBROMACULAR
DEGENERATION. SCIENCE 135* 789-791, 1962.

DANES, B. S. AND BEARN, A. G.* METACHROMASIA AND SKIN-FIBROBLAST CULTURES IN
JUVENILE FAMILIAL AMAUROTIC IDIOCY. LANCET 2* 855-856, 1968.

DAYAN, A. D. AND TRICKEY, R. J.* THYROID INVOLVEMENT IN JUVENILE AMAUROTIC
IDIOCY (BATTEN'S DISEASE). LANCET 2* 296-297, 1970.

EDGAR, G. W. AND POST, P. J.* AMAUROTIC IDIOCY AND EPILEPSY. EPILEPSIA 4* 241-
260, 1963.

GONATAS, N. K., TERRY, R. D., WINKLER, R., KOREY, S. R., GOMEZ, C. J. AND STEIN, A.* A CASE OF JUVENILE LIPIDOSIS* THE SIGNIFICANCE OF ELECTRON MICROSCOPIC AND BIOCHEMICAL OBSERVATIONS OF A CEREBRAL BIOPSY. J. NEUROPATH. EXP. NEUROL. 22* 557-580, 1963.

HARLEM, O. K.* JUVENILE CEREBRORETINAL DEGENERATION (SPIELMEYER-VOGT). AM. J. DIS. CHILD. 100* 918-923, 1960.

LEVENSON, J., LINDAHL-KIESSLING, K. AND RAYNER, S.* CARNOSINE EXCRETION IN JUVENILE AMAUROTIC IDIOCY. LANCET 2* 756-757, 1964.

MCKUSICK, V. A. AND COLLEAGUES* MEDICAL GENETICS 1962. J. CHRONIC DIS. 16* 457-634, 1963. (FIG. 33).

RAYNER, S.* JUVENILE AMAUROTIC IDIOCY IN SWEDEN WITH PARTICULAR REFERENCE TO THE OCCURRENCE OF VACUOLES IN THE LYMPHOCYTES OF HOMO- AND HETEROZYGOTES. UPPSALA* UNIVERSITY OF UPPSALA, 1962.

RAYNER, S.* JUVENILE AMAUROTIC IDIOCY IN SWEDEN. PROC. 11TH INTERN. CONG. GENET., THE HAUGE, 1963. P. 283.

SEITELBERGER, F., JACOB, H. AND SCHNABEL, R.* THE MYOCLONIC VARIANT OF CEREBRAL LIPIDOSIS. IN, ARONSON, S. M. AND VOLK, B. W. (EDS.)* INBORN DISORDERS OF SPHINGOLIPID METABOLISM. OXFORD* PERGANON PRESS, 1967. PP. 43-74.

SJOGREN, T.* DIE JUVENILE AMAUROTISCHE IDIOTIE. KLINISCHE UND ERBLICHKEITS MEDIZINISCHE UNTERSUCHUNGEN. HEREDITAS 14* 197-426, 1931.

STROUTH, J. C., ZEMAN, W. AND MERRITT, A. D.* LEUKOCYTE ABNORMALITIES IN FAMILIAL AMAUROTIC IDIOCY. NEW ENG. J. MED. 274* 36-38, 1966.

ZEMAN, W. AND DONAHUE, S.* FINE STRUCTURE OF THE LIPID BODIES IN JUVENILE AMAUROTIC IDIOCY. ACTA NEUROPATH. 3* 144-149, 1963.

ZEMAN, W. AND STROUTH, J. C.* LEUKOCYTIC HYPERGRANULATION VERSUS LYMPHOCYTIC VACUOLIZATION AS MARKERS FOR HETEROZYGOTES AND WITH BATTEN-SPIELMEYER-VOGT DISEASE. IN, ARONSON, S. M. AND VOLK, B. W. (EDS.)* INBORN DISORDERS OF SPHINGO-LIPID METABOLISM. OXFORD* PERGAMON PRESS, 1967. PP. 475-484.

R
E
C
E
S
S
I
V
E

20430 AMAUROTIC IDIOCY, ADULT TYPE

THE EXISTENCE OF THIS TYPE IS QUESTIONABLE, IN THE OPINION OF SOME. THE CASE OF KUFS (1925) HAD ONSET AT AGE 26 AND DEATH AT AGE 38. FINE, BARRON AND HIRANO (1960) FOUND REPORTS OF 18 COMPLETE HISTOLOGIC DESCRIPTIONS. CASES WITH THE ANATOMIC CHARACTERISTICS LISTED FOR THE JUVENILE FORM MAY HAVE LATE ONSET, MAKING IT POSSIBLE THAT THE ADULT AND JUVENILE FORMS ARE IN FACT ONE ENTITY (ZEMAN AND HOFFMAN, 1962). CHOU AND THOMPSON (1970) REPORTED THE MORPHOLOGIC CHANGES IN A MAN WHO WAS WELL UNTIL AGE 17 AND DIED AT AGE 32. A SISTER WAS SAID TO HAVE DIED OF A SIMILAR CLINICAL PICTURE (SEIZURES, INTELLECTUAL DETERIORATION, LACK OF MOTOR CONTROL, DEVELOPMENT OF ATHETOID MOVEMENTS). THE PARENTS WERE WELL AND WERE RELATED AS FIRST COUSINS.

CHOU, S. M. AND THOMPSON, H. G.* ELECTRON MICROSCOPY OF STORAGE CYTOSOMES IN KUFS' DISEASE. ARCH. NEUROL. 23* 489-501, 1970.

FINE, D. I., BARRON, K. D. AND HIRANO, A.* CENTRAL NERVOUS SYSTEM LIPIDOSIS IN AN ADULT WITH ATROPHY OF THE CEREBELLAR GRANULAR LAYER. A CASE REPORT. J. NEUROL. 19* 355-369, 1960.

KUFS, H.* UBER EINE SPATFORM DER AMAURTISCHEN IDIOTIE UND IHRE HEREDOFAMILIAREN GRUNDLAGEN. ZBL. GES. NEUROL. PSYCHIAT. 95* 169-188, 1925.

ZEMAN, W. AND HOFFMAN, J.* JUVENILE AND LATE FORMS OF AMAUROTIC IDIOCY IN ONE FAMILY. J. NEUROL. NEUROSURG. PSYCHIAT. 25* 352-362, 1962.

*20440 AMAUROTIC IDIOCY, CONGENITAL FORM

NORMAN AND WOOD (1941) DESCRIBED A SINGLE CASE, A FEMALE INFANT WHO DIED AT 18 DAYS. THE PARENTS WERE NOT RELATED. (TAY-SACHS DISEASE DOES NOT BECOME EVIDENT BEFORE THREE MONTHS AT THE EARLIEST.) IN THIS CASE THE INTRACELLULAR GRANULAR INCLUSIONS WERE INSOLUBLE. TWO OTHER SIBS HAD SIMILAR CLINICAL AND HISTOLOGIC FINDINGS (BROWN AND COLLEAGUES, 1954). ANOTHER CASE MAY BE THAT OF EPSTEIN (1917) IN WHICH MANIFESTATION APPEARED IN THE SECOND WEEK OF POSTNATAL LIFE. HAGBERG ET AL. (1965) FOUND A DISIALOGANGLIOSIDE, G(D3), NOT PREVIOUSLY IDENTIFIED, IN TISSUE FROM CONGENITAL AMAUROTIC IDIOCY.

BROWN, N. J., CORNER, B. D. AND DODGSON, M. C. H.* A SECOND CASE IN THE SAME FAMILY OF CONGENITAL FAMILIAL CEREBRAL LIPOIDOSIS RESEMBLING AMAUROTIC FAMILY IDIOCY. ARCH. DIS. CHILD. 29* 48-54, 1954.

EPSTEIN, J.* AMAUROTIC FAMILY IDIOCY. NEW YORK J. MED. 106* 887-889, 1917.

HAGBERG, B., HULTQVIST, G., OHMAN, R. AND SVENNERHOLM, L.* CONGENITAL AMAUROTIC IDIOCY. ACTA PAEDIAT. SCAND. 54* 116-130, 1965.

NORMAN, R. M. AND WOOD, N.* A CONGENITAL FORM OF AMAUROTIC FAMILY IDIOCY. J. NEUROL. PSYCHIAT. 4* 175-190, 1941.

20450 AMAUROTIC IDIOCY, LATE INFANTILE TYPE (JANSKY-BIELSCHOWSKY)

NO FUNDUS CHANGE OR OPTIC ATROPHY IS OBSERVED. THE CHERRY RED SPOT IS TYPICAL OF THE INFANTILE FORM (TAY-SACHS) AND RETINITIS PIGMENTOSA IS TYPICAL OF THE JUVENILE FORM (SPIELMEYER-VOGT-BATTEN). MORE CEREBELLAR INVOLVEMENT OCCURS IN THE LATE INFANTILE FORM THAN IN THE OTHERS. HASSIN (1926) REVIEWED THE PATHOLOGY. SEITELBERGER, VOGEL AND STEPAN (1957) COLLECTED 28 CASES FROM THE WORLD'S LITERATURE. ON THE BASIS OF ELECTRON MICROSCOPIC FINDINGS GONATAS ET AL. (1968) SUGGESTED THAT TWO CASES THEY STUDIED AND 4 CASES REPORTED BY OTHERS REPRESENTED A DIFFERENT TYPE OF LATE INFANTILE AMAUROTIC IDIOCY. SOME CASES REPORTED AS THIS ENTITY MAY BE INSTANCES OF GENERALIZED GANGLIOSIDOSIS (DONAHUE ET AL., 1967).

DONAHUE, S., ZEMAN, W. AND WATANABE, I.* ELECTRON MICROSCOPIC OBSERVATIONS IN BATTEN'S DISEASE. IN, ARONSON, S. M. AND VOLK, B. W. (EDS.)* INBORN DISORDERS OF SPHINGOLIPID METABOLISM. OXFORD* PERGAMON PRESS, 1967. PP. 3-22.

GONATAS, N. K., GAMBETTI, P. AND BAIRD, H.* A SECOND TYPE OF LATE INFANTILE AMAUROTIC IDIOCY WITH MULTILAMELLAR CYTOSOMES. J. NEUROPATH. EXP. NEUROL. 27* 371-389, 1968.

HASSIN, G. B.* AMAUROTIC FAMILY IDIOCY* LATE INFANTILE TYPE (BIELSCHOWSKY) WITH THE CLINICAL PICTURE OF DECEREBRATE RIGIDITY. ARCH. NEUROL. PSYCHIAT. 16* 708-727, 1926.

SEITELBERGER, F., VOGEL, G. AND STEPAN, H.* SPATINFANTILE AMAUROTISCHE IDIOTIE. ARCH. PSYCHIAT. NERVENKR. 196* 154-190, 1957.

VOLK, B. W., WALLACE, B. J., SCHNECK, L. AND SAIFER, A.* LATE INFANTILE AMAUROTIC IDIOCY. ULTRAMICROSCOPIC AND HISTOCHEMICAL STUDIES ON A CASE. ARCH. PATH. 78* 483-500, 1964.

*20460 AMAUROTIC IDIOCY, LATE INFANTILE, WITH MULTILAMELLAR CYTOSOMES

ELFENBEIN AND CANTOR (1969) SUGGESTED THIS DESIGNATION, BASED ON THE STRIKING MORPHOLOGIC FEATURE, FOR A DISORDER WITH ONSET BETWEEN 2 AND A HALF AND 4 YEARS, SEIZURES, MYOCLONUS, DEMENTIA, BLINDNESS WITH PIGMENTARY CHANGES IN THE FUNDUS. THEY NOTED FAMILIAL OCCURRENCE AS DID ALSO RICHARDSON AND BORNHOFEN (1968) AND GONATAS ET AL. (1968).

ELFENBEIN, I. B. AND CANTOR, H. E.* LATE INFANTILE AMAUROTIC IDIOCY WITH MULTILAMELLAR CYTOSOMES* AN ELECTRON MICROSCOPIC STUDY. J. PEDIAT. 75* 253-264, 1969.

GONATAS, N. K., GAMBETTI, P. AND BAIRD, H.* A SECOND TYPE OF LATE INFANTILE AMAUROTIC IDIOCY WITH MULTILAMELLAR CYTOSOMES. J. NEUROPATH. EXP. NEUROL. 27* 371-389, 1968.

RICHARDSON, M. E. AND BORNHOFEN, J. H.* EARLY CHILDHOOD CEREBRAL LIPIDOSIS WITH PROMINENT MYOCLONUS. ULTRASTRUCTURAL AND HISTOCHEMICAL STUDIES OF A CEREBRAL BIOPSY. ARCH. NEUROL. 18* 34-43, 1968.

*20470 AMELOGENESIS IMPERFECTA, PIGMENTED HYPOMATURATION TYPE

FOR A GENERAL DISCUSSION OF THIS AND OTHER GENETIC ABNORMALITIES OF THE TEETH AND RELATED STRUCTURES SEE WITKOP (1965). ONLY TWO FAMILIES HAVE BEEN STUDIED. IN ONE A BROTHER AND SISTER WERE AFFECTED. PARENTS AND MORE REMOTE RELATIVES WERE UNAFFECTED. THE PARENTS WERE FIRST COUSINS ONCE REMOVED. BOTH THE PRIMARY AND THE SECONDARY DENTITION WERE AFFECTED. THE TEETH HAD A SHINEY AGAR JELLY APPEARANCE AND THE ENAMEL WAS SOFTER THAN NORMAL. THE USUAL RADIOGRAPHIC CONTRAST BETWEEN ENAMEL AND DENTINE WAS LACKING. HISTOLOGICALLY A BROWN PIGMENT WHICH IS PROBABLY NOT DERIVED FROM BLOOD PIGMENTS BUT IS OF UNKNOWN NATURE WAS DEMONSTRABLE IN THE MIDDLE LAYERS OF ENAMEL.

WITKOP, C. J.* GENETIC DISEASE OF THE ORAL CAVITY. IN, TIECKE, R. W. (ED.)* ORAL PATHOLOGY. NEW YORK* MCGRAW-HILL, 1965.

20480 AMINOACIDURIA WITH MENTAL DEFICIENCY, DWARFISM, MUSCULAR DYSTROPHY, OSTEOPORO-SIS AND ACIDOSIS

STRANSKY, BAYANI-SIOSON, AND LEE (1962) DESCRIBED A FAMILY IN WHICH 5 OF 7 SIBS HAD THIS COMBINATION. THE MOTHER AND TWO NORMAL SIBS HAD MILD AMINOACIDURIA.

STRANSKY, E., BAYANI-SIOSON, P. S. AND LEE, W.* A PECULIAR TYPE OF FAMILIAL MENTAL DEFICIENCY, PROBABLY DUE TO METABOLIC DISTURBANCE. A PRELIMINARY REPORT. PHILIPP. MED. ASS. J. 38* 903-908, 1962.

DE SOUZA (1963) REPORTED 4 AFFECTED SIBS (1 MALE, 3 FEMALE). ONSET WAS BETWEEN 10 AND 13 YEARS. THE LESIONS WERE MAINLY AROUND THE JOINTS AND WERE BULLOUS IN NATURE.

DE SOUZA, A. R.* AMILOIDOSE CUTANEA BULHOSA FAMILIAL. OBSERVACAO DE 4 CASOS. REV. HOSP. CLIN. FAC. MED. S. PAULO 18* 413-417, 1963.

20500 AMYOTONIA CONGENITA (OPPENHEIM'S DISEASE)

MUCH UNCERTAINTY EXISTS AS TO WHAT OPPENHEIM HAD IN MIND AND WHAT THIS ENTITY IS - IF INDEED IT EXISTS AT ALL. THE BEST DISCUSSION IS THAT OF GREENFIELD, CORNMAN AND SHY (1958) UNDER THE HEADING OF 'THE FLOPPY INFANT.' WHEN THE PRIMARY DEFECT RESIDES IN THE SPINAL CORD THE CONDITION IS INFANTILE MUSCULAR ATROPHY (Q.V.), OTHERWISE KNOWN AS WERDNIG-HOFFMANN DISEASE OR INFANTILE SPINAL AMYOTROPHY. POSSIBLY THE TERM AMYOTONIA CONGENITA SHOULD BE RESERVED FOR THOSE CONDITIONS IN WHICH THE PRIMARY ABNORMALITY RESIDES IN MUSCLE AND THE DISORDER IS ESSENTIALLY NON-PROGRESSIVE. CERTAINLY THERE ARE MULTIPLE CAUSES, E.G., GLYCOGEN STORAGE DISEASE, THE ATONIC-ASTATIC SYNDROME OF FOERSTER, AND THE CONGENITAL NONPROGRES- SIVE MYOPATHY (Q.V.) DESCRIBED BY BATTEN AND BY TURNER. NEMALINE MYOPATHY AND CENTRAL CORE DISEASES (Q.V.) ARE OTHER ENTITIES PRODUCING FLOPPY INFANTS.

GREENFIELD, J. G., CORNMAN, T. AND SHY, G. M.* THE PROGNOSTIC VALUE OF THE MUSCLE BIOPSY IN THE 'FLOPPY INFANT.' BRAIN 81* 461-484, 1958.

*20510 AMYOTROPHIC LATERAL SCLEROSIS, JUVENILE

IN AN AMISH ISOLATE WE (GRAGG ET AL., 1971)HAVE OBSERVED TWO BROTHERS WITH ONSET IN THE FIRST DECADE OF THE ALS SYMPTOM COMPLEX* DISTAL MUSCULAR ATROPHY, INCREASED DEEP TENDON REFLEXES, SPASTICITY AND FASCICULATIONS. REFSUM AND SKILLICON (1954) DESCRIBED THE SAME PICTURE IN TWO BROTHERS AND A SISTER. ONSET WAS BETWEEN 3 AND 5 YEARS. THEY STATED THAT THE CONDITION WAS INDISTINGUISHABLE FROM AMYOTROPHIC LATERAL SCLEROSIS.

GRAGG, G. W., FOGELSON, M. H. AND ZWIRECKI, R. J.* JUVENILE AMYOTROPHIC LATERAL SCLEROSIS IN TWO BROTHERS FROM AN INBRED COMMUNITY. IN, BERGSMA, D. (ED.)* CLINICAL DELINEATION OF BIRTH DEFECTS. VII. NERVOUS SYSTEM. BALTIMORE* WILLIAMS AND WILKINS, 1971.

REFSUM, S. AND SKILLICON, S. A.* AMYOTROPHIC FAMILIAL SPASTIC PARAPLEGIA. NEUROLOGY 4* 40-47, 1954.

20520 AMYOTROPHIC LATERAL SCLEROSIS, JUVENILE, WITH DEMENTIA

HOFFMANN (1894) DESCRIBED SLOWLY PROGRESSIVE JUVENILE AMYOTROPHIC LATERAL SCLEROSIS WITH CONCOMITANTLY PROGRESSIVE DEMENTIA IN 4 SIBS. STAAL AND WENT (1968) DESCRIBED 7 SIBS (OUT OF 15), OFFSPRING OF A FIRST COUSIN MARRIAGE, AFFECTED BY THE SAME DISORDER. THREE BOYS AND 4 GIRLS WERE AFFECTED. DEATH HAD OCCURRED IN 5 OF 7 SIBS AT INTERVALS VARYING FROM 9 TO 21 YEARS AFTER ONSET OF SYMPTOMS WHICH STARTED AT ABOUT AGE 10 YEARS.

HOFFMANN, J.* UEBER EINEN EIGENARTIGEN SYMPTOMENCOMPLEX, EINE COMBINATION VON ANGENBORENEM SCHWACHSINN MIT PROGRESSIVER MUSKELATROPHIE, ALS WEITEREN BEITRAG ZU DEN ERBLICHEN NERVENKRANKHEITEN. DEUTSCH. Z. NERVENHEILK. 6* 150-166, 1894.

STAAL, A. AND WENT, L. N.* JUVENILE AMYOTROPHIC LATERAL SCLEROSIS-DEMENTIA COMPLEX IN A DUTCH FAMILY. NEUROLOGY 18* 800-806, 1968.

*20530 ANALBUMINEMIA

ANALBUMINEMIA IS A COMPLETELY RECESSIVE CONDITION. SERUM ALBUMIN HAS A NORMAL LEVEL IN HETEROZYGOTES. THE HOMOZYGOTES HAVE REMARKABLY LITTLE INCONVENIENCE ATTRIBUTABLE TO THE LACK OF SERUM ALBUMIN. THE DISORDER WAS FIRST REPORTED IN 1954 BY BENNHOLD AND COLLEAGUES OF TUBINGEN. IT MUST BE VERY RARE. SEE REVIEW BY OTT (1962). WHETHER THE MUTATION IS AT THE SAME LOCUS AS THOSE RESPONSIBLE FOR THE ELECTROPHORETIC VARIANTS OF ALBUMIN (SEE DOMINANT CATALOG) IS UNKNOWN.

BENNHOLD, H. AND KALLEE, E.* COMPARATIVE STUDIES ON THE HALF-LIFE OF 1131 LABELLED ALBUMINS AND NONRADIOACTIVE HUMAN SERUM ALBUMIN IN A CASE OF ANALBUMINE- MIA. J. CLIN. INVEST. 38* 863-872, 1959.

BENNHOLD, H., PETERS, H. AND ROTH, E.* UBER EINEN FALL VON KOMPLETTER ANALBU- MINAEMIE OHNE WESENTLICHE KLINISCHE KRANKHEITSZEICHEN. VERH. DEUTSCH. GES. INN. MED. 60* 630-634, 1954.

OTT, H.* ANALBUMINEMIA. IN, ERBLICHE STOFFWECHSELKRANKHEITEN. LINNEWEH, F. (ED.)* MUNICH* URBAN AND SCHWARZENBERG, 1962. P. 44.

*20540 ANALPHALIPOPROTEINEMIA (TANGIER DISEASE)

THE DISORDER HAS BEEN FOUND AMONG INHABITANTS OF TANGIER ISLAND IN THE CHESAPEAKE

BAY, MOST OF WHOM ARE DESCENDANTS OF FIRST SETTLERS OF 1686. CHARACTERISTICS ARE VERY LARGE TONSILS WHICH HAVE A VERY CHARACTERISTIC GROSS AND HISTOLOGIC APPEARANCE, ENLARGED LIVER, SPLEEN AND LYMPH NODES, AND HYPOCHOLESTEROLEMIA. THE THYMUS IS LOADED WITH LIPID WHICH CAN BE SHOWN TO CONSIST OF CHOLESTEROL ESTERS. HETEROZYGOTES SHOW LOW ALPHA-LIPOPROTEINS IN THE SERUM. OTHER AFFECTED FAMILIES HAVE BEEN DISCOVERED IN MISSOURI AND IN KENTUCKY. IN BRITAIN KOCEN ET AL. (1967) DESCRIBED THE CONDITION IN A 37 YEAR OLD AIR FORCE CORPORAL WHO SHOWED WIDESPREAD DISSOCIATED LOSS OF PAIN AND TEMPERATURE SENSATION AND PROGRESSIVE MUSCLE WASTING AND WEAKNESS. THEY COMMENTED THAT WHEREAS THE CHARACTERISTIC PHARYNGEAL APPEARANCE HAD BEEN THE PRESENTING FEATURE IN CHILDREN, ADOLESCENTS HAD PRESENTED WITH RELAPSING PERIPHERAL NEUROPATHY AND ADULTS WITH HYPERSPLENISM OR WITH PRECOCIOUS CORONARY ARTERY DISEASE. ENGEL ET AL. (1967) FOUND RECURRENT NEUROPATHY AND INTESTINAL LIPID STORAGE AS FEATURES.

ENGEL, W. K., DORMAN, J. D., LEVY, R. I. AND FREDRICKSON, D. S.* NEUROPATHY IN TANGIER DISEASE. ALPHA-LIPOPROTEIN DEFICIENCY MANIFESTING AS FAMILIAL RECURRENT NEUROPATHY AND INTESTINAL LIPID STORAGE. ARCH. NEUROL. 17* 1-9, 1967.

FREDRICKSON, D. S.* FAMILIAL HIGH DENSITY LIPOPROTEIN DEFICIENCY* TANGIER DISEASE. IN, STANBURY, J. B., WYNGAARDEN, J. B. AND FREDRICKSON, D. S. (EDS.)* THE METABOLIC BASIS OF INHERITED DISEASE. NEW YORK* MCGRAW-HILL, 1966 (2ND ED.). PP. 486-508.

FREDRICKSON, D. S.* THE INHERITANCE OF HIGH DENSITY LIPOPROTEIN DEFICIENCY (TANGIER DISEASE). J. CLIN. INVEST 43* 228-236, 1964.

KOCEN, R. S., LLOYD, J. K., LASCELLES, P. T., FOSBROOKE, A. AND WILLIAMS, D.* FAMILIAL ALPHA-LIPOPROTEIN DEFICIENCY (TANGIER DISEASE) WITH NEUROLOGICAL ABNORMALITIES. LANCET 1* 1341-1345, 1967.

20550 ANAL-SACRAL ANOMALIES

AARONSON (1970) DESCRIBED TWO BROTHERS AND A SISTER WITH ANTERIOR SACRAL MENINGOCELE, ANAL CANAL DUPLICATION CYST AND COVERED ANUS. THE PARENTS WERE NOT RELATED.

AARONSON, I.* ANTERIOR SACRAL MENINGOCELE, ANAL CANAL DUPLICATION CYST AND COVERED ANUS OCCURRING IN ONE FAMILY. J. PEDIAT. SURG. 5* 559-563, 1970.

20560 ANEMIA AND TRIPHALANGEAL THUMBS

AASE AND SMITH (1969) OBSERVED 2 BROTHERS WITH CONGENITAL ANEMIA AND TRIPHALANGEAL THUMBS. IN ONE, VENTRICULAR SEPTAL DEFECT WAS THOUGHT TO BE PRESENT. THE SHOULDERS WERE NARROW AND SLOPING. THEY CONSIDERED IT AN ENTITY DISTINCT FROM FANCONI'S PANMYELOPATHY, THROMBOCYTOPENIA WITH ABSENT RADIUS, AND THE HOLT-ORAM SYNDROME.

AASE, J. M. AND SMITH, D. W.* CONGENITAL ANEMIA AND TRIPHALANGEAL THUMBS* A NEW SYNDROME. J. PEDIAT. 74* 471-474, 1969.

20570 ANEMIA, AUTOIMMUNE HEMOLYTIC

DOBBS (1965) REPORTED BROTHER AND SISTER WITH *COOMBS POSITIVE* HEMOLYTIC ANEMIA. ANOTHER SISTER SEEMS TO HAVE DIED OF AUTOIMMUNE HEMOLYTIC ANEMIA. POSITIVE LATEX FIXATION, POSITIVE WASSERMANN TEST AND NEGATIVE T. PALLIDUM TEST WAS FOUND IN BOTH PARENTS AND THE FATHER HAD HYPERGAMMAGLOBULINEMIA. OTHERS HAVE REPORTED FAMILIAL AUTOIMMUNE HEMOLYTIC ANEMIA WITH ABNORMALITIES OF GAMMA GLOBULIN.

DOBBS, C. E.* FAMILIAL AUTO-IMMUNE HEMOLYTIC ANEMIA. ARCH. INTERN. MED. 116* 273-276, 1965.

FIALKOW, P. J., FUDENBERG, H. AND EPSTEIN, W. V.* *ACQUIRED* ANTIBODY HEMOLYTIC ANEMIA AND FAMILIAL ABERRATIONS IN GAMMA GLOBULINS. AM. J. MED. 36* 188-199, 1964.

KISSMEYER-NIELSEN, F., HANSEN, K. AND KIELER, J.* IMMUNO-HEMOLYTIC ANEMIA WITH FAMILIAL OCCURRENCE. ACTA MED. SCAND. 144* 35-39, 1952.

20580 ANEMIA, CHLORAMPHENICOL-INDUCED

NAGAO AND MAUER (1969) DESCRIBED IDENTICAL TWINS WITH CHLORAMPHENICOL-INDUCED APLASTIC ANEMIA. DAMESHEK (1969), IN AN ACCOMPANYING EDITORIAL, REVIEWED EVIDENCE FOR A GENETIC SUSCEPTIBILITY TO DRUG-INDUCED BONE MARROW SUPPRESSION.

DAMESHEK, W.* CHLORAMPHENICOL APLASTIC ANEMIA IN IDENTICAL TWINS - A CLUE TO PATHOGENESIS. (EDITORIAL) NEW ENG. J. MED. 281* 42-43, 1969.

NAGAO, T. AND MAUER, A. M.* CONCORDANCE FOR DRUG-INDUCED APLASTIC ANEMIA IN IDENTICAL TWINS. NEW ENG. J. MED. 281* 7-11, 1969.

20590 ANEMIA, CONGENITAL HYPOPLASTIC, OF BLACKFAN AND DIAMOND (CHRONIC CONGENITAL AREGENERATIVE ANEMIA, ERYTHROGENESIS IMPERFECTA, *PURE RED CELL ANEMIA*)

FAMILIAL CASES HAVE BEEN REPORTED BY BURGERT, KENNEDY AND PEASE (1954) AND BY DIAMOND, ALLEN AND MAGILL (1961). THIS DISORDER IS SOMETIMES ENCOUNTERED IN THE NEWBORN, IS PROGRESSIVE AND IS NON-REGENERATIVE. THERE IS NO ERYTHROBLASTOSIS, HEMOLYSIS OR HEPATOSPLENOMEGALY (UNTIL MANY TRANSFUSIONS HAVE BEEN GIVEN). LEUKOCYTES AND PLATELETS ARE USUALLY NORMAL. OCCASIONALLY CORTISONE IS EFFECTIVE. IN SOME AN ABNORMALITY OF TRYPTOPHANE METABOLISM, MANIFESTED BY URINARY EXCRETION OF ANTHRANILIC ACID, HAS BEEN FOUND. HIRSCHMAN ET AL. (1969) REPORTED TWO BROTHERS WITH APLASTIC ANEMIA SIMILAR TO FANCONI ANEMIA BUT WITHOUT ASSOCIATED CONGENITAL ANOMALIES. BOTH RESPONDED TO ANDROGEN THERAPY. BOTH SHOWED INCREASED CHROMOSOMAL BREAKAGE AS IN FANCONI ANEMIA. ONE HAD A STABLE TRANSLOCATION CHROMOSOME IN BONE MARROW CELLS. THE OTHER'S SKIN FIBROBLASTS SHOWED INCREASED SUSCEPTIBILITY TO 'MALIGNANT' TRANSFORMATION BY SV40 VIRUS, AS IN FANCONI ANEMIA. SKIN FIBROBLASTS OF THE MOTHER AND A SISTER, BOTH NORMAL, ALSO SHOWED INCREASED SUSCEPTIBILITY TO 'MALIGNANT' TRANSFORMATION. THE FATHER WAS, IT SEEMS, NOT STUDIED FROM THIS POINT OF VIEW.

ALTMAN, K. I. AND MILLER, G.* A DISTURBANCE OF TRYPTOPHAN METABOLISM IN CONGENITAL HYPOPLASTIC ANEMIA. NATURE 172* 868 ONLY, 1953.

BLOOM, G. E., WARNER, S., GERALD, P. S. AND DIAMOND, L. K.* CHROMOSOME ABNORMALITIES IN CONSTITUTIONAL APLASTIC ANEMIA. NEW ENG. J. MED. 274* 8-14, 1966.

BURGERT, E. O., JR., KENNEDY, R. L. J. AND PEASE, G. L.* CONGENITAL HYPOPLASTIC ANEMIA. PEDIATRICS 13* 218-226, 1954.

DIAMOND, L. K., ALLEN, D. W. AND MAGILL, F. B.* CONGENITAL (ERYTHROID) HYPOPLASTIC ANEMIA* A 25 YEAR STUDY. AM. J. DIS. CHILD. 102* 403-415, 1961.

HIRSCHMAN, R. J., SHULMAN, N. R., ABUELO, J. G. AND WHANG-PENG, J.* CHROMOSOMAL ABERRATIONS IN TWO CASES OF INHERITED APLASTIC ANEMIA WITH UNUSUAL CLINICAL FEATURES. ANN. INTERN. MED. 71* 107-117, 1969.

KASS, A. AND SUNDAL, A.* ANAEMIA HYPOPLASTICA CONGENITA (ANAEMIA TYPUS JOSEPHS-DIAMOND-BLACKFAN). REPORT OF A CASE TREATED WITH ADRENOCORTICOTROPIN WITH EFFECT. ACTA PAEDIAT. 42* 265-274, 1953.

PEARSON, H. A. AND CONE, T. E., JR.* CONGENITAL HYPOPLASTIC ANEMIA. PEDIATRICS 19* 192-200, 1957.

R
E
C   *20600 ANEMIA, FAMILIAL PYRIDOXINE-RESPONSIVE
E
S   UNLIKE THE CLINICALLY SIMILAR DISORDER REPORTED BY COOLEY AND BY RUNDLES AND FALLS
S   AND TRANSMITTED AS AN X-LINKED RECESSIVE, THE CONDITION IN THE FAMILY DESCRIBED BY
I   COTTON AND HARRIS (1962) WAS CLEARLY AUTOSOMAL RECESSIVE.
V
E
COTTON, H. B. AND HARRIS, J. W.* FAMILIAL PYRIDOXINE-RESPONSIVE ANEMIA. (ABSTRACT) J. CLIN. INVEST. 41* 1352 ONLY, 1962.

20610 ANEMIA, HYPOCHROMIC MICROCYTIC

SHAHIDI, NATHAN AND DIAMOND (1964) DESCRIBED HYPOCHROMIC MICROCYTIC ANEMIA IN A BROTHER AND SISTER OF FRENCH-CANADIAN EXTRACTION. AN ERROR IN IRON METABOLISM WAS CHARACTERIZED BY HIGH SERUM IRON, MASSIVE HEPATIC IRON DEPOSITION AND ABSENCE OF STAINABLE BONE MARROW IRON STORES. NO DEFECT IN TRANSFERRIN OR IN THE QUALITATIVE ASPECTS OF HEME SYNTHESIS COULD BE SHOWN. THE PARENTS AND TWO OTHER SIBS WERE NORMAL. DESPITE ADEQUATE TRANSFERRIN-IRON COMPLEX, DELIVERY OF IRON TO THE ERYTHROID BONE MARROW WAS APPARENTLY INSUFFICIENT FOR THE DEMANDS OF HEMOGLOBIN SYNTHESIS.

SHAHIDI, N. T., NATHAN, D. G. AND DIAMOND, L. K.* IRON DEFICIENCY ANEMIA ASSOCIATED WITH AN ERROR OF IRON METABOLISM IN TWO SIBLINGS. J. CLIN. INVEST. 43* 510-521, 1964.

20620 ANEMIA, NONSPHEROCYTIC HEMOLYTIC

SELWYN AND DACIE (1954) ORIGINALLY DIVIDED THIS GROUP INTO TYPE I AND II, ACCORDING TO WHETHER AUTOHEMOLYSIS WAS OR WAS NOT CORRECTED BY ADDITION OF GLUCOSE AND ADENOSINE TO THE INCUBATION SYSTEM. THIS STILL HAS SOME USEFULNESS IN INITIAL STUDY OF CASES. A DEFECT IN GLYCOLYSIS WAS SPECULATED IN TYPE II CASES. PYRUVATE KINASE DEFICIENCY AND TRIOSEPHOSPHATE ISOMERASE DEFICIENCY FALL INTO THIS GROUP WHEREAS GLUCOSE-6-PHOSPHATE DEHYDROGENASE DEFICIENCY (X-LINKED) AND HB ZURICH ARE IN THE TYPE I CATEGORY.

DESFORGES, J. F.* ERTHROCYTE METABOLISM IN HEMOLYSIS. NEW ENG. J. MED. 273* 1310-1321, 1965.

SELWYN, J. G. AND DACIE, J. V.* AUTOHEMOLYSIS AND OTHER CHANGES RESULTING FROM THE INCUBATION IN VITRO OF RED CELLS FROM PATIENTS WITH CONGENITAL HEMOLYTIC ANEMIA. BLOOD 9* 414-438, 1954.

20630 ANEMIA, NONSPHEROCYTIC HEMOLYTIC, ASSOCIATED WITH ABNORMALITY OF RED-CELL

IN A POLISH-BORN JEWISH FAMILY, DANON ET AL. (1962) DESCRIBED AN ELECTRON MICROSCOPIC ABNORMALITY OF THE RED-CELL MEMBRANE WHICH PROBABLY WAS RESPONSIBLE FOR SUSCEPTIBILITY TO HEMOLYSIS ON EXPOSURE TO DRUGS AND POSSIBLY VIRUSES. TWO SISTERS HAD SIMILAR FINDINGS. QUESTIONABLE ANOMALY WAS FOUND IN THE PROBAND'S SON.

DANON, D., DE VRIES, A., DJALDETTI, M. AND KIRSCHMANN, C.* EPISODES OF ACUTE HAEMOLYTIC ANAEMIA IN A PATIENT WITH FAMILIAL ULTRASTRUCTURAL ABNORMALITY OF THE RED-CELL MEMBRANE. BRIT. J. HAEMAT. 8* 274-282, 1962.

20640 ANEMIA, NONSPHEROCYTIC HEMOLYTIC, POSSIBLY DUE TO DEFECT IN PORPHYRIN METABO-LISM

FROM BERNE, TONZ, MEREU AND KASER (1961) REPORTED TWO BROTHERS, AGE 7 AND 14 YEARS, WITH HEMOLYTIC DISEASE ALREADY MANIFEST IN THE FIRST WEEKS OF LIFE. CHRONIC JAUNDICE, SEVERE ANEMIA AND SPLENOMEGALY WERE FEATURES. SPLENECTOMY WAS OF SOME BENEFIT. SEVERAL ENZYMES OF THE ERYTHROCYTE WERE NORMAL, BUT PYRUVATE KINASE ACTIVITY WAS NOT MEASURED. THE URINE CONSISTENTLY SHOWED AN INCREASED AMOUNT OF PORPHOBILINOGEN AND DELTA-AMINOLEVULINIC ACID. A DEFECT IN PORPHYRIN METABOLISM (I.E., HEME SYNTHESIS) WAS SUGGESTED. SINCE THE ANCESTORS OF THE AMISH CASES OF PYRUVATE KINASE DEFICIENCY (Q.V.) FIRST REPORTED BY BOWMAN AND PROCOPIO ORIGINATED IN THE CANTON BERNE, STUDIES OF PYRUVATE KINASE ARE PARTICULARLY PERTINENT.

TONZ, O., MEREU, T. AND KASER, H.* FAMILIARE, NICHT-SPHAROCYTARE HAMOLYTISCHE ANAMIE MIT AUSSCHEIDUNG VON PORPHYRINPRAKURSOREN. HELV. PAEDIAT. ACTA 16* 111-133, 1961.

20650 ANENCEPHALY

PENROSE (1957) CONCLUDED THAT RECESSIVE CASES EXIST. MULTIPLE AFFECTED SIBS WERE REPORTED BY SEVERAL AUTHORS, E.G., IFFY (1963) WHO OBSERVED THREE AFFECTED SIBS AND QUOTED THE DESCRIPTION BY MARTIN (1840) OF 6 AFFECTED SIBS. A STRIKING GEOGRAPHIC VARIATION MAY BE IN PART DUE TO ETHNIC GENETIC DIFFERENCES (MASTERSON, 1962). CONCORDANTLY AFFECTED PRESUMABLY MONOZYGOTIC TWINS WERE REPORTED BY TABER AND ELWELL (1960), JOSEPHSON AND WALLER (1933) AND LABATE AND CALVELLI (1952). DISCORDANCE IN MONOZYGOTIC TWINS WAS REPORTED BY GREBE (1949), AND PEDLOW (1961) AND LITT AND STRAUSS (1935). HORNE'S PATIENT (1958) HAD 4 ANENCEPHALIC OFFSPRING OF WHICH THE LAST WAS SIRED BY A MAN OTHER THAN THE HUSBAND. IN SINGLE FAMILIES, (STEVENSON, 1960* MARTIN, 1840) SIX SIBS HAVE BEEN AFFECTED. DUMOULIN AND GORDON (1959) REPORTED A PATIENT WHO IN ADDITION TO PRODUCING 3 NORMAL AND 2 ANENCEPHALIC INFANTS HAD UNIOVULAR TWINS, ONE OF WHICH WAS ANENCEPHALIC. RECORD AND MCKEOWN (1950) ESTIMATED THAT THE EMPIRIC RISK OF RECURRENCE IS ABOUT 2 PERCENT. YEN AND MACMAHON (1968) STUDIED THE RECURRENCE OF ANENCEPHALY IN FAMILIES AND CONCLUDED THAT THE FINDINGS WERE EXPLAINED BY A PERSISTENT ENVIRONMENTAL FACTOR AS ADEQUATE-LY AS BY GENETIC FACTORS. CHRISTAKOS AND SIMPSON (1969) DESCRIBED ANENCEPHALY IN THREE SIBS.

RECESSIVE

CHRISTAKOS, A. C. AND SIMPSON, J. L.* ANENCEPHALY IN THREE SIBLINGS. OBSTET. GYNEC. 33* 267-270, 1969.

COLEMAN, J. U.* REPEAT ANENCEPHALY. CANAD. MED. ASS. J. 79* 395-397, 1958.

DUMOULIN, J. G. AND GORDON, M. E.* ANENCEPHALY IN TWINS. J. OBSTET. GYNAEC. BRIT. COMM. 66* 964-968, 1959.

GREBE, H.* ANENCEPHALIE BEI EINEM PAARLING VON EINEIIGEN ZWILLINGEN. VIRCHOW. ARCH. PATH. ANAT. 316* 116-124, 1949.

HORNE, H. W.* ANENCEPHALY IN FOUR CONSECUTIVE PREGNANCIES. REPORT OF A CASE. FERTIL. STERIL. 9* 67-68, 1958.

IFFY, L.* THRICE RECURRING ANENCEPHALUS. BRIT. J. CLIN. PRACT. 17* 83-84, 1963.

JOSEPHSON, J. E. AND WALLER, K. B.* ANENCEPHALY IN IDENTICAL TWINS. CANAD. MED. ASS. J. 29* 34-37, 1933.

LABATE, J. S. AND CALVELLI, G. J., JR.* ANENCEPHALIC TWINS WITH RUPTURE OF THE UTERUS. NEW YORK J. MED. 52* 2662 ONLY, 1952.

LITT, S. AND STRAUSS, H. A.* MONOAMNIOTIC TWINS, ONE NORMAL, OTHER ANENCEPHA-LIC* MULTIPLE TRUE KNOTS IN CORDS. AM. J. OBSTET. GYNEC. 30* 728-730, 1935.

MARTIN, J.* SUCCESSION OF MONSTROUS BIRTHS OCCURRING IN THE SAME FEMALE. MED. EXAM. 5* 23, 1840.

MASTERSON, J. G.* EMPIRIC RISK, GENETIC COUNSELING AND PREVENTIVE MEASURES IN ANENCEPHALY. ACTA GENET. STATIST. MED. 12* 219-229, 1962.

PEDLOW, P. R. B.* ANENCEPHALY IN A MONO-AMNIOTIC TWIN. BRIT. MED. J. 2* 997-998, 1961.

PENROSE, L. S.* GENETICS OF ANENCEPHALY. J. MENT. DEFIC. RES. 1* 4-15, 1957.

RECORD, R. G. AND MCKEOWN, T.* CONGENITAL MALFORMATION OF THE CENTRAL NERVOUS SYSTEM. III. RISK OF MALFORMATION IN SIBS OF MALFORMED INDIVIDUALS. BRIT. J. PREV. SOC. MED. 4* 217-220, 1950.

STEVENSON, A. C.* THE RELATION OF HYDRAMNIOS WITH CONGENITAL MALFORMATIONS. IN, WOLSTENHOLME, G. E. W. AND O'CONNOR, C. M. (EDS.)* CIBA FOUNDATION SYMPOSIUM ON CONGENITAL MALFORMATIONS. BOSTON* LITTLE, BROWN AND CO., 1960. P. 259.

TABER, K. W. AND ELWELL, W. J., JR.* MONOZYGOTIC ANENCEPHALIC TWINS. MARYLAND MED. J. 9* 14 ONLY, 1960.

YEN, S. AND MACMAHON, B.* GENETICS OF ANENCEPHALY AND SPINA BIFIDA.Q LANCET 2* 623-626, 1968.

*20660 ANHIDROSIS

ANHIDROTIC ECTODERMAL DYSPLASIA IS USUALLY INHERITED AS AN X-LINKED DISORDER. MAHLOUDJI AND LIVINGSTON (1967) DESCRIBED AN IRANIAN SIBSHIP IN WHICH A BOY AND TWO GIRLS HAD ANHIDROSIS WITHOUT DENTAL, FACIAL, BRAIN OR OTHER ANOMALIES CHARACTERISTIC OF THE X-LINKED DISORDER. THE PARENTS WERE FIRST COUSINS. SEE ECTODERMAL DYSPLASIA, ANHIDROTIC, IN THIS CATALOG.

MAHLOUDJI, M. AND LIVINGSTON, K. E.* FAMILIAL AND CONGENITAL SIMPLE ANHIDROSIS. AM. J. DIS. CHILD. 113* 477-479, 1967.

20670 ANIRIDIA, CEREBELLAR ATAXIA AND MENTAL DEFICIENCY

GILLESPIE (1965) DESCRIBED BROTHERS AND SISTERS WITH THIS COMBINATION WHICH HAS APPARENTLY NOT BEEN REPORTED PREVIOUSLY, ALTHOUGH CEREBELLAR ATAXIA, MENTAL DEFICIENCY AND CONGENITAL CATARACTS ARE KNOWN IN THE MARINESCO-SJOGREN SYNDROME. IT IS LIKELY THAT GILLESPIE'S PATIENTS REPRESENT A SEPARATE MUTATION. THE KARYOTYPE WAS NORMAL IN HIS PATIENTS.

GILLESPIE, F. D.* ANIRIDIA, CEREBELLAR ATAXIA, AND OLIGOPHRENIA IN SIBLINGS. ARCH. OPHTHAL. 73* 338-341, 1965.

20680 ANONYCHIA

RECESSIVE INHERITANCE IS NOT FIRMLY ESTABLISHED AND, IF IT EXISTS, MUST BE RARE. LITTMAN AND LEVIN (1964) OBSERVED AN AFFECTED BROTHER AND SISTER WITH NO OTHER ANOMALY AND WITH NO AFFECTED RELATIVES. TIMMER AND WILDERVANCK (1969) DESCRIBED CONGENITAL COMPLETE ANONYCHIA IN A GIRL WHOSE PARENTS WERE SOMEWHAT MORE CLOSELY RELATED THAN SECOND COUSINS.

LITTMAN, A. AND LEVIN, S.* ANONYCHIA AS A RECESSIVE AUTOSOMAL TRAIT IN MAN. J. INVEST. DERM. 42* 177-178, 1964.

TIMMER, J. AND WILDERVANCK, L. S.* ANONYCHIA CONGENITA TOTALIS VAN VINGERS EN TENSEN. NEDERL. T. GENEESK. 113* 395-397, 1969.

*20690 ANOPHTHALMOS, TRUE OR PRIMARY

THIS ANOMALY IS DUE TO FAILURE OF FORMATION OF THE OPTIC PIT. ONLY THE ECTODERMAL ELEMENTS ARE MISSING. IT IS ALWAYS BILATERAL. IN ALMOST ALL INSTANCES THE PARENTS ARE RELATED. FOR EXAMPLE, CECCHETTO (1920) REPORTED A PEDIGREE IN WHICH TWO BROTHERS, EACH MARRIED TO A FIRST COUSIN, HAD A CHILD WITH BILATERAL ANOPHTHA-LMOS. THE COMMON GRANDPARENTS WERE ALSO FIRST COUSINS. HESSELBERG (1951) REPORTED AFFECTED CHILDREN FROM FIRST COUSIN PARENTS. SORSBY (1934) DISCOVERED EARLY REPORTS OF AFFECTED SIBS WITH NORMAL PARENTS. ASHLEY (1947) REPORTED AFFECTED JAPANESE BROTHER AND SISTER. SOMETIMES DIFFERENTIATION OF EXTREME MICROPHTHALMOS (Q.V.) FROM ANOPHTHALMOS IS DIFFICULT.

ASHLEY, L. M.* BILATERAL ANOPHTHALMOS IN A BROTHER AND SISTER. J. HERED. 38* 174-176, 1947.

CECCHETTO, E.* DELL'ANOFTALMO CONGENITO FAMILIARE. ARCH. OTTAL. 27* 114-119, 1920.

HESSELBERG, C.* CONGENITAL BILATERAL ANOPHTHALMIA. ACTA OPHTHAL. 29* 183-189, 1951.

JOSEPH, R.* A PEDIGREE OF ANOPHTHALMOS. BRIT. J. OPHTHAL. 41* 541-543, 1957.

SORSBY, A.* ANOPHTHALMOS* UNPUBLISHED MANUSCRIPT BY JAMES BRIGGS GIVING FIRST ACCOUNT OF FAMILIAL OCCURRENCE OF CONDITION. BRIT. J. OPHTHAL. 18* 469-472, 1934.

20700 ANOSMIA FOR ISOBUTYRIC ACID

R
E
C
E
S
S
I
V
E

AMOORE (1967) STUDIED ANOSMIA FOR THE SWEAT-LIKE ODOR OF ISOBUTYRIC ACID. THE FREQUENCY WAS ABOUT 2.5 PERCENT. NO FAMILY STUDIES WERE REPORTED. BY ANALOGY TO DALTONISM, HE SUGGESTED IT BE CALLED DAVISM IN HONOR OF ALFRED DAVIS WHO DESCRIBED IT.

AMOORE, J. E.* SPECIFIC ANOSMIA* A CLUE TO THE OLFACTORY CODE. NATURE 214* 1095-1098, 1967.

20710 ANOTIA AND MEATAL ATRESIA

ELLWOOD ET AL. (1968) DESCRIBED TWO SIBS WITH BILATERAL ANOTIA AND MEATAL ATRESIA. IN A SECOND UNRELATED FAMILY, ONE SIB HAD UNILATERAL MICROTIA AND BILATERAL MEATAL ATRESIA WHEREAS THE OTHER HAD UNILATERAL MICROTIA AND MEATAL ATRESIA.

ELLWOOD, L. C., WINTER, S. T. AND DAR, H.* FAMILIAL MICROTIA WITH MEATAL ATRESIA IN TWO SIBSHIPS. J. MED. GENET. 5* 289-291, 1968.

20720 ANTITHROMBIN III DEFICIENCY

DEFICIENCY OF ANTITHROMBIN III LEADS TO AN INCREASED TENDENCY TO THROMBOEMBOLISM. VON KAULLA (1970), WHO HAS STUDIED THIS BLOOD FACTOR (VON KAULLA AND VON KAULLA, 1967), STATES THAT THE DEFICIENCY "CAN BE HEREDITARY" BUT THIS IS NOT FULLY EXPLORED.

VON KAULLA, E. AND VON KAULLA, K. N.* ANTITHROMBIN III AND DISEASES. AM. J. CLIN. PATH. 48* 69-80, 1967.

20730 ANTITHROMBIN, FAMILIAL HEMORRHAGIC DIATHESIS DUE TO

BROWN AND COLLEAGUES (1963) HAVE DESCRIBED A HEMORRHAGIC DIATHESIS APPARENTLY DUE TO THE PRESENCE OF AN ANTITHROMBIN AS THE PRIMARY DEFECT. THE DISORDER OCCURRED IN A MOHAWK INDIAN KINDRED. RECESSIVE INHERITANCE IS NOT COMPLETELY CERTAIN.

BROWN, G. M., DIAMANT, N. E., GALBRAITH, P. R. AND WILSON, W. E. C.* A FAMILIAL HEMORRHAGIC DIATHESIS DUE TO AN ANTITHROMBIN. BLOOD 21* 298-305, 1963.

*20740 ANTITRYPSIN DEFICIENCY OF PLASMA

LAURELL AND ERIKSSON (1963) DESCRIBED ABSENCE OF ALPHA-1-ANTITRYPSIN FROM THE PLASMA IN PATIENTS WITH DEGENERATIVE LUNG DISEASE LEADING TO DEATH IN MIDDLE LIFE. FAMILY STUDIES INDICATE RECESSIVE INHERITANCE. THE HETEROZYGOTES ARE FREE OF DISEASE BUT CAN BE IDENTIFIED CHEMICALLY. SEVERAL WORKERS HAVE CONFIRMED THESE FINDINGS. OF 12 PATIENTS WITH DESTRUCTIVE LUNG DISEASE PRESENT PRIOR TO AGE FORTY, TWO WERE JUDGED BY TARKOFF ET AL. (1968) TO BE HOMOZYGOUS FOR THE DEFICIEN-CY AND ONE HETEROZYGOUS. AMONG 103 PATIENTS WITH OBSTRUCTIVE LUNG DISEASE KUEPPERS ET AL. (1969) FOUND 5 HOMOZYGOTES AND 25 HETEROZYGOTES FOR THE DEFICIENCY GENE. THEY SUGGESTED THAT ESPECIALLY IN MALES HETEROZYGOSITY MAY PREDISPOSE TO CHRONIC OBSTRUCTIVE LUNG DISEASE. LIEBERMAN (1969) PRESENTED EVIDENCE INDICATING THAT HETEROZYGOTES ALSO HAVE A PREDISPOSITION TO LUNG DISEASE. THE IMPORTANCE OF PROMPT TREATMENT OF RESPIRATORY INFECTIONS AND AVOIDANCE OF PROTEOLYTIC AEROSOLS, SMOKING AND EMPLOYMENT ENTAILING EXPOSURE TO RESPIRATORY IRRITANTS WAS EMPHASIZED AS PREVENTIVE MEASURES IN THESE FAMILIES. BELL (1970) POINTED OUT THAT THE EMPHYSEMATOUS CHANGES INVOLVE PRIMARILY THE LOWER LUNG FIELDS. GANS ET AL. (1969) DESCRIBED FAMILIAL INFANTILE LIVER CIRRHOSIS IN PRESUMED HOMOZYGOTES FOR ALPHA(1)-TRYPSIN DEFICIENCY.

BELL, R. S.* THE RADIOGRAPHIC MANIFESTATIONS OF ALPHA-1 ANTITRYPSIN DEFICIENCY. AN IMPORTANT RECOGNIZABLE PATTERN OF CHRONIC OBSTRUCTIVE PULMONARY DISEASE (COPD). RADIOLOGY 95* 19-24, 1970.

ERIKSSON, S.* STUDIES IN ALPHA 1-ANTITRYPSIN DEFICIENCY. ACTA MED. SCAND. 177 (SUPPL. 432)* 1-85, 1965.

FALK, G. A. AND BRISCOE, W. A.* ALPHA-1-ANTITRYPSIN DEFICIENCY IN CHRONIC OBSTRUCTIVE PULMONARY DISEASE. (EDITORIAL) ANN. INTERN. MED. 72* 427-429, 1970.

FALK, G. A. AND BRISCOE, W. A.* CHRONIC OBSTRUCTIVE PULMONARY DISEASE AND HETEROZYGOUS ALPHA-1-ANTITRYPSIN DEFICIENCY. (EDITORIAL) ANN. INTERN. MED. 72* 595-596, 1970.

GANS, H., SHARP, H. L. AND TANS, B. H.* ANTIPROTEASE DEFICIENCY AND FAMILIAL INFANTILE LIVER CIRRHOSIS. SURG. GYNEC. OBSTET. 129* 289-299, 1969.

HEPPER, N. G., BLACK, L. F., GLEICH, G. J. AND KUEPPERS, F.* THE PREVALENCE OF ALPHA(1)-ANTITRYPSIN DEFICIENCY IN SELECTED GROUPS OF PATIENTS WITH CHRONIC OBSTRUCTIVE LUNG DISEASE. MAYO CLIN. PROC. 44* 697-710, 1969.

KUEPPERS, F., BRISCOE, W. A. AND BEARN, A. G.* HEREDITARY DEFICIENCY OF SERUM ALPHA 1-ANTITRYPSIN. SCIENCE 146* 1678-1679, 1964.

KUEPPERS, F., FALLAT, R. AND LARSON, R. K.* OBSTRUCTIVE LUNG DISEASES AND ALPHA-ANTITRYPSIN DEFICIENCY GENE HETEROZYGOSITY. SCIENCE 165* 899-901, 1969.

LAURELL, C. B. AND ERIKSSON, S.* THE ELECTROPHORETIC ALPHA-1-GLOBULIN PATTERN OF SERUM IN ALPHA-1-ANTITRYPSIN DEFICIENCY. SCAND. J. CLIN. LAB. INVEST. 15* 132-140, 1963.

LIEBERMAN, J.* HETEROZYGOUS AND HOMOZYGOUS ALPHA-1-ANTITRYPSIN DEFICIENCY IN PATIENTS WITH PULMONARY EMPHYSEMA. NEW ENG. J. MED. 281* 279-284, 1969.

LOPEZ, V., OETLIKER, O., COLOMBO, J. P. AND BUTLER, R.* EIN FALL VON FAMILIAREM ALPHA-1-ANTITRYPSIN-MANGEL. HELV. PAEDIAT. ACTA 19* 296-303, 1964.

PIERCE, J. A., EISEN, A. Z. AND DHINGRA, H. K.* RELATIONSHIP OF ANTITRYPSIN DEFICIENCY TO THE PATHOGENESIS OF EMPHYSEMA. TRANS. ASS. AM. PHYS. 82* 87-97, 1969.

SHARP, H. L., BRIDGES, R. A., KRIVIT, W. AND FREIER, E. F.* CIRRHOSIS ASSO-CIATED WITH ALPHA-1-ANTITRYPSIN DEFICIENCY* A PREVIOUSLY UNRECOGNIZED INHERITED DISORDER. J. LAB. CLIN. MED. 73* 934-939, 1969.

TALAMO, R. C., ALLEN, J. D., KAHAN, M. G. AND AUSTEN, K. F.* HEREDITARY ALPHA (1)-ANTITRYPSIN DEFICIENCY. NEW ENG. J. MED. 278* 345-351, 1968.

TARKOFF, M. P., KUEPPERS, F. AND MILLER, W. F.* PULMONARY EMPHYSEMA AND ALPHA(1)-ANTITRYPSIN DEFICIENCY. AM. J. MED. 45* 220-228, 1968.

TOWNLEY, R. G., RYNING, F., LYNCH, H. AND BRODY, A. W.* OBSTRUCTIVE LUNG DISEASE IN HEREDITARY ALPHA-1-ANTITRYPSIN DEFICIENCY. J.A.M.A. 214* 325-331, 1970.

20750 ANUS, IMPERFORATE

FAMILIES WITH MULTIPLE AFFECTED SIBS, BOTH MALE AND FEMALE, HAVE BEEN REPORTED (VAN GELDER AND KLOEPFER, 1961* WINKLER AND WEINSTEIN, 1970). SEE X-LINKED CATALOG.

VAN GELDER, D. W. AND KLOEPFER, H. W.* FAMILIAL ANORECTAL ANOMALIES. PEDIA-TRICS 27* 334-336, 1961.

WINKLER, J. M. AND WEINSTEIN, E. D.* IMPERFORATE ANUS AND HEREDITY. J. PEDIAT. SURG. 5* 555-558, 1970.

R
E
C
E
S
S
I
V
E

20760 AORTIC ARCH SYNDROME ("YOUNG FEMALE ARTERITIS," "PULSELESS DISEASE," OR TAKAYASU'S ARTERITIS)

WE HAVE OBSERVED JAPANESE SISTERS WITH AORTIC ARCH SYNDROME. THIS COMMON DISEASE IN JAPANESE IS NOT STRIKINGLY FAMILIAL. THE RACIAL CONCENTRATION OF CASES IS NOT NECESSARILY GENETIC. THE DISEASE IS RELATIVELY FREQUENT THROUGHOUT THE ORIENT, FOR EXAMPLE IN INDIA AMONG CAUCASOID PEOPLE OF THAT COUNTRY. SEVERAL STUDIES SUGGEST AN AUTOIMMUNE BASIS. A MODEST FAMILIAL AGGREGATION MAY HAVE THE SAME BASIS AS THAT OBSERVED IN OTHER TYPES OF POSSIBLE AUTOIMMUNE DISEASE, SUCH AS HASHIMOTO'S STRUMA (Q.V.).

HIRSCH, M. S., AIKAT, B. K. AND BASU, A. K.* TAKAYASU'S ARTERITIS. REPORT OF FIVE CASES WITH IMMUNOLOGIC STUDIES. BULL. HOPKINS HOSP. 115* 29-64, 1964.

IKEDA, M.* IMMUNOLOGIC STUDIES ON TAKAYASU'S ARTERITIS. JAP. CIR. J. 30* 87-89, 1966.

ITO, I.* AORTITIS SYNDROME WITH REFERENCE TO DETECTION OF ANTI-AORTA ANTIBODY FROM PATIENTS' SERA. JAP. CIRC. J. 30* 75-78, 1966.

*20770 APLASIA CUTIS CONGENITA (CONGENITAL DEFECT OF SKIN, CONGENITAL DEFECT OF SKULL AND SCALP)

THE SCALP IS THE MOST FREQUENT SITE. LESIONS ON THE TRUNK OR EXTREMITIES APPEAR AS AREAS IN WHICH THE ABSENT SKIN IS REPRESENTED BY A THIN TRANSPARENT MEMBRANE THROUGH WHICH UNDERLYING STRUCTURES ARE VISIBLE. BONE UNDERLYING THE INVOLVED SKIN, ESPECIALLY SKULL, SHOWS A DISTURBANCE OF DEVELOPMENT. THIS AND THE SITE OF PREDILECTION LEADS TO THE DESIGNATION "CONGENITAL DEFECT OF SKULL AND SCALP" SOMETIMES USED. RECESSIVE INHERITANCE IS SUGGESTED BY THE FINDINGS IN SOME FAMILIES* GEDDA ET AL. (1963) REPORTED THE CONDITION IN A BOY AND GIRL FROM CONSANGUINEOUS PARENTS. IN OTHER FAMILIES DOMINANT INHERITANCE WITH REDUCED PENETRANCE IS EQUALLY POSSIBLE (RAUSCHKOLB AND ENRIQUEZ, 1962). A DEFECT IN THE SKIN OF THE SCALP IS SOMETIMES FOUND IN CASES OF D1 TRISOMY (LEE, 1964) AND THOSE OF DELETION OF CHROMOSOME 4 OR 5 (HIRSCHHORN ET AL., 1965). A SIMILAR CONDITION WITH ABSENCE DEFECT OF THE LIMBS IS DESCRIBED IN THE CATALOG OF DOMINANTS.

DE VINK, L. P. H. J.* KONGENITALER HAUTDEFEKT BEI EINEM NEUGEBORENEN. ARCH. GYNAEK. 167* 291-299, 1938.

GEDDA, L., MURATORE, A. AND BERNARDI, A.* LA GANGRENA ASETTICA DELLA TECA CRANICA COME APLASIA CIRCOSCRITTA EREDITARIA DEL NEONATO. ACTA GENET. MED. GEM. 12* 117-133, 1963.

341-358, 1931.

HIRSCHHORN, K., COOPER, H. L. AND FIRSCHEIN, I. L.* DELETION OF SHORT ARMS OF
CHROMOSOME 4-5 IN A CHILD WITH DEFECTS OF MIDLINE FUSION. HUMANGENETIK 1* 479-
482, 1965.

LEE, C. S. N.* BALTIMORE, MD.* PERSONAL COMMUNICATION, 1964.

RAUSCHKOLB, R. R. AND ENRIQUEZ, S. I.* APLASIA CUTIS CONGENITA. ARCH. DERM.
86* 54-57, 1962.

ROGATZ, J. L. AND DAVIDSON, H.* CONGENITAL DEFECT OF SKIN IN NEWBORN INFANT.
AM. J. DIS. CHILD. 65* 916-919, 1943.

*20780 ARGININEMIA

TERHEGGEN ET AL. (1969) DESCRIBED TWO SISTERS, AGED 18 MONTHS AND 5 YEARS, WITH
SPASTIC PARAPLEGIA, EPILEPTIC SEIZURES AND SEVERE MENTAL RETARDATION. THE PARENTS
WERE RELATED. ARGININE LEVELS WERE HIGH IN THE BLOOD AND SPINAL FLUID OF THE
PATIENTS AND SHOWED INTERMEDIATE ELEVATIONS IN BOTH PARENTS AND TWO HEALTHY SIBS.
ARGINASE ACTIVITY IN RED CELLS WAS VERY LOW IN THE PATIENTS AND INTERMEDIATE IN
LEVELS IN THE PARENTS. THE OBSERVATION THAT RESEARCH WORKERS WITH THE SHOPE VIRUS
HAVE LOW BLOOD ARGININE LED TO THE USE OF SHOPE VIRUS IN THIS DISORDER (RODGERS,
1970). THE ABILITY OF THIS DNA VIRUS TO RESTORE ARGINASE ACTIVITY IN THE AFFECTED
CHILDREN AND THE CLINICAL EFFECTS OF SAGERS, 1970). THE ABILITY OF THIS DNA VIRUS
TO RESTORE ARGINASE ACTIVITY IN THE AFFECTED CHILDREN AND THE CLINICAL EFFECTS OF
SOME REMAIN TO BE DETERMINED.

TERHEGGEN, H. G., SCHWENK, A., LOWENTHAL, A., VAN SANDE, M. AND COLOMBO, J. P.*
ARGININAEMIA WITH ARGINASE DEFICIENCY. (LETTER) LANCET 2* 748-749, 1969.

TERHEGGEN, H. G., SCHWENK, A., LOWENTHAL, A., VAN SANDE, M. AND COLOMBO, J. P.*
HYPERARGINAMIE MIT ARGINASEDEFEKT. EINE NEUE FAMILIARE STOFFWECHSELSTORUNG. Z.
KINDERHEILK. 107* 298-323, 1970.

ROGERS, S.* OAK RIDGE, TENN.* PERSONAL COMMUNICATION, 1970.

*20790 ARGININOSUCCINICACIDURIA

ONSET IS IN THE FIRST WEEKS OF LIFE. FEATURES INCLUDE MENTAL AND PHYSICAL
RETARDATION, LIVER ENLARGEMENT, SKIN LESIONS, DRY AND BRITTLE HAIR SHOWING
TRICHORRHEXIS NODOSA MICROSCOPICALLY AND FLUORESCING RED, CONVULSIONS AND EPISODIC
UNCONSCIOUSNESS. BRITTLE HAIR MAY BE FOUND ONLY ON A LOW PROTEIN DIET (CORYELL ET
AL., 1964), BECAUSE THIS HAS NOT BEEN AN IMPRESSIVE FEATURE IN THIS COUNTRY. THE
PATIENTS CANNOT MAKE ARGININE WHICH, HOWEVER, IS PROBABLY SUPPLIED ADEQUATELY BY
THE USUAL DIET IN THE U.S. IN BRITAIN, WHERE THE AVERAGE PROTEIN INTAKE IS LESS
AMPLE, HAIR CHANGES ARE THE RULE. LEWIS AND MILLER (1970) DESCRIBED THE NEUROPA-
THOLOGIC CHANGES. ASTROCYTE TRANSFORMATION TO ALZHEIMER TYPE II GLIA MAY BE A
CONSISTENT FEATURE OF ANY FORM OF HYPERAMMONEMIA. POSTMORTEM LIVER SHOWED MARKED
DEFICIENCY OF ARGININOSUCCINATELYASE.

CORYELL, M. E., HALL, W. K., THEVAOS, T. G., WELTER, D. A., GATZ, A. J.,
HORTON, B. F., SISSCN, B. D., LOOPER, J. W., JR. AND FARROW, R. T.* FAMILIAL STUDY
OF HUMAN ENZYME DEFECT, ARGININOSUCCINIC ACIDURIA. BIOCHEM. BIOPHYS. RES. COMMUN.
14* 307-312, 1964.

EFRON, M. L.* DISEASES OF THE UREA CYCLE* ARGININOSUCCINIC ACIDURIA. IN,
STANBURY, J. B., WYNGAARDEN, J. B. AND FREDRICKSON, D. S. (EDS.)* THE METABOLIC
BASIS OF INHERITED DISEASE. NEW YORK* MCGRAW-HILL, 1966 (2ND ED.). PP. 393-408.

KINT, J. AND CARTON, D.* DEFICIENT ARGININOSUCCINASE ACTIVITY IN BRAIN IN
ARGININOSUCCINICACIDURIA. (LETTER) LANCET 2* 635 ONLY, 1968.

LEVIN, B.* ARGINOSUCCINIC ACIDURIA. AM. J. DIS. CHILD. 113* 162-165, 1967.

LEVIN, B., MACKAY, H. M. AND OBERHOLZER, V. G.* ARGININOSUCCINIC ACIDURIA. AN
INBORN ERROR OF AMINO ACID METABOLISM. ARCH. DIS. CHILD. 36* 622-632, 1961.

LEWIS, P. D. AND MILLER, A. L.* ARGININOSUCCINIC ACIDURIA. CASE REPORT WITH
NEUROPATHOLOGICAL FINDINGS. BRAIN 93* 413-422, 1970.

MOSER, H. W., EFRON, M. L., BROWN, H., DIAMOND, R. AND NEUMANN, C. G.*
ARGININOSUCCINIC ACIDURIA* REPORT OF TWO CASES AND DEMONSTRATION OF INTERMITTENT
ELEVATION OF BLOOD AMMONIA. AM. J. MED. 42* 9-26, 1967.

*20800 ARTERIAL CALCIFICATION, GENERALIZED, OF INFANCY

THIS LESION HAS BEEN NOTED IN MULTIPLE SIBS (HUNT AND LEYS, 1957* MENTON AND
FETTERMAN, 1948). IT MAY BE FUNDAMENTALLY A DEFECT OF ELASTIC FIBER. CALCIFICA-
TION OCCURS PARTICULARLY IN THE INTERNAL ELASTIC LAMINA. MATERIAL WITH THE
STAINING PROPERTIES OF MUCOPOLYSACCHARIDE ACCUMULATES AROUND THE ELASTIC FIBERS.

FINE CALCIUM INCRUSTATION OF THE LAMINA IS THE MINIMAL LESION. LATER THE LAMINA IS RUPTURED AND OCCLUSIVE CHANGES IN THE INTIMA TAKE PLACE. DEATH FROM MYOCARDIAL INFARCTION USUALLY OCCURS IN THE FIRST SIX MONTHS. CALCIFICATION IN A PERIPHERAL ARTERY WITH EKG CHANGES OF OCCLUSIVE CORONARY ARTERY DISEASE SUGGESTS THE DIAGNOSIS. WITZLEBEN (1970) SUGGESTED THAT CALCIFICATION HAS BEEN OVEREMPHASIZED AND IS REALLY ONLY A SECONDARY PHENOMENON. 'INFANTILE CORONARY SCLEROSIS' IS TOO RESTRICTIVE IN ITS TOPOGRAPHIC IMPLICATIONS. HE SUGGESTED 'OCCLUSIVE INFANTILE ARTERIOPATHY' AS THE PREFERED TERM.

HUNT, A. C. AND LEYS, D. G.* GENERALIZED ARTERIAL CALCIFICATION IN INFANCY. BRIT. MED. J. 1* 385-386, 1957.

MCKUSICK, V. A.* HERITABLE DISORDERS OF CONNECTIVE TISSUE. ST. LOUIS* C. V. MOSBY CO., 1960 (2ND ED.). PP. 310-311 AND FIG. 103.

MENTON, M. L. AND FETTERMAN, G. G.* CORONARY SCLEROSIS IN INFANCY. REPORT OF THREE AUTOPSIED CASES, TWO IN SIBLINGS. AM. J. CLIN. PATH. 18* 805-810, 1948.

MORAN, J. J. AND BECKER, S. M.* IDIOPATHIC ARTERIAL CALCIFICATION OF INFANCY* REPORT OF 2 CASES OCCURRING IN SIBLINGS, AND REVIEW OF THE LITERATURE. AM. J. CLIN. PATH. 31* 517-529, 1959.

WITZLEBEN, C. L.* IDIOPATHIC INFANTILE ARTERIAL CALCIFICATION - A MISNOMER.Q AM. J. CARDIOL. 26* 305-309, 1970.

20810 ARTHROGRYPOSIS MULTIPLEX CONGENITA

LIKE AMYOTONIA CONGENITA, ARTHROGRYPOSIS IS REALLY A SYNDROME. GENETIC FORMS SEEM TO BE RARE. SEVERAL DISCORDANT MONOZYGOTIC TWIN PAIRS HAVE BEEN DESCRIBED. THE POSSIBILITY OF INFECTION OF THE FETUS BY A VIRUS WITH NEUROMYAL TROPISM (E.G., COCKSACKIE) SHOULD BE INVESTIGATED EPIDEMIOLOGICALLY, VIROLOGICALLY AND IMMUNOLO-GICALLY.
FRISCHKNECHT AND COLLEAGUES (1960) DESCRIBED THREE AFFECTED SIBS AND SUGGESTED INSTEAD OF ARTHROGRYPOSIS THE DESIGNATION 'NEUROARTHROMYODYSPLASIA' BECAUSE AT AUTOPSY CHANGES WERE FOUND TO INVOLVE THE SPINAL CORD AND THE BETZ CELLS. SWINYARD (1963) HAS ALSO REPORTED FAMILIAL CASES. WEISSMAN AND COLLEAGUES (1963) DESCRIBED AN ARTHROGRYPOSIS-LIKE PICTURE CONSISTING OF FLEXION CONTRACTURES AT THE ELBOWS OR KNEES AND NO DISLOCATION OF THE HIPS. BARGETON ET AL. (1961) REPORTED AUTOPSY FINDINGS IN ONE OF TWO BROTHERS, THE OFFSPRING OF FIRST COUSIN PARENTS. THE PRIMARY LESIONS WERE NEUROLOGIC. EK (1958) HAD AFFECTED SISTERS. IN ADDITION TO THE FORMS OF ARTHROGRYPOSIS DUE TO LOSS OF MOTOR NEURONS IN THE ANTERIOR HORN OF THE SPINAL CORD AND DUE TO CONGENITAL MUSCULAR DYSTROPHY, BARGETON ET AL. (1961) DESCRIBED A THIRD TYPE WHICH IS FAMILIAL AND CHARACTERIZED BY FOCAL COLLAGENOUS PROLIFERATION IN THE ANTERIOR SPINAL ROOTS. PENA ET AL. (1968) STUDIED TWO PUERTO RICAN FAMILIES, EACH WITH TWO AFFECTED CHILDREN. AT LEAST ONE OF THE FOUR AFFECTED CHILDREN WAS FEMALE. THE ACCUMULATED EXPERIENCE APPEARS TO INDICATE THE EXISTENCE OF AT LEAST ONE FORM OF RECESSIVELY INHERITED ARTHROGRYPOSIS (HENCE THE ASTERISK). PROBABLY THESE REPRESENT ONLY A SMALL PROPORTION OF THE WHOLE. SRIVASTAVA (1968) REPORTED AS ARTHROGRYPOSIS TWO BROTHERS WITH MULTIPLE HEMIVERTEBRAE AND FUSION OF SEVERAL VERTEBRAL BODIES. FLEXION CONTRACTURE OF THE ELBOWS AND KNEES WAS PRESENT. HOWEVER, ARTHROGRYPOSIS DOES NOT SEEM A JUSTIFIED DIAGNOSIS. LAITINEN AND HIRVENSALO (1966) OBSERVED AFFECTED SIBS. THREE SIBS WERE APPARENTLY AFFECTED IN A FAMILY REPORTED BY PENA ET AL. (1968). HISTOLOGIC ABNORMALITIES WERE FOUND IN THE SPINAL CORD. LEBENTHAL ET AL. (1970) REPORTED FURTHER OBSERVATIONS OF THE KINDRED STUDIED BY WEISSMAN ET AL. THEY FOUND 23 CASES IN AN INBRED ARAB GROUP AND CONCLUDED THAT THE DISORDER IS OF THE MYOPATHIC TYPE IN THESE CASES. SIX OF THE PATIENTS HAD CONGENITAL HEART DISEASE. THE DRACHMAN HYPOTHESIS THAT ARTHROGRYPOSIS IS CAUSED BY IMMOBILIZATION OF FETAL LIMBS DURING THE PERIOD OF FORMATION OF JOINTS RECEIVED SUPPORT FROM THE FINDING OF ARTHROGRYPOSIS IN THE OFFSPRING OF A WOMAN WHO RECEIVED TUBOCURARINE IN EARLY PREGNANCY FOR TREATMENT OF TETANUS (JAGO, 1970).

R
E
C
E
S
S
I
V
E

BARGETON, E., NEZELOF, C., GURAN, P. AND JOB, J.-C.* ETUDE ANATOMIQUE D'UN CAS D'ARTHROGRYPOSE MULTIPLE CONGENITALE ET FAMILIALE. REV. NEUROL. 104* 479-489, 1961.

DRACHMAN, D. B. AND BANKER, B. Q.* ARTHROGRYPOSIS MULTIPLEX CONGENITA. CASE DUE TO DISEASE OF THE ANTERIOR HORN CELLS. ARCH. NEUROL. 5* 77-93, 1961.

DRACHMAN, D. B. AND COULOMBRE, A. J.* EXPERIMENTAL CLUBFOOT AND ARTHROGRYPOSIS MULTIPLEX CONGENITA. LANCET 2* 523-526, 1962.

EK, J. I.* CEREBRAL LESIONS IN ARTHROGRYPOSIS MULTIPLEX CONGENITA. ACTA PAEDIAT. 47* 302-316, 1958.

FRISCHKNECHT, W., BIANCHI, L. AND PILLERI, G.* FAMILIARE ARTHROGRYPOSIS MULTIPLEX CONGENITA. HELV. PAEDIAT. ACTA 15* 259-279, 1960.

JAGO, R. H.* ARTHROGRYPOSIS FOLLOWING TREATMENT OF MATERNAL TETANUS WITH MUSCLE RELAXANTS. CASE REPORT. ARCH. DIS. CHILD. 45* 277-279, 1970.

LAITINEN, O. AND HIRVENSALO, M.* ARTHROGRYPOSIS MULTIPLEX CONGENITA. ANN.

LEBENTHAL, E., SHOCHET, S. B., ADAM, A., SEELENFREUND, M., FRIED, A., NAJENSON, T., SANDBANK, V. AND MATOTH, Y.* ARTHROGRYPOSIS MULTIPLEX CONGENITA - 23 CASES IN AN ARAB KINDRED. PEDIATRICS 46* 891-899, 1970.

PENA, C. E., MILLER, F., BUDZILOVICH, G. N. AND FEIGIN, I.* ARTHROGRYPOSIS MULTIPLEX CONGENITA* REPORT OF TWO CASES OF A RADICULAR TYPE WITH FAMILIAL INCIDENCE. NEUROLOGY 18* 926-930, 1968.

SRIVASTAVA, R. N.* ARTHROGRYPOSIS MULTIPLEX CONGENITA. CASE REPORT OF TWO SIBLINGS. CLIN. PEDIAT. 7* 691-694, 1968.

SWINYARD, C. A.* MULTIPLE CONGENITAL CONTRACTURES (ARTHROGRYPOSIS) NATURE OF THE SYNDROME AND HEREDITARY CONSIDERATIONS. PROC. SEC. INTERN. CONG. HUM. GENET. (ROME, SEPT. 6-12, 1961.) 3* 1397-1398, 1963.

WEISSMAN, S. L., KHERMOSH, C. AND ADAM, A.* ARTHROGRYPOSIS IN AN ARAB FAMILY. IN, GOLDSCHMIDT, E. (ED.)* GENETICS OF MIGRANT AND ISOLATE POPULATIONS. BALTIMORE* WILLIAMS AND WILKINS, 1963. P. 313.

*20820 ARTHROGRYPOSIS-LIKE DISORDER

PETAJAN ET AL. (1969) DESCRIBED AN ARTHROGRYPOSIS-LIKE SYNDROME IN THE ESKIMO. THEY CALLED IT KUSKOKWIM DISEASE FOR THE KUSKOKWIM DELTA AREA WHERE IT WAS OBSERVED. MULTIPLE JOINT CONTRACTURES AFFECTED PREDOMINANTLY THE KNEES AND ANKLES WITH ATROPHY AND COMPENSATORY HYPERTROPHY OF ASSOCIATED MUSCLE GROUPS. THE FAMILIAL PATTERN STRONGLY SUGGESTED AUTOSOMAL RECESSIVE INHERITANCE.

PETAJAN, J. H., MOMBERGER, G. L., AASE, J. AND WRIGHT, D. G.* ARTHROGRYPOSIS SYNDROME (KUSKOKWIM DISEASE) IN THE ESKIMO. J.A.M.A. 209* 1481-1486, 1969.

WRIGHT, D. G. AND AASE, J.* THE KUSKOKWIM SYNDROME* AN INHERITED FORM OF ARTHROGRYPOSIS IN THE ALASKAN ESKIMO. THE CLINICAL DELINEATION OF BIRTH DEFECTS. III. LIMB MALFORMATIONS. NEW YORK* NATIONAL FOUNDATION, 1969. PP. 91-95.

20830 ASCITES, CHYLOUS

LEE AND YOUNG (1953) DESCRIBED CHYLOUS ASCITES IN TWO FEMALE SIBS UNDER ONE YEAR OF AGE. ONE ALSO HAD SWELLING OF ONE ARM EVIDENT AT ONE WEEK AND THE ENTIRE BODY SOMEWHAT LATER AND DEVELOPED BILATERAL GLAUCOMA IN THE FIRST 6 MONTHS OF LIFE. BOTH THIS PATIENT AND THE YOUNGER SISTER HAD SPONTANEOUS CLEARING OF THE MANIFESTATIONS. CHYLOUS ASCITES AND CHYLOUS PLEURAL EFFUSIONS PROBABLY OCCUR AT TIMES WITH HEREDITARY LYMPHEDEMA, BUT THIS CONDITION IN ITS VARIOUS FORMS IS USUALLY DOMINANT.

LEE, C.-H. AND YOUNG, J. R.* CHYLOUS ASCITES IN SIBLINGS. J. PEDIAT. 42* 83-86, 1953.

*20840 ASPARTYLGLYCOSAMINURIA

IN A 32 YEAR OLD FEMALE AND HER 20 YEAR OLD BROTHER WITH MENTAL RETARDATION POUITT ET AL. (1968) FOUND URINARY EXCRETION OF ABNORMAL AMOUNTS OF 2-ACETAMIDO-1-(BETA PRIME-L-ASPARTAMIDO)-1, 2-DIDEOXYGLUCOSE. AN ENZYME RESPONSIBLE FOR HYDROLYZING THIS COMPOUND IS NORMALLY PRESENT IN SEMINAL FLUID BUT WAS ABSENT IN THAT OF THE BROTHER. A GENERALIZED LACK OF THIS ENZYME WAS POSTULATED. BOTH SIBS HAD THICK SAGGING SKIN OF THE CHEEKS, A FINDING NOT PRESENT IN NORMAL MEMBERS OF THE FAMILY. PALO AND MATTSSON (1970) REPORTED 11 CASES. THE PARENTS OF ONE PATIENT WERE FIRST COUSINS. THEY ESTIMATED THAT THERE ARE AT LEAST 130 CASES IN THE TOTAL POPULATION OF 4.5 MILLION IN FINLAND. PKU HAS A VERY LOW INCIDENCE IN FINLAND (PALO, 1967). OTHER RECESSIVE DISORDERS WHICH SEEM TO HAVE A RELATIVELY HIGH FREQUENCY IN FINLAND INCLUDE CONGENITAL NEPHROSIS (Q.V.). THE FINNISH CASES SHOWED, IN ADDITION TO SEVERE MENTAL RETARDATION, SAGGING CHEEKS, BROAD NOSE AND FACE, SHORT NECK, CRANIAL ASYMMETRY, SCOLIOSIS, PERIODIC HYPERACTIVITY, AND VACUOLATED LYMPHOCYTES. DIARRHEA AND FREQUENT INFECTIONS WERE PROBLEMS IN INFANCY. THIS DISORDER WAS FIRST REPORTED BY JENNER AND POUITT (1967).

PALO, J. AND MATTSSON, K.* ELEVEN NEW CASES OF ASPARTYLGLYCOSAMINURIA. J. MENT. DEFIC. RES. 14* 168-173, 1970.

PALO, J.* PREVALENCE OF PHENYLKETONURIA AND SOME OTHER METABOLIC DISORDERS AMONG MENTALLY RETARDED PATIENTS IN FINLAND. ACTA NEUROL. SCAND. 43* 573-579, 1967.

POUITT, R. J., JENNER, F. A. AND MERSKEY, H.* ASPARTYLGLYCOSAMINURIA* AN INBORN ERROR OF METABOLISM ASSOCIATED WITH MENTAL DEFECT. LANCET 2* 253-255, 1968.

20850 ASPHYXIATING THORACIC DYSTROPHY OF THE NEWBORN (JEUNE'S SYNDROME THORACIC-PELVIC-PHALANGEAL DYSTROPHY)

MOST CASES HAVE A FATAL OUTCOME IN THE NEWBORN PERIOD. INVOLVEMENT OF THE RIB CAGE IS RESPONSIBLE FOR ASPHYXIA. CHANGES HERE AND IN THE EXTREMITIES ARE RATHER

SIMILAR TO THOSE OF THE ELLIS-VAN CREVELD SYNDROME. INDEED POLYDACTYLY WAS PRESENT IN A CASE OF PIRNAR AND NEUHAUSER (1966). THE LATTER AUTHORS OBSERVED THREE AFFECTED BROTHERS. DYSPLASIA OF THE FINGERNAILS IS NOT PRESENT IN THIS CONDITION. CHRONIC NEPHRITIS IS A COMPLICATION (WAHLERS, 1966). HANISSIAN ET AL. (1967) REPORTED TWO FAMILIES EACH WITH TWO AFFECTED BROTHERS. ONE FAMILY WAS NEGRO. THESE AUTHORS THOUGHT THE FAMILY REPORTED BY SHAPIRA ET AL. (1965) HAD THIS CONDITION. LANGER (1968) POINTED OUT THAT IN THOSE CASES WITH POLYDACTYLY DIFFERENTIATION FROM ELLIS-VAN CREVELD SYNDROME MAY NOT BE POSSIBLE ON RADIOLOGIC GROUNDS ALONE. POLYDACTYLY IS AN INCONSTANT FEATURE OF THIS AND WHEN PRESENT USUALLY AFFECTS THE FEET ALSO. (POLYDACTYLY OF THE HANDS IS A CONSTANT FEATURE IN EVC BUT THE FEET ARE UNCOMMONLY AFFECTED.) NAIL DYSPLASIA AND PECULIAR UPPER LIP (FEATURES OF EVC) ARE NOT SEEN IN THIS CONDITION. THE MAIN VISCERAL ABNORMALITY IS RENAL IN THIS CONDITION, WHEREAS IT IS CARDIAC IN EVC. SHOKEIR (1970) DESCRIBED FIVE RELATED AFFECTED PERSONS OF NORWEGIAN EXTRACTION. CYSTIC RENAL CHANGES (POTTER'S TYPE IV) WERE DESCRIBED.

HANISSIAN, A. S., RIGGS, W. W., JR. AND THOMAS, D. A.* INFANTILE THORACIC DYSTROPHY - A VARIANT OF ELLIS-VAN CREVELD SYNDROME. J. PEDIAT. 71* 855-864, 1967.

HERDMAN, R. C. AND LANGER, L. O.* THE THORACIC ASPHYXIANT DYSTROPHY AND RENAL DISEASE. AM. J. DIS. CHILD. 116* 192-201, 1968.

JEUNE, M., BERAUD, C. AND CARRON, R.* DYSTROPHIE THORACIQUE ASPHYXIANTE DE CARACTERE FAMILIAL. ARCH. FRANC. PEDIAT. 12* 886-891, 1955.

LANGER, L. O., JR.* THORACIC-PELVIC-PHALANGEAL DYSTROPHY* ASPHYXIATING THORACIC DYSTROPHY OF THE NEWBORN, INFANTILE THORACIC DYSTROPHY. RADIOLOGY 91* 447-456, 1968.

MAROTEAUX, P. AND SAVART, P.* LA DYSTROPHIE THORACIQUE ASPHYXIANTE* ETUDE RADIOLOGIQUE ET RAPPORTS AVEC LE SYNDROME D'ELLIS ET VAN CREVELD. ANN. RADIOL. 7* 332-338, 1964.

PIRNAR, T. AND NEUHAUSER, E. B. D.* ASPHYXIATING THORACIC DYSTROPHY OF THE NEWBORN. AM. J. ROENTGEN. 98* 358-364, 1966.

SHAPIRA, E., FISCHEL, E., MOSES, S. AND LEVIN, S.* SYNDROME OF INCOMPLETE REGIONAL ACHONDROPLASIA (ILIUM AND RIBS) WITH ABDOMINAL MUSCLE DYSPLASIA. ARCH. DIS. CHILD. 40* 694-697, 1965.

SHOKEIR, M. H. K.* ASPHYXIATING THORACIC CHONDRODYSTROPHY* ASSOCIATION WITH URINARY MALFORMATIONS AND EVIDENCE FOR HETEROZYGOUS EXPRESSION. (ABSTRACT) AM. J. HUM. GENET. 22* 18A-19A, 1970.

WAHLERS* CITED BY LENZ, W.* SYMPOSION UBER GENERALISIERTE ANOMALIEN DES SKELETES. MSCHR. KINDERHEILK. 114* 157-158, 1966.

20860 ASTHMA, SHORT STATURE AND ELEVATED IGA

SLY AND HEIMLICH (1967) REPORTED IDENTICAL FEMALE TWINS WITH THIS COMBINATION. THE MOTHER AND SOME OF THE SIBS WERE THOUGHT ALSO TO HAVE ABNORMALITIES OF IMMUNOGLOBULINS.

SLY, R. M. AND HEIMLICH, E. M.* IDENTICAL TWINS WITH SHORT STATURE, ELEVATED IGA AND ASTHMA. ANN. ALLERG. 25* 578-586, 1967.

20870 ATAXIA WITH MYOCLONUS EPILEPSY AND PRESENILE DEMENTIA

IN A BROTHER AND SISTER, SKRE AND LOKEN (1970) DESCRIBED A DISORDER WITH CLINICAL FEATURES OF FRIEDREICH'S ATAXIA AND IN THE LATE STAGES MYOCLONUS EPILEPSY AND PROGRESSIVE DEMENTIA. NEUROPATHOLOGIC STUDIES SHOWED SPINOCEREBELLAR DEGENERATION AS IN FRIEDREICH'S ATAXIA, CEREBRAL INVOLVEMENT AS IN SUBACUTE PRESENILE DEMENTIA, AND PERIPHERAL NEUROPATHY AS IN CHARCOT-MARIE-TOOTH'S DISEASE.

SKRE, H. AND LOKEN, A. C.* MYOCLONUS EPILEPSY AND SUBACUTE PRESENILE DEMENTIA IN HEREDO-ATAXIA. A CLINICAL, ELECTROENCEPHALOGRAPHIC, AND PATHOLOGICAL STUDY WITH A DISCUSSION OF CLASSIFICATION AND ETIOLOGY. ACTA NEUROL. SCAND. 46* 18-42, 1970.

*20880 ATAXIA, INTERMITTENT, WITH PYRUVATE DECARBOXYLASE DEFICIENCY

BLASS ET AL. (1970) DESCRIBED A DEFICIENCY OF PYRUVATE DECARBOXYLASE IN AN 8 YEAR OLD BOY WHO HAD SUFFERED 2 TO 6 EPISODES OF ATAXIA EACH YEAR SINCE THE AGE OF 16 MONTHS. MOST ATTACKS FOLLOWED NONSPECIFIC FEBRILE ILLNESS OR OTHER STRESSES. CHORIOATHETOSIS AS WELL AS CEREBELLAR ATAXIA WAS PRESENT DURING THE EPISODES. SERUM PYRUVIC ACID AND ALANINE LEVELS WERE ELEVATED. THE FATHER'S FIBROBLASTS AND LEUKOCYTES SHOWED PARTIALLY DEFECTIVE PYRUVATE DECARBOXYLASE AND VALUES IN THE MOTHER WERE AT THE LOWER LIMIT OF NORMAL.

BLASS, J. P., AVIGAN, J. AND UHLENDORF, B. W.* A DEFECT IN PYRUVATE DECARBOXY-LASE IN A CHILD WITH AN INTERMITTENT MOVEMENT DISORDER. J. CLIN. INVEST. 49* 423-

R
E
C
E
S
S
I
V
E

*20890 ATAXIA-TELANGIECTASIA

THE FEATURES ARE PROGRESSIVE CEREBELLAR ATAXIA, TELANGIECTASES ESPECIALLY OF THE
CONJUNCTIVA, AND PRONENESS TO SINOPULMONARY INFECTION. THE NATURE OF THE BASIC
DEFECT IS A MYSTERY. A DEFECT OF THE IMMUNE MECHANISM AND HYPOPLASIA OF THE
THYMUS IS DEMONSTRATED. IN TWO AMISH SIBSHIPS, OF WHICH THE FOUR PARENTS SHARED A
COMMON ANCESTRAL COUPLE, ATAXIA TELANGIECTASIA OCCURRED IN ONE AND SWISS-TYPE
AGAMMAGLOBULINEMIA (Q.V.) IN THE SECOND, SUGGESTING TO MCKUSICK AND CROSS (1966) A
POSSIBLE RELATIONSHIP OF THESE TWO DISORDERS OF THE IMMUNE MECHANISM. PATIENTS
WITH THIS DISORDER TEND TO DEVELOP LYMPHATIC MALIGNANCY. HECHT ET AL. (1966)
OBSERVED LYMPHOCYTIC LEUKEMIA IN PATIENTS WITH ATAXIA-TELANGIECTASIA. A NON-
LEUKEMIC SIB AND TWO UNRELATED PATIENTS WITH ATAXIA-TELANGIECTASIA HAD MULTIPLE
CHROMOSOMAL BREAKS AND IMPAIRED RESPONSIVENESS TO PHYTOHEMAGGLUTININ. LEUKEMIA
AND CHROMOSOMAL ABNORMALITIES OCCUR IN AT LEAST TWO OTHER MENDELIAN DISORDERS,
FANCONI'S PANCYTOPENIA AND BLOOM'S DISEASE. TELENGIECTASES CAN BE INCONSPICUOUS
AND PATIENTS MAY BE DIAGNOSED AS 'FRIEDREICH'S ATAXIA' FOR MANY YEARS. THE OLDEST
PATIENTS KNOWN TO ME ARE NOW 41 AND 37 YEARS OLD. HAERER ET AL. (1969) DESCRIBED
A NEGRO SIBSHIP OF 12, OF WHOM 5 HAD ATAXIA-TELANGIECTASIA, OF WHOM 2 DIED OF
MUCINOUS ADENOCARCINOMA OF THE STOMACH AT AGES 21 AND 19 YEARS. HAGBERG ET AL.
(1970) DESCRIBED A DISORDER SUGGESTING ATAXIA-TELANGIECTASIA IN ALL RESPECTS
EXCEPT THAT NO TELANGIECTASES WERE PRESENT. TWO SIBS WITH UNRELATED PARENTS WERE
AFFECTED. ALTHOUGH THEY CONSIDERED IT A DISTINCT ENTITY, THE EVIDENCE IS NOT
COMPLETELY CONVINCING. THE POSSIBILITY OF HETEROALLELES AT THE ATAXIA-TELANGIEC-
TASIA LOCI MIGHT BE SUGGESTED.

AMMANN, A. J., CAIN, W. A., ISHIZAKA, K., HONG, R. AND GOOD, R. A.* IMMUNOGLO-
BULIN E DEFICIENCY IN ATAXIA-TELANGIECTASIA. NEW ENG. J. MED. 281* 469-472, 1969.

BODER, E. AND SEDGWICK, R. P.* ATAXIA-TELANGIECTASIA* A FAMILIAL SYNDROME OF
PROGRESSIVE CEREBELLAR ATAXIA, OCULOCUTANEOUS TELANGIECTASIA AND FREQUENT
PULMONARY INFECTION. PEDIATRICS 21* 526-554, 1958.

FEIGIN, R. D., VIETTI, T. J., WYATT, R. G., KAUFMAN, D. G. AND SMITH, C. H.*
ATAXIA TELANGIECTASIA WITH GRANULOCYTOPENIA. J. PEDIAT. 77* 431-438, 1970.

HAERER, A. F., JACKSON, J. F. AND EVERS, C. G.* ATAXIA-TELANGIECTASIA WITH
GASTRIC ADENOCARCINOMA. J.A.M.A. 210* 1884-1887, 1969.

HAGBERG, A., HANSSON, O., LEDIN, S. AND NILSSON, K.* FAMILIAL ATAXIC DIPLEGIA
WITH DEFICIENT CELLULAR IMMUNITY. ACTA PAEDIAT. SCAND. 59* 545-550, 1970.

HECHT, F., KOLER, R. D., RIGAS, D. A., DAHNKE, G. S., CASE, M. P., TISDALE, V.
AND MILLER, R. W.* LEUKEMIA AND LYMPHOCYTES IN ATAXIA-TELANGIECTASIA. (LETTER)
LANCET 2* 1193 ONLY, 1966.

KOREIN, J., STEINMAN, P. A. AND SENZ, E. H.* ATAXIA-TELANGIECTASIA* REPORT OF A
CASE AND REVIEW OF THE LITERATURE. ARCH. NEUROL. 4* 272-280, 1961.

LISKER, R. AND COBO, A.* CHROMOSOME BREAKAGE IN ATAXIA-TELANGIECTASIA.
(LETTER) LANCET 1* 618 ONLY, 1970.

MCKUSICK, V. A. AND CROSS, H. E.* ATAXIA-TELANGIECTASIA AND SWISS-TYPE
AGAMMAGLOBULINEMIA. TWO GENETIC DISORDERS OF THE IMMUNE MECHANISM IN RELATED
AMISH SIBSHIPS. J.A.M.A. 195* 739-745, 1966.

MILLER, M. E. AND CHATTEN, J.* OVARIAN CHANGES IN ATAXIA TELANGIECTASIA. ACTA
PAEDIAT. SCAND. 56* 559-561, 1967.

PETERSON, R. D. A., KELLY, W. D. AND GOOD, R. A.* ATAXIA-TELANGIECTASIA* ITS
ASSOCIATION WITH A DEFECTIVE THYMUS, IMMUNOLOGICAL-DEFICIENCY DISEASE AND
MALIGNANCY. LANCET 1* 1189-1193, 1964.

REYE, C. AND MOSMAN, N. S. W.* ATAXIA-TELANGIECTASIA. AM. J. DIS. CHILD. 99*
238-247, 1960.

SCHALCH, D. S., MCFARLIN, D. E. AND BARLOW, M. H.* UNUSUAL FORM OF DIABETES
MELLITUS IN ATAXIA TELANGIECTASIA. NEW ENG. J. MED. 282* 1396-1401, 1970.

SHUSTER, J., HART, Z., STIMSON, C. W., BROUGH, A. J. AND POULIK, M. D.* ATAXIA-
TELANGIECTASIA WITH CEREBELLAR TUMOR. PEDIATRICS 37* 776-786, 1966.

SOURANDER, P., BONNEVIER, J. O. AND OLSSON, Y.* A CASE OF ATAXIA-TELANGIECTASIA
WITH LESIONS IN THE SPINAL CORD. ACTA NEUROL. SCAND. 42* 354-366, 1966.

TADJOEDIN, M. K. AND FRASER, F. C.* HEREDITY OF ATAXIA-TELANGIECTASIA (LOUIS-
BAR SYNDROME). AM. J. DIS. CHILD. 110* 64-68, 1965.

20900 ATAXIC DIPLEGIA AND DEFECTIVE CELLULAR IMMUNITY

HAGBERG ET AL. (1970) DESCRIBED AFFECTED BROTHER AND SISTER. THE SISTER HAD

R
E
C
E
S
S
I
V
E

VACCINIA GANGRENOSA, AT AGE 15 MONTHS, WHICH WAS SUCCESSFULLY DRUG-TREATED. SHE DIED OF GENERALIZED VARICELLA AT AGE FOUR AND ONE HALF. THE BROTHER DIED AT FIVE OF BRAIN ABSCESS.

HAGBERG, B., HANSSON, O., LIDEN, S. AND NILSSON, K.* FAMILIAL ATAXIC DIPLEGIA WITH DEFICIENT CELLULAR IMMUNITY. A NEW CLINICAL ENTITY. ACTA PAEDIAT. SCAND. 59* 545-550, 1970.

*20910 ATONIC-ASTATIC SYNDROME OF FOERSTER

MANIFESTATIONS ARE OLIGOPHRENIA, PRONOUNCED MUSCULAR HYPOTONIA, STATIC ATAXIA, ASTASIA, ABASIA AND SLOW, MONOTONOUS SPEECH. VAN ROSSUM (1959) DESCRIBED AN AFFECTED BROTHER AND SISTER FROM CONSANGUINEOUS PARENTS. CONSANGUINITY HAS BEEN DESCRIBED IN TWO OTHER REPORTS.

VAN ROSSUM, A.* FOERSTER'S ATONIC-ASTATIC SYNDROME. RECENT NEUROLOGICAL RESEARCH, ELSEVIER, 1959.

20920 ATOPIC HYPERSENSITIVITY

ASTHMA, HAY FEVER AND ECZEMA ARE EMBRACED BY THIS TERM. THE GENETICS IS CERTAINLY NOT SIMPLE. TIPS (1954) THOUGHT THAT EACH OF THE THREE FORMS OF ATOPY IS DETERMINED BY HOMOZYGOSITY AT A SINGLE AND SEPARATE LOCUS.

RAJKA, G.* PRURIGO BESNIER (ATOPIC DERMATITIS) WITH SPECIAL REFERENCE TO THE ROLE OF ALLERGIC FACTORS. I. THE INFLUENCE OF ATOPIC HEREDITARY FACTORS. ACTA DERMATOVENER. 40* 285-306, 1960.

TIPS, R. L.* A STUDY OF THE INHERITANCE OF ATOPIC HYPERSENSITIVITY IN MAN. AM. J. HUM. GENET. 6* 328-343, 1954.

*20930 ATRANSFERRINEMIA

HEILMEYER AND COLLEAGUES (1961) DESCRIBED TOTAL ABSENCE OF TRANSFERRIN IN A 7 YEAR OLD GIRL WHOSE PRESENTING COMPLAINT WAS SEVERE HYPOCHROMIC ANEMIA. DEATH OCCURRED FROM HEART FAILURE. SEVERE HEMOSIDEROSIS OF THE HEART AND LIVER WAS FOUND AT AUTOPSY. LOW NORMAL TRANSFERRIN LEVELS WERE FOUND IN BOTH PARENTS, WHO WERE NOT KNOWN TO BE RELATED (PERSONAL COMMUNICATION).

HEILMEYER, L., KELLER, W., VIVELL, O., KEIDERLING, W., BETKE, K., WOHLER, F. AND SCHULTZE, H. E.* CONGENITAL TRANSFERRIN DEFICIENCY IN A SEVEN-YEAR-OLD GIRL. GERMAN MED. MONTHLY 6* 385-389, 1961.

HEILMEYER, L., KELLER, W., VIVELL, O., KEIDERLING, W., BETKE, K., WOHLER, F. AND SCHULTZE, H. E.* KONGENITALE ATRANSFERRINAMIE BEI EINEM SIEBEN JAHRE ALTEN KIND. DEUTSCH. MED. WSCHR. 86* 1745-1751, 1961.

20940 ATRIAL SEPTAL DEFECT, PRIMUM TYPE

YAO ET AL. (1968) OBSERVED FOUR SIBS WITH ATRIAL SEPTAL DEFECT OF THE PRIMUM TYPE. FIVE OTHER SIBS AND THE PARENTS WERE NORMAL. FAMILIAL AGGREGATION OF SECUNDUM ASD HAS BEEN REPORTED RATHER FREQUENTLY (E.G., NORA AND MEYER, 1966), BUT THE EXPERIENCE OF YAO ET AL. IS UNUSUAL.

NORA, J. J. AND MEYER, T. C.* FAMILIAL NATURE OF CONGENITAL HEART DISEASE. PEDIATRICS 37* 329-334, 1966.

YAO, J., THOMPSON, M. W., TRUSLER, G. A. AND TRIMBLE, A. S.* FAMILIAL ATRIAL SEPTAL DEFECT OF THE PRIMUM TYPE* A REPORT OF FOUR CASES IN ONE SIBSHIP. CANAD. MED. ASS. J. 98* 218-219, 1968.

*20950 ATRICHIA WITH PAPULAR LESIONS

ALMOST COMPLETE ABSENCE OF HAIR AND PAPILLARY LESIONS OVER MOST OF THE BODY WERE FEATURES. THE PATIENTS ARE BORN WITH HAIR WHICH FALLS OUT AND IS NOT REPLACED. HISTOLOGIC STUDIES SHOW MALFORMATION OF THE HAIR FOLLICLES. DAMSTE AND PRAKKEN (1954) DESCRIBED A KINDRED IN WHICH THREE SISTERS AND TWO SONS OF THEIR MOTHER'S FIRST COUSIN WERE AFFECTED. LOEWENTHAL AND PRAKKEN (1961) DESCRIBED ANOTHER CASE, THE DAUGHTER OF THIRD COUSINS.

DAMSTE, T. J. AND PRAKKEN, J. R.* ATRICHIA WITH PAPULAR LESIONS* VARIANT OF CONGENITAL ECTODERMAL DYSPLASIA. DERMATOLOGICA 108* 114-122, 1954.

LOEWENTHAL, L. J. A. AND PRAKKEN, J. R.* ATRICHIA WITH PAPULAR LESIONS. DERMATOLOGICA 122* 85-89, 1961.

20960 ATRIOVENTRICULAR DISSOCIATION

WAGNER AND HALL (1967) REPORTED TWO BROTHERS AND A SISTER WITH CONGENITAL ATRIOVENTRICULAR DISSOCIATION. THEY EMPHASIZED THAT THIS IS DISTINCT FROM A-V BLOCK. IN DISSOCIATION THE ABNORMALITY SEEMS TO BE "LAZY" SINO-ATRIAL PACEMAKER WITH THE A-V NODE TAKING OVER INTERMITTENTLY BY DEFAULT. IN A-V BLOCK AN

WAGNER, C. W., JR. AND HALL, R. J.* CONGENITAL FAMILIAL ATRIOVENTRICULAR DISSOCIATION* REPORT OF THREE SIBLINGS. AM. J. CARDIOL. 19* 593-596, 1967.

*20970 ATROPHODERMIA VERMICULATA (FOLLICULITIS ULERYTHEMATOSA, ATROPHODERMA RETICULATA, HONEYCOMB ATROPHY, ATROPHODERMIA RETICULATA SYMMETRICA FACIEI, ETC.)

THE SKIN CHANGES ARE USUALLY LIMITED TO THE FACE AND CONSIST OF SYMMETRICAL SMALL CROWDED AREAS OF SKIN ATROPHY PRODUCING PITS WITH SHARP EDGES AND AN OVERALL WORM-EATEN APPEARANCE. ASSOCIATION WITH CONGENITAL HEART BLOCK, COARCTATION OF THE AORTA AND OTHER DEFECTS HAS BEEN DESCRIBED BY KOOIJ AND VENTER (1959) AND CAROL AND COLLEAGUES (1940) REPORTED FAMILIAL OCCURRENCE WITH HEART ANOMALY.

CAROL, W. L. L., GODFRIED, E. G., PRAKKEN, J. R. AND PRICK, J. J. G.* V. RECKLINGHAUSENSCHE NEUROFIBROMATOSIS, ATROPHODERMIA VERMICULATA UND KONGENITALE HERZANOMALIE ALS HAUPTKENNZEICHEN EINES FAMILIAR-HEREDITAREN SYNDROMS. DERMATOLOGICA 81* 345-365, 1940.

KOOIJ, R. AND VENTER, J.* ATROPHODERMIA VERMICULATA WITH UNUSUAL LOCALISATION AND ASSOCIATED CONGENITAL ANOMALIES. DERMATOLOGIA 118* 161-167, 1959.

MACKEE, G. M. AND CIPOLLARO, A. C.* FOLLICULITIS ULERYTHEMATOSA RETICULATA. ARCH. DERM. SYPH. 57* 281-292, 1948.

SAVATARD, L.* HONEYCOMB ATROPHY. BRIT. J. DERM. 55* 259-266, 1943.

20980 AUSTRALIA ANTIGEN

BLUMBERG ET AL. (1965) DESCRIBED AN ANTIGEN IN THE SERUM OF AN AUSTRALIAN ABORIGINE WHICH REACTED WITH AN ANTIBODY IN CERTAIN HEMOPHILIC PATIENTS WHO HAD RECIEVED MULTIPLE TRANSFUSIONS. THE SAME ANTIGEN APPEARED IN THE SERUM OF SOME LEUKEMIA PATIENTS. THE POSSIBLE HEREDITARY NATURE OF THE ANTIGEN REMAINS TO BE PROVED. BLUMBERG ET AL. (1966) FOUND REASONABLY GOOD AGREEMENT OF FAMILY DATA WITH THE EXPECTATIONS THAT INDIVIDUALS HOMOZYGOUS FOR A GENE TENTATIVELY DESIGNATED AU(1) HAVE THE ANTIGEN DETECTABLE BY DOUBLE DIFFUSION METHODS, WHEREAS PERSONS HETEROZYGOUS FOR THE GENE OR LACKING IT ENTIRELY DO NOT HAVE THE ANTIGEN. BLUMBERG ET AL. (1967) FOUND THAT THE AUSTRALIA ANTIGEN IS MORE COMMON IN PATIENTS WITH LEPROMATOUS LEPROSY THAN IN PATIENTS WITH TUBERCULOID LEPROSY OR IN NON-LEPROSY CONTROLS. ASSOCIATION WITH HEPATITIS HAS ALSO BEEN DEMONSTRATED. AU(1) HAS BEEN FOUND IN THE SERUM OF 38-58 PERCENT OF PATIENTS WITH ACUTE HEPATITIS (LONDON ET AL., 1969) BUT IN LESS THAN 0.1 PERCENT OF HEALTHY NORTH AMERICANS. THE VIRAL NATURE OF THE AUSTRALIA ANTIGEN IS SUGGESTED BY ELECTRON-MICROSCOPIC STUDIES (BAYER ET AL., 1968). WITH FLUORESCENT ANTIBODY TECHNIQUES AU(1) HAS BEEN DETECTED CONSISTENTLY IN THE NUCLEI OF LIVER CELLS FROM HEPATITIS PATIENTS WITH AU(1) IN THEIR SERUM (MILLMAN ET AL., 1969). AUSTRALIA ANTIGEN IS FOUND IN THE SERA OF PATIENTS WITH ACUTE AND CHRONIC HEPATITIS AND MAY ACTUALLY BE A FORM OF VIRUS. IT IS VERY COMMON IN TROPICAL AREAS AND PERSONS IN THESE AREAS WITH THE ANTIGEN APPEAR TO BE HEPATITIS CARRIERS. THE ANTIGEN IS DETECTED BY IMMUNODIFFUSION IN AGAR GEL (OUCHTERLONY METHOD). FAMILY STUDIES BY BLUMBERG ET AL. (1969) SUGGESTED RECESSIVE INHERITANCE OF SUSCEPTIBILITY TO INFECTION AS MANIFESTED BY PRESENCE OF THE AUSTRALIA ANTIGEN.

R
E
C
E
S
S
I
V
E

ALTER, H. J. AND BLUMBERG, B. S.* FURTHER STUDIES ON A *NEW HUMAN* ISOPRECIPITIN SYSTEM (AUSTRALIA ANTIGEN). BLOOD 27* 297-309, 1966.

BAYER, M. E., BLUMBERG, B. S. AND WERNER, B.* PARTICLES ASSOCIATED WITH AUSTRALIA ANTIGEN IN THE SERA OF PATIENTS WITH LEUKAEMIA, DOWN'S SYNDROME AND HEPATITIS. NATURE 218* 1057-1059, 1968.

BLUMBERG, B. S., ALTER, H. J. AND VISNICH, S.* A *NEW* ANTIGEN IN LEUKEMIA SERA. J.A.M.A. 191* 541-546, 1965.

BLUMBERG, B. S., FRIEDLAENDER, J. S., WOODSIDE, A., SUTNICK, A. I. AND LONDON, W. T.* HEPATITIS AND AUSTRALIA ANTIGEN* AUTOSOMAL RECESSIVE INHERITANCE OF SUSCEPTIBILITY TO INFECTION IN HUMANS. PROC. NAT. ACAD. SCI. 62* 1108-1115, 1969.

BLUMBERG, B. S., MELARTIN, L., GUINTO, R. S. AND WERNER, B.* FAMILY STUDIES OF A HUMAN SERUM ISOANTIGEN SYSTEM (AUSTRALIA ANTIGEN). AM. J. HUM. GENET. 18* 594-608, 1966.

BLUMBERG, B. S., MELARTIN, L., LECHAT, M. AND GUINTO, R. S.* ASSOCIATION BETWEEN LEPROMATOUS LEPROSY AND AUSTRALIA ANTIGEN. LANCET 2* 173-176, 1967.

BLUMBERG, B. S., SUTNICK, A. I. AND LONDON, W. T.* AUSTRALIA ANTIGEN AS A HEPATITIS VIRUS. VARIATION IN HOST RESPONSE. AM. J. MED. 48* 1-8, 1970.

LONDON, W. T., SUTNICK, A. I. AND BLUMBERG, B. S.* AUSTRALIA ANTIGEN AND ACUTE VIRAL HEPATITIS. ANN. INTERN. MED. 70* 55-59, 1969.

MILLMAN, I., ZAVATONE, V., GERSTLEY, B. J. S. AND BLUMBERG, B. S.* AUSTRALIA ANTIGEN DETECTED THE NUCLEI OF LIVER CELLS OF PATIENTS WITH VIRAL HEPATITIS BY THE

FLOURESCENT ANTIBODY TECHNIQUE. NATURE 222* 181-184, 1969.

WRIGHT, R., MCCOLLUM, R. W. AND KLATSKIN, G.* AUSTRALIA ANTIGEN IN ACUTE AND CHRONIC LIVER DISEASE. LANCET 2* 117-121, 1969.

*20990 BARDET-BIEDL SYNDROME

AMMANN (1970) POINTED OUT THAT THE SYNDROME USUALLY CALLED LAURENCE-MOON-BIEDL-BARDET SYNDROME (MENTAL RETARDATION, PIGMENTARY RETINOPATHY, POLYDACTYLY, OBESITY, HYPOGENITALISM) WAS PRESENT IN BIEDL (1922) AND BARDET'S (1920) PATIENTS, BUT THAT THOSE OF LAURENCE AND MOON HAD A DISTINCT DISORDER WITH PARAPLEGIA AND WITHOUT POLYDACTYLY AND OBESITY (SEE LAURENCE-MOON SYNDROME). AS INDICATED BY AMMANN'S STUDY, RESIDUAL HETEROGENEITY MAY EXIST EVEN AFTER THE LAURENCE-MOON SYNDROME IS SEPARATED OFF. CLEARLY BIEMOND SYNDROME II (IRIS COLOBOMA, HYPOGENITALISM, OBESITY, POLYDACTYLY AND MENTAL RETARDATION) IS DISTINCT, AS IS ALSO ALSTROM'S SYNDROME (RETINITIS PIGMENTOSA, OBESITY, DIABETES MELLITUS AND PERCEPTIVE DEAFNESS).

AMMANN, F.* INVESTIGATIONS CLINIQUES ET GENETIQUES SUR LE SYNDROME DE BARDET-BIEDL EN SUISSE. J. GENET. HUM. 18 (SUPPL.)* 1-310, 1970.

BARDET, G.* SUR UN SYNDROME D'OBESITE INFANTILE AVEC POLYDACTYLIE ET RETINITE PIGMENTAIRE. (CONTRIBUTION A L'ETUDE DES FORMES CLINIQUE DE L'OBESITE HYPOPHY-SAIRE). THESIS, PARIS, NO. 479, 1920.

BELL, J.* THE LAURENCE-MOON SYNDROME. IN, PENROSE, L. S. (ED.)* TREASURY OF HUMAN INHERITANCE. CAMBRIDGE* UNIV. PRESS, VOL. 5 (PART III)* 51-96, 1958.

BIEDL, A.* EIN GESCHWISTERPAAR MIT ADIPOSO-GENITALER DYSTROPHIE. DEUTSCH. MED. WSCHR. 48* 1630 ONLY, 1922.

CICCARELLI, E. C. AND VESELL, E. S.* LAURENCE-MOON-BIEDL SYNDROME. REPORT OF AN UNUSUAL FAMILY. AM. J. DIS. CHILD. 101* 519-524, 1961.

KALBIAN, V. V.* LAURENCE-MOON-BIEDL SYNDROME IN AN ARAB BOY* FAMILIAL INCIDENCE. J. CLIN. ENDOCR. 16* 1622-1625, 1956.

R
E
C
E
S
S
I
V
E

*21000 BEHR'S SYNDROME (BEHR'S COMPLICATED FORM OF INFANTILE HEREDITARY OPTIC ATROPHY)

BEHR'S DESCRIPTION WAS PUBLISHED IN 1909. ONSET IS IN EARLY INFANCY AND THE FEATURES ARE (1) BILATERAL OPTIC ATROPHY, WITH FIELD DEFECTS, GENERALLY TEMPORAL AND RARELY COMPLETE, (2) NEUROLOGIC SIGNS (INCREASED TENDON REFLEXES, BABINSKI SIGN, SLIGHT INCOORDINATION WITH ATAXIA AND SPASTIC GAIT, MENTAL DEFICIENCY, NYSTAGMUS), AND (3) STATIC CONDITION FOR MANY YEARS FOLLOWING A PERIOD OF PROGRESSION. INVOLVEMENT OF MULTIPLE BROTHERS AND SISTERS WITH NORMAL PARENTS AND PARENTAL CONSANGUINITY SUGGESTS RECESSIVE INHERITANCE. VAN BOGAERT AND ANDRE-VAN LEEUWEN (1942) REPORTED NECROPSY FINDINGS, BUT IN THEIR PEDIGREE MILD MANIFESTATIONS WERE EVIDENT IN HETEROZYGOTES.

BEHR, C.* DIE KOMPLIZIERTE, HEREDITARFAMILIARE OPTIKUSATROPHIE DES KINDESALTERS* EIN BISHER NICHT BESCHRIEBENER SYMPTOMKOMPLEX. KLIN. MBL. AUGENHEILK. 47* 138-160, 1909.

FRANCESCHETTI, A. AND BAMATTER, F.* ATROPHIE OPTIQUE INFANTILE ASSOCIEE A DES TROUBLES GENERAUX (SYNDROME DE BEHR). SCHWEIZ. MED. WSCHR. 21* 285-286, 1940.

VAN BOGAERT, L. AND ANDRE-VAN LEEUWEN, M.* PREMIERE OBSERVATION ANATOMO-CLINIQUE DE L'ATROPHIE OPTIQUE HEREDOFAMILIALE COMPLIQUEE DE BEHR. BULL. ACAD. ROY. MED. BELG. 7* 218-225, 1942.

21010 BETA-AMINOISOBUTYRIC ACID (BAIB), URINARY EXCRETION OF

BAIB IS A NON-PROTEIN AMINO ACID, I.E. IT IS NOT A CONSTITUENT AMINO ACID OF ANY PROTEIN. NOT ONLY IS THE URINARY EXCRETION OF BAIB A GENETIC TRAIT, BUT ALSO IT IS EXCRETED IN LEUKEMIA AND BY MONGOLOID IDIOTS (WRIGHT, FINK, 1957). YANAI ET AL. (1969), FROM AN EXTENSIVE STUDY IN JAPAN, CONCLUDED THAT HIGH EXCRETION IS RECESSIVE. HETEROZYGOTES EXCRETED MORE BAIB THAN DID HOMOZYGOUS LOW EXCRETORS.

DE GROUCHY, J. AND SUTTON, H. E.* A GENETIC STUDY OF BETA-AMINOISOBUTYRIC ACID EXCRETION. AM. J. HUM. GENET. 9* 76-80, 1957.

GARTLER, S. M., FIRSCHEIN, I. L. AND KRAUS, B. S.* AN INVESTIGATION INTO THE GENETICS AND RACIAL VARIATION OF BAIB EXCRETION. AM. J. HUM. GENET. 9* 200-207, 1957.

WRIGHT, S. W. AND FINK, K.* THE EXCRETION OF BETA-AMINOISOBUTYRIC ACID IN NORMAL, MONGOLOID MENTALLY AND NON-MONGOLOID DEFECTIVE CHILDREN. AM. J. MENT. DEFIC. 61* 530-533, 1957.

YANAI, J., KAKIMOTO, Y., TSUJIO, T. AND SANO, I.* GENETIC STUDY OF BETA-AMINOISOBUTYRIC ACID EXCRETION BY JAPANESE. AM. J. HUM. GENET. 21* 115-132, 1969.

LIKE MAPLE SYRUP URINE DISEASE AND ISOVALERIC ACIDEMIA THIS IS AN INBORN ERROR OF THE LEUCINE DEGRADATION PATHWAY. THE PATIENT HAD NO TENDENCY TO METABOLIC ACIDOSIS, A FEATURE OF THE OTHER TWO CONDITIONS. THE MAIN MANIFESTATIONS WERE MUSCULAR HYPOTONIA AND ATROPHY, PROBABLY OF SPINAL ORIGIN. THE DISORDER WAS GRADUALLY PROGRESSIVE DESPITE A DIET WHICH REDUCED EXCRETION OF THE ABNORMAL METABOLITES. A SINGLE PATIENT WAS STUDIED. THE TWO PARENTS AND TWO SIBS EXCRETED ONE OF THE ABNORMAL METABOLITES AND WERE JUDGED TO BE HETEROZYGOUS. TANAKA AND ISSELBACHER (1970) SUPPORTED THE SUGGESTION THAT THE METABOLIC BLOCK IS AT THE STAGE OF BETA-METHYLCROTONYL COA CARBOXYLASE (ONE OF SEVERAL ENZYMES WHICH CONTAIN BIOTIN AS AN ESSENTIAL FUNCTIONAL GROUP) BY SHOWING THAT IN THE EXPERIMENTAL ANIMAL BIOTIN DEFICIENCY IS ACCOMPANIED BY BETA-HYDROXYISOVALERIC ACIDURIA.

ELDJARN, L., JELLUM, E., STOKKE, O., PANDE, H. AND WAALER, P. E.* BETA-HYDROXYISOVALERIC ACIDURIA AND BETA-METHYLCROTONYLGLYCINURIA* A NEW INBORN ERROR OF METABOLISM. (LETTER) LANCET 1* 521-522, 1970.

TANAKA, K. AND ISSELBACHER, K. J.* EXPERIMENTAL BETA-HYDROXYISOVALERIC ACIDURIA INDUCED BY BIOTIN DEFICIENCY. (LETTER) LANCET 2* 930-931, 1970.

21030 BIEMOND'S CONGENITAL AND FAMILIAL ANALGESIA

BIEMOND (1955) DESCRIBED 11 YEAR OLD FRATERNAL TWINS (MALE AND FEMALE) WITH LOSS OF PAIN SENSATION, DIMINISHED TOUCH AND TEMPERATURE SENSE, AND ABSENT TENDON REFLEXES. POSTMORTEM SHOWED DEFICIENT DEVELOPMENT IN THE POSTERIOR ROOT GANGLIA, GASSERIAN GANGLION, POSTERIOR ROOTS, POSTERIOR HORNS OF THE SPINAL GRAY MATTER AND POSTERIOR COLUMNS. THE SPINOTHALAMIC TRACTS COULD NOT BE DEMONSTRATED. IN A CHILD (D.D., 762247) INCORRECTLY DIAGNOSED AS DYSAUTONOMIA, FREYTAG AND LINDENBERG (1967) FOUND 'ABSENCE OF POSTERIOR ASCENDING TRACTS, SEVERE REDUCTION IN THE NUMBER OF NEURONS IN PERIPHERAL SENSORY AND AUTONOMIC GANGLIA AND A HYPOPLASIA OF THE PYRAMIDAL TRACTS.'

BIEMOND, A.* INVESTIGATION OF THE BRAIN IN A CASE OF CONGENITAL AND FAMILIAL ANALGESIA. PROC. 11TH INTERN. CONG. NEUROPATH. LONDON* SEPT.. 1955.

FREYTAG, E. AND LINDENBERG, R.* NEUROPATHOLOGIC FINDINGS IN PATIENTS OF A HOSPITAL FOR THE MENTALLY DEFICIENT. A SURVEY OF 359 CASES. JOHNS HOPKINS MED. J. 121* 379-392, 1967.

21040 BIFID NOSE (MEDIAN FISSURE OF NOSE, MEDIAN CLEFT NOSE)

KHOO BOO-CHAI (1965) DESCRIBED 3 CASES IN SIBS OF ASIATIC INDIAN DESCENT. ESSER (1939) REPORTED FOUR AFFECTED SIBS (2 MALES, 2 FEMALES) AND AN AFFECTED MALE FIRST COUSIN. OCULAR HYPERTELORISM (SOMETIMES A DOMINANT) IS OCCASIONALLY ASSOCIATED WITH BIFID NOSE BUT THE GENETICS OF THE COMBINATION IS UNKNOWN.

ESSER, E.* MEDIAN FISSURE OF THE NOSE. PLAST. CHIR. 1* 40-50, 1939.

GLANZ, S.* HYPERTELORISM AND THE BIFID NOSE. STH. MED. J. 59* 631-635, 1966.

KHOO BOO-CHAI* THE BIFID NOSE, WITH REPORT OF 3 CASES IN SIBLINGS. PLAST. RECONSTR. SURG. 36* 626-628, 1965.

21050 BILIARY ATRESIA, EXTRAHEPATIC

KRAUSS (1964) NOTED THE REPORTS OF 5 SIBSHIPS IN WHICH TWO OR MORE SIBS WERE AFFECTED. RENAL AND CARDIAC MALFORMATIONS WERE ASSOCIATED IN KRAUSS' CASES. SWEET (1932) FOUND 3 CASES IN ONE FAMILY AND TWO OF THE 3 HAD RIGHT VENTRICULAR HYPERTROPHY (ONE WITH VSD AND PDA). OTHER FAMILIAL CASES HAVE BEEN REPORTED BY HOPKINS (1941), RUMBER (1961) AND WHITTEN (1952).

HOPKINS, N. K.* CONGENITAL ABSENCE OF COMMON DUCT* THREE CASES IN ONE FAMILY. J. LANCET 61* 90-91, 1941.

KRAUSS, A. N.* FAMILIAL EXTRAHEPATIC BILIARY ATRESIA. J. PEDIAT. 65* 933-937, 1964.

RUMBER, W.* UBER DIE KONGENITALE GALLENWEGSATRESIE ZUM FAMILIAREN VORKOMMEN UND ZUR GENESE DIESER FEHLBILDUNG. ARCH. KINDERHEILK. 164* 238-248, 1961.

SWEET, L. K.* CONGENITAL MALFORMATION OF THE BILE DUCTS. A REPORT OF THREE CASES IN ONE FAMILY. J. PEDIAT. 1* 496-501, 1932.

WHITTEN, W. W. AND ADIE, G. C.* CONGENITAL BILIARY ATRESIA. REPORT OF THREE CASES* TWO OCCURRING IN ONE FAMILY. J. PEDIAT. 40* 539-548, 1952.

*21060 BIRD-HEADED DWARF (NANOCEPHALY OR SECKEL'S TYPE DWARFISM)

THIS CONDITION WAS GIVEN ITS TWO NAMES BY VIRCHOW. SECKEL (1960) PRODUCED THE DEFINITIVE PUBLICATION BASED ON TWO PERSONALLY OBSERVED CASES AND THIRTEEN RELIABLE PLUS ELEVEN LESS RELIABLE CASES FROM THE LITERATURE. IN ADDITION TO

R
E
C
E
S
S
I
V
E

DWARFISM OF 'LOW BIRTH WEIGHT' TYPE, THE FEATURES ARE SMALL HEAD, LARGE EYES, BEAKLIKE PROTRUSION OF THE NOSE, NARROW FACE AND RECEDING LOWER JAW. MENTAL RETARDATION IS NOT AS MARKED AS MIGHT BE EXPECTED IN VIEW OF THE VERY SMALL BRAIN. MULTIPLE OCCURRENCE IN THE SAME SIBSHIP, INCREASED FREQUENCY OF PARENTAL CONSAN-GUINITY, OCCURRENCE IN BOTH SEXES AND NORMAL PARENTS SUGGEST AUTOSOMAL RECESSIVE INHERITANCE. AFFECTED SISTERS WERE REPORTED BY BLACK (1961). HARPER ET AL. (1967) REPORTED BROTHER AND SISTER WHO STRIKINGLY RESEMBLED SECKEL'S CASES 1 AND 2, TWO OTHER REPORTED CASES AND THE THREE SIBS REPORTED BY MCKUSICK ET AL. (1967).

BLACK, J.* LOW BIRTH WEIGHT DWARFISM. ARCH. DIS. CHILD. 36* 633-644, 1961.

HARPER, R. G., ORTI, E. AND BAKER, R. K.* BIRD-HEADED DWARFS (SECKEL'S SYNDROME). A FAMILIAL PATTERN OF DEVELOPMENTAL, DENTAL, SKELETAL, GENITAL AND CENTRAL NERVOUS SYSTEM ANOMALIES. J. PEDIAT. 70* 799-804, 1967.

MCKUSICK, V. A., MAHLOUDJI, M., ABBOTT, M. H., LINDENBERG, R. AND KEPAS, D.* SECKEL'S BIRD-HEADED DWARFISM. NEW ENG. J. MED. 277* 279-286, 1967.

SECKEL, H. P. G.* BIRD-HEADED DWARFS. STUDIES IN DEVELOPMENTAL ANTHROPOLOGY INCLUDING HUMAN PROPORTIONS. SPRINGFIELD, ILL.* CHARLES C THOMAS, 1960.

21070 BIRD-HEADED DWARFISM, MONTREAL TYPE

IN MONTREAL FITCH ET AL. (1970) DESCRIBED A PATIENT WITH A FORM OF BIRD-HEADED DWARFISM CLEARLY DISTINCT FROM SECKEL'S TYPE. SIGNS OF PREMATURE SENILITY, NAMELY PREMATURE GRAYING AND LOSS OF SCALP HAIR, REDUNDANT AND WRINKLED SKIN OF THE PALMS. OTHER FEATURES INCLUDED MENTAL RETARDATION, PTOSIS AND CRYPTORCHIDISM. BIRTH WEIGHT WAS NORMAL. ALTHOUGH SOME FEATURES SUGGESTED THE SYNDROMES OF WERNER, SECKEL, HALLERMANN-STREIFF, NOONAN, ETC., THE AUTHORS CONSIDERED THAT DIFFERENCES FROM ALL THESE EXISTED JUSTIFYING ITS LISTING AS A SEPARATE ENTITY. WE (SMITH ET AL., 1970) AGREE, HAVING OBSERVED AN AFFECTED BROTHER AND SISTER, AND PROPOSE AUTOSOMAL RECESSIVE INHERITANCE. TO TAKE CARE OF THE PROBLEM OF NOMENCLA-TURE I SUGGEST WE BORROW THE PRACTICE OF THE HEMOGLOBINOLOGISTS AND CALL THIS THE MONTREAL TYPE OF BIRD-HEADED DWARFISM.

FITCH, N., PINSKY, L. AND LACHANCE, R. C.* A FORM OF BIRD-HEADED DWARFISM WITH FEATURES OF PREMATURE SENILITY. AM. J. DIS. CHILD. 120* 260-264, 1970.

SMITH, W. K. AND MCKUSICK, V. A.* BALTIMORE, UNPUBLISHED OBSERVATIONS, 1970.

21080 BLOOD GROUPS

ALL BLOOD GROUPS ARE CO-DOMINANT WITH RARE EXCEPTIONS. BLOOD TYPE A(1) IS DOMINANT TO BLOOD TYPE A(2), SO THAT THE A(1) A(2) HETEROZYGOTE TYPES AS A(1). A(1), A(2) AND B BLOOD TYPES ARE DOMINANT TO BLOOD TYPE O. THE BOMBAY PHENOTYPE (Q.V.) IS DUE TO A RECESSIVE GENE. IN ADDITION VARIOUS BLOOD GROUP PHENOTYPES WHICH ARE THOUGHT TO BE THE RESULT OF GENETIC DELETION BEHAVE AS RECESSIVES. THESE INCLUDE THE RH - PHENOTYPE WITH NO RH ANTIGENS (VOS ET AL., 1961) AND THE K(O) PHENOTYPE IN WHICH NO ANTIGEN OF THE KELL SYSTEM IS DEMONSTRABLE (NUNN ET AL., 1966). EXAMPLES ARE ALSO KNOWN IN THE DUFFY AND LUTHERAN SYSTEMS.

NUNN, H. D., GILES, C. M. AND DORMANDY, K. M.* A SECOND EXAMPLE OF ANTI-KU IN A PATIENT WHO HAS THE RARE KELL PHENOTYPE, K(O). VOX SANG. 11* 611-619, 1966.

VOS, G. H., VOS, D., KIRK, R. L. AND SANGER, R.* A SAMPLE OF BLOOD WITH NO DETECTABLE RH ANTIGENS. LANCET 1* 14-15, 1961.

*21090 BLOOM'S SYNDROME (DWARFISM WITH SKIN CHANGES)

THE DWARFISM IS OF THE 'LOW BIRTH WEIGHT' TYPE, I.E., ALTHOUGH FULL TERM THE CHILD IS ABNORMALLY SMALL. THE CUTANEOUS FEATURE IS RASH FROM SENSITIVITY TO SUNLIGHT. SZALAY (1963) PROVIDED THE FIRST EVIDENCE OF A GENETIC BASIS. HE DESCRIBED (1) AN ISOLATED CASE, THE CHILD OF FIRST COUSIN PARENTS, AND (2) TWO AFFECTED SIBS. MULTIPLE SEEMINGLY NON-SPECIFIC CHROMOSOMAL BREAKS HAVE BEEN OBSERVED IN THESE CASES AS IN FANCONI'S ANEMIA (Q.V.) AND MAY BE RELATED CAUSALLY TO THE HIGH FREQUENCY OF LEUKEMIA (GERMAN ET AL., 1965). NINE OF 13 FAMILIES WERE JEWISH. LANDAU ET AL. (1966) DESCRIBED A PATIENT WHOSE PARENTS WERE SECOND COUSINS AND WHO SHOWED LOW GAMMA-A AND GAMMA-M SERUM PROTEINS. FERRARA ET AL. (1967) DESCRIBED THE DISEASE IN A 'CHINESE-AMERICAN.' TWELVE OF 21 FAMILIES FIRST DISCOVERED WITH BLOOM'S SYNDROME WERE ASKENAZIC AND IN THESE ONLY ONE PARENTAL COUPLE WAS CONSANGUINEOUS. ON THE OTHER HAND, 6 OF THE OTHER 9 NON-JEWISH UNIONS WERE CONSANGUINEOUS. THE JEWISH GENE APPEARED TO HAVE ORIGINATED IN A LOCAL AREA OF EASTERN EUROPE. IN A LATER TABULATION OF CASES, GERMAN (1969) FOUND THAT 10 OF 21 FAMILIES WERE ASHKENAZIC.

BLOOM, D.* THE SYNDROME OF CONGENITAL TELANGIECTATIC ERYTHEMA AND STUNTED GROWTH. J. PEDIAT. 68* 103-113, 1966.

FERRARA, A., FONTANA, V. J. AND NUMSEN, G.* BLOOM'S SYNDROME IN ORIENTAL MALE. NEW YORK J. MED. 67* 3258-3262, 1967.

GERMAN, J.* BLOOM'S SYNDROME. I. GENETICAL AND CLINICAL OBSERVATIONS IN THE

R
E
C
E
S
S
I
V
E

GERMAN, J., ARCHIBALD, R. AND BLOOM, D.* CHROMOSOMAL BREAKAGE IN A RARE AND PROBABLY GENETICALLY DETERMINED SYNDROME OF MAN. SCIENCE 148* 506-507, 1965.

LANDAU, J. W., SASAKI, M. S., NEWCOMER, V. D. AND NORMAN, A.* BLOOM'S SYNDROME. THE SYNDROME OF TELANGIECTATIC ERYTHEMA AND GROWTH RETARDATION. ARCH. DERM. 94* 687-694, 1966.

SAWITSKY, A., BLOOM, D. AND GERMAN, J.* CHROMOSOMAL BREAKAGE AND ACUTE LEUKEMIA IN CONGENITAL TELANGIECTATIC ERYTHEMA AND STUNTED GROWTH. ANN. INTERN. MED. 65* 487-495, 1966.

SZALAY, G. C.* DWARFISM WITH SKIN MANIFESTATIONS. J. PEDIAT. 62* 686-695, 1963.

21100   BLUE DIAPER SYNDROME (FAMILIAL HYPERCALCEMIA WITH NEPHROCALCINOSIS AND INDICANURIA)

HYPERCALCEMIA AND NEPHROCALCINOSIS ARE ASSOCIATED WITH A DEFECT IN THE INTESTINAL TRANSPORT OF TRYPTOPHAN. BACTERIAL DEGRADATION OF THE TRYPTOPHAN LEADS TO EXCESSIVE INDOLE PRODUCTION AND THUS TO INDICANURIA WHICH, ON OXIDATION TO INDIGO BLUE, CAUSES A PECULIAR BLUISH DISCOLORATION OF THE DIAPER. DRUMMOND, MICHAEL, ULSTROM AND GOOD (1964) REPORTED TWO AFFECTED BROTHERS. ALTHOUGH ALMOST CERTAINLY RECESSIVE, THE DISORDER COULD BE X-LINKED.

DRUMMOND, K. N., MICHAEL, A. F., ULSTROM, R. A. AND GOOD, R. A.* THE BLUE DIAPER SYNDROME* FAMILIAL HYPERCALCEMIA WITH NEPHROCALCINOSIS AND INDICANURIA. A NEW FAMILIAL DISEASE, WITH DEFINITION OF THE METABOLIC ABNORMALITY. AM. J. MED. 37* 928-948, 1964.

*21110 BOMBAY PHENOTYPE

ALL HUMAN BLOODS, WITH EXCEEDINGLY RARE EXCEPTIONS, CARRY THE RED CELL H ANTIGEN. IT IS PRESENT IN GREATEST AMOUNT ON TYPE O RED CELLS AND LEAST ON (A1B) CELLS. THE ANTIGEN IS NOW REGARDED AS AN INTERMEDIATE STAGE IN A SERIES OF SYNTHESES ENDING, IN THE PRESENCE OF THE A OR B GENES, IN THE PRODUCTION OF THE CORRESPON-DING A AND B ANTIGENS. THE FIRST EXAMPLES OF BLOOD COMPLETELY LACKING H WERE FOUND IN BOMBAY BY BHENDE AND COLLEAGUES (1952). THESE INDIVIDUALS ARE RECOGNIZED BY THE PRESENCE OF ANTI-H IN THE SERUM, IN ADDITION TO ANTI-A AND ANTI-B, AS IN TYPE O PERSONS. BY FAMILY STUDIES LEVINE AND COLLEAGUES (1955) AND ALOYSIA ET AL. (1961) SHOWED THAT THE BOMBAY PHENOTYPE, CALLED BY THEM OH, IS DUE TO THE PRESENCE IN HOMOZYGOUS STATE OF A RARE RECESSIVE GENE. YUNIS ET AL. (1969) FOUND SEVEN AFFECTED PERSONS IN THREE GENERATIONS INCLUDING A HOMOZYGOUS X HETEROZYGOUS MATING. THEY PROPOSED THAT THERE ARE TWO KINDS OF BOMBAY GENOTYPES.

R
E
C
E
S
S
I
V
E

ALOYSIA, M., GELB, A. G., FUDENBERG, H., HAMPER, J., TIPPETT, P. AND RACE, R. R.* THE EXPECTED 'BOMBAY' GROUP O(H-A1) AND O(H-A2). TRANSFUSION 1* 212-217, 1961.

BHENDE, Y. M., DESHPANDE, C. K., BHATIA, H. M., SANGER, R., RACE, R. R., MORGAN, W. T. J. AND WATKINS, W. M.* A 'NEW' BLOOD GROUP CHARACTER RELATED TO THE ABO SYSTEM. LANCET 1* 903-904, 1952.

HRUBISKO, M., LALUHA, J., MERGANCOVA, O. AND ZAKOVICOVA, S.* NEW VARIANTS IN THE ABOH BLOOD GROUP SYSTEM DUE TO INTERACTION OF RECESSIVE GENES CONTROLLING THE FORMATION OF H ANTIGEN IN ERYTHROCYTES* THE 'BOMBAY-LIKE' PHENOTYPES O HM, OB HM, OAB HM. VOX SANG. 19* 113-122, 1970.

LEVINE, P., ROBINSON, E., CELANO, M., BRIGGS, O. AND FALKINBURG, L.* GENE INTERACTION RESULTING IN SUPPRESSION OF BLOOD GROUP SUBSTANCE B. BLOOD 10* 1100-1108, 1955.

YUNIS, E. J., SVARDAL, J. M. AND BRIDGES, R. A.* GENETICS OF THE BOMBAY PHENOTYPE. BLOOD 33* 124-132, 1969.

21120 BOWEN'S SYNDROME OF MULTIPLE MALFORMATIONS

BOWEN AND COLLEAGUES (1964) DESCRIBED TWO FAMILIES, EACH WITH TWO SIBS DISPLAYING FEATURES SUGGESTING AUTOSOMAL TRISOMY, PARTICULARLY TRISOMY 17-18. HOWEVER, NO CHROMOSOMAL ABNORMALITY WAS IDENTIFIED. CARDINAL FEATURES WERE FAILURE TO THRIVE, ABSENT OR WEAK SUCKING AND SWALLOWING, FINGER FLEXION, CONGENITAL GLAUCOMA, MALFORMED EARS, SMALL MANDIBLE, HEART MALFORMATIONS, ENLARGED CLITORIS, HYPOSPA-DIAS, AGENESIS OF THE CORPUS CALLOSUM AND DEATH AT AN EARLY AGE. NO PARENTAL CONSANGUINITY WAS DEMONSTRATED IN EITHER FAMILY. ONE FAMILY WAS NEGRO, THE OTHER WHITE. SEE FRASER'S SYNDROME FOR A COMPARABLE, ALTHOUGH SEEMINGLY DISTINCT, SYNDROME OF MALFORMATIONS IN SIBS. IT NOW SEEMS CLEAR THAT THE SECOND OF THE FAMILIES REPORTED BY BOWEN ET AL., THAT CONTRIBUTED BY ZELLWEGER, HAD CEREBRO-HEPATO-RENAL SYNDROME (Q.V.). THE NATURE OF THE DEFECT IN THE FIRST FAMILY IS NOT CERTAIN.

BOWEN, P., LEE, C. N. S., ZELLWEGER, H. AND LINDENBURG, R.* A FAMILIAL SYNDROME

21130 BOWING OF LEGS, ANTERIOR, WITH DWARFISM (WEISMANN-NETTER SYNDROME* TOXOPACHYOS-
TEOSE DIAPHYSAIRE TIBIO-PERONIERE)

THE PRESENTING MANIFESTATIONS ARE DWARFISM AND SABRE SHINS. MENTAL RETARDATION,
MILD UPPER EXTREMITY INVOLVEMENT AND DURAL CALCIFICATION. FAMILIAL INCIDENCE HAS
BEEN NOTED BY LARCAN ET AL. (1963). HOEFNAGEL (1969) AND KEATS AND ALAVI (1970)
HAVE REPORTED CASES IN THIS COUNTRY.

HOEFNAGEL, D.* MALFORMATION SYNDROMES WITH MENTAL DEFICIENCY. THE CLINICAL
DELINEATION OF BIRTH DEFECTS. II. MALFORMATION SYNDROMES. NEW YORK* NATIONAL
FOUNDATION, 1969. PP. 11-14.

KEATS, T. E. AND ALAVI, M. S.* TOXOPACHYOSTEOSE DIAPHYSAIRE TIBIO-PERONIERE
(WEISMANN-NETTER SYNDROME). AM. J. ROENTGEN. 109* 568-574, 1970.

KREWER, B.* DYSMORPHIE JAMBIERE DE WEISMANN-NETTER (TOXO-PACHY-OSTEOSE
DIAPHYSAIRE TIBIO-PERONIERE) CHEZ DEUX VRAIS JUMEAUX. PRESSE MED. 69* 419-420,
1961.

LARCAN, A., CAYOTTE, J. L., GAUCHER, A. AND BERTHEAU, J. M.* LA TOXOPACHYOS-
TEOSE DE WEISMANN-NETTER. ANN. MED. 2* 1724-1732, 1963.

21140 BRONCHIECTASIS

DANIELSON ET AL. (1967) FOUND 4 OF 5 SIBS (2 MALE, 2 FEMALE) AFFECTED WITH
BRONCHIECTASIA OF THE MIDDLE LOBE.

DANIELSON, G. K., HANSON, C. W. AND COOPER, E. C.* MIDDLE LOBE BRONCHIECTASIS.
REPORT OF AN UNUSUAL FAMILIAL OCCURRENCE. J.A.M.A. 201* 605-608, 1967.

21150 BULBAR PALSY, PROGRESSIVE, OF CHILDHOOD (FAZIO-LONDE'S DISEASE)

LONDE (1894) REPORTED AFFECTED 5 AND 6 YEAR OLD BROTHERS WHOSE PARENTS WERE FIRST
COUSINS. MARINESCO (1915) DESCRIBED IT IN A 12 YEAR OLD GIRL AND HER 8 YEAR OLD
BROTHER. PYRAMIDAL TRACTS WERE NOT INVOLVED. FAZIO'S CASES ARE SAID (GOMEZ,
CLERMONT, BERNSTEIN, 1962) TO HAVE BEEN A MOTHER AND HER FOUR AND ONE HALF YEAR
OLD SON. SEE AMYOTROPHIC LATERAL SCLEROSIS.

GOMEZ, M. R., CLERMONT, V. AND BERNSTEIN, J.* PROGRESSIVE BULBAR PARALYSIS IN
CHILDHOOD (FAZIO-LONDE'S DISEASE). REPORT OF A CASE WITH PATHOLOGIC EVIDENCE OF
NUCLEAR ATROPHY. ARCH. NEUROL. 6* 317-323, 1962.

LONDE, P.* PARALYSIE BULBAIRE PROGRESSIVE, INFANTILE ET FAMILIALE. REV. MED.
14* 212-254, 1894.

MARINESCO, G.* SUR DEUX CAS DE PARALYSIE BULBAIRE PROGRESSIVE INFANTILE ET
FAMILIALE. COMP. REND. SOC. BIOL. 78* 481-483, 1915.

*21160 BYLER'S DISEASE (FATAL INTRAHEPATIC CHOLESTASIS)

IN THE OLD ORDER AMISH, CLAYTON AND HIS COLLEAGUES (1965) HAVE DEMONSTRATED A
VARIETY OF INTRAHEPATIC CHOLESTASIS WHICH LEADS TO DEATH IN THE FIRST DECADE OF
LIFE. IT APPEARS TO BE DIFFERENT FROM THE MORE BENIGN TYPE OF INTRAHEPATIC
CHOLESTASIS (Q.V.). FEATURES ARE (1) EARLY ONSET OF LOOSE, FOUL-SMELLING STOOLS,
(2) 'ATTACKS' OF JAUNDICE POSSIBLY RELATED TO INFECTION, (3) HEPATOSPLENOMEGALY,
(4) DWARFISM AND (5) IN 4 OF 6 CASES, DEATH BETWEEN 17 MONTHS AND 8 YEARS. ONE
MOTHER HAD EXTREME PRURITUS WITHOUT JAUNDICE IN THE LAST TRIMESTER OF EACH OF 4
PREGNANCIES. TWO FATHERS HAD REDUCED MAXIMUM EXCRETION OF BSP. CHOLESTYRAMINE, A
BILE-SALT-SEQUESTERING EXCHANGE RESIN, REDUCED THE HYPERBILIRUBINEMIA. BECAUSE
THE BILE SHOWED AN INCREASED PROPORTION OF DIHYDROXY BILE SALTS, AS WELL AS THE
EARLY ONSET OF CHANGES IN THE STOOL AND THE RESPONSE TO CHOLESTYRAMINE, A DEFECT
IN BILE SALT METABOLISM WAS POSTULATED. SERUM CHOLESTEROL WAS LOW. A FAMILIAL
CHOLESTATIC DISORDER WHICH IS PROBABLY DIFFERENT WAS STUDIED BY KAYE (SEE KAYE'S
DISEASE). THE SAME CONDITION WAS PROBABLY DESCRIBED BY GRAY AND SAUNDERS (1966)
IN TWO SISTERS, OFFSPRING OF UNRELATED PARENTS (MOTHER WELSH, FATHER IRISH), WHO
DIED UNDER 3 YEARS OF AGE. TOUSSAINT AND GROS (1966) REPORTED AFFECTED BROTHERS.
THE SAME CONDITION MAY HAVE BEEN PRESENT IN THE PATIENT REPORTED BY HIROOKA AND
OHNO (1968).

CLAYTON, R. J., IBER, F. L., RUEBNER, B. H. AND MCKUSICK, V. A.* BYLER'S
DISEASE. FATAL FAMILIAL INTRAHEPATIC CHOLESTASIS IN AN AMISH KINDRED. (ABSTRACT)
J. PEDIAT. 67* 1025-1028, 1965.

GRAY, O. P. AND SAUNDERS, R. A.* FAMILIAL INTRAHEPATIC CHOLESTATIC JAUNDICE IN
INFANCY. ARCH. DIS. CHILD. 41* 320-328, 1966.

HIROOKA, M. AND OHNO, T.* A CASE OF FAMILIAL INTRAHEPATIC CHOLESTASIS. TOHOKU
J. EXP. MED. 94* 293-306, 1968.

JUBERG, R. C., HOLLAND-MORITZ, R. M., HENLEY, K. S. AND GONZALEZ, C. F.*

38* 819-836, 1966.

TOUSSAINT, W. AND GROS, H.* FAMILIARER ICTERUS DURCH INTRAHEPATISCHE CHOLES-
TASE. DEUTSCH. Z. VERDAU. STOFFWECHSELKR. 26* 23-31, 1966.

21170 B12-BINDING ALPHA GLOBULIN, DEFICIENCY OF

IN TWO PUERTO RICAN-CORSICAN BROTHERS IN THEIR 40'S, LOW VITAMIN B12 AND LOW B12-
BINDING ALPHA GLOBULIN WERE FOUND IN THE BLOOD. NO SYMPTOMS WERE ATTRIBUTABLE
THERETO. THREE CHILDREN OF ONE OF THE MEN HAD NORMAL VALVES.

CARMEL, R. AND HERBERT, V.* DEFICIENCY OF VITAMIN B12-BINDING ALPHA GLOBULIN IN
TWO BROTHERS. BLOOD 33* 1-12, 1969.

21180 CALCIFICATION OF JOINTS AND ARTERIES

SHARP (1954) DESCRIBED A FAMILY IN WHICH TWO OF FOUR SIBS FROM A FIRST COUSIN
MARRIAGE DISPLAYED CALCIFICATION OF JOINT STRUCTURES AND ARTERIES OF AN UNUSUAL
TYPE. THE REMAINING TWO SIBS AND THE SON AND DAUGHTER OF ONE OF THE SEVERELY
AFFECTED SIBS SEEMED TO SHOW A MILDER FORM OF THE DISORDER AFFECTING ONLY
ARTERIES. TWO PREVIOUSLY REPORTED SPORADIC CASES WERE NOTED.

SHARP, J.* HEREDO-FAMILIAL VASCULAR AND ARTICULAR CALCIFICATION. ANN. RHEUM.
DIS. 13* 15-27, 1954.

*21190 CALCINOSIS, TUMORAL, WITH HYPERPHOSPHATEMIA

BALDURSSON ET AL. (1969) OBSERVED FOUR AFFECTED SIBS OUT OF TWELVE IN A NEGRO
FAMILY. HYPERPHOSPHATEMIA WAS DOCUMENTED AS EARLY AS TWENTY-ONE MONTHS OF AGE IN
ONE OF THEM IN WHOM TUMORAL CALCINOSIS APPEARED AT FOUR YEARS. A MAJORITY OF THE
CASES OF THIS CONDITION REPORTED IN THE ANGLO-AMERICAN LITERATURE HAVE BEEN IN
NEGROES. OTHER FAMILIAL CASES HAVE BEEN REPORTED BY BARTON AND REEVES (1961) AND
HARKESS AND PETERS (1967). DODGE, TRAVIS AND ASSEMI (1965) DESCRIBED THREE SIBS
WITH HETEROTOPIC CALCIFICATION, HYPERPHOSPHATEMIA, UNRESPONSIVENESS TO PARATHYROID
HORMONE, AND ELEVATED RENAL TUBULAR MAXIMUM FOR PHOSPHATE REABSORPTION. STIGMATA
OF ALBRIGHT'S OSTEODYSTROPHY (X-LINKED) WERE NOT PRESENT. SOME REPORTED PATIENTS
HAVE HAD ANGIOID STREAKS OF THE RETINA (MCPHAUL, ENGEL, 1961). THIS IS CONSISTENT
WITH THE VIEW THAT ANGIOID STREAKS IN PSEUDOXANTHOMA ELASTICUM, SICKLE CELL ANEMIA
AND PAGET'S DISEASE ARE DUE TO A BRITTLE STATE OF BRUCH'S MEMBRANE PRODUCED BY
DEPOSITION OF CALCIUM, IRON AND PERHAPS OTHER CATIONS. GHORMLEY (1942) REPORTED
MULTIPLE AFFECTED SIBS. MCPHAUL AND ENGEL (1961) REPORTED AFFECTED BROTHERS AND
IN ANOTHER FAMILY THE PROBAND'S PATERNAL GRANDFATHER WAS THOUGHT TO HAVE BEEN
AFFECTED AND HE WAS RELATED TO A FAMILY REPORTED AS PSEUDOXANTHOMA ELASTICUM.
FROM BEIRUT NAJJAR ET AL. (1968) DESCRIBED TWO SIBS WITH PERIARTICULAR CALCIFIED
MASSES, INCREASED BLOOD PHOSPHORUS, NORMAL BLOOD CALCIUM, CLACIFIED VESSELS AND
SKIN CHANGES OF PXE. THE PARENTS MAY HAVE BEEN RELATED. AN AUNT WAS SAID TO HAVE
HETEROTOPIC CALCIFICATION. I SUSPECT THAT THIS IS A DISORDER DISTINCT FROM
ORDINARY PXE, ALTHOUGH WITH MANY SIMILAR FEATURES. IN A REVIEW OF THE RADIOLOGIC
FINDINGS OF PXE, JAMES ET AL. (1969) PICTURED A LARGE CALCIFIED MASS IN THE REGION
OF THE ELBOW. THE PATIENT PROBABLY HAD THE ENTITY DISCUSSED HERE.

R
E
C
E
S
S
I
V
E

BALDURSSON, H., EVANS, E. B., DODGE, W. F. AND JACKSON, W. T.* TUMORAL
CALCINOSIS WITH HYPERPHOSPHATEMIA. A REPORT OF A FAMILY WITH INCIDENCE IN FOUR
SIBLINGS. J. BONE JOINT SURG. 51B* 913-925, 1969.

BARTON, D. L. AND REEVES, R. J.* TUMORAL CALCINOSIS. REPORT OF 3 CASES AND
REVIEW OF THE LITERATURE. AM. J. ROENTGEN. 86* 351-358, 1961.

DODGE, W. F., TRAVIS, L. B. AND ASSEMI, M.* FAMILIAL HETEROTOPIC CALCIFICATION
AND HYPERPHOSPHATEMIA UNRESPONSIVE TO PARATHYROID EXTRACT. (ABSTRACT) J. PEDIAT.
67* 944-945, 1965.

GHORMLEY, R. K.* MULTIPLE CALCIFIED BURSAE AND CALCIFIED CYSTS IN SOFT TISSUES.
TRANS. WEST. SURG. ASS. 51* 292-309, 1942.

HARKESS, J. W. AND PETERS, H. J.* TUMORAL CALCINOSIS. A REPORT OF SIX CASES.
J. BONE JOINT SURG. 49A* 721-731, 1967.

JAMES, A. E., JR., EATON, S. B., BLAZEK, J. V., DONNER, M. W. AND REEVES, R.
J.* ROENTGEN FINDINGS IN PSEUDOXANTHOMA ELASTICUM (PXE). AM. J. ROENTGEN. 106*
642-647, 1969.

MCPHAUL, J. J., JR. AND ENGEL, F. L.* HETEROTOPIC CALCIFICATION, HYPERPHOSPHA-
TEMIA AND ANGIOID STREAKS OF THE RETINA. AM. J. MED. 31* 488-492, 1961.

NAJJAR, S. S., FARAH, F. S., KURBAN, A. K., MELHEM, R. E. AND KHATCHADOURIAN,
A. K.* TUMORAL CALCINOSIS AND PSEUDOXANTHOMA ELASTICUM. J. PEDIAT. 72* 243-247,
1968.

21200 CANCER OF THE BREAST, FAMILIAL

CADY (1970) DESCRIBED A FAMILY IN WHICH THREE SISTERS HAD BILATERAL BREAST CANCER. TOGETHER WITH REPORTS IN THE LITERATURE, THIS SUGGESTED TO HIM THE EXISTENCE OF FAMILIES WITH A PARTICULAR TENDENCY TO EARLY ONSET AND BILATERAL BREAST CANCER. THE GENETIC BASIS MIGHT, OF COURSE, BE MULTIFACTORIAL.

CADY, B.* FAMILIAL BILATERAL CANCER OF THE BREAST. ANN. SURG. 172* 264-272, 1970.

21210 CARDIO-AUDITORY SYNDROME OF SANCHEZ CASCOS

A NEW CARDIO-AUDITORY SYNDROME WAS FOUND IN 12 DEAF CHILDREN BY SANCHEZ CASCOS ET AL. (1969). ALL BUT 2 HAD X-RAY EVIDENCE OF LEFT VENTRICULAR HYPERTROPHY, MOST HAD ELECTROCARDIOGRAPHIC CHANGES OF BIVENTRICULAR HYPERTROPHY AND MOST SHOWED A HIGH PROPORTION OF WHORLS IN THE DERMATOGLYPHS. ONE OF THE 12 WAS A GIRL. ONE OF THE PARENTAL PAIRS WAS CONSANGUINEOUS. SIX OF THE 12 WERE IN 3 SIBSHIPS.

SANCHEZ CASCOS, A., SANCHEZ-HARGUINDEY, L. AND DE RABAGO, P.* CARDIO-AUDITORY SYNDROMES. CARDIAC AND GENETIC STUDY OF 511 DEAF-MUTE CHILDREN. BRIT. HEART J. 31* 26-33, 1969.

*21220 CARNOSINEMIA

PERRY ET AL. (1967) DESCRIBED TWO UNRELATED CHILDREN WITH A PROGRESSIVE NEUROLOGIC DISORDER CHARACTERIZED BY SEVERE MENTAL DEFECT AND MYOCLONIC SEIZURES. BOTH EXCRETED CARNOSINE IN THE URINE, EVEN WHEN ALL SOURCE OF THE DIPEPTIDE WAS EXCLUDED FROM THE DIET. BOTH HAD UNUSUALLY HIGH CONCENTRATIONS OF HOMOCARNOSINE IN THE CEREBROSPINAL FLUID. WHEN FED A DIETARY SOURCE OF ANSERINE, THE CHILDREN EXCRETED ANSERINE IN THE URINE BUT NOT ITS HYDROLYSIS PRODUCT, METHYLHISTIDINE. PERRY ET AL. SUGGESTED THAT ONE AND PERHAPS BOTH HAD A DEFECT IN CARNOSINASE ACTIVITY. ONE CHILD, OF GERMAN AND DUTCH ANCESTRY, WAS THE OFFSPRING OF FIRST-COUSIN PARENTS. THE OTHER CHILD WAS OF CHINESE ANCESTRY. PERRY ET AL. (1968) FOUND THAT THE ENZYME OF NORMAL HUMAN SERUM THAT HYDROLYZES THE DIPEPTIDES CARNOSINE AND ANSERINE INTO THEIR CONSTITUENT AMINO ACIDS WAS ALMOST ABSENT IN THE TWO PATIENTS. NO COMMENT WAS MADE ON THE LEVEL OF ENZYME IN THE PARENTS. CARNOSINE IS A DIPEPTIDE OF ALANINE AND HISTIDINE. SCRIVER ET AL. (1968) COMMENTED ON THE POSSIBLE RELATIONSHIP OF THE MENTAL RETARDATION THAT OCCURS WITH HYPER-BETA-CARNOSINEMIA (Q.V.) AND PHENYLKETONURIA. IN THE CASE OF THE AFFECTED DUTCH CHILD REPORTED BY HEESWIJK ET AL. (1969) THE PARENTS WERE CONSANGUINEOUS AND SHOWED DECREASED SERUM CARNOSINASE ACTIVITY.

HEESWIJK, P. J., TRIJBELS, J. M. F., SCHRETLEN, A. M., MUNSTER, P. J. J. AND MONNENS, L. A. H.* A PATIENT WITH A DEFICIENCY OF SERUM-CARNOSINASE ACTIVITY. ACTA PAEDIAT. SCAND. 58* 584-592, 1969.

PERRY, T. L., HANSEN, S. AND LOVE, D.* SERUM-CARNOSINASE DEFICIENCY IN CARNOSINAEMIA. LANCET 1* 1229-1230, 1968.

PERRY, T. L., HANSEN, S., TISCHLER, B., BUNTING, R. AND BERRY, K.* CARNOSINE-MIA* METABOLIC DISORDER WITH NEUROLOGIC DISEASE AND MENTAL DEFECT. NEW ENG. J. MED. 277* 1219-1227, 1967.

SCRIVER, C. R., ALLEN, R. J., TOURTELLOTTE, W. W., ADRIAENSSENS, K., LOWENTHAL, A. AND MARDENS, Y.* CARNOSINAEMIA. (LETTER) LANCET 1* 1249 ONLY, 1968.

*21230 CARTILAGE-HAIR HYPOPLASIA

THIS DISORDER WAS FIRST RECOGNIZED AS A SYNDROME IN THE OLD ORDER AMISH, A RELIGIOUS ISOLATE, BUT HAS MORE RECENTLY BEEN IDENTIFIED IN OTHER GROUPS. THE SKELETAL FEATURE IS SHORT-LIMBED DWARFISM. BY X-RAY THE CHANGES ARE OF THE TYPE CALLED METAPHYSEAL DYSOSTOSIS BY THE RADIOLOGISTS. BIOPSY SHOWS HYPOPLASIA OF CARTILAGE TO BE THE NATURE OF THE ABNORMALITY. THE HAIR IS FINE, SPARSE AND LIGHT-COLORED. MICROSCOPICALLY IT HAS AN ABNORMALLY SMALL CALIBER. AUTOSOMAL RECESSIVE INHERITANCE SEEMS QUITE CERTAIN ALTHOUGH PENETRANCE IS REDUCED (WHEN DWARFISM IS TAKEN AS THE PHENOTYPE FOR ASCERTAINMENT). THE RELATIONSHIP OF THE SYNDROME DESCRIBED BY BURGERT, DOWER AND TAUXE (1965), WITH AREGENERATIVE ANEMIA AND CELIAC SYNDROME, IS UNCLEAR. UNEXPLAINED FEATURES PRESENT IN SOME CASES INCLUDE ANEMIA, MALABSORPTION, HIRSCHSPRUNG'S DISEASE, AND SUSCEPTIBILITY TO CHICKEN POX. SOME OF THESE FEATURES RESEMBLE THOSE OF THE PATIENTS WITH PANCREATIC INSUFFICIENCY AND NEUTROPENIA REPORTED BY BURKE ET AL. (1967) AND SOME OF THEIR PATIENTS HAD METAPHYSEAL CHANGES. SEE ALSO THE REPORTS OF BURGERT ET AL. (1965) AND OF THEODOROU AND ADAMS (1963).

BURGERT, E. O., JR., DOWER, J. C. AND TAUXE, W. N.* A NEW SYNDROME - AREGENERATIVE ANEMIA, MALABSORPTION (CELIAC), DYSCHONDROPLASIA AND HYPERPHOSPHATEMIA. (ABSTRACT) J. PEDIAT. 67* 711-712, 1965.

BURKE, V., COLEBATCH, J. H., ANDERSON, C. M. AND SIMONS, M. J.* ASSOCIATION OF PANCREATIC INSUFFICIENCY AND CHRONIC NEUTROPENIA IN CHILDHOOD. ARCH. DIS. CHILD. 42* 147-157, 1967.

COUPE, R. L. AND LOWRY, R. B.* ABNORMALITY OF THE HAIR IN CARTILAGE-HAIR HYPOPLASIA. DERMATOLOGICA 141* 329-334, 1970.

R
E
C
E
S
S
I
V
E

HALLE, M. A., COLLIPP, P. J. AND ROGINSKY, M.* CARTILAGE-HAIR HYPOPLASIA IN CHILDHOOD. NEW YORK J. MED. 70* 2705-2708, 1970.

LOWRY, R. B., WOOD, B. J., BIRKBECK, J. A. AND PADWICK, P. H.* CARTILAGE-HAIR HYPOPLASIA. A RARE AND RECESSIVE CAUSE OF DWARFISM. CLIN. PEDIAT. 9* 44-46, 1970.

LUX, S. E., JOHNSTON, R. B., JR., AUGUST, C. S., SAY, B., PENCHASZADEH, V. B., ROSEN, F. S. AND MCKUSICK, V. A.* NEUTROPENIA AND ABNORMAL CELLULAR IMMUNITY IN CARTILAGE-HAIR HYPOPLASIA. NEW ENG. J. MED. 282* 234-236, 1970.

MCKUSICK, V. A., ELDRIDGE, R., HOSTETLER, J. A., EGELAND, J. A. AND RUANGWIT, U.* DWARFISM IN THE AMISH. II. CARTILAGE-HAIR HYPOPLASIA. BULL. HOPKINS HOSP. 116* 285-326, 1965.

THEODOROU, S. D. AND ADAMS, J.* AN UNUSUAL CASE OF METAPHYSIAL DYSPLASIA. J. BONE JOINT SURG. 45B* 364-369, 1963.

*21240 CATARACT AND CONGENITAL ICHTHYOSIS

PINKERTON (1958) DESCRIBED JAPANESE SIBS WITH CORTICAL CATARACT AND ICHTHYOSIS. THE PARENTS WERE NOT AFFECTED BY EITHER DISORDER AND WERE NOT RELATED. JANCKE (1950) REPORTED THREE AFFECTED SISTERS.

JANCKE, G.* CATARACTA SYNDERMATOTICA UND ICHTHYOSIS CONGENITA. KLIN. MBL. AUGENHEILK. 117* 286-290, 1950.

PINKERTON, O. D.* CATARACT ASSOCIATED WITH CONGENITAL ICHTHYOSIS. ARCH. OPHTHAL. 60* 393-396, 1958.

*21250 CATARACT, CONGENITAL OR JUVENILE

CATARACT OCCURS AS A FEATURE OF SEVERAL OF THE OTHER ENTITIES IN THIS CATALOG* GALACTOSEMIA, CEREBRAL CHOLESTERINOSIS, CHONDRODYSTROPHIA CALCIFICANS CONGENITA, CONGENITAL AMAUROSIS, ROTHMUND'S SYNDROME, MARINESCO-SJOGREN SYNDROME, CROME'S SYNDROME, REFSUM'S SYNDROME, RETINITIS PIGMENTOSA, ETC. IN ADDITION CATARACT SOMETIMES OCCURS AS AN ISOLATED DEFECT WITH RECESSIVE INHERITANCE. FOR EXAMPLE, SAEBO (1949) STUDIED 17 FAMILIES WITH CASES OF CONGENITAL OR JUVENILE CATARACTS. TWO OR MORE SIBS WERE AFFECTED IN 8 FAMILIES. IN 9 FAMILIES THE PARENTS WERE RELATED, BEING FIRST-COUSINS IN 5. IN ONE FAMILY THE PROBAND HAD RETINITIS PIGMENTOSA (Q.V.), OF WHICH CATARACT IS A KNOWN COMPLICATION. IN ANOTHER FAMILY THE PROBAND HAD RETINITIS PIGMENTOSA AND DEAFMUTISM (USHER'S SYNDROME, Q.V.). RECESSIVELY INHERITED CATARACT SEEMS TO BE UNUSUALLY FREQUENT IN JAPAN (NAKAJIMA, 1964).

FRANCOIS, J.* HEREDITY IN OPHTHALMOLOGY. ST. LOUIS* C. V. MOSBY CO., 1961. P. 356.

GIANFERRARI, L., CRESSERI, A. AND MALTARELLO, A.* RICERCHE SULLA EREDITARIETA DELL'IDROFTALMO E DELLA CATARATTA CONGENITA IN PAESI DELLE PREALPI OROBICHE. ACTA GENET. MED. GEM. 3* 1-15, 1954.

JOSEPH, R.* CONGENITAL TOTAL CATARACT - POSSIBLY RECESSIVE. BRIT. J. OPHTHAL. 41* 444-445, 1957.

KLEIN, D.* CATARACTE CONGENITALE FAMILIALE* CONSANGUINITE DES PARENTS. J. GENET. HUM. 5* 283-284, 1956.

NAKAJIMA, A.* POPULATION GENETIC STUDY OF BLINDING DISEASES IN JAPAN. PROC. 2ND. INTERN. CONG. HUM. GENET., ROMÉ, 1961. VOL. 3, P. 1961, 1964.

SAEBO, J.* AN INVESTIGATION INTO THE MODE OF HEREDITY OF CONGENITAL AND JUVENILE CATARACTS. BRIT. J. OPHTHAL. 33* 601-629, 1949.

21260 CATARACT, NUCLEAR

ALTHOUGH USUALLY INHERITED AS A DOMINANT (Q.V.), NUCLEAR CATARACT MAY BE INHERITED AS A RECESSIVE IN THE PEDIGREES REPORTED BY RADOS (1947) AND OTHERS.

RADOS, A.* CENTRAL PULVERULENT (DISCOID) CATARACT AND ITS HEREDITARY TRANSMIS-SION. ARCH. OPHTHAL. 38* 57-77, 1947.

21270 CATARACT, TOTAL NUCLEAR

ALTHOUGH USUALLY INHERITED AS A DOMINANT (Q.V.), 'RECESSIVE PEDIGREES' ARE REPORTED.

BANE, W. M.* CONGENITAL CATARACTS. AM. J. OPHTHAL. 27* 651 ONLY, 1944.

SAEBO, J.* AN INVESTIGATION INTO THE MODE OF HEREDITY OF CONGENITAL AND JUVENILE CATARACTS. BRIT. J. OPHTHAL. 33* 601-629, 1949.

WAGNER, H.* RECESSIVE VERERBTER ANGEBORENER STAR. KLIN. MBL. AUGENHEILK. 104* 337-338, 1940.

*21280 CEPHALIN LIPIDOSIS

FROM ENGLAND BAAR AND HICKMANS (1956) REPORTED ON A BROTHER AND SISTER WITH MENTAL RETARDATION AND SLOW DETERIORATION, MARKED SPLENOMEGALY WITH ABSENCE OF GLANDULAR INVOLVEMENT OR BONE CHANGES, AND DEATH AT 4 AND 6 YEARS. THE RETICULOENDOTHELIAL CELLS OF THE LIVER AND SPLEEN AND THE NERVE CELLS OF THE CEREBRAL CORTEX AND SPINAL CORD SHOWED EXTENSIVE LIPID DEPOSITION. THE LIPID WAS IDENTIFIED AS INOSAMINE PHOSPHATIDE. NO SIMILAR CASES HAD BEEN PREVIOUSLY REPORTED.

BAAR, H. S. AND HICKMANS, E. M.* CEPHALIN-LIPIDOSIS* A NEW DISORDER OF LIPID METABOLISM. ACTA MED. SCAND. 155* 49-64, 1956.

21290 CEREBELLAR ATAXIA, INFANTILE, WITH PROGRESSIVE EXTERNAL OPHTHALMOPLEGIA

IN THE FAMILY DESCRIBED BY FRANCESCHETTI AND COLLEAGUES (1945) FOUR OF FIVE SIBS HAD CEREBELLAR ATAXIA (WHICH WAS CONSIDERED TO BE OF THE PIERRE MARIE TYPE) COMBINED WITH OPHTHALMOPLEGIA. THE PARENTS WERE NORMAL AND NOT RELATED.

FRANCESCHETTI, A., DE MORSIER, G. AND KLEIN, D.* UBER EINE NEUE MIT OPHTHALMOP-LEGIA EXTERNA PROGRESSIVA KOMBINIERTE INFANTILE FORM VON ZEREBELLARER HEREDOATAXIE (P. MARIE) BEI VIER GESCHWISTERN. ARCH. KLAUS STIFT. VERERBUNGSFORCH. 20 (SUPPL.)* 59-81, 1945.

21300 CEREBELLAR HYPOPLASIA

TWO PAIRS OF AFFECTED SIBS HAVE BEEN REPORTED (CROUZON, 1929* SARROUY ET AL., 1957). IN ADDITION NORMAN AND URICH (1958) NOTED PARENTAL CONSANGUINITY IN AN ISOLATED CASE. SEE CEREBELLO-PARENCHYMAL ATROPHY IV.

CROUZON, O.* ATROPHIE CEREBELLEUSE IDIOTIQUE, IN ETUDES SUR LES MALADIES FAMILIALES NERVEUSES ET DYSTROPHIQUES. PARIS, 1929. PP. 90-111.

FRIEDE, R. L.* ARRESTED CEREBELLAR DEVELOPMENT, A TYPE OF CEREBELLAR DEGENERA-TION IN AMAUROTIC IDIOCY. J. NEUROL. NEUROSURG. PSYCHIAT. 27* 41-45, 1964.

NORMAN, R. M. AND URICH, H.* CEREBELLAR HYPOPLASIA ASSOCIATED WITH SYSTEMIC DEGENERATION IN EARLY LIFE. J. NEUROL. NEUROSURG. PSYCHIAT. 21* 159-166, 1958.

SARROUY, C., RAFFI, A. AND BOINEAU, N.* A PROPOS DE DEUX CAS D*HYPOPLASIC CEREBELLEUSE DANS UNE MEME FRATRIE. ARCH. FRANC. PEDIAT. 14* 449-460, 1957.

21310 CEREBELLO-PARENCHYMAL DISORDER II (CPD II LATE ONSET RECESSIVE TYPE)

ATAXIA AND DYSARTHRIA DEVELOPED IN THE FOURTH OR FIFTH DECADES OF LIFE. RICHTER (1940) DESCRIBED THREE AFFECTED SIBS AND THORPE (1935) DESCRIBED TWO. AUTOPSIES SHOWED ABSENT PURKINJE CELLS BUT ONLY MILD LOSS OF GRANULE CELLS AND DENTATE NEURONES. THE INFERIOR OLIVARY NUCLEI AND THE PONS WERE NORMAL.

RICHTER, R.* CLINICO-PATHOLOGIC STUDY OF PARENCHYMATOUS CORTICAL CEREBELLAR ATROPHY* REPORT OF FAMILIAL CASE. J. NERV. MENT. DIS. 91* 37-46, 1940.

THORPE, F. T.* FAMILIAL DEGENERATION OF THE CEREBELLUM IN ASSOCIATION WITH EPILEPSY. A REPORT OF TWO CASES, ONE WITH PATHOLOGICAL FINDINGS. BRAIN 58* 97-114, 1935.

21320 CEREBELLO-PARENCHYMAL DISORDER III (CPD III CONGENITAL CEREBELLAR GRANULAR CELL HYPOPLASIA AND MENTAL RETARDATION)

JERVIS (1954) ALSO OBSERVED THE DISORDER IN BOTH OF MONOZYGOTIC TWINS. MENTAL DEFICIENCY AND CEREBELLAR ATAXIA ARE CONGENITAL. THE CEREBELLUM IS SMALL WITH SEVERE LOSS OF GRANULE CELLS AND WITH HETEROTOPIC PURKINJE CELLS. INFECTION OF THE FETAL RAT BY RAT VIRUS (MARGOLIS AND KELHAM, 1968) AND OF THE FETAL KITTEN BY PANLEUKOPENIA VIRUS (KELHAM AND MARGOLIS, 1966) RESULTS IN A SIMILAR PICTURE OF GRANULE CELL HYPOPLASIA. NORMAN (1940) DESCRIBED THREE AFFECTED SIBS IN ONE FAMILY AND TWO IN ANOTHER. SCHERER (1933) DESCRIBED TWO AFFECTED SIBS AND JERVIS (1950), THREE AFFECTED SIBS.

JERVIS, G. A.* CONCORDANT PRIMARY ATROPHY OF CEREBELLAR GRANULES IN MONOZYGOTIC TWINS. ACTA GENET. MED. GEM. 3* 153-162, 1954.

JERVIS, G. A.* EARLY FAMILIAL CEREBELLAR DEGENERATION. (REPORT OF THREE CASES IN ONE FAMILY). J. NERV. MENT. DIS. 111* 398-407, 1950.

KELHAM, L. AND MARGOLIS, G.* VIRAL ETIOLOGY OF SPONTANEOUS ATAXIA OF CATS. AM. J. PATH. 48* 991-1011, 1966.

MARGOLIS, G. AND KILHAM, L.* VIRUS-INDUCED CEREBELLAR HYPOPLASIA. RES. PUBL. ASS. RES. NERV. MENT. DIS. 44* 113-146, 1968.

NORMAN, R. M.* PRIMARY DEGENERATION OF THE GRANULAR LAYER OF THE CEREBELLUM* AN UNUSUAL FORM OF FAMILIAL CEREBELLAR ATROPHY OCCURRING IN EARLY LIFE. BRAIN 63* 365-379, 1940.

SCHERER, H. J.* BEITRAGE ZUR PATHOLOGISCHEN ANATOMIE DES KLEINHIRNS* GENUINE KLEINHERN ATROPHIEN. ZBL. NEUROL. PSYCHIAT. 145* 335-405, 1933.

21330 CEREBELLO-PARENCHYMAL DISORDER IV (CPD IV* CEREBELLAR VERMIS AGENESIS)

DE HAENE (1955) COLLECTED FROM THE LITERATURE 4 CASES OF TOTAL AND 7 CASES OF PARTIAL AGENESIS OF THE VERMIS OF THE CEREBELLUM, AND ADDED THE ONLY FAMILIAL EXAMPLE* 3 BROTHERS (ONE AUTOPSY) DIED AT AGE 4-8 YEARS, THE ILLNESS BEING CHARACTERIZED BY TREMOR AND HYPOTONIA. ANDERMANN (1968) TELLS ME OF 4 FRENCH-CANADIAN SIBS WITH THIS CONDITION. RESPIRATION WAS CHARACTERIZED BY ALTERNATING HYPERPNEA AS IN CHEYNE-STOKES RESPIRATION. JOUBERT ET AL. (1969) DESCRIBED FOUR FRENCH-CANADIAN SIBS WITH THIS ABNORMALITY. BY AUTOPSY OR PNEUMOENCEPHALOGRAM THE VERMIS WAS SHOWN TO BE COMPLETELY OR PARTIALLY ABSENT IN ALL FOUR. ONE ALSO HAD AN OCCIPITAL MENINGOMYELOCELE. SYMPTOMS INCLUDED EPISODIC HYPERPNEA, ABNORMAL EYE MOVEMENTS AND PSYCHOMOTOR RETARDATION. THE OLDEST LIVING SIB WAS 8 YEARS OLD. THE PARENTS WERE DISTANTLY RELATED. SEE CEREBELLAR HYPOPLASIA.

DE HAENE, A.* AGENESIE PARTIELLE DU VERMIS DU CERVELET A CARACTERE FAMILIAL. ACTA NEUROL. BELG. 55* 622-628, 1955.

JOUBERT, M., EISENRING, J. J., ROBB, J. P. AND ANDERMANN, F.* FAMILIAL AGENESIS OF THE CEREBELLAR VERMIS. A SYNDROME OF EPISODIC HYPERPNEA, ABNORMAL EYE MOVEMENTS, ATAXIA, AND RETARDATION. NEUROLOGY 19* 813-825, 1969.

21340 CEREBELLO-PARENCHYMAL DISORDER V (CPA V* SPINODENTATE ATROPHY* DYSSYNERGIA CEREBELLARIS MYOCLONICA OF HUNT)

RAMSEY HUNT (1921) DESCRIBED TWIN BROTHERS WITH A CEREBELLAR DISTURBANCE COMBINED WITH SEVERE MYOCLONIC JERKS BOUGHT ON BY MUSCULAR EFFORT. AUTOPSY IN ONE OF THEM WHO DIED AT AGE 36 YEARS SHOWED MARKED LOSS OF DENTATE NEURONES AND THEIR FIBERS IN THE SUPERIOR CEREBELLAR PEDUNCLES. HUNT DESCRIBED SEVERAL OTHER CASES WITH AFFECTED RELATIVES AND WITHOUT AUTOPSY.

HUNT, J. R.* DYSSYNERGIA CEREBELLARIS MYOCLONICA - PRIMARY ATROPHY OF THE DENTATE SYSTEM* A CONTRIBUTION TO THE PATHOLOGY AND SYMPTOMATOLOGY OF THE CEREBELLUM. BRAIN 44* 490-538, 1921.

21350 CEREBRAL ANGIOPATHY, DYSHORIC

RICHARD AND COLLEAGUES (1965) STUDIED THE BRAIN OF 18 MEMBERS OF 8 FAMILIES IN WHICH ONE MEMBER HAD HISTOLOGICALLY CONFIRMED ANGIOPATHY. OF 6 SIBSHIPS STUDIED, 5 HAD MORE THAN ONE AFFECTED SIB. PARENT-CHILD PAIRS WERE STUDIED BUT IN NO INSTANCE WERE BOTH INVOLVED. THIS CONDITION, DESCRIBED BY OPPENHEIM, IS CHARAC-TERIZED BY ARTERIOLOCAPILLARY DEGENERATION PARTICULARLY IN THE OCCIPITAL CORTEX AND THE CALCARINE AREA.

RICHARD, J., DE AJURIAGUERRA, J. AND CONSTANTINIDIS, J.* L'INCIDENCE FAMILIALE DE L'ANGIOPATHIE DYSHORIQUE DU CORTEX CEREBRAL. INT. J. NEUROPSYCHIAT. 1* 118-124, 1965.

21360 CEREBRAL CALCIFICATION, NON-ARTERIOSCLEROTIC

THIS CONDITION WAS PROBABLY FIRST DESCRIBED BY FAHR IN 1930. MELCHIOR, BENDA AND YAKOVLEV (1960) DESCRIBED FAMILIES WITH AFFECTED SIBS, 3 OUT OF 10 IN ONE AND 2 OUT OF 4 IN THE SECOND. THE CLINICAL EVOLUTION IS THAT OF A DEGENERATIVE RATHER THAN A DEVELOPMENTAL DISORDER. PROGRESSIVE DETERIORATION OF MENTALITY AND LOSS OF MOTOR ACCOMPLISHMENTS TAKE PLACE AND SYMMETRICAL SPASTIC PARALYSIS AND SOMETIMES ATHETOSIS APPEAR, PROGRESSING TO A DECEREBRATE STATE. THE HEAD IS SMALL AND ROUND. OPTIC ATROPHY MAY BE PRESENT. MINERAL DEPOSITS ARE DISTRIBUTED THROUGHOUT THE CEREBRAL CORTEX, BASAL GANGLIA, DENTATE NUCLEUS, SUBTHALAMUS AND RED NUCLEUS WITH CELL LOSS IN THESE AREAS. CALCIFICATION PROBABLY OCCURS IN AREAS OF DEMYELINATION AND LIPID DEPOSITION. HALLERVORDEN (1950) OBSERVED SIBS AS DID ALSO BEYME (1945) AND FOLEY (1951). JERVIS (1954) DESCRIBED THE PATHOLOGIC FINDINGS IN TWO CASES WHO WERE MICROCEPHALIC IDIOTS WITH MUSCULAR HYPERTONICITY AND CHOREO-ATHETOSIS. CALCIFICATION WAS FOUND IN THE BASAL GANGLIA, CEREBELLUM AND CEREBRAL CORTEX AND THE CENTRUM OVALE SHOWED EXTENSIVE DEMYELINATION. BOWMAN (1954) DESCRIBED TWO AFFECTED MALE SIBS. ONE DIED AT 33 MONTHS AND ONE AT 31 MONTHS. CALCIFICATION WAS DEMONSTRATED AT AUTOPSY BUT NOT BY X-RAY DURING LIFE. LOWENTHAL (1948) REVIEWED 32 CASES IN THE LITERATURE OF WHICH 3 WERE FAMILIAL. IN SOME CASES HYPOPARATHYROIDISM MAY BE PRESENT. PILLERI (1966) REPORTED CLINICO-ANATOMIC STUDIES OF A 64 YEAR OLD MALE WITH FAHR'S DISEASE, OR NONARTERIOSCLEROTIC, IDIOPATHIC INTRACEREBRAL CALCIFICATION OF THE BLOOD VESSELS. THE DISORDER WAS DIAGNOSED RADIOLOGICALLY IN THREE GENERATIONS OF THE FAMILY. CLINICAL FEATURES INCLUDED FITS, PYRAMIDAL SYMPTOMS, CEREBELLAR DYSARTHRIA AND PSYCHIC CHANGES. CALCIFICATION INVOLVED THE MEDIA AND ADVENTITIA OF BRAIN VESSELS OF ALL SIZES AND CALCIUM CONCRETIONS LAY FREE IN THE TISSUES. MALE-TO-MALE TRANSMISSION WAS NOT PROVED. ALMOST CERTAINLY MORE THAN ONE GENETIC VARIETY OF NON-ARTERIOSCLEROTIC CEREBRAL CALCIFICATION EXISTS. BABBITT ET AL. (1968) DESCRIBED THIS DISORDER,

R
E
C
E
S
S
I
V
E

CALLED BY THEM 'FAMILIAL CEREBROVASCULAR FERROCALCINOSIS' IN TWO SISTERS AND A BROTHER.

BEYME, F.* UBER DAS GEHIRN EINER FAMILIAR OLIGOPHRENEN MIT SYMMETRISCHEN KALKABLAGERUNGEN BESONDERS IN DEN STAMMGANGLIEN. SCHWEIZ. ARCH. NEUROL. PSYCHIAT. 56* 161-190, 1945.

BABBITT, D. P., TANG, T., DOBBS, J. AND BERK, R.* IDIOPATHIC FAMILIAL CEREBRO-VASCULAR FERROCALCINOSIS (FAHR'S DISEASE) AND REVIEW OF DIFFERENTIAL DIAGNOSIS OF INTRACRANIAL CALCIFICATION IN CHILDREN. AM. J. ROENTGEN. 105* 352-358, 1968.

BOWMAN, M. S.* FAMILIAL OCCURRENCE OF 'IDIOPATHIC' CALCIFICATION OF CEREBRAL CAPILLARIES. AM. J. PATH. 30* 87-97, 1954.

FAHR, T.* IDIOPATHISCHE VERKALKUNG DER HIRNGEFASSE. ZBL. ALLG. PATH. 50* 129-133, 1930.

FOLEY, J.* CALCIFICATION OF THE CORPUS STRIATUM AND DENTATE NUCLEI OCCURRING IN A FAMILY. J. NEUROL. NEUROSURG. PSYCHIAT. 14* 253-261, 1951.

HALLEVORDEN, I.* UBER DIFFUSE SYMMETRISCHE KALKABLAGERUNGEN BEI EINEM KRANKHEI-TSBILD MIT MIKROCEPHALIE UND MENINGOENCEPHALITIS. ARCH. PSYCHIAT. 184* 579-600, 1950.

JERVIS, G. A.* MICROCEPHALY WITH EXTENSIVE CALCIUM DEPOSITS AND DEMYELINATION. J. NEUROPATH. EXP. NEUROL. 13* 318-329, 1954.

LOWENTHAL, A.* LA CALCIFICATION VASCULAIRE INTRACEREBRALE NON ARTERIOSCLEREUSE DE FAHR. EST-ELLE LA MANIFESTATION CEREBRALE D'UNE PERTURBATION DES FONCTIONS PARATHYROIDIENNES.Q ACTA NEUROL. PSYCHIAT. BELG. 48* 613-631, 1948.

MELCHIOR, J. C., BENDA, C. E. AND YAKOVLEV, P. I.* FAMILIAL IDIOPATHIC CEREBRAL CALCIFICATIONS IN CHILDHOOD. AM. J. DIS. CHILD. 99* 787-803, 1960.

PILLERI, G.* A CASE OF MORBUS FAHR (NON ARTERIOSCLEROTIC, IDIOPATHIC INTRACERE-BRAL CALCIFICATION OF THE BLOOD VESSELS) IN THREE GENERATIONS. A CLINICO-ANATOMICAL CONTRIBUTION. PSYCHIAT. NEUROL. 152* 43-58, 1966.

RECESSIVE

*21370 CEREBRAL CHOLESTERINOSIS (CEREBROTENDINOUS XANTHOMATOSIS)

VAN BOGAERT AND COLLEAGUES (1937) DESCRIBED AFFECTED COUSINS. ONSET WAS AT AGE 12 OR 13 YEARS. WHEN EXAMINED IN THEIR 30'S THE PATIENTS DEMONSTRATED CEREBELLOPYRA-MIDAL SIGNS, MYOCLONUS OF THE SOFT PALATE, MENTAL DEBILITY, CATARACTS, XANTHELAS-MATA AND TENDON XANTHOMATA. AT AUTOPSY MANY DEPOSITS WERE FOUND IN THE WHITE MATTER OF THE CEREBELLUM AND THE CEREBRAL PEDUNCLES. MENKES ET AL. (1968) DESCRIBED BROTHER AND SISTER, AGES 60 AND 57 YEARS, RESPECTIVELY. THE BROTHER HAD SLOWLY PROGRESSIVE ATAXIA IN LATER YEARS. CATARACTS WERE REMOVED IN HIS 20'S AND HE HAD ENLARGED ACHILLES TENDONS FROM CHILDHOOD. SERUM CHOLESTEROL WAS NORMAL. HE DIED OF MYOCARDIAL INFARCTION. THE CEREBELLAR WHITE MATTER WAS DEMYELINATED AND CONTAINED CHOLESTEROL DEPOSITS. THE SISTER HAD HAD PROGRESSIVE ENLARGEMENT OF ACHILLES TENDONS, MINIMAL MENTAL RETARDATION AND UNSTEADINESS OF GAIT. BILATERAL CATARACTS WERE REMOVED AT AGE 24 YEARS. SERUM CHOLESTEROL WAS NORMAL. MENKES AND HIS COLLEAGUES (1968) SPECULATED THAT THE DEFECT CONCERNS TRANSPORT OF CHOLESTEROL OUT OF CELLS. CHOLESTEROL CAN BE SYNTHESIZED IN MANY TISSUES BUT OXIDATION IS VIRTUALLY LIMITED TO THE LIVER. WHEREAS TENDON XANTHOMATA AND CATARACTS MAY APPEAR EARLY, NEUROLOGIC IMPAIRMENT MAY BE A LATE DEVELOPMENT. PHILIPPART AND VAN BOGAERT (1969) GAVE FOLLOW-UP ON A MEMBER OF THE FIRST FAMILY DESCRIBED BY VAN BOGAERT. THE DISORDER IS CHARACTERIZED BY PROGRESSIVE CEREBELLAR ATAXIA AFTER PUBERTY, JUVENILE CATARACTS, SYSTEMIC SPINAL CORD INVOLVEMENT AND A PSEUDOBULBAR PHASE LEADING TO DEATH. THE DEPOSITED MATERIAL IS CHOLESTANOL. THE DIAGNOSIS CAN BE MADE BY DEMONSTRATING CHOLESTANOL IN ABNORMAL AMOUNTS IN THE SERUM AND TENDON OF PERSONS SUSPECTED OF BEING AFFECTED.

GIAMPALMO, A.* LES LIPIDOSES CHOLESTERINIQUES DU SYSTEME NERVEUX. ACTA NEUROL. BELG. 54* 786-808, 1954.

MENKES, J. H., SCHIMSCHOCK, J. R. AND SWANSON, P. D.* CEREBROTENDINOUS XANTHOMATOSIS* THE STORAGE OF CHOLESTANOL WITHIN THE NERVOUS SYSTEM. ARCH. NEUROL. 19* 47-53, 1968.

PHILIPPART, M. AND VAN BOGAERT, L.* CHOLESTANOLOSIS (CEREBROTENDINOUS XANTHOMA-TOSIS). A FOLLOW-UP STUDY ON THE ORIGINAL FAMILY. ARCH. NEUROL. 21* 603-610, 1969.

SCHIMSCHOCK, J. R., ALVORD, E. C., JR. AND SWANSON, P. D.* CEREBROTENDINOUS XANTHOMATOSIS* CLINICAL AND PATHOLOGICAL STUDIES. ARCH. NEUROL. 18* 688-698, 1968.

SCHNEIDER, C.* UBER EINE EIGENARTIGE HIRNERKRANKUNG (VASKULARE LIPOIDOSE). ALLG. Z. PSYCHIAT. 104* 144-163, 1936.

VAN BOGAERT, L., SCHERER, H. J. AND EPSTEIN, E.* UNE FORME CEREBRAE DE LA

VAN BOGAERT, L., SCHERER, H. J., FROEHLICH, A. AND EPSTEIN, E.* UNE DEUXIEME OBSERVATION DE CHOLESTERINOSE TENDINEUSE SYMETRIQUE AVEC SYMPTOMES CEREBRAUX. ANN. MED. 42* 69-101, 1937.

21380 CEREBRAL GIGANTISM (SOTOS' SYNDROME)

EXCEPT FOR A CONCORDANT SET OF IDENTICAL TWINS (HOOK AND REYNOLDS, 1967), MOST CASES HAVE BEEN SPORADIC. (I HAVE OBSERVED THE CASE OF AN AFFECTED BOY WHOSE FATHER, NOT AVAILABLE FOR STUDY, IS DESCRIBED AS HAVING SIMILAR FEATURES.) THE REPORTED CASES MAY REPRESENT NEW DOMINANT MUTATIONS. LARGE SIZE WITH LARGE HANDS AND FEET ARE PRESENT FROM BIRTH. GROWTH IS RAPID IN THE FIRST YEARS OF LIFE BUT FINAL HEIGHT MAY NOT BE EXCESSIVE. BONE AGE IS ADVANCED. THE SKULL IS LARGE WITH MODERATE PROGNATHISM. MILD DILATION OF THE CEREBRAL VENTRICLES, NONSPECIFIC EEG CHANGES AND SEIZURES HAVE BEEN OBSERVED. POOR COORDINATION AND MENTAL RETARDATION ARE FEATURES. THE DIFFERENTIAL DIAGNOSIS SHOULD INCLUDE THE XYY SYNDROME. BEJAR ET AL. (1970) STUDIED TWO PATIENTS FINDING ABNORMAL DERMATOGLYPHICS, NORMAL GROWTH HORMONE LEVELS, AND HIGH LEVELS OF VALINE, ISOLEUCINE AND LEUCINE IN THE BLOOD. THE GLYCINE-TO-VALINE RATIO SEEMED PARTICULARLY USEFUL IN DISTINGUISHING PATIENTS FROM CONTROLS. HOOFT ET AL. (1968) DESCRIBED CEREBRAL GIGANTISM IN TWO FIRST COUSINS.

BEJAR, R. L., SMITH, G. F., PARK, S., SPELLACY, W. N., WOLFSON, S. L. AND NYHAN, W. L.* CEREBRAL GIGANTISM* CONCENTRATIONS OF AMINO ACIDS IN PLASMA AND MUSCLE. J. PEDIAT. 76* 105-111, 1970.

HOOFT, C., SCHOTE, H. AND VAN HOOVER, G.* FAMILIAL CEREBRAL GIGANTISM. ACTA PAEDIAT. BELG. 22* 173-186, 1968.

HOOK, E. B. AND REYNOLDS, J. W.* CEREBRAL GIGANTISM* ENDOCRINOLOGICAL AND CLINICAL OBSERVATIONS OF SIX PATIENTS INCLUDING A CONGENITAL GIANT, CONCORDANT MONOZYGOTIC TWINS, AND A CHILD WHO ACHIEVED ADULT GIGANTIC SIZE. J. PEDIAT. 70* 900-914, 1967.

SOTOS, J. F., DODGE, P. R., MUIRHEAD, D., CRAWFORD, J. D. AND TALBOT, N. B.* CEREBRAL GIGANTISM IN CHILDHOOD. A SYNDROME OF EXCESSIVELY RAPID GROWTH WITH ACROMEGALIC FEATURES AND A NONPROGRESSIVE NEUROLOGIC DISORDER. NEW ENG. J. MED. 271* 109-116, 1964.

STEPHENSON, J. N., MELLINGER, R. C. AND MANSON, G.* CEREBRAL GIGANTISM. PEDIATRICS 41* 130-138, 1968.

21390 CEREBRAL SCLEROSIS LIKE PELIZAEUS-MERZBACHER DISEASE

FAHMY ET AL. (1969) OBSERVED A BROTHER AND SISTER (OUT OF A SIBSHIP OF 11), OFFSPRING OF FIRST COUSIN PARENTS, WHO HAD A SLOWLY PROGRESSIVE NEUROLOGIC DISORDER BEGINNING ITS MANIFESTATIONS IN EARLY CHILDHOOD. ELECTRON MICROSCOPIC STUDIES OF SURAL NERVE SHOWED UNIQUE ROD-SHAPED BODIES IN SCHWANN CELLS. THE CLINICAL PICTURE WAS SIMILAR TO THAT OF THE PELIZAEUS-MERZBACHER SYNDROME, AN X-LINKED DISORDER.

FAHMY, A., CARTER, T., PAULSON, G. AND NANCE, W. E.* A 'NEW' FORM OF HEREDITARY CEREBRAL SCLEROSIS. ARCH. NEUROL. 20* 468-478, 1969.

21400 CEREBRO-COSTO-MANDIBULAR SYNDROME

IN A FEMALE AND TWO MALE SIBS, MCNICHOLL ET AL. (1970) DESCRIBED A SYNDROME OF MENTAL RETARDATION, PALATAL DEFECTS (SHORT HARD PALATE WITH CENTRAL HOLE, ABSENT SOFT PALATE, ABSENT UVULA), MICROGNATHIA, GLOSSOPTOSIS, SEVERE COSTOVERTEBRAL ABNORMALITIES. A BARKING COUGH IN ONE SUGGESTED TRACHEAL CARTILAGE ABNORMALITY AS IN THE CASE OF SMITH ET AL. (1966) WHICH BORE OTHER SIMILARITIES.

MCNICHOLL, B., EGAN-MITCHELL, B., MURRAY, J. P., DOYLE, J. F., KENNEDY, J. D. AND CROME, L.* CEREBRO-COSTO-MANDIBULAR SYNDROME. A NEW FAMILIAL DEVELOPMENTAL DISORDER. ARCH. DIS. CHILD. 45* 421-424, 1970.

SMITH, D. W., THEILER, K. AND SCHACHENMANN, G.* RIB-GAP DEFECT WITH MICROGNA-THIA, MALFORMED TRACHEAL CARTILAGES, AND REDUNDANT SKIN* A NEW PATTERN OF DEFECTIVE DEVELOPMENT. J. PEDIAT. 69* 799-803, 1966.

*21410 CEREBRO-HEPATO-RENAL SYNDROME (ZELLWEGER SYNDROME)

SMITH, OPITZ AND INHORN (1965) DESCRIBED A CAUCASIAN BROTHER AND SISTER WHO DIED AT 8 AND 10 WEEKS OF AGE WITH ABERRANT DEVELOPMENT OF THE SKULL, FACE, EARS, EYES, HANDS AND FEET, POLYCYSTIC KIDNEYS WITH ADEQUATE FUNCTIONAL RENAL PARENCHYMA AND INTRAHEPATIC BILIARY DYSGENESIS. JAUNDICE DEVELOPED BEFORE DEATH. THE KARYOTYPE WAS NORMAL. PASSARGE AND MCADAMS (1967) DESCRIBED 5 SISTERS OUT OF A SIBSHIP OF 13 WITH SEVERE, GENERALIZED HYPOTONIA AND ABSENT MORO RESPONSE, CHARACTERISTIC CRANIOFACIAL ABNORMALITIES, CORTICAL RENAL CYSTS AND HEPATOMEGALY. THE BRAIN IN TWO STUDIED HISTOLOGICALLY SHOWED SUDANOPHILIC LEUKODYSTROPHY. THE AUTHORS CONSIDERED THIS TO BE THE SAME ENTITY AS THAT REPORTED BY SMITH, OPITZ AND INHORN

(1965) AND PERHAPS THE SAME AS THAT DESCRIBED BY BOWEN ET AL. (1964). THEY PROPOSED CEREBRO-HEPATO-RENAL SYNDROME AS AN APPROPRIATE DESIGNATION. BOWEN ET AL. (1964) DESCRIBED TWO FAMILIES EACH WITH TWO SIBS WHO DISPLAYED AN UNUSUAL MALFORMATION SYNDROME. OPITZ ET AL. (1969) DESCRIBED FURTHER CASES, SUGGESTED THAT ONLY ONE OF THE TWO SETS OF SIBS (THAT CONTRIBUTED BY ZELLWEGER) HAD THE CEREBRO-HEPATO-RENAL SYNDROME, AND MADE THE IMPORTANT OBSERVATION THAT SERUM IRON LEVEL AND IRON BINDING CAPACITY WERE HIGH IN ONE WELL-STUDIED CASE AND SHOULD PROVIDE AN EASY METHOD FOR DIAGNOSIS OF THIS DISORDER. A DEFECT IN THE PLACENTAL IRON TRANSFER MECHANISM WAS POSTULATED. CHONDRAL CALCIFICATION, MOST MARKED IN THE PATELLAS, IS A FEATURE POINTED OUT BY POZNANSKI ET AL. (1970). THE CHANGE IS SOMEWHAT LIKE THAT OF CHONDRODYSTROPHIA CALCIFICANS CONGENITA.

BOWEN, P., LEE, C. S. N., ZELLWEGER, H. AND LINDENBURG, R.* A FAMILIAL SYNDROME OF MULTIPLE CONGENITAL DEFECTS. BULL. JOHNS HOPKINS HOSP. 114* 402-414, 1964.

OPITZ, J. M., ZURHEIN, G. M., VITALE, L., SHAHIDI, N. T., HOWE, J. J., CHOU, S. M., SHANKLIN, D. R., SYBERS, H. D., DOOD, A. R. AND GERRITSEN, T.* THE ZELLWEGER SYNDROME (CEREBRO-HEPATO-RENAL SYNDROME). THE CLINICAL DELINEATION OF BIRTH DEFECTS. II. MALFORMATION SYNDROMES. NEW YORK* NATIONAL FOUNDATION, 1969. PP. 144-160.

PASSARGE, E. AND MCADAMS, A. J.* CEREBRO-HEPATO-RENAL SYNDROME. A NEWLY RECOGNIZED HEREDITARY DISORDER OF MULTIPLE CONGENITAL DEFECTS, INCLUDING SUDANO-PHILIC LEUKODYSTROPHY, CIRRHOSIS OF THE LIVER, AND POLYCYSTIC KIDNEYS. J. PEDIAT. 71* 691-702, 1967.

POZNANSKI, A. K., NOSANCHUK, J. S., BAUBLIS, J. AND HOLT, J. F.* THE CEREBRO-HEPATO-RENAL SYNDROME (CHRS)* (ZELLWEGER'S SYNDROME). AM. J. ROENTGEN. 109* 313-322, 1970.

SMITH, D. W., OPITZ, J. M. AND INHORN, S. L.* A SYNDROME OF MULTIPLE DEVELOP-MENTAL DEFECTS INCLUDING POLYCYSTIC KIDNEYS AND INTRAHEPATIC BILIARY DYSGENESIS IN 2 SIBLINGS. J. PEDIAT. 67* 617-624, 1965.

21420 CEROID STORAGE DISEASE

OPPENHEIMER AND ANDREWS (1959) REPORTED TWO CASES* (1), A WHITE 4 YEAR OLD MALE FROM WEST VIRGINIA (B2644* AUT. 24455) WHO DIED FROM LIVER FAILURE AND HAD CEROID DEPOSITS OF LIVER, SPLEEN AND INTESTINAL MUCOSA* AND (2), A WHITE 22 MONTH OLD FEMALE WHO AT AUTOPSY HAD CEROID LIMITED LARGELY TO HEPATIC MACROPHAGES. LANDING AND SHIRKEY (1957) DESCRIBED TWO CHILDREN WHO MAY HAVE HAD THE SAME DISORDER. NO EVIDENCE FOR OR AGAINST A GENETIC BASIS IS AVAILABLE.

LANDING, B. H. AND SHIRKEY, H. S.* A SYNDROME OF RECURRENT INFECTION AND INFILTRATION OF VISCERA BY PIGMENTED LIPID HISTIOCYTES. PEDIATRICS 20* 431-447, 1957.

OPPENHEIMER, E. H. AND ANDREWS, E. C., JR.* CEROID STORAGE DISEASE IN CHILD-HOOD. PEDIATRICS 23* 1091-1102, 1959.

21430 CERVICAL VERTEBRAL FUSION

C5-C6 FUSION MAY BE RECESSIVELY INHERITED. LUBS, GUNDERSON AND GREENSPAN (1963) FOUND TWO OF ELEVEN SIBS WITH THIS TYPE OF FUSION AND A THIRD WITH NARROWING OF THE INTERSPACE. THE PARENTS WERE PROBABLY CONSANGUINEOUS.

GUNDERSON, C. H., GREENSPAN, R. H., GLASER, G. H. AND LUBS, H. A., JR.* THE KLIPPEL-FEIL SYNDROME* GENETIC AND CLINICAL REEVALUATION OF CERVICAL FUSION. MEDICINE 46* 491-512, 1967.

LUBS, H. A., JR., GUNDERSON, C. H. AND GREENSPAN, R. H.* GENETIC REEVALUATION OF FUSED CERVICAL VERTEBRAE (KLIPPEL-FEIL ANOMALY). CLIN. RES. 11* 179 ONLY, 1963.

*21440 CHARCOT-MARIE-TOOTH PERONEAL MUSCULAR ATROPHY

THE AUTOSOMAL RECESSIVE FORM IS LESS FREQUENT THAN THE DOMINANT AND X-LINKED RECESSIVE FORMS. THIS IS ONE OF THE CONDITIONS USED BY ALLAN (1939) TO ILLUSTRATE THE "LAW" THAT RECESSIVE DISORDERS ARE MORE SEVERE THAN DOMINANT ONES AND THAT X-LINKED DISORDERS TEND TO BE INTERMEDIATE IN SEVERITY. THIS DISORDER MAY BE UNUSUALLY FREQUENT IN THE HILL FOLK OF THE WESTERN PART OF NORTH CAROLINA WHERE ALLAN WORKED. CONTRARY TO THE USUAL RARITY OF THE RECESSIVE FORM, HE FOUND 8 YOUNG GIRLS WITH THE DISORDER IN THE NORTH CAROLINA ORTHOPEDIC HOSPITAL WHICH CATERED TO PATIENTS UNDER THE AGE OF 16 YEARS. THE EIGHT CAME FROM SIX FAMILIES WITH BOTH PARENTS NORMAL. IN 4 OF THE 6 FAMILIES THE PARENTS WERE COUSINS. IN TWO BROTHERS AND THEIR NEPHEW (SON OF A SISTER), ROSENBERG AND CHUTORIAN (1967) FOUND THE COMBINATION OF PROGRESSIVE POLYNEUROPATHY SUGGESTING CHARCOT-MARIE-TOOTH DISEASE WITH DEAFNESS AND VISUAL IMPAIRMENT DUE TO DEGENERATION OF THE ACOUSTIC AND OPTIC NERVES. THIS SYNDROME WAS DESCRIBED IN JAPANESE BROTHER AND SISTER BY IWASHITA ET AL. (1970) THEREBY EXCLUDING X-LINKED INHERITANCE IF THE SAME DISORDER AS THAT DESCRIBED BY ROSENBERG AND CHUTORIAN (1967) WAS IN FACT PRESENT. ALTHOUGH THE RELATIONSHIP OF THE AFFECTED MALES IS CONSISTENT WITH X-LINKED RECESSIVE

RECESSIVE

ALLAN, W.* RELATION OF HEREDITARY PATTERN TO CLINICAL SEVERITY AS ILLUSTRATED
BY PERONEAL ATROPHY. ARCH. INTERN. MED. 63* 1123-1131, 1939.

IWASHITA, H., INOUE, N., ARAKI, S. AND KUROIWA, Y.* OPTIC ATROPHY, NEURAL
DEAFNESS, AND DISTAL NEUROGENIC AMYOTROPHY. REPORT OF A FAMILY WITH TWO AFFECTED
SIBLINGS. ARCH. NEUROL. 22* 357-364, 1970.

ROSENBERG, R. N. AND CHUTORIAN, A.* FAMILIAL OPTICOACOUSTIC NERVE DEGENERATION
AND POLYNEUROPATHY. NEUROLOGY 17* 827-832, 1967.

*21450 CHEDIAK-HIGASHI SYNDROME

THE FEATURES ARE DECREASED PIGMENTATION OF HAIR AND EYES, CALLED PARTIAL ALBINISM,
PHOTOPHOBIA, NYSTAGMUS, LARGE EOSINOPHILIC, PEROXIDASE-POSITIVE INCLUSION BODIES
IN THE MYELOBLASTS AND PROMYELOCYTES OF THE BONE MARROW, NEUTROPENIA, ABNORMAL
SUSCEPTIBILITY TO INFECTION AND PECULIAR MALIGNANT LYMPHOMA. DEATH OCCURS BEFORE
THE AGE OF 7 YEARS. HERMANSKY AND PUDLAK (1959) DESCRIBED TWO UNRELATED ALBINOS
WITH LIFE-LONG BLEEDING TENDENCY AND PECULIAR PIGMENTED RETICULAR CELLS IN THE
BONE MARROW. ONE WAS MALE, ONE FEMALE, BOTH WERE 33 YEARS OLD. THIS MAY
REPRESENT A DISTINCT ENTITY, POSSIBLY INHERITED AS A RECESSIVE. (SEE ALBINISM
WITH HEMORRHAGIC DIATHESIS AND PIGMENTED RETICULO-ENDOTHELIAL CELLS.)
KRITZLER AND COLLEAGUES (1964) FOUND THE KARYOTYPE NORMAL IN A 16 YEAR OLD
PATIENT. GLYCOLIPID INCLUSIONS WERE DESCRIBED IN HISTIOCYTES, RENAL TUBULAR
EPITHELIUM AND NEURONS. HETEROZYGOTES WERE IDENTIFIABLE BY THE PRESENCE OF A
GRANULAR ANOMALY OF THE LYMPHOCYTES. THE PATIENT DIED OF MASSIVE GASTROINTESTINAL
HEMORRHAGE.
PADGETT ET AL. (1964) DESCRIBED THE CHEDIAK-HIGASHI SYNDROME IN MINK AND
CATTLE. IN THESE SPECIES ALSO IT IS AUTOSOMAL RECESSIVE. LEUKEMIA AND LYMPHOMA
HAVE BEEN OBSERVED (EFRATI, JONAS, 1958).
WINDHORST, ZELICKSON AND GOOD (1966) FOUND LARGE LYSOSOMAL GRANULES IN
LEUKOCYTES AND GIANT MELANOSOMES IN MELANOCYTES. FOR THIS REASON LEADER ET AL.
(1966) HAVE REFERRED TO THE CONDITION AS "HEREDITARY LEUKOMELANOPATHY."

CHEDIAK, M.* NOUVELLE ANOMALIE LEUCOCYTAIRE DE CARACTERE CONSTITUTIONNEL ET
FAMILIAL. REV. HEMAT. 7* 362-367, 1952.

EFRATI, P. AND JONAS, W.* CHEDIAK'S ANOMALY OF LEUKOCYTES IN MALIGNANT LYMPHOMA
ASSOCIATED WITH LEUKEMIC MANIFESTATIONS* CASE REPORT WITH NECROPSY. BLOOD 13*
1063-1073, 1958.

GILLOON, J. R., PEASE, G. L. AND MILLS, S. D.* CHEDIAK-HIGASHI ANOMALY OF THE
LEUKOCYTES. REPORT OF A CASE. MAYO CLIN. PROC. 35* 635-640, 1960.

HERMANSKY, F. AND PUDLAK, P.* ALBINISM ASSOCIATED WITH HEMORRHAGIC DIATHESIS
AND UNUSUAL PIGMENTED RETICULAR CELLS IN THE BONE MARROW* REPORT OF TWO CASES WITH
HISTOCHEMICAL STUDIES. BLOOD 14* 162-169, 1959.

KANFER, J. N., BLUME, R. S., YANKEE, R. A. AND WOLFF, S. M.* SPHINGOLIPID
METABOLISM IN LEUKOCYTES IN CHEDIAK-HIGASHI SYNDROME. NEW ENG. J. MED. 279* 410-
413, 1968.

KRITZLER, R. A., TERNER, J. Y., LINDENBAUM, J., MAGIDSON, J., WILLIAMS, R.,
PREISIG, R. AND PHILLIPS, G. B.* CHEDIAK-HIGASHI SYNDROME. CYTOLOGIC AND SERUM
LIPID OBSERVATIONS IN A CASE AND FAMILY. AM. J. MED. 36* 583-594, 1964.

LEADER, R. W., PADGETT, G. A. AND GORHAM, J. R.* HEREDITARY LEUKOMELANOPATHY
(CHEDIAK-HIGASHI SYNDROME OF MAN, MINK AND CATTLE). IN, D. C. GAJDUSEK, C. J.
GIBBS, JR. AND M. ALPERS (EDS.). SLOW, LATENT AND TEMPERATE VIRUS INFECTIONS.
PP. 393-399, 1966.

PADGETT, G. A., LEADER, R. W., GORHAM, J. R. AND O'MARY, C. C.* THE FAMILIAL
OCCURRENCE OF THE CHEDIAK-HIGASHI SYNDROME IN MINK AND CATTLE. GENETICS 49* 505-
512, 1964.

PAGE, A. R., BERENDES, H., WARNER, J. AND GOOD, R. A.* THE CHEDIAK-HIGASHI
SYNDROME. BLOOD 20* 330-343, 1962.

SADAN, N., YAFFE, D., ROZENSZAJN, L. AND EFRATI, P.* CHEDIAK'S DISEASE*
CLINICAL, CYTOLOGICAL AND HEREDITARY ASPECTS. (ABSTRACT) ISRAEL J. MED. SCI. 1*
850 ONLY, 1965.

SPENCER, W. H. AND HOGAN, M. J.* OCULAR MANIFESTATIONS OF CHEDIAK-HIGASHI
SYNDROME. REPORT OF A CASE WITH HISTOPATHOLOGIC EXAMINATION OF OCULAR TISSUES.
AM. J. OPHTHAL. 50* 1197-1203, 1962.

STEGMAIER, O. C. AND SCHNEIDER, L. A.* CHEDIAK-HIGASHI SYNDROME* DERMATOLOGIC
MANIFESTATIONS. ARCH. DERM. 91* 1-8, 1965.

TAY, C. H., LOPEZ, C. G. AND LAZARUS, A. R.* THE CHEDIAK-HIGASHI SYNDROME.

RECESSIVE

MED. J. AUST. 2* 1024-1028, 1970.

WHITE, J. G.* THE CHEDIAK-HIGASHI SYNDROME* A POSSIBLE LYSOSOMAL DISEASE. BLOOD 28* 143-156, 1966.

WINDHORST, D. B., WHITE, J. G., ZELICKSON, A. S., CLAWSON, C. C., DENT, P. B., POLLARA, B. AND GOOD, R. A.* THE CHEDIAK-HIGASHI ANOMALY AND THE ALEUTIAN TRAIT IN MINK* HOMOLOGOUS DEFECTS OF LYSOSOMAL STRUCTURE. ANN. N.Y. ACAD. SCI. 155* 818-846, 1968.

WINDHORST, D. B., ZELICKSON, A. S. AND GOOD, R. A.* CHEDIAK-HIGASHI SYNDROME* HEREDITARY GIGANTISM OF CYTOPLASMIC ORGANELLES. SCIENCE 151* 81-83, 1966.

21460 CHEILOSIS-SEBORRHEA-AMINOACIDURIA

MENANO AND HIS COLLEAGUES (1960), OF LISBON, DESCRIBED A CHILD FROM HEALTHY AND APPARENTLY UNRELATED PARENTS WHO HAD CHEILOSIS-LIKE MUCOSAL AND CUTANEOUS LESIONS, SEBORRHEIC DERMATITIS AND AMINOACIDURIA. A BROTHER AND THE MOTHER HAD SIMILAR AMINOACIDURIA BUT WERE FREE OF THE OTHER MANIFESTATIONS. UNTIL FURTHER OBSERVATIONS ARE REPORTED, THE NATURE OF THIS SYNDROME, IF SUCH IT IS, REMAINS UNCLEAR.

MENANO, H., RELVAS, M. E., FERRAZ, F., HALPERN, M. AND TEIXEIRA, F.* CHEILOSIS-LIKE MUCOUS AND CUTANEOUS LESIONS, SEBORRHEIC DERMATITIS AND HEREDITARY AMINOACIDURIA. HELV. PAEDIAT. ACTA 15* 487-494, 1960.

*21470 CHLORIDE DIARRHEA, FAMILIAL

VOLUMINOUS WATERY STOOLS CONTAINING AN EXCESS OF CHLORIDE ARE PRESENT FROM A FEW WEEKS OF AGE. THE CHILDREN ARE OFTEN PREMATURE AND HYDRAMNIOS MAY COMPLICATE PREGNANCY. POTASSIUM CHLORIDE IS THE MAIN THERAPY. PASTERNACK AND PERHEENTUPA (1966) DESCRIBED VASCULAR CHANGES RESEMBLING THOSE OF HYPERTENSIVE ANGIOPATHY IN SEVEN CHILDREN AGES 1 TO 42 MONTHS AT THE TIME OF BIOPSY. ALL WERE NORMOTENSIVE. KIDNEY AND MUSCLE WERE BIOPSIED. THIS DISORDER WAS DESCRIBED FIRST BY GAMBLE ET AL. (1945) AND DARROW (1945). BOTH SEXES HAVE BEEN AFFECTED AND TWO SIBS APPEAR TO HAVE BEEN AFFECTED IN SEVERAL FAMILIES (KELSEY, 1954* PERHEENTUPA ET AL., 1965).

DARROW, D. C.* CONGENITAL ALKALOSIS WITH DIARRHEA. J. PEDIAT. 26* 519-532, 1945.

GAMBLE, J. L., FAHEY, K. R., APPLETON, J. AND MACLACHLAN, E. A.* CONGENITAL ALKALOSIS WITH DIARRHEA. J. PEDIAT. 26* 509-518, 1945.

KELSEY, W. M.* CONGENITAL ALKALOSIS WITH DIARRHEA. AM. J. DIS. CHILD. 88* 344-347, 1954.

PASTERNACK, A. AND PERHEENTUPA, J.* HYPERTENSIVE ANGIOPATHY IN FAMILIAL CHLORIDE DIARRHOEA. LANCET 2* 1047-1049, 1966.

PERHEENTUPA, J., EKLUND, J. AND KOJO, N.* FAMILIAL CHLORIDE DIARRHOEA ('CONGENITAL ALKALOSIS WITH DIARRHOEA'). ACTA PAEDIAT. SCAND. 159 (SUPPL.)* 119-120, 1965.

YSSING, M. AND FRIIS-HANSEN, B.* CONGENITAL ALKALOSIS WITH DIARRHEA. ACTA PAEDIAT. SCAND. 55* 341-344, 1966.

21480 CHOANAL ATRESIA, POSTERIOR

THIS IS A THREAT TO LIFE BECAUSE YOUNG INFANTS CANNOT ESTABLISH THE HABIT OF MOUTH BREATHING. RANSOME (1964) FOUND 12 FAMILIES WITH TWO OR MORE MEMBERS AFFECTED. ONE OF THESE, IN WHICH 4 OF 5 SIBS WERE AFFECTED, WAS DESCRIBED BY HIM. MOST CASES OF MULTIPLE AFFECTED RELATIVES HAVE CONCERNED SIBS. HOWEVER, THE FIRST REPORTED, THAT BY LANG (1912), INVOLVED IN ADDITION TO THE PROBAND, THE MOTHER, SISTER AND MATERNAL AUNT AND PERHAPS A BROTHER. FENDEL (1966) DESCRIBED AFFECTED SIBS. GRAHNE AND KALTIOKALLIO (1966) OBSERVED AFFECTED SISTERS. THE CONDITION IS SAID TO OCCUR TWICE AS OFTEN IN GIRLS AS IN BOYS AND MORE FREQUENTLY IN THE RIGHT SIDE THAN THE LEFT SIDE.

DIRLEWANGER, A.* HEREDITARES VORKOMMEN VON CHOANALATRESIEN. PRACT. OTORHENOLARYNG. 28* 211-218, 1966.

FENDEL, K.* ZUR FAMILIAREN HAUFUNG DER ANGEBORENEN CHOANALATRESIE. Z. LARYNG. RHINOL. OTOL. 45* 67-73, 1966.

GRAHNE, B. AND KALTIOKALLIO, K.* CONGENITAL CHOANAL ATRESIS AND ITS HEREDITY. ACTA OTOLARYNG. 62* 193-200, 1966.

LANG, J.* UEBER CHOANENATRESIE (HEREDITAT DERSELBEN). MSCHR. OHRENHEILK. 46* 970-1001, 1912.

RANSOME, J.* FAMILIAL INCIDENCE OF POSTERIOR CHOANAL ATRESIA. J. LARYNG. 78* 551-554, 1964.

R
E
C
E
S
S
I
V
E

IN A NORWEGIAN KINDRED AAGENAES ET AL. (1970) DESCRIBED A SYNDROME OF HEREDITARY RECURRENT CHOLESTASIS AND LYMPHEDEMA. JAUNDICE BECAME EVIDENT SOON AFTER BIRTH AND RECURRED IN EPISODES THROUGHOUT LIFE. EDEMA IN THE LEGS BEGAN AT ABOUT SCHOOL AGE AND PROGRESSED. IT WAS SHOWN TO BE DUE TO HYPOPLASIA OF THE LYMPHATIC VESSELS OF THE LEGS. SIXTEEN INDIVIDUALS IN 7 INTERCONNECTED SIBSHIPS APPEAR TO HAVE BEEN AFFECTED. ONE INSTANCE AFFECTED MOTHER AND DAUGHTER MAY HAVE RESULTED FROM THE FACT THAT THE FATHER WAS A HETEROZYGOTE.

AAGENAES, O., CUDERMAN, B., SIGSTAD, H., LEONARD, A. S., KRIVIT, W. AND SHARP, H. L.* CLINICAL AND EXPERIMENTAL RELATIONSHIPS BETWEEN CHOLESTASIS AND ABNORMAL HEPATIC LYMPHATICS. (ABSTRACT) PEDIAT. RES. 4* 377 ONLY, 1970.

AAGENAES, O., SIGSTAD, H. AND BJORN-HANSEN, R.* LYMPHOEDEMA IN HEREDITARY RECURRENT CHOLESTASIS FROM BIRTH. ARCH. DIS. CHILD. 45* 690-695, 1970.

SHARP, H. L. AND KRIVIT, W.* HEREDITARY LYMPHEDEMA AND OBSTRUCTIVE JAUNDICE. J. PEDIAT. 78* 491-496, 1971.

21500 CHOLESTEROL ESTER STORAGE DISEASE OF LIVER

SCHIFF ET AL. (1968) DESCRIBED CHOLESTEROL ESTER STORAGE DISEASE OF THE LIVER IN TEEN-AGE BROTHER AND SISTER WHOSE LIVERS WERE ORANGE IN COLOR. FOUR YOUNGER SIBS SHOWED MILDER CHANGES. THE PARENTS WERE NOT RELATED TO THEIR KNOWLEDGE.

SCHIFF, L., SCHUBERT, W. K., MCADAMS, A. J., SPIEGEL, E. L. AND O'DONNELL, J. F.* HEPATIC CHOLESTEROL ESTER STORAGE DISEASE, A FAMILIAL DISORDER. I. CLINICAL ASPECTS. AM. J. MED. 44* 538-546, 1968.

*21510 CHONDRODYSPLASIA PUNCTATA (CHONDRODYSTROPHIA CALCIFICANS CONGENITA, CHONDRODYS-
       TROPHIA CALCIFICANS PUNCTATA, CONRADI'S DISEASE)

THIS IS A RARE DISORDER OF THE BONES OF THE FETUS AND NEWBORN, CHARACTERIZED BY THE PRESENCE OF STIPPLED FOCI OF CALCIFICATION WITHIN HYALINE CARTILAGE AND ASSOCIATED WITH DWARFING, CONGENITAL CATARACT AND VARIOUS MALFORMATIONS. SEVERAL FAMILIES OF AFFECTED SIBS ARE REPORTED AND THE FREQUENCY OF PARENTAL CONSANGUINITY IS RATHER HIGH. DOUBTLESSLY THERE ARE A NUMBER OF DIFFERENT ENTITIES WHICH HAVE THE SAME CARTILAGINOUS CHANGES, E.G., ROSENFIELD ET AL. (1962) FOUND THEM IN A CASE OF TRISOMY 18. THE EVOLUTION OF THIS DISORDER OF EARLY LIFE INTO MULTIPLE EPIPHYSEAL DYSPLASIA WAS OBSERVED BY SILVERMAN (1961) AND THE INHERITANCE SEEMS TO BE DOMINANT. THUS IT IS POSSIBLE THAT A QUITE DIFFERENT ENTITY IS REPRESENTED. SKIN CHANGES LIKE ICHTHYOSIFORM ERYTHRODERMA HAVE BEEN REPORTED, AS WELL AS CONTRACTURES. MELNICK (1965) OBSERVED A CASE IN THE OFFSPRING OF A FATHER-DAUGHTER MATING. FIFTEEN YEAR FOLLOW-UP WAS PROVIDED BY COMINGS ET AL. (1968). CATARACT AND RADIOLOGIC CHANGES OF CHONDRODYSTROPHIA CALCIFICANS CONGENITA OCCUR IN SOME CASES OF THE CEREBRO-HEPATO-RENAL SYNDROME OF ZELLWEGER (Q.V.). SADDLE NOSE SECONDARY TO INVOLVEMENT OF THE FACIAL BONES IS PRESENT IN ABOUT 40 PERCENT OF CASES ACCORDING TO FRITSCH AND MANZKE (1963). IN AUSTRALIA THIS FEATURE HAS LED TO THE CONDITION BEING CALLED THE KOALA BEAR SYNDROME (DANKS, 1970). IT WAS THE SUGGESTION OF A GROUP CONVENED IN PARIS BY THE EUROPEAN SOCIETY OF PEDIATRIC RADIOLOGY THAT THE DISORDER BE CALLED CHONDRODYSPLASIA PUNCTATA (MAROTEAUX, 1970). SPRANGER ET AL. (1970) CONCLUDED THAT PUNCTATA INTRA- AND EXTRACARTILAGINOUS CALCIFICATION MAY BE FOUND IN A VARIETY OF HEREDITARY AND NONHEREDITARY CONDI-TIONS. PUNCTATE CALCIFICATIONS MAY OCCUR, FOR EXAMPLE, IN ZELLWEGER'S SYNDROME (Q.V.). THEY SUGGESTED THAT ZELLWEGER'S SYNDROME WAS PRESENT IN THE CASES REPORTED AS INSTANCES OF CHONDRODYSTROPHIA CALCIFICANS BY DE LANGE AND JANSSEN (1949), GEKLE (1963), PHILIPS (CASE 2, 1957), AND PUTSCHAR (1951). IN ONE, THE CONRADI-HUNERMANN TYPE, CALCIFICATION IS PREDOMINANTLY EPIPHYSEAL, THE CHANGES MAY BE ASYMMETRICAL PRODUCING A SHORT LEG FOR EXAMPLE. IT IS IN THIS FORM THAT IS ASSOCIATED WITH CHARACTERISTIC FACIES, WITH CATARACT IN ABOUT 18 PERCENT AND WITH SKIN CHANGES IN ABOUT 28 PERCENT. ELEVATED PATERNAL AGE IN SPORADIC CASES SUGGESTS A DOMINANT FORM. A FEW INSTANCES OF PARENTAL CONSANGUINITY SUPPORTS RECESSIVE INHERITANCE. THE SECOND FORM IS CALLED RHIZOMELIC TYPE BECAUSE OF SEVERE, SYMMETRICAL PROXIMAL SHORTENING OF THE LIMBS. THERE ARE MARKED METAPHY-SEAL CHANGES, CATARACTS IN ABOUT 72 PERCENT OF CASES, SKIN CHANGES IN ABOUT 27 PERCENT. INHERITANCE IS CLEARLY RECESSIVE.

ALLANSMITH, M. AND SENZ, E.* CHONDRODYSTROPHIA CONGENITA PUNCTATA (CONRADI'S DISEASE). AM. J. DIS. CHILD. 100* 109-116, 1960.

BODIAN, E. L.* SKIN MANIFESTATIONS OF CONRADI'S DISEASE. CHONDRODYSTROPHIA CONGENITA PUNCTATA. ARCH. DERM. 94* 743-748, 1966.

COMINGS, D. E., PAPAZIAN, C. AND SCHOENE, H. R.* CONRADI'S DISEASE (CHONDRODYS-TROPHIA CALCIFICANS CONGENITA, CONGENITAL STIPPLED EPIPHYSES). J. PEDIAT. 72* 63-69, 1968.

DANKS, D. M.* MELBOURNE, AUSTRALIA* PERSONAL COMMUNICATION, 1970.

DE LANGE, C. AND JANSSEN, T.* CONGENITAL CHONDRODYSTROPHIA CALCIFICANS OF INFANT IN ASSOCIATION WITH OTHER ABNORMALITIES* CASE. MSCHR. KINDERGENEESK. 17*

FRASER, F. C. AND SCRIVER, J. B.* A HEREDITARY FACTOR IN CHONDRODYSTROPHIA CALCIFICANS CONGENITA. NEW ENG. J. MED 250* 272-277, 1954.

FRITSCH, H. AND MANZKE, H.* BEITRAG ZUR CHONDRODYSTROPHIA CALCIFICANS CONNATA (CONRADI-HUNERMANN-SYNDROM). ARCH. KINDERHEILK. 169* 235-254, 1963.

GEKLE, D.* EIN BEITRAG ZUM PROBLEM DER CHONDRODYSTROPHIA CALCIFICANS CONGENITA. ARCH. KINDERHEILK. 169* 267-273, 1963.

JOSEPHSON, B. M. AND ORIATTI, M. D.* CHONDRODYSTROPHIA CALCIFICANS CONGENITA* REPORT OF A CASE AND REVIEW OF THE LITERATURE. PEDIATRICS 28* 425-435, 1961.

MAROTEAUX, P.* NOMENCLATURE INTERNATIONALE DES MALADIES OSSEUSES CONSTITU-TIONELLES. ANN. RADIOL. 13* 455-464, 1970.

MELNICK, J. C.* CHONDRODYSTROPHIA CALCIFICANS CONGENITA (CHONDRODYSPLASIA EPIPHYSIALIS PUNCTATA, STIPPLED EPIPHYSES). AM. J. DIS. CHILD. 110* 218-225, 1965.

PHILIPS, L. I.* CHONDRODYSTROPHIA CALCIFICANS CONGENITA. NEW ZEAL. J. MED. 56* 22-27, 1957.

PUTSCHAR, W. G. J.* CHONDRODYSTROPHIA CALCIFICANS CONGENITA (DYSPLASIA EPIPHYSIALIS PUNCTATA). BULL. HOSP. JOINT DIS. 11* 514-527, 1951.

ROSENFIELD, R. L., BREIBART, S., ISAACS, H., KLEVIT, H. D. AND MELLMAN, W. J.* TRISOMY OF CHROMOSOMES 13-15 AND 17-18* ITS ASSOCIATION WITH INFANTILE ARTERIOSC-LEROSIS. AM. J. MED. SCI. 244* 763-779, 1962.

SILVERMAN, F. N.* DYSPLASIES EPIPHYSAIRES* ENTITE PROTEIFORME. ANN. RADIOL. 4* 833-867, 1961.

SPRANGER, J. W., OPITZ, J. M. AND BIDDER, V.* HETEROGENEITY OF CHONDRODYSPLASIA PUNCTATA. HUMANGENETIK 11* 190-212, 1971.

TASKER, W. G., MASTRI, A. R. AND GOLD, A. P.* CHONDRODYSTROPHIA CALCIFICANS CONGENITA (DYSPLASIA EPIPHYSALIS PUNCTATA). RECOGNITION OF THE CLINICAL PICTURE. AM. J. DIS. CHILD. 119* 122-127, 1970.

21520 CHONDRODYSTROPHY, JOINT DISLOCATION, GLAUCOMA, AND MENTAL RETARDATION

THESE WERE THE FEATURES OF TWO SISTERS, AGES 8 AND 20 MONTHS, REPORTED BY DESBUQUOIS ET AL. (1966). DISLOCATION OF THE PATELLAE AND HIPS WAS PRESENT. DWARFING WAS SEVERE.

DESBUQUOIS, G., GRENIER, B., MICHEL, J. AND ROSSIGNOL, C.* NANISME CHONDRODYS-TROPHIQUE AVEC OSSIFICATION ANARCHIQUE ET POLY-MALFORMATIONS CHEZ DEUX SOEURS. ARCH. FRANC. PEDIAT. 23* 573-587, 1966.

21530 CHONDROSARCOMA

SCHAJOWICZ AND BESSONE (1967) DESCRIBED THREE BROTHERS WHO RESPECTIVELY DEVELOPED CHONDROSARCOMA OF THE PELVIC BONE AT 18 YEARS, OF THE FIBULA AND FEMUR AT 16 YEARS AND OF THE FEMUR AT 17 YEARS. TWO BROTHERS AND A SISTER WERE LIVING AND WELL. KARYOTYPES WERE NORMAL. SEE OSTEOGENIC SARCOMA.

SCHAJOWICZ, F. AND BESSONE, J. E.* CHONDROSARCOMA IN 3 BROTHERS. A PATHOLOGI-CAL AND GENETIC STUDY. J. BONE JOINT SURG. 49A* 129-141, 1967.

21540 CHORDOMA

FOOTE AND OTHERS (1958) DESCRIBED MIDDLE-AGED BROTHER AND SISTER WITH SACRO-COCCYGEAL CHORDOMA. RECURRENCE AND METASTASES OCCURRED IN BOTH.

FOOTE, R. F., ABLIN, G. AND HALL, W.* CHORDOMA IN SIBLINGS. CALIF. MED. 88* 383-386, 1958.

21550 CHOROIDAL SCLEROSIS

WAARDENBURG (1952) DESCRIBED CENTRAL CHOROIDAL SCLEROSIS IN TWO DAUGHTERS OF A FIRST COUSIN MARRIAGE. MANY OTHERS HAVE REPORTED SIBS WITH CENTRAL CHOROIDAL SCLEROSIS AND SEVERAL INSTANCES OF PARENTAL CONSANGUINITY ARE ON RECORD (E.G., SORSBY AND CRICK, 1953).

SORSBY, A. AND CRICK, R. P.* CENTRAL AREOLAR CHOROIDAL SCLEROSIS. BRIT. J. OPHTHAL. 37* 129-139, 1953.

WAARDENBURG, P. J.* ANGIO-SCLEROSE FAMILIALE DE LA CHOROIDE. J. GENET. HUM. 1* 83-93, 1952.

R
E
C
E
S
S
I
V
E

ASIDE FROM WILSON'S DISEASE, TYPE IV GLYCOGEN STORAGE DISEASE AND GALACTOSEMIA (Q.V.), WELL KNOWN CAUSES OF FAMILIAL CIRRHOSIS, FAMILIES WITH MULTIPLE AFFECTED SIBS AND NORMAL PARENTS HAVE BEEN OBSERVED (IBER, MADDREY, 1965). THE GROUP IS PROBABLY HETEROGENEOUS AND IN SOME INSTANCES NON-GENETIC FACTORS MAY BE RESPONSIBLE FOR THE FAMILIAL AGGREGATION. IBER AND MADDREY (1965) REVIEWED 13 REPORTED FAMILIES AND 8 OF THEIR OWN, EACH WITH TWO OR MORE AFFECTED MEMBERS. THEY POINTED OUT THAT WITH ONE EXCEPTION THE MULTIPLE CASES WERE IN THE SAME GENERATION. WITHIN A GIVEN FAMILY AGE OF ONSET, CLINICAL COURSE AND BIOPSY FINDINGS WERE VERY SIMILAR BUT THERE WERE WIDE DIFFERENCES BETWEEN FAMILIES. ALSO SEE WILSON'S DISEASE AND INTRAHEPATIC CHOLESTASIS. BABER (1956) DESCRIBED CASES OF CONGENITAL CIRRHOSIS WITH GENERALIZED AMINOACIDURIA. SOME OF THESE PATIENTS MAY BE EXAMPLES OF WILSON'S DISEASE. OTHERS MAY HAVE TYROSINEMIA (ZETTERSTROM 1963, GENTZ ET AL., 1965). SEE TYROSINEMIA. IN INDIA, SO-CALLED INDIAN CHILDHOOD CIRRHOSIS (SEN'S SYNDROME) AFFECTS MULTIPLE SIBS (CHAUDHURI AND CHAUDHURI, 1965).

BABER, M. D.* CASE OF CONGENITAL CIRRHOSIS OF THE LIVER WITH RENAL TUBULAR DEFECTS AKIN TO THOSE IN THE FANCONI SYNDROME. ARCH. DIS. CHILD. 31* 335-339, 1956.

CHAUDHURI, A. AND CHAUDHURI, K. C.* THE KARYOTYPE IN INFANTILE CIRRHOSIS OF THE LIVER (SEN'S SYNDROME). INDIAN J. PEDIAT. 32* 209-218, 1965.

GENTZ, J., JAGENBURG, R. AND ZETTERSTROM, R.* TYROSINEMIA* AN INBORN ERROR OF TYROSINE METABOLISM WITH CIRRHOSIS OF THE LIVER AND MULTIPLE RENAL TUBULAR DEFECTS. J. PEDIAT. 66* 670-696, 1965.

IBER, F. L. AND MADDREY, W. C.* FAMILIAL HEPATIC DISEASES WITH CIRRHOSIS OR WITHOUT PORTAL HYPERTENSION. PROGR. LIVER DIS. 2* 290-302, 1965.

MADDREY, W. C. AND IBER, F. L.* FAMILIAL CIRRHOSIS. A CLINICAL AND PATHOLOGICAL STUDY. ANN. INTERN. MED. 61* 667-679, 1964.

MILLER, M. C.* FAMILIAL CIRRHOSIS WITH HEPATOMA. AM. J. DIG. DIS. 12* 633-638, 1967.

ZETTERSTROM, R.* TYROSINOSIS. ANN. N.Y. ACAD. SCI. 111* 220-226, 1963.

*21570 CITRULLINURIA

SEVERE VOMITING SPELLS BEGINNING AT THE AGE OF 9 MONTHS AND MENTAL RETARDATION WERE FEATURES OF THE FIRST CASE, OFFSPRING OF FIRST COUSIN PARENTS. MCMURRAY AND COLLEAGUES (1962) FOUND CITRULLINE IN VERY HIGH CONCENTRATION IN SERUM, SPINAL FLUID AND URINE. THE AMINO ACID GETS ITS NAME FROM ITS HIGH CONCENTRATION IN THE WATERMELON CITRULLUS VULGARIS. VISAKORPI (1962) ALSO DESCRIBED A CASE OF CITRULLINURIA. VOMITING AND AMMONIA INTOXICATION ARE OTHER MANIFESTATIONS. THE ENZYME DEFECT IS THOUGHT TO CONCERN ARGININOSUCCINIC ACID SYNTHETASE.

MCMURRAY, W. C., MOHYUDDIN, F., ROSSITER, R. J., RATHBUN, J. C., VALENTINE, G. H., KOEGLER, S. J. AND ZARFAS, D. E.* CITRULLINURIA* A NEW AMINOACIDURIA ASSOCIATED WITH MENTAL RETARDATION. LANCET 1* 138 ONLY, 1962.

MCMURRAY, W. C., RATHBUN, J. C., MOHYUDDIN, F. AND KOEGLER, S. J.* CITRULLINURIA. PEDIATRICS 32* 347-357, 1963.

MOHYUDDIN, F., RATHBUN, J. C. AND MCMURRAY, W. C.* STUDIES ON AMINO ACID METABOLISM IN CITRULLINURIA. AM. J. DIS. CHILD. 113* 152-156, 1967.

MORROW, G., III., BARNESS, L. A. AND EFRON, M. L.* CITRULLINEMIA WITH DEFECTIVE UREA PRODUCTION. PEDIATRICS 40* 565-574, 1967.

TEDESCO, T. A. AND MELLMAN, W. J.* ARGININOSUCCINATE SYNTHETASE ACTIVITY AND CITRULLINE METABOLISM IN CELLS CULTURED FROM A CITRULLINEMIC SUBJECT. PROC. NAT. ACAD. SCI. 57* 829-834, 1967.

VISAKORPI, J. K.* CITRULLINURIA. (LETTER) LANCET 1* 1357-1358, 1962.

21580 CLEFT LARYNX, POSTERIOR

ZACHARY AND EMERY (1961) REPORTED THREE CASES OF LACK OF FUSION OF THE POSTERIOR LARYNX AND PERSISTENCE OF COMMON TRACHEOESOPHAGUS. TWO OF THESE WERE SIBS, THE MOTHER HAVING TWO OTHER NORMAL CHILDREN. ONE WAS MALE, THE SEX OF THE SECOND WAS NOT STATED. IN SPORADIC CASES MALES AND FEMALES ARE AFFECTED ABOUT EQUALLY OFTEN. FINLAY (1949) AND CROOKS (1954) DESCRIBED A FAMILY OF 5 GIRLS, FOUR OF WHOM HAD LARYNGEAL STRIDOR. AT LEAST TWO HAD CLEFT LARYNX. ORDINARY TRACHEO-ESOPHAGEAL FISTULA SHOWS LITTLE FAMILIAL AGGREGATION.

CROOKS, J.* NON-INFLAMMATORY LARYNGEAL STRIDOR IN INFANTS. ARCH. DIS. CHILD. 29* 12-17, 1954.

FINLAY, H. V. L.* FAMILIAL CONGENITAL STRIDOR. ARCH. DIS. CHILD. 24* 219-223,

R
E
C
E
S
S
I
V
E

ZACHARY, R. B. AND EMERY, J. L.* FAILURE OF SEPARATION OF LARYNX AND TRACHEA FROM THE ESOPHAGUS. PERSISTENT ESOPHAGOTRACHEA. SURGERY 49* 525-529, 1961.

21590 CLEFT LIP WITH OR WITHOUT CLEFT PALATE

AS AN ISOLATED MALFORMATION CLEFT LIP WITH OR WITHOUT CLEFT PALATE BEHAVES AS AN ENTITY DISTINCT FROM CLEFT PALATE ALONE (Q.V.). IT APPEARS TO HAVE COMPLEX GENETICS. CURTIS, FRASER AND WARBURTON (1961) ESTIMATED THAT THE RISK OF RECURRENCE IN SUBSEQUENTLY BORN CHILDREN IS 4 PERCENT IF ONE CHILD HAS IT, 4 PERCENT IF ONE PARENT HAS IT, 17 PERCENT IF ONE PARENT AND ONE CHILD HAS IT AND 9 PERCENT IF TWO CHILDREN HAVE IT. THE SYNDROME OF CLEFT LIP WITH OR WITHOUT CLEFT PALATE IN ASSOCIATION WITH MUCOUS PITS OF THE LOWER LIP IS INHERITED AS AN AUTOSOMAL DOMINANT.

CURTIS, E. J., FRASER, F. C. AND WARBURTON, D.* CONGENITAL CLEFT LIP AND PALATE. AM. J. DIS. CHILD. 102* 853-857, 1961.

21600 CLEFT LIP, MEDIAN, WITH POSTAXIAL POLYDACTYLY

THURSTON (1909) DESCRIBED TWO HINDU BROTHERS WITH MEDIAN CLEFT OF THE UPPER LIP ASSOCIATED WITH POSTAXIAL POLYDACTYLY (COMPLETELY FORMED EXTRA DIGITS) OF BOTH HANDS AND FEET. THE PARENTS WERE NORMAL. CONSANGUINITY WAS NOT COMMENTED ON. THIS COULD BE EITHER AUTOSOMAL OR X-LINKED RECESSIVE.

THURSTON, E. O.* A CASE OF MEDIAN HARE-LIP ASSOCIATED WITH OTHER MALFORMATIONS. LANCET 2* 996-997, 1909.

21610 CLEFT LIP-PALATE WITH ABNORMAL THUMBS AND MICROCEPHALY

JUBERG AND HAYWARD (1968) DESCRIBED A SYNDROME WITH ORAL, CRANIAL AND DIGITAL MANIFESTATIONS IN 5 OF 6 CHILDREN OF NORMAL, UNRELATED PARENTS. TWO BROTHERS HAD CLEFT LIP AND PALATE, MICROCEPHALY, HYPOPLASIA AND DISTAL PLACEMENT OF THE THUMBS AND ELBOW DEFORMITIES LIMITING EXTENSION. ONE OF THE BROTHERS HAD TOE ANOMALIES AS DID 3 OF THE 4 SISTERS. AMONG THE SISTERS MICROCEPHALY, STIFF THUMBS AND FORME FRUSTE CLEFT LIP WERE OBSERVED.

JUBERG, R. C. AND HAYWARD, J. R.* A NEW FAMILIAL SYNDROME OF ORAL, CRANIAL, AND DIGITAL ANOMALIES. J. PEDIAT. 74* 755-762, 1968.

21620 CLEFT PALATE ALONE

CLEFT PALATE AS AN ISOLATED MALFORMATION BEHAVES AS AN ENTITY DISTINCT FROM CLEFT LIP WITH OR WITHOUT CLEFT PALATE. CURTIS, FRASER AND WARBURTON (1961) ESTIMATED THAT THE RISK OF RECURRENCE IN SUBSEQUENTLY BORN CHILDREN IS ABOUT 2 PERCENT IF ONE CHILD HAS IT, 6 PERCENT IF ONE PARENT HAS IT AND 15 PERCENT IF ONE PARENT AND ONE CHILD HAVE IT. AS FOR CLEFT LIP WITH OR WITHOUT CLEFT PALATE, AS WELL AS MANY OTHER RELATIVELY FREQUENT CONGENITAL MALFORMATIONS, THE GENETICS IS APPARENTLY COMPLEX.

CURTIS, E. J., FRASER, F. C. AND WARBURTON, D.* CONGENITAL CLEFT LIP AND PALATE. AM. J. DIS. CHILD. 102* 853-857, 1961.

21630 CLEFT PALATE, DEAFNESS, OLIGODONTIA

IN A SIBSHIP OF SWEDISH EXTRACTION, GORLIN ET AL. (1971) OBSERVED TWO SISTERS WITH CLEFT SOFT PALATE, SEVERE OLIGODONTIA OF THE DECIDUOUS TEETH, NO PERMANENT DENTITION, BILATERAL CONDUCTIVE DEAFNESS DUE TO FIXATION OF THE FOOTPLATE OF THE STAPES, SHORT HALLUCES WITH WIDE SPACE BETWEEN THE FIRST AND SECOND TOES, AND COALITION OF BONES IN THE FOOT.

GORLIN, R. J., SCHLORF, R. A. AND PAPARELLA, M. M.* CLEFT PALATE, STAPES FIXATION AND OLIGODONTIA. THE CLINICAL DELINEATION OF BIRTH DEFECTS. X. THE ENDOCRINE SYSTEM. BALTIMORE* WILLIAMS AND WILKINS, 1971.

*21640 COCKAYNE SYNDROME

MACDONALD, FITCH AND LEWIS (1960) DESCRIBED AFFECTION OF 3 OUT OF 5 SIBS. CHARACTERISTICS ARE DWARFISM, PRECOCIOUSLY SENILE APPEARANCE, PIGMENTARY RETINAL DEGENERATION, OPTIC ATROPHY, DEAFNESS, MARBLE EPIPHYSES IN SOME DIGITS, SENSITIVITY TO SUNLIGHT AND MENTAL RETARDATION. THE MOST STRIKING PEDIGREE IS THAT OF PADDISON, MOOSSY, DERBES AND KLOEPFER (1963). NEILL AND DINGWALL (1950) DESCRIBED A PROGERIA-LIKE SYNDROME CHARACTERIZED BY DWARFISM, MICROCEPHALY, SEVERE MENTAL RETARDATION, 'PEPPER-AND-SALT' CHORIORETINITIS, AND INTRACRANIAL CALCIFICATION. THE PARENTS WERE NOT CLOSELY RELATED. IT NOW SEEMS LIKELY THAT THE DIAGNOSIS WAS THE COCKAYNE SYNDROME. DEATH FROM EARLY ATHEROSCLEROSIS OCCURRED IN THESE SIBS AS IN PROGERIA (NEILL, 1966). NORMAN (1963) EXAMINED THE BRAIN OF THE TWO SIBS. MASSIVE PERICAPILLARY CALCIFICATION WAS PRESENT IN THE PUTAMINA, THALAMI AND CEREBELLAR WHITE MATTER SUPERFICIAL TO THE DENTATE NUCLEI. IN THE LARGER VESSELS THE CALCIFICATION WAS MAINLY IN THE ADVENTITIAL COAT. IN 1971, THROUGH THE COURTESY OF KLOEPFER, I HAD AN OPPORTUNITY TO SEE TWO AFFECTED MALES, THEN AGES 29

R
E
C
E
S
S
I
V
E

AND 24, FROM THIS PEDIGREE. THEY WERE MARKEDLY DWARFED WITH "HOLLOW EYES." THEY COULD NOT CLOSE THE EYES COMPLETELY SO THAT SEVERE CORNEAL CHANGES CONTRIBUTED TO THE VISUAL IMPAIRMENT. HEAD AND BODY HAIR WAS OF NORMAL MALE QUALITY AND DISTRIBUTION. THE FACE REQUIRED SHAVING SEVERAL TIMES A WEEK.

COTTON, R. B., KEATS, T. E. AND MCCOY, E. E.* ABNORMAL BLOOD GLUCOSE REGULATION IN COCKAYNE'S SYNDROME. PEDIATRICS 46* 54-60, 1970.

FUJIMOTO, W. Y., GREENE, M. L. AND SEEGMILLER, J. E.* COCKAYNE'S SYNDROME* REPORT OF A CASE WITH HYPERLIPOPROTEINEMIA, HYPERINSULINEMIA, RENAL DISEASE, AND NORMAL GROWTH HORMONE. J. PEDIAT. 75* 881-884, 1969.

LANNING, M. AND SIMILA, S.* COCKAYNE'S SYNDROME. REPORT OF A CASE WITH NORMAL INTELLIGENCE. Z. KINDERHEILK. 109* 70-75, 1970.

MACDONALD, W. B., FITCH, K. D. AND LEWIS, I. C.* COCKAYNE'S SYNDROME* AN HEREDO-FAMILIAL DISORDER OF GROWTH AND DEVELOPMENT. PEDIATRICS 25* 997-1007, 1960.

MOOSA, A. AND DUBOWITZ, V.* PERIPHERAL NEUROPATHY IN COCKAYNE'S SYNDROME. ARCH. DIS. CHILD. 45* 674-677, 1970.

NEILL, C. A. AND DINGWALL, M. M.* A SYNDROME RESEMBLING PROGERIA* A REVIEW OF TWO CASES. ARCH. DIS. CHILD. 25* 213-223, 1950.

NEILL, C. A.* BALTIMORE, MD.* PERSONAL COMMUNICATION, 1966.

NORMAN, R. M. AND TINGEY, A. H.* SYNDROME OF MICRENCEPHALY, STRIO-CEREBELLAR CALCIFICATIONS, AND LEUCODYSTROPHY. J. NEUROL. NEUROSURG. PSYCHIAT. 29* 157-163, 1966.

NORMAN, R. M.* MALFORMATIONS OF THE NERVOUS SYSTEM, BIRTH INJURY AND DISEASES OF EARLY LIFE. IN, BLACKWOOD AND OTHERS (EDS.)* GREENFIELD'S NEUROPATHOLOGY. BALTIMORE* WILLIAMS AND WILKINS, 1963. P. 350.

PADDISON, R. M., MOOSSY, J., DERBES, V. J. AND KLOEPFER, W.* COCKAYNE'S SYNDROME. A REPORT OF FIVE NEW CASES WITH BIOCHEMICAL, CHROMOSOMAL, DERMATOLOGIC, GENETIC AND NEUROPATHOLOGIC OBSERVATIONS. DERM. TROP. 2* 195-203, 1963.

ROWLATT, U.* COCKAYNE'S SYNDROME. REPORT OF CASE WITH NECROPSY FINDINGS. ACTA NEUROPATH. 14* 52-61, 1969.

21650 COFFIN SYNDROME

COFFIN (1968) DESCRIBED THREE UNRELATED INSTITUTIONALIZED CHILDREN WITH A DISORDER CHARACTERIZED BY (1) SMALL SIZE AT BIRTH, (2) SEVERELY RETARDED SOMATIC GROWTH AND MENTAL DEVELOPMENT, (3) SLENDER HABITUS, (4) CHARACTERISTIC FACIES WITH PROMINENT FOREHEAD AND EYES, INFANTILE MOUTH WITH DOWNTURNED CORNERS AND LOW-SET, SIMPLIFIED PINNAE, (5) LAX JOINTS, (6) SPASTIC TETRAPLEGIA, (7) CONVULSIONS IN INFANCY, (8) FREQUENT RESPIRATORY INFECTIONS, AND (9) RETARDED BONE AGE. ONE HAD CLEFT PALATE AND TETRALOGY OF FALLOT. NEITHER A GENETIC NOR AN EXOGENOUS CAUSE WAS EVIDENT, ALTHOUGH COFFIN WAS IMPRESSED WITH THE VARIETY OF DRUGS TAKEN BY THE MOTHERS DURING GESTATION. IN A FOLLOW-UP NOTE, COFFIN AND WILSON (1971) REPORTED THAT, ALTHOUGH TWO LABORATORIES HAD REPORTED THE CHROMOSOMES TO BE NORMAL, RESTUDY SHOWED PARTIAL DELETION OF THE SHORT ARM OF A NO. 4 CHROMOSOME (4 P-), THE CHARACTERISTIC FINDING IN THE WOLF-HIRSCHHORN SYNDROME (1965) IN TWO OF THE THREE SIBS. THE CHROMOSOMES OF BOTH PARENTS WERE NORMAL.

COFFIN, G. S. AND WILSON, M. G.* WOLF-HIRSCHHORN SYNDROME. AM. J. DIS. CHILD. 121* 265 ONLY, 1971.

COFFIN, G. S.* A SYNDROME OF RETARDED DEVELOPMENT WITH CHARACTERISTIC AP-PEARANCE. AM. J. DIS. CHILD. 115* 698-702, 1968.

HIRSCHHORN, K., COOPER, H. L. AND FIRSCHEIN, I. L.* DELETION OF SHORT ARMS OF CHROMOSOME 4-5 IN A CHILD WITH DEFECTS OF MIDLINE FUSION. HUMANGENETIK 1* 479-482, 1965.

WOLF, U., REINWEIN, H. AND PORSCH, R.* DEFIZIENZ AN DEN KUZEN ARMEN EINS CHROMOSOMS NR. 4. HUMANGENETIK 1* 397-413, 1965.

21660 COLLAGENOMA, FAMILIAL CUTANEOUS

HENDERSON ET AL. (1968) DESCRIBED THREE BROTHERS WITH NUMEROUS SKIN NODULES ON THE BACK. THESE CONSISTED OF THICKENED DERMIS DUE TO INCREASED COLLAGENOUS TISSUE. ONE BROTHER HAD IDIOPATHIC MYOCARDOPATHY, A SECOND HAD ATROPHY OF THE LEFT IRIS AND SEVERE HIGH FREQUENCY SENSORINEURAL HEARING LOSS, AND THE THIRD HAD RECURRENT VASCULITIS. THUS, THE CUTANEOUS ABNORMALITY MAY BE MERELY PART OF A SYSTEMIC DISORDER. IT SEEMS NOT TO HAVE BEEN PREVIOUSLY REPORTED.

HENDERSON, R. R., WHEELER, C. E., JR. AND ABELE, D. C.* FAMILIAL CUTANEOUS COLLAGENOMA. ARCH. DERM. 98* 23-27, 1968.

THIS IS A DESCRIPTIVE TERM APPROPRIATE TO THE APPEARANCE OF THE NEWBORN WITH A NUMBER OF CONDITIONS INVOLVING X-LINKED ICHTHYOSIS, BULLOUS AND NON-BULLOUS ICHTHYOSIFORM ERYTHRODERMIA, SJOGREN-LARSSON SYNDROME, AND ICHTHYOSIS CONGENITA.

21680 COLOBOMA OF MACULA AND SKELETAL ANOMALIES

PHILLIPS AND GRIFFITHS (1969) DESCRIBED A BROTHER AND SISTER WITH BILATERAL MACULAR COLOBOMA, CLEFT PALATE, HALLUX VALGUS AND OTHER ABNORMALITIES. THE PARENTS WERE NOT RELATED. THE OCULAR TRAIT WAS LIKE THAT DESCRIBED BY SORSBY AS A DOMINANT AND LISTED HERE AS 'COLOBOMA OF THE MACULA WITH TYPE B BRACHYDACTYLY' (Q.V.). ALTHOUGH DIGITAL ABNORMALITIES WERE PRESENT IN THE SIBS REPORTED BY PHILLIPS AND GRIFFITHS, THEY WERE OF RELATIVELY MILD TYPE AND DIFFERENT NATURE THAN THOSE IN SORSBY'S FAMILY.

PHILLIPS, C. I. AND GRIFFITHS, D. L.* MACULAR COLOBOMA AND SKELETAL ABNORMALITY. BRIT. J. OPHTHAL. 53* 346-349, 1969.

*21690 COLOR BLINDNESS, TOTAL

THE BRITISH EXPRESSION 'DAY-BLINDNESS' IS A GOOD ONE BECAUSE THE CONES ARE MISSING AND THE SUBJECTS SEE BETTER AT NIGHT. THIS TERM IS PARALLEL TO NIGHT-BLINDNESS. THE LARGEST PEDIGREE IS THAT OF A FAMILY RESIDING ON THE ISLAND OF FUR IN THE LIMFJORD IN THE NORTH OF DENMARK (HOLM AND LODBERG, 1940* FRANCESCHETTI, FRANCOIS AND BABEL, 1963).

FRANCESCHETTI, A., FRANCOIS, J. AND BABEL, J.* LES HEREDO-DEGENERESCENCES CHORIO-RETINIENNES (DEGENERESCENCES TAPETO-RETINIENNES) PARIS* MASSON, 2* 1252-1254, 1963.

HANHART, E.* UBER DEN ZUSAMMENHANG 48 NEUER BEOBACHTUNGEN VON TOTALER FARBENBLINDHEIT (ACROMATOPSIE) MIT DEN 21 BISHER PUBLIZIERTEN SCHWEIZER FALLEN UND DIE HALDANESCHE LOKALISATION DES BETREFFENDEN GENS IM X-CHROMOSOM. ARCH. KLAUS STIFT. VERERBUNGSFORCH. 23* 465 ONLY, 1948.

HARRISON, R., HOEFNAGEL, D. AND HAYWARD, J. N.* CONGENITAL TOTAL COLOR BLINDNESS. ARCH. OPHTHAL. 64* 685-692, 1960.

HOLM, E. AND LODBERG, C. V.* FAMILY WITH TOTAL COLOUR-BLINDNESS. ACTA OPHTHAL. 18* 224-258, 1940.

*21700 COMPLEMENT COMPONENT C-PRIME-2, DEFICIENCY OF

KLEMPERER ET AL. (1966, 1967) FOUND MULTIPLE AFFECTED PERSONS IN A KINDRED. NO GENE PRODUCT WAS DETECTED IN THOSE WITH THE DEFICIENCY (HOMOZYGOTES). IN HETEROZYGOTES A PARTIAL DEFICIENCY OF C-PRIME-2 WAS FOUND. RESTUDY OF SILVERSTEIN'S FAMILY DEMONSTRATED IDENTICAL FINDINGS. NONE OF THE HOMOZYGOTES HAVE BEEN UNDULY SENSITIVE TO BACTERIAL INFECTION OR HAD OTHER EVIDENT ABNORMALITY. BY MEANS OF MONOSPECIFIC ANTISERUM, POLLEY (1968) SHOWED THAT HOMOZYGOTES HAVE NO SECOND COMPONENT OF COMPLEMENT AND HETEROZYGOTES HAVE AN INTERMEDIATE AMOUNT. THUS, THE DEFECT IS FAILURE OF SYNTHESIS RATHER THAN SYNTHESIS OF AN INACTIVE ANALOG. SEE VARIANTS OF C2 IN DOMINANT CATALOG. THESE MAY CONCERN ONE AND THE SAME LOCUS. IT WAS THE RECOMMENDATION OF A NOMENCLATURE CONFERENCE SPONSORED BY W.H.O. (1968) THAT THE 'PRIME' BE DROPPED AND THAT IN THE ORDER OF THEIR REACTIONS THE COMPLEMENT COMPONENTS BE DESIGNATED C1, C2, C3, C4, C5, C6, C7, C8, C9.

AUSTEN, K. F.* INBORN ERRORS OF THE COMPLEMENT SYSTEM OF MAN. NEW ENG. J. MED. 276* 1363-1367, 1967.

AUSTEN, K. F., BECKER, E. L., BERO, C. E., BORSOS, T., DALMASSO, A. P. AND DA SILVA, D.* NOMENCLATURE OF COMPLEMENT. BULL. WORLD HEALTH ORGAN. 39* 935-938, 1968.

KLEMPERER, M. R., AUSTEN, K. F. AND ROSEN, F. S.* HEREDITARY DEFICIENCY OF SECOND COMPONENT OF COMPLEMENT (C-PRIME-2) IN MAN* FURTHER OBSERVATIONS ON A SECOND KINDRED. J. IMMUNOL. 98* 72-78, 1967.

KLEMPERER, M. R., WOODWORTH, H. C., ROSEN, F. S. AND AUSTEN, K. F.* HEREDITARY DEFICIENCY OF SECOND COMPONENT OF COMPLEMENT (C-PRIME-2) IN MAN. J. CLIN. INVEST. 45* 880-890, 1966.

POLLEY, M. J.* INHERITED C-PRIME-2 DEFICIENCY IN MAN* LACK OF IMMUNOCHEMICALLY DETECTABLE C-PRIME-2 PROTEIN IN SERUMS FROM DEFICIENT INDIVIDUALS. SCIENCE 161* 1149-1151, 1968.

RUDDY, S. AND AUSTEN, K. F.* INHERITED ABNORMALITIES OF THE COMPLEMENT SYSTEM IN MAN. IN, STEINBERG, A. G. AND BEARN, A. G. (EDS.)* PROGRESS IN MEDICAL GENETICS, CHAPTER 3 VOL. 7, 1970. PP. 69-95.

SILVERSTEIN, A. M.* ESSENTIAL HYPOCOMPLEMENTEMIA. REPORT OF A CASE. BLOOD 16* 1338-1341, 1960.

R
E
C
E
S
S
I
V
E

TEMTAMY (1966) COULD FIND NO EVIDENCE OF A CLEAR OR SIMPLE GENETIC BASIS. SINCE THE WORK OF STREETER (1930) THE CAUSATIVE ROLE OF AMNIOTIC BANDS HAS BEEN DISCOUNTED AND THE MALFORMATIONS, BOTH THE BANDS AND THE ASSOCIATED ABSENCE DEFORMITIES, ARE THOUGHT TO RESULT FROM TISSUE NECROSIS PROBABLY ON A VASCULAR BASIS. HOWEVER, THE WORK OF TORPIN (1968) MAKES A MODIFIED FORM OF THE AMNIOTIC BAND THEORY PLAUSIBLE. A CONSIDERABLE BODY OF OBSERVATIONS INDICATES THAT RUPTURE OF THE AMNION AND CONSTRICTION OF MEMBERS WHICH ARE DISPLACED THROUGH HOLES IN THE AMNION ARE INVOLVED. AMPUTATED PARTS HAVE BEEN RECOVERED IN SOME INSTANCES.

STREETER, G. L.* FOCAL DEFICIENCIES IN FETAL TISSUES AND THEIR RELATION TO INTRA UTERINE AMPUTATION. CONTRIB. EMBRYOL. CARNEGIE INST. WASHINGTON 22* (NO. 126) 1-144, 1930.

TEMTAMY, S. A.* GENETIC FACTORS IN HAND MALFORMATIONS. PH. D. THESIS, JOHNS HOPKINS UNIVERSITY, 1966.

TORPIN, R.* FETAL MALFORMATIONS CAUSED BY AMNION RUPTURE DURING GESTATION. SPRINGFIELD, ILL.* CHARLES C THOMAS, 1968.

21720 CONVULSIVE DISORDER, FAMILIAL, WITH PRENATAL OR EARLY ONSET

IN UTERO ONSET WAS NOTED BY BADR EL-DIN (1960), WHO DESCRIBED THE CONDITION IN SIBS AS A FAMILIAL CONVULSIVE DISORDER. OTHER FEATURES WERE MENTAL RETARDATION, GENERALIZED HYPERTONUS, REFLEX MYOCLONUS AND DEATH IN THE FIRST YEAR. WINKELMAN AND MOORE (1942) DESCRIBED A SINGLE CASE WITH ANTENATAL ONSET. LIU AND SYLVESTER (1960) REPORTED A DISORDER BEGINNING NEAR OR BEFORE BIRTH AND CHARACTERIZED BY MENTAL DETERIORATION, FITS, SPASTICITY, PARALYSIS, DEAFNESS AND BLINDNESS. THE PARENTS WERE NOT RELATED AND TWO BROTHERS WERE AFFECTED. THE CONDITION COULD, OF COURSE, BE X-LINKED AS WELL AS AUTOSOMAL RECESSIVE. SEE ALSO JOSEPH'S SYNDROME, WHICH HAS CONVULSIONS OF EARLY ONSET AS ONE FEATURE. INTRAUTERINE CONVULSIONS ALSO OCCUR IN PYRIDOXINE DEPENDENCY (BEJSOVEC ET AL., 1967), WHICH IS DISCUSSED ELSEWHERE.

BADR EL-DIN, M. K.* A FAMILIAL CONVULSIVE DISORDER WITH AN UNUSUAL ONSET DURING INTRAUTERINE LIFE. A CASE REPORT. J. PEDIAT. 56* 655-657, 1960.

BEJSOVEC, M., KULENDA, Z. AND PONCA, E.* FAMILIAL INTRAUTERINE CONVULSIONS IN PYRIDOXINE DEPENDENCY. ARCH. DIS. CHILD. 42* 201-207, 1967.

LIU, M. C. AND SYLVESTER, P. E.* FAMILIAL DIFFUSE PROGRESSIVE ENCEPHALOPATHY. ARCH. DIS. CHILD. 35* 345-351, 1960.

WINKELMAN, N. W. AND MOORE, M. T.* PROGRESSIVE DEGENERATIVE ENCEPHALOPATHY (REPORT OF CASE IN INFANCY WITH ANTENATAL ONSET SIMULATING 'SWAYBACK' OF LAMBS). J. NEUROPATH. EXP. NEUROL. 1* 127 ONLY, 1942.

*21730 CORNEA PLANA

IN 1925 FELIX DESCRIBED TWO AFFECTED BROTHERS FROM AN UNCLE-NIECE MATING. IN 1961 FORSIUS REPORTED A STUDY IN FINLAND IN WHICH 19 CASES WERE FOUND IN 9 FAMILIES IN PATTERNS CONSISTENT WITH AUTOSOMAL RECESSIVE INHERITANCE.

FELIX, C. H.* CONGENITALE FAMILIARE CORNEA PLANA. KLIN. MBL. AUGENHEILK. 74* 710-716,, SPRINGFIELD, ILL.* 1925. (PEDIGREE, FIG. 345, P. 448 OF WAARDENBURG, P. J., FRANCESCHETTI, A. AND KLEIN, D. (EDS.)* GENETICS AND OPHTHALMOLOGY, VOL. I. CHARLES C THOMAS, 1961.)

FORSIUS, H.* STUDIEN UBER CORNEA PLANA CONGENITA BEI 19 KRANKEN IN 9 FAMILIEN. ACTA OPHTHAL. 39* 203-221, 1961.

21740 CORNEAL DYSTROPHY AND PERCEPTIVE DEAFNESS

HARBOYAN ET AL. (1971) DESCRIBED THREE SIBS FROM A CONSANGUINEOUS MATING WITH LATE ONSET PERCEPTIVE DEAFNESS AND CORNEAL CLOUDING LIKE THAT OF CONGENITAL HEREDITARY CORNEAL DYSTROPHY (Q.V.).

HARBOYAN, G., MAMO, J., DER KALOUSTIAN, V. AND KARAM, F.* CONGENITAL CORNEAL DYSTROPHY. PROGRESSIVE SENSORINEURAL DEAFNESS IN A FAMILY. ARCH. OPHTHAL. 85* 27-32, 1971.

*21750 CORNEAL DYSTROPHY, BAND-SHAPED (BAND KERATOPATHY)

STREIFF AND ZWAHLEN (1946) OBSERVED THE RARE HEREDITARY FORM OF BAND-SHAPED CORNEAL DYSTROPHY IN THREE OF 9 CHILDREN OF A FIRST-COUSIN MATING. THE OPACITY BEGAN AT PUBERTY IN TWO BUT WAS ALREADY PRESENT AT BIRTH IN THE THIRD. THE OPACITY FORMS A WELL-DELIMITED BAND ACROSS THE CORNEA AT THE LEVEL OF THE PUPIL AND OCCUPYING THE REGION OF THE PALPEBRAL FISSURE. IT IS DENSER CENTRALLY AND CONSISTS OF MANY SMALL GRAYISH ELEMENTS LIKE TAPIOCA GRAINS. CORNEAL DIAGRAMS AND THE PEDIGREE ARE REPRODUCED BY WAARDENBURG (1961). BAND KERATOPATHY MAY OCCUR IN HYPERCALCEMIA, STILL'S JUVENILE ARTHRITIS, TUBEROUS SCLEROSIS, FANCONI'S SYNDROME,

RECESSIVE

HYPOPHOSPHATASIA, ETC. BROTHER AND SISTER, AGES 11 AND 16, WERE REPORTED BY FUCHS (1939). ON THE OTHER HAND FATHER AND SON WERE REPORTED BY GLEES (1950).

FUCHS, A.* UBER PRIMARE GURTELFORMIGE HORNHAUTTRUBUNG. KLIN. MBL. AUGENHEILK. 103* 300-309, 1939.

GLEES, M.* UBER FAMILIARES AUFTRETEN DER PRIMAREN BANDFORMIGEN HORNHAUTDE-GENERATION. KLIN. MBL. AUGENHEILK. 116* 185-187, 1950.

STREIFF, E. B. AND ZWAHLEN, P.* UNE FAMILLE AVEC DEGENERESCENCE EN BANDELETTE DE LA CORNEE. OPHTHALMOLOGICA III* 129-134, 1946. (SEE ALSO FIG. 392 IN, WAARDENBURG, P. J., FRANCESCHETTI, A. AND KLEIN, D. (EDS.)* GENETICS AND OPHTHAL-MOLOGY. SPRINGFIELD, ILL.* CHARLES C THOMAS, 1* 485 ONLY, 1961.).

21760 CORNEAL DYSTROPHY, CENTRAL TYPE

FRANCOIS (1958) DESCRIBED A BROTHER AND SISTER, AGES 50 AND 35, RESPECTIVELY, WITH WHAT HE CONSIDERED TO BE A 'NEW' TYPE OF HEREDITARY CORNEAL DYSTROPHY. THEY REFERRED TO IT AS 'DYSTROPHIE CORNEENNE NUAGEUSE CENTRALE.'

FRANCOIS, J.* L'HEREDITE EN OPHTHALMOLOGIE. PARIS* MASSON, 1958.

*21770 CORNEAL DYSTROPHY, CONGENITAL HEREDITARY

MAUMENEE (1960) REPORTED SEVERAL CASES IN WHICH FAMILY HISTORIES SUGGESTED RECESSIVE INHERITANCE. IN EACH OF TWO FAMILIES A BROTHER AND SISTER WERE AFFECTED. ONE WAS A NEGRO FAMILY (L. M. 644879 AND F. M. 644875) AND THE OTHER WAS A WEST VIRGINIAN WHITE FAMILY (J. M. 354118 AND W. M. 354126). IN VIEW OF THE DEGREE OF CORNEAL CLOUDING, VISION IS OFTEN REMARKABLY GOOD. REDMOND (1946) DESCRIBED 3 AFFECTED DAUGHTERS OF NORMAL BUT CONSANGUINEOUS PARENTS.

MAUMENEE, A. E.* CONGENITAL HEREDITARY CORNEAL DYSTROPHY. AM. J. OPHTHAL. 50* 1114-1124, 1960.

REDMOND, S. P.* THREE SISTERS SHOWING CONGENITAL OPACITIES IN THE CORNEA. TRANS. OPHTHAL. SOC. U.K. 66* 367-368, 1946.

WAARDENBURG, P. J., FRANCESCHETTI, A. AND KLEIN, D. S. (EDS.)* IN, GENETICS AND OPHTHALMOLOGY. SPRINGFIELD, ILL.* CHARLES C THOMAS, 1* 485 ONLY, 1961.

*21780 CORNEAL DYSTROPHY, MACULAR TYPE (GROENOUW'S TYPE II)

THE DIFFERENTIATION FROM THE GRANULAR AND LATTICE TYPES (SEE DOMINANT CATALOG) WAS DISCUSSED BY JONES AND ZIMMERMAN (1961). ONSET OCCURS IN THE FIRST DECADE, USUALLY BETWEEN AGES 5 AND 9. THE DISORDER IS PROGRESSIVE. MINUTE, GRAY, PUNCTATE OPACITIES DEVELOP. CORNEAL SENSITIVITY IS USUALLY REDUCED. PAINFUL ATTACKS WITH PHOTOPHOBIA, FOREIGN BODY SENSATIONS, AND RECURRENT EROSIONS OCCUR IN MOST PATIENTS. ACID MUCOPOLYSACCHARIDES ARE DEMONSTRABLE IN CORNEAL FIBROBLASTS. KLINTWORTH AND VOGEL (1964) SUGGESTED THAT THIS IS A LOCALIZED MUCOPOLYSACCHARIDE.

BLUM, J. D.* RELATIONS ENTRE LES DEGENERESCENCES HEREDO-FAMILIALES ET LES OPACITIES CONGENITALES DE LA CORNEE (ETUDE CLINIQUE ET GENEALOGIQUE). OPHTHALMO-LOGICA 109* 123-136, 1944.

GOLDBERG, M. F., MAUMENEE, A. E., AND MCKUSICK, V. A.* CORNEAL DYSTROPHIES ASSOCIATED WITH ABNORMALITIES OF MUCOPOLYSACCHARIDE METABOLISM. ARCH. OPHTHAL. 74* 516-520, 1965.

JONES, S. T. AND ZIMMERMAN, L. E.* HISTOPATHOLOGIC DIFFERENTIATION OF GRANULAR, MACULAR AND LATTICE DYSTROPHIES OF THE CORNEA. AM. J. OPHTHAL. 51* 394-410, 1961.

KLINTWORTH, G. K. AND VOGEL, F. S.* MACULAR CORNEAL DYSTROPHY. AN INHERITED ACID MUCOPOLYSACCHARIDE STORAGE DISEASE OF THE CORNEAL FIBROBLAST. AM. J. PATH. 45* 565-586, 1964.

21790 CORNELIA DE LANGE SYNDROME (TYPUS DEGENERATIVUS AMSTELODAMENSIS)

IN 1933 IN AMSTERDAM, CORNELIA DE LANGE DESCRIBED TWO INFANT GIRLS WITH MENTAL DEFICIENCY AND OTHER FEATURES. THE FACIES ARE CURIOUS, WITH EYEBROWS GROWING ACROSS THE BASE OF THE NOSE (SYNOPHRYS), HAIR GROWING WELL DOWN ONTO THE FOREHEAD, AND LOW ON THE NECK, UNUSUALLY LONG EYELASHES, DEPRESSED BRIDGE OF NOSE WHICH HAS UPTILTED TIP AND FORWARD-DIRECTED NOSTRILS, SMALL WIDELY SPACED TEETH, SMALL HEAD AND LOW-SET EARS. 'THE HANDS ARE CHARACTERISTIC, WITH FLAT SPADE-LIKE APPEARANCE AND SHORT TAPERING FINGERS, THE FIFTH ESPECIALLY SO AND CURVED INWARDS. A SINGLE DEEP TRANSVERSE CREASE WAS SEEN OVER THE PALMS' (SCHLESINGER AND COLLEAGUES, 1963). THE THUMBS APPEAR TO ARISE FROM A POSITION ABNORMALLY FAR PROXIMAL. THE THENAR EMINENCE IS INCONSPICUOUS SO THAT THE THUMB SUGGESTS A LOBSTER CLAW. LARGE JOINTS SHOW LIMITATION OF MOTION. AT TIMES ABSENCE DEFORMITY, USUALLY OF ONE ARM ONLY, IS SEVERE SO THAT ONLY A SINGLE FINGER REMAINS ON A SHORT ARM. A CASE WAS REPORTED BY ULLRICH (1951).
IN SOME INSTANCES (E.G., BORGHI ET AL., 1954), MULTIPLE SIBS HAVE BEEN AFFECTED WITH BOTH PARENTS NORMAL. ALTHOUGH PTACEK ET AL. (1963) SUGGESTED

R
E
C
E
S
S
I
V
E

DOMINANT INHERITANCE, OPITZ (1964) LATER THOUGHT RECESSIVE INHERITANCE LIKELY. NO
CHROMOSOMAL ABNORMALITY HAS BEEN RELATED TO THE SYNDROME. THE LARGE NUMBER OF
DE LANGE CASES FOUND TO HAVE ONE OR ANOTHER TYPE OF CHROMOSOMAL ABERRATION MAY BE
FORTUITOUS, MAY INDICATE A PREDISPOSITION TO CHROMOSOMAL CHANGE INDUCED IN SOME
WAY BY A POINT MUTATION (AS IN BLOOM'S SYNDROME AND IN FANCONI PANMYELOPATHY), OR
MAY INDEED HAVE CAUSE-AND-EFFECT RELATIONSHIP. ACCORDING TO CRAIG AND LUZZATTI
(1965), 11 OUT OF 38 PATIENTS IN WHOM THE CHROMOSOMES HAVE BEEN STUDIED SHOWED
ABNORMALITIES. THEY FELT THIS WAS MORE THAN CHANCE ASSOCIATION. FALEK, SCHMIDT
AND JERVIS (1966) DESCRIBED THREE AFFECTED SIBS AND THEIR AFFECTED FIRST COUSINS.
PATIENTS SHOWED 46 CHROMOSOMES WITH LOSS OF ONE SMALL ACROCENTRIC OF THE G GROUP
AND AN ADDITIONAL METACENTRIC CHROMOSOME RESEMBLING, BUT SOMEWHAT SMALLER THAN,
THE 16TH CHROMOSOME. SIX PHENOTYPICALLY NORMAL RELATIVES INCLUDING ONE PARENT OF
EACH OF THE TWO AFFECTED SIBSHIPS HAD THE SAME ANOMALOUS CHROMOSOME AS THE
AFFECTED CHILDREN BUT IN ADDITION AN APPARENT DELETION OF ONE CHROMOSOME 3. THE
AUTHORS SUGGESTED THAT THE CORNELIA DE LANGE SYNDROME IS DUE TO EXCESSIVE
CHROMOSOME 3 MATERIAL. THE ANOMALOUS CHROMOSOME WAS INTERPRETED AS COMBINING ONE
G CHROMOSOME WITH A FRAGMENT FROM ONE CHROMOSOME 3. MCARTHUR AND EDWARDS (1967)
FOUND NORMAL CHROMOSOMES IN ALL 20 OF THEIR CASES. HOWEVER, THEY EXPRESSED THE
OPINION THAT THE CONDITION IS MOST LIKELY RELATED TO A CHROMOSOMAL DEFICIENCY
WHICH IS NOT USUALLY DETECTABLE. THIS WOULD EXPLAIN BOTH THE USUAL SPORADIC
NATURE AND THE OCCASIONAL FAMILIAL OCCURRENCE. BROHOLM ET AL. (1968) DESCRIBED A
PATIENT WITH CORNELIA DE LANGE SYNDROME AND A B-D TRANSLOCATION INHERITED FROM THE
NORMAL MOTHER. THE PATIENT WAS THOUGHT TO BE PARTIALLY TRISOMIC FOR A GROUP D
CHROMOSOME. PASHAYAN ET AL. (1969) CONCLUDED THAT THE RECESSIVE HYPOTHESIS CAN BE
REJECTED. THE EMPIRIC RECURRENCE RISK IN A SIB OF AN AFFECTED CHILD WAS ESTIMATED
TO BE BETWEEN 2 AND 5 PERCENT. FAMILIAL OCCURRENCE AND PARENTAL CONSANGUINITY
WERE NOTED BY PEARCE ET AL. (1967). OPITZ (1971) FOUND NORMAL PARENTAL AGE
(AVERAGE PATERNAL AND MATERNAL AGE 30.6 AND 28.9 YEARS, RESPECTIVELY), SUGGESTING
A NEW DOMINANT MUTATION.

    BORGHI, A., GIUSTI, G. AND BIGOZZI, U.* NANISMO DEGENERATIVO TIPO DI AMSTERDAM
(TYPUS AMSTELODAMENSIS - MALATTIA DI CORNELIA DE LANGE)* PRESENTAZIONE DI UN CASO
E CONSIDERAZIONI DI ORDINE GENETICO. ACTA GENET. MED. GEM. 3* 365-372, 1954.

    BROHOLM, K.-A., EEG-OLOFSSON, O. AND HALL, B.* AN INHERITED CHROMOSOME
ABERRATION IN A GIRL WITH SIGNS OF DE LANGE SYNDROME. ACTA PAEDIAT. SCAND. 57*
547-552, 1968.

    CRAIG, A. P. AND LUZZATTO, L.* TRANSLOCATION IN DE LANGE'S SYNDROME. LANCET 2*
445-446, 1965.

    DE LANGE, C.* SUR UN TYPE NOUVEAU DE DEGENERATION (TYPUS AMSTELODAMENSIS).
ARCH. MED. ENF. 36* 713-719, 1933.

    FALEK, A., SCHMIDT, R. AND JERVIS, G. A.* FAMILIAL DE LANGE SYNDROME WITH
CHROMOSOME ABNORMALITIES. PEDIATRICS 37* 92-101, 1966.

    MCARTHUR, R. G. AND EDWARDS, J. H.* DE LANGE SYNDROME* REPORT OF 20 CASES.
CANAD. MED. ASS. J. 96* 1185-1198, 1967.

    OPITZ, J. M.* COMMENT. IN, GELLIS, S. S. (ED.)* YEAR BOOK OF PEDIATRICS, 1971.
CHICAGO* YEAR BOOK MEDICAL PUBLISHERS, 1971. P. 489.

    OPITZ, J. M., SEGAL, A. T., LEHRKE, R. L., NADLER, H. L.* THE ETIOLOGY OF THE
BRACHMANN-DE LANGE SYNDROME. BIRTH DEFECTS REPRINT SERIES, NATIONAL FOUNDATION -
MARCH OF DIMES, 1964. PP. 22-23.

    PASHAYAN, H., WHELAN, D., GUTTMAN, S. AND FRASER, F. C.* VARIABILITY OF THE
DE LANGE SYNDROME* REPORT OF 3 CASES AND GENETIC ANALYSIS OF 54 FAMILIES. J.
PEDIAT. 75* 853-858, 1969.

    PAYNE, H. W. AND MAEDA, W. K.* THE CORNELIA DE LANGE SYNDROME* CLINICAL AND
CYTOGENETIC INTERPRETATIONS. CANAD. MED. ASS. J. 93* 577-586, 1965.

    PEARCE, P. M., PITT, D. B. AND ROBOZ, P.* SIX CASES OF THE DE LANGE'S SYNDROME*
PARENTAL CONSANGUINITY IN TWO. MED. J. AUST. 1* 502-506, 1967.

    PTACEK, L. J., OPITZ, J. M., SMITH, D. W., GERRITSEN, T. AND WAISMAN, H. A.*
THE CORNELIA DE LANGE SYNDROME. J. PEDIAT. 63* 1000-1020, 1963.

    SCHLESINGER, B., CLAYTON, B., BODIAN, M. AND JONES, K. V.* TYPUS DEGENERATIVUS
AMSTELODAMENSIS. ARCH. DIS. CHILD. 38* 349-357, 1963.

    SMITH, G. F.* A STUDY OF THE DERMATOGLYPHS IN THE DE LANGE SYNDROME. J. MENT.
DEFIC. RES. 10* 241-247, 1966.

    ULLRICH, O.* TYPUS AMSTELODAMENSIS (CORNELIA DE LANGE). ERGEBN. INN. MED.
KINDERHEILK. 2* 454-458, 1951.

21800 CORPUS CALLOSUM, AGENESIS OF

NAIMAN AND FRASER (1955) DESCRIBED TWO SISTERS AND ZIEGLER (1958) DESCRIBED TWO

BROTHERS WITH AGENESIS OF THE CORPUS CALLOSUM ASSOCIATED WITH MENTAL AND PHYSICAL RETARDATION. AN X-LINKED FORM (Q.V.) DESCRIBED BY MENKES ET AL. HAD ADDITIONAL DEVELOPMENTAL ABNORMALITIES OF THE BRAIN.

NAIMAN, J. AND FRASER, F. C.* AGENESIS OF THE CORPUS CALLOSUM. A REPORT OF TWO CASES IN SIBLINGS. ARCH. NEUROL. PSYCHIAT. 74* 182-185, 1955.

ZIEGLER, E.* BOSARTIGE FAMILIARE FRUHINFANTILE KRAMPFKRANKHEIT, TEILWEISE VERBUNDEN MIT FAMILIARER BALKENAPLASIE. HELV. PAEDIAT. ACTA 13* 169-184, 1958.

*21810 CRANIAL NERVES, CONGENITAL PARESIS OF

STARK (1940) OBSERVED CONGENITAL WEAKNESS OF CRANIAL NERVES III, IV AND VII IN TWO SISTERS AND A BROTHER FROM A CONSANGUINEOUS MATING. THOMAS (1898) DESCRIBED CONGENITAL FACIAL PARALYSIS IN TWO BROTHERS WHO ALSO HAD MALFORMED EXTERNAL EARS. CADWALADER (1922) REPORTED AFFECTED SIBS FROM A FIRST COUSIN MARRIAGE.

CADWALADER, W. B.* TWO CASES OF AGENESIS (CONGENITAL PARALYSIS) OF THE CRANIAL NERVES. AM. J. MED. SCI. 163* 744-748, 1922.

HENDERSON, J. L.* THE CONGENITAL FACIAL DIPLEGIA SYNDROME* CLINICAL FEATURES, PATHOLOGY AND AETIOLOGY. A REVIEW OF 61 CASES. BRAIN 62* 381-403, 1939.

STARK, T.* UEBER KONGENITALE UND PROGRESSIVE OPHTHALMOPLEGIEN (UNTER BERUCKSTI-GUNG DES *INFANTILEN MOEBIUSSCHEN KERNSCHWUNDS*). ZBL. GES. OPHTHAL. 43* 148-149, 1940.

THOMAS, H. M.* CONGENITAL FACIAL PARALYSIS. J. NERV. MENT. DIS. 25* 571-593, 1898.

21820 CRANIAL NERVES, RECURRENT PARESIS OF

IN THE OFFSPRING OF JEWISH FIRST COUSINS, CURRIE (1970) DESCRIBED 4 SIBS (3 BROTHERS AND A SISTER) OF 5 WHO SUFFERED RECURRENT EPISODES OF BELL'S PALSY AND EXTERNAL OPHTHALMOPLEGIA. ALL 4 HAD BELL'S PALSY TO A TOTAL OF 7 EPISODES. THREE HAD A TOTAL OF 4 EPISODES OF OCULAR PALSY. ONE BROTHER HAD PROVED DIABETES AND ONE HAD LATENT DIABETES. ONE HAD POLYCYTHEMIA. THE EPISODES WERE CHARACTERISTIC OF THOSE IN DIABETICS. THE LACK OF IRIDOPLEGIA WITH THE THIRD NERVE PALSY DISTINGUISHES THE OCULAR PALSY FROM THAT OF BERRY ANEURYSM. THIS IS PROBABLY JUST A CHANCE FAMILIAL AGGREGATION OF CRANIAL NEUROPATHY IN DIABETES.

CURRIE, S.* FAMILIAL OCULOMOTOR PALSY WITH BELL'S PALSY. BRAIN 93* 193-198, 1970.

*21830 CRANIODIAPHYSEAL DYSPLASIA

CRANIAL AND FACIAL HYPEROSTOSIS RESULTS IN A CHARACTERISTIC CLINICAL AND RADIOGRA-PHIC APPEARANCE. THE DIAPHYSES OF THE BONES ARE GENERALLY EXPANDED. HALLIDAY (1949) AND STRANSKY (1962) REPORTED ISOLATED CASES VERY SIMILAR IN FINDINGS. FACIAL AND CRANIAL THICKENING AND DISTORTION ARE PARTICULARLY STRIKING IN THIS FORM. MOST CASES HAVE BEEN MENTALLY RETARDED. UNLIKE THE SITUATION IN THE CRANIOMETAPHYSEAL DYSPLASIAS (Q.V.), THE LONG BONES DO NOT SHOW METAPHYSEAL FLARING BUT SHOW DIAPHYSEAL ENDOSTOSIS AND A SHAPE LIKE A POLICEMAN'S NIGHTSTICK. AFFECTED MALE AND FEMALE SIBS WERE REPORTED BY DE SOUZA (1927) AND THE PARENTS OF HALLIDAY'S CASE (1949) WERE RELATED. JOSEPH ET AL. (1958), WHO FIRST SUGGESTED THE DESIGNATION OF PROGRESSIVE CRANIO-DIAPHYSEAL DYSPLASIA, DESCRIBED A PATIENT WITH A PICTURE THEY CONSIDERED IDENTICAL TO THAT DESCRIBED BY HALLIDAY.

DE SOUZA, O.* LEONTIASIS OSSEA. PORTO ALEGRE (BRAZIL) FACULDADE DE MED. REV. DOS. CURSOS. 13* 47-54, 1927.

HALLIDAY, J.* RARE CASE OF BONE DYSTROPHY. BRIT. J. SURG. 37* 52-63, 1949.

JOSEPH, R., LEFEBVRE, J., GUY, E. AND JOB, J. C.* DYSPLASIE CRANIO-DIAPHYSAIRE PROGRESSIVE. SES RELATIONS AVEC LA DYSPLASIE DIAPHYSAIRE PROGRESSIVE DE CAMURATI-ENGELMANN. ANN. RADIOL. 1* 477-490, 1958.

STRANSKY, E., MABILANGAN, L. AND LARA, R. T.* ON PAGET'S DISEASE WITH LEONTIA-SIS OSSEA AND HYPOTHYREOSIS, STARTING IN EARLY CHILDHOOD. ANN. PAEDIAT. 199* 399-408, 1962.

*21840 CRANIOMETAPHYSEAL DYSPLASIA

BOTH DOMINANT AND RECESSIVE FORMS HAVE BEEN IDENTIFIED. THE RECESSIVE FORM IS MORE SEVERE THAN THE DOMINANT FORM. NASAL OBSTRUCTION IS USUALLY COMPLETE AND INVOLVEMENT OF CRANIAL NERVES IS THE RULE. CASE 4 OF JACKSON ET AL. (1954) WAS BLIND FROM OPTIC ATROPHY AT 15 MONTHS. DEAFNESS AND FACIAL PALSY ARE THE RULE. AFFECTED SIBS WERE DESCRIBED BY MILLARD ET AL. (1967) AND BY LEHMANN (1957) AND PARENTAL CONSANGUINITY WAS RECORDED BY LIEVRE AND FISCHGOLD (1956).

JACKSON, W. P. U., HANELIN, J. AND ALBRIGHT, F.* METAPHYSEAL DYSPLASIA, EPIPHYSEAL DYSPLASIA, DIAPHYSEAL DYSPLASIA, AND RELATED CONDITIONS* FAMILIAL

R
E
C
E
S
S
I
V
E

LEHMANN, E. C. H.* FAMILIAL OSTEODYSTROPHY OF THE SKULL AND FACE. J. BONE
JOINT SURG. 39B* 313-315, 1957.

LIEVRE, J. A. AND FISCHGOLD, H.* LEONTIASIS OSSEA CHEZ L'ENFANT (OSTEOPETROSE
PARTIELLE PROBABLE). PRESSE MED. 64* 763-765, 1956.

MILLARD, D. R., MAISELS, D. D., BATSTONE, J. H. F. AND YATES, B. W.* CRANIOFA-
CIAL SURGERY IN CRANIOMETAPHYSEAL DYSPLASIA. AM. J. SURG. 113* 615-621, 1967.

21850 CRANIOSTENOSIS

IN THE AMISH OF HOLMES COUNTY (OHIO), CROSS (1969) OBSERVED MULTIPLE CASES OF
CRANIOSTENOSIS IN A PEDIGREE PATTERN CONSISTENT WITH AUTOSOMAL RECESSIVE INHERI-
TANCE. MOST OTHER REPORTS HAVE SUGGESTED DOMINANT INHERITANCE (Q.V.). HOWEVER,
DUGUID (1929) FOUND IT IN 4 SIBS. GILLOT ET AL. (1960) FOUND CRANIOSTENOSIS IN A
BROTHER AND SISTER WHOSE PARENTS AND THREE SIBS WERE UNAFFECTED. GAUDIER ET AL.
(1967) REVIEWED THE SUBJECT AND REPORTED A SERIES OF CASES WHICH INCLUDED AN
AFFECTED BROTHER AND SISTER. CRANIOSTENOSIS IS A FEATURE OF HYPOPHOSPHATASIA
(Q.V.). ARMENDARES (1967) ALSO CONCLUDED THAT INHERITANCE IS RECESSIVE.

ARMENDARES, S.* THE INHERITANCE OF CRANIOSTENOSIS* STUDY OF THIRTEEN FAMILIES.
MEETING, AM. SOC. HUM. GENET., TORONTO, DEC. 1-3, 1967.

CROSS, H. E. AND OPITZ, J.* CRANIOSYNOSTOSIS IN THE AMISH. J. PEDIAT. 75*
1037-1044, 1969.

DUGUID, H.* AN INSTANCE OF FAMILIAL SCAPHOCEPHALY. J. MENT. SCI. 75* 704-706,
1929.

GAUDIER, B., LAINE, E., FONTAINE, G., CASTIER, C. AND FARRIAUX, J.-P.* LES
CRANIOSYNOSTOSES (ETUDE DE VINGT OBSERVATIONS). ARCH. FRANC. PEDIAT. 24* 775-792,
1967.

GILLOT, F., MARCHIONI, J. AND REIBEL, C.* CRANIOSTENOSE FAMILIALE. PEDIATRIE
15* 695-697, 1960.

21860 CRANIOSYNOSTOSIS WITH RADIAL DEFECTS

BALLER (1950) DESCRIBED A FEMALE WITH OXYCEPHALY AND ABSENT RADIUS. THE PARENTS
WERE THIRD COUSINS. GEROLD (1959) DESCRIBED A BROTHER AND SISTER, AGED 16 YEARS
AND 2 DAYS, WITH TOWER SKULL, RADIAL APLASIA AND SLIGHT ULNAR HYPOPLASIA.

BALLER, F.* RADIUSAPLASIE UND INZUCHT. Z. MENSCHL. VERERB. KONSTITUTIONSL. 29*
782-790, 1950.

GEROLD, M.* FRAKTURHEILUNG BEI EINEM SELTENEN FALL KONGENITALER ANOMALIE DER
OBEREN GLIEDMASSEN. (HEALING OF A FRACTURE IN AN UNUSUAL CASE OF CONGENITAL
ANOMALY OF THE UPPER EXTREMITIES). ZBL. CHIR. 84* 831-834, 1959.

*21870 CRETINISM, ATHYREOTIC

ATHYREOTIC CRETINISM IS NOT AS CLEARLY MENDELIZING AS IS GOITROUS CRETINISM.
THERE IS SOME FAMILIAL AGGREGATION WHICH MAY BE OF THE SAME TYPE AS IS SEEN WITH
MANY COMMON CONGENITAL MALFORMATIONS. IT IS NOTEWORTHY THAT WHETHER GOITER IS
PRESENT OR NOT IS DEPENDENT ON AGE AND TREATMENT. UNDER CERTAIN CIRCUMSTANCES A
PATIENT WHO HAS THE SAME DEFECT AS IN ONE OF THE TYPES OF GOITROUS CRETINISM MAY
APPEAR TO BE ATHYREOTIC (BEIERWALTES, 1964). BLIZZARD AND OTHERS (1960) HAVE
SUGGESTED THAT MATERNAL AUTOANTIBODIES MAY BE RESPONSIBLE FOR DESTRUCTION OF THE
FETAL THYROID. THEY OBSERVED THE BIRTH OF TWO SUCCESSIVE CRETINS FROM A MOTHER
WITH ANTIBODIES. ANTIBODIES WERE IMPLICATED IN THE FAMILIAL CASES OF SUTHERLAND
ET AL. (1960). THIS COULD BE A NON-GENETIC MECHANISM OF FAMILIAL OCCURRENCE OF
ATHYREOTIC CRETINISM. ALTHOUGH USUALLY THESE CASES, LIKE THOSE OF PANHYPOPITUI-
TARISM, ARE SPORADIC, IN 152 CASES IN WILKINS' CLINIC ONE PAIR OF SIBS WAS FOUND
(1965). AINGER AND KELLEY (1955) REPORTED THREE SIBS, AND SUTHERLAND AND
COLLEAGUES (1960) THREE SIBS. FEMALES ARE AFFECTED ABOUT TWICE AS OFTEN AS MALES.
MYOTONIA AND MUSCULAR PSEUDOHYPERTROPHY OCCUR IN SOME OF THESE PATIENTS, THE SO-
CALLED KOCHER-DEBRE-SEMELAIGNE SYNDROME. ATHYREOTIC CRETINISM IS PROBABLY AS
HETEROGENEOUS A CATEGORY AS GOITROUS CRETINISM. THE JUSTIFICATION FOR MARKING
THIS ITEM WITH AN ASTERISK COMES FROM THE EVIDENCE THAT AT LEAST ONE FORM OF
ATHYREOTIC CRETINISM IS INHERITED AS A RECESSIVE. IN AN INBRED AMISH GROUP (CROSS
AND COLLEAGUES, 1968), WE HAVE OBSERVED TWO SISTERS WITH CRETINISM AND THE KOCHER-
DEBRE-SEMELAIGNE SYNDROME. ALTHOUGH NO THYROID WAS PALPABLE, SENSITIVE SCANNING
TECHNIQUES SHOWED THE PRESENCE OF A SMALL AMOUNT OF THYROID TISSUE IN THE NECK.
THUS, 'AGOITROUS CRETINISM' IS A BETTER DESIGNATION THAN ATHYREOTIC CRETINISM.
GREIG ET AL. (1966) DESCRIBED TWO PAIRS OF MONOZYGOTIC TWINS WITH THE CO-TWINS
BOTH AFFECTED IN EACH CASE. ONE PAIR WAS CONSIDERED ATHYREOTIC AND THE OTHER HAD
RESIDUAL THYROID AND ECTOPIC TISSUE, RESPECTIVELY. IN ANOTHER INSTANCE A MOTHER
AND CHILD WERE AFFECTED. THE FATHER WAS UNKNOWN AND PRESUMABLY INCEST WAS

POSSIBLE, MAKING RECESSIVE INHERITANCE LIKELY IN THAT INSTANCE ALSO. THE AUTHORS REFERRED TO THE CONDITION AS THYROID DYSGENESIS.

AINGER, L. E. AND KELLEY, V. C.* FAMILIAL ATHYREOTIC CRETINISM* REPORT OF 3 CASES. J. CLIN. ENDOCR. 15* 469-475, 1955.

BEIERWALTES, W. H.* GENETICS OF THYROID DISEASE. IN, HAZARD, J. B. AND SMITH, D. E. (EDS.)* THE THYROID. BALTIMORE* WILLIAMS AND WILKINS, 1964.

BLIZZARD, R. M., CHANDLER, R. W., LANDING, B. H., PETTIT, M. D. AND WEST, C. D.* MATERNAL AUTOIMMUNIZATION TO THYROID AS A PROBABLE CAUSE OF ATHYROTIC CRETINISM. NEW ENG. J. MED. 263* 327-336, 1960.

CROSS, H. E., HOLLANDER, C. S., RIMOIN, D. L. AND MCKUSICK, V. A.* FAMILIAL AGOITROUS CRETINISM ACCOMPANIED BY MUSCULAR HYPERTROPHY. PEDIATRICS 41* 413-420, 1968.

GREIG, W. R., HENDERSON, A. S., BOYLE, J. A., MCGIRR, E. M. AND HUTCHISON, J. H.* THYROID DYSGENESIS IN TWO PAIRS OF MONOZYGOTIC TWINS AND IN A MOTHER AND CHILD. J. CLIN. ENDOCR. 26* 1309-1316, 1966.

NAJJAR, S. S. AND NACHMAN, H. S.* THE KOCHER-DEBRE-SEMELAIGNE SYNDROME. HYPOTHYROIDISM WITH MUSCULAR 'HYPERTROPHY.' J. PEDIAT. 66* 901-908, 1965.

SUTHERLAND, J. M., ESSELBORN, V. M., BURKET, R. L., SKILLMAN, T. B. AND BENSON, J. T.* FAMILIAL NONGOITROUS CRETINISM APPARENTLY DUE TO MATERNAL ANTITHYROID ANTIBODY. NEW ENG. J. MED. 263* 336-341, 1960.

WILKINS, L.* DIAGNOSIS AND TREATMENT OF ENDOCRINE DISORDERS IN CHILDHOOD AND ADOLESCENCE. SPRINGFIELD, ILL.* CHARLES C THOMAS, 1965 (3RD ED.).

*21880 CRIGLER-NAJJAR SYNDROME

R
E
C
E
S
S
I
V
E

INTENSE JAUNDICE APPEARS IN THE FIRST DAYS OF LIFE AND PERSISTS THEREAFTER. SOME AFFECTED INFANTS DIE IN THE FIRST WEEKS OR MONTHS OF LIFE WITH KERNICTERUS. OTHERS HAVE SURVIVED WITH LITTLE OR NO NEUROLOGIC DEFECT. THE LEVEL OF BILIRUBIN IN THE BLOOD IS IN THE VICINITY OF 20 MG PERCENT WITH MOST OF IT INDIRECT REACTING. CHILDS, SIDBURY AND MIGEON (1959) CONCLUDED THAT TESTS USING SODIUM SALICYLATE SHOW IMPAIRMENT OF GLUCURONIDE CONJUGATION IN HETEROZYGOTES. ONE OF THE AFFECTED SIBSHIPS IN THE INBRED KINDRED REPORTED BY CRIGLER AND NAJJAR (1952) INCLUDED A CASE OF MORQUIO SYNDROME. DIRECT DEMONSTRATION OF THE ENZYME DEFECT WAS PROVIDED BY SZABO AND COLLEAGUES (1962). THE SAME GROUP FOUND REDUCED URINARY EXCRETION OF MENTHOL FOLLOWING ORAL LOADING DOSE IN BOTH PARENTS, THREE GRAND-PARENTS AND SIX SIBS OF A CASE. THE VALUES WERE MIDWAY BETWEEN THOSE OF NORMAL CONTROLS AND THE VERY LOW VALUES OBSERVED IN AFFECTED PERSONS. BOTH PARENTS HAD NORMAL BILIRUBIN TOLERANCE TESTS. BILIRUBIN IS LINKED TO GLUCURONIC ACID BY AN ESTER BOND WHEREAS MENTHOL AND OTHER TEST SUBSTANCES, SUCH AS PARA-AMINOPHENOL, SALICYLAMIDE AND 4-METHYL UMBELLIFERONE, HAVE AN ETHER BOND. SUGAR (1961) DESCRIBED A PATIENT WHO SURVIVED TO ADULTHOOD, MARRIED AND HAD TWO CHILDREN OF WHICH ONE WAS SEVERELY AFFECTED. FURTHER INSIGHT INTO THE NATURAL HISTORY OF THIS DISEASE WAS AFFORDED BY THE OBSERVATIONS OF BLUMENSCHEIN ET AL. (1968). A MALE MEMBER OF THE KINDRED ORIGINALLY STUDIED BY CRIGLER AND NAJJAR WAS NORMAL, APART FROM HIS JAUNDICE, FOR ALL HIS LIFE UNTIL AGE 16 WHEN HE DEVELOPED NEUROLOGIC DISABILITY PROGRESSING TO DEATH AFTER 6 MONTHS. GARDNER AND KONIGSMARK (1969) DESCRIBED THE HISTOPATHOLOGIC FINDINGS IN THAT PATIENT. SEE HYPERBILIRUBINEMIA, ARIAS TYPE, IN DOMINANT CATALOG FOR DISCUSSION OF ANOTHER DEFECT INVOLVING GLUCURONYL TRANSFERASE. BLUMENSCHEIN ET AL. (1968) DESCRIBED THE CLINICAL FEATURES. SOME PRESUMED CASES OF CRIGLER-NAJJAR SYNDROME HAVE BEEN SAID TO RESPOND TO PHENOBARBITAL WITH LOWERING OF SERUM BILIRUBIN (KARON ET AL., 1970). SERUM BILIRUBIN CONCENTRATIONS OF NEWBORN INFANTS CAN BE REDUCED BY EXPOSURE TO SUNLIGHT OR ARTIFICIAL BLUE LIGHT. THIS MEASURE WAS FOUND EFFECTIVE IN A CASE OF PRESUMED CRIGLER-NAJJAR SYNDROME (KARON ET AL., 1970).

BLUMENSCHEIN, S. D., KALLEN, R. J., STOREY, B., NATZSCHKA, J. C., ODELL, G. B. AND CHILDS, B.* FAMILIAL NONHEMOLYTIC JAUNDICE WITH LATE ONSET OF NEUROLOGICAL CHANGE. PEDIATRICS 42* 786-792, 1968.

CHILDS, B., SIDBURY, J. E. AND MIGEON, C. J.* GLUCURONIC ACID CONJUGATION BY PATIENTS WITH FAMILIAL NONHEMOLYTIC JAUNDICE AND THEIR RELATIVES. PEDIATRICS 23* 903-913, 1959.

CRIGLER, J. F., JR. AND NAJJAR, V. A.* CONGENITAL FAMILIAL NONHEMOLYTIC JAUNDICE WITH KERNICTERUS. PEDIATRICS 10* 169-179, 1952.

GARDNER, W. A., JR. AND KONIGSMARK, B. W.* FAMILIAL NONHEMOLYTIC JAUNDICE* BILIRUBINOSIS AND ENCEPHALOPATHY. PEDIATRICS 43* 365-376, 1969.

KARON, M., IMACH, D. AND SCHWARTZ, A.* EFFECTIVE PHOTOTHERAPY IN CONGENITAL NONOBSTRUCTIVE, NONHEMOLYTIC JAUNDICE. NEW ENG. J. MED. 282* 377-380, 1970.

SUGAR, P.* FAMILIAL NONHEMOLYTIC JAUNDICE. CONGENITAL WITH KERNICTERUS. ARCH. INTERN. MED. 108* 121-127, 1961.

SYNDROME BY THE MENTHOL TEST. ACTA PAEDIAT. ACAD. SCI. HUNG. 4* 153-158, 1963.

SZABO, L., KOVACS, Z. AND EBREY, P.* CONGENITAL NON-HAEMOLYTIC JAUNDICE. (LETTER) LANCET 1* 322 ONLY, 1962.

*21890 CROME'S SYNDROME

CROME, DUCKETT AND FRANKLIN (1963) DESCRIBED TWO FEMALE INFANTS WITH AN IDENTICAL DISORDER - CONGENITAL CATARACTS, EPILEPTIC FITS, MENTAL RETARDATION, SMALL STATURE, AND DEATH (AT 4 AND 8 MONTHS). POSTMORTEM SHOWED RENAL TUBULAR NECROSIS AND ENCEPHALOPATHY. THE PARENTS WERE FIRST COUSINS. SIMILARITIES TO MARINESCO-SJOGREN SYNDROME (Q.V.), AND TO LOWE'S SYNDROME WERE POINTED OUT. THE LATTER IS AN X-LINKED RECESSIVE. THE FORMER IS AUTOSOMAL RECESSIVE BUT RENAL CHANGE HAS NOT BEEN DESCRIBED AND SURVIVAL TO A LATER AGE IS USUAL.

CROME, L., DUCKETT, S. AND FRANKLIN, A. W.* CONGENITAL CATARACTS, RENAL TUBULAR NECROSIS AND ENCEPHALOPATHY IN TWO SISTERS. ARCH. DIS. CHILD. 38* 505-515, 1963.

21900 CRYPTOPHTHALMOS WITH OTHER MALFORMATIONS

IN EACH OF THE TWO SIBSHIPS FRASER (1962) OBSERVED TWO SISTERS AFFECTED AT BIRTH BY VARIOUS COMBINATIONS* (A) CRYPTOPHTHALMOS (B) ABSENT OR MALFORMED LACRIMAL DUCTS (C) MIDDLE AND OUTER EAR MALFORMATIONS (D) HIGH PALATE (E) CLEAVAGE ALONG THE MIDPLANE OF NARES AND TONGUE (F) HYPERTELORISM (G) LARYNGEAL STENOSIS (H) SYNDACTYLY (I) WIDE SEPARATION OF SYMPHYSIS PUBIS (J) DISPLACEMENT OF UMBILICUS AND NIPPLES (K) PRIMITIVE MESENTRY OF SMALL BOWEL (L) MALDEVELOPED KIDNEYS (M) FUSION OF LABIA AND ENLARGEMENT OF CLITORIS (N) BICORNUATE UTERUS AND MALFORMED FALLOPIAN TUBES. IN EACH SIBSHIP ONE SISTER WAS STILLBORN AND THE OTHER VIABLE. SEX CHROMATIN WAS POSITIVE IN BOTH SURVIVING INFANTS. NEITHER SET OF PARENTS WAS CONSANGUINEOUS. SEE BOWEN SYNDROME FOR A COMPARABLE BUT PROBABLY DISTINCT SYNDROME OF MULTIPLE CONGENITAL MALFORMATIONS.
GUPTA AND SAXEMA (1962) REPORTED CRYPTOPHTHALMOS IN TWO OFFSPRING OF CONSANGUINEOUS PARENTS. IN ONE IT WAS UNILATERAL AND DEATH OCCURED AT 1 MONTH. IN THE SECOND THE CRYPTOPHTHALMOS WAS BILATERAL AND WAS ACCOMPANIED BY CONGENITAL DEAFNESS, UNDESCENDED TESTES, SMALL PENIS WITH HYPOSPADIAS AND OTHER DEFORMITIES. THE OLDER LITERATURE ON CRYPTOPHTHALMOS WITH ASSOCIATED MALFORMATIONS IS REVIEWED BY DUKE-ELDER (1963). FRANCOIS (1969) DESCRIBED AFFECTED BROTHER AND SISTER AND GAVE A COMPREHENSIVE REVIEW POINTING OUT THE RATHER FREQUENT EXAMPLES OF PARENTAL CONSANGUINITY (ABOUT 15 PERCENT OF CASES) AND OF FAMILIAL CASES. SYNDACTYLY IS A FEATURE OF MANY OF THE CASES.

DUKE-ELDER, S.* SYSTEM OF OPHTHALMOLOGY, NORMAL AND ABNORMAL DEVELOPMENT. ST. LOUIS* C. V. MOSBY CO. 3* (PART 2) 1963. PP. 829-834.

FRANCOIS, J.* SYNDROME MALFORMATIF AVEC CRYPTOPHTALMIE. ACTA GENET. MED. GEM. 18* 18-50, 1969.

FRASER, G. R.* OUR GENETICAL 'LOAD.' A REVIEW OF SOME ASPECTS OF GENETICAL VARIATION. ANN. HUM. GENET. 25* 387-415, 1962.

FRASER, G. R.* XX CHROMOSOMES AND RENAL AGENESIS. (LETTER) LANCET 1* 1427 ONLY, 1966.

GUPTA, S. P. AND SAXEMA, R. C.* CRYPTOPHTHALMOS. BRIT. J. OPHTHAL. 46* 629-632, 1962.

*21910 CUTIS LAXA

GOLTZ, HULT, GOLDFARB AND GORLIN (1965) DESCRIBED AFFECTED BROTHERS AND SUGGESTED RECESSIVE INHERITANCE BECAUSE OF OTHER REPORTED INSTANCES OF AFFECTED SIBS AS WELL AS PARENTAL CONSANGUINITY. ONE CHILD HAD MULTIPLE DIVERTICULA (ESOPHAGUS, DUODENUM, ILEUM, BLADDER). THE OTHER HAD PULMONARY EMPHYSEMA AND DIED AT 18 MONTHS FROM COR PULMONALE. THE AUTHORS SUGGESTED 'GENERALIZED ELASTOLYSIS' AS A MORE SATISFACTORY DESIGNATION. DEATH FROM PULMONARY EMPHYSEMA WAS ALSO DESCRIBED BY CHRISTIAENS ET AL. (1954). HAYDEN ET AL. (1968) DESCRIBED A 4 YEAR OLD PATIENT WITH CUTIS LAXA AND CONGENITAL PULMONARY ARTERY STENOSIS. A DEFICIENCY OF ELASTIC FIBERS IN THE SKIN WAS REPORTED. HAJJAR AND JOYNER (1968) DESCRIBED A 6 MONTH OLD PUERTO RICAN CHILD WITH ADVANCED PULMONARY EMPHYSEMA. SERUM COPPER LEVEL WAS LOW AND URINARY EXCRETION HIGH, CONSISTENT WITH THE THEORY THAT DEFICIENCY OF SERUM COPPER PRODUCES A LOW ELASTASE INHIBITOR SUBSTANCE WITH INCREASED DESTRUCTION OF ELASTIC FIBERS (GOLTZ ET AL., 1965). THE NEGRO PATIENT OF MAXWELL AND ESTERLY (1969) HAD PULMONARY EMPHYSEMA. HERNIAS HAVE BEEN AN IMPORTANT FEATURE OF MANY CASES (SCHREIBER AND TILLEY, 1961* CASHMAN, 1957* GOLTZ ET AL., 1965).

BEIGHTON, P., BULL, J. C. AND EDGERTON, M. T.* PLASTIC SURGERY IN CUTIS LAXA. BRIT. J. PLAST. SURG. 23* 285-290, 1970.

CASHMAN, M. E.* CUTIS LAXA. PROC. ROY. SOC. MED. 50* 719-720, 1957.

CHRISTIAENS, L., MARCHAND-ALPHANT, A. AND FOVET, A.* EMPHYSEME CONGENITAL ET CUTIX LAXA. PRESSE MED. 62* 1799-1801, 1954.

GOLTZ, R. W., HULT, A. M., GOLDFARB, M. AND GORLIN, R. J.* CUTIS LAXA, A MANIFESTATION OF GENERALIZED ELASTOLYSIS. ARCH. DERM. 92* 373-387, 1965.

HAJJAR, B. A. AND JOYNER, E. N.* CONGENITAL CUTIS LAXA WITH ADVANCED CARDIOPUL-MONARY DISEASE. J. PEDIAT. 73* 116-119, 1968.

HAYDEN, J. G., TALNER, N. S. AND KLAUS, S. N.* CUTIS LAXA ASSOCIATED WITH PULMONARY ARTERY STENOSIS. J. PEDIAT. 72* 506-509, 1968.

MAXWELL, E. AND ESTERLY, N. B.* CUTIS LAXA. AM. J. DIS. CHILD. 117* 479-482, 1969.

SCHREIBER, M. M. AND TILLEY, J. C.* CUTIS LAXA. ARCH. DERM. 84* 266-272, 1961.

21920 CUTIS LAXA WITH BONE DYSTROPHY

FITTKE (1942) DESCRIBED A TEN AND ONE HALF MONTH OLD FEMALE WHOSE SKIN FROM BIRTH HAD BEEN IN LOOSE REDUNDANT FOLDS. THE FACE WAS SPARED, HOWEVER. ON STRETCHING, THE SKIN RETURNED ONLY SLOWLY TO ITS ORIGINAL POSITION. THE SKELETAL SYSTEM SHOWED WIDELY PERSISTENT FONTANELLES, SLIGHT OXYCEPHALY, AND DISLOCATION OF ONE HIP. THE PARENTS WERE NOT KNOWN TO BE RELATED BUT LIVED IN THE AREA OF EUROPE WHERE MOST PERSONS WERE RELATED IN SOME DEGREE. THE MOTHER, AGE 25 YEARS, HAD LONG SUFFERED FROM 'WEAK KNEE JOINTS.' AN 8 YEAR OLD COUSIN OF THE PROBAND SHOWED THE SAME SKIN CHANGES, AS WELL AS PIGEON BREAST, STATIC SCOLIOSIS, AND FLAT FEET. THE FONTANELLES HAD NOT CLOSED UNTIL THE THIRD YEAR. THE CASE OF DEBRE ET AL. (1937) MAY BE IDENTICAL.

DEBRE, R., MARIE, J. AND SERINGE, P.* 'CUTIS LAXA' AVEC DYSTROPHIES OSSEUSES. BULL. SOC. MED. HOP. PARIS 53* 1038-1039, 1937.

FITTKE, H.* UBER EINE UNGEWOHNLICHE FORM 'MULTIPLER ERBABARTUNG' (CHALODERMIE UND DYSOSTOSE). Z. KINDERHEILK. 63* 510-523, 1942.

21930 CUTIS VERTICIS GYRATA AND MENTAL DEFICIENCY

MCDOWALL (1893) FIRST DESCRIBED THIS ASSOCIATION WHICH MAY NOT BE RARE SINCE AKESSON (1964) FOUND 47 CASES IN A SURVEY OF INSTITUTIONALIZED MENTAL DEFECTIVES IN SWEDEN. SEE ACROMEGALOID CHANGES, ETC., IN DOMINANT CATALOG.

AKESSON, H. O.* CUTIS VERTICIS GYRATA AND MENTAL DEFICIENCY IN SWEDEN. I. EPIDEMIOLOGIC AND CLINICAL ASPECTS. ACTA MED. SCAND. 175* 115-127, 1964.

AKESSON, H. O.* CUTIS VERTICIS GYRATA AND MENTAL DEFICIENCY IN SWEDEN. II. GENETIC ASPECTS. ACTA MED. SCAND. 177* 459-464, 1965.

MCDOWALL, T. W.* CASE OF ABNORMAL DEVELOPMENT OF THE SCALP. J. MENT. SCI. 39* 62-64, 1893.

21940 CYANOSIS AND HEPATIC DISEASE

SILVERMAN ET AL. (1968) OBSERVED 2 CHILDREN, BROTHER AND SISTER, WHO DEVELOPED DYSPNEA, CYANOSIS AND DIGITAL CLUBBING 11 AND 18 MONTHS AFTER EPISODES OF HEPATITIS. PULMONARY ARTERIOVENOUS FISTULAE TOO SMALL TO BE DEMONSTRATED BY ANGIOGRAPHY WERE POSTULATED.

SILVERMAN, A., COOPER, M. D., MOLLER, J. H. AND GOOD, R. A.* SYNDROME OF CYANOSIS, DIGITAL CLUBBING, AND HEPATIC DISEASE IN SIBLINGS. J. PEDIAT. 72* 70-80, 1968.

*21950 CYSTATHIONINURIA

DURING A SURVEY BY PAPER CHROMATOGRAPHY OF AMINO ACIDS IN THE URINE OF PATIENTS IN AN INSTITUTION FOR MENTAL DEFECTIVES, HARRIS, PENROSE AND THOMAS (1959) DISCOVERED A CASE WITH ABNORMAL EXCRETION OF CYSTATHIONINE. AN INBORN ERROR INVOLVING THE CLEAVAGE OF CYSTATHIONINE TO GIVE CYSTEINE AND HOMOSERINE WAS SUGGESTED. THE SUBJECT WAS A SEVERELY RETARDED FEMALE AGED 64 YEARS AT THE TIME OF STUDY. ANOTHER CASE WAS STUDIED AT THE NEW YORK HOSPITAL. OTHER CLINICAL MANIFESTATIONS HAVE BEEN CLUBFOOT, DEVELOPMENTAL DEFECTS ABOUT THE EARS, CONVULSIONS AND THROMBOCYTOPENIA. URINARY LITHIASIS ALSO OCCURS. FRIMPTER (1965) HAS SHOWN THAT THE DEFECT INVOLVES CYSTATHIONASE WHICH DOES NOT PROPERLY BIND ITS COENZYME, PYRIDOXAL PHOSPHATE. IN VITRO STUDIES SUGGESTED THAT HIGH PYRIDOXINE WOULD BE THERAPEUTICALLY BENEFICIAL. MONGEAU ET AL. (1967) DESCRIBED THE CASE OF A 2 YEAR OLD BOY WITH NORMAL MENTALITY, THROMBOCYTOPENIA AND URINARY CALCULI. THE RELATION OF THE LATTER TWO FEATURES TO THE METABOLIC DEFECT WAS PROBLEMATICAL. BOTH PARENTS (WHO WERE APPARENTLY UNRELATED) SHOWED CYSTATHIONINURIA AFTER METHIONINE LOADING TEST. WITH ADMINISTRATION OF PYRIDOXINE, CYSTATHIONINURIA WAS DIMINISHED IN THE PROBAND. SCHNEIDERMAN (1967) STUDIED TWO MENTALLY RETARDED BROTHERS WHO EXCRETED LARGE AMOUNTS OF CYSTATHIONINE AFTER METHIONINE INGESTION. THE MOTHER AND ANOTHER BROTHER EXCRETED LESSER BUT ABNORMAL AMOUNTS AFTER METHIONINE LOADING. THE FATHER WAS NOT TESTED. PERRY ET AL. (1968) DISCOVERED CYSTATHIONINURIA IN A BROTHER AND SISTER WHEN THE BROTHER'S URINE WAS BY CHANCE SUBJECTED TO 2-DIMEN-SIONAL PAPER CHROMATOGRAPHY FOR AMINO ACIDS. BOTH CHILDREN WERE NORMAL. THE

R
E
C
E
S
S
I
V
E

PARENTS EXCRETED CYSTATHIONINE ONLY AFTER METHIONINE LOADING. THE AUTHORS SUGGESTED THAT MENTAL DEFECT AND OTHER DISORDERS REPORTED IN ASSOCIATION WITH CYSTATHIONINURIA MAY HAVE BEEN COINCIDENTAL. WHELAN AND SCRIVER (1968) ALSO FOUND CYSTATHIONINURIA AS AN APPARENTLY BENIGN INBORN ERROR. THE CASE OF TADA ET AL. (1968) DID NOT RESPOND TO B6.

FRIMPTER, G. W.* CYSTATHIONINURIA* NATURE OF THE DEFECT. SCIENCE 149* 1095-1096, 1965.

FRIMPTER, G. W.* CYSTATHIONINURIA. IN, STANBURY, J. B., WYNGAARDEN, J. B. AND FREDRICKSON, D. S. (EDS.)* THE METABOLIC BASIS OF INHERITED DISEASE. NEW YORK* MCGRAW-HILL, 1966 (2ND ED.). PP. 409-419.

FRIMPTER, G. W., HAYMOVITZ, A. AND HORWITH, M.* CYSTATHIONINURIA. NEW ENG. J. MED. 268* 333-339, 1963.

HARRIS, H., PENROSE, L. S. AND THOMAS, D. H. H.* CYSTATHIONINURIA. ANN. HUM. GENET. 23* 442-453, 1959.

MONGEAU, J.-G., HILGARTNER, M., WORTHEN, H. G., AND FRIMPTER, G. W.* CYSTA-THIONINURIA* STUDY OF AN INFANT WITH NORMAL MENTALITY, THROMBOCYTOPENIA, AND RENAL CALCULI. J. PEDIAT. 69* 1113-1120, 1967.

PERRY, T. L., HARDWICK, D. F., HANSEN, S., LOVE, D. L. AND ISRAELS, S.* CYSTATHIONINURIA IN TWO HEALTHY SIBLINGS. NEW ENG. J. MED. 278* 590-592, 1968.

SCHNEIDERMAN, L. J.* LATENT CYSTATHIONINURIA. J. MED. GENET. 4* 260-263, 1967.

SCOTT, C. R., DASSELL, S. W., CLARK, S. H., CHIANG-TENG, C. AND SWEDBERG, K. R.* CYSTATHIONINEMIA* A BENIGN GENETIC CONDITION. J. PEDIAT. 76* 571-577, 1970.

SHAW, K. N. F., LIEBERMAN, E., KOCH, R. AND DONNELL, G. N.* CYSTATHIONINURIA. AM. J. DIS. CHILD. 113* 119-128, 1967.

TADA, K., YOSHIDA, T., YOKOYAMA, Y., SATO, T., NAKAGAWA, H. AND ARAKAWA, T.* CYSTATHIONINURIA NOT ASSOCIATED WITH VITAMIN B6 DEPENDENCY* A PROBABLY NEW TYPE OF CYSTATHIONINURIA. TOHOKU J. EXP. MED. 95* 235-242, 1968.

WHELAN, D. T. AND SCRIVER, C. R.* CYSTATHIONINURIA AND RENAL IMINOGLYCINURIA IN A PEDIGREE. A PERSPECTIVE ON COUNSELING. NEW ENG. J. MED. 278* 924-927, 1968.

21960 CYSTIC DISEASE OF LUNG

A STRIKINGLY HIGH FREQUENCY OF CYSTIC DISEASE OF THE LUNG HAS BEEN OBSERVED IN "ORIENTAL" (NON-ASHKENAZI) JEWS IN ISRAEL, PARTICULARLY IN YEMENITES (RACZ ET AL., 1965). THE DISEASE MANIFESTS ITSELF RELATIVELY EARLY IN LIFE, EVEN IN THE FIRST DECADE IN SOME AND RECURRENT INFECTION IS THE PRINCIPAL FEATURE. FAMILY STUDIES HAVE NOT BEEN REPORTED. SEE FIBROCYSTIC PULMONARY DYSPLASIA IN THE DOMINANT CATALOG. THE GENETICS OF THIS DISORDER IS UNCLEAR. HOWEVER, THE OBSERVATIONS OF A RELATIVELY HIGH FREQUENCY IN ORIENTAL JEWS IN ISRAEL (BAUM ET AL., 1966) AND IN THE MAORI OF NEW ZEALAND (HINDS, 1958) ARE NOTEWORTHY.

BAUM, G. L., RACZ, I., BUBIS, J. J., MOLHO, M. AND SHAPIRO, B. L.* CYSTIC DISEASE OF THE LUNG. REPORT OF EIGHTY-EIGHT CASES, WITH AN ETHNOLOGIC RELATION-SHIP. AM. J. MED. 40* 578-602, 1966.

HINDS, J. R.* BRONCHIECTASIS IN THE MAORI. NEW ZEAL. MED. J. 57* 328-332, 1958.

RACZ, I. AND BAUM, G. L.* THE RELATIONSHIP OF ETHNIC ORIGIN TO THE PREVALENCE OF CYSTIC LUNG DISEASE IN ISRAEL. A PRELIMINARY REPORT. AM. REV. RESP. DIS. 91* 552-555, 1965.

*21970 CYSTIC FIBROSIS (MUCOVISCIDOSIS)

MANIFESTATIONS RELATE NOT ONLY TO THE DISRUPTION OF EXOCRINE FUNCTION OF THE PANCREAS BUT ALSO TO INTESTINAL GLANDS (MECONIUM ILEUS), BILIARY TREE (BILIARY CIRRHOSIS), BRONCHIAL GLANDS (CHRONIC BRONCHO-PULMONARY INFECTION WITH EMPHYSEMA), AND SWEAT GLANDS (HIGH SWEAT ELECTROLYTE WITH DEPLETION IN A HOT ENVIRONMENT).
ATTEMPTING TOTAL ASCERTAINMENT OF CASES IN WHITE CHILDREN BORN ALIVE IN OHIO DURING THE YEARS 1950 THROUGH 1953, STEINBERG AND BROWN (1960) ESTIMATE THE PHENOTYPE FREQUENCY TO BE ABOUT 1 IN 3,700, A VALUE ONLY ABOUT ONE-FOURTH THAT OF SOME EARLIER ESTIMATES. CYSTIC FIBROSIS EVEN AT THIS LOWER ESTIMATE IS THE MOST FREQUENT LETHAL GENETIC DISEASE OF CHILDHOOD. THE GENE FREQUENCY WAS ESTIMATED TO BE ABOUT .016 AND ABOUT 3 PERCENT OF WHITE PERSONS ARE HETEROZYGOTES. IN CONNECTICUT HONEYMAN AND SIKER (1965) ARRIVED AT HIGHER ESTIMATES OF 1 IN 489 (MAXIMAL) AND 1 IN 1863 (MINIMAL).
ROBERTS (1960) COLLECTED FAMILY DATA WHICH APPEARED TO HIM INCONSISTENT WITH THE QUARTER RATIO EXPECTED OF A RECESSIVE TRAIT. BULMER (1961) POINTED OUT, HOWEVER, THAT WHEN PROPER CORRECTION IS MADE FOR ASCERTAINMENT BIAS THE OBSERVED PROPORTIONS MAY AGREE WITH THOSE EXPECTED FOR A RECESSIVE TRAIT. RECESSIVE INHERITANCE WAS FIRST SHOWN BY LOWE, MAY AND REED (1949). THE OBSERVATION OF

SPOCK ET AL. (1967) THAT PATIENTS HAVE A FACTOR IN SERUM WHICH INHIBITS THE ACTION OF CILIA IN EXPLANTS OF RABBIT TRACHEAL MUCOSA MAY PROVE VERY IMPORTANT. SERUM FROM HETEROZYGOTES CONTAINED AN AMOUNT OF THE FACTOR INTERMEDIATE BETWEEN NONE (THE NORMAL SITUATION) AND THE LEVEL IN PATIENTS. DANES AND BEARN (1968) FOUND, IN SKIN FIBROBLASTS FROM BOTH HOMOZYGOTES AND HETEROZYGOTES, CYTOPLASMIC INTRAVE-SICULAR METACHROMASIA OF A TYPE READILY DISTINGUISHED FROM THAT OF MUCOPOLYSAC-CHARIDOSES. SMITH ET AL. (1968) FOUND CYSTIC FIBROSIS IN A CHILD WITH CRI-DU-CHAT SYNDROME. ONLY THE MOTHER WAS HETEROZYGOUS BY SPOCK TEST. THEY SUGGESTED THAT LOSS OF PART OF THE SHORT ARM OF THE CHROMOSOME 5 DERIVED FROM THE FATHER HAD OCCURRED AND THAT THE DELETED PORTION CARRIES THE CYSTIC FIBROSIS LOCUS. DANES AND BEARN (1968) FOUND VESICULAR METACHROMASIA IN THE FIBROBLASTS OF BOTH PARENTS SUGGESTING THAT THE REPORTED EXPERIENCE CANNOT BE TAKEN AS EVIDENCE OF LOCALIZA-TION OF THE CF GENE ON THE SHORT ARM OF CHROMOSOME 5. DANES AND BEARN (1969) DESCRIBED A MORPHOLOGIC CHANGE IN THE FIBROBLASTS AND FURTHERMORE SUGGESTED THAT HOMOZYGOSITY AT EITHER OF TWO DIFFERENT LOCI CAN PRODUCE CYSTIC FIBROSIS. IN TYPE I THE FIBROBLAST SHOW DISCRETE METACHROMATIC CYTOPLASMIC VESICLES AND NORMAL MUCOPOLYSACCHARIDE CONTENT. IN TYPE II, FIBROBLAST METACHROMASIA IS PRESENT IN BOTH VESICLES AND GRANULES AND IS EVENLY DISTRIBUTED THROUGH THE CYTOPLASM* MUCOPOLYSACCHARIDE CONTENT OF THE CELLS IS MARKEDLY INCREASED. KAPLAN ET AL. (1968) FOUND THAT MALES WITH CYSTIC FIBROSIS ARE INFERTILE BECAUSE OF FAILURE OF NORMAL DEVELOPMENT OF THE VAS DEFERENS. OPPENHEIMER AND ESTERLY (1969) CONCLUDED THAT THE CHANGES IN THE TRANSPORT DUCTS OF THE MALE GENITAL SYSTEM ARE RESPONSIBLE FOR INFERTILITY AND ARE NOT A DEVELOPMENTAL ANOMALY BUT DEGENERATIVE CHANGE DUE TO OBSTRUCTION LIKE THAT WHICH OCCURS IN THE PANCREAS AND SALIVARY GLANDS. FORMERLY KNOWN AS CYSTIC FIBROSIS OF THE PANCREAS, THIS ENTITY HAS INCREASINGLY BEEN LABELLED SIMPLY 'CYSTIC FIBROSIS.' OPPENHEIMER ET AL. (1970) SUGGESTED THAT CHARACTERISTICS OF CERVICAL MUCUS MAY ACCOUNT FOR INFERTILITY IN FEMALES WITH CYSTIC FIBROSIS.

BRUSILOW, S. W.* CYSTIC FIBROSIS IN ADULTS. ANN. REV. MED. 21* 99-104, 1970.

BULMER, M. G.* FIBROCYSTIC DISEASE OF THE PANCREAS* A COMMENT. ANN. HUM. GENET. 25* 163-164, 1961.

DANES, B. S. AND BEARN, A. G.* A GENETIC CELL MARKER IN CYSTIC FIBROSIS OF THE PANCREAS. LANCET 1* 1061-1063, 1968.

DANES, B. S. AND BEARN, A. G.* CYSTIC FIBROSIS OF THE PANCREAS. A STUDY IN CELL CULTURE. J. EXP. MED. 129* 775-794, 1969.

DANES, B. S. AND BEARN, A. G.* CYSTIC FIBROSIS* AN IMPROVED METHOD FOR STUDYING WHITE BLOOD-CELLS IN CULTURE. (LETTER) LANCET 2* 437 ONLY, 1969.

DANES, B. S. AND BEARN, A. G.* CYSTIC FIBROSIS* DISTRIBUTION OF MUCOPOLYSAC-CHARIDES IN FIBROBLAST CULTURES. BIOCHEM. BIOPHYS. RES. COMMUN. 36* 919-924, 1969.

DANES, B. S. AND BEARN, A. G.* LOCALISATION OF THE CYSTIC-FIBROSIS GENE. (LETTER) LANCET 2* 1303 ONLY, 1968.

DANKS, D. M., ALLAN, J. AND ANDERSON, C. M.* A GENETIC STUDY OF FIBROCYSTIC DISEASE OF THE PANCREAS. ANN. HUM. GENET. 28* 323-356, 1965.

DI SANT'AGNESE, P. A. AND TALAMO, R. C.* PATHOGENESIS AND PHYSIOPATHOLOGY OF CYSTIC FIBROSIS OF THE PANCREAS* FIBROCYSTIC DISEASE OF THE PANCREAS (MUCO-VISCIDOSIS). NEW ENG. J. MED. 277* 1287-1274 AND 1344-1352, 1967.

HARRIS, R. L. AND RILEY, H. D., JR.* CYSTIC FIBROSIS IN THE AMERICAN INDIAN. PEDIATRICS 41* 733-738, 1968.

HONEYMAN, M. S. AND SIKER, E.* CYSTIC FIBROSIS OF THE PANCREAS* AN ESTIMATE OF THE INCIDENCE. AM. J. HUM. GENET. 17* 461-465, 1965.

KAPLAN, E., SHWACHMAN, H., PERLMUTTER, A. D., RULE, A., KHAW, K.-T. AND HOLSCLAW, D. S.* REPRODUCTIVE FAILURE IN MALES WITH CYSTIC FIBROSIS. NEW ENG. J. MED. 279* 65-69, 1968.

LOBECK, C. C.* CYSTIC FIBROSIS OF THE PANCREAS. IN, STANBURY, J. B., WYNGAAR-DEN, J. B. AND FREDRICKSON, D. S. (EDS.)* THE METABOLIC BASIS OF INHERITED DISEASE. NEW YORK* MCGRAW-HILL, 1966 (2ND ED.). PP. 1300-1317.

LOWE, C. U., MAY, C. D. AND REED, S. C.* FIBROSIS OF THE PANCREAS IN INFANTS AND CHILDREN* A STATISTICAL STUDY OF CLINICAL AND HEREDITARY FEATURES. AM. J. DIS. CHILD. 78* 349-374, 1949.

MANGOS, J. A. AND MCSHERRY, N. R.* STUDIES ON THE MECHANISM OF INHIBITION OF SODIUM TRANSPORT IN CYSTIC FIBROSIS OF THE PANCREAS. PEDIAT. RES. 2* 378-384, 1968.

OPPENHEIMER, E. H. AND ESTERLY, J. R.* OBSERVATIONS ON CYSTIC FIBROSIS OF THE PANCREAS. V. DEVELOPMENTAL CHANGES IN THE MALE GENITAL SYSTEM. J. PEDIAT. 75* 806-811, 1969.

RECESSIVE

OPPENHEIMER, E. H. AND ESTERLY, J. R.* OBSERVATIONS ON CYSTIC FIBROSIS OF THE PANCREAS. VI. THE UTERINE CERVIX. J. PEDIAT. 77* 991-995, 1970.

OPPENHEIMER, E. H., CASE, A. L., ESTERLY, J. R. AND ROTHBERG, R. M.* CERVICAL MUCUS IN CYSTIC FIBROSIS* A POSSIBLE CAUSE OF INFERTILITY. AM. J. OBSTET. GYNEC. 108* 673-674, 1970.

ROBERTS, G. B. S.* FAMILIAL INCIDENCE OF FIBROCYSTIC DISEASE OF THE PANCREAS. ANN. HUM. GENET. 24* 127-135, 1960.

SMITH, D. W., DOCTER, J. M., FERRIER, P. E., FRIAS, J. L. AND SPOCK, A.* POSSIBLE LOCALISATION OF THE GENE FOR CYSTIC FIBROSIS OF THE PANCREAS TO THE SHORT ARM OF CHROMOSOME 5. LANCET 2* 309-312, 1968.

SPOCK, A., HEICK, H. M. C., CRESS, H. AND LOGAN, W. S.* ABNORMAL SERUM FACTOR IN PATIENTS WITH CYSTIC FIBROSIS OF THE PANCREAS. PEDIAT. RES. 1* 173-177, 1967.

STEINBERG, A. G. AND BROWN, D. C.* ON THE INCIDENCE OF CYSTIC FIBROSIS OF THE PANCREAS. AM. J. HUM. GENET. 12* 416-424, 1960.

WRIGHT, S. W. AND MORTON, N. E.* GENETIC STUDIES ON CYSTIC FIBROSIS IN HAWAII. AM. J. HUM. GENET. 20* 157-162, 1968.

21980 CYSTINOSIS I (EARLY ONSET NEPHROPATHIC TYPE INFANTILE TYPE)

THE FACT THAT PLASMA LEVELS ARE WELL BELOW SATURATION INDICATES THAT THE DEFECT IS A CELLULAR ONE. WITHIN THE CELL CYSTINE IS COMPARTMENTALIZED WITH ACID PHOSPHA- TASE AND IS MEMBRANE-BOUND AS DEMONSTRATED BY ELECTRONMICROSCOPY. FERRITIN ACCUMULATES IN THE SAME ORGANELLE WHICH APPEARS TO BE THE LYSOSOME. AN ABNORMALI- TY IN HETEROZYGOTES WAS DEMONSTRATED BY SCHNEIDER ET AL. (1967) WHO FOUND THE CONCENTRATION OF FREE CYSTINE TO BE ABOUT 6 TIMES NORMAL IN THE LEUKOCYTES OF PARENTS OF PATIENTS. THE FEATURES RESULTING FROM ACCUMULATION OF CYSTINE IN THE KIDNEY ARE THOSE OF THE FANCONI SYNDROME (Q.V.). TEREE ET AL. (1970) STUDIED TWO MALE SIBS WITH CYSTINOSIS PHYSIOLOGICALLY AND ANATOMICALLY. MICRODISSECTION OF THE KIDNEY TUBULES SUGGESTED THAT THE MORPHOLOGIC ABNORMALITY OF THE PROXIMAL TUBULE IS 'ACQUIRED' AND PROGRESSIVE. MAHONEY ET AL. (1970) FOUND THAT RENAL TRANSPLANTS IN FOUR CHILDREN WITH CYSTINOSIS DID NOT DEVELOP GLOMERULAR AND TUBULAR EPITHELIAL CELLULAR CHANGES OF CYSTINOSIS.

MAHONEY, C. P., STRIKER, G. E., HICKMAN, R. O., MANNING, G. B. AND MARCHIORO, T. L.* RENAL TRANSPLANTATION FOR CHILDHOOD CYSTINOSIS. NEW ENG. J. MED. 283* 397- 402, 1970.

SCHNEIDER, J. A., BRADLEY, K. AND SEEGMILLER, J. E.* INCREASED CYSTINE IN LEUKOCYTES FROM INDIVIDUALS HOMOZYGOUS AND HETEROZYGOUS FOR CYSTINOSIS. SCIENCE 157* 1321-1322, 1967.

SCHULMAN, J. D., FUJIMOTO, W. Y., BRADLEY, K. H. AND SEEGMILLER, J. E.* IDENTIFICATION OF HETEROZYGOUS GENOTYPE FOR CYSTINOSIS IN UTERO BY A NEW PULSE- LABELING TECHNIQUE* PRELIMINARY REPORT. J. PEDIAT. 77* 468-470, 1970.

TEREE, T. M., FRIEDMAN, A. B., KENT, L. M. AND FETTERMAN, G. H.* CYSTINOSIS AND PROXIMAL TUBULAR NEPHROPATHY IN SIBLINGS. PROGRESSIVE DEVELOPMENT OF THE PHYSIOLOGICAL AND ANATOMICAL LESION. AM. J. DIS. CHILD. 119* 481-487, 1970.

WEINBERG, T.* CYSTINE STORAGE DISEASE. REPORT OF A CASE. AM. J. CLIN. PATH. 29* 54-60, 1958.

WORTHEN, H. G. AND GOOD, R. A.* THE DE TONI-FANCONI SYNDROME WITH CYSTINOSIS* CLINICAL AND METABOLIC STUDY OF TWO CASES IN A FAMILY AND A CRITICAL REVIEW OF THE NATURE OF THE SYNDROME. AM. J. DIS. CHILD. 100* 653-688, 1960.

21990 CYSTINOSIS II (LATE ONSET NEPHROPATHIC TYPE JUVENILE OR ADOLESCENT TYPE)

THIS FORM OF CYSTINE NEPHROPATHY MANIFESTS ITSELF FIRST AT AGE 10 OR 12 YEARS WITH PROTEINURIA DUE TO GLOMERULAR DAMAGE RATHER THAN WITH THE MANIFESTATIONS OF TUBULAR DAMAGE WHICH OCCUR FIRST IN CYSTINOSIS I. THERE IS NO EXCESS AMINOACI- DURIA AND STATURE IS NORMAL. PHOTOPHOBIA, LATE DEVELOPMENT OF PIGMENTARY RETINOPATHY AND CHRONIC HEADACHES ARE FEATURES. WHITE CELLS SHOW HIGH CYSTINE CONTENT IN HETEROZYGOTES FOR CYSTINOSIS II, JUST AS THEY DO IN CYSTINOSIS I.

22000 CYSTINOSIS III (BENIGN TYPE ADULT TYPE)

A BENIGN FORM OF CYSTINOSIS HAS BEEN DESCRIBED IN A FEW CASES. FOR EXAMPLE, LEITMAN ET AL. (1966) OBSERVED THREE AFFECTED SIBS FROM COUSIN PARENTS. THE AGES OF PATIENTS WERE 53, 50 AND 42 YEARS. CRYSTALS OF CYSTINE WERE DEMONSTRATED IN THE CORNEA, BUFFY COAT OF THE BLOOD AND BONE MARROW. NO AMINOACIDURIA OR IMPAIRMENT OF RENAL FUNCTION WAS FOUND. COGAN ET AL. (1958) ALSO HAD AN ASYMP- TOMATIC ADULT WITH CYSTINE DEMONSTRABLE IN CORNEA AND BONE MARROW. ALTHOUGH THE PATIENTS WITH ADULT CYSTINOSIS SHOW CHARACTERISTIC CRYSTALS IN THE CORNEA, CONJUNCTIVA, CIRCULATING WHITE CELLS AND BONE MARROW, NO EVIDENCE OF RENAL TUBULAR DYSFUNCTION IS FOUND. SOME REPORTED CASES OF FAMILIAL CRYSTALLINE CORNEAL

R
E
C
E
S
S
I
V
E

DYSTROPHY MAY BE EXAMPLES OF THIS CONDITION. DEPOSITS RESEMBLING THOSE OF CYSTINOSIS OCCUR IN THE CORNEA IN PATIENTS WITH DYSPROTEINEMIA SUCH AS IN MULTIPLE MYELOMA (BURKI, 1958). SCHNEIDER ET AL. (1968) REPORTED STUDIES OF 3 FURTHER ADULT CYSTINOSIS CASES. THE INTRACELLULAR DEPOSITS OF FREE CYSTINE APPEAR TO BE UNAVAILABLE FOR SUSTAINING NORMAL METABOLISM SINCE FIBROBLASTS FROM EITHER THE CHILDHOOD OR THE ADULT TYPE ARE NOT VIABLE IN A CYSTINE-FREE MEDIUM. THE INTRACELLULAR CONTENT OF CYSTINE IS LOWER IN THE ADULT FORM THAN IN THE CHILDHOOD FORM, YET HIGHER THAN IN THE HETEROZYGOTE FOR THE CHILDHOOD FORM. RETINAL LESIONS OCCUR IN THE CHILDHOOD FORM BUT NOT THE ADULT FORM AND MAY BE RESPONSIBLE FOR THE PHOTOPHOBIA WHICH IS MUCH MORE A FEATURE OF THE CHILDHOOD FORM. AN ABNORMALITY IN HETEROZYGOTES WAS DEMONSTRATED BY SCHNEIDER ET AL. (1967) WHO FOUND THE CONCENTRA- TION OF FREE CYSTINE TO BE ABOUT 6 TIMES NORMAL IN THE LEUKOCYTES OF PARENTS OF PATIENTS. BRUBAKER ET AL. (1970) DESCRIBED BROTHER AND SISTER, AGES 16 AND 11 YEARS, RESPECTIVELY. SINCE THEY HAD NO PROTEINURIA OR OTHER CLINICAL ABNORMALITY EXCEPT FOR CRYSTALLINE CORNEAL DEPOSITS, THEIR DISORDER FITS THE 'ADULT' TYPE RATHER THAN THE JUVENILE OR ADOLESCENT TYPE.

BRUBAKER, R. F., WONG, V. G., SCHULMAN, J. D., SEEGMILLER, J. E. AND KUWABARA, T.* BENIGN CYSTINOSIS. THE CLINICAL, BIOCHEMICAL AND MORPHOLOGIC FINDINGS IN A FAMILY WITH TWO AFFECTED SIBLINGS. AM. J. MED. 49* 546-550, 1970.

BURKI, E.* A CASE OF CORNEAL CHANGES IN MULTIPLE MYELOMA (PLASMACYTOMA) - UBER HORNHAUTVERANDERUNGER BEI EINEM FALL VON MULTIPLEM MYELOM (PLASMOCYTOM). OPHTHALMOLOGICA 135* 565-572, 1958.

BURKI, E. AND ROHNER, M.* EIN SELTENER FALL VON KRISTALLINER HORNHAUTDEGENERA- TION. A RARE CASE OF CRYSTALLINE CORNEAL DEGENERATION. OPHTHALMOLOGICA 129* 211- 217, 1955.

COGAN, D. G., KUWABARA, T., HURLBUT, C. S. AND MCMURRAY, V.* FURTHUR OBSERVA- TIONS ON CYSTINOSIS IN THE ADULT. J.A.M.A. 166* 1725-1726, 1958.

LEITMAN, P. S., FRAZIER, P. D., WONG, V. G., SHOTTON, D. AND SEEGMILLER, J. E.* ADULT CYSTINOSIS - A BENIGN DISORDER. AM. J. MED. 40* 511-517, 1966.

SCHNEIDER, J. A., BRADLEY, K. AND SEEGMILLER, J. E.* INCREASED CYSTINE IN LEUKOCYTES FROM INDIVIDUALS HOMOZYGOUS AND HETEROZYGOUS FOR CYSTINOSIS. SCIENCE 157* 1321-1322, 1967.

SCHNEIDER, J. A., WONG, V., BRADLEY, K. AND SEEGMILLER, J. E.* BIOCHEMICAL COMPARISONS OF THE ADULT AND CHILDHOOD FORMS OF CYSTINOSIS. NEW ENG. J. MED. 279* 1253-1257, 1968.

R
E
C
E
S
S
I
V
E

*22010 CYSTINURIA I, II, III (AT LEAST 3 ALLELES AT ONE LOCUS)

IN CYSTINURIA I THE HOMOZYGOTE EXCRETES RELATIVELY LARGE AMOUNTS OF CYSTINE, LYSINE, ARGININE AND ORNITHINE IN THE URINE. HETEROZYGOTES (E.G., PARENTS) HAVE NO ABNORMAL AMINOACIDURIA. URINARY STONES FORM IN ALL THREE TYPES OF CYSTINURIA BECAUSE OF THE LIMITED SOLUBILITY OF THIS AMINO ACID.
CYSTINURIA II IS INCOMPLETELY RECESSIVE BECAUSE HETEROZYGOTES HAVE A MODERATE DEGREE OF AMINOACIDURIA, MAINLY CYSTINE AND LYSINE, AND MAY OCCASIONALLY FORM CYSTINE STONES. OBSERVATIONS IN KINDREDS IN WHICH BOTH CYSTINURIA I AND CYS- TINURIA II ARE SEGREGATING DEMONSTRATE THAT THE GENES FOR THESE ARE ALLELIC (HERSHKO ET AL., 1965).
IN CYSTINURIA III, INTESTINAL TRANSPORT OF ALL DIBASIC AMINO ACIDS IS RETAINED BY HETEROZYGOTES AND HOMOZYGOTES EXCRETE CYSTINE IN SLIGHT EXCESS.
ROSENBERG (1966) AND OTHERS OBSERVED FAMILIES IN WHICH PERSONS DOUBLY HETEROZYGOUS (I-II, I-III, OR II-III) HAD FULL-BLOWN CYSTINURIA. THE FINDINGS ARE BEST EXPLAINED ON THE BASIS OF ALLELISM OF THE GENES RESPONSIBLE FOR THE 3 TYPES. SCRIVER ET AL. (1970) PRESENTED EVIDENCE INDICATING THAT CYSTINURIA PATIENTS ARE AT INCREASED RISK FOR IMPAIRED CEREBRAL FUNCTION.

BOSTROM, H. AND TOTTIE, K.* CYSTINURIA IN SWEDEN. II. THE INCIDENCE OF HOMOZYGOUS CYSTINURIA IN SWEDISH SCHOOL CHILDREN. ACTA PAEDIAT. 48* 345-352, 1959.

BOSTROM, H.* CYSTINURIA IN SWEDEN III. THE PROGNOSIS OF HOMOZYGOUS CYSTINURIA. ACTA CHIR. SCAND. 116* 287-295, 1959.

FARISS, B. L. AND KOLB, F. O.* FACTORS INVOLVED IN CRYSTAL FORMATION IN CYSTINURIA. REDUCTION IN CYSTINE CYSTALLURIA WITH CHLORDIAZEPOXIDE AND DURING NEPHROTIC SYNDROME. J.A.M.A. 205* 846-848, 1968.

HARRIS, H., MITTWOCH, U., ROBSON, E. B. AND WARREN, F. L.* PHENOTYPES AND GENOTYPES IN CYSTINURIA. ANN. HUM. GENET. 20* 57-91, 1955.

HERSHKO, C., BEN-AMI, E., PACIORKOVSKI, J. AND LEVIN, N.* ALLELOMORPHISM IN CYSTINURIA. PROC. TEL. HASHOMER. HOSP. 4* 21-23, 1965.

KNOX, W. E.* CYSTINURIA. IN, STANBURY, J. B., WYNGAARDEN, J. B. AND FREDRICK- SON, D. S. (EDS.)* THE METABOLIC BASIS OF INHERITED DISEASE. NEW YORK* MCGRAW- HILL, 1966 (2ND ED.). PP. 1262-1282.

TINURIA. AM. J. HUM. GENET. 10* 3-32, 1958.

ROSENBERG, L. E.* CYSTINURIA* GENETIC HETEROGENEITY AND ALLELISM. SCIENCE 154* 1341-1343, 1966.

ROSENBERG, L. E., DOWNING, S., DURANT, J. L. AND SEGAL, S.* CYSTINURIA* BIOCHEMICAL EVIDENCE FOR THREE GENETICALLY DISTINCT DISEASES. J. CLIN. INVEST. 45* 365-371, 1966.

ROSENBERG, L. E., DURANT, J. L. AND HOLLAND, J. M.* INTESTINAL ABSORPTION AND RENAL EXTRACTION OF CYSTINE AND CYSTEINE IN CYSTINURIA. NEW ENG. J. MED. 273* 1239-1245, 1965.

SCRIVER, C. R., WHELAN, D. T., CLOW, C. L. AND DALLAIRE, L.* CYSTINURIA* INCREASED PREVALENCE IN PATIENTS WITH MENTAL DISEASE. NEW ENG. J. MED. 283* 783-786, 1970.

*22020 DANDY-WALKER SYNDROME

THE PRIMARY DEFECT IS ATRESIA OF THE FORAMINA OF LUSCHKA AND MAGENDIE. THE FOURTH VENTRICLE BECOMES DILATED INTO A LARGE CYST IN THE POSTERIOR FOSSA. CLEMENT BENDA (1954) APPARENTLY INTRODUCED THE DESIGNATION DANDY-WALKER SYNDROME. FURTHERMORE HE REPORTED FAMILIAL OCCURRENCE. D'AGOSTINO, KERNOHAN AND BROWN (1963) FOUND THE CONDITION IN SIBS WHO ALSO HAD POLYCYSTIC KIDNEYS.

BENDA, C. E.* THE DANDY-WALKER SYNDROME OR THE SO-CALLED ATRESIA OF THE FORAMEN OF MAGENDIE. J. NEUROPATH. EXP. NEUROL. 13* 14-29, 1954.

D'AGOSTINO, A. N., KERNOHAN, J. W. AND BROWN, J. R.* THE DANDY-WALKER SYNDROME. J. NEUROPATH. EXP. NEUROL. 22* 450-470, 1963.

22030 DEAFMUTISM AND FAMILIAL MYOCLONUS EPILEPSY

LATHAM AND MUNRO (1937) REPORTED A FAMILY IN WHICH THE PARENTS WERE SECOND COUSINS AND 5 OUT OF 8 SIBS HAD CONGENITAL DEAFNESS WITH MYOCLONUS EPILEPSY WHICH BEGAN AT AGE 10-12 YEARS. PROBABLY NO OTHER SUCH FAMILIES HAVE BEEN REPORTED. SEE MYOCLONUS, CEREBELLAR ATAXIA AND DEAFNESS.

LATHAM, A. D. AND MUNRO, T. A.* FAMILIAL MYOCLONUS EPILEPSY ASSOCIATED WITH DEAF-MUTISM IN A FAMILY SHOWING OTHER PSYCHOBIOLOGICAL ABNORMALITIES. ANN. EUGEN. 8* 166-175, 1937.

*22040 DEAFMUTISM AND FUNCTIONAL HEART DISEASE (PROLONGED QT INTERVAL IN EKG AND SUDDEN DEATH)

IN THE REPORT OF LEVINE AND WOODWORTH (1958) NO NOTE ON PARENTAL CONSANGUINITY WAS RECORDED. THERE WAS BUT ONE CASE, THE PROBAND, IN THE FAMILY. IN JERVELL AND LANGE-NIELSEN'S REPORT (1957) 4 OF 6 CHILDREN WERE DESCRIBED AS AFFECTED AND THE PARENTS WERE NOT RELATED. FRASER, FROGGATT AND MURPHY (1964) ESTIMATED THAT THE PREVALENCE IN CHILDREN AGES 4-15 IN ENGLAND, WALES AND IRELAND IS BETWEEN 1.6 AND 6 PER MILLION. THEY SUGGESTED THAT HETEROZYGOUS PERSONS MAY SHOW SLIGHT OR MODERATE PROLONGATION OF THE QT INTERVAL. ALSO SEE VENTRICULAR FIBRILLATION IN DOMINANT CATALOG. IN STUDIES OF THE TEMPORAL BONES OF TWO CHILDREN WHO DIED WITH THIS CONDITION, FRIEDMANN, FRASER AND FROGGATT (1966) FOUND A STRIKING ANOMALY IN THE FORM OF PAS-POSITIVE HYALINE NODULES THROUGHOUT BOTH THE COCHLEAR AND THE VESTIBULAR PORTIONS OF THE MEMBRANOUS LABYRINTH IN, OR ADJACENT TO, THE TERMINAL VESSELS OF THE VASCULAR STRIA.

FRASER, G. R. AND FROGGATT, P.* THE SYNDROME OF CONGENITAL DEAFNESS WITH ABNORMAL ELECTROCARDIOGRAM. HEREDITY 15* 454, 1960.

FRASER, G. R., FROGGATT, P. AND JAMES, T. N.* CONGENITAL DEAFNESS ASSOCIATED WITH ELECTROCARDIOGRAPHIC ABNORMALITIES, FAINTING ATTACKS AND SUDDEN DEATH. QUART. J. MED. 33* 361-385, 1964.

FRASER, G. R., FROGGATT, P. AND MURPHY, T.* GENETICAL ASPECTS OF THE CARDIOAU-DITORY SYNDROME OF JERVELL AND LANGE-NIELSEN (CONGENITAL DEAFNESS AND ELECTROCAR-DIOGRAPHIC ABNORMALITIES). ANN. HUM. GENET. 28* 133-157, 1964.

FRIEDMANN, I., FRASER, G. R. AND FROGGATT, P.* PATHOLOGY OF THE EAR IN THE CARDIOAUDITORY SYNDROME OF JERVELL AND LANGE-NIELSEN (RECESSIVE DEAFNESS WITH ELECTROCARDIOGRAPHIC ABNORMALITIES). J. LARYNG. 80* 451-470, 1966.

JERVELL, A. AND LANGE-NIELSEN, F.* CONGENITAL DEAF-MUTISM, FUNCTIONAL HEART DISEASE WITH PROLONGATION OF Q-T INTERVAL AND SUDDEN DEATH. AM. HEART J. 54* 59-68, 1957.

LEVINE, S. A. AND WOODWORTH, C. R.* CONGENITAL DEAF-MUTISM, PROLONGED QT INTERVAL, SYNCOPAL ATTACKS AND SUDDEN DEATH. NEW ENG. J. MED. 259* 412-417, 1958.

22050 DEAFMUTISM AND ONYCHODYSTROPHY

FEINMESSER AND ZELIG (1961) REPORTED TWO AFFECTED SISTERS FROM A CONSANGUINEOUS MATING. THE ASSOCIATION MIGHT, OF COURSE, BE MERELY THE COINCIDENCE OF TWO RARE RECESSIVES. GOODMAN ET AL. (1969) OBSERVED MOTHER AND SON WITH SENSORINEURAL DEAFNESS AND ONYCHODYSTROPHY. THE FATHER ALSO HAD SENSORINEURAL DEAFNESS, PRESUMABLY OF A TYPE DIFFERENT FROM THAT IN HIS WIFE. IN THE MOTHER THE RIGHT THUMB WAS TRIPHALANGIC. THE LEFT THUMB WAS BIPHALANGIC BUT A RUDIMENTARY THIRD PHALANX APPEARED TO BE FUSED WITH THE MIDDLE PHALANX. THIS MAY BE A DOMINANT TRAIT DISTINCT FROM THAT REPORTED BY FEINMESSER AND ZELIG (1961). WALBAUM ET AL. (1970) DESCRIBED A BROTHER AND SISTER WITH MENTAL RETARDATION, PERCEPTIVE DEAFNESS, DYSPLASIA OF THE FINGER NAILS, TRIPHALANGEAL THUMBS, HYPOPLASIA OF THE TERMINAL PHALANGES, AND "DECAPSALIDIC" FINGERPRINTS, I.E., AN ARCH PATTERN ON EACH FINGER. THE PARENTS WERE NORMAL AND UNRELATED. THEY POINTED OUT SIMILARITIES TO THE CASES OF FEINMESSER AND ZELIG (1961) AND OF GOODMAN ET AL. (1969).

FEINMESSER, M. AND ZELIG, S.* CONGENITAL DEAFNESS ASSOCIATED WITH ONYCHODYSTRO-PHY. ARCH. OTOLARYNG. 74* 507-508, 1961.

GOODMAN, R. M., LOCKAREFF, S. AND GWINUP, G.* HEREDITARY CONGENITAL DEAFNESS WITH ONYCHODYSTROPHY. ARCH. OTOLARYNG. 90* 474-477, 1969.

WALBAUM, R., FONTAINE, G., LIENHARDT, J. AND PIQUET, J. J.* SURDITE FAMILIALE AVEC OSTEO-ONYCHO-DYSPLASIE. J. GENET. HUM. 18* 101-108, 1970.

22060 DEAFMUTISM AND SPLIT HANDS AND FEET

WILDERVANCK (1963) OBSERVED THE ASSOCIATION IN TWO SONS OF UNRELATED PARENTS. BIRCH-JENSEN (1949) MENTIONED A SPORADIC CASE OF THE ASSOCIATION. G. R. FRASER (PERSONAL COMMUNICATION) HAS SEEN A BROTHER AND SISTER WITH THIS COMBINATION.

BIRCH-JENSEN, A.* CONGENITAL DEFORMITIES OF THE UPPER EXTREMITIES. OP. EX. DOMO BIOL. HERED. HUM. U. HAFNIENSIS. 19* 1949.

WILDERVANCK, L. S.* DEAFNESS ASSOCIATED WITH SPLIT HANDS AND FEET IN TWO SIBLINGS. A NEW SYNDROME. PROC. 11TH. INTERN. CONG. GENET., THE HAGUE, 1963. PP. 286-287.

R
E
C
E
S
S
I
V
E

*22070 DEAFMUTISM I (CONGENITAL DEAFNESS)

BECAUSE OF THE PRESENCE OF DEAFNESS FROM BIRTH SPEECH DOES NOT DEVELOP UNLESS THE AFFECTED CHILD HAS SPECIAL TRAINING, HENCE THE POPULAR TERM DEAF-MUTISM FOR CONGENITAL DEAFNESS. MANY, ESPECIALLY THOSE INVOLVED IN TEACHING THE DEAF, DISAPPROVE OF THE TERM AND APPROPRIATELY SO BECAUSE MUTISM IS NOT AN IMMUTABLE PART OF THE PHENOTYPE.
FRASER (1964) ESTIMATED THAT HALF OF SEVERE CHILDHOOD DEAFNESS WAS DUE TO SIMPLE MENDELIAN INHERITANCE AND THAT 87 PERCENT OF THIS GROUP IS AUTOSOMAL RECESSIVE. THREE RECESSIVE SYNDROMES WERE IDENTIFIABLE* PENDRED'S SYNDROME (10 PERCENT OF THE HEREDITARY GROUP), USHER'S SYNDROME (2 PERCENT) AND DEAFNESS WITH UNIQUE EKG CHANGES (1 PERCENT). THE EXISTENCE OF SEVERAL GENETIC FORMS IS SUPPORTED BY THE DIVERSITY OF FINDINGS IN THE EARS OF DEAF-MUTES. ORMEROD (1960) RECOGNIZED THE FOLLOWING TYPES, BEGINNING WITH THE MOST COMPLETE FORM OF DEAFNESS* (1) MICHEL TYPE - COMPLETE LACK OF DEVELOPMENT OF INTERNAL EAR. (2) MONDINI-ALEXANDER TYPE - DEVELOPMENT ONLY OF A SINGLE NERVED TUBE REPRESENTING THE COCHLEA AND SIMILAR IMMATURITY OF THE VESTIBULAR CANALS. (3) BING-SIEBENMANN TYPE - BONEY LABYRINTH WELL FORMED BUT MEMBRANOUS PART AND PARTICULARLY THE SENSE ORGAN POORLY DEVELOPED. THIS TYPE IS OFTEN ASSOCIATED WITH RETINITIS PIGMENTOSA AND-OR MENTAL RETARDATION. (4) SCHEIBE COCHLEO-SACCULAR TYPE. IN THIS FORM, WHICH IS THE MOST FREQUENT ONE, THE VESTIBULAR PART IS DEVELOPED AND FUNCTIONING. MALFORMATION IS RESTRICTED TO THE MEMBRANOUS COCHLEA AND SACCULE. THIS TYPE OCCURS IN WAARDENBURG'S SYNDROME, A DOMINANT. (5) SIEBENMANN TYPE - CHANGES MAINLY IN MIDDLE EAR AND OFTEN DUE TO THYROID HORMONE DEFICIENCY. THE MIDDLE EAR IS INVOLVED IN MYXOMATOUS CHANGE WHICH MAY BE EMBRYONIC PERSISTENCE. (6) MICROTIA AND ATRESIA OF THE MEATUS - ABNORMALITY LIMITED TO THE EXTERNAL EAR.
BY INGENIOUS MATHEMATICAL ANALYSIS MORTON (1960) HAS ARRIVED AT THE CONCLU-SION THAT RECESSIVE INHERITANCE IS RESPONSIBLE FOR 68 PERCENT OF CONGENITAL DEAFNESS, THAT HOMOZYGOSITY AT ANY ONE OF 35 LOCI CAN RESULT IN THIS PHENOTYPE AND THAT 16 PERCENT OF THE NORMAL POPULATION ARE CARRIERS OF A GENE FOR DEAF-MUTISM.
AS EARLY AS 1862 BOUDIN NOTED THE ASSOCIATION BETWEEN CONSANGUINITY AND DEAF-MUTISM.

BOUDIN, M.* DE LA NECESSITE DES CROISEMENTS, ET DU DANGER DES UNIONS CONSAN-GUINS DANS L'ESPECE HUMAINE ET PARMI LES ANIMAUX. REC. MED. CHIR. ET PHARM. MILIT. 7* 193-197, 1862.

CHUNG, C. S., ROBINSON, O. W. AND MORTON, N. E.* A NOTE ON DEAFMUTISM. ANN. HUM. GENET. 23* 357-366, 1959.

DERAEMAEKER, R.* RECESSIVE CONGENITAL DEAFNESS IN A NORTH BELGIAN PROVINCE. ACTA GENET. STATIST. MED. 10* 295-304, 1960.

FRASER, G. R.* PROFOUND CHILDHOOD DEAFNESS. J. MED. GENET. 1* 118-151, 1964.

HANHART, E.* DIE "SPORADISCHE" TAUBSTUMMHEIT ALS PROTOTYP EINER EINFACHREZESSI-

LINDENOV, H.* THE ETIOLOGY OF DEAF-MUTISM WITH SPECIAL REFERENCE TO HEREDITY.
OP. EX. DOMO BIOL. HERED. HUM. U. HAFNIENSIS. 8* 1-268, 1945.

MORTON, N. E.* THE MUTATIONAL LOAD DUE TO DETRIMENTAL GENES IN MAN. AM. J.
HUM. GENET. 12* 348-364, 1960.

ORMEROD, F. C.* THE PATHOLOGY OF CONGENITAL DEAFNESS. J. LARYNG. 74* 919-950,
1960.

SLATIS, H. M.* COMMENTS ON THE INHERITANCE OF DEAF MUTISM IN NORTHERN IRELAND.
ANN. HUM. GENET. 22* 153-157, 1957.

STEVENSON, A. C. AND CHEESEMAN, E. A.* HEREDITARY DEAF MUTISM, WITH PARTICULAR
REFERENCE TO NORTHERN IRELAND. ANN. HUM. GENET. 20* 177-231, 1956.

*22080 DEAFMUTISM II (CONGENITAL DEAFNESS)

DIRECT GENETIC EVIDENCE FOR THE EXISTENCE OF AT LEAST TWO NON-ALLELIC, RECESSIVE,
PHENOTYPICALLY INDISTINGUISHABLE FORMS OF DEAFMUTISM IS PROVIDED BY THE RATHER
FREQUENT PEDIGREES OF THE TYPE REPORTED BY STEVENSON AND CHEESEMAN (1956). IN
ONLY 5 OF 32 HEREDITARY DEAF BY HEREDITARY DEAF MATINGS WERE ALL CHILDREN DEAF.
FROM THIS THE AUTHORS CONCLUDED THAT THERE ARE PROBABLY SIX SEPARATE LOCI FOR
RECESSIVE DEAFMUTISM ASSUMING THAT THE MUTANT GENES AT EACH HAVE A SIMILAR
FREQUENCY. SEE COMMENTS OF SLATIS (1957). CHUNG, ROBINSON AND MORTON (1959) ALSO
SUPPORTED THE NOTION OF MULTIPLE RECESSIVE FORMS OF DEAFMUTISM. THE EXISTENCE AS
LISTED BELOW OF NO FEWER THAN SIX RECESSIVE SYNDROMES WITH DEAFMUTISM AS THE MAIN
FEATURE BUT WITH VARIOUS ASSOCIATED FEATURES IS FURTHER CORROBORATION. MENGEL ET
AL. (1968) PRESENTED AN INSTRUCTIVE PEDIGREE IN WHICH TWO CONGENITAL DEAF PARENTS
HAD ALL NORMAL-HEARING OFFSPRING. ONE PARENT CAME FROM A MENNONITE GROUP WITH
NUMEROUS CASES OF CONGENITAL DEAFNESS IN A RECESSIVE PATTERN. THE OTHER PARENT
CAME FROM AN AMISH GROUP WHICH ALSO CONTAINED SEVERAL PERSONS WITH APPARENTLY
RECESSIVELY INHERITED CONGENITAL DEAFNESS.

CHUNG, C. S., ROBINSON, O. W. AND MORTON, N. E.* A NOTE ON DEAF MUTISM. ANN.
HUM. GENET. 23* 357-366, 1959.

MENGEL, M. C., KONIGSMARK, B. W. AND MCKUSICK, V. A.* TWO TYPES OF CONGENITAL
RECESSIVE DEAFNESS. EYE EAR NOSE THROAT MONTHLY 48* 301-305, 1968.

SLATIS, H. M.* COMMENTS ON THE INHERITANCE OF DEAF MUTISM IN NORTHERN IRELAND.
ANN. HUM. GENET. 22* 153-157, 1958.

STEVENSON, A. C. AND CHEESEMAN, E. A.* HEREDITARY DEAF MUTISM, WITH PARTICULAR
REFERENCE TO NORTHERN IRELAND. ANN. HUM. GENET. 20* 177-231, 1956.

22090 DEAFMUTISM WITH TOTAL ALBINISM

ZIPRKOWSKI AND ADAM (1964) DESCRIBED A SEPHARDIC JEWISH FAMILY FROM MOROCCO IN
WHICH TWO CHILDREN IN EACH OF TWO FAMILIES WITH CONSANGUINEOUS PARENTS HAD THE
ASSOCIATION MENTIONED. THE TWO SIBSHIPS ARE RELATED TO EACH OTHER AND SHARED A
PAIR OF GREAT-GREAT-GRANDPARENTS IN COMMON. IN ONE SIBSHIP THREE SIBS OF THE TWO
DOUBLY AFFECTED SIBS HAD ONLY CONGENITAL DEAFNESS. THUS IT IS NOT COMPLETELY
CERTAIN THAT THE ASSOCIATION IS A MONOMERIC SYNDROME. DOMINANT AND X-LINKED
RECESSIVE FORMS OF CONGENITAL DEAFNESS WITH ALBINISM, TOTAL OR PARTIAL, WERE
REVIEWED BY THESE AUTHORS.

ZIPRKOWSKI, L. AND ADAM, A.* RECESSIVE TOTAL ALBINISM AND CONGENITAL DEAFMU-
TISM. ARCH. DERM. 89* 151-155, 1964.

22100 DEAFMUTISM, SEMILETHAL

PFANDLER (1960) STUDIED DEAF-MUTISM IN SEVERAL POPULATIONS OF SWITZERLAND AND
FOUND THAT THE PROPORTION OF AFFECTED SIBS WAS FAR LESS THAN THE EXPECTED 0.25
(6.25 TO 16.7 PERCENT). HE SUGGESTED THAT A SEMILETHAL EFFECT OF THE GENE COULD
EXPLAIN THE FINDINGS. THE DATA SHOWED A DEFICIENCY OF DEAF-MUTE FEMALES. AN
ALTERNATIVE HYPOTHESIS - THE NECESSARY COINCIDENCE OF HOMOZYGOSITY AT TWO SEPARATE
LOCI - DID NOT FIT THE DATA SATISFACTORILY. MENTAL DEFECT AND HYPOGONADISM ALSO
OCCURRED IN THESE CASES. IT IS POSSIBLE THAT THIS SERIES WAS CONTAMINATED BY
SPORADIC CASES OF NON-GENETIC OR NON-RECESSIVE CAUSATION.

PFANDLER, U.* UNE FORME SEMILETALE DE LA SURDIMUTITE RECESSIVE DANS DIFFERENTES
POPULATIONS DE LA SUISSE ORIENTALE. BULL. ACAD. SUISSE SCI. MED. 16* 255-277,
1960.

22110 DEAFNESS AND ATOPIC DERMATITIS

KONIGSMARK ET AL. (1968) OBSERVED COCHLEAR DEAFNESS AND ATYPICAL ATOPIC DERMATITIS
IN TWO BROTHERS AND A SISTER. THE ATYPICAL FEATURES OF ATOPIC DERMATITIS WERE
SOMEWHAT LATE ONSET (9-11 YEARS) AND LOCATION ON THE HANDS AND FOREARMS.

KONIGSMARK, B. W., HOLLANDER, M. B. AND BERLIN, C. I.* FAMILIAL NEURAL HEARING LOSS AND ATOPIC DERMATITIS. J.A.M.A. 204* 953-957, 1968.

22120 DEAFNESS, COCHLEAR, WITH MYOPIA AND INTELLECTUAL IMPAIRMENT

ELDRIDGE ET AL. (1968), IN A SURVEY OF MENTAL RETARDATION IN AN INBRED AMISH COMMUNITY, OBSERVED FOUR OF SEVEN SIBS IN A FAMILY (2 MALES, 2 FEMALES) WITH THE ABOVE COMBINATION. THE EXTENT OF INTELLECTUAL IMPAIRMENT WAS DIFFICULT TO EVALUATE. SENSORY DEPRIVATION MIGHT BE A MAIN FACTOR.

ELDRIDGE, R., BERLIN, C. I., MONEY, J. W. AND MCKUSICK, V. A.* COCHLEAR DEAFNESS, MYOPIA, AND INTELLECTUAL IMPAIRMENT IN AN AMISH FAMILY. A NEW SYNDROME OF HEREDITARY DEAFNESS. ARCH. OTOLARYNG. 88* 49-54, 1968.

*22130 DEAFNESS, CONDUCTIVE, WITH MALFORMED EXTERNAL EAR

IN TWO SIBSHIPS IN A MENNONITE ISOLATE, MENGEL ET AL. (1969) OBSERVED 6 PERSONS WITH CONDUCTIVE DEAFNESS AND MALFORMED, LOW-SET EXTERNAL EAR. THE FOUR PARENTS SHARED A COMMON ANCESTRAL COUPLE. AT OPERATION MALFORMATION OF THE OSSICLES WAS DEMONSTRATED IN THE MIDDLE EAR. MENTAL RETARDATION AND HYPOGONADISM MAY BE ADDITIONAL FEATURES.

MENGEL, M. C., KONIGSMARK, B. W., BERLIN, C. I. AND MCKUSICK, V. A.* CONDUCTIVE HEARING LOSS AND MALFORMED LOW-SET EARS, AS A POSSIBLE RECESSIVE SYNDROME. J. MED. GENET. 6* 14-21, 1969.

22140 DEAFNESS, NERVE TYPE, MESENTERIC DIVERTICULA OF SMALL BOWEL, AND PROGRESSIVE NEUROPATHY

HIRSCHOWITZ ET AL. (1971) DESCRIBED THREE SISTERS FROM A SIBSHIP OF SIX, WHO HAD PROGRESSIVE NERVE DEAFNESS BEGINNING AT 8, 3 AND 9 YEARS, RESPECTIVELY, AND BECOMING COMPLETE OR NEARLY COMPLETE BY AGES 10, 5 AND 18 YEARS. VESTIBULAR FUNCTION REMAINED NORMAL. PROGRESSIVE SENSORY NEUROPATHY WITHOUT PERIPHERAL TROPHIC CHANGES WAS ALSO PRESENT. TACHYCARDIA AND LOSS OF THE CAROTID SINUS REFLEX MAY INDICATE INVOLVEMENT OF THE CARDIAC VAGUS. INVOLVEMENT OF THE VAGUS NERVE LED TO PROGRESSIVE LOSS OF GASTRIC MOTILITY. TWO OF THE SISTERS WERE DEMONSTRATED TO HAVE MULTIPLE DIVERTICULA WITH JEJUNOILEAL ULCERATION FROM WHICH THE ELDEST SISTER DIED AT AGE 18 YEARS. MALABSORPTION OF FAT AND INTESTINAL LOSS OF SERUM PROTEIN OCCURRED. A SURVIVING SISTER HAD MARKED ACANTHOSIS NIGRICANS. THIS APPEARS TO BE AN ENTITY DISTINCT FROM OTHERS SUCH AS REFSUM'S SYNDROME AND HEREDITARY SENSORY RADICULAR NEUROPATHY (Q.V.).

HIRSCHOWITZ, B. I., GROLL, A. AND CEBALLOS, R.* HEREDITARY NERVE DEAFNESS IN 3 SISTERS WITH ABSENT GASTRIC MOTILITY, SMALL BOWEL DIVERTICULITIS AND ULCERATION AND PROGRESSIVE SENSORY NEUROPATHY. IN PRESS, 1971.

22150 DEAFNESS, NEURAL, CONGENITAL MODERATE

KONIGSMARK ET AL. (1970) DESCRIBED CONGENITAL MODERATE NEURAL HEARING LOSS IN THREE SIBSHIPS WITH APPARENT RECESSIVE INHERITANCE. THEY CONCLUDED THAT THIS TYPE HAD NOT BEEN DESCRIBED PREVIOUSLY.

KONIGSMARK, B. W., MENGEL, M. C. AND HASKINS, H.* FAMILIAL CONGENITAL MODERATE NEURAL HEARING LOSS. J. LARYNG. 84* 495-505, 1970.

22160 DEAFNESS, NEURAL, EARLY ONSET

MENGEL ET AL. (1967) FOUND SEVERE DEAFNESS IN 16 MEMBERS OF A KINDRED. BY HISTORY ALL WERE BORN WITH AT LEAST SOME HEARING BUT SUFFERED PROGRESSIVE SEVERE LOSS IN LATER CHILDHOOD. SONOGRAPHIC AND SPEECH ANALYSIS GAVE FURTHER EVIDENCE OF SOME HEARING IN EARLY CHILDHOOD. AUDIOLOGIC TESTS SUGGESTED COCHLEAR LOCATION OF THE DEFECT. ALTHOUGH SUCCESSIVE GENERATIONS WERE AFFECTED IN SOME INSTANCES, CONSANGUINITY AND RECESSIVE INHERITANCE WERE THOUGHT TO ACCOUNT FOR THE FINDING.

MENGEL, M. C., KONIGSMARK, B. W., BERLIN, C. I. AND MCKUSICK, V. A.* RECESSIVE EARLY-ONSET NEURAL DEAFNESS. ACTA OTOLARYNG. 64* 313-326, 1967.

22170 DEAFNESS, NEURAL, WITH ATYPICAL ATOPIC DERMATITIS

KONIGSMARK ET AL. (1968) FOUND THIS COMBINATION IN 3 OF 4 SIBS. THE ATOPIC DERMATITIS WAS ATYPICAL IN LATE AGE OF ONSET AND DISTRIBUTION (ULNAR ASPECTS OF FOREARMS AND ANTECUBITAL FOSSAE). THE HEARING LOSS WAS COCHLEAR, WAS FIRST NOTED BETWEEN AGES 3 AND 5 YEARS AND WAS SUFFICIENTLY MILD THAT IT CAUSED NO DIFFICULTY IN SCHOOL.

KONIGSMARK, B. W., HOLLANDER, M. B. AND BERLIN, C. I.* FAMILIAL NEURAL HEARING LOSS AND ATOPIC DERMATITIS. J.A.M.A. 204* 953-957, 1968.

*22180 DERMO-CHONDRO-CORNEAL DYSTROPHY OF FRANCOIS

THE FEATURES ARE (1) SKELETAL DEFORMITY OF THE HANDS AND FEET, (2) XANTHOMATOUS NODULES ON THE PINNAE, DORSAL SURFACE OF THE METACARPOPHALANGEAL AND INTERPHALAN-

R
E
C
E
S
S
I
V
E

GEAL JOINTS, POSTERIOR SURFACE OF THE ELBOWS, NOSE, ETC., AND (3) CORNEAL DYSTROPHY. FRANCOIS (1949) OBSERVED TWO AFFECTED SIBS AND THE PARENTS OF JENSEN'S CASE WERE RELATED. REMKY AND ENGELBRECHT (1967) DESCRIBED THE DISORDER IN BOTH OF UNLIKE-SEX TWINS. THEY IDENTIFIED A HYPERCHOLESTEROLEMIC EARLY STAGE, INVOLVEMENT OF THE ENTIRE SKELETON EXCEPT THE VERTEBRAE AND SKULL AND ABNORMAL EEG WITH SEIZURES.

FRANCOIS, J. AND DETRAIT, C.* DYSTROPHIE DERMO-CHONDRO-CORNEENNE FAMILIALE. ANN. PAEDIAT. 174* 145-174, 1950.

FRANCOIS, J.* DYSTROPHIE DERMO-CHONDRO-CORNEENNE FAMILIALE. ANN. OCULIST. 182* 409-442, 1949.

JENSEN, V. J.* DERMO-CHONDRO-CORNEAL DYSTROPHY* REPORT OF A CASE. ACTA OPHTHAL. 36* 71-78, 1958.

REMKY, H. AND ENGELBRECHT, G.* DYSTROPHIA DERMO-CHONDRO-CORNEALIS (FRANCOIS). KLIN. MBL. AUGENHEILK. 151* 319-331, 1967.

WIEDEMANN, H.-R.* ZUR FRANCOIS'SCHEN KRANKHEIT. AERZTL. WSCHR. 13* 905-909, 1958.

22190 DETACHMENT OF RETINA, CONGENITAL

NORRIE'S DISEASE, AN X-LINKED CONDITION, IS A FORM OF CONGENITAL, SOLID DETACHMENT OF THE RETINA. AN AUTOSOMAL RECESSIVE FORM OF CONGENITAL RETINAL DETACHMENT IS SUGGESTED BY THE REPORTS OF WEVE (1938) AND OF JOANNIDES AND PROTONOTARIOS (1965).

JOANNIDES, T. AND PROTONOTARIOS, P.* DECOLLEMENT FACIFORME DE LE RETINE CHEZ UN FRERE ET UNE SOEUR. ANN. OCULIST. 198* 904-911, 1965.

WEVE, H.* ABLATIO FALCIFORMIS CONGENITA (RETINAL FOLD). BRIT. J. OPHTHAL. 22* 456-470, 1938.

22200 DIABETES INSIPIDUS

X-LINKED AND AUTOSOMAL DOMINANT FORMS OF DIABETES INSIPIDUS ARE KNOWN IN MAN. AUTOSOMAL RECESSIVE DIABETES INSIPIDUS DUE TO A DEFECT IN VASOPRESSIN SYNTHESIS BY THE POSTERIOR PITUITARY IS KNOWN IN THE RAT (VALTIN ET AL., 1965).

VALTIN, H., SAWYER, W. H. AND SOKOL, H. W.* NEUROHYPOPHYSIAL PRINCIPLES IN RATS HOMOZYGOUS AND HETEROZYGOUS FOR HYPOTHALAMIC DIABETES INSIPIDUS (BRATTLEBORO STRAIN). ENDOCRINOLOGY 77* 701-706, 1965.

R
E
C
E
S
S
I
V
E

22210 DIABETES MELLITUS

ALTHOUGH THE IMPORTANT GENETIC FACTOR IN DIABETES IS OBVIOUS, THE MODE OF INHERITANCE IS OBSCURE. RECESSIVE, DOMINANT AND MULTIFACTORIAL HYPOTHESES HAVE BEEN ADVANCED. MULTIPLE DISTINCT ENTITIES PROBABLY EXIST UNDER THIS HEADING. NILSSON (1964) COMMENTED ON THE DIFFICULTIES OF DISTINGUISHING DOMINANT AND RECESSIVE INHERITANCE WHEN GENE FREQUENCY IS HIGH. HE CONSIDERED MOST LIKELY AUTOSOMAL RECESSIVE INHERITANCE WITH A GENE FREQUENCY OF ABOUT 0.30 AND A LIFE-TIME PENETRANCE OF ABOUT 70 PERCENT FOR MALES AND 90 PERCENT FOR FEMALES. A GENE FREQUENCY OF ABOUT 0.05 AND A PENETRANCE OF 25-30 PERCENT WOULD BE REQUIRED TO ACCOUNT FOR THE FINDINGS ON A DOMINANT HYPOTHESIS. USING SYNALBUMIN INSULIN ANTAGONISM AS A TEST, VALLANCE-OWEN (1966) STUDIED 9 FAMILIES CONTAINING 16 OVERT CASES OF DIABETES MELLITUS AND CONCLUDED THAT THE STATE OF SYNALBUMIN POSITIVITY IS A DOMINANT.

NEEL, J. V., FAJANS, S. S., CONN, J. W. AND DAVIDSON, R. T.* DIABETES MELLITUS. GENETICS AND EPIDEMIOLOGY OF CHRONIC DISEASES. NEEL, J. V., SHAW, M. W. AND SHULL, W. J. (EDS.)* WASHINGTON, D. C.* GOVERNMENT PRINTING OFFICE, 1965.

NILSSON, S. E.* ON THE HEREDITY OF DIABETES MELLITUS AND ITS INTERRELATIONSHIP WITH SOME OTHER DISEASES. ACTA GENET. STATIST. MED. 14* 97-124, 1964.

PYKE, D. A.* THE GENETICS OF DIABETES. POSTGRAD. MED. J. 46* 604-606, 1970.

RENOLD, A. E. AND CAHILL, G. F., JR.* DIABETES MELLITUS. IN, STANBURY, J. B., WYNGAARDEN, J. B. AND FREDRICKSON, D. S. (EDS.)* THE METABOLIC BASIS OF INHERITED DISEASE. NEW YORK* MCGRAW-HILL, 1966 (2ND ED.). PP. 69-108.

SIMPSON, N. E.* MULTIFACTORIAL INHERITANCE. A POSSIBLE HYPOTHESIS FOR DIABETES. DIABETES 13* 462-471, 1964.

VALLANCE-OWEN, J.* THE INHERITANCE OF ESSENTIAL DIABETES MELLITUS FROM STUDIES OF SYNALBUMIN INSULIN ANTAGONIST. DIABETOLOGIA 2* 248-252, 1966.

22220 DIABETES MELLITUS AND DIABETES INSIPIDUS

RAITI, PLOTKIN AND NEWNS (1963) REPORTED TWO SISTERS WITH BOTH DIABETES MELLITUS AND DIABETES INSIPIDUS. THE ASSOCIATION IN THE SAME PATIENT IS RARE AND NO OTHER

INSTANCE OF FAMILIAL OCCURRENCE OF THE ASSOCIATION HAS BEEN REPORTED. DIABETES MELLITUS DEVELOPED AT AGE 9 AND AGE 5 YEARS. AUTOSOMAL RECESSIVE INHERITANCE WAS SUGGESTED. HISTOCYTOSIS X IS AN 'ACQUIRED' CAUSE OF DOUBLE DIABETES.

HURLEY, P. J., HITCHCOCK, G. C. AND WILSON, J. D.* HISTOCYTOSIS X AND DOUBLE DIABETES. AUST. ANN. MED. 16* 250-254, 1967.

RAITI, S., PLOTKIN, S. AND NEWNS, G. H.* DIABETES MELLITUS AND INSIPIDUS IN TWO SISTERS. BRIT. MED. J. 2* 1625-1629, 1963.

22230 DIABETES MELLITUS, JUVENILE, WITH OPTIC ATROPHY

HEARING LOSS ALSO OCCURS IN SOME CASES. WOLFRAM AND WAGENER (1938) FOUND JUVENILE DIABETES MELLITUS AND OPTIC ATROPHY IN 4 OF 8 SIBS. TYRER (1943) OBSERVED THREE AFFECTED OUT OF 8 SIBS. TYRER (1943) OBSERVED THREE AFFECTED OUT OF 4 OFFSPRINGS OF A FIRST COUSIN MARRIAGE. ROSE ET AL. (1966) REVIEWED THESE AND OTHER REPORTS AND DESCRIBED SEVERAL CASES INCLUDING TWO UNRELATED CASES, EACH THE SONS OF A CONSANGUINEOUS MATING. THEY SUGGESTED THAT HOMOZYGOSITY FOR A GENE WITH PLEIOTRO-PIC EFFECTS MAY BE INVOLVED AND THAT BECAUSE OF CLINICAL HETEROGENEITY MORE THAN ONE LOCUS MAY BE INVOLVED. ALL SEVEN PATIENTS DESCRIBED BY ROSE ET AL. (1966) WERE MALE. AFFECTED FEMALES WERE DESCRIBED BY OTHERS, E.G., WOLFRAM AND TYRER. RORSMAN AND SODERSTROM (1967) DESCRIBED A FAMILY IN WHICH THREE SISTERS AND A BROTHER DEVELOPED DIABETES MELLITUS AND OPTIC ATROPHY IN THEIR TEENS. IN ONE THE OPTIC ATROPHY APPEARED BEFORE THE DIABETES MELLITUS. DIABETES MELLITUS, DIABETES INSIPIDUS AND OPTIC ATROPHY WERE ASSOCIATED IN A FAMILY RECENTLY STUDIED HERE (D.R., 1264444). STARNES AND WELSH (1970) NOTED ASSOCIATION OF RENAL CALCULI. THE STONES WERE PREDOMINANTLY CALCIUM OXALATE IN ONE CASE.

RORSMAN, G. AND SODERSTROM, N.* OPTIC ATROPHY AND JUVENILE DIABETES MELLITUS WITH FAMILIAL OCCURRENCE. ACTA MED. SCAND. 182* 419-425, 1967.

ROSE, F. C., FRASER, G. R., FRIEDMANN, A. I. AND KOHNER, E. M.* THE ASSOCIATION OF JUVENILE DIABETES MELLITUS AND OPTIC ATROPHY* CLINICAL AND GENETICAL ASPECTS. QUART. J. MED. 35* 385-405, 1966.

STARNES, C. W. AND WELSH, J. D.* INTESTINAL SUCRASE-ISOMALTASE DEFICIENCY AND RENAL CALCULI. NEW ENG. J. MED. 282* 1023-1024, 1970.

TYRER, J.* A CASE OF INFANTILISM WITH GOITRE, DIABETES MELLITUS, MENTAL DEFECT AND BILATERAL PRIMARY OPTIC ATROPHY. MED. J. AUST. 2* 398-401, 1943.

WOLFRAM, D. J. AND WAGENER, H. P.* DIABETES MELLITUS AND SIMPLE OPTIC ATROPHY AMONG SIBLINGS* REPORT OF FOUR CASES. PROC. MAYO CLIN. 13* 715-718, 1938.

22240 DIAPHRAGM, UNILATERAL AGENESIS OF

PASSARGE ET AL. (1968) REPORTED UNILATERAL AGENESIS OF THE DIAPHRAGM IN A BROTHER AND SISTER AND FOUND FOUR REPORTS OF MULTIPLE AFFECTED SIBS IN THE LITERATURE.

PASSARGE, E., HALSEY, H. AND GERMAN, J.* UNILATERAL AGENESIS OF THE DIAPHRAGM. HUMANGENETIK 5* 226-230, 1968.

TEN KATE, L. P. AND ANDERS, G. J. P. A.* UNILATERAL AGENESIS OF THE DIAPHRAGM. (LETTER) HUMANGENETIK 8* 366-367, 1970.

22250 DIASTEMATOMYELIA

IN THIS CONDITION THE SPINAL CORD IS DIVIDED LONGITUDINALLY IN THE ANTERO-POSTERIOR PLANE BY A FIBROUS OR BONY STRUCTURE. THE CASES ARE USUALLY ISOLATED BUT AFFECTED SISTERS WERE REPORTED BY KAPSALAKIS (1964).

KAPSALAKIS, Z.* DIASTEMATOMYELIA IN TWO SISTERS. J. NEUROSURG. 21* 66-67, 1964.

*22260 DIASTROPHIC DWARFISM

THE PATIENTS SHOW SCOLIOSIS, A FORM OF CLUBBED FOOT BILATERALLY, MALFORMED PINNAE WITH CALCIFICATION OF THE CARTILAGE, PREMATURE CALCIFICATION OF THE COSTAL CARTILAGES AND CLEFT PALATE IN SOME CASES. PARTICULARLY CHARACTERISTIC IS THE 'HITCH HICKER' THUMB DUE TO DEFORMITY OF THE FIRST METATARSAL. THE TERM DIASTRO-PHIC WAS BORROWED BY LAMY AND MAROTEAUX (1960) FROM GEOLOGY* DIASTROPHISM IS THE PROCESS OF BENDING OF THE EARTH'S CRUST BY WHICH MOUNTAINS, CONTINENTS, OCEAN BASINS, ETC., ARE FORMED. CASES HAVE BEEN DESCRIBED UNDER MANY DIFFERENT DESIGNATIONS IN THE PAST. SEE THE CASE DESCRIBED BY MAU (1958) IN HIS SECTION ON 'MULTIPLE CONGENITAL MALFORMATIONS AND CONTRACTURES.' THESE CASES HAVE FREQUENTLY BEEN PLACED IN THE WASTEBASKET OF ARTHROGRYPOSIS MULTIPLEX CONGENITA IN HOSPITAL DIAGNOSTIC FILES. MANY CASES OF SO-CALLED ACHONDROPLASIA WITH CLUBFOOT ARE EXAMPLES OF DIASTROPHIC DWARFISM (E.G. KITE, 1964). THE FOOT DEFORMITY IS RELATIVELY REFRACTORY TO SURGICAL TREATMENT. LANGER (1967) REFERS TO AN ENTITY WHICH PHENOTYPICALLY IS A MILD FORM OF DIASTROPHIC DWARFISM AS 'DIASTROPHIC VARIANT.' BONEY CHANGES ARE QUALITATIVELY SIMILAR BUT LESS SEVERE. SOFT TISSUE CHANGES ARE ABSENT OR MILD AND THE CLUBFOOT IS NOT AS RESISTANT TO TREATMENT AS IN

R
E
C
E
S
S
I
V
E

(1963) AND JAGER AND REFIOR (1969). KNOWN TO ME ARE TWO AFFECTED WOMEN EACH OF
WHOM HAD A NORMAL CHILD DELIVERED BY CAESARIAN AND A 50 YEAR OLD AFFECTED MAN WITH
TWO NORMAL TEEN-AGE DAUGHTERS.

JAGER, M. AND REFIOR, H. J.* DIASTROPHISCHER ZWERGWUCHS. Z. ORTHOP. 106* 830-
840, 1969.

KITE, J. H.* THE CLUBFOOT. NEW YORK* GRUNE AND STRATTON, 210-218, 1964.

LAMY, M. AND MAROTEAUX, P.* LA NANISME DIASTROPHIQUE. PRESSE MED. 68* 1977-
1980, 1960.

LANGER, L. O., JR.* DIASTROPHIC DWARFISM IN EARLY INFANCY. AM. J. ROENTGEN.
93* 399-404, 1965.

LANGER, L. O., JR.* MINNEAPOLIS, MINN.* PERSONAL COMMUNICATION, 1967.

MAU, H.* WESEN UND BEDEUTUNG DER ENCHONDRALEN DYSOSTOSEN. STUTTGART* GEORG
THIEME VERLAG, 1958. P. 108 FF.

MCKUSICK, V. A. AND MILCH, R. A.* THE CLINICAL BEHAVIOR OF GENETIC DISEASE*
SELECTED ASPECTS. CLIN. ORTHOP. 33* 22-39, 1964.

TAYBI, H.* DIASTROPHIC DWARFISM. RADIOLOGY 80* 1-10, 1963.

*22270 DIBASICAMINOACIDURIA II

OYANAGI ET AL. (1970) DESCRIBED SEVERE MENTAL RETARDATION, PHYSICAL RETARDATION,
MILD INTESTINAL MALABSORPTION SYNDROME, AND INCREASED URINARY EXCRETION OF LYSINE,
ORNITHINE AND ARGININE IN TWO JAPANESE SISTERS WITH SECOND COUSIN PARENTS.
CYSTINE EXCRETION WAS ALWAYS WITHIN NORMAL LIMITS. THIS DISORDER SEEMS TO BE
PARTICULARLY FREQUENT IN FINLAND. KEKOMAKI ET AL. (1967) DESCRIBED AN AFFECTED
MALE AGE 23 YEARS AND HIS AFFECTED 15 YEAR OLD SISTER. BOTH REFUSED PROTEIN-RICH
FOOD. INSTITUTION OF COW'S MILK AT AGE 1 YEAR RESULTED IN PROLONGED WATERY
DIARRHEA AND RETARDATION OF PHYSICAL DEVELOPMENT. WITH INCREASE IN PROTEIN IN HIS
TEENS THE MALE GREW BUT MENTAL FUNCTION DETERIORATED AND TYPICAL ATTACKS OF STUPOR
AND ASTERIXIS OCCURRED, ACCOMPANIED BY HYPERAMMONEMIA. THE LIVER WAS ENLARGED AND
FATTY. IN THEIR FIRST REPORT IN 1965, PERHEENTUPA AND VISAKORPI DESCRIBED TWO
AFFECTED INFANT SIBS. BLOOD UREA IS LOW. LYSINE AND ARGININE ARE INCREASED IN
THE URINE. IN A GROUP OF CHILDREN INCLUDING SEVERAL PAIRS OF SIBS ONE OF WHICH
HAD CONSANGUINEOUS PARENTS, KEKOMAKI ET AL. (1967) DESCRIBED VOMITING, DIARRHEA,
FAILURE TO THRIVE, HEPATOMEGALY, DIFFUSE CIRRHOSIS, LOW BLOOD UREA, HYPERAMMONEMIA
AND LEUKOPENIA. SYMPTOMS WERE AGGRAVATED BY HIGH PROTEIN INTAKE AND RELIEVED BY
PROTEIN RESTRICTION. AN EXCESS OF ORNITHINE ARGININE AND LYSINE, BUT NOT OF
CYSTINE, WAS EXCRETED IN THE URINE. INTESTINAL ABSORPTION OF ARGININE AND LYSINE
WAS NORMAL. A LOW CONCENTRATION OF ARGININE RELATIVE TO LYSINE IN BODY FLUIDS WAS
THOUGHT RESPONSIBLE FOR THE HYPERAMMONEMIA AND REDUCED UREA SYNTHESIS. AN
ASYMPTOMATIC DIBASICAMINOACIDURIA BEHAVING AS A DOMINANT WAS DESCRIBED IN FRENCH-
CANADIANS BY WHELAN AND SCRIVER (1968). SEE HYPERAMMONEMIA.

KEKOMAKI, M., TOIVAKKA, E., HAKKINEN, V. AND SALASPURO, M.* FAMILIAL PROTEIN
INTOLERANCE WITH DEFICIENT TRANSPORT OF BASIC AMINO ACIDS. ACTA MED. SCAND. 183*
357-359, 1968.

KEKOMAKI, M., VISAKORPI, J. K., PERHEENTUPA, J. AND SAXEN, L.* FAMILIAL PROTEIN
INTOLERANCE WITH DEFICIENT TRANSPORT OF BASIC AMINO ACIDS. AN ANALYSIS OF 10
PATIENTS. ACTA PAEDIAT. SCAND. 56* 617-630, 1967.

OYANAGI, K., MIURA, R. AND YAMANOUCHI, T.* CONGENITAL LYSINURIA* A NEW
INHERITED TRANSPORT DISORDER OF DIBASIC AMINO ACIDS. J. PEDIAT. 77* 259-266,
1970.

PERHEENTUPA, J. AND VISAKORPI, J. K.* PROTEIN INTOLERANCE WITH DEFICIENT
TRANSPORT OF BASIC AMINO ACIDS. ANOTHER INBORN ERROR OF METABOLISM. LANCET 2*
813-816, 1965.

WHELAN, D. T. AND SCRIVER, C. R.* HYPERDIBASICAMINOACIDURIA* AN INHERITED
DISORDER OF AMINO ACID TRANSPORT. PEDIAT. RES. 2* 523-534, 1968.

*22280 DIPHOSPHOGLYCERATE MUTASE DEFICIENCY OF ERYTHROCYTE, ANEMIA DUE TO

SCHROTER (1965) DESCRIBED SEVERE HEMOLYTIC ANEMIA IN AN INFANT. ALTHOUGH THE
PROBAND'S BLOOD COULD NOT BE STUDIED BECAUSE OF MULTIPLE TRANSFUSIONS, THE
ERYTHROCYTES OF THE CONSANGUINEOUS PARENTS, THE SISTER AND THE FATHER'S MOTHER
SHOWED ACTIVITY OF 2,3-DIPHOSPHOGLYCERATE MUTASE ABOUT HALF OF NORMAL. THE FAMILY
OF BOWDLER AND PRANKERD (1964) IS PUZZLING IN THAT FATHER AND SON HAD HEMOLYTIC
ANEMIA FOR WHICH SPLENECTOMY WAS PERFORMED. IN FATHER AND SON, LABIE ET AL.
(1970) FOUND A DECREASE IN DPGM BY ABOUT 50 PERCENT. AN INCREASE IN OXYGEN
AFFINITY OF HEMOGLOBIN WAS OBSERVED. SCHROTER (1965) OBSERVED HETEROZYGOTES IN 3
GENERATIONS INCLUDING BOTH PARENTS OF A HOMOZYGOUS CHILD WITH HEMOLYTIC ANEMIA.

RECESSIVE

BOWDLER, A. J. AND PRANKERD, T. A. J.* STUDIES IN CONGENITAL NON-SPHEROCYTIC HAEMOLYTIC ANAEMIAS WITH SPECIFIC ENZYME DEFECTS. ACTA HAEMAT. 31* 65-78, 1964.

LABIE, D., LEROUX, J. P., NAJMAN, A. AND REYROLLE, C.* FAMILIAL DIPHOSPHOGLY-CERATEMUTASE DEFICIENCY. INFLUENCE ON THE OXYGEN AFFINITY CURVES OF HEMOGLOBIN. FEBS LETTERS 9* 37-40, 1970.

LOHR, G. W. AND WALLER, H. D.* ZUR BIOCHEMIE EINIGER ANGEBORENER HAMOLYTISCHER ANAMIEN. FOLIA HAEMAT. 8* 377-397, 1963.

SCHROTER, W.* KONGENITALE NICHTSPHAROCYTARE HAMOLYTISCHE ANAMIE BEI 2,3-DIPHOSPHOGLYCERATMUTASE-MANGEL DER ERYTHROCYTEN IM FRUHEN SAUGLINGSALTER. KLIN. WSCHR. 43* 1147-1153, 1965.

22290 DISACCHARIDE INTOLERANCE I (CONGENITAL SUCROSE-ISOMALTOSE MALABSORPTION CONGENITAL SUCROSE INTOLERANCE)

DAHLQVIST (1967) GAVE A USEFUL REVIEW OF THE SMALL INTESTINAL DISACCHARIDASES IN MAN. HE RECOGNIZES SIX OF THESE, SO PRESUMABLY SIX UNITARY DEFECTS PLUS MANY COMBINED DEFECTS MIGHT OCCUR. THE SIX ARE MALTASE IA, MALTASE IB (INVERTASE), MALTASE II, MALTASE III, LACTASE (WHICH MAY BE TWO ENZYMES) AND TREHALASE. MALTOSE AND LACTOSE ARE WELL TOLERATED IN 'SUCROSE INTOLERANCE.' PRESUMABLY THE DEFECT CONCERNS INTESTINAL INVERTASE. SEE DURAND (1964) FOR A SYMPOSIUM ON THIS WHOLE GROUP OF DISORDERS. PETERSON AND HERBER (1967) FOUND THAT INTESTINAL SUCRASE DEFICIENCY IS A CAUSE OF DIARRHEA IN ADULTS AND PRESENT IN A FREQUENCY OF ALMOST 0.2 PERCENT. ENZYME OF FUNGAL ORIGIN IS EFFECTIVE TREATMENT. INVOLVEMENT OF MULTIPLE SIBS (KERRY AND TOWNLEY, 1965) AND CONSANGUINEOUS PARENTS (JANSEN ET AL., 1965) SUPPORT RECESSIVE INHERITANCE. HOMOZYGOTES HAVE SEVERE ENZYME DEFICIENCY WITH CLINICAL SYMPTOMS THROUGHOUT LIFE. HETEROZYGOTES HAVE INTERME-DIATE ENZYME VALUES AND NO SYMPTOMS IN ADULTHOOD, BUT MAY HAVE MILD SYMPTOMS IN INFANCY. RATHER NUMEROUS EXAMPLES OF AFFECTED SIBS AND SEVERAL INSTANCES OF CONSANGUINEOUS PARENTS ARE RECORDED. A FORM SYMPTOMATIC IN ADULTS AND LATE IN ONSET WAS DESCRIBED BY JANSEN ET AL. (1965).

BRUNT, P. W. AND MCKUSICK, V. A.* FAMILIAL DYSAUTONOMIA. A REPORT OF GENETIC AND CLINICAL STUDIES, WITH A REVIEW OF THE LITERATURE. MEDICINE 49* 343-374, 1970.

DAHLQVIST, A.* LOCALIZATION OF THE SMALL-INTESTINAL DISACCHARIDASES. AM. J. CLIN. NUTR. 20* 81-88, 1967.

DAVIDSON, M.* DISACCHARIDE INTOLERANCE. PEDIAT. CLIN. N. AM. 14* 93-107, 1967.

DURAND, P. (ED.)* DISORDERS DUE TO INTESTINAL DEFECTIVE CARBOHYDRATE DIGESTION AND ABSORPTION. (SYMPOSIUM) ROME, 1964.

HOLZEL, A.* SUGAR MALABSORPTION DUE TO DEFICIENCIES OF DISACCHARIDASE ACTIVI-TIES AND OF MONOSACCHARIDE TRANSPORT. ARCH. DIS. CHILD. 42* 341-352, 1967.

JANSEN, W., QUE, G. S. AND VEEGER, W.* PRIMARY COMBINED SACCHARASE AND ISOMALTASE DEFICIENCY. REPORT OF TWO ADULT SIBLINGS OF CONSANGUINEOUS PARENTAGE. ARCH. INTERN. MED. 116* 879-885, 1965.

KERRY, K. R. AND TOWNLEY, R. R. W.* GENETIC ASPECTS OF INTESTINAL SUCRASE-ISOMALTASE DEFICIENCY. AUST. PAEDIAT. J. 1* 223-235, 1965.

PETERSON, M. L. AND HERBER, R.* INTESTINAL SUCRASE DEFICIENCY. TRANS. ASS. AM. PHYSICIANS 80* 275-283, 1967.

PRADER, A. AND AURICCHIO, S.* DEFECTS OF INTESTINAL DISACCHARIDE ABSORPTION. ANN. REV. MED. 16* 345-358, 1965.

*22300 DISACCHARIDE INTOLERANCE II (CONGENITAL LACTOSE INTOLERANCE)

CELLOBIOSE INTOLERANCE WOULD BE EXPECTED AS WELL AS THAT FOR LACTOSE. SUCROSE, MALTOSE AND STARCH ARE WELL TOLERATED. AFFECTED SIBS WERE DESCRIBED BY HOLZEL ET AL. (1959), WEIJERS AND VAN DE KAMER (1964), AND LAUNIALA ET AL. (1969). NO INSTANCE OF PARENTAL CONSANGUINITY HAS BEEN REPORTED AND NO STIGMA OF HETEROZYGO-SITY HAS BEEN NOTED. IN A BREASTFED INFANT WHO DEVELOPED WATERY DIARRHEA ON THE THIRD DAY OF LIFE, LEVIN ET AL. (1970) DEMONSTRATED ABSENT LACTASE IN A SPECIMEN OF DUODENAL MUCOSA WHICH WAS HISTOLOGICALLY NORMAL AND SHOWED NORMAL MALTASE ISOMALTASE AND SUCRASE ACTIVITIES. CONVINCING DIRECT DEMONSTRATION OF ABSENT LACTASE IN BIOPSIES OBTAINED IN INFANCY, HAS BEEN ACHIEVED ONLY TWICE BEFORE, ACCORDING TO THE AUTHORS. A SISTER OF THE PROBAND WAS PROBABLY IDENTICALLY AFFECTED.

DAHLQVIST, A.* SPECIFICITY OF THE HUMAN INTESTINAL DISACCHARIDASES AND IMPLICATIONS FOR HEREDITARY DISACCHARIDE INTOLERANCE. J. CLIN. INVEST. 41* 463-470, 1962.

DARLING, S., MORTENSEN, O. AND SONDERGAARD, G.* LACTOSURIA AND AMINO-ACIDURIA IN INFANCY* A NEW INBORN ERROR OF METABOLISM.Q ACTA PAEDIAT. 49* 281-290, 1960.

R
E
C
E
S
S
I
V
E

HOLZEL, A., SCHWARZ, V. AND SUTCLIFFE, K. W.* DEFECTIVE LACTOSE ABSORPTION CAUSING MALNUTRITION IN INFANCY. LANCET 1* 1126-1128, 1959.

LAUNIALA, K., PERHEENTUPA, J. AND HALLMAN, N.* CONGENITAL SUGAR MALABSORPTION. IN, GARDNER, L. I. (ED.)* ENDOCRINE AND GENETIC DISEASES OF CHILDHOOD. PHILADEL-PHIA* W. B. SAUNDERS CO., 1969. PP. 830-843.

LEVIN, B., ABRAHAM, J. M., BURGESS, E. A. AND WALLIS, P. G.* CONGENITAL LACTOSE MALABSORPTION. ARCH. DIS. CHILD. 45* 173-177, 1970.

WEIJERS, H. A. AND VAN DE KAMER, J. H.* FERMENTATIVE DIARRHOEAS. IN, DURAND, P. (ED.)* DISORDERS DUE TO INTESTINAL DEFECTIVE CARBOHYDRATE DIGESTION AND ABSORPTION. ROME* IL PENSIERO SCIENTIFICO, 1964.

*22310 DISACCHARIDE INTOLERANCE III (ADULT LACTASE DEFICIENCY)

SEVERAL STUDIES (CUATRECASAS ET AL., 1965* FRIEDLAND, 1965) OF THE ORAL LACTOSE TOLERANCE TEST HAVE FOUND DIARRHEA AND FLAT BLOOD-GLUCOSE CURVES IN A CONSIDERABLE PROPORTION OF ADULTS, ESPECIALLY IN NEGROES. INTESTINAL LACTASE ACTIVITY IS LOST WITH AGE IN RATS, PIGS AND RABBITS. MAN MAY BE POLYMORPHIC WITH REGARD TO THE LOSS OR RETENTION OF LACTASE ACTIVITY IN ADULTHOOD. THE GENETIC CONTROL OF THIS AND ITS RELATIONSHIP TO LACTASE DEFICIENCY EVIDENT IN INFANCY (SEE DISACCHARIDE INTOLERANCE III) HAS NOT BEEN WORKED OUT. LACTOSE INTOLERANCE IS MUCH MORE FREQUENT IN NEGROES THAN IN CAUCASOIDS (BAYLESS AND ROSENSWEIG, 1966). ISOLATED LACTASE DEFICIENCY OF ADULTHOOD IS ALSO MORE FREQUENT IN THE AMERICAN INDIAN THAN CAUCASIANS (WELSH ET AL., 1967). LACTOSE INTOLERANCE IS ALSO PRESENT IN A GREAT MAJORITY OF ADULT ORIENTALS (HUANG AND BAYLESS, 1968). THE INTOLERANCE USUALLY FIRST APPEARS IN THE LATE TEENS. PERHAPS THIS REPRESENTS FAILURE OF DEVELOPMENT OF A NORMAL POST-WEANING LACTOSE DIGESTING SYSTEM. COOK (1967) FOUND THAT THE DEFICIENCY DEVELOPED IN THE FIRST FOUR YEARS AND SOMETIMES IN THE FIRST 6 MONTHS IN AFRICANS. ROSENSWEIG ET AL. (1967) FOUND THREE GROUPS AS TO LACTASE LEVEL AND SUGGESTED THAT THESE CORRESPOND TO THREE GENOTYPES. SOME HETEROZYGOTES IN THEIR CLASSIFICATION HAD MILK AND LACTOSE INDUCED SYMPTOMS. WORK OF SEMENZA ET AL. (1965) SUGGESTS THE EXISTENCE OF TWO SEPARATE LACTASES WHICH MAY BE UNDER SEPARATE GENETIC CONTROL.

THE FORM OF INTESTINAL LACTASE DEFICIENCY PRESENT IN ADULTS WAS CALLED PRIMARY HYPOLACTASIA BY FERGUSON AND MAXWELL (1967) AS CONTRASTED WITH HEREDITARY ALACTASIA, THE DISORDER CAUSING DIARRHEA IN INFANCY (SEE DISACCHARIDE INTOLERANCE III). THESE AUTHORS DESCRIBED AFFECTED BROTHER AND SISTER. IN PATIENTS WITH INTESTINAL MALABSORPTION (E.G. TROPICAL SPRUE) GRAY ET AL. (1969) FOUND THAT, OF THE TWO LACTASES WITH DIFFERENT PH OPTIMA FOUND IN NORMAL INTESTINE, ONLY ENZYME I WITH A PH OPTIMUM OF 6.0 AND MOLECULAR WEIGHT OF 280,000 WAS ABSENT. SIMILAR STUDIES IN ADULT INTESTINAL LACTASE DEFICIENCY WITHOUT MALABSORPTION ARE INDI-CATED. BAER (1970) SUGGESTED THAT THE DEVELOPMENT OF YOGURT WAS A COMPENSATION FOR THE INTESTINAL LACTASE DEFICIENCY IN COUNTRIES WITH A LARGE FREQUENCY OF THE DISORDER. WELSH (1970) REVIEWED REPORTS OF A HIGH FREQUENCY IN AMERICAN NEGROES, AFRICANS, ASIANS, GREEK CYPRIOTS, AUSTRALIAN ABORIGINES AND SOUTH AMERICAN INDIANS. FERGUSON AND MAXWELL (1967) OBSERVED TWO AFFECTED CHILDREN WITH NORMAL PARENTS. THE FAMILY DATA OF WELSH (1970) INDICATE A GENETIC BASIS BUT GIVE NO CONCLUSIVE INDICATION OF THE MODE OF INHERITANCE.

BAER, D.* LACTASE DEFICIENCY AND YOGURT. SOCIAL BIOL. 17* 143 ONLY, 1970.

BAYLESS, T. M. AND ROSENSWEIG, N. S.* A RACIAL DIFFERENCE IN INCIDENCE OF LACTASE DEFICIENCY. A SURVEY OF MILK INTOLERANCE AND LACTASE DEFICIENCY IN HEALTHY ADULT MALES. J.A.M.A. 197* 968-972, 1966.

BAYLESS, T. M. AND ROSENSWEIG, N. S.* INCIDENCE AND IMPLICATIONS OF LACTASE DEFICIENCY AND MILK INTOLERANCE IN WHITE AND NEGRO POPULATIONS. JOHNS HOPKINS MED. J. 121* 54-64, 1967.

BRYANT, G. D., CHU, Y. K. AND LOVITT, R.* INCIDENCE AND AETIOLOGY OF LACTOSE INTOLERANCE. MED. J. AUST. 1* 1285-1288, 1970.

COOK, G. C.* LACTASE ACTIVITY IN NEWBORN AND INFANT BAGANDA. BRIT. MED. J. 1* 527-530, 1967.

CUATRECASAS, P., LOCKWOOD, D. H. AND CALDWELL, J. R.* LACTASE DEFICIENCY IN THE ADULT. A COMMON OCCURRENCE. LANCET 1* 14-18, 1965.

DE RITIS, F., BALESTRIERI, G. G., RUGGIERO, G., FILOSA, E. AND AURICCHIO, S.* HIGH FREQUENCY OF LACTASE ACTIVITY DEFICIENCY IN SMALL BOWEL OF ADULTS IN THE NEAPOLITAN AREA. ENZYM. BIOL. CLIN. 11* 263-267, 1970.

FERGUSON, A. AND MAXWELL, J. D.* GENETIC AETIOLOGY OF LACTOSE INTOLERANCE. LANCET 2* 188-190, 1967.

FRIELAND, N.* *NORMAL* LACTOSE TOLERANCE TEST. ARCH. INTERN. MED. 116* 886-888, 1965.

GILAT, T., KUHN, R., GELMAN, E. AND MIZRAHY, O.* LACTASE DEFICIENCY IN JEWISH COMMUNITIES IN ISRAEL. AM. J. DIG. DIS. 15* 895-904, 1970.

GRAY, G. M., SANTIAGO, N. A., COLVER, E. H. AND GENEL, M.* INTESTINAL BETA-GALACTOSIDASES. II. BIOCHEMICAL ALTERATION IN HUMAN LACTASE DEFICIENCY. J. CLIN. INVEST. 48* 729-735, 1969.

HUANG, S.-S. AND BAYLESS, T. M.* LACTOSE INTOLERANCE IN HEALTHY CHILDREN. NEW ENG. J. MED. 276* 1283-1287, 1967.

HUANG, S.-S. AND BAYLESS, T. M.* MILK AND LACTOSE INTOLERANCE IN HEALTHY ORIENTALS. SCIENCE 160* 83-84, 1968.

JUSSILA, J., ISOKOSKI, M. AND LAUNIALA, K.* PREVALENCE OF LACTOSE MALABSORPTION IN A FINNISH RURAL POPULATION. SCAND. J. GASTROENT. 5* 49-56, 1970.

ROSENSWEIG, N. S., HUANG, S.-S. AND BAYLESS, T. M.* TRANSMISSION OF LACTOSE INTOLERANCE. (LETTER) LANCET 2* 777 ONLY, 1967.

SEMENZA, G., AURICCHIO, S. AND RUBINO, A.* MULTIPLICITY OF HUMAN INTESTINAL DISACCHARIDASES. I. CHROMATOGRAPHIC SEPARATION OF MALTASES AND OF TWO LACTASES. BIOCHIM. BIOPHYS. ACTA 96* 487-497, 1965.

WELSH, J. D.* ISOLATED LACTASE DEFICIENCY IN HUMANS* REPORT ON 100 PATIENTS. MEDICINE 49* 257-277, 1970.

WELSH, J. D., ROHRER, V., KNUDSEN, K. B. AND PAUSTIAN, F. F.* ISOLATED LACTASE DEFICIENCY* CORRELATION OF LABORATORY STUDIES AND CLINICAL DATA. ARCH. INTERN. MED. 120* 261-269, 1967.

22320 DISSEMINATED SCLEROSIS (MULTIPLE SCLEROSIS)

MACKAY AND MYRIANTHOPOULOS (1966) FOUND THAT CONCORDANCE IS SLIGHTLY HIGHER IN MONOZYGOTIC THAN IN DIZYGOTIC TWINS AND THAT MULTIPLE SCLEROSIS IS ABOUT 20 TIMES MORE FREQUENT AMONG RELATIVES OF PROBANDS THAN IN THE GENERAL POPULATION. THE FREQUENCY DECLINED AS THE RELATIONSHIP TO THE PROBAND BECAME MORE REMOTE. THEY CONCLUDED THAT THE FAMILY DATA CONSISTENT WITH AUTOSOMAL RECESSIVE INHERITANCE WITH REDUCED PENETRANCE BUT THAT EXOGENOUS FACTORS MUST BE VERY STRONG. ON THE OTHER HAND, THE CONCORDANCE RATE IN MONOZYGOTIC TWINS IS SO LOW THAT IT IS DIFFICULT TO THINK THAT GENETIC FACTORS ARE OF GREAT IMPORTANCE. THERE APPEAR TO BE RARE FORMS OF MULTIPLE SCLEROSIS OR MULTIPLE SCLEROSIS-LIKE DISEASES WHICH ARE GENETIC.

MACKAY, R. P. AND MYRIANTHOPOULOS, N. C.* MULTIPLE SCLEROSIS IN TWINS AND THEIR RELATIVES. FINAL REPORT. ARCH. NEUROL. 15* 449-462, 1966.

MYRIANTHOPOULOS, N. C. AND MACKAY, R. P.* MULTIPLE SCLEROSIS IN TWINS AND THEIR RELATIVES* GENETIC ANALYSIS OF FAMILY HISTORIES. ACTA GENET. 10* 33-47, 1960.

22330 DISSEMINATED SCLEROSIS WITH NARCOLEPSY

EKBOM (1966) DESCRIBED FOUR FAMILIES IN WHICH MULTIPLE MEMBERS HAD MULTIPLE SCLEROSIS. IN 3 OF THE 4 FAMILIES ONE OR MORE AFFECTED PERSONS ALSO HAD NARCOLEPSY. NO CONSANGUINITY WAS FOUND.

EKBOM, K.* FAMILIAL MULTIPLE SCLEROSIS ASSOCIATED WITH NARCOLEPSY. ARCH. NEUROL. 15* 337-344, 1966.

22340 DUODENAL ATRESIA

MISHALANY ET AL. (1970) DESCRIBED TWO CHILDREN WITH DUODENAL ATRESIA, ALL FOUR PARENTS OF WHOM WERE DESCENDENTS FROM ONE COUPLE, BEING RELATED AS FIRST COUSINS. SEE JEJUNAL ATRESIA.

MISHALANY, H. G., DER KALOUSTIAN, V. M. AND GHANDOUR, M.* FAMILIAL CONGENITAL DUODENAL ATRESIA. PEDIATRICS 46* 629-632, 1970.

22350 DWARFISM, LOW BIRTH-WEIGHT TYPE, WITH UNRESPONSIVENESS TO GROWTH HORMONE

VAN GEMUND ET AL. (1969) DESCRIBED TWO BOYS WHO WERE OFFSPRING OF FIRST COUSIN PARENTS AND 'SMALL FOR DATES' AT BIRTH SHOWED MARKED DWARFISM, SEVERE MENTAL RETARDATION, AND CONGENITAL DEAFNESS. ONE RELATIVE WAS CONGENITALLY DEAF WITH NORMAL STATURE AND INTELLECT. A MATERNAL UNCLE WAS AN IMBECILE AND DWARFED WITHOUT DEAFNESS. INSULIN-INDUCED HYPOGLYCEMIA EVOKED EXCESSIVELY HIGH LEVELS OF IMMUNOREACTIVE HGH. THEY DID NOT SHOW INCREASED SENSITIVITY TO FATTY ACID LEVELS. ORALLY ADMINISTERED GLUCOSE SUPPRESSED HGH AND EVOCATED INSULIN SECRETION. EXOGENOUS HGH DID NOT DECREASE URINARY NITROGEN EXCRETION OR INCREASE URINARY HYDROXYPROLINE EXCRETION. GROWTH PROMOTING EFFECTS OF EXOGENOSIS TESTOSTERONE WERE INTACT. UNRESPONSIVENESS TO SOMATOTROPIC EFFECTS OF HGH WERE POSTULATED. THE CONSANGUINITY SUGGESTS AUTOSOMAL RECESSIVE INHERITANCE. SINCE A MATERNAL UNCLE HAD DWARFISM AND MENTAL RETARDATION, X-LINKED RECESSIVE INHERITANCE IS A POSSIBILITY.

VAN GEMUND, J. J., LAURENT DE ANGULO, M. S. AND VANGELDEREN, H. H.* FAMILIAL PRENATAL DWARFISM WITH ELEVATED SERUM IMMUNO-REACTIVE GROWTH HORMONE LEVELS AND

22360 DWARFISM, "SNUB-NOSED" TYPE

LEVI (1910) DESCRIBED A VARIETY OF LOW BIRTH WEIGHT DWARFS WITH NORMAL PROPORTIONS AS "MICROSOMIE ESSENTIELLE." BLACK (1961) REFERRED TO THEM AS "SNUB-NOSED DWARFS." VERSCHUER AND CONRADI (1938) SUGGESTED RECESSIVE INHERITANCE. THE LOW BIRTH WEIGHT IS PROBABLY NOT WELL DOCUMENTED AND THESE MAY BE INSTANCES OF SEXUAL ATELEIOSIS (Q.V.).

BLACK, J.* LOW BIRTH WEIGHT DWARFISM. ARCH. DIS. CHILD. 36* 633-644, 1961.

LEVI, E.* CONTRIBUTION A LA CONNAISSANCE DE LA MICROSOMIE ESSENTIELLE HEREDO-FAMILIALE* DISTINCTION DE CETTE FORME CLINIQUE D'AVEC LES NANISMES, LES INFANTI-LISMES ET LES FORMES MIXTES DE CES DIFFERENTES DYSTROPHIES. N. ICONOG. SALPET. 23* 522-570, 1910.

VON VERSCHUER, O. F. AND CONRADI, L.* EINE SIPPE MIT REZESSIV ERBLICHEM PRIMORDIALEM ZWERGWUCHS. Z. MENSCHL. VERERB. KONSTITUTIONSL. 22* 261-267, 1938.

22370 DWARFISM, TYPE UNCLEAR

SEVERAL REPORTS OF CASES ANSWERING THIS DESCRIPTION COULD PROBABLY BE FOUND. ONE, A PERSONAL CASE IN WHICH RECESSIVE INHERITANCE WAS STRONGLY SUGGESTED, IS SHOWN IN FIG. 35 OF MCKUSICK ET AL. (1963).

MCKUSICK, V. A. AND COLLEAGUES* MEDICAL GENETICS 1962. J. CHRONIC DIS. 16* 457-634, 1963.

22380 DYGGVE-MELCHIOR-CLAUSEN DISEASE

AMONG THE CHILDREN FROM UNCLE-NIECE MARRIAGE IN GREENLAND, DYGGVE ET AL. (1962) FOUND THREE CHILDREN WITH A CONDITION RESEMBLING HURLER SYNDROME AND MORQUIO SYNDROME IN SOME RESPECTS. THE FINGERS WERE CLAWED WITH LIMITATION IN EXTENSION. THE PATIENTS WERE MENTALLY RETARDED AND THE URINE SHOWED MUCOPOLYSACCHARIDE. THE SPINE SHOWED GENERALIZED PLATYSPONDYLY. IRREGULARITIES OF THE ILIAC CREST GAVE AN APPEARANCE OF A LACE BORDER AROUND IT. THE PATIENT SHOWN IN FAMILY 12 (PLATE XII) OF HOBAEK'S NORWEGIAN STUDY IS PROBABLY IDENTICAL.

DYGGVE, H. V., MELCHIOR, J. C. AND CLAUSEN, J.* MORQUIO-ULLRICH'S DISEASE. AN INBORN ERROR OF METABOLISM.Q ARCH. DIS. CHILD. 37* 525-534, 1962.

HOBAEK, A.* PROBLEMS OF HEREDITARY CHONDRODYSPLASIAS. OSLO, NORWAY* OSLO U. PRESS, 1961.

*22390 DYSAUTONOMIA (RILEY-DAY SYNDROME)

FEATURES ARE LACK OF TEARING, EMOTIONAL LABILITY, PAROXYSMAL HYPERTENSION, INCREASED SWEATING, COLD HANDS AND FEET, CORNEAL ANESTHESIA, ERYTHEMATOUS BLOTCHING OF THE SKIN, AND DROOLING. ALMOST ALL CASES ARE ASHKENAZI JEWS. BROWN, BEAUCHEMIN AND LINDE (1964) DESCRIBED THE PATHOLOGICAL FINDINGS IN TWO JEWISH SIBS WITH THIS DISEASE, NAMELY, DEMYELINATION IN THE MEDULLA, PONTINE RETICULAR FORMATION AND DORSO-LONGITUDINAL TRACTS, AND DEGENERATION, PIGMENTATION AND LOSS OF CELLS IN AUTONOMIC GANGLIA. YATSU AND ZUSSMAN (1964) PROVIDED FOLLOW-UP ON ONE OF THE 5 CASES REPORTED BY RILEY AND DAY IN 1949. THE PATIENT DIED SUDDENLY AT AGE 31. IN ISRAEL, AS IN THE UNITED STATES, MOST CASES ARE ASHKENAZIC JEWS FROM POLAND (GOLDSTEIN-NIEVIAZHSKI AND WALLIS, 1966). RARE NON-JEWISH CASES HAVE BEEN WELL DOCUMENTED (BURKE, 1966). CONDITIONS WHICH HAVE BEEN CONFUSED WITH DYSAU-TONOMIA INCLUDE BIEMOND'S CONGENITAL AND FAMILIAL ANALGESIA AND NEUROPATHY, CONGENITAL SENSORY, WITH ANHIDROSIS.

AGUAYO, A. J., NAIR, C. P. V. AND BRAY, G. M.* PERIPHERAL NERVE ABNORMALITIES IN THE RILEY-DAY SYNDROME. FINDINGS IN A SURAL NERVE BIOPSY. ARCH. NEUROL. 24* 106-116, 1971.

BROWN, W. J., BEAUCHEMIN, J. A. AND LINDE, L. M.* A NEUROPATHOLOGICAL STUDY OF FAMILIAL DYSAUTONOMIA (RILEY-DAY SYNDROME) IN SIBLINGS. J. NEUROL. NEUROSURG. PSYCHIAT. 27* 131-139, 1964.

BRUNT, P. W. AND MCKUSICK, V. A.* FAMILIAL DYSAUTONOMIA. A REPORT OF GENETIC AND CLINICAL STUDIES, WITH A REVIEW OF THE LITERATURE. MEDICINE 49* 343-374, 1970.

BURKE, V.* FAMILIAL DYSAUTONOMIA. AUST. PAEDIAT. J. 2* 58-63, 1966.

GITLOW, S. E., BERTANI, L. M., WILK, E., LI, B. L. AND DZIEDZIC, S.* EXCRETION OF CATECHOLAMINE METABOLITES BY CHILDREN WITH FAMILIAL DYSAUTONOMIA. PEDIATRICS 46* 513-522, 1970.

GOLDSTEIN-NIEVIAZHSKI, C. AND WALLIS, K.* RILEY-DAY SYNDROME (FAMILIAL DYSAUTONOMIA). SURVEY OF 27 CASES. ANN. PAEDIAT. 206* 188-194, 1966.

R
E
C
E
S
S
I
V
E

HUTCHISON, J. H. AND HAMILTON, W.* FAMILIAL DYSAUTONOMIA IN TWO SIBLINGS. LANCET 1* 1216-1218, 1962.

MCKENDRICK, T.* FAMILIAL DYSAUTONOMIA. ARCH. DIS. CHILD. 33* 465-468, 1958.

MCKUSICK, V. A., NORUM, R. A., FARKAS, H. J., BRUNT, P. W. AND MAHLOUDJI, M.* THE RILEY-DAY SYNDROME - OBSERVATIONS ON GENETICS AND SURVIVORSHIP. ISRAEL J. MED. SCI. 3* 372-379, 1967.

PEARSON, J., FINEGOLD, M. J. AND BUDZILOVICH, G.* THE TONGUE AND TASTE IN FAMILIAL DYSAUTONOMIA. PEDIATRICS 45* 739-745, 1970.

RILEY, C. M.* FAMILIAL AUTONOMIC DYSFUNCTION. J.A.M.A. 149* 1532-1535, 1952.

YATSU, F. AND ZUSSMAN, W.* FAMILIAL DYSAUTONOMIA (RILEY-DAY SYNDROME). CASE REPORT WITH POST-MORTEM FINDINGS OF A PATIENT AT AGE 31. ARCH. NEUROL. 10* 459-463, 1964.

22400 DYSAUTONOMIA-LIKE DISORDER

SCHMIDT ET AL. (1970) CONCLUDED THAT THE DISORDER THEY OBSERVED IN TWO DAUGHTERS OF A SEPHARDIC UNCLE-NEICE MARRIAGE WAS A DISORDER DISTINCT FROM FAMILIAL DYSAUTONOMIA, WHICH, OF COURSE, OCCURS MAINLY IN ASHKENAZIC JEWS. IN THESE PATIENTS MENTAL RETARDATION AND NORMAL TASTE, FUNGIFORM PAPILLAE, HISTAMINE TEST AND URINARY VMA EXCRETION DIFFERENTIATE THE CONDITION. SEE NEUROPATHY, CONGENITAL SENSORY, WITH ANHIDROSIS, ANOTHER DYSAUTONOMIA LIKE CONDITION.

SCHMIDT, R., ALKAN, W. J., MOSES, S. W., MUNDEL, G. AND ROIZEN, S.* A CLINICAL ENTITY SIMULATING FAMILIAL DYSAUTONOMIA IN A NORTH AFRICAN JEWISH FAMILY. J. PEDIAT. 76* 283-288, 1970.

*22410 DYSERYTHROPOIETIC ANEMIA

THE TWO FAMILIES REPORTED BY VERWILGHEN ET AL. (1969) APPARENTLY HAD A DISTINCT FORM OF CONGENITAL DYSERYTHROPOIETIC ANEMIA.

VERWILGHEN, R., VERHAEGEN, H., WAUMANS, P. AND BEERT, J.* INEFFECTIVE ERYTHRO-POIESIS WITH MORPHOLOGICALLY ABNORMAL ERYTHROBLASTS AND UNCONJUGATED HYPERBILIRU-BINAEMIA. BRIT. J. HAEMAT. 17* 27-33, 1969.

22420 DYSGENESIS MESODERMALIS CORNEAE ET SCLERAE

BERTELSEN (1968) DESCRIBED A BROTHER AND SISTER WITH FIRST COUSIN PARENTS AND MARKEDLY BLUE SCLERAE AND THIN CORNEA. IN THE GIRL, RUPTURE OF THE CORNEA OCCURRED IN BOTH EYES AFTER SLIGHT INDIRECT TRAUMA. MEGALOCORNEA, DEEP ANTERIOR CHAMBERS AND SEVERE MYOPIA WERE PRESENT. NO SIGNS OF OSTEOGENESIS IMPERFECTA WERE PRESENT IN THE PATIENTS OR FAMILY.

BERTELSEN, T. I.* DYSGENESIS MESODERMALIS CORNEAE ET SCLERAE. RUPTURE OF BOTH CORNEAE IN A PATIENT WITH BLUE SCLERAE. ACTA OPHTHAL. 46* 486-491, 1968.

*22430 DYSOSTEOSCLEROSIS

SPRANGER ET AL. (1968) USED THIS TERM TO DISTINGUISH A SYNDROME CHIEFLY CHARAC-TERIZED BY OSTEOSCLEROSIS AND PLATYSPONDYLY. THE AFFECTED CHILDREN ARE USUALLY SHORT AND HAVE A TENDENCY TO FRACTURE. CRANIAL NERVE COMPRESSION OCCURS IN SOME. MACULAR ATROPHY OF THE SKIN, FLATTENED FINGERNAILS, AND POORLY CALCIFIED OR CHALKY ENAMEL HAS BEEN NOTED. THE CALVARIUM, ESPECIALLY IN THE FRONTAL AREA, AND THE BASE OF THE SKULL ARE SCLEROTIC. THE VERTEBRAL BODIES ARE FLATTENED, DEFORMED AND DIFFUSELY DENSE. WHILE THE REST OF THE LONG BONES ARE SCLEROTIC, WIDELY SPLAYED SUBMETAPHYSEAL PORTIONS ARE CLEAR WITH IRREGULARLY COARSE TRABECULAR PATTERN. AFFECTED SIBS HAVE BEEN REPORTED BY ELLIS (1934), FIELD (1939) AND STEHR (1942). PARENTAL CONSANGUINITY WAS NOTED BY SPRANGER ET AL. (1968) AND BY ELLIS (1934) AND FIELD (1939).

ELLIS, R. W. B.* OSTEOPETROSIS (MARBLE BONES* ALBERS-SCHONBERG'S DISEASE* OSTEOSCLEROSIS FRAGILIS GENERALISATA* CONGENITAL OSTEOSCLEROSIS). PROC. ROY. SOC. MED. 27* 1563-1571, 1934.

FIELD, C. E.* ALBERS-SCHONBERG DISEASE. ATYPICAL CASE. PROC. ROY. SOC. MED. 32* 320-324, 1939.

SPRANGER, J., ALBRECHT, C., ROHWEDDER, H. J. AND WIEDEMANN, H. R.* DIE DYSOSTEOSKLEROSE* EINE SONDER FORM DER GENERALISIERTEN OSTEOSKEROSE. FORTSCHR. ROENTGENSTR. 109* 504-512, 1968.

STEHR, L.* PATHOGENESE UND KLINIK DER OSTEOSKLEROSEN. ARCH. ORTHOP. UNFALL-CHIR. 41* 156-182, 1942.

22440 DYSOSTOSIS, ENCHONDRAL, OF NIERHOFF-HUBNER TYPE

THE FEATURES ARE MICROMELIA WITH NORMAL STATURE AT BIRTH, SOMETIMES MICROCEPHALY,

R
E
C
E
S
S
I
V
E

RIBS.   OF 6 SIBS, 3, A FEMALE AND 2 MALES, DIED AT THE AGE OF A FEW WEEKS. ALL SHOWED CLONIC CONVULSIONS, AND AT AUTOPSY LEPTOMENINGEAL HEMORRHAGES.

RUPPRECHT, E. AND DORFEL, E.* ENCHONDRALE DYSOSTOSE TYP NIERHOFF-HUBNER BEI 3 GESCHWISTERN. ARCH. KINDERHEILK. 173* 64-73, 1966.

*22450 DYSTONIA MUSCULORUM DEFORMANS

SANTANGELO (1934) OBSERVED 3 OF 5 CHILDREN AFFECTED, FROM A MARRIAGE OF UNAFFECTED SECOND COUSINS. ELDRIDGE (1967) CONCLUDED, FROM A STUDY OF A LARGE SERIES OF CASES AND THEIR FAMILIES IN THE UNITED STATES THAT A RECESSIVE FORM IS PARTICULAR-LY FREQUENT IN JEWS AND DIFFERS FROM THE AUTOSOMAL DOMINANT FORM IN EARLIER AGE OF ONSET AND MORE CONSISTENT GRADE OF SEVERITY. ELDRIDGE ET AL. (1970) PRESENTED EVIDENCE FAVORING INCREASED INTELLIGENCE IN THIS DISORDER. IF A DEFINITE ALTHOUGH PERHAPS MORE DIFFICULT TO DEMONSTRATE SUPERIORITY OF INTELLIGENCE WERE TO OCCUR IN HETEROZYGOTES, THE RELATIVELY HIGH FREQUENCY OF THE DYSTONIA GENE IN JEWS MIGHT HAVE ITS EXPLANATION THEREIN.

ELDRIDGE, R.* BETHESDA, MD.* PERSONAL COMMUNICATION, 1967.

ELDRIDGE, R., HARLAN, A., COOPER, I. S. AND RIKLAN, M.* SUPERIOR INTELLIGENCE IN RECESSIVELY INHERITED TORSION DYSTONIA. LANCET 1* 65-67, 1970.

SANTANGELO, G.* CONTRIBUTO CLINICO ALLA CONOSCENZA DELLE FORME FAMILIARI DELLA DYSBASIA LORDOTICA PROGRESSIVA (SPASMO DI TORSIONE). G. PSYCHIAT. NEUROPAT. 62* 52-77, 1934.

22460 DYSTONIA, PERIODIC

SMITH AND HEERSEMA (1941) OBSERVED EPISODIC DYSTONIC MOVEMENTS OF 5-10 SECONDS DURATION INDUCED BY MOVEMENT IN THREE UNRELATED SIBSHIPS OF POLISH AND LITHUANIAN EXTRACTION.   FOUR, ONE AND TWO SIBS WERE AFFECTED. SEE FAMILIAL PAROXYSMAL CHOREO-ATHETOSIS FOR A SOMEWHAT SIMILAR CONDITION INHERITED AS A DOMINANT. ALSO SEE DYSTONIA IN THE DOMINANT CATALOG.

SMITH, L. A. AND HEERSEMA, P. H.* PERIODIC DYSTONIA. PROC. MAYO CLIN. 16* 842-846, 1941.

22470 EBSTEIN'S ANOMALY

GUERON ET AL. (1966) DESCRIBED A BROTHER AND SISTER WITH EBSTEIN'S ANOMALY. EBSTEIN'S ANOMALY, A CONGENITAL MALFORMATION OF THE HEART, WHICH CONSISTS OF DOWNWARD PLACEMENT OF THE TRICUSPID VALVE SUCH THAT PART OF THE RIGHT VENTRICLE BECOMES INCORPORATED INTO THE PRE-TRICUSPID CHAMBER. ASSOCIATED DEFORMITY OF THE TRICUSPID LEAFLETS AND DEFECT OF THE ATRIAL SEPTUM ARE FREQUENT. DONEGAN ET AL. (1968) FOUND EBSTEIN'S ANOMALY IN A 6 YEAR OLD BOY AND HIS MATERNAL UNCLE. GOUFFAULT ET AL. (1960) FOUND EBSTEIN'S MALFORMATION IN ONE SIB AND A COMPARABLE DEFORMITY OF THE MITRAL VALVE IN A SISTER. THE SAME COMBINATION OF EBSTEIN'S ANOMALY IN ONE SIB AND COMPARABLE MITRAL ANOMALY IN ANOTHER WAS APPARENTLY PRESENT IN THE FAMILY REPORTED BY YAMAUCHI AND CAYLER (1964).

DONEGAN, C. C., JR., MOORE, M. M., WILEY, T. M., JR., HERNANDEZ, F. A., GREEN, J. R., JR. AND SCHIEBLER, G. L.* FAMILIAL EBSTEIN'S ANOMALY OF THE TRICUSPID VALVE. AM. HEART J. 75* 375-379, 1968.

GOUFFAULT, J., LEDAMANY, L. AND LENEGRE, J.* UN TYPE PARTICULIER D'ANOMALIE CONGENITALE DE LA VALVE MITRALE. ARCH. MAL. COEUR. 53* 1175-1181, 1960.

GUERON, M., HIRSCH, M., STERN, J., COHEN, W. AND LEVY, M. J.* FAMILIAL EBSTEIN'S ANOMALY WITH EMPHASIS ON THE SURGICAL TREATMENT. AM. J. CARDIOL. 18* 105-111, 1966.

YAMAUCHI, T. AND CAYLER, G. G.* EBSTEIN'S ANOMALY IN THE NEONATE. A CLINICAL STUDY OF THREE CASES OBSERVED FROM BIRTH THROUGH INFANCY. AM. J. DIS. CHILD. 107* 165-172, 1964.

22480 ECTODERMAL DYSPLASIA AND NEURISENSORY DEAFNESS

MIKAELIAN ET AL. (1970) DESCRIBED BROTHER AND SISTER WHOSE PARENTS WERE FIRST COUSINS AND WHO HAD HIDROTIC ECTODERMAL DYSPLASIA, SENSORINEURAL HEARING LOSS (DUE PROBABLY TO A DEFECT OF THE CELLS OF ORGAN OF CORTI WHICH ARE OF ECTODERMAL ORIGIN) AND CONTRACTURE OF THE FIFTH FINGERS. THE SISTER ALSO HAD THORACIC SCOLIOSIS.

MIKAELIAN, D. O., DER KALOUSTIAN, V. M., SHAHIN, N. A. AND BARSOUMIAN, V. M.* CONGENITAL ECTODERMAL DYSPLASIA WITH HEARING LOSS. ARCH. OTOLARYNG. 92* 85-89, 1970.

*22490 ECTODERMAL DYSPLASIA, ANHIDROTIC

A RARE AUTOSOMAL RECESSIVE FORM OF ANHIDROTIC ECTODERMAL DYSPLASIA IS SUGGESTED BY

THE FINDINGS OF PASSARGE, NUZUM AND SCHUBERT (1966) IN INBRED PEOPLE OF EASTERN KENTUCKY. PHENOTYPICALLY THE FEATURES WERE INDISTINGUISHABLE FROM THOSE IN MALES WITH THE X-LINKED FORM. THE EXISTENCE OF AN AUTOSOMAL RECESSIVE FORM IS FURTHER SUPPORTED STRONGLY BY THE REPORT BY GORLIN ET AL. (1970) OF A FEMALE WITH THE FULL-BLOWN SYNDROME AND BY THEIR REVIEW OF REPORTED CASES IN FEMALES AND OF PARENTAL CONSANGUINITY.

CRUMP, I. A. AND DANKS, D. M.* HYPOHIDROTIC ECTODERMAL DYSPLASIA. A STUDY OF SWEAT PORES IN THE X-LINKED FORM AND IN A FAMILY WITH PROBABLE AUTOSOMAL RECESSIVE INHERITANCE. J. PEDIAT. 78* 466-473, 1971.

GORLIN, R. J., OLD, T. AND ANDERSON, V. E.* HYPOHIDROTIC ECTODERMAL DYSPLASIA IN FEMALES. A CRITICAL ANALYSIS AND ARGUMENT FOR GENETIC HETEROGENEITY. Z. KINDERHEILK. 108* 1-11, 1970.

PASSARGE, E., NUZUM, C. T. AND SCHUBERT, W. K.* ANHIDROTIC ECTODERMAL DYSPLASIA AS AUTOSOMAL RECESSIVE TRAIT IN AN INBRED KINDRED. HUMANGENETIK 3* 181-185, 1966.

*22500 ECTODERMAL DYSPLASIA, CLEFT LIP AND PALATE, HAND AND FOOT DEFORMITY AND MENTAL RETARDATION

ROSSELLI AND GULIENETTI (1961) DESCRIBED FOUR PATIENTS WITH ANHIDROSIS, HYPOTRI-CHOSIS, MICRODONTIA, DYSPLASIA OF NAILS, CLEFT LIP AND PALATE, DEFORMITY OF THE FINGERS AND TOES, AND MALFORMATION IN THE GENITOURINARY SYSTEM. POPLITEAL AND PERINEAL PTERYGIUM WAS ALSO DESCRIBED. SYNDACTYLY WAS THE PREDOMINANT DIGITAL DEFORMITY. TWO WERE BROTHER AND SISTER WHOSE PARENTS WERE SECOND COUSINS. A FAMILY OBSERVED BY BOWEN HAD 3 AFFECTED SIBS OUT OF 10. CLEFT LIP AND PALATE, POPLITEAL PTERYGIUM AND DIGITAL AND GENITAL ANOMALIES ALSO OCCUR APPARENTLY AS A DOMINANT (Q.V.).

BOWEN, P.* EDMONTON, ALBERTA, CANADA* PERSONAL COMMUNICATION, 1967.

ROSSELLI, D. AND GULIENETTI, R.* ECTODERMAL DYSPLASIA. BRIT. J. PLAST. SURG. 14* 190-204, 1961.

22510 ECTOPIA LENTIS

AN AUTOSOMAL RECESSIVE FORM OF UNCOMPLICATED ECTOPIA LENTIS MAY OCCUR. THIS IS NOT AS WELL ESTABLISHED, HOWEVER, AS IS ECTOPIA LENTIS WITH ECTOPIA OF THE PUPIL (Q.V.). SEE ALSO WEILL-MARCHESANI SYNDROME AND HOMOCYSTINURIA.

MCKUSICK, V. A.* PRIMORDIAL DWARFISM AND ECTOPIA LENTIS. AM. J. HUM. GENET. 7* 189-198, 1955.

*22520 ECTOPIA LENTIS ASSOCIATED WITH ECTOPIA OF THE PUPIL

THE LENS AND THE PUPIL ARE USUALLY DISPLACED IN OPPOSITE DIRECTIONS. WHETHER SIMPLE ECTOPIA LENTIS IS AN ENTITY SEPARATE FROM THIS IS SOMEWHAT DOUBTFUL SINCE SIMPLE AND 'ASSOCIATED' FORMS ARE SAID TO OCCUR IN THE SAME FAMILY (FRANCESCHETTI, 1927* DIETHELM, 1947). THE RECESSIVE INHERITANCE OF COMBINED ECTOPIA LENTIS AND ECTOPIA PUPILLAE HAS BEEN WELL ESTABLISHED (SIEMENS, 1920).

DIETHELM, W.* UBER ECTOPIA LENTIS OHNE ARACHNODAKTYLIE UND IHRE BEZIEHUNGEN ZUR ECTOPIA LENTIS ET PUPILLAE. OPHTHALMOLOGIA 114* 16-32, 1947.

FRANCESCHETTI, A.* ECTOPIA LENTIS ET PUPILLAE CONGENITA ALS REZESSIVES ERBLEIDEN UND IHRE MANIFESTIERUNG DURCH KONSANGUINITAT. KLIN. MBL. AUGENHEILK. 78* 351-362, 1927.

FRANCOIS, J.* HEREDITY IN OPHTHALMOLOGY. ST. LOUIS* C. V. MOSBY CO., 1961. P. 164, FIG. 101.

SIEMENS, H. W.* UEBER DIE AETIOLOGIE DER ECTOPIA LENTIS ET PUPILLAE. GRAEFE. ARCH. OPHTHAL. 109* 359-383, 1920.

WAARDENBURG, P. J.* UEBER DAS ERBLICHKEITSMOMENT BEI DER ANGEBORENEN EKTOPIE DER PUPILLE UND DER LINSE. GENETICA 6* 337-382, 1924.

22530 ECTRODACTYLY (ABSENCE OF FINGERS) (SEE SPLIT-HAND)

KLEIN (1932) DESCRIBED AN AFFECTED BOY AND GIRL BORN FROM THE MATING BETWEEN A MAN AND THE DAUGHTER OF HIS HALF-BROTHER. WHEN HEREDITARY, THIS TRAIT USUALLY BEHAVES AS A DOMINANT.

KLEIN, I. J.* HEREDITARY ECTRODACTYLISM IN SIBLINGS. AM. J. DIS. CHILD. 43* 136-142, 1932.

22540 EHLERS-DANLOS SYNDROME

BEIGHTON (1970) RAISED THE POSSIBILITY OF AN AUTOSOMAL RECESSIVE FORM OF THE EHLERS-DANLOS SYNDROME, IN WHICH SKIN AND JOINT CHANGES LIKE THOSE OF THE DOMINANT FORM OCCUR BUT IN ADDITION SERIOUS OCULAR COMPLICATIONS, PARTICULARLY RETINAL

R
E
C
E
S
S
I
V
E

DETACHMENT, ARE A CONSPICUOUS FEATURE. HE DESCRIBED AFFECTED BROTHER AND SISTER WITH NORMAL PARENTS. THE AFFECTED MALE HAD FOUR UNAFFECTED CHILDREN.

BEIGHTON, P.* SERIOUS OPHTHALMOLOGICAL COMPLICATIONS IN THE EHLERS-DANLOS SYNDROME. BRIT. J. OPHTHAL. 54* 263-268, 1970.

*22550 ELLIS-VAN CREVELD SYNDROME (CHONDROECTODERMAL DYSPLASIA)

THE LARGEST PEDIGREE IS THAT OBSERVED BY MCKUSICK AND COLLEAGUES (1964) IN AN INBRED RELIGIOUS ISOLATE, THE OLD ORDER AMISH, IN LANCASTER COUNTY, PENNSYLVANIA. ALMOST AS MANY PERSONS ARE KNOWN IN THIS ONE KINDRED AS ARE REPORTED IN ALL THE MEDICAL LITERATURE. FEATURES ARE DWARFISM WITH MOST STRIKING SHORTENING IN THE DISTAL PART OF THE EXTREMITIES, POLYDACTYLY, FUSION OF THE HAMATE AND CAPITATE BONES OF THE WRIST, DYSTROPHY OF THE FINGERNAILS, CHANGE IN THE UPPER LIP VARIOUSLY CALLED 'PARTIAL HARE-LIP,' 'LIP-TIE,' ETC., AND CARDIAC MALFORMATION, USUALLY SEPTAL DEFECTS AND OFTEN SINGLE ATRIUM. MESOECTODERMAL DYSPLASIA SEEMS A BETTER DESIGNATION THAN CHONDROECTODERMAL DYSPLASIA.

ALVAREZ-BORJA, A.* ELLIS-VAN CREVELD SYNDROME. REPORT OF TWO CASES. PEDIA-TRICS 26* 301-309, 1960.

DONLAN, M. A., MURPHY, J. J. AND BRAKEL, C. A.* ELLIS-VAN CREVELD SYNDROME ASSOCIATED WITH COMPLETE SITUS INVERSUS. CLIN. PEDIAT. 8* 366-368, 1969.

DOUGLAS, W. F., SCHONHOLTZ, G. J. AND GEPPERT, L. J.* CHONDROECTODERMAL DYSPLASIA (ELLIS-VAN CREVELD SYNDROME). AM. J. DIS. CHILD. 97* 473-478, 1959.

HIROKAWA, K. AND SUZUKI, S.* ELLIS-VAN CREVELD SYNDROME* REPORT OF AN AUTOPSY CASE. ACTA PATH. JAP. 17* 139-143, 1967.

HUSSON, G. S. AND PARKMAN, P.* CHONDROECTODERMAL DYSPLASIA (ELLIS-VAN CREVELD SYNDROME) WITH A COMPLEX CARDIAC MALFORMATION. PEDIATRICS 28* 285-292, 1961.

MCKUSICK, V. A., EGELAND, J. A., ELDRIDGE, R. AND KRUSEN, D. E.* DWARFISM IN THE AMISH. I. THE ELLIS-VAN CREVELD SYNDROME. BULL. HOPKINS HOSP. 115* 306-336, 1964.

WALLS, W. L., ALTMAN, D. H. AND WINSLOW, O. P.* CHONDROECTODERMAL DYSPLASIA (ELLIS-VAN CREVELD SYNDROME). REPORT OF A CASE AND REVIEW OF THE LITERATURE. AM. J. DIS. CHILD. 98* 242-248, 1959.

R
E
C
E
S
S
I
V
E

22560 EMG SYNDROME (EXOPHTHALMOS-MACROGLOSSIA-GIGANTISM SYNDROME BECKWITH-WIEDEMANN SYNDROME)

THE ENLARGED TONGUE, TOGETHER WITH OMPHALOCELE OR OTHER UMBILICAL ABNORMALITIES, PERMITS RECOGNITION OF THE DISORDER AT BIRTH. BECAUSE MANY OF THE AFFECTED INFANTS HAVE HYPOGLYCEMIA IN THE FIRST DAYS OF LIFE, ANTICIPATION OF THIS COMPLICATION CAN PREVENT SERIOUS NEUROLOGIC SEQUELAE. VISCEROMEGALY, ADRENOCORTI-CAL CYTOANEGALY AND DYSPLASIA OF THE RENAL MEDULLA ARE CONSPICUOUS FEATURES. ADRENAL CARCINOMA OR NEPHROBLASTOMA OCCURS WITH INCREASED FREQUENCY. WIEDEMANN (1964) REPORTED THREE AFFECTED SIBS AND IRVING (1967) OBSERVED A FAMILY WITH TWO AFFECTED SIBS AND AN AFFECTED SECOND COUSIN. I HAVE SEEN THIS DISORDER IN A NEGRO CHILD AND THORBURN ET AL. (1970) DESCRIBED 6 CASES IN JAMAICAN NEGROES AND ESTIMATED AN INCIDENCE OF 1 IN 13,700 BIRTHS.

BECKWITH, J. B.* MACROGLOSSIA, OMPHALOCELE, ADRENAL CYTOMEGALY, GIGANTISM, AND HYPERPLASTIC VISCEROMEGALY. THE CLINICAL DELINEATION OF BIRTH DEFECTS. II. MALFORMATION SYNDROMES. NEW YORK* NATIONAL FOUNDATION, 1969. PP. 188-196.

FILIPPI, G. AND MCKUSICK, V. A.* THE BECKWITH-WIEDEMANN SYNDROME (THE EXOMPHA-LOS-MACROGLOSSIA-GIGANTISM SYNDROME)* REPORT OF TWO CASES AND REVIEW OF THE LITERATURE. MEDICINE 49* 279-298, 1970.

IRVING, I. M.* THE 'E.M.G.' SYNDROME (EXOMPHALOS, MACROGLOSSIA, GIGANTISM). PROGR. PEDIAT. SURG. 1* 1-16, 1970.

IRVING, I. M.* EXAMPHALOS WITH MACROGLOSSIA* A STUDY OF ELEVEN CASES. J. PEDIAT. SURG. 2* 499-507, 1967.

THORBURN, M. J., WRIGHT, E. S., MILLER, C. G. AND SMITH-READ, E. H. M.* EXOMPHALOS-MACROGLOSSIA-GIGANTISM SYNDROME IN JAMAICAN INFANTS. AM. J. DIS. CHILD. 119* 316-321, 1970.

WIEDEMANN, H.-R.* COMPLEXE MALFORMATIF FAMILIAL AVEC HERNIE OMBILICALE ET MACROGLOSSIE--UN 'SYNDROME NOUVEAU'.Q J. GENET. HUM. 13* 223-232, 1964.

WIEDEMANN, H.-R.* DAS EMG-SYNDROME* EXOMPHALOS, MAKROGLOSSIE, GIGANTISMUS UND KOHLENHYDRATSTOFF-WECHSEL-STORUNG. Z. KINDERHEILK. 106* 171-185, 1969.

WIEDEMANN, H.-R., SPRANGER, J., MOGHAREI, M., KUBLER, W., TOLKSDORF, M., BONTEMPS, M., DRESCHER, J. AND GUNSCHERA, H.* UBER DAS SYNDROM EXOMPHALOS-MAKROGLOSSIE-GIGANTISMUS, UBER GENERALISIERTE MUSKELHYPERTROPHIE, PROGRESSIVE

LIPODYSTROPHIE UND MIESCHER-SYNDROM IM SINNE DIENCEPHALER SYNDROME. Z. KINDER-HEILK. 102* 1-36, 1968.

22570 ENCEPHALOMALACIA, MULTILOCULAR

CROME AND WILLIAMS (1960) OBSERVED MULTILOCULAR ENCEPHALOMALACIA IN AN INFANT WHO DIED AT ONE MONTH OF AGE. A SIB WAS LIVING AT AGE 6 YEARS BUT MAY HAVE HAD THE SAME ABNORMALITY MANIFESTED BY MICROCEPHALY, SPASTIC DIPLEGIA AND IDIOCY. IT IS NOT CERTAIN THAT THIS IS A DISTINCT ENTITY.

CROME, L. AND WILLIAMS, C.* THE PROBLEM OF FAMILIAL MULTILOCULAR ENCEPHALOMALA-CIA. ACTA PAEDIAT. 49* 175-184, 1960.

22580 ENCEPHALOPATHY OF INFANCY AND CHILDHOOD, DEGENERATIVE FAMILIAL

DEGENERATIVE FAMILIAL ENCEPHALOPATHIES OF INFANCY AND CHILDHOOD ARE PROBABLY OF MANY TYPES. BOTH CLINICALLY AND PATHOLOGICALLY THEY CONSTITUTE A CONFUSED GROUP. CLINICAL FEATURES HAVE OFTEN BEEN PICKED OUT FOR DESIGNATING AND CLASSIFYING THEM, E.G., CONVULSIONS, BLINDNESS, MYOCLONUS, SPASTICITY, ETC. THESE ARE AN UNSATISFA-CTORY BASIS. HOWEVER, MYOCLONUS OCCURS, FOR EXAMPLE, IN MANY TYPES OF INFANTILE ENCEPHALOPATHY AND THE NAME MYOCLONIC EPILEPSY SHOULD BE RESERVED FOR THE SPECIFIC ENTITY DESCRIBED BY UNVERRICHT AND LUNDBORG AND CHARACTERIZED PATHOLOGICALLY BY AMYLOID INTRACELLULAR INCLUSIONS CALLED LAFORA BODIES.
IT IS POSSIBLE, WITH FULL CLINICAL, GENETIC, HISTOLOGIC AND CHEMICAL DATA, TO DIFFERENTIATE THE FOLLOWING TYPES* 1. INFANTILE AMAUROTIC FAMILY IDIOCY, OR TAY-SACHS DISEASE 2. METACHROMATIC LEUKOENCEPHALOPATHY 3. INFANTILE SUBACUTE NECROTIZING ENCEPHALOPATHY 4. SPONGY DEGENERATION 5. HALLERVORDEN-SPATZ DISEASE 6. SEITELBERGER'S INFANTILE NEUROAXONAL DYSTROPHY 7. KRABBE'S GLOBOID CELL SCLEROSIS. THE FOLLOWING CONDITIONS ARE NOT YET ESTABLISHED AS DISTINCT ENTITIES* 1. JOSEPH'S SYNDROME 2. SPASTIC PSEUDOSCLEROSIS 3. MULTILOCULAR ENCEPHALOMALACIA 4. SUDANOPHILIC CEREBRAL SCLEROSIS

22590 ENCEPHALOPATHY, PROGRESSIVE, WITH DISTURBANCE OF LINOLENIC ACID METABOLISM

IN A SINGLE CHILD WITH UNRELATED PARENTS, HAGBERG ET AL. (1968) DESCRIBED AN APPARENTLY NEW ENTITY, CHARACTERIZED BY MENTAL RETARDATION, LOSS OF SPEECH, MINOR MOTOR SEIZURES, REGRESSION OF MOTOR DEVELOPMENT, AND ATAXIA. HISTOLOGICALLY THE BRAIN SHOWED TOTAL DERANGEMENT OF CORTICAL CYTOARCHITECTURE, SEVERE DEGENERATION OF WHITE MATTER AND DEPOSITS OF GRANULAR MATERIAL SUGGESTING FREE FATTY ACIDS AND UNSATURATED FATTY ACIDS. BIOCHEMICAL STUDIES SHOWED A DISTURBANCE OF LINOLENIC ACID METABOLISM.

HAGBERG, B., SOURANDER, P. AND SVENNERHOLM, L.* LATE INFANTILE PROGRESSIVE ENCEPHALOPATHY WITH DISTURBED POLY-UNSATURATED FAT METABOLISM. ACTA PAEDIAT. SCAND. 57* 495-499, 1968.

*22600 ENDOCARDIAL FIBROELASTOSIS

THE REPORTS OF ENDOCARDIAL FIBROELASTOSIS IN SIBS INCLUDE THOSE OF VESTERMARK (1962), WINTER AND COLLEAGUES (1960), ZANKER AND FISHER (1960) AND MCKUSICK AND COLLEAGUES (1962). MOLLER ET AL. (1966) DESCRIBED ENDOCARDIAL FIBROELASTOSIS IN A YOUNG WOMAN WHO DIED OF HEART FAILURE DURING THE POSTPARTUM PERIOD AND IN THE CHILD WHO WAS BORN OF THAT PREGNANCY AND DIED AT 11 MONTHS OF AGE. EITHER GENETIC CAUSATION OR VIRAL INFECTION WAS SUGGESTED. AMONG THE CHILDREN OF FIRST COUSIN PARENTS RAFINSKI ET AL. (1967) OBSERVED THREE WHO DIED OF ENDOCARDIAL FIBROELASTO-SIS AT AGES OF 10, 11 AND 13 YEARS, WHICH IS LONGER SURVIVAL THAN IS USUAL. ALTHOUGH THE ACCUMULATED EXPERIENCE STRONGLY SUPPORTS THE EXISTENCE OF AN AUTOSOMAL RECESSIVE VARIETY OF ENDOCARDIAL FIBROELASTOSIS, MANY CASES MAY OCCUR ON A NON-GENETIC BASIS.

MCKUSICK, V. A. AND COLLEAGUES* MEDICAL GENETICS 1961. J. CHRONIC DIS. 15* 417-572, 1962 (FIG. 18).

MOLLER, J. H., FISCH, R. O., FROM, A. H. L. AND EDWARDS, J. E.* ENDOCARDIAL FIBROELASTOSIS OCCURRING IN A MOTHER AND SON. PEDIATRICS 38* 918-921, 1966.

RAFINSKI, T., GOLENIA, A., WOZNIEWICZ, B. AND WLAD, S.* FAMILIAL ENDOCARDIAL FIBROELASTOSIS. J. PEDIAT. 70* 574-576, 1967.

VESTERMARK, S.* PRIMARY ENDOCARDIAL FIBROELASTOSIS IN SIBLINGS. ACTA PAEDIAT. 51* 94-96, 1962.

WINTER, S. T., MOSES, W. S., COHEN, N. J. AND NAFTALIN, J. M.* PRIMARY ENDOCARDIAL FIBROELASTOSIS IN TWO SISTERS. AM. J. DIS. CHILD. 99* 529-533, 1960.

ZANKER, T. AND FISHER, R. S.* ENDOCARDIAL FIBROELASTOSIS IN SIBLINGS. MARYLAND MED. J. 9* 60-65, 1960.

22610 ENDOCARDIAL FIBROELASTOSIS AND COARCTATION OF ABDOMINAL AORTA

HALLIDIE-SMITH AND OLSEN (1968) DESCRIBED A GIRL AND HER TWO AFFECTED BROTHERS. MITRAL REGURGITATION WAS PRESENT. THE PARENTS WERE NOT RELATED.

R
E
C
E
S
S
I
V
E

HALLIDIE-SMITH, K. A. AND OLSEN, E. G. J.* ENDOCARDIAL FIBRO-ELASTOSIS, MITRAL INCOMPETENCE, AND COARCTATION OF ABDOMINAL AORTA. A REPORT OF 3 SIBS. BRIT. HEART J. 30* 850-858, 1968.

*22620 ENTEROKINASE DEFICIENCY

HADORN ET AL. (1969) DESCRIBED A FEMALE INFANT WITH DIARRHEA, FAILURE TO THRIVE AND HYPOPROTEINEMIC EDEMA WHO WAS SHOWN TO HAVE DEFICIENCY OF THE INTESTINAL ENTEROKINASE WHICH ACTIVATES PANCREATIC PROTEOLYTIC ENZYMES (TRYPSIN, CHYMOTRYPSIN AND CARBOXYPEPTIDASE-A). THE PARENTS WERE NOT STUDIED.

HADORN, B., TARLOW, M. J., LLOYD, J. AND WOLFF, O. H.* INTESTINAL ENTEROKINASE DEFICIENCY. LANCET 1* 812-813, 1969.

TARLOW, M. J., HADORN, B., ARTHURTON, M. W. AND LLOYD, J. K.* INTESTINAL ENTEROKINASE DEFICIENCY. A NEWLY-RECOGNIZED DISORDER OF PROTEIN DIGESTION. ARCH. DIS. CHILD. 45* 651-655, 1970.

22630 ENTEROPATHY, PROTEIN-LOSING

IN THE FAMILY DESCRIBED BY SHEBA ET AL. (1968) INHERITANCE APPEARED CLEARLY TO BE AUTOSOMAL RECESSIVE. INTESTINAL LYMPHANGIECTASIA WAS SUSPECTED BUT NOT PROVED.

SHEBA, C., SHAMI, M., FRAND, M., THEODOR, E. AND ROTEM, Y.* FAMILIAL PROTEIN LOSING ENTEROPATHY. PROC. TEL-HASHOMER HOSP. 7* 62-66, 1968.

22640 EPIDERMODYSPLASIA VERRUCIFORMIS

SULLIVAN AND ELLIS (1939) FOUND THAT OF THE 16 PREVIOUSLY REPORTED FAMILIES, FOUR HAD CONSANGUINEOUS PARENTS. THE LESIONS OFTEN RESEMBLE VERRUCAE PLANAE. THE MUCOUS MEMBRANES, HAIR AND NAILS ARE NOT AFFECTED. MALIGNANT DEGENERATION, USUALLY OF THE SUPERFICIAL BASAL CELL TYPE, IS FREQUENT. CHARACTERISTIC CHANGES IN THE EPIDERMAL CELLS WITH PECULIAR VACUOLIZATION ARE OBSERVED.
ELLIS (1953) STATED THAT THIS DISORDER OCCURS MOST FREQUENTLY IN ORIENTALS. IT IS BY NO MEANS PROVED THAT THIS IS A MENDELIZING DISORDER. THE VIEW THAT EPIDERMODYSPLASIA VERRUCIFORMIS IS AN EXTENSIVE FORM OF VIRAL VERRUCAE PLANAE IS SUPPORTED BY SUCCESSFUL AUTOINNOCULATION AND HETEROINNOCULATION EXPERIMENTS. LUTZ (1957) WHO WAS ONE OF THE FIRST TO DESCRIBE THE CONDITION, ACCEPTED THAT IT IS NOT AN ENTITY BUT SUGGESTED THAT GENETIC PREDISPOSITION MAY ACCOUNT FOR THE EXTENSI- VENESS OF THE ERUPTION OF WARTS. FAMILIAL AGGREGATION WAS DESCRIBED BY MIDANA (1949) AND BY JABLONSKA ET AL. (1966). HERMANN (1955) FOUND PARENTAL CONSANGUINI- TY. BAKER (1968) AS WELL AS OTHERS DEMONSTRATED, BY ELECTRON MICROSCOPY, PARTICLES SUGGESTING PAPOVA VIRUS.

R
E
C
E
S
S
I
V
E

BAKER, H.* EPIDERMODYSPLASIA VERRUCIFORMIS WITH ELECTRON MICROSCOPIC DEMONSTRA- TION OF VIRUS. PROC. ROY. SOC. MED. 61* 589-590, 1968.

ELLIS, F.* IN DISCUSSION OF BARKER AND SACHS. ARCH. DERM. 67* 443-455, 1953.

HERMANN, H.* EPIDERMODYSPLASIA VERRUCIFORMIS* ERB- UND ERSCHEINUNGSBILD. Z. MENSCHL. VERERB. KONSTITUTIONSL. 32* 409-417, 1955.

JABLONSKA, S. AND FORMAS, I.* WEITERE POSITIVE ERGEBNISSE MIT AUTO- UND HETEROINOKULATION BEI EPIDERMODYSPLASIA VERRUCIFORMIS LEWANDOWSKY-LUTZ. DERMATO- LOGICA 118* 86-93, 1959.

JABLONSKA, S., FABJANSKA, L. AND FORMAS, I.* ON THE VIRAL ETIOLOGY OF EPIDERMO- DYSPLASIA VERRUCIFORMIS. DERMATOLOGICA 132* 369-385, 1966.

LUTZ, W.* ZUR EPIDERMODYSPLASIA VERRUCIFORMIS. DERMATOLOGICA 115* 309-314, 1957.

MIDANA, A.* SULLA QUESTIONE DEI RAPPORTI TRA EPIDERMODYSPLASIA VERRUCIFORMIS E VERRUCOSI GENERALIZZATA. DERMATOLOGICA 99* 1-23, 1949.

SULLIVAN, M. AND ELLIS, F. A.* EPIDERMODYSPLASIA VERRUCIFORMIS (LEWANDOWSKY AND LUTZ). ARCH. DERM. SYPH. 40* 422-432, 1939.

*22650 EPIDERMOLYSIS BULLOSA DYSTROPHICA NEUROTROPHICA (EPIDERMOLYSIS BULLOSA WITH CONGENITAL DEAFNESS)

THIS 'NEW' ENTITY WAS DELINEATED BY GEDDE-DAHL (1970). THE FEATURES ARE ONSET OF LOCALIZED TRAUMATIC BLISTERING IN LATE CHILDHOOD OR ADOLESCENCE, ONSET OF NAIL MANIFESTATIONS SEVERAL YEARS BEFORE THE SKIN MANIFESTATIONS, DIFFUSE AND SLOWLY PROGRESSIVE SKIN ATROPHY OF HANDS, FEET, ELBOWS, KNEES, PALMS AND SOLES WITH LOSS OF DERMAL RIDGE PATTERN OF FINGERS, OCCASIONAL BLISTERING OF ORAL MUCOSA AND CONGENITAL, SLOWLY PROGRESSIVE PERCEPTIVE DEAFNESS.

GEDDE-DAHL, T., JR.* EPIDERMOLYSIS BULLOSA. A CLINICAL, GENETIC AND EPIDEMIO- LOGICAL STUDY. OSLO, NORWAY, 1970.

*22660 EPIDERMOLYSIS BULLOSA DYSTROPHICA

THERE MAY BE FIVE VARIETIES OF EPIDERMOLYSIS BULLOSA (DAVISON, 1965) - (1) DOMINANT EPIDERMOLYSIS BULLOSA SIMPLEX, (2) DOMINANT EPIDERMOLYSIS BULLOSA OF COCKAYNE, (3) DOMINANT EPIDERMOLYSIS BULLOSA DYSTROPHICA, (4) RECESSIVE EPIDERMOLYSIS BULLOSA DYSTROPHICA, AND (5) RECESSIVE EPIDERMOLYSIS BULLOSA LETALIS. THIS SEVERE AND DESTRUCTIVE FORM OF EPIDERMOLYSIS BULLOSA MAY BE PRESENT AT BIRTH OR APPEARS IN INFANCY. HANDS, FEET, ELBOWS AND KNEES ARE SITES OF PREDILECTION. BULLAE ALSO DEVELOP ON THE MUCOSAL SURFACES AND EVEN THE CONJUNCTIVA AND CORNEA MAY BE INVOLVED. THE IMPRESSIVE KINDRED REPORTED BY HOFMAN IS DIAGRAMMED ON PAGE 279 OF VON VERSCHUER (1959).

BOOK, J.* FREQUENCE DE MUTATION DE LA CHONDRODYSTROPHIE ET DE L'EPIDERMOLYSE BULLEUSE DANS UNE POPULATION DU SUD DE LA SUEDE. J. GENET. HUM. 1* 24-26, 1952.

DAVISON, B. C. C.* EPIDERMOLYSIS BULLOSA. J. MED. GENET. 2* 233-242, 1965.

HEINRICHSBAUER, F.* EIN WEITERER BEITRAG ZUR FRAGE ANGEBORENER HAUTDEFEKTE. (UBER EIN FAMILIARES LETALES KRANKHEITSBILD MIT BLASENBILDUNG UND ANGEBORENEN DEFEKTEN DER HAUT). ARCH. GYNAEK. 134* 673-692, 1928.

ROBINSON, M. M.* EPIDERMOLYSIS BULLOSA HEREDITARIA. UROL. CUTAN. REV. 50* 545-561, 1946.

SCHNYDER, U. W. AND EICHHOFF, D.* ZUR KLINIK UND GENETIK DER DOMINANT-DYSTROPHISCHEN EPIDERMOLYSIS BULLOSA HEREDITARIA. ARCH. DERM. 218* 62-90, 1963.

SORSBY, A. (ED.)* CLINICAL GENETICS. ST. LOUIS* C. V. MOSBY CO., 1953. P. 136.

SORSBY, A., ROBERTS, J. A. F. AND BRAIN, R. T.* ESSENTIAL SHRINKING OF CONJUNCTIVA IN HEREDITARY AFFECTION ALLIED TO EPIDERMOLYSIS BULLOSA. DOCUM. OPHTHAL. 5-6* 118-150, 1951.

VON VERSCHUER, O. F.* GENETIK DES MENSCHEN. LEHRBUCH DER HUMANGENETIK. BERLIN* URBAN AND SCHWARZENBERG, 1959.

*22670 EPIDERMOLYSIS BULLOSA LETALIS

RECESSIVE

ROBERTS AND COLLEAGUES (1960) DESCRIBED THREE CASES IN BRANCHES OF A FRENCH-CANADIAN FAMILY FROM AN AREA IN NOVA SCOTIA WITH MUCH INBREEDING. THE INFANTS WERE BORN WITH BULLOUS LESIONS AND DIED AT 20, 24 AND 42 DAYS, RESPECTIVELY, DESPITE METICULOUS NURSING CARE, ANTIBIOTICS, CORTICOSTEROIDS AND INCREASED DIETARY PROTEIN. LOSS OF SERUM PROTEIN AND ELECTROLYTES AND DERMAL SEPSIS SEEMED TO HAVE BEEN RESPONSIBLE FOR DEATH.
KLUNKER (1963) THOUGHT IT DOUBTFUL THAT THE TWO FORMS OF EPIDERMOLYSIS BULLOSA HERE LISTED ARE SEPARATE AND DISTINCT. EVEN IF DISTINCT, THEIR ALLELIC VERSUS NON-ALLELIC RELATIONSHIP IS, OF COURSE, UNKNOWN. DAVISON (1965) ALSO FOUND 'LETHAL' CASES IN THE SAME SIBSHIP AS CASES WITH THE DYSTHROPHIC FORM. CROSS ET AL. (1968) STUDIED AN EXTENSIVELY INVOLVED KINDRED. THE CONSISTENTLY LETHAL BEHAVIOR SUGGESTS THAT IT MAY INDEED BE DISTINCT. CONGENITAL ABSENCE OF SKIN IN LOCALIZED AREAS IS PROBABLY DUE TO INTRAUTERINE TRAUMA AND BULLAE. THE HANDS AND FEET ARE RELATIVELY SPARED. EXCEPT FOR DYSTROPHIC NAILS THE PATIENTS CAN COMPLETELY RECOVER AFTER AGE TWO YEARS IF THERAPY WITH MASSIVE STEROIDS AND PREVENTION AND THERAPY OF INFECTIONS ARE ADEQUATE.

BERGENHOLTZ, A. AND OLSSON, O.* EPIDERMOLYSIS BULLOSA HEREDITARIA. I. EPIDERMOLYSIS BULLOSA HEREDITARIA LETALIS. A SURVEY OF THE LITERATURE AND REPORT OF 11 CASES. ACTA DERMATOVENER. 48* 220-241, 1968.

CROSS, H. E., WELLS, R. S. AND ESTERLY, J. R.* INHERITANCE IN EPIDERMOLYSIS BULLOSA LETALIS. J. MED. GENET. 5* 189-196, 1968.

DAVISON, B. C. C.* EPIDERMOLYSIS BULLOSA. J. MED. GENET. 2* 233-242, 1965.

KLUNKER, W.* ZUR NOSOLOGISCHEN STELLUNG DER EPIDERMOLYSIS BULLOSA HEREDITARIA LETALIS HERLITZ (MIT KASUISTIK). ARCH. KLIN. EXP. DERM. 216* 74-100, 1963.

ROBERTS, M. H., HOWELL, D. R. S., BRAMHALL, J. L. AND REUBNER, B.* EPIDERMOLYSIS BULLOSA LETALIS* REPORT OF THREE CASES WITH PARTICULAR REFERENCE TO THE HISTOPATHOLOGY OF THE SKIN. PEDIATRICS 25* 283-290, 1960.

22680 EPILEPSY, PHOTOGENIC, SPASTIC DIPLEGIA AND MENTAL RETARDATION

DALY, SIEKERT AND BURKE (1959) FOUND 3 OF 4 SIBS AFFECTED.

DALY, D., SIEKERT, R. G. AND BURKE, E. C.* A VARIETY OF FAMILIAL LIGHT SENSITIVE EPILEPSY. ELECTROENCEPH. CLIN. NEUROPHYSIOL. 11* 141-145, 1959.

22690 EPIPHYSEAL DYSPLASIA

JUBERG AND HOLT (1968) DESCRIBED THREE SISTERS AND A BROTHER WITH MULTIPLE EPIPHYSEAL DYSPLASIA. THE PARENTS WERE NORMAL AND NOT RELATED. THIS EXPERIENCE AND SOME REPORTED IN THE LITERATURE, INCLUDING INSTANCES OF PARENTAL CONSANGUINI-

JUBERG, R. C. AND HOLT, J. F.* INHERITANCE OF MULTIPLE EPIPHYSEAL DYSPLASIA, TARDA. AM. J. HUM. GENET. 20* 549-563, 1968.

22700 ERYTHEMA OF ACRAL REGIONS

IN A BROTHER AND SISTER AND A PATERNAL FIRST COUSIN OF THEIRS, BRYAN AND COSKEY (1967) DESCRIBED AN ASYMPTOMATIC ERYTHEMATOUS, PAPULAR AND PLACQUE-LIKE ERYTHEMA APPEARING IN INFANCY AND INVOLVING THE EXTERNAL EARS AND EXTREMITIES. IN THE SIBSHIP OF THE AFFECTED SIBS, FOUR HAD CLUBFOOT AND DENTAL ANOMALIES.

BRYAN, H. G. AND COSKEY, R. J.* FAMILIAL ERYTHEMA OF ACRAL REGIONS. ARCH. DERM. 95* 483-486, 1967.

22710 ERYTHRODERMIA DESQUAMATIVA OF LEINER

SIMON, BECKER AND WIEDEMANN (1965) DESCRIBED THREE MALE SIBS WITH ERYTHRODERMA, SEVERE DIARRHEA AND REDUCED RESISTANCE TO INFECTION. DEATH OCCURRED AT THE AGE OF 2, 6 AND 9 MONTHS. POSTMORTEM FINDINGS INCLUDED LYMPHATIC HYPOPLASIA AND INCREASE IN RETICULAR CELLS OF THE LYMPH NODES.

SIMON, C., BECKER, V. AND WIEDEMANN, H.-R.* UBER EIN UNTER DEM BILDE DER ERYTHRODERMIA DESQUAMATIVA LEINER VERLAUFENES TODLICHES LEIDEN BEI DREI BRUDERN. Z. KINDERHEILK. 94* 12-24, 1965.

*22720 EUNUCHOIDISM, FAMILIAL HYPOGONADOTROPHIC

IN SOME FAMILIES BOTH MALES AND FEMALES ARE AFFECTED (BIBEN AND GORDAN, 1955) AND ONLY MEMBERS OF ONE GENERATION (HURXTHAL, 1943). LE MARQUAND (1954) DESCRIBED THREE AFFECTED BROTHERS AND TWO AFFECTED SISTERS IN THE SAME FAMILY. THE PARENTS WERE NOT RELATED. IT IS LIKELY THAT THERE IS A RECESSIVELY INHERITED MONOTROPIC PITUITARY DEFECT, LIMITED TO GONADOTROPIN, COMPARABLE TO THE MONOTROPIC DEFECT OF GROWTH HORMONE DEMONSTRATED IN SEXUAL ATELIOTIC DWARFS ('MIDGETS'). EWER (1968) OBSERVED AFFECTED BROTHER AND 2 SISTERS FROM A MARRIAGE OF SECOND COUSINS ONCE REMOVED. ANOTHER SIB, A MALE, DECEASED, WAS PROBABLY AFFECTED. ABSENCE OF SECONDARY SEX CHARACTERISTICS AND RELATIVELY LONG EXTREMITIES WERE THE ONLY FINDINGS. CLOMIPHENE ADMINISTRATION HAS NO EFFECT (EWER, 1968).

BIBEN, R. L. AND GORDAN, G. S.* FAMILIAL HYPOGONADOTROPIC EUNUCHOIDISM. J. CLIN. ENDOCRIN. 15* 931-942, 1955.

EWER, R. W.* FAMILIAL MONOTROPIC PITUITARY GONADOTROPIN INSUFFICIENCY. J. CLIN. ENDOCR. 28* 783-788, 1968.

HURXTHAL, L. M.* SUBLINGUAL USE OF TESTOSTERONE IN 7 CASES OF HYPOGONADISM* REPORT OF 3 CONGENITAL EUNUCHOIDS OCCURRING IN ONE FAMILY. J. CLIN. ENDOCR. 3* 551-556, 1943.

LE MARQUAND, H. S.* CONGENITAL HYPOGONADOTROPHIC HYPOGONADISM IN FIVE MEMBERS OF A FAMILY, THREE BROTHERS AND TWO SISTERS. PROC. ROY. SOC. MED. 47* 442-446, 1954.

22730 FACTOR V AND FACTOR VIII, COMBINED DEFICIENCY OF

CONGENITAL HEMORRHAGIC DISORDERS CHARACTERIZED BY DEFICIENCY OF TWO CLOTTING FACTORS COMPRISE A DISPUTED GROUP. COMBINED DEFICIENCY OF FACTORS V AND VIII IS SUPPORTED BY RELATIVELY CONVINCING LABORATORY DATA. SEVEN PATIENTS IN 5 FAMILIES HAVE BEEN DESCRIBED. AT LEAST THREE OF FIVE PARENTAL MATINGS WERE CONSANGUINEOUS (JONES ET AL., 1962).

JONES, J. H., RIZZA, C. R., HARDISTY, R. M., DORMANDY, K. M., AND MACPHERSON, J. C.* COMBINED DEFICIENCY OF FACTOR V AND FACTOR VIII (ANTIHEMOPHILIC GLOBULIN). A REPORT OF THREE CASES. BRIT. J. HEAMAT. 8* 120-128, 1962.

22740 FACTOR V DEFICIENCY (OWREN'S PARAHEMOPHILIA LABILE FACTOR DEFICIENCY)

THE DIAGNOSIS OF THIS HEMORRHAGIC DIATHESIS IS MADE BY THE PROLONGED ONE-STAGE PROTHROMBIN TIME WHICH IS COMPLETELY CORRECTED BY THE ADDITION OF FRESH DEPROTH-ROMBINIZED RABBIT PLASMA. BLEEDING TIMES AND CLOTTING TIMES ARE CONSISTENTLY PROLONGED. CLINICAL BLEEDING IS USUALLY MILD. HETEROZYGOTES HAVE LOWERED LEVELS OF FACTOR V BUT PROBABLY NEVER HAVE ABNORMAL BLEEDING. PARENTAL CONSANGUINITY WAS DESCRIBED BY KINGSLEY (1954), AND BY SEIBERT, MARGOLIUS AND RATNOFF (1958).

FRIEDMAN, I. A., QUICK, A. J., HIGGINS, F., HUSSEY, C. V. AND HICKEY, M. E.* HEREDITARY LABILE FACTOR (FACTOR V) DEFICIENCY. J.A.M.A. 175* 370-374, 1961.

KINGSLEY, C. S.* FAMILIAL FACTOR V DEFICIENCY* THE PATTERN OF HEREDITY. QUART. J. MED. 23* 323-329, 1954.

SEIBERT, R. H., MARGOLIUS, A., JR. AND RATNOFF, O. D.* OBSERVATIONS ON HEMOPHILIA, PARAHEMOPHILIA AND COEXISTENT HEMOPHILIA AND PARAHEMOPHILIA.

ALTERATIONS IN THE PLATELETS AND THE THROMBOPLASTIN GENERATION TEST. J. LAB. CLIN. MED. 52* 449-462, 1958.

*22750 FACTOR VII DEFICIENCY (HYPOPROCONVERTINEMIA)

RECESSIVE INHERITANCE IS ESTABLISHED BY THE DEMONSTRATION OF LOWER-THAN-NORMAL LEVELS OF FACTOR VII IN BOTH PARENTS (KUPFER, HANNA AND KINNE, 1960). SEE REVIEW BY MARDER AND SHULMAN (1964).

GLUECK, H. I. AND SUTHERLAND, J. M.* INHERITED FACTOR-VII DEFECT IN NEGRO FAMILY. PEDIATRICS 27* 204-213, 1961.

HITZIG, W. H. AND ZOLLINGER, W.* KONGENITALEN FAKTOR-VII MANGEL. FAMILIENUNTER-SUCHUNG UND PHYSIOLOGISCHE STUDIEN UBER DEN FAKTOR VII. HELV. PAEDIAT. ACTA 13* 189-203, 1958.

KUPFER, H. G., HANNA, B. L. AND KINNE, D. R.* CONGENITAL FACTOR VII DEFICIENCY WITH NORMAL STUART ACTIVITY* CLINICAL, GENETIC AND EXPERIMENTAL OBSERVATIONS. BLOOD 15* 146-163, 1960.

MARDER, V. J. AND SHULMAN, N. R.* CLINICAL ASPECTS OF CONGENITAL FACTOR VII DEFICIENCY. AM. J. MED. 37* 182-194, 1964.

*22760 FACTOR X DEFICIENCY (DEFICIENCY OF STUART-PROWER FACTOR)

THE BLEEDING TENDENCY IS MANIFESTED BY PROLONGED NASAL AND MUCOSAL HEMORRHAGE, MENORRHAGIA, HEMATURIA AND OCCASIONALLY HEMARTHROSIS. MR. STUART AND MISS. PROWER WERE THE FIRST PERSONS SHOWN TO HAVE THIS ABNORMALITY. MR. STUART WAS THE PRODUCT OF AN AUNT-NEPHEW MATING. GIROLAMI ET AL. (1970) DESCRIBED A HEMORRHAGIC DISORDER WHICH MAY BE THE RESULT OF AN ABNORMAL FACTOR X.

BACHMANN, F.* FAMILIENUNTERSUCHUNGEN BEIM KONGENITALEN STUART-PROWER-FACTOR MANGEL. ARCH. KLAUS STIFT. VERERBUNGSFORSCH. 33* 27-78, 1958.

GIROLAMI, A., MOLARO, G., LAZZARIN, N., SCARPA, R. AND BRUNETTI, A.* CONGENITAL HAEMORRHAGIC CONDITION SIMILAR BUT NOT IDENTICAL TO FACTOR X DEFICIENCY. A HAEMORRHAGIC STATE DUE TO AN ABNORMAL FACTOR X.Q SCAND. J. HAEMAT. 7* 91-99, 1970.

GIROLAMI, A., MOLARO, G., LAZZARIN, N., SCARPA, R. AND BRUNETTI, A.* A *NEW* CONGENITAL HAEMORRHAGIC CONDITION DUE TO THE PRESENCE OF AN ABNORMAL FACTOR X (FACTOR X FRIULI)* STUDY OF A LARGE KINDRED. BRIT. J. HAEMAT. 19* 179-192, 1970.

ROOS, J. AND HUIZINGA, J.* GENETIC INVESTIGATION OF THE STUART COAGULATION DEFECT. ACTA GENET. STATIST. MED. 9* 115-122, 1959.

*22770 FANCONI SYNDROME I (CHILDHOOD AND INFANTILE FORM WITHOUT CYSTINOSIS)

THE MAIN FEATURES OF THE FANCONI SYNDROME ARE RICKETS OR OSTEOMALACIA, WHICH IS RESISTANT TO VITAMIN D IN THE USUAL DOSES, GLUCOSURIA, GENERALIZED AMINOACIDURIA AND HYPERPHOSPHATURIA IN SPITE OF NORMAL OR REDUCED PLASMA CONCENTRATIONS OF THESE SUBSTANCES, AND USUALLY CHRONIC ACIDOSIS, HYPOURICEMIA AND HYPOKALEMIA. CLAY, DARMADY AND HAWKINS (1953) DESCRIBED A CHARACTERISTIC SWAN-NECK DEFORMITY OF THE PROXIMAL RENAL TUBULE. IN AN IRAQI JEWISH FAMILY, KLAJMAN AND ARBER (1967) FOUND GLYCOSURIA AND AMINOACIDURIA IN A WOMAN AND HER SON. HER HUSBAND WAS A FIRST COUSIN. TWO OTHER SONS HAD GLYCOSURIA, AMINOACIDURIA AND LOW SERUM ALKALINE PHOSPHATASE. ANOTHER SON HAD ONLY GLYCOSURIA AND TWO OTHER SONS HAD ONLY LOW ALKALINE PHOSPHATASE. A PHENOCOPY OF THE GENETIC FANCONI SYNDROME IS PRODUCED BY INGESTION OF DEGRADED (*OUTDATED*) TETRACYCLINE (BRODEHL ET AL., 1968).

BRODEHL, J., GELLISSEN, K., HAGGE, W. AND SCHUMACHER, H.* REVERSIBLES RENALES FANCONI-SYNDROM DURCH TOXISCHES ABBAUPRODUKT DES TETRAZYKLINS. HELV. PAEDIAT. ACTA 23* 373-383, 1968.

CLAY, R. D., DARMADY, E. M. AND HAWKINS, M.* THE NATURE OF THE RENAL LESION IN THE FANCONI SYNDROME. J. PATH. BACT. 65* 551-558, 1953.

HARRISON, H. E.* THE FANCONI SYNDROME. J. CHRONIC DIS. 7* 346-355, 1958.

KLAJMAN, A. AND ARBER, I.* FAMILIAL GLYCOSURIA AND AMINO-ACIDURIA ASSOCIATED WITH LOW SERUM ALKALINE PHOSPHATASE. ISRAEL J. MED. SCI. 3* 392-396, 1967.

LEAF, A.* THE SYNDROME OF OSTEOMALACIA, RENAL GLYCOSURIA, AMINO-ACIDURIA AND INCREASED PHOSPHORUS CLEARANCE (THE FANCONI SYNDROME). IN, STANBURY, J. B., WYNGAARDEN, J. B. AND FREDRICKSON, D. S. (EDS.)* THE METABOLIC BASIS OF INHERITED DISEASE. NEW YORK* MCGRAW-HILL, 1966 (2ND ED.). PP. 1205-1220.

*22780 FANCONI SYNDROME II (*ADULT* FORM WITHOUT CYSTINOSIS)

DENT AND HARRIS'S FAMILY (1956) IS THE MOST CONVINCING FOR RECESSIVE INHERITANCE. FOUR OUT OF FIVE SIBS WERE AFFECTED. THE DISEASE PRESENTS AT ABOUT AGE 40. THE BONES BECOME TENDER AND SHOW *LOOSER ZONES* BY X-RAY. LOSS OF HEIGHT AND MUSCLE

R
E
C
E
S
S
I
V
E

AS IN THE CHILDHOOD FORM. NO CYSTINOSIS IS DEMONSTRABLE. SERUM PHOSPHORUS IS LOW
AND PHOSPHATASE ELEVATED. HUNT ET AL. (1966) DESCRIBED A FAMILY IN WHICH PERSONS
IN FOUR GENERATIONS APPEAR TO HAVE HAD RETARDED GROWTH, RICKETS, HYPOPHOSPHATEMIA,
HYPOKALEMIA, ACIDOSIS, AMINOACIDURIA, PROTEINURIA AND GLYCOSURIA. AUTOPSY AND
BIOPSIES SHOWED NO CYSTINE DEPOSITS IN TISSUES. INHERITANCE WAS THOUGHT TO BE
DOMINANT.

DENT, C. E. AND HARRIS, H.* HEREDITARY FORMS OF RICKETS AND OSTEOMALACIA. J.
BONE JOINT SURG. 38B* 204-226, 1956.

HUNT, D. D., STEARNS, G., MCKINLEY, J. B., FRONING, E., HICKS, P. AND BONFIG-
LIO, M.* LONG-TERM STUDY OF A FAMILY WITH FANCONI SYNDROME WITHOUT CYSTINOSIS (DE
TONI-DEBRE-FANCONI SYNDROME). AM. J. MED. 40* 492-510, 1966.

WILSON, D. R. AND YENDT, E. R.* TREATMENT OF THE ADULT FANCONI SYNDROME WITH
ORAL PHOSPHATE SUPPLEMENTS AND ALKALI. REPORT OF TWO CASES ASSOCIATED WITH
NEPHROLITHIASIS. AM. J. MED. 35* 487-511, 1963.

*22790 FANCONI'S PANCYTOPENIA (CONSTITUTIONAL INFANTILE PANMYELOPATHY)

USUALLY ALL MARROW ELEMENTS ARE AFFECTED WITH ANEMIA, LEUKOPENIA AND THROMBOPENIA.
PIGMENTARY CHANGES IN THE SKIN AND MALFORMATIONS OF THE HEART, KIDNEY AND
EXTREMITIES (APLASIA OF THE RADIUS, THUMB DEFORMITY) ARE ASSOCIATED FEATURES.
LEUKEMIA IS A FATAL COMPLICATION (GARRIGA AND CROSBY, 1959) AND MAY OCCUR IN
FAMILY MEMBERS LACKING FULL-BLOWN FEATURES. THIS PARTICULAR POINT MUTATION
APPARENTLY PREDISPOSES TO MULTIPLE CHROMOSOMAL BREAKS (BLOOM ET AL., 1966).
BLOOM'S SYNDROME (Q.V.) IS ANOTHER SINGLE GENE DISORDER ACCOMPANIED BY CHROMOSOMAL
BREAKAGE AND PREDISPOSITION TO LEUKEMIA. LOHR ET AL. (1965) IN TWO BROTHERS AND A
THIRD UNRELATED PATIENT FOUND MARKED REDUCTION OF RED CELL, LEUKOCYTE AND PLATELET
HEXOKINASE ACTIVITY. THIS IS APPARENTLY A DIFFERENT DEFECT FROM THE HEXOKINASE
DEFICIENCY (Q.V.) WHICH IS LIMITED TO RED CELLS AND WHICH RESULTS IN HEMOLYTIC
ANEMIA ALONE. A CONSISTENT DEFECT IN HEXOKINASE CANNOT BE CONSIDERED AS PROVED
(BRUNETTI ET AL., 1966). RADIUS-PLATELET HYPOPLASIA (Q.V.) IS A SEPARATE ENTITY.
ZAIZOV ET AL. (1969) DESCRIBED TWO SISTERS AND A BROTHER WITH PANCYTOPENIA LIKE
THAT OF FANCONI'S SYNDROME BUT WITHOUT CONGENITAL MALFORMATIONS. CHROMOSOMAL
CHANGES LIKE THOSE OF FANCONI'S SYNDROME WERE PRESENT AND PATCHY AREAS OF
HYPERPIGMENTATION WERE NOTED IN TWO OF THE SIBS.

BLOOM, G. E., WARNER, S., GERALD, P. S. AND DIAMOND, L. K.* CHROMOSOME
ABNORMALITIES IN CONSTITUTIONAL APLASTIC ANEMIA. NEW ENG. J. MED. 274* 8-14,
1966.

BRUNETTI, P., NEUCI, G. G., VACCARO, R., PUXEDDU, A. AND MIGLIORINI, E.*
FANCONI'S ANAEMIA. (LETTER) LANCET 2* 1194-1195, 1966.

FANCONI, G.* FAMILIAL CONSTITUTIONAL PANMYELOCYTOPATHY, FANCONI'S ANEMIA (F.
A.). I. CLINICAL ASPECTS. SEMINARS HEMAT. 4* 233-240, 1966.

GARRIGA, S. AND CROSBY, W. H.* THE INCIDENCE OF LEUKEMIA IN FAMILIES OF
PATIENTS WITH HYPOPLASIA OF THE MARROW. BLOOD 14* 1008-1014, 1959.

LOHR, G. W., WALLER, H. D., ANSCHUTZ, F. AND KNOPP, A.* BIOCHEMISCHE DEFEKTE IN
DEN BLUTZELLEN BEI FAMILIARER PANMYELOPATHIE (TYP FANCONI). HUMANGENETIK 1* 383-
387, 1965.

MCDONALD, R. AND GOLDSCHMIDT, B.* PANCYTOPENIA WITH CONGENITAL DEFECTS
(FANCONI'S ANAEMIA). ARCH. DIS. CHILD. 35* 367-372, 1960.

SCHMID, W.* FAMILIAL CONSTITUTIONAL PANMYELOCYTOPATHY, FANCONI'S ANEMIA (F.
A.). II. A DISCUSSION OF THE CYTOGENETIC FINDINGS IN FANCONI'S ANEMIA. SEMINARS
HEMAT. 4* 241-249, 1967.

SCHMID, W., SCHARER, K., BAUMANN, T. AND FANCONI, G.* CHROMOSOMENBRUCHIGKEIT
BEI DER FAMILIAREN PANMYELOPATHIE (TYPUS FANCONI). SCHWEIZ. MED. WSCHR. 95* 1461-
1464, 1965.

SWIFT, M. R. AND HIRSCHHORN, K.* FANCONI'S ANEMIA* INHERITED SUSCEPTIBILITY TO
CHROMOSOME BREAKAGE IN VARIOUS TISSUES. ANN. INTERN. MED. 65* 496-503, 1966.

ZAIZOV, R., MATOTH, Y. AND MAMON, Z.* FAMILIAL APLASTIC ANAEMIA WITHOUT
CONGENITAL MALFORMATIONS. ACTA PAEDIAT. SCAND. 58* 151-156, 1969.

*22800 FARBER'S LIPOGRANULOMATOSIS

IN THE FEW REPORTED CASES MANIFESTATIONS APPEARED IN THE FIRST FEW WEEKS OF LIFE
AND CONSISTED OF IRRITABILITY, HOARSE CRY AND NODULAR, ERYTHEMATOUS SWELLINGS OF
THE WRISTS AND OTHER SITES, PARTICULARLY THOSE SUBJECT TO TRAUMA. SEVERE MOTOR
AND MENTAL RETARDATION IS EVIDENT. DEATH OCCURS BY 2 YEARS OF AGE. THE HISTOLO-
GIC APPEARANCE IS GRANULOMATOUS. IN THE NERVOUS SYSTEM BOTH NEURONES AND GLIAL
CELLS ARE SWOLLEN WITH STORED MATERIAL WITH THE CHARACTERISTICS OF NONSULFONATED
ACID MUCOPOLYSACCHARIDE (ABUL-HAJ AND COLLEAGUES, 1962). PARENTAL CONSANGUINITY

HAS BEEN IDENTIFIED IN NO INSTANCE. HOWEVER, IN ONE CASE PARENTS HAD THE SAME FAMILY NAME IN ANCESTORS, AND TWO OF 3 FAMILIES SEEN AT CHILDREN'S HOSPITAL, BOSTON, WERE OF PORTUGUESE EXTRACTION. THE FAMILY WITH TWO AFFECTED SIBS HAD FATHER FROM THE AZORES ISLANDS AND MOTHER FROM THE MADEIRA ISLANDS. THE PARENTS OF THE OTHER FAMILY WERE BOTH BORN IN THE AZORES (CROCKER ET AL., 1967). CLAUSEN ET AL. (1970) PROPOSED THAT AN ENZYMATIC DEFECT IN GLYCOLIPID DEGRADATION IS THE BASIC FAULT.

ABUL-HAJ, S. K., MARTZ, D. G., DOUGLAS, W. F. AND GEPPERT, L. J.* FARBER'S DISEASE. REPORT OF A CASE WITH OBSERVATIONS ON ITS HISTIOGENESIS AND NOTES ON THE NATURE OF THE STORED MATERIAL. J. PEDIAT. 61* 221-232, 1962.

CLAUSEN, J. AND RAMPINI, S.* CHEMICAL STUDIES OF FARBER'S DISEASE. ACTA NEUROL. SCAND. 46* 313-322, 1970.

CROCKER, A. C., COHEN, J. AND FARBER, S.* THE 'LIPOGRANULOMATOSIS' SYNDROME* REVIEW, WITH REPORT OF PATIENT SHOWING MILD INVOLVEMENT. IN, ARONSON, S. M. AND VOLK, B. W. (EDS.)* INBORN DISORDERS OF SPHINGOLIPID METABOLISM. OXFORD* PERGAMON PRESS, 1967. PP. 485-503.

FARBER, S., COHEN, J. AND UZMAN, L. L.* LIPOGRANULOMATOSIS* A NEW LIPO-GLYCO-PROTEIN 'STORAGE' DISEASE. J. MOUNT SINAI HOSP. N.Y. 24* 816-837, 1957.

22810 FATTY METAMORPHOSIS OF VISCERA

PEREMANS ET AL. (1967) DESCRIBED A SIBSHIP OF 14 CHILDREN, OFFSPRING OF FIRST COUSINS ONCE REMOVED, AMONG WHOM 5 CHILDREN SHOWED PROGRESSIVE MUSCULAR HYPOTONIA, LETHARGY, COMA AND DEATH IN THE FIRST DAYS OF LIFE. A SIXTH CHILD WAS FOUND TO HAVE HYPOCALCEMIA AND HYPOGLYCEMIA. AT AUTOPSY, THE HEART, LIVER AND KIDNEYS WERE GROSSLY VERY PALE AND HISTOLOGICALLY THESE AND OTHER ORGANS SHOWED LOADING OF PARENCHYMAL CELLS WITH SUDANOPHILIC MATERIAL. AUTOPSY IN TWO OF THE OTHER INFANTS ALSO SHOWED PALLOR OF VISCERA. THE RELATIONSHIP TO THE CONDITION DESCRIBED BY UTIAN ET AL. (1964) AND REYE ET AL. (1963) WAS UNCLEAR. SATRAN ET AL. (1969) DESCRIBED TWO BROTHERS AND A SISTER WHO DIED AT AGES 4 DAYS, 19 DAYS AND 12 WEEKS OF FATTY LIVER DISEASE MARKED BY A SEVERE HEMORRHAGIC DISORDER. THEY SUGGESTED THAT THE DISORDER REPORTED BY PEREMANS ET AL. (1966) MAY BE THE SAME.

R
E
C
E
S
S
I
V
E

PEREMANS, J., DEGRAEF, P. J., STRUBBE, G. AND DE BLOCK, G.* FAMILIAL METABOLIC DISORDER WITH FATTY METAMORPHOSIS OF THE VISCERA. J. PEDIAT. 69* 1108-1112, 1967.

REYE, R. D. K., MORGAN, G. AND BARAL, J.* ENCEPHALOPATHY AND FATTY DEGENERATION OF THE VISCERA. A DISEASE ENTITY IN CHILDREN. LANCET 2* 749-752, 1963.

SATRAN, L., SHARP, H. L., SCHENKEN, J. R. AND KRIVIT, W.* FATAL NEONATAL HEPATIC STEATOSIS* A NEW FAMILIAL DISORDER. J. PEDIAT. 75* 39-46, 1969.

UTIAN, H. L., WAGNER, J. M. AND SICHEL, R. J. S.* WHITE LIVER DISEASE. LANCET 2* 1043-1045, 1964.

22820 FEMUR-FIBULA-ULNA (FFU) SYNDROME

NEITHER FAMILIAL OCCURRENCE NOR ASSOCIATED EXOGENOUS FACTORS HAVE BEEN IDENTIFIED. WHEN CASES OF FEMORAL DEFECTS ASSOCIATED WITH MALFORMATIONS OF THE ARMS ARE COLLECTED, A HIGHLY SPECIFIC PATTERN OF RARE ARM DEFECTS ARE FOUND, SUCH AS AMELIA, PEROMELIA AT THE LOWER END OF THE HUMERUS, HUMERORADIAL SYNOSTOSIS, DEFECTS OF THE ULNA AND ULNAR RAYS (KUHNE ET AL., 1967). THIS DISORDER HAS BEEN CALLED PFFD (PROXIMAL FOCAL FEMORAL DEFICIENCY) IN THIS COUNTRY.

KUHNE, D., LENZ, W., PETERSEN, D. AND SCHONENBERG, H.* DEFEKT VON FEMUR UND FIBULA MIT AMELIE, PEROMELIE ODER ULNAREN STRAHLDEFEKTEN DER ARME. EIN SYNDROM. HUMANGENETIK 3* 244-263, 1967.

22830 FERTILE EUNUCH

MCCULLAGH, BECK AND SCHAFFENBURG'S (1953) PATIENT HAD A BROTHER WITH EUNUCHOIDAL FEATURES WHO REFUSED EXAMINATION. A DEFICIENCY OF ICSH (INTERSTITIAL CELL STIMULATING HORMONE) WAS POSTULATED. LUTEINIZING HORMONE (LH) IN THE MALE IS ALSO KNOWN AS ICSH (INTERSTITIAL CELL STIMULATING HORMONE). THE CLINICAL PICTURE IS ONE OF ANDROGENIC INSUFFICIENCY WITH 'NORMAL' SPERMATOGENESIS. THE SEMEN SHOWS ABNORMALITIES OF SPERM COUNT, MORPHOLOGY AND MOBILITY BUT AT LEAST TWO PATIENTS ARE SAID TO HAVE FATHERED CHILDREN. ISOLATED DEFICIENCY OF LH, IN THE PRESENCE OF NORMAL CONCENTRATIONS OF FSH, WAS DOCUMENTED BY RADIO-IMMUNO-ASSAY BY FAIMAN ET AL. (1968).

FAIMAN, C., HOFFMAN, D. L., RYAN, R. J. AND ALBERT, A.* THE 'FERTILE EUNUCH' SYNDROME* DEMONSTRATION OF ISOLATED LUTEINIZING HORMONE DEFICIENCY BY RADIO-IMMUNO-ASSAY TECHNIQUE. MAYO CLIN. PROC. 43* 661-667, 1968.

MCCULLAGH, E. P., BECK, J. C. AND SCHAFFENBURG, C. A.* SYNDROME OF EUNUCHOIDISM WITH SPERMIOGENESIS, NORMAL URINARY FSH AND LOW OR NORMAL ICSH* ('FERTILE EUNUCHS'). J. CLIN. ENDOCR. 13* 489-509, 1953.

HERMAN ET AL. (1969) DESCRIBED TWIN BROTHERS OF LEBANESE EXTRACTION WITH PERSIS-
TENT FEVER OF 102 DEGREES F. WITHOUT DIURNAL VARIATION. THE FAMILY CONTAINED
MULTIPLE CONSANGUINEOUS MARRIAGES. HORMONAL AND SWEAT STUDIES YIELDED NORMAL
FINDINGS. ADRENOSTEROID AND URONIC ACIDS WHICH INHIBIT BETA-GLUCURONIDASE
DECREASED THE TEMPERATURE. THE AUTHORS SUGGESTED THAT BETA-GLUCURONIDASE IS
IMPORTANT IN CONTROLLING THE LEVEL OF FREE INTRAHEPATIC ETIOCHOLANOLONE AND THAT
THESE PATIENTS HAD AN ABNORMALITY OF THE ENZYME SUCH THAT IT IS MORE ACTIVE,
PERHAPS BECAUSE OF UNDERSENSITIVITY TO NATURAL INHIBITORS.

HERMAN, R. H., OVERHOLT, E. L. AND HAGLER, L.* FAMILIAL LIFE-LONG PERSISTENT
FEVER OF UNKNOWN ORIGIN RESPONDING TO DEXAMETHASONE AND URONIC ACIDS. AM. J. MED.
46* 142-153, 1969.

*22850 FIBRIN-STABILIZING FACTOR (FIBRINASE, OR FACTOR XIII) DEFICIENCY

SEVERAL FAMILIES HAVE BEEN REPORTED FROM SWITZERLAND AND FINLAND. WOUND HEALING
IS POOR. HEMORRHAGE FROM THE UMBILICAL CORD AND INTRACRANIAL HEMORRHAGE HAVE BEEN
OBSERVED. BY MEANS OF A TECHNIQUE WITH ENHANCED SENSITIVITY, DUCKERT (1964)
DEMONSTRATED PARTIAL DEFICIENCY IN PRESUMPTIVE HETEROZYGOTES. UREA-SOLUBILITY OF
THE FIBRIN CLOT IS AN IN VITRO CHARACTERISTIC. ALL THE *USUAL* CLOTTING TESTS ARE
NORMAL, BUT THE DIAGNOSIS IS MADE EASILY BY THE UREA SOLUBILITY TEST. BUTTEN
(1967) DESCRIBED A CASE BOTH OF WHOSE PARENTS AS WELL AS SEVERAL OTHER RELATIVES
WERE BY TEST APPARENTLY HETEROZYGOUS. FISHER ET AL. (1966) DESCRIBED AN AFFECTED
MOROCCAN WOMAN WHO WAS OFFSPRING OF AN UNCLE-NIECE MATING. PARENTS AND SIBS WERE
APPARENTLY NORMAL. RATNOFF AND STEINBERG (1968) POINTED OUT THAT, ALTHOUGH THE
EVIDENCE FOR AUTOSOMAL RECESSIVE INHERITANCE IN SOME FAMILIES IS QUITE CONVINCING,
THE POSSIBILITY OF X-LINKED RECESSIVE INHERITANCE IN OTHER FAMILIES IS SUGGESTED
BY THE DATA. ZAHIR (1969) OBSERVED AN AFFECTED FEMALE THE OFFSPRING OF A FIRST
COUSIN MARRIAGE. BOTH PARENTS HAD LOW FACTOR XIII LEVELS.

AMRIS, C. J. AND RANEK, L.* A CASE OF FIBRIN-STABILIZING FACTOR (FSF) DEFICIEN-
CY. THROMB. DIATH. HAEMORRH. 14* 332-340, 1965.

BUTTEN, A. F. H.* CONGENITAL DEFICIENCY OF FACTOR XIII (FIBRIN-STABILIZING
FACTOR). REPORT OF A CASE AND REVIEW OF THE LITERATURE. AM. J. MED. 43* 751-761,
1967.

DUCKERT, F.* FACTOR XIII DEFICIENCY. PROC. 10TH INTERN. CONGR. SOC. HAEMATOL.,
STOCKHOLM, 1964.

DUCKERT, F., JUNG, E. AND SHMERLING, D. H.* A HITHERTO UNDESCRIBED CONGENITAL
HAEMORRHAGIC DIATHESIS PROBABLY DUE TO FIBRIN STABILIZING FACTOR DEFICIENCY.
THROMB. DIATH. HAEMORRH. 5* 179-186, 1960.

FISHER, S., RIKOVER, M. AND NAOR, S.* FACTOR 13 DEFICIENCY WITH SEVERE
HEMORRHAGIC DIATHESIS. BLOOD 28* 34-39, 1966.

IKKALA, E. AND NEVANLINNA, H. R.* CONGENITAL DEFICIENCY OF FIBRIN STABILIZING
FACTOR. THROMB. DIATH. HAEMORRH. 7* 567-571, 1962.

LORAND, L., URAYAMA, T., ATENCIO, A. C. AND HSIA, D. Y.-Y.* INHERITANCE OF
DEFICIENCY OF FIBRIN-STABILIZING FACTOR (FACTOR XIII). AM. J. HUM. GENET. 22* 89-
95, 1970.

RATNOFF, O. D. AND STEINBERG, A. G.* INHERITANCE OF FIBRIN-STABILIZING-FACTOR
DEFICIENCY. LANCET 1* 25-26, 1968.

SHMERLING, D. H., JUNG, E. AND DUCKERT, F.* EINE NEUE FAMILIARE KOAGULOPATHIE
INFOLGE MANGELS AN FIBRINSTABILISIERENDEM FAKTOR. HELV. PAEDIAT. ACTA 15* 471-
478, 1960.

ZAHIR, M.* CONGENITAL DEFICIENCY OF FIBRIN-STABILIZING FACTOR. REPORT OF A
CASE AND FAMILY STUDY. J.A.M.A. 207* 751-753, 1969.

R
E
C
E
S
S
I
V
E

22860 FIBROMATOSIS, JUVENILE

BOTH MALES AND FEMALES ARE AFFECTED AND IN AT LEAST TWO INSTANCES (DRESCHER ET
AL., 1967* ENJOJI ET AL., 1968) TWO AFFECTED SIBS HAVE BEEN REPORTED. THE
DISORDER IS CHARACTERIZED BY MULTIPLE SUBCUTANEOUS TUMORS, PARTICULARLY OF THE
SCALP, APPEARING AT ABOUT AGE 2 YEARS AND SLOWLY GROWING, CAUSING DEFORMITIES.
NODULAR OR DIFFUSE HYPERTROPHY OF THE GUMS IS ALSO OBSERVED. THE TUMORS RECUR
AFTER REMOVAL. HISTOLOGICALLY THEY DEMONSTRATE AN ABUNDANCE OF HOMOGENEOUS,
AMORPHOUS, ACIDOPHILIC GROUND SUBSTANCE IN WHICH SPINDLE SHAPED CELLS FORM MINUTE
STREAKS.

DRESCHER, E., WOYKE, S., MARKIEWICZ, C. AND TEGI, S.* JUVENILE FIBROMATOSIS IN
SIBLINGS (FIBROMATOSIS HYALINICA MULTIPLEX JUVENILIS). J. PEDIAT. SURG. 2* 427-
430, 1967.

ENJOJI, M., KATO, N., KAMIKARZURU, K. AND ARIMA, E.* JUVENILE FIBROMATOSIS OF

THE SCALP IN SIBLINGS. ACTA MED. UNIV. KAGOSHIMA (SUPPL. 10)* 145-151, 1968.

WOYKE, S., WENANCJUSZ, D. AND OLSZEWSKI, W.* ULTRASTRUCTURE OF A FIBROMATOSIS HYALINICA MULTIPLEX JUVENILIS. CANCER 26* 1157-1168, 1970.

22870 FIBROMUSCULAR HYPERPLASIA OF THE RENAL ARTERIES

THIS CHANGE, LEADING TO HYPERTENSION, OCCURS ALMOST ONLY IN FEMALES, MANIFESTING ITSELF IN EARLY ADULTHOOD AS A RULE. HANSEN, HOLTEN AND THORBERG (1965) REPORTED AFFECTED SISTERS. A 25 YEAR OLD PATIENT WITH THIS ANOMALY HAD A HYPERTENSIVE 22 YEAR OLD BROTHER (WOOD, BORGES, 1963). OTHER VISCERAL ARTERIES ARE AFFECTED IN SOME PATIENTS. HALPERN, SANFORD AND VIAMONTE (1965) DESCRIBED AFFECTED SISTERS BUT GAVE NO INFORMATION ON THE PARENTS OR OTHER SIBS.

HALPERN, M. M., SANFORD, H. S. AND VIAMONTE, M., JR.* RENAL-ARTERY ABNORMALITIES IN THREE HYPERTENSIVE SISTERS. PROBABLE FAMILIAL FIBROMUSCULAR HYPERPLASIA. J.A.M.A. 194* 512-513, 1965.

HANSEN, J., HOLTEN, C. AND THORBERG, J. V.* HYPERTENSION IN TWO SISTERS CAUSED BY SO-CALLED FIBROMUSCULAR HYPERPLASIA OF THE RENAL ARTERIES. ACTA MED. SCAND. 178* 461-474, 1965.

NAJAFI, H.* FIBROMUSCULAR HYPERPLASIA OF THE EXTERNAL ILIAC ARTERIES. AN UNUSUAL CAUSE OF INTERMITTENT CLAUDICATION. ARCH. SURG. 92* 394-396, 1966.

WOOD, C. AND BORGES, F. J.* PERIMUSCULAR FIBROSIS OF RENAL ARTERIES WITH HYPERTENSION. ARCH. INTERN. MED. 112* 79-91, 1963.

22880 FIBROSCLEROSIS, MULTIFOCAL

COMINGS ET AL. (1967) REPORTED TWO BROTHERS, OFFSPRING OF A FIRST COUSIN MARRIAGE, WHO HAD DIFFERENT COMBINATIONS OF RETROPERITONEAL FIBROSIS, MEDIASTINAL FIBROSIS, SCLEROSING CHOLANGITIS, RIEDEL'S SCLEROSING THYROIDITIS AND PSEUDOTUMOR OF THE ORBIT. ONE OF THE BROTHERS HAD FIBROTIC CONTRACTURE OF THE FINGERS.

COMINGS, D. E., SKUBI, K. B., VAN EYES, J. AND MOTULSKY, A. G.* FAMILIAL MULTIFOCAL FIBROSCLEROSIS. FINDINGS SUGGESTING THAT RETROPERITONEAL FIBROSIS, MEDIASTINAL FIBROSIS, SCLEROSING CHOLANGITIS, RIEDEL'S THYROIDITIS AND PSEUDOTUMOR OF THE ORBIT MAY BE DIFFERENT MANIFESTATIONS OF A SINGLE DISEASE. ANN. INTERN. MED. 66* 884-892, 1967.

22890 FIBULA APLASIA AND COMPLEX BRACHYDACTYLY

THIS SYNDROME SEEMS TO HAVE BEEN DESCRIBED ONLY BY GREBE (1955) WHO REPORTED A BROTHER AND SISTER, FROM A FIRST COUSIN MARRIAGE, WHO HAD SHORTENING OF VARIOUS METACARPALS, SMALL CARPALS, TRAPEZOID MIDDLE PHALANX OF THE INDEX FINGER, WITH RADIAL DEVIATION, ALMOST COMPLETE ABSENCE OF THE FIBULA BILATERALLY AND TIBIO-TARSAL DISLOCATION (VOLKMANN'S DEFORMITY). THE TOES WERE SHORT AND LATERALLY DEVIATED.

GREBE, H.* CHONDRODYSPLASIE. ROME* INT. GREG. MENDEL, 1955. PP. 300-303.

22900 FLETCHER FACTOR DEFICIENCY

HATHAWAY ET AL. (1965) DESCRIBED A KENTUCKY KINDRED IN WHICH FOUR SIBS OF THE NAME FLETCHER SHOWED A PREVIOUSLY UNDESCRIBED COAGULATION DEFECT. ALTHOUGH THEY HAD NO ABNORMAL BLEEDING TENDENCY, THEIR BLOOD SHOWED MUCH PROLONGED ACTIVATED PARTIAL THROMBOPLASTIN TIME AND DELAYED THROMBOPLASTIN GENERATION BUT NORMAL PROTHROMBIN TIME. PLASMAS DEFICIENT IN FACTOR VIII, IX, XI AND XII CORRECTED THE ABNORMALITY. HATTERSLEY AND HAYSE (1970) REPORTED THREE UNRELATED CASES.

HATHAWAY, W. E., BELHASEN, L. P. AND HATHAWAY, H. S.* EVIDENCE FOR A NEW PLASMA THROMBOPLASTIN FACTOR. I. CASE REPORT, COAGULATION STUDIES AND PHYSIOCHEMICAL PROPERTIES. BLOOD 26* 521-532, 1965.

HATTERSLEY, P. G. AND HAYSE, D.* FLETCHER FACTOR DEFICIENCY* A REPORT OF THREE UNRELATED CASES. BRIT. J. HAEMAT. 18* 411-416, 1970.

*22910 FORMIMINOTRANSFERASE DEFICIENCY

MENTAL RETARDATION IS THE MAIN CLINICAL FEATURE. THE FERRIC CHLORIDE TEST IS POSITIVE DUE TO FORMIMINOGLUTAMIC ACID IN THE URINE. THE FEATURES ARE MARKED MENTAL AND PHYSICAL RETARDATION, ANEMIA, MEGALOBLASTIC BONE MARROW AND BIOCHEMICAL EVIDENCE OF DISTURBED FOLIC ACID METABOLISM. TWO RELATED PATIENTS, BOTH JAPANESE, HAVE BEEN DESCRIBED. VERY LARGE AMOUNTS OF FIGLU WERE EXCRETE IN THE URINE. THE LEVEL OF FOLIC ACID IN THE BLOOD IS INCREASED. HYPERFOLICACIDEMIA FOLLOWED HISTIDINE LOADING. THE SINGLE CASE DESCRIBED BY ARAKAWA ET AL. (1965) HAD HYPERSEGMENTATION OF THE NUCLEI OF NEUTROPHILS. THIS MAY HAVE BEEN FORTUITOUS ASSOCIATION OF AN INDEPENDENT TRAIT, SINCE THE FATHER AND HIS SISTER AND MOTHER SHOWED THE SAME FINDING BUT WERE OTHERWISE NORMAL. SEE UNDRITZ ANOMALY, A DOMINANT.

R
E
C
E
S
S
I
V
E

ARAKAWA, T. S., FUJII, M. AND OHARA, K.* ERYTHROCYTE FORMIMINOTRANSFERASE ACTIVITY IN FORMININOTRANSFERASE DEFICIENCY SYNDROME. TOHOKU J. EXP. MED. 88* 195-202, 1966.

ARAKAWA, T. S., OHARA, K., TAKAHASHI, Y., OGASAWARA, J., HAYASHI, T., CHIBA, R., WADA, Y., TADA, K., MIZUNO, T., OKAMURA, T. AND YOSHIDA, T.* FORMIMINOTRANS-FERASE-DEFICIENCY SYNDROME* A NEW INBORN ERROR OF FOLIC ACID METABOLISM. ANN. PAEDIAT. 205* 1-11, 1965.

ARAKAWA, T. S., TAMURA, T., HIGASHI, O., OHARA, K., TANNO, K., HONDA, Y., NARISAWA, K., KONNO, T., WADA, Y., SATO, Y. AND MIZUNO, T.* FORMININOTRANSFERASE DEFICIENCY SYNDROME ASSOCIATED WITH MEGALOBLASTIC ANEMIA RESPONSIVE TO PYRIDOXINE OR FOLIC ACID. TOHOKU J. EXP. MED. 94* 3-16, 1968.

*22920 FRAGILITAS OCULI (CORNEAL FRAGILITY, KERATOGLOBUS, BLUE SCLERAE) WITH JOINT HYPEREXTENSIBILITY

A SEEMINGLY DISTINCTIVE DISORDER WITH CLEARLY AUTOSOMAL RECESSIVE INHERITANCE HAS BEEN DESCRIBED BY STEIN ET AL. (1968) IN TWO TUNISIAN JEWISH BROTHERS WITH CONSANGUINEOUS PARENTS. HYAMS ET AL. (1969) IN A TUNISIAN JEWISH BOY WHO MAY BE RELATED TO THE PATIENTS OF STEIN ET AL. (1968) BECAUSE *THE TWO FAMILIES COME FROM THE SAME TOWN IN TUNISIA,* BY BADTKE (1941) IN TWO SISTERS WITH RELATED PARENTS FROM SOUTH TYROL, BY TUCKER IN A BROTHER AND SISTER WITH FIRST COUSIN PARENTS, AND BY ARKIN IN A 17 YEAR OLD BOY. THE FEATURES INCLUDE BLUE SCLERAE* LARGE CLOUDY, THIN, BULGING CORNEA, NOTED FROM EARLY IN LIFE, AND MIMICKING BUPHTHALMOS BUT ACCOMPANIED BY NORMAL INTRAOCULAR PRESSURE* FRAGILITY OF THE CORNEA WITH REPEATED RUPTURE* DENTAL ABNORMALITIES SOMEWHAT LIKE THOSE OF OSTEOGENESIS IMPERFECTA* ABNORMAL PROCLIVITY TO FRACTURE OF BONES* LONG SLENDER HYPEREXTENSIBLE FINGERS* HERNIA. THE TUMISIAN CASES OF STEIN ET AL. (1968) AND HYAMS (1969) HAD RED HAIR, A SUFFICIENTLY UNUSUAL FINDING IN THIS GROUP TO SUGGEST TO THE AUTHORS THAT IT IS A PART OF THE SYNDROME. IN KERATOGLOBUS THE THINNING OF THE CORNEA IS GENERALIZED OR IN THE PERIPHERY, WHEREAS IN KERATOCONUS IT IS MAINLY CENTRAL.

ARKIN, W.* BLUE SCLERAS WITH KERATOGLOBUS. AM. J. OPHTHAL. 58* 678-682, 1964.

BADTKE, G.* UEBER EINEN EIGENARTIGEN FALL VON KERATOKONUS UND BLAUEN SKLEREN BEI GESCHWISTERN. KLIN. MBL. AUGENHEILK. 106* 585-592, 1941.

HYAMS, S. W., KAR, H. AND NEUMANN, E.* BLUE SCLERAE AND KERATOGLOBUS. OCULAR SIGNS OF A SYSTEMIC CONNECTIVE TISSUE DISORDER. BRIT. J. OPHTHAL. 53* 53-58, 1969.

STEIN, R., LAZAR, M. AND ADAM, A.* BRITTLE CORNEA. A FAMILIAL TRAIT ASSOCIATED WITH BLUE SCLERA. AM. J. OPHTHAL. 66* 67-69, 1968.

R
E
C
E
S
S
I
V
E

*22930 FRIEDREICH'S ATAXIA

THIS IS ONE OF THE RARE HEREDITARY SPINOCEREBELLAR DEGENERATIONS. THE SPINOCERE-BELLAR TRACTS, DORSAL COLUMNS, PYRAMIDAL TRACTS AND, TO A LESSER EXTENT, THE CEREBELLUM AND MEDULLA ARE INVOLVED. THE DISORDER IS USUALLY MANIFEST BEFORE ADOLESCENCE AND IS GENERALLY CHARACTERIZED BY INCOORDINATION OF LIMB MOVEMENTS, DYSARTHRIA, NYSTAGMUS, DIMINISHED OR ABSENT TENDON REFLEXES, BABINSKI'S SIGN, IMPAIRMENT OF POSITION AND VIBRATORY SENSES, SCOLIOSIS, PES CAVUS AND HAMMER TOE. THE TRIAD OF HYPOACTIVE KNEE AND ANKLE JERKS, SIGNS OF PROGRESSIVE CEREBELLAR DYSFUNCTION AND PRE-ADOLESCENT ONSET IS COMMONLY REGARDED AS SUFFICIENT FOR DIAGNOSIS. CARDIAC MANIFESTATIONS ARE CONSPICUOUS IN SOME CASES (BOYER, CHISHOLM AND MCKUSICK, 1962). HEWER (1968) FOUND THAT ONE-HALF OF 82 FATAL CASES OF FRIEDREICH'S ATAXIA DIED OF HEART FAILURE AND NEARLY THREE-QUARTERS HAD EVIDENCE OF CARDIAC DYSFUNCTION IN LIFE. 23 PERCENT HAD DIABETES AND 4 DEVELOPED DIABETIC KETOSIS TERMINALLY. ONE CASE HAD AN AFFECTED PARENT. AGE AT DEATH VARIED FROM THE FIRST (3 CASES) TO THE EIGHTH (1 CASE) DECADE WITH A MEAN OF 36.6 YEARS.

BOYER, S. H., CHISHOLM, A. W. AND MCKUSICK, V. A.* CARDIAC ASPECTS OF FRIE-DREICH'S ATAXIA. CIRCULATION 25* 493-505, 1962.

HARTMAN, J. M. AND BOOTH, R. W.* FRIEDREICH'S ATAXIA* A NEUROCARDIAC DISEASE. AM. HEART J. 60* 716-720, 1960.

HECK, A. F.* A STUDY OF NEURAL AND EXTRANEURAL FINDINGS IN A LARGE FAMILY WITH FRIEDREICH'S ATAXIA. J. NEUROL. SCI. 1* 226-255, 1964.

HEWER, R. L.* STUDY OF FATAL CASES OF FRIEDREICH'S ATAXIA. BRIT. MED. J. 3* 649-652, 1968.

HUGHES, J. T., BROWNELL, B. AND HEWER, R. L.* THE PERIPHERAL SENSORY PATHWAY IN FRIEDREICH'S ATAXIA. AN EXAMINATION BY LIGHT AND ELECTRON MICROSCOPY OF THE POSTERIOR NERVE ROOTS, POSTERIOR ROOT GANGLIA, AND PERIPHERAL SENSORY NERVES IN CASES OF FRIEDREICH'S ATAXIA. BRAIN 91* 803-818, 1969.

KOENNICKE, W.* FRIEDREICHSCHE ATAXIE UND TAUBSTUMMHEIT. ZBL. GES. NEUROL. PSYCHIAT. 53* 161-164, 1919-20.

GORLIN (1969) DESCRIBED A MALE PATIENT WITH EXTRAORDINARILY MARKED FRONTAL HYPEROSTOSIS GIVING GREAT PROMINENCE TO THE SUPRACILIARY RIDGES, UNDERDEVELOPED MANDIBLE, CRYPTORCHIDISM, SUBLUXATED RADIAL HEADS, AND METAPHYSEAL DYSPLASIA LIKE THAT IN PYLE'S DISEASE (METAPHYSEAL DYSPLASIA). NOTHING IS KNOWN OF ITS GENETICS. THIS MAY BE THE DISORDER PRESENT IN THE CASE DESCRIBED BY WALKER (1969). STRIKING OVERGROWTH OF BONE IN THE SUPERCILIARY REGION WAS REPAIRED BY REMOVAL OF EXCESS BONE.

GORLIN, R. J. AND COHEN, M. M., JR.* FRONTOMETAPHYSEAL DYSPLASIA. A NEW SYNDROME. AM. J. DIS. CHILD. 118* 487-494, 1969.

WALKER, B. A.* A CRANIODIAPHYSEAL DYSPLASIA OR CRANIOMETAPHYSEAL DYSPLASIA.Q THE CLINICAL DELINEATION OF BIRTH DEFECTS. IV. SKELETAL DYSPLASIAS. NEW YORK* NATIONAL FOUNDATION, 1969. PP. 298-300.

22950 FRUCTOSE AND GALACTOSE INTOLERANCE

IN 1961 DORMANDY AND PORTER REPORTED THE ABOVE COMBINATION IN TWO SISTERS. UNLIKE FRUCTOSE INTOLERANCE PATIENTS, BOTH WERE FOND OF CANDY AND SHOWED NO NAUSEA OR VOMITING AFTER FRUCTOSE INGESTION. BOTH GALACTOSE AND FRUCTOSE INDUCED SEVERE HYPOGLYCEMIA. GALACTOSE-1-PHOSPHATE URIDYL TRANSFERASE, THE ENZYME DEFICIENT IN GALACTOSEMIA, WAS NORMAL. IN BOTH PATIENTS SERUM INSULIN BY IMMUNO-ASSAY WAS IN THE SAME HIGH RANGE AS IS FOUND IN PATIENTS WITH BETA ISLET CELL ADENOMAS (SAMOLS AND DORMANDY, 1963).

DORMANDY, T. L. AND PORTER, R. J.* FAMILIAL FRUCTOSE AND GALACTOSE INTOLERANCE. LANCET 1* 1189-1194, 1961.

SAMOLS, E. AND DORMANDY, T. L.* INSULIN RESPONSE TO FRUCTOSE AND GALACTOSE. LANCET 1* 478-479, 1963.

*22960 FRUCTOSE INTOLERANCE, HEREDITARY (FRUCTOSEMIA)

R
E
C
E
S
S
I
V
E

MOST OF THE RECOGNIZED CASES HAVE BEEN SEVERELY ILL INFANTS WITH RECURRENT HYPOGLYCEMIA AND VOMITING, OCCURRING AT THE TIME OF WEANING WHEN FRUCTOSE OR SUCROSE IS ADDED TO THE DIET AND RESULTING IN MARKED MALNUTRITION. HOWEVER, A THREE YEAR OLD BROTHER OF A SEVERELY AFFECTED INFANT WAS FOUND TO HAVE HEPATOMEGA-LY AND HYPOGLYCEMIC SHOCK WAS PRECIPITATED BY AN ORAL TEST DOSE OF FRUCTOSE, ALTHOUGH HE WAS CLINICALLY HEALTHY (PERHEENTUPA AND PITKANEN, 1962). HE HAD A MARKED AVERSION TO SWEETS AND FRUIT. FROESCH ET AL. (1963) DESCRIBED TWO ADULTS, AGES 33 AND 39 YEARS, WITH THE SAME CONDITION. IN ADDITION TO THE AVERSION TO FRUCTOSE-CONTAINING FOODS, REMARKABLE ABSENCE OF DENTAL CARIES WAS NOTED. THE DEFECT RESIDES IN THE LIVER ALDOLASE, WHICH SPLITS FRUCTOSE-1-PHOSPHATE. BY ANALOGY TO GALACTOSEMIA THE TERM FRUCTOSEMIA WAS SUGGESTED BY LEVIN ET AL. (1963). THE PATIENT REPORTED BY MASS ET AL. (1966) HAD RENAL TUBULAR ACIDOSIS AS AN INDEPENDENT RECESSIVE (Q.V.) OR AS A COMPLICATION OF THE FRUCTOSEMIA. WOLF ET AL. (1959) RECORDED CASES IN FATHER AND SON BUT THE MOTHER MAY HAVE BEEN HETEROZYGOUS. SWALES AND SMITH (1956) DESCRIBED AN AFFECTED 21 YEAR OLD MAN. EVIDENCE FOR GENETIC HETEROGENEITY WAS CONSIDERED CONVINCING BY LEVIN ET AL. (1968). BOTH STRUCTURAL AND CONTROLLER MUTATIONS MAY EXIST, AS WELL AS MORE THAN ONE TYPE OF STRUCTURAL MUTATION. ONE OF THEIR CASES AND A PREVIOUSLY REPORTED ONE HAD A NEAR NORMAL RATIO OF FRUCTOSE-1-PHOSPHATE ALDOLASE TO FRUCTOSE DIPHOSPHATE ALDOLASE, SUGGESTING A CONTROLLER MUTATION. KOHLIN AND MELIN (1968) REPORTED ADULT CASES. PERHEENTUPA AND RAIVIO (1967) DISCUSSED HYPERURICEMIA IN THIS DISORDER.

CORNBLATH, M., ROSENTHAL, I. M., REISNER, S. H., WYBREGT, S. H. AND CRANE, R. K.* HEREDITARY FRUCTOSE INTOLERANCE. NEW ENG. J. MED. 269* 1271-1278, 1963.

FROESCH, E. R., WOLF, H. P., BAITSCH, H., PRADER, A. AND LABHART, A.* HEREDI-TARY FRUCTOSE INTOLERANCE* AN INBORN DEFECT OF HEPATIC FRUCTOSE-1-PHOSPHATE SPLITTING ALDOLASE. AM. J. MED. 34* 151-167, 1963.

KOHLIN, P. AND MELIN, K.* HEREDITARY FRUCTOSE INTOLERANCE IN FOUR SWEDISH FAMILIES. ACTA PAEDIAT. SCAND. 57* 24-32, 1968.

KRANHOLD, J. F., LOH, D. AND MORRIS, R. C., JR.* RENAL FRUCTOSE-METABOLIZING ENZYMES* SIGNIFICANCE IN HEREDITARY FRUCTOSE INTOLERANCE. SCIENCE 165* 402-403, 1969.

LEVIN, B., OBERHOLZER, V. G., SNODGRASS, G. J. A. I., STIMMLER, L. AND WILMERS, M. J.* FRUCTOSAEMIA. AN INBORN ERROR OF FRUCTOSE METABOLISM. ARCH. DIS. CHILD. 38* 220-230, 1963.

LEVIN, B., SNODGRASS, G. J. A. I., OBERHOLZER, V. G., BURGESS, E. A. AND DOBBS, R. H.* FRUCTOSAEMIA* OBSERVATIONS ON SEVEN CASES. AM. J. MED. 45* 826-838, 1968.

MASS, R. E., SMITH, W. R. AND WALSH, J. R.* THE ASSOCIATION OF HEREDITARY FRUCTOSE INTOLERANCE AND RENAL TUBULAR ACIDOSIS. AM. J. MED. SCI. 251* 516-523, 1966.

NIKKILA, E. A., SOMERSALO, O., PITKANEN, E. AND PERHEENTUPA, J.* HEREDITARY FRUCTOSE INTOLERANCE, AN INBORN DEFICIENCY OF LIVER ALDOLASE COMPLEX. METABOLISM 11* 727-731, 1962.

PERHEENTUPA, J. AND PITKANEN, E.* SYMPTOMLESS HEREDITARY FRUCTOSE INTOLERANCE. (LETTER) LANCET 1* 1358-1359, 1962.

PERHEENTUPA, J. AND RAIVIO, K.* FRUCTOSE-INDUCED HYPERURICAEMIA. LANCET 2* 528-531, 1967.

RENNERT, O. M. AND GREER, M.* HEREDITARY FRUCTOSEMIA. NEUROLOGY 20* 421-425, 1970.

SWALES, J. D. AND SMITH, A. D. M.* ADULT FRUCTOSE INTOLERANCE. QUART. J. MED. 35* 455-473, 1966.

WOLF, H., ZSCHOCKE, D., WEDEMEYER, F. W. AND HUBNER, W.* ANGEBORENE HEREDITARE FRUCTOSE-INTOLERANZ. KLIN. WSCHR. 37* 693-696, 1959.

*22970 FRUCTOSE-1, 6-DIPHOSPHATASE, HEPATIC DEFICIENCY OF

BAKER AND WINEGRAD (1970) DESCRIBED A GIRL WITH HYPOGLYCEMIA AND METABOLIC ACIDOSIS ON FASTING. THE DEFECT WAS IMPAIRED GLUCONEOGENESIS DUE TO DEFICIENCY OF HEPATIC FRUCTOSE-1, 6-DIPHOSPHATASE. A SIB HAD DIED OF A CLINICALLY SIMILAR AILMENT.

BAKER, L. AND WINEGRAD, A. I.* FASTING HYPOGLYCAEMIA AND METABOLIC ACIDOSIS ASSOCIATED WITH DEFICIENCY OF HEPATIC FRUCTOSE-1, 6-DIPHOSPHATASE ACTIVITY. LANCET 2* 13-16, 1970.

*22980 FRUCTOSURIA

THIS IS A BENIGN, ASYMPTOMATIC DEFECT OF INTERMEDIARY METABOLISM. THERE IS NO EVIDENCE OF A RENAL DEFECT. THE ENZYME INVOLVED IS THOUGHT TO BE HEPATIC FRUCTOKINASE.

FROESCH, E. R.* ESSENTIAL FRUCTOSURIA AND HEREDITARY FRUCTOSE INTOLERANCE. IN, STANBURY, J. B., WYNGAARDEN, J. B. AND FREDRICKSON, D. S. (EDS.)* THE METABOLIC BASIS OF INHERITED DISEASE. NEW YORK* MCGRAW-HILL, 1966 (2ND ED.). PP. 124-140.

LASKER, M.* ESSENTIAL FRUCTOSURIA. HUM. BIOL. 13* 51-63, 1941.

22990 FUCHS ATROPHIA GYRATA CHORIOIDEAE ET RETINAE

THIS VERY RARE DISORDER IS CHARACTERIZED BY SLOWLY PROGRESSIVE ATROPHY OF THE CHOROID, PIGMENT EPITHELIUM AND RETINA. FRANCOIS AND HIS COLLEAGUES OBSERVED A PATIENT BORN OF A CONSANGUINEOUS MARRIAGE IN WHOM ALDER'S ANOMALY OF THE LEUKO-CYTES WAS PRESENT NOT ONLY IN THE PATIENT BUT ALSO IN BOTH PARENTS AND IN OTHER MEMBERS OF THE FAMILY THROUGH FOUR GENERATIONS. THESE WORKERS SUGGESTED THAT THE LEUKOCYTE ANOMALY IS A HETEROZYGOUS EXPRESSION OF THE GENE WHICH IN THE HOMOZYGOUS STATE PRODUCES FUCHS* ATROPHY. IN A LATER PUBLICATION, HOWEVER, FRANCOIS ET AL. (1966) REPORTED FAILURE TO FIND THE ALDER ANOMALY IN 9 PATIENTS WITH THE EYE ANOMALY.

FRANCOIS, J.* HEREDITY IN OPHTHALMOLOGY. ST. LOUIS* C. V. MOSBY CO., 1961.

FRANCOIS, J.* PROGRESS IN MEDICAL GENETICS. IN, STEINBERG, A. G. AND BEARN, A. G. (EDS.)* NEW YORK* GRUNE AND STRATTON, 2* 1962.

FRANCOIS, J., BARBIER, F. AND DE ROUCK, A.* A PROPOS DES CONDUCTEURS DU GENE DE L'ATROPHIA GYRATA CHORIOIDEAE ET RETINAE DE FUCHS. ACTA GENET. MED. GEM. 15* 34-35, 1966.

FRANCOIS, J., BARBIER, F. AND DE ROUCK, A.* LES CONDUCTEURS DU GENE DE L'ATROPHIA GYRATA CHORIOIDEAE ET RETINAE DE FUCHS (ANOMALIE D'ALDER). ACTA GENET. MED. GEM. 9* 74-91, 1960.

*23000 FUCOSIDOSIS

IN THE HURLER SYNDROME AND RELATED CONDITIONS, ENLARGEMENT OF LYSOSOMES IN THE LIVER SUGGESTED A DEFECT IN AN ACID HYDROLASE. VAN HOOF AND HERS (1968) FOUND A DEFICIENCY OF ALPHA-FUCOSIDASE ACTIVITY IN THE LIVER OF PATIENTS WITH A HURLER-LIKE DISORDER DESCRIBED BY DURAND ET AL. (1967, 1968). FUCOSE ACCUMULATED IN ALL TISSUES (DURAND ET AL., 1968). THE PATIENT OF BERNARD ET AL. (1966) WAS FEMALE. DURAND ET AL. (1968) CALLED THE CONDITION FUCOSIDOSIS. THE BELGIAN PATIENT STUDIED BY LOEB ET AL. (1969) IS PROBABLY RELATED TO THE TWO ITALIAN PATIENTS REPORTED BY DURAND ET AL. (1969).

DURAND, P., BORRONE, C. AND DELLA CELLA, G.* FUCOSIDOSIS. J. PEDIAT. 75* 665-674, 1969.

DURAND, P., BORRONE, C., DELLA CELLA, G. AND PHILIPPART, M.* FUCOSIDOSIS.

(LETTER) LANCET 1* 1198 ONLY, 1968.

DURAND, P., PHILIPPART, M., BORRONE, C. AND DELLA CELLA, G.* A NEW GLYCOLIPID STORAGE DISEASE. (ABSTRACT) PEDIAT. RES. 1* 416 ONLY, 1967.

LEROY, J. G.* FUCOSIDOSIS.Q (LETTER) LANCET 2* 408-409, 1968.

LOEB, H., TONDEUR, M., JONNIAUX, G., MOCKEL-POHL, S. AND VAMOS-HURWITZ, E.* BIOCHEMICAL AND ULTRASTRUCTURAL STUDIES IN A CASE OF MUCOPOLYSACCHARIDOSIS F (FUCOSIDOSIS). HELV. PAEDIAT. ACTA 24* 519-537, 1969.

VAN HOOF, F. AND HERS, H. G.* MUCOPOLYSACCHARIDOSIS BY ABSENCE OF ALPHA-FUCOSIDASE. (LETTER) LANCET 1* 1198 ONLY, 1968.

23010 FUNDUS FLAVIMACULATUS

THIS IS PROBABLY A GENETIC DISORDER AND PROBABLY AUTOSOMAL RECESSIVE. KLEIN AND KRILL (1967) OBSERVED A *FAMILIAL INCIDENCE . . . IN 10 OF 27 PATIENTS.* THE 10 FAMILIAL CASES INCLUDED FOUR PAIRS OF AFFECTED SIBS WITH OSTENSIBLY NORMAL PARENTS WHO WERE, HOWEVER, NOT EXAMINED IN MOST INSTANCES. NO PARENTAL CONSANGUINITY WAS DESCRIBED. IN ONE INSTANCE THE FATHER AND TWO DAUGHTERS WERE AFFECTED. IN THE INSTANCE OF AN AFFECTED BROTHER AND SISTER, THE FATHER WAS NEGRO AND THE MOTHER WHITE. THUS THE INHERITANCE IS IN DOUBT. THIS DISORDER DERIVES ITS NAME FROM THE OCCURRENCE OF MANY YELLOW SPOTS RATHER UNIFORMLY DISTRIBUTED OVER THE FUNDUS.

KLEIN, B. A. AND KRILL, A. E.* FUNDUS FLAVIMACULATUS* CLINICAL, FUNCTIONAL AND HISTOPATHOLOGIC OBSERVATIONS. AM. J. OPHTHAL. 64* 3-23, 1967.

*23020 GALACTOKINASE DEFICIENCY

IN TWO SIBS OF A CONSANGUINEOUS GYPSY FAMILY, GITZELMANN (1967) FOUND JUVENILE CATARACT RELATED TO GALACTOKINASE DEFICIENCY. FANCONI HAD PREVIOUSLY REPORTED THE CASES AS INSTANCES OF *GALACTOSE DIABETES.* GALACTOSE-1-PHOSPHATE URIDYLTRANS-FERASE ACTIVITY IN RED CELL WAS NORMAL. NO MENTAL RETARDATION WAS PRESENT. SEVERAL CLOSE RELATIVES HAD REDUCED RED CELL GALACTOKINASE ACTIVITY SUGGESTING THAT THEY ARE HETEROZYGOTES. MENTAL RETARDATION WAS PRESENT IN SOME OF COTTON*S CASES (1967). IN BUFFALO, N.Y., MAYES AND GUTHRIE (1968) FOUND 6 HETEROZYGOTES AMONG 642 PERSONS. THE ETHNIC EXTRACTION WAS NOT GIVEN.

COTTON, J.-B.* DEFICIT HEREDITAIRE EN GALACTOKINASE. PEDIATRIE 22* 609-611, 1967.

GITZELMANN, R.* HEREDITARY GALACTOKINASE DEFICIENCY, A NEWLY RECOGNIZED CAUSE OF JUVENILE CATARACTS. PEDIAT. RES. 1* 14-23, 1967.

MAYES, J. S. AND GUTHRIE, R.* DETECTION OF HETEROZYGOTES FOR GALACTOKINASE DEFICIENCY IN A HUMAN POPULATION. BIOCHEM. GENET. 2* 219-230, 1968.

THALHAMMER, O., GITZELMANN, R. AND PANTLITSCHKO, M.* HYPERGALACTOSEMIA AND GALACTOSURIA DUE TO GALACTOKINASE DEFICIENCY IN A NEW BORN. PEDIATRICS 42* 441-445, 1968.

23030 GALACTORRHEA

WIDER ET AL. (1969) DESCRIBED 3 SISTERS WITH NON-PUERPERAL GALACTORRHEA OCCURRING AFTER TREATMENT WITH ORAL CONTRACEPTIVE. ALTHOUGH ALL 3 HAD OLIGO-OVULATION THE EVIDENCE SUGGESTED INDEPENDENT CONTROL OF OVULATION AND LACTATION* GALACTORRHEA CONTINUED IN ONE SISTER WHILE SHE TOOK AN ORAL CONTRACEPTIVE CONTAINING ESTROGEN-PROGESTERONE WHILE PRESUMABLY SUPPRESSED PRODUCTION OF PLASMA GONADOTROPIA BY MEASURES WHICH STIMULATED THE RELEASE OF GONADOTROPINS. TWO OF THE SISTERS CONCEIVED AFTER OVULATIONS WHICH OCCURRED DESPITE CONTINUING OVULATION.

WIDER, J. A., MARSHALL, J. R. AND ROSS, G. T.* FAMILIAL GALACTORRHEA IN THREE SISTERS WITH OLIGO-OVULATIONS. J.A.M.A. 209* 669-671, 1969.

*23040 GALACTOSEMIA

CARDINAL FEATURES ARE HEPATOMEGALY, CATARACTS AND MENTAL RETARDATION. THE DEFECT CONCERNS GALACTOSE-1-PHOSPHATE URIDYL TRANSFERASE. BEUTLER, BALUDA, STURGEON AND DAY (1965) HAVE SUGGESTED THAT SOME PERSONS WITH INTERMEDIATE LEVELS OF THE ENZYME ARE NOT HETEROZYGOTES FOR THE USUAL GALACTOSEMIA BUT RATHER ARE HOMOZYGOTES FOR WHAT THEY TERM THE DUARTE VARIANT. HETEROZYGOTES FOR THIS VARIANT HAVE ABOUT 75 PERCENT NORMAL ACTIVITY. THIS NEW FORM WAS DISCOVERED IN THE COURSE OF A SCREENING PROGRAM. ANOTHER TYPE OF GALACTOSEMIA HAS BEEN CALLED THE NEGRO VARIANT. THE DIFFERENCE IN BEHAVIOR OF THE METABOLISM OF GALACTOSE IN THOSE PATIENTS MAY BE DUE TO THE DEVELOPMENT OF AN ALTERNATIVE PATHWAY (CUATRECASAS AND SEGAL, 1966). OTHER RELEVANT OBSERVATIONS ON THE NEGRO VARIANT WERE REPORTED BY BAKER ET AL. (1967), MELLMAN ET AL. (1965), AND HSIA (1967). MELLMAN ET AL. (1965) SHOWED THAT THE HETEROZYGOUS PARENTS OF THE NEGRO VARIANT SHOW NEARLY NORMAL ENZYME LEVELS IN WHITE CELLS WHEREAS CLASSICALLY GALACTOSEMIC HETEROZYGOTES HAVE ABOUT 50 PERCENT ACTIVITY IN BOTH RED CELLS AND WHITE CELLS. HETEROGENEITY WAS DEMONSTRATED BY THE STUDIES OF SEGAL AND CUATRECASAS (1968). IN MASSACHUSETTS

R
E
C
E
S
S
I
V
E

SHIH ET AL. (1971), ON THE BASIS OF A SCREENING OF NEWBORNS, FOUND ONLY TWO CASES OF GALACTOSEMIA AMONG 374,341 BIRTHS. BOTH INFANTS DIED WITH ESCHERICHIA COLI SEPSIS IN THE NEONATAL PERIOD.

BAKER, L., MELLMAN, W. J., TEDESCO, T. A. AND SEGAL, S.* GALACTOSEMIA* SYMPTOMATIC AND ASYMPTOMATIC HOMOZYGOTES IN ONE NEGRO SIBSHIP. J. PEDIAT. 68* 551-558, 1967.

BEUTLER, E., BALUDA, M. C., STURGEON, P. AND DAY, R.* A NEW GENETIC ABNORMALITY RESULTING IN GALACTOSE-1-PHOSPHATE URIDYLTRANSFERASE DEFICIENCY. LANCET 1* 353-354, 1965.

CUATRECASAS, P. AND SEGAL, S.* GALACTOSE CONVERSION TO D-XYLULOSE* AN ALTERNATE ROUTE OF GALACTOSE METABOLISM. SCIENCE 153* 549-550, 1966.

DAWSON, S. P., HICKMAN, R. O. AND KELLEY, V. C.* GALACTOSEMIA. A GENETIC STUDY OF FOUR GENERATIONS BY ENZYME ASSAY. AM. J. DIS. CHILD. 100* 69-73, 1960.

GITZELMANN, R., POLEY, J. R. AND PRADER, A.* PARTIAL GALACTOSE-1-PHOSPHATE URIDYLTRANSFERASE DEFICIENCY DUE TO A VARIANT ENZYME. HELV. PAEDIAT. ACTA 22* 252-257, 1967.

HSIA, D. Y.-Y.* GALACTOSEMIA. (CONFERENCE, 1967). SPRINGFIELD, ILL* CHARLES C THOMAS, 1969.

HSIA, D. Y.-Y.* CLINICAL VARIANTS OF GALACTOSEMIA. METABOLISM 16* 419-437, 1967.

ISSELBACHER, K.* GALACTOSEMIA. IN, STANBURY, J. B., WYNGAARDEN, J. B. AND FREDRICKSON, D. S. (EDS.)* THE METABOLIC BASIS OF INHERITED DISEASE. NEW YORK* MCGRAW-HILL, 1966 (2ND ED.). PP. 178-188.

MELLMAN, W. J., TEDESCO, T. A. AND BAKER, L.* A NEW GENETIC ABNORMALITY. (LETTER) LANCET 1* 1395-1396, 1965.

NADLER, H. L., CHACKO, C. M. AND RACHMELER, M.* INTERALLELIC COMPLEMENTATION IN HYBRID CELLS DERIVED FROM HUMAN DIPLOID STRAINS DEFICIENT IN GALACTOSE-1-PHOSPHATE URIDYL TRANSFERASE ACTIVITY. PROC. NAT. ACAD. SCI. 67* 976-982, 1970.

SEGAL, S. AND CUATRECASAS, P.* THE OXIDATION OF C(14) GALACTOSE BY PATIENTS WITH CONGENITAL GALACTOSEMIA. EVIDENCE FOR A DIRECT OXIDATIVE PATHWAY. AM. J. MED. 44* 340-347, 1968.

SHIH, V. E., LEVY, H. L., KAROLKEWICZ, V., HOUGHTON, S., EFRON, M. L., ISSELBACHER, K. J., BEUTLER, E. AND MACCREADY, R. A.* GALACTOSEMIA SCREENING OF NEWBORNS IN MASSACHUSETTS. NEW ENG. J. MED. 284* 753-757, 1971.

WALKER, F. A., HSIA, D. Y.-Y., SLATIS, H. M. AND STEINBERG, A. G.* GALACTOSE-MIA* A STUDY OF TWENTY-SEVEN KINDREDS IN NORTH AMERICA. ANN. HUM. GENET. 25* 287-311, 1962.

R
E
C
E
S
S
I
V
E

*23050 GANGLIOSIDOSIS, GENERALIZED GM(1), TYPE I

LANDING (1964) FIRST DESCRIBED THIS ENTITY WHICH HAS BEEN VARIOUSLY CALLED *HURLER VARIANT,* *PSEUDO-HURLER DISEASE,* AND *TAY-SACHS DISEASE WITH VISCERAL INVOLVE-MENT.* O'BRIEN ET AL. (1965) SUGGESTED THE DESIGNATION *GENERALIZED GANGLIOSIDO-SIS.* THE FEATURES ARE (1) SEVERE CEREBRAL DEGENERATION LEADING TO DEATH WITHIN THE FIRST TWO YEARS OF LIFE, (2) ACCUMULATION OF GANGLIOSIDE IN NEURONS, AND IN HEPATIC, SPLENIC AND OTHER HISTIOCYTES, AND IN RENAL GLOMERULAR EPITHELIUM, AND (3) THE PRESENCE OF SKELETAL DEFORMITIES RESEMBLING HURLER'S DISEASE. THE GANGLIOSIDE STORED IS DIFFERENT FROM THAT IN TAY-SACHS DISEASE. IT WAS IDENTIFIED AS A GM(1) GANGLIOSIDE BY O'BRIEN ET AL. (1965). SCOTT ET AL. (1967) DESCRIBED AFFECTED SIBS. RENAL BIOPSY SHOWED STORAGE OF AN ACID MUCOPOLYSACCHARIDE RATHER THAN A GLYCOLIPID IN VACUOLES OF THE GLOMERULAR EPITHELIUM. THE VACUOLES WERE THOUGHT TO REPRESENT LYSOSOMES. THEY SUGGESTED THAT NEURO-VISCERAL LIPIDOSIS OR GENERALIZED GANGLIOSIDOSIS, AS IT HAS BEEN CALLED, MAY BE CLOSELY RELATED TO THE HURLER SYNDROME WHICH IT RESEMBLES CLINICALLY AND RADIOLOGICALLY. OKADA AND O'BRIEN (1968) DEMONSTRATED THAT BETA-GALACTOSIDASE DEFICIENCY IS THE FUNDAMENTAL FAULT IN GENERALIZED GANGLIOSIDOSIS. THE SAME ENZYME CLEAVES THE TERMINAL GALACTOSE FROM THE OLIGOSACCHARIDE MOIETY OF GM(1) AND BREAKS DOWN MUCOPOLYSAC-CHARIDE. GROSSMAN AND DANES (1968) DEMONSTRATED X-RAY FEATURES RESEMBLING THOSE OF HURLER SYNDROME, INCREASED SYNTHESIS AND STORAGE OF MUCOPOLYSACCHARIDES BY SKIN FIBROBLASTS, AND MARKED METACHROMASIA OF FIBROBLASTS IN BOTH PARENTS SUPPORTING AUTOSOMAL RECESSIVE INHERITANCE. CAFFEY (1951) PROBABLY DESCRIBED THE FIRST CASES, INTERPRETING THEM AS GARGOYLISM WITH PRENATAL ONSET. O'BRIEN (1969) FOUND THAT ALL THREE ISOENZYMES OF ACID BETA-GALACTOSIDASE, A, B AND C, WERE GROSSLY DEFICIENT IN ALL TISSUES.

CAFFEY, J.* GARGOYLISM (HUNTER-HURLER DISEASE, DYSOSTOSIS MULTIPLEX, LIPOCHON-DRODYSTROPHY)* PRENATAL AND NEONATAL BONE LESIONS AND THEIR EARLY POSTNATAL EVOLUTION. BULL. HOSP. JOINT DIS. 12* 38-66, 1951.

EMERY, J. M., GREEN, W. R., WYLLIE, R. G. AND HOWELL, R. R.* G(M1)-GANGLIOSIDO-SIS. ARCH. OPHTHAL. 85* 177-187, 1971.

GROSSMAN, H. AND DANES, B. S.* NEUROVISCERAL STORAGE DISEASE* FEATURES AND MODE OF INHERITANCE. AM. J. ROENTGEN. 103* 149-153, 1968.

LANDING, B. H., SILVERMAN, F. N., CRAIG, J. M., JACOBY, M. D., LAHEY, M. E. AND CHADWICK, D. L.* FAMILIAL NEUROVISCERAL LIPIDOSIS. AN ANALYSIS OF EIGHT CASES OF A SYNDROME PREVIOUSLY REPORTED AS 'HURLER-VARIANT,' 'PSEUDO-HURLER DISEASE' AND 'TAY-SACHS DISEASE WITH VISCERAL INVOLVEMENT.' AM. J. DIS. CHILD. 108* 503-522, 1964.

MACBRINN, M. C., OKADA, S., HO, M. W., HU, C. C. AND O'BRIEN, J. S.* GENERA-LIZED GANGLIOSIDOSIS* IMPAIRED CLEAVAGE OF GALACTOSE FROM A MUCOPOLYSACCHARIDE AND A GLYCOPROTEIN. SCIENCE 163* 946-947, 1969.

O'BRIEN, J.* GENERALIZED GANGLIOSIDOSIS. J. PEDIAT. 75* 167-186, 1969.

O'BRIEN, J. S., STERN, M. B., LANDING, B. H., O'BRIEN, J. K. AND DONNELL, G. N.* GENERALIZED GANGLIOSIDOSIS* ANOTHER INBORN ERROR OF GANGLIOSIDE METABOLISM.Q AM. J. DIS. CHILD. 109* 338-346, 1965.

OKADA, S. AND O'BRIEN, J. S.* GENERALIZED GANGLIOSIDOSIS* BETA-GALACTOSIDASE DEFICIENCY. SCIENCE 160* 1002-1004, 1968.

SCOTT, C. R., LAGUNOFF, D. AND TRUMP, B. F.* FAMILIAL NEURO-VISCERAL LIPIDOSIS. J. PEDIAT. 71* 357-366, 1967.

THOMAS, G. H.* BETA-D-GALACTOSIDASE IN HUMAN URINE* DEFICIENCY IN GENERALIZED GANGLIOSIDOSIS. J. LAB. CLIN. MED. 74* 725-731, 1969.

*23060 GANGLIOSIDOSIS, GENERALIZED GM(1), TYPE II, OR JUVENILE TYPE

THIS DISORDER DIFFERS CLINICALLY AND CHEMICALLY FROM TYPE I. ONLY B AND C ISOENZYMES OF BETA-GALACTOSIDASE ARE DEFICIENT (O'BRIEN, 1969). GM(1) GANGLIO-SIDES ACCUMULATE IN THE BRAIN BUT NOT IN THE VISCERA. INSTEAD THE VISCERA SHOW EXCESSIVE AMOUNTS OF UNDERSULFATED KERATANSULFATE-LIKE MUCOPOLYSACCHARIDE (SUZUKI ET AL., 1969* FIRST PATIENT). THE PATIENTS OF KINT ET AL. (1969) AND WOLFE ET AL. (1970) APPARENTLY HAD TYPE II GM(1)-GANGLIOSIDOSIS. CLINICALLY THE DISORDER DEVELOPS LATER THAN TYPE I GANGLIOSIDOSIS. WHEREAS TYPE I IS USUALLY EVIDENT AT BIRTH AND THE AFFECTED INFANT RARELY SURVIVES BEYOND THE AGE OF TWO YEARS, CLINICAL SYMPTOMS DO NOT DEVELOP IN TYPE II UNTIL THE SECOND YEAR OF LIFE AND SURVIVAL TO 10 YEARS HAS BEEN OBSERVED. THE INITIAL DESCRIPTION WAS MADE BY DERRY ET AL. (1968) IN TWO SIBS OF FRENCH-CANADIAN ANCESTRY.

DERRY, D. M., FAWCETT, J. S., ANDERMANN, F. AND WOLFE, L. S.* LATE INFANTILE SYSTEMIC LIPIDOSIS (MAJOR MONOSIALOGANGLIOSIDOSIS DELINEATION OF TWO TYPES). NEUROLOGY 18* 340-347, 1968.

KINT, J. A., DACREMONT, G. AND VLIETINCK, R.* TYPE II GM(1) GANGLIOSIDOSIS.Q LANCET 2* 108-109, 1969.

O'BRIEN, J. S.* FIVE GANGLIOSIDOSIS. (LETTER) LANCET 2* 805 ONLY, 1969.

SUZUKI, K., SUZUKI, K. AND KAMOSHITA, S.* CHEMICAL PATHOLOGY OF GM(1)-GANGLIO-SIDOSIS (GENERALIZED GANGLIOSIDOSIS). J. NEUROPATH. EXP. NEUROL. 28* 25-73, 1969.

WOLFE, L. S., CALLAHAN, J., FAWCETT, J. S., ANDERMANN, F. AND SCRIVER, C. R.* GM(1)-GANGLIOSIDOSIS WITHOUT CHONDRODYSTROPHY OR VISCEROMEGALY. NEUROLOGY 20* 23-43, 1970.

*23070 GANGLIOSIDOSIS, GM(2), TYPE III, OR JUVENILE TYPE

SIX PATIENTS IN FOUR FAMILIES HAVE BEEN OBSERVED (SUZUKI ET AL., 1970* O'BRIEN, 1971). ALL HAVE BEEN OF NON-JEWISH ORIGIN, AS IN THE CASE OF SANDHOFF'S DISEASE (TYPE II GM(2)-GANGLIOSIDOSIS). ONSET OCCURS WITH ATAXIA BETWEEN AGES 2 AND 6 YEARS. THEREAFTER DETERIORATION TO DECEREBRATE RIGIDITY TAKES PLACE. BLINDNESS OCCURRED LATE IN THE COURSE IN ONLY SOME PATIENTS, UNLIKE THE SITUATION IN TAY-SACHS' AND SANDHOFF'S DISEASES IN WHICH BLINDNESS IS AN INVARIABLE AND EARLY DEVELOPMENT. DEATH USUALLY OCCURS BETWEEN AGES 5 AND 15 YEARS. THE DISORDER IS PROBABLY OFTEN MISDIAGNOSED BATTEN-SPIELMEYER-VOGT DISEASE. THE DEFECT IN THIS DISORDER IS A PARTIAL DEFICIENCY OF HEXOSAMINIDASE A, THE COMPONENT DEFICIENT IN TAY-SACHS DISEASE.

O'BRIEN, J. S.* GANGLIOSIDE STORAGE DISEASES. IN, HARRIS, H. (ED.)* ADVANCES IN HUMAN GENETICS, 1971.

SUZUKI, K., SUZUKI, K., RAPIN, I., SUZUKI, Y. AND ISHII, N.* JUVENILE GM(2)-GANGLIOSIDOSIS. CLINICAL VARIANT OF TAY-SACHS DISEASE OR A NEW DISEASE. NEUROLOGY 20* 190-204, 1970.

SUZUKI, Y. AND SUZUKI, K.* PARTIAL DEFICIENCY OF HEXOSAMINIDASE COMPONENT A IN

R
E
C
E
S
S
I
V
E

*23080 GAUCHER'S DISEASE TYPE I (NON-CEREBRAL, JUVENILE)

THE SEVERAL FORMS OF GAUCHER'S DISEASE ARE CEREBROSIDE LIPIDOSES. THE DISEASE HAS
BEEN DIAGNOSED AS EARLY AS THE FIRST WEEK OF LIFE AND AS LATE AS 86 YEARS. THE
CLASSIFICATION FOLLOWED HERE IS THAT OF KNUDSON AND KAPLAN (1962). AN INSTRUCTIVE
PEDIGREE WAS REPORTED BY HERRLIN AND HILLBORG (1962). SERUM ACID PHOSPHATASE
(WHICH UNLIKE THE PROSTATIC ENZYME IS NOT INHIBITED BY L-TARTRATE) IS ELEVATED.
WIEDEMANN AND COLLEAGUES (1965) FOUND TYPICAL GAUCHER CELLS IN THE BONE MARROW OF
TWO CLINICALLY NORMAL PARENTS AND A NORMAL SISTER OF TWO AFFECTED CHILDREN AND IN
THE TWO CLINICALLY NORMAL PARENTS AND TWO NORMAL SISTERS OF AN AFFECTED YOUNG MAN.
BRADY ET AL. (1965) DEMONSTRATED A DEFICIENCY OF GLUCOCERBROSIDE-SPLITTING ENZYME
IN THE SPLEEN OF GAUCHER'S DISEASE. THIS ENZYME, NORMALLY PRESENT IN LARGE
AMOUNTS IN THE SPLEEN, IS THOUGHT TO BE INVOLVED IN THE BREAK-DOWN OF GLOBOSIDE,
AN IMPORTANT LIPOID CONSTITUENT OF RED CELLS. DANES AND BEARN (1968) FOUND GIANT
FIBROBLASTS CONTAINING METACHROMATIC MATERIAL IN BOTH AFFECTED PERSONS AND
HETEROZYGOTES FOR THE CHRONIC NONCEREBRAL FORM.

    BRADY, R. O.* THE SPHINGOLIPIDOSES. NEW ENG. J. MED. 275* 312-318, 1966.

    BRADY, R. O., KANFER, J. N. AND SHAPIRO, D.* METABOLISM OF GLUCOCEREBROSIDES.
II. EVIDENCE OF AN ENZYMATIC DEFICIENCY IN GAUCHER'S DISEASE. BIOCHEM. BIOPHYS.
RES. COMMUN. 18* 221-225, 1965.

    CROCKER, A. C. AND LANDING, B. H.* PHOSPHATASE STUDIES IN GAUCHER'S DISEASE.
METABOLISM 9* 341-362, 1960.

    DANES, B. S. AND BEARN, A. G.* GAUCHER'S DISEASE* A GENETIC DISEASE DETECTED IN
SKIN FIBROBLAST CULTURES. SCIENCE 161* 1347-1348, 1968.

    DAVIES, G. T. AND FOREMAN, H. M.* HAEMORRHAGIC PERICARDIAL EFFUSION IN ADULT
GAUCHER'S DISEASE. BRIT. HEART J. 32* 855-858, 1970.

    FREDRICKSON, D. S.* CEREBROSIDE LIPIDOSIS* GAUCHER'S DISEASE. IN, STANBURY, J.
B., WYNGAARDEN, J. B. AND FREDRICKSON, D. S. (EDS.)* THE METABOLIC BASIS OF
INHERITED DISEASE. NEW YORK* MCGRAW-HILL, 1966 (2ND ED.). PP. 565-585.

    HERRLIN, K.-M. AND HILLBORG, P. O.* NEUROLOGICAL SIGNS IN A JUVENILE FORM OF
GAUCHER'S DISEASE. ACTA PAEDIAT. 51* 137-154, 1962.

    HSIA, D. Y.-Y., NAYLOR, J. AND BIGLER, J. A.* GAUCHER'S DISEASE* REPORT OF TWO
CASES IN FATHER AND SON AND REVIEW OF THE LITERATURE. NEW ENG. J. MED. 261* 164-
169, 1959.

    KAMPINE, J. P., BRADY, R. O. AND KANFER, J. N.* DIAGNOSIS OF GAUCHER'S DISEASE
AND NIEMANN-PICK DISEASE WITH SMALL SAMPLES OF VENOUS BLOOD. SCIENCE 155* 86-88,
1967.

    KNUDSON, A. G., JR. AND KAPLAN, W. D.* GENETICS OF THE SPHINGOLIPIDOSES. IN,
AARONSON, S. M. AND VOLK, B. W. (EDS.)* CEREBRAL SPHINGOLIPIDOSES. A SYMPOSIUM ON
TAY-SACHS DISEASE. NEW YORK* ACADEMIC PRESS. PP. 395-411, 1962.

    WIEDEMANN, H.-R., GERKEN, H., GRAUCOB, E. AND HANSEN, H.-G.* RECOGNITION OF
HETEROZYGOSITY IN SPHINGOLIPIDOSES. (LETTER) LANCET 1* 1283 ONLY, 1965.

*23090 GAUCHER'S DISEASE TYPE II (INFANTILE, CEREBRAL)

THIS FORM DOES NOT SHOW A PREPONDERANT JEWISH INCIDENCE. WE HAVE OBSERVED NEGRO
CASES. DRUKKER ET AL. (1970) DESCRIBED A CASE IN A SEPHARDIC JEWISH INFANT. THE
DISORDER LED TO DEATH AT THE AGE 48 HOURS FROM INTRACRANIAL HEMORRHAGE. DEATH
USUALLY OCCURS BEFORE THE AGE OF ONE YEAR. ENLARGEMENT OF THE ABDOMIN FROM
HEPATOSPLENOMEGALY AND NEUROLOGIC SIGNS SUCH AS RETROFLEXION OF THE HEAD,
STRABISMUS, DYSPHAGIA, CHOKING SPELLS AND HYPERTONICITY ARE FEATURES.

    DRUKKER, A., SACKS, M. I. AND GATT, S.* THE INFANTILE FORM OF GAUCHER'S DISEASE
IN AN INFANT OF JEWISH SEPHARDIC ORIGIN. PEDIATRICS 45* 1017-1023, 1970.

*23100 GAUCHER'S DISEASE TYPE III (JUVENILE AND ADULT, CEREBRAL)

HEMATOLOGIC ABNORMALITIES WITH HYPERSPLENISM, BONE LESIONS, SKIN PIGMENTATION AND
PINGUECULAE OCCUR IN THIS FORM. THIS TYPE IS PARTICULARLY FREQUENT IN JEWS. FOR
REFERENCES, SEE GAUCHER'S DISEASE, TYPE I. PARTIAL MANIFESTATION IN HETEROZYGOTES
HAS LED SOME TO PROPOSE DOMINANT INHERITANCE. DESNICK ET AL. (1971) DEMONSTRATED
THAT BOTH HOMOZYGOTES AND HETEROZYGOTES CAN BE IDENTIFIED BY CHEMICAL ANALYSIS OF
THE SEDIMENT FROM A 24-HOUR URINE COLLECTION. INDIVIDUAL NEUTRAL GLYCOSPHINGOLI-
PIDS WERE SEPARATED BY THIN-LAYER CHROMATOGRAPHY AND QUANTITATIVELY ESTIMATED BY
GAS-LIQUID CHROMATOGRAPHY. OTHER GLYCOSPHINGOLIPIDOSES WHICH COULD BE DIAGNOSED
BY THIS METHOD INCLUDED KRABBE'S LEUKODYSTROPHY, LACTOSYLCERAMIDOSIS, FABRY'S
DISEASE, SANDHOFF'S DISEASE AND METACHROMATIC LEUKODYSTROPHY. BEUTLER ET AL.
(1971) DEMONSTRATED DEFICIENCY OF BETA-GLUCOSIDASE ACTIVITY IN FIBROBLASTS FROM
HOMOZYGOTES WITH THE ADULT FORM OF GAUCHER'S DISEASE AND FOUND AN INTERMEDIATE

R
E
C
E
S
S
I
V
E

BEUTLER, E. AND KUHL, W.* THE DIAGNOSIS OF THE ADULT TYPE OF GAUCHER'S DISEASE AND ITS CARRIER STATE BY DEMONSTRATION OF DEFICIENCY OF BETA-GLUCOSIDASE ACTIVITY IN PERIPHERAL BLOOD LEUKOCYTES. J. LAB. CLIN. MED. 76* 747-755, 1970.

BEUTLER, E., KUHL, W., TRINIDAD, F., TEPLITZ, R. AND NADLER, H.* BETA-GLUCOSI-DASE ACTIVITY IN FIBROBLASTS FROM HOMOZYGOTES AND HETEROZYGOTES FOR GAUCHER'S DISEASE. AM. J. HUM. GENET. 23* 62-66, 1971.

DESNICK, R. J., DAWSON, G., DESNICK, S. J., SWEELEY, C. C. AND KRIVIT, W.* DIAGNOSIS OF GLYCOSPHINGOLIPIDOSES BY URINARY-SEDIMENT ANALYSIS. NEW ENG. J. MED. 284* 739-744, 1971.

*23110 GIANT CELL HEPATITIS, NEONATAL

INCREASED PARENTAL CONSANGUINITY SUGGESTED AUTOSOMAL RECESSIVE INHERITANCE. HOWEVER, ONLY 12 OF 71 SIBS OF INDEX CASES WERE ALSO AFFECTED. IT WAS SUGGESTED THAT IN SOME WITH THE APPROPRIATE GENOTYPE THE DISEASE IS MANIFESTED SO SEVERELY OR SO MILDLY THAT THE DIAGNOSIS IS NOT MADE. AN APPARENT EXCESS OF AFFECTED MALES MAY BE FURTHER EVIDENCE OF FAILURE OF MANIFESTATION OF THE GENOTYPE. ALTERNATIVE-LY THE CASES ANALYZED MAY INCLUDE MORE THAN ONE DISEASE.

CASSADY, G., MORRISON, A. B. AND COHEN, M. M.* FAMILIAL 'GIANT-CELL HEPATITIS' IN INFANCY. CLINICAL, PATHOLOGIC, AND GENETIC STUDIES ON A LARGE FAMILY. AM. J. DIS. CHILD. 107* 456-469, 1964.

DANKS, D. AND BODIAN, M.* A GENETIC STUDY OF NEONATAL OBSTRUCTIVE JAUNDICE. ARCH. DIS. CHILD. 38* 378-390, 1960.

23120 GLAUCOMA WITH ELEVATED EPISCLERAL VENOUS PRESSURES

IN MOTHER AND DAUGHTER AND PROBABLY IN THE MOTHER'S FATHER, MINAS AND PODOS (1968) OBSERVED OPEN ANGLE GLAUCOMA WITH ELEVATED EPISCLERAL VENOUS PRESSURE, MANIFEST BY DILATED EPISCLERAL VEINS.

MINAS, T. F. AND PODOS, S. M.* FAMILIAL GLAUCOMA ASSOCIATED WITH ELEVATED EPISCLERAL VENOUS PRESSURE. ARCH. OPHTHAL. 80* 202-208, 1968.

*23130 GLAUCOMA, CONGENITAL (BUPHTHALMOS)

THE OCULAR GLOBE IS USUALLY LARGE AS A RESULT OF THE INCREASED INTRA-OCULAR PRESSURE DATING FROM INTRAUTERINE LIFE, HENCE THE TERM BUPHTHALMOS, MEANING 'OX EYE.' IN ONLY ABOUT HALF OF CASES ARE BOTH EYES INVOLVED AND MALES ARE AFFECTED SOMEWHAT MORE OFTEN THAN FEMALES. THE CANAL OF SCHLEMM IS PRESENT AND COMMUNI-CATES NORMALLY WITH THE VEINS AS IS PROVED BY DEMONSTRABLE FILLING OF THE CANAL WITH BLOOD WHEN THE JUGULAR VEINS ARE COMPRESSED. THE DEFECT IS THOUGHT TO INVOLVE THE PERMEABILITY OF THE TRABECULUM TO AQUEOUS HUMOR. AUTOSOMAL RECESSIVE INHERITANCE IS QUITE CERTAIN IN A SIGNIFICANT PROPORTION OF CASES. THE SYNDROME OF CONGENITAL GLAUCOMA WITH MENTAL RETARDATION AND DECREASED RENAL AMMONIUM PRODUCTION (LOWE'S SYNDROME) IS INHERITED AS AN X-LINKED RECESSIVE. AUTOSOMAL RECESSIVE GLAUCOMA OCCURS IN THE RABBIT (HANNA ET AL., 1962).

BARKAN, O. AND FERGUSON, W. J., JR.* CONGENITAL GLAUCOMA. PEDIAT. CLIN. N. AM. 5* 225-229, 1958.

GRAHAM, M. V. AND CRICK, R. P.* BILATERAL CONGENITAL BUPHTHALMOS IN TWO SISTERS. BRIT. J. OPHTHAL. 42* 370-371, 1958.

HANNA, B. L., SAWIN, P. B. AND SHEPPARD, L. B.* RECESSIVE BUPHTHALMOS IN THE RABBIT. GENETICS 47* 519-529, 1962.

WESTERLUND, E.* CLINICAL AND GENETIC STUDIES ON THE PRIMARY GLAUCOMA DISEASES. OP. EX. DOMO BIOL. HERED. HUM. U. HAFNIENSIS 12* 11-207, 1947.

23140 GLAUCOMA, CONGENITAL, WITH MENTAL RETARDATION

WE HAVE OBSERVED THREE SIBS (2 MALES, 1 FEMALE) WITH CONGENITAL GLAUCOMA AND SEVERE MENTAL RETARDATION (214487, 261714). ONE OF THE MALES, THE OLDEST OF THE 3 AFFECTED SIBS, DIED AT AGE 32 OF CORONARY OCCLUSION.

*23150 GLAUCOMA, JUVENILE

THERE IS SOME QUESTION WHAT SHOULD BE CLASSIFIED AS JUVENILE GLAUCOMA. MOST CASES MAY BE EITHER CONGENITAL GLAUCOMA WITH LATE ONSET OR OPEN-ANGLE OR CLOSED-ANGLE GLAUCOMA WITH EARLY ONSET. WAARDENBURG (1950) SUGGESTED THAT RECESSIVE INHERI-TANCE OF SOME CASES OF GLAUCOMA IS PROVED BY (1) A HIGH FREQUENCY OF PARENTAL CONSANGUINITY, (2) THE PRESENCE OF THE DISEASE IN ABOUT 25 PERCENT OF SIBS OF PROBANDS, (3) THE PRESENCE OF THE DISEASE IN ALL CHILDREN OF A MARRIAGE BETWEEN TWO AFFECTED PERSONS, AND (4) THE OCCURRENCE OF GLAUCOMA IN COLLATERALS OF BOTH PARENTS IN SOME FAMILIES. BEIGUELMAN AND PRADO (1963) REPORTED A BRAZILIAN PEDIGREE AS CONVINCING EVIDENCE FOR RECESSIVE INHERITANCE OF JUVENILE GLAUCOMA.

R
E
C
E
S
S
I
V
E

BEIGUELMAN, B. AND PRADO, D.* RECESSIVE JUVENILE GLAUCOMA. J. GENET. HUM. 12* 53-54, 1963.

WAARDENBURG, P. J.* UBER DAS FAMILIARE VORKOMMEN UND DEN ERBGANG DES PRAESENI-LEN UND SENILEN GLAUKOMS. GENETICA 25* 79-125, 1950.

*23160 GLUCOSE-GALACTOSE MALABSORPTION

A PICTURE CLINICALLY INDISTINGUISHABLE FROM INTESTINAL DISACCHARIDASE DEFICIENCY IS PRODUCED BY INTESTINAL MONOSACCHARIDASE DEFICIENCY. BECAUSE OF THE DEFICIENCY GLUCOSE AND GALACTOSE ARE NOT ABSORBED. FRUCTOSE AND XYLOSE ARE NORMALLY ABSORBED. THIS DISORDER IS A TRANSPORT DEFECT. IN VITRO THE INTESTINAL MUCOSA IS INCAPABLE OF TAKING UP GLUCOSE EVEN TO THE CONCENTRATION OF THE MEDIUM. OCCUR-RENCE IN BOTH SEXES, FAMILIAL INCIDENCE, AND AT LEAST THREE INSTANCES OF PARENTAL CONSANGUINITY ARE CONSISTENT WITH AUTOSOMAL RECESSIVE INHERITANCE.

ANDERSON, C. M., KERRY, K. R. AND TOWNLEY, R. R. W.* AN INBORN DEFECT OF INTESTINAL ABSORPTION OF CERTAIN MONOSACCHARIDES. ARCH. DIS. CHILD. 40* 1-6, 1965.

ELSAS, L. J., HILLMAN, R. E., PATTERSON, J. H. AND ROSENBERG, L. E.* RENAL AND INTESTINAL HEXOSE TRANSPORT IN FAMILIAL GLUCOSE-GALACTOSE MALABSORPTION. J. CLIN. INVEST. 49* 576-585, 1970.

LINDQUIST, B., MEEUWISSE, G. AND MELIN, K.* OSMOTIC DIARRHOEA IN GENETICALLY TRANSMITTED GLUCOSE-GALACTOSE MALABSORPTION. ACTA PEDIAT. 52* 217-219, 1963.

MEEUWISSE, G. W.* GLUCOSE-GALACTOSE MALABSORPTION. STUDIES ON THE INTERMEDIATE CARBOHYDRATE METABOLISM. HELVET. PAEDIAT. ACTA 25* 13-24, 1970.

MEEUWISSE, G. W. AND DAHLQVIST, A.* GLUCOSE-GALACTOSE MALABSORPTION. A STUDY WITH BIOPSY OF THE SMALL INTESTINAL MUCOSA. ACTA PAEDIAT. SCAND. 57* 273-280, 1968.

SCHNEIDER, A. J., KINTNER, W. B. AND STIRLING, C. E.* GLUCOSE-GALACTOSE MALABSORPTION. REPORT OF A CASE WITH AUTORADIOGRAPHIC STUDIES OF A MUCOSAL BIOPSY. NEW ENG. J. MED. 274* 305-312, 1966.

*23170 GLUTATHIONE PEROXIDASE DEFICIENCY, HEMOLYTIC ANEMIA DUE TO

NECHELES ET AL. (1968) OBSERVED HEMOLYTIC DISEASE OF THE NEWBORN WITH HYPERBILIRU-BINEMIA AND HEINZ BODIES, ASSOCIATED WITH PARTIAL DEFICIENCY OF RED CELL GLUTA-THIONE PEROXIDASE. THE CLINICAL MANIFESTATIONS WERE SELF-LIMITED AND EVIDENCE OF HEMOLYSIS HAD DISAPPEARED BY 3 MONTHS OF AGE, ALTHOUGH THE ENZYME DEFICIENCY PERSISTED. SIBS WERE AFFECTED IN SOME INSTANCES AND ONE PARENT HAD COMPARABLY DEPRESSED ENZYME LEVEL AND A HISTORY OF NEONATAL JAUNDICE. NECHELES ET AL. (1969) FOUND LOW LEVELS OF GLUTATHIONE PEROXIDASE IN AN 18 YEAR OLD PUERTO RICAN MALE WITH COMPENSATED HEMOLYTIC ANEMIA. BOTH PARENTS AND ONE SIB HAD INTERMEDIATE ENZYME LEVELS.

BOIVIN, P., GALAND, C. AND HAKIM, J.* ANEMIE HEMOLYTIQUE AVEC DEFICIT EN GLUTATHION-PEROXYDASE CHEZ UN ADULTE. ENZYMOL. BIOL. CLIN. 10* 68-80, 1969.

NECHELES, T. F., BOLES, T. A. AND ALLEN, D. M.* ERYTHROCYTE GLUTATHIONE-PEROXIDASE DEFICIENCY AND HEMOLYTIC DISEASE OF THE NEWBORN INFANT. J. PEDIAT. 72* 319-324, 1968.

NECHELES, T. F., MALDONADO, N., BARQUET-CHEDIAK, A. AND ALLEN, D. M.* HOMOZY-GOUS ERYTHROCYTE GLUTATHIONE-PEROXIDASE DEFICIENCY* CLINICAL AND BIOCHEMICAL STUDIES. BLOOD 33* 164-169, 1969.

NECHELES, T. F., STEINBERG, M. H. AND CAMERON, D.* ERYTHROCYTE GLUTATHIONE-PEROXIDASE DEFICIENCY. BRIT. J. HAEMAT. 19* 605-612, 1970.

STEINBERG, M., BRAUER, M. J. AND NECHELES, T. F.* ACUTE HEMOLYTIC ANEMIA ASSOCIATED WITH ERYTHROCYTE GLUTATHIONE-PEROXIDASE DEFICIENCY. ARCH. INTERN. MED. 125* 302-303, 1970.

*23180 GLUTATHIONE REDUCTASE, HEMOLYTIC ANEMIA DUE TO DEFICIENCY OF, IN RED CELLS

LOHR AND WALLER (1962) OBSERVED A *NEW* FORM OF ENZYME-DEFICIENCY HEMOLYTIC ANEMIA. GLUTATHIONE REDUCTASE WAS DEFICIENT. REDUCED GLUTATHIONE (GSH) WAS LOW AS A CONSEQUENCE. (THIS CONDITION IS APPARENTLY DISTINCT FROM THAT DESCRIBED BY OORT ET AL. (1961) IN WHICH GSH WAS ALSO LOW, BUT GLUCOSE-6-PHOSPHATE DEHYDRO-GENASE AND GLUTATHIONE REDUCTASE WERE NORMAL.) LOHR (1963) HAS OBSERVED 10 HOMOZYGOTES AND 5 HETEROZYGOTES IN A FAMILY DISTRIBUTION CONSISTENT WITH AUTOSOMAL RECESSIVE INHERITANCE. BLUME ET AL. (1968) STUDIED A KINDRED WITH MANY PERSONS WHO WERE DEMONSTRABLY HETEROZYGOUS BY CHEMICAL TEST. ALTHOUGH ASYMPTOMATIC HETEROZYGOTES WERE IDENTIFIED BY THE LEVEL OF GLUTATHIONE REDUCTASE IN THE RED CELLS, ELECTROPHORESIS OF THE ENZYME AND HEINZ BODY TEST. THE ENZYME IS STRUC-TURALLY ABNORMAL. HAMPEL ET AL. (1969) FOUND A MARKEDLY INCREASED FREQUENCY OF CHROMOSOMAL ABERRATIONS IN A PATIENT WITH PANCYTOPENIA AND ABSENT GR-II BAND IN

THE ELECTROPHEROGRAM. THE MOTHER WAS HEMATOLOGICALLY NORMAL BUT HAD ABSENT GR-II BAND AND A MODERATE INCREASE IN THE FREQUENCY OF CHROMOSOMAL ABERRATIONS. ADDITION OF CHLORAMPHENICOL TO THE CULTURES INCREASED THE NUMBER OF DAMAGED CHROMOSOMES IN BOTH THE MOTHER AND THE SON.

BLUME, K. G., GOTTWIK, M., LOHR, G. W. AND RUDIGER, H. W.* FAMILIENUNTERSUCHUN-GEN ZUM GLUTATHIONREDUKTASEMANGEL MENSCHLICHER ERYTHROCYTEN. HUMANGENETIK 6* 163-170, 1968.

CARSON, P. E., BREWER, G. J. AND ICKES, C.* DECREASED GLUTATHIONE REDUCTASE WITH SUSCEPTIBILITY TO HEMOLYSIS. (ABSTRACT) J. LAB. CLIN. MED. 58* 804 ONLY, 1961.

HAMPEL, K. E., LOHR, G. W., BLUME, K. G. AND RUDIGER, H. W.* SPONTANE UND CHLORAMPHENICOLINDUZIERTE CHROMOSOMENMUTATIONEN UND BIOCHEMISCHE BEFUNDE BEI ZWEI FALLEN MIT GLUTATHIONREDUKTASEMANGEL (NAD(P)H* GLUTATHIONE OXIDOREDUCTASE, E.C.1.6.4.2). HUMANGENETIK 7* 305-313, 1969.

KURZ, R. AND HOHENWALLNER, W.* FAMILIARER GLUTATHIONREDUKTASEMANGEL UND STORUNG DER GLUTATHIONSYNTHESE IM ERYTHROZYTEN. HELV. PAEDIAT. ACTA 25* 542-552, 1970.

LOHR, G. W. AND WALLER, H. D.* EINE NEUE ENZYMOPENISCHE HAMOLYTISCHE ANAMIE MIT GLUTATHIONREDUKTASE-MANGEL. MED. KLIN. 57* 1521-1525, 1962.

LOHR, G. W. AND WALLER, H. D.* ZUR BIOCHEMIE EINIGER ANGEBORENER HAMOLYTISCHER ANAMIEN. FOLIA HAEMAT. 8* 377-397, 1963.

LOHR, G. W.* MARBURG, AUSTRALIA* PERSONAL COMMUNICATION, 1963.

OORT, M., LOOS, J. H. AND PRINS, H. K.* HEREDITARY ABSENCE OF REDUCED GLUTA-THIONE IN THE ERYTHROCYTES - A NEW CLINICAL AND BIOCHEMICAL ENTITY. VOX SANG. 6* 370-373, 1961.

*23190 GLUTATHIONE SYNTHETASE DEFICIENCY OF ERYTHROCYTES, HEMOLYTIC ANEMIA DUE TO

R
E
C
E
S
S
I
V
E

MOHLER ET AL. (1970) DESCRIBED A MAN OF SCOTTISH EXTRACTION WITH HEMOLYTIC ANEMIA DUE TO DEFICIENCY OF GLUTATHIONE SYNTHETASE. (TWO SEPARATE ENZYMES ARE INVOLVED IN GLUTATHIONE SYNTHESIS. THE COUPLING OF GLUTAMIC ACID AND CYSTEINE IS CATALYZED BY GLUTAMYL-CYSTEINE SYNTHETASE AND GLYCINE IS ADDED TO FORM THE TRIPEPTIDE THROUGH THE ENZYMATIC ACTION OF GLUTATHIONE SYNTHETASE.) FOUR CHILDREN OF THE PROBAND, ONE OF THREE OF HIS SIBS AND BOTH PARENTS HAD INTERMEDIATE LEVELS OF ENZYME. PRESUMABLY THE FAMILY OF OORT ET AL. (1961) AND OF PRINS ET AL. (1966) HAD THE SAME CONDITION AS DID ALSO THAT OF BOIVIN ET AL. (1966). IN THE FAMILY REPORTED BY PRINS AND COLLEAGUES (1963), THREE OUT OF 12 SIBS FROM CONSANGUINEOUS (SECOND COUSIN) PARENTS HAD ABSENCE OF GLUTATHIONE IN THE ERYTHROCYTES. THE CLINICAL PICTURE WAS THAT OF NONSPHEROCYTIC HEMOLYTIC ANEMIA. GLYOXYLASE ACTIVITY, WHICH IS DEPENDENT ON GLUTATHIONE AS A COFACTOR, WAS ALSO DEFICIENT. OTHER ENZYMES WERE INCREASED, PRESUMABLY DUE TO THE YOUNGER AVERAGE AGE OF ERYTHROCYTES. IN A LATER REPORT ON THE KINDRED 5 CASES IN 2 SIBSHIPS WITH ALL 4 PARENTS TRACED TO A COMMON ANCESTRAL COUPLE WERE DESCRIBED. GLUTATHIONE (GAMMA-GLUTAMYL-CYSTEINYL-GLYCINE) WAS LESS THAN 10 PERCENT OF NORMAL IN PRESUMED HOMOZYGOTES.

BOIVIN, P., GALAND, C., ANDRE, R. AND DEBRAY, J.* ANEMIES HEMOLYTIQUES CONGENITALES AVEC DEFICIT ISOLE EN GLUTATHION REDUIT PAR DEFICIT EN GLUTATHION SYNTHETASE. NOUV. REV. FRANC. HEMAT. 6* 859-865, 1966.

MOHLER, D. N., MAJERUS, P. W., MINNICH, V., HESS, C. E. AND GARRICK, M. D.* GLUTATHIONE SYNTHETASE DEFICIENCY AS A CAUSE OF HEREDITARY HEMOLYTIC DISEASE. NEW ENG. J. MED. 283* 1253-1257, 1970.

OORT, M., LOOS, J. A. AND PRINS, H. K.* HEREDITARY ABSENCE OF REDUCED GLUTA-THIONE IN THE ERYTHROCYTES - A NEW CLINICAL AND BIOCHEMICAL ENTITY. VOX SANG. 6* 370-373, 1961.

PRINS, H. K., OORT, M., LOOS, J. A., ZURCHER, C. AND BECKERS, T.* CONGENITAL NONSPHEROCYTIC HEMOLYTIC ANEMIA, ASSOCIATED WITH GLUTATHIONE DEFICIENCY OF THE ERYTHROCYTES. HEMATOLOGIC, BIOCHEMICAL AND GENETIC STUDIES. BLOOD 27* 145-166, 1966.

ZURCHER, C.* GLUTATHIONE DEFICIENCY. IN, BEUTLER, E. (ED.)* HEREDITARY DISORDERS OF ERYTHROCYTE METABOLISM. NEW YORK* GRUNE AND STRATTON, 1967.

23200 GLYCINEMIA (HYPERGLYCINEMIA WITH KETOACIDOSIS AND LEUKOPENIA) PROPIONICACIDE-MIA

THE FEATURES ARE EPISODIC VOMITING, LETHARGY AND KETOSIS, NEUTROPENIA, PERIODIC THROMBOCYTOPENIA, HYPOGAMMAGLOBULINEMIA, DEVELOPMENTAL RETARDATION AND INTOLERANCE TO PROTEIN. OUTSTANDING CHEMICAL FEATURES ARE HYPERGLYCINEMIA AND HYPERGLY-CINURIA. THIS DISORDER IS NOT TO BE CONFUSED WITH HEREDITARY GLYCINURIA WHICH HAS BEEN DESCRIBED ONLY IN ONE FAMILY (DE VRIES ET AL. 1957) AND IS PRESUMABLY TRANSMITTED AS A DOMINANT BECAUSE AFFECTED MEMBERS OCCURRED IN THREE SUCCESSIVE

GENERATIONS. (THE POSSIBILITY OF QUASI-DOMINANT PEDIGREE PATTERN SHOULD BE INVESTIGATED BY INQUIRY INTO THE POSSIBILITY OF CONSANGUINITY AND THE PRESENCE OF A PARTIAL DEFECT IN THE PRESUMABLY NORMAL SPOUSES.) THE DEFECT RESIDES IN THE RENAL TUBULE. TO AVOID CONFUSION AND TO PARALLEL THE USAGE WITH GALACTOSEMIA, I PREFER TO CALL THIS DISEASE GLYCINEMIA AND THE DISORDER IN THE BULGARIAN-JEWISH FAMILY GLYCINURIA, PARALLELING THE USAGE WITH CYSTINURIA. SORIANO ET AL. (1967) SUGGESTED THAT IN THE DISORDER FIRST DESCRIBED BY CHILDS ET AL. (1961) A GENERALIZED DEFECT IN UTILIZATION OF AMINO ACIDS RESULTS IN EXCESSIVE DEAMINATION OF CERTAIN AMINO ACIDS IN MUSCLE, WITH CONSEQUENT HYPERAMMONEMIA AND KETOACIDOSIS. IN A SECOND GROUP OF PATIENTS WHOSE DISORDER IS ALSO TERMED HYPERGLYCINEMIA, KETOACIDOSIS, NEUTROPENIA AND THROMBOCYTOPENIA HAVE NOT BEEN OBSERVED AND GLYCINE IS THE ONLY AMINO ACID PRESENT IN EXCESS IN SERUM AND URINE. SEE HYPERGLYCINEMIA, ISOLATED. ALSO SEE METHYLMALONIC ACIDURIA. HSIA ET AL. (1969) DEMONSTRATED DEFICIENT PROPIONATE CARBOXYLATION AS THE BASIC DEFECT IN KETOTIC HYPERGLYCINEMIA. IN A MALE PAKISTANI OFFSPRING OF FIRST COUSIN PARENTS, GOMPERTZ ET AL. (1970) DESCRIBED ACIDOSIS AND KETOSIS DUE TO PROPIONICACIDEMIA, LEADING TO DEATH AT 8 DAYS. A SIB HAD DIED AT 2 WEEKS OF AGE WITH METABOLIC ACIDOSIS AND KETONURIA. THE DEFECT WAS FOUND TO INVOLVE MITOCHONDRIAL PROPIONYL COA CARBOXYLASE. THE SAME CONDITION WAS DESCRIBED BY HOMMES ET AL. (1968). HSIA ET AL. (1971) SHOWED THAT 'KETOTIC HYPERGLYCINEMIA' IS THE SAME AS PROPIONICACIDEMIA AND IS THE RESULT OF A DEFECT IN PROPIONYL-COA CARBOXYLASE. THEY STUDIED FIBROBLASTS FROM A SISTER OF THE BOY IN WHOM THIS DISORDER WAS FIRST DESCRIBED BY CHILDS ET AL. (1961). CLINICAL AND BIOCHEMICAL SIMILARITIES BETWEEN THE CONDITION AND METHYLMALONICACIDURIA HAD SUGGESTED THAT IT ALSO HAD A DEFECT IN THE PROPIONATE-METHYLMALONATE-SUCCINATE PATHWAY. GOMPERTZ ET AL. (1970) FOUND THE SAME ENZYME DEFECT IN PROPIONICACIDEMIA.

CHILDS, B., NYHAN, W. L., BORDEN, M., BARD, L. AND COOKE, R. E.* IDIOPATHIC HYPERGLYCINEMIA AND HYPERGLYCINURIA* A NEW DISORDER OF AMINO ACID METABOLISM. PEDIATRICS 27* 522-538, 1961.

DE VRIES, A., KOCHWA, S., LAZEBNIK, J., FRANK, M. AND DJALDETTI, M.* GLYCINURIA, A HEREDITARY DISORDER ASSOCIATED WITH NEPHROLITHIASIS. AM. J. MED. 23* 408-415, 1957.

GOMPERTZ, D., BAU, D. C. K., STORRS, C. N., PETERS, T. J. AND HUGHES, E. A.* LOCALISATION OF ENZYMIC DEFECT IN PROPIONICACIDAEMIA. LANCET 1* 1140-1143, 1970.

HOMMES, F. A., KUIPERS, J. R. G., ELEMA, J. D., JANSEN, J. F. AND JONXIS, J. H. P.* PROPIONICACIDEMIA, A NEW INBORN ERROR OF METABOLISM. PEDIAT. RES. 2* 519-524, 1968.

HSIA, Y. E., SCULLY, K. J. AND ROSENBERG, L. E.* DEFECTIVE PROPIONATE CARBOXYLATION IN KETOTIC HYPERGLYCINAEMIA. LANCET 1* 757-758, 1969.

HSIA, Y. E., SCULLY, K. J. AND ROSENBERG, L. E.* INHERITED PROPIONYL-COA CARBOXYLASE DEFICIENCY IN 'KETOTIC HYPERGLYCINEMIA.' J. CLIN. INVEST. 50* 127-130, 1971.

NYHAN, W. L.* TREATMENT OF HYPERGLYCINEMIA. AM. J. DIS. CHILD. 113* 129-133, 1967.

NYHAN, W. L., BORDEN, M. AND CHILDS, B.* IDIOPATHIC HYPERGLYCINEMIA* A NEW DISORDER OF AMINO-ACIDS METABOLISM. II. THE CONCENTRATIONS OF OTHER AMINO-ACIDS IN THE PLASMA AND THEIR MODIFICATION BY THE ADMINISTRATION OF LEUCINE. PEDIATRICS 27* 539-550, 1961.

NYHAN, W. L., CHISOLM, J. J., JR. AND EDWARDS, R. O., JR.* IDIOPATHIC HYPERGLYCINURIA. III. REPORT OF A SECOND CASE. J. PEDIAT. 62* 540-545, 1963.

RAMPINI, S., VISCHER, D., CURTIUS, H. C., ANDERS, P. W., TANCREDI, F., FRISCHKNECHT, W. AND PRADER, A.* HEREDITARE HYPERGLYCINAMIE. HELV. PAEDIAT. ACTA 22* 135-159, 1967.

SORIANO, J. R., TAITZ, L. S., FINBERG, L. AND EDELMANN, C. M., JR.* HYPERGLYCINEMIA WITH KETOACIDOSIS AND LEUKOPENIA. PEDIATRICS 39* 818-828, 1967.

WYNGAARDEN, J. B. AND SEGAL, S.* THE HYPERGLYCINURIAS. IN, STANBURY, J. B., WYNGAARDEN, J. B. AND FREDRICKSON, D. S. (EDS.)* THE METABOLIC BASIS OF INHERITED DISEASE. NEW YORK* MCGRAW-HILL, 1966 (2ND ED.). PP. 341-352.

23210 GLYCOGEN STORAGE DISEASE LIMITED TO HEART (ANTOPOL'S DISEASE)

IN 1940 ANTOPOL AND COLLEAGUES DESCRIBED TWO BROTHERS WHO DIED IN THE SECOND DECADE OF LIFE WITH HEART FAILURE AND SHOWED AT AUTOPSY, IN ONE SO STUDIED, GLYCOGEN STORAGE DISEASE LIMITED TO THE MYOCARDIUM. MEHRIZI AND OPPENHEIMER (1960) REPORTED TWO RELATED CASES WHICH APPEAR TO REPRESENT THE IDENTICAL DISEASE (J.H.H. CASES B46872 AND A70767). ANTOPOL'S CASE HAD EXCESSIVE DEPOSITS OF GLYCOGEN IN SKELETAL MUSCLE ALSO AND COMMENTS ON SKELETAL MUSCLE WERE NOT MADE IN THE CASES OF MEHRIZI AND OPPENHEIMER. THUS, IT IS NOT CERTAIN THAT THIS ENTITY IS DISTINCT FROM ONE OF THE OTHER GLYCOGENOSES.

ANTOPOL, W., BOAS, E. P., LEVISON, W. AND TUCHMAN, L. R.* CARDIAC HYPERTROPHY CAUSED BY GLYCOGEN STORAGE DISEASE IN A 15-YEAR-OLD BOY. AM. HEART J. 20* 546-556, 1940.

MEHRIZI, A. AND OPPENHEIMER, E. H.* HEART FAILURE ASSOCIATED WITH UNUSUAL DEPOSITION OF GLYCOGEN IN THE MYOCARDIUM. BULL. HOPKINS HOSP. 107* 329-336, 1960.

23220 GLYCOGEN STORAGE DISEASE I (VON GIERKE'S DISEASE HEPATORENAL FORM OF GLYCOGEN STORAGE DISEASE* GLUCOSE-6-PHOSPHATASE DEFICIENCY* HEPATORENAL GLYCOGENOSIS)

THE LIVER AND KIDNEY ARE INVOLVED. THE BASIC DEFECT RESIDES IN GLUCOSE-6-PHOSPHATASE. HYPOGLYCEMIA IS A MAJOR PROBLEM. LIPIDEMIA ALSO OCCURS AND MAY LEAD TO XANTHOMA FORMATION. RARE SURVIVAL TO ADULTHOOD HAS BEEN OBSERVED. HYPERURICE-MIA HAS BEEN OBSERVED IN A CONSIDERABLE NUMBER OF PATIENTS AND IN SOME CLINICAL GOUT HAS OCCURRED. INHIBITED TUBULAR SECRETION OF URIC ACID DUE TO HYPERLACTICA-CIDEMIA AND KETONEMIA HAS BEEN POSTULATED. SENIOR AND LORIDAN (1968) FOUND THAT THE EFFECTS OF GLYCEROL ADMINISTERED BY MOUTH ON LEVELS OF GLUCOSE AND OF LACTATE, TOGETHER WITH THE RESPONSE TO EPINEPHRINE OR GLUCAGON PERMITTED DIFFERENTIATION OF THE SEVERAL TYPES OF HEPATIC GLYCOGENOSIS (I, II, III AND IV). THEY PROPOSED THE EXISTENCE OF A SECOND TYPE OF VON GIERKE'S DISEASE IN WHICH, ALTHOUGH GLUCOSE-6-PHOSPHATASE ACTIVITY IS PRESENT OR IN VITRO ASSAY, GLUCOSE IS NOT LIBERATED FROM GLUCOSE-6-PHOSPHATE IN VIVO. THEY REFERRED TO THIS AS 'FUNCTIONAL DEFICIENCY OF G6P.' THEY POINTED OUT THAT SOME MUTANTS IN NEUROSPORA SHOW IMPAIRED ENZYME FUNCTION IN THE INTACT FUNGUS DESPITE NORMAL ACTIVITY IN HOMOGENATES. THE GLYCOGEN STORAGE DISEASES REPRESENT A NOTABLE EXAMPLE OF GENETIC HETEROGENEITY. GLYCOGENOSIS I IN PARTICULAR ILLUSTRATES PLEIOTROPISM WITH SIMULATION OF PRIMARY GOUT AND XANTHOMATOSIS.

FIELD, R. A.* GLYCOGEN DEPOSITION DISEASE. IN, STANBURY, J. B., WYNGAARDEN, J. B. AND FREDRICKSON, D. S. (EDS.)* THE METABOLIC BASIS OF INHERITED DISEASE. NEW YORK* MCGRAW-HILL, 1966 (2ND ED.). PP. 141-177.

FINE, R. N., WILSON, W. A. AND DONNELL, G. N.* RETINAL CHANGES IN GLYCOGEN STORAGE DISEASE TYPE I. AM. J. DIS. CHILD. 115* 328-331, 1968.

HOWELL, R. R.* THE GLYCOGEN STORAGE DISEASES. IN, STANBURY, J. B., WYNGAARDEN, J. B. AND FREDRICKSON, D. S. (EDS.)* THE METABOLIC BASIS OF INHERITED DISEASE. NEW YORK* MCGRAW-HILL, 1970 (3RD ED.).

HOWELL, R. R.* THE INTERRELATIONSHIP OF GLYCOGEN STORAGE DISEASE AND GOUT. ARTH. RHEUM. 8* 780-785, 1965.

SENIOR, B. AND LORIDAN, L.* FUNCTIONAL DIFFERENTIATION OF GLYCOGENOSES OF THE LIVER* WITH RESPECT TO THE USE OF GLYCEROL. NEW ENG. J. MED. 279* 965-970, 1968.

SENIOR, B. AND LORIDAN, L.* LIVER GLYCOGENOSES* METABOLISM OF INTRAVENOUSLY ADMINISTERED GLYCEROL. NEW ENG. J. MED. 279* 958-965, 1968.

SIDBURY, J. B., JR.* THE GENETICS OF THE GLYCOGEN STORAGE DISEASE. IN, STEINBERG, A. G. AND BEARN, A. G. (EDS.)* PROGRESS IN MEDICAL GENETICS. GRUNE AND STRATTON, VOL. 4, 1965. PP. 32-58.

23230 GLYCOGEN STORAGE DISEASE II (POMPE'S DISEASE CARDIAC FORM OF GENERALIZED GLYCOGENOSIS* CARDIOMEGALIA GLYCOGENICA DIFFUSA* ETC.)

THE DEFECT INVOLVES ACID-ALPHA-1,4-GLUCOSIDASE AND INVOLVEMENT IS GENERALIZED. THE AFFECTED CHILDREN ARE PROSTRATE, APPEAR IMBECILIC, AND ARE MARKEDLY HYPOTONIC WITH LARGE HEARTS. THE TONGUE IS ENLARGED. NEUROLOGIC DISORDERS MAY RESULT FROM EXTENSIVE CNS INVOLVEMENT. THE LIVER IS RARELY ENLARGED (EXCEPT AS A RESULT OF HEART FAILURE) AND HYPOGLYCEMIA AND ACIDOSIS DO NOT OCCUR AS THEY DO IN TYPE I. SEE FIELD, R. A.* LOC. CIT. POMPE'S DISEASE MAY BE OF MORE THAN ONE TYPE. IN THE CLASSICAL CASES DEATH OCCURS IN THE FIRST YEAR AND CARDIAC INVOLVEMENT IS STRIKING. INDEED, POMPE REPORTED THIS CONDITION IN 1932 AS 'IDIOPATHIC HYPERTRO-PHY OF THE HEART' AND 'CARDIOMEGALIA GLYCOGENICA' IS A SYNONYM. HOWEVER, SMITH, ZELLWEGER AND AFIFI (1967) REPORTED A BOY WITH AMYOTONIC FORM OF DISEASE AND SURVIVAL TO THE AGE OF ALMOST 11 YEARS. THE HEART WAS NOT INVOLVED SIGNIFICANTLY. ALPHA-1, 4-GLUCOSIDASE WAS ABSENT FROM LIVER AND MUSCLE. THERE WERE HEAVY GLYCOGEN DEPOSITS AND AN ANOMALOUS POLYSACCHARIDE WITH SHORT OUTER CHAINS WAS IDENTIFIED. SMITH, AMICK AND SIDBURY (1966) REPORTED A SIMILAR CASE IN A BOY WHO SURVIVED TO THE AGE OF 4.5 YEARS. ALTHOUGH THIS FORM OF GLYCOGEN STORAGE DISEASE HAS LONG BEEN KNOWN, THE ENZYME DEFECT WAS ELUCIVE. THE ABOVE NAMED ENZYME, ALSO CALLED ACID MALTASE, IS A LYSOSOMAL ENZYME WITH A PH OPTIMUM OF 4.5-5. WHEREAS THE GLYCOGEN IS DISTRIBUTED RATHER UNIFORMLY IN THE CYTOPLASM IN THE OTHER GLYCOGENOSES, IT IS ENCLOSED IN LYSOSOMAL MEMBRANES IN THIS FORM. HUDGSON ET AL. (1968) REPORTED THE CASE OF A PORTUGESE GIRL WHO DIED AT AGE 19 AND THAT OF A LIVING 44 YEAR OLD HOUSEWIFE. OTHER EXPERIENCES SUGGESTING THE EXISTENCE OF MORE THAN ONE TYPE OF GLYCOGENOSIS II WERE REPORTED BY SWAIMAN ET AL. (1968). ZELLWEGER ET AL. (1965) DESCRIBED BROTHERS AGE 15 AND 4.5 YEARS WITH MINIMAL MANIFESTATIONS LIMITED TO SKELETAL MUSCLE. A DEFICIENCY OF MUSCLE ALPHA-1,4-GLUCOSIDASE WAS DEMONSTRATED. MUSCLE SHOWED ABNORMAL ACCUMULATIONS OF GLYCOGEN. A MATERNAL UNCLE MAY HAVE BEEN AFFECTED ALSO. MUSCLE ENZYME STUDIES IN THE PARENTS MIGHT DIFFERENTIATE AUTOSOMAL FROM X-LINKED INHERITANCE.

R
E
C
E
S
S
I
V
E

HIRSCHHORN, K., NADLER, H. L., WAITHE, W. I., BROWN, B. I. AND HIRSCHHORN, R.* POMPE'S DISEASE* DETECTION OF HETEROZYGOTES BY LYMPHOCYTE STIMULATION. SCIENCE 166* 1632-1633, 1969.

HUDGSON, P., GARDNER-MEDWIN, D., WORSFOLD, M., PENNINGTON, R. J. T. AND WALTON, J. N.* ADULT MYOPATHY FROM GLYCOGEN STORAGE DISEASE DUE TO ACID MALTASE DEFICIEN-CY. BRAIN 91* 435-462, 1968.

SMITH, H. L., AMICK, L. D. AND SIDBURY, J. B., JR.* TYPE II GLYCOGENOSIS. AM. J. DIS. CHILD. 3* 475-481, 1966.

SMITH, J., ZELLWEGER, H. AND AFIFI, A. K.* MUSCULAR FORM OF GLYCOGENOSIS, TYPE II (POMPE). NEUROLOGY 17* 537-549, 1967.

SWAIMAN, K. F., KENNEDY, W. R. AND SAULS, H. S.* LATE INFANTILE ACID MALTASE DEFICIENCY. ARCH. NEUROL. 18* 642-648, 1968.

ZELLWEGER, H., BROWN, B. I., MCCORMICK, W. F. AND JUN-BI, T.* A MILD FORM OF MUSCULAR GLYCOGENOSIS IN TWO BROTHERS WITH ALPHA-1,4-GLUCOSIDASE DEFICIENCY. ANN. PAEDIAT. 205* 413-437, 1965.

23240 GLYCOGEN STORAGE DISEASE III (FORBES' DISEASE CORI'S DISEASE* LIMIT DEXTRINO-SIS)

LIVER AND HEART MUSCLE SHOW PREDOMINANT EFFECTS. THE DEFECT CONCERNS DEBRANCHER ENZYME (AMYLO-1, 6-GLUCOSIDASE). THE CLINICAL FEATURES ARE SOMEWHAT LIKE TYPE I BUT MILDER AND INVOLVEMENT OF HEART AND SKELETAL MUSCLE ADDS OTHER FEATURES. IN ISRAEL 73 PERCENT OF GLYCOGEN STORAGE DISEASE WAS OF THIS TYPE AND ALL WERE NON-ASHKENAZI, BEING MAINLY OF NORTH AFRICAN EXTRACTION, IN WHICH GROUP THE MINIMAL ESTIMATE OF FREQUENCY WAS 1 IN 5,420 (LEVIN ET AL., 1967). SEE FIELD, R. A.* LOC. CIT.

GARANCIS, J. C., PANARES, R. R., GOOD, T. A. AND KUZMA, J. F.* TYPE III GLYCOGENOSIS. A BIOCHEMICAL AND ELECTRON MICROSCOPIC STUDY. LAB. INVEST. 22* 468-477, 1970.

LEVIN, S., MOSES, S. W., CHAYOTH, R., JADOGA, N. AND STEINITZ, K.* GLYCOGEN STORAGE DISEASE IN ISRAEL. A CLINICAL, BIOCHEMICAL AND GENETIC STUDY. ISRAEL J. MED. SCI. 3* 397-410, 1967.

WAALER, P. E., GARATUN-TJELDSTO, O. AND MOE, P. J.* GENETIC STUDIES IN GLYCOGEN STORAGE DISEASE TYPE III. ACTA PAEDIAT. SCAND. 59* 529-535, 1970.

23250 GLYCOGEN STORAGE DISEASE IV (ANDERSEN'S DISEASE BRANCHER DEFICIENCY* AMYLOPEC-TINOSIS* FAMILIAL CIRRHOSIS WITH DEPOSITION OF ABNORMAL GLYCOGEN)

THE LIVER SHOWS THE MAIN INVOLVEMENT, RESULTING FROM A DEFECT OF AMYLO(1,4 TO 1,6) TRANSGLUCOSIDASE (BRANCHER ENZYME). VERY FEW CASES HAVE BEEN IDENTIFIED BUT THE EVIDENCE OF RECESSIVE INHERITANCE IS STRONG* AFFECTED SIBS, PARENTAL CONSANGUINI-TY, PARTIAL ENZYME DEFICIENCY IN BOTH PARENTS. LEVIN ET AL. (1968) DESCRIBED A CASE OF THIS RARE FORM OF GLYCOGENOSIS, ALTERNATIVELY CALLED AMYLOPECTINOSIS. IT IS DISTINGUISHED FROM THE MORE COMMON TYPES BY EARLY DEVELOPMENT OF CIRRHOSIS WITH PORTAL HYPERTENSION, ENDING IN SEVERE LIVER FAILURE, AS WELL AS POSITIVE RESULTS IN THE SIMPLE TEST WITH IODINE (FORMATION OF A BLUE COLORED COMPLEX OF GLYCOGEN AND IODINE).

FIELD, R. A.* LOC. CIT.

HOWELL, R. R.* LOC. CIT., 1970.

LEVIN, B., BURGESS, E. A. AND MORTIMER, P. E.* GLYCOGEN STORAGE DISEASE TYPE IV, AMYLOPECTINOSIS. ARCH. DIS. CHILD. 43* 548-555, 1968.

SCHOCHET, S. S., JR., MCCORMICK, W. F. AND ZELLWEGER, H.* TYPE IV GLYCOGENOSIS (AMYLOPECTINOSIS). ARCH. PATH. 90* 354-363, 1970.

23260 GLYCOGEN STORAGE DISEASE V (MCARDLE'S DISEASE MYOPHOSPHORYLASE DEFICIENCY GLYCOGENOSIS)

SKELETAL MUSCLE IS INVOLVED EXCLUSIVELY IN A DEFICIENCY OF MUSCLE PHOSPHORYLASE. THE DISORDER MAY PRESENT AS INTERMITTENT MYOGLOBINURIA. A. S. (718935) IS A JOHNS HOPKINS HOSPITAL CASE OF THE DISEASE. MCARDLE'S ORIGINAL PATIENT WAS A 30 YEAR OLD MAN WHO EXPERIENCED FIRST PAIN AND THEN WEAKNESS AND STIFFNESS WITH EXERCISE OF ANY MUSCLE INCLUDING THE MASSETERS. SYMPTOMS DISAPPEARED PROMPTLY WITH REST. BLOOD LACTATE DOES NOT INCREASE AFTER EXERCISE.
     A DEFICIENCY OF PHOSPHOFRUCTOKINASE (SEE GLYCOGEN STORAGE DISEASE VII) PRODUCES THE SAME CLINICAL PICTURE. THIS IS NOT SURPRISING SINCE THE ENZYME DEFICIENCY RESULTS IN INABILITY TO METABOLIZE THROUGH FRUCTOSE TO LACTOSE. A DIFFERENT CONDITION MAY HAVE BEEN REPORTED BY DI SANT'AGNESE AND COLLEAGUES (1962) IN A TWO-AND-ONE-HALF-YEAR-OLD CHILD WITH HYPOTONIA AND PALATAL PARALYSIS WITHOUT CARDIOMEGALY OR HEPATOMEGALY. STRIATED MUSCLE SHOWED AN EXCESSIVE ACCUMULATION OF GLYCOGEN WHICH HAD NORMAL CHEMICAL STRUCTURE. DEBRANCHER ENZYME WAS NORMAL.

UNFORTUNATELY PHOSPHORYLASE ACTIVITY WAS NOT DETERMINED. THE POSSIBILITY OF MORE THAN ONE FORM OF MUSCLE PHOSPHORYLASE DEFICIENCY IS ALSO SUGGESTED BY THE CASE OF MELLICK, MAHLER AND HUGHES (1962).

THIS IS A CAUSE OF MYOGLOBINURIA. THE PHASES OF THE DISEASE ARE (1) IN CHILDHOOD AND ADOLESCENCE, INTERMITTENT DARK URINE, (2) IN EARLY ADULT LIFE, CRAMPING MUSCLE PAIN ON EXERTION, OCCASIONALLY FOLLOWED BY TRANSIENT MYOGLO-BINURIA, AND (3) IN THE FOURTH (OR FIFTH) DECADE, PERSISTENT AND PROGRESSIVE WEAKNESS AND WASTING OF MUSCLE, WITH ABSENT OR RARE MYOGLOBINURIA. ENGEL, EYERMAN AND WILLIAMS (1963) OBSERVED ONSET OF FIRST MANIFESTATIONS AT AGE 49 IN A SISTER AND BROTHER. THE SISTER HAD PROGRESSIVE GENERALIZED MUSCULAR WEAKNESS WITHOUT CRAMPS AND HAD COMPLETE ABSENCE OF ENZYME. THE BROTHER HAD MUSCLE CRAMPS AFTER EXERCISE AND ABOUT 35 PERCENT NORMAL ACTIVITY OF PHOSPHORYLASE. NEITHER HAD MYOGLOBINURIA. DAWSON, SPONG AND HARRINGTON (1968) SUGGESTED A TEST FOR DETECTION OF ASYMPTOMATIC HETEROZYGOTES BASED ON THE DEVELOPMENT OF BRIEF PAINFUL CRAMPS DURING EXERCISE.

DAWSON, D. M., SPONG, F. L. AND HARRINGTON, J. F.* MCARDLE'S DISEASE* LACK OF MUSCLE PHOSPHORYLASE. ANN. INTERN. MED. 69* 229-236, 1968.

DI SANT'AGNESE, P. A., ANDERSON, D. H. AND METCALF, K. M.* GLYCOGEN STORAGE DISEASE OF THE MUSCLES. J. PEDIAT. 61* 438-442, 1962.

ENGEL, W. K., EYERMAN, E. L. AND WILLIAMS, H. E.* LATE-ONSET TYPE OF SKELETAL-MUSCLE PHOSPHORYLASE DEFICIENCY. A NEW FAMILIAL VARIETY WITH COMPLETELY AND PARTIALLY AFFECTED SUBJECTS. NEW ENG. J. MED. 268* 135-137, 1963.

FIELD, R. A.* GLYCOGEN DEPOSITION DISEASE. IN, STANBURY, J. B., WYNGAARDEN, J. B. AND FREDRICKSON, D. S. (EDS.)* THE METABOLIC BASIS OF INHERITED DISEASE. NEW YORK* MCGRAW-HILL, 1966 (2ND ED.). PP. 156-207.

LEHOCZKY, T., HALASY, M., SIMON, G. AND HARMOS, G.* GLYCOGENIC MYOPATHY. A CASE OF SKELETAL MUSCLE-GLYCOGENOSIS IN TWINS. J. NEUROL. SCI. 2* 366-384, 1965.

MELLICK, R. S., MAHLER, R. F. AND HUGHES, B. P.* MCARDLE'S SYNDROME. PHOS-PHORYLASE-DEFICIENT MYOPATHY. LANCET 1* 1045-1048, 1962.

ROWLAND, L. P., LOVELACE, R. E., SCHOTLAND, D. L., ARAKI, S. AND CARMEL, P.* THE CLINICAL DIAGNOSIS OF MCARDLE'S DISEASE. IDENTIFICATION OF ANOTHER FAMILY WITH DEFICIENCY OF MUSCLE PHOSPHORYLASE. NEUROLOGY 16* 93-100, 1966.

SCHMID, R. AND HAMMAKER, L.* HEREDITARY ABSENCE OF MUSCLE PHOSPHORYLASE (MCARDLE'S SYNDROME). NEW ENG. J. MED. 264* 223-225, 1961.

SCHMID, R. AND MAHLER, R.* CHRONIC PROGRESSIVE MYOPATHY WITH MYOGLOBINURIA* DEMONSTRATION OF A GLYCOGENOLYTIC DEFECT IN THE MUSCLE. J. CLIN. INVEST. 38* 2044-2058, 1959.

R
E
C
E
S
S
I
V
E

23270 GLYCOGEN STORAGE DISEASE VI (HERS' DISEASE PHOSPHORYLASE DEFICIENCY GLYCOGEN-STORAGE DISEASE OF LIVER)

THE CLINICAL PICTURE IS ONE OF MILD TO MODERATE HYPOGLYCEMIA, MILD KETOSIS, GROWTH RETARDATION AND PROMINENT HEPATOMEGALY. HEART AND SKELETAL MUSCLE ARE NOT AFFECTED. THE PROGNOSIS SEEMS TO BE EXCELLENT. WALLIS ET AL. (1966) DETERMINED ERYTHROCYTE GLYCOGEN CONCENTRATION AND LEUKOCYTE PHOSPHORYLASE ACTIVITY IN 17 MEMBERS OF 4 GENERATIONS OF THE FAMILY OF A BOY WITH BIOPSY-PROVED GLYCOGEN STORAGE DISEASE OF TYPE VI. THE FINDINGS CLEARLY INDICATE AUTOSOMAL RECESSIVE INHERITANCE. HERS AND VAN HOOF (1968) SUGGESTED THAT TYPE VI IS A "WAITING ROOM" FROM WHICH NEW ENTITIES WILL BE SEPARATED IN THE FUTURE. THE CLASS WILL BE RESERVED FOR THOSE WITH LIVER PHOSPHORYLASE DEFICIENCY AS THE PRIMARY DEFECT. DEFICIENCY OF PHOSPHORYLASE KINASE IS AN X-LINKED DEFECT (SEE GLYCOGEN STORAGE DISEASE VIII IN THE X-LINKED CATALOG).

HERS, H. G. AND VAN HOOF, F.* GLYCOGEN STORAGE DISEASES* TYPE II AND TYPE VI GLYCOGENOSIS. IN, DICKENS, F., RANDLE, P. J. AND WHELAN, W. J. (EDS.)* CARBOHY-DRATE METABOLISM AND ITS DISORDERS. NEW YORK* ACADEMIC PRESS, 1968.

HERS, H. G.* ETUDES ENZYMATIQUES SUR FRAGMENTS HEPATIQUES* APPLICATION A LA CLASSIFICATION DES GLYCOGENOSES. REV. INT. HEPAT. 9* 35-55, 1959.

WALLIS, P. G., SIDBURY, J. B., JR. AND HARRIS, R. C.* HEPATIC PHOSPHORYLASE DEFECT. STUDIES ON PERIPHERAL BLOOD. AM. J. DIS. CHILD. 111* 278-282, 1966.

WILLIAMS, H. E. AND FIELD, J. B.* LOW LEUKOCYTE PHOSPHORYLASE IN HEPATIC PHOSPHORYLASE-DEFICIENT GLYCOGEN STORAGE DISEASE. J. CLIN. INVEST. 40* 1841-1845, 1961.

*23280 GLYCOGEN STORAGE DISEASE VII (PHOSPHOFRUCTOKINASE DEFICIENCY GLYCOGEN DISEASE OF MUSCLE)

LAYZER ET AL. (1967) PROVIDED STRONG EVIDENCE FOR RECESSIVE INHERITANCE BY DEMONSTRATING PARTIAL DEFICIENCY OF ENZYME ACTIVITY IN ERYTHROCYTES OF BOTH PARENTS OF AN AFFECTED 18 YEAR OLD MALE. PARENTS WERE NOT KNOWN TO BE RELATED.

THE ONLY PREVIOUSLY DISCRIBED FAMILY WAS THAT REPORTED FROM JAPAN BY TARUI ET AL. (1967). MUSCLE CRAMPS WITH EXERTION AND MYGLOBINURIA WITH EXTREME EXERTION ARE FEATURES AS IN MCARDLE'S DISEASE (GLYCOGEN STORAGE DISEASE V). THAT THE CLINICAL MANIFESTATIONS ARE IDENTICAL IS NOT SURPRISING SINCE IN BOTH PRODUCTION OF LACTATE IS INTERFERED WITH.

LAYZER, R. B., ROWLAND, L. P. AND RANNEY, H. M.* MUSCLE PHOSPHOFRUCTOKINASE DEFICIENCY. ARCH. NEUROL. 17* 512-523, 1967.

NISHIKAWA, M., TSUKIYAMA, K., ENOMOTO, T., TARUI, S., OKUNO, G., UEDA, K., IKURA, T., TSUJII, T., SUGASE, T., SUDA, M. AND TANAKA, T.* A NEW TYPE OF SKELETAL MUSCLE GLYCOGENOSIS DUE TO PHOSPHOFRUCTOKINASE DEFICIENCY. PROC. JAP. ACAD. 41* 350-353, 1965.

TARUI, S., OKUNO, G., IKURA, Y. AND SHIMA, K.* PHOSPHOFRUCTOKINASE DEFICIENCY IN SKELETAL MUSCLE* A NEW TYPE OF GLYCOGENOSIS. BIOCHEM. BIOPHYS. RES. COMMUN. 19* 517-523, 1967.

23290 GLYCOPROTEIN STORAGE DISEASE

ZUGIBE ET AL. (1969) DESCRIBED A 52 YEAR OLD MAN WITH GOUT AND MARKED SPLENOMEGA-LY. RETICULOENDOTHELIAL CELLS IN THE SPLEEN AND BONE MARROW CONTAINED LARGE EOSINOPHILIC GRANULES WHEN STAINED WITH HEMATOXYLIN AND EOSIN. URINARY HEXOSAMINE LEVELS WERE ELEVATED IN THE PROBAND AND SOME CLOSE RELATIVES.

ZUGIBE, F. T., GILBERT, E. F. AND GAZIANO, D.* GLYCOPROTEIN STORAGE DISEASE, A NEW ENTITY. AM. J. MED. 47* 135-140, 1969.

23300 GLYCOPROTEIN* LACK OF BETA(2)-GLYCOPROTEIN I

HAUPT ET AL. (1968) DESCRIBED A FAMILY IN WHICH TWO BROTHERS HAD COMPLETE ABSENCE OF WHAT THEY TERMED BETA(2)-GLYCOPROTEIN I. BOTH PARENTS, A SISTER, AND BOTH CHILDREN OF ONE OF THE BROTHERS HAD HALF-NORMAL LEVELS OF THE PROTEIN.

HAUPT, H., SCHWICK, H. G. AND STORIKO, K.* UBER EINEN ERBLICHEN BETA(2)-GLYCOPROTEIN I-MANGEL. HUMANGENETIK 5* 291-293, 1968.

*23310 GLYCOSURIA, RENAL (ALSO SEE FANCONI SYNDROME)

THIS TRAIT HAS OFTEN BEEN CONSIDERED A DOMINANT (HJARNE, 1927). ALTHOUGH IT IS INCOMPLETELY RECESSIVE, I.E. HETEROZYGOTES MAY SHOW MILD GLYCOSURIA, CONSISTENT HEAVY GLYCOSURIA IS A FEATURE OF THE HOMOZYGOTE (KHACHADURIAN, 1964). THE PHYSIOLOGIC DEFECT IS LOW RENAL THRESHOLD FOR GLUCOSE. THE CLINICAL PICTURE IS LOSS OF 50-60 GMS. OF GLUCOSE IN THE URINE DAILY DESPITE A NORMAL GLUCOSE TOLERANCE TEST. A RELATION TO DIABETES MELLITUS HAS BEEN SUSPECTED BUT NOT COMPLETELY ESTABLISHED. MONASTERIO ET AL. (1964) DID MICRODISSECTION AND ELECTRON MICROSCOPY IN TWO CASES. ABNORMALITY WAS LIMITED TO THE PROXIMAL TUBULES WHICH SHOWED VACUOLIZATION, ACCUMULATION OF ABNORMAL PAS-POSITIVE MATERIAL AND CHANGES IN THE BRUSH BORDER. ELSAS AND ROSENBERG (1969) CLARIFIED THE SITUATION BY POINTING OUT THAT TYPE A (LOW THRESHOLD AND LOW GLUCOSE TM) AND TYPE B (LOW THRESHOLD BUT NORMAL TM) MAY BE OBSERVED IN THE SAME FAMILY, THAT BOTH PARENTS MAY BE COMPLETELY NORMAL OR MAY SHOW ABNORMALITY IN THE RENAL TUBULAR TRANSPORT OF GLUCOSE, AND THAT DEFECTIVE REABSORPTION OF GLUCOSE BY THE KIDNEY NEED NOT BE ACCOMPANIED BY ABNORMALITIES IN INTESTINAL GLUCOSE TRANSPORT. SEVERAL DIFFERENT MUTATIONS ARE PROBABLY INVOLVED IN RENAL GLYCOSURIA, AS IN THE CASE IN CYSTINURIA.

ELSAS, L. J. AND ROSENBERG, L. E.* FAMILIAL RENAL GLYCOSURIA* A GENETIC REAPPRAISAL OF HEXOSE TRANSPORT BY KIDNEY AND INTESTINE. J. CLIN. INVEST. 48* 1845-1854, 1969.

ELSAS, L. J., HILLMAN, R. E., PATTERSON, J. H. AND ROSENBERG, L. E.* RENAL AND INTESTINAL HEXOSE TRANSPORT IN FAMILIAL GLUCOSE-GALACTOSE MALABSORPTION. J. CLIN. INVEST. 49* 576-585, 1970.

GJONE, E.* IDIOPATISK RENAL GLYKOSURIA IN 3 GENERATIONER WITH HIGH INCIDENCE. NORD. MED. 59* 306-307, 1958.

HJARNE, V.* STUDY OF ORTHOGLYCAEMIC GLYCOSURIA WITH PARTICULAR REFERENCE TO ITS HEREDITABILITY. ACTA MED. SCAND. 67* 422-571, 1927.

KHACHADURIAN, A. K. AND KHACHADURIAN, L. A.* THE INHERITANCE OF RENAL GLYCO-SURIA. AM. J. HUM. GENET. 16* 189-194, 1964.

KRANE, S. M.* RENAL GLYCOSURIA. IN, STANBURY, J. B., WYNGAARDEN, J. B. AND FREDRICKSON, D. S. (EDS.)* THE METABOLIC BASIS OF INHERITED DISEASE. NEW YORK* MCGRAW-HILL, 1966 (2ND ED.). PP. 1221-1229.

MONASTERIO, G., OLIVER, J., MUIESAN, G., PARDELLI, G., MARINOZZI, V. AND MACDOWELL, M.* RENAL DIABETES AS A CONGENITAL TUBULAR DYSPLASIA. AM. J. MED. 37* 44-61, 1964.

23320 GLYOXALASE II (HYDROXYACYL-GLUTATHIONE HYDROLASE) DEFICIENCY

VALENTINE ET AL. (1970) DESCRIBED A FAMILY IN WHICH HOMOZYGOTES AND HETEROZYGOTES FOR DEFICIENCY OF GLYOXALASE II (HYDROXYACYL-GLUTATHIONE HYDROLASE) COULD BE DEMONSTRATED IN THREE GENERATIONS OF A FAMILY. HOMOZYGOTES HAD NO CLINICAL OR HEMATOLOGIC ABNORMALITY AND ELLIPTOCYTOSIS (WHICH WAS SEGREGATING INDEPENDENTLY IN THE FAMILY) WAS NOT WORSENED BY THE PRESENCE OF THE ENZYME DEFECT.

VALENTINE, W. N., PAGLIA, D. E., NEERHOUT, R. C. AND KONRAD, P. N.* ERYTHROCYTE GLYOXALASE II DEFICIENCY WITH COINCIDENTAL HEREDITARY ELLIPTOCYTOSIS. BLOOD 36* 797-808, 1970.

*23330 GONADAL DYSGENESIS, XX TYPE

ELLIOTT, SANDLER AND RABINOWITZ (1959) REPORTED THE CONDITION IN 3 SISTERS WHO HAD NORMAL STATURE AND SEX CHROMATIN BUT HAD NEVER MENSTRUATED AND HAD SEVERE OSTEOPOROSIS. THE PARENTS WERE FIRST COUSINS IN THE CASE OF THE TWO AFFECTED SISTERS (WITH NORMAL STATURE AND SEX-CHROMATIN POSITIVITY) REPORTED BY KLOTZ, MERGER AND AVRIL (1956). CHRISTAKOS ET AL. (1969) OBSERVED GONADAL DYSGENESIS IN THREE SISTERS WHOSE PARENTS WERE SECOND COUSINS. EACH HAD A NORMAL FEMALE 46-XX KAROTYPE. SOMATIC FEATURES OF TURNER'S SYNDROME WERE NOT FOUND. ALL THREE HAD ELEVATED GONADOTROPINS AND LAPAROTOMY ON THE TWO OLDER SISTERS SHOWED STREAK GONADS AND UNSTIMULATED MULLERIAN STRUCTURES. GONADAL DYSGENESIS, OFTEN WITH SOMATIC ABNORMALITIES, HAS BEEN REPORTED IN SIBS BY SEVERAL OTHER AUTHORS AND IN SOME OF THESE REPORTS THE PARENTS WERE CONSANGUINEOUS. SIMPSON AND GERMAN (1970) POINTED OUT THAT ONLY AFFECTED SIBS HAVE BEEN DESCRIBED AND PARENTAL CONSANGUINITY IS FREQUENT.

BOCZKOWSKI, K.* PURE GONADAL DYSGENESIS AND OVARIAN DYSPLASIA IN SISTERS. AM. J. OBSTET. GYNEC. 106* 626-628, 1970.

CHRISTAKOS, A. C., SIMPSON, J. L., YOUNGER, J. B. AND CHRISTIAN, C. D.* GONADAL DYSGENESIS AS AN AUTOSOMAL RECESSIVE CONDITION. AM. J. OBSTET. GYNEC. 104* 1027-1030, 1969.

ELLIOTT, G. A., SANDLER, A. AND RABINOWITZ, D.* GONADAL DYSGENESIS IN THREE SISTERS. J. CLIN. ENDOCR. 19* 995-1003, 1959.

KLOTZ, H. P., MERGER, R. AND AVRIL, J.* SYNDROME DE TURNER CHEZ DEUX SOEURS ISSUES DE COUSIN GERMAINS. CONSIDERATION PATHOGENIQUES. ANN. ENDOCR. 17* 43-46, 1956.

PEREZ-BALLESTER, B., GREENBLATT, R. B. AND BYRD, J. R.* FAMILIAL GONADAL DYSGENESIS. AM. J. OBSTET. GYNEC. 107* 1262-1263, 1970.

SIMPSON, J. L. AND GERMAN, J.* GENETIC ASPECTS OF GONADAL DYSGENESIS ASSOCIATED WITH NORMAL CHROMOSOMAL COMPLEMENTS. (ABSTRACT) AM. J. HUM. GENET. 22* 24A ONLY, 1970.

23340 GONADAL DYSGENESIS, XX TYPE, WITH DEAFNESS

TWO FAMILIES HAVE BEEN REPORTED IN WHICH MULTIPLE MEMBERS WITH XX GONADAL DYSGENESIS ALL HAD DEAFNESS AS WELL SUGGESTING THE EXISTENCE OF TWO RECESSIVE FORMS OF THIS DISORDER (CHRISTAKOS ET AL., 1969* PEREZ-BALLESTER ET AL., 1970).

CHRISTAKOS, A. C., SIMPSON, J. L., YOUNGER, J. B. AND CHRISTIAN, C. D.* GONADAL DYSGENESIS AS AN AUTOSOMAL RECESSIVE CONDITION. AM. J. OBSTET. GYNEC. 104* 1027-1030, 1969.

PEREZ-BALLESTER, B., GREENBLATT, R. B. AND BYRD, J. R.* FAMILIAL GONADAL DYSGENESIS. AM. J. OBSTET. GYNEC. 107* 1262-1263, 1970.

23350 GORLIN'S SYNDROME (CRANIOFACIAL DYSOSTOSIS, HYPERTRICHOSIS, HYPOPLASIA OF LABIA MAJORA, DENTAL AND EYE ANOMALIES, PATENT DUCTUS ARTERIOSUS, NORMAL INTELLIGENCE)

GORLIN, CHAUDHRY AND MOSS (1960) DESCRIBED SISTERS WITH THIS COMBINATION OF FEATURES. THE PARENTS WERE NOT KNOWN TO BE RELATED. THE SAME SISTERS WERE REPORTED BY FEINBERG (1960) AS INSTANCES OF THE WEILL-MARCHESANI SYNDROME (Q.V.), WHICH IS CLEARLY AN INCORRECT DIAGNOSIS.

FEINBERG, S. B.* CONGENITAL MESODERMAL DYSMORPHO-DYSTROPHY (BRACHYMORPHIC TYPE). RADIOLOGY 74* 218-224, 1960.

GORLIN, R. J., CHAUDHRY, A. P. AND MOSS, M. L.* CRANIOFACIAL DYSOSTOSIS, PATENT DUCTUS ARTERIOSUS, HYPERTRICHOSIS, HYPOPLASIA OF LABIA MAJORA, DENTAL AND EYE ANOMALIES - A NEW SYNDROME.Q J. PEDIAT. 56* 778-785, 1960.

23360 GRANULOCYTOPENIA WITH IMMUNOGLOBULIN ABNORMALITY

LONSDALE ET AL. (1967) DESCRIBED THREE BROTHERS WHO DIED AT AGES 12 MONTHS, 6 YEARS, AND 41 MONTHS FROM OVERWHELMING INFECTION. THE BONE MARROW PICTURE INDICATED MATURATION ARREST AND IN TWO PATIENTS EPISODES OF LEUKOCYTOSIS OF UNKNOWN CAUSE PUNCTUATED THE COURSE. TOTAL GAMMA GLOBULINS WERE LOW IN THE SERUM.

R
E
C
E
S
S
I
V
E

LONSDALE, D., DEODHAR, S. D. AND MERCER, R. D.* FAMILIAL GRANULOCYTOPENIA AND
ASSOCIATED IMMUNOGLOBULIN ABNORMALITY. REPORT OF THREE CASES IN YOUNG BROTHERS.
J. PEDIAT. 71* 790-801, 1967.

*23370 GRANULOMATOUS DISEASE DUE TO LEUKOCYTE MALFUNCTION

IN ADDITION TO THE WELL-ESTABLISHED X-LINKED FORM, AN AUTOSOMAL RECESSIVE FORM
APPEARS TO EXIST. BAEHNER AND NATHAN (1968) OBSERVED A 17 YEAR OLD FEMALE,
OFFSPRING OF FIRST COUSINS, WHO SHOWED A CLINICAL COURSE AND LEUKOCYTE BEHAVIOR IN
VITRO LIKE THOSE IN AFFECTED MALES WITH THE X-LINKED DISEASE. CHROMOSOMES WERE
NORMAL. THE NITRO BLUE TETRAZOLIUM TEST OF LEUKOCYTES WAS NORMAL IN ALL RELA-
TIVES. AZIMI ET AL. (1968), FURTHERMORE, DESCRIBED THREE NEGRO SISTERS WITH THE
SAME ABNORMALITY. IN BOTH FAMILIES, PARENTS SHOWED NORMAL LEUKOCYTE FUNCTION.
OTHER FEMALE PATIENTS HAVE BEEN REPORTED. HOLMES ET AL. (1970) PRESENTED EVIDENCE
THAT LEUKOCYTE GLUTATHIONE PEROXIDASE ACTIVITY IS DEFECTIVE IN FEMALES WITH
CHRONIC GRANULOMATOUS DISEASE. DEFICIENCY OF RED CELL GLUTATHIONE PEROXIDASE
LEADS TO HEMOLYTIC ANEMIA, A FEATURE ABSENT IN THE PRESENT CASES.

AZIMI, P. H., BODENBENDER, J. G., HINTZ, R. L. AND KONTRAS, S. B.* CHRONIC
GRANULOMATOUS DISEASE IN THREE FEMALE SIBLINGS. J.A.M.A. 206* 2865-2870, 1968.

BAEHNER, R. L. AND NATHAN, D. G.* QUANTITATIVE NITROBLUE TETRAZOLIUM TEST IN
CHRONIC GRANULOMATOUS DISEASE. NEW ENG. J. MED. 278* 971-976, 1968.

HOLMES, B., PARK, B. H., MALAEVISTA, S. E., QUIE, P. G., NELSON, D. L. AND
GOOD, R. A.* CHRONIC GRANULOMATOUS DISEASE IN FEMALES. A DEFICIENCY OF LEUKOCYTE
GLUTATHIONE PEROXIDASE. NEW ENG. J. MED. 283* 217-221, 1970.

23380 GROUPED PIGMENTATION OF THE MACULA

GROUPED PIGMENTATION OF THE RETINA LIMITED STRICTLY TO THE FOVEAL AREA WAS
DESCRIBED BY LOEWENSTEIN AND STEEL (1941) AND BY CHAN (1951). FORGACS AND BOZIN
(1966) REPORTED THE FIRST FAMILIAL INCIDENCE, TWO AFFECTED SISTERS. THEY
COMPLAINED OF METAMORPHOPSIA AND SHOWED PIGMENTED SPOTS SURROUNDED BY A CLEAR HALO
IN THE FOVEAL AREA. FORSIUS (1970) DOUBTED THAT THE DISORDER IN THE SISTERS WAS
GROUPED PIGMENTATION OF THE MACULA AND POINTED TO THE LACK OF FAMILIAL INCIDENCE
IN SEVERAL STUDIES INCLUDING HIS OWN. FURTHERMORE, HE FOUND NO PARENTAL CONSAN-
GUINITY. HE CONCLUDED THAT THE ANOMALY IS THE RESULT OF AN EMBRYONIC ACCIDENT.

CHAN, E.* MELANOSIS RETINAE. CHINESE MED. J. 69* 431-432, 1951.

FORGACS, J. AND BOZIN, I.* MANIFESTATION FAMILIALE DE PIGMENTATIONS GROUPEES DE
LA REGION MACULAIRE. OPHTHALMOLOGICA 152* 364-368, 1966.

FORSIUS, H., ERIKSSON, A., NUUTILA, A., VAINIO-MATTILA, B. AND KRAUSE, U.* A
GENETIC STUDY OF THREE RARE RETINAL DISORDERS* DYSTROPHIA RETINAE DYSACUSIS
SYNDROME, X-CHROMOSOMAL RETINOSCHISIS AND GROUPED PIGMENTS OF THE RETINA. THE
CLINICAL DELINEATION OF BIRTH DEFECTS. VIII. EYE. BALTIMORE* WILLIAMS AND
WILKINS, 1970.

LOEWENSTEIN, A. AND STEEL, J.* SPECIAL CASE OF MELANOSIS FUNDI* BILATERAL
CONGENITAL GROUP PIGMENTATION OF THE CENTRAL AREA. BRIT. J. OPHTHAL. 25* 417-423,
1941.

R
E
C
E
S
S
I
V
E

23390 GYNECOMASTIA, HEREDITARY

SOME FAMILIES SUGGEST AUTOSOMAL RECESSIVE INHERITANCE BECAUSE OF INVOLVEMENT OF
TWO OR MORE BROTHERS WITH BOTH PARENTS NORMAL BUT CONSANGUINEOUS. HOWEVER,
BECAUSE OF MALE LIMITATION THE RECESSIVE PATTERN COULD RESULT BY CHANCE OF
TRANSMISSION THROUGH FEMALES FOR SEVERAL GENERATIONS.

LJUNGBERG, T.* HEREDITARY GYNAECOMASTIA. ACTA MED. SCAND. 168* 371-379, 1960.

*23400 HAGEMAN FACTOR DEFICIENCY

NO SYMPTOMS OCCUR. THE DEFICIENCY IS USUALLY DISCOVERED BECAUSE OF THE PRACTICE
IN SOME HOSPITALS OF ROUTINELY PERFORMING WHOLE BLOOD CLOTTING TIMES BEFORE
SURGICAL OPERATIONS (MCCAIN, CHERNOFF AND GRAHAM, 1959). RATNOFF AND STEINBERG
(1962) ANALYZED DATA ON 55 CASES IN 37 FAMILIES. PARENTAL CONSANGUINITY WAS
PRESENT IN AT LEAST TWO INSTANCES. SOME HETEROZYGOTES SHOW PARTIAL DEFICIENCY.
THE JAPANESE CASE REPORTED BY MIWA ET AL. (1968) HAD FIRST COUSIN PARENTS. JOSSO
AND DE GROUCHY (1968) PRESENTED EVIDENCE THAT THE HAGEMAN LOCUS MAY BE ON THE
SHORT ARM OF A GROUP C CHROMOSOME, PROBABLY NO. 6. EGEBERG (1970) DESCRIBED FOUR
NORWEGIAN FAMILIES WITH DEFICIENT FACTOR XII (ABOUT HALF NORMAL). UNLIKE THE
USUAL EXPERIENCE OF NO ABNORMALITY, THEY SHOWED A SLIGHT TO MODERATE BLEEDING
TENDENCY AND A HIGH INCIDENCE OF CEREBRAL APOPLEXY OCCURRING AT A RELATIVELY EARLY
AGE. SOME OF THE PATIENTS HAD ATTACKS OF LOCAL EDEMA, SEVERE HEADACHE, ABDOMINAL
PAIN AND VARIOUS FORMS OF ALLERGY.

EGEBERG, O.* FACTOR XII DEFECT AND HEMORRHAGE. EVIDENCE FOR A NEW TYPE OF
HEREDITARY HEMOSTATIC DISORDER. THROMB. DIATH. HAEMORRH. 23* 432-440, 1970.

JOSSO, F. AND DE GROUCHY, J.* LOCALISATION PROBABLE D'UN LOCUS HAGEMAN (FACTEUR XII) SUR UN AUTOSOME. ANN. GENET. 11* 95-97, 1968.

MCCAIN, K. F., CHERNOFF, A. I. AND GRAHAM, J. B.* ESTABLISHMENT OF THE INHERITANCE OF HAGEMAN DEFECT AS AN AUTOSOMAL RECESSIVE TRAIT. HEMOPHILIA AND OTHER HEMORRHAGIC STATES. BRINKHOUS, K. M. (ED.)* CHAPEL HILL* UNIVERSITY OF NORTH CAROLINA PRESS, 1959. PP. 179-191.

MIWA, S., ASAI, I., TSUKADA, T., SHIMIZU, M., TERAMURA, K. AND SUNAGA, Y.* HAGEMAN FACTOR DEFICIENCY. REPORT OF A CASE FOUND IN A JAPANESE GIRL. ACTA HAEMAT. 39* 36-41, 1968.

RATNOFF, O. D. AND STEINBERG, A. G.* FURTHER STUDIES ON THE INHERITANCE OF HAGEMAN TRAIT. J. LAB. CLIN. MED. 59* 980-985, 1962.

RATNOFF, O. D., BUSSE, R. J., JR. AND SHEON, R. P.* THE DEMISE OF JOHN HAGEMAN. NEW ENG. J. MED. 279* 760-761, 1968.

THOMPSON, J. H., JR., SPITTEL, J. A., JR., PASCUZZI, C. A. AND OWEN, C. A., JR.* LABORATORY AND GENETIC OBSERVATIONS IN ANOTHER FAMILY WITH HAGEMAN TRAIT. MAYO CLIN. PROC. 35* 421-427, 1960.

23410 HALLERMANN-STREIFF SYNDROME

THIS IS ALSO CALLED THE DYSCEPHALIC SYNDROME OF FRANCOIS. THE FEATURES ARE BIRD-LIKE FACIES WITH HYPOPLASTIC MANDIBLE AND BEAKED NOSE, PROPORTIONAL DWARFISM, HYPOTRICHOSIS, MICROPHTHALMIA AND CONGENITAL CATARACT. TEETH ARE ALREADY PRESENT AT BIRTH. AFFECTED MONOZYGOTIC TWINS AND AFFECTED SIBS ARE KNOWN. SOME OF THE FEATURES SUGGEST BIRD-HEAD DWARFISM (Q.V.). FORSIUS AND DE LA CHAPELLE (1964) FOUND NORMAL CHROMOSOMES IN TWO CASES. THE ONLY REPORTED FAMILIAL CASES MAY BE THOSE OF BUENO (1966) WHO FOUND THIS SYNDROME IN TWO OUT OF THREE SIBS RESULTING FROM A CONSANGUINEOUS MARRIAGE. KARYOTYPES WERE NORMAL. ON THE OTHER HAND FRASER AND FRIEDMANN (1967) SUPPORTED DOMINANT INHERITANCE WITH ALMOST ALL CASES BEING THE RESULT OF FRESH MUTATION. THEY POINTED TO THE PROBABLE CASES IN FATHER AND DAUGHTER REPORTED BY GUYARD ET AL. (1962). DENTAL FEATURES WERE DISCUSSED BY CASPERSEN AND WARBURG (1968).

R
E
C
E
S
S
I
V
E

BUENO, M.* SINDROME DE HALLERMAN-STREIFF-FRANCOIS. A PROPOSITO DE UNA PRESENTACION FAMILIAR. BOLL. SOC. VASCO-NAVARRA 1* 21-35, 1966.

CARONES, A. V.* FRANCOIS'S DYSCEPHALIC SYNDROME. OPHTHALMOLOGICA 142* 510-518, 1961.

CASPERSEN, I. AND WARBURG, M.* HALLERMANN-STREIFF SYNDROME. ACTA OPHTHAL. 46* 385-390, 1968.

FALLS, H. F. AND SCHULL, W. J.* HALLERMANN-STREIFF SYNDROME. A DYSCEPHALY WITH CONGENITAL CATARACTS AND HYPOTRICHOSIS. ARCH. OPHTHAL. 63* 409-420, 1960.

FRASER, G. R. AND FRIEDMANN, A. I.* THE CAUSES OF BLINDNESS IN CHILDHOOD. A STUDY OF 776 CHILDREN WITH SEVERE VISUAL HANDICAPS. BALTIMORE* JOHNS HOPKINS PRESS, 1967. P. 89.

FORSIUS, H. AND DE LA CHAPELLE, A.* DYSCEPHALIA OCULO-MANDIBULO-FACIALIS. TWO CASES IN WHICH THE CHROMOSOMES WERE STUDIED. ANN. PAEDIAT. FENN. 10* 280-287, 1964.

GUYARD, M., PERDRIEL, G. AND CERUTI, F.* ON 2 CASES OF CRANIAL DYSOSTOSIS WITH 'BIRD HEAD.' BULL. SOC. OPHTAL. FRANC. 62* 443-447, 1962.

HOEFNAGEL, D. AND BENIRSCHKE, K.* DYSCEPHALIA MANDIBULO-OCULO-FACIALIS (HALLERMANN-STREIFF SYNDROME). ARCH. DIS. CHILD. 40* 57-61, 1965.

*23420 HALLERVORDEN AND SPATZ, SYNDROME OF

THE ORIGINAL DESCRIPTION BY THE AUTHORS WHOSE NAMES ARE ATTACHED TO THIS SYNDROME CONCERNED A SIBSHIP OF 12 IN WHICH 5 SISTERS SHOWED CLINICALLY INCREASING DYSARTHRIA AND PROGRESSIVE DEMENTIA, AND AT AUTOPSY BROWN DISCOLORATION OF THE GLOBUS PALLIDUS AND SUBSTANTIA NIGRA WAS OBSERVED. FAMILIAL CASES HAVE BEEN REPORTED BY OTHERS AS WELL. ABOUT 30 CASES HAD BEEN REPORTED BY MEYER (1958). CLINICALLY THE CONDITION IS CHARACTERIZED BY PROGRESSIVE RIGIDITY, FIRST IN THE LOWER AND LATER IN THE UPPER EXTREMITIES. AN EQUINOVARUS DEFORMITY OF THE FOOT HAS BEEN THE FIRST SIGN IN SEVERAL CASES. INVOLUNTARY MOVEMENTS OF CHOREIC OR ATHETOID TYPE SOMETIMES PRECEDE OR ACCOMPANY RIGIDITY. BOTH INVOLUNTARY MOVEMENTS AND RIGIDITY MAY INVOLVE MUSCLES SUPPLIED BY CRANIAL NERVES, RESULTING IN DIFFICULTIES IN ARTICULATION AND SWALLOWING. MENTAL DETERIORATION AND EPILEPSY OCCUR IN SOME. ONSET IS IN THE FIRST OR SECOND DECADE AND DEATH USUALLY BEFORE THE AGE OF 30 YEARS.

HALLERVORDEN, J. AND SPATZ, H.* EIGENARTIGE ERKRANKUNG IM EXTRAPYRAMIDALEN SYSTEM MIT BESONDERER BETEILIGUNG DES GLOBUS PALLIDUS UND DER SUBSTANTIA NIGRA. EIN BEITRAG ZU DEN BEZIEHUNGEN ZWISCHEN DIESEN BEIDEN ZENTREN. ZBL. GES. NEUROL.

MEYER, A.* THE HALLERVORDEN-SPATZ SYNDROME. IN, GREENFIELD, J. G. (ED.)* NEUROPATHOLOGY. LONDON* EDWARD ARNOLD LTD., 1958. P. 525 FF.

23430 HALO NEVI (LEUKODERMA ACQUISITUM CENTRIFUGUM OF SUTTON)

CHISA (1965) REPORTED AFFECTED BROTHER AND SISTER AND KOPF, MORRILL AND SILBERBERG (1965) HAD AFFECTED SISTERS.

CHISA, N.* MULTIPLE HALO NEVI IN SIBLINGS. ARCH. DERM. 92* 404-405, 1965.

KOPF, A. W., MORRILL, S. D. AND SILBERBERG, I.* BROAD SPECTRUM OF LEUKODERMA ACQUISITUM CENTRIFUGUM. ARCH. DERM. 92* 14-35, 1965.

*23450 HARTNUP'S DISEASE

FIRST DESCRIBED BY BARON, DENT, HARRIS, HART AND JEPSON (1956), THIS DISORDER IS CHARACTERIZED BY A PELLAGRA-LIKE LIGHT-SENSITIVE RASH, CEREBELLAR ATAXIA, EMOTIONAL INSTABILITY AND AMINOACIDURIA. THE DEFECT INVOLVES THE INTESTINAL AND RENAL TRANSPORT OF CERTAIN NEUTRAL ALPHA-AMINO ACIDS (SCRIVER, 1965). IN THE UNITED STATES, CASES OF THE FULL-BLOWN CLINICAL DISORDER ARE NOT SEEN, PROBABLY BECAUSE OF SUPER-ADEQUATE DIET. POMEROY ET AL. (1968) REPORTED THE FIRST INSTANCE OF AFFECTED PERSONS (ONE MALE, ONE FEMALE) WHO HAD CHILDREN. IN COLOMBIA LOPEZ ET AL. (1969) DESCRIBED TWO AFFECTED BROTHERS WHOSE PARENTS WERE DOUBLE SECOND COUSINS. TWO OTHER DECEASED BROTHERS WERE PROBABLY AFFECTED ALSO. GENETIC HETEROGENEITY PROBABLY EXISTS BECAUSE CASES HAVE BEEN DESCRIBED IN WHICH ONLY THE URINARY CHARACTERISTICS OF HARTNUP'S DISEASE WERE PRESENT, AND NO EVIDENCE OF AN INTESTINAL TRANSPORT DEFECT (SRIKANTIA ET AL., 1964). SEAKINS AND ERSSER (1967) DESCRIBED A PATIENT IN WHOM THE INTESTINAL TRANSPORT DEFECT WAS PARTIALLY EVIDENT ONLY UNDER LOADING CONDITIONS. LYSINE TRANSPORT WAS IMPAIRED, WHEREAS HISTIDINE TRANSPORT WAS NOT.

BARON, D. N., DENT, C. E., HARRIS, H., HART, E. W. AND JEPSON, J. B.* HEREDI-TARY PELLAGRA-LIKE SKIN RASH WITH TEMPORARY CEREBELLAR ATAXIA, CONSTANT RENAL AMINO-ACIDURIA AND OTHER BIZARRE BIOCHEMICAL FEATURES. LANCET 2* 421-433, 1956.

BORRIE, P. F. AND LEWIS, C. A.* HARTNUP DISEASE. PROC. ROY. SOC. MED. 55* 231-232, 1962.

JEPSON, J. B.* HARTNUP DISEASE. IN, STANBURY, J. B., WYNGAARDEN, J. B. AND FREDRICKSON, D. S. (EDS.)* THE METABOLIC BASIS OF INHERITED DISEASES. NEW YORK* MCGRAW-HILL, 1966 (2ND ED.). PP. 1283-1299.

LOPEZ, G. F., VELEZ, A. H. AND TORO, G. G.* HARTNUP DISEASE IN TWO COLOMBIAN SIBLINGS. NEUROLOGY 19* 71-76, 1969.

MILNE, M. D., CRAWFORD, M. A., GIRAO, C. B. AND LOUGHRIDGE, L. W.* THE METABOLIC DISORDER IN HARTNUP DISEASE. QUART. J. MED. 29* 407-421, 1960.

POMEROY, J., EFRON, M. L., DAYMAN, J. AND HOEFNAGEL, D.* HARTNUP DISORDER IN A NEW ENGLAND FAMILY. NEW ENG. J. MED. 278* 1214-1216, 1968.

SCRIVER, C. R.* HARTNUP DISEASE. A GENETIC MODIFICATION OF INTESTINAL AND RENAL TRANSPORT OF CERTAIN NEUTRAL ALPHA-AMINO ACIDS. NEW ENG. J. MED. 273* 530-532, 1965.

SEAKINS, J. W. AND ERSSER, R. S.* EFFECTS OF AMINO ACID LOADS ON A HEALTHY INFANT WITH THE BIOCHEMICAL FEATURES OF HARTNUP DISEASE. ARCH. DIS. CHILD. 42* 682-688, 1967.

SRIKANTIA, S. G., VENKATACHALAM, P. S. AND REDDY, V.* CLINICAL AND BIOCHEMICAL FEATURES OF A CASE OF HARTNUP DISEASE. BRIT. MED. J. 1* 282-285, 1964.

23460 HEART BLOCK AND OPHTHALMOPLEGIA

ROSS ET AL. (1969) DESCRIBED THE ASSOCIATION OF CHRONIC PROGRESSIVE EXTERNAL OPHTHALMOPLEGIA AND COMPLETE HEART BLOCK AND NOTED FOUR EARLIER REPORTS OF THE SAME. APPARENTLY NO FAMILIAL CASES HAVE BEEN REPORTED. ROSENBERG ET AL. (1968) REVIEWED SYNDROMES INVOLVING OPHTHALMOPLEGIA.

ROSENBERG, R. N., SCHOTLAND, D. L., LOVELACE, R. E. AND ROWLAND, L. P.* PROGRESSIVE OPHTHALMOPLEGIA* REPORT OF CASES. ARCH. NEUROL. 19* 362-376, 1968.

ROSS, A., LIPSCHUTZ, D., AUSTIN, J. AND SMITH, J., JR.* EXTERNAL OPHTHALMOPLE-GIA AND COMPLETE HEART BLOCK. NEW ENG. J. MED. 280* 313-315, 1969.

*23470 HEART BLOCK, CONGENITAL

A RATHER LARGE NUMBER OF FAMILIES WITH MULTIPLE AFFECTED SIBS AND NORMAL PARENTS HAVE BEEN REPORTED. LATTA AND CRITTENDEN (1964) STUDIED THE HEARTS OF TWO SIBS (THE 7TH AND 8TH OFFSPRING) WHO DIED NEONATALLY OF CONGENITAL HEART BLOCK. IN

NEITHER WAS AN ATRIOVENTRICULAR NODE FOUND, NOR WERE MYOCARDIAL FIBERS PRESENT IN THE LOWER PART OF THE INTERATRIAL SEPTUM. BOTH HEARTS SHOWED FOCI OF CALCIFICATION, FIBROSIS, INCREASED VASCULARIZATION AND A FEW SMALL ACCUMULATIONS OF INFLAMMATORY CELLS. THUS, FETAL INFECTION COULD HAVE BEEN RESPONSIBLE. IN ANOTHER FAMILY CRITTENDEN, LATTA AND TICINOVICH (1964) DESCRIBED FOUR OF EIGHT SIBS WITH CONGENITAL HEART BLOCK. A FIFTH MAY HAVE BEEN AFFECTED. ONE DIED AT AGE 14 AND THE OTHERS DIED IN THE NEONATAL PERIOD. THE PARENTS WERE NORMAL AND OF CZECHOSLOVAKIAN ANCESTRY. NO MENTION OF CONSANGUINITY WAS MADE.

AYLWARD, R. D.* CONGENITAL HEART-BLOCK. THE OCCURRENCE OF TWO CASES OF CONGENITAL HEART-BLOCK IN ONE FAMILY IS SO UNUSUAL AS TO DESERVE BEING PLACED ON RECORD. BRIT. MED. J. 1* 943 ONLY, 1928.

CRITTENDEN, I. H., LATTA, H. AND TICINOVICH, D. A.* FAMILIAL CONGENITAL HEART BLOCK. AM. J. DIS. CHILD. 108* 104-108, 1964.

LATTA, H. AND CRITTENDEN, I. H.* ACQUIRED LESIONS OF THE CONDUCTION SYSTEM IN FAMILIAL CONGENITAL HEART BLOCK. LAB. INVEST. 13* 214-221, 1964.

LYNCH, R. J. AND ENGLE, M. A.* FAMILIAL CONGENITAL COMPLETE HEART BLOCK. AM. J. DIS. CHILD. 102* 210-217, 1961.

OSLER, W.* ON THE SO-CALLED STOKES-ADAMS DISEASE (SLOW PULSE WITH SYNCOPAL ATTACKS). LANCET 2* 516-524, 1903.

WALLGREN, G. AND AGORIO, E.* CONGENITAL COMPLETE A-V BLOCK IN THREE SIBLINGS. ACTA PAEDIAT. 49* 49-56, 1960.

23480 HEMANGIOMATOSIS, CUTANEOUS, WITH ASSOCIATED FEATURES

GLUSZCZ, POLIS AND WALESZKOWSKI (1963) DESCRIBED FOUR SIBS WITH CUTANEOUS HEMANGIOMATOSIS, ACROCYANOSIS, HYPERFLEXIBILITY OF JOINTS AND PHIMOSIS. SOME SHOWED SLIGHT ABNORMALITIES OF THE VERTEBRAL BODIES AND OCULAR HYPERTELORISM. IN TWO (A FEMALE AGE 15 AND A MALE AGE 19) TUMORS RESEMBLING CEREBELLAR ANGIOBLASTOMA OF VON HIPPEL-LINDAU'S DISEASE WERE REMOVED FROM THE CERVICO-THORACIC PORTION OF THE SPINAL CANAL.

R
E
C
E
S
S
I
V
E

GLUSZCZ, A., POLIS, Z. AND WALESZKOWSKI, J.* FAMILIAL SYNDROME OF GENERAL DYSPLASIA OF THE CONNECTIVE TISSUE AND OF THE VASCULAR SYSTEM ASSOCIATED WITH ANGIOBLASTOMA OF THE SPINAL CANAL. POL. MED. J. 2* 924-936, 1963.

*23490 HEMERALOPIA, ESSENTIAL, WITH HIGH GRADE MYOPIA

GASSLER'S INSTRUCTIVE PEDIGREE OF AN INBRED SWISS KINDRED (1925) WITH NIGHT BLINDNESS AND MYOPIA IS REPRODUCED BY FRANCOIS (1961). (THE TERM HEMERALOPIA WHICH LITERALLY MEANS 'DAY BLINDNESS,' IS A MISNOMER. NYCTALOPIA IS THE PROPER TERM.)

FRANCOIS, J.* HEREDITY IN OPHTHALMOLOGY. ST. LOUIS* C. V. MOSBY CO., 1961. P. 400, FIG. 368.

GASSLER, V. J.* UBER EINE BIS JETZT NICHT BEKANNTE RECESSIVE VERKNUPFUNG VON HOCHGRADIGER MYOPIE MIT ANGEBORENER HEMERALOPIE. ARCH. KLAUS STIFT. VERERBUNGS-FORSCH. 1* 259-272, 1925.

23500 HEMIHYPERTROPHY

FRAUMENI ET AL. (1967) DESCRIBED AFFECTED BROTHER AND SISTER AND RECORDED THAT THEIR MATERNAL UNCLE WAS SAID TO HAVE HAD ONE LEG LONGER THAN THE OTHER SINCE CHILDHOOD. THEY REVIEWED 6 OTHER EXAMPLES OF FAMILIAL OCCURRENCE. THESE INCLUDED INSTANCES OF SUCCESSIVE GENERATIONS AFFECTED.

FRAUMENI, J. F., JR., GEISER, C. F. AND MANNING, M. D.* WILMS' TUMOR AND CONGENITAL HEMIHYPERTROPHY* REPORT OF FIVE NEW CASES AND REVIEW OF LITERATURE. PEDIATRICS 40* 886-899, 1967.

23510 HEMOCHROMATOSIS, IDIOPATHIC NEONATAL (OR PERINATAL) GIANT CELL HEPATITIS

FEINBERG (1960) REPORTED TWO PAIRS OF MALE SIBS AND LAURENDEAU, HILL AND MANNING (1961) OBSERVED TWO AFFECTED SISTERS. THE DISORDER IS SOMETIMES LOOSELY LABELED 'NEONATAL HEPATITIS.'

FEINBERG, R.* PERINATAL IDIOPATHIC HEMOCHROMATOSIS* GIANT CELL HEPATITIS INTERPRETED AS AN INBORN ERROR OF METABOLISM. AM. J. CLIN. PATH. 33* 480-491, 1960.

LAURENDEAU, T., HILL, J. E. AND MANNING, G. B.* IDIOPATHIC NEONATAL HEMOCHROMATOSIS IN SIBLINGS. AN INBORN ERROR OF METABOLISM. ARCH. PATH. 72* 410-423, 1961.

*23520 HEMOCHROMATOSIS, JUVENILE

DEBRE AND COLLEAGUES (1958) CONCLUDED THAT THE BIOCHEMICAL DEFECT OF IDIOPATHIC

HEMOCHROMATOSIS IS PRESENT IN HETEROZYGOTES AND THAT WHETHER THE DISEASE DEVELOPS IS DEPENDENT ON OTHER INFLUENCES ON IRON METABOLISM. THEY SUGGEST THAT JUVENILE HEMOCHROMATOSIS RESULTING FROM CONSANGUINEOUS MARRIAGES MAY REPRESENT THE HOMOZYGOUS STATE OF THE GENE. THE PEDIGREE OF NUSSBAUMER, PLATTNER AND RYWLIN (1952) IS REPRODUCED BY SORSBY (1953). THE INHERITANCE OF THE USUAL ADULT HEMOCHROMATOSIS IS PROBABLY DOMINANT (WILLIAMS, SCHEUER, SHERLOCK, 1962).

DEBRE, R., DREYFUS, J.-C., FREZAL, J., LABIE, D., LAMY, M., MAROTEAUX, P., SCHAPIRA, F. AND SCHAPIRA, G.* GENETICS OF HAEMOCHROMATOSIS. ANN. HUM. GENET. 23* 16-30, 1958.

FELTS, J. H., NELSON, J. R., HERNDON, C. N. AND SPURR, C. L.* HEMOCHROMATOSIS IN TWO YOUNG SISTERS. CASE STUDIES AND A FAMILY SURVEY. ANN. INTERN. MED. 67* 117-123, 1967.

NUSSBAUMER, T., PLATTNER, H. C. AND RYWLIN, A.* HEMOCHROMATOSE JUVENILE CHEZ TROIS SOEURS ET UN FRERE AVEC CONSANGUINITE DES PARENTS* ETUDE ANATOMOCLINIQUE ET GENETIQUE DU SYNDROME ENDOCRINOHEPATO-MYOCARDIQUE. J. GENET. HUM. 1* 53-59, 1952.

SORSBY, A. (ED.)* CLINICAL GENETICS. ST. LOUIS* C. V. MOSBY CO., 1953. P. 206.

WILLIAMS, R., SCHEUER, P. J. AND SHERLOCK, S.* THE INHERITANCE OF IDIOPATHIC HAEMOCHROMATOSIS. A CLINICAL AND LIVER BIOPSY STUDY OF 16 FAMILIES. QUART. J. MED. 31* 249-265, 1962.

23530 HEMOGLOBIN A2, COMPLETE ABSENCE OF

THIS OCCURS IN THE HOMOZYGOTE FOR THE *PERSISTENT FETAL HEMOGLOBIN GENE,* FOR THE HB LEPORE GENE, OR FOR THE DELTA THALASSEMIA GENE.

23540 HEMOLYTIC-UREMIC SYNDROME

IN TWO SISTERS, HAGGE AND COLLEAGUES (1967) FOUND INTRAVASCULAR HEMOLYSIS, THROMBOCYTOPENIA AND AZOTEMIA. REPEATED ATTACKS ENDING IN RENAL FAILURE AND DEATH AT AGE 8 YEARS. THE SECOND RECOVERED COMPLETELY AFTER ONE ATTACK. CONCORDANT MONOZYGOTIC TWINS HAVE ALSO BEEN REPORTED (CAMPBELL AND CARRE, 1965). THE FEATURES ARE ACUTE RENAL FAILURE, THROMBOCYTOPENIA AND HEMOLYTIC ANEMIA ASSOCIATED WITH DISTORTED ERYTHROCYTES (*BURR CELLS*). GIANANTONIO ET AL. (1968) OBSERVED 75 CASES IN ARGENTINA WHERE THE DISORDER SEEMS UNUSUALLY FREQUENT AND ASSEMBLED SOME EVIDENCE FOR VIRAL ETIOLOGY. AT ANY RATE MENDELIAN INHERITANCE OF A SIGNIFICANT PROPORTION OF CASES SEEMS VERY UNLIKELY. CHAN ET AL. (1969) FOUND THE DISORDER IN TWO ADOPTED, UNRELATED SIBS.

RECESSIVE

CAMPBELL, S. AND CARRE, I. J.* FATAL HAEMOLYTIC URAEMIC SYNDROME AND IDIOPATHIC HYPERLIPAEMIA IN MONOZYGOTIC TWINS. ARCH. DIS. CHILD. 40* 654-658, 1965.

CHAN, J. C. M., ELEFF, M. G. AND CAMPBELL, R. A.* THE HEMOLYTIC-UREMIC SYNDROME IN NONRELATED ADOPTED SIBLINGS. J. PEDIAT. 75* 1050-1053, 1969.

GIANANTONIO, C. A., VITACCO, M., MENDILAHARZU, F. AND GALLO, G.* THE HEMOLYTIC-UREMIC SYNDROME. RENAL STATUS OF 76 PATIENTS AT LONG-TERM FOLLOW-UP. J. PEDIAT. 72* 757-765, 1968.

HAGGE, W. W., HOLLEY, K. E., BURKE, E. C. AND STICKLER, G. B.* HEMOLYTIC-UREMIC SYNDROME IN TWO SIBLINGS. NEW ENG. J. MED. 277* 138-139, 1967.

23550 HEMOSIDEROSIS, PULMONARY, WITH DEFICIENCY OF GAMMA-A GLOBULIN

IDIOPATHIC PULMONARY HEMOSIDEROSIS HAS NOT BEEN SHOWN TO BE FAMILIAL. THAT A GENERALIZED DYSFUNCTION OF THE MACROPHAGES SYSTEM MAY BE INVOLVED IN SOME CASES - AND THAT THE DEFECT MAY BE GENETICALLY DETERMINED - IS SUGGESTED BY THE FINDING IN SOME CASES OF DEFICIENCY OF GAMMA-A GLOBULIN AND OF HISTOLOGIC ALTERATIONS IN THE LYMPHORETICULAR ORGANS COMPATIBLE WITH AN IMMUNE DEFICIENCY DISORDER.

KRIEGER, I. AND BROUGH, J. A.* GAMMA-A DEFICIENCY AND HYPOCHROMIC ANEMIA DUE TO DEFECTIVE IRON MOBILIZATION. NEW ENG. J. MED. 276* 886-894, 1967.

*23560 HERMAPHRODITISM, TRUE

MILNER ET AL. (1958) REPORTED TWO *BROTHERS* WHO HAD HYPOSPADIAS AND BOTH TESTICULAR AND OVARIAN TISSUE BILATERALLY. FAMILIAL CASES HAVE ALSO BEEN REPORTED BY ROSENBERG, CLAYTON AND HSU (1963), WHO FOUND A NORMAL FEMALE KARYOTYPE IN SEVERAL TISSUES EXAMINED.

MILNER, W. A., GARLICK, W. B., FINK, A. J. AND STEIN, A. A.* TRUE HERMAPHRODITE SIBLINGS. J. UROL. 79* 1003-1009, 1958.

ROSENBERG, H. S., CLAYTON, G. W. AND HSU, T. C.* FAMILIAL TRJE HERMAPHRODISM. J. CLIN. ENDOCR. 23* 203-206, 1963.

*23570 HEXOKINASE DEFICIENCY HEMOLYTIC ANEMIA

VALENTINE ET AL. (1967) DESCRIBED A CHILD WITH ANEMIA PRESENT FROM BIRTH AND DEFICIENCY OF RED CELL HEXOKINASE. THE FATHER AND ONE SIB HAD LOW LEVELS. THE MOTHER'S LEVEL WAS ALSO LOW BUT WITHIN THE RANGE OF NORMAL. THE DEFICIENCY APPARENTLY DID NOT INVOLVE LEUKOCYTES AND PLATELETS AND IS DIFFERENT FROM THE HEXOKINASE DEFICIENCY IDENTIFIED IN FANCONI'S PANCYTOPENIA (Q.V.).

KEITT, A. S.* HEMOLYTIC ANEMIA WITH IMPAIRED HEXOKINASE ACTIVITY. J. CLIN. INVEST. 48* 1997-2007, 1969.

VALENTINE, W. N., OSKI, F. A., PAGLIA, D. E., BAUGHAN, M. A., SCHNEIDER, A. S. AND NAIMAN, J. L.* HEREDITARY HEMOLYTIC ANEMIA WITH HEXOKINASE DEFICIENCY. ROLE OF HEXOKINASE IN ERYTHROCYTE AGING. NEW ENG. J. MED. 276* 1-11, 1967.

*23575 HEXOSEPHOSPHATE ISOMERASE DEFICIENCY HEMOLYTIC ANEMIA

PAGLIA ET AL. (1969) FOUND DEFICIENCY OF RED CELL AND LEUKOCYTE GLUCOSEPHOSPHATE ISOMERASE IN 3 SIBS WITH HEMOLYTIC ANEMIA. THE ANEMIA WAS AMELIORATED BY SPLENECTOMY. HETEROZYGOTES COULD BE IDENTIFIED

PAGLIA, D. E., HOLLAND, P., BAUGHAN, M. A. AND VALENTINE, W. N.* OCCURRENCE OF DEFECTIVE HEXOSEPHOSPHATE ISOMERIZATION IN HUMAN ERYTHROCYTES AND LEUKOCYTES. NEW ENG. J. MED. 280* 66-71, 1969.

*23580 HISTIDINEMIA

A FALSE POSITIVE FERRIC CHLORIDE URINE TEST FOR PHENYLKETONURIA OCCURS IN THESE CASES. OF NOTE IS THE OCCURRENCE OF A PIN-POINTED CEREBRAL DEFECT INVOLVING SPEECH. A MAJORITY OF CASES SHOW RETARDATION, HOWEVER, AND TREATMENT WITH HISTIDINE-RESTRICTION IS WORTHWHILE IN THE OPINION OF WADMAN ET AL. (1967). THE CASES REPORTED BY WOODY ET AL. (1965) HAD A PARTIAL HISTIDASE DEFICIENCY, INDICATING HETEROGENEITY IN THIS CONDITION. ROSENBLATT ET AL. (1970) DESCRIBED HISTIDINEMIA DISCOVERED IN A 17 YEAR OLD FRENCH-CANADIAN GIRL AFTER RENAL TRANSPLANT FOR CHRONIC GLOMERULONEPHRITIS. THE HISTIDASE ACTIVITY OF THE TRANSPLANTED KIDNEY WAS NOT ADEQUATE TO CORRECT THE METABOLIC DEFECT.

AUERBACH, V. H., DIGEORGE, A. M., BALDRIDGE, R. C., TOURTELLOTTE, C. D. AND BRIGHAM, M. P.* HISTIDINEMIA* A DEFICIENCY IN HISTIDASE RESULTING IN THE URINARY EXCRETION OF HISTIDINE AND OF IMIDAZOLEPYRUVIC ACID. J. PEDIAT. 60* 487-497, 1962.

LA DU, B. N.* HISTIDINEMIA* CURRENT STATUS. AM. J. DIS. CHILD. 113* 88-92, 1967.

LA DU, B. N., HOWELL, R. R., JACOBY, G. A., SEEGMILLER, J. E., SOBER, E. K., ZANNONI, V. G., CANBY, J. P. AND ZIEGLER, L. K.* CLINICAL AND BIOCHEMICAL STUDIES ON TWO CASES OF HISTIDINEMIA. PEDIATRICS 32* 216-227, 1963.

ROSENBLATT, D., MOHYUDDIN, F. AND SCRIVER, C. R.* HISTIDINEMIA DISCOVERED BY URINE SCREENING AFTER RENAL TRANSPLANTATION. PEDIATRICS 46* 47-53, 1970.

WADMAN, S. K., VAN SPRANG, F. J., VAN STEKELENBURG, G. K. AND DE BREE, P. K.* THREE NEW CASES OF HISTIDINEMIA. CLINICAL AND BIOCHEMICAL DATA. ACTA PAEDIAT. SCAND. 56* 485-492, 1967.

WOODY, N. C., SNYDER, C. H. AND HARRIS, J. A.* HISTIDINEMIA. AM. J. DIS. CHILD. 110* 606-613, 1965.

*23590 HISTIOCYTOSIS, FAMILIAL LIPOCHROME

IN THREE SISTERS IN A SIBSHIP OF 9 FORD AND COLLEAGUES (1962) OBSERVED LIPOCHROME GRANULATION OF THE HISTIOCYTES, PULMONARY INFILTRATION, HYPERGLOBULINEMIA, TRANSIENT POLYARTHRITIS AND SUSCEPTIBILITY TO INFECTION. NO ABNORMALITY WAS SEEN IN PLASMA CELLS OR LYMPHOCYTES. THE HYPERGLOBULINEMIA INVOLVED GAMMA- AND ALPHA (2)-GLOBULINS. THE AUTHORS SUGGESTED THAT THE PRIMARY DEFECT CAUSED THE LIPOCH-ROME DEPOSITION AND THAT THE OTHER FEATURES WERE SECONDARY TO THE DEPOSITS. THE AGES OF THE SISTERS WERE 26, 21 AND 16 YEARS. PINCUS AND KLEBANOFF (1971) DEMONSTRATED A DEFECT IN THE CONVERSION OF IODIDE TO A TRICHLOROACETIC-ACID-PRECIPITABLE FORM BY PHAGOCYTIZING LEUKOCYTES. A DEFECT WAS ALSO SHOWN IN CHRONIC GRANULOMATOUS DISEASE AND IN MYELOPEROXIDASE DEFICIENCY BUT NOT IN JOB'S SYNDROME.

FORD, D. K., PRICE, G. E., CULLING, C. F. A. AND VASSAR, P. S.* FAMILIAL LIPOCHROME PIGMENTATION OF HISTIOCYTES WITH HYPERGLOBULINEMIA, PULMONARY INFILTRA-TION, SPLENOMEGALY, ARTHRITIS AND SUSCEPTIBILITY TO INFECTION. AM. J. MED. 33* 478-489, 1962.

PINCUS, S. H. AND KLEBANOFF, S. J.* QUANTITATIVE LEUKOCYTE IODINATION. NEW ENG. J. MED. 284* 744-750, 1971.

23600 HODGKIN'S DISEASE

MANIGAND AND COLLEAGUES (1964) DESCRIBED A BROTHER AND SISTER WITH HODGKIN'S DISEASE AND REVIEWED THE LITERATURE ON FAMILIAL OCCURRENCE.

R
E
C
E
S
S
I
V
E

*23610 HOLOPROSENCEPHALY, FAMILIAL ALOBAR (ARHINENCEPHALY)

DEMYER, ZEMAN AND PALMER (1963) DESCRIBED TWO SISTERS WITH ALOBAR HOLOPROSENCEPHA-
LY ASSOCIATED WITH MEDIAN CLEFT LIP AND PALATE. A PATERNAL AUNT MAY HAVE BEEN
IDENTICALLY AFFECTED. CHROMOSOMES WERE NORMAL. HOLOPROSENCEPHALY WITH A
DIFFERENT ARRAY OF EXTRA-CEPHALIC MALFORMATIONS OCCURS WITH 13-15 TRISOMY. HINTZ
ET AL. (1968) ALSO OBSERVED AFFECTED SIBS. COHEN AND GORLIN (1969) DESCRIBED A
CHIPPEWA INDIAN SIBSHIP IN WHICH ONE SIB HAD CYCLOPIA AND FOUR OTHERS HAD CLEFT
LIP AND-OR PALATE. THE PARENTS WERE RELATED. CONSANGUINITY WAS ALSO NOTED IN THE
CASES OF KLOPSTOCK (1921) AND GREBE (1954). DEMYER (1963) POINTED OUT THAT THERE
IS A SPECTRUM OF HOLOPROSENCEPHALIC DISORDERS REPRESENTING IMPAIRED MIDLINE
CLEAVAGE OF THE EMBRYONIC FOREBRAIN. IN CYCLOPIA, THE MOST EXTREME FORM, A SINGLE
EYE GLOBE WITH VARYING DEGREES OF DOUBLING OF INTRINSIC OCULAR STRUCTURES, ARHINIA
AND A BLIND-ENDING PROBOSCIS LOCATED ABOVE THE MEDIAN EYE ARE FOUND. IN ETHMOCE-
PHALY THE FEATURES ARE EXTREME ORBITAL HYPOTELORISM, ARHINIA, AND A BLIND-ENDED
PROBOSCIS LOCATED BETWEEN THE EYES. IN CEBOCEPHALY, ORBITAL HYPOTELORISM IS
ASSOCIATED WITH SINGLE-NOSTRIL NOSE. PREMAXILLARY AGENESIS IS CHARACTERIZED BY A
MEDIAN PSEUDOCLEFT, AGENESIS OF NASAL BONES AND PRIMARY PALATE, AND OCULAR
HYPOTELORISM. ALOBAR HOLOPROSENCEPHALY, CEBOCEPHALY, AND PREMAXILLARY AGENESIS.
ELLIS (1865) REPORTED TWINS WITH CYCLOPS. KLOPSTOCK (1921) REPORTED TWO BROTHERS.
THREE CHILDREN WERE AFFECTED IN THE FAMILY REPORTED BY DOMINOK AND KIRCHMAIR
(1961). PFITZER AND MUNTEFERING (1968) OBSERVED 4 AFFECTED CHILDREN WHOSE MOTHERS
WERE RELATIVES AND HAD THE SAME ANOMALOUS KARYOTYPE, THOUGHT TO REPRESENT BALANCED
TRANSLOCATION. DALLAIRE ET AL. (1971) DESCRIBED MULTIPLE AFFECTED PERSONS IN
SEVERAL DIFFERENT SIBSHIPS OF A FRENCH-CANADIAN KINDRED.

COHEN, M. M., JR. AND GORLIN, R. J.* GENETIC CONSIDERATIONS IN A SIBSHIP OF
CYCLOPIA AND CLEFTS. THE CLINICAL DELINEATION OF BIRTH DEFECTS. II. MALFORMA-
TION SYNDROMES. NEW YORK* NATIONAL FOUNDATION, 1969. PP. 113-118.

DALLAIRE, L., FRASER, F. C. AND WIGLESWORTH, F. W.* FAMILIAL HOLOPROSENCEPHALY.
THE CLINICAL DELINEATION OF BIRTH DEFECTS. XI. OROFACIAL STRUCTURES. BALTIMORE*
WILLIAMS AND WILKINS, 1971.

DEMYER, W., ZEMAN, W. AND PALMER, C. D.* FAMILIAL ALOBAR HOLOPROSENCEPHALY
(ARHINENCEPHALY) WITH MEDIAN CLEFT LIP AND PALATE. REPORT OF PATIENT WITH 46
CHROMOSOMES. NEUROLOGY 13* 913-918, 1963.

DOMINOK, G. W. AND KIRCHMAIR, H.* FAMILIAL INCIDENCE OF MALFORMATIONS OF THE
ARHINENCEPHALIA GROUP. Z. KINDERHEILK. 85* 19-30, 1961.

ELLIS, R.* ON A RARE FORM OF TWIN MONSTROSITY. TRANS. OBSTET. SOC. 7* 160-164,
1865.

GREBE, H.* FAMILIENBEFUNDE BEI LATALEN ANOMALIEN DER KORPERFORM. ACTA. GENET.
MED. GEM. 3* 93-111, 1954.

HINTZ, R. L., MENKING, M. AND SOTOS, J. F.* FAMILIAL HOLOPROSENCEPHALY WITH
ENDOCRINE DYSGENESIS. J. PEDIAT. 72* 81-87, 1968.

KLOPSTOCK, A.* FAMILIARES VORKOMMEN VON CYKLOPIE UND ARRHINENCEPHALIE. MSCHR.
GEBURTSH. GYNAK. 56* 59-71, 1921.

PFITZER, P. AND MUNTEFERING, H.* CYCLOPISM AS A HEREDITARY MALFORMATION.
NATURE 217* 1071-1072, 1968.

*23620 HOMOCYSTINURIA

THIS DISORDER WAS DISCOVERED IN 1962, INDEPENDENTLY BY GERRITSEN, VAUGHN AND
WAISMAN IN MADISON, WIS., AND BY CARSON ET AL. IN BELFAST, NORTHERN IRELAND. THE
PATIENTS OF BOTH GROUPS WERE STUDIED BECAUSE OF MENTAL RETARDATION. IT IS NOW
KNOWN THAT ABOUT ONE-THIRD OF SUBJECTS HAVE NORMAL INTELLIGENCE. ECTOPIA LENTIS
IS A CONSTANT FEATURE IN PATIENTS OVER AGE 10 BUT BECAUSE OF ITS PROGRESSIVE
NATURE MAY BE ABSENT IN YOUNGER PATIENTS. SKELETAL FEATURES SUGGESTING MARFAN
SYNDROME, GENERALIZED OSTEOPOROSIS AND THROMBOTIC LESIONS OF ARTERIES AND VEINS
ARE OTHER FEATURES. METHIONINE AS WELL AS HOMOCYSTINE IS ELEVATED IN THE URINE.
THE DEFECT CONCERNS CYSTATHIONINE SYNTHETASE. SEE SULFO-CYSTEINURIA. THE
DISORDER HAS BEEN OBSERVED IN JAPAN (TADA ET AL., 1967) AND IN PERSONS OF MANY
DIFFERENT ETHNIC EXTRACTIONS LIVING IN THE UNITED STATES (SCHIMKE ET AL., 1965).
SPAETH AND BARBOUR (1967) DESCRIBED A SILVER-NITROPRUSSIDE TEST WHICH IS ALMOST
COMPLETELY SPECIFIC FOR HOMOCYSTINE. UHLENDORF AND MUDD (1968) FOUND THAT
FIBROBLASTS DERIVED FROM SKIN AND CELLS IN AMNIOTIC FLUID, GROWN IN TISSUE
CULTURE, HAVE CYSTATHIONINE SYNTHETASE ACTIVITY, ALTHOUGH THE ENZYME IS NOT
DETECTABLE IN INTACT NORMAL SKIN. FIBROBLASTS GROWN FROM THE SKIN OF HOMOCYS-
TINURIC PERSONS ARE DEFICIENT IN THE ENZYME. THE OBSERVATIONS OF RATNOFF (1968)
MAY HAVE BEARING ON THE MECHANISM OF THE THROMBOTIC ACCIDENTS. CAREY ET AL.
(1968) POINTED OUT THAT 27 CASES HAD BEEN FOUND IN IRELAND. CAREY ET AL. (1968)
SUGGESTED THAT FOLIC ACID IN PHARMACOLOGIC DOSES IS THERAPEUTICALLY VALUABLE IN
THIS DISEASE. DECREASE IN URINARY EXCRETION OF HOMOCYSTINE AND INCREASE IN

R
E
C
E
S
S
I
V
E

METHIONINE WAS NOTED DURING TREATMENT. KELLY AND COPELAND (1968) SUGGEST THAT THERE IS AN ALTERNATIVE PATHWAY FOR METABOLISM OF HOMOCYSTEINE THROUGH HOMOLAN-THIONINE.

BARBER, G. W. AND SPAETH, G. L.* PYRIDOXINE THERAPY IN HOMOCYSTINURIA. (LETTER) LANCET 1* 337 ONLY, 1967.

CAREY, M. C., DONOVAN, D. E., FITZGERALD, O. AND MCAULEY, F. D.* HOMOCYS-TINURIA. A CLINICAL AND PATHOLOGICAL STUDY OF NINE SUBJECTS IN SIX FAMILIES. AM. J. MED. 45* 7-25, 1968.

CAREY, M. C., FENNELLY, J. J. AND FITZGERALD, O.* HOMOCYSTINURIA. II. SUBNORMAL SERUM FOLATE LEVELS, INCREASED FOLATE CLEARANCE AND EFFECTS OF FOLIC ACID THERAPY. AM. J. MED. 45* 26-31, 1968.

CARSON, N. A. J. AND NEILL, D. W.* METABOLIC ABNORMALITIES DETECTED IN A SURVEY OF MENTALLY BACKWARD INDIVIDUALS IN NORTHERN IRELAND. ARCH. DIS. CHILD. 37* 505-513, 1962.

CARSON, N. A. J., CUSWORTH, D. C., DENT, C. E., FIELD, C. M. B., NEILL, D. W. AND WESTALL, R. G.* HOMOCYSTINURIA* A NEW INBORN ERROR OF METABOLISM ASSOCIATED WITH MENTAL DEFICIENCY. ARCH. DIS. CHILD. 38* 425-436, 1963.

FIELD, C. M. B., CARSON, N. A. J., CUSWORTH, D. C., DENT, C. E. AND NEILL, D. W.* HOMOCYSTINURIA, A NEW DISORDER OF METABOLISM. (ABSTRACT) PROC. 10TH INTERN. CONGR. PEDIAT., LISBON, 1962. PP. 274-275.

FRIMPTER, G. W.* HOMOCYSTINURIA* VITAMIN B6 DEPENDENT OR NOT.Q (EDITORIAL) ANN. INTERN. MED. 71* 209-211, 1969.

GERRITSEN, T., VAUGHN, J. G. AND WAISMAN, H. A.* THE IDENTIFICATION OF HOMOCYSTINE IN THE URINE. BIOCHEM. BIOPHYS. RES. COMMUN. 9* 493-496, 1962.

HOOFT, C., CARTON, D. AND SAMYN, W.* PYRIDOXINE TREATMENT IN HOMOCYSTINURIA. (LETTER) LANCET 1* 1384 ONLY, 1967.

KAESER, A. C., RODNIGHT, R. AND ELLIS, B. A.* PSYCHIATRIC AND BIOCHEMICAL ASPECTS OF A CASE OF HOMOCYSTINURIA. J. NEUROL. NEUROSURG. PSYCHIAT. 32* 88-93, 1969.

KELLY, S. AND COPELAND, W.* PRELIMINARY REPORT* A HYPOTHESIS IN THE HOMOCYS-TINURIC'S RESPONSE TO PYRIDOXINE. METABOLISM 17* 794-795, 1968.

KOMROWER, G. M.* DIETARY TREATMENT OF HOMOCYSTINURIA. AM. J. DIS. CHILD. 113* 98-100, 1967.

MCCULLY, K. S. AND RAGSDALE, B. D.* PRODUCTION OF ARTERIOSCLEROSIS BY HOMOCYS-TINURIA. AM. J. PATH. 61* 1-12, 1970.

MUDD, S. H., EDWARDS, W. A., LOEB, P. M., BROWN, M. S. AND LASTER, L.* HOMOCYSTINURIA DUE TO CYSTATHIONINE SYNTHASE DEFICIENCY* THE EFFECT OF PYRIDOXINE. J. CLIN. INVEST. 49* 1762-1773, 1970.

MUDD, S. H., LEVY, H. L., ABELES, R. H.* A DERANGEMENT IN B12 METABOLISM LEADING TO HOMOCYSTINEMIA, CYSTATHIONINEMIA AND METHYLMALONIC ACIDURIA. BIOCHEM. BIOPHYS. RES. COMMUN. 35* 121-126, 1969.

PERRY, T. L., HANSEN, S., LOVE, D. L., CRAWFORD, L. E. AND TISCHLER, B.* TREATMENT OF HOMOCYSTINURIA WITH A LOW-METHIONINE DIET, SUPPLEMENTAL CYSTINE AND A METHYL DONOR. LANCET 2* 474-478, 1968.

RATNOFF, O. D.* ACTIVATION OF HAGEMAN FACTOR BY L-HOMOCYSTINE. SCIENCE 162* 1007-1009, 1968.

SCHIMKE, R. N., MCKUSICK, V. A., HUANG, T. AND POLLACK, A. D.* HOMOCYSTINURIA* STUDIES OF 20 FAMILIES WITH 38 AFFECTED MEMBERS. J.A.M.A. 193* 711-719, 1965.

SHIH, V. E. AND EFRON, M. L.* PYRIDOXINE-UNRESPONSIVE HOMOCYSTINURIA. FINAL DIAGNOSIS OF MGH CASE 19471, 1933. NEW ENG. J. MED. 283* 1206-1208, 1970.

SHIPMAN, R. T., TOWNLEY, R. R. W. AND DANKS, D. M.* HOMOCYSTINURIA, ADDISONIAN PERNICIOUS ANAEMIA, AND PARTIAL DELETION OF A G CHROMOSOME. LANCET 2* 693-694, 1969.

SPAETH, G. L. AND BARBER, G. W.* PREVALENCE OF HOMOCYSTEINURIA AMONG THE MENTALLY RETARDED* EVALUATION OF A SPECIFIC SCREENING TEST. PEDIATRICS 40* 586-589, 1967.

TADA, K., YOSHIDA, T., HIRONO, H. AND ARAKAWA, T.* HOMOCYSTINURIA* AMINO ACID PATTERN OF THE LIVER. TOHOKU J. EXP. MED. 92* 325-332, 1967.

UHLENDORF, B. W. AND MUDD, S. H.* CYSTATHIONINE SYNTHASE IN TISSUE CULTURE

RECESSIVE

WONG, P. K. W., SCHWARZ, V. AND KOMROWER, G. M.* THE BIOSYNTHESIS OF CYSTA-
THIONINE IN PATIENTS WITH HOMOCYSTINURIA. PEDIAT. RES. 2* 149-160, 1968.

*23630 HOOFT'S DISEASE

HOOFT (1962) OF GHENT, BELGIUM, DESCRIBED A FAMILY IN WHICH TWO SISTERS HAD
RETARDED PHYSICAL DEVELOPMENT, ERYTHEMATO-SQUAMOUS ERUPTION, OPAQUE LEUKONYCHIA,
MENTAL RETARDATION AND LOW SERUM LIPIDS. ONE HAD TAPETORETINAL DEGENERATION.
ACANTHOCYTOSIS AND DISTURBANCE OF INTESTINAL ABSORPTION (SEE ABETALIPOPROTEINEMIA)
WERE NOT PRESENT.

FRANCOIS, J. AND DE BLOND, R.* DEGENERESCENCE TAPETO-RETINIENNE ASSOCIEE A UN
SYNDROME HYPOLIPIDEMIQUE. ACTA GENET. MED. GEM. 12* 145-157, 1963.

HOOFT, C., DE LAEY, P., HERPOL, J., DE LOORE, F. AND VERBEECK, J.* FAMILIAL
HYPOLIPIDAEMIA AND RETARDED DEVELOPMENT WITHOUT STEATORRHOEA. ANOTHER INBORN
ERROR OF METABOLISM.Q HELV. PAEDIAT. ACTA 17* 1-23, 1962.

23640 HUMERORADIAL SYNOSTOSIS

IN TWO OF 3 SONS OF THIRD COUSIN PARENTS KEUTEL ET AL. (1970) DESCRIBED HUMERORA-
DIAL SYNOSTOSIS. NO PRECISELY IDENTICAL CASES WERE FOUND IN THE LITERATURE.

KEUTEL, J., KINDERMANN, I. AND MOCKEL, H.* EINE WAHRSCHEINLICH AUTOSOMAL
RECESSIV VERERBTE SKELETMISSBILDUNG MIT HUMERORADIALSYNOSTOSE. HUMANGENETIK 9*
43-53, 1970.

*23650 HYALOIDEO-TAPETORETINAL DEGENERATION OF FAVRE

FAVRE (1958) DESCRIBED BROTHER AND SISTER AND RICCI (1960) ADDED A CASE. THIS IS
TO BE DISTINGUISHED FROM X-LINKED RETINOSCHISIS AND FROM AUTOSOMAL DOMINANT
HYALOIDEO-RETINAL DEGENERATION (Q.V.). IT IS CHARACTERIZED BY A LIQUEFIED
VITREOUS BODY WITH PRERETINAL BAND-SHAPED STRUCTURES (VEIL), MACULAR CHANGES IN
THE FORM OF RETINOSCHISIS OR EDEMA AND PIGMENTARY DEGENERATION OF THE RETINA WITH
HEMERALOPIA AND EXTINGUISHED ELECTRORETINOGRAM. CATARACT IS A COMPLICATION.

FAVRE, M.* A PROPOS DE DEUX CAS DE DEGENERESCENCE HYALOIDEORETINIENNE. TWO
CASES OF HYALOID-RETINAL DEGENERATION. OPHTHALMOLOGICA 135* 604-609, 1958.

RICCI, A.* CLINIQUE ET TRANSMISSION GENETIQUE DES DIFFERENTES FORMES DE
DEGENERESCENCES VITREO-RETINIENNES. OPHTHALMOLOGICA 139* 338-342, 1960.

*23660 HYDROCEPHALUS

THIS ABNORMALITY CAN, OF COURSE, HAVE MANY CAUSES SUCH AS ARNOLD-CHIARI MALFORMA-
TION, ATRESIA OF FORAMEN OF MAGENDIE, STENOSIS OF AQUEDUCT OF SYLVIUS (AN X-LINKED
TRAIT), TOXOPLASMOSIS, HYDRANENCEPHALY, ETC. FURTHERMORE, IT DEVELOPS IN INFANCY
OR CHILDHOOD IN ACHONDROPLASIA (A DOMINANT) AND IN HURLER'S DISEASE. SCHOCKAERT
AND JANSSENS (1952) OBSERVED FOUR SIBS, INCLUDING A FEMALE, WITH HYDROCEPHALUS.
ABDUL-KARIM ET AL. (1964) REPORTED TWO INSTANCES OF CONSANGUINEOUS UNIONS EACH OF
WHICH RESULTED IN THREE AFFECTED SIBS. I HAVE KNOWLEDGE OF AN AMISH FAMILY IN
WHICH ONE FEMALE AND TWO MALE SIBS HAVE HYDROCEPHALUS. MEHNE'S FAMILY (1961) WAS
NON-AMISH, LIVING IN INDIANA. BORLE (1953) REVIEWED THE INSTANCES OF FAMILIAL
HYDROCEPHALUS AND GELLMAN (1959) REVIEWED THOSE OF HYDROCEPHALUS IN TWINS. A SEX-
LINKED RECESSIVE VARIETY OF STENOSIS OF THE AQUEDUCT OF SYLVIUS HAS BECOME
FAMILIAR IN RECENT YEARS THROUGH THE WORK OF EDWARDS (1961).

ABDUL-KARIM, R., ILIYA, F. AND ISKANDAR, G.* CONSECUTIVE HYDROCEPHALUS. REPORT
OF TWO CASES. OBSTET. GYNEC. 24* 376-378, 1964.

BORLE, A.* SUR L'ETIOLOGIE DE L'HYDROCEPHALIE CONGENITALE A PROPOS D'UN CAS
D'HYDROCEPHALIE CONCORDANTE CHEZ DES JUMEAUX UNIVITELLINS. J. GENET HUM. 2* 157-
202, 1953.

EDWARDS, J. H.* THE SYNDROME OF SEX-LINKED HYDROCEPHALUS. ARCH. DIS. CHILD.
36* 486-493, 1961.

GELLMAN, V.* CONGENITAL HYDROCEPHALUS IN MONOVULAR TWINS. ARCH. DIS. CHILD.
34* 274-276, 1959.

MEHNE, R. G.* THREE HYDROCEPHALIC NEWBORNS - EACH OF A SUCCESSIVE PREGNANCY OF
A WHITE FEMALE. ARCH. PEDIAT. 78* 67-71, 1961.

SCHOCKAERT, R. AND JANSSENS, J.* HYDROCEPHALIES CONGENITALES REPETEES.
BRUXELLES MED. 32* 2011-2019, 1952.

*23670 HYDROMETROCOLPOS

THIS MALFORMATION DEVELOPS AS A RESULT OF TRANSVERSE VAGINAL MEMBRANE AND

R
E
C
E
S
S
I
V
E

EXCESSIVE CERVICAL SECRETIONS IN RESPONSE TO MATERNAL HORMONE. MCKUSICK AND COLLEAGUES (1964) HAVE EVIDENCE THAT AT LEAST ONE FORM IS INHERITED AS AN AUTOSOMAL RECESSIVE. BIRTH OF ANOTHER AFFECTED FEMALE IN A THIRD SIBSHIP CLOSELY RELATED TO ONE OF THE TWO REPORTED IN 1964 FURTHER STRENGTHENS THE CONCLUSION (MCKUSICK ET AL., 1968). HYDROMETROCOLPOS HAS BEEN DESCRIBED IN THE ELLIS-VAN CREVELD SYNDROME (AKOUN AND BAGARD, 1956). DANGY ET AL. (1971) FOUND HYDROMETRO-COLPOS SECONDARY TO VAGINAL ATRESIA AND BILATERAL POSTAXIAL HEXADACTYLY IN AN OFFSPRING OF FIRST COUSIN PARENTS.

AKOUN, R. AND BAGARD, M.* LA MALADIE E'ELLIS-VAN CREVELD. ALGERIE MED. 60* 769-772, 1956.

DANGY, C. I., APTEKAR, R. G. AND CANN, H. M.* HEREDITARY HYDROMETROCOLPOS WITH POLYDACTYLY IN INFANCY. PEDIATRICS 47* 138-141, 1971.

MCKUSICK, V. A., BAUER, R. L., KOOP, C. E. AND SCOTT, R. B.* HYDROMETROCOLPOS AS A SIMPLY INHERITED MALFORMATION. J.A.M.A. 189* 813-816, 1964.

MCKUSICK, V. A., WEILBAECHER, R. G. AND GRAGG, G. W.* RECESSIVE INHERITANCE OF A CONGENITAL MALFORMATION SYNDROME. J.A.M.A. 204* 113-118, 1968.

23680 HYDROXYKYNURENINURIA

KOMROWER, ET AL. (1964) DESCRIBED A FEMALE PATIENT, AN ONLY CHILD, WHO EXCRETED LARGE AMOUNTS OF KYNURENINE, 3-HYDROXYKYNURENINE AND XANTHURENIC ACID IN THE URINE. ABSENCE OF KYNURENINASE WAS POSTULATED RESULTING IN A BLOCK IN THE PATHWAY FROM TRYPTOPHAN TO NICOTINIC ACID. UNDER THESE CIRCUMSTANCES TRYPTOPHAN IS NO LONGER A SOURCE OF NICOTINIC ACID AND DEFICIENCY OF THE VITAMIN CAN DEVELOP. THE MOTHER EXCRETED 3-4 TIMES NORMAL AMOUNTS OF XANTHURENIC ACID. THE FATHER'S EXCRETION WAS AT THE UPPER LIMIT OF NORMAL.

KOMROWER, G. M. AND WESTALL, R.* HYDROXYKYNURENINURIA. AM. J. DIS. CHILD. 113* 77-80, 1967.

KOMROWER, G. M., WILSON, V., CLAMP, J. R. AND WESTALL, R. G.* HYDROXY-KYNURENINURIA. A CASE OF ABNORMAL TRYPTOPHANE METABOLISM PROBABLY DUE TO A DEFICIENCY OF KYNURENINASE. ARCH. DIS. CHILD. 39* 250-256, 1964.

R
E
C
E
S
S
I
V
E

*23690 HYDROXYLYSINURIA

BENSON ET AL. (1969) DESCRIBED HYDROXYLYSINURIA IN A 19 YEAR OLD MAN AND HIS 16 YEAR OLD SISTER WHO HAD MYOCLONIC AND MAJOR MOTOR SEIZURES AND WERE MENTALLY RETARDED. THE PARENTS WERE RELATED. THE CLINICAL FEATURES WERE SIMILAR IN A PATIENT REPORTED BY PARKER ET AL. (1970).

BENSON, P. F., SWIFT, P. N. AND YOUNG, V. K.* HYDROXYLYSINURIA. (ABSTRACT) ARCH. DIS. CHILD. 44* 134-135, 1969.

PARKER, C. E., SHAW, K. N. F., JACOBS, E. E. AND GUTENSTEIN, M.* HYDROXYLY-SINURIA. (LETTER) LANCET 1* 1119-1120, 1970.

*23700 HYDROXYPROLINEMIA

MENTAL RETARDATION AND MICROSCOPIC HEMATURIA ARE CLINICAL FEATURES. A DEFECT IN HYDROXYPROLINE OXIDASE IS PROPOSED (EFRON, BIXBY, PRYLES, 1965). PRIOR TO THE DISCOVERY OF THIS DISORDER THE SAME ENZYMES WERE THOUGHT TO BE INVOLVED IN PROLINE AND HYDROXYPROLINE BREAKDOWN. (SEE HYPERPROLINEMIA.) EVEN WHEN ONLY ONE CASE WAS REPORTED, A FEMALE, THIS CONDITION WAS THOUGHT TO BE AN AUTOSOMAL RECESSIVE BECAUSE OF ITS NATURE AS AN INBORN ERROR OF METABOLISM AND BECAUSE THE PARENTS WERE THOUGHT TO HAVE BEEN SIBS. PELKONEN AND KIVIRIKKO (1970) DESCRIBED HYDROXY-PROLINEMIA IN A BROTHER AND SISTER. NO CLINICAL ABNORMALITY WAS PRESENT AND THE AUTHORS SUGGESTED THAT HYDROXYPROLINEMIA IS LIKE CYSTATHIONINURIA A 'NON-DISEASE.'

EFRON, M. L., BIXBY, E. M. AND PRYLES, C. V.* HYDROXYPROLINEMIA. II. A RARE METABOLIC DISEASE DUE TO DEFICIENCY OF ENZYME 'HYDROXYPROLINE OXIDASE.' NEW ENG. J. MED. 272* 1299-1309, 1965.

PELKONEN, R. AND KIVIRIKKO, K. I.* HYDROXYPROLINEMIA* AN APPARENTLY HARMLESS FAMILIAL METABOLIC DISORDER. NEW ENG. J. MED. 283* 451-456, 1970.

SCRIVER, C. R.* MEMBRANE TRANSPORT IN DISORDERS OF IMINO-ACID METABOLISM. AM. J. DIS. CHILD. 113* 170-174, 1967.

23710 HYMEN, IMPERFORATE

MCILROY AND WARD (1930) REPORTED THREE SISTERS AGES 20, 16 AND 14 WHO HAD NOT MENSTRUATED AND ALL HAD IMPERFORATE HYMEN. THE TWO OLDER SIBS HAD HEMATOCOLPOS. HYDROMETROCOLPOS OF CONGENITAL TYPE (Q.V.) IS DUE TO TRANSVERSE VAGINAL SEPTUM DIFFERENT FROM THE HYMEN.

MCILROY, L. AND WARD, I. V.* THREE CASES OF IMPERFORATE HYMEN OCCURRING IN ONE FAMILY. PROC. ROY. SOC. MED. 23* 633-634, 1930.

RUSSELL (1962) DESCRIBED TWO COUSINS WITH CHRONIC AMMONIA INTOXICATION AND MENTAL DETERIORATION. BY LIVER BIOPSY THE ACTIVITY OF HEPATIC ORNITHINE TRANSCARBAMYLASE WAS SHOWN TO BE VERY LOW. A DEFECT IS PRESUMED TO BE PRESENT IN UREA SYNTHESIS AT THE LEVEL OF CONVERSION OF ORNITHINE TO CITRULLINE. (SEE ALSO LYSINE INTOLERENCE AND CITRULLINURIA.) FOUR FORMS OF HYPERAMMONEMIA CORRESPONDING TO EACH OF THE ENZYMES REQUIRED FOR THE KREBS-HENSELEIT UREA CYCLE HAVE NOW BEEN RECOGNIZED. THE GENETIC INTERPRETATION OF ORNITHINE TRANSCARBAMYLASE DEFICIENCY IS COMPLICATED BY THE REPORT OF LEVIN ET AL. (1969) OF A TYPICALLY AFFECTED FEMALE INFANT WHOSE MOTHER HAD AN AVERSION TO PROTEIN AND RAISED PLASMA AMMONIA LEVELS, WHEREAS THE FATHER WAS NORMAL. THE AUTHORS POINTED TO THE RARITY OF MALE CASES OF THE CONDITION. IN ANOTHER INFANT, A MALE, LEVIN ET AL. (1969) FOUND WHAT THEY CONSIDERED A VARIANT OF THE USUAL HYPERAMMONEMIA DUE TO ORNITHINE TRANSCARBAMYLASE DEFICIENCY, PRESUMABLY DUE TO A DIFFERENT ENZYMATIC CHANGE. ENZYME ACTIVITY WAS 25 PERCENT OF NORMAL, RATHER THAN 5-7 PERCENT OF NORMAL AS IN OTHER CASES, AND OTHER PROPERTIES OF THE ENZYME SHOWED DIFFERENCES FROM THE NORMAL. THE CLINICAL PICTURE WAS MILDER THAN IN THE USUAL CASES. BRUTON ET AL. (1970) DESCRIBED ASTROCYTE TRANSFORMATION TO ALZHEIMER TYPE II GLIA, A FEATURE OF ANY FORM OF HYPERAMMONEMIA.

BRUTON, C. J., CORSELLIS, J. A. N. AND RUSSELL, A.* HEREDITARY HYPERAMMONAEMIA. BRAIN 93* 423-434, 1970.

HERRIN, J. T. AND MCCREDIE, D. A.* PERITONEAL DIALYSIS IN THE REDUCTION OF BLOOD AMMONIA LEVELS IN A CASE OF HYPERAMMONAEMIA. ARCH. DIS. CHILD. 44* 149-151, 1969.

HOPKINS, I. J., CONNELLY, J. F., DAWSON, A. G., HIRD, F. J. R. AND MADDISON, T. G.* HYPERAMMONAEMIA DUE TO ORNITHINE TRANSCARBAMYLASE DEFICIENCY. ARCH. DIS. CHILD. 44* 143-148, 1969.

LEVIN, B., ABRAHAM, J. M., OBERHOLZER, V. G. AND BURGESS, E. A.* HYPERAMMONAE-MIA* A DEFICIENCY OF LIVER ORNITHINE TRANSCARBAMYLASE. OCCURRENCE IN MOTHER AND CHILD. ARCH. DIS. CHILD. 44* 152-161, 1969.

RUSSELL, A., LEVIN, B., OBERHOLZER, V. G. AND SINCLAIR, L.* HYPERAMMONAEMIA. A NEW INSTANCE OF AN INBORN ENZYMATIC DEFECT OF THE BIOSYNTHESIS OF UREA. LANCET 2* 699-700, 1962.

*23730 HYPERAMMONEMIA II (CARBAMYL PHOSPHATE SYNTHETASE DEFICIENCY)

A SECOND TYPE OF HYPERAMMONEMIA HAS A DEFECT IN THE PRECEDING STEP OF THE UREA CYCLE, INVOLVING CARBAMYL PHOSPHATE SYNTHETASE. SERUM UREA NITROGEN MAY BE VERY LOW IN THESE CASES. THE PATIENTS SHOW AN AMAZING TOLERANCE TO HIGH AMMONIA LEVELS. DEFECTS IN THE AMMONIA CYCLE ARE ESPECIALLY LIKELY TO BE ACCOMPANIED BY AMMONIA INTOXICATION. DEFECTS HAVE BEEN IDENTIFIED AT 4 OF THE 5 STEPS. SEE CITRULLINEMIA AND ARGININOSUCCINACIDURIA. A REMARKABLE FEATURE OF PATIENTS WITH THESE DISORDERS IS THEIR DISLIKE OF PROTEIN-CONTAINING FOODS, A PHENOMENON AKIN TO THE AVOIDANCE OF MILK BY GALACTOSEMICS.

EFRON, M. L.* DISEASES OF THE UREA CYCLE. IN, STANBURY, J. B., WYNGAARDEN, J. B. AND FREDRICKSON, D. S. (EDS.)* THE METABOLIC BASIS OF INHERITED DISEASE. NEW YORK* MCGRAW-HILL, 1966 (2ND ED.). PP. 393-408.

FREEMAN, J. M., NICHOLSON, J. F., SCHIMKE, R. T., ROWLAND, L. P. AND CARTER, S.* CONGENITAL HYPERAMMONEMIA* ASSOCIATION WITH HYPERGLYCINEMIA AND DECREASED LEVELS OF CARBAMYL PHOSPHATE SYNTHETASE. ARCH. NEUROL. 23* 430-437, 1970.

23740 HYPER-BETA-ALANINEMIA

SCRIVER, PUESCHEL AND DAVIES (1966) DESCRIBED A SOMNOLENT CONVULSING MALE INFANT WHO HAD HYPER-BETA-ALANINEMIA. BETA AMINO ACIDS (BETA-ALANINE, BETA-AMINO-ISOBUTYRIC ACID AND TAURINE) WERE EXCRETED IN EXCESS IN THE URINE, AS A RESULT PROBABLY OF AN INTERACTION BETWEEN BETA-ALANINE AND A SPECIFIC CELLULAR TRANSPORT SYSTEM WITH PREFERENCE FOR BETA-AMINO COMPOUNDS. GABA (GAMMA-AMINO-BUTYRIC ACID) WAS ALSO PRESENT IN THE URINE BUT THIS WAS INDEPENDENT OF PLASMA LEVELS OF ALANINE. POSTMORTEM TISSUES HAD ELEVATED LEVELS OF BETA-ALANINE AND CARNOSINE. THE AUTHORS SUGGESTED A DEFECT IN BETA-ALANINE-ALPHA-KETOGLUTARATE TRANSAMINASE WHICH COULD EXPAND THE FREE BETA-ALANINE POOL AND INCREASE TISSUE CARNOSINE. BETA ALANINE IS A CENTRAL NERVOUS SYSTEM DEPRESSANT. INHIBITION OF GABA TRANSAMINASE AND DISPLACEMENT OF GABA FROM CENTRAL NERVOUS SYSTEM BINDING SITES MAY ACCOUNT FOR GABA-URIA AND CONVULSIONS. THE PARENTS WERE HEALTHY AND NOT RELATED. THREE HALF SIBS WERE NORMAL. ONE INFANT DIED FOUR HOURS AFTER BIRTH WITH *BREATHING TROUBLE.* A FIFTH PREGNANCY ENDED IN MISCARRIAGE.

SCRIVER, C. R., PUESCHEL, S. AND DAVIES, E.* HYPER-BETA-ALANINEMIA ASSOCIATED WITH BETA-AMINOACIDURIA AND GAMMA-AMINOBUTYRICACIDURIA, SOMNOLENCE AND SEIZURES. NEW ENG. J. MED. 274* 635-643, 1966.

*23750 HYPERBILIRUBINEMIA II (DUBIN-JOHNSON SYNDROME)

THE USEFULNESS OF INBRED GROUPS FOR THE STUDY OF RARE RECESSIVES IS NICELY ILLUSTRATED BY THIS DISORDER WHICH OCCURS WITH A MINIMAL FREQUENCY OF 1 PER 1300 AMONG IRANIAN JEWS (SHANI ET AL., 1970). THE CHARACTERISTICS OF THE DISORDER ARE HYPERBILIRUBINEMIA DEPOSITION OF MELANIN (OR AT LEAST MELANIN-LIKE PIGMENT) IN OTHERWISE NORMAL LIVER CELLS, IN SOME HEPATOMEGALY AND ABDOMINAL PAIN, PROLONGED RETENTION OF SULFOBROMOPHTHALEIN (WHICH MAY SHOW A HIGHER CONCENTRATION AT 60 TO 90 MINUTES THAT AT 45 MINUTES) AND OTHERWISE NORMAL LIVER FUNCTION.

SHANI ET AL. (1970) STUDIED 101 PATIENTS WITH THE DUBIN-JOHNSON SYNDROME (DJS) ASCERTAINED IN ISRAEL BETWEEN 1955 AND 1969. AGE AT ONSET OF JAUNDICE VARIED FROM 10 WEEKS TO 56 YEARS. PENETRANCE IS REDUCED IN FEMALES. SIXTY-FOUR OF THE CASES WERE IRANIAN JEWS. PARENTS OF AFFECTED SIBSHIPS WERE CONSANGUINEOUS IN 45 PERCENT OF CASES AS COMPARED WITH A FREQUENCY OF 26 PERCENT AMONG IRANIAN JEWS GENERALLY. SEGREGATION ANALYSIS YIELDED RESULTS CONSISTENT WITH AUTOSOMAL RECESSIVE INHERITANCE WITH REDUCED PENETRANCE. THE AUTHORS SUGGESTED THAT MINOR ABNORMALITIES MAY OCCUR IN HETEROZYGOTES. THIS SUGGESTION IS SUPPORTED BY THE FINDINGS OF BUTT ET AL. (1966), WHO PERFORMED AN EXTENSIVE FAMILY STUDY WITH LIVER BIOPSIES AND OTHER EXAMINATIONS IN MANY RELATIVES.

IN THE ISRAEL GROUP OF CASES OF DJS, SELIGSOHN ET AL. (1970) REPORTED A STRIKING ASSOCIATION WITH DEFICIENCY OF FACTOR VII. THE ASSOCIATION WAS LIMITED TO IRANIAN JEWS. I WONDER IF THIS MAY NOT INDICATE THAT THE DJS AND FACTOR VII LOCI ARE CLOSELY LINKED AND THAT THE TWO MUTANT GENES ARE IN COUPLING IN A MAJORITY OF THE IRANIAN JEWISH GROUP, NOT HAVING YET ATTAINED EQUILIBRIUM OF LINKAGE PHASE. BEFORE THE REPORT OF SHANI ET AL. (1970), THE DUBIN-JOHNSON SYNDROME HAS BEEN DESCRIBED TWICE IN MOTHER AND SON (BEKER AND READ, 1958* WOLF ET AL., 1960), BUT AT LEAST 7 INSTANCES OF MULTIPLE AFFECTED SIBS WITH NORMAL PARENTS ARE ON RECORD (DU AND ROGERS, 1967). FURTHERMORE, CALDERON AND GOLDGRABER (1961) DESCRIBED A PERUVIAN PATIENT WHOSE PARENTS WERE FIRST COUSINS. DU AND ROGERS (1967) DESCRIBED THREE AFFECTED SISTERS WHOSE CLINICALLY NORMAL PARENTS WERE FIRST COUSINS ONCE REMOVED. THREE OFFSPRING OF ONE AFFECTED SISTER HAD NORMAL LIVERS (BY INSPECTION AT LAPAROTOMY IN 2 AND BY AUTOPSY IN THE THIRD).

BEKER, S. AND READ, A. E.* FAMILIAL DUBIN-JOHNSON SYNDROME. GASTROENTEROLOGY 35* 387-389, 1958.

BUTT, H. R., ANDERSON, E., FOULK, W. T., BAGGENSTOSS, A. H., SCHOENFIELD, L. J. AND DICKSON, E. R.* STUDIES OF CHRONIC IDIOPATHIC JAUNDICE (DUBIN-JOHNSON SYNDROME). II. EVALUATION OF A LARGE FAMILY WITH THE TRAIT. GASTROENTEROLOGY 51* 619-630, 1966.

CALDERON, A. AND GOLDGRABER, M. B.* CHRONIC IDIOPATHIC JAUNDICE* A CASE REPORT. GASTROENTEROLOGY 40* 244-247, 1961.

DU, J. N. H. AND ROGERS, A. G.* DUBIN-JOHNSON SYNDROME* A FAMILY WITH THREE AFFECTED SISTERS. CANAD. MED. ASS. J. 97* 1225-1226, 1967.

SELIGSOHN, U., SHANI, M., RAMOT, B., ADAM, A. AND SHEBA, C.* DUBIN-JOHNSON SYNDROME IN ISRAEL. II. ASSOCIATION WITH FACTOR-VII DEFICIENCY. QUART. J. MED. 39* 569-584, 1970.

SHANI, M., SELIGSOHN, U., GILON, E., SHEBA, C. AND ADAM, A.* DUBIN-JOHNSON SYNDROME IN ISRAEL. I. CLINICAL, LABORATORY, AND GENETIC ASPECTS OF 101 CASES. QUART. J. MED. 39* 549-567, 1970.

WOLF, R. L., PIZETTE, M., RICHMAN, A., DREILING, D. A., JACOBS, W., FERNANDEZ, O. AND POPPER, H.* CHRONIC IDIOPATHIC JAUNDICE. A STUDY OF TWO AFFLICTED FAMILIES. AM. J. MED. 28* 32-41, 1960.

*23780 HYPERBILIRUBINEMIA, SHUNT

ISRAELS, SUDERMAN AND RITZMANN (1959) DESCRIBED WHAT THEY CALLED SHUNT HYPERBI-LIRUBINEMIA* EXCESS BILIRUBIN APPEARS TO BE DERIVED FROM A SOURCE OTHER THAN CIRCULATING ERYTHROCYTES, THROUGH AN ALTERNATIVE PATHWAY OF BILIRUBIN PRODUCTION. CLINICAL MANIFESTATIONS - JAUNDICE AND SPLENOMEGALY - HAVE THEIR ONSET IN THE SECOND DECADE. THEY OBSERVED THREE AFFECTED SIBS AND A FOURTH CASE IN MENNONITES LIVING IN CANADA. THE AUTHORS SUGGESTED THAT THESE PATIENTS MIGHT BE RELATED TO THOSE DESCRIBED BY KALK (1955) OF KASSEL, WHICH IS NOT FAR FROM KREFELD, WHICH FORMERLY WAS A GERMAN MENNONITE CENTER. ISRAELS AND HIS COLLEAGUES (1963) CONFIRMED THEIR EARLIER WORK THAT THE UNDERLYING MECHANISM IS AN INCREASED PRODUCTION OF BILIRUBIN FROM THE EARLY BREAKDOWN OF HEME OR ITS PRECURSORS. THE LIVER APPEARS TO BE CAPABLE OF DIRECT SYNTHESIS OF BILIRUBIN ('EARLY LABELLING BILIRUBIN') WITHOUT THE INTERMEDIACY OF HEMOGLOBIN. THE CONDITION MAY BE RATHER FREQUENT. IT SHOULD BE SUSPECTED WHENEVER FECAL UROBILINOGEN IS MARKEDLY INCREASED IN THE ABSENCE OF SIGNS OF HEMOLYSIS.

ISRAELS, L. G., SUDERMAN, H. J. AND RITZMANN, S. E.* HYPERBILIRUBINEMIA DUE TO AN ALTERNATE PATH OF BILIRUBIN PRODUCTION. AM. J. MED. 27* 693-702, 1959.

ISRAELS, L. G., YAMAMOTO, T., SKANDERBEG, J. AND ZIPURSKY, A.* SHUNT BILIRUBIN* EVIDENCE FOR TWO COMPONENTS. SCIENCE 139* 1054-1055, 1963.

KALK, H. AND WILDHIRT, E.* DIE POSTHEPATITISCHE HYPERBILIRUBINAMIE. Z. KLIN. MED. 153* 354-387, 1955.

23790 HYPERBILIRUBINEMIA, TRANSIENT FAMILIAL NEONATAL

THE   CAUSE MAY BE STEROIDAL SUBSTANCES IN THE PLASMA AND MILK OF THE MOTHER WHICH
INHIBIT CONJUGATION OF BILIRUBIN (LUCEY, ARIAS AND MCKAY, 1960). THE SAME
CONDITION MAY BE PRESENT IN YEMENITE JEWS (SHEBA). OCCASIONALLY, SEVERE NEONATAL
UNCONJUGATED HYPERBILIRUBINEMIA OCCURS WITHOUT EVIDENT ETIOLOGIC EXPLANATION.
LUCEY, ARIAS AND MCKAY (1960) AND ARIAS AND COLLEAGUES (1965) SUGGESTED THAT SOME
OF THESE CASES MAY HAVE A FAMILIAL BASIS. THE LATTER AUTHORS FOUND, FURTHERMORE,
A HIGH LEVEL OF A MATERNAL SERUM SUBSTANCE WHICH INHIBITS FORMATION OF THE
GLUCURONIDE OF DIRECT-REACTING BILIRUBIN AND O-AMINOPHENOL BY RAT LIVER SLICES AND
HOMOGENATES. THE INHIBITOR WAS PRESENT IN THESE MOTHERS IN CONCENTRATIONS FOUR TO
TEN TIMES THAT IN OTHER PREGNANT MOTHERS. THE INHIBITOR IS PROBABLY A PROGESTA-
TIONAL STEROID. (THIS ENTITY IS DISTINCT FROM THE SEVERE AND PROLONGED UNCONJU-
GATED HYPERBILIRUBINEMIA WHICH OCCURS IN BREAST-FED BUT NOT IN BOTTLE-FED INFANTS
OF MOTHERS WHOSE BREAST MILK CONTAINS A STEROL WHICH INHIBITS HEPATIC GLUCURONYL
TRANSFERASE ACTIVITY IN VITRO. THE LATTER STATE MAY ALSO HAVE A GENETIC BASIS.)
ARIAS AND COLLEAGUES (1965) MADE REFERENCE TO OBSERVATIONS ON FIVE MOTHERS WHO
GAVE BIRTH TO A TOTAL OF 16 INFANTS, EACH OF WHOM HAD SEVERE TRANSIENT NEONATAL
HYPERBILIRUBINEMIA. THREE OF THE 16 DIED OF KERNICTERUS AND ONE WAS LEFT WITH
QUADRIPLEGIC CEREBRAL PALSY. THE MOTHERS DO NOT SHOW HYPERBILIRUBINEMIA, PROBABLY
BECAUSE OF A LARGE FUNCTIONAL RESERVE. THIS IS AN INTERESTING GENETIC DISEASE OF
WHICH THERE ARE FEW EXAMPLES - ONE IN WHICH THE GENOTYPE OF THE MOTHER IS
RESPONSIBLE FOR THE DISEASE IN THE INFANT. ANOTHER EXAMPLE IS MENTAL RETARDATION
IN THE OFFSPRING OF WOMEN WITH PHENYLKETONURIA (MABRY, ET AL., 1963). THE ETHNIC
BACKGROUND OF THESE MOTHERS AND THE PRESENCE OR ABSENCE OF CONSANGUINITY IN THEIR
PARENTS WOULD BE OF INTEREST. TRANSIENT NONHEMOLYTIC UNCONJUGATED HYPERBILIRU-
BINEMIA IS OBSERVED IN BREAST-FED BUT NOT BOTTLE-FED BABIES OF MOTHERS WHOSE
BREAST MILK CONTAINS PREGNANE-3 (ALPHA), 20 (BETA)-DIOL THAT COMPETITIVELY
INHIBITS HEPATIC GLUCURONYL TRANSFERASE ACTIVITY IN VITRO. SERUM FROM THESE
MOTHERS CONTAINS NO MORE INHIBITORY SUBSTANCE THAN DOES NORMAL PREGNANCY SERUM.
KERNICTERUS HAS NOT BEEN OBSERVED, PROBABLY BECAUSE SEVERE JAUNDICE DOES NOT
DEVELOP UNTIL THE 7TH TO 10TH DAY, WHEN THE INFANT'S BLOOD-BRAIN BARRIER HAS
BECOME RELATIVELY IMPERMEABLE TO UNCONJUGATED BILIRUBIN. THIS IS ANOTHER
PHENOTYPE OF THE INFANT WHICH IS DEPENDENT ON THE MATERNAL GENOTYPE.

ARIAS, I. M. AND GARTNER, L. M.* PRODUCTION OF UNCONJUGATED HYPERBILIRUBINAEMIA
IN FULL-TERM NEW-BORN INFANTS FOLLOWING ADMINISTRATION OF PREGNANE-3 (ALPHA), 20
(BETA)-DIOL. NATURE 203* 1292-1293, 1964.

ARIAS, I. M., GARTNER, L. M., SEIFTER, S. AND FURMAN, M.* PROLONGED NEONATAL
UNCONJUGATED HYPERBILIRUBINEMIA ASSOCIATED WITH BREAST FEEDING AND A STEROID,
PREGNANE-3 (ALPHA), 20 (BETA)-DIOL, IN MATERNAL MILK THAT INHIBITS GLUCURONIDE
FORMATION IN VITRO. J. CLIN. INVEST. 43* 2037-2047, 1964.

ARIAS, I. M., WOLFSON, S., LUCEY, J. F. AND MCKAY, R. J., JR.* TRANSIENT
FAMILIAL NEONATAL HYPERBILIRUBINEMIA. J. CLIN. INVEST. 44* 1442-1450, 1965.

LUCEY, J. F., ARIAS, I. M. AND MCKAY, R. J., JR.* TRANSIENT FAMILIAL NEONATAL
HYPERBILIRUBINEMIA. AM. J. DIS. CHILD. 100* 787-789, 1960.

MABRY, C. C., DENNISTON, J. C., NELSON, T. L. AND NELSON, C. D.* MATERNAL
PHENYLKETONURIA* A CAUSE OF MENTAL RETARDATION IN CHILDREN WITHOUT THE METABOLIC
DEFECT. NEW ENG. J. MED. 269* 1404-1408, 1963.

NEWMAN, A. J. AND GROSS, S.* HYPERBILIRUBINEMIA IN BREAST-FED INFANTS.
PEDIATRICS 32* 995-1001, 1963.

SHEBA, C.* TEL-AVIV, ISRAEL* PERSONAL COMMUNICATION, 1964.

23800 HYPERCALCEMIA, IDIOPATHIC

SUSPICION OF A GENETIC BASIS OF HYPERCALCEMIA WAS PROVIDED BY THE FAMILY REPORTED
FIRST IN 1959 AND LATER IN 1963. TWO SISTERS WERE AFFECTED. THE AUTHORS (SMITH
ET AL., 1959, KENNY ET AL., 1963) SUGGESTED THAT THE DEFECT MAY CONCERN VITAMIN D
INACTIVATION. THE PARENTS HAD NORMAL SERUM CALCIUM LEVELS. THE MOTHER, BUT NOT
THE FATHER, BECAME HYPERCALCEMIC WITH A SMALL DOSE OF ADDED VITAMIN D (BLIZZARD,
1963, EHRHARDT AND MONEY, 1967). IT IS POSSIBLE, THEREFORE, THAT THE CONDITION IS
DOMINANT, NOT RECESSIVE.
HOOFT AND HIS COLLEAGUES (1961) DESCRIBED A FAMILY IN WHICH A CHILD HAD
IDIOPATHIC HYPERCALCEMIA AND THE FATHER HAD SARCOIDOSIS WITH HYPERCALCEMIA. SEE
DISCUSSION OF HYPERCALCEMIA IN CONNECTION WITH SUPRAVALVAR AORTIC STENOSIS IN THE
DOMINANT CATALOG. ALTHOUGH BOTH AORTIC AND PULMONARY STENOSIS OCCUR WITH BOTH
RUBELLA AND HYPERCALCEMIA, AORTIC STENOSIS IS MORE FREQUENT WITH HYPERCALCEMIA AND
PULMONARY STENOSIS WITH RUBELLA (VARGHESE ET AL., 1969).

BLIZZARD, R. M.* BALTIMORE, MD.* PERSONAL COMMUNICATION, 1963.

EHRHARDT, A. A. AND MONEY, J.* HYPERCALCEMIA - A FAMILY STUDY OF PSYCHOLOGIC
FUNCTIONING. JOHNS HOPKINS MED. J. 121* 14-20, 1967.

HOOFT, C., VERMASSEN, A., EECKELS, R. AND VANHEULE, R.* FAMILIAL INCIDENCE OF HYPERCALCEAMIA. EXTREME HYPERSENSITIVITY TO VITAMIN D IN AN INFANT WHOSE FATHER SUFFERED FROM SARCOIDOSIS. HELV. PAEDIAT. ACTA 16* 199-210, 1961.

KENNY, F. M., ACETO, T., JR., PURISCH, M., HARRISON, H. E., HARRISON, H. C. AND BLIZZARD, R. M.* METABOLIC STUDIES IN A PATIENT WITH IDIOPATHIC HYPERCALCEMIA OF INFANCY. J. PEDIAT. 62* 531-537, 1963.

SMITH, D. W., BLIZZARD, R. M. AND HARRISON, H. E.* IDIOPATHIC HYPERCALCEMIA. A CASE REPORT WITH ASSAYS OF VITAMIN D IN THE SERUM. PEDIATRICS 24* 258-269, 1959.

VARGHESE, P. J., IZUKAWA, T. AND ROWE, R. D.* SUPRAVALVULAR AORTIC STENOSIS AS PART OF RUBELLA SYNDROME, WITH DISCUSSION OF PATHOGENESIS. BRIT. HEART J. 31* 59-62, 1969.

23810 HYPERCALCIURIA

DE LUCA AND GUZZETTA (1965) REPORTED FOUR BROTHERS, THE PRODUCTS OF THEIR MOTHER'S FIRST FOUR PREGNANCIES, WITH HYPERCALCIURIA. TWO YOUNGER SIBS, GIRLS, WERE NORMAL. THE PARENTS WERE NOT RELATED. A DEFECT OF THE RENAL TUBULE WAS POSTU-LATED. WHETHER GENETIC AND, IF SO, WHETHER AUTOSOMAL ARE NOT PROVED.

DE LUCA, R. AND GUZZETTA, F.* IDIOPATHIC HYPERCALCIURIA IN CHILDREN. OBSERVA-TIONS IN 4 BROTHERS. PEDIATRIA 73* 613-640, 1965.

23820 HYPERCYSTINURIA

A RENAL TUBULAR DEFECT LIMITED TO CYSTINE AND THEREFORE DISTINCT FROM THAT IN THE SEVERAL FORMS OF CLASSICAL CYSTINURIA WAS DESCRIBED BY BRODEHL ET AL. (1967). TWO SIBS WERE AFFECTED. THE PARENTS WERE NOT RELATED.

BRODEHL, J., GELLISSEN, K. AND KOWALEWSKI, S.* ISOLIERTER DEFEKT DER TUBULAREN CYSTIN-RUCKRESORPTION IN EINER FAMILIE MIT IDIOPATHISCHEM HYPOPARATHYROIDISMUS. KLIN. WSCHR. 45* 38-40, 1967.

*23830 HYPERGLYCINEMIA, ISOLATED

R
E
C
E
S
S
I
V
E

UNLIKE GLYCINEMIA WITH KETOACIDOSIS AND LEUKOPENIA (Q.V.), EPISODIC KETOACIDOSIS WITH VOMITING, NEUTROPENIA AND THROMBOCYTOPENIA DO NOT OCCUR AND GLYCINE IS THE ONLY AMINO ACID ELEVATED IN SERUM AND URINE. GLYCINE IS THE ONLY AMINO ACID HARMFUL TO THESE PATIENTS. SOME HAVE DIED IN THE NEWBORN PERIOD AFTER A COURSE CHARACTERIZED BY LETHARGY, WEAK CRY, GENERALIZED HYPOTONIA, ABSENT REFLEXES, AND PERIODIC MYOCLONIC JERKS (BALFE ET AL., 1965). THE FEW WHO ATTAIN AN OLDER AGE SHOW SEVERE MENTAL RETARDATION (MABRY AND KARAM, 1963* GERRITSEN ET AL., 1965). SIBS WITH THIS CONDITION HAVE BEEN REPORTED. GERRITSEN ET AL. (1965) DESCRIBED ABNORMALLY LOW OXALATE EXCRETION IN THE URINE AND POSTULATED A DEFECT IN GLYCINE OXIDASE. TADA ET AL. (1969) CONCLUDED THAT THE PRIMARY LESION IN HYPERGLYCINEMIA OF THE NON-KETOTIC VARIETY IS IN THE GLYSINE CLEAVAGE REACTION.

BALFE, J. W., LEVISON, H., HANLEY, W. B., JACKSON, S. H. AND SASS-KORTSAK, A.* HYPERGLYCINEMIA AND GLYCINURIA IN A NEWBORN. (ABSTRACT) CANAD. MED. ASS. J. 92* 347 ONLY, 1965.

GERRITSEN, T., KAVEGGIA, E. AND WAISMAN, H. A.* A NEW TYPE OF IDIOPATHIC HYPERGLYCINEMIA WITH HYPO-OXALURIA. PEDIATRICS 36* 882-891, 1965.

MABRY, C. C. AND KARAM, F. A.* IDIOPATHIC HYPERGLYCINEMIA AND HYPERGLYCINURIA. (ABSTRACT) STH. MED. J. 56* 1444 ONLY, 1963.

TADA, K., NARISAWA, K., YOSHIDA, T., KONNA, T., YOKOYAMA, Y., NAKAGAWA, H., TANNO, K., MOCHIZUKI, K. AND ARAKAWA, T.* HYPERGLYCINEMIA* A DEFECT IN GLYCINE CLEAVAGE REACTION. TOHOKU J. EXP. MED. 98* 289-296, 1969.

23840 HYPERLIPIDEMIA V (FAMILIAL HYPERPREBETALIPOPROTEINEMIA, CARBOHYDRATE-INDUCIBLE HYPERLIPEMIA)

THE CHOLESTEROL IS NOT AS MARKEDLY ELEVATED AS IN TYPE III. TRIGLYCERIDES ARE MARKEDLY ELEVATED. LIKE TYPE III, THE HYPERLIPEMIA IS CARBOHYDRATE-INDUCIBLE, PHLA IS NORMAL AND THE GLUCOSE TOLERANCE TEST MAY BE ABNORMAL.

23850 HYPERLIPIDEMIA VI (FAMILIAL HYPERCHYLOMICRONEMIA WITH HYPERPREBETALIPOPROTEINE-MIA, MIXED HYPERLIPEMIA, COMBINED FAT AND CARBOHYDRATE-INDUCED HYPERLIPEMIA)

ON A REGULAR DIET BOTH CHYLOMICRA AND PRE-BETA-LIPOPROTEINS ARE INCREASED. ALPHA-AND BETA-LIPOPROTEINS ARE NORMAL OR LOW. FEATURES ARE OCCULT OR MILD DIABETES MELLITUS, BOUTS OF ABDOMINAL PAIN, AND ERUPTIVE XANTHOMA. FREDRICKSON AND LEES (1966) OBSERVED PARENTAL CONSANGUINITY. HENCE, THIS MAY BE A RECESSIVE.

FREDRICKSON, D. S. AND LEES, R. S.* FAMILIAL HYPERLIPOPROTEINEMIA. IN, STANBURY, J. B., WYNGAARDEN, J. B. AND FREDRICKSON, D. S. (EDS.)* THE METABOLIC BASIS OF INHERITED DISEASE. NEW YORK* MCGRAW-HILL, 1966 (2ND ED.). PP. 429-485.

NIXON, J. C., MARTIN, W. G., KALAB, M. AND MONAHAN, G. J.* TYPE V HYPERLIPOPRO-
TEINEMIA. A STUDY OF A PATIENT AND FAMILY. CLIN. BIOCHEM. 2* 389-398, 1969.

23860 HYPERLIPOPROTEINEMIA I (FAMILIAL HYPERCHYLOMICRONEMIA, IDIOPATHIC HYPERLIPERMIA
OF BURGER-GRUTZ TYPE, ESSENTIAL FAMILIAL HYPERLIPEMIA)

HOLT AND HIS COLLEAGUES (1939) FIRST REPORTED THE FAMILIAL OCCURRENCE OF THIS
SYNDROME.   BOGGS AND COLLEAGUES (1957) DESCRIBED THREE AFFECTED SIBS FROM A FIRST
COUSIN MATING.   MASSIVE HYPERCHYLOMICRONEMIA OCCURS WHEN THE PATIENT IS ON A
NORMAL DIET AND DISAPPEARS COMPLETELY IN A FEW DAYS ON FAT-FREE FEEDING. ON A
NORMAL DIET ALPHA AND BETA LIPOPROTEINS ARE LOW. A DEFECT IN REMOVAL OF CHYLOMI-
CRONS (FAT INDUCTION) AND OF OTHER TRIGLYCERIDE-RICH LIPOPROTEINS (CARBOHYDRATE
INDUCTION) IS PRESENT. DECREASED PLASMA POSTHEPARINLIPOLYTIC ACTIVITY (PHLA) IS
DEMONSTRATED.   LOW TISSUE ACTIVITY OF LIPOPROTEIN LIPASE IS SUSPECTED.   THE FULL
BLOWN DISEASE, MANIFESTED BY ATTACKS OF ABDOMINAL PAIN, HEPATOSPLENOMEGALY,
ERUPTIVE XANTHOMAS, AND LACTESCENCE OF THE PLASMA, IS A RECESSIVE.   HETEROZYGOTES
MAY SHOW SLIGHT HYPERLIPEMIA AND REDUCED PHLA. PRECOCIOUS ATHEROSCLEROSIS SEEMS
NOT TO BE A FEATURE. THIS CONDITION WAS CALLED FAT-INDUCED HYPERTRIGLYCERIDEMIA
BY NEVIN AND SLACK (1968).

BERGER, H., RICHTER, A., GILARDI, A. AND WAGNER, H.* ESSENTIAL FAMILIAL
HYPERLIPAEMIA IN A 2-YEAR-OLD CHILD. ANN. PAEDIAT. 199* 445-466, 1962.

BOGGS, J. D., HSIA, D. Y.-Y., MAIS, R. F. AND BIGLER, J. A.* THE GENETIC
MECHANISM OF IDIOPATHIC HYPERLIPEMIA. NEW ENG. J. MED. 257* 1101-1108, 1957.

FRANKLIN, S. M.* SPLENOMEGALY WITH LIPAEMIA. PROC. ROY. SOC. MED. 30* 711
ONLY, 1937.

FREDRICKSON, D. S. AND LEES, R. S.* HYPERLIPOPROTEINEMIA. IN, STANBURY, J. B.,
WYNGAARDEN, J. B. AND FREDRICKSON, D. S. (EDS.)* THE METABOLIC BASIS OF INHERITED
DISEASE. NEW YORK* MCGRAW-HILL, 1966 (2ND ED.). PP. 429-485.

HOLT, L. E., JR., AYLWARD, F. X. AND TIMBERS, H. G.* IDIOPATHIC FAMILIAL
LIPEMIA. BULL. HOPKINS HOSP. 64* 279-314, 1939.

NEVIN, N. C. AND SLACK, J.* HYPERLIPIDAEMIC XANTHOMATOSIS II* MODE OF INHERI-
TANCE IN 55 FAMILIES WITH ESSENTIAL HYPERLIPIDAEMIA AND XANTHOMATOSIS. J. MED.
GENET. 5* 9-28, 1968.

WESSLER, S. AND AVIOLI, L. A.* FAMILIAL HYPERLIPOPROTEINEMIA. J.A.M.A. 207*
929-937, 1969.

*23870 HYPERLYSINEMIA

GHADIMI ET AL. (1965) FOUND HYPERLYSINEMIA IN TWO UNRELATED MENTALLY RETARDED
PATIENTS.   THE LEVEL OF LYSINE IN THE CSF WAS ALSO ELEVATED. BLOOD LEVELS ROSE
ABNORMALLY WITH LYSINE LOADING. A BLOCK IN THE METABOLISM OF LYSINE WAS POSTU-
LATED.   THE PATIENTS WERE AGED 2 AND 27 YEARS. IMPAIRED SEXUAL DEVELOPMENT, LAX
LIGAMENTS AND MUSCLES, CONVULSIONS IN EARLY LIFE AND PERHAPS MILD ANEMIA WERE
FEATURES.   WOODY (1964) FOUND ELEVATED LYSINE IN THE BLOOD AND SPINAL FLUID OF A
PHYSICALLY AND MENTALLY RETARDED GIRL WITH CONVULSIONS, MUSCULAR AND LIGAMENTOUS
ASTHENIA, AND NORMOCYTIC, NORMOCHROMIC ANEMIA WHICH RESPONDED TO DIETARY RESTRIC-
TION OF LYSINE. THIS WORKER SUGGESTED THAT INCORPORATION OF LYSINE INTO PROTEIN
WAS DEFECTIVE.   AN OSTENSIBLY NORMAL COUSIN ALSO HAD HYPERLYSINURIA.   THE PARENTS
OF THE PROBAND WERE RELATED. DANCIS ET AL. (1969) DEMONSTRATED REDUCED LYSINE-
KETOGLUTARATE REDUCTASE ACTIVITY IN SKIN FIBROBLASTS FROM 3 AFFECTED SIBS.   IN
VIEW OF THE LIGAMENTOUS LAXITY, IT IS OF INTEREST THAT SUBLUXATION OF THE LENSES
DEVELOPED IN SOME OF THE PATIENTS (WOODY, 1971). THE HYPERLYSINEMIA IN THE CASES
STUDIED BY DAVIS ET AL. (1969) WAS MORE MARKED THAN THAT IN OTHER REPORTED CASES
SUCH AS THAT OF GHADIMI ET AL. (1965) YET THE LATTER CASES WERE MORE SEVERELY
RETARDED.   THE RELATIONSHIP TO THESE OTHER REPORTED CASES AND TO THE ENTITY
DISCUSSED ELSEWHERE AS LYSINE INTOLERANCE AWAITS ELUCIDATION. SACCHAROPINURIA
(CARSON ET AL., 1968) IS PRESUMABLY A DISTINCT DISORDER INVOLVING THE LYSINE
METABOLIC PATHWAY AND SHOWING HYPERLYSINEMIA. ONE OF THE CASES OF GHADIMI ET AL.
(1965) WAS THE PRODUCT OF FATHER-DAUGHER INCEST. WOODY'S CASES ARE INBRED
LOUISIANA CAJUNS.

CARSON, N. A. J., SCALLY, B. G., NEILL, D. W. AND CARRE, I. J.* SACCHARO-
PINURIA* A NEW BORN ERROR OF LYSINE METABOLISM. NATURE 218* 679 ONLY, 1968.

CHOREMIS, C., YANNOKOS, D., PAPADATOS, C. AND BAROUTSOU, E.* OSTEITIS DEFORMANS
(PAGET'S DISEASE) IN AN 11-YEAR-OLD BOY. HELV. PAEDIAT. ACTA 13* 185-188, 1958.

DANCIS, J., HUTZLER, J., COX, R. P. AND WOODY, N. C.* FAMILIAL HYPERLYSINEMIA
WITH LYSINE-KETOGLUTARATE REDUCTASE INSUFFICIENCY.   J. CLIN. INVEST. 48* 1447-
1452, 1969.

GHADIMI, H., BINNINGTON, V. I. AND PECORA, P.* HYPERLYSINEMIA ASSOCIATED WITH
MENTAL RETARDATION. NEW ENG. J. MED. 273* 723-729, 1965.

SMITH, T. H., HOLLAND, M. G. AND WOODY, N. C.* OCULAR ABNORMALITIES IN

ASSOCIATION WITH HYPERLYSINEMIA. (ABSTRACT) TRANS. AM. ACAD. OPHTHAL. OTOLARYNG. 74* 895, 1970.

SWOBODA, H.* HYPEROSTOSIS CORTICALIS DEFORMANS JUVENILIS* UNGEWOHNLICHE GENERALISIERTE OSTEOPATHIE BEI ZWEI GESCHWISTERN. HELV. PAEDIAT. ACTA 13* 292-312, 1958.

WOODY, N. C.* HYPERLYSINEMIA. AM. J. DIS. CHILD. 108* 543-553, 1964.

WOODY, N. C.* NEW ORLEANS, LA.* PERSONAL COMMUNICATION, 1971.

WOODY, N. C., HUTZLER, J. AND DANCIS, J.* FURTHER STUDIES OF HYPERLYSINEMIA. AM. J. DIS. CHILD. 112* 577-580, 1960.

23880 HYPERMETABOLISM DUE TO DEFECT IN MITOCHONDRIA

LUFT AND COLLEAGUES (1962) OBSERVED A 35 YEAR OLD PATIENT WITH A BMR OF 150 TO 200 PERCENT SINCE AT LEAST 7 YEARS OF AGE, YET NORMAL THYROID FUNCTION. STUDIES OF MITOCHONDRIA FROM SKELETAL MUSCLE SHOWED A DEFECT OF COUPLING BETWEEN OXIDATION AND PHOSPHORYLATION. THE PARENTS WERE NOT RELATED AND NO OTHER CASES WERE RECOGNIZED IN THE FAMILY. HOWEVER, THE POSSIBILITY OF A GENETIC BASIS WAS RAISED.

LUFT, R., IKKOS, D., PALMIERI, G., ERNSTER, L. AND AFZELIUS, B.* A CASE OF SEVERE HYPERMETABOLISM OF NONTHYROID ORIGIN WITH A DEFECT IN THE MAINTENANCE OF MITOCHONDRIAL RESPIRATORY CONTROL* A CORRELATED CLINICAL, BIOCHEMICAL, AND MORPHOLOGICAL STUDY. J. CLIN. INVEST. 41* 1776-1804, 1962.

23890 HYPERMETHIONINEMIA

PERRY ET AL. (1965) DESCRIBED THREE SIBS (2 FEMALES AND A MALE) IN ONE SIBSHIP WHO DIED IN THE THIRD MONTH AFTER AN ILLNESS CHARACTERIZED BY IRRITABILITY AND PROGRESSIVE SOMNOLENCE, AND TERMINALLY BY A TENDENCY TO BLEED AND HYPOGLYCEMIA. A PECULIAR ODOR WAS NOTED. PATHOLOGIC CHANGES INCLUDED HEPATIC CIRRHOSIS, RENAL TUBULAR DILATATION AND PANCREATIC ISLET HYPERTROPHY. BIOCHEMICAL STUDIES SHOWED GENERALIZED AMINOACIDURIA, VERY MARKED ELEVATION OF METHIONINE IN THE SERUM AND A DISPROPORTIONATELY HIGH URINARY EXCRETION OF METHIONINE. ALPHA-KETO-GAMMA-METHIOLBUTYRIC ACID WAS PRESENT IN THE URINE AND MAY ACCOUNT FOR THE PECULIAR ODOR. THE HYPERTROPHY OF THE ISLETS OF LANGERHANS WAS PROBABLY DUE TO STIMULATION BY METHIONINE OR ONE OF ITS METABOLITES. IT SEEMS LIKELY THAT THE DISORDER WAS TYROSINEMIA (Q.V.) SINCE HYPERMETHIONINEMIA OCCURS SECONDARY TO LIVER FAILURE IN THAT CONDITION (SCRIVER ET AL., 1967).

PERRY, T. L., HARDWICK, D. F., DIXON, G. H., DOLMAN, C. L. AND HANSEN, S.* HYPERMETHIONINEMIA* A METABOLIC DISORDER ASSOCIATED WITH CIRRHOSIS, ISLET CELL HYPERPLASIA, AND RENAL TUBULAR DEGENERATION. PEDIATRICS 36* 236-250, 1965.

SCRIVER, C. R., LAROCHELLE, J. AND SILVERBERG, M.* HEREDITARY TYROSINEMIA AND TYROSYLURIA IN A FRENCH CANADIAN GEOGRAPHIC ISOLATE. AM. J. DIS. CHILD. 113* 41-46, 1967.

*23900 HYPEROSTOSIS CORTICALIS DEFORMANS JUVENILIS (JUVENILE PAGET'S DISEASE, CHRONIC CONGENITAL IDIOPATHIC HYPERPHOSPHATASEMIA)

CAFFEY (1961) AND RUBIN (1964) PRESENTED CASES. BAKWIN AND EIGER (1956) AND BAKWIN, GOLDEN AND FOX (1964) DESCRIBED A FAMILIAL DISORDER MANIFESTING ITSELF FROM EARLY IN LIFE BY LARGE HEAD AND EXPANDED AND BOWED EXTREMITIES. ALKALINE PHOSPHATASE WAS ELEVATED. THE LONG BONES ARE GREATLY EXPANDED WITH OSTEOPOROSIS AND COARSE TRABECULATIONS. THE CALVARIUM IS MARKEDLY THICKENED WITH ISLANDS OF INCREASED BONE DENSITY. MUSCULAR WEAKNESS MAY BE STRIKING. IN BAKWIN'S FAMILY TWO SISTERS WERE SEVERELY AFFECTED. THE PARENTS WERE FIRST COUSINS AND THE MOTHER WAS MILDLY AFFECTED. THE FINDINGS IN HER WOULD PROBABLY HAVE ESCAPED DETECTION IF X-RAYS HAD NOT BEEN MADE. THE AUTHORS THOUGHT THIS TO BE THE SAME AS THE CONDITION DESCRIBED IN TWO SISTERS BY SWOBODA (1958) AS HYPEROSTOSIS CORTICALIS DEFORMANS JUVENILIS AND BY CHOREMIS ET AL. (1958) AS PAGET'S DISEASE IN AN 11 YEAR OLD BOY. OF INTEREST IS THE PRESENCE OF ANGIOID STREAKS IN ONE OF BAKWIN'S PATIENTS. FANCONI (1964) DESCRIBED THE X-RAY AND HISTOLOGIC CHANGES IN A YOUNG BRAZILIAN MALE AND SUGGESTED THE DESIGNATION OSTEOCHALASIA DESMALIS FAMILIARIS. SINCE THE BASIC DISORDER IS UNKNOWN, ANOTHER LABEL IS NOT WARRANTED. THE CONDITION CALLED FAMILIAL OSTEOECTASIA BY STEMMERMANN (1966) APPEARS TO BE THE SAME. HIS CASES WERE IN BROTHER AND SISTER, AGE 2 AND 3, OF PUERTO RICAN ANCESTRY. BAKWIN, GOLDEN AND FOX (1964) OBSERVED THIS DISORDER IN TWO SISTERS OF PUERTO RICAN PARENTAGE. BOTH HAD RETINAL DEGENERATION. IN ONE THE CHANGES INCLUDED ANGIOID STREAKS. BROTHER AND SISTER OF MIXED HAWAIIAN, FILIPINO AND PUERTO RICAN ANCESTRY WERE DESCRIBED BY EYRING AND EISENBERG (1968). FRAGILE BONES, PREMATURE LOSS OF TEETH AND DWARFISM WERE FEATURES. INCREASED BONE FORMATION AND DESTRUCTION WERE THOUGHT TO BE PRESENT. BOTH ACID AND ALKALINE PHOSPHATASES AND LEUCINE AMINO PEPTIDASE WERE ELEVATED. INCREASED HYDROXYPROLINE IN BLOOD AND URINE AND HYPERURICEMIA WERE ALSO DEMONSTRATED.

BAKWIN, H. AND EIGER, M. S.* FRAGILE BONES AND MACROCRANIUM. J. PEDIAT. 49* 558-564, 1956.

R
E
C
E
S
S
I
V
E

BAKWIN, H., GOLDEN, A. AND FOX, S.* FAMILIAL OSTEOECTASIA WITH MACROCRANIUM. AM. J. ROENTGEN. 91* 609-617, 1964.

EYRING, E. J. AND EISENBERG, E.* CONGENITAL HYPERPHOSPHATASIA. A CLINICAL, PATHOLOGICAL, AND BIOCHEMICAL STUDY OF TWO CASES. J. BONE JOINT SURG. 50A* 1099-1117, 1968.

CAFFEY, J.* PEDIATRIC X-RAY DIAGNOSIS. CHICAGO* YEAR BOOK MEDICAL PUBLISHERS, (4TH ED.) 1961.

FANCONI, G., MOREIRA, G., UEHLINGER, E. AND GIEDION, A.* OSTEOCHALASIA DESMALIS FAMILIARIS. HYPEROSTOSIS CORTICALIS DEFORMANS JUVENILES, CHRONIC IDIOPATHIC HYPERPHOSPHATASIA AND MACROCRANIUM. HELV. PAEDIAT. ACTA 19* 279-295, 1964.

RUBIN, P.* CHRONIC IDIOPATHIC HYPERPHOSPHATASEMIA, CONGENITAL. (SYNDROME* JUVENILE PAGET'S DISEASE, HYPEROSTOSIS CORTICALIS DEFORMANS JUVENILES, HYPERPHOS-PHATASIA). DYNAMIC CLASSIFICATION OF BONE DYSPLASIAS. CHICAGO* YEAR BOOK MEDICAL PUBLISHERS, 1964. PP. 340-344.

STEMMERMANN, G. N.* AN HISTOLOGIC AND HISTOCHEMICAL STUDY OF FAMILIAL OSTEOEC-TASIA (CHRONIC IDIOPATHIC HYPERPHOSPHATASIA). AM. J. PATH. 48* 641-651, 1966.

23910 HYPEROSTOSIS CORTICALIS GENERALISATA (VAN BUCHEM'S DISEASE HYPERPHOSPHATASEMIA TARDA)

VAN BUCHEM AND COLLEAGUES (1962) FOUND OSTEOSCLEROSIS OF THE SKULL, MANDIBLE, CLAVICLES, RIBS AND DIAPHYSIS OF THE LONG BONES BEGINNING DURING PUBERTY AND SOMETIMES LEADING TO OPTIC ATROPHY AND PERCEPTIVE DEAFNESS FROM NERVE PRESSURE. THE SAME DISORDER WAS PROBABLY REPORTED EARLIER BY GARLAND (1946) AS 'GENERALIZED LEONTIASIS OSSEA' AND BY HALLIDAY (1949) AS BONE DYSTROPHY.

GARLAND, L. H.* GENERALIZED LEONTIASIS OSSEA. AM. J. ROENTGEN. 55* 37-43, 1946.

HALLIDAY, J.* A RARE CASE OF BONE DYSTROPHY. BRIT. J. SURG. 37* 52-63, 1949.

VAN BUCHEM, F. S. P., HADDERS, H. N., HANSEN, J. F. AND WOLDRING, M. G.* HYPEROSTOSIS CORTICALIS GENERALISATA* REPORT OF SEVEN CASES. AM. J. MED. 33* 387-397, 1962.

23920 HYPERPARATHYROIDISM, NEONATAL FAMILIAL PRIMARY

HILLMAN AND COLLEAGUES (1964) DESCRIBED NEONATAL PRIMARY HYPERPARATHYROIDISM IN TWO MALE SIBS, OFFSPRING OF FIRST COUSIN PARENTS. PHILIPS (1948) HAD EARLIER REPORTED ONE OF THE SIBS.

HILLMAN, D. A., SCRIVER, C. R., PEDVIS, S. AND SHRAGOVITCH, I.* NEONATAL FAMILIAL PRIMARY HYPERPARATHYROIDISM. NEW ENG. J. MED. 270* 483-490, 1964.

PHILIPS, R. N.* PRIMARY DIFFUSE PARATHYROID HYPERPLASIA IN AN INFANT OF FOUR MONTHS. PEDIATRICS 2* 428-434, 1948.

*23930 HYPERPHOSPHATASIA WITH MENTAL RETARDATION

THREE SIBS AND A FIRST COUSIN HAD SEVERE MENTAL RETARDATION, SEIZURES, VARIOUS NEUROLOGIC ABNORMALITIES AND GREATLY ELEVATED ALKALINE PHOSPHATASE. BOTH PAIRS OF PARENTS WERE CONSANGUINEOUS. THE ALKALINE PHOSPHATASE PRESENT IN EXCESS SEEMED TO BE OF HEPATIC ORIGIN.

MABRY, C. C., BAUTISTA, A., KIRK, R. F. H., DUBILIER, L. D., BRAUNSTEIN, H. AND KOEPKE, J. A.* FAMILIAL HYPERPHOSPHATASIA WITH MENTAL RETARDATION, SEIZURES, AND NEUROLOGIC DEFICITS. J. PEDIAT. 77* 74-85, 1970.

23940 HYPERPIPECOLATEMIA

IN A CHILD WITH A DEGENERATIVE NEUROLOGICAL DISEASE AND HEPATOMEGALY, GATFIELD ET AL. (1968) FOUND GROSSLY ELEVATED BLOOD CONCENTRATIONS OF PIPECOLIC ACID WITH MILD GENERALIZED AMINOACIDURIA. PIPECOLIC ACID IS AN INTERMEDIATE IN LYSINE CATABO-LISM. HOWEVER, THE PATIENT SHOWED NO DELAY IN CLEARING LYSINE FROM THE BLOOD, INDICATING AS DOES OTHER EVIDENCE THAT THE MAIN LYSINE CATABOLIC PATHWAY IS NOT IN A PIPECOLIC ACID. AUTOPSY REVEALED WIDESPREAD DEMYELINATION IN THE CENTRAL NERVOUS SYSTEM.

GATFIELD, P. D., TALLER, E., HINTON, G. G., WALLACE, A. C., ABDELNOUR, G. M. AND HAUST, M. D.* HYPERPIPECOLATEMIA* A NEW METABOLIC DISORDER ASSOCIATED WITH NEUROPATHY AND HEPATOMEGALY* A CASE STUDY. CANAD. MED. ASS. J. 99* 1215-1233, 1968.

*23950 HYPERPROLINEMIA, TYPE I

SCRIVER, SCHAFER AND EFRON (1961) AND SCHAFER, SCRIVER AND EFRON (1962) DESCRIBED A FAMILY IN WHICH THE MALE PROBAND AND THREE SIBS HAD ELEVATED PLASMA LEVELS OF L-

PROLINE. PROBABLY THE ANOMALY BORE NO RELATION TO TWO OTHER GENETIC DEFECTS IN THE SAME FAMILY* FAMILIAL NEPHROPATHY AND PHOTOGENIC EPILEPSY. THE AMINO-ACIDURIA INCLUDES HYDROXYPROLINE AND GLYCINE AS WELL AS PROLINE, PRESUMABLY BECAUSE THESE THREE AMINO ACIDS SHARE A RENAL TUBULAR ACTIVE TRANSPORT MECHANISM WHICH IS OVERLOADED BY THE HIGH LEVEL OF PROLINE IN THE GLOMERULAR FILTRATE. TWO TYPES OF HYPERPROLINEMIA APPEAR TO EXIST. IN TYPE I REFERRED TO ABOVE THE DEFECT INVOLVES THE ENZYME PROLINE OXIDASE (EFRON, 1965). RENAL ABNORMALITIES OCCUR IN THIS FORM. IN TYPE II, CHARACTERIZED BY MENTAL RETARDATION AND CONVULSIONS, THE ENZYME DEFECT CONCERNS DELTA 1- PYRROLINE-5-CARBOXYLATE (PC) DEHYDROGENASE AND THE SUBSTANCE NORMALLY ACTED ON BY THIS ENZYME IS EXCRETED IN THE URINE. THE FAMILY OF EFRON (1965) WAS ITALIAN. THAT OF SCRIVER ET AL. (1961) AND SCHAFER ET AL. (1962) WAS SCOTCH-IRISH. PERRY ET AL. (1968) REPORTED HYPERPROLINEMIA OF TYPE I IN TWO GENERATIONS OF A CONSANGUINEOUS AMERICAN INDIAN FAMILY. HEREDITARY RENAL ABNORMALITIES OCCURRED IN MEMBERS OF 3 GENERATIONS. THE PROBAND LATER DEVELOPED WILMS* TUMOR. MARKED ELEVATIONS OF PLASMA PROLINE OCCUR IN HOMOZYGOTES AND NORMAL OR MODERATELY ELEVATED LEVELS IN HETEROZYGOTES, IN THE VIEW OF THE AUTHORS. BOTH GENOTYPES ARE ACCOMPANIED BY RENAL ABNORMALITIES. MENTAL RETARDATION IS NOT A FEATURE OF TYPE I HYPERPROLINEMIA. GOYER ET AL. (1968) OBSERVED HEREDITARY NEPHRITIS, NEUROSENSORY HEARING LOSS, PROLINURIA AND ICHTHYOSIS IN VARIOUS COMBINATIONS IN 23 MEMBERS OF A KINDRED. THE RELATION TO THE HYPERPROLINURIAS AND TO ALPORT*S SYNDROME IS NOT CLEAR. THE PATIENT REPORTED BY ROKKONES ET AL. (1968) HAD UNCLE-NIECE PARENTS. SELKOE (1969) DESCRIBED A SECOND TYPE OF HYPERPROLINEMIA WITH ONLY MILD MENTAL RETARDATION AND WITHOUT RENAL DISEASE. THE ENZYME INVOLVED SEEMS TO BE DELTA PRIME-PYRROLINE-5-CARBOXYLIC ACID DEHYDROGENASE. EMERY ET AL. (1968) DESCRIBED AN AFFECTED 18 YEAR OLD GIRL WHO WAS MENTALLY RETARDED AND HAD A RETARDED SISTER WHO HAD DIED PROBABLY OF THE SAME DISORDER.

EFRON, M. L.* DISORDERS OF PROLINE AND HYDROXYPROLINE METABOLISM. IN, STANBURY, J. B., WYNGAARDEN, J. B. AND FREDRICKSON, D. S. (EDS.)* THE METABOLIC BASIS OF INHERITED DISEASE. NEW YORK* MCGRAW-HILL, 1966 (2ND ED.). PP. 376-392.

EFRON, M. L.* FAMILIAL HYPERPROLINEMIA. REPORT OF SECOND CASE, ASSOCIATED WITH CONGENITAL RENAL MALFORMATION, HEREDITARY HEMATURIA AND MILD MENTAL RETARDATION, WITH DEMONSTRATION OF ENZYME DEFECT. NEW ENG. J. MED. 272* 1243-1254, 1965.

EMERY, F. A., GOLDIE, L. AND STERN, J.* HYPERPROLINAEMIA TYPE 2. J. MENT. DEFIC. RES. 12* 187-195, 1968.

GOYER, R. A., REYNOLDS, J., JR., BURKE, J. AND BURKHOLDER, P.* HEREDITARY RENAL DISEASE WITH NEUROSENSORY HEARING LOSS, PROLINURIA AND ICHTHYOSIS. AM. J. MED. SCI. 256* 166-179, 1968.

PERRY, T. L., HARDWICK, D. F., LOWRY, R. B. AND HANSEN, S.* HYPERPROLINAEMIA IN TWO SUCCESSIVE GENERATIONS OF A NORTH AMERICAN INDIAN FAMILY. ANN. HUM. GENET. 31* 401-408, 1968.

ROKKONES, T. AND LOKEN, A. C.* CONGENITAL RENAL DYSPLASIA, RETINAL DYSPLASIA AND MENTAL RETARDATION ASSOCIATED WITH HYPERPROLINURIA AND HYPER-OH-PROLINURIA. ACTA PAEDIAT. SCAND. 57* 225-229, 1968.

SCHAFER, I. A., SCRIVER, C. R. AND EFRON, M. L.* FAMILIAL HYPERPROLINEMIA, CEREBRAL DYSFUNCTION AND RENAL ANOMALIES OCCURRING IN A FAMILY WITH HEREDITARY NEPHROPATHY AND DEAFNESS. NEW ENG. J. MED. 267* 51-60, 1962.

SCRIVER, C. R., SCHAFER, I. A. AND EFRON, M. L.* NEW RENAL TUBULAR AMINO-ACID TRANSPORT SYSTEM AND A NEW HEREDITARY DISORDER OF AMINO-ACID METABOLISM. NATURE 192* 672-673, 1961.

SELKOE, D. J.* FAMILIAL HYPERPROLINEMIA AND MENTAL RETARDATION. A SECOND METABOLIC TYPE. NEUROLOGY 19* 494-502, 1969.

*23961 HYPERPROLINEMIA, TYPE II

SEE ABOVE.

23960 HYPERSEROTONEMIA

SOUTHREN ET AL. (1959) DESCRIBED A 49 YEAR OLD WOMAN WHO FROM EARLY CHILDHOOD HAD SEVERE RAGE REACTIONS WITH EPISODES OF FLUSHING OF THE FACE, NECK AND ARMS. HAND TREMOR, SLURRED SPEECH AND ATAXIA BEGAN AT AGE 32. BLOOD SEROTONIN WAS MARKEDLY ELEVATED. 5-HYDROXYINDOLEACETIC ACID WAS NORMAL IN THE URINE BUT INCREASED AFTER ADMINISTRATION OF SEROTONIN. ADMINISTRATION OF RESERPINE AGGRAVATED THE SYMPTOMS.

SOUTHREN, A. L., WARNER, R. R. P., CHRISTOFF, N. I. AND WEINER, H. E.* AN UNUSUAL NEUROLOGIC SYNDROME ASSOCIATED WITH HYPERSEROTONEMIA. NEW ENG. J. MED. 260* 1265-1268, 1959.

23970 HYPERTELORISM, CRYPTORCHIDISM, DIGITAL CONTRACTURES, STERNAL DEFORMITY, AND OSTEOCHONDRITIS DISSECANS

THIS COMBINATION OF ABNORMALITIES HAS BEEN NOTED IN TWO BROTHERS. OSTEOCHONDRITIS DISSECANS OCCURRED AT MULTIPLE SITES (KNEE, ELBOW, ETC.). EARLY FUSION OF THE

R
E
C
E
S
S
I
V
E

MANUBRIUM AND CORPUS STERNI OCCURRED. THE EARS WERE FLOPPY. FAMILIAL OSTEOCHON-DRITIS DISSECANS HAVE BEEN THOUGHT TO BE DOMINANT (Q.V.). PTOSIS WAS PRESENT IN ONE OF THE BROTHERS. GORLIN (1967) HAS SHOWN ME A FAMILY IN WHICH TWO BOYS AND THEIR MOTHER HAVE MANIFESTATIONS LIKE THOSE IN THE SIBS REPORTED BY HANLEY ET AL. (1967). THE BOYS HAD DIFFERENT FATHERS. HENCE, THE INHERITANCE MAY BE DOMINANT. WELCH (1970) HAS EVALUATED TWO BROTHERS WITH THIS SYNDROME.

GORLIN, R. J.* MINNEAPOLIS, MINN.* PERSONAL COMMUNICATION, 1967.

HANLEY, W. B., MCKUSICK, V. A. AND BARRANCO, F. T.* OSTEOCHONDRITIS DISSECANS WITH ASSOCIATED MALFORMATIONS IN TWO BROTHERS. A REVIEW OF FAMILIAL ASPECTS. J. BONE JOINT SURG. 49A* 925-937, 1967.

WELCH, J. P.* HALIFAX, NOVA SCOTIA* PERSONAL COMMUNICATION, 1971.

23980 HYPERTELORISM, MICROTIA, FACIAL CLEFTING (HMC) SYNDROME

BIXLER, CHRISTIAN AND GORLIN (1969) DESCRIBED TWO SISTERS WHO HAD HYPERTELORISM, MICROTIA, AND CLEFTING OF THE LIP, PALATE AND NOSE. IN ADDITION, THEY SHOWED PSYCHOMOTOR RETARDATION, ATRETIC AUDITORY CANALS, MICROCEPHALY, AND ECTOPIC KIDNEYS. BOTH HAD CONGENITAL HEART MALFORMATIONS, AS DID ALSO SEVERAL RELATIVES ON THE MOTHER'S SIDE. THE PARENTS WERE NORMAL AND UNRELATED.

BIXLER, D., CHRISTIAN, J. C. AND GORLIN, R. J.* HYPERTELORISM, MICROTIA AND FACIAL CLEFTING* A NEW INHERITED SYNDROME. THE CLINICAL DELINEATION OF BIRTH DEFECTS. II. MALFORMATION SYNDROMES. NEW YORK* NATIONAL FOUNDATION, 1969. PP. 77-81.

EDGERTON, M. T., UDVARHELYI, G. B. AND KNOX, D. L.* THE SURGICAL CORRECTION OF OCULAR HYPERTELORISM. ANN. SURG. 172* 473-496, 1970.

23990 HYPERTROPHIC NEUROPATHY AND CATARACT

GOLD AND HOGENKUIS (1968) OBSERVED THIS COMBINATION IN 2 SISTERS AND THEIR BROTHER OF HINDU EXTRACTION. SPINAL FLUID PROTEIN WAS MODERATELY ELEVATED. SEVERE DISTAL SENSORY AND MOTOR LOSS WAS PRESENT.

GOLD, G. N. AND HOGENKUIS, L. A. H.* HYPERTROPHIC INTERSTITIAL NEUROPATHY AND CATARACTS. NEUROLOGY 18* 526-533, 1968.

24000 HYPERURICEMIA, INFANTILE, WITH ABNORMAL BEHAVIOR AND NORMAL HYPOXANTHINE GUANINE PHOSPHORIBOSYL TRANSFERASE

NYHAN ET AL. (1969) REPORTED A 3 YEAR OLD BOY WITH MENTAL RETARDATION, DYSPLASTIC TEETH, FAILURE TO CRY WITH TEARS, ABSENT SPEECH AND AUTISTIC BEHAVIOR. HGPT WAS NORMAL, WHEREAS THE ACTIVITY OF ADENINE PHOSPHORIBOSYLTRANSFERASE WAS INCREASED. NOTHING IS KNOWN ABOUT ITS GENETICS.

NYHAN, W. L., JAMES, J. A., TEBERG, A. J., SWEETMAN, L. AND NELSON, L. G.* A NEW DISORDER OF PURINE METABOLISM WITH BEHAVIORAL MANIFESTATIONS. J. PEDIAT. 74* 20-27, 1969.

24010 HYPERURICEMIA, LIPODYSTROPHY AND NEUROLOGIC DEFECT

MEADOR (1966) HAS INFORMED ME OF THREE SIBS (2 FEMALE, 1 MALE), WHOSE PARENTS ARE PROBABLY RELATED AND WHO SHOW LOSS OF FAT ON THE LOWER PART OF THE BODY WITH ABUNDANT FAT ON THE UPPER PART, ESPECIALLY AROUND THE NECK, PYRAMIDAL TRACT DISEASE, PES CAVUS, AND HYPERURICEMIA WITH CLINICAL GOUT. THE APPROXIMATE AGES WERE 28, 24 AND 18.

MEADOR, C.* BIRMINGHAM, ALA.* PERSONAL COMMUNICATION, 1966.

*24020 HYPOADRENOCORTICISM, FAMILIAL

THE ISOLATED FORM IS LESS FREQUENT THAN THAT COMBINED WITH OTHER ENDOCRINOPATHY, PARTICULARLY HYPOPARATHYROIDISM. A NOTEWORTHY FEATURE IS THE LACK OF HYPOALDOS-TERONISM (STEMPFEL AND ENGEL, 1960* SHEPARD, LANDING AND MASON, 1959). ANDROGEN METABOLISM COULD NOT BE TESTED. THESE CASES MAY WELL HAVE A DEFECT LIMITED TO CORTICOID METABOLISM. SOME OF THESE CASES MAY WITH MORE VALIDITY BE CLASSED AS ADRENAL UNRESPONSIVENESS TO ACTH (Q.V.). BERLIN (1952) REPORTED ADDISON'S DISEASE IN BROTHER AND SISTER, THE LATTER HAVING ALSO PERNICIOUS ANEMIA. BROCHNER-MORTENSEN (1956) DESCRIBED ADDISON'S DISEASE IN TWO BROTHERS AND TWO OF THEIR MATERNAL UNCLES. MEAKIN, NELSON AND THORN (1959) DESCRIBED TWO BROTHERS WITH ONSET OF ADRENAL INSUFFICIENCY AT AGE 3-4 YEARS. ADDISON'S DISEASE FALLS INTO THE SAME CATEGORY AS PERNICIOUS ANEMIA, SYSTEMIC LUPUS ERYTHEMATOSUS, MYASTHENIA GRAVIS, HASHIMOTO'S THYROIDITIS, ATHYREOTIC CRETINISM, IN WHICH AN AUTOIMMUNE BASIS IS SUGGESTED BY SOME EVIDENCE AND IN WHICH FAMILIAL AGGREGATION OCCURS. IN ALL THESE CONDITIONS, THE ROLE OF A SINGLE GENETIC LOCUS IN ETIOLOGY IS UNCLEAR. WILLIAMS AND FREEMAN (1965) REPORTED ADRENAL CORTICAL HYPOFUNCTION WITHOUT SALT LOSS IN 3 OF 4 CHILDREN OF SECOND COUSIN PARENTS. O'DONOHOE AND HOLLAND (1968) DESCRIBED AUTOPSY-PROVEN ADRENAL HYPOPLASIA IN A SISTER OF TWO AFFECTED MALES. LEMLI AND SMITH (1968) REPORTED AFFECTED SISTERS.

BERLIN, R.* ADDISON'S DISEASE. FAMILIAL INCIDENCE AND OCCURRENCE IN ASSOCIA-
TION WITH PERNICIOUS ANEMIA. ACTA MED. SCAND. 144* 1-6, 1952.

BOYD, J. F. AND MACDONALD, A. M.* ADRENAL CORTICAL HYPOPLASIA IN SIBLINGS.
ARCH. DIS. CHILD. 35* 561-568, 1960.

BROCHNER-MORTENSEN, K.* FAMILIAL OCCURRENCE OF ADDISON'S DISEASE. ACTA MED.
SCAND. 156* 205-209, 1956.

LEMLI, L. AND SMITH, D. W.* IDIOPATHIC ADRENAL INSUFFICIENCY IN TWO SIBLINGS.
MAANDSCHR. KINDERGENEESK. 34* 63, 1968.

LOURIA, D. B., SHANNON, D., JOHNSON, G., CAROLINE, L., OKAS, A. AND TASCHDJIAN,
C.* THE SUSCEPTIBILITY TO MONILIASIS IN CHILDREN WITH ENDOCRINE HYPOFUNCTION.
TRANS. ASS. AM. PHYSICIANS 80* 236-249, 1967.

MEAKIN, J. W., NELSON, D. H. AND THORN, G. W.* ADDISON'S DISEASE IN TWO
BROTHERS. J. CLIN. ENDOCR. 19* 726-731, 1959.

MITCHELL, R. G. AND RHANEY, K.* CONGENITAL ADRENAL HYPOPLASIA IN SIBLINGS.
LANCET 1* 488-492, 1959.

O'DONOHOE, N. V. AND HOLLAND, P. D. J.* FAMILIAL CONGENITAL ADRENAL HYPOPLASIA.
ARCH. DIS. CHILD. 43* 717-723, 1968.

SHEPARD, T. H., LANDING, B. H. AND MASON, D. G.* FAMILIAL ADDISON'S DISEASE*
CASE REPORTS OF TWO SISTERS WITH CORTICOID DEFICIENCY UNASSOCIATED WITH HYPOALDOS-
TERONISM. AM. J. DIS. CHILD. 97* 154-162, 1959.

STEMPFEL, R. S., JR. AND ENGEL, F. L.* A CONGENITAL, FAMILIAL SYNDROME OF
ADRENOCORTICAL INSUFFICIENCY WITHOUT HYPOALDOSTERONISM. J. PEDIAT. 57* 443-451,
1960.

WILLIAMS, H. E. AND FREEMAN, M.* PRIMARY FAMILIAL ADDISON'S DISEASE. AUST.
PEDIAT. J. 1* 93-97, 1965.

R
E
C *24030 HYPOADRENOCORTICISM, WITH HYPOPARATHYROIDISM AND SUPERFICIAL MONILIASIS
E
S
S MONILIASIS USUALLY PRECEDES SYMPTOMS AND SIGNS OF ENDOCRINOPATHY. FURTHERMORE,
I HYPOPARATHYROIDISM USUALLY REVEALS ITSELF BEFORE ADRENAL INSUFFICIENCY. SEE
V HYPOPARATHYROIDISM.
E   AN INFECTIOUS ETIOLOGY WAS SUGGESTED BY KUNIN AND COLLEAGUES (1963) WHO
POINTED OUT THAT HEPATITIS HAS OCCURRED IN A NUMBER OF THESE CASES BEFORE THE
DEVELOPMENT OF ENDOCRINOPATHY.
       HUNG, MIGEON AND PARROTT (1963) FOUND CIRCULATING ADRENAL ANTIBODIES IN TWO
SIBS WITH ADDISON'S DISEASE. A THIRD SIB HAD DIED FROM ADDISON'S DISEASE. ONE OF
THE AFFECTED SIBS ALSO HAD HYPOPARATHYROIDISM, PERNICIOUS ANEMIA AND SUPERFICIAL
MONILIASIS. THE AUTHORS SUGGESTED THE DISORDER MAY NOT BE INHERITED AS A SIMPLE
MENDELIAN RECESSIVE BUT MAY BE AUTO-IMMUNE IN NATURE. SHANNON ET AL. (1966) MADE
THE NOVEL SUGGESTION THAT A GENETIC DEFECT OF THE INTEGUMENT IS PRIMARY AND
PREDISPOSES TO DEVELOPMENT OF CHRONIC MONILIASIS, AND THAT AN ABSORPTION PRODUCT
OF CANDIDA ALBICANS ACTS DIRECTLY AS A TOXIN OR INDIRECTLY AS A CROSS-REACTING
ANTIGEN TO GIVE PROGRESSIVE TISSUE DAMAGE. IF TRUE, THE THEORY MAKES IT URGENT TO
ERADICATE THE FUNGUS FROM THESE PATIENTS. HETEROGENEITY IN THIS GROUP OF CASES
(ADDISON'S DISEASE WITHOUT HYPOPARATHYROIDISM, ADDISON'S DISEASE WITH HYPOPARA-
THYROIDISM, HYPOPARATHYROIDISM WITHOUT ADDISON'S DISEASE, SCHMIDT'S SYNDROME) WAS
SUGGESTED BY THE ANALYSIS OF SPINNER ET AL. (1968). FOZ ET AL. (1970) MADE A
BRIEF NOTE OF A SIBSHIP, OFFSPRING OF FIRST-COUSIN PARENTS, CONTAINING TWO FEMALE
SIBS WITH IDIOPATHIC ADDISON'S DISEASE. ONE ALSO HAD PRIMARY HYPOPARATHYROIDISM
AND ONE HAD ORAL CANDIDIASIS.

CRAIG, J. M., SCHIFF, L. H. AND BOONE, J. E.* CHRONIC MONILIASIS ASSOCIATED
WITH ADDISON'S DISEASE. AM. J. DIS. CHILD. 89* 669-684, 1955.

FOZ, M., MIRADA, A. AND GUARDIA, J.* ENDOCRINE DISORDERS IN A FAMILY. (LETTER)
LANCET 2* 269 ONLY, 1970.

GASS, J. D. M.* THE SYNDROME OF KERATOCONJUNCTIVITIS, SUPERFICIAL MONILIASIS,
IDIOPATHIC HYPOPARATHYROIDISM AND ADDISON'S DISEASE. AM. J. OPHTHAL. 54* 660-674,
1962.

HIEKKALA, H.* IDIOPATHIC HYPOPARATHYROIDISM, ADRENAL INSUFFICIENCY AND
MONILIASIS IN CHILDREN. ANN. PAEDIAT. FENN. 10* 213-222, 1964.

HUNG, W., MIGEON, C. J. AND PARROTT, R. H.* A POSSIBLE AUTOIMMUNE BASIS FOR
ADDISON'S DISEASE IN THREE SIBLINGS, ONE WITH IDIOPATHIC HYPOPARATHYROIDISM,
PERNICIOUS ANEMIA AND SUPERFICIAL MONILIASIS. NEW ENG. J. MED. 269* 658-663,
1963.

KENNY, F. M. AND HOLLIDAY, M. D.* HYPOPARATHYROIDISM, MONILIASIS, ADDISON'S AND
HASHIMOTO'S DISEASE. HYPERCALCEMIA TREATED WITH INTRAVENOUSLY ADMINISTERED SODIUM
SULFATE. NEW ENG. J. MED. 271* 708-713, 1964.

KUNIN, A. S., MACKAY, B. R., BURNS, S. L. AND HALBERSTAM, M. J.* THE SYNDROME
OF HYPOPARATHYROIDISM AND ADRENOCORTICAL INSUFFICIENCY, A POSSIBLE SEQUEL OF
HEPATITIS* CASE REPORT AND REVIEW OF THE LITERATURE. AM. J. MED. 34* 856-866,
1963.

SHANNON, D. C., JOHNSON, G. AND AUSTEN, K. F.* GENETIC AND CLINICAL ASPECTS OF
THE SYNDROME OF CHRONIC MONILIASIS AND ENDOCRINE DEFICITS. SOC. PEDIAT. RES.
(APRIL 29-30, 1966) 101 ONLY, 1966.

SPINNER, M. W., BLIZZARD, R. M. AND CHILDS, B.* CLINICAL AND GENETICALLY
HETEROGENEITY IN IDIOPATHIC ADDISON'S DISEASE AND HYPOPARATHYROIDISM. J. CLIN.
ENDOCR. 28* 795-804, 1968.

SWEETNAM, W. P.* JUVENILE FAMILIAL ENDOCRINOPATHY. LANCET 1* 463-465, 1966.

WHITAKER, J. A., LANDING, B. H., ESSELBORN, V. M. AND WILLIAMS, R. R.* SYNDROME
OF FAMILIAL JUVENILE HYPOADRENOCORTICISM, HYPOPARATHYROIDISM AND SUPERFICIAL
MONILIASIS. J. CLIN. ENDOCR. 16* 1374-1387, 1956.

*24040 HYPOASCORBEMIA

AS FAR AS IS KNOWN, ALL MEN LACK THE ABILITY TO SYNTHESIZE ASCORBIC ACID, THROUGH
LACK OF THE ENZYME L-GULONOLACTONE OXIDASE WHICH MOST OTHER MAMMALS POSSESS. AS
STONE (1967) POINTS OUT HYPOASCORBEMIA IS AN INBORN ERROR OF METABOLISM.
BORROWING A TERM FROM THE BLOOD GROUPS WE MIGHT SAY THAT IT IS A *PUBLIC* INBORN
ERROR OF METABOLISM. THE MECHANISM WHEREBY AN ORGANISM LOSES A PARTICULAR
METABOLIC FUNCTION WHICH IS OF NO USE IN A PARTICULAR ENVIRONMENTAL WAS DISCUSSED
BY KING AND JUKES (1969). THE ACCUMULATION OF RANDOM MUTATIONS IS THE GENE FOR
THE RELEVANT ENZYME MIGHT BE EXPECTED TO DESTROY THE FUNCTIONAL CAPACITY OF THE
ENZYME, MOST MUTATIONS BEING DISRUPTIVE. IF THE ENZYME IS NOT REQUIRED IN THE
PARTICULAR ENVIRONMENT, THE CONSTRAINT OF SELECTION IS REMOVED. PRIMATES AND THE
GUINEA PIG, BY THIS HYPOTHESIS, HAVE LOST THE CAPACITY TO SYNTHESIZE ASCORBIC ACID
BECAUSE OF THE ADEQUACY OF DIETARY INTAKE. AN INTRASPECIES EXAMPLE OF THIS
PHENOMENON MAY BE THE LOSS OF ADULT INTESTINAL LACTASE IN PEOPLE WHO DO NOT
CONSUME MILK.

KING, J. L. AND JUKES, T. H.* NON-DARWINIAN EVOLUTION. SCIENCE 164* 788-798,
1969.

PAULING, L.* EVOLUTION AND THE NEED FOR ASCORBIC ACID. PROC. NAT. ACAD. SCI.
67* 1643-1648, 1970.

STONE, I.* THE GENETIC DISEASE, HYPOASCORBEMIA. A FRESH APPROACH TO AN ANCIENT
DISEASE AND SOME OF ITS MEDICAL IMPLICATIONS. ACTA GENET. MED. GEM. 16* 52-62,
1967.

*24050 HYPOGAMMAGLOBULINEMIA (SEE ALSO AGAMMAGLOBULINEMIA, NETHERTON'S DISEASE)

WOLLHEIM (1961) DESCRIBED TWO FEMALES WITH *ACQUIRED* HYPOGAMMAGLOBULINEMIA WHO
CAME FROM DIFFERENT PARTS OF SWEDEN BUT WERE REMOTELY RELATED. HE SUGGESTED THAT
A RECESSIVE GENETIC FACTOR MAY BE INVOLVED IN *ACQUIRED* HYPOGAMMAGLOBULINEMIA.
KAMIN ET AL. (1968) FOUND THAT PHYTOHEMAGGLUTININ-INDUCED INCORPORATION OF
LABELLED PRECURSORS INTO DNA AND RNA BY LYMPHOCYTES IS SIGNIFICANTLY DIMINISHED IN
CELLS OF ADULTS WITH SO-CALLED *ACQUIRED* AGAMMAGLOBULINEMIA. THE DIFFERENCE WAS
INDEPENDANT OF THE CHARACTERISTICS OF THE CULTURE-MEDIUM, INDICATING A CELLULAR
ABNORMALITY. THEY SUGGESTED THAT THIS IS THE FIRST LABORATORY TEST THAT DETECTS
THE CARRIER STATE IN A GENETICALLY DETERMINED DISORDER THAT BECOMES MANIFEST IN
ADULT LIFE.

CHARACHE, P., ROSEN, F. S., JANEWAY, C. A., CRAIG, J. M. AND ROSENBERG, H. A.*
ACQUIRED AGAMMAGLOBULINEMIA IN SIBLINGS. LANCET 1* 234-237, 1965.

KAMIN, R. M., FUDENBERG, H. H. AND DOUGLAS, S. D.* A GENETIC DEFECT IN
ACQUIRED AGAMMAGLOBULINEMIA. PROC. NAT. ACAD. SCI. 60* 881-885, 1968.

WOLLHEIM, F. A.* INHERITED *ACQUIRED* HYPOGAMMAGLOBULINAEMIA. LANCET 1* 316-
317, 1961.

WOLLHEIM, F. A.* PRIMARY *ACQUIRED* HYPOGAMMAGLOBULINEMIA* GENETIC DEFECT OR
ACQUIRED DISEASE.Q IN, IMMUNOLOGIC DEFICIENCY DISEASES IN MAN (BIRTH DEFECTS
ORIGINAL ARTICLE SERIES, VOL. IV, NO. 1). NEW YORK* NATIONAL FOUNDATION, 1968.

*24060 HYPOGLYCEMIA DUE TO DEFICIENCY OF GLYCOGEN SYNTHETASE IN THE LIVER

IN A WELL STUDIED FAMILY, LEWIS, SPENCER-PEET AND STEWART (1963) DEMONSTRATED THAT
INFANTILE HYPOGLYCEMIA WAS DUE TO A DEFICIENCY OF GLYCOGEN SYNTHETASE IN THE
LIVER. THE CASES WERE PROBABLY OF THE SAME TYPE AS THOSE REPORTED BY BROBERGER
AND ZETTERSTROM (1961) BECAUSE URINARY EXCRETION OF CATECHOLAMINES WAS NOT
INFLUENCED BY HYPOGLYCEMIA. THE OBSERVATIONS OF LEWIS ET AL. (1963) ARE PARTICU-
LARLY CONVINCING EVIDENCE FOR AUTOSOMAL RECESSIVE INHERITANCE OF THIS ONE FORM,
ALTHOUGH IRON-CLAD PROOF AWAITS DEMONSTRATION OF A PARTIAL DEFICIENCY IN BOTH
PARENTS. SEE FRUCTOSE-1,6-PHOSPHATASE, HEPATIC DEFICIENCY OF (ANOTHER CAUSE OF

R
E
C
E
S
S
I
V
E

BROBERGER, O. AND ZETTERSTROM, R.* HYPOGLYCEMIA WITH AN INABILITY TO INCREASE THE EPINEPHRINE SECRETION IN INSULIN-INDUCED HYPOGLYCEMIA. J. PEDIAT. 59* 215-222, 1961.

LEWIS, G. M., SPENCER-PEET, J. AND STEWART, K. M.* INFANTILE HYPOGLYCAEMIA DUE TO INHERITED DEFICIENCY OF GLYCOGEN SYNTHETASE IN LIVER. ARCH. DIS. CHILD. 38* 40-48, 1963.

24070 HYPOGLYCEMIA WITH ABSENT PANCREATIC ALPHA CELLS

MCQUARRIE ET AL. (1950) OBSERVED THE CONDITIONS IN SIBS. GOTLIN AND SILVER (1970) MEASURED HIGH INSULIN LEVELS.

GOTLIN, R. W. AND SILVER, H. K.* NEONATAL HYPOGLYCAEMIA, HYPERINSULINISM, AND ABSENCE OF PANCREATIC ALPHA-CELLS. (LETTER) LANCET 2* 1346 ONLY, 1970.

MCQUARRIE, I., BELL, E. T., ZIMMERMAN, B. AND WRIGHT, W. S.* DEFICIENCY OF ALPHA CELLS OF PANCREAS AS POSSIBLE ETIOLOGICAL FACTOR IN FAMILIAL HYPOGLYCEMOSIS. (ABSTRACT) FED. PROC. 9* 337 ONLY, 1950.

*24080 HYPOGLYCEMIA, LEUCINE INDUCED

SEVERAL TYPES OF FAMILIAL INFANTILE HYPOGLYCEMIA HAVE BEEN REPORTED, INCLUDING THOSE PRECIPITATED BY LEUCINE (COCHRANE ET AL., 1956* DIGEORGE AND AUERBACH, 1960). EBBIN ET AL. (1967) OBSERVED SYMPTOMATIC HYPOGLYCEMIA WITH LEUCINE SENSITIVITY IN A MOTHER AND DAUGHTER. OTHER CASES OF ADULTS WITH LEUCINE SENSITIVITY HAVE HAD ISLET ADENOMAS WHICH APPARENTLY WERE NOT PRESENT IN THIS CASE, HOWEVER.

COCHRANE, W. A., PAYNE, W. W., SIMPKISS, M. J. AND WOOLF, L. I.* FAMILIAL HYPOGLYCEMIA PRECIPITATED BY AMINO ACIDS. J. CLIN. INVEST. 35* 411-422, 1956.

DIGEORGE, A. M. AND AUERBACH, V. H.* LEUCINE-INDUCED HYPOGLYCEMIA* A REVIEW AND SPECULATIONS. AM. J. MED. SCI. 240* 792-801, 1960.

EBBIN, A. J., HUNTLEY, C. AND TRANQUADA, R. E.* SYMPTOMATIC LEUCINE SENSITIVITY IN A MOTHER AND DAUGHTER. METABOLISM 16* 926-932, 1967.

MCQUARRIE, I.* IDIOPATHIC SPONTANEOUSLY OCCURRING HYPOGLYCEMIA IN INFANTS. CLINICAL SIGNIFICANCE OF PROBLEMS AND TREATMENT. AM. J. DIS. CHILD. 87* 399-428, 1954.

R
E
C
E
S
S
I
V
E

24090 HYPOGLYCEMIA, NEONATAL, SIMULATING FOETOPATHIA DIABETICA

HANSSON AND REDIN (1963) OBSERVED TWO FEMALE OFFSPRING FROM FIRST-COUSIN PARENTS WHO HAD NEONATAL HYPOGLYCEMIA AND AN APPEARANCE LIKE CUSHING'S DISEASE. ALTHOUGH THESE FEATURES SUGGESTED THOSE OF THE BABY BORN OF A DIABETIC MOTHER, THE GLUCOSE TOLERANCE TEST WAS NORMAL IN THE MOTHER.

HANSSON, G. AND REDIN, B.* FAMILIAL NEONATAL HYPOGLYCEMIA. A SYNDROME RESEMBLING FOETOPATHIA DIABETICA. ACTA PAEDIAT. 52* 145-152, 1963.

24100 HYPOGONADISM WITH LOW-GRADE MENTAL DEFICIENCY AND MICROCEPHALY

KRAUS-RUPPERT (1958) DESCRIBED THREE BROTHERS FROM A CONSANGUINEOUS MATING. SYNDACTYLY OF THE SECOND TO FOURTH TOES AND EUNUCHOIDISM WERE ALSO PRESENT. THE TESTES SHOWED NO SPERMATOGENESIS AND THE INTERSTITIUM WAS OCCUPIED MAINLY BY CONNECTIVE TISSUE.

KRAUS-RUPPERT, R.* ZUR FRAGE EREBTER DIENCEPHALER STORUNGEN (INFANTILER EUNUCHOIDISMUS SOWIE MIKROCEPHALIE BEI RECESSIVEM ERBGANG). Z. MENSCHL. VERERB. KONSTITUTIONSL. 34* 643-656, 1958.

24110 HYPOGONADISM, MALE

FAMILIAL MALE HYPOGONADISM IS A HIGHLY HETEROZYGOUS CATEGORY FROM WHICH SOME DISORDERS SUCH AS REIFENSTEIN'S SYNDROME, KALLMAN'S SYNDROME, ISOLATED GONADOTRO-PIN DEFICIENCY AND SOME OTHER ENTITIES CAN BE SEPARATED PRESENTLY. THE PRESENCE OF AN AUTOSOMAL RECESSIVE FORM IS SUGGESTED BY THE OCCURRENCE OF PARENTAL CONSANGUINITY (NOWAKOWSKI AND LENZ, 1961). FERRIMAN (1954) DESCRIBED A POSSIBLY DISTINCT FORM IN TWO SONS OF FIRST-COUSIN PARENTS. FIRST DEGREE HYPOSPADIAS, SMALL PENIS, GYNECOMASTIA, MARKEDLY DIMINISHED SECONDARY SEXUAL CHARACTERS AND NORMAL SIZED TESTES WERE DESCRIBED. IN ALL EXCEPT THE PARENTAL CONSANGUINITY SUGGESTING RECESSIVE INHERITANCE, THE DISORDER RESEMBLES REIFENSTEIN SYNDROME CLINICALLY.

FERRIMAN, D. G.* FAMILIAL HYPOGONADISM. PROC. ROY. SOC. MED. 47* 439-442, 1954.

NOWAKOWSKI, H. AND LENZ, W.* GENETIC ASPECTS IN MALE HYPOGONADISM. RECENT

*24120 HYPOKALEMIC ALKALOSIS (BARTTER'S SYNDROME)

BARTTER'S SYNDROME (BARTTER ET AL., 1962) IS AN UNUSUAL FORM OF SECONDARY HYPERALDOSTERONISM IN WHICH HYPERTROPHY AND HYPERPLASIA OF THE JUXTAGLOMERULAR CELLS ARE ASSOCIATED WITH NORMAL BLOOD PRESSURE AND HYPOKALEMIC ALKALOSIS IN THE ABSENCE OF EDEMA. CANNON ET AL. (1968) REVIEWED THE SUBJECT AND POINTED OUT THAT AFFECTED TWINS WERE REPORTED BY CAMPBELL ET AL. (1966) AND AFFECTED SIBS BY TRYGSTAD ET AL. (1967). EVIDENCE FOR A PRIMARY DEFECT IN MEMBRANE TRANSPORT WAS PRESENTED BY GARDNER ET AL. (1970), ON THE BASIS OF STUDIES OF SODIUM CONTENT AND OUTFLUX OF ERYTHROCYTES. SUTHERLAND ET AL. (1970) DESCRIBED THE DISORDER IN THREE SIBS (INCLUDING A PAIR OF FEMALE TWINS) AND IN THE OFFSPRING OF AN INCESTUOUS (FATHER-DAUGHTER) MATING. ARANT ET AL. (1970) REPORTED ON TWO BROTHERS WITH FEATURES OF BARTTER'S SYNDROME BUT WITH SEVERE AZOTEMIA AT THE ONSET AND IN ONE OF THEM RENAL OSTEODYSTROPHY. RENAL BIOPSY SHOWED ONLY MILD HYPERPLASIA OF JUXTAGLOMERULAR CELLS AND SEVERE GLOMERULONEPHRITIS.

ARANT, B. S., BRACKETT, N. C., JR., YOUNG, R. B. AND STILL, W. J. S.* CASE STUDIES OF SIBLINGS WITH JUXTAGLOMERULAR HYPERPLASIA AND SECONDARY ALDOSTERONISM ASSOCIATED WITH SEVERE AZOTEMIA AND RENAL RICKETS - BARTTER'S SYNDROME OR DISEASE.Q PEDIATRICS 46* 344-361, 1970.

BARTTER, F. C., PRONOVE, P., GELL, J. R., JR. AND MACCARDLE, R. C.* HYPERPLASIA OF THE JUXTAGLOMERULAR COMPLEX WITH HYPERALDOSTERONISM AND HYPOKALEMIC ALKALOSIS. A NEW SYNDROME. AM. J. MED. 33* 811-828, 1962.

CAMPBELL, R. A., BLAIR, H. R., KLEVIT, H. D. AND GOODNIGHT, S. H.* HYPOKALEMIC ALKALOSIS AND NORMOPIESIS WITH ELEVATED ALDOSTERONE EXCRETION IN AN 8-YEAR-OLD TWIN GIRL. (ABSTRACT) SOC. PEDIAT. RES., ATLANTIC CITY, 1966. P. 111.

CANNON, P. J., LEEMING, J. M., SOMMERS, S. C., WINTERS, R. W. AND LARAGH, J. H.* JUXTAGLOMERULAR CELL HYPERPLASIA AND SECONDARY HYPERALDOSTERONISM (BARTTER'S SYNDROME)* A RE-EVALUATION OF THE PATHOPHYSIOLOGY. MEDICINE 47* 107-131, 1968.

GARDNER, J., LAPEY, A., SIMOPOULOS, A. AND BRAVO, E.* EVIDENCE FOR A PRIMARY DISTURBANCE OF MEMBRANE TRANSPORT IN BARTTER'S SYNDROME AND LIDDLE'S SYNDROME. (ABSTRACT) J. CLIN. INVEST. 49* 32A ONLY, 1970.

SUTHERLAND, L. E., HARTROFT, P., BALIS, J. V., BAILEY, J. D. AND LYNCH, M. J.* BARTTER'S SYNDROME. A REPORT OF FOUR CASES, INCLUDING THREE IN ONE SIBSHIP, WITH COMPARATIVE HISTOLOGIC EVALUATION OF THE JUXTAGLOMERULAR APPARATUSES AND GLOMERULI. ACTA PAEDIAT. SCAND. (SUPPL. 201)* 24, 1970.

TRYGSTAD, C. W., MANGOS, J. A., HANSEN, M. R. AND LOBECK, C. C.* FAMILIAL HYPOKALEMIC ALKALOSIS WITH GROWTH FAILURE. AM. PEDIAT. SOC., ATLANTIC CITY, 1967. P. 66.

R
E
C
E
S
S
I
V
E

24130 HYPOMAGNESEMIA, PRIMARY

FRIEDMAN, HATCHER AND WATSON (1967) DESCRIBED CONVULSIONS IN INFANTS IN THE NEONATAL PERIOD. PRIMARY HYPOMAGNESEMIA DUE POSSIBLY TO A DEFECT IN INTESTINAL ABSORPTION WAS THOUGHT TO BE PRESENT. ASSOCIATED HYPOCALCEMIA WAS CORRECTED BY ADMINISTRATION OF MAGNESIUM ALONE. THE GENETIC BASIS OF THE DEFECT WAS SUGGESTED BY ITS PERSISTENCE OVER A PERIOD OF MONTHS AND BY THE FACT THAT THE PARENTS WERE FIRST COUSINS.

FRIEDMAN, M., HATCHER, G. AND WATSON, L.* PRIMARY HYPOMAGNESAEMIA WITH SECONDARY HYPOCALCAEMIA IN AN INFANT. LANCET 1* 703-705, 1967.

24140 HYPOPARATHYROIDISM

SOME REPORTS SUGGEST RECESSIVE INHERITANCE. AFFECTED SIBS WERE BORN OF CONSANGUINEOUS PARENTS (SUTPHIN ET AL., 1943* CHAPTAL ET AL., 1960). BRONSKY ET AL. (1968) DESCRIBED TWO BROTHERS WHO DEVELOPED IDIOPATHIC HYPOPARATHYROIDISM WHEN 11 AND 21 YEARS OLD. A SISTER, WHO DIED WHEN 19 YEARS OLD, MAY ALSO HAVE BEEN AFFECTED. SIX OTHER FAMILIES, IN WHICH MORE THAN ONE MEMBER WAS AFFECTED, WERE FOUND IN THE LITERATURE. CONGENITAL ABSENCE OF THE PARATHYROID AND THYMUS GLANDS (III AND IV PHARYNGEAL POUCH SYNDROME, OR DIGEORGE SYNDROME, Q.V.) IS ALWAYS A SPORADIC CONDITION (TAITZ ET AL., 1966). FAMILIAL CASES OF SUTPHIN ET AL. (1943) SHOWED MONILIASIS ALSO (SEE HYPOADRENOCORTICISM WITH HYPOPARATHYROIDISM AND SUPERFICIAL MONILIASIS).

BRONSKY, D., KIAMKO, R. T. AND WALDSTEIN, S. S.* FAMILIAL IDIOPATHIC HYPOPARATHYROIDISM. J. CLIN. ENDOCR. 28* 61-65, 1968.

CHAPTAL, J., JEAN, R., BONNET, H., GUILLAUMOT, R. AND MOREL, G.* HYPOPARATHYROIDIE FAMILIALE. ETUDES CLINIQUE, BIOLOGIQUE ET THERAPEUTIQUE. ARCH. FRANC. PEDIAT. 17* 866-878, 1960.

SUTPHIN, A., ALBRIGHT, F. AND MCCUNE, D. J.* FIVE CASES (THREE IN SIBLINGS) OF IDIOPATHIC HYPOPARATHYROIDISM ASSOCIATED WITH MONILIASIS. J. CLIN. ENDOCR. 3*

TAITZ, L. S., ZARATE-SALVADOR, C. AND SCHWARTZ, E.* CONGENITAL ABSENCE OF THE PARATHYROID AND THYMUS GLANDS IN AN INFANT (III AND IV PHARYNGEAL POUCH SYNDROME). PEDIATRICS 38* 412-418, 1966.

*24150 HYPOPHOSPHATASIA (PHOSPHOETHANOLAMINURIA)

IN MOST CASES HYPOPHOSPHATASIA IS A GRAVE AND USUALLY FATAL DISORDER OF INFANCY. HOWEVER, BETHUNE AND DENT (1960) DESCRIBED TWO SISTERS IN THEIR 40'S WITH SKELETAL TROUBLE DATING FROM CHILDHOOD. THIS MAY BE THE SAME DISORDER AS THE GRAVE ONE OF INFANCY, FOR WE MAY JUST NOW BE RECOGNIZING THE SPECTRUM OF SEVERITY WHICH THE DISEASE CAN SHOW. THE HETEROZYGOTE CAN BE RECOGNIZED BY LOW SERUM LEVELS OF ALKALINE PHOSPHATASE (RATHBUN ET AL., 1961). PIMSTONE, EISENBERG AND SILVERMAN (1966) POINTED OUT THAT PREMATURE SHEDDING OF TEETH MAY BE THE ONLY OVERT MANIFESTATION. ALMOST CERTAINLY SEVERAL GENETICALLY DISTINCT TYPES OF HYPOPHOS-PHATASIA EXIST BUT THE DETAILS HAVE NOT BEEN FULLY ELUCIDATED. THREE MORE OR LESS DISTINCT TYPES CAN BE IDENTIFIED* (1) TYPE 1 WITH ONSET IN UTERO OR IN EARLY POSTNATAL LIFE, CRANIOSTENOSIS, SEVERE SKELETAL ABNORMALITIES, HYPERCALCEMIA, DEATH IN THE FIRST YEAR OR SO OF LIFE. (2) TYPE 2 WITH LATER, MORE GRADUAL DEVELOPMENT OF SYMPTOMS, MODERATELY SEVERE 'RACHITIC' SKELETAL CHANGES AND PREMATURE LOSS OF TEETH. (3) TYPE 3 WITH NO SYMPTOMS, THE CONDITION BEING DETERMINED ON ROUTINE STUDIES. EISENBERG AND PIMSTONE (1967) DESCRIBED A 50 YEAR OLD WOMAN WITH HYPOPHOSPHATASIA BUT PROVIDED NO FAMILY DATA. IN 1940 MACEY REPORTED TWO BROTHERS WITH VERY LOW VALUES FOR SERUM PHOSPHATASE WHO HAD 'RICKETS' IN CHILDHOOD AND FEMORAL PSEUDOFRACTURES IN ADULTHOOD. O'DUFFY (1970) REPORTED ON THE OCCURRENCE OF ATTACKS OF MONOARTHRITIS AND WIDE-SPREAD CALCIFICATION OF ARTICULAR CARTILAGE IN A 51 YEAR OLD WOMAN WITH HYPOPHOSPHATASIA.

BARTTER, F. C.* HYPOPHOSPHATASIA. IN, STANBURY, J. B., WYNGAARDEN, J. B. AND FREDRICKSON, D. S. (EDS.)* THE METABOLIC BASIS OF INHERITED DISEASE. NEW YORK* MCGRAW-HILL, 1966 (2ND ED.). PP. 1015-1023.

BETHUNE, J. E. AND DENT, C. E.* HYPOPHOSPHATASIA IN THE ADULT. AM. J. MED. 28* 615-622, 1960.

EISENBERG, E. AND PIMSTONE, B.* HYPOPHOSPHATASIA IN AN ADULT. A CASE REPORT. CLIN. ORTHOP. 52* 199-212, 1967.

MACEY, H. B.* MULTIPLE PSEUDOFRACTURES* REPORT OF A CASE. PROC. STAFF MEET. MAYO CLINIC 15* 789-791, 1940.

O'DUFFY, J. D.* HYPOPHOSPHATASIA ASSOCIATED WITH CALCIUM PYROPHOSPHATE DIHYDRATE DEPOSITS IN CARTILAGE. REPORT OF A CASE. ARTHRITIS RHEUM. 13* 381-388, 1970.

PIMSTONE, B., EISENBERG, E. AND SILVERMAN, S.* HYPOPHOSPHATASIA* GENETIC AND DENTAL STUDIES. ANN. INTERN. MED. 65* 722-729, 1966.

RATHBUN, J. C., MACDONALD, J. W., ROBINSON, H. M. C. AND WANKLIN, J. M.* HYPOPHOSPHATASIA* A GENETIC STUDY. ARCH. DIS. CHILD. 36* 540-542, 1961.

TEREE, T. M. AND KLEIN, L.* HYPOPHOSPHATASIA* CLINICAL AND METABOLIC STUDIES. J. PEDIAT. 72* 41-50, 1968.

24160 HYPOPROTEINEMIA, HYPERCATABOLIC

WALDMANN ET AL. (1968) DESCRIBED TWO SIBS, A 34 YEAR OLD WOMAN AND 17 YEAR OLD MAN, WHO WERE PRODUCTS OF A FIRST-COUSIN MARRIAGE AND SHOWED MARKED REDUCTION OF SERUM IGG AND OF ALBUMIN. IGM AND IGA WERE NORMAL OR SLIGHTLY ELEVATED. THE RATE OF CATABOLISM OF IGG WAS INCREASED FIVE FOLD OVER THE NORMAL. EXCESSIVE GASTROIN-TESTINAL LOSS WAS EXCLUDED AS THE CAUSE OF THE HYPOPROTEINEMIA.

WALDMANN, T. A.* DISORDERS OF IMMUNOGLOBULIN METABOLISM. NEW ENG. J. MED. 281* 1170-1177, 1969.

WALDMANN, T. A., MILLER, E. J. AND TERRY, W. D.* HYPERCATABOLISM OF IGG AND ALBUMIN* A NEW FAMILIAL DISORDER. (ABSTRACT) CLIN. RES. 16* 45 ONLY, 1968.

*24170 HYPOPROTHROMBINEMIA

IN THE REPORT OF JOSSO AND COLLEAGUES (1962) TWO OFFSPRING OF A FIRST-COUSIN MATING WERE AFFECTED. DEBASTOS, RENO AND CORREA (1964) DESCRIBED THREE AFFECTED SIBS WITH CONSANGUINEOUS PARENTS. A FOURTH SIB DIED OF UMBILICAL BLEEDING. IN A PATIENT REPORTED BY QUICK AND HUSSEY (1962), LANCHANTIN ET AL. (1968) FOUND NO IDENTIFIABLE PROTEIN THUS DISTINGUISHING THE DISORDER FROM THAT IN WHICH IMMUNOAS-SAYABLE BUT BIOLOGICALLY INACTIVE PROTEIN IS PRESENT (SEE DYSPROTHROMBINEMIA).

DEBASTOS, O., RENO, R. S. AND CORREA, O. T.* A STUDY OF THREE CASES OF FAMILIAL CONGENITAL HYPOPROTHROMBINEMIA (FACTOR II DEFICIENCY). THROMB. DIATH. HAEMORRH. 11* 497-505, 1964.

JOSSO, P., PROU-WARTELLE, O. AND SOULIER, J. P.* ETUDE D*UN CAS D*HYPOPROTHROM-BINEMIE CONGENITALE. NOUV. REV. FRANC. HEMAT. 2* 647-672, 1962.

KATTLOVE, H. E., SHAPIRO, S. S. AND SPIVACK, M.* HEREDITARY PROTHROMBIN DEFICIENCY. NEW ENG. J. MED. 282* 57-61, 1970.

LANCHANTIN, G. F., HART, D. W., FRIEDMANN, J. A., SAAVEDRA, N. V. AND MEHL, J. W.* AMINO ACID COMPOSITION OF HUMAN PLASMA PROTHROMBIN. J. BIOL. CHEM. 243* 5479-5485, 1968.

POOL, J. G., DESAI, R. AND KROPATKIN, M.* SEVERE CONGENITAL HYPOPROTHROMBINEMIA IN A NEGRO BOY. THROMB. DIATH. HAEMORRH. 8* 235-240, 1962.

QUICK, A. J. AND HUSSEY, C. V.* HEREDITARY HYPOPROTHROMBINEMIAS. LANCET 1* 173-177, 1962.

24180 HYPOTHALAMIC HAMARTOMAS

HYPOTHALAMIC HAMARTOMAS WERE OBSERVED IN SIBS AND IN COUSINS (MARCUSE ET AL., 1953).

MARCUSE, P. M., BURGER, R. A. AND SALMON, G. W.* HAMARTOMA OF THE HYPOTHALAMUS. REPORT OF TWO CASES WITH ASSOCIATED DEVELOPMENTAL DEFECTS. J. PEDIAT. 43* 301-308, 1953.

*24190 HYPOTRICHOSIS ('HAIRLESSNESS')

ISOLATED ALOPECIA OR HYPOTRICHOSIS IS RARE. THE DISORDER IS CHARACTERIZED BY FAILURE TO REPLACE THE INTRAUTERINE HAIR WHICH IS SHED SHORTLY BEFORE OR AFTER BIRTH. PUBIC AND AXILLARY HAIR DO NOT DEVELOP AT PUBERTY. NO ABNORMALITY OF TEETH, NAILS OR SWEAT GLANDS IS PRESENT. SLY AND TREISTER (1967) OBSERVED THE CONDITION IN 6 OF 13 SIBS. THIS AND 13 PREVIOUSLY REPORTED FAMILIES SUPPORTED AUTOSOMAL RECESSIVE INHERITANCE. RECESSIVE HAIRLESSNESS HAS BEEN OBSERVED IN THE DEER MOUSE, HOUSE MOUSE, RAT AND RABBIT.

SLY, W. S. AND TREISTER, M.* ISOLATED CONGENITAL HYPOTRICHOSIS* RECESSIVE HAIRLESSNESS IN MAN. TO BE PUBLISHED.

24200 HYPOTRICHOSIS, SYNDACTYLY AND RETINITIS PIGMENTOSA

ALBRECTSEN AND SVENDSEN (1956) REPORTED BROTHER AND SISTER, OFFSPRING OF FIRST COUSIN PARENTS WITH THIS COMBINATION. THE BOY SHOWED PARTIAL ECTRODACTYLY AS WELL AS SYNDACTYLY.

ALBRECTSEN, B. AND SVENDSEN, I. B.* HYPOTRICHOSIS, SYNDACTYLY AND RETINAL DEGENERATION IN TWO SIBLINGS. ACTA DERMATOVENER. 36* 96-101, 1956.

*24210 ICHTHYOSIFORM ERYTHRODERMA, BROCQ'S CONGENITAL, NON-BULLOUS FORM

IN THE CASE OF WILE (1924) THREE MALES WERE AFFECTED. THEY WERE THE OFFSPRING OF MATINGS IN WHICH TWO BROTHERS MARRIED TWO SISTERS, WHO WERE THEIR FIRST COUSINS. THE SUBJECT WAS REVIEWED BY MACKEE AND ROSEN (1917). ARCE AND BERCHMANS (1969) DESCRIBED ICHTHYOSIFORM DERMATOSIS IN 13 MEMBERS OF AN INBRED BRAZILIAN KINDRED.
HEIMENDINGER AND SCHNYDER (1962) DISTINGUISHED TWO TYPES OF CONGENITAL ICHTHYOSIFORM ERYTHRODERMA, ONE INHERITED AS AN AUTOSOMAL DOMINANT AND THE OTHER AS AN AUTOSOMAL RECESSIVE TRAIT. THE RECESSIVE FORM IS NON-BULLOUS AND IS ASSOCIATED WITH GROWTH RETARDATION, OLIGOPHRENIA, SPASTIC PARALYSIS, GENITAL HYPOPLASIA, HYPOTRICHIA AND SHORTENED LIFE-EXPECTANCY. IN THE AUTOSOMAL DOMINANT OR BULLOUS FORM (Q.V.), HOWEVER, LIFE-EXPECTANCY IS NOT SHORTENED AND THE ASSOCIATED SYMPTOMS INCLUDE ONLY SEBORRHEA OF THE HEAD AND PROBABLY POLYDIPSIA. BOTH TYPES BEGIN AT BIRTH AND ARE LOCALIZED MOSTLY ON THE FLEXOR SURFACES. FOR CLASSIFICATION OF THE ICHTHYOSES, SEE ICHTHYOSES IN THE DOMINANT CATALOG.

ARCE, B. AND BERCHMANS, M.* AN ICHTHYOSIFORM DERMATOSIS WITH CLINICAL FORMS OF CONGENITAL ICHTHYOSIFORM ERYTHRODERMA AND ICHTHYOSIS VULGARIS. HUM. HERED. 19* 121-125, 1969.

HEIMENDINGER, J. AND SCHNYDER, U. W.* BULLOSE *ERYTHRODERMIE ICHTHYOSIFORME CONGENITALE* IN ZWEI GENERATIONEN. HELV. PAEDIAT. ACTA 17* 47-55, 1962.

MACKEE, G. M. AND ROSEN, I.* ERYTHRODERMIE CONGENITALE ICHTHYOSIFORME* REPORT OF A CASE WITH A DISCUSSION OF THE CLINICAL AND HISTOLOGICAL FEATURES AND A REVIEW OF THE LITERATURE. J. CUTAN. DIS. 35* 235-251, AND 511-540, 1917.

WILE, U. J.* FAMILIAL STUDY OF THREE UNUSUAL CASES OF CONGENITAL ICHTHYOSIFORM ERYTHRODERMIA. ARCH. DERM. SYPH. 10* 487-498, 1924.

*24220 ICHTHYOSIFORM ERYTHRODERMA, UNILATERAL, WITH EPSILATERAL MALFORMATIONS ESPECIAL ABSENCE DEFORMITY OF LIMBS

FALEK ET AL. (1968) DESCRIBED SIBS WITH THE COMBINATION AND OTHER FAMILIAL CASES ARE KNOWN.

R
E
C
E
S
S
I
V
E

CULLEN, S. I., HARRIS, D. E., CARTER, C. H. AND REED, W. B.* CONGENITAL UNILATERAL ICHTHYOSIFORM ERYTHRODERMA. ARCH. DERM. 99* 724-729, 1969.

FALEK, A., HEATH, C. W., JR., EBBIN, A. J. AND MCLEAN, W. R.* UNILATERAL LIMB AND SKIN DEFORMITIES WITH CONGENITAL HEART DISEASE IN TWO SIBLINGS* A LETHAL SYNDROME. J. PEDIAT. 73* 910-913, 1968.

*24230 ICHTHYOSIS CONGENITA (LAMELLAR EXFOLIATION, OR DESQUAMATION OF THE NEWBORN, COLLODION FETUS, ETC.)

THE INFANT WITH THIS DISORDER MAY DIE OF COMPLICATIONS (SEPSIS, PROTEIN AND ELECTROLYTE LOSS) IN THE FIRST MONTHS OF LIFE OR THE SKIN DISORDER MAY HEAL COMPLETELY. SOMETIMES A CONDITION LIKE ORDINARY ICHTHYOSIS SIMPLEX IS PRESENT FOR THE REST OF THE PATIENT'S LIFE. (SEE PICTURE, SORSBY, 1953.) NIX ET AL. (1963) DESCRIBED 9 CASES AMONG 22 OFFSPRINGS OF THREE COUPLES OF GERMAN EXTRACTION. ALL SIX PARENTS HAD A COMMON ANCESTRAL COUPLE. THEY CONCLUDED THAT THE *HARLEQUIN FETUS* IS THE RESULT OF A SEPARATE RECESSIVE GENE.

BELISARIO, C. AND PANERO, C.* SU DI UN CASO DI *COLLODION-SKIN.* RIV. CLIN. PEDIAT. 69* 312-324, 1962.

NIX, T. E., JR., KLOEPFER, H. W. AND DERBES, V. J.* ICHTHYOSIS, LAMELLAR EXFOLIATIVE TYPE. DERM. TROP. 2* 142-152, 1963.

SHELMIRE, J. B., JR.* LAMELLAR EXFOLIATION OF THE NEWBORN. ARCH. DERM. 71* 471-475, 1955.

SMEENK, G.* TWO FAMILIES WITH COLLODION BABIES. BRIT. J. DERM. 78* 81-86, 1966.

SORSBY, A. (ED.)* CLINICAL GENETICS. ST. LOUIS* C. V. MOSBY CO. 1953. P. 136.

VON REUSS, A. R.* THE DISEASES OF THE NEWBORN. NEW YORK* WILLIAM AND WOOD CO., 1922.

24240 ICHTHYOSIS CONGENITA WITH BILIARY ATRESIA

GOULD (1854) DESCRIBED TWO SIBS WITH THIS COMBINATION.

GOULD, A. A.* ICHTHYOSIS IN AN INFANT* HEMORRHAGE FROM UMBILICUS* DEATH. AM. J. MED. SCI. 27* 356 ONLY, 1854.

24250 ICHTHYOSIS, CONGENITAL, *HARLEQUIN FETUS* TYPE

NIX ET AL. (1963) CLAIMED THAT THIS IS A RECESSIVE DISORDER DISTINCT FROM THE LAMELLAR EXFOLIATIVE TYPE OF CONGENITAL ICHTHYOSIS. IT CARRIES A MORE GRAVE PROGNOSIS (SHELMIRE, 1955). EVIDENCE FOR RECESSIVE INHERITANCE WAS PROVIDED BY SEVERAL FAMILY REPORTS (BUSTAMANTE AND TEJEDA, 1950* KINGERY, 1926* LATTUADA AND PARKER, 1951* SMITH, 1880* THOMSON AND WAKELEY, 1921).

BUSTAMENTE, W. AND TEJEDA, M.* ICHTHYOSIS FETALIS GRAVIS IN TWO SUCCESSIVE PREGNANCIES. J. PEDIAT. 36* 501-504, 1950.

KINGERY, L. B.* ICHTHYOSIS CONGENITA WITH UNUSUAL COMPLICATIONS. ARCH. DERM. SYPH. 13* 90-105, 1926.

LATTUADA, H. P. AND PARKER, M. S.* CONGENITAL ICHTHYOSIS. AM. J. SURG. 82* 236-239, 1951.

NIX, T. E., JR., KLOEPFER, H. W. AND DERBES, V. J.* ICHTHYOSIS, LAMELLAR EXFOLIATIVE TYPE. DERM. TROP. 2* 142-152, 1963.

SHELMIRE, J. B., JR.* LAMELLAR EXFOLIATION OF NEWBORN. ARCH. DERM. 71* 471-475, 1955.

SMITH, R. W.* A CASE OF INTRAUTERINE ICHTHYOSIS. AM. J. OBSTET. GYNEC. 13* 458-461, 1880.

THOMSON, M. S. AND WAKELEY, C. P. G.* THE HARLEQUIN FOETUS. J. OBSTET. GYNEC. BRIT. EMP. 28* 190-203, 1921.

*24260 IMINOGLYCINURIA

THE IMINO ACIDS, PROLINE AND HYDROXYPROLINE, SHARE A RENAL TUBULAR REABSORPTIVE MECHANISM WITH GLYCINE. ROSENBERG ET AL., (1968) FOUND INCREASED AMOUNTS OF ALL THREE SUBSTANCES IN THE URINE OF A 6 YEAR OLD BOY WITH CONGENITAL NERVE DEAFNESS. BOTH PARENTS HAD HYPERGLYCINURIA WITHOUT IMINOACIDURIA. NO DEFECT IN INTESTINAL TRANSPORT OF THESE SUBSTANCES WAS FOUND. THESE AUTHORS, AS WELL AS WHELAN AND SCRIVER (1968) CONCLUDED THAT IMINOGLYCINURIA IS THE HOMOZYGOUS FORM OF THE TRAIT THAT PRESENTS AS HYPERGLYCINURIA IN THE HETEROZYGOTE. IT IS, A BENIGN INBORN ERROR OF AMINO ACID TRANSPORT. SEE ALSO HYPERPROLINEMIA, HYDROXYPROLINEMIA, GLYCINEMIA AND GLYCINURIA. GENETIC HETEROGENEITY IN IMINOGLYCINURIA IS SUGGESTED

R
E
C
E
S
S
I
V
E

BY THE FACTS THAT SOME APPARENT HOMOZYGOTES SHOW A DEFECT IN INTESTINAL ABSORPTION OF L-PROLINE WHEREAS OTHERS DO NOT (GOODMAN ET AL., 1967* SCRIVER, 1968), AND THAT SOME OBLIGATE HETEROZYGOTES SHOW HYPERGLYCINURIA WITH GLYCINE LOADING, WHEREAS OTHERS DO NOT (SCRIVER, 1968). SCRIVER (1968) OBSERVED THE INSTRUCTIVE CASE OF AN APPARENT HOMOZYGOTES CHILD WHOSE FATHER HAD HYPERGLYCINURIA AND MOTHER DID NOT. HE SUGGESTED THAT THIS CHILD WAS A 'COMPOUND' CARRYING TO DIFFERENT MUTANT ALLELES. SIMILAR COMPOUNDS FOR CYSTINURIA HAVE BEEN OBSERVED. SCRIVER ALSO SUGGESTED PLAUSIBLY THAT GLYCINURIA (Q.V. IN DOMINANT CATALOG) IS THE HETEROZYGOUS STATE OF IMINOGLYCINURIA. IMINOGLYCINURIA MAY BE MORE FREQUENT IN ASHKENAZIC JEWS THAN OTHERS.

GOODMAN, S. I., MCINTYRE, C. A., JR. AND O'BRIEN, D.* IMPAIRED INTESTINAL TRANSPORT OF PROLINE IN A PATIENT WITH FAMILIAL IMINOACIDURIA. J. PEDIAT. 71* 246-249, 1967.

ROSENBERG, L. E., DURANT, J. L. AND ELSAS, L. J.* FAMILIAL IMINOGLYCINURIA* AN INBORN ERROR OF RENAL TUBULAR TRANSPORT. NEW ENG. J. MED. 278* 1407-1413, 1968.

SCRIVER, C. R.* RENAL TUBULAR TRANSPORT OF PROLINE, HYDROXYPROLINE, AND GLYCINE. III. GENETIC BASIS FOR MORE THAN ONE MODE OF TRANSPORT IN HUMAN KIDNEY. J. CLIN. INVEST. 47* 823-835, 1968.

WHELAN, D. T. AND SCRIVER, C. R.* CYSTATHIONINURIA AND RENAL IMINOGLYCINURIA IN A PEDIGREE. A PERSPECTIVE ON COUNSELING. NEW ENG. J. MED. 278* 924-927, 1968.

24270 IMMUNE DEFECT DUE TO ABSENCE OF THYMUS

THE POSSIBILITY OF A SEPARATE ENTITY DISTINCT FROM BRUTON TYPE AGAMMAGLOBULINEMIA IN WHICH THE TONSILLAR SYSTEM IS ABSENT AND FROM SWISS-TYPE AGAMMAGLOBULINEMIA (Q.V.) IN WHICH BOTH THE THYMUS AND THE TONSILLAR SYSTEMS ARE ABSENT HAS BEEN POSTULATED BY COOPER, PETERSON AND GOOD (1965). IN THIS ENTITY THE DEFECT MAY BE LIMITED TO THE THYMUS SYSTEM WHICH IS RESPONSIBLE FOR CELLULAR IMMUNITY. THE CASES OF ALLIBONE ET AL. (1964) AND NEZELOF ET AL. (1964) MAY BE EXAMPLES. FULGINITI ET AL. (1967) OBSERVED TWO SISTERS IN ONE FAMILY AND A BROTHER AND SISTER IN ANOTHER FAMILY, WITH THYMIC DYSPLASIA (SIMILAR TO THAT SEEN IN SWISS-TYPE AGAMMAGLOBULINEMIA), LYMPHOPENIA AND NORMAL IMMUNOGLOBULINS. THREE DIED BEFORE AGE 2 YEARS OF RECURRENT PSEUDOMONAS AND MONILIA INFECTIONS. THE LIVING CHILD DISPLAYED IMPAIRED DELAYED HYPERSENSITIVITY. NO SKIN REACTIONS TO MUMPS, PARAINFLUENZA OR MONILIA ANTIGENS WERE OBSERVED. REPEATED ATTEMPTS TO PRODUCE SENSITIVITY TO FLUORODINITROBENZENE FAILED AND A SKIN GRAFT FROM THE MOTHER SHOWED NO SKIN REJECTION. NEZELOF ET AL. (1964) FIRST REPORTED THIS SYNDROME. SOME OF THESE PATIENTS HAVE CHANGES OF METAPHYSEAL DYSOSTOSIS (FULGINITI ET AL., 1967), SUGGESTING A RELATIONSHIP TO CARTILAGE-HAIR HYPOPLASIA (Q.V.) IN WHICH SUSCEPTIBILITY TO VIRAL INFECTIONS MAY BE PRESENT. FURTHERMORE A PATIENT THOUGHT TO HAVE SWISS-TYPE AGAMMAGLOBULINEMIA HAD 'ACHONDROPLASIA' (MCKUSICK AND CROSS, 1966). THIS ASSOCIATION OF DWARFISM PROBABLY REPRESENTS A DISTINCT ENTITY (SEE 'ACHONDROPLASIA' WITH SWISS-TYPE AGAMMAGLOBULINEMIA). NAHMIAS ET AL. (1967) OBSERVED MARKED SUSCEPTIBILITY TO MEASLES WITH DEATH FROM GIANT CELL PNEUMONIA. AUTOPSY SHOWED PLASMA CELLS BUT NO SMALL LYMPHOCYTES AND NO THYMUS. IN THE NEGRO SIBSHIP THEY DESCRIBED 3 GIRLS AND 1 BOY WHO WERE DEFINITELY AFFECTED AND ANOTHER GIRL MAY HAVE BEEN AFFECTED. HUMORAL IMMUNITY IS NORMAL BUT CELLULAR IMMUNITY IS DEFICIENT, FINDINGS PRECISELY OPPOSITE TO THOSE OF CONGENITAL AGAMMAGLOBULINEMIA (KRETSCHMER ET AL., 1968).

RECESSIVE

ALLIBONE, E. C., GOLDIE, W. AND MARMION, B. P.* PNEUMOCYSTIS CARINII PNEUMONIA AND PROGRESSIVE VACCINIA IN SIBLINGS. ARCH. DIS. CHILD. 39* 26-34, 1964.

COOPER, M. D., PETERSON, R. D. A. AND GOOD, R. A.* A NEW CONCEPT OF THE CELLULAR BASIS OF IMMUNITY. (ABSTRACT) J. PEDIAT. 67* 907-908, 1965.

FULGINITI, V. A., HATHAWAY, W. E., PEARLMAN, D. S. AND KEMPE, C. H.* AGAMMAGLO-BULINEMIA AND ACHONDROPLASIA. (LETTER) BRIT. MED. J. 1* 242 ONLY, 1967.

FULGINITI, V. A., HATHAWAY, W. E., PEARLMAN, D. S., BLACKBURN, W. R., REIQUAM, C. W., GITHENS, J. H., CLAMAN, H. N. AND KEMPE, C. H.* DISSOCIATION OF DELAYED-HYPERSENSITIVITY AND ANTIBODY-SYNTHESIZING CAPACITIES IN MAN. REPORT OF TWO SIBSHIPS WITH THYMIC DYSPLASIA, LYMPHOID TISSUE DEPLETION, AND NORMAL IMMUNOGLOBU-LINS. LANCET 2* 5-8, 1967.

KRETSCHMER, R., SAY, B., BROWN, D. AND ROSEN, F. S.* CONGENITAL APLASIA OF THE THYMUS GLAND (DIGEORGE'S SYNDROME). NEW ENG. J. MED. 279* 1295-1301, 1968.

MCKUSICK, V. A. AND CROSS, H. E.* ATAXIA-TELANGIECTASIA AND SWISS-TYPE AGAMMAGLOBULINEMIA. TWO GENETIC DISORDERS OF THE IMMUNE MECHANISMS IN RELATED AMISH SIBSHIPS. J.A.M.A. 195* 739-745, 1966.

MILLER, M. E. AND SCHIEKEN, R. M.* THYMIC DYSPLASIA. A SEPARATE ENTITY FROM 'SWISS AGAMMAGLOBULINEMIA.' AM. J. MED. SCI. 253* 741-750, 1967.

NAHMIAS, A. J., GRIFFITH, D., SALBURY, C. AND YOSHIDA, K.* THYMIC APLASIA* WITH LYMPHOPENIA, PLASMA CELLS, AND NORMAL IMMUNOGLOBULINS. J.A.M.A. 201* 729-734, 1967.

NEZELOF, C., JAMMET, M.-L., LORTHOLARY, P., LABRUNE, B. AND LAMY, M.* L'HYPOP-LASIE HEREDITAIRE DU THYMUS* SA PLACE ET SA RESPONSABILITE DANS UNE OBSERVATION D'APLASIE LYMPHOCYTAIRE, NORMOPLASMOCYTAIRE ET NORMOGLOBULINEMIQUE DU NOURRISSON. ARCH. FRANC. PEDIAT. 21* 897-920, 1964.

*24280 IMMUNE DEFECT WITH LYMPHOTOXIC FACTOR

KRETSCHMER ET AL. (1969) DESCRIBED A BROTHER AND SISTER WHO DIED IN CHILDHOOD WITH AN ILLNESS CHARACTERIZED BY RECURRENT INFECTIONS, ECZEMA AND EPISODIC LYMPHOPENIA. THE BOY SHOWED DYSGAMMAGLOBULINEMIA, IMPAIRED CELLULAR IMMUNITY AND IMMUNOLOGIC AMNESIA LIKE THAT IN ANIMALS TREATED WITH ANTILYMPHOCYTE SERUM. A COMPLEMENT-DEPENDENT LYMPHOTOXIC FACTOR WAS DEMONSTRATED IN THE BOY'S SERUM DURING AN EPISODE OF LYMPHOPENIA. POSTMORTEM EXAMINATION IN BOTH SHOWED DEPLETION OF SMALL LYMPHOCYTE FROM THYMUS-DEPENDENT AREAS OF PERIPHERAL LYMPHOID ORGANS. THE AUTOSOMAL INHERITANCE AND LACK OF THROMBOCYTOPENIA DISTINGJISH THIS DISORDER FROM THE WISKOTT-ALDRICH SYNDROME (Q.V.). AT LEAST 9 OTHER CASES HAVE BEEN REPORTED (E.G., STOOP ET AL., 1962).

KRETSCHMER, R., AUGUST, C. S., ROSEN, F. S. AND JANEWAY, C. A.* RECURRENT INFECTIONS, EPISODIC LYMPHOPENIA AND IMPAIRED CELLULAR IMMUNITY* FURTHER OBSERVA-TIONS ON 'IMMUNOLOGIC AMNESIA' IN TWO SIBLINGS. NEW ENG. J. MED. 281* 285-290, 1969.

STOOP, J. W., BALLIEUX, R. E. AND WEYERS, H. A.* PARAPROTEINEMIA WITH SECONDARY IMMUNE GLOBULIN DEFICIENCY IN INFANTS. PEDIATRICS 29* 97-104, 1962.

24290 INDOLYLACROYL GLYCINURIA WITH MENTAL RETARDATION

MELLMAN ET AL. (1963) FOUND INDOLYLACROYL GLYCINURIA IN THE URINE OF FIVE MENTALLY RETARDED SIBS. THE MOTHER ALSO EXCRETED THE SUBSTANCE. TRYPTOPHANE LOADING ORALLY OR INTRAVENOUSLY DID NOT INCREASE THE EXCRETION BUT ORAL NEOMYCIN CAUSED DISAPPEARANCE OF THE SUBSTANCE FROM THE URINE IN FOUR OF THE FIVE SIBS. THE SUBSTANCE WOULD APPEAR TO BE DERIVED FROM THE BOWEL WHERE IT IS PROBABLY A PRODUCT OF BACTERIAL ACTION AND MAY FIND ITS WAY INTO THE BLOOD AND URINE BECAUSE OF A SPECIFIC TRANSMUCOSAL TRANSPORT DEFECT AS IN HARTNUP'S DISEASE.

MELLMAN, W. J., BARNESS, L. A., TEDESCO, T. A. AND BESSELMAN, D.* INDOLYLACROYL GLYCINE EXCRETION IN A FAMILY WITH MENTAL RETARDATION. CLIN. CHIM. ACTA 8* 843-847, 1963.

24300 INSENSITIVITY TO PAIN (INDIFFERENCE TO PAIN CONGENITAL ANALGIA) (ALSO SEE NEUROPATHY, SENSORY. ALSO SEE BIEMOND'S CONGENITAL AND FAMILIAL ANALGESIA)

SALDANHA AND HIS COLLEAGUES (1964) DESCRIBED TWO FAMILIES. IN ONE THREE BROTHERS OUT OF TEN SIBS AND IN THE OTHER TWO SIBS OUT OF ELEVEN WERE AFFECTED. THE PARENTS OF THE PROBANDS WERE NORMAL AND IN ONE CASE WERE CONSANGUINEOUS (F=0.0703). RECESSIVE INHERITANCE WAS PROPOSED. HOWEVER, A CHROMOSOMAL ABERRATION (MOSAICISM) WAS ALSO DETECTED (BECAK ET AL. 1963). INSENSITIVITY TO PAIN IS A FEATURE OF FAMILIAL DYSAUTONOMIA (Q.V.) WITH WHICH THIS PURE FORM SHOULD NOT BE CONFUSED.
SOME CASES CLASSED AS INSENSITIVITY TO PAIN MAY HAVE CONGENITAL SENSORY NEUROPATHY, WHICH MAY BE MERELY A MILD FORM OF ACRO-OSTEOLYSIS (Q.V.). WHEN FAMILIAL, SENSORY NEUROPATHY IS SAID TO SHOW DOMINANT INHERITANCE. WINKELMANN, LAMBERT AND HAYLES (1962) REVIEWED THE SUBJECT OF CONGENITAL ABSENCE OF PAIN WITH A USEFUL DISCUSSION OF DIFFERENTIAL DIAGNOSIS.
FANCONI AND FERRAZZINI (1957) DESCRIBED AN AFFECTED BROTHER AND SISTER FROM CONSANGUINEOUS PARENTS AND PARENTAL CONSANGUINITY HAS BEEN NOTED IN OTHER CASES (THIEMANN, 1961). SALDANHA, SCHMIDT AND LEON (1964) DESCRIBED TWO FAMILIES WITH THREE OUT OF 10 OFFSPRING OF UNRELATED PARENTS IN ONE AND TWO AFFECTED IN THE SECOND WITH FIRST-COUSIN PARENTS. ALTHOUGH THE PATIENTS DO NOT REACT TO PAINFUL STIMULI, THEY ARE OTHERWISE NEUROLOGICALLY NORMAL. ABSENT CORNEAL REFLEXES AND SLIGHT MENTAL RETARDATION HAVE ALSO BEEN DESCRIBED. IN SEVERAL BUT NOT ALL OF THESE PATIENTS, BECAK, BECAK AND ANDRADE (1964) FOUND MOSAICISM OF CELLS WITH NORMAL KARYOTYPE AND CELLS TRISOMIC FOR A CHROMOSOME IN THE 13-15 GROUP. GILLEY AND COLLEAGUES (1964) DESCRIBED 2 AFFECTED SIBS WHO WERE BORN OF NORMAL PARENTS AND WERE NORMALLY INTELLIGENT. BERTOYE AND COLLEAGUES (1964) OBSERVED THE DISORDER IN THE CHILD OF CONSANGUINEOUS PARENTS. IN A CASE OF INDIFFERENCE TO PAIN REPORTED BY OGDEN ET AL. (1959) THE PARENTS WERE FIRST COUSINS. BLAU AND MUTTON (1967) COULD DEMONSTRATE NO CHROMOSOMAL ABNORMALITY. SILVERMAN AND GILDEN (1959) DESCRIBED A FAMILY IN WHICH TWO OF EIGHT CHILDREN OF CONSANGUINEOUS PARENTS WERE AFFECTED. GAUDIER ET AL. (1969) DESCRIBED AFFECTED BROTHERS.

BECAK, W., BECAK, M. L. AND ANDRADE, J. D.* A GENETICAL INVESTIGATION OF CONGENITAL ANALGESIA. I. CYTOGENETIC STUDIES. ACTA GENET. STATIST. MED. 14* 133-142, 1964.

BECAK, W., BECAK, M. L. AND SCHMIDT, B. J.* CHROMOSOME TRISOMY OF GROUP 13-15 IN TWO CASES OF GENERALISED CONGENITAL ANALGESIA. (LETTER) LANCET 1* 664-665, 1963.

BERTOYE, A., CARRON, R., ROSENBERG, D., COTTON, J.-B. AND MICHEL, M.* A PROPOS D'UNE OBSERVATION D'INDIFFERENCE CONGENITALE A LA DOULEUR (ANALGESIE CONGENITALE

RECESSIVE

BLAU, J. N. AND MUTTON, D. E.* CHROMOSOME STUDIES IN THE *SENSORY SYNDROME.*
ACTA GENET. 17* 226-233, 1967.

BOURLAND, A. AND WINKELMANN, R. K.* STUDY OF CUTANEOUS INNERVATION IN CONGENI-
TAL ANESTHESIA. ARCH. NEUROL. 14* 223-227, 1966.

FANCONI, G. AND FERRAZZINI, F.* KONGENITALE ANALGIE (KONGENITALE GENERALISIERTE
SCHMERZINDIFFERENZ). HELV. PAEDIAT. ACTA 12* 79-115, 1957.

GAUDIER, B., BOURLOND, A., NUYTS, J.-P., RYCKEWAERT, P. H., LEFEBVRE, P. AND
RYCKEWAERT-SANDOR, L.* L'INDIFFERENCE CONGENITALE A LA DOULEUR. A PROPOS DE DEUX
NOUVELLES OBSERVATIONS. ARCH. FRANC. PEDIAT. 26* 1027-1040, 1969.

GILLY, R., CHEVALLIER, G., FORAY, G., RAMBAUD, G. AND RAVEAU, J.* INDIFFERENCE
CONGENITALE A LA DOULEUR. OBSERVATION FAMILIALE, PARTICULARITES CLINIQUES ET
BIOLOGIQUES. PEDIATRIE 19* 609-614, 1964.

OGDEN, T. E., ROBERT, F. AND CARMICHAEL, E. A.* SOME SENSORY SYNDROMES IN
CHILDREN* INDIFFERENCE TO PAIN AND SENSORY NEUROPATHY. J. NEUROL. NEUROSURG.
PSYCHIAT. 22* 267-276, 1959.

SALDANHA, P. H., SCHMIDT, B. J. AND LEON, N.* A GENETICAL INVESTIGATION OF
CONGENITAL ANALGESIA. II. CLINICO-GENETICAL STUDIES. ACTA GENET. STATIST. MED.
14* 143-158, 1964.

SILVERMAN, F. N. AND GILDEN, J. J.* CONGENITAL INSENSITIVITY TO PAIN. A
NEUROLOGIC SYNDROME WITH BIZARRE SKELETAL LESIONS. RADIOLOGY 72* 176-190, 1959.

THIEMANN, H. H.* ANALGIA CONGENITA (ANGEBORENE UNIVERSELLE SCHMERZINDIFFERENZ).
ARCH. KINDERHEILK. 164* 255-262, 1961.

WINKELMANN, R. K., LAMBERT, E. H. AND HAYLES, A. B.* CONGENITAL ABSENCE OF
PAIN. REPORT OF A CASE AND EXPERIMENTAL STUDIES. ARCH. DERM. 85* 325-339, 1962.

24310 INTERNAL CAROTID ARTERIES, HYPOPLASIA OF

AUSTIN AND STEARS (1971) REPORTED HYPOPLASIA OF BOTH INTERNAL CAROTID ARTERIES IN
TWO AND POSSIBLY THREE BROTHERS FROM A SIBSHIP OF 11. SYMPTOMS BEGAN AT AGES 18,
30 AND 33 YEARS AND WERE ATTRIBUTABLE TO CEREBRAL ISCHEMIA. ONE BECAME DEMENTED.

AUSTIN, J. H. AND STEARS, J. C.* FAMILIAL HYPOPLASIA OF BOTH INTERNAL CAROTID
ARTERIES. ARCH. NEUROL. 24* 1-10, 1971.

24320 INTRACRANIAL HYPERTENSION, IDIOPATHIC

BUCHHEIT ET AL. (1969) DESCRIBED TWO SISTERS WITH IDIOPATHIC INTRACRANIAL
HYPERTENSION WITH PAPILLEDEMA (PSEUDOTUMOR CEREBRI).

BUCHHEIT, W. A., BURTON, C., HAAG, B. AND SHAW, D.* FAMILIAL PAPILLEDEMA AND
IDIOPATHIC INTRACRANIAL HYPERTENSION. NEW ENG. J. MED. 280* 938-942, 1969.

24330 INTRAHEPATIC CHOLESTASIS

KUHN (1963) DESCRIBED TWO TEEN-AGE BROTHERS WITH REPEATED ATTACKS OF JAUNDICE
ACCOMPANIED BY ITCHING AND HEPATOMEGALY. PROGRESSION TO BILIARY CIRRHOSIS WAS
SUSPECTED IN ONE. HE SUGGESTED THAT THE SAME CONDITION WAS DESCRIBED BY TYGSTRUP
(1960) IN TWO DISTANTLY RELATED 15 YEAR OLD BOYS LIVING IN A SMALL VILLAGE IN THE
FAROE ISLANDS. ONSET IN THESE WAS IN THE FIRST TWO YEARS OF LIFE. CHOLESTASIS
WAS DEMONSTRATED BY LIVER BIOPSY AND DIRECT CHOLANGIOGRAPHY. KAYE (1965) STUDIED
THREE SIBS WITH INTRAHEPATIC CHOLESTASIS IN WHICH ITCHING PREDATED JAUNDICE WHICH
BEGAN BY 2 OR 3 YEARS. ONE SIB DIED AT ABOUT 7 YEARS OF AGE AND 2 WERE STILL
ALIVE AT AGES OF ABOUT 10 AND 5. CHOLESTYRAMINE HAD NO BENEFIT. SOMAYAJI ET AL.
(1968) REPORTED SISTERS WHO DEVELOPED CHOLESTATIC JAUNDICE FOLLOWING THE TAKING OF
AN ORAL CONTRACEPTIVE AGENT. ONE OF THEM HAD HAD PRURITUS DURING THE LATTER PART
OF EACH OF THREE PREGNANCIES. INTRAHEPATIC CHOLESTASIS OF PREGNANCY HAS BEEN
REPORTED IN SISTERS BY SVANBORG AND OHLSSON, CAHILL (SGO 114* 545, 1962) AND FAST
AND ROULSTON (1964). MOTHER AND TWO DAUGHTERS WERE AFFECTED IN THE REPORT OF
HOLZBACH AND SANDERS (1965). MOTHERS OF PATIENTS WITH BYLER'S DISEASE (Q.V.) HAD
SEVERE PRURITUS IN LATE PREGNANCY RAISING THE POSSIBILITY THAT CHOLESTASIS OF
PREGNANCY MAY BE A MANIFESTATION OF THE HETEROZYGOUS STATE OF THE GENE WHICH IN
THE HOMOZYGOTE PRODUCES A FATAL FORM OF CHOLESTASIS (MCKUSICK AND CLAYTON, 1968).

CAHILL, K. M.* HEPATITIS IN PREGNANCY. SURG. GYNEC. OBSTET. 114* 545-552,
1962.

DA SILVA, L. C. AND DE BRITO, T.* BENIGN RECURRENT INTRAHEPATIC CHOLESTASIS IN
TWO BROTHERS. A CLINICAL LIGHT AND ELECTRON MICROSCOPY STUDY. ANN. INTERN. MED.
65* 330-341, 1966.

FAST, B. B. AND ROULSTON, T. M.* IDIOPATHIC JAUNDICE OF PREGNANCY. AM. J.

R
E
C
E
S
S
I
V
E

OBSTET. GYNEC. 88* 314-321, 1964.

HOLZBACH, R. T. AND SANDERS, J. H.* RECURRENT INTRAHEPATIC CHOLESTASIS OF PREGNANCY. OBSERVATIONS ON PATHOGENESIS. J.A.M.A. 193* 542-544, 1965.

KAYE, R.* COMMENTS. J. PEDIAT. 67* 1027-1028, 1965.

KUHN, H. A.* INTRAHEPATIC CHOLESTASIS IN TWO BROTHERS. GERMAN MED. MONTHLY 8* 185-188, 1963.

MCKUSICK, V. A. AND CLAYTON, R. J.* CHOLESTASIS OF PREGNANCY. (LETTER) NEW ENG. J. MED. 278* 566 ONLY, 1968.

SOMAYAJI, B. N., PATON, A., PRICE, J. H., HARRIS, A. W. AND FLEWETT, T. H.* NORETHISTERONE JAUNDICE IN TWO SISTERS. BRIT. MED. J. 2* 281-283, 1968.

SVANBORG, A. AND OHLSSON, S.* RECURRENT JAUNDICE OF PREGNANCY. A CLINICAL STUDY OF TWENTY-TWO CASES. AM. J. MED. 27* 40-49, 1959.

TYGSTRUP, N.* INTERMITTENT POSSIBLY FAMILIAL INTRAHEPATIC CHOLESTATIC JAUNDICE. LANCET 1* 1171-1172, 1960.

*24340 ISONIAZID (INH) INACTIVATION

THE ANTI-TUBERCULOSIS AGENT, INH, IS RENDERED THERAPEUTICALLY INACTIVE BY ACETYLATION. MOST, PERHAPS ALL POPULATIONS OF THE WORLD ARE POLYMORPHIC FOR 'RAPID INACTIVATION' VERSUS 'SLOW INACTIVATION.' THE 'SLOW INACTIVATOR' PERSON IS HOMOZYGOUS. THE RAPID INACTIVATOR PERSON MAY BE EITHER HOMOZYGOUS OR HETEROZY- GOUS. SUNAHARA'S METHOD PERMITS SEPARATION OF THE HOMOZYGOTES AND HETEROZYGOTES, I.E., THREE GENOTYPES IN ALL. THE RAPID VS. SLOW ACETYLATION OF SULFADIAZINE IN RABBITS (FRYMOYER AND JACOX, 1963) IS SIMILAR. THE POLYMORPHISM IN ACETYLATION EXTENDS TO THE ACETYLATION OF SULFAMETHAZINE WHICH CAN BE USED AS A TEST (PARKER, 1969).

EVANS, D. A. P., MANLEY, K. A. AND MCKUSICK, V. A.* GENETIC CONTROL OF ISONIAZID METABOLISM IN MAN. BRIT. MED. J. 2* 485-491, 1960.

FRYMOYER, J. W. AND JACOX, R. F.* STUDIES OF GENETICALLY CONTROLLED SULFADIA- ZINE ACETYLATION IN RABBIT LIVERS* POSSIBLE IDENTIFICATION OF THE HETEROZYGOUS TRAIT. J. LAB. CLIN. MED. 62* 905-909, 1963.

PARKER, J. M.* HUMAN VARIABILITY IN THE METABOLISM OF SULFAMETHAZINE. HUM. HERED. 19* 402-409, 1969.

SCHLOOT, W. AND GOEDDE, H. W.* STUDIES ON THE POLYMORPHISM OF ISONIAZID (INH) ACETYLATION IN RHESUS MONKEYS (MACACA MULATTA). ACTA GENET. STATIST. MED. 18* 394-398, 1968.

SUNAHARA, S., URANO, M. AND OGAWA, M.* GENETICAL AND GEOGRAPHIC STUDIES ON ISONIAZID INACTIVATION. SCIENCE 134* 1530-1531, 1961.

*24350 ISOVALERICACIDEMIA

BUDD ET AL. (1967) OBSERVED BROTHER AND SISTER WHO STARTING BEFORE AGE 6 MONTHS SHOWED RETARDED PSYCHOMOTOR DEVELOPMENT, A PECULIAR ODOR RESEMBLING SWEATY FEET, AN AVERSION TO DIETARY PROTEIN, AND PERNICIOUS VOMITING, LEADING TO ACIDOSIS AND COMA. THE ODOR IS DUE TO ISOVALERIC ACID, AN INTERMEDIARY OF LEUCINE. THE DEFECT CONCERNS IVA-CO A DEHYDROGENASE. THE UNUSUAL SMELL WAS IDENTIFIED AS ISOVALERIC ACID BY EXPERTS OF THE ARTHUR D. LITTLE CO., INDUSTRIAL CONSULTANTS, CAMBRIDGE, MASS. IN THE METABOLIC PATHWAYS THIS DISORDER IS CLOSELY RELATED TO MAPLE SYRUP URINE DISEASE. SEE ALSO SIDBURY SYNDROME.

BUDD, M. A., TANAKA, K., HOLMES, L. B., EFRON, M. L., CRAWFORD, J. D. AND ISSELBACHER, K. J.* ISOVALERIC ACIDEMIA* CLINICAL FEATURE OF A NEW GENETIC DEFECT OF LEUCINE METABOLISM. NEW ENG. J. MED. 277* 321-327, 1967.

EFRON, M. L.* ISOVALERIC ACIDEMIA. AM. J. DIS. CHILD. 113* 74-76, 1967.

NEWMAN, C. G. H., WILSON, B. D. R., CALLAGHAN, P. AND YOUNG, L.* NEONATAL DEATH ASSOCIATED WITH ISOVALERICACIDAEMIA. LANCET 2* 439-441, 1967.

TANAKA, K., BUDD, M. A., EFRON, M. L. AND ISSELBACHER, K. J.* ISOVALERIC ACIDEMIA* A NEW GENETIC DEFECT OF LEUCINE METABOLISM. PROC. NAT. ACAD. SCI. 56* 236-242, 1966.

TANAKA, K., ORR, J. AND ISSELBACHER, K. J.* IDENTIFICATION OF B-HYDROXYISOVA- LERIC ACID IN THE URINE OF A PATIENT WITH ISOVALERIC ACIDEMIA. BIOCHIM. BIOPHYS. ACTA 152* 638-641, 1968.

*24360 JEJUNAL ATRESIA ('APPLE PEEL' SYNDROME)

IN THIS CONDITION, BECAUSE OF AGENESIS OF THE MESENTERY, THE DISTAL SMALL BOWEL

COMES STRAIGHT OFF THE CAECUM AND TWISTS AROUND THE MARGINAL ARTERY, SUGGESTING A MAYPOLE OR APPLE PEEL AT OPERATION. MISHALANY AND NAJJAR (1968) OBSERVED 3 AFFECTED OUT OF 16 LIVEBORN OFFSPRING OF FIRST COUSIN PARENTS AND BLYTH AND DICKSON (1969) OBSERVED TWO AFFECTED SIBS IN EACH OF TWO FAMILIES. SEE DUODENAL ATRESIA.

BLYTH, H. AND DICKSON, J. A. S.* APPLE PEEL SYNDROME (CONGENITAL INTESTINAL ATRESIA). A FAMILY STUDY OF SEVEN INDEX PATIENTS. J. MED. GENET. 6* 275-277, 1969.

MISHALANY, H. G. AND NAJJAR, F. B.* FAMILIAL JEJUNAL ATRESIA* THREE CASES IN ONE FAMILY. J. PEDIAT. 73* 753-755, 1968.

*24370 JOB'S SYNDROME

THE BOOK OF JOB RECORDS THAT *SATAN . . . . . SMOTE JOB WITH SORE BOILS FROM THE SOLE OF HIS FOOT UNTO HIS CROWN* (JOB 2*7). FOR THIS REASON DAVIS ET AL. (1966) GAVE THE NAME JOB'S SYNDROME TO DISORDER AFFECTING TWO UNRELATED GIRLS. BOTH HAD HAD LIFE-LONG HISTORIES OF INDOLENT (*COLD*) STAPHYLOCOCCAL ABSCESSES. A DEFECT IN LOCAL RESISTANCE TO STAPHYLOCCAL INFECTION WAS SUGGESTED. THOMPSON (1968) INFORMED ME OF AFFECTED SIBS IN A SOUTHERN ITALIAN FAMILY WITH POSSIBLY CONSANGUINEOUS PARENTS. THESE PATIENTS LIKE DAVIS' HAD FAIR SKIN AND RED HAIR. SHERRY (1968) OBSERVED A NEGRO CHILD WITH CHARACTERISTIC FEATURES BUT THE USUAL NEGRO HAIR. TWO SISTERS WITH JOE'S SYNDROME REPORTED BY DAVIS ET AL. IN 1966 WERE REPORTED BY WHITE ET AL. (1969) TO HAVE NORMAL LEUKOCYTE FUNCTIONS WHICH ARE DEFECTIVE IN CHRONIC GRANULOMATOUS DISEASE. BANNATYNE ET AL. (1969) DESCRIBED TWO AFFECTED SISTERS WHOSE PARENTS WERE SECOND COUSINS. DESPITE THE FACT THAT THEIR PARENTS WERE DARK-SKINNED AND DARK-HAIRED SOUTHERN ITALIAN IMMIGRANTS, THE PROBAND HAD RED HAIR, FAIR SKIN AND REDDISH-BROWN EYES. A SISTER WAS CLINICALLY WELL BUT HAD A MILD LEUKOCYTE DEFECT DEMONSTRATED IN VITRO AND HAD RED HAIR.

BANNATYNE, R. M., SKOWRON, P. N. AND WEBER, J. L.* JOB'S SYNDROME, A VARIANT OF CHRONIC GRANULOMATOUS DISEASE. J. PEDIAT. 75* 236-242, 1969.

DAVIS, S. D., SCHALLER, J. AND WEDGWOOD, R. J.* JOB'S SYNDROME. RECURRENT, *COLD,* STAPHYLOCOCCAL ABSCESSES. LANCET 1* 1013-1015, 1966.

SHERRY, M. N.* WASHINGTON, D.C.* PERSONAL COMMUNICATION, 1968.

THOMPSON, M. W.* TORONTO, CANADA* PERSONAL COMMUNICATION, 1968.

WHITE, L. R., IANNETTA, A., KAPLAN, E. L., DAVIS, S. D. AND WEDGWOOD, R. J.* LEUKOCYTES IN JOB'S SYNDROME. (LETTER) LANCET 1* 630 ONLY, 1969.

24380 JOINT LAXITY (ARTHROCHALASIS MULTIPLEX CONGENITA)

EXTREME JOINT LAXITY WITH MULTIPLE RECURRENT JOINT DISLOCATIONS WAS OBSERVED IN THREE SIBS, THE OFFSPRING OF THIRD COUSIN PARENTS (MCKUSICK, 1966). THE PARENTS WERE SAID TO BE UNAFFECTED BUT WERE NOT EXAMINED. IT IS POSSIBLE THAT THIS IS THE SAME ENTITY THAT IS LISTED IN THE DOMINANT CATALOG (ONE OR BOTH PARENTS BEING IN FACT AFFECTED). EPICANTHUS, DEPRESSED NASAL BRIDGE, MICROGNATHIA AND DIAPHRAGMATIC HERNIA OCCUR IN SOME OF THESE PATIENTS BUT LACK OF SKIN CHANGES (BRUISABILITY, FRAGILITY, ETC.) DISTINGUISHES THIS CONDITION FROM THE EHLERS-DANLOS SYNDROME. THE DISORDER WAS OBSERVED BY CAPOTORTI AND ANTONELLI (1966) IN AN INBRED KINDRED. SEE LARSEN'S SYNDROME.

CAPOTORTI, L. AND ANTONELLI, M.* SINDROME DI EHLERS-DANLOS. QUATTRO CASI ACCERTATI E DUE PROBABLI IN UNA FAMIGLIA CON PIU MATRIMONI FRA CONSANGUINEI. ACTA GENET. MED. GEM. 15* 273-295, 1966.

HASS, J. AND HASS, R.* ARTHROCHALASIS MULTIPLEX CONGENITA. CONGENITAL FLACCIDITY OF THE JOINTS. J. BONE JOINT SURG. 40A* 663-674, 1958.

MCKUSICK, V. A.* HERITABLE DISORDERS OF CONNECTIVE TISSUE. ST. LOUIS* C. V. MOSBY CO., 1966 (3RD ED.). FIGS. 5-11.

24390 JORDANS' ANOMALY OF LEUKOCYTES

JORDANS (1953) FOUND FAT-CONTAINING CYTOPLASMIC VACUOLES IN THE LEUKOCYTES OF TWO BROTHERS WITH PROGRESSIVE MUSCULAR DYSTROPHY. ROZENSZAJN ET AL. (1966) FOUND THEM IN TWO SISTERS WITH ICHTHYOSIS.

JORDANS, G. H. W.* THE FAMILIAL OCCURRENCE OF FAT CONTAINING VACUOLES IN THE LEUKOCYTES DIAGNOSED IN TWO BROTHERS SUFFERING FROM DYSTROPHIA MUSCULORUM PROGRESSIVA (ERB). ACTA MED. SCAND. 145* 419-423, 1953.

ROZENSZAJN, L., KLAJMAN, A., YAFFE, D. AND EFRATI, P.* JORDANS' ANOMALY IN WHITE BLOOD CELLS. REPORT OF CASE. BLOOD 28* 258-265, 1966.

24400 JOSEPH'S SYNDROME

THE FEATURES ARE CONVULSIONS OF EARLY ONSET, ELEVATED SPINAL FLUID PROTEIN,

R
E
C
E
S
S
I
V
E

AMINOACIDURIA (PROLINE, HYDROXYPROLINE, GLYCINE). SEVERAL DISORDERS, E.G., MAPLE SYRUP URINE DISEASE, WOULD FIT THIS SYNDROME. IT IS NOT CLEAR THAT IT IS A DISTINCT ENTITY.

JONXIS, J. H. P.* HEREDITARY AMINOACIDURIA. IN, STEINBERG, A. G. AND BEARN, A. G. (EDS.)* PROGRESS IN MEDICAL GENETICS. NEW YORK* GRUNE AND STRATTON, 2* 1962.

JOSEPH, R., RIBIERRE, M., JOB, J.-C. AND GIRAULT, M.* MALADIE FAMILIALE ASSOCIANT DES CONVULSIONS A DEBUT TRES PRECOCE, UNE HYPERALBUMINORACHIE ET UNE HYPERAMINOACIDURIE. ARCH. FRANC. PEDIAT. 15* 374-387, 1958.

24410 JUMPING FRENCHMAN OF MAINE (SEE ALSO HYPER-REFLEXIA, HEREDITARY)

BEARD (1878) FIRST STUDIED THIS DISORDER, AN EXAGGERATED STARTLE REFLEX. STEVENS (1966) HAS WRITTEN ON IT. BEARD THOUGHT IT FAMILIAL AND A DISORDER PARTICULARLY OF FRENCH CANADIANS. STEVENS CITED A PERSONAL COMMUNICATION DESCRIBING FIVE AFFECTED SIBS, OFFSPRING OF A FRENCH CANADIAN FISHING GUIDE IN WEDGPORT, NOVA SCOTIA.

BEARD, G. M.* REMARKS UPON 'JUMPERS OR JUMPING FRENCHMEN.' J. NERV. MENT. DIS. 5* 526, 1878.

STEVENS, H.* JUMPING FRENCHMEN OF MAINE. ARCH. NEUROL. 12* 311-314, 1966.

24420 KALLMANN SYNDROME (HYPOGONADOTROPIC HYPOGONADISM AND ANOSMIA)

THIS ENTITY IS DISCUSSED ALSO IN THE X-LINKAGE CATALOG. MIDLINE CRANIAL ANOMALIES (CLEFT LIP, CLEFT PALATE AND IMPERFECT FUSION) ARE ALSO FEATURES. ROSEN (1965) EXAMINED A LARGE KINDRED WITH A HIGH RATE OF CONSANGUINITY AND FOUND 5 CASES OF HYPOGONADISM, 3 OF ANOSMIA AND 6 OF MIDLINE ANOMALIES. TWO PERSONS HAD TWO DEFECTS AND 2 SHOWED ALL THREE. BOTH MALES AND FEMALES WERE AFFECTED AND THE PEDIGREE SUGGESTED AUTOSOMAL RECESSIVE INHERITANCE. TAGATZ ET AL. (1970) DESCRIBED THREE UNRELATED FEMALES WITH HYPOGONADOTROPIC HYPOGONADISM AND ANOSMIA. NO RELATIVE WAS AFFECTED AND THE PARENTS IN EACH CASE WERE UNRELATED. INDUCTION OF OVULATION WITH RESULTING NORMAL TERM PREGNANCY WAS ACHIEVED IN TWO OF THE PATIENTS WITH EXOGENOUS GONADOTROPINS.

R
E
C
E
S
S
I
V
E

ROSEN, S. W.* THE SYNDROME OF HYPOGONADISM, ANOSMIA AND MIDLINE CRANIAL ANOMALIES. PROC. 47TH MEET. ENDOCR. SOC., 1965.

TAGATZ, G., FIALKOW, P. J., SMITH, D. AND SPADONI, L.* HYPOGONADOTROPIC HYPOGONADISM ASSOCIATED WITH ANOSMIA IN THE FEMALE. NEW ENG. J. MED. 283* 1326-1329, 1970.

24430 KALLMANN SYNDROME WITH FACIAL CLEFTING

ROSEN (1965) PRESENTED EVIDENCE FOR A RECESSIVE FORM OF KALLMANN SYNDROME (HYPOGONADOTROPHIC HYPOGONADISM AND ANOSMIA) WHICH HAS FACIAL CLEFTING AS AN ADDITIONAL FEATURE. ROSEN'S PATIENTS CAME FROM A CONSANGUINEOUS FRENCH-CANADIAN FAMILY. THE SAME OR A RELATED DISORDER MAY BE THAT REPORTED BY HINTZ ET AL. (1968).

HINTZ, R. L., MENKING, M. AND SOTOS, J. F.* FAMILIAL HOLOPROSENCEPHALY WITH ENDOCRINE DYSGENESIS. J. PEDIAT. 72* 81-87, 1968.

ROSEN, S. W.* THE SYNDRCME OF HYPOGONADISM, ANOSMIA AND MIDLINE CRANIAL ANOMALIES. PROC. 47TH MEETING ENDOCR. SOC., 1965.

*24440 KARTAGENER'S SYNDROME (DEXTROCARDIA, BRONCHIECTASIS AND SINUSITIS)

KARTAGENER AND STUCKI (1962) FOUND 334 CASES IN THE LITERATURE AND ADDED TWO MORE. GORHAM AND MERSELIS (1959) CONCLUDED THAT THE DISORDER IS INHERITED AS A RECESSIVE WITH INCOMPLETE PENETRANCE. FAMILY STUDIES WERE DONE BY KNOX, MURRAY AND STRANG (1960) AND BY COOK ET AL. (1962). KNOX ET AL. (1960) SUGGESTED LINKAGE WITH THE RHESUS LOCUS. PROBABLY ALL FAMILIAL CASES HAVE BEEN CONFINED TO SIBS, ALTHOUGH TORGERSEN (1947) SUGGESTED DOMINANT INHERITANCE. MORENO ET AL. (1965) FOUND THE FULL SYNDROME IN TWO OF 5 OFFSPRING OF FIRST-COUSIN PARENTS. ANOTHER SIB HAD BRONCHIECTASIS AS DID ALSO THE FATHER AND THE OTHER TWO CHILDREN WERE 'CHRONIC COUGHERS.' HOLMES ET AL. (1968) FOUND LOW SERUM LEVELS OF GAMMA A GLOBULIN IN SOME CASES.

COOK, C. D., GELLER, F., HUTCHISON, G. B., GERALD, P. S. AND ALLEN, F. H., JR.* BLOOD GROUPING IN THREE FAMILIES WITH KARTAGENER'S SYNDROME. AM. J. HUM. GENET. 14* 290-294, 1962.

GORHAM, G. W. AND MERSELIS, J. G., JR.* KARTAGENER'S TRIAD* A FAMILY STUDY. BULL. HOPKINS HOSP. 104* 11-16 1959.

HARTLINE, J. V. AND ZELKOWITZ, P. S.* KARTAGENER'S SYNDROME IN CHILDHOOD. AM. J. DIS. CHILD. 121* 349-352, 1971.

HOLMES, L. B., BLENNERHASSETT, J. B. AND AUSTEN, K. F.* A REAPPRAISAL OF

KARTAGENER, M. AND STUCKI, P.* BRONCHIECTASIS WITH SITUS INVERSUS. ARCH. PEDIAT. 79* 193-207, 1962.

KNOX, G., MURRAY, S. AND STRANG, L.* A FAMILY WITH KARTAGENER'S SYNDROME* LINKAGE DATA. ANN. HUM. GENET. 24* 137-140, 1960.

LOGAN, W. D., JR., ABBOTT, O. A. AND HATCHER, C. R., JR.* KARTAGENER'S TRIAD. DIS. CHEST 48* 613-616, 1965.

MORENO, J., ORTEGA, L. AND MONTERO, E.* SINDROME DE KARTAGENER. REFERENCIA DE DOS CASOS FAMILIARES CON ANALYSIS CITOGENETICO. AN. DESARROLLO 13* 207-213, 1965.

TORGERSEN, J.* TRANSPOSITION OF VISCERA-BRONCHIECTASIS, AND NASAL POLYPS. A GENETICAL ANALYSIS AND CONTRIBUTIONS TO THE PROBLEM OF CONSTITUTION. ACTA RADIOL. 28* 17-24, 1947.

24450 KERATOCONUS

HAMILTON (1938) CLAIMED THAT CERTAIN OF HIS PEDIGREES STRONGLY SUPPORTED AUTOSOMAL RECESSIVE INHERITANCE. KERATOCONUS IS A FEATURE OF AMAUROSIS CONGENITA (Q.V.). INDEED IT IS AN OCCASIONAL FEATURE OF MONGOLISM. IN THIS AND OTHER CONDITIONS INCLUDING AMAUROSIS CONGENITA OF LEBER, EYE RUBBING MAY BE AN IMPORTANT FACTOR IN THE CAUSATION OF KERATOCONUS. IT IS UNPROVED THAT KERATOCONUS OCCURS AS AN ISOLATED MENDELIZING DISORDER.

HAMILTON, J. B.* SIGNIFICANCE OF HEREDITY IN OPHTHALMOLOGY. PRELIMINARY SURVEY OF HEREDITARY EYE DISEASES IN TASMANIA. BRIT. J. OPHTHAL. 22* 83-108, 1938.

VAN DER HOEVE, J.* VERERBBARKEIT DES KERATOKONUS. Z. AUGENHEILK. 52* 321-336, 1924.

24460 KERATOCONUS POSTICUS CIRCUMSCRIPTUS

HANEY AND FALLS (1961) DESCRIBED AFFECTED BROTHER AND SISTER WITH ASSOCIATED MANIFESTATIONS IN THE FORM OF RETARDED MENTAL AND PHYSICAL GROWTH, HYPERTELORISM, CORNEAL NEBULAE, SHORT 'BULL NECK,' STUBBY LIMBS AND DIGITS. THEY QUOTED THE FOLLOWING DESCRIPTION OF THE CORNEAL LESION* '.....THE APPEARANCE ONE MIGHT EXPECT IF INTO THE POSTERIOR SURFACE OF A PLASTIC CORNEA ONE HAD EXCAVATED A SUBSIDIARY SMALL BASIN-LIKE DEPRESSION BY PRESSING INTO IT A MARBLE OF MUCH SMALLER CURVATURE THAN THAT OF THE CORNEAL SURFACE ITSELF.' THE PARENTS DENIED CONSANGUINITY. CURIOUSLY THE AUTHORS SUGGESTED AUTOSOMAL DOMINANT INHERITANCE WITH POOR PENE-TRANCE. IT IS TRUE THAT JACOBS (1957) REPORTED KERATOCONUS POSTICUS IN FATHER AND SON. HE MADE NO MENTION OF ASSOCIATED MANIFESTATIONS.

HANEY, W. P. AND FALLS, H. F.* THE OCCURRENCE OF CONGENITAL KERATOCONUS POSTICUS CIRCUMSCRIPTUS IN TWO SIBLINGS PRESENTING A PREVIOUSLY UNRECOGNIZED SYNDROME. AM. J. OPHTHAL. 52* 53-57, 1961.

JACOBS, H. B.* POSTERIOR CONICAL CORNEA. BRIT. J. OPHTHAL. 41* 31-39, 1957.

*24480 KERATOSIS PALMO-PLANTARIS WITH CORNEAL DYSTROPHY

THE NAMES OF RICHNER (1938) AND HANHART (1948) ARE ASSOCIATED WITH THIS DISORDER. THE PARENTS OF HANHART'S PATIENT (1947) WERE SECOND COUSINS. RICHNER (1938) DESCRIBED SKIN LESIONS IN BROTHER AND SISTER. ONLY THE BROTHER HAD CORNEAL LESIONS. WAARDENBURG (1961) DESCRIBED CHILDREN OF A FIRST COUSIN MARRIAGE, ONE WITH THE FULL SYNDROME AND ONE WITH ONLY CORNEAL CHANGES. HANHART'S PATIENTS (1947) ALSO HAD SEVERE MENTAL AND SOMATIC RETARDATION. THE PEDIGREE HE REPORTED IS REPRODUCED BY WAARDENBURG. VENTURA ET AL. (1965) DESCRIBED THE SYNDROME IN TWO SONS OF FIRST COUSIN PARENTS.

HANHART, E.* NEUE SONDERFORMEN VON KERATOSIS PALMO-PLANTARIS, U.A. EINE REGELMASSIG-DOMINANTE MIT SYSTEMATISIERTEN LIPOMEN, FERNER 2 EINFACH-REZESSIVE MIT SCHWACHSINN UND Z.T. MIT HORNHAUTVERANDERUNGEN DES AUGES (EKTODERMATOSYNDROM). DERMATOLOGICA 94* 286-308, 1947.

VENTURA, G., BIASINI, G. AND PETROZZI, M.* CHERATOMIA PALMOPLANTARE DISSIPATUM ASSOCIATO A LESIONI CORNEALI IN DUE FRATELLI. BOLL. OCULIST. 44* 497-510, 1965.

WAARDENBURG, P. J., FRANCESCHETTI, A. AND KLEIN, D.* IN, GENETICS AND OPHTHAL-MOLOGY. SPRINGFIELD, ILL.* CHARLES C THOMAS, 1* 515-517, 1961.

*24500 KERATOSIS PALMO-PLANTARIS WITH PERIODONTOPATHIA (PAPILLON-LEFEVRE SYNDROME)

BOTH THE MILK TEETH AND THE PERMANENT TEETH ARE LOST PREMATURELY. THE SKIN LESIONS ARE VERY SIMILAR OR IDENTICAL TO THOSE OF MAL DE MELEDA (Q.V.). GORLIN, SEDANO AND ANDERSON (1964) SUGGESTED THAT CALCIFICATION OF THE DURA MATER IS A THIRD COMPONENT OF THE SYNDROME. SCHOPF ET AL. (1971) DESCRIBED KERATOSIS PALMO-PLANTARIS WITH HYPODONTIA, HYPOTRICHOSIS AND CYSTS OF THE EYELIDS IN SISTERS WHOSE PARENTS WERE FIRST COUSINS. THE DECIDUOUS TEETH WERE LOST EARLY AND THE PERMANENT

434

DENTITION IN ONE PATIENT CONSISTED ONLY OF TWO INCISORS AND A MOLAR. PALMO-PLANTAR KERATOSIS AND FRAGILITY OF THE NAILS BEGAN AT ABOUT AGE 12. AT AGE 25 THE HEAD HAIR BECAME SPARCE AND BODY HAIR WAS LOST COMPLETELY. CYSTS OF BOTH UPPER AND LOWER EYELIDS WERE NOTED AT AGE 60. THE CYSTS WERE THOUGHT TO BE DERIVED FROM THE GLANDS OF MOLL. THIS MAY BE THE PAPILLON-LEFEVRE SYNDROME.

GORLIN, R. J., SEDANO, H. AND ANDERSON, V. E.* THE SYNDROME OF PALMAR-PLANTAR HYPERKERATOSIS AND PREMATURE PERIODONTAL DESTRUCTION OF THE TEETH. A CLINICAL AND GENETIC ANALYSIS OF THE PAPILLON-LEFEVRE SYNDROME. J. PEDIAT. 65* 895-908, 1964.

GREITHER, A.* KERATOSIS PALMO-PLANTARIS MIT PERIODONTOPATHIE (PAPILLON-LEFEVRE). DERMATOLOGICA 119* 248-263, 1959.

JANSEN, L. H. AND DEKKER, G.* HYPERKERATOSIS PALMO-PLANTARIS WITH PERIODONTOSIS (PAPILLON-LEFEVRE). DERMATOLOGICA 113* 207-219, 1956.

SCHOPF, E., SCHULZ, H.-J. AND PASSARGE, E.* SYNDROME OF CYSTIC EYELIDS, PALMO-PLANTAR KERATOSIS, HYPODONTIA AND HYPOTRICHOSIS AS A POSSIBLE AUTOSOMAL RECESSIVE TRAIT. THE CLINICAL DELINEATION OF BIRTH DEFECTS. XII. SKIN, HAIR AND NAILS. BALTIMORE* WILLIAMS AND WILKINS, 1971.

ZIPRKOWSKI, L., RAYMON, Y. AND BRISH, M.* HYPERKERATOSIS PALMOPLANTARIS WITH PERIODONTOSIS (PAPILLON-LEFEVRE). ARCH. DERM. 88* 207-209, 1963.

24510 KETOACIDURIA WITH MENTAL DEFICIENCY AND OTHER FEATURES (RICHARDS-RUNDLE SYNDROME)

RICHARDS AND RUNDLE (1959) DESCRIBED A FAMILY IN WHICH 5 OF 13 OFFSPRING OF A MARRIAGE OF FIRST COUSINS ONCE REMOVED HAD KETOACIDURIA, MENTAL RETARDATION, UNDER-DEVELOPMENT OF SECONDARY SEX CHARACTERISTICS, DEAFNESS, ATAXIA, AND PERIPHERAL MUSCLE WASTING. SEE ALSO THE REPORT OF MATTHEWS (1950). THE CONDITION PROGRESSED IN CHILDHOOD BUT EVENTUALLY BECAME STATIC. IT REPRESENTED NO RISK TO LIFE. RICHARDS AND RUNDLE FOUND IN THE LITERATURE A DESCRIPTION OF A BROTHER AND SISTER WHO PROBABLY HAD THE SAME CONDITION (KOENNECKE, 1920).

KOENNECKE, W.* FRIEDREICHSCHE ATAXIE UND TAUBSTUMMHEIT. Z. NEUROL. PSYCHIAT. 53* 161-165, 1920.

MATTHEWS, W. B.* FAMILIAL ATAXIA, DEAF-MUTISM, AND MUSCULAR WASTING. J. NEUROL. PSYCHIAT. 13* 307-311, 1950.

RICHARDS, B. W. AND RUNDLE, A. T.* A FAMILIAL HORMONAL DISORDER ASSOCIATED WITH MENTAL DEFICIENCY, DEAF MUTISM AND ATAXIA. J. MENT. DEFIC. RES. 3* 33-55, 1959.

R
E
C
E
S
S
I
V
E

*24520 KRABBE'S DISEASE (GLOBOID CELL SCLEROSIS)

ONSET OCCURS AT 4-6 MONTHS OF AGE. DEFINITIVE DIAGNOSIS IN THIS DISORDER WHICH CLINICALLY CAN BE SO SIMILAR TO SEVERAL OTHER ENCEPHALOPATHIES OF INFANCY, IS MADE BY FINDING CHARACTERISTIC 'GLOBOID CELLS' IN BRAIN TISSUE. NELSON AND COLLEAGUES (1963) OBSERVED THREE AFFECTED SIBS. A SOMEWHAT SIMILAR STATE HAS BEEN DESCRIBED IN ADULTS BY FERRARO (1927), BUT THIS MAY BE A GENETICALLY DISTINCT CONDITION. SEE DISCUSSION OF MENKES (1963). D'AGOSTINO ET AL (1963) CONCLUDED THAT THE INITIAL HISTOLOGIC MANIFESTATION OF THE DISEASE IS THE PRESENCE OF PAS-POSITIVE MATERIAL EXTRACELLULARLY AND CERITHIN MICROGLIAL CELLS, WHICH LATER APPEAR AS GLOBOID CELLS. FIRST COUSIN PARENTS WERE NOTED BY VAN GEHUCHTEN (1956). MANY HAVE DESCRIBED AFFECTED SIBS. FERRARO (1927) DESCRIBED A POSSIBLY RELATED DISORDER IN THREE ADULT SIBS. ALTHOUGH DEFICIENCY OF CEREBROSIDE-SULFATIDE SULFOTRANSFERASE WAS EARLIER REPORTED IN KRABBE'S DISEASE (BACHHAWAT ET AL., 1967), SUZUKI AND SUZUKI (1970) FOUND DEFICIENCY OF GALACTOCEREBROSIDE BETA-GALACTOSIDASE WHICH THEY FELT IS ETIOLOGIC AND BETTER ACCOUNTS FOR THE MORPHOLOGIC AND BIOCHEMICAL FEATURES OF THE DISORDER. SUZUKI ET AL. (1971) HAS SUCCEEDED IN DEMONSTRATING AN INTERMEDIATE LEVEL OF ACTIVITY OF GALACTOCEREBROSIDE BETA-GALACTOSIDASE IN SERUM, WHITE CELLS AND FIBROBLASTS OF HETEROZYGOTES.

AUSTIN, J.* STUDIES IN GLOBOID (KRABBE) LEUKODYSTROPHY. I. THE SIGNIFICANCE OF LIPID ABNORMALITIES IN WHITE MATTER IN 8 GLOBOID AND 13 CONTROL PATIENTS. ARCH. NEUROL. 9* 207-231, 1963.

AUSTIN, J., SUZUKI, K., ARMSTRONG, D., BRADY, R., BACHHAWAT, B. K., SCHLENKER, J. AND STUMPF, D.* STUDIES IN GLOBOID (KRABBE) LEUKODYSTROPHY (GLD). V. CONTROLLED ENZYMIC STUDIES IN TEN HUMAN CASES. ARCH. NEUROL. 23* 502-512, 1970.

BACHHAWAT, B. K., AUSTIN, J. AND ARMSTRONG, D.* A CEREBROSIDE SULPHOTRANSFERASE DEFICIENCY IN A HUMAN DISORDER OF MYELIN. BIOCHEM. J. 104* 15C-17C, 1967.

D'AGOSTINO, A. N., SAYRE, G. P. AND HAYLES, A. B.* KRABBE'S DISEASE. GLOBOID CELL TYPE OF LEUKODYSTROPHY. ARCH. NEUROL. 8* 82-96, 1963.

FERRARO, A.* FAMILIAL FORM OF ENCEPHALITIS PERIAXIALIS DIFFUSA. J. NERV. MENT. DIS. 66* 329-354, 1927.

KRABBE, K.* A NEW FAMILIAL INFANTILE FORM OF DIFFUSE BRAIN-SCLEROSIS. BRAIN

39* 74-114, 1916.

MENKES, J. H.* METABOLIC DISEASE OF THE NERVOUS SYSTEM. IN, BRENNEMANN, J. (ED.)* PRACTICE OF PEDIATRICS. HAGERSTOWN* W. F. PRYOR CO. 4* 1963.

NELSON, E., AUREBECK, G., OSTERBERG, K., BERRY, J., JABBOUR, J. T. AND BORNHOFEN, J.* ULTRASTRUCTURAL AND CHEMICAL STUDIES ON KRABBE'S DISEASE. J. NEUROPATH. EXP. NEUROL. 22* 414-434, 1963.

NORMAN, R. M., OPPENHEIMER, D. R. AND TINGEY, A. H.* HISTOLOGICAL AND CHEMICAL FINDINGS IN KRABBE'S LEUCODYSTROPHY. J. NEUROL. NEUROSURG. PSYCHIAT. 24* 223-232, 1961.

SUZUKI, K. AND SUZUKI, Y.* GLOBOID CELL LEUCODYSTROPHY (KRABBE'S DISEASE)* DEFICIENCY OF GALACTOCEREBROSIDE BETA-GALACTOSIDASE. PROC. NAT. ACAD. SCI. 66* 302-309, 1970.

SUZUKI, Y. AND SUZUKI, K.* KRABBE'S GLOBOID CELL LEUKODYSTROPHY* DEFICIENCY OF GALACTOCEREBROSIDASE IN SERUM, LEUKOCYTES, AND FIBROBLASTS. SCIENCE 171* 73-74, 1971.

VAN GEHUCHTEN, P.* SUR L'ORIGINE DES CELLULES GLOBOIDES DANS UN CAS DE SCLEROSE DIFFUSE. REV. NEUROL. 94* 253-258, 1956.

24530 KURU

REPRODUCTION OF THE DISEASE CLINICALLY AND HISTOPATHOLOGICALLY IN CHIMPANZEES INJECTED WITH MATERIAL FROM THE BRAIN OF HUMAN CASES (GAJDUSEK ET AL., 1966) SEEMS TO ESTABLISH KURU AS BEING DUE TO A 'SLOW VIRUS.' WHETHER SIGNIFICANT GENETIC FACTORS ARE ALSO INVOLVED REMAINS UNCERTAIN. 'SCRAPIE' IS A CHRONIC NEUROLOGIC DISEASE OF SHEEP IN WHICH A 'SLOW VIRUS' HAS BEEN DEMONSTRATED BUT GENETIC FACTORS MAY ALSO BE INVOLVED. BENNETT ET AL. (1959) HAD SUGGESTED THAT AFFECTED MALES WERE HOMOZYGOUS AND AFFECTED FEMALES EITHER HOMOZYGOUS OR HETEROZYGOUS FOR A SINGLE GENE FOR KURU.

BECK, E., DANIEL, P. M., ALPERS, M., GAJDUSEK, D. C. AND GIBBS, C. J., JR.* EXPERIMENTAL 'KURU' IN CHIMPANZEES. A PATHOLOGICAL REPORT. LANCET 2* 1056-1059, 1966.

BENNETT, J. H., RHODES, F. A. AND ROBSON, H. N.* A POSSIBLE GENETIC BASIS FOR KURU. AM. J. HUM. GENET. 11* 169-187, 1959.

GAJDUSEK, D. C., GIBBS, C. J., JR. AND ALPERS, M.* EXPERIMENTAL TRANSMISSION OF A KURU-LIKE SYNDROME TO CHIMPANZEES. NATURE 209* 794-796, 1966.

GAJDUSEK, D. C., GIBBS, C. J., JR. AND ALPERS, M.* TRANSMISSION AND PASSAGE OF EXPERIMENTAL 'KURU' TO CHIMPANZEES. SCIENCE 155* 212-214, 1967.

*24540 LACTIC ACIDOSIS, FAMILIAL INFANTILE

ERICKSON (1965) REPORTED AFFECTED BROTHER AND SISTER WITH RELATIVES WHO DIED IN INFANCY PERHAPS OF THE SAME CONDITION. THE DIAGNOSIS IS SUGGESTED BY DISCREPANCY BETWEEN TOTAL CATIONS AND ANIONS IN THE BLOOD. MENTAL RETARDATION IS PRESENT. TREATMENT CONSISTS OF REPLACING GLUCOSE WITH GALACTOSE AND OF ADMINISTERED BICARBONATE. LACTIC ACIDOSIS OCCURS IN GLYCOGEN STORAGE DISEASE I (Q.V.). WORSLEY ET AL. (1965) DESCRIBED TWO BROTHERS WHO PRESENTED IN THE SECOND YEAR OF LIFE WITH ATAXIA, MUSCLE TWITCHING AND INTERMITTENT HYPERPNEA AT REST. THE CONDITION PROGRESSED WITH MENTAL DETERIORATION, LOSS OF SCALP HAIR AND DEATH ABOUT 6 MONTHS AFTER ONSET. WIDESPREAD NECROTIZING ENCEPHALOPATHY WAS FOUND AT AUTOPSY. SPONTANEOUS INCREASES IN LACTIC ACID IN THE BLOOD WERE APPARENTLY RESPONSIBLE FOR THE HYPERPNEA. RENAL AMINOACIDURIA AND LOWERED SERUM PHOSPHATE WERE ALSO FOUND. THEY SUGGESTED THAT THIS IS THE FIRST DESCRIPTION OF FAMILIAL LACTIC ACIDOSIS IN YOUNG CHILDREN. HAWORTH, FORD AND YOUNOSZAI (1967) DESCRIBED AN AMERICAN INDIAN FAMILY IN WHICH THREE SIBS WERE MENTALLY RETARDED AND HAD CONVULSIONS, OTHER NEUROLOGIC ABNORMALITIES, MUSCULAR HYPOTONIA, OBESITY AND SIGNS AND SYMPTOMS OF METABOLIC ACIDOSIS. BLOOD LACTATE AND PYRUVATE LEVELS WERE ELEVATED. FIVE OTHER INDIANS DIED BEFORE 2 YEARS OF AGE WITH SYMPTOMS SUGGESTING THE SAME DISORDER.

ERICKSON, R. J.* FAMILIAL INFANTILE LACTIC ACIDOSIS. J. PEDIAT. 66* 1004-1016, 1965.

HAWORTH, J. C., FORD, J. D. AND YOUNOSZAI, M. K.* FAMILIAL CHRONIC ACIDOSIS DUE TO AN ERROR IN LACTATE AND PYRUVATE METABOLISM. CANAD. MED. ASS. J. 97* 773-779, 1967.

WORSLEY, H. E., BROOKFIELD, R. W., ELWOOD, J. S., NOBLE, R. L. AND TAYLOR, W. H.* LACTIC ACIDOSIS WITH NECROTIZING ENCEPHALOPATHY IN TWO SIBS. ARCH. DIS. CHILD. 40* 492-501, 1965.

24550 LACTOSYL CERAMIDOSIS

DAWSON, G. AND STEIN, A. O.* LACTOSYL CERAMIDOSIS* CATABOLIC ENZYME DEFECT OF

RECESSIVE

*24560 LARSEN'S SYNDROME

LARSEN, SCHOTTSTAEDT AND BOST (1950) CALLED ATTENTION TO A SYNDROME OF MULTIPLE
CONGENITAL DISLOCATIONS AND CHARACTERISTIC FACIES (PROMINENT FOREHEAD, DEPRESSED
NASAL BRIDGE, WIDE-SPACED EYES). CLUBFOOT, BILATERAL DISLOCATION OF ELBOWS, HIPS
AND KNEES (MOST CHARACTERISTICALLY, ANTERIOR DISLOCATION OF THE TIBIA ON THE
FEMUR), AND SHORT METACARPALS WITH CYLINDRICAL FINGERS LACKING THE USUAL TAPERING
WERE THE SKELETAL FEATURES OF NOTE. CLEFT PALATE, HYDROCEPHALUS AND ABNORMALITIES
OF SPINAL SEGMENTATION WERE FOUND IN SOME. THESE AUTHORS FOUND NO SIMILAR CASES
IN THE FAMILIES. SEE P. 126 OF GORLIN AND PINDBORG (1964). SEVERAL INSTANCES OF
MULTIPLE AFFECTED SIBS ARE KNOWN TO ME. STEEL (1966) HAS OBSERVED THREE AFFECTED
SIBS AND RIMOIN (1970) SHOWED ME A FAMILY WITH MULTIPLE AFFECTED SIBS. THE SIBS
REPORTED BY BLOCK AND PECK (1965) MAY HAVE HAD THIS CONDITION, CONGENITAL
DISLOCATION OF THE KNEES WITH UNILATERAL CATARACT AND UNILATERAL UNDESCENDED
TESTIS WAS PRESENT IN A NEWBORN MALE. A SISTER WAS BORN WITH BILATERAL DISLOCA-
TION OF THE KNEES AND HIPS AND CLEFT PALATE. ONE OF THE EARLIEST REPORTS MAY HAVE
BEEN THAT OF MCFARLAND (1929). LATTA ET AL. (1971) MADE A POINT OF A JUXTACAL-
CANEAL ACCESSORY BONE WHICH MAY BE SPECIFIC FOR THIS ENTITY. THE MOTHER OF THEIR
PATIENT HAD A SADDLE NOSE WHICH DEVELOPED AT AGE 18 AFTER TENNIS-BALL TRAUMA.
AUTOSOMAL DOMINANT INHERITANCE IS SUGGESTED BY MCFARLANE'S REPORT (1947) OF A
WOMAN WITH SADDLE NOSE, CONGENITAL DISLOCATION OF THE KNEES AND HYPEREXTENSIBILITY
OF THE ELBOWS. BY EACH OF THREE CIFFERENT MATES SHE PRODUCED AN AFFECTED CHILD
WITH BILATERAL KNEE DISLOCATIONS.

BLOCH, C. AND PECK, H. M.* BILATERAL CONGENITAL DISLOCATION OF THE KNEES. J.
MT. SINAI HOSP. 32* 607-614, 1965.

GORLIN, R. J. AND PINDBORG, J. J.* SYNDROMES OF THE HEAD AND NECK. NEW YORK*
BLAKISTON DIVISION, MCGRAW-HILL BOOK CO., 1964.

LARSEN, L. J., SCHOTTSTAEDT, E. R. AND BOST, F. C.* MULTIPLE CONGENITAL
DISLOCATIONS ASSOCIATED WITH CHARACTERISTIC FACIAL ABNORMALITY. J. PEDIAT. 37*
574-581, 1950.

LATTA, R. J., GRAHAM, C. B., AASE, J., SCHAM, S. M. AND SMITH, D. W.* LARSEN'S
SYNDROME* A SKELETAL DYSPLASIA WITH MULTIPLE JOINT DISLOCATIONS AND UNUSUAL
FACIES. J. PEDIAT. 78* 291-298, 1971.

MCFARLANE, A. L.* A REPORT ON FOUR CASES OF CONGENITAL GENU RECURVATUM
OCCURRING IN ONE FAMILY. BRIT. J. SURG. 34* 388-391, 1947.

MCFARLAND, B. L.* CONGENITAL DISLOCATION OF THE KNEE. J. BONE JOINT SURG. 11*
281-285, 1929.

RIMOIN, D. L.* ST. LOUIS, MO.* PERSONAL COMMUNICATION, 1970.

STEEL, H. M.* PHILADELPHIA, PENN.* PERSONAL COMMUNICATION, 1966.

24570 LARYNGEAL ABDUCTOR PARALYSIS

PLOTT (1964) DESCRIBED THREE BROTHERS WITH PERMANENT CONGENITAL LARYNGEAL ABDUCTOR
PARALYSIS AND MENTAL DEFICIENCY. A FOURTH MALE SIB SUSPECTED OF HAVING BEEN
AFFECTED DIED PERINATALLY. DYSGENESIS OF THE NUCLEUS AMBIGUUS WAS CONSIDERED
LIKELY. X-LINKED RECESSIVE INHERITANCE IS, OF COURSE, POSSIBLE.

PLOTT, D.* CONGENITAL LARYNGEAL-ABDUCTOR PARALYSIS DUE TO NUCLEUS AMBIGUUS
DYSGENESIS IN THREE BROTHERS. NEW ENG. J. MED. 271* 593-597, 1964.

*24580 LAURENCE-MOON SYNDROME

THE FEATURES IN THE FOUR SIBS REPORTED BY LAURENCE AND MOON (1866) AND LATER BY
HUTCHINSON (1882, 1900) WERE MENTAL RETARDATION, PIGMENTARY RETINOPATHY, HYPOGENI-
TALISM AND SPASTIC PARAPLEGIA. IT REPRESENTS AN ENTITY DISTINCT FROM THAT
DESCRIBED BY BARDET AND BIEDL (SEE BARDET-BIEDL SYNDROME). UNFORTUNATELY MOST
AUTHORS HAVE ADOPTED THE DESIGNATION SUGGESTED BY SOLIS-COHEN AND WEISS (1925),
LAURENCE-MOON-BIEDL-BARDET SYNDROME. THE LAURENCE-MOON SYNDROME (STRICTU SENSU)
IS THE SAME AS THE DISORDER REPORTED BY KAPUSCINSKI (1934). THE FAMILY REPORTED
BY BOWEN ET AL. (1965) PROBABLY HAD THIS SYNDROME.

BOWEN, P., FERGUSON-SMITH, M. A., MOSIER, D., LEE, C. S. N. AND BUTLER, H. G.*
THE LAURENCE-MOON SYNDROME. ASSOCIATION WITH HYPOGONADOTROPHIC HYPOGONADISM AND
SEX-CHROMOSOME ANEUPLOIDY. ARCH. INTERN. MED. 116* 598-604, 1965.

HUTCHINSON, J.* ON RETINITIS PIGMENTOSA AND ALLIED AFFECTIONS, AS ILLUSTRATING
THE LAWS OF HEREDITY. OPHTHAL. REV. 1* 2-7 AND 26-30, 1882.

HUTCHINSON, J.* SLOWLY PROGRESSIVE PARAPLEGIA AND DISEASE OF THE CHOROIDS WITH
DEFECTIVE INTELLECT AND ARRESTED SEXUAL DEVELOPMENT. ARCH. SURG. 11* 118-122,
1900.

KAPUSCINSKI, W.* UBER FAMILIARE ADERHAUTENTARTUNG MIT ATAKTISCHEN STORUNGEN. BER. DTSCH. OPHTHAL. GES. 50* 13-19, 1934.

LAURENCE, J. Z. AND MOON, R. C.* FOUR CASES OF RETINITIS PIGMENTOSA OCCURRING IN THE SAME FAMILY AND ACCOMPANIED BY GENERAL IMPERFECTION OF DEVELOPMENT. OPHTHAL. REV. 2* 32-41, 1866.

SOLIS-COHEN, S. AND WEISS, E.* DYSTROPHIA ADIPOSOGENITALIS WITH ATYPICAL RETINITIS PIGMENTOSA AND MENTAL DEFICIENCY* THE LAURENCE-BIEDL SYNDROME. AM. J. MED. SCI. 169* 489-505, 1925.

STIGGELBOUT, T.* THE (LAURENCE MOON) BARDET BIEDL SYNDROME. ASSEN, THE NETHERLANDS* VAN GORCUM, 1969.

24590 LECITHIN CHOLESTEROL ACETYLTRANSFERASE (LCAT) DEFICIENCY (NORUM*S DISEASE)

IN NORWAY NORUM AND GJONE (1967) DESCRIBED A POSSIBLY "NEW" ERROR OF LIPID METABOLISM IN SISTERS WITH NORMOCHROMIC ANEMIA, PROTEINURIA AND CORNEAL DEPOSITS OF LIPID. TOTAL SERUM CHOLESTEROL WAS ELEVATED, ALMOST ALL OF IT BEING FREE CHOLESTEROL. LACK OF PLASMA CHOLESTEROL-LECITHIN ACYLTRANSFERASE WAS POSTULATED. GJONE AND NORUM (1968) REPORTED THE CLINICAL FEATURES IN 3 ADULT SISTERS WHO SHOWED ONLY TRACES OF ESTERIFIED CHOLESTEROL IN THE SERUM. ALL HAD PROTEINURIA AND ANEMIA. TOTAL CHOLESTEROL, TRIGLYCERIDE AND PHOSPHOLIPID WERE INCREASED. LYSOLECITHIN OF SERUM WAS DECREASED. FOAM CELLS WERE PRESENT IN THE BONE MARROW AND IN THE GLOMERULAR TUFTS OF THE KIDNEY. THE TONSILS WERE NORMAL. THE LIVER WAS NOT ENLARGED AND THERE WAS NO EVIDENCE OF LIVER DISEASE WHICH MIGHT ACCOUNT FOR A DEFECT IN CHOLESTEROL ESTERIFICATION.

GJONE, E. AND NORUM, K. R.* FAMILIAL SERUM CHOLESTEROL ESTER DEFICIENCY. CLINICAL STUDY OF A PATIENT WITH A NEW SYNDROME. ACTA MED. SCAND. 183* 107-112, 1968.

GJONE, E., TORSVIK, H. AND NORUM, K. R.* FAMILIAL PLASMA CHOLESTEROL ESTER DEFICIENCY. A STUDY OF ERYTHROCYTES. SCAND. J. CLIN. LAB. INVEST. 21* 327-332, 1968.

NORUM, K. R. AND GJONE, E.* FAMILIAL SERUM-CHOLESTEROL ESTERIFICATION FAILURE. A NEW INBORN ERROR OF METABOLISM. BIOCHIM. BIOPHYS. ACTA 144* 698-700, 1967.

*24600 LEG, ABSENCE DEFORMITY OF, WITH CONGENITAL CATARACT

IN TWO DISTANTLY RELATED AMISH BOYS, MCKUSICK ET AL. (1968) OBSERVED ABSENCE DEFORMITY OF ONE LEG, CONGENITAL CATARACT AND PROGRESSIVE SCOLIOSIS. ALL FOUR PARENTS SHARED AT LEAST TWO ANCESTRAL COUPLES IN COMMON.

MCKUSICK, V. A., WEILBAECHER, R. G. AND GRAGG, G. W.* RECESSIVE INHERITANCE OF A CONGENITAL MALFORMATION SYNDROME. J.A.M.A. 204* 113-118, 1968.

R
E
C
E
S
S
I
V
E

24610 LEIOMYOMATA OF SKIN

KLOEPFER AND COLLEAGUES (1958) DESCRIBED THREE HALF-FIRST-COUSINS WITH MULTIPLE LEIOMYOMATA OF THE SKIN. THE PARENTS AND COMMON GRANDPARENT WERE NOT KNOWN TO BE AFFECTED, BUT ALL CRITICAL INDIVIDUALS WERE NOT EXAMINED. IN THIS TYPE OF ANOMALY ONE WOULD, AS THE AUTHORS POINT OUT, ANTICIPATE DOMINANT INHERITANCE, PROBABLY WITH REDUCED PENETRANCE.

KLOEPFER, H. W., KRAFCHUK, J., DERBES, V. AND BURKS, J.* HEREDITARY MULTIPLE LEIOMYOMA OF THE SKIN. AM. J. HUM. GENET. 10* 48-52, 1958.

*24620 LEPRECHAUNISM

AMONG THE CHILDREN OF SECOND COUSINS ONCE REMOVED, DONOHUE AND UCHIDA (1954) OBSERVED TWO SISTERS WITH THE FOLLOWING FEATURES - APPARENT CESSATION OF GROWTH AT ABOUT THE SEVENTH MONTH OF GESTATION, PECULIAR FACIES CREATING A GNOMELIKE APPEARANCE AND LEADING TO THE DESIGNATION, AND SEVERE ENDOCRINE DISTURBANCE INDICATED BY EMACIATION, ENLARGEMENT OF BREASTS AND CLITORIS AND HISTOLOGIC CHANGES IN THE OVARIES, PANCREAS AND BREASTS. THREE ABORTIONS (ONE AT 4 MONTHS, THE OTHERS EARLIER) HAD BEEN EXPERIENCED BY THIS MOTHER. THE PATIENTS DIED AT 46 AND 66 DAYS OF AGE, RESPECTIVELY. PATTERSON AND WATKINS (1962) DESCRIBED A PROBABLE CASE IN A MALE. THE FOUR PREVIOUSLY DESCRIBED CASES HAD BEEN FEMALE. FOLLOW-UP OBSERVATIONS (PATTERSON, 1969) SUGGEST THAT THIS MAY HAVE BEEN A DIFFERENT DISORDER. THERE WERE CLINICAL SIGNS OF CUSHING*S DISEASE AND AT AUTOPSY THE ADRENALS WERE FOUND TO BE MUCH ENLARGED. BEFORE THE PATIENT DIED AT THE AGE OF ALMOST 8 YEARS, SEVERE CHANGES IN THE BONES, OF AN UNUSUAL TYPE, HAD DEVELOPED. SERUM ALKALINE PHOSPHATASE WAS ALWAYS LOW, BUT NO PHOSPHOETHANOLAMINE WAS DEMONSTRATED IN THE URINE. TWO AFFECTED SISTERS WERE REPORTED BY LAKATOS AND COLLEAGUES (1963). SALMON AND WEBB (1963) OBSERVED CONSANGUINEOUS PARENTS OF A CASE. DEKABAN (1965) FOUND NORMAL CHROMSOMES. SEE SEIP SYNDROME.

DEKABAN, A.* METABOLIC AND CHROMOSOMAL STUDIES IN LEPRECHAUNISM. ARCH. DIS. CHILD. 40* 632-636, 1965.

DONOHUE, W. L. AND UCHIDA, I.* LEPRECHAUNISM* A EUPHUISM FOR A RARE FAMILIAL DISORDER. J. PEDIAT. 45* 505-519, 1954.

EVANS, P. R.* LEPRECHAUNISM. ARCH. DIS. CHILD. 30* 479-483, 1955.

KUHLKAMP, F. AND HELWIG, H.* DAS KRANKHEITSBILD DES KONGENITALEN DYSENDOKRINIS-MUS ODER LEPRECHAUNISMUS. Z. KINDERHEILK. 109* 50-63, 1970.

LAKATOS, I., KALLO, A. AND SZIJARTO, L.* LEPRECHAUNISM (DONOHUE SYNDROME). ORV. HETIL. 104* 1075-1080, 1963.

PATTERSON, J. H. AND WATKINS, W. L.* LEPRECHAUNISM IN A MALE INFANT. J. PEDIAT. 60* 730-739, 1962.

PATTERSON, J. H.* PRESENTATION OF A PATIENT WITH LEPRECHAUNISM. THE CLINICAL DELINEATION OF BIRTH DEFECTS. IV. SKELETAL DYSPLASIAS. NEW YORK* NATIONAL FOUNDATION, 1969. PP. 117-121.

SALMON, M. A. AND WEBB, J. N.* DYSTROPHIC CHANGES ASSOCIATED WITH LEPRECHAUNISM IN MALE INFANT. ARCH. DIS. CHILD. 38* 530-535, 1963.

SUMMITT, R. L. AND FAVARA, B. E.* LEPRECHAUNISM (DONOHUE'S SYNDROME)* A CASE REPORT. J. PEDIAT. 74* 601-610, 1969.

24630 LEPROSY, VULNERABILITY TO

BEIGUELMAN (1968) REVIEWED THE EVIDENCE FOR AN INHERITED BASIS OF VULNERABILITY TO LEPROSY AND THE FAMILIAL PATTERN OF THE MITSUDA (LATE LEPROMIN) REACTION. THE FOLLOWING OBSERVATIONS SUGGEST THE HERITABILITY OF LEPROSY* (1) THE DISEASE FAILS TO MANIFEST ITSELF IN MOST EXPOSED PERSONS, EVEN HEAVILY EXPOSED PERSONS. (2) THE FREQUENCY OF LEPROSY AMONG RELATIVES OF INDEX CASES IS HIGHER WHEN THE SUBJECTS ARE FROM A CONSANGUINEOUS MARRIAGE. (3) DIFFERENT RACIAL STOCKS LIVING IN THE SAME AREA SHOW DIFFERENT PREVALENCE RATES. (4) EVEN IN POPULATIONS WITH A HIGH FREQUENCY, FAMILIAL AGGREGATION IS DEMONSTRABLE, I.E., THE DISTRIBUTION IN SIBSHIPS IS NOT RANDOM. (5) THE DISTRIBUTION OF POLAR TYPES (TYPICAL LEPROMATOUS OR MALIGNANT VERSUS TYPICAL TUBERCULOID OR BENIGN) IS NOT AT RANDOM AMONG AFFECTED SIB PAIRS. (6) ONE POLAR FORM CANNOT BE CONVERTED INTO THE OTHER BY ENVIRONMENTAL AGENTS. BEIGUELMAN AND QUAGLIATO (1965) STUDIED THE FAMILIAL DISTRIBUTION OF THE MITSUDA REACTION AND PRESENTED EVIDENCE WHICH CAN BE INTERPRETED AS SUPPORTING MONOGENIC DETERMINATION.

BEIGUELMAN, B. AND QUAGLIATO, R.* NATURE AND FAMILIAL CHARACTER OF THE LEPROMIN REACTIONS. INT. J. LEPROSY 33* 800-807, 1965.

BEIGUELMAN, B.* SOME REMARKS ON THE GENETICS OF LEPROSY RESISTANCE. ACTA GENET. MED. GEM. 17* 584-594, 1968.

*24640 LETTERER-SIWE DISEASE

KLOEPFER 1971 HAS AN UNPUBLISHED PEDIGREE OF AN INBRED KINDRED SUGGESTING AUTOSOMAL RECESSIVE INHERITANCE. CHRISTIE AND COLLEAGUES (1954) DESCRIBED THE DISEASE IN SIBS WHO WERE NEVER IN CONTACT, THUS TENDING TO DISCREDIT AN INFECTIOUS HYPOTHESIS. ROGERS AND BENSON (1962) REPORTED AFFECTED SIBS AND REVIEWED THE LITERATURE. FALK AND GELLEI (1963) ALSO OBSERVED A FAMILY.
SCHOECK, PETERSON AND GOOD (1963) DESCRIBED TWO SIBS WITH LETTERER-SIWE DISEASE (ACUTE DISSEMINATED HISTIOCYTOSIS X). TEN OTHER FAMILIES WITH MULTIPLE AFFECTED SIBS WERE REVIEWED, INCLUDING FARQUHAR'S 'FAMILIAL HEMOPHAGOCYTIC RETICULOSIS' (Q.V.) AND NELSON'S 'GENERALIZED LYMPHOHISTIOCYTIC INFILTRATION' (Q.V.), WHICH SCHOECK AND HIS COLLEAGUES SUGGEST ARE ALL THE SAME ENTITY. IN A SURVEY OF DEATHS FROM LETTERER-SIWE DISEASE IN A FIVE YEAR PERIOD IN THE U.S., GLASS AND MILLER (1968) FOUND FIVE SIB PAIRS AMONG 270 DEATHS, A PAIR OF CONCOR-DANT LIKE-SEX TWINS, AND A PEAK OF MORTALITY UNDER 1 YEAR OF AGE.

CHRISTIE, A., BATSON, R., SHAPIRO, J., RILEY, H. D., LAUGHMILLER, R. AND STAHLMAN, M.* ACUTE DISSEMINATED (NON-LIPID) RETICULOENDOTHELIOSIS. ACTA PAEDIAT. 43 (SUPPL. 100)* 65-76, 1954.

FALK, W. AND GELLEI, B.* LETTERER-SIWE DISEASE (NON-LIPOID RETICULOENDOTHELIO-SIS). IN, GOLDSCHMIDT, E. (ED.)* GENETICS OF MIGRANT AND ISOLATE POPULATIONS. BALTIMORE* WILLIAMS AND WILKINS, 1963. P. 312. (SEE ALSO, THE FAMILIAL OCCURRENCE OF LETTERER-SIWE DISEASE. ACTA PAEDIAT. 46* 471-480, 1957.)

GLASS, A. G. AND MILLER, R. W.* U.S. MORTALITY FROM LETTERER-SIWE DISEASE, 1960-1964. PEDIATRICS 42* 364-367, 1968.

JUBERG, R. C., KLOEPFER, H. W. AND OBERMAN, H. A.* GENETIC DETERMINATION OF ACUTE DISSEMINATED HISTIOCYTOSIS X (LETTERER-SIWE SYNDROME). PEDIATRICS 45* 753-765, 1970.

KLOEPFER, H. W.* NEW ORLEANS, LA.* PERSONAL COMMUNICATION, 1971.

ROGERS, D. L. AND BENSON, T. E.* FAMILIAL LETTERER-SIWE DISEASE. REPORT OF A

R
E
C
E
S
S
I
V
E

CASE. J. PEDIAT. 60* 550-554, 1962.

SCHOECK, V. W., PETERSON, R. D. A. AND GOOD, R. A.* FAMILIAL OCCURRENCE OF
LETTERER-SIWE DISEASE. PEDIATRICS 32* 1055-1063, 1963.

*24650 LEUKOMELANODERMA, INFANTILISM, MENTAL RETARDATION, HYPODONTIA, HYPOTRICHOSIS

IN THE FAMILY REPORTED BY BERLIN (1961) TWO MALES AND TWO FEMALES WERE AFFECTED
OUT OF 12 OFFSPRING OF A COUSIN MARRIAGE.

BERLIN, C.* CONGENITAL GENERALIZED MELANOLEUCODERMA ASSOCIATED WITH HYPODONTIA,
HYPOTRICHOSIS, STUNTED GROWTH AND MENTAL RETARDATION OCCURRING IN TWO BROTHERS AND
TWO SISTERS. DERMATOLOGICA 123* 227-243, 1961.

*24660 LIPASE, CONGENITAL ABSENCE OF PANCREATIC

SHELDON (1964) DESCRIBED TWO UNRELATED SIBSHIPS WITH A BROTHER AND SISTER IN ONE
AND TWO BROTHERS IN ANOTHER SHOWING CONGENITAL ABSENCE OF PANCREATIC LIPASE. REY
ET AL. (1966) DESCRIBED A SINGLE CASE. IN NONE WERE THE PARENTS RELATED.

REY, J., FREZAL, J., ROYER, P. AND LAMY, M.* L'ABSENCE CONGENITALE DE LIPASE
PANCREATIQUE. ARCH. FRANC. PEDIAT. 23* 5-14, 1966.

SHELDON, W.* CONGENITAL PANCREATIC LIPASE DEFICIENCY. ARCH. DIS. CHILD. 39*
268-271, 1964.

24670 LIPID TRANSPORT DEFECT OF INTESTINE

ANDERSON ET AL. (1961), LAMY ET AL. (1967) AND SILVERBERG ET AL. (1968) DESCRIBED
CASES. TWO BROTHERS WERE AFFECTED (LAMY ET AL., 1967). PARENTAL CONSANGUINITY
WAS NOTED BY SILVERBERG ET AL. (1968). INTESTINAL SYMPTOMS AND A FAILURE OF FAT
TRANSPORT OCCUR AS IN ABETALIPOPROTEINEMIA BUT NEITHER ACANTHOCYTOSIS OR NEURO-
OCULAR SYMPTOMS OCCUR AND LOW-DENSITY LIPOPROTEINS ARE PRESENT IN THE PLASMA. AS
IN ABETALIPOPROTEINEMIA, THERE IS FAILURE OF CHYLOMICRON FORMATION. THE NATURE OF
THE DEFECT IS UNKNOWN, AS IS ALSO THE GENETIC RELATIONSHIP TO ABETALIPOPROTEINE-
MIA, E.G. WHETHER THE GENES ARE ALLELIC.

ANDERSON, C. M., TOWNLEY, R. R., FREEMAN, M. AND JOHANSEN, P.* UNUSUAL CAUSES
OF STEATORRHOEA IN INFANCY AND CHILDHOOD. MED. J. AUST. 2* 617-622, 1961.

LAMY, M., FREZAL, J., REY, J., JOS, J., NEZELOF, C., HERRAULT, A. AND COHEN-
SOLAL, J.* DIARRHEE CHRONIQUE PAR TROUBLE DU TRANSFERT INTRA-CELLULAIRE DES
LIPIDES. ARCH. FRANC. PEDIAT. 24* 1079 ONLY, 1967.

SILVERBERG, M., KESSLER, J., NEUMANN, P. Z. AND WIGLESWORTH, F. W.* AN
INTESTINAL LIPID TRANSPORT DEFECT. A POSSIBLE VARIANT OF HYPO-BETA-LIPOPROTEINE-
MIA. (ABSTRACT) GASTROENTEROLOGY 54* 1271-1272, 1968.

24680 LIPIDOSIS, JUVENILE DYSTONIC

DELEON ET AL. (1969) DESCRIBED TWO FEMALES AND A MALE IN A NEGRO KINDRED WITH A
JUVENILE FORM OF CEREBRAL LIPIDOSIS. CLINICAL FEATURES WERE ONSET BETWEEN AGE 4
AND 9 YEARS, DEMENTIA PROGRESSING TO COMPLETE AMENTIA AND AN AKINETIC MUTE STATE,
GRAND MAL AND MINOR MOTOR SEIZURES, PROGRESSIVE DYSTONIA OF POSTURE WITH TENDENCY
TO FLEXION OF THE ARMS, HYPEREXTENSION OF THE SPINE AND EXTENSION OF THE LEGS, BUT
WITHOUT TORSION DYSTONIA, CLUMSINESS AND MILD ATYPICAL ATAXIA, SOME INTENTION
TREMOR AND ATHETOSIS, GRASP REFLEXES AND SEVERE REFLEX TRISMUS IN THE FINAL
STAGES, TENDENCY TO HYPERREFLEXIA BUT PRESERVATION OF FAIR STRENGTH AND NORMAL
PLANTAR REFLEXES UNTIL LATE. NOTABLY ABSENT WERE RETINAL DEGENERATION, MYOCLONUS,
PROMINENT PYRAMIDAL OR BULBAR INVOLVEMENT AND HEPATOSPLENOMEGALY. IN ONE CASE
FOAM HISTIOCYTES WERE DEMONSTRATED IN THE BONE MARROW. CEREBRAL SPHINGOLIPIDS IN
BIOPSY-OBTAINED MATERIAL WERE NORMAL. ELECTRONMICROSCOPIC FINDINGS SUPPORTED THE
DISTINCTNESS OF THIS ENTITY (ELFENBEIN, 1968). THE CASE REPORTED BY KIDD (1967)
IS THOUGHT TO BE IDENTICAL.

DELEON, G. A., KABACK, M. M., ELFENBEIN, I. B., PERCY, A. K. AND BRADY, R. O.*
JUVENILE DYSTONIA LIPIDOSIS. JOHNS HOPKINS MED. J. 125* 62-77, 1969.

ELFENBEIN, I. B.* DYSTONIC JUVENILE IDIOCY WITHOUT AMAUROSIS. A NEW SYNDROME.
JOHNS HOPKINS MED. J. 123* 205-221, 1968.

KIDD, M.* AN ELECTRONMICROSCOPIC STUDY OF A CASE OF ATYPICAL CEREBRAL LIPIDO-
SIS. ACTA NEUROPATH. 9* 70-78, 1967.

24690 LIPOCALCIGRANULOMATOSIS (LIPOIDO-CALCINOSIS, LIPOID CALCAREOUS GOUT)

COLLARD (1966) DESCRIBED 2 AFFECTED SISTERS IN A SIBSHIP OF 5. CALCIFICATION OF
THE MEDIA WAS LIMITED TO ARTERIES OF THE LEG. THE PARENTS WERE NORMAL AND
UNRELATED. LARGE CALCIFIED TOPHUS-LIKE NODULES WERE SITUATED AROUND THE JOINTS OF
THE FINGERS AND TOES. ALTHOUGH RHEUMATIC SYMPTOMS HAD BEGUN AT AGE 20 IN BOTH,
THE SISTERS WERE IN THEIR 50'S AT THE TIME OF REPORT.

RECESSIVE

COLLARD, M.* UNE FORME FAMILIALE DE LIPOCALCIGRANULOMATOSE AVEC CALCINOSE ARTERIELLE. J. RAIDOL. ELECTR. 47* 31-40, 1966.

TEUTSCHLAENDER, O.* DIE LIPOIDO-CALCINOSIS ODER LIPOIDKALKGICHT (LIPOCALCINO-GRANULOMATOSE). BEITR. PATH. ANAT. 110* 402-432, 1949.

24700 LIPODYSTROPHY AND CYSTIC ANGIOMATOSIS

BRUNZELL ET AL. (1963) DESCRIBED 5 NEGRO SIBS (OUT OF 12) WITH CONGENITAL GENERALIZED LIPODYSTROPHY AND SYSTEMIC CYSTIC ANGIOMATOSIS. THE QUESTION IS WHETHER THIS IS DISTINCT FROM CONGENITAL LIPODYSTROPHY, OR SEIP'S SYNDROME (Q.V.).

BRUNZELL, J. D., SHANKLE, S. W. AND BETHUNE, J. E.* CONGENITAL GENERALIZED LIPODYSTROPHY ACCOMPANIED BY SYSTEMIC CYSTIC ANGIOMATOSIS. ANN. INTERN. MED. 69* 501-516, 1968.

*24710 LIPOID PROTEINOSIS OF URBACH AND WIETHE (LIPOPROTEINOSIS, HYALINOSIS CUTIS ET MUCOSAE)

THE ASSOCIATION OF EARLY HOARSENESS WITH AN UNUSUAL SKIN ERUPTION SUGGESTS THIS DIAGNOSIS. CUTANEOUS AND MUCOSAL INFILTRATIONS MAY TAKE PROTEAN FORMS. LIPIDS OF THE BLOOD MAY BE ELEVATED. DEFINITIVE INFORMATION ON THE BIOLOGICAL BEHAVIOR, E.G., AGE OF ONSET, PROGNOSIS, ETC., IS NOT AVAILABLE. MOST OF THE CASES HAVE BEEN DESCRIBED ON AN AD HOC BASIS BY DERMATOLOGISTS OR LARYNGOLOGISTS. MULTIPLE CASES, MALE AND FEMALE, IN SIBSHIPS AND FREQUENT PARENTAL CONSANGUINITY MAKE RECESSIVE INHERITANCE VERY LIKELY. I KNOW OF A FAMILY IN WHICH MOTHER AND CHILDREN ARE AFFECTED. HOWEVER, CONSANGUINITY OF THE MOTHER AND HER SPOUSE IS SUSPECTED. PAPULAR INFILTRATION OF THE MARGIN OF THE LIDS PRODUCING 'ITCHY EYES,' AND INFILTRATION IN THE TONGUE AND ITS FRENULUM, IN THE LARYNX LEADING TO HOARSENESS AND IN THE SKIN (E.G., ELBOWS AND AXILLA) IS CHARACTERISTIC. ERYTHRO-POIETIC PROTOPORPHYRIA (Q.V.) IS SOMETIMES MIS-DIAGNOSED LIPOID PROTEINOSIS. THE GENE IS SAID TO BE UNUSUALLY FREQUENT IN SOUTH AFRICA. A DISTURBANCE IN MUCOPOLY-SACCHARIDE METABOLISM WAS SUGGESTED BY MOYNAHAN (1966). IN THE FAMILY REPORTED BY ROSENTHAL AND DUKE (1967) MOTHER AND 3 SONS AND A DAUGHTER WERE AFFECTED BUT THE FATHER WAS A FIRST COUSIN OF THE MOTHER. THUS, QUASI-DOMINANT PEDIGREE PATTERN RESULTING FROM CONSANGUINITY IS LIKELY. ALMOST A QUARTER OF ALL REPORTED CASES OF LIPOID PROTEINOSIS HAVE BEEN IN RESIDENTS OF SOUTH AFRICA. RECESSIVE INHERITANCE IS WELL DOCUMENTED BY THE STUDY OF GORDON ET AL. (1969) OF NUMEROUS CASES IN AN INBRED SOUTH AFRICAN COMMUNITY.

R
E
C
E
S
S
I
V
E

BEUREY, J., NEIMANN, N., PIERSON, M., TRIDON, P., SAPELIER AND MEDLIN, P.* MALADIE DURBACH-WIETHE FAMILIALE AVEC INDIFFERENCE A LA DOULEUR. ARCH. BELG. DERM. SYPH. 19* 310-312, 1964.

BLODI, F. C., WHINERY, R. D. AND HENDRICKS, C. A.* LIPID-PROTEINOSIS (URBACH-WIETHE) INVOLVING THE LIDS. TRANS. AM. OPHTHAL. SOC. 58* 155-166, 1960.

BURNETT, J. W. AND MARCY, S. M.* LIPOID PROTEINOSIS. AM. J. DIS. CHILD. 105* 81-84, 1963.

CAPLAN, R. M.* LIPOID PROTEINOSIS* A REVIEW INCLUDING SOME NEW OBSERVATIONS. UNIV. MICH. MED. BULL. 28* 365-377, 1962.

DE SOUZA AND PATRICIO* IN L'HEREDITE EN MEDECINE. TOURAINE, A. (ED.)* PARIS* MASSON AND CIE., 1955. P. 232. FIG. 137.

GORDON, H., GORDON, W. AND BOTHA, V.* LIPOID PROTEINOSIS IN AN INBRED NAMAQUA-LAND COMMUNITY. LANCET 1* 1032-1035, 1969.

HEWSON, S. E.* LIPIDPROTEINOSIS (URBACH-WIETHE SYNDROME). BRIT. J. OPHTHAL. 47* 242-245, 1963.

HEYL, T.* GENEALOGY OF LIPOID PROTEINOSIS. (LETTER) LANCET 2* 162-163, 1969.

LAYMON, C. W. AND HILL, E. M.* AN APPRAISAL OF HYALINOSIS CUTIS ET MUCOSAE. ARCH. DERM. 75* 55-65, 1957.

MOYNAHAN, E. J.* HYALINOSIS CUTIS ET MUCOSAE (LIPOID PROTEINOSIS). DEMONSTRA-TION OF A NEW DISORDER OF MACOPOLYSACCHARIDE METABOLISM. PROC. ROY. SOC. MED. 59* 1125-1126, 1966.

ROSENTHAL, A. R. AND DUKE, J. R.* LIPOID PROTEINOSIS* CASE REPORT OF DIRECT LINEAL TRANSMISSION. AM. J. OPHTHAL. 64* 1120-1124, 1967.

SCOTT, F. P. AND FINDLAY, G. H.* HYALINOSIS CUTIS ET MUCOSAE (LIPOID PROTEINO-SIS). S. AFR. MED. J. 34* 189-195, 1960.

URBACH, E. AND WIETHE, C.* LIPOIDOSIS CUTIS ET MUCOSAE. VIRCHOW. ARCH. PATH. ANAT. 273* 285-319, 1929.

*24720 LISSENCEPHALY SYNDROME

LISSENCEPHALY MEANS "SMOOTH BRAIN," I.E., BRAIN WITHOUT CONVOLUTIONS OR GYRI. MILLER (1963) DESCRIBED THIS CONDITION IN A BROTHER AND SISTER WHO WERE THE FIFTH AND SIXTH CHILDREN OF UNRELATED PARENTS. THE FEATURES WERE MICROCEPHALY, SMALL MANDIBLE, BIZARRE FACIES, FAILURE TO THRIVE, RETARDED MOTOR DEVELOPMENT, DYSPHAGIA, DECORTICATE AND DECEREBRATE POSTURES, AND DEATH AT 3 AND 4 MONTHS. AUTOPSY SHOWED ANOMALIES OF THE BRAIN, KIDNEY, HEART AND GASTROINTESTINAL TRACT. THE BRAINS WERE SMOOTH WITH LARGE VENTRICLES AND A HISTOLOGIC ARCHITECTURE MORE LIKE NORMAL FETAL BRAIN OF 3-4 MONTHS GESTATION. DIEKER ET AL. (1969) DESCRIBED TWO AFFECTED BROTHERS AND AN AFFECTED FEMALE MATERNAL FIRST COUSIN. THEY ALSO EMPHASIZED THAT THIS SHOULD BE TERMED THE LISSENCEPHALY SYNDROME BECAUSE MALFORMATIONS OF THE HEART, KIDNEYS AND OTHER ORGANS ARE ASSOCIATED, AS WELL AS POLYDACTYLY, UNUSUAL FACIAL APPEARANCE.

REZNIK AND ALBERCA-SERRANO (1964) DESCRIBED TWO BROTHERS WITH CONGENITAL HYPERTELORISM, MENTAL DEFECT, INTRACTABLE EPILEPSY, PROGRESSIVE SPASTIC PARAPLEGIA AND DEATH AT AGES 19 AND 9 YEARS. THE MOTHER SHOWED HYPERTELORISM AND SHORT-LIVED EPILEPTIFORM ATTACKS. AUTOPSY SHOWED LISSENCEPHALY WITH MASSIVE NEURONAL HETEROTOPIES AND LARGE VENTRICULAR CAVITIES OF EMBRYONIC TYPE. (THE FINDINGS IN THE MOTHER MAKE X-LINKED RECESSIVE INHERITANCE A POSSIBILITY.) THE PATIENTS OF REZNIK AND ALBERCA-SERRANO (1964) MAY HAVE SUFFERED FROM A DISORDER DISTINCT FROM THAT OF MILLER (1963) AND DIEKER ET AL. (1969). ALL THESE CASES ARE IDIOTS. NONE LEARNED TO SPEAK. THEY MAY WALK BY 3 TO 5 YEARS BUT SPASTIC DIPLEGIA WITH SPASTIC GAIT IS EVIDENT. AS IN OTHER FORMS OF STATIONARY FORE-BRAIN DEVELOPMENTAL ANOMALIES, DECEREBRATE POSTURING WITH HEAD RETRACTION EMERGES IN THE FIRST YEAR OF LIFE.

DIEKER, H., EDWARDS, R. H., ZURHEIN, G., CHOU, S. M., HARTMAN, H. A. AND OPITZ, J. M.* THE LISSENCEPHALY SYNDROME. THE CLINICAL DELINEATION OF BIRTH DEFECTS. II. MALFORMATION SYNDROMES. NEW YORK* NATION FOUNDATION, 1969. PP. 53-64.

MILLER, J. Q.* LISSENCEPHALY IN 2 SIBLINGS. NEUROLOGY 13* 841-850, 1963.

REZNIK, M. AND ALBERCA-SERRANO, R.* FORME FAMILIALE D'HYPERTELORISME AVEC LISSENCEPHALIE SE PRESENTANT CLINIQUEMENT SOUS FORME D'UNE ARRIERATION MENTALE AVEC EPILEPSIE ET PARAPLEGIE SPASMODIQUE. J. NEUROL. SCI. 1* 40-58, 1964.

24730 LIVER CANCER

KAPLAN AND COLE (1965) DESCRIBED PRIMARY LIVER CANCER IN 3 BROTHERS. RECESSIVE INHERITANCE IS, OF COURSE, NOT PROVED. X-LINKED RECESSIVE INHERITANCE IS AS PLAUSIBLE AS AUTOSOMAL RECESSIVE.

KAPLAN, L. AND COLE, S. L.* FRATERNAL PRIMARY HEPATOCELLULAR CARCINOMA IN THREE MALES, ADULT SIBLINGS. AM. J. MED. 39* 305-311, 1965.

24740 LOW BIRTH WEIGHT DWARFISM WITH SKELETAL DYSPLASIA

TAYBI AND LINDER (1967) DESCRIBED BROTHER AND SISTER, OF ITALIAN EXTRACTION WITH FIRST COUSIN PARENTS, WHO HAD LOW BIRTH WEIGHT DWARFISM, DYSPLASIA OF THE OSSEOUS SKELETON INCLUDING THE SKULL, MICROCEPHALY, AND DEATH AT AGES 1 MONTH AND 1 YEAR. AUTOPSY WAS DONE IN BOTH. EXTENSIVE MALFORMATION OF THE BRAIN WAS PRESENT.

TAYBI, H. AND LINDER, D.* CONGENITAL FAMILIAL DWARFISM WITH CEPHALOSKELETAL DYSPLASIA. RADIOLOGY 89* 275-281, 1967.

24750 LYMPHOHISTIOCYTIC INFILTRATION, GENERALIZED

NELSON AND COLLEAGUES (1961) CLAIM THAT THE DISORDER THEY DESCRIBE IS QUITE DIFFERENT FROM LETTERER-SIWE DISEASE (Q.V.) AND PRESUMABLY ALSO FROM HISTOPHAGOCYTIC (OR HEMOPHAGOCYTIC) RETICULOSIS (Q.V.). CHEDIAK-HIGASHI SYNDROME (Q.V.) HAS ONLY PARTIAL SIMILARITY. MOZZICONACCI AND COLLEAGUES (1965) DESCRIBED TWO BROTHERS, AGES 6 AND 8, WITH THIS FATAL DISEASE CHARACTERIZED BY HIGH AND IRREGULAR FEVER, HEPATOSPLENOMEGALY, PURPURA, AND LATER JAUNDICE, POLYNEURITIS, MENINGEAL REACTION, CHOKED DISKS, MODERATE ANEMIA AND SEVERE GRANULOCYTOPENIA.

LANDING, B. H., STRAUSS, L., CROCKER, A. C., BRAUNSTEIN, H., HENLEY, W. L., WILL, J. R. AND SANDERS, M.* THROMBOCYTOPENIC PURPURA WITH HISTIOCYTOSIS OF THE SPLEEN. NEW ENG. J. MED. 265* 572-576, 1961.

MOZZICONACCI, P., NEZELOF, C., ATTAL, C., GIRARD, F., PHAM-HUU-TRUNG, (NI)., WEIL, J., DESBUQUOIS, B. AND GADOT, M.* LA LYMPHO-HISTIOCYTOSE FAMILIALE. ARCH. FRANC. PEDIAT. 22* 385-408, 1965.

NELSON, P., SANTAMARIA, A., OLSON, R. L. AND NAYAK, N. C.* GENERALIZED LYMPHOHISTIOCYTIC INFILTRATION. A FAMILIAL DISEASE NOT PREVIOUSLY DESCRIBED AND DIFFERENT FROM LETTERER-SIWE DISEASE AND CHEDIAK-HIGASHI SYNDROME. PEDIATRICS 27* 931-950, 1961.

24760 LYMPHOHISTIOCYTOSIS OF NERVOUS SYSTEM

PRICE ET AL. (1971) DESCRIBED FOUR OUT OF 12 SIBS WITH A PROGRESSIVE NEUROLOGIC DISEASE CHARACTERIZED BY DIFFUSE LYMPHOHISTIOCYTIC INFILTRATIONS OF THE CENTRAL NERVOUS SYSTEM IN ASSOCIATION WITH MULTIPLE FOCI OF PARENCHYMAL DESTRUCTION. THE

RANGE OF AGE AT DEATH WAS 15 MONTHS TO 12 YEARS. THE SPINAL FLUID SHOWED PLEOCYTOSIS AND INCREASED PROTEIN. HISTOLOGICALLY THE DISORDER RESEMBLED FAMILIAL HEMOPHAGOCYTIC RETICULOSIS OR FAMILIAL ERYTHROPHAGOCYTIC LYMPHOHISTIOCYTOSIS BUT UNLIKE THESE CONDITIONS THE PROCESS WAS LARGELY CONFIRMED TO THE CNS.

PRICE, D. L., WOOLSEY, J. E., ROSMAN, N. P. AND RICHARDSON, E. P., JR.* FAMILIAL LYMPHOHISTIOCYTOSIS OF THE NERVOUS SYSTEM. ARCH. NEUROL. 24* 270-283, 1971.

24770 LYMPHOID SYSTEM DETERIORATION, PROGRESSIVE

SEEGER ET AL. (1970) DESCRIBED BROTHER AND SISTER WITH A *NEW* IMMUNOLOGIC DISORDER, CHARACTERIZED BY DEFECTIVE CELLULAR AND HUMORAL IMMUNITY, ASSOCIATED BONE MARROW APLASIA, DEFICIENCY OF IGG AND IGM WITH NORMAL IGA. ONE PATIENT DEVELOPED GRAFT-VERSUS-HOST REACTION AS A COMPLICATION OF BLOOD TRANSFUSION. LYMPHOPENIA AND CANDIDIASIS DEVELOPED. THE PROGRESSIVE NATURE BEGINNING IN THE SECOND YEAR OF LIFE WAS EMPHASIZED.

SEEGER, R. C., AMMANN, A. J., GOOD, R. A. AND HONG, R.* PROGRESSIVE LYMPHOID SYSTEM DETERIORATION* A NEW FAMILIAL LYMPHOPENIC IMMUNOLOGICAL DEFICIENCY DISEASE. CLIN. EXP. IMMUN. 6* 169-180, 1970.

*24780 LYMPHOPENIC HYPERGAMMAGLOBULINEMIA, ANTIBODY DEFICIENCY, AUTO-IMMUNE HEMOLYTIC ANEMIA AND GLOMERULONEPHRITIS

SCHALLER ET AL., (1966) DESCRIBED AN INFANT WITH THESE FEATURES PLUS MARKED LYMPHOID HYPOPLASIA, ABSENCE OF LYMPHOID ELEMENTS AND HASSALL'S CORPUSCLES FROM THYMUS AND PLASMOCYTOSIS. SHE DIED AT 6 MONTHS WITH PNEUMOCYSTIS CARINII PNEUMONIA. TWO SIBS SUCCUMBED APPARENTLY FROM THE SAME AILMENT.

SCHALLER, J., DAVIS, S. D., CHING, Y. C., LAGUNOFF, D., WILLIAMS, C. P. S. AND WEDGWOOD, R. J.* HYPERGAMMAGLOBULINAEMIA, ANTIBODY DEFICIENCY, AUTOIMMUNE HAEMOLYTIC ANAEMIA, AND NEPHRITIS IN AN INFANT WITH A FAMILIAL LYMPHOPENIC IMMUNE DEFECT. LANCET 2* 825-829, 1966.

*24790 LYSINE INTOLERANCE

R
E
C
E
S
S
I
V
E

COLOMBO AND COLLEAGUES (1964) DESCRIBED EPISODIC VOMITING, RIGIDITY AND COMA IN AN INFANT, RELIEVED BY LOW PROTEIN DIET. DURING COMA, AMMONIA WAS HIGH IN THE BLOOD AND THE AMINO ACIDS LYSINE AND ARGININE WERE ALSO HIGH. DEFECT IN DEGRADATION OF LYSINE WAS PROPOSED. LYSINE IS A POTENT COMPETITIVE INHIBITOR OF ARGINASE. AS A RESULT UREA SYNTHESIS AND AMMONIA DETOXICATION ARE INTERFERED WITH. COLOMBO ET AL. (1967) DEMONSTRATED A DEFECT IN L-LYSINE* NAD-OXIDO-REDUCTASE ACTIVITY IN LIVER. THIS APPARENTLY IS RESPONSIBLE FOR ACCUMULATION OF LYSINE. HYPERLYSINEMIA (Q.V.) IS A SEPARATE ENTITY.

COLOMBO, J. P., BURGI, W., RICHTERICH, R. AND ROSSI, E.* CONGENITAL LYSINE INTOLERANCE WITH PERIODIC AMMONIA INTOXICATION* A DEFECT IN L-LYSINE DEGRADATION. METABOLISM 16* 910-925, 1967.

COLOMBO, J. P., RICHTERICH, R., DONATH, A., SPAHR, A. AND ROSSI, E.* CONGENITAL LYSINE INTOLERANCE WITH PERIODIC AMMONIA INTOXICATION. LANCET 1* 1014-1015, 1964.

COLOMBO, J. P., VASSELLA, F., HUMBEL, R. AND BURGI, W.* LYSINE INTOLERANCE WITH PERIODIC AMMONIA INTOXICATION. AM. J. DIS. CHILD. 113* 138-141, 1967.

24800 MACROCEPHALY

WALSH (1957) DESCRIBED THREE AFFECTED SIBS WITH NORMAL PARENTS. AT LEAST TWO OF THE THREE WERE FEMALE. MENTAL DEFECT AND OPTIC ATROPHY WERE PRESENT. IN ANOTHER FAMILY TWO SIBS MAY HAVE BEEN AFFECTED. OF COURSE, A LARGE HEAD OCCURS WITH HYDROCEPHALUS AND WITH GARGOYLISM AND IS ALSO A FEATURE OF CANAVAN'S DISEASE. WEIL (1933) DESCRIBED THE CASE OF A MALE IN WHICH AT AUTOPSY THE BRAIN (AT AGE 7 YEARS) WEIGHED 1856 GM. THE PRECENTRAL AREA WAS UNDERDEVELOPED AS WERE ALSO SKELETAL MUSCULATURE AND THE ADRENAL MEDULLAS. MENTAL DEVELOPMENT HAD BEEN NORMAL UNTIL AGE 6. A BROTHER HAD A LARGE HEAD BUT WAS WELL AT AGE 12 YEARS. THE POSSIBILITY OF X-LINKED RECESSIVE MACROCEPHALY WAS RAISED BY WAISMAN (1967). DIFFERENTIATION FROM X-LINKED STENOSIS OF THE AQUEDUCT OF SYLVIUS IS NECESSARY.

WAISMAN, H. A.* MADISON, WIS.* PERSONAL COMMUNICATION, 1967.

WALSH, F. B.* CLINICAL NEURO-OPHTHALMOLOGY. BALTIMORE* WILLIAMS AND WILKINS, 1957 (2ND ED.). PP. 402-404.

WEIL, A.* MEGALENCEPHALY WITH DIFFUSE GLIOBLASTOMATOSIS OF THE BRAIN STEM AND THE CEREBELLUM. ARCH. NEUROL. PSYCHIAT. 30* 795-809, 1933.

24810 MACROSOMIA ADIPOSA CONGENITA

CHRISTIANSEN (1929) DESCRIBED A DANISH KINDRED IN WHICH 7 INFANTS (6 FEMALES, 1 MALE), THE OFFSPRING OF SISTERS BY PRESUMABLY UNRELATED HUSBANDS, DEVELOPED GROSS OBESITY BEGINNING SOON AFTER BIRTH. PRECOCIOUS SKELETAL DEVELOPMENT WAS EVIDENT

IN THE OSSIFICATION CENTERS AND TEETH. MARKED VORACITY WAS A FEATURE. RELATIVE EOSINOPHILIA AND LOW VITALITY WITH DEATH OF FIVE OF THE CHILDREN IN THE FIRST YEAR WERE NOTED. ADRENOCORTICAL ADENOMAS WERE FOUND AT AUTOPSY. THE NATURE OF THE DISORDER IS OBSCURE.

CHRISTIANSEN, T.* MACROSOMIA ADIPOSA CONGENITA. A NEW DYSENDOCRINE SYNDROME OF FAMILIAL OCCURRENCE. ENDOCRINOLOGY 13* 149-163, 1929.

*24820 MACULAR DEGENERATION OF THE RETINA

DEGENERATION LIMITED TO THE MACULAR AREA OF THE RETINA WAS DESCRIBED IN MULTIPLE SIBS BY FORD (1961) AND BY WALSH (1957). TYPICALLY ONSET IS IN EARLY OR MIDDLE CHILDHOOD. SOMETIMES THE CONDITION HAS BEEN CALLED CENTRAL RETINITIS PIGMENTOSA OR RETINITIS PIGMENTOSA WITH MACULAR INVOLVEMENT. HOWEVER, ORDINARY RETINITIS PIGMENTOSA DOES NOT AFFECT THE MACULA. HOMOZYGOSITY AT ANY ONE OF SEVERAL LOCI IS PROBABLY CAPABLE OF PRODUCING THIS PHENOTYPE.

FORD, F. R.* DISEASES OF THE NERVOUS SYSTEM IN INFANCY, CHILDHOOD AND ADOLES-CENCE. SPRINGFIELD, ILL.* CHARLES C THOMAS, 1961. PP. 358-359.

WALSH, F. B.* CLINICAL NEURO-OPHTHALMOLOGY. BALTIMORE* WILLIAMS AND WILKINS, 1957 (2ND ED.). PP. 673-674.

WRIGHT, R. E.* FAMILIAL MACULAR DEGENERATION. BRIT. J. OPHTHAL. 19* 160-165, 1935.

*24830 MAL DE MELEDA (KERATOSIS PALMO-PLANTARIS TRANSGRADIENS OF SIEMENS)

CONGENITAL SYMMETRICAL CORNIFICATION OF THE PALMS AND SOLES WITH ICHTHYOTIC CHANGES ELSEWHERE CHARACTERIZE THIS DISORDER WHICH DERIVES ITS NAME FROM ITS RELATIVELY HIGH FREQUENCY AMONG INHABITANTS OF THE ISLAND OF MELEDA, DALMATIA, YUGOSLAVIA. BOSNJAKOVIC (1938) STUDIED THE FAMILY IN MLJET (OR MELEDA). SCHNYDER ET AL. (1969) PROVIDED MORE RECENT OBSERVATIONS. HYPERHIDROSIS, PERIORAL ERYTHEMA AND LICHENOID PLAQUES WERE ALSO NOTED.

BOSNJAKOVIC, S.* VERERBUNGSVERHALTNISSE BEI DER SOG. KRANKHEIT VON MLJET ('MAL DE MELEDA'). ACTA DERMATOVENEN. 19* 88-122, 1938.

NILES, H. D. AND KLUMPP, M. M.* MAL DE MELEDA* REVIEW OF THE LITERATURE AND REPORT OF FOUR CASES. ARCH. DERM. SYPH. 39* 409-421, 1939.

SALAMON, T. AND LAZOVIC, O.* CONTRIBUTION AU PROBLEME DE LA MALADIE DE MLJET (MAL DE MELEDA). J. GENET. HUM. 10* 172-201, 1961.

SCHNYDER, U. W., FRANCESCHETTI, A. T., CESZAROVIC, B. AND SEGEDIN, J.* LA MALADIE DE MELEDA AUTOCHTONE. ANN. DERM. SYPH. 96* 517-530, 1969.

R
E
C
E
S
S
I
V
E

24840 MANDIBULOFACIAL DYSOSTOSIS WITH MENTAL DEFICIENCY

JANCAR (1961) DESCRIBED A FAMILY WITH POSSIBLE RECESSIVE INHERITANCE. THE CHANGES IN THE HEAD WERE REMINISCENT OF THOSE OF TRISOMY 17-18. HOWEVER, IN ONE OF THE AFFECTED MALES NO ABNORMALITY OF THE CHROMOSOMES WAS DETECTED.

JANCAR, J.* MANDIBULO-FACIAL DYSOSTOSIS (BERRY-FRANCESCHETTI SYNDROME). J. IRISH MED. ASS. 48* 145-148, 1961.

24850 MANNOSIDOSIS

OCKERMAN (1967) DESCRIBED A BOY WHO REPRESENTED AN ISOLATED CASE OF AN APPARENTLY 'NEW' DISORDER. SUSCEPTIBILITY TO INFECTION, VOMITING, COARSE FEATURES, MACROG-LOSSIA, FLAT NOSE, LARGE CLUMSY EARS, WIDELY SPACED TEETH, LARGE HEAD, BIG HANDS AND FEET, TALL STATURE, SLIGHT HEPATOSPLENOMEGALY, MUSCULAR HYPOTONIA, LUMBAR GIBBUS, RADIOGRAPHIC SKELETAL ABNORMALITIES, DILATED CEREBRAL VENTRICLES, LENTICULAR OPACITIES, HYPOGAMMAGLOBULINEMIA, 'STORAGE CELLS' IN THE BONE MARROW, AND VACUOLATED LYMPHOCYTES IN THE BONE MARROW AND BLOOD WERE FEATURES. HISTOLOGIC STUDY SHOWED STORAGE OF MATERIAL (NOT ACID MUCOPOLYSACCHARIDE) IN CEREBRAL CORTEX, BRAIN STEM, SPINAL MEDULLA, NEUROHYPOPHYSIS, RETINA AND MYENTERIC PLEXUS. TOTAL MANNOSE IN THE LIVER WAS STRIKINGLY INCREASED. ALPHA-MANNOSIDASE ACTIVITY IN ALL TISSUES STUDIED WAS ABNORMALLY LOW WHEREAS OTHER ACID HYDROLASES HAD HIGHER ACTIVITIES THAN NORMAL. ONLY ONE PATIENT HAS BEEN OBSERVED. HE DIED AT THE AGE OF FOUR AND ONE HALF YEARS DURING AN ATTACK OF INCREASED INTRACRANIAL PRESSURE.

HULTBERG, B.* PROPERTIES OF ALPHA-MANNOSIDASE IN MANNOSIDOSIS. SCAND. J. CLIN. LAB. INVEST. 26* 155-160, 1970.

KJELLMANN, B., GAMSTORP, I., BRUN, A., OCKERMAN, P. A. AND PALMGREN, B.* MANNOSIDOSIS* A CLINICAL AND HISTOPATHOLOGIC STUDY. J. PEDIAT. 75* 366-373, 1969.

OCKERMAN, P. A.* A GENERALIZED STORAGE DISORDER RESEMBLING HURLER'S SYNDROME. LANCET 2* 239-241, 1967.

OCKERMAN, P. A.* MANNOSIDOSIS* ISOLATION OF OLIGOSACCHARIDE STORAGE MATERIAL

FROM BRAIN. J. PEDIAT. 75* 360-365, 1969.

*24860 MAPLE SYRUP URINE DISEASE (BRANCHED-CHAIN KETOACIDURIA)

FEATURES ARE MENTAL AND PHYSICAL RETARDATION, FEEDING PROBLEMS AND A MAPLE SYRUP
ODOR TO THE URINE. THE KETO ACIDS OF LEUCINE, ISOLEUCINE AND VALINE ARE PRESENT
IN THE URINE, SUGGESTING A BLOCK IN OXIDATIVE DECARBOXYLATION. A MILD VARIANT HAS
BEEN REPORTED WHICH MAY BE A SEPARATE ENTITY (MORRIS ET AL., 1961). THE KETO ACID
OF ISOLEUCINE (ALPHA-KETO-BETA-METHYLVALINIC ACID) IS RESPONSIBLE FOR THE
CHARACTERISTIC ODOR. IN TWO SIBS OF EACH OF TWO FAMILIES, DANCIS, HUTZLER AND
ROKKONES (1967) OBSERVED A VARIANT OF MSUD. THE CHILDREN SUFFERED FROM A
TRANSIENT NEUROLOGIC DISORDER ASSOCIATED WITH ELEVATION OF BRANCHED-CHAIN AMINO
ACIDS AND THEIR KETO ACIDS IN, AND A DISTINCTIVE ODOR TO, THE URINE. LATE ONSET
OF SYMPTONS AND CLINICAL NORMALITY BETWEEN ATTACKS DIFFERENTIATED THE CONDITION
FROM REGULAR MSUD. HOWEVER, ONE SIB OF EACH FAMILY DIED DURING AN ATTACK. THE
LEVEL OF LEUKOCYTE KETO ACID DECARBOXYLASE ACTIVITY SEEMED TO BE HIGHER THAN IN
THE CLASSIC FORM OF THE DISEASE. ONE MUST TAKE THE LYMPHOCYTE COUNT INTO ACCOUNT
IN TESTING FOR HETEROZYGOTES. THE RELEVANT ENZYME IS IN THE LYMPHOCYTES AND
LYMPHOCYTOPENIA OR LYMPHOCYTOSIS CAN GIVE FALSE POSITIVE OR FALSE NEGATIVE TESTS
FOR HETEROZYGOSITY. TWO NORWEGIAN FAMILIES WITH THE INTERMITTENT FORM WERE
DESCRIBED BY GOEDDE ET AL. (1970). IN THIS FORM ONLY ONE PARENT SHOWS DECREASED
ENZYME ACTIVITY, AS A RULE. SCHULMAN ET AL. (1970) DESCRIBED A PATIENT AFFECTED
WITH A VARIANT.

DANCIS, J. AND LEVITZ, M.* MAPLE SYRUP URINE DISEASE (BRANCHED CHAIN KE-
TONURIA). IN, STANBURY, J. B., WYNGAARDEN, J. B. AND FREDRICKSON, D. S. (EDS.)*
THE METABOLIC BASIS OF INHERITED DISEASE. NEW YORK* MCGRAW-HILL, 1966 (2ND ED.).
PP. 353-365.

DANCIS, J., HUTZLER, J. AND LEVITZ, M.* THE DIAGNOSIS OF MAPLE SYRUP DISEASE
(BRANCHED CHAIN KETOACIDURIA) BY THE IN VITRO STUDY OF THE PERIPHERAL LEUKOCYTE.
PEDIATRICS 32* 234-238, 1963.

DANCIS, J., HUTZLER, J. AND ROKKONES, T.* INTERMITTENT BRANCHED-CHAIN KE-
TONURIA. VARIANT OF MAPLE-SYRUP-URINE DISEASE. NEW ENG. J. MED. 276* 84-89,
1967.

DANCIS, J., LEVITZ, M. AND WESTALL, R. G.* MAPLE SYRUP URINE DISEASE* BRANCHED-
CHAIN KETOACIDURIA. PEDIATRICS 25* 72-79, 1960.

GOEDDE, H. W., LANGENBECK, U. AND BRACKERTZ, D.* DETECTION OF HETEROZYGOTES IN
MAPLE SYRUP URINE DISEASE* ROLE OF LYMPHOCYTE COUNT. HUMANGENETIK 6* 189-190,
1968.

GOEDDE, H. W., LANGENBECK, U., BRACKERTZ, D., KELLER, W., ROKKONES, T.,
HALVORSEN, S., KIIL, R. AND MERTON, B.* CLINICAL AND BIOCHEMICAL-GENETIC ASPECTS
OF INTERMITTENT BRANCHED-CHAIN KETOACIDURIA. REPORT OF TWO SCANDINAVIAN FAMILIES.
ACTA PAEDIAT. SCAND. 59* 83-87, 1970.

KIIL, R. AND ROKKONES, T.* LATE MANIFESTING VARIANT OF BRANCHED-CHAIN KETOACI-
DURIA* (MAPLE SYRUP URINE DISEASE). ACTA PAEDIAT. 53* 356-364, 1964.

MORRIS, M. D., FISHER, D. A. AND FISER, R.* LATE-ONSET BRANCHED-CHAIN KETOACI-
DURIA* (MAPLE SYRUP URINE DISEASE). J. LANCET 86* 149-152, 1966.

MORRIS, M. D., LEWIS, B. D., DOOLAN, P. D. AND HARPER, H. A.* CLINICAL AND
BIOCHEMICAL OBSERVATIONS ON AN APPARENTLY NONFATAL VARIANT OF BRANCHED-CHAIN
KETOACIDURIA (MAPLE SYRUP URINE DISEASE). PEDIATRICS 28* 918-923, 1961.

NORTON, P. M., ROITMAN, E., SNYDERMAN, S. E. AND HOLT, L. E., JR.* A NEW
FINDING IN MAPLE-SYRUP-URINE DISEASE. LANCET 1* 26-27, 1962.

SCHULMAN, J. D., LUSTBERG, T. J., KENNEDY, J. L., MUSELES, M. AND SEEGMILLER,
J. E.* A NEW VARIANT OF MAPLE SYRUP URINE DISEASE (BRANCHED CHAIN KETOACIDURIA).
CLINICAL AND BIOCHEMICAL EVALUATION. AM. J. MED. 49* 118-124, 1970.

SNYDERMAN, S. E.* THE THERAPY OF MAPLE SYRUP URINE DISEASE. AM. J. DIS. CHILD.
113* 68-73, 1967.

WOODY, N. C. AND HARRIS, J. A.* FAMILY SCREENING STUDIES IN MAPLE SYRUP URINE
DISEASE (BRANCHED-CHAIN KETOACIDURIA). J. PEDIAT. 66* 1042-1048, 1965.

24870 MARDEN-WALKER SYNDROME

MARDEN AND WALKER (1966) DESCRIBED AN INFANT WITH BLEPHAROPHIMOSIS, MICROGNATHIA,
IMMOBILE FACIES, KYPHOSCOLIOSIS, LIMB CONTRACTURES, PIGEON BREAST AND ARACHNODAC-
TYLY. THERE WAS MICROCYSTIC DISEASE OF THE KIDNEY. THE INFANT DIED AT THREE
MONTHS OF AGE. IN SOME RESPECTS THE CASE RESEMBLED THE SIBS WITH MYOTONIA
MYOPATHY, ETC. (Q.V.) DESCRIBED BY ABERFELD ET AL. (1965).

MARDEN, P. M. AND WALKER, W. A.* A NEW GENERALIZED CONNECTIVE TISSUE SYNDROME.
J. PEDIAT. 112* 225-228, 1966.

R
E
C
E
S
S
I
V
E

CEREBELLAR ATAXIA, CONGENITAL CATARACTS, RETARDED SOMATIC AND MENTAL MATURATION ARE THE CARDINAL FEATURES. ALTER AND HIS COLLEAGUES (1962) SUGGESTED THE DESIGNATION "HEREDITARY OLIGOPHRENIC CEREBELLOLENTAL DEGENERATION." GARLAND AND MOORHOUSE (1953) PUBLISHED A STRIKING PEDIGREE. A DOMINANTLY INHERITED SYNDROME OF CATARACT AND ATAXIA IS ALSO KNOWN. IN A BOY ALMOST 5 YEARS OLD FRANCESCHETTI ET AL. (1966) FOUND THE BRAIN LESIONS LIMITED ALMOST EXCLUSIVELY TO THE CEREBELLUM WHICH SHOWED MASSIVE CORTICAL ATROPHY. MANY OF THE PURKINJE CELLS WHICH REMAINED WERE VACUOLATED OR BINUCLEATED.

ALTER, M., TALBERT, O. R. AND CROFFEAD, G.* CEREBELLAR ATAXIA, CONGENITAL CATARACTS AND RETARDED SOMATIC AND MENTAL MATURATION. REPORT OF CASES OF MARINES-CO-SJOGREN SYNDROME. NEUROLOGY 12* 836-847, 1962.

FRANCESCHETTI, A., KLEIN, D., WILDI, E. AND TODOROV, A.* LE SYNDROME DE MARINESCO-SJOGREN. PREMIERE VERIFICATION ANATOMIQUE. ARCH. SUISSES NEUR. NEUROCHIR. PSYCHIAT. 97* 234-240, 1966.

GARLAND, H. AND MOORHOUSE, D.* AN EXTREMELY RARE RECESSIVE HEREDITARY SYNDROME INCLUDING CEREBELLAR ATAXIA, OLIGOPHRENIA, CATARACT, AND OTHER FEATURES. J. NEUROL. NEUROSURG. PSYCHIAT. 16* 110-116, 1953.

SJOGREN, T.* HEREDITARY CONGENITAL SPINOCEREBELLAR ATAXIA ACCOMPANIED BY CONGENITAL CATARACT AND OLIGOPHRENIA. A GENETIC AND CLINICAL INVESTIGATION. CONFIN. NEUROL. 10* 293-308, 1950.

SJOGREN, T.* HEREDITARY CONGENITAL SPINOCEREBELLAR ATAXIA COMBINED WITH CONGENITAL CATARACT AND OLIGOPHRENIA. ACTA PSYCHIAT. NEUROL. SCAND. 46 (SUPPL.)* 286-289, 1947.

TODOROV, A.* LE SYNDROME DE MARINESCO-SJOGREN PREMIERE ETUDE ANATOMO-CLINIQUE. J. GENET. HUM. 14* 197-233, 1965.

*24890 MAST SYNDROME

IN AN OHIO AMISH ISOLATE CROSS AND MCKUSICK (1967) FOUND 20 CASES OF A RECESSIVELY INHERITED FORM OF PRESENILE DEMENTIA WHICH THEY TERMED MAST SYNDROME. ONSET IN THE LATE TEENS OR TWENTIES AND SLOW PROGRESSION WITH DEVELOPMENT OF SPASTIC PARAPARESIS AND BASAL GANGLION MANIFESTATIONS WERE FEATURES.

CROSS, H. E. AND MCKUSICK, V. A.* THE MAST SYNDROME* A RECESSIVELY INHERITED FORM OF PRESENILE DEMENTIA WITH MOTOR DISTURBANCES. ARCH. NEUROL. 16* 1-13, 1967.

*24900 MECKEL SYNDROME

THIS CONDITION IS ALSO CALLED DYSENCEPHALIA SPLANCHNOCYSTICA AND GRUBER'S SYNDROME (1934). OPITZ AND HOWE (1969) SUGGESTED IT BE CALLED MECKEL'S SYNDROME BECAUSE OF MECKEL'S CLEAR DESCRIPTION (1822). ALTHOUGH A GREAT VARIETY OF MALFORMATIONS HAVE BEEN OBSERVED AND NO SINGLE MALFORMATION IS INVARIABLY PRESENT OR UNIQUE TO MECKEL'S SYNDROME, A FREQUENT AND PARTICULARLY MEMORABLE COMBINATION IS SLOPING FOREHEAD, POSTERIOR EXENCEPHALOCELE, POLYDACTYLY AND POLYCYSTIC KIDNEYS. DEATH OCCURS IN THE PERINATAL PERIOD. NUMEROUS EXAMPLES OF AFFECTED SIBS, CONCORDANCE IN PRESUMEDLY MONOZYGOTIC TWINS (STOCKARD, 1921), ROUGHLY EQUAL OCCURRENCE IN MALES AND FEMALES, AND PARENTAL CONSANGUINITY IN SOME INSTANCES (TUCKER ET AL., 1966* WALBAUM ET AL., 1967) MAKE AUTOSOMAL RECESSIVE INHERITANCE QUITE CERTAIN. SEE EDITORIAL (1970) FOR BIOGRAPHICAL INFORMATION ON MECKEL. SIMOPOULOS ET AL. (1967) DESCRIBED THREE MALE SIBS WITH POLYCYSTIC KIDNEYS, INTERNAL HYDROCEPHALUS AND POSTAXIAL POLYDACTYLY. THE PARENTS WERE NOT RELATED.

EDITORIAL* JOHANN FRIEDRICH MECKEL, THE YOUNGER (1781-1833). J.A.M.A. 214* 138-139, 1970.

GRUBER, G. B.* BEITRAGE ZUR FRAGE "GEKOPPELTER" MISSBILDUNGEN. (AKROCEPHALO-SYNDACTYLIE UND DYSENCEPHALIA SPLANCHNOCYSTICA). BEITR. PATH. ANAT. 93* 459-476, 1934.

MECKEL, J. F.* BESCHREIBUNG ZWEIER DURCH SEHR AHNLICHE BILDUNGSABWEICHUNGEN ENTSTELLTER GESCHWISTER. DEUTSCH. ARCH. PHYSIOL. 7* 99-172, 1822.

OPITZ, J. M. AND HOWE, J. J.* THE MECKEL SYNDROME (DYSENCEPHALIA SPLANCHNOCYS-TICA, THE GRUBER SYNDROME). THE CLINICAL DELINEATION OF BIRTH DEFECTS. II. MALFORMATION SYNDROMES. NEW YORK* NATIONAL FOUNDATION, 1969. PP. 167-179.

SIMOPOULOS, A. P., BRENNAN, G. G., ALWAN, A. AND FIDIS, N.* POLYCYSTIC KIDNEYS, INTERNAL HYDROCEPHALUS AND POLYDACTYLISM IN NEWBORN SIBLINGS. PEDIATRICS 39* 931-934, 1967.

STOCKARD, C. R.* DEVELOPMENTAL RATE AND STRUCTURAL EXPRESSION* AN EXPERIMENTAL STUDY OF TWINS, "DOUBLE MONSTERS" AND SINGLE DEFORMITIES, AND THE INTERACTION AMONG EMBRYONIC ORGANS DURING THEIR ORIGIN AND DEVELOPMENT. AM. J. ANAT. 28* 115-277, 1921.

TUCKER, C. C., FINLEY, S. C., TUCKER, E. S. AND FINLEY, W. H.* ORAL-FACIAL-DIGITAL SYNDROME, WITH POLYCYSTIC KIDNEYS AND LIVER* PATHOLOGICAL AND CYTOGENETIC STUDIES. J. MED. GENET. 3* 145-147, 1966.

WALBAUM, R., DEHAENE, P. AND DUTHOIT, F.* POLYDACTYLIE FAMILIALE AVEC DYSPLASIE NEURO-CRANIENNE. ANN. GENET. 10* 39-41, 1967.

*24910 MEDITERRANEAN FEVER, FAMILIAL

THIS DISEASE OCCURS MAINLY IN ARMENIANS AND SEPHARDIC JEWS (THOSE WHO LEFT SPAIN DURING THE INQUISITION AND SETTLED IN VARIOUS COUNTRIES BORDERING THE MEDITER-RANEAN). FEATURES INCLUDE SHORT RECURRENT BOUTS OF FEVER ACCOMPANIED BY PAIN IN THE ABDOMEN, CHEST OR JOINTS AND AN ERYSIPELAS-LIKE ERYTHEMA. THE SEDIMENTATION RATE IS INCREASED, BUT THE WHITE COUNT IS USUALLY NORMAL. MANY OF THE PATIENTS HAVE BEEN SUBJECTED TO ONE OR MORE NEEDLESS LAPAROTOMIES. AMYLOIDOSIS IS A COMPLICATION AND MAY DEVELOP WITHOUT OVERT CRISES OF THE ABOVE DESCRIPTION. SOHAR AND HIS COLLEAGUES (1967) ESTIMATED THAT IN SOME JEWISH GROUPS THE PHENOTYPE FREQUENCY IS 1 IN 2720 AND THAT THE MINIMAL ESTIMATES FOR GENE FREQUENCY AND HETEROZYGOTE FREQUENCY ARE 1 IN 52 AND 1 IN 26, RESPECTIVELY. THE POSSIBILITY THAT THE DISORDER IN ARMENIANS IS DISTINCT FROM THAT IN SEPHARDIC JEWS IS SUGGESTED BY THE ALLEGED RARITY OF AMYLOIDOSIS AND EFFICACY OF LOW-FAT DIET IN ARMENIAN CASES. THIS CONDITION IS CALLED *FAMILIAL PAROXYSMAL PERITONITIS* BY SIEGAL (1964) WHO WAS THE FIRST TO DELINEATE THE DISORDER CLEARLY IN THIS COUNTRY AND WHO HAS OBSERVED RATHER NUMEROUS CASES IN ASHKENAZI JEWS. THE NUMBER OF ASHKENAZIC CASES OBSERVED IN ISRAEL BY SOHAR ET AL. (1967) IS SUFFICIENT TO MAKE IT NOT SURPRISING THAT A FAIR NUMBER OF CASES ARE OBSERVED IN THE LARGE ASHKENAZIC GROUP IN THE UNITED STATES. IN TURKEY MANY CASES OF FMF ARE OBSERVED IN PERSONS WITHOUT KNOWN ARMENIAN ANCESTRY (SOKMEN, 1959).
UNDER THE DESIGNATION PERIODIC PERITONITIS REIMANN ET AL. (1954) REPORTED PRESUMABLY THE SAME DISORDER IN 20 PERSONS IN 5 GENERATIONS OF AN ARMENIAN FAMILY LIVING IN THE NEAR EAST. A *SKIPPED GENERATION* OCCURRED IN TWO INSTANCES. THIS MAY BE AN INSTANCE OF QUASI-DOMINANCE RESULTING FROM FREQJENT MARRIAGE OF HOMOZYGOUS AFFECTED WITH HETEROZYGOTES. UNDER THE TERM PERIODIC PERITONITIS, REIMANN ET AL. (1954) DESCRIBED MANY CASES FROM LEBANON, MOST OF THEM ARMENIAN. IN ONE REMARKABLE FAMILY, SURVIVORS OF THE SEIGE OF MUSA DAGH, 20 AFFECTED PERSONS IN FIVE GENERATIONS. THERE WERE 3 INSTANCES OF SKIPS IN THE PEDIGREE. CONCEIVAB-LY HIGH GENE FREQUENCY AND SMALL BREEDING GROUP CAN ACCOUNT FOR THE FINDINGS. CERTAINLY THE DISTRIBUTION OF CASES IN THE UNITED STATES IS MUCH MORE SUGGESTIVE OF RECESSIVE THAN OF DOMINANT INHERITANCE. REICH AND FRANKLIN (1970) DESCRIBED A 79 YEAR OLD SICILIAN WITH INTESTINAL AMYLOIDOSIS WHOSE DAUGHTER AND GRANDAUGHTER HAD ATTACKS OF FEVER AND ABDOMINAL PAIN. THE ITALIAN EXTRACTION, LONG SURVIVAL AND 3 GENERATION INVOLVEMENT IS UNUSUAL FOR FMF.

R
E
C
E
S
S
I
V
E

DORMER, A. E. AND HALE, J. F.* FAMILIAL MEDITERRANEAN FEVER, A CAUSE OF PERIODIC FEVER. BRIT. MED. J. 1* 87-89, 1962.

EHRENFELD, E. N., ELIAKIM, M. AND RACHMILEWITZ, M.* RECURRENT POLYSEROSITIS (FAMILIAL MEDITERRANEAN FEVER* PERIODIC DISEASE). A REPORT OF FIFTY-FIVE CASES. AM. J. MED. 31* 107-123, 1961.

HELLER, H., SOHAR, E., GAFNI, J. AND HELLER, J.* AMYLOIDOSIS IN FAMILIAL MEDITERRANEAN FEVER. ARCH. INTERN. MED. 107* 539-550, 1961.

HURWICH, B. J., SCHWARTZ, J. AND GOLDFARB, S.* RECORD SURVIVAL OF SIBLINGS WITH FAMILIAL MEDITERRANEAN FEVER, PHENOTYPES 1 AND 2. ARCH. INTERN. MED. 125* 308-311, 1970.

LAWRENCE, J. S. AND MELLINKOFF, S. M.* FAMILIAL MEDITERRANEAN FEVER. TRANS. ASS. AM. PHYSICIANS 72* 111-121, 1959.

OZDEMIR, A. I. AND SOKMEN, C.* FAMILIAL MEDITERRANEAN FEVER AMONG THE TURKISH PEOPLE. AM. J. GASTROENT. 51* 311-316, 1969.

REICH, C. B. AND FRANKLIN, E. C.* FAMILIAL MEDITERRANEAN FEVER IN AN ITALIAN FAMILY. ARCH. INTERN. MED. 125* 337-340, 1970.

REIMANN, H. A., MOADIE, J., SEMERDIJIAN, S. AND SAHYOUN, P. F.* PERIODIC PERITONITIS-HEREDITY AND PATHOLOGY. REPORT OF SEVENTY-TWO CASES. J.A.M.A. 154* 1254-1259, 1954.

SIEGAL, S.* FAMILIAL PAROXYSMAL POLYSEROSITIS. ANALYSIS OF FIFTY CASES. AM. J. MED. 36* 893-918, 1964.

SOHAR, E., GAFNI, J., PRAS, M., AND HELLER, H.* FAMILIAL MEDITERRANEAN FEVER. A SURVEY OF 470 CASES AND REVIEW OF LITERATURE. AM. J. MED. 43* 227-253, 1967.

SOKMEN, C.* COMMENT. TRANS. ASS. AM. PHYSICIANS 72* 120-121, 1959.

24920 MEGACOLON, AGANGLIONIC (HIRSCHSPRUNG*S DISEASE)

IN MICE AGANGLIONIC MEGACOLON IS ASSOCIATED WITH PIEBALD TRAIT AND INHERITED APPARENTLY AS AN AUTOSOMAL RECESSIVE (BIELSCHOWSKY AND SCHOFIELD, 1962). WE KNOW

OF A HUMAN CASE OF HETEROCHROMIA IRIDIS AND MEGACOLON (R.C., 943266), CONGENITAL DEAFNESS ALSO BEING PRESENT. BOGGS AND KIDD (1958) DESCRIBED SIBS WITH ABSENCE OF THE INNERVATION OF THE ENTIRE INTESTINAL TRACT BELOW THE LIGAMENT OF TREITZ. IT IS NOTEWORTHY THAT BODIAN AND CARTER (1963) FOUND THAT IN HIRSCHSPRUNG'S DISEASE, OF WHICH BOGGS AND KIDD'S CASES REPRESENT A VARIETY, CASES WITH EXTENSIVE INVOLVEMENT OF THE GUT WERE MORE LIKELY TO BE FAMILIAL. FOR THE SERIES OF HIRSCHSPRUNG'S DISEASE AS A WHOLE THEY COULD NOT DEMONSTRATE SIMPLE MENDELIAN INHERITANCE. HIRSCHSPRUNG'S DISEASE IS PROBABLY MULTIFACTORIAL (POLYGENETIC) IN ITS CAUSATION. ALL MULTIFACTORIAL TRAITS HAVE A 'SLIDING' RISK. NOT ONLY DOES THE RECURRENCE RISK INCREASE AS THE NUMBER OF AFFECTED SIBS INCREASES, BUT IT ALSO IS GREATER WHEN INVOLVEMENT IS MORE SEVERE. THUS IT IS NOT UNEXPECTED THAT CASES WITH MORE EXTENSIVE INVOLVEMENT ARE MORE LIKELY TO BE FAMILIAL. PASSARGE (1967) ARRIVED AT A SIMILAR CONCLUSION. EMPIRIC RISK FIGURES WERE AS FOLLOWS* 7.2 PERCENT FOR THE SIBS OF AN AFFECTED FEMALE, 2.6 PERCENT FOR THE SIBS OF AN AFFECTED MALE. AGANGLIONIC MEGACOLON IS CLEARLY A HETEROGENEOUS CATEGORY. IT IS A FREQUENT FINDING IN CASES OF TRISOMY 21 (MONGOLISM). SIX OF 63 PROBANDS IN THE PASSARGE (1967) STUDY WERE CASES OF MONGOLISM.

BIELSCHOWSKY, M. AND SCHOFIELD, G. C.* STUDIES ON MEGACOLON IN PIEBALD MICE. AUST. J. EXP. BIOL. MED. SCI. 40* 395-403, 1962.

BODIAN, M. AND CARTER, C. O.* A FAMILY STUDY OF HIRSCHSPRUNG'S DISEASE. ANN. HUM. GENET. 26* 261-277, 1963.

BOGGS, J. D. AND KIDD, J. M.* CONGENITAL ABNORMALITIES OF INTESTINAL INNERVA-TION* ABSENCE OF INNERVATION OF JEJUNUM, ILEUM AND COLON IN SIBLINGS. PEDIATRICS 21* 261-266, 1958.

LANE, P. W.* ASSOCIATION OF MEGACOLON WITH TWO RECESSIVE SPOTTING GENES IN THE MOUSE. J. HERED. 57* 29-31, 1966.

PASSARGE, E.* THE GENETICS OF HIRSCHSPRUNG'S DISEASE. EVIDENCE FOR HETERO-GENEOUS ETIOLOGY AND A STUDY OF SIXTY-THREE FAMILIES. NEW ENG. J. MED. 276* 138-143, 1967.

*24930 MEGALOBLASTIC ANEMIA RESPONSIVE TO FOLIC ACID, ATAXIA, MENTAL RETARDATION AND CONVULSIONS

LUHBY ET AL. (1965) OBSERVED AFFECTED SISTERS. ABSORPTION OF FOLIC ACID FROM THE INTESTINAL TRACT WAS MARKEDLY DEFECTIVE. PARENTERAL ADMINISTRATION OF FOLIC ACID CORRECTED THE ANEMIA.

LUHBY, A. L., COOPERMAN, J. M. AND PESCI-BOUREL, A.* A NEW INBORN ERROR OF METABOLISM* FOLIC ACID RESPONSIVE MEGALOBLASTIC ANEMIA, ATAXIA, MENTAL RETARDA-TION, AND CONVULSIONS. J. PEDIAT. 67* 1052 ONLY, 1965.

24940 MELANOSIS, NEUROCUTANEOUS

THIS RARE CONDITION, ASSOCIATED SKIN AND MENINGEAL PIGMENTATION, IS POTENTIALLY HIGHLY MALIGNANT. DEATH USUALLY OCCURS IN EARLY CHILDHOOD. NO CERTAIN EVIDENCE OF A MENDELIAN BASIS HAS BEEN FOUND. THE CONDITION IS THOUGHT TO BE A CONGENITAL DYSPLASIA OF THE NEURAL CREST.

FOX, H., EMERY, J. L., GOODBODY, R. A. AND YATES, P. O.* NEURO-CUTANEOUS MELANOSIS. ARCH. DIS. CHILD. 39* 508-516, 1964.

REED, W. B., BECKER, S. W., SR., BECKER, S. W., JR. AND NICKEL, W. R.* GIANT PIGMENTED NEVI MELANOMA, AND LEPTOMENINGEAL MELANOCYTOSIS* A CLINICAL AND HISTOPATHOLOGICAL STUDY. ARCH. DERM. 91* 100-119, 1965.

TVETEN, L.* PRIMARY MENINGEAL MELANOSIS. A CLINICO-PATHOLOGICAL REPORT OF TWO CASES. ACTA PATH. MICROBIOL. SCAND. 63* 1-10, 1965.

24950 MENTAL RETARDATION

MENTAL RETARDATION IS A LEADING FEATURE OF MANY PHENOTYPES LISTED HERE, E.G., AMAUROTIC IDIOCY, CYSTATHIONINURIA, GALACTOSEMIA, HYPERGLYCINEMIA, KETOACIDURIA WITH MENTAL DEFICIENCY AND OTHER FEATURES, AMINOACIDURIA AND OTHER FEATURES, ANIRIDIA, ATONIA-ASTATIC SYNDROME, CEREBELLAR ATROPHY, CUTIS VERTICIS GYRATA, MEGALOBLASTIC ANEMIA, HOMOCYSTINURIA, THE LAURENCE-MOON-BIEDL SYNDROME, MICROCE-PHALY, PHENYLKETONURIA, THE SJOGREN-LARSSON SYNDROME, SMITH SYNDROME, THE MUCOPOLYSACCHARIDOSES, METHEMOGLOBINEMIA AND THE SEVERAL DEFECTS OF THYROID HORMONE SYNTHESIS. IN ADDITION, STUDIES IN MENTAL INSTITUTIONS SUCH AS THOSE OF PRIEST AND COLLEAGUES (1961) AND OF WRIGHT AND COLLEAGUES (1959) SHOW THAT MENTAL RETARDATION OF UNCLASSIFIED TYPE OCCURS IN MULTIPLE SIBS IN A CONSIDERABLE NUMBER OF CASES. SOME OF THESE DOUBTLESS REPRESENT RARE RECESSIVE DISORDERS. STUDY OF THIS GROUP MAY REVEAL 'NEW' RECESSIVE DISEASES. SEE TRICHOMEGALY, ETC.
BREG (1962) HAS IN HIS CLASSIFICATION OF MENTAL DEFECT A WASTE-BASKET GROUP, 'HEREDITARY CEREBRAL MALDEVELOPMENT, NOT CLINICALLY CLASSIFIABLE.' MOST OF THESE CASES ARE, HE THINKS, AUTOSOMAL RECESSIVE DISORDERS. TWO OR MORE SIBS SHOW INTELLECTUAL IMPAIRMENT, USUALLY IN THE LOW OR MIDDLE GRADE RANGE WITHOUT OTHER CLINICAL OR LABORATORY MANIFESTATIONS THAT PERMIT FURTHER CLASSIFICATION. AMONG

3,500 ADMISSIONS TO AN INSTITUTION FOR MENTAL DEFECTIVES HE FOUND 53 CASES HE SO CLASSIFIED. IN THE SAME GROUP 25 CASES OF PHENYLKETONURIA, 3 OF GOITROUS CRETINISM, 39 OF CEREBRAL DEGENERATIVE DISEASES (INCLUDING THE LIPIDOSES AND SCLEROSES) AND 20 OF PRIMARY MICROCEPHALY WERE OBSERVED.

THE STUDY OF CARSON AND NEILL (1962) IS ILLUSTRATIVE OF THE TYPE OF CHEMICAL INVESTIGATIONS WHICH CAN BE USED TO DETECT METABOLIC ERRORS IN AN INBRED POPULATION AND SPECIFICALLY IN CASES OF MENTAL RETARDATION. MCMURRAY (1962) ALSO REVIEWED THE BIOCHEMICAL DEFECTS THAT HAVE BEEN IDENTIFIED IN PATIENTS WITH MENTAL RETARDATION.

MORTON (1960) ARRIVED AT THE CONCLUSION THAT HOMOZYGOSITY AT ANY ONE OF 69 LOCI MAY RESULT IN LOW-GRADE MENTAL DEFECT, THAT ABOUT 8 PERCENT OF SUCH CASES ARE RECESSIVE AND THAT ABOUT A THIRD OF NORMAL PERSONS ARE HETEROZYGOUS FOR A GENE FOR LOW-GRADE MENTAL DEFECT. AN ESTIMATE OF 114 LOCI WAS ARRIVED AT BY DEWEY, BARRAI, MORTON AND MI (1965). KARLSSON AND COLLEAGUES (1961) USED THE SAME APPROACH OF STUDYING FAMILIES WITH MULTIPLE AFFECTED SIBS. IN THE FAMILY REPORTED BY FRIEDMAN AND ROY (1944) ALL 6 CHILDREN OF PARENTS WHO WERE FIRST COUSINS ONCE REMOVED BUT OF NORMAL INTELLIGENCE WERE SEVERELY RETARDED WITH INTERNAL STRABISMUS, HYPERACTIVE TENDON REFLEXES AND POSITIVE BABINSKIS. THE MOTHER WAS SAID TO HAVE AN ABNORMAL ELECTROENCEPHALOGRAM, NYSTAGMUS AND EXTERNAL STRABISMUS. MATERNAL PHENYLKETONURIA (Q.V.) CAN RESULT IN MENTAL RETARDATION IN MULTIPLE SIBS AND THE MOTHER MAY APPEAR NORMAL. DEKABAN (1958) DESCRIBED A FAMILY IN WHICH BOTH PARENTS HAD UNDIFFERENTIATED MENTAL RETARDATION AS DID ALSO ALL THREE OF THEIR CHILDREN. A BROTHER OF THE FATHER WAS ALSO RETARDED. ALL FOUR GRANDPARENTS WERE OF NORMAL INTELLIGENCE. HE SUGGESTED THAT AN ACCUMULATION OF PEDIGREES IN WHICH BOTH PARENTS ARE AFFECTED WOULD HELP ELUCIDATE THE CATEGORY OF UNDIFFERENTIATED MENTAL RETARDATION.

BREG, W. R.* GENETIC ASPECTS OF MENTAL RETARDATION. QUART. REV. PEDIAT. 17* 9-23, 1962.

CARSON, N. A. J. AND NEILL, D. W.* METABOLIC ABNORMALITIES DETECTED IN A SURVEY OF MENTALLY BACKWARD INDIVIDUALS IN NORTHERN IRELAND. ARCH. DIS. CHILD. 37* 505-513, 1962.

DEKABAN, A. S.* MENTAL DEFICIENCY. RECESSIVE TRANSMISSION TO ALL CHILDREN BY PARENTS SIMILARLY AFFECTED. ARCH. NEUROL. PSYCHIAT. 79* 123-131, 1958.

DEWEY, W. J., BARRAI, I., MORTON, N. E. AND MI, M. P.* RECESSIVE GENES IN SEVERE MENTAL DEFECT. AM. J. HUM. GENET. 17* 237-256, 1965.

FRIEDMAN, A. P. AND ROY, J. E.* AN UNUSUAL FAMILIAL SYNDROME. J. NERV. MENT. DIS. 99* 42-44, 1944.

KARLSSON, J. L., KIHARA, H., GRANT, J. AND NELSON, T. L.* METABOLIC DISORDERS LEADING TO MENTAL DEFICIENCY. I. SCREENING FOR EXCESSIVE URINARY EXCRETION OF NITROGENOUS COMPOUNDS. J. MENT. DEFIC. RES. 5* 17-29, 1961.

MCMURRAY, W. C.* BIOCHEMICAL GENETICS AND MENTAL RETARDATION. CANAD. MED. ASS. J. 87* 486-490, 1962.

MORTON, N. E.* THE MUTATIONAL LOAD DUE TO DETRIMENTAL GENES IN MAN. AM. J. HUM. GENET. 12* 348-364, 1960.

PRIEST, J. H., THULINE, H. C., LAVECK, G. D. AND JARVIS, D. B.* AN APPROACH TO GENETIC FACTORS IN MENTAL RETARDATION. STUDIES OF FAMILIES CONTAINING AT LEAST TWO SIBLINGS ADMITTED TO A STATE INSTITUTION FOR THE RETARDED. AM. J. MENT. DEFIC. 66* 42-50, 1961.

WRIGHT, S. W., TARJAN, G. AND EYER, L.* INVESTIGATION OF FAMILIES WITH TWO OR MORE MENTALLY DEFECTIVE SIBLINGS* CLINICAL OBSERVATIONS. AM. J. DIS. CHILD. 97* 445-456, 1959.

24960 MENTAL RETARDATION SYNDROME (MIETENS-WEBER TYPE)

MIETENS AND WEBER (1966) DESCRIBED, IN 4 OF SIX OFFSPRING OF UNAFFECTED PARENTS, A SYNDROME CONSISTING OF MENTAL RETARDATION, CORNEAL OPACITY, NYSTAGMUS, STRABISMUS, SMALL PINCHED NOSE, FLEXION CONTRACTURE OF THE ELBOWS, DISLOCATION OF HEAD OF RADIUS, ABNORMALLY SHORT ULNA AND RADIUS, AND CLINODACTYLY. THE PARENTS WERE SECOND COUSINS.

MIETENS, C. AND WEBER, H.* A SYNDROME CHARACTERIZED BY CORNEAL OPACITY, NYSTAGMUS, FLEXION CONTRACTURE OF THE ELBOWS, GROWTH FAILURE, AND MENTAL RETARDATION. J. PEDIAT. 69* 624-629, 1966.

*24970 MESOMELIC DWARFISM OF THE HYPOPLASTIC ULNA, FIBULA AND MANDIBLE TYPE

IN THE COURSE OF STUDIES OF INBRED GROUPS IN NORTHERN SWEDEN, BOOK OBSERVED A SEVERE FORM OF CHONDRODYSTROPHY WHICH MAY BE DIFFERENT FROM OTHERS LISTED HERE. THE PARENTS OF THE PROBAND WERE FIRST COUSINS. HETEROZYGOTES IN THIS KINDRED WERE SHORT (THE FATHER WAS 160 CM AND THE MOTHER 150 CM) AND HAD RELATIVELY SHORT FINGERS AND BROAD HANDS, BUT OTHERWISE WERE NOT STRIKINGLY ABNORMAL. CHONDROHYPOPLASIA WAS THE DESIGNATION BOOK USED FOR THE HETEROZYGOTES. BOOK (1950) THOUGHT

R
E
C
E
S
S
I
V
E

THE DISORDER MOST CLOSELY RESEMBLED THAT IN THE H FAMILY REPORTED BY BRAILSFORD (1935). IN THIS FAMILY CHILDREN OF NORMAL BUT SHORT PARENTS WERE AFFECTED. BLOCKEY AND LAWRIE (1963) DESCRIBED 2 AFFECTED SIBS (A BROTHER AND A SISTER), THE OFFSPRING OF NORMAL PARENTS. THERE WAS NO MENTION OF PARENTAL CONSANGUINITY. THE LIMB MALFORMATION IS SEVERE APLASIA OR HYPOPLASIA OF THE ULNA AND FIBULA, THICKENED AND CURVED RADIUS AND TIBIA. OTHER THAN DISPLACEMENT DEFORMITIES OF THE HANDS AND FEET, THEIR SKELETAL STRUCTURES ARE NORMAL. THIS ENTITY CAN BE DESIGNATED MICROMELIC DWARFISM. BLOCKEY AND LAWRIE (1963), MISTAKENLY I THINK, CONSIDERED THEIR CASES INSTANCES OF NIEVERGELT'S SYNDROME, A DOMINANT (Q.V.). LANGER (1967) STUDIED TWO CASES AND REFERRED TO THE ENTITY AS "MESOMELIC DWARFISM OF THE HYPOPLASTIC ULNA, FIBULA, MANDIBLE TYPE." HYPOPLASIA OF THE MANDIBLE WAS A FEATURE NOT EMPHASIZED IN OTHER REPORTS. MESOMELIC IS A NON-SPECIFIC TERM WHICH REFERS TO SHORTENING MOST STRIKING IN THE FOREARM AND LOWER LEG. THIS IS A CHARACTERISTIC OF DYSCHONDROSTEOSIS (Q.V.) AND OF THE ELLIS-VAN CREVELD SYNDROME (Q.V.). ALSO SEE MICROMELIC DWARFISM.

BLOCKEY, N. J. AND LAWRIE, J. H.* AN UNUSUAL SYMMETRICAL DISTAL LIMB DEFORMITY IN SIBLINGS. J. BONE JOINT SURG. 45B* 745-747, 1963.

BOOK, J. A.* A CLINICAL AND GENETICAL STUDY OF DISTURBED SKELETAL GROWTH (CHONDROHYPOPLASIA). HEREDITAS 36* 161-180, 1950.

BRAILSFORD, J. F.* DYSTROPHIES OF THE SKELETON. BRIT. J. RADIOL. 8* 533-569, 1935.

LANGER, L. O., JR.* MESOMELIC DWARFISM OF THE HYPOPLASTIC ULNA, FIBULA, MANDIBLE TYPE. RADIOLOGY 89* 654-660, 1967.

24980 METACHROMATIC LEUKODYSTROPHY AND AMAUROTIC IDIOCY, COMBINED FEATURES OF

MOSSAKOWSKI, MATHIESON AND CUMINGS (1961) FOUND THREE AFFECTED SIBS IN A FRENCH-CANADIAN FAMILY IN WHOM HISTOLOGIC AND CHEMICAL FEATURES OF BOTH DISEASES WERE PRESENT.

MOSSAKOWSKI, M., MATHIESON, G. AND CUMINGS, J. N.* ON THE RELATIONSHIP OF METACHROMATIC LEUCODYSTROPHY AND AMAUROTIC IDIOCY. BRAIN 84* 585-604, 1961.

24990 METACHROMATIC LEUKODYSTROPHY WITH MUCOPOLYSACCHARIDURIA

IN A BROTHER AND SISTER, BISCHEL, AUSTIN AND KEMENY (1966) DESCRIBED A VARIANT TYPE OF MLD IN WHICH ACID POLYSACCHARIDE, MAINLY HEPARITIN SULFATE, WAS FOUND IN EXCESS IN THE BRAIN, KIDNEY AND URINE. THE PATIENTS DIED AT THE AGES 11 AND 12.

BISCHEL, M., AUSTIN, J. AND KEMENY, M.* METACHROMATIC LEUKODYSTROPHY (MLD). VII. ELEVATED SULFATE ACID POLYSACCHARIDE LEVELS IN URINE AND POSTMORTEM TISSUE. ARCH. NEUROL. 15* 13-28, 1966.

*25000 METACHROMATIC LEUKODYSTROPHY, ADULT

AT LEAST TWO FORMS OF METACHROMATIC LEUKODYSTROPHY (MLD) CAN BE DISTINGUISHED. THE LATE INFANTILE FORM HAS ITS ONSET BEFORE AGE 30 MONTHS AND THE ADULT FORM BEGINS AFTER AGE 16. IN ADDITION, ONSET WAS BETWEEN 4 AND 15 YEARS IN A GROUP DIFFICULT TO CLASSIFY. IN THE ADULT FORM INITIAL SYMPTOMS HAVE USUALLY BEEN PSYCHIATRIC LEADING TO A DIAGNOSIS OF SCHIZOPHRENIA. DISORDERS OF MOVEMENT AND POSTURE APPEAR LATE. DIFFERENCES FROM THE LATE INFANTILE FORM ALSO INCLUDE ABILITY TO DEMONSTRATE METACHROMATIC MATERIAL IN PARAFFIN- OR CELLOIDIN-EMBEDDED SECTIONS IN THE ADULT FORM AND PROBABLY GREATER SULFATIDE EXCESS IN THE GRAY THAN IN THE WHITE MATTER IN THIS FORM. THE RELATION OF THE ADULT FORM TO THE PRESUMED X-LINKED CEREBRAL SCLEROSIS OF SCHOLZ (Q.V.) IS UNCLEAR. THE GALLBLADDER IS USUALLY NON-FUNCTIONAL. BETTS ET AL. (1968) DESCRIBED A MAN WHO WAS 28 WHEN ADMITTED TO A PSYCHIATRIC HOSPITAL FOR "ACUTE SCHIZOPHRENIA" AND 35 WHEN HE DIED OF BRONCHOPNEUMONIA. MULLER ET AL. (1969) AND PILZ AND MULLER (1969) DESCRIBED TWO UNRELATED WOMEN WITH THIS DISORDER. AFFECTED SIBS WERE RECORDED BY AUSTIN ET AL. (1968), AMONG OTHERS.

AUSTIN, J., ARMSTRONG, D., FOUCH, S., MITCHELL, C., STUMPF, D., SHEARER, L. AND BRINER, O.* METACHROMATIC LEUKODYSTROPHY (MLD). VIII. MLD IN ADULTS* DIAGNOSIS AND PATHOGENESIS. ARCH. NEUROL. 18* 225-240, 1968.

BETTS, T. A., SMITH, W. T. AND KELLY, R. E.* ADULT METACHROMATIC LEUKODYSTROPHY (SULPHATIDE LIPIDOSIS) SIMULATING ACUTE SCHIZOPHRENIA. REPORT OF A CASE. NEUROLOGY 18* 1140-1142, 1968.

MULLER, D., PILZ, H. AND TER MEULEN, V.* STUDIES ON ADULT METACHROMATIC LEUKODYSTROPHY. I. CLINICAL, MORPHOLOGICAL AND HISTOCHEMICAL OBSERVATIONS IN TWO CASES. J. NEUROL. SCI. 9* 567-584, 1969.

PILZ, H. AND MULLER, D.* STUDIES ON ADULT METACHROMATIC LEUKODYSTROPHY. II. BIOCHEMICAL ASPECTS OF ADULT CASES OF METACHROMATIC LEUKODYSTROPHY. J. NEUROL. SCI. 9* 585-595, 1969.

SOURANDER, P. AND SVENNERHOLM, L.* SULPHATIDE LIPIDOSIS IN THE ADULT WITH THE

CLINICAL PICTURE OF PROGRESSIVE ORGANIC DEMENTIA WITH EPILEPTIC SEIZURES. ACTA NEUROPATH. 1* 384-396, 1962.

VAN BOGAERT, L. V. AND DEWULF, A.* DIFFUSE PROGRESSIVE LEUKODYSTROPHY IN THE ADULT WITH PRODUCTION OF METACHROMATIC DEGENERATIVE PRODUCTS (ALZHEIMER-BARON-CINI). ARCH. NEUROL. PSYCHIAT. 42* 1083-1097, 1939.

25010 METACHROMATIC LEUKODYSTROPHY, INFANTILE (METACHROMATIC LEUKOENCEPHALOPATHY METACHROMATIC FORM OF DIFFUSE CEREBRAL SCLEROSIS* SULFATIDE LIPIDOSIS)

THIS CONDITION WAS FIRST DESCRIBED BY GREENFIELD IN 1933. ONSET IS USUALLY IN THE SECOND YEAR OF LIFE AND DEATH OCCURS BEFORE FIVE YEARS IN MOST. CLINICAL FEATURES ARE MOTOR SYMPTOMS, RIGIDITY, MENTAL DETERIORATION AND IN SOME CONVULSIONS. EARLY DEVELOPMENT IS NORMAL BUT ONSET OCCURS BEFORE 30 MONTHS OF AGE. THE CEREBROSPINAL FLUID PROTEIN IS USUALLY OVER 100 MG. PERCENT.
GALACTOSPHINGOSULFATIDES STRONGLY METACHROMATIC, DOUBLY REFRACTILE IN POLARIZED LIGHT AND PINK WITH PAS ARE FOUND IN EXCESS IN THE WHITE MATTER OF THE CENTRAL NERVOUS SYSTEM, IN THE KIDNEY AND IN THE URINARY SEDIMENT (AUSTIN, 1960). THE DEFECT MAY CONCERN THE LYSOSOMAL ENZYME ARYL SULFATASE-A (AUSTIN, ET AL. 1964). MASTERS ET AL. (1964) DESCRIBED FOUR CASES IN TWO FAMILIES. PROGRESSIVE PHYSICAL AND MENTAL DETERIORATION BEGAN A FEW MONTHS AFTER BIRTH. MEGACOLON WITH ATTACKS OF ABDOMINAL DISTENSION WAS OBSERVED. SUFFICIENT DIFFERENCE FROM THE USUAL CASES EXISTED AS TO SUGGEST TO THE AUTHORS THAT MORE THAN ONE ENTITY IS ENCOMPASSED BY METACHROMATIC LEUKODYSTROPHY. A CURIOUS FEATURE OF LATER BEDRIDDEN STAGES OF THE DISEASE IS MARKED GENU RECURVATUM. THE FIRST MANIFESTATIONS APPEARING BEFORE THE SECOND BIRTHDAY, INCLUDE HYPOTONIA, MUSCLE WEAKNESS AND UNSTEADY GAIT, SUGGESTING A MYOPATHY OR NEUROPATHY. AUSTIN'S TEST TO DEMONSTRATE ABSENCE OF ARYLSULFATASE A (ASA) ACTIVITY IN THE URINE IS USEFUL IN THE EARLY DIAGNOSIS (GREENE ET AL., 1967). SINCE THE METACHROMATIC MATERIAL IS CEREBROSIDE SULFATE, MLD IS A SULFATIDE LIPIDOSIS. SEE SULFATIDOSIS, JUVENILE, FOR A DISORDER WHICH COMBINES FEATURES OF A MUCOPOLYSACCHARIDOSIS WITH THOSE OF METACHROMATIC LEUKODYSTROPHY. STUMPF ET AL. (1971) PRESENTED EVIDENCE TO SUGGEST THAT THE ABNORMALITY IN ARYLSULFATASE A IS QUALITATIVELY DIFFERENT IN THE LATE INFANTILE AND JUVENILE FORMS OF METACHROMATIC LEUKODYSTROPHY. KABACK AND HOWELL (1970) DEMONSTRATED PROFOUND DEFICIENCY OF ARYLSULFATASE A IN CULTURED SKIN FIBROBLASTS OF PATIENTS AND AN INTERMEDIATE DEFICIENCY IN CARRIERS. NORMALLY ENZYME LEVELS WERE LOW IN MID-TRIMESTER AMNIOTIC CELLS* HENCE HOMOZYGOTES CANNOT BE RELIABLY IDENTIFIED BY AMNIOCENTESIS.

R
E
C
E
S
S
I
V
E

AUSTIN, J. H.* METACHROMATIC FORM OF DIFFUSE CEREBRAL SCLEROSIS. III. SIGNIFICANCE OF SULFATIDE AND OTHER LIPID ABNORMALITIES IN WHITE MATTER AND KIDNEY. NEUROLOGY 10* 470-483, 1960.

AUSTIN, J. H.* SOME RECENT FINDINGS IN LEUKODYSTROPHIES AND IN GARGOYLISM. IN, ARONSON, S. M. AND VOLK, B. W. (EDS.)* INBORN DISORDERS OF SPHINGOLIPID METABO-LISM. OXFORD* PERGAMON PRESS, 1967. PP. 359-387.

AUSTIN, J., MCAFEE, D. AND SHEARER, L.* METACHROMATIC FORM OF DIFFUSE CEREBRAL SCLEROSIS. IV. LOW SULFATASE ACTIVITY IN THE URINE OF NINE LIVING PATIENTS WITH METACHROMATIC LEUKODYSTROPHY (MLD). ARCH. NEUROL. 12* 447-455, 1965.

AUSTIN, J., MCAFEE, D., ARMSTRONG, D., O'ROURKE, M., SHEARER, L. AND BACHHAWAT, B.* ABNORMAL SULPHATASE ACTIVITIES IN TWO HUMAN DISEASES (METACHROMATIC LEUKODYS-TROPHY AND GARGOYLISM). BIOCHEM. J. 93* 15C-17C, 1964.

BLACK, J. W. AND CUMINGS, J. N.* INFANTILE METACHROMATIC LEUKODYSTROPHY. J. NEUROL. NEUROSURG. PSYCHIAT. 24* 233-239, 1961.

CRAVIOTO, H., O'BRIEN, J., LOCKWOOD, R., KASTEN, F. H. AND BOOKER, J.* METACHROMATIC LEUKODYSTROPHY (SULFATIDE LIPIDOSES) CULTURED IN VITRO. SCIENCE 156* 243-245, 1967.

GREENE, H., HUG, G. AND SCHUBERT, W. K.* ARYLSULFATASE A IN THE URINE AND METACHROMATIC LEUKODYSTROPHY. J. PEDIAT. 71* 709-711, 1967.

GREENFIELD, J. G.* FORM OF PROGRESSIVE CEREBRAL SCLEROSIS IN INFANTS ASSOCIATED WITH PRIMARY DEGENERATION OF INTERFASCICULAR GLIA. PROC. ROY. SOC. MED. 26* 690-697, 1933.

HAGBERG, B., SOURANDER, P. AND SVENNERHOLM, L.* SULFATIDE LIPIDOSIS IN CHILDHOOD. AM. J. DIS. CHILD. 104* 644-656, 1962.

JERVIS, G. A.* INFANTILE METACHROMATIC LEUKODYSTROPHY* (GREENFIELD'S DISEASE). J. NEUROPATH. EXP. NEUROL. 19* 323-341, 1960.

KABACK, M. M. AND HOWELL, R. R.* INFANTILE METACHROMATIC LEUKODYSTROPHY* HETEROZYGOTE DETECTION IN SKIN FIBROBLASTS AND POSSIBLE APPLICATIONS TO INTRAU-TERINE DIAGNOSIS. NEW ENG. J. MED. 282* 1336-1340, 1970.

MASTERS, P. L., MACDONALD, W. B., RYAN, M. M. P. AND CUMINGS, J. N.* FAMILIAL LEUCODYSTROPHY. ARCH. DIS. CHILD. 39* 345-355, 1964.

MOSER, H. W. AND LEES, M.* SULFATIDE LIPIDOSIS* METACHROMATIC LEUKODYSTROPHY. IN, STANBURY, J. B., WYNGAARDEN, J. B. AND FREDRICKSON, D. S. (EDS.)* THE METABOLIC BASIS OF INHERITED DISEASE. NEW YORK* MCGRAW-HILL, 1966 (2ND ED.). PP. 539-564.

PERCY, A. K. AND BRADY, R. O.* METACHROMATIC LEUKODYSTROPHY* DIAGNOSIS WITH SAMPLES OF VENOUS BLOOD. SCIENCE 161* 594-595, 1968.

STUMPF, D. AND AUSTIN, J.* METACHROMATIC LEUKODYSTROPHY (MLD). IX. QUALITA-TIVE AND QUANTITATIVE DIFFERENCES IN URINARY ARYLSULFATASE A IN DIFFERENT FORMS OF MLD. ARCH. NEUROL. 24* 117-124, 1971.

25020 METACHROMATIC LEUKODYSTROPHY, JUVENILE

SCHUTTA ET AL. (1966) RECOGNIZED A FORM OF METACHROMATIC LEUKODYSTROPHY WITH ONSET BETWEEN AGES 4 AND 10 YEARS, AS COMPARED WITH THE MORE FREQUENT LATE INFANTILE FORM WITH ONSET BETWEEN AGES 12 AND 24 MONTHS. LYON ET AL. (1961) DESCRIBED AFFECTED BROTHERS WITH ONSET AT 7 YEARS AND AT 4 YEARS AND WITH MARKED ELEVATION OF PROTEIN IN THE CEREBROSPINAL FLUID.

LYON, G., ARTHUIS, M. AND THIEFFRY, S.* LEUCODYSTROPHIE METACHROMATIQUE INFANTILE FAMILIALE. ETUDE DE DEUX OBSERVATIONS, DONT UNE AVEC EXAMEN ANATOMIQUE ET CHIMIQUE. REV. NEUROL. 104* 508-533, 1961.

SCHUTTA, H. S., PRATT, R. T. C., METZ, H., EVANS, K. A. AND CARTER, C. O.* A FAMILY STUDY OF THE LATE INFANTILE AND JUVENILE FORMS OF METACHROMATIC LEUKODYS-TROPHY. J. MED. GENET. 3* 86-91, 1966.

25030 METAPHYSEAL DYSOSTOSIS, PENA TYPE

PENA (1965) AND LENZ (1967) DESCRIBED AFFECTED SIBS, THE PARENTS BEING NORMAL. THE METAPHYSES OF THE LONG BONES HAD AN EXTENSIVE SPONGE-LIKE APPEARANCE RADIOLO-GICALLY AND SHOWED HISTOLOGICALLY NUMEROUS ISLANDS OF CARTILAGE REMINISCENT OF ENCHONDROMATOSIS. VAANDRAGER (1960) DESCRIBED CONCORDANT ONE-EGG TWINS. KOZLOWSKI AND SIKORSKA (1970) DESCRIBED A CASE.

KOZLOWSKI, K. AND SIKORSKA, B.* DYSPLASIA METAPHYSARIA, TYP, VAANDRAGER-PENA. Z. KINDERHEILK. 108* 165-170, 1970.

LENZ, W.* DIAGNOSIS IN MEDICAL GENETICS. IN, CROW, J. F. AND NEEL, J. V. (EDS.)* PROC. 3RD. INTERN. CONG. HUM. GENET., SEPT. 1966. BALTIMORE* JOHNS HOPKINS PRESS, 1967. PP. 29-36.

PENA, J.* DISOSTOSIS METAFISARIA. UNA REVISION. CON APORTACION DE UNA OBSERCACION FAMILIAR. UNA FORMA NUEVA DE LA ENFERMEDAD.Q RADIOLOGIA 47* 3-22, 1965.

VAANDRAGER, G. J.* METAFYSAIRE DYSOSTOSIS.Q NEDERL. T. GENEESK. 104* 547-552, 1960.

25040 METAPHYSEAL DYSOSTOSIS, SPAHR TYPE

SPAHR AND SPAHR-HARTMANN (1961) DESCRIBED FOUR SIBS WITH METAPHYSEAL DYSOSTOSIS. THE PARENTS WERE NORMAL BUT CONSANGUINEOUS. BOWING OF THE LEGS WAS STRIKING AND AT LEAST ONE REQUIRED BILATERAL OSTEOTOMY.

SPAHR, A. AND SPAHR-HARTMANN, I.* DYSOSTOSE METAPHYSAIRE FAMILIALE. ETUDE DE 4 CAS DANS UNE FRATRIE. HELV. PAEDIAT. ACTA 16* 836-849, 1961.

25050 METAPHYSEAL MODELING ABNORMALITY, SKIN LESIONS AND SPASTIC PARAPLEGIA

ROY, MAROTEAUX ET AL. (1968) DESCRIBED A 14 YEAR OLD GIRL WITH DEFECTIVE METAPHY-SEAL MODELING AS IN PYLE'S DISEASE, INCREASED BONE DENSITY, PLAQUE-LIKE SKIN LESIONS, AND SIGNS OF SPASTIC PARAPLEGIA. THE PARENTS WERE NOT RELATED.

ROY, C., MAROTEAUX, P., KREMP, L., COURTECUISSE, V. AND ALAGILLE, D.* UN NOUVEAU SYNDROME OSSEUX AVEC ANOMALIES CUTANEES ET TROUBLES NEUROLOGIQUES. ARCH. FRANC. PEDIAT. 25* 893-906, 1968.

*25060 METATROPIC DWARFISM

MAROTEAUX, SPRANGER AND WIEDEMANN (1966) DESCRIBED A CHONDRODYSTROPHY WHICH AT BIRTH IS LIKELY TO BE CALLED ACHONDROPLASIA BECAUSE OF THE SHORT LIMBS AND LATER IN LIFE MORQUIO SYNDROME BECAUSE OF THE RELATIVELY SHORT SPINE AND SEVERE SCOLIOSIS. THE DESIGNATION FOR THE CONDITION WAS CHOSEN TO CONVEY THE CHANGE OR REVERSAL IN BODY PROPORTIONS. THE MANIFESTATIONS ARE ALREADY PRESENT AT BIRTH, WITH GENERALIZED EPI-METAPHYSEAL DISTURBANCE OF OSSIFICATION. KYPHOSCOLIOSIS IS PROGRESSIVE AND SEVERE. ANISOSPONDYLY, HALBERD-SHAPED PELVIS AND HYPERPLASTIC FEMORAL TROCHANTERS ARE FEATURES. THE COCCYX IS UNUSUALLY LONG RESULTING IN A TAIL. AT BIRTH IT MAY BE CALLED HYPERPLASTIC TYPE OF ACHONDROPLASIA. THE ENDS OF THE FEMURS AND HUMERI ARE TRUMPETED. THE TWO BROTHERS REPORTED BY MICHAIL ET AL. (1956) PROBABLY HAD THIS CONDITION WHICH APPEARS TO BE AUTOSOMAL RECESSIVE. THE

R
E
C
E
S
S
I
V
E

DISORDER DESCRIBED BY KNIEST (1952) HAS SOME SIMILARITY TO METATROPIC DWARFISM BUT MUST BE CONSIDERED A SEPARATE ENTITY WHICH MIGHT BE CALLED METATROPHIC DWARFISM, TYPE II, OR KNIEST SYNDROME.

JENKINS, P., SMITH, M. B., MCKINNELL, J. S.* METATROPIC DWARFISM. BRIT. J. RADIOL. 43* 561-565, 1970.

KNIEST, W.* ZUR ABGRENZUNG DER DYSOSTOSIS ENCHONDRALIS VON DER CHONDRODYSTRO-PHIE. Z. KINDERHEILK. 43* 633-640, 1952.

LAROSE, J. H. AND GAY, B. B., JR.* METATROPIC DWARFISM. AM. J. ROENTGEN. 106* 156-161, 1969.

MAROTEAUX, P., SPRANGER, J. AND WIEDEMANN, H.-R.* DER METATROPISCHE ZWERGWUCHS. ARCH. KINDERHEILK. 173* 211-226, 1966.

MICHAIL, J., MATSOVKAS, J., THEODOROU, S. AND HOULIARAS, K.* MALADIE DE MORQUIO (OSTEOCHONDRODYSTROPHIE POLYEPIPHYSAIRE DEFORMANTE) CHEZ DEUX FRERES. HELV. PAEDIAT. ACTA 11* 403-413, 1956.

*25070 METHEMOGLOBIN REDUCTASE (TPNH-) (DEFICIENCY OF NADPH-DEPENDENT METHEMOGLOBIN REDUCTASE)

IN RECESSIVELY INHERITED METHEMOGLOBINEMIA (SEE BELOW), DPNH-METHEMOGLOBIN REDUCTASE IS DEFICIENT. SASS ET AL. (1967) FOUND A NEGRO MALE WITH TPNH-METHEMOG-LOBIN REDUCTASE DEFICIENCY. THE CASE WAS DETECTED WHEN THE PATIENT'S RED CELLS WERE FOUND TO BE ABNORMAL WITH THE METHYLENE-BLUE SCREENING TEST WHICH IS ORDINARILY AN INDICATION OF G6PD-DEFICIENCY BUT BY ACTUAL ASSAY G6PD ACTIVITY WAS FOUND NORMAL. ADMINISTRATION OF PRIMAQUINE FOR 30 DAYS PRODUCED NO HEMOLYSIS. FIVE CLOSE RELATIVES INCLUDING THE MOTHER HAD INTERMEDIATE LEVELS OF TPNH-METHEMOGLOBIN REDUCTASE CONSISTENT WITH HETEROZYGOUS STATUS. THE FATHER WAS DEAD. AS ONE WOULD PREDICT FROM KNOWLEDGE OF THE RELATIVE ACTIVITIES OF THE TPNH- AND DPNH-METHEMOGLOBIN REDUCTASES, METHEMOGLOBINEMIA WAS NOT PRESENT IN THE PRESUMED HOMOZYGOTE. BLOOM AND ZARKOWSKY (1970) ALSO REPORTED SUCH A PATIENT.

BLOOM, G. E. AND ZARKOWSKY, H. S.* HETEROGENEITY OF THE ENZYME DEFECT IN CONGENITAL METHEMOGLOBINEMIA. NEW ENG. J. MED. 281* 919-922, 1970.

SASS, M. D., CARUSO, C. J. AND FARHANGI, M.* TPNH-METHEMOGLOBIN REDUCTASE DEFICIENCY* A NEW RED-CELL ENZYME DEFECT. J. LAB. CLIN. MED. 70* 760-767, 1967.

25080 METHEMOGLOBINEMIA DUE TO DEFICIENCY OF METHEMOGLOBIN-REDUCTASE (DIAPHORASE) DEFICIENCY OF NADPH-DEPENDENT METHEMOGLOBIN REDUCTASE

THIS DISORDER DEMONSTRATES VERY WELL THAT THE CLINICAL DISORDERS RESULTING FROM ENZYME DEFICIENCIES, I.E., INBORN ERRORS OF METABOLISM, ARE INHERITED AS RECES-SIVES, WHEREAS STRUCTURAL DEFECTS, SUCH AS BRACHYDACTYLY AND STRUCTURAL ANOMALIES OF NONENZYMATIC PROTEINS, ARE USUALLY INHERITED AS DOMINANTS. THE FORM OF METHEMOGLOBIN WITH ELECTROPHORETICALLY ATYPICAL HEMOGLOBIN (OF WHICH THERE ARE SEVERAL TYPES) IS DOMINANT (SEE HB M).
MENTAL DEFICIENCY OCCURS ONLY WITH THE ENZYME-DEFICIENT RECESSIVE FORM OF THE DISORDER (HITZENBERGER, 1932* WORSTER-DROUGHT, WHITE AND SARGENT, 1953* JAFFE, 1963).
MULLER AND COLLEAGUES (1963) DESCRIBED 3 SIBS WITH METHEMOGLOBINEMIA. THEY SHOWED DEFICIENT ABILITY OF ERYTHROCYTES TO UTILIZE GLUCOSE FOR METHEMOGLOBIN REDUCTION BUT NORMAL REDUCTION OF LACTATE. THEY CONCLUDED THAT TWO ENZYME-DEFICIENT FORMS OF METHEMOGLOBINEMIA MAY EXIST JUST AS THERE ARE TWO METHEMOGLO-BIN-REDUCING SYSTEMS NORMALLY PRESENT IN RED CELLS, VIZ., NICOTINAMIDE-ADENINE DINUCLEOTIDE PHOSPHATE (NADPH2) REDUCTASE OR NICOTINAMIDE-ADENINE DINUCLEOTIDE (NADH2) REDUCTASE. MULLER ET AL. (1963) SUGGESTED THAT THEIR FAMILY SUFFERED FROM A DEFECT IN THE FORMER SYSTEM. THE ENZYME TYPE OF METHEMOGLOBINEMIA HAS UNPRECE-DENTEDLY HIGH FREQUENCY IN THE ATHABASKAN INDIANS (ESKIMOS) OF ALASKA (SCOTT, 1960* SCOTT ET AL., 1963). BALSAMO, HARDY AND SCOTT (1964) ALSO OBSERVED DIAPHORASE DEFICIENCY IN NAVAJO INDIANS. SINCE THE NAVAJO INDIANS AND THE ATHABASKAN INDIANS OF ALASKA ARE THE SAME LINGUISTIC STOCK, THE FINDING MAY ILLUSTRATE THE USEFULNESS OF RARE RECESSIVE GENES IN TRACING RELATIONSHIPS OF ETHNIC GROUPS. OZSOYLU (1967) REPORTED ENZYME-DEFICIENCY METHEMOGLOBINEMIA IN 3 GENERATIONS AND PROPOSED DOMINANT INHERITANCE. HOWEVER, CONSANGUINITY WAS PRESENT TO ACCOUNT FOR A QUASI-DOMINANT PATTERN. THE AUTHOR THOUGHT THIS POSSIBILITY WAS EXCLUDED BY A NORMAL DIAPHORASE ACTIVITY IN TWO INDIVIDUALS WHO WOULD NEED TO BE HETEROZYGOTES TO ACCOUNT FOR THE PATTERN. ENTEROGENOUS METHEMOGLOBINEMIA MIGHT BE CONFUSED WITH THE GENETIC FORM. ROSSI ET AL. (1966) DESCRIBED A CASE WITH METHEMOGLOBINEMIA FOR 14 YEARS BEFORE CURE BY A COURSE OF NEOMYCIN. WEST ET AL. (1967) PROVIDED ELECTROPHORETIC EVIDENCE OF ANOMALOUS ENZYME STRUCTURE IN A CASE OF METHEMOGLOBINEMIA. COHEN ET AL. (1968) SUGGESTED THAT METHEMOGLOBINEMIA INDUCED BY MALARIAL PROPHYLAXIS (BY CHLOROQUINE, PRIMAQUINE AND DIAMINO-DIPHENYL-SULFONE) WAS AN INDICATION OF THE PRESENCE OF THE HETEROZYGOUS STATE. ELECTRO-PHORETIC VARIANTS OF NADH DIAPHORASE WITHOUT METHEMOGLOBINEMIA HAVE ALSO BEEN FOUND, WITH A FAMILY PATTERN CONSISTENT WITH CO-DOMINANT INHERITANCE. BLOOM AND ZARKOWSKY (1970) DESCRIBED THREE VARIETIES* TOTAL ABSENCE OF DETECTABLE ENZYME ACTIVITY, DECREASED QUANTITIES OF PRESUMABLY NORMAL ENZYME AND DECREASED QUANTI-TIES OF STRUCTURALLY VARIANT ENZYME. THEY ADDED TWO NEW STRUCTURAL VARIANTS OF

R
E
C
E
S
S
I
V
E

(1967).   TREATMENT   WITH   METHYLENE BLUE (100-300 MG. ORALLY PER DAY) OR ASCORBIC
ACID (500   MG.   A DAY) IS OF COSMETIC VALUE (WALLER, 1970).   ADDITIONAL ELECTRO-
PHORETIC   VARIANTS   OF RED CELL NADH DIAPHORASE WERE DESCRIBED BY HOPKINSON ET AL.
(1970).

BALSAMO, P., HARDY, W. R. AND SCOTT, E. M.* HEREDITARY METHEMOGLOBINEMIA DUE TO
DIAPHORASE DEFICIENCY IN NAVAJO INDIANS. J. PEDIAT. 65* 928-930, 1964.

BLOOM,   G.   E.   AND   ZARKOWSKY,   H.   S.* HETEROGENEITY OF THE ENZYME DEFECT IN
CONGENITAL METHEMOGLOBINEMIA. NEW ENG. J. MED. 281* 919-922, 1970.

CAWEIN, M., BEHLEN, C. H., LAPPAT, E. J. AND COHN, J. E.* HEREDITARY DIAPHORASE
DEFICIENCY AND METHEMOGLOBINEMIA. ARCH. INTERN. MED. 113* 578-585, 1964.

COHEN,   R. J., SACHS, J. R., WICKER, D. J. AND CONRAD, M. E.* METHEMOGLOBINEMIA
PROVOKED   BY   MALARIAL   CHEMOPROPHYLAXIS   IN VIETNAM. NEW ENG. J. MED. 279* 1127-
1131, 1968.

FIALKOW,   P.   J.,   BROWDER,   J.   A.,   SPARKES, R. S. AND MOTULSKY, A. G.* MENTAL
RETARDATION   IN   METHEMOGLOBINEMIA DUE TO DIAPHORASE DEFICIENCY.   NEW ENG. J. MED.
273* 840-845, 1965.

GIBLETT,   E.   R. AND DETTER, J. C.* INHERITED NADH DIAPHORASE VARIATION WITHOUT
METHEMOGLOBINEMIA. AM. SOC. HUM. GENET., SAN FRANCISCO, OCT., 1969.

HITZENBERGER,   K.* AUTOTOXIC   CYANOSIS DUE TO INTRAGLOBULAR METHEMOGLOBINEMIA.
WEIN. ARCH. MED. 23* 85-96, 1932.

HOPKINSON,   D.   A.,   CORNEY,   G., COOK, P. J. L., ROBSON, E. B. AND HARRIS, H.*
GENETICALLY DETERMINED ELECTROPHORETIC VARIANTS OF HUMAN RED CELL NADH DIAPHORASE.
ANN. HUM. GENET. 34* 1-10, 1970.

HSIEH, H.-S. AND JAFFE, E. R.* ELECTROPHORETIC AND FUNCTIONAL VARIANTS OF NADH-
METHEMOGLOBIN REDUCTASE IN HEREDITARY METHOMOGLOBINEMIA. J. CLIN. INVEST. 50*
196-202, 1971.

JAFFE,   E. R.* THE REDUCTION OF METHEMOGLOBIN IN ERYTHROCYTES OF A PATIENT WITH
CONGENITAL   METHEMOGLOBINEMIA,   SUBJECTS   WITH   ERYTHROCYTE   GLUCOSE-6-PHOSPHATE
DEHYDROGENASE DEFICIENCY, AND NORMAL INDIVIDUALS. BLOOD 21* 561-572, 1963.

KAPLAN,   J.-C.   AND   BEUTLER,   E.* ELECTROPHORESIS OF RED CELL NADH- AND NADPH-
DIAPHORASES   IN   NORMAL   SUBJECTS   AND PATIENTS WITH CONGENITAL METHEMOGLOBINEMIA.
BIOCHEM. BIOPHYS. RES. COMMUN. 29* 605-610, 1967.

MULLER,   J.,   MURAWSKI,   K.,   SZYMANOWSKA,   Z., KOZIOROWSKI, A. AND RADWAN, L.*
HEREDITARY   DEFICIENCY OF NADPH 2-METHAEMOGLOBIN REDUCTASE. ACTA MED. SCAND. 173*
243-247, 1963.

OZSOYLU, S.* HEREDITARY METHEMOGLOBINEMIC CYANOSIS DUE TO DIAPHORASE DEFICIENCY
IN THREE SUCCESSIVE GENERATIONS. ACTA HAEMAT. 37* 276-283, 1967.

ROSSI, E. C., BRYAN, G. T., SCHILLING, R. F. AND CLATANOFF, D. V.* REMISSION OF
CHRONIC   METHEMOGLOBINEMIA   FOLLOWING   NEOMYCIN THERAPY. AM. J. MED. 40* 440-447,
1966.

SCOTT, E. M. AND WRIGHT, R. C.* THE ABSENCE OF CLOSE LINKAGE OF METHEMOGLOBINE-
MIA AND OTHER LOCI. AM. J. HUM. GENET. 21* 194-195, 1969.

SCOTT,   E.   M.* THE RELATIONSHIP OF DIAPHORASE OF HUMAN ERYTHROCYTES TO INHERI-
TANCE OF METHEMOGLOBINEMIA. J. CLIN. INVEST. 39* 1176-1179, 1960.

SCOTT,   E.   M.,   LEWIS,   M.,   KAITA, H., CHOWN, B. AND GIBLETT, E. R.* THE ABSENCE
OF   CLOSE   LINKAGE   OF METHEMOGLOBINEMIA AND BLOOD GROUP LOCI. AM. J. HUM. GENET.
15* 493-494, 1963.

TOWNES,   P.   L.   AND   MORRISON, M.* INVESTIGATION OF THE DEFECT IN A VARIANT OF
HEREDITARY METHEMOGLOBINEMIA. BLOOD 19* 60-74, 1962.

WALLER, H. D.* INHERITED METHEMOGLOBINEMIA (ENZYME DEFICIENCIES). HUMANGENETIK
9* 217-218, 1970.

WEST,   C.   A.,   GOMPERTS,   B.   D.,   HUEHNS, E. R., KESSEL, I. AND ASHBY, J. R.*
DEMONSTRATION   OF   AN   ENZYME VARIANT IN A CASE OF CONGENITAL METHAEMOGLOBINAEMIA.
BRIT. MED. J. 4* 212-214, 1967.

WORSTER-DROUGHT,   C.,   WHITE,   J.   C. AND SARGENT, F.* FAMILIAL, IDIOPATHIC
METHAEMOGLOBINAEMIA ASSOCIATED WITH MENTAL DEFICIENCY AND NEUROLOGICAL ABNORMALI-
TIES. BRIT. MED. J. 2* 114-118, 1953.

*25090 METHIONINE MALABSORPTION SYNDROME

THE MANIFESTATIONS IN THE PATIENT DESCRIBED BY HOOFT ET AL. (1968) WERE DIARRHEA, CONVULSIONS, PECULIAR SMELL, AND MENTAL RETARDATION. BOTH PARENTS AND THREE SIBS SHOWED ABNORMAL EXCRETION OF ALPHA-HYDROXYBUTYRIC ACID AFTER METHIONINE LOAD, A PRESUMED MANIFESTATION OF HETEROZYGOSITY. THEY CONSIDERED THIS DISORDER DIFFERENT FROM 'OASTHOUSE DISEASE' OF SMITH AND STRANG.

HOOFT, C., CARTON, D., SNOECK, J., TIMMERMANS, J., ANTENER, I., VAN DER HENDE, C. AND OYAERT, W.* FURTHER INVESTIGATIONS IN THE METHIONINE MALABSORPTION SYNDROME. HELV. PAEDIAT. ACTA 23* 334-349, 1968.

*25100 METHYLMALONICACIDURIA I

ROSENBERG ET AL. (1968) DESCRIBED AN 8 MONTH OLD BOY WITH PROFOUND METABOLIC ACIDOSIS, DEVELOPMENTAL RETARDATION AND AN UNUSUAL BIOCHEMICAL TRIAD* METHYLMA-LONIC ACIDURIA, LONG CHAIN KETONURIA AND INTERMITTENT HYPERGLYCINEMIA. VALINE, ISOLEUCINE OR HIGH PROTEIN INTAKE ACCENTUATED THE BIOCHEMICAL ABNORMALITIES. ROSENBERG ET AL. (1968) PRESENTED INDIRECT EVIDENCE THAT THE DEFECT CONCERNS METHYLMALONYL-COA ISOMERASE, A VITAMIN B12 DEPENDENT ENZYME WHICH CONVERTS METHYLMALONYL-COA TO SUCCINYL-COA. FURTHERMORE THEY FOUND THAT THEIR PATIENT RESPONDED TO VITAMIN B12 ADMINISTRATION. THUS, IN SOME BUT NOT ALL PATIENTS, THE CHARACTERISTIC AND POTENTIALLY LETHAL EPISODES OF KETOACIDOSIS CAN BE AVOIDED. BARNESS ET AL. (1968) ALSO POINTED OUT THAT SOME CASES OF METHYLMALONIC ACIDURIA RESPOND TO VITAMIN B12 AND OTHERS DO NOT. FURTHERMORE, OF THOSE NOT RESPONSIVE TO B12, SOME HAVE HYPERGLYCINEMIA AND SOME DO NOT. THE CONVERSION OF METHYLMALONATE TO SUCCINATE INVOLVES TWO ENZYMES ONLY ONE OF WHICH IS B12-DEPENDENT. MORROW ET AL. (1969) PROVIDED ENZYMATIC PROOF OF TWO FORMS OF THE DISEASE. METHYLMALONYL-CO A CARBONYLMUTASE ACTIVITY WAS ESSENTIALLY ABSENT FROM THE LIVER IN A VITAMIN B12-UNRESPONSIVE CASE, WHEREAS IN A VITAMIN B12-RESPONSIVE CASE THE LIVER SHOWED IN VITRO NORMAL ENZYMATIC ACTIVITY WITH ADDED COENZYME AND ESSENTIALLY NO ACTIVITY WITHOUT ADDED COENZYME.

BARNESS, L. A. AND MORROW, G., III* METHYLMALONIC ACIDURIA - A NEWLY DISCOVERED INBORN ERROR. ANN. INTERN. MED. 69* 633-635, 1968.

HSIA, Y. E., LILLJEQVIST, A.-C. AND ROSENBERG, L. E.* VITAMIN B12-DEPENDENT METHYLMALONIC ACIDURIA AMINO ACID TOXICITY, LONG CHAIN KETONURIA, AND PROTECTIVE EFFECT OF VITAMIN B12. PEDIATRICS 46* 497-507, 1970.

MORROW, G., III, BARNESS, L. A., CARDINALE, G. J., ABELES, R. H. AND FLAKS, J. G.* CONGENITAL METHYLMALONIC ACIDEMIA* ENZYMATIC EVIDENCE FOR TWO FORMS OF THE DISEASE. PROC. NAT. ACAD. SCI. 63* 191-197, 1969.

OBERHOLZER, V. G., LEVIN, B., BURGESS, E. A. AND YOUNG, W. F.* METHYLMALONIC ACIDURIA. AN INBORN ERROR OF METABOLISM LEADING TO CHRONIC METABOLIC ACIDOSIS. ARCH. DIS. CHILD. 42* 492-504, 1967.

ROSENBERG, L. E., LILLJEQVIST, A.-C. AND HSIA, Y. E.* METHYLMALONIC ACIDURIA* AN INBORN ERROR LEADING TO METABOLIC ACIDOSIS, LONG-CHAIN KETONURIA AND HYPERGLY-CINEMIA. NEW ENG. J. MED. 278* 1319-1322, 1968.

ROSENBERG, L. E., LILLJEQVIST, A.-C. AND HSIA, Y. E.* METHYLMALONIC ACIDURIA* METABOLIC BLOCK LOCALIZATION AND VITAMIN B12 DEPENDENCY. SCIENCE 162* 805-807, 1968.

*25110 METHYLMALONICACIDURIA II

SEE METHYLMALONICACIDURIA I FOR EVIDENCE OF THE EXISTENCE OF TWO ENZYMATICALLY DISTINCT FORMS OF METHYLMALONICACIDURIA.

*25120 MICROCEPHALY

MICROCEPHALY IS A HETEROGENEOUS STATE (COWIE, 1960). CARE MUST BE TAKEN TO DISTINGUISH MICROCEPHALY SECONDARY TO DEGENERATIVE BRAIN DISORDER FROM TRUE MICROCEPHALY WHICH IS INHERITED AS AN AUTOSOMAL RECESSIVE. MICROCEPHALY IS PRODUCED, FURTHERMORE, BY EXPOSURE OF THE HUMAN FETUS TO X-RAYS (PLUMMER, 1952). IN TRUE MICROCEPHALY THERE IS NO NEUROLOGIC DEFECT AND NO SKELETAL OR OTHER MALFORMATION. A WELL-INTEGRATED EXTROVERT PERSONALITY IS MAINTAINED. IN THE NETHERLANDS THE FREQUENCY OF TRUE MICROCEPHALY WAS PLACED AT ABOUT 1 IN 250,000 BY VAN DEN BOSCH (1959). THE MOST EXTENSIVE PEDIGREE YET REPORTED IS THAT ASSEMBLED BY KLOEPFER AND COLLEAGUES (1964). THE CONSISTENT ASSOCIATION OF CHORIORETINOPA-THY IN THE MICROCEPHALIC PATIENTS REPORTED BY MCKUSICK ET AL. (1966) MAY INDICATE THE EXISTENCE OF A SEPARATE ENTITY. SCHMIDT ET AL. (1968) OBSERVED THE SAME ASSOCIATION IN MULTIPLE MEMBERS OF A FAMILY.

BRANDON, M. G. W., KIRMAN, B. H. AND WILLIAMS, C. E.* MICROCEPHALY IN ONE OF MONOZYGOUS TWINS. ARCH. DIS. CHILD. 34* 56-59, 1959.

COWIE, V.* THE GENETICS AND SUB-CLASSIFICATION OF MICROCEPHALY. J. MENT. DEFIC. RES. 4* 42-47, 1960.

DAVIES, H. AND KIRMAN, B. H.* MICROCEPHALY. ARCH. DIS. CHILD. 37* 623-627, 1962.

RECESSIVE

COMBINATA UND DAS HERDWEISE VORKOMMEN DER MIKROCEPHALIA VERA IN SCHWEIZER
ISOLATEN. ACTA GENET. MED. GEM. 7* 445-524, 1958.

KLOEPFER, H. W., PLATOU, R. V. AND HANSCHE, W. J.* MANIFESTATIONS OF A
RECESSIVE GENE FOR MICROCEPHALY IN A POPULATION ISOLATE. J. GENET. HUM. 13* 52-
59, 1964.

KOCH, G.* GENETICS OF MICROCEPHALY IN MAN. ACTA GENET. MED. GEM. 8* 75-86,
1959.

KOMAI, T., KISHIMOTO, K. AND OZAKI, Y.* GENETIC STUDY OF MICROCEPHALY BASED ON
JAPANESE MATERIAL. AM. J. HUM. GENET. 7* 51-65, 1955.

MCKUSICK, V. A., STAUFFER, M., KNOX, D. L. AND CLARK, D. B.* CHORIORETINOPATHY
WITH HEREDITARY MICROCEPHALY. ARCH. OPHTHAL. 75* 597-600, 1966.

PLUMMER, G.* ANOMALIES OCCURRING IN CHILDREN EXPOSED IN UTERO TO THE ATOMIC
BOMB IN HIROSHIMA. PEDIATRICS 10* 687-693, 1952.

SCHMIDT, B., JAEGER, W. AND NEUBAUER, H.* EIN MIKROZEPHALIE-SYNDROME MIT
ATYPISCHER TAPETORETINALER DEGENERATION BEI 3 GESCHWISTERN. KLIN. MBL. AUGEN-
HEILK. 150* 188-196, 1968.

VAN DEN BOSCH, J.* MICROCEPHALY IN THE NETHERLANDS* A CLINICAL AND GENETICAL
STUDY. ANN. HUM. GENET. 23* 91-116, 1959.

25130 MICROCEPHALY, HIATUS HERNIA AND NEPHROTIC SYNDROME

GALLOWAY AND MOWAT (1968) OBSERVED A BROTHER AND SISTER WITH THIS COMBINATION.
DEATH FROM NEPHROSIS OCCURRED AT 20 AND 28 MONTHS, RESPECTIVELY. PARENTAL
CONSANGUINITY COULD NOT BE DEMONSTRATED.

GALLOWAY, W. H. AND MOWAT, A. P.* CONGENITAL MICROCEPHALY WITH HIATUS HERNIA
AND NEPHROTIC SYNDROME IN TWO SIBS. J. MED. GENET. 5* 319-321, 1968.

25140 MICROCOLON

CARESANO AND BORGHI (1966) DESCRIBED MICROCOLON IN TWO NEWBORN MALES OF AN ITALIAN
FAMILY. MICROCOLON OCCURS WITH AGANGLIOSIS OF THE ENTIRE COLON AND PART OF THE
SMALL INTESTINE AND WITH OBSTRUCTION OF THE SMALL INTESTINE AS IN CONGENITAL
ATRESIA OR MECONIUM ILEUS. THUS, A FAMILIAL AGGREGATION OF MICROCOLON MIGHT
RESULT FROM THE WELL-KNOWN OCCURRENCE OF MECONIUM ILEUS WITH CYSTIC FIBROSIS OF
THE PANCREAS. LEE AND MACMILLAN (1950) CLAIM THAT IT CAN RARELY BE CONSIDERED A
PRIMARY ENTITY.

CARESANO, A. AND BORGHI, A.* IL MICROCOLON* A PROPITO DI DUE OSSERVAZIONI NELLA
MEDESIMA FAMIGLIA. QUAD. RADIOL. 31* 173-185, 1966.

HUNT, H. B.* ROENTGENOLOGICAL ASPECTS OF THE CONGENITALLY SMALL COLON AND OF
INTESTINAL OCCLUSIONS* WITH REPORT OF FIVE CASES. AM. J. ROENTGEN. 41* 564-574,
1939.

LEE, C. M., JR. AND MACMILLAN, B. G.* THE FALLACY IN THE DIAGNOSIS OF MICROCO-
LON IN THE NEWBORN. RADIOLOGY 55* 807-813, 1950.

25150 MICROPHTHALMIA AND MENTAL DEFICIENCY

THIS COMBINATION SUGGESTS NORRIE'S DISEASE, AN X-LINKED DISORDER (Q.V.). SJOGREN
AND LARSSON (1949) DESCRIBED THE ASSOCIATION AS AN AUTOSOMAL RECESSIVE SYNDROME.
PINSKY ET AL. (1965) DESCRIBED THREE SISTERS WITH MICROPHTHALMOS, SEVERE MENTAL
RETARDATION AND SPASTIC CEREBRAL PALSY.

PINSKY, L., DIGEORGE, A. M., HARLEY, R. D. AND BAIRD, H. W., III* MICROPHTHAL-
MOS, CORNEAL OPACITY, MENTAL RETARDATION, AND SPASTIC CEREBRAL PALSY. AN
OCULOCEREBRAL SYNDROME. J. PEDIAT. 67* 387-398, 1965.

SJOGREN, T. AND LARSSON, T.* MICROPHTHALMOS AND ANOPHTHALMOS WITH OR WITHOUT
COINCIDENT OLIGOPHRENIA. A CLINICAL AND GENETIC-STATISTICAL STUDY. ACTA
PSYCHIAT. NEUROL. SCAND. 56 (SUPPL.)* 1-103, 1949.

*25160 MICROPHTHALMOS

GILL AND HARRIS (1959) REPORTED A FAMILY WITH TWO CASES OF MICROPHTHALMOS, IN THE
PROBAND AND IN HER GREAT-AUNT. WOLFF (1930) DESCRIBED A FAMILY OF 10 CHILDREN
WHOSE PARENTS WERE FIRST COUSINS AND AMONG WHOM 3 MALES AND TWO FEMALES HAD
MICROPHTHALMOS, HIGH GRADE HYPEROPIA (UP TO +20D) AND GLAUCOMA. IN EXTREME
INSTANCES DIFFERENTIATION FROM ANOPHTHALMOS (Q.V.) MAY BE IMPOSSIBLE WITHOUT
HISTOLOGIC STUDY. THE EYE IS GENERALLY SMALL WITHOUT GROSS CONGENITAL MALFORMA-
TIONS. HOLST (1950) OBSERVED 6 CASES IN TWO RELATED SIBSHIPS. NANOPHTHALMOS IS A
SYNONYM FOR MICROPHTHALMOS. BOTH DOMINANT AND RECESSIVE FORMS ARE KNOWN.

RECESSIVE

ASHLEY, L. M.* BILATERAL ANOPHTHALMOS IN BROTHER AND SISTER. J. HERED. 38* 174-176, 1947.

GILL, E. G. AND HARRIS, R. B.* CONGENITAL MICROPHTHALMOS WITH CYST FORMATION. VIRGINIAN MED. MONTHLY 86* 33-36, 1959.

HOLST* BLINDHETSARSAKER I NORGE (OSLO), 1950. CITED BY SORSBY, A.* SYSTEM OF OPHTHALMOLOGY, NORMAL AND ABNORMAL DEVELOPMENT. ST. LOUIS* C.V. MOSBY CO., 3* (PART 2) 1963. P. 490.

JOSEPH, R.* A PEDIGREE OF ANOPHTHALMOS. BRIT. J. OPHTHAL. 41* 541-543, 1957.

MCMILLAN, L.* ANOPHTHALMIA AND MALDEVELOPMENT OF THE EYES* FOUR CASES IN THE SAME FAMILY. BRIT. J. OPHTHAL. 5* 121-122, 1921.

WOLFF, E.* A MICROPHTHALMIC FAMILY. PROC. ROY. SOC. MED. 23 (PART I)* 623-626, 1930.

25170 MICROPHTHALMOS WITH HYPERMETROPIA, RETINAL DEGENERATION, MACROPHAKIA AND DENTAL ANOMALIES

IN A SIBSHIP OF 7 WITHOUT PARENTAL CONSANGUINITY, FRANCESCHETTI AND GERNET (1965) FOUND FOUR (THREE MALES, ONE FEMALE) WITH MARKED MICROPHTHALMOS, DIAGNOSED WITH THE ECHOGRAM (ULTRASONOGRAM), WITH CORNEA OF NORMAL SIZE. ASSOCIATED FEATURES WERE HIGH GRADE HYPERMETROPIA, MACROPHAKIA, RETINAL DEGENERATION AND DENTAL ANOMALIES. TWO HAD GLAUCOMA.

FRANCESCHETTI, A. AND GERNET, H.* DIAGNOSTIC ULTRASONIQUE D'UNE MICROPHTALMIE SANS MICROCORNEE, AVEC MACROPHAKIE, HAUTE HYPERMETROPIE ASSOCIEE A UNE DEGENERESCENCE TAPETO-RETINIENNE, UNE DISPOSITION GLAUCOMATEUSE ET DES ANOMALIES DENTAIRES (NOUVEAU SYNDROME FAMILIAL). ARCH. OPHTAL. (PARIS) 25* 105-116, 1965.

25180 MICROTIA WITH MEATAL ATRESIA

ELLWOOD ET AL. (1968) REPORTED (1) BROTHER AND SISTER WITH BILATERAL ANOTIA WITH MEATAL ATRESIA AND (2) TWO BROTHERS, ONE WITH UNILATERAL MICROTIA AND BILATERAL MEATAL ATRESIA AND THE OTHER WITH UNILATERAL MICROTIA AND MEATAL ATRESIA. THE FIRST SIBSHIP HAD HAD FIRST COUSIN PARENTS. THE EVIDENCE FOR RECESSIVE INHERITANCE IS INCONCLUSIVE.

ELLWOOD, L. C., WINTER, S. T. AND DAR, H.* FAMILIAL MICROTIA WITH MEATAL ATRESIA IN TWO SIBSHIPS. J. MED. GENET. 5* 289-291, 1968.

25190 MITOCHONDRIAL ABNORMALITIES WITH MYOPATHY

SEVERAL PROBABLY DISTINCT MYOPATHIES WITH MORPHOLOGIC AND-OR BIOCHEMICAL ABNORMALITIES OF THE MITOCHONDRIA HAVE BEEN DESCRIBED. (SEE HYPERMETABOLISM DUE TO DEFECT IN MITOCHONDRIA. SEE PLEOCONIAL MYOPATHY. SEE MYOPATHY WITH GIANT ABNORMAL MITOCHONDRIA.) COLEMAN ET AL. (1967) DESCRIBED TWO PATIENTS WITH PROGRESSIVE PROXIMAL AND SUBSEQUENTLY DISTAL MUSCLE FATIGABILITY AND WEAKNESS AT AGES 5 TO 10 YEARS. UNUSUALLY LARGE MITOCHONDRIA, WITH HIGH ACTIVITIES OF OXIDATIVE ENZYMES, AND ABNORMAL ACCUMULATION OF NEUTRAL FAT WERE DEMONSTRATED BY MUSCLE BIOPSY. THE MUSCLE MITOCHONDRIA CONTAINED ANOMALOUS QUADRILAMINAR STRUCTURES (PRICE ET AL., 1967). VAN WIJNGAARDEN ET AL. (1967) GAVE A FOLLOW-UP ON THE PATIENT OF LUFT ET AL. (SEE HYPERMETABOLISM DUE TO DEFECT IN MITOCHONDRIA) AND DESCRIBED ANOTHER CASE OF MYOPATHY WITH MITOCHONDRIAL ABNORMALITY.

COLEMAN, R. F., NIENHUIS, A. W., BROWN, W. J., MUNSAT, T. L. AND PEARSON, C. M.* NEW MYOPATHY WITH MITOCHONDRIAL ENZYME HYPERACTIVITY. J.A.M.A. 199* 624-630, 1967.

PRICE, H. M., GORDON, G. B., MUNSAT, T. L. AND PEARSON, C. M.* MYOPATHY WITH ATYPICAL MITOCHONDRIA IN TYPE I SKELETAL MUSCLE FIBERS. A HISTOCHEMICAL AND ULTRASTRUCTURAL STUDY. J. NEUROPATH. EXP. NEUROL. 26* 475-497, 1967.

VAN WIJNGAARDEN, G. K., BETHLEM, J., MEIJER, A. E. F. H., HULSMANN, W. C. AND FELTKAMP, C. A.* SKELETAL MUSCLE DISEASE WITH ABNORMAL MITOCHONDRIA. BRAIN 90* 577-592, 1967.

25200 MITOCHONDRIAL MYOPATHY WITH SALT CRAVING

SPIRO ET AL. (1970) DESCRIBED A 13 YEAR OLD BOY WHO WAS FLOPPY AT BIRTH AND SHOWED DELAYED MOTOR MILESTONES WAS FOUND TO HAVE SEVERE SALT CRAVING AND NON-PROGRESSIVE MYOPATHY. ULTRASTRUCTURAL ABNORMALITIES CONSISTING OF INCREASED NUMBERS OF LARGE MITOCHONDRIA ALIGNED WITH LIPID BODIES WERE NOTED IN BIOPSIED SKELETAL MUSCLE FIBERS. NO OTHER MEMBERS OF THE FAMILY WERE AFFECTED.

SPIRO, A. J., PRINEAS, J. W. AND MOORE, C. L.* A NEW MITOCHONDRIAL MYOPATHY IN A PATIENT WITH SALT CRAVING. ARCH. NEUROL. 22* 259-269, 1970.

*25210 MOHR SYNDROME

RECESSIVE

OTTO L. MOHR (1941) DESCRIBED A FAMILY IN WHICH FOUR MALES OF A SIBSHIP OF FIVE
BOYS AND TWO GIRLS SHOWED A SYNDROME WHICH WAS DETAILED IN THE CASE OF ONE
AFFECTED MALE WHOM HE PERSONALLY OBSERVED. THE FEATURES WERE POLY-, SYN-, AND
BRACHYDACTYLY, LOBATE TONGUE WITH PAPILLIFORM PROTUBERANCES, HIGH ARCHED PALATE,
ANGULAR FORM OF THE ALVEOLAR PROCESS OF THE MANDIBLE, SUPERNUMERARY SUTURES IN THE
SKULL, AND AN EPISODIC NEUROMUSCULAR DISTURBANCE. THREE OF THE FOUR AFFECTED
MALES HAD DIED PRIOR TO THE TIME OF REPORT. ONE OF THESE HAD CLEFT PALATE. NO
SIMILARLY AFFECTED PERSONS IN PREVIOUS GENERATIONS WERE KNOWN. THE PARENTS WERE
NOT RELATED. MOHR SUGGESTED THAT THE SYNDROME IS DUE TO A RECESSIVE, SUB-LETHAL,
X-LINKED GENE. OBVIOUSLY THE EVIDENCE FOR THIS SUGGESTION WAS FEEBLE. CLAUSSEN
(1946) PROVIDED A FOLLOW-UP OF THE KINDRED WITH DESCRIPTION OF AN AFFECTED MALE
COUSIN. FURTHERMORE, THE PARENTS OF THE NEW CASE WERE RELATED. HE SUGGESTED
AUTOSOMAL RECESSIVE INHERITANCE, WHICH SEEMS TO BE SUPPORTED BY GORLIN'S (1967)
OBSERVATION OF THE SAME SYNDROME IN TWO SISTERS. IN SEVERAL RESPECTS THE MOHR
SYNDROME RESEMBLES ORAL-FACIAL-DIGITAL SYNDROME. RIMOIN AND EDGERTON (1967)
DESCRIBED THREE AFFECTED SIBS (TWO MALE, ONE FEMALE) AND SUGGESTED THAT THIS MIGHT
BE CALLED THE ORAL-FACIAL-DIGITAL SYNDROME II. IN ADDITION TO THE DIFFERENT MODE
OF INHERITANCE, THE MOHR SYNDROME SHOWS NONE OF THE SKIN AND HAIR CHANGES OF THE
X-LINKED ORAL-FACIAL-DIGITAL SYNDROME I BUT DOES SHOW CONDUCTIVE HEARING LOSS AND
BILATERAL HALLUCAL POLYSYNDACTYLY NOT PRESENT IN OFD I.

CLAUSSEN, O.* ET ARVELIG SYNDROM OMFATTENDE TUNGEMISSDANNELSE OG POLYDAKTYLI.
NORD. MED. 30* 1147-1151, 1946.

GORLIN, R. J.* MINNEAPOLIS, MINN.* PERSONAL COMMUNICATION, 1967.

MOHR, O. L.* A HEREDITARY LETHAL SYNDROME IN MAN. AVH. NORSKE VIDENSKAD. OSLO
14* 1-18, 1941.

RIMOIN, D. L. AND EDGERTON, M. T.* GENETIC AND CLINICAL HETEROGENEITY IN THE
ORAL-FACIAL-DIGITAL SYNDROMES. J. PEDIAT. 71* 94-102, 1967.

25220 MONILETHRIX

EXTENSIVELY AFFECTED KINDREDS WITH THE PATTERN OF DOMINANT INHERITANCE HAVE BEEN
REPORTED. HOWEVER, HANHART (1955) CLAIMED RECESSIVE INHERITANCE FOR A KINDRED HE
STUDIED, AND WORKING ALSO IN ZURICH SALAMON AND SCHNYDER (1962) SUGGESTED THAT ONE
OUT OF FIVE FAMILIES MIGHT HAVE A RECESSIVE FORM OF THE DISORDER. RECESSIVE
INHERITANCE CANNOT BE CONSIDERED AS PROVED, HOWEVER.

HANHART, E.* ERSTMALIGER HINWEIS AUF DAS VORKOMMEN EINES MONOHYBRIDREZESSIVEN
ERBGANGS BEI MONILETHRIX (MONILETRICHOSIS). ARCH. KLAUS STIFT. VERERBUNGSFORSCH.
30* 1-11, 1955.

SALAMON, T. AND SCHNYDER, U. W.* UBER DIE MONILETHRIX. ARCH. KLIN. EXP. DERM.
215* 105-136, 1962.

*25230 MORQUIO SYNDROME, NON-KERATOSULFATE-EXCRETING TYPE

SOME PATIENTS HAVE A DISORDER QUALITATIVELY LIKE MUCOPOLYSACCHARIDOSIS IV (Q.V.)
BUT MILDER. SLIGHT CORNEAL CLOUDING OCCURS. THIS IS THE CONDITION PRESENT IN THE
PATIENT SHOWN BY MCKUSICK (1960, P. 91). THE PATIENT HAS A NORMAL CHILD. TWO
MALE FIRST COUSINS ARE IDENTICALLY AFFECTED. THESE PATIENTS COME FROM AN INBRED
EARLY AMERICAN GROUP IN WHICH AT LEAST 4 OTHER RARE RECESSIVES HAVE BEEN FOUND*
CRIGLER-NAJJAR SYNDROME, HOMOCYSTINURIA, BIRD-HEADED DWARFISM, AND METACHROMATIC
LEUKODYSTROPHY. MANY FORMS OF SPONDYLOEPIPHYSEAL DYSPLASIA HAVE BEEN INCORRECTLY
LABELLED MORQUIO SYNDROME. THERE ARE, HOWEVER, SOME CASES WHICH SEEM LEGITIMATELY
TERMED MORQUIO SYNDROME IN WHICH KERATOSULFATE IS NOT EXCRETED IN THE URINE. THE
CONDITION OR CONDITIONS IN THIS GROUP OF PATIENTS MAY STILL BE THE RESULT OF A
DISTURBANCE IN MUCOPOLYSACCHARIDE METABOLISM. DANES AND BEARN (1967) STUDIED 8
FAMILIES, EACH WITH AT LEAST ONE CASE OF MORQUIO SYNDROME. IN 6 FAMILIES WITH THE
DISORDER LIMITED TO THE SKELETON NO METACHROMASIA WAS FOUND IN FIBROBLASTS. IN
ONE OF THE OTHER FAMILIES CORNEAL CLOUDING, REILLY BODIES AND SEVERE MENTAL
RETARDATION ACCOMPANIED THE SKELETAL FEATURES AND IN A SECOND 'SHOE-SHAPED' SELLA
TURCICA AND WIDENED LUMERAL SHAFTS ACCOMPANIED THE USUAL FEATURES OF MORQUIO
SYNDROME. BOTH THESE TWO FAMILIES DID SHOW FIBROBLAST METACHROMASIA. IN ADDITION
TO THE MORQUIO SYNDROME WITH KERATOSULFATE EXCRETION (SEE MUCOPOLYSACCHARIDOSIS
TYPE IV) SOME CASES WITH MILDER CHANGES AND LONGER SURVIVAL FALL INTO NO OTHER
CATEGORY. MILD CLOUDING OF THE CORNEA DEVELOPS LATE. PATIENT E. M. (JHH 695487)
PROBABLY HAS THIS CONDITION (MCKUSICK, 1966). SHE HAS BORNE A CHILD WHO IS
NORMAL. TWO MALE COUSINS HAVE THE SAME CONDITION. THEY COME FROM AN INBRED EARLY
AMERICAN GROUP THAT ALSO HAS CASES OF SECKEL'S BIRD-HEADED DWARFISM, HOMOCYS-
TINURIA, METACHROMATIC LEUKODYSTROPHY, CRIGLER-NAJJAR SYNDROME AND HYDROCEPHALUS.

DANES, B. S. AND BEARN, A. G.* CELLULAR METACHROMASIA, A GENETIC MARKER FOR
STUDYING THE MUCOPOLYSACCHARIDOSES. LANCET 1* 241-243, 1967.

MCKUSICK, V. A.* HERITABLE DISORDERS OF CONNECTIVE TISSUE. ST. LOUIS* C. V.
MOSBY CO., 1960 (2ND ED.).

MCKUSICK, V. A.* HERITABLE DISORDERS OF CONNECTIVE TISSUE. ST. LOUIS* C. V.
MOSBY CO., 1966 (3RD ED.).

IN THE TERMINOLOGY, CLASSIFICATION, AND NUMBERING OF THIS CATEGORY, I HAVE
FOLLOWED SPRANGER AND WIEDEMANN (1970). MUCOLIPIDOSIS I WAS FORMERLY CALLED
LIPOMUCOPOLYSACCHARIDOSIS. THE DISORDER IS CHARACTERIZED BY MILD HURLER-LIKE
MANIFESTATIONS WITH MODERATE MENTAL RETARDATION, NO EXCESS MUCOPOLYSACCHARIDURIA
AND PECULIAR INCLUSIONS OF THE FIBROBLASTS. SPRANGER AND WIEDEMANN (1970)
OBSERVED THREE AFFECTED SIBS AND PARENTAL CONSANGUINITY IN ONE INSTANCE. THEY
SUGGESTED THAT THE SIBS DESCRIBED BY PINCUS ET AL. (1967) HAD THIS DISORDER AS DID
THE PATIENT REPORTED BY SANFILIPPO ET AL. (1962). SEE CASE OF LOEB ET AL. (1969).

LOEB, H., TEPPEL, M. AND CREMER, N.* CLINICAL, BIOCHEMICAL AND ULTRASTRUCTURAL
STUDIES OF AN ATYPICAL FORM OF MUCOPOLYSACCHARIDOSIS. ACTA PAEDIAT. 58* 220-228,
1969.

PINCUS, J. H., ROSSI, J. P. AND DAROFF, R. B.* DELAYED DEVELOPMENT OF DISTURBED
MUCOPOLYSACCHARIDE METABOLISM IN A HURLER VARIANT. ARCH. NEUROL. 16* 244-253,
1967.

SANFILIPPO, S. J., YUNIS, J. AND WORTHEN, H. G.* AN UNUSUAL STORAGE DISEASE
RESEMBLING THE HURLER-HUNTER SYNDROME. (ABSTRACT) AM. J. DIS. CHILD. 104* 553
ONLY, 1962.

SPRANGER, J. AND WIEDEMANN, H.-R.* THE GENETIC MUCOLIPIDOSES. DIAGNOSIS AND
DIFFERENTIAL DIAGNOSIS. HUMANGENETIK 9* 113-139, 1970.

SPRANGER, J., WIEDEMANN, H.-R., TOLKSDORF, M., GRAUCOB, E. AND CAESAR, R.*
LIPOMUCOPOLYSACCHARIDOSE* EINE NEUE SPEICHERKRANKHEIT. Z. KINDERHEILK. 103* 285-
306, 1968.

*25250 MUCOLIPIDOSIS II (I-CELL DISEASE)

THIS IS A HURLER-LIKE CONDITION WITH SEVERE CLINICAL AND RADIOLOGIC FEATURES,
PECULIAR FIBROBLAST INCLUSIONS AND NO EXCESSIVE MUCOPOLYSACCHARIDURIA. CONGENITAL
DISLOCATION OF THE HIP, THORACIC DEFORMITIES, HERNIA AND HYPERPLASTIC GUMS ARE
EVIDENT SOON AFTER BIRTH. RETARDED PSYCHOMOTOR DEVELOPMENT, CLEAR CORNEAS,
RESTRICTED JOINT MOBILITY ARE OTHER FEATURES. LEROY ET AL. (1969) FIRST DESCRIBED
THIS CONDITION. BOTH SEXES HAVE BEEN AFFECTED, SIBS WERE AFFECTED IN TWO FAMILIES
AND THE PARENTS OF ONE OF THE PATIENTS OF SPRANGER AND WIEDEMANN (1970) WERE FIRST
COUSINS. ABNORMAL INCLUSIONS WERE FOUND IN THE FIBROBLASTS OF SOME HETEROZYGOTES
(LEROY ET AL., 1969).

DEMARS, R. I. AND LEROY, J.* THE REMARKABLE CELLS CULTURED FROM A HUMAN WITH
HURLER'S SYNDROME. AN APPROACH TO VISUAL SELECTION FOR IN VITRO GENETIC STUDIES.
IN VITRO 2* 107, 1967.

LEROY, J. G. AND DEMARS, R. I.* MUTANT ENZYMATIC AND CYTOLOGICAL PHENOTYPES IN
CULTURED HUMAN FIBROBLASTS. SCIENCE 157* 804-806, 1967.

LEROY, J. G., DEMARS, R. I. AND OPITZ, J. M.* I-CELL DISEASE. THE CLINICAL
DELINEATION OF BIRTH DEFECTS. IV. SKELETAL DYSPLASIAS. NEW YORK* NATIONAL
FOUNDATION, 1969. PP. 174-185.

SPRANGER, J. W. AND WIEDEMANN, H.-R.* THE GENETIC MUCOLIPIDOSES. DIAGNOSIS AND
DIFFERENTIAL DIAGNOSIS. HUMANGENETIK 9* 113-139, 1970.

*25260 MUCOLIPIDOSIS III (PSEUDO-HURLER POLYDYSTROPHY)

UNDER THE DESIGNATION 'PSEUDO POLYDYSTROPHIE DE HURLER,' MAROTEAUX AND LAMY (1966)
DESCRIBED 4 CASES WITH MANY OF THE FEATURES OF THE HURLER SYNDROME BUT A MUCH
SLOWER CLINICAL EVOLUTION AND NO MUCOPOLYSACCHARIDURIA. THE BONE MARROW CONTAINED
CELLS REMINISCENT OF THOSE IN THE HURLER SYNDROME BUT VACUOLES WERE EMPTY.
HYPOPLASIA OF THE ODONTOID WAS NOTED IN AT LEAST ONE CASE. THE AUTHORS POINTED
OUT THAT THIS IS PROBABLY THE SAME CONDITION AS THAT IN A PATIENT LISTED AMONG
'CASES DEFYING CLASSIFICATION' IN THE REPORT OF MCKUSICK ET AL. (1965). IT IS
PLAUSIBLE THAT THERE SHOULD BE GENETIC DEFECTS OF MUCOPOLYSACCHARIDE METABOLISM
WITHOUT MUCOPOLYSACCHARIDURIA AND THIS IS PROBABLY AN EXAMPLE. IT HOLDS A
RELATIONSHIP TO MUCOPOLYSACCHARIDOSIS I COMPARABLE TO THE RELATIONSHIP OF THE NON-
KERATOSULFATE-EXCRETING MORQUIO SYNDROME TO MUCOPOLYSACCHARIDOSIS IV. I HAVE TWO
BROTHER-SISTER PAIRS AMONG THE SIX PATIENTS WITH THIS DISORDER WHOM I HAVE STUDIED
IN DETAIL. SEVERAL OTHER PATIENTS ARE KNOWN TO ME. THE SIBS REPORTED BY
STEINBACH ET AL. (1968) APPEAR TO HAVE HAD THIS CONDITION.

MAROTEAUX, P. AND LAMY, M.* LA PSEUDO-POLYDYSTROPHIE DE HURLER. PRESSE MED.
74* 2889-2892, 1966.

MCKUSICK, V. A., KAPLAN, D., WISE, D., HANLEY, W. B., SUDDARTH, S. B., SEVICK,
M. E. AND MAUMANEE, A. E.* THE GENETIC MUCOPOLYSACCHARIDOSES. MEDICINE 44* 445-
483, 1965.

STEINBACH, H. L., PREGER, L., WILLIAMS, H. E. AND COHEN, P.* THE HURLER
SYNDROME WITHOUT ABNORMAL MUCOPOLYSACCHARIDURIA. RADIOLOGY 90* 472-478, 1968.

R
E
C
E
S
S
I
V
E

NOT ONLY ARE SPECIAL STUDIES SUCH AS THOSE BY THE METHODS OF NEUFELD REVEALING HETEROGENEITY WITHIN SEVERAL OF THE SIX MAIN TYPES OF MUCOPOLYSACCHARIDOSIS BUT ALSO SOME FORMS REMAIN UNCLASSIFIED. FOR EXAMPLE, HORTON AND SCHIMKE (1970) DESCRIBED BROTHER AND SISTER, AGES 13 AND 11, WITH FEATURES LIKE PSEUDO-HURLER POLYDYSTROPHY (MUCOLIPIDOSIS III) BUT WITH MUCOPOLYSACCHARIDES (BOTH CHONDROITIN SULFATE B AND HEPARITIN SULFATE) IN THE URINE IN AMOUNTS ABOUT 10 TO 15 TIMES THE NORMAL. INTELLIGENCE WAS NORMAL. BROWN AND KUWABARA (1970) OBSERVED TWO SISTERS, AGES 5 AND 13 YEARS, WITH HURLER-LIKE FACIES, SWOLLEN FINGERS, DWARFED STATURE, SEVERE PROGRESSIVE JOINT DESTRUCTION AND PECULIAR PROGRESSIVE PERIPHERAL ANNULAR CORNEAL OF CALCIFICATION. THE PARENTS WERE PUERTO RICAN FIRST COUSINS. FIBROB-LASTS SHOWED METACHROMASIA AND INCREASED MUCOPOLYSACCHARIDE. URINARY MUCOPOLYSAC-CHARIDE WAS NORMAL. HIGH DOSES OF VITAMINS SEEMED TO BE BENEFICIAL.

BROWN, S. I. AND KUWABARA, T.* PERIPHERAL CORNEAL OPACITIES AND SKELETAL DEFORMITIES. A NEWLY RECOGNIZED ACID MUCOPOLYSACCHARIDOSIS SIMULATING RHEUMATOID ARTHRITIS. ARCH. OPHTHAL. 83* 667-677, 1970.

HORTON, W. A. AND SCHIMKE, R. N.* A NEW MUCOPOLYSACCHARIDOSIS. J. PEDIAT. 77* 252-258, 1970.

25280 MUCOPOLYSACCHARIDOSIS TYPE I (HURLER SYNDROME GARGOYLISM)

THE AUTOSOMAL RECESSIVE FORM IS MORE FREQUENT THAN TYPE II, WHICH IS X-LINKED, HAS NO CLOUDING OF THE CORNEA AND PURSUES A SLOWER COURSE. IN TWO CASES PRESUMABLY OF THIS TYPE, AUSTIN ET AL. (1964) FOUND AN INCREASE IN ACTIVITY OF THE LYSOSOMAL ENZYME ARYLSULPHATASE-B IN LIVER, KIDNEY AND BRAIN. DANES AND BEARN (1965) FOUND THAT CELLULAR ACCUMULATION OF MUCOPOLYSACCHARIDES PERSISTS IN CULTURED FIBROB-LASTS. FRATANTONI, HALL AND NEUFELD (1968) SHOWED THAT THE ACCUMULATION RESULTS FROM INEFFICIENT DEGRADATION OF INTRACELLULAR MUCOPOLYSACCHARIDE RATHER THAN EXCESSIVE SYNTHESIS OR REDUCED SECRETION. FURTHERMORE THEY FOUND THAT MIXING OF FIBROBLASTS FROM HURLER AND HUNTER PATIENTS CAUSES MUTUAL CORRECTION OF THE INTRACELLULAR ACCUMULATION OF MUCOPOLYSACCHARIDES. MEDIUM IN WHICH CELLS OF THE OTHER TYPE OR NORMAL CELLS HAD BEEN INCUBATED WAS ALSO EFFECTIVE IN CORRECTING THE DEFECT. THUS, ISOLATION AND IDENTIFICATION OF THE CORRECTIVE FACTOR IN THE MEDIUM OPENS UP POSSIBILITIES OF CLARIFYING THE NORMAL MECHANISMS OF MPS DEGRADATION, AS WELL AS THERAPY. DIFFERENTIATION OF THE SANFILIPPO SYNDROME (MPS III) FROM THE HURLER AND HUNTER SYNDROMES IS ALSO POSSIBLE BY THIS MIXED CULTURE METHOD. NEUHAUSER ET AL. (1968) CONCLUDED THAT SUBARACHNOID CYSTS ARE OFTEN RESPONSIBLE FOR THE ENLARGED SELLA IN THE HURLER SYNDROME. IF THE MUTATION RATES ARE THE SAME AND THE HETEROZYGOTES FOR BOTH CONDITIONS HAVE NO REPRODUCTIVE ADVANTAGE OR DISADVANTAGE, THE HUNTER SYNDROME SHOULD BE ONE AND ONE HALF TIMES MORE FREQUENT AMONG NEWBORNS THAN THE HURLER SYNDROME (MCKUSICK, 1970). OBSERVATIONS PROBABLY DOES NOT AGREE WITH EXPECTATION. IMPROVEMENT, CLINICAL AND CHEMICAL, WITH PLASMA INFUSIONS HAS BEEN CLAIMED (DI FERRANTE ET AL., 1971). RESULTS OF TREATMENT WITH PURIFIED PREPARATIONS OF NEUFELD'S CORRECTION FACTOR ARE EAGERLY AWAITED.

RECESSIVE

AUSTIN, J., MCAFEE, D., ARMSTRONG, D., O'ROURKE, M., SHEARER, L. AND BACHHAWAT, B.* ABNORMAL SULPHATASE ACTIVITIES IN TWO HUMAN DISEASES (METACHROMATIC LEUCODYS-TROPHY AND GARGOYLISM). BIOCHEM. J. 93* 15C-17C, 1964.

DANES, B. S. AND BEARN, A. G.* HURLER'S SYNDROME* DEMONSTRATION OF AN INHERITED DISORDER OF CONNECTIVE TISSUE IN CELL CULTURE. SCIENCE 149* 987-989, 1965.

DANES, B. S., QUEENAN, J. T., GADOW, E. C., AND CEDERQUIST, L. L.* ANTENATAL DIAGNOSIS OF MUCOPOLYSACCHARIDOSES. (LETTER) LANCET 1* 946-947, 1970.

DI FERRANTE, N., NICHOLS, B. L., DONNELLY, P. V., NERI, G., HRGOVCIC, R. AND BERGLUND, R. K.* INDUCED DEGRADATION OF GLYCOSAMINOGLYCANS IN HURLER'S AND HUNTER'S SYNDROMES BY PLASMA INFUSIONS. PROC. NAT. ACAD. SCI. 68* 303-307, 1971.

FOLEY, K. M., DANES, B. S. AND BEARN, A. G.* WHITE BLOOD CELL CULTURES IN GENETIC STUDIES ON THE HUMAN MUCOPOLYSACCHARIDOSES. SCIENCE 164* 424-426, 1969.

FRATANTONI, J. C., HALL, C. W. AND NEUFELD, E. F.* HURLER AND HUNTER SYNDROMES* MUTUAL CORRECTION OF THE DEFECT IN CULTURED FIBROBLASTS. SCIENCE 162* 570-572, 1968.

FRATANTONI, J. C., HALL, C. W. AND NEUFELD, E. F.* THE DEFECT IN HURLER'S AND HUNTER'S SYNDROMES* FAULTY DEGRADATION OF MUCOPOLYSACCHARIDE. PROC. NAT. ACAD. SCI. 60* 699-706, 1968.

FRATANTONI, J. C., NEUFELD, E. F., UHLENDORF, B. W. AND JACOBSON, C. B.* INTRAUTERINE DIAGNOSIS OF THE HURLER AND HUNTER SYNDROMES. NEW ENG. J. MED. 280* 686-688, 1969.

HO, M. W. AND O'BRIEN, J. S.* HURLER'S SYNDROME* DEFICIENCY OF A SPECIFIC BETA GALACTOSIDASE ISOENZYME. SCIENCE 165* 611-613, 1969.

LEROY, J. G. AND CROCKER, A. C.* STUDIES ON THE GENETICS OF THE HURLER-HUNTER SYNDROME. IN, ARONSON, S. M. AND VOLK, B. W. (EDS.)* INBORN DISORDERS OF

SPHINGOLIPID METABOLISM. OXFORD* PERGAMON PRESS, 1967. PP. 455-473.

MACBRINN, M., OKADA, S., WOOLLACOTT, M., PATEL, V., HO, M. W., TAPPEL, A. L. AND O'BRIEN, J. S.* BETA-GALACTOSIDASE DEFICIENCY IN THE HURLER SYNDROME. NEW ENG. J. MED. 281* 338-343, 1969.

MANLEY, G. AND HAWKSWORTH, J.* DIAGNOSIS OF HURLER'S SYNDROME IN THE HOSPITAL LABORATORY AND THE DETERMINATION OF ITS GENETIC TYPE. ARCH. DIS. CHILD. 41* 91-96, 1966.

MCKUSICK, V. A.* HERITABLE DISORDERS OF CONNECTIVE TISSUE. ST. LOUIS* C. V. MOSBY CO., 1966 (3RD. ED.).

MCKUSICK, V. A.* RELATIVE FREQUENCY OF THE HUNTER AND HURLER SYNDROMES. NEW ENG. J. MED. 283* 853-854, 1970.

NEUFELD, E. F. AND FRATANTONI, J. C.* INBORN ERRORS OF MUCOPOLYSACCHARIDE METABOLISM. FAULTY DEGRADATIVE MECHANISMS ARE IMPLICATED IN THIS GROUP OF HUMAN DISEASES. SCIENCE 169* 141-146, 1970.

NEUHAUSER, E. B., GRISCOM, N. T. AND GILLES, F. H.* ARACHNOID CYSTS IN THE HURLER-HUNTER SYNDROME. ANN. RADIOL. (PARIS) 11* 453-469, 1968.

SCHAFER, I. A., SULLIVAN, J. C., SVEJCAR, J., KOFOED, J. AND ROBERTSON, W. B.* STUDY OF THE HURLER SYNDROME USING CELL CULTURE* DEFINITION OF THE BIOCHEMICAL PHENOTYPE AND THE EFFECT OF ASCORBIC ACID ON THE MUTANT CELL. J. CLIN. INVEST. 47* 321-328, 1968.

SCHAFER, I. A., SULLIVAN, J. C., SVEJCAR, J., KOFOED, J. AND ROBERTSON, W. B.* VITAMIN C-INDUCED INCREASE OF DERMATAN SULFATE IN CULTURED HURLER'S FIBROBLASTS. SCIENCE 153* 1008-1010, 1966.

*25290 MUCOPOLYSACCHARIDOSIS TYPE III (SANFILIPPO SYNDROME)

R
E
C
E
S
S
I
V
E

IN THIS VARIETY ONLY HEPARITIN SULFATE IS EXCRETED IN THE URINE. THE CLINICAL FEATURES ARE SEVERE MENTAL DEFECT WITH RELATIVELY MILD SOMATIC FEATURES (MODERATE-LY SEVERE CLAW HAND AND VISCEROMEGALY, LITTLE OR NO CORNEAL CLOUDING OR SKELETAL, E.G., VERTEBRAL, CHANGE). THE PRESENTING PROBLEM MAY BE MARKED OVERACTIVITY, DESTRUCTIVE TENDENCIES AND OTHER BEHAVIORAL ABERRATIONS IN A CHILD OF 4 TO 6. MAROTEAUX (1966) REPORTED A KINDRED IN WHICH THREE SEPARATE CONSANGUINEOUS MARRIAGES RESULTED IN A TOTAL OF FOUR CASES. THE RADIOLOGIC FINDINGS IN THE SKELETON ARE RELATIVELY MILD AND CONSIST OF PERSISTENT BICONVEXITY OF THE VERTEBRAL BODIES, ABSENT HYDROCEPHALUS AND VERY THICK CALVARIUM.

LANGER, L. O.* THE RADIOGRAPHIC MANIFESTATIONS OF THE HS-MUCOPOLYSACCHARIDOSIS OF SANFILIPPO, WITH DISCUSSION OF THIS CONDITION IN RELATION TO THE OTHER MUCOPOLYSACCHARIDOSES AND A CLASSIFICATION OF THESE FUNDAMENTALLY SIMILAR ENTITIES. ANN. RADIOL. 7* 315-325, 1964.

MAROTEAUX, P., FREZAL, J., TAHBAZ-ZADEH AND LAMY, M.* UNE OBSERVATION FAMILIALE D'OLIGOPHRENIE POLYDYSTROPHIQUE. J. GENET. HUM. 15* 93-102, 1966.

MCKUSICK, V. A., KAPLAN, D., WISE, D., HANLEY, W. B., SUDDARTH, S. B., SEVICK, M. E. AND MAUMANEE, A. E.* THE GENETIC MUCOPOLYSACCHARIDOSES. MEDICINE 44* 445-483, 1965.

SANFILIPPO, S. J., PODOSIN, R., LANGER, L. AND GOOD, R. A.* MENTAL RETARDATION ASSOCIATED WITH ACID MUCOPOLYSACCHARIDURIA (HEPARITIN SULFATE TYPE). J. PEDIAT. 63* 837-838, 1963.

SPRANGER, J., TELLER, W., KOSENOW, W., MURKEN, J. AND ECKERT-HUSEMAN, E.* DIE HS-MUCOPOLYSACCHARIDOSE VON SANFILIPPO (POLYDYSTROPHE OLIGOPHRENIE). BERICHT UBER 10 PATIENTEN. Z. KINDERHEILK. 101* 71-84, 1967.

WALLACE, B. J., KAPLAN, D., ADACHI, M., SCHNECK, L. AND VOLK, B. W.* MUCOPOLY-SACCHARIDOSIS TYPE III. MORPHOLOGIC AND BIOCHEMICAL STUDIES OF TWO SIBLINGS WITH SANFILIPPO SYNDROME. ARCH. PATH. 82* 462-473, 1966.

*25300 MUCOPOLYSACCHARIDOSIS TYPE IV (MORQUIO SYNDROME)

IT SEEMS LIKELY THAT THE CONDITION DESCRIBED IN 1929 BY MORQUIO IN MONTEVIDEO AND BRAILSFORD IN BIRMINGHAM, ENG., WAS THE ENTITY IN WHICH WE NOW RECOGNIZE THE OCCURRENCE OF CORNEAL CLOUDING, AORTIC VALVE DISEASE AND URINARY EXCRETION OF KERATOSULFATE. BETWEEN 1929 AND 1959 A MISCELLANY OF SKELETAL DISORDERS WAS INCLUDED IN THE MORQUIO CATEGORY. THESE INCLUDED VARIOUS TYPES OF SPONDYLO-EPIPHYSEAL DYSPLASIA AND MULTIPLE EPIPHYSEAL DYSPLASIA. IN THE LATE 1950'S WHEN MUCOPOLYSACCHARIDURIA AND EXTRA-SKELETAL FEATURES WERE RECOGNIZED, THE EPONYM MORQUIO-ULLRICH WAS PROPOSED. IT SEEMS PERFERABLE, HOWEVER, TO RETAIN THE DESIGNATION MORQUIO SYNDROME FOR THIS CONDITION AND TO SEPARATE OUT THE SIMULATING CONDITIONS WHICH REPRESENT ENTITIES DISTINCT FROM THAT DESCRIBED BY MORQUIO AND BRAILSFORD. THIS AND SOME OTHER FORMS OF SPONDYLOEPIPHYSEAL DYSPLASIA ARE PRONE TO THE DANGEROUS COMPLICATIONS OF ATLANTO-AXIAL DISLOCATION, DUE TO HYPOPLASIA OF

BLAW, M. E. AND LANGER, L. O.* SPINAL CORD COMPRESSION IN MORQUIO-BRAILSFORD'S DISEASE. J. PEDIAT. 74* 593-600, 1969.

GREENBERG, A. D.* ATLANTO-AXIAL DISLOCATIONS. BRAIN 91* 655-684, 1968.

LANGER, L. O., JR. AND CAREY, L. S.* THE ROENTGENOGRAPHIC FEATURES OF THE KS MUCOPOLYSACCHARIDOSIS OF MORQUIO (MORQUIO-BRAILFORD'S DISEASE). AM. J. ROENTGEN. 97* 1-20, 1966.

LINKER, A., EVANS, L. R. AND LANGER, L. O.* MORQUIO'S DISEASE AND MUCOPOLYSAC-CHARIDE EXCRETION. J. PEDIAT. 77* 1039-1047, 1970.

MAROTEAUX, P. AND LAMY, M.* OPACITES CORNEENNES ET TROUBLES METABOLIQUES DANS LA MALADIE DE MORQUIO. REV. FRANC. ETUD. CLIN. BIOL. 6* 481-483, 1961.

PEDRINI, V., LENNZI, L. AND ZAMTOTTI, V.* ISOLATION AND IDENTIFICATION OF KERATOSULPHATE IN URINE OF PATIENTS AFFECTED BY MORQUIO-JLLRICH DISEASE. PROC. SOC. EXP. BIOL. MED. 110* 847-849, 1962.

ROBINS, M. M., STEVENS, H. F. AND LINKER, A.* MORQUIO'S DISEASE* AN ABNORMALITY OF MUCOPOLYSACCHARIDE METABOLISM. J. PEDIAT. 62* 881-889, 1963.

VON NOORDEN, G. K., ZELLWEGER, H. AND PONSETI, I. V.* OCULAR FINDINGS IN MORQUIO-ULLRICH'S DISEASE. ARCH. OPHTHAL. 64* 585-591, 1960.

ZELLWEGER, H., PONSETI, I. V., PEDRINI, V., STAMLER, F. S. AND VON NOORDEN, G. K.* MORQUIO-ULLRICH'S DISEASE. REPORT OF 2 CASES. J. PEDIAT. 59* 549-561, 1961.

*25310 MUCOPOLYSACCHARIDOSIS TYPE V (SCHEIE'S SYNDROME, LATE HURLER'S SYNDROME, ETC.)

STIFF JOINTS, CLOUDING OF THE CORNEA MOST DENSE PERIPHERALLY, SURVIVAL TO A LATE AGE WITH LITTLE IF ANY IMPAIRMENT OF INTELLECT, AND AORTIC REGURGITATION ARE FEATURES. CHONDROITIN SULFATE B IS EXCRETED IN THE URINE IN EXCESS. THE SECOND CASE OF EMERIT ET AL. (1966) WAS PROBABLY OF THIS TYPE. THE PARENTS WERE SECOND COUSINS. THE FACIES AND HANDS WERE CHARACTERISTIC AND AORTIC REGURGITATION WAS PRESENT. THE PATIENT, A 32 YEAR OLD FEMALE, HAD A SON WITH TRICUSPID ATRESIA AND SITUS INVERSUS. THE SISTERS, AGES 47 AND 55, REPORTED BY KOSKENOJA AND SUVANTO (1959) PROBABLY HAD THIS CONDITION. THE CASE OF POULET (1968) WITH TWO AFFECTED COUSINS WAS PROBABLY SCHEIE'S SYNDROME. WEISMANN AND NEUFELD (1970) FOUND SURPRISINGLY NO CROSS-CORRECTION OF SCHEIE AND HURLER FIBROBLASTS, BUT THE EXPECTED CROSS-CORRECTION OF SCHEIE FIBROBLASTS WITH THOSE FROM SANFILIPPO AND HUNTER PATIENTS. THE POSSIBLE INTERPRETATIONS INCLUDE ALLELISM OF THE TWO GENES, EITHER DIFFERENT AMINO ACIDS SUBSTITUTED AT THE SAME SITE IN THE CISTRON WITH DIFFERENT CHANGES IN THE PROPERTIES OF THE PRODUCT PROTEIN (ENZYME) AS IN HB S AND HB C, OR AMINO ACIDS SUBSTITUTED AT DIFFERENT SITES IN THE SAME CISTRON, AGAIN WITH QUITE DIFFERENT EFFECTS ON THE PROPERTIES OF THE PRODUCT PROTEIN, AS IN HB S AND HB M(SASKATOON). IN THE LATTER SITUATION, THE TERM HETEROALLELE IS SOMETIMES USED. IT IS THEORETICALLY POSSIBLE THAT SOME OF THE PHENOTYPICALLY OVERLAPPING, 'NEW' MUCOPOLYSACCHARIDOSES THAT ARE BEING DESCRIBED ARE EXAMPLES OF SO-CALLED COMPOUNDS OF HETEROALLELES, COMPARABLE TO THE SC SITUATION. IN SUCH INSTANCES THE PARENTS WOULD NOT BE EXPECTED TO BE CONSANGUINEOUS.

RECESSIVE

EMERIT, I., MAROTEAUX, P. AND VERNANT, P.* DEUX OBSERVATIONS DE MUCOPOLYSAC-CHARIDOSE AVEC ATTEINTE CARDIO-VASCULAIRE. ARCH. FRANC. PEDIAT. 23* 1075-1087, 1966.

KOSKENOJA, M. AND SUVANTO, E.* GARGOYLISM* REPORT OF ADULT FORM WITH GLAUCOMA IN TWO SISTERS. ACTA OPHTHAL. 37* 234-240, 1959.

POULET, J.* MUCOPOLYSACCHARIDOSE DU TYPE HURLER I SANS DETERIORATION MENTALE CHEZ UN ADULTE ET SES DEUX GERMAINS. SEM. HOP. PARIS 44* 2545-2554, 1968.

SCHEIE, H. G., HAMBRICK, G. W., JR. AND BARNESS, L. A.* A NEWLY RECOGNIZED FORME FRUSTE OF HURLER'S DISEASE (GARGOYLISM). AM. J. OPHTHAL. 53* 753-769, 1962.

WEISMANN, V. AND NEUFELD, E. F.* SCHEIE AND HURLER SYNDROMES* APPARENT IDENTITY OF THE BIOCHEMICAL DEFECT. SCIENCE 169* 72-74, 1970.

*25320 MUCOPOLYSACCHARIDOSIS TYPE VI (MAROTEAUX-LAMY SYNDROME)

THE CLINICAL CHARACTERISTICS ARE STRIKING OSSEOUS AND CORNEAL CHANGES (LIKE THOSE OF MPS I) WITHOUT INTELLECTUAL IMPAIRMENT. ONLY (OR PREDOMINANTLY) CHONDROITIN SULFATE B IS EXCRETED IN THE URINE.

GOLDBERG, M. F., SCOTT, C. I. AND MCKUSICK, V. A.* HYDROCEPHALUS AND PAPILLEDE-MA IN THE MAROTEAUX-LAMY SYNDROME (MUCOPOLYSACCHARIDOSIS TYPE VI). AM. J. OPHTHAL. 69* 969-975, 1970.

MAROTEAUX, P. AND LAMY, M.* HURLER'S DISEASE, MORQUIO'S DISEASE, AND RELATED MUCOPOLYSACCHARIDOSES. J. PEDIAT. 67* 312-323, 1965.

MAROTEAUX, P., LEVEQUE, B., MARIE, J. AND LAMY, M.* UNE NOUVELLE DYSOSTOSE AVEC ELIMINATION URINAIRE DE CHONDROITINE-SULFATE B. PRESSE MED. 71* 1849-1852, 1963.

*25330 MUSCULAR ATROPHY, INFANTILE (WERDNIG-HOFFMANN)

THE AGE OF ONSET IS THE MAIN FEATURE DISTINGUISHING THE INFANTILE (WERDNIG-HOFFMANN) AND JUVENILE (KUGELBERG-WELANDER) TYPES.

MARQUARDT, MACLOWRY AND PERRY (1962), AMONG OTHERS, HAVE DESCRIBED THE DISORDER IN TWINS. BRANDT (1949) REPORTED THE LARGEST SINGLE STUDY, INVOLVING 112 CASES IN 70 FAMILIES. SEGREGATION ANALYSIS YIELDED RESULTS CONSISTENT WITH AUTOSOMAL RECESSIVE INHERITANCE. ALMOST 6 PERCENT OF PARENTS WERE CONSANGUINEOUS, A VALUE 8 TIMES THAT IN CONTROLS. IN 51 OF 112, THE SPINAL TYPE WAS PROVED. IN 2 OR 3 THE MYOPATHIC TYPE WAS PROVED. IN 59 THE TYPE WAS NOT DETERMINED. WERDNIG-HOFFMANN PARALYSIS WAS PRESENT IN SEVERAL MEMBERS OF THE INBRED GROUP OF SCOTTISH TINKERS WITH FAMILIAL GOITER (SEE THYROID HORMONOGENESIS, GENETIC DEFECT IN, IV). HOGENHUIS ET AL. (1967) REPORTED SPECIAL STUDIES OF A CHINESE FAMILY IN WHICH 4 OF 8 SIBS SUCCUMBED TO WERDNIG-HOFFMANN DISEASE.

BRANDT, S.* HEREDITARY FACTORS IN INFANTILE PROGRESSIVE MUSCULAR ATROPHY. STUDY OF ONE-HUNDRED AND TWELVE CASES IN SEVENTY FAMILIES. AM. J. DIS. CHILD. 78* 226-236, 1949.

BRANDT, S.* WERDNIG-HOFFMANN'S INFANTILE PROGRESSIVE MUSCULAR ATROPHY. OP. EX. DOMO BIOL. HERED. HUM. U. HAFNIENSIS 22* 1-328, 1950.

GAMSTORP, I.* PROGRESSIVE SPINAL MUSCULAR ATROPHY WITH ONSET IN INFANCY OR EARLY CHILDHOOD. ACTA PAEDIAT. SCAND. 56* 408-423, 1967.

HANHART, E.* DIE INFANTILE PROGRESSIVE SPINALE MUSKELATROPHIE (WERDNIG-HOFFMANN) ALS EINFACH-REZESSIVE, SUBLETALE MUTATION AUF GRUND VON 29 FALLEN IN 14 SIPPEN. HELV. PAEDIAT. ACTA 1* 110-133, 1945.

HOGENHUIS, L. A., SPAULDING, S. W. AND ENGEL, W. K.* NEURONAL RNA METABOLISM IN INFANTILE SPINAL MUSCULAR ATROPHY (WERDNIG-HOFFMANN'S DISEASE) STUDIED BY RADIOAUTOGRAPHY* A NEW TECHNIC IN THE INVESTIGATION OF NEUROLOGICAL DISEASE. J. NEUROPATH. EXP. NEUROL. 26* 335-341, 1967.

MARQUARDT, J. E., MACLOWRY, J. AND PERRY, R. E.* INFANTILE PROGRESSIVE SPINAL MUSCULAR ATROPHY IN IDENTICAL NEGRO TWINS. NEW ENG. J. MED. 267* 386-388, 1962.

*25340 MUSCULAR ATROPHY, JUVENILE (KUGELBERG-WELANDER)

KUGELBERG AND WELANDER (1956) FOUND 5 AFFECTED CHILDREN AMONG THE 12 OFFSPRING OF NORMAL PARENTS* TWO OF THE FIVE WERE MONOZYGOTIC TWINS. SPIRA (1963) DESCRIBED 7 AFFECTED MEMBERS IN TWO SIBSHIPS OF A FAMILY. IN EACH CASE THE AFFECTED PERSONS WERE OFFSPRING OF A FIRST COUSIN MARRIAGE. LEVY AND WITTIG (1962) DESCRIBED PROXIMAL MUSCULAR ATROPHY IN TWO HALF-BROTHERS, WITH ONSET AT 13 AND 16 YEARS. ONSET IS USUALLY BETWEEN 2 AND 17 YEARS. ATROPHY AND WEAKNESS OF PROXIMAL LIMB MUSCLES, PRIMARILY IN THE LEGS, IS FOLLOWED BY DISTAL INVOLVEMENT. USUALLY THE CASES ARE DIAGNOSED AS LIMB-GIRDLE MUSCULAR DYSTROPHY UNTIL THEY ARE STUDIED FULLY. TWITCHINGS (FASCICULATIONS) ARE AN IMPORTANT DIFFERENTIATING SIGN. MUSCULAR BIOPSY AND ELECTROMYOGRAPHY SHOW THE TRUE NATURE OF THE PROCESS AS A LOWER MOTOR NEURONE DISEASE. FURUKAWA ET AL. (1968) REPORTED TWO FAMILIES, EACH WITH AFFECTED BROTHER AND SISTER. THE PARENTS IN ONE WERE FIRST COUSINS. THEY POINTED OUT THAT IN THEIR CASES AS WELL AS THOSE IN THE LITERATURE THE SYMPTOMS OF FEMALE PATIENTS WERE MILD AND THE CLINICAL COURSE SLOW WHEREAS MALE SIBS WERE SEVERELY AFFECTED. THEY INTERPRETED THIS AS SEX-INFLUENCE. A DOMINANT FORM REPRESENTED BY THE MOTHER AND TWO CHILDREN DESCRIBED BY FORD (1961) MAY ALSO EXIST AND THIS MAY BE THE SAME AS WHAT HAS BEEN TERMED SCAPULOPERONEAL AMYOTROPHY (Q.V.).

FORD, F. R.* DISEASES OF THE NERVOUS SYSTEM IN INFANCY, CHILDHOOD AND ADOLES-CENCE. SPRINGFIELD, ILL.* CHARLES C THOMAS, 1961. P. 390.

FURUKAWA, T., NAKAO, K., SUGITA, H. AND TSUKAGOSHI, H.* KUGELBERG-WELANDER DISEASE, WITH PARTICULAR REFERENCE TO SEX-INFLUENCED MANIFESTATIONS. ARCH. NEUROL. 19* 156-162, 1968.

FURUKAWA, T., TSUKAGOSHI, H., SUGITA, H., KONDO, K. AND TSUBAKI, T.* CLINICAL AND GENETIC CONSIDERATIONS ON KUGELBERG-WELANDER'S DISEASE. CLIN. NEUROL. 6* 148-155, 1966.

HAUSMANOWA-PETRUSEWICZ, I., SOBKOWICZ, H., ZIELINSKA, S. AND DOBOSZ, I.* APROPOS OF HEREDOFAMILIAL JUVENILE MUSCULAR ATROPHY. SCHWEIZ. ARCH. NEUROL. PSYCHIAT. 90* 255-267, 1962.

KUGELBERG, E. AND WELANDER, L.* HEREDOFAMILIAL JUVENILE MUSCULAR ATROPHY SIMULATING MUSCULAR DYSTROPHY. ARCH. NEUROL. PSYCHIAT. 75* 500-509, 1956.

LEVY, J. A. AND WITTIG, E. O.* FAMILIAL PROXIMAL MUSCULAR ATROPHY. NEUROPSI-QUIATRIA 20* 233-237, 1962.

R
E
C
E
S
S
I
V
E

MEADOWS, J. C., MARSDEN, C. D. AND HARRIMAN, D. G. F.* CHRONIC SPINAL MUSCULAR ATROPHY IN ADULTS. I. THE KUGELBERG-WELANDER SYNDROME. J. NEUROL. SCI. 9* 527-550, 1969.

SMITH, J. B. AND PATEL, A.* THE WOHLFART-KUGELBERG-WELANDER DISEASE. REVIEW OF THE LITERATURE AND REPORT OF A CASE. NEUROLOGY 15* 469-473, 1965.

SPIRA, R.* NEUROGENIC, FAMILIAL, GIRDLE TYPE MUSCULAR ATROPHY (CLINICAL ELECTROMYOGRAPHIC AND PATHOLOGICAL STUDY). CONFIN. NEUROL. 23* 245-255, 1963.

25350 MUSCULAR ATROPHY, PROGRESSIVE

ASANO AND COLLEAGUES (1960) DESCRIBED A FORM OF DISTAL MUSCULAR ATROPHY BEGINNING IN THE FIRST YEAR OF LIFE. FEATURES INCLUDE IMPAIRED SENSIBILITY IN THE FEET, DYSARTHRIA, CHOREIC MOVEMENTS OF ARMS AND FACE, PARTIAL OPTIC ATROPHY, SCOLIOSIS, INCONTINENCE, MENTAL DEFICIENCY AND INCREASED DEEP TENDON REFLEXES.

ASANO, N. AND COLLEAGUES* A PECULIAR TYPE OF PROGRESSIVE MUSCULAR ATROPHY. JAP. J. HUM. GENET. 5* 139, 1960.

*25360 MUSCULAR DYSTROPHY I (LIMB-GIRDLE, PELVO-FEMORAL OR LEYDEN-MOEBIUS TYPE)

THE LIMB-GIRDLE TYPE OF MUSCULAR DYSTROPHY HAS ITS ONSET USUALLY IN CHILDHOOD BUT SOMETIMES IN MATURITY OR MIDDLE AGE. INVOLVEMENT IS FIRST EVIDENT IN EITHER THE PELVIC OR, LESS FREQUENTLY, THE SHOULDER GIRDLE, OFTEN WITH ASYMMETRY OF WASTING WHEN THE UPPER LIMBS ARE FIRST INVOLVED. SPREAD FROM THE LOWER TO THE UPPER LIMBS OR VICE VERSA OCCURS WITHIN TWENTY YEARS. PSEUDOHYPERTROPHY OF THE CALVES *IS UNCOMMON BUT MAY BE COUNTERFEITED BY A STOCKY BUILD OR WASTING OF THE VASTI* (CHUNG AND MORTON, 1959). THE RATE OF PROGRESSION IS VARIABLE. SEVERE DISABILITY WITH INABILITY TO WALK IS SEEN WITHIN 20-30 YEARS OF ONSET. CONTRACTURES AND FACIAL WEAKNESS OCCUR ONLY LATE IN SOME CASES. AGE AT DEATH SHOWS A WIDE SPREAD WITH THE LARGEST NUMBER DYING IN MIDDLE LIFE.
ONLY 59 PERCENT OF CASES OF LIMB-GIRDLE MUSCULAR DYSTROPHY COULD, IN THE ANALYSIS OF CHUNG AND MORTON (1959), BE ASCRIBED TO AUTOSOMAL RECESSIVE INHERITANCE. THE REMAINDER WERE SPORADIC CASES OF UNKNOWN ETIOLOGY. BY AN INGENIOUS MATHEMATICAL ANALYSIS MORTON (1960) CONCLUDED THAT HOMOZYGOSITY AT EITHER OF TWO LOCI MAY RESULT IN LIMB-GIRDLE MUSCULAR DYSTROPHY AND THAT ABOUT 1.6 PERCENT OF THE NORMAL POPULATION IS HETEROZYGOUS FOR A LIMB-GIRDLE MUSCULAR DYSTROPHY GENE.
PFANDLER (1950) REPORTED AN EXTENSIVE SWISS PEDIGREE WHICH WAS REPRODUCED BY TOURAINE (1955). JACKSON AND CAREY (1961) FOUND THE SAME TYPE OF MUSCULAR DYSTROPHY IN THE DESCENDANTS OF SWISS IMMIGRANTS IN A RELIGIOUS ISOLATE (AMISH) IN INDIANA. CARDIAC INVOLVEMENT IN BROTHER AND SISTER WITH THIS TYPE WAS NOTED BY FELSCH ET AL. (1966).

R
E
C
E
S
S
I
V
E

CHUNG, C. S. AND MORTON, N. E.* DISCRIMINATION OF GENETIC ENTITIES IN MUSCULAR DYSTROPHY. AM. J. HUM. GENET. 11* 339-359, 1959.

FELSCH, G., HOFFMEYER, O. AND RICHTER, G.* HERZBETEILUNG BEI DYSTROPHIA MUSCULORUM PROGRESSIVA (ERB). Z. GES. INN. MED. 21* 73-79, 1966.

JACKSON, C. E. AND CAREY, J. H.* PROGRESSIVE MUSCULAR DYSTROPHY* AUTOSOMAL RECESSIVE TYPE. PEDIATRICS 28* 77-84, 1961.

JACKSON, C. E. AND STREHLER, D. A.* LIMB-GIRDLE MUSCULAR DYSTROPHY* CLINICAL MANIFESTATIONS AND DETECTION OF PRECLINICAL DISEASE. PEDIATRICS 41* 495-502, 1968.

MORTON, N. E. AND CHUNG, C. S.* FORMAL GENETICS OF MUSCULAR DYSTROPHY. AM. J. HUM. GENET. 11* 360-379, 1959.

MORTON, N. E.* THE MUTATIONAL LOAD DUE TO DETRIMENTAL GENES IN MAN. AM. J. HUM. GENET. 12* 348-364, 1960.

PFANDLER, U.* EINE EINFACH REZESSIVE FORM DER DYSTROPHIA MUSCULORUM PROGRESSIVA MIT EINER SIPPENSTAMMTAFEL AUS DEM EMMENTAL (SCHWEIZ). DEUTSCH. MED. WSCHR. 75* 1221-1225, 1950.

TOURAINE, A.* L'HEREDITE EN MEDECINE. PARIS* MASSON, 1955. P. 710.

*25370 MUSCULAR DYSTROPHY II (RESEMBLING X-LINKED DUCHENNE MUSCULAR DYSTROPHY)

AUTOSOMAL RECESSIVE INHERITANCE OF MUSCULAR DYSTROPHY RESEMBLING THE X-LINKED DUCHENNE TYPE HAS BEEN REPORTED BY KLOEPFER AND TALLEY (1958), DUBOWITZ (1960) AND SKYRING AND MCKUSICK (1961), AMONG OTHERS. ONSET BEFORE 5 YEARS, CONFINEMENT TO WHEELCHAIR BY 12 YEARS AND DEATH USUALLY BEFORE 20 YEARS CHARACTERIZE THE COURSE. PSEUDOHYPERTROPHY IS PRESENT. SKYRING AND MCKUSICK (1961) SUGGESTED THAT THE SIGNS OF CARDIAC INVOLVEMENT PRESENT IN THE X-LINKED FORM MAY BE LACKING IN THE AUTOSOMAL VARIETY. IN 1971, THROUGH THE COURTESY OF KLOEPFER, I HAD AN OPPORTUNITY TO RESTUDY TWO AFFECTED MEMBERS, A BROTHER AND SISTER (IX,22 AND IX,23 OF THE ORIGINAL PEDIGREE), REPORTED BY KLOEPFER AND TALLEY (1958). THEY WERE THEN 30 AND 27 YEARS OLD, RESPECTIVELY, AND HAD EVIDENCE OF CARDIAC INVOLVEMENT WITH CHRONIC CONGESTIVE HEART FAILURE IN THE GIRL AND ARRHYTHMIA WITH CORONARY SINUS RHYTHM BY

ELECTROCARDIOGRAM IN THE MALE. THE GIRL HAD TWO CHILDREN OF AGES 6 AND 4 YEARS.

DUBOWITZ, V.* PROGRESSIVE MUSCULAR DYSTROPHY OF THE DUCHENNE TYPE IN FEMALES AND ITS MODE OF INHERITANCE. BRAIN 83* 432-439, 1960.

KLOEPFER, H. W. AND TALLEY, C.* AUTOSOMAL RECESSIVE INHERITANCE OF DUCHENNE-TYPE MUSCULAR DYSTROPHY. ANN. HUM. GENET. 22* 138-143, 1958.

SKYRING, A. AND MCKUSICK, V. A.* CLINICAL, GENETIC AND ELECTROCARDIOGRAPHIC STUDIES IN CHILDHOOD MUSCULAR DYSTROPHY. AM. J. MED. SCI. 242* 534-547, 1961.

25380 MUSCULAR DYSTROPHY, CONGENITAL PROGRESSIVE, WITH MENTAL RETARDATION

PARENTAL CONSANGUINITY WAS PRESENT IN 6 FAMILIES STUDIED BY FUKUYAMA ET AL. (1960). IN TWO SIBSHIPS MULTIPLE CASES WERE OBSERVED.

FUKUYAMA, F., KAWOZURA, M. AND HARUNA, H.* A PECULIAR FORM OF CONGENITAL MUSCULAR DYSTROPHY* REPORT OF 15 CASES. PEDIATRICA 44* 5, 1960.

*25390 MUSCULAR DYSTROPHY, CONGENITAL, PRODUCING ARTHROGRYPOSIS

PEARSON AND FOWLER (1963) DESCRIBED NON-PROGRESSIVE MYOPATHY IN SIBS, PRODUCING THE ARTHROGRYPOSIS SYNDROME (Q.V.). A SIMILAR SITUATION MAY HAVE EXISTED IN THE FAMILY REPORTED BY BANKER ET AL. (1957) AND POSSIBLY THE SAME CONDITION WAS REPORTED BY LOWENTHAL AS MYOSCLEROSIS (Q.V.). THUS, CONGENITAL MYOPATHY MAY PRODUCE IN INFANCY THE PICTURE OF ARTHROGRYPOSIS OR THAT OF AMYOTONIA CONGENITA (SEE MYOPATHY, CONGENITAL, BATTEN-TURNER TYPE).

BANKER, B. Q., VICTOR, M. AND ADAMS, R. D.* ARTHROGRYPOSIS MULTIPLEX DUE TO CONGENITAL MUSCULAR DYSTROPHY. BRAIN 80* 319-334, 1957.

PEARSON, C. M. AND FOWLER, W. G., JR.* HEREDITARY NON-PROGRESSIVE MUSCULAR DYSTROPHY INDUCING ARTHROGRYPOSIS SYNDROME. BRAIN 86* 75-88, 1963.

25400 MUSCULAR DYSTROPHY, CONGENITAL, WITH INFANTILE CATARACT AND HYPOGONADISM

R
E
C
E
S
S
I
V
E

BASSOE (1956) DESCRIBED A SYNDROME OF CONGENITAL MUSCULAR DYSTROPHY INFANTILE CATARACT, AND HYPOGONADISM (IN FEMALES OVARIAN AGENESIS, IN MALES KLINEFETTER'S SYNDROME). SEVEN PERSONS LIVING IN A SMALL, ISOLATED NORWEGIAN VILLAGE WERE IDENTIFIED.

BASSOE, H. H.* FAMILIAL CONGENITAL MUSCULAR DYSTROPHY WITH GONADAL DYSGENESIS. J. CLIN. ENDOCR. 16* 1614-1621, 1956.

25410 MUSCULAR DYSTROPHY, CONGENITAL, WITH RAPID PROGRESSION

IN ADDITION TO THE SLOWLY PROGRESSIVE CONGENITAL MYOPATHY (Q.V.) DESCRIBED BY BATTEN AND TURNER, CONGENITAL MUSCULAR DYSTROPHY PRODUCING ARTHROGRYPOSIS, AND THAT ASSOCIATED WITH MENTAL RETARDATION, CONGENITAL AND RAPIDLY PROGRESSIVE MUSCULAR DYSTROPHY WAS REPORTED BY DE LANGE (1937) IN THREE MEMBERS OF EACH OF TWO SIBSHIPS RELATED AS SECOND COUSINS. THE CONDITION DESCRIBED BY SHORT (1963) AND BY WHARTON (1965) MAY BE THE SAME.

DE LANGE, C.* STUDIEN UBER ANGEBORENE LAHMUNGEN BZW. ANGEBORENE HYPOTONIE. ACTA PAEDIAT. 20 (SUPPL. III)* 1-51, 1937.

SHORT, J. K.* CONGENITAL MUSCULAR DYSTROPHY. A CASE REPORT WITH AUTOPSY FINDINGS. NEUROLOGY 13* 526-530, 1963.

WHARTON, B. A.* AN UNUSUAL VARIETY OF MUSCULAR DYSTROPHY. LANCET 1* 248-249, 1965.

25420 MYASTHENIA GRAVIS

ACCORDING TO CELESIA (1965), THE DISEASE HAS BEEN LIMITED TO ONE GENERATION IN 18 OF THE 22 REPORTED FAMILIES WITH MULTIPLE CASES. IN THE OTHER FOUR FAMILIES 2 GENERATIONS WERE AFFECTED. THE FAMILIAL FORM USUALLY AFFECTS YOUNG CHILDREN OR ADOLESCENTS AND ONSET IN ADULTHOOD IS RARE. THE FAMILIAL FORM IS, FURTHERMORE, STATIC OR ONLY SLOWLY PROGRESSIVE. WALSH AND HOYT (1959) AND ROTHBART (1937) EACH REPORTED A FAMILY WITH FOUR AFFECTED BROTHERS. AFFECTED BROTHER-SISTER PAIRS HAVE BEEN REPORTED BY TENG AND OSSERMAN (1956) AND CELESIA (1965) AMONG OTHERS. AFFECTED PARENT AND OFFSPRING WERE REPORTED BY FOLDES AND MCNALL (1960), AMONG OTHERS. KURLAND AND ALTER (1961) REVIEWED THE REPORTS OF FAMILIAL AGGREGATION AND TWIN CASES AND CONCLUDED THAT 'THERE IS AS YET INSUFFICIENT EVIDENCE TO SUGGEST THAT GENETIC FACTORS ARE OF SIGNIFICANCE IN THE ETIOLOGY OF MYASTHENIA GRAVIS.' KOTT AND BORNSTEIN (1969) OBSERVED FOUR AFFECTED SIBS. IT SEEMS LIKELY THAT A SMALL PROPORTION OF CASES ARE MENDELIAN. THE CHARACTERISTICS ARE ONSET IN THE FIRST YEAR OF LIFE, GOOD RESPONSE TO ANTI-CHOLINESTERASE DRUGS, GOOD PROGNOSIS AND ABSENCE OF ANTIMUSCLE ANTIBODIES IN THE SERUM. PARENTAL CONSANGUINITY HAS BEEN REPORTED IN AT LEAST TWO INSTANCES OF MULTIPLE AFFECTED SIBS.

CELESIA, G. G.* MYASTHENIA GRAVIS IN TWO SIBLINGS. ARCH. NEUROL. 12* 206-210,

FOLDES, F. F. AND MCNALL, P. G.* UNUSUAL FAMILIAL OCCURRENCE OF MYASTHENIA GRAVIS. J.A.M.A. 174* 418-420, 1960.

KOTT, E. AND BORNSTEIN, B.* FAMILIAL EARLY INFANTILE MYASTHENIA GRAVIS WITH A 15-YEAR FOLLOW-UP. J. NEUROL. SCI. 8* 573-578, 1969.

KURLAND, L. T. AND ALTER, M.* CURRENT STATUS OF THE EPIDEMIOLOGY AND GENETICS OF MYASTHENIA GRAVIS. MYASTHENIA GRAVIS (SECOND INTERNATIONAL SYMPOSIUM PROCEE-DINGS). VIETS, H. R. (ED.)* SPRINGFIELD, ILL.* CHARLES C THOMAS, 1961. PP. 307-336.

ROTHBART, H. B.* MYASTHENIA GRAVIS IN CHILDREN* ITS FAMILIAL INCIDENCE. J.A.M.A. 108* 715-717, 1937.

TENG, P. AND OSSERMAN, K. E.* STUDIES IN MYASTHENIA GRAVIS* NEONATAL AND JUVENILE TYPES. J. MOUNT SINAI HOSP. N.Y. 23* 711-727, 1956.

WALSH, F. B. AND HOYT, W. F.* EXTERNAL OPHTHALMOPLEGIA AS PART OF CONGENITAL MYASTHENIA IN SIBLINGS* MYASTHENIA GRAVIS IN CHILDREN* REPORT OF FAMILY SHOWING CONGENITAL MYASTHENIA. AM. J. OPHTHAL. 47* 28-34, 1959.

WARRIER, C. B. AND PILLAI, T. D.* FAMILIAL MYASTHENIA GRAVIS. BRIT. MED. J. 3* 839-840, 1967.

25430 MYASTHENIC MYOPATHY

JOHNS, DREIFUSS, CROWLEY AND FAKADEJ (1966) DESCRIBED A SIBSHIP OF 8 OF WHOM 4 (2 MALES, 2 FEMALES) DEVELOPED IN ADOLESCENCE A PROXIMAL MYOPATHY INVOLVING THE PECTORAL AND PELVIC GIRDLES. BY 10 YEARS AFTER ONSET THEY SHOWED A PROMINENT MYASTHENIC REACTION AND GOOD RESPONSE TO CHOLINESTERASE INHIBITORS. ELECTROMYO-GRAPHIC FINDINGS WERE TYPICAL OF MYASTHENIA GRAVIS.

JOHNS, T. R., DREIFUSS, F. E., CROWLEY, W. J. AND FAKADEJ, A. V.* FAMILIAL NONPROGRESSIVE MYASTHENIC MYOPATHY. (ABSTRACT) NEUROLOGY 16* 307 ONLY, 1966.

25440 MYCOSIS FUNGOIDES

IN BROTHER AND SISTER, SANDBANK AND KATZENELLENBOGEN (1968) OBSERVED MYCOSIS FUNGOIDES. FEW REPORTS OF FAMILIAL OCCURRENCE HAVE APPEARED. CAMERON (1933) REPORTED THE CONDITION IN MOTHER AND DAUGHTER.

CAMERON, O. J.* MYCOSIS FUNGOIDES IN MOTHER AND IN DAUGHTER. ARCH. DERM. 27* 232-236, 1933.

SANDBANK, M. AND KATZENELLENBOGEN, I.* MYCOSIS FUNGOIDES OF PROLONGED DURATION IN SIBLINGS. ARCH. DERM. 98* 620-627, 1968.

25450 MYELOMA, MULTIPLE

LEONCINI AND KORNGOLD (1964) DESCRIBED MULTIPLE MYELOMA IN TWO SISTERS AND REVIEWED THE LITERATURE ON FAMILIAL CASES. THOMAS (1964) OBSERVED MYELOMA IN A BROTHER AND SISTER. ALEXANDER AND BENNINGHOFF (1965) DESCRIBED 3 AFFECTED NEGRO SIBS. AFFECTED SIBS HAVE BEEN REPORTED BY A NUMBER OF OTHER AUTHORS. AXELSSON AND HALLEN (1965) FOUND TWO FAMILIES, ONE WITH TWO AND ONE WITH THREE SIBS, SHOWING HIGH M-COMPONENT ON A LARGE POPULATION SURVEY IN SWEDEN. IN A THIRD FAMILY TWO PERSONS WITH HIGH M-COMPONENT WERE MORE REMOTELY RELATED. THESE 7 WERE FROM A TOTAL GROUP OF 59 (OUT OF 7918) FOUND TO HAVE M-COMPONENT. THEIR CONDITION WAS CONSIDERED TO BE A VARIETY OF ESSENTIAL BENIGN MONOCLONAL HYPERGAMMAGLOBULINE-MIA. MANSON (1961) REPORTED AFFECTED SISTERS, ONE OF WHOM ALSO HAD PERNICIOUS ANEMIA. MYELOMA HAS ALSO BEEN OBSERVED IN FATHER AND SON (NADEAU ET AL., 1956). BERLIN ET AL. (1968) DESCRIBED FAMILIAL OCCURRENCE OF M-COMPONENTS. WHITEHOUSE (1971) OBSERVED AFFECTED BROTHER AND SISTER.

ALEXANDER, L. L. AND BENNINGHOFF, D. L.* FAMILIAL MULTIPLE MYELOMA. J. NAT. MED. ASS. 57* 471-475, 1965.

AXELSSON, U. AND HALLEN, J.* FAMILIAL OCCURRENCE OF PATHOLOGICAL SERUM-PROTEINS OF DIFFERENT GAMMA-GLOBULIN GROUPS. LANCET 2* 369-370, 1965.

BERLIN, S.-O., ODEBERG, H. AND WEINGART, L.* FAMILIAL OCCURRENCE OF M-COM-PONENTS. ACTA MED. SCAND. 183* 347-350, 1968.

HERRELL, W. E., RUFF, J. D. AND BAYRD, E. D.* MULTIPLE MYELOMA IN SIBLINGS. J.A.M.A. 167* 1485-1487, 1958.

LEONCINI, D. L. AND KORNGOLD, L.* MULTIPLE MYELOMA IN 2 SISTERS. AN IMMUNOCHE-MICAL STUDY. CANCER 17* 733-737, 1964.

MANSON, D. I.* MULTIPLE MYELOMA IN SISTERS. SCOT. MED. J. 6* 188 ONLY, 1961.

R
E
C
E
S
S
I
V
E

NADEAU, L. A., MAGALINI, S. I. AND STEFANINI, M.* FAMILIAL MULTIPLE MYELOMA. ARCH. PATH. 61* 101-106, 1956.

THOMAS, T. F.* MULTIPLE MYELOMA IN SIBLINGS. NEW YORK J. MED. 64* 2096-2099, 1964.

WHITEHOUSE, S.* BALTIMORE, MD.* PERSONAL COMMUNICATION, 1971.

*25460 MYELOPEROXIDASE DEFICIENCY

LEHRER AND CLINE (1969) FOUND NO DETECTABLE ACTIVITY OF THE LYSOSOMAL ENZYME MYELOPEROXIDASE (MPO) IN NEUTROPHILS AND MONOCYTES OF A PATIENT WITH DISSEMINATED CANDIDIASIS. OTHER GRANULE-ASSOCIATED ENZYMES WERE NORMAL. LEUKOCYTES FROM ONE OF THE PROBAND'S SISTERS ALSO SHOWED NO MPO ACTIVITY. LEUKOCYTES FROM THE PROBAND'S FOUR SONS SHOWED ABOUT ONE-THIRD NORMAL LEVELS. THE PROBAND AND HIS RELATIVES HAD NOT EXPERIENCED FREQUENT OR UNUSUAL BACTERIAL INFECTIONS. SALMON ET AL. (1970) DEMONSTRATED IMMUNOLOGICALLY ABSENCE OF MPO PROTEIN, AT LEAST ABSENCE OF CROSS-REACTING MATERIAL, IN HOMOZYGOTES. EOSINOPHILIC PEROXIDASE, WHICH IS CHEMICALLY DISTINCT FROM MLO WAS NORMAL.

LEHRER, R. I. AND CLINE, M. J.* LEUKOCYTE MYELOPEROXIDASE DEFICIENCY AND DISSEMINATED CANDIDIASIS* THE ROLE OF MYELOPEROXIDASE IN RESISTANCE TO CANDIDA INFECTION. J. CLIN. INVEST. 48* 1478-1488, 1969.

SALMON, S. E., CLINE, M. J., SCHULTZ, J. AND LEHRER, R. I.* MYELOPEROXIDASE DEFICIENCY* IMMUNOLOGIC STUDY OF A GENETIC LEUKOCYTE DEFECT. NEW ENG. J. MED. 282* 250-253, 1970.

25470 MYELOPROLIFERATIVE DISEASE

RANDALL, ET AL. (1965) OBSERVED A SEVERE MYELOPROLIFERATIVE DISORDER WITH FEATURES RESEMBLING CHRONIC OR SUBACUTE MYELOID LEUKEMIA IN 9 CHILDREN RELATED AS FIRST OR SECOND COUSINS. TWO CHILDREN RECOVERED COMPLETELY AFTER A CHRONIC ILLNESS OF 10-12 YEARS. NO CONSISTENT CHROMOSOMAL ABERRATION WAS FOUND. LOW LEUKOCYTE ALKALINE PHOSPHATASE WAS FOUND IN ALL AFFECTED CHILDREN AND IN 18 OF 20 ASYMPTOMATIC RELATIVES.

RANDALL, D. L., REIQUAM, C. W., GITHENS, J. H. AND ROBINSON, A.* FAMILIAL MYELOPROLIFERATIVE DISEASE. A NEW SYNDROME CLOSELY SIMULATING MYELOGENOUS LEUKEMIA IN CHILDHOOD. AM. J. DIS. CHILD. 110* 479-500, 1965.

*25480 MYOCLONIC EPILEPSY OF UNVERRICHT AND LUNDBORG

R
E
C
E
S
S
I
V
E

THE ONSET, OCCURRING BETWEEN 6 AND 13 YEARS OF AGE, IS CHARACTERIZED BY CONVUL-SIONS. MYOCLONUS BEGINS 1 TO 5 YEARS LATER. THE TWITCHINGS OCCUR PREDOMINANTLY IN THE PROXIMAL MUSCLES OF THE EXTREMITIES AND ARE BILATERALLY SYMMETRICAL, ALTHOUGH ASYNCHRONOUS. AT FIRST SMALL, THEY BECOME LATE IN THE CLINICAL COURSE SO VIOLENT THAT THE VICTIM IS THROWN TO THE FLOOR. MENTAL DETERIORATION AND EVENTUALLY DEMENTIA DEVELOP. SIGNS OF CEREBELLAR ATAXIA ARE PRESENT LATE IN THE COURSE, WHICH USUALLY IS 10 TO 20 YEARS IN DURATION. NOAD AND LANCE (1960) DESCRIBED MYOCLONIC EPILEPSY WITH CEREBELLAR ATAXIA IN SEVERAL OFFSPRING OF A MATING OF FIRST COUSINS ONCE REMOVED.
STEVENSON POINTED OUT, IN A DISCUSSION OF GENETIC ASPECTS OF THE STUDY BY HARRIMAN AND MILLAR (1955), THAT LUNDBORG'S STUDY IS 'OF CONSIDERABLE HISTORIC INTEREST IN HUMAN GENETICS.' LUNDBORG'S DATA WERE USED TO DEMONSTRATE CLEARLY FOR THE FIRST TIME THE PATTERN OF SIMPLE RECESSIVE INHERITANCE IN MAN. THE STATISTI-CAL ANALYSIS WAS DONE FIRST BY WEINBERG (1912) AND LATER BY BERNSTEIN (1929).
MYOCLONIC EPILEPSY IS A SYMPTOM OF A NUMBER OF THE CNS DISORDERS LISTED IN THIS CATALOG, INCLUDING AMAUROTIC IDIOCY AND THE VARIOUS DEGENERATIVE DISORDERS. IN FACT, MYOCLONUS OCCURS WITH MOST BRAIN DISEASES OF CHILDREN. FOR EXAMPLE, THE SIBS REPORTED BY MORSE (1949) AS MYOCLONIC EPILEPSY WERE REPORTED BY FORD, LIVINGSTON AND PRYLES (1951) AS 'FAMILIAL DEGENERATION OF THE CEREBRAL GRAY MATTER IN CHILDHOOD.' IN THE SPECIFIC ENTITY WHICH DESERVES TO BE CALLED MYOCLONIC EPILEPSY AND WHICH IS REPRESENTED BY THE CASES OF UNVERRICHT (1891) AND LUNDBORG (1913), INTRACELLULAR LAFORA BODIES SUGGESTING AMYLOID ARE FOUND IN THE BRAIN AND SIMILAR INCLUSIONS IN THE CELLS OF THE HEART AND LIVER (HARRIMAN AND MILLAR, 1955). THE LAFORA MATERIAL HAS THE PROPERTIES OF AN ACID MUCOPOLYSACCHARIDE. YOKOI ET AL. (1968) ARRIVED AT A PRELIMINARY CONCLUSION THAT THE LAFORA BODY IS POLYGLYCOSAN IN NATURE. THEY PICTURED THE EXISTENCE OF AN ENZYME DEFECT WHICH LEADS TO DEPOSITION OF POLYGLUCOSANS NEAR THEIR SITE OF SYNTHESIS IN THE AGRANULAR ENDOPLASMIC RETICULUM. SCHWARZ AND YANOFF (1965) DESCRIBED A BROTHER AND SISTER, OFFSPRING OF A ONE AND ONE HALF COUSIN MARRIAGE, WITH THIS DISEASE. SEIZURES BEGAN AT AGE 15 IN THE BOY WITH SLOWLY PROGRESSIVE MOTOR AND MENTAL DETERIORATION TO DEATH AT AGE TWENTY THREE AND ONE HALF YEARS. THE SISTER'S SEIZURES BEGAN AT AGE 14 AND PROGRESSION TO DEMENTIA AND BLINDNESS OCCURRED, WITH DEATH AT AGE 19. INTRA AND EXTRACELLULAR LAFORA BODIES WERE FOUND IN THE CNS, RETINA, AXIS CYLINDERS OF SPINAL NERVES, HEART MUSCLE, LIVER CELLS AND STRIATED MUSCLE FIBERS. DIAGNOSIS BY LIVER BIOPSY OR MUSCLE BIOPSY WAS PROPOSED. VOGEL, HAFNER AND DIEBOLD (1965) HAVE SUGGESTED THE EXISTENCE OF TWO RECESSIVELY INHERITED TYPES, BOTH OF WHICH SHOW LAFORA BODIES* (1) THE UNVERRICHT OR 'CLASSICAL' TYPE HAS A RELATIVELY MALIGNANT COURSE WITH EARLY DEATH. (2) THE LUNDBORG TYPE PURSUES A RELATIVELY BENIGN COURSE WITH DEATH AT A LATER STAGE. KRAUS-RUPPERT ET AL. (1970)

ALSO THOUGHT THAT THE LUNDBORG AND UNVERRICHT TYPES ARE DISTINGUISHABLE.
SEE ALSO DEAF-MUTISM WITH FAMILIAL MYOCLONUS EPILEPSY. BY THIS CLASSIFICA-
TION THE CASE OF JANEWAY ET AL. (1967) PROBABLY REPRESENTED UNVERRICHT'S TYPE
(ALTHOUGH THE AUTHORS THOUGHT OTHERWISE). THERE IS ALSO AN AUTOSOMAL DOMINANT
TYPE (WITHOUT LAFORA BODIES). FLUHARTY ET AL. (1970) DESCRIBED IN CULTURED
FIBROBLASTS BODIES WHICH MAY BE THE EQUIVALENT OF THE LAFORA BODY OBSERVED
HISTOLOGICALLY.

FORD, F. R., LIVINGSTON, S. AND PRYLES, C. V.* FAMILIAL DEGENERATION OF
CEREBRAL GRAY MATTER IN CHILDHOOD, WITH CONVULSIONS, MYOCLONUS, SPASTICITY,
CEREBELLAR ATAXIA, CHOREOATHETOSIS, DEMENTIA, AND DEATH IN STATUS EPILEPTICUS*
DIFFERENTIATION OF INFANTILE AND JUVENILE TYPES. J. PEDIAT. 39* 33-43, 1951.

FLUHARTY, A. L., PORTER, M. T., HIRSH, G. A., PEVIDA, E. AND KIHARA, H.*
METACHROMASIA IN FIBROBLASTS FROM A PATIENT WITH LAFORA'S DISEASE. (LETTER)
LANCET 2* 109-110, 1970.

HARRIMAN, D. G. F. AND MILLAR, J. H. D.* PROGRESSIVE FAMILIAL MYOCLONIC
EPILEPSY IN 3 FAMILIES* ITS CLINICAL FEATURES AND PATHOLOGICAL BASIS. BRAIN 78*
325-349, 1955.

JANEWAY, R., RAVENS, J. R., PEARCE, L. A., ODOR, D. L. AND SUZUKI, K.*
PROGRESSIVE MYOCLONUS EPILEPSY WITH LAFORA INCLUSION BODIES. I. CLINICAL,
GENETIC, HISTOPATHOLOGIC AND BIOCHEMICAL ASPECTS. ARCH. NEUROL. 16* 565-582,
1967.

KRAUS-RUPPERT, R., OSTERTAG, B. AND HAFNER, H.* A STUDY OF THE LATE FORM (TYPE
LUNDBORG) OF PROGRESSIVE MYOCLONIC EPILEPSY. J. NEUROL. SCI. 11* 1-16, 1970.

LUNDBORG, H. B.* DER ERBGANG DER PROGRESSIVEN MYOKLONUS-EPILEPSIE. (MYOKLONIE-
EPILEPSIE UNVERRICHT'S FAMILIARE MYOKLONIE). ZBL. GES NEUROL. PSYCHIAT. 9* 353-
358, 1912.

LUNDBORG, H. B.* DIE PROGRESSIVE MYOKLONUS-EPILEPSIE (UNVERRICHT'S MYOKLONIE).
UPSALA* ALMQVIST AND WIKSELL, 8* 567-570, 1903.

LUNDBORG, H. B.* MEDIZINISCH-BIOLOGISCHE FAMILIENFORSCHUNGEN INNERHALB EINES
2232 KOPFIGEN BAUERNGESCHLECHTES IN SCHWEDEN. JENA* FISCHER, 1913.

MORSE, W. I.* HEREDITARY MYOCLONUS EPILEPSY* TWO CASES WITH PATHOLOGICAL
FINDINGS. BULL. HOPKINS HOSP. 84* 116-134, 1949.

NOAD, K. B. AND LANCE, J. W.* FAMILIAL MYOCLONIC EPILEPSY AND ITS ASSOCIATION
WITH CEREBELLAR DISTURBANCE. BRAIN 83* 618-630, 1960.

SCHWARZ, G. A. AND YANOFF, M.* LAFORA'S DISEASE, DISTINCT CLINICO-PATHOLOGIC
FORM OF UNVERRICHT'S SYNDROME. ARCH. NEUROL. 12* 172-188, 1965.

UNVERRICHT, H.* DIE MYOCLONIE. BERLIN* FRANZ DEUTICKE, 1891.

VOGEL, F., HAFNER, H. AND DIEBOLD, K.* ZUR GENETIK DER PROGRESSIVEN MYOKLONUSE-
PILEPSIEN (UNVERRICHT-LUNDBORG). HUMANGENETIK 1* 437-475, 1965.

YANOFF, M. AND SCHWARTZ, G. A.* LAFORA'S DISEASE* A DISTINCT GENETICALLY
DETERMINED FORM OF UNVERRICHT'S SYNDROME. J. GENET. HUM. 14* 235-244, 1965.

YOKOI, S., AUSTIN, J., WITMER, F. AND SAKAI, M.* STUDIES IN MYOCLONUS EPILEPSY
(LAFORA BODY FORM). I. ISOLATION AND PRELIMINARY CHARACTERIZATION OF LAFORA
BODIES IN TWO CASES. ARCH. NEUROL. 19* 15-33, 1968.

R
E
C
E
S
S
I
V
E

25500 MYOPATHY PRODUCING CONGENITAL OPHTHALMOPLEGIA AND *FLOPPY BABY* SYNDROME

HURWITZ ET AL. (1969) DESCRIBED AFFECTED BROTHER AND SISTER. THEY AND BOTH
PARENTS HAD AMINOACIDURIA WHICH WAS OF UNCERTAIN RELATIONSHIP TO THE MYOPATHY.
CLINICALLY THE MYOPATHY MOST RESEMBLED THAT DESCRIBED BY BATTEN AND TURNER (SEE
MYOPATHY, CONGENITAL). OPHTHALMOPLEGIA AND FLOPPINESS ALSO OCCUR WITH MYOTUBULAR
MYOPATHY (SEE MYOPATHY, CENTRONUCLEAR) BUT THIS ENTITY WAS EXCLUDED BY THE MUSCLE
BIOPSY IN THE CASES OF HURWITZ ET AL. (1969).

HURWITZ, L. J., CARSON, N. A. J., ALLEN, I. V. AND CHOPRA, J. S.* CONGENITAL
OPHTHALMOPLEGIA, FLOPPY BABY SYNDROME, MYOPATHY AND AMINOACIDURIA. REPORT OF A
FAMILY. J. NEUROL. NEUROSURG. PSYCHIAT. 32* 495-508, 1969.

25510 MYOPATHY WITH ABNORMAL LIPID METABOLISM

BRADLEY ET AL. (1969) DESCRIBED THE CASE OF A 25 YEAR OLD WOMAN, OFFSPRING OF
FIRST-COUSIN PARENTS, WITH MYOPATHY INVOLVING THE MUSCLES OF THE NECK AND PROXIMAL
LIMBS. MUSCLE BIOPSY SHOWED INTERFIBRILLAR AND SUBSARCOLEMMAL VACUOLES, BY
HISTOCHEMICAL STUDY NORMAL TYPE-II MUSCLE FIBERS WITH EXCESSIVE NEUTRAL FAT AND
FREE FATTY ACIDS IN TYPE-I FIBERS, AND BY ELECTRON MICROSCOPY DEGENERATE MITOCHON-
DRIA. THE DEFECT MAY RESIDE IN THE PATHWAY OF FREE FATTY ACID OXIDATION. A
SPECIFIC LIPASE MAY BE DEFICIENT. ENGEL ET AL. (1970) DESCRIBED IDENTICAL TWIN

SISTERS, AGED 18 YEARS, WHO FROM EARLY CHILDHOOD HAD HAD MUSCLE ACHEING WITH MYOGLOBINURIA, SOMETIMES INDUCED BY EXERCISE. FASTING OR HIGH FAT, CARBOHYDRATE, ISOCALORIE DIET INDUCED MUSCLE ACHES, MARKED RISE IN THE SERUM LEVEL OF MUSCLE ENZYMES, AND NO KETONEMIA OR KETONURIA. SINCE ADMINISTRATION OF MEDIUM-CHAIN TRIGLYCERIDES PRODUCED THE EXPECTED NORMAL KETONEMIA AND KETONURIA, A DEFECT IN LONG-CHAIN FATTY ACID UTILIZATION WAS POSTULATED. A DEFECT IN AN ENERGY SOURCE TO MUSCLE WAS APPARENTLY RESPONSIBLE FOR THE SYMPTOMS. POSSIBLE IMPLICATION OF THE CARNITINE SYSTEM WAS SUGGESTED BY BRESSLER (1970).

BRADLEY, W. G., HUDGSON, P., GARDNER-MEDWIN, D. AND WALTON, J. N.* MYOPATHY ASSOCIATED WITH ABNORMAL LIPID METABOLISM IN SKELETAL MUSCLE. LANCET 1* 495-498, 1969.

BRESSLER, R.* CARNITINE AND THE TWINS. (EDITORIAL) NEW ENG. J. MED. 282* 745-746, 1970.

ENGEL, W. K., VICK, N. A., GLUECK, C. J. AND LEVY, R. I.* A SKELETAL-MUSCLE DISORDER ASSOCIATED WITH INTERMITTENT SYMPTOMS AND A POSSIBLE DEFECT OF LIPID METABOLISM. NEW ENG. J. MED. 282* 697-704, 1970.

25520 MYOPATHY, CENTRONUCLEAR (MYOTUBULAR MYOPATHY)

SHER ET AL. (1967) DESCRIBED TWO NEGRO SISTERS SUFFERING FROM GENERALIZED WEAKNESS AND WASTING. IN 80 TO 98 PERCENT OF MUSCLE FIBERS NUMEROUS NUCLEI WERE SITUATED CENTRALLY. LITTLE DEGENERATIVE CHANGE WAS EVIDENT IN THE MUSCLES. THE ASYMPTOMATIC MOTHER SHOWED A MIXTURE OF SMALL, CENTRALLY NUCLEATED FIBERS AND NORMAL FIBERS. CLINICALLY, THE MYOPATHY BEGAN EARLY IN LIFE AND PROGRESSED SLOWLY, RESULTING IN MARKED PTOSIS, GENERALIZED MUSCULAR ATROPHY AND SCOLIOSIS. AN ISOLATED CASE WAS REPORTED BY SPIRO ET AL. (1966) WHO CALLED IT MYOTUBULAR MYOPATHY. IN THE DEVELOPMENT OF SKELETAL MUSCLE A *MYOTUBULAR* STAGE WITH CENTRALLY LOCATED NUCLEI OCCURS IN UTERO AT ABOUT 10 WEEKS OF AGE. SPIRO ET AL. (1966) THOUGHT THIS DISEASE MAY REPRESENT PERSISTENCE OF FETAL MUSCLE. PEARSON ET AL. (1967) DESCRIBED A FEMALE PATIENT WITH EVIDENCE OF MYOPATHY FROM BIRTH. THE MOTHER, ALTHOUGH CLINICALLY NORMAL, SHOWED MINOR HISTOLOGIC ABNORMALITIES OF SKELETAL MUSCLE. KARPATI ET AL. (1970) DESCRIBED WHAT MAY BE THE SAME DISORDER IN MOTHER AND DAUGHTER. BRADLEY ET AL. (1970) DESCRIBED AFFECTED NEGRO BROTHERS WITH WEAKNESS BEGAN AT 8 AND 15 YEARS OF AGE AND DEATH AT 34 YEARS OF AGE IN BOTH. HETEROGENEITY IS SUGGESTED BY THE DESCRIPTION OF X-LINKED RECESSIVE INHERITANCE (Q.V.). BRADLEY ET AL. (1970) CONCLUDED THAT THE DISORDER IS A DEGENERATION, NOT A MATURATION ARREST.

BRADLEY, W. G., PRICE, D. L. AND WATANABE, C. K.* FAMILIAL CENTRONUCLEAR MYOPATHY. J. NEUROL. NEUROSURG. PSYCHIAT. 33* 687-693, 1970.

KARPATI, G., CARPENTER, S. AND NELSON, R. F.* TYPE I MUSCLE FIBRE ATROPHY AND CENTRAL NUCLEI* A RARE FAMILIAL NEUROMUSCULAR DISEASE. J. NEUROL. SCI. 10* 489-500, 1970.

PEARSON, C. M., COLEMAN, R. F., FOWLER, W. M., JR., MOMMAERTS, W. F. H. M., MUNSAT, T. L. AND PETER, J. B.* SKELETAL MUSCLE* BASIC AND CLINICAL ASPECTS AND ILLUSTRATIVE NEW DISEASES. ANN. INTERN. MED. 67* 614-650, 1967.

SHER, J. H., RIMALOVSKI, A. B., ATHANASSIADES, T. J. AND ARONSON, S. M.* FAMILIAL CENTRONUCLEAR MYOPATHY* A CLINICAL AND PATHOLOGICAL STUDY. NEUROLOGY 17* 727-742, 1967.

SPIRO, A. J., SHY, G. M. AND GONATAS, N. K.* MYOTUBULAR MYOPATHY. ARCH. NEUROL. 14* 1-14, 1966.

*25530 MYOPATHY, CONGENITAL (BATTEN-TURNER TYPE)

BATTEN (1910) AND LATER TURNER (1949, 1962) PROVIDED 50 YEARS* OBSERVATIONS ON A FAMILY IN WHICH 6 SIBS PRESENTED IN INFANCY THE PICTURE OF *AMYOTONIA CONGENITA* AND LATER IN LIFE A NON-PROGRESSIVE MYOPATHY. THE PARENTS WERE NOT RELATED.

BATTEN, F. E.* THE MYOPATHIES OR MUSCULAR DYSTROPHIES* A CRITICAL REVIEW. QUART. J. MED. 3* 313-328, 1910.

TURNER, J. W. A. AND LEES, F.* CONGENITAL MYOPATHY - A FIFTY-YEAR FOLLOW-UP. BRAIN 85* 733-740, 1962.

TURNER, J. W. A.* ON MYOTONIA CONGENITA. BRAIN 72* 25-34, 1949.

25540 MYOPATHY, WITH GIANT ABNORMAL MITOCHONDRIA

SHY AND GONATAS (1964) OBSERVED AN 8 YEAR OLD CHILD WITH HYPOTONIA AND PROXIMAL WEAKNESS. CYTOCHEMICAL AND ELECTRON-MICROSCOPIC STUDIES OF MUSCLE SHOWED LARGE BIZARRE MITOCHONDRIA. VASCULAR SMOOTH MUSCLE, LEUCOCYTES AND INTRAMYAL NERVES DID NOT SHOW THESE CHANGES. THE PATIENT'S BASAL METABOLIC RATE WAS NORMAL. THIS AND THE MORPHOLOGIC FINDINGS WERE DIFFERENT FROM THE CASE OF LUFT ET AL. (SEE HYPERMETABOLISM DUE TO DEFECT IN MITOCHONDRIA). A SISTER HAD DIED AT 18 MONTHS OF AGE OF WHAT WAS DIAGNOSED WERDNIG-HOFFMANN DISEASE. D*AGOSTINO ET AL. (1968)

R
E
C
E
S
S
I
V
E

RETARDATION. MITOCHONDRIA OF EXCESSIVE SIZE AND NUMBER WERE FOUND. THIS WAS, THEN, BOTH MEGACONIAL AND PLEOCONIAL.

D'AGOSTINO, A. N., ZITER, F. A., ROLLISON, M. L. AND BRAY, P. F.* FAMILIAL MYOPATHY WITH ABNORMAL MUSCLE MITOCHONDRIA. ARCH. NEUROL. 18* 388-401, 1968.

SHY, G. M. AND GONATAS, N. K.* HUMAN MYOPATHY WITH GIANT ABNORMAL MITOCHONDRIA. SCIENCE 145* 493-496, 1964.

SHY, G. M., GONATAS, N. K. AND PEREZ, M.* TWO CHILDHOOD MYOPATHIES WITH ABNORMAL MITOCHONDRIA* I. MEGACONIAL MYOPATHY. II. PLEOCONIAL MYOPATHY. BRAIN 89* 133-158, 1966.

25550 MYOPIA, INFANTILE SEVERE

FOR DISCUSSION OF POSSIBLE RECESSIVE INHERITANCE BASED ON THE OCCURRENCE IN OFFSPRING OF CONSANGUINEOUS MATINGS, SEE WAARDENBURG (1963).

WAARDENBURG, P. J., FRANCESCHETTI, A. AND KLEIN, D.* IN, GENETICS AND OPHTHAL-MOLOGY. SPRINGFIELD, ILL.* CHARLES C THOMAS, 2* 1246-1248, 1963.

25560 MYOSCLEROSIS, CONGENITAL, OF LOWENTHAL

LOWENTHAL (1954) DESCRIBED SYMMETRICAL CONGENITAL CONTRACTURES OF THE JOINTS IN 4 SIBS, OFFSPRING OF NORMAL PARENTS. SCLEROSIS OF BOTH MUSCLE AND SKIN WAS THOUGHT TO BE PRESENT. SEE MUSCULAR DYSTROPHY, CONGENITAL, PRODUCING ARTHROGRYPOSIS.

LOWENTHAL, A.* UN GROUPE HEREDODEGENERATIF NOUVEAU* LES MYOSCLEROSES HEREDOFA-MILIALES. ACTA NEUROL. BELG. 54* 155-165, 1954.

*25570 MYOTONIA, GENERALIZED

BECKER (1966) CONCLUDED THAT A RECESSIVE FORM OF MYOTONIA IS MORE FREQUENT THAN THE DOMINANT MYOTONIA CONGENITA OF THOMSEN. SEGREGATION RATIOS AND THE FREQUENCY OF PARENTAL CONSANGUINITY SUGGESTED RECESSIVE INHERITANCE. THE RECESSIVE FORM IS APPARENTLY NOT CONGENITAL BUT BEGINS USUALLY AT AGE 4-6 YEARS. THE INVOLVEMENT IS MORE SEVERE THAN IN THOMSEN'S DISEASE. WINTERS (1970) DESCRIBED MYOTONIA CONGENITA IN TWO BROTHERS AND A SISTER WITH NORMAL PARENTS.

BECKER, P. E.* GENERALIZED MYOTONIA OF RECESSIVE INHERITANCE. PROC. THIRD INTERN. CONG. HUM. GENET. (CHICAGO, SEPT. 5-10, 1966).

BECKER, P. E.* ZUR GENETIK DER MYOTONIEN. IN, KUHN, E. (ED.)* PROGRESSIVE MUSKELODYSTROPHIE, MYOTONIE, MYASTHENIE. BERLIN* SPRINGER-VERLAG, 1966. PP. 247-255.

WINTERS, J. L. AND MCLAUGHLIN, L. A.* MYOTONIA CONGENITA. A REVIEW OF FOUR CASES. J. BONE JOINT SURG. 52A* 1345-1350, 1970.

*25580 MYOTONIC MYOPATHY, DWARFISM, CHONDRODYSTROPHY, AND OCULAR AND FACIAL ABNORMALI-TIES

ABERFELD, HINTERBUCHNER AND SCHNEIDER (1965) DESCRIBED BROTHER AND SISTER WITH AN APPARENTLY PROGRESSIVE DISORDER CHARACTERIZED BY MYOTONIC MYOPATHY, DYSTROPHY OF EPIPHYSEAL CARTILAGES, JOINT CONTRACTURES, BLEPHAROPHIMOSIS, MYOPIA, PIGEON BREAST. THIS REPORT ILLUSTRATES THE CONFUSION THAT CAN BE CREATED BY MULTIPLE REPORTS OF THE SAME FAMILY. ALTHOUGH NOT NOTED BY ABERFELD ET AL. (1965) IN THEIR REPORT WHICH FOCUSED ON NEUROLOGIC ASPECTS, THE SAME SIBS HAD PREVIOUSLY BEEN REPORTED BY SCHWARTZ AND JAMPEL (1962) WHO FOCUSED ATTENTION ON THE BLEPHAROPHIMO-SIS. MEREU ET AL. (1969) DESCRIBED AFFECTED BROTHER AND SISTER WITH UNRELATED PARENTS. ABERFELD ET AL. (1970) REPORTED BROTHER AND SISTER. HUTTENLOCHER ET AL. (1969) DESCRIBED AFFECTED BROTHER AND SISTER. THEY POSTULATED A MEMBRANE DEFECT WITH INABILITY TO MAINTAIN A PROPER GRADIENT OF SODIUM AND POTASSIUM. ABNORMALLY LOW MUSCLE POTASSIUM WAS FOUND. PROCAINE AMIDE THERAPY HELPED MUSCLE FUNCTION.

ABERFELD, D. C., NAMBA, T., VYE, M. V. AND GROB, D.* CHONDRODYSTROPHIC MYOTONIA* REPORT OF TWO CASES. MYOTONIC DWARFISM, DIFFUSE BONE DISEASE, AND UNUSUAL OCULAR AND FACIAL ABNORMALITIES. ARCH. NEUROL. 22* 455-462, 1970.

ABERFELD, D. C., HINTERBUCHNER, L. P. AND SCHNEIDER, M.* MYOTONIA, DWARFISM, DIFFUSE BONE DISEASE AND UNUSUAL OCULAR AND FACIAL ABNORMALITIES (A NEW SYNDROME). BRAIN 88* 313-322, 1965.

HUTTENLOCHER, P. R., LANDWIRTH, J., HANSON, V., GALLAGHER, B. B. AND BENSCH, K.* OSTEO-CHONDRO-MUSCULAR DYSTROPHY. A DISORDER MANIFESTED BY MULTIPLE SKELETAL DEFORMITIES, MYOTONIA, AND DYSTROPHIC CHANGES IN MUSCLE. PEDIATRICS 44* 945-958, 1969.

MEREU, T. R., PORTER, I. H. AND HUG, G.* MYOTONIA, SHORTNESS OF STATURE, AND HIP DYSPLASIA. AM. J. DIS. CHILD. 117* 470-478, 1969.

SCHWARTZ, O. AND JAMPEL, R. S.* CONGENITAL BLEPHAROPHIMOSIS ASSOCIATED WITH A UNIQUE GENERALIZED MYOPATHY. ARCH. OPHTHAL. 68* 52-57, 1962.

25590 MYXEDEMA

HALL (1965) DESCRIBED FIVE FAMILIES IN WHICH 14 CASES OF MYXEDEMA OCCURRED IN ADDITION TO THE FIVE PROBANDS. IN ONE OF THESE, A CASE OF THYROTOXICOSIS WAS ALSO OBSERVED AND IN EACH OF TWO FAMILIES A RELATIVE HAD NON-TOXIC GOITER. A SIXTH PROBAND HAD A DAUGHTER WITH THYROTOXICOSIS. IN THE FAMILIES OF 32 OTHER PATIENTS WITH MYXEDEMA NO THYROID DYSFUNCTION WAS DETECTED. ENVIRONMENTAL FACTORS, SUCH AS VIRAL INFECTION, CANNOT BE EXCLUDED IN THE CAUSATION OF SUCH FAMILIAL AGGREGATION. HOWEVER, THE FINDINGS WERE CONSIDERED COMPATIBLE WITH SEX-INFLUENCED RECESSIVE INHERITANCE AND ALSO WITH THE PREVIOUS SUGGESTION OF A GENETIC RELATIONSHIP OF MYXEDEMA TO HYPERTHYROIDISM AND TO NON-TOXIC GOITER. IN ONE FAMILY *BILATERAL INHERITANCE OF THYROID DISEASE* WAS DEMONSTRATED.

HALL, P. F.* FAMILIAL OCCURRENCE OF MYXEDEMA. J. MED. GENET. 2* 173-180, 1965.

*25600 NECROTIZING ENCEPHALOPATHY, INFANTILE SUBACUTE

THE MAIN PATHOLOGY IS GRAY MATTER DEGENERATION WITH FOCI OF NECROSIS AND CAPILLARY PROLIFERATION IN THE BRAIN STEM. FEIGIN AND WOLF (1954) OBSERVED TWO AFFECTED SIBS FROM A CONSANGUINEOUS MATING. BECAUSE OF SIMILARITY TO WERNICKE'S ENCEPHALO-PATHY, THEY SUGGESTED THAT A GENETIC DEFECT IN SOME WAY RELATED TO THIAMINE WAS PRESENT. JOHNS HOPKINS CASES INCLUDE K.L.M. (B5346* PATH 24642), WHO HAD AN AFFECTED SIB AND IS REFERRED TO BY FORD (1960). CLARK (1964) PICTURED THE HISTOPATHOLOGY OF THIS CASE. THIS MAY BE THE SAME CONDITION AS LACTIC ACIDOSIS OF INFANCY (Q.V.), WHICH LEADS TO NECROTIZING ENCEPHALOPATHY. THIS CONDITION WAS FIRST DESCRIBED BY LEIGH (1951). THE MAIN BIOCHEMICAL FINDINGS ARE HIGH PYRUVATE AND LACTATE IN THE BLOOD AND SLIGHTLY LOW GLUCOSE LEVELS IN BLOOD AND CSF. HOMMES ET AL. (1968), WHO STUDIED A FAMILY WITH THREE AFFECTED SIBS, CONCLUDED THAT GLUCONEOGENESIS IS IMPAIRED. ABSENCE OF PYRUVATE CARBOXYLASE IN THE LIVER WAS DEMONSTRATED AND THIS WAS SUGGESTED AS THE BASIC DEFECT. CLAYTON ET AL. (1967) DEMONSTRATED THERAPEUTIC BENEFIT OF LIPOIC ACID. COOPER ET AL. (1969, 1970) FOUND THAT PATIENTS WITH SNE ELABORATE A FACTOR FOUND IN THE BLOOD AND URINE WHICH INHIBITS THE SYNTHESIS OF THIAMINE TRIPHOSPHATE (TTP) IN BRAIN TISSUE. THE ENZYME RESPONSIBLE FOR TTP SYNTHESIS IS CALLED THIAMINE PYROPHOSPHATE-ADENOSINE TRIPHOS-PHATE PHOSPHORYL TRANSFERASE. TTP IS COMPLETELY ABSENT IN POSTMORTEM BRAIN. AN ASSAY FOR THE INHIBITOR OF TTP SYNTHESIS CAN BE PERFORMED ON URINE OR BLOOD FOR DIAGNOSTIC PURPOSES.

CLARK, D. B.* INFANTILE SUBACUTE NECROTIZING ENCEPHALOPATHY. IN, NELSON, W. E. (ED.)* TEXTBOOK OF PEDIATRICS. PHILADELPHIA* W. B. SAUNDERS, 1964 (8TH ED.).

CLAYTON, B. E., DOBBS, R. H. AND PATRICK, A. D.* LEIGH'S SUBACUTE NECROTIZING ENCEPHALOPATHY* CLINICAL AND BIOCHEMICAL STUDY, WITH SPECIAL REFERENCE TO THERAPY WITH LIPOATE. ARCH. DIS. CHILD. 42* 467-478, 1967.

COOPER, J. R., ITOKAWA, Y. AND PINCUS, J. H.* THIAMINE TRIPHOSPHATE DEFICIENCY IN SUBACUTE NECROTIZING ENCEPHALOMYELOPATHY. SCIENCE 164* 74-75, 1969.

COOPER, J. R., PINCUS, J. H., ITOKAWA, Y. AND PIROS, K.* EXPERIENCE WITH PHOSPHORYL TRANSFERASE INHIBITION IN SUBACUTE NECROTIZING ENCEPHALOMYELOPATHY. NEW ENG. J. MED. 283* 793-795, 1970.

DAVID, R. B., GOMEZ, M. R. AND OKAZAKI, H.* NECROTIZING ENCEPHALOMYELOPATHY (LEIGH). DEVELOP. MED. CHILD. NEUROL. 12* 436-445, 1970.

FEIGIN, I. AND WOLF, A.* A DISEASE IN INFANTS RESEMBLING CHRONIC WERNICKE'S ENCEPHALOPATHY. J. PEDIAT. 45* 243-263, 1954.

FORD, F. R.* A DISEASE RESEMBLING WERNICKE'S ENCEPHALOPATHY (FEIGEN AND WOLF). DISEASES OF THE NERVOUS SYSTEM IN INFANCY, CHILDHOOD AND ADOLESCENCE. SPRING-FIELD, ILL.* CHARLES C THOMAS, 1960. (4TH ED.). PP. 407-410.

HOMMES, F. A., POLMAN, H. A. AND REERINK, J. D.* LEIGH'S ENCEPHALOMYELOPATHY* AN INBORN ERROR OF GLUCONEOGENESIS. ARCH. DIS. CHILD. 43* 423-426, 1968.

LEIGH, D.* SUBACUTE NECROTIZING ENCEPHALOMYELOPATHY IN AN INFANT. J. NEUROL. NEUROSURG. PSYCHIAT. 14* 216-221, 1951.

RICHTER, R. B.* INFANTILE SUBACUTE NECROTIZING ENCEPHALOPATHY WITH PREDILECTION FOR THE BRAIN STEM. J. NEUROPATH. EXP. NEUROL. 16* 281-307, 1957.

*25610 NEPHRONOPHTHISIS, FAMILIAL JUVENILE

LIKE SEVERAL OTHER MENDELIZING DISORDERS, THIS ONE WAS FIRST DESCRIBED BY FANCONI AND HIS COLLEAGUES (1951). IN THE VARIOUS REPORTS ANEMIA, POLYURIA, POLYDIPSIA, ISOSTHENURIA AND DEATH IN UREMIA HAVE BEEN FEATURES. HYPERTENSION AND PROTEINURIA ARE CONSPICUOUS IN THEIR ABSENCE. SYMMETRICAL DESTRUCTION OF THE KIDNEYS INVOLVING BOTH TUBULES AND GLOMERULI (WHICH WERE HYALINIZED) ARE OBSERVED. THE AGE AT DEATH RANGES FROM ABOUT 4 TO ABOUT 15 YEARS. VON SYDOW AND RANSTROM (1962)

R
E
C
E
S
S
I
V
E

OBSERVED PARENTAL CONSANGUINITY. MANGOS ET AL. (1964) THOUGHT DECREASED URINE CONCENTRATING ABILITY MIGHT BE A MANIFESTATION OF HETEROZYGOTES. HERDMAN ET AL. (1967) DESCRIBED MEDULLARY CYSTIC DISEASE IN 7 AND 5 YEAR OLD SIBS AND IN A 7 YEAR OLD BOY WHOSE SISTER HAD DIED OF THE DISEASE. THEY WERE IMPRESSED WITH THE PROBABLE IDENTITY OF MEDULLARY CYSTIC DISEASE AND FAMILIAL NEPHRONOPHTHISIS. MONGEAU AND WORTHEN (1967) CAME TO THE SAME CONCLUSION, AS DID ALSO STRAUSS AND SOMMERS (1967) WHO WITH HUMOR COMMENTED THAT THOSE WHO GAVE THE NAME OF MEDULLARY CYSTS OF THE KIDNEY FOCUSED "ATTENTION ON THE HOLE AS THE CHARACTERISTIC FEATURE OF THE DOUGHNUT RATHER THAN ON THE KIND OF DOUGH ENCLOSING THE HOLE." EVEN THOUGH ONE FORM OF MEDULLARY CYSTIC DISEASE MAY BE THE SAME AS JUVENILE NEPHRONOPHTHISIS, IT IS CLEAR THAT A SEPARATE FORM OF POLYCYSTIC KIDNEY, MEDULLARY TYPE (Q.V.), INHERITED AS A DOMINANT, ALSO EXISTS. THE SIBSHIP REPORTED BY MEIER AND HESS (1965) HAD FIRST COUSIN PARENTS AND APPARENTLY INDEPENDENT INHERITANCE OF TWO RECESSIVES, RETINITIS PIGMENTOSA AND NEPHRONOPHTHISIS.

ALEXANDER, F. AND CAMPBELL, S.* FAMILIAL UREMIC MEDULLARY CYSTIC DISEASE. PEDIATRICS 45* 1024-1028, 1970.

BROBERGER, O., WINBERG, J. AND ZETTERSTROM, R.* JUVENILE NEPHRONOPHTHISIS. I. A GENETICALLY DETERMINED NEPHROPATHY WITH HYPOTONIC POLYURIA AND AZOTAEMIA. ACTA PAEDIAT. 49* 470-479, 1960.

FANCONI, G., HANHART, E., VON ALBERTINI, A., UHLINGER, E., DOLIVO, G. AND PRADER, A.* DIE FAMILIARE JUVENILE NEPHRONOPHTHISE. (DIE IDIOPATHISCHE PARENCHY- MATOSE). HELV. PAEDIAT. ACTA 6* 1-49, 1951.

GISELSON, N., HEINEGARD, D., HOLMBERG, C.-G., LINDBERG, L.-G., LINDSTEDT, E., LINDSTEDT, G. AND SCHERSTEN, B.* RENAL MEDULLARY CYSTIC DISEASE OR FAMILIAL JUVENILE NEPHRONOPHTHISIS* A RENAL TUBULAR DISEASE. AM. J. MED. 48* 174-184, 1970.

HACKZELL, G. AND LUNDMARK, C.* FAMILIAL JUVENILE NEPHRONOPHTHISIS. ACTA PAEDIAT. 47* 428-440, 1958.

HERDMAN, R. C., GOOD, R. A. AND VERNIER, R. L.* MEDULLARY CYSTIC DISEASE IN TWO SIBLINGS. AM. J. MED. 43* 335-344, 1967.

MANGOS, J. A., OPITZ, J. M., LOBECK, C. C. AND COOKSON, D. V.* FAMILIAL JUVENILE NEPHRONOPHTHISIS. AN UNRECOGNIZED RENAL DISEASE IN THE UNITED STATES. PEDIATRICS 34* 337-345, 1964.

MEIER, D. A. AND HESS, J. W.* FAMILIAL NEPHROPATHY WITH RETINITIS PIGMENTOSA* A NEW OCULORENAL SYNDROME IN ADULTS. AM. J. MED. 39* 58-69, 1965.

MONGEAU, J.-G. AND WORTHEN, H. G.* NEPHRONOPHTHISIS AND MEDULLARY CYSTIC DISEASE. AM. J. MED. 43* 345-355, 1967.

STRAUSS, M. B. AND SOMMERS, S. C.* MEDULLARY CYSTIC DISEASE AND FAMILIAL JUVENILE NEPHRONOPHTHISIS. CLINICAL AND PATHOLOGICAL IDENTITY. NEW ENG. J. MED. 277* 863-864, 1967.

VON SYDOW, G. AND RANSTROM, S.* FAMILIAL JUVENILE NEPHRONOPHTHISIS. ACTA PAEDIAT. 51* 561-574, 1962.

25620 NEPHROSIS WITH DEAFNESS AND URINARY TRACT AND OTHER MALFORMATIONS

BRAUN AND BAYER (1962) DESCRIBED A SIBSHIP OF 12 CONTAINING 5 AFFECTED BROTHERS. TWO BROTHERS, 5 SISTERS AND BOTH PARENTS WERE NORMAL. PARENTAL CONSANGUINITY WAS DENIED. WHEREAS TWO OF THE AFFECTED SIBS HAD URINARY TRACT AND DIGITAL ANOMALIES, BIFID UVULA, NEPHROSIS AND DEAFNESS, ONE BROTHER WAS DEAF AND HAD DIGITAL ANOMALIES ONLY, AND 2 BROTHERS HAD NEPHROSIS ONLY. THE DIGITAL ANOMALY CONSISTED OF SHORT AND BIFID DISTAL PHALANGES OF THUMBS AND BIG TOES, FOR WHICH NO PHOTO- GRAPHS OR ROENTGENOGRAMS WERE PUBLISHED. DEAFNESS WAS CONDUCTIVE, WITH NO MALFORMATIONS OF THE MIDDLE EAR BONE (ONE OF THE AFFECTED SIBS WAS AUTOPSIED). A FEMALE RELATIVE WAS KNOWN TO BE DEAF. THE AUTHOR SUGGESTED EITHER AUTOSOMAL RECESSIVE OR X-LINKED DOMINANT INHERITANCE (THE MOTHER HAD RENAL COMPLICATION AND HYPERTENSION DURING HER PREGNANCIES) OF THIS SYNDROME, WHICH WAS NOT PREVIOUSLY DESCRIBED IN THE LITERATURE.

BRAUN, F. C., JR. AND BAYER, J. F.* FAMILIAL NEPHROSIS ASSOCIATED WITH DEAFNESS AND CONGENITAL URINARY TRACT ANOMALIES IN SIBLINGS. J. PEDIAT. 60* 33-41, 1962.

*25630 NEPHROSIS, CONGENITAL

WHEREAS THE USUAL IDIOPATHIC NEPHROTIC SYNDROME OF CHILDHOOD ALMOST NEVER HAS ITS ONSET BEFORE THE AGE OF 18 MONTHS, CONGENITAL NEPHROSIS SHOWS ITSELF IN THE FIRST DAYS OR WEEKS OF LIFE. FURTHERMORE, THE FAMILIAL OCCURRENCE INCLUDING PARENTAL CONSANGUINITY IS THAT OF AN AUTOSOMAL RECESSIVE TRAIT. OTHERWISE THE CLINICAL, CHEMICAL AND PATHOLOGIC FEATURES ARE IDENTICAL WITH THOSE OF THE IDIOPATHIC CONDITION. A LARGE SERIES OF CASES WAS COLLECTED BY HALLMAN AND HJELT (1959) IN FINLAND AND BY VERNIER, BRUNSON AND GOOD (1957) AND WORTHEN, VERNIER AND GOOD (1959) IN MINNESOTA, WHERE MANY PERSONS OF FINNISH EXTRACTION LIVE. THE LATTER

GROUP WAS IMPRESSED WITH THE HIGH FREQUENCY OF MATERNAL TOXEMIA IN THESE CASES. GILES ET AL. (1957) HAVE REPORTED TWO AFFECTED SIBS FROM A FIRST COUSIN MARRIAGE AND A THIRD CASE, THE CHILD OF COUSINS. ONGRE (1961) DESCRIBED SIBS WITH NEPHROSIS STARTING IN THE NEONATAL PERIOD AND WITH CYSTIC-LIKE DILATION OF RENAL TUBULES. IT IS LIKELY THAT THIS IS NOT CONGENITAL CYSTIC DISEASE BUT RATHER CONGENITAL NEPHROSIS, AS IN THE OTHER SERIES MENTIONED. CONGENITAL HEART DISEASE WAS ALSO PRESENT IN THE CASES REPORTED BY FOURNIER ET AL. (1963). THIS DISORDER SEEMS TO HAVE A RELATIVELY HIGH FREQUENCY IN FINLAND (NORIO ET AL., 1964). MCCROY AND COLLEAGUES (1966) SUGGESTED THAT FAMILIAL NEPHROSIS IS OF TWO TYPES. ONE SIMULATES THE SPORADIC FORM OF CHILDHOOD NEPHROSIS AND IS SEPARABLE ONLY BY THE OCCURRENCE OF NEPHROSIS IN MORE THAN ONE FAMILY MEMBER. THE OTHER, MOST PROPERLY CALLED CONGENITAL, OR PERHAPS EVEN BETTER NEONATAL, NEPHROSIS IS CLEARLY DIFFEREN-TIATED BY EARLY AGE OF ONSET, LACK OF RESPONSIVENESS TO THERAPY, POOR PROGNOSIS AND DISTINCTIVE MORPHOLOGIC CHANGES.

FOURNIER, A., PAGET, M., PAULI, A. AND DEVIN, P.* SYNDROMES NEPHROTIQUES FAMILIAUX. SYNDROME NEPHROTIQUE ASSOCIE A UNE CARDIOPATHIE CONGENITALE CHEZ QUATRE SOEURS. PEDIATRIE 18* 677-685, 1963.

GILES, H. M., PUGH, R. C. B., DARMADY, E. M., STRANACK, F. AND WOOLF, L. I.* THE NEPHROTIC SYNDROME IN EARLY INFANCY* A REPORT OF 3 CASES. ARCH. DIS. CHILD. 32* 167-180, 1957.

HALLMAN, N. AND HJELT, L.* CONGENITAL NEPHROTIC SYNDROME. J. PEDIAT. 55* 152-162, 1959.

HALLMAN, N., HJELT, L. AND AHVENAINEN, E. K.* NEPHROTIC SYNDROME IN NEWBORN AND YOUNG INFANTS. ANN. PAEDIAT. FENN. 2* 227-241, 1956.

HALLMAN, N., NORIO, R. AND KOUVALAINEN, K.* MAIN FEATURES OF THE CONGENITAL NEPHROTIC SYNDROME. ACTA PAEDIAT. SCAND. 172 (SUPPL.)* 75-78, 1967.

MCCROY, W. W., SHIBUYA, M. AND WORTHEN, H. G.* HEREDITARY RENAL GLOMERULAR DISEASE IN INFANCY AND CHILDHOOD. ADVANCES PEDIAT. 14* 253-280, 1966.

NORIO, R.* HEREDITY IN THE CONGENITAL NEPHROTIC SYNDROME. A GENETIC STUDY OF 57 FINNISH FAMILIES WITH A REVIEW OF REPORTED CASES. ANN. PAEDIAT. FENN. 12 (SUPPL. 27)* 1-94, 1966.

NORIO, R., HJELT, L. AND HALLMAN, N.* CONGENITAL NEPHROTIC SYNDROME* AN INHERITED DISEASE.Q A PRELIMINARY REPORT. ANN. PAEDIAT. FENN. 10* 223-227, 1964.

ONGRE, A. A.* NEPHROTIC SYNDROME WITH CYST-LIKE DILATIONS OF RENAL TUBULES* REPORT OF 2 CASES IN SIBLINGS IN EARLY INFANCY. ACTA PATH. MICROBIOL. SCAND. 51* 1-8, 1961.

VERNIER, R. L., BRUNSON, J. AND GOOD, R. A.* STUDIES ON FAMILIAL NEPHROSIS. I. CLINICAL AND PATHOLOGIC STUDY OF FOUR CASES IN A SINGLE FAMILY. AM. J. DIS. CHILD. 93* 469-485, 1957.

WORTHEN, H. G., VERNIER, R. L. AND GOOD, R. A.* INFANTILE NEPHROSIS* CLINICAL BIOCHEMICAL, AND MORPHOLOGIC STUDIES OF THE SYNDROME. AM. J. DIS. CHILD. 98* 731-748, 1959.

R
E
C
E
S
S
I
V
E

25640 NERVOUS SYSTEM DISORDER RESEMBLING REFSUM'S DISEASE AND HURLER'S DISEASE

SHY ET AL. (1967) DESCRIBED A 21 YEAR OLD NEGRO GIRL WITH PROGRESSIVE PTOSIS, EXTERNAL OPHTHALMOPLEGIA, RETINITIS PIGMENTOSA, ATAXIA, ABSENT DEEP TENDON REFLEXES, ELEVATED CEREBROSPINAL FLUID PROTEIN, AND HISTOLOGIC FEATURES COMPATIBLE WITH EITHER HURLER'S SYNDROME (MPS I) OR WITH REFSUM'S DISEASE. NEITHER PHYTANIC ACID NOR MUCOPOLYSACCHARIDE WAS FOUND IN EXCESS IN THE TISSUES, HOWEVER.

GONATAS, N. K.* A GENERALIZED DISORDER OF NERVOUS SYSTEM, SKELETAL MUSCLE AND HEART RESEMBLING REFSUM'S DISEASE AND HURLER'S SYNDROME. II. ULTRASTRUCTURE. AM. J. MED. 42* 169-178, 1967.

SHY, G. M., SILBERBERG, D. H., APPEL, S. H., MISHKIN, M. M. AND GODFREY, E. H.* A GENERALIZED DISORDER OF NERVOUS SYSTEM, SKELETAL MUSCLE AND HEART RESEMBLING REFSUM'S DISEASE AND HURLER'S SYNDROME. I. CLINICAL, PATHOLOGIC AND BIOCHEMICAL CHARACTERISTICS. AM. J. MED. 42* 163-168, 1967.

*25650 NETHERTON'S DISEASE

THE FEATURES ARE 'BAMBOO HAIR' (TRICHORRHEXIS NODOSA, OR, BECAUSE OF THE NODES, INVAGINATA), CONGENITAL ICHTHYOSIFORM ERYTHRODERMA AND ATOPIC DIATHESIS. IT HAS BEEN OBSERVED ALMOST ONLY IN FEMALES. THE PARENTS OF WILKINSON, CURTIS AND HAWK'S PATIENT (1964) WERE THIRD COUSINS. THEY SUGGESTED THAT THE DISORDER IS AN AUTOSOMAL RECESSIVE INBORN ERROR OF METABOLISM. THEIR PATIENT ALSO HAD HYPOGAMMA-GLOBULINEMIA. STANKLER AND COCHRANE (1967) DESCRIBED AFFECTED SISTERS OF ITALIAN EXTRACTION. PORTER AND STARKE (1968) REPORTED AN AFFECTED MALE. SEVERAL MALES IN THE FAMILY INCLUDING THE PROBAND HAD HISTOLOGICALLY TYPICAL X-LINKED ICHTHYOSIS AND THE RELATIONSHIP OF THESE MALES WAS CONSISTENT WITH X-LINKAGE.

PORTER, P. S. AND STARKE, J. C.* NETHERTON'S SYNDROME. ARCH. DIS. CHILD. 43*
319-322, 1968.

STANKLER, L. AND COCHRANE, T.* NETHERTON'S DISEASE IN TWO SISTERS. BRIT. J.
DERM. 79* 187-196, 1967.

WILKINSON, R. D., CURTIS, G. H. AND HAWK, W. A.* NETHERTON'S DISEASE* TRICHORR-
HEXIS INVAGINATA (BAMBOO HAIR) CONGENITAL ICHTHYOSIFORM ERYTHRODERMA AND THE
ATOPIC DIATHESIS. A HISTOPATHOLOGIC STUDY. ARCH. DERM. 89* 46-54, 1964.

*25660 NEUROAXONAL DYSTROPHY, INFANTILE (SEITELBERGER)

THE DEGENERATIVE ENCEPHALOPATHY DESCRIBED FIRST BY SEITELBERGER (1952) IS SIMILAR
TO, BUT NOT IDENTICAL WITH, HALLERVORDEN-SPATZ DISEASE (Q.V.). VISCERAL CHANGES
WERE DESCRIBED BY COWEN AND OLMSTEAD (1963) AND BY SANDBANK (1965). THE CHANGES
IN THE BRAIN ARE WIDESPREAD FOCAL SWELLING AND DEGENERATION OF AXONS WITH
SCATTERED 'SPHEROIDS' (COWEN, OLMSTEAD, 1963). CROME AND WELLER (1965) DESCRIBED
A BROTHER AND SISTER WHO DIED AT 12 AND 18 MONTHS, RESPECTIVELY, WITH MENTAL
RETARDATION, PARALYSIS AND EPILEPSY.

COWEN, D. AND OLMSTEAD, E. V.* INFANTILE NEUROAXONAL DYSTROPHY. J. NEUROPATH.
EXP. NEUROL. 22* 175-236, 1963.

CROME, L. AND WELLER, S. D. V.* INFANTILE NEUROAXONAL DYSTROPHY. ARCH. DIS.
CHILD. 40* 502-507, 1965.

NAKAI, H., LANDING, B. H. AND SCHUBERT, W. K.* SEITELBERGER'S SPASTIC AMAUROTIC
AXONAL IDIOCY. REPORT OF A CASE IN A 9-YEAR-OLD BOY WITH COMMENT ON VISCERAL
MANIFESTATION. PEDIATRICS 25* 441-449, 1960.

SANDBANK, V.* INFANTILE NEUROAXONAL DYSTROPHY. ARCH. NEUROL. 12* 155-159,
1965.

25670 NEUROBLASTOMA

DODGE AND BENNER (1945) REPORTED A BROTHER AND SISTER WITH NEUROBLASTOMA OF THE
ADRENAL MEDULLA. THE FATHER AND 3 OF HIS 5 SIBS IN THE REPORT OF CHATTEN AND
VOORHESS (1967) HAD CAFE-AU-LAIT SPOTS. GRIFFIN AND BOLANDE (1969) DESCRIBED TWO
SISTERS WITH CONGENITAL DISSEMINATED NEUROBLASTOMA. IN BOTH REGRESSION OF THE
RETROPERITONEAL TUMORS TO FIBROCALCIFIC RESIDUES AND MATURATION TO GANGLIONEUROMA
WERE OBSERVED. IN ONE OF THEM, METASTATIC NODULES IN THE SKIN MATURED TO
GANGLIONEUROMAS AND BY PROGRESSIVE LOSS OF GANGLION CELLS CAME TO RESEMBLE
NEUROFIBROMAS CLOSELY. A 15 YEAR OLD SISTER SHOWED BY X-RAY, A SMALL FOCUS OF
ADRENAL CALCIFICATION. THESE SISTERS WERE MENTIONED IN THE REPORT OF CHATTEN AND
VOORHESS (1967).

CHATTEN, J. AND VOORHESS, M. L.* FAMILIAL NEUROBLASTOMA. REPORT OF A KINDRED
WITH MULTIPLE DISORDERS, INCLUDING NEUROBLASTOMAS IN FOUR SIBLINGS. NEW ENG. J.
MED. 277* 1230-1236, 1967.

DODGE, H. J. AND BENNER, M. C.* NEUROBLASTOMA OF THE ADRENAL MEDULLA IN
SIBLINGS. ROCKY MOUNTAIN MED. J. 42* 35-38, 1945.

GRIFFIN, M. E. AND BOLANDE, R. P.* FAMILIAL NEUROBLASTOMA WITH REGRESSION AND
MATURATION TO GANGLIONEUROFIBROMA. PEDIATRICS 43* 377-382, 1969.

*25680 NEUROPATHY, CONGENITAL SENSORY, WITH ANHIDROSIS

PINSKY AND DIGEORGE (1966) DESCRIBED THREE MENTALLY RETARDED CHILDREN, OF WHICH
TWO WERE SIBS, WITH RECURRENT EPISODES OF UNEXPLAINED FEVER, REPEATED TRAUMATIC
AND THERMAL INJURIES AND SELF-MUTILATING BEHAVIOR. SWEATING COULD NOT BE ELICITED
BY THERMAL, PAINFUL, EMOTIONAL OR CHEMICAL STIMULI. HISTAMINE EVOKED NO AXONE
FLARE. SUBCUTANEOUS ADMINISTRATION OF MECHOLYL OR NEOSTIGMINE IN DOSES CAPABLE OF
PRODUCING LACRIMATION IN NORMAL CHILDREN, FAILED TO DO SO IN THE PRESENT PATIENTS,
DESPITE THEIR OCCASIONAL SPONTANEOUS LACRIMATION. ONE WAS FEMALE AND TWO MALES.
SWANSON (1963) DESCRIBED THE SAME SYNDROME IN TWO MALE SIBS. SWANSON, BUCHAN AND
ALVORD (1963) DESCRIBED THE HISTOLOGIC FINDINGS, NAMELY ABSENCE OF LISSAUER'S
TRACT (THIN MYELINATED AFFERENT FIBERS) AND SMALL DORSAL ROOT AXONS. SINCE BOTH
DORSAL ROOT AND SYMPATHETIC GANGLIA DERIVE FROM THE NEURAL CREST, THEY THOUGHT A
UNIFIED ANATOMICAL BASIS MIGHT BE PROVIDED. DYSAUTONOMIA (Q.V.) HAS BEEN
INCORRECTLY DIAGNOSED IN SOME CASES. BIEMOND'S CONGENITAL AND FAMILIAL ANALGESIA
(Q.V.) IS ANOTHER CONDITION SOMETIMES CONFUSED WITH DYSAUTONOMIA. WOLFE AND
HENKIN (1970) REFERRED TO THE DISORDER IN PINSKY AND DIGEORGE'S SIBS AS TYPE II
FAMILIAL DYSAUTONOMIA. THEY SUGGESTED THAT IT IS THE SAME AS THE DISORDER
REPORTED IN TWO SIBS OF EACH OF TWO FAMILIES BY SWANSON (1963) AND BY VASSELLA ET
AL. (1968).

BROWN, J. W. AND PODOSIN, R.* A SYNDROME OF THE NEURAL CREST. ARCH. NEUROL.
15* 294-301, 1966.

PINSKY, L. AND DIGEORGE, A. M.* CONGENITAL FAMILIAL SENSORY NEUROPATHY WITH
ANHIDROSIS. J. PEDIAT. 68* 1-13, 1966.

SWANSON, A. G.* CONGENITAL INSENSITIVITY TO PAIN WITH ANHIDROSIS. A UNIQUE SYNDROME IN TWO MALE SIBLINGS. ARCH. NEUROL. 8* 299-306, 1963.

SWANSON, A. G., BUCHAN, G. C. AND ALVORD, E. D., JR.* ABSENCE OF LISSAUER'S TRACT AND SMALL DORSAL ROOT AXONS IN FAMILIAL, CONGENITAL, UNIVERSAL INSENSITIVITY TO PAIN. TRANS. AM. NEUROL. ASS. 88* 99-103, 1963.

VASSELLA, F., EMRICH, H. M., KRAUS-RUPPERT, R., AUFDERMAUR, F. AND TONZ, O.* CONGENITAL SENSORY NEUROPATHY WITH ANHIDROSIS. ARCH. DIS. CHILD. 43* 124-130, 1968.

WOLFE, S. M. AND HENKIN, R. I.* ABSENCE OF TASTE IN TYPE II FAMILIAL DYSAU-TONOMIA* UNRESPONSIVENESS TO METHACHOLINE DESPITE THE PRESENCE OF TASTE BUDS. J. PEDIAT. 77* 103-108, 1970.

*25690 NEUROPATHY, PROGRESSIVE SENSORY, OF CHILDREN

JOHNSON AND SPALDING (1964) DESCRIBED SENSORY NEUROPATHY IN TWO BOYS, AGED 10 YEARS AND 15 YEARS, EACH OF WHOM HAD CONSANGUINEOUS PARENTS. THE DISORDER BEGAN IN EARLY CHILDHOOD, PROGRESSED SLOWLY, INVOLVED ALL MODALITIES OF SENSATION WITH NO DISTURBANCE OF MOTOR AND AUTONOMIC FUNCTION, AND WAS PREDOMINANTLY DISTAL WITH LATE INVOLVEMENT OF THE TRUNK. LOSS OF DIGITS AND CHARCOT JOINTS AT THE ANKLES RESULTED. THE DISORDER IS DIFFERENTIATED FROM CONGENITAL INDIFFERENCE TO PAIN BY INVOLVEMENT OF ALL SENSORY MODALITIES, PRESERVATION OF SENSATION INCLUDING PAIN PROXIMALLY, LOSS OF TENDON REFLEXES, GRADUAL PROGRESSION, AND PERIPHERAL NERVE DEGENERATION. IT IS DIFFERENTIATED FROM HEREDITARY SENSORY RADICULAR NEUROPATHY BY ITS MODE OF INHERITANCE (RECESSIVE, NOT DOMINANT), EARLY AGE OF ONSET AND ULTIMATE INVOLVEMENT OF THE TRUNK. THE PATIENT REPORTED BY OGDEN ET AL. (1959) AS PROGRESSIVE SENSORY RADICULAR NEUROPATHY OF DENNY-BROWN WAS PROBABLY THIS CONDITION BECAUSE SYMPTOMS BEGAN AT LEAST AS EARLY AS 1 YEAR AND THE PARENTS WERE FIRST COUSINS. HADDOW ET AL. (1970) DESCRIBED A BROTHER AND SISTER, OFFSPRING OF NONCONSANGUINEOUS PARENTS (MOTHER, IRISH* FATHER, FRENCH-CANADIAN), WITH NON-PROGRESSIVE SENSORY DEFECT LEADING TO EXTENSIVE DAMAGE TO THE FINGERS. THE CASES OF HADDOW ET AL. (1970) HAD LOW SPINAL FLUID PROTEIN, SUFFERED FROM UNEXPLAINED CHRONIC DIARRHEA IN EARLY LIFE. THEY SUGGESTED THAT THE DISORDER IN THE FRENCH-CANADIAN FAMILY DESCRIBED BY HOULD AND VERRET (1967) WAS THE SAME, EVEN THOUGH ONSET WAS NOT UNTIL THE MIDDLE OF THE FIRST DECADE.

HADDOW, J. E., SHAPIRO, S. R. AND GALL, D. G.* CONGENITAL SENSORY NEUROPATHY IN SIBLINGS. PEDIATRICS 45* 651-655, 1970.

HOULD, F. AND VERRET, S.* NEUROPATHIE RADICULAIRE HEREDITAIRE AVEC PERTES DE SENSIBILITE* ETUDE D'UNE FAMILLE CANADIENNE-FRANCAISE. LAVAL MED. 38* 454-459, 1967.

JOHNSON, R. H. AND SPALDING, J. M. K.* PROGRESSIVE SENSORY NEUROPATHY IN CHILDREN. J. NEUROL. NEUROSURG. PSYCHIAT. 27* 125-130, 1964.

OGDEN, T. E., ROBERT, F. AND CARMICHAEL, E. A.* SOME SENSORY SYNDROMES IN CHILDREN* INDIFFERENCE TO PAIN AND SENSORY NEUROPATHY. J. NEUROL. NEUROSURG. PSYCHIAT. 22* 267-276, 1959.

25700 NEUROVISCERAL STORAGE DISEASE WITH CURVILINEAR BODIES

DUFFY ET AL. (1968) DESCRIBED A SINGLE CASE OF A 6 YEAR OLD BOY WITH A NEUROVIS-CERAL STORAGE DISEASE WITH CURVILINEAR BODIES DEMONSTRATED INTRACELLULARLY BY ELECTRON MICROSCOPY. THE DIAGNOSIS WAS POSSIBLE IN VITAM BY RECTAL OR OTHER VISCERAL BIOPSY. CHEMICAL STUDIES SHOWED THIS IS NOT A GANGLIOSIDOSIS.

DUFFY, P. E., KORNFELD, M. AND SUZUKI, K.* NEUROVISCERAL STORAGE DISEASE WITH CURVILINEAR BODIES. J. NEUROPATH. EXP. NEUROL. 27* 351-370, 1968.

25710 NEUTROPENIA, LETHAL CONGENITAL, WITH EOSINOPHILIA

ANDREWS, MCCLELLAN AND SCOTT (1960) DESCRIBED TWO AFFECTED SIBS. THE PARENTS WERE NOT KNOWN TO BE RELATED.

ANDREWS, J. P., MCCLELLAN, J. T. AND SCOTT, C. H.* LETHAL CONGENITAL NEUTRO-PENIA WITH EOSINOPHILIA OCCURRING IN TWO SIBLINGS. AM. J. MED. 29* 358-362, 1960.

*25720 NIEMANN-PICK DISEASE (SPHINGOMYELIN LIPIDOSIS)

LIPID, MAINLY SPHINGOMYELIN, ACCUMULATES IN RETICULOENDOTHELIAL AND OTHER CELL TYPES THROUGHOUT THE BODY. THE ACCUMULATION IN GANGLION CELLS OF THE CENTRAL NERVOUS SYSTEM LEADS TO CELL DEATH. HEPATOSPLENOMEGALY, RETARDED PHYSICAL AND MENTAL GROWTH AND SEVERE NEUROLOGIC DISTURBANCES ARE FEATURES. SYMPTOMS USUALLY DEVELOP BY 6 MONTHS AND DEATH OCCURS BY THREE YEARS OF AGE. HOWEVER, RECENT PUBLICATIONS (CROCKER AND FARBER, 1958* FORSYTHE, MCKEOWN AND NEILL, 1959) MAKE IT CLEAR THAT THE BIOLOGICAL BEHAVIOR CAN BE MORE WIDELY VARIABLE THAN THE LAST STATEMENT MIGHT SUGGEST AND THAT SURVIVAL TO ADULTHOOD IS POSSIBLE IF AN EARLY CRITICAL PERIOD IS SURVIVED. KNUDSON AND KAPLAN (1962) EMPHASIZED THE EXISTENCE OF DIFFERENT GROUPS AND SUGGESTED THAT THREE TYPES CAN BE DISTINGUISHED*

R
E
C
E
S
S
I
V
E

INFANTILE CEREBRAL, JUVENILE CEREBRAL AND NON-CEREBRAL TYPES. WIEDEMANN AND
COLLEAGUES (1965) FOUND LARGE STORAGE CELLS IN THE BONE MARROW OF BOTH CLINICALLY
NORMAL PARENTS OF A SIBSHIP WITH SEVERAL AFFECTED CHILDREN. THE PARENTS WERE
FIRST COUSINS. ABOUT 40 PERCENT OF CASES ARE JEWISH. A POSSIBLE VARIANT STUDIED
BY CROCKER AND FARBER (1958) AND BY FREDRICKSON (1966) OCCURS IN PATIENTS OF
FRENCH-CANADIAN EXTRACTION, COMING FROM THE VICINITY OF YARMOUTH, NOVA SCOTIA.
THE COURSE IS PROTRACTED WITH SLOW PROGRESSION OF NEUROLOGIC ABNORMALITIES TO
SEVERE DISABILITY. JAUNDICE IS A PROMINENT FEATURE. PFANDLER (1953) DESCRIBED
NON-JEWISH SWISS BROTHERS (OUT OF 14 SIBS) WHO DIED AT AGES 29 AND 33 YEARS.
TERRY ET AL. (1954) DESCRIBED THE SPORADIC CASE OF A JEWISH MALE WHO DIED AT AGE
51 YEARS. IT SEEMS POSSIBLE THAT THESE ARE INSTANCES OF A SEPARATE DISORDER.
HETEROGENEITY WAS ALSO EMPHASIZED BY LOWDEN ET AL. (1967) WHO DESCRIBED NON-JEWISH
SIBS WITH BOTH CLINICAL AND CHEMICAL DIFFERENCES FROM THE USUAL DISEASE. IN THE
CLASSIC INFANTILE TYPE BRADY ET AL. (1966) DEMONSTRATED THAT THE BIOCHEMICAL
DEFECT IS A DEFICIENT ACTIVITY OF THE ENZYME WHICH CATALYZES CLEAVAGE OF SPHIN-
GOMYELIN TO PHOSPHORYLCHOLINE AND CERAMIDE. UHLENDORF ET AL. (1967) FOUND THAT
THE METABOLIC DEFECT PERSISTS IN CELL CULTURE. SPECIFICALLY INCREASED SPHINGOMYE-
LIN WAS DEMONSTRATED IN CELLS FROM BONE MARROW, SKIN AND AMNION. THE LAST MAKES
PRENATAL DIAGNOSIS POSSIBLE. ABOUT 85 PERCENT OF PATIENTS FALL INTO CROCKER'S
GROUP A, WITH DEATH BEFORE AGE 3 YEARS. IN GROUP B, THE VISCERAL OR 'CHRONIC'
FORM, PATIENTS REMAIN FREE OF NEUROLOGIC MANIFESTATIONS DESPITE MASSIVE VISCERAL
INVOLVEMENT. IN BOTH FORMS A DEFICIENCY OF SPHINGOMYELINASE HAS BEEN DEMONS-
TRATED. PATIENTS IN GROUP C HAVE A SLOWER PROGRESSION OF CLINICAL SYMPTOMS. CNS
SYMPTOMS APPEAR BETWEEN 2 AND 4 YEARS. SPASTICITY IS STRIKING AND SEIZURES,
PARTICULARLY MYOCLONIC JERKS, ARE COMMON. GROUP D (THE 'NOVA SCOTIAN TYPE' OF
CROCKER) ALSO HAS SLOW PROGRESSION. NEUROLOGIC ABNORMALITIES BEGIN IN EARLY OR
MIDDLE CHILDHOOD. THE BIOCHEMICAL ABNORMALITIES OF GROUPS C AND D ARE LESS
CLEARLY KNOWN THAN THOSE OF GROUPS A AND B. FIVE DISTINCT FORMS OF NIEMANN-PICK
DISEASE ARE DISTINGUISHED* THE CLASSICAL INFANTILE FORM (TYPE A OF CROCKER), THE
VISCERAL FORM (TYPE B), THE SUBACUTE OR JUVENILE FORM (TYPE C), THE NOVA SCOTIAN
VARIANT (TYPE D), AND THE ADULT FORM (TERRY ET AL., 1954* LYNN AND TERRY, 1964).
SCHNEIDER AND KENNEDY (1967) FOUND THAT SPHINGOMYELINASE IS DEFICIENT ONLY IN THE
INFANTILE AND VISCERAL FORMS. CROCKER (1961) PROVIDED THE DELINEATION OF THE
FIRST FOUR TYPES.

BRADY, R. O.* THE SPHINGOLIPIDOSES. NEW ENG. J. MED. 275* 312-318, 1966.

BRADY, R. O., KANFER, J. N., MOCK, M. B. AND FREDRICKSON, D. S.* THE METABOLISM
OF SPHINGOMYELIN. II. EVIDENCE OF AN ENZYMATIC DEFICIENCY IN NIEMANN-PICK
DISEASE. PROC. NAT. ACAD. SCI. 55* 366-369, 1966.

CROCKER, A. C. AND FARBER, S.* NIEMANN-PICK DISEASE* A REVIEW OF EIGHTEEN
PATIENTS. MEDICINE 37* 1-95, 1958.

CROCKER, A. C.* THE CEREBRAL DEFECT IN TAY-SACHS DISEASE AND NIEMANN-PICK
DISEASE. J. NEUROCHEM. 7* 69-80, 1961.

FORSYTHE, W. I., MCKEOWN, E. F. AND NEILL, D. W.* THREE CASES OF NIEMANN PICK'S
DISEASE IN CHILDREN. ARCH. DIS. CHILD. 34* 406-409, 1959.

FREDRICKSON, D. S.* SPHINGOMYELIN LIPIDOSIS* NIEMANN-PICK DISEASE. IN,
STANBURY, J. B., WYNGAARDEN, J. B. AND FREDRICKSON, D. S. (EDS.)* THE METABOLIC
BASIS OF INHERITED DISEASE. NEW YORK* MCGRAW-HILL, 1966 (2ND ED.). PP. 586-617.

KAMPINE, J. P., BRADY, R. O. AND KANFER, J. N.* DIAGNOSIS OF GAUCHER'S DISEASE
AND NIEMANN-PICK DISEASE WITH SMALL SAMPLES OF VENOUS BLOOD. SCIENCE 155* 86-88,
1967.

KNUDSON, A. G., JR. AND KAPLAN, W. D.* GENETICS OF THE SPHINGOLIPIDOSES. IN,
AARONSON, S. M. AND VOLK, B. W. (EDS.)* CEREBRAL SPHINGOLIPIDOSES. A SYMPOSIUM ON
TAY-SACHS DISEASE. NEW YORK* ACADEMIC PRESS, 1962. PP. 395-411.

LOWDEN, J. A., LARAMEE, M. A. AND WENTWORTH, P.* THE SUBACUTE FORM OF NIEMANN-
PICK DISEASE. ARCH. NEUROL. 17* 230-237, 1967.

LYNN, R. AND TERRY, R. D.* LIPID HISTOCHEMISTRY AND ELECTRON MICROSCOPY IN
ADULT NIEMANN-PICK DISEASE. AM. J. MED. 37* 987-994, 1964.

PFANDLER, U.* NOUVELLES CONCEPTIONS SUR L'HEREDITE ET LA PATHOGENIE DE LA
MALADIE DE NIEMANN-PICK. HELV. MED. ACTA 20* 216-241, 1953.

PHILIPPART, M., MARTIN, L., MARTIN, J. J. AND MENKES, J. H.* NIEMANN-PICK
DISEASE. MORPHOLOGIC AND BIOCHEMICAL STUDIES IN THE VISCERAL FORM WITH LATE
CENTRAL NERVOUS SYSTEM INVOLVEMENT (CROCKER'S GROUP C). ARCH. NEUROL. 20* 227-
238, 1969.

SCHNEIDER, P. B. AND KENNEDY, E. P.* SPHINGOMYELINASE IN NORMAL HUMAN SPLEENS
AND IN SPLEENS FROM SUBJECTS WITH NIEMANN-PICK DISEASE. J. LIPID RES. 8* 202-209,
1967.

TERRY, R., SPERRY, W. M. AND BRODOFF, B.* ADULT LIPIDOSIS RESEMBLING NIEMANN-
PICK'S DISEASE. AM. J. PATH. 30* 263-285, 1954.

UHLENDORF, B. W., HOLTZ, A. I., MOCK, M. B. AND FREDRICKSON, D. S.* PERSISTENCE OF A METABOLIC DEFECT IN TISSUE CULTURES DERIVED FROM PATIENTS WITH NIEMANN-PICK DISEASE. IN, ARONSON, S. M. AND VOLK, B. W. (EDS.)* INBORN DISORDERS OF SPHINGO-LIPID METABOLISM. OXFORD* PERGAMON PRESS, 1967. PP. 443-453.

WIEDEMANN, H.-R., GERKEN, H., GRAUCOB, E. AND HANSEN, H.-G.* RECOGNITION OF HETEROZYGOSITY IN SPHINGOLIPIDOSES. (LETTER) LANCET 1* 1283 ONLY, 1965.

25730 NON-DISJUNCTION

THE POSSIBILITY OF RECESSIVE GENES PREDISPOSING TO NON-DISJUNCTION WAS EXAMINED BY KWITEROVICH ET AL. (1966) BY DETERMINING THE FREQUENCY OF MONGOLISM IN AN INBRED AMISH POPULATION AND BY MATSUNAGA (1966) AND FORSSMAN AND AKESSON (1966) WHO INVESTIGATED THE FREQUENCY OF INBREEDING AMONG MOTHERS OF CASES OF MONGOLISM. ALL THREE STUDIES GAVE NO SUGGESTION OF INBREEDING EFFECT. THIS, DESPITE WORK OF GOWEN (1933) INDICATING SUCH AN EFFECT IN DROSOPHILA MELANOGASTER AND SUGGESTIVE EARLIER WORK WITH MONGOLISM. HIRSCHHORN AND HSU (1969) DESCRIBED TWO SISTERS WITH XYY-XY-XO MOSAICISM WHOSE BROTHER HAD XYY-XY MOSAICISM. THE PARENTS WERE SECOND COUSINS. SEE ALSO SATELLITE ASSOCIATION RESULTING IN FAMILIAL CHROMOSOMAL MOSAICISM. THE OCCURRENCE OF MULTIPLE CASES OF VARIOUS ANEUPLOID STATES IN THE SAME SIBSHIP OR KINDRED HAS BEEN INTERPRETED BY SOME AS INDICATING A FAMILIAL, PRESUMABLY GENETIC, TENDENCY TO ANAPHASE LOSS OR NONDISJUNCTION (E.G. BOCZKOWSKI ET AL., 1969). HSU ET AL. (1970) DESCRIBED A FAMILY OF PORTUGUESE EXTRACTION IN WHICH TWO SISTERS HAD 45, X-46, XY-47, XYY MOSAICISM AND A BROTHER HAD 46, XY-47, XYY MOSAICISM. A THIRD SISTER SHOWED 5 PERCENT ABERRANT CELLS (EXTRA B GROUP CHROMOSOME, EXTRA SMALL ACROCENTRIC, MISSING C GROUP CHROMOSOME). THE PARENTS WERE SECOND COUSINS. THE AUTHORS POSTULATED AN AUTOSOMAL RECESSIVE GENE WHICH PREDISPOSES THE HOMOZYGOTE TO *MITOTIC INSTABILITY.* OTHERS HAVE PROPOSED A DOMINANT FACTOR FOR NONDISJUNCTION. SEE SATELLITE ASSOCIATION, ETC. BEADLE (1932) DESCRIBED IN MAIZE A RECESSIVE GENE *STICKY* WHICH PREDISPOSED TO MITOTIC NONDISJUNCTION. LEWIS AND GENCARELLA (1952) DESCRIBED A SIMILAR RECESSIVE MUTATION IN DROSOPHILA.

BEADLE, G. W.* A GENE FOR STICKY CHROMOSOMES IN ZEA MAYS. Z. IND. ABSTAM. VERERBUNGSL. 63* 195-217, 1932.

R
E
C
E
S
S
I
V
E

BOCZKOWSKI, K., HERMAN, E. AND JEDRZEJEWSKI, M.* THE PRESENCE OF TURNER'S SYNDROME WITH 45, X KARYOTYPE IN TWO GENERATIONS. AM. J. OBSTET. GYNEC. 103* 597-599, 1969.

GOLDSTEIN, A., HAUSKNECHT, R., HSU, L. Y., BRENDLER, H. AND HIRSCHHORN, K.* SEX CHROMOSOME MOSAICISM IN 3 SIBS. CLINICAL AND PATHOLOGIC ASPECTS. AM. J. OBSTET. GYNEC. 107* 108-115, 1970.

GOWEN, J. W.* MEIOSIS AS A GENETIC CHARACTER IN DROSOPHILA MELANOGASTER. J. EXP. ZOOL. 65* 83-106, 1933.

HSU, L. Y. F., HIRSCHHORN, K., GOLDSTEIN, A. AND BARCINSKI, M. A.* FAMILIAL CHROMOSOMAL MOSAICISM, GENETIC ASPECTS. ANN. HUM. GENET. 33* 343-349, 1970.

HIRSCHHORN, K. AND HSU, L. Y.* SEX CHROMOSOME MOSAICISM IN INDIVIDUALS WITH A Y CHROMOSOME. THE CLINICAL DELINEATION OF BIRTH DEFECTS. V. PHENOTYPIC ASPECTS OF CHROMOSOMAL ABERRATIONS. NEW YORK* NATIONAL FOUNDATION, 1969. PP. 19-23.

KWITEROVICH, P. O., JR., CROSS, H. E. AND MCKUSICK, V. A.* MONGOLISM IN AN INBRED POPULATION. BULL. HOPKINS HOSP. 119* 268-275, 1966.

LEWIS, E. B. AND GENCARELLA, W.* CLARET AND NON-DISJUNCTION IN DROSOPHILA MELANOGASTER. (ABSTRACT) GENETICS 37* 600-601, 1952.

MATSUNAGA, E.* DOWN'S SYNDROME AND MATERNAL INBREEDING. ACTA GENET. MED. GEM. 15* 224-229, 1966.

PENROSE, L. S.* MONGOLISM. BRIT. MED. BULL. 17* 184-189, 1961.

25740 NYSTAGMUS

FOR EVIDENCE OF AUTOSOMAL RECESSIVE INHERITANCE OF AN ISOLATED VARIETY OF NYSTAGMUS, SEE REVIEW BY WAARDENBURG (1962), INCLUDING PEDIGREES (WAARDENBURG, 1963).

WAARDENBURG, P. J.* DE GENETICA MEDICA. ROME* L. GEDDA (ED.) 6* 100 ONLY, 1962.

WAARDENBURG, P. J., FRANCESCHETTI, A. AND KLEIN, D. (EDS.)* IN, GENETICS AND OPHTHALMOLOGY. SPRINGFIELD, ILL.* CHARLES C THOMAS, 2* 1043 ONLY, 1963.

2575(OBESITY-HYPOVENTILATION SYNDROME (PICKWICKIAN SYNDROME)

FALSETTI AND COLLEAGUES (1964) DESCRIBED AFFECTED BROTHER AND SISTER. THE FEATURES ARE OBESITY, CYANOSIS, SOMNOLENCE, MUSCULAR TWITCHING AND PERIODIC BREATHING.

*25760 OCULAR MYOPATHY WITH CURARE SENSITIVITY

IN AN INBRED KINDRED OF SOUTH INDIA, MATHEW ET AL. (1970) OBSERVED 9 PERSONS WITH
STATIC OPHTHALMOPARESIS BEGINNING IN CHILDHOOD. OROPHARYNGEAL WEAKNESS WAS NOT
ASSOCIATED BUT LIMB WEAKNESS WAS NOTED IN 2. THERE WAS NO RESPONSE TO NEOSTIGMINE
OR ECHOPHONIUM, AND THE RESPONSE TO TETANIC STIMULATION OF THE ULNAR NERVE WAS
NORMAL. THE AUTHORS FOR THESE REASONS REGARDED THE CONDITION AS AN OCULAR
MYOPATHY AND NOT A FORM OF MYASTHENIA GRAVIS, DESPITE THE FACT THAT ALL SUBJECTS
WERE AS SENSITIVE TO TUBOCURARINE AS PATIENTS WITH MYASTHENIA GRAVIS. THE
PEDIGREE IS CONVINCINGLY THAT OF AN AUTOSOMAL RECESSIVE. TWO ASYMPTOMATIC
PRESUMED HETEROZYGOTES SHOWED SENSITIVITY TO TUBOCURARINE.

MATHEW, N. T., JACOB, J. C. AND CHANDY, J.* FAMILIAL OCULAR MYOPATHY WITH
CURARE SENSITIVITY. ARCH. NEUROL. 22* 68-74, 1970.

25770 OCULO-AURICULO-VERTEBRAL DYSPLASIA (OAV SYNDROME* GOLDENHAR SYNDROME)

THE FEATURES ARE (1) COLOBOMA OF THE EYELID AND DERMOID OF THE CONJUNCTIVA, (2)
ACCESSORY AURICULAR APPENDAGES ANTERIOR TO THE EAR, AND (3) VERTEBRAL ANOMALIES.
THE ZYGOMATIC ARCHES ARE HYPOPLASTIC, PRODUCING ABSENCE OF THE USUAL MALAR
EMINENCES, AND THE MANDIBLE IS HYPOPLASTIC AS IN MANDIBULO-FACIAL DYSOSTOSIS
(Q.V.) WITH WHICH THE OAV SYNDROME IS SOMETIMES CONFUSED. SARAUX, GRIGNON AND
DHERMY (1963) DESCRIBED 2 AFFECTED SISTERS BORN OF HEALTHY, UNRELATED PARENTS.
THE KARYOTYPE WAS NORMAL. PROTO AND SCULLICA (1966) DESCRIBED THE CONDITION IN A
FATHER AND HIS SON AND DAUGHTER. THE MOTHER WAS A FIRST COUSIN OF THE FATHER. A
PATIENT POSSIBLY WITH THE SAME CONDITION WAS OBSERVED BY FRASER (1957) TO HAVE
ACRO-OSTEOLYSIS OF THE TERMINAL PHALANGES. SUMMITT (1969) DESCRIBED A KINDRED
WITH MANY AFFECTED PERSONS IN AN AUTOSOMAL DOMINANT PATTERN INCLUDING MALE-TO-MALE
TRANSMISSION. NOTABLE VARIABILITY IN THE CLINICAL PICTURE WAS DESCRIBED. WHITE
(1969) DESCRIBED A GIRL WITH SOME OF THE FEATURES OF GOLDENHAR'S SYNDROME. SHE
SHOWED EPIBULBAR DERMOID, NASAL FISTULA NEAR NOSTRIL, AND NASAL SEPTUM AND IN THE
MOUTH BEHIND THE PHILTRUM. KRAUSE (1970) DESCRIBED AFFECTED BROTHER AND SISTER.
THE PROBAND HAD A HEMANGIOMA OF THE SCALP. SARAUX ET AL. (1963) DESCRIBED
AFFECTED SISTERS.

FRASER, G. R.* ADELAIDE, AUSTRALIA* PERSONAL COMMUNICATION, 1967.

GOLDENHAR, M.* ASSOCIATIONS MALFORMATIVES DE L'OEIL ET DE L'OREILLE. EN
PARTICULIER, LE SYNDROME* DERMOIDE EPIBULBAIRE-APPENDICES AURICULAIRES - FISTULA
AURIS CONGENITA ET SES RELATIONS AVEC LA DYSOSTOSE MANDIBULO-FACIALE. J. GENET.
HUM. 1* 243-282, 1952.

GORLIN, R. J. AND PINDBORG, J. J.* OCULOAURICULOVERTEBRAL DYSPLASIA. IN,
SYNDROMES OF THE HEAD AND NECK. NEW YORK* BLACKISTON DIVISION, MCGRAW-HILL BOOK
CO., 1964. PP. 419-426.

KRAUSE, U.* THE SYNDROME OF GOLDENHAR AFFECTING TWO SIBLINGS. ACTA OPHTHAL.
48* 494-499, 1970.

PROTO, F. AND SCULLICA, L.* CONTRIBUTO ALLO STUDIO DELLA EREDITARIETA DIE
DERMOIDI EPIBULBARI. ACTA GENET. MED. GEM. 15* 351-363, 1966.

SARAUX, H., GRIGNON, J.-L. AND DHERMY, P.* A PROPOS D'UNE OBSERVATION FAMILIALE
DE SYNDROME DE FRANCESCHETTI-GOLDENHAR. BULL. SOC. OPHTAL. FRANC. 63* 705-707,
1963.

SUMMITT, R. L.* FAMILIAL GOLDENHAR SYNDROME. THE CLINICAL DELINEATION OF BIRTH
DEFECTS. II. MALFORMATION SYNDROMES. NEW YORK* NATIONAL FOUNDATION, 1969. PP.
106-109.

WHITE, J. H.* OCULO-NASAL DYSPLASIA. J. GENET. HUM. 17* 107-114, 1969.

*25780 OCULOCEREBRAL SYNDROME WITH HYPOPIGMENTATION

CROSS, MCKUSICK AND BREEN (1967) DESCRIBED A FAMILY IN WHICH FOUR SIBS, TWO MALE
AND TWO FEMALE, HAD CUTANEOUS HYPOPIGMENTATION, SEVERE OCULAR ANOMALIES, AND
CEREBRAL DEFECT MANIFESTED BY SPASTICITY, MENTAL AND PHYSICAL RETARDATION AND
ATHETOID MOVEMENTS.

CROSS, H. E., MCKUSICK, V. A. AND BREEN, W.* A NEW OCULOCEREBRAL SYNDROME WITH
HYPOPIGMENTATION. J. PEDIAT. 70* 398-406, 1967.

25790 OCULO-OSTEO-CUTANEOUS SYNDROME

TUOMAALA AND HAAPANEN (1968) DESCRIBED TWO SISTERS AND A BROTHER WITH SIMILAR
ANOMALIES OF THE EYES (STRABISMUS, MYOPIA, DISTICHIASIS), BONES (SHORT STATURE,
BRACHYDACTYLY, HYPOPLASTIC MAXILLA), AND SKIN (SCANTY HAIR, HYPOPIGMENTATION).
THE PATIENTS WERE ALL MENTALLY RETARDED.

TUOMAALA, P. AND HAAPANEN, E.* THREE SIBLINGS WITH SIMILAR ANOMALIES IN THE EYES, BONES AND SKIN. ACTA OPHTHAL. 46* 365-371, 1968.

25800 ODOR, PECULIAR

A PECULIAR ODOR IN ASSOCIATION WITH MENTAL RETARDATION IS A VALUABLE CLUE TO THE PRESENCE OF A METABOLIC DEFECT, WITNESS MAPLE SYRUP URINE DISEASE, ISOVALERICACI-DEMIA, PHENYLKETONURIA, SIDBURY SYNDROME, OASTHOUSE URINE DISEASE, METHIONINE MALABSORPTION.

*25810 OGUCHI'S DISEASE

THE CHARACTERISTICS ARE CONGENITAL, STATIC HEMERALOPIA AND DIFFUSE YELLOW OR GRAY COLORATION OF THE FUNDUS. AFTER 2 OR 3 HOURS IN TOTAL DARKNESS, THE NORMAL COLOR OF THE FUNDUS RETURNS. THE CONDITION IS MORE FREQUENT IN JAPANESE. SEE HEMERALO-PIA FOR A COMMENT ON THE USE OF THIS TERM.

CACCAMISE, W. C.* CONGENITAL NONPROGRESSIVE NIGHT BLINDNESS. BULL. U.S. ARMY MED. DEPT. 9* 920-928, 1949.

FRANCESCHETTI, A. AND CHOME-BERCIOUX, N.* FUNDUS ALBIPUNCTATUS CUM HEMERALOPIE (CAS STATIONNAIRE DEPUIS 49 ANS). OPHTHALMOLOGICA 121* 185-193, 1951.

FRANCOIS, J., VERRIEST, G. AND DE ROUCK, A.* LA MALADIE D'OGUCHI. OPHTHALMOLO-GICA 131* 1-40, 1956.

KLEIN, B. A.* A CASE OF SO-CALLED OGUCHI'S DISEASE IN THE U.S.A. AM. J. OPHTHAL. 22* 953-955, 1939.

25820 OLIVER SYNDROME (POSTAXIAL POLYDACTYLY AND MENTAL RETARDATION)

OLIVER (1940) DESCRIBED TWO FEMALE AND ONE MALE OFFSPRING OF A COUSIN MARRIAGE WITH THIS COMBINATION.

OLIVER, C. P.* RECESSIVE POLYDACTYLISM ASSOCIATED WITH MENTAL DEFICIENCY. J. HERED. 31* 365-367, 1940.

25830 OLIVOPONTOCEREBELLAR ATROPHY II (OPCA II, FICKLER-WINKLER TYPE)

ASIDE FROM THE DIFFERENT MODE OF INHERITANCE, OPCA II DIFFERS FROM OPCA I (Q.V.) IN A LACK OF INVOLUNTARY MOVEMENTS AND OF SENSORY CHANGES.

FICKLER, A.* KLINISCHE UND PATHOLOGISCH-ANATOMISCHE BEITRAG ZU DEN ERKRANKUNGEN DES KLEINHIRNS. DEUTSCH. Z. NERVENHEILK. 41* 306-375, 1911.

WINKLER, C.* A CASE OF OLIVO-PONTINE CEREBELLAR ATROPHY AND OUR CONCEPTIONS OF NEO- AND PALAIO-CEREBELLUM. SCHWEIZ. ARCH. NEUROL. PSYCHIAT. 13* 684-702, 1923.

*25840 OPHTHALMOPLEGIA TOTALIS WITH PTOSIS AND MIOSIS

FOR EVIDENCE SUPPORTING THE EXISTENCE OF AN AUTOSOMAL RECESSIVE FORM, SEE WAARDENBURG (1962, 1963).

WAARDENBURG, P. J.* DE GENETICA MEDICA. ROME* L. GEDDA (ED.) 6* 100 ONLY, 1962.

WAARDENBURG, P. J., FRANCESCHETTI, A. AND KLEIN, D.* IN, GENETICS AND OPHTHAL-MOLOGY. SPRINGFIELD, ILL.* CHARLES C THOMAS, 2* 78 ONLY, 1963.

25850 OPTIC ATROPHY, CONGENITAL OR EARLY INFANTILE

THIS DISORDER SHOULD BE DISTINGUISHED FROM CONGENITAL AMAUROSIS (TAPETORETINAL DYSPLASIA). KJER (1959) REVIEWED THE SUBJECT OF AN AUTOSOMAL RECESSIVE FORM IN CONNECTION WITH HIS STUDY OF A DOMINANT FORM. RECENT REPORTS ARE FEW IN NUMBER. PARENTAL CONSANGUINITY WAS NOTED IN EARLIER REPORTS.

KJER, P.* INFANTILE OPTIC ATROPHY WITH DOMINANT MODE OF INHERITANCE* A CLINICAL AND GENETIC STUDY OF 19 DANISH FAMILIES. ACTA OPHTHAL. 54 (SUPPL.)* 1-147, 1959.

25860 OPTIC ATROPHY, NERVE DEAFNESS, AND DIABETES MELLITUS

SHAW AND DUNCAN (1958) DESCRIBED TWO SISTERS AND A NIECE WITH OPTIC ATROPHY, NERVE DEAFNESS AND DIABETES MELLITUS. ALL THREE FEATURES HAD THEIR ONSET IN THE FIRST YEAR OF LIFE.

ROSE, F. C., FRASER, G. R., FRIEDMANN, A. I. AND KOHNER, E. M.* THE ASSOCIATION OF JUVENILE DIABETES MELLITUS AND OPTIC ATROPHY* CLINICAL AND GENETICAL ASPECTS. QUART. J. MED. 35* 385-405, 1966.

SHAW, D. A. AND DUNCAN, L. J. P.* OPTIC ATROPHY AND NERVE DEAFNESS IN DIABETES MELLITUS. J. NEUROL. PSYCHIAT. 21* 47-49, 1958.

R
E
C
E
S
S
I
V
E

MULLER AND ZEMAN (1965) REPORTED TWO BROTHERS WITH DEGENERATION OF THE OPTIC,
COCHLEAR, DENTATE AND MEDIAL LEMNISCAL SYSTEMS. THE CLINICAL PICTURE COULD BE
CORRELATED. SEVEN OTHER CASES ARE NOW KNOWN. BLINDNESS WITH OPTIC ATROPHY,
DEAFNESS, LITTLE OR NO SPEECH, SPASTICITY AND DEATH BEFORE AGE 10 WERE FEATURES.

MULLER, J. AND ZEMAN, W.* DEGENERESCENCE SYSTEMATISEE OPTICO-COCHLEO-DENTELEE.
ACTA NEUROPATH. 5* 26-39, 1965.

25880 ORAL SENSIBILITY, DISTURBANCE OF

BOSMA (1965) HAS STUDIED A CONDITION IN WHICH BECAUSE OF SENSORY PROBLEM IN THE
MOUTH THE PATIENT REMAINS INFANTILE IN ORAL CONFIGURATION AND FUNCTION. THE
LABIAL GATE REMAINS INFANTILE WITH DROOLING, AND NIPPLE (SUCKLE) FEEDING ONLY IS
PRACTICED, EVEN IN THE ADULT. ONE EXPECTS THE LABIAL GATE FUNCTION TO DEVELOP BY
AGE 22-24 MONTHS. TWO-POINT DISCRIMINATION IS DEFECTIVE IN THE MOUTH. THE
PATIENTS APPEAR TO HAVE FACIAL DIPLEGIA. THE SMILE IS TRANSVERSE AS IN DYSAU-
TONOMIA.   OFTEN THE PATIENT STANDS WITH THE HEAD BACK TO PREVENT DROOLING, AND IN
SOME INSTANCES THE SALIVARY GLANDS HAVE BEEN REMOVED. MINOR NEUROLOGIC DEFECTS
MAY BE DEMONSTRABLE ELSEWHERE SUCH AS IN THE HANDS WHERE A SENSORY TYPE OF
INCOORDINATION IS DEMONSTRABLE. ONE 19 YEAR OLD FEMALE HAS MARRIED. NO FAMILIAL
CASES HAVE IN FACT BEEN IDENTIFIED BUT FEW CASES ARE KNOWN.

BOSMA, J. F.* BETHESDA, MD.* PERSONAL COMMUNICATION, 1965.

BOSMA, J. F., GROSSMAN, R. C. AND KAVANAGH, J. F.* A SYNDROME OF IMPAIRMENT OF
ORAL PERCEPTION. IN, BOSMA, J. F. (ED.)* SYMPOSIUM ON ORAL SENSATION AND
PERCEPTION. SPRINGFIELD, ILL.* CHARLES C THOMAS, 1967. PP. 318-335.

*25890 OROTICACIDURIA

THE FEATURES (HUGULEY ET AL., 1959) ARE MEGALOBLASTIC ANEMIA WHICH IS UNRESPONSIVE
TO VITAMIN B12 AND FOLIC ACID, HYPOCHROMIC, MICROCYTIC CIRCULATING ERYTHROCYTES
WHICH DO NOT CHANGE WITH ADMINISTRATION OF IRON OR PYRIDOXINE, LARGE AMOUNTS OF
OROTIC ACID IN THE URINE, AND CORRECTION OF ANEMIA WITH REDUCTION IN OROTIC ACID
EXCRETION WHEN URIDYLIC ACID AND CYTIDYLIC ACID WERE ADMINISTERED. FALLON AND
COLLEAGUES (1964) HAVE EXTENSIVELY STUDIED THE HETEROZYGOTES IN THE FIRST FAMILY
DESCRIBED (HUGULEY ET AL., 1959). A SECOND FAMILY HAS BEEN DISCOVERED IN NEW
ZEALAND AND A THIRD IN TEXAS (HAGGARD, LOCKHART, 1965). IN THE LAST PATIENT
URINARY OBSTRUCTION WAS PRODUCED BY THE HIGH URINARY EXCRETION OF OROTIC ACID.
ROGERS ET AL. (1968) DESCRIBED ANOTHER CASE, FROM NORTH CAROLINA. ROGERS AND
PORTER (1968) DEVISED A SCREENING TEST WHICH IS EFFECTIVE IN DETECTING EITHER
HOMOZYGOTES OR HETEROZYGOTES.

R
E
C
E
S
S
I
V
E

BECROFT, D. M. O., PHILLIPS, L. I. AND SIMMONDS, A.* HEREDITARY OROTIC
ACIDURIA* LONG-TERM THERAPY WITH URIDINE AND A TRIAL OF URACIL. J. PEDIAT. 75*
885-891, 1969.

FALLON, H. J., SMITH, L. H., GRAHAM, J. B. AND BURNETT, C. H.* A GENETIC STUDY
OF HEREDITARY OROTIC ACIDURIA. NEW ENG. J. MED. 270* 878-881, 1964.

HAGGARD, M. E. AND LOCKHART, L. H.* HEREDITARY OROTIC ACIDURIA, A DISORDER OF
PYRIMIDINE METABOLISM RESPONSIVE TO URIDINE THERAPY. (ABSTRACT) J. PEDIAT. 67*
906 ONLY, 1965.

HUGULEY, C. M., JR., BAIN, J. A., RIVERS, S. L. AND SCOGGINS, R. B.* REFRACTORY
MEGALOBLASTIC ANEMIA ASSOCIATED WITH EXCRETION OF OROTIC ACID. BLOOD 14* 615-634,
1959.

ROGERS, L. E. AND PORTER, F. S.* HEREDITARY OROTIC ACIDURIA. II. A URINARY
SCREENING TEST. PEDIATRICS 42* 423-428, 1968.

ROGERS, L. E., WARFORD, L. R., PATTERSON, R. B. AND PORTER, F. S.* HEREDITARY
OROTIC ACIDURIA. I. A NEW CASE WITH FAMILY STUDIES. PEDIATRICS 42* 415-422,
1968.

SMITH, L. H., JR.* HEREDITARY OROTIC ACIDURIA-PYRIMIDINE AUXOTROPHISM IN MAN.
(EDITORIAL) AM. J. MED. 38* 1-6, 1965.

SMITH, L. H., JR., HUGULEY, C. M., JR. AND BAIN, J. A.* HEREDITARY OROTIC
ACIDURIA. IN, STANBURY, J. B., WYNGAARDEN, J. B. AND FREDRICKSON, D. S. (EDS.)*
THE METABOLIC BASIS OF INHERITED DISEASE. NEW YORK* MCGRAW-HILL, 1966 (2ND ED.).
PP. 739-758.

TUBERGEN, D. G., KROOTH, R. S. AND HEYN, R. M.* HEREDITARY OROTIC ACIDURIA WITH
NORMAL GROWTH AND DEVELOPMENT. AM. J. DIS. CHILD. 118* 864-870, 1969.

*25900 OSTEOARTHROPATHY OF SCHINZ AND FURTWAENGLER

IN 1928, IN FREIBURG, GERMANY, SCHINZ AND FURTWAENGLER DESCRIBED A SIBSHIP OF 11,
THE OFFSPRING OF A FIRST COUSIN MARRIAGE, IN WHICH A MAN THEN 29 YEARS OLD AND

THREE OF HIS SISTERS WERE IDENTICALLY AFFECTED BY A DISORDER OF WHICH A STRIKING FEATURE WAS STIFF JOINTS. FLEXION CONTRACTURE IN THE FINGERS AND TOES WAS COMBINED WITH REDUCED MOBILITY IN THE ANKLES, WRISTS, KNEES, ELBOWS, HIPS, SHOULDERS AND SPINE. THE FACE WAS RED WITH SOMEWHAT PROMINENT FOREHEAD, BROAD NOSE AND FLESHY TONGUE. INTELLIGENCE WAS NORMAL. UMBILICAL HERNIA WAS PRESENT IN THE MALE, WHOSE HEIGHT WAS 61.4 INCHES. X-RAYS SHOWED THICK SKULL, SHORT POSTERIOR CRANIAL FOSSA AND PROMINENT EXTERNAL AND INTERNAL OCCIPITAL PROTU-BERANCE. A STRIKING FEATURE WAS EXTENSIVE DESTRUCTION OR DISTURBANCE IN THE DEVELOPMENT OF THE CARPAL AND TARSAL BONES. IN 1934 HORSCH DESCRIBED A SISTER FROM THE SAME SIBSHIP. ALL FEATURES INCLUDING THOSE IN THE CARPAL AND TARSAL BONES WERE IDENTICAL. THE BROTHER WAS RESTUDIED WITH DESCRIPTION OF CYSTS IN THE HEAD OF THE HUMERUS AND THE EPIPHYSIS OF THE RADIUS AND DIGITS. LANGER, KRONEN-BERG AND GORLIN (1966) DESCRIBED A 61 YEAR OLD MALE WHO APPEARED TO HAVE THE SAME DISORDER, INCLUDING CHANGES IN THE JOINTS, CARPAL AND TARSAL BONES, AND CORNEA. THE URINE CONTAINED NO EXCESS OF ACID MUCOPOLYSACCHARIDE BUT DID HAVE AN EXCESS OF A GLYCOPROTEIN. MANY OF THE FEATURES RESEMBLE THOSE OF THE HUNTER SYNDROME (MPS II) AND OF SCHEIE'S SYNDROME (MPS V), AND SPRANGER (1970) THINKS THAT SCHINZ CASES HAD SCHEIE'S SYNDROME BUT IT IS LIKELY THAT THIS IS A SEPARATE ENTITY. (HUNTER SYNDROME IS X-LINKED.) THE SKELETAL CHANGES ARE SOMEWHAT LIKE THOSE OF THE DOMINANT DISORDER, HEREDITARY PROGRESSIVE ARTHRO-OPHTHALMOPATHY.

HORSCH, K.* UBER HEREDITARE DEGENERATIVE OSTEOARTHROPATHIE. ARCH. ORTHOP. UNFALLCHIR. 34* 536-540, 1934.

LANGER, L. O., JR., KRONENBERG, R. S. AND GORLIN, R. J.* A CASE SIMULATING HURLER SYNDROME OF UNUSUAL LONGEVITY, WITHOUT ABNORMAL MUCOPOLYSACCHARIDURIA. A PROPOSED CLASSIFICATION OF THE VARIOUS FORMS OF THE SYNDROME AND SIMILAR DISEASES. AM. J. MED. 40* 448-457, 1966.

SCHINZ, H. R. AND FURTWAENGLER, A.* ZUR KENNTNIS EINER HEREDITAREN OSTEO-ARTHROPATHIE MIT REZEZSIVEM EREGANG. DEUTSCH. Z. CHIR. 207* 398-416, 1928.

SCHMIDT, R.* EINE BISHER NICHT BESCHRIEBENE FORM FAMIL HORNHAUTENARTUNG IN VERBINDUNG MIT OSTROARTHROPATHIE. KLIN. MBL. AUGENGEILK. 100* 616-620, 1938.

SPRANGER, J.* MADISON, WIS.* PERSONAL COMMUNICATION, 1970.

R
E
C
E
S
S
I
V
E

25910 OSTEOARTHROPATHY, FAMILIAL IDIOPATHIC, OF CHILDHOOD

CURRARINO ET AL. (1961) AND CHAMBERLAIN ET AL. (1965) REPORTED A NEGRO FAMILY IN WHICH THREE SISTERS HAD A FORM OF OSTEOARTHROPATHY SEEMINGLY DISTINCT FROM PACHYDERMOPERIOSTOSIS (Q.V.). THE SALIENT FEATURES WERE CLUBBING OF THE FINGERS, ECZEMATOUS SKIN ERUPTION, PERIOSTEAL NEW BONE FORMATION, AND DEFECTS OF THE CRANIAL BONES RESULTING IN WIDE FONTANELLES. CREMIN (1970) DESCRIBED A CASE.

CHAMBERLAIN, D. S., WHITAKER, J. AND SILVERMAN, F. N.* IDIOPATHIC OSTEOARTHRO-PATHY AND CRANIAL DEFECTS IN CHILDREN (FAMILIAL IDIOPATHIC OSTEOARTHROPATHY). AM. J. ROENTGEN. 93* 408-415, 1965.

CREMIN, B. J.* FAMILIAL IDIOPATHIC OSTEOARTHROPATHY OF CHILDREN* A CASE REPORT AND PROGRESS. BRIT. J. RADIOL. 43* 568-570, 1970.

CURRARINO, G., TIERNEY, R. C., GIESEL, R. G. AND WEIHL, C.* FAMILIAL IDIOPATHIC OSTEOARTHROPATHY. AM. J. ROENTGEN. 85* 633-644, 1961.

25920 OSTEOCHONDROSIS DEFORMANS TIBIAE, FAMILIAL INFANTILE TYPE

OSTEOCHONDROSIS DEFORMANS TIBIAE IS ALSO CALLED TIBIA VARA, OR BLOUNT'S DISEASE. BLOUNT (1937) DISTINGUISHED INFANTILE AND JUVENILE FORMS. SEVASTIKOGLOU AND ERIKSSON (1967) OBSERVED FOUR AFFECTED WITH THE INFANTILE FORM IN A SIBSHIP OF 6 CHILDREN. TWO OF THE AFFECTED WERE IDENTICAL TWINS. SEE TIBIA VARA IN DOMINANT CATALOG.

BLOUNT, W. P.* TIBIA VARA* OSTEOCHONDROSIS DEFORMANS TIBIAE. J. BONE JOINT SURG. 19* 1-29, 1937.

SEVASTIKOGLOU, J. A. AND ERIKSSON, J.* FAMILIAL INFANTILE OSTEOCHONDROSIS DEFORMANS TIBIAE. IDIOPATHIC TIBIA VARA. A CASE REPORT. ACTA ORTHOP. SCAND. 38* 81-87, 1967.

25930 OSTEODYSTROPHY AND MENTAL RETARDATION

RUVALCABA ET AL. (1971) DESCRIBED TWO BROTHERS, BORN TO UNRELATED PARENTS, WHO SHOWED MENTAL RETARDATION, SHORT STATURE, MICROCEPHALY, PECULIAR FACIES WITH HOOKED NOSE AND SMALL MOUTH, NARROW THORACIC CAGE WITH PECTUS CARINATUM HYPOPLAS-TIC GENITALIA, HYPOPLASTIC 'ONION SKIN' CUTANEOUS LESIONS AND SKELETAL DEFORMITIES INCLUDING SHORT METATARSALS AND METACARPALS AND EPIPHYSITIS OF THE SPINE. BECAUSE TWO FEMALE MATERNAL COUSINS SHOWED SOME OF THE SAME FEATURES, X-LINKED SEMI-DOMINANT INHERITANCE WAS CONSIDERED. ONE OF THE GIRLS SEEM TO HAVE BEEN FULLY AFFECTED, HOWEVER. SHE DIED AT AGE 17 YEARS WITH CONGENITAL HYDROCEPHALUS AND THE DANDY-WALKER ANOMALY.

SMARS, BECKMAN AND BOOK (1961), MCKUSICK AND COLLEAGUES (1961), AWWAAD AND REDA (1960) AND OTHERS HAVE DESCRIBED FAMILIES WITH TWO OR MORE AFFECTED SIBS FROM OSTENSIBLY NORMAL PARENTS. SUCH IS PROBABLY TO BE EXPECTED OF A DOMINANT TRAIT WITH WIDE EXPRESSIVITY AND DOES NOT REQUIRE A RECESSIVE EXPLANATION. HANHART (1951), HOWEVER, DESCRIBED A KINDRED WITH AFFECTED MEMBERS IN FIVE SIBSHIPS. HERE INCOMPLETE DOMINANCE IS NOT SO SATISFACTORY AN EXPLANATION. IN ALL SUCH STUDIES CARE MUST BE TAKEN NOT TO CONFUSE HYPOPHOSPHATASIA FOR OSTEOGENESIS IMPERFECTA. KAPLAN AND BALDINO (1953) DESCRIBED A KINDRED DERIVED FROM AN INBRED, ARABIC-SPEAKING, POLYGAMOUS SECT CALLED THE MOZABITES, LIVING IN SOUTHERN ALGERIA. NINE CASES OCCURRED IN FOUR SIBSHIPS AMONG THE DESCENDANTS AND LAPLANE ET AL. (1959) AND KAPLAN ET AL. (1958), IN A FOLLOW-UP OF THE SAME KINDRED DESCRIBED 19 CASES. PARENTAL CONSANGUINITY WAS NOTED BY SEVERAL AUTHORS, INCLUDING FREUND AND LEHMACHER (1954) AND ROHWEDDER (1953) WHO DESCRIBED A CASE IN WHICH THE PARENTS WERE BROTHER AND SISTER.

MEYER (1955) REPORTED 'ATYPICAL OSTEOGENESIS IMPERFECTA' IN SEVERAL OF THE 11 OFFSPRING OF A MENTALLY DEFECTIVE WOMAN BY HER OWN FATHER. MANIFESTATIONS WERE SPONTANEOUS FRACTURES, GENERALIZED OSTEOPOROSIS, AND WORMIAN BONES IN THE AREA OF THE LAMBDOIDAL SUTURES. BLUE SCLERAE AND DEAFNESS WERE NOT PRESENT. MORPHOLOGI-CALLY THESE APPEAR TO BE TWO FORMS OF OI CONGENITA, A THIN BONED AND A BROAD-BONED TYPE. THE LATTER IS WELL ILLUSTRATED BY THE MALE AND FEMALE SIBS REPORTED BY REMIGIO AND GRINVALSKY (1970). ONE HAD DISLOCATED LENSES, AORTIC COARCTATION, AND BASOPHILIC AND MUCOID CHANGES IN THE CONNECTIVE TISSUE OF THE HEART VALVES AND AORTA. THE OTHER HAD LESS PRONOUNCED CHANGES OF THE SAME NATURE IN THE AORTA. PARENTAL CONSANGUINITY WAS DENIED. THE BROAD-BONED TYPE IS ALSO ILLUSTRATED IN FIG. 6-3 BY MCKUSICK (1966) AND THE THIN-BONE TYPE IN FIG. 6-5.

AWWAAD, S. AND REDA, M.* OSTEOGENESIS IMPERFECTA* REVIEW OF LITERATURE AND A REPORT ON THREE CASES. ARCH. PEDIAT. 77* 280-290, 1960.

FREUND, R. AND LEHMACHER, K.* BEITRAG ZUR VERERBUNG DER OSTEOGENESIS IMPERFEC-TA. GEBURTSH. FRAUENHEILK. 14* 171-177, 1954.

GOLDFARB, A. A. AND FORD, D., JR.* OSTEOGENESIS IMPERFECTA CONGENITA IN CONSECUTIVE SIBLINGS. J. PEDIAT. 44* 264-268, 1954.

HANHART, E.* UBER EINE NEUE FORM VON OSTEOPSATHYROSIS CONGENITA MIT EINFACH-REZESSIVEM, SOWIE 4 NEUE SIPPEN MIT DOMINANTEM ERBGANG UND DIE FRAGE DER VERERBUNG DER SOG. OSTEOGENESIS IMPERFECTA. ARCH. KLAUS STIFT. VERERBUNGSFORSCH. 26* 426-437, 1951.

IBSEN, K. H.* DISTINCT VARIETIES OF OSTEOGENESIS IMPERFECTA. CLIN. ORTHOP. 50* 279-290, 1967.

KAPLAN, M. AND BALDINO, C.* DYSPLASIE PERIOSTALE PARAISSANT FAMILIALE ET TRANSMISE SUIVANT LE MODE MENDELIEN RECESSIF. ARCH. FRANC. PEDIAT. 10* 943-950, 1953.

KAPLAN, M., LAPLANE, M. R., DEBRAY, P. AND LASFARGUES, G.* SUR L'HEREDITE DE LA DYSPLASIE PERIOSTALE COMPLEMENT A LA COMMUNICATION DE M. KAPLAN ET C. BALDINO. ARCH. FRANC. PEDIAT. 15* 1097-1101, 1958.

LAPLANE, M. R., LASFARGUES, G. AND DEBRAY, P.* ESSAI DE CLASSIFICATION GENETIQUE DES OSTEOGENESES IMPARFAITES. PRESSE MED. 67* 893-895, 1959.

MCKUSICK, V. A. AND COLLEAGUES* MEDICAL GENETICS 1960. J. CHRONIC DIS. 434-435, 1961. (FIG 50).

MCKUSICK, V. A.* HERITABLE DISORDERS OF CONNECTIVE TISSUE. ST. LOUIS* C. V. MOSBY CO., 1966 (3RD ED.).

MEYER, H.* ATYPICAL OSTEOGENESIS IMPERFECTA* LOBSTEIN'S DISEASE. ARCH. PEDIAT. 72* 182-186, 1955.

REMIGIO, P. A. AND GRINVALSKY, H. T.* OSTEOGENESIS IMPERFECTA CONGENITA* ASSOCIATION WITH CONSPICUOUS EXTRASKELETAL CONNECTIVE TISSUE DYSPLASIA. AM. J. DIS. CHILD. 119* 524-528, 1970.

ROHWEDDER, H. J.* EIN BEITRAG ZUR FRAGE DES ERBGANGES DER OSTEOGENESIS IMPERFECTA VROLIK. ARCH. KINDERHEILK. 147* 256-262, 1953.

SCHRODER, G.* EINE KLINISCH-ERBBIOLOGISCHE UNTERSUCHUNG DES KRANKENGUTES IN WESTFALEN. SCHATZUNG DER MUTATIONSRATEN FUR DEN REGIERUNGSBEZIRK MUNSTER (WESTFALEN). Z. MENSCHL. VERERB. KONSTITUTIONSL. 37* 632-676, 1964.

SMARS, G., BECKMAN, L. AND BOOK, J. A.* OSTEOGENESIS IMPERFECTA AND BLOOD GROUPS. ACTA GENET. STATIST. MED. 11* 133-136, 1961.

ZEITOUN, M. M., IBRAHIM, A. H. AND KASSEM, A. S.* OSTEOGENESIS IMPERFECTA CONGENITA IN DIZYGOTIC TWINS. ARCH. DIS. CHILD. 38* 289-291, 1963.

R
E
C
E
S
S
I
V
E

HARMON AND MORTON (1966) REPORTED OSTEOGENIC SARCOMA IN 4 SIBS, WITH ONSET AT 15, 20, 11 AND 22 YEARS. ON THE OTHER HAND, EPSTEIN AND BIXLER (1970) OBSERVED OSTEOGENIC SARCOMA IN A FATHER AND DAUGHTER. SEE CHONDROSARCOMA.

EPSTEIN, L. I., BIXLER, D. AND BENNETT, J. E.* AN INCIDENT OF FAMILIAR CANCER* INCLUDING 3 CASES OF OSTEOGENIC SARCOMA. CANCER 25* 889-891, 1970.

HARMON, T. P. AND MORTON, K. S.* OSTEOGENIC SARCOMA IN FOUR SIBLINGS. J. BONE JOINT SURG. 48B* 493-498, 1966.

*25960 OSTEOLYSIS, HEREDITARY MULTICENTRIC

AMONG THE OFFSPRING OF DOUBLE SECOND COUSINS, TORG ET AL. (1969) DESCRIBED A NEW SKELETAL DISORDER TO WHICH THEY GAVE THE ABOVE DESIGNATION. IN ADDITION TO COLLAPSE AND RESORPTION OF THE CARPAL AND TARSAL BONES, THERE WERE OSTEOPOROSIS, CORTICAL THINNING AND INCREASED CALIBER OF THE TUBULAR AND LONG BONES. CLINICAL-LY, THE DISORDER WAS CHARACTERIZED BY FUSIFORM ENLARGEMENT OF THE DIGITS AND FLEXION CONTRACTURES OF THE KNEES, HIP AND ELBOWS.

TORG, J. S., DIGEORGE, A. M., KIRKPATRICK, J. A., JR. AND MARTINEZ TRUJILLO, M.* HEREDITARY MULTICENTRIC OSTEOLYSIS WITH RECESSIVE TRANSMISSION* A NEW SYNDROME. J. PEDIAT. 75* 243-252, 1969.

*25970 OSTEOPETROSIS ('MARBLE BONES,' ALBERS-SCHONBERG DISEASE)

THE FEATURES ARE MACROCEPHALY, PROGRESSIVE DEAFNESS AND BLINDNESS, HEPATOSPLENOME-GALY AND SEVERE ANEMIA BEGINNING IN EARLY INFANCY OR IN FETAL LIFE. THE CONDITION RESULTS FROM DEFECTIVE RESORPTION OF IMMATURE BONE. BY X-RAY THE DIAGNOSIS MAY BE MADE BEFORE BIRTH OF THE AFFECTED FETUS.
ENELL AND PEHRSON DESCRIBED 2 SIBS AND A COUSIN AFFECTED WITH THE EARLY SEVERE FORM IN A HIGHLY INBRED KINDRED. AN AUTOSOMAL DOMINANT FORM IS MORE BENIGN. OSTEOSCLEROSIS ALSO OCCURS IN PYCNODYSOSTOSIS, IN VAN BUCHEM'S DISEASE AND IN ENGELMANN'S DISEASE. SEE HYPEROSTOSES. SIMILARITIES TO THE GREY-LETHAL MUTATION IN THE MOUSE, WHICH SEEMS TO BE A THYROCALCITONIN EXCESS DISEASE, HAS STIMULATED SEARCH FOR ABNORMALITY OF THIS HORMONE IN OSTEOPETROSIS AND OTHER OSTEOSCLEROTIC CONDITIONS. THE OCCURRENCE OF HYPOCALCEMICA AND EVEN TETANY IN CASES OF OSTEOPETROSIS (E.G., J.H.H. 1208323) IS CONSISTENT WITH A THYROCALCITONIN DISORDER. KEITH (1968) PRESENTED EVIDENCE SUGGESTING THAT PRIMARY RETINAL ATROPHY, NOT OPTIC ATROPHY FROM NERVE PRESSURE, OCCURS IN OSTEOPETROSIS. MOE AND SKJAEVELAND (1969) DESCRIBED BENEFICIAL EFFECTS OF CORTISONE.

ENELL, H. AND PEHRSON, M.* STUDIES ON OSTEOPETROSIS. I. CLINICAL REPORT OF THREE CASES WITH GENETIC CONSIDERATIONS. ACTA PAEDIAT. 47* 279-287, 1958.

HANHART, E. AND SCHACKERMANN, (NI)* IN, WAARDENBURG, P. J., FRANCESCHETTI, A. AND KLEIN, D. (EDS.)* GENETICS AND OPHTHALMOLOGY. SPRINGFIELD, ILL.* CHARLES C THOMAS, 1* 336 ONLY, 1960.

HANHART, E.* UEBER DIE GENETIK DER EINFACH-REZESSIVEN FORMEN DER MARMORKNOCHEN-KRANKHEIT UND ZWEI ENTSPRECHENDE STAMMBAUME AUS DER SCHWEIZ. HELV. PAEDIAT. ACTA 3* 113-125, 1948.

KEITH, C. G.* RETINAL ATROPHY IN OSTEOPETROSIS. ARCH. OPHTHAL. 79* 234-241, 1968.

MOE, P. J. AND SKJAEVELAND, A.* THERAPEUTIC STUDIES IN OSTEOPETROSIS* REPORT OF FOUR CASES. ACTA PAEDIAT. SCAND. 58* 593-600, 1969.

TIPS, R. L. AND LYNCH, H. T.* MALIGNANT CONGENITAL OSTEOPETROSIS RESULTING FROM A CONSANGUINEOUS MARRIAGE. ACTA PAEDIAT. 51* 585-588, 1962.

25980 OSTEOPOROSIS, JUVENILE

IDIOPATHIC OSTEOPOROSIS OF CHILDHOOD OR ADOLESCENCE WITHOUT BLUE SCLERAE AND OTHER STIGMATA OF OSTEOGENESIS IMPERFECTA IS OCCASIONALLY OBSERVED AND SOMETIMES MORE THAN ONE SIB IS AFFECTED. THIS MAY BE A DISTINCT RECESSIVELY INHERITED ENTITY. THE CONDITION DESCRIBED BY CHOWERS AND COLLEAGUES (1962) MAY FALL INTO THIS CATEGORY BUT THE PRESENCE OF AMINOACIDURIA AND LOW SERUM URIC ACID MAKES A RENAL TUBULAR DEFECT OF THE FANCONI TYPE LIKELY.

BERGLUND, G. AND LINDQUIST, B.* OSTEOPENIA IN ADOLESCENCE. CLIN. ORTHOP. 17* 259-264, 1960.

CHOWERS, I., CZACZKES, J. W., EHRENFELD, E. N. AND LANDAU, S.* FAMILIAL AMINOACIDURIA IN OSTEOGENESIS IMPERFECTA. J.A.M.A. 181* 771-775, 1962.

DENT, C. E. AND FRIEDMAN, M.* IDIOPATHIC JUVENILE OSTEOPOROSIS. QUART. J. MED. 34* 177-210, 1965.

JACKSON, W. P. U.* OSTEOPOROSIS OF UNKNOWN CAUSE IN YOUNGER PEOPLE. IDIOPATHIC

R
E
C
E
S
S
I
V
E

*25990 OXALOSIS I

THE CONDITION IS CHARACTERIZED BY A CONTINUOUS HIGH URINARY OXALATE EXCRETION AND
PROGRESSIVE BILATERAL OXALATE UROLITHIASIS AND NEPHROCALCINOSIS. EXTRA-RENAL
DEPOSITS OF OXALATE OCCUR IN LATER STAGES. DEATH FROM RENAL FAILURE OCCURS IN
CHILDHOOD OR EARLY ADULT LIFE. (SEE DOMINANT CATALOG FOR DESCRIPTION OF OXALATE
URINARY CALCULI FOLLOWING MALE-LIMITED AUTOSOMAL DOMINANT PEDIGREE PATTERN.)
WILLIAMS AND SMITH (1968) WERE ABLE TO DISTINGUISH TWO DISTINCT GENETIC DISORDERS
AMONG CASES OF PRIMARY HYPEROXALURIA. THE LARGEST PROPORTION HAD GLYCOLIC
ACIDURIA AND HYPEROXALURIA, MARKED REDUCTION IN METABOLISM OF C14-LABELED
GLYOXYLATE OR GLYCOLATE TO CARBON DIXIODE, INCREASED CONVERSION OF GLYOXYLATE TO
URINARY GLYCOLATE AND A DEFECT OF THE ENZYME SOLUBLE 2-OXO-GLUTARATE* GLYOXYLATE
CARBOLIGASE. OTHER PATIENTS WITH PRIMARY HYPEROXALURIA EXCRETED NORMAL AMOUNTS OF
GLYCOLIC ACID BUT LARGE AMOUNTS OF L-GLYCERIC ACID, A COMPOUND NOT PREVIOUSLY
FOUND IN BIOLOGICAL MATERIAL. IN THIS FORM THE DEFECT IS THOUGHT TO RESIDE IN THE
ENZYME D-GLYCERIC DEHYDROGENASE (GLYOXYLATE REDUCTASE). PRESUMABLY TWO SEPARATE
GENETIC LOCI ARE INVOLVED. KLAUWERS ET AL. (1969) DEMONSTRATED THAT, AS IN
CYSTINOSIS, RENAL TRANSPLANTATION IS UNSUCCESSFUL BECAUSE THE DONOR KIDNEY BECOMES
INVOLVED WITH FUNCTIONAL FAILURE. LINDENMAYER (1970) REPORTED ON FOUR CASES OF
OXALOSIS IN THREE SIBSHIPS. FIVE OF THE SIX PARENTS HE COULD TRACE TO A COMMON
ANCESTRAL COUPLE BORN IN THE 1700'S.   A USEFUL REVIEW OF PUBLISHED CASES WAS
PROVIDED.

   DENT, C. E. AND STAMP, T. C. B.* TREATMENT OF PRIMARY HYPEROXALURIA. ARCH.
DIS. CHILD. 45* 735-745, 1970.

   FREDERICK, E. W., RABKIN, M. T., RICHIE, R. H., JR. AND SMITH, L. H., JR.*
STUDIES ON PRIMARY HYPEROXALURIA. I. IN VIVO DEMONSTRATION OF A DEFECT IN
GLYOXYLATE METABOLISM. NEW ENG. J. MED. 269* 821-829, 1963.

   HOCKADAY, T. D. R., CLAYTON, J. E. AND SMITH, L. H., JR.* THE METABOLIC ERROR
IN PRIMARY HYPEROXALURIA. ARCH. DIS. CHILD. 40* 485-491, 1965.

   KLAUWERS, J., WOLF, P. L. AND COHN, R.* RENAL TRANSPLANTATION IN PRIMARY
OXALOSIS. J.A.M.A. 209* 551 ONLY, 1969.

   KOCH, J., STOKSTAD, E. L., WILLIAMS, H. E. AND SMITH, L. H., JR.* DEFICIENCY OF
2-OXO-GLUTARATE* GLYOXYLATE CARBOLIGASE ACTIVITY IN PRIMARY HYPEROXALURIA. PROC.
NAT. ACAD. SCI. 57* 1123-1129, 1967.

   LIBAN, E.* OXALOSIS IN A TRIPOLITANIAN KINSHIP. IN, GOLDSCHMIDT, E. (ED.)*
GENETICS OF MIGRANT AND ISOLATE POPULATIONS. BALTIMORE* WILLIAMS AND WILKINS,
1963. P. 303.

   LINDENMAYER, J.-P.* L'HEREDITE DANS L'OXALOSE FAMILIALE. J. GENET. HUM. 18*
31-44, 1970.

   WILLIAMS, H. E. AND SMITH, L. H., JR.* L-GLYCERIC ACIDURIA* NEW GENETIC VARIANT
OF PRIMARY HYPEROXALURIA. NEW ENG. J. MED. 278* 233-239, 1968.

   WYNGAARDEN, J. B. AND ELDER, T. D.* PRIMARY HYPEROXALURIA AND OXALOSIS. IN,
STANBURY, J. B., WYNGAARDEN, J. B. AND FREDRICKSON, D. S. (EDS.)* THE METABOLIC
BASIS OF INHERITED DISEASE. NEW YORK* MCGRAW-HILL, 1966 (2ND ED.). PP. 189-212.

*26000 OXALOSIS II

SEE ABOVE FOR EVIDENCE FOR TWO SEPARATE TYPES OF HYPEROXALURIA WHICH ARE DISTINCT
BIOCHEMICALLY AND PRESUMABLY ARE THE RESULT OF MUTATION AT SEPARATE LOCI.
WILLIAMS AND SMITH (1971) PRESENTED EVIDENCE THAT IN THIS FORM OF HYPEROXALURIA
HYDROXYPYRUVATE, PRESENT IN EXCESS BECAUSE OF DEFICIENCY IN THE ENZYME WHICH
CONVERTS IT TO D-GLYCERATE, STIMULATES OXIDATION OF GLYCOLATE TO OXYLATE AND
DECREASES REDUCTION OF GLYOXYLATE TO GLYCOLATE. THIS IS A NOVEL EXPLANATION FOR
THE PHENOTYPIC CONSEQUENCES OF A GANODIAN INBORN ERROR OF METABOLISM.

   WILLIAMS, H. E. AND SMITH, L. H., JR.* HYPEROXALURIA IN L-GLYCERIC ACIDURIA*
POSSIBLE PATHOGENETIC MECHANISM. SCIENCE 171* 390-391, 1971.

26010 PA POLYMORPHISM OF ALPHA-2-GLOBULIN

A POLYMORPHISM OF ALPHA-2-GLOBULIN WAS DEMONSTRATED BY MACLAREN ET AL. (1966)
USING THE OUCHTERLONY METHOD OF IMMUNODIFFUSION AND ANTISERUM PRODUCED IN SHEEP.
ABOUT 18 PERCENT OF MALES AND YOUNG FEMALES ARE POSITIVE. ALL WOMEN IN LATE
PREGNANCY AND WOMAN TAKING THE CONTRACEPTIVE AGENT ENOVID ARE POSITIVE. THE
DESIGNATION PA WAS GIVEN FOR THIS REASON AND MEANS 'PREGNANCY ASSOCIATED.' CORD
BLOODS ARE NEGATIVE. FAMILY DATA BEST FITTED THE VIEW THAT PA-1-POSITIVITY IS AN
AUTOSOMAL RECESSIVE TRAIT. THUS, THIS SYSTEM IS A DISTINCTLY UNUSUAL ONE FROM
SEVERAL POINTS OF VIEW. HAPTOGLOBIN AND THE GC PROTEIN ARE ALSO ALPHA-2-GLOBU-
LINS.

   MACLAREN, J. A., REID, D. E., KONUGRES, A. A. AND ALLEN, F. H., JR.* PA 1, A

R
E
C
E
S
S
I
V
E

NEW INHERITED ALPHA-2-GLOBULIN OF HUMAN SERUM.   VOX SANG. 11* 553-560, 1966.

26020 PALLIDAL DEGENERATION, PROGRESSIVE, WITH RETINITIS PIGMENTOSA

WINKELMAN (1932) DESCRIBED THIS COMBINATION IN TWO BROTHERS. THE EARLY ONSET RETINITIS PIGMENTOSA PROGRESSED TO BLINDNESS. PROGRESSIVE RIGIDITY OF EXTRAPYRA-MIDAL TYPE AND DYSARTHRIA WERE FEATURES. THE PYRAMIDAL TRACTS WERE, BY BOTH CLINICAL AND PATHOLOGIC EVIDENCE, UNAFFECTED, AND THERE WERE NO SENSORY CHANGES. ONE BROTHER DIED AT AGE 24 YEARS. DESTRUCTION OF THE PALLIDA AND RETICULAR PORTIONS OF THE SUBSTANTIA NIGRA WERE DEMONSTRATED. X-LINKED INHERITANCE IS, OF COURSE, POSSIBLE.

WINKELMAN, N. W.* PROGRESSIVE PALLIDAL DEGENERATION. A NEW CLINICOPATHOLOGIC SYNDROME. ARCH. NEUROL. PSYCHIAT. 27* 1-21, 1932.

*26030 PALLIDO-PYRAMIDAL SYNDROME

DAVISON (1954) DESCRIBED 5 AFFECTED CASES IN 3 FAMILIES. IN ONE FAMILY A BROTHER AND SISTER WITH FIRST-COUSIN PARENTS WERE AFFECTED AND IN ANOTHER FAMILY A BROTHER AND SISTER WITH UNCLE-NIECE PARENTS WERE AFFECTED. THE ILLNESS BEGAN IN THE SECOND OR EARLY THIRD DECADE WITH THE PICTURE OF PARALYSIS AGITANS AND PYRAMIDAL TRACT SIGNS. AUTOPSY (DAVISON, 1954) SHOWED PALLOR OF THE PALLIDAL SEGMENTS, THINNING OF THE ANSA LENTICULARIS, SLIGHT SHRINKAGE AND CELLULAR CHANGE IN THE SUBSTANTIA NIGRA AND EARLY DEMYELINATION OF THE PYRAMIDS AND CROSSED PYRAMIDAL TRACTS. ONE OF DAVISON'S CASES HAD BEEN PREVIOUSLY REPORTED BY RAMSEY HUNT (1917). TREMOR AND RIGIDITY OF PARALYSIS AGITANS TYPE BEGAN AT AGE 13. CLINICAL-LY, WILSON'S DISEASE WAS CONSIDERED LIKELY FOR A TIME. THE PATIENT SURVIVED UNTIL AGE 65 YEARS. THE SAME DISORDER MAY HAVE BEEN DESCRIBED AS FAMILIAL PROGRESSIVE PALLIDUM ATROPHY, IN SIX SIBS, BY LANGE AND POPPE (1963). LANGE ET AL. (1970) GAVE INFORMATION ON THE AUTOPSY FINDINGS.

DAVISON, C.* PALLIDO-PYRAMIDAL DISEASE. J. NEUROPATH. EXP. NEUROL. 13* 50-59, 1954.

HUNT, J. R.* PROGRESSIVE ATROPHY OF THE GLOBUS PALLIDUS (PRIMARY ATROPHY OF THE PALLIDAL SYSTEM). A SYSTEM OF THE PARALYSIS AGITANS TYPE, CHARACTERIZED BY ATROPHY OF THE MOTOR CELLS OF THE CORPUS STRIATUM. A CONTRIBUTION TO THE FUNCTIONS OF THE CORPUS STRIATUM. BRAIN 40* 58-148, 1917.

JELLINGER, K.* PROGRESSIV PALLIDUM ATROPHIE. J. NEUROL. SCI. 6* 19-44, 1968.

LANGE, E. AND POPPE, W.* KLINISCHER BEITRAG ZUM KRANKHEITSBILD DER PROGRESSIVEN PALLIDUMATROPHIE (VAN BOGAERT). PSYCHIAT. NEUROL. 146* 176-192, 1963.

LANGE, E., POPPE, W. AND SCHOLTZE, P.* FAMILIAL PROGRESSIVE PALLIDUM ATROPHY. EUROP. NEUROL. 3* 265-257, 1970.

*26040 PANCREATIC INSUFFICIENCY AND BONE MARROW DYSFUNCTION (SHWACHMAN SYNDROME)

SHWACHMAN ET AL. (1964) DESCRIBED A SYNDROME OF PANCREATIC INSUFFICIENCY (SUGGES-TING CYSTIC FIBROSIS OF THE PANCREAS BUT WITH NORMAL SWEAT ELECTROLYTES AND NO RESPIRATORY DIFFICULTIES) AND PANCYTOPENIA. ONE SIBSHIP CONTAINED TWO AFFECTED BROTHERS AND AN AFFECTED FEMALE. THE SAME SYNDROME WAS DESCRIBED BY NEZELOF AND WATCHI (1961) AND MORE RECENTLY BY OTHER AUTHORS SUCH AS PRINGLE, YOUNG AND HAWORTH (1968). GOLDSTEIN (1968) AND OTHERS BEFORE HIM CALLED THIS CONDITION CONGENITAL LIPOMATOSIS OF THE PANCREAS. HE DESCRIBED ONE AFFECTED OF A PAIR OF FRATERNAL TWIN GIRLS. AFFECTED SIBS WERE REFERRED TO BY BURKE ET AL. (1967) AND PRINGLE ET AL. (1968) OBSERVED ASSOCIATED SKELETAL CHANGES OF THE METAPHYSEAL DYSOSTOSIS TYPE. THESE ARE OF INTEREST BECAUSE OF THE DIGESTIVE ABNORMALITIES (NOT YET WELL CHARACTERIZED) AND HEMATOLOGIC CHANGES IN CARTILAGE-HAIR HYPOPLASIA (Q.V.), A FORM OF METAPHYSEAL DYSOSTOSIS.

BODIAN, M., SHELDON, W. AND LIGHTWOOD, R.* CONGENITAL HYPOPLASIA OF THE EXOCRINE PANCREAS. ACTA PAEDIAT. 53* 282-293, 1964.

BURKE, V., COLEBATCH, J. H., ANDERSON, C. M. AND SIMONS, M. J.* ASSOCIATION OF PANCREATIC INSUFFICIENCY AND CHRONIC NEUTROPENIA IN CHILDHOOD. ARCH. DIS. CHILD. 42* 147-157, 1967.

GOLDSTEIN, R.* CONGENITAL LIPOMATOSIS OF THE PANCREAS. MALABSORPTION, DWARFISM, LEUKOPENIA WITH RELATIVE GRANULOCYTOPENIA AND THROMBOCYTOPENIA. CLIN. PEDIAT. 7* 419-422, 1968.

NEZELOF, C. AND WATCHI, M.* L'HYPOPLASIE CONGENITALE LIPOMATEUSE DU PANCREAS EXOCRINE CHEZ L'ENFANT. (DEUX OBSERVATIONS ET REVUE DE LA LITTERATURE). ARCH. FRANC. PEDIAT. 18* 1135-1172, 1961.

PRINGLE, E. M., YOUNG, W. F. AND HAWORTH, E. M.* SYNDROME OF PANCREATIC INSUFFICIENCY, BLOOD DYSCRASIA AND METAPHYSEAL DYSPLASIA. PROC. ROY. SOC. MED. 61* 776-777, 1968.

SAINT-MARTIN, J., FOURNET, J.-P., CHARLES, J., SCHAISON, G., NODOT, A., MEYER,

R
E
C
E
S
S
I
V
E

B. AND VIALATTE, J.* EXTERNAL PANCREATIC INSUFFICIENCY WITH CHRONIC GRANULOPENIA* A NEW CASE WITH OSSEOUS ABNORMALITIES. ARCH. FRANC. PEDIAT. 26* 861-871, 1969.

SHMERLING, D. H., PRADER, A., HITZIG, W. H., GIEDION, A., HADORN, B. AND KUHNI, M.* SYNDROME OF EXOCRINE PANCREATIC INSUFFICIENCY, NEUTROPENIA, METAPHYSEAL DYSOSTOSIS AND DWARFISM. HELV. PAEDIAT. ACTA 24* 547-575, 1969.

SHWACHMAN, H., DIAMOND, L. K., OSKI, F. A. AND KHAW, K. T.* THE SYNDROME OF PANCREATIC INSUFFICIENCY AND BONE MARROW DYSFUNCTION. J. PEDIAT. 65* 645-663, 1964.

26050 PAPILLOMA OF CHOROID PLEXUS

KOMMINOTH ET AL. (1965) OBSERVED INTRAVENTRICULAR PAPILLOMA OF THE CHOROID PLEXUS IN A 2 YEAR OLD BOY AND HIS 4 YEAR OLD SISTER.

KOMMINOTH, R., WORINGER, E., BAUMGARTNER, J., BRAUN, J. P. AND LE MAISTRE, D.* PAPILLOME INTRAVENTRICULAIRE FAMILIAL. CARACTERISTIQUES ANGIOGRAPHIQUES. NEUROCHIRURGIE 11* 267-272, 1965.

26060 PELIZAEUS-MERZBACHER DISEASE, INFANTILE ACUTE TYPE

NISENBAUM, SANDBANK AND KOHN (1965) DESCRIBED A FAMILY IN WHICH 6 OF 7 SIBS DIED IN THE FIRST MONTHS OF LIFE. THE PARENTS, YEMENITE JEWS, WERE APPARENTLY UNRELATED. ALL SIX AFFECTED CHILDREN WERE BORN PREMATURELY AT BIRTH WEIGHTS OF 1350 TO 2200 G. COMPLETE NEUROPATHOLOGIC STUDY WAS PERFORMED IN ONE CASE. SINCE THIS IS CLEARLY NOT THE CONDITION DESCRIBED BY PELIZAEUS AND MERZBACHER, THE APPROPRIATENESS OF USING THIS EPONYM CAN BE QUESTIONED. VOMITING BEGINNING AT 1-3 WEEKS AFTER BIRTH AND PROGRESSING TO CONTINUOUS PROJECTILE VOMITING WAS THE MAIN FEATURE.

NANCE, W. E.* NASHVILLE, TENN.* PERSONAL COMMUNICATION, 1968.

NISENBAUM, C., SANDBANK, V. AND KOHN, R.* PELIZAEUS-MERZBACHER DISEASE, 'INFANTILE ACUTE TYPE.' REPORT OF A FAMILY. ANN. PAEDIAT. 204* 365-376, 1965.

26070 PENDRED SYNDROME (HEREDITARY GOITER AND DEAFNESS)

THE THYROID IS ENLARGED. THE SUBJECTS ARE USUALLY EUTHYROID BUT OCCASIONALLY MAY BE HYPOTHYROID. PERCHLORATE ADMINISTERED AFTER RADIOIODINE CAUSED DISCHARGE OF IODINE IN THE HOMOZYGOTES AND NOT IN CONTROLS (FRASER, MORGANS, TROTTER, 1960). THE DEAFNESS IS PERCEPTIVE IN TYPE AND SOMETIMES DEFECTIVE VESTIBULAR FUNCTION IS ASSOCIATED. THE DEAFNESS IS NOT CAUSED BY HYPOTHYROIDISM BUT IS RATHER A SECOND EXPRESSION OF THE SAME GENETIC DEFECT. BATSAKIS AND NISHIYAMA (1962) ESTIMATED THAT PENDRED'S SYNDROME ACCOUNTS FOR 1 TO 10 PERCENT OF HEREDITARY DEAFNESS. THERE APPEAR TO BE AT LEAST TWO DISTINCT VARIETIES OF PENDRED'S SYNDROME, BECAUSE HOLLANDER AND HIS COLLEAGUES (1964) FOUND A DEFECT INVOLVING NOT AN INADEQUATE IODINATION OF TYROSINE BUT APPARENTLY THE CONDENSATION OF IODOTYROSINES TO FORM IODOTHYRONINES. FRASER (1965) ESTIMATED THE FREQUENCY IN THE BRITISH ISLES TO BE ABOUT 0.000075. JOHNSEN (1958) OBSERVED QUASI-DOMINANT INHERITANCE THROUGH THREE GENERATIONS BECAUSE OF MARRIAGE OF AFFECTED PERSONS. BECAUSE OF THE UNCERTAINTY AS TO WHETHER ORGANIFICATION DEFECT WITH DEAFNESS IS DIFFERENT FROM ORGANIFICATION DEFECT WITHOUT DEAFNESS, NO ASTERISK IS USED HERE. SEE THYROID HORMONOGENESIS, GENETIC DEFECT IN, IIB.

BATSAKIS, J. G. AND NISHIYAMA, R. H.* DEAFNESS WITH SPORADIC GOITER* PENDRED'S SYNDROME. ARCH. OTOLARYNG. 76* 401-406, 1962.

DERAEMAEKER, R.* CONGENITAL DEAFNESS AND GOITER. AM. J. HUM. GENET. 8* 253-256, 1956.

FISHMAN, J., FRASER, F. C., WATANABE, M., SODHI, H. S. AND BECK, J. C.* FAMILIAL NERVE DEAFNESS AND GOITRE. CANAD. MED. ASS. J. 83* 889-892, 1960.

FRASER, G. R.* ASSOCIATION OF CONGENITAL DEAFNESS WITH GOITRE (PENDRED'S SYNDROME). A STUDY OF 207 FAMILIES. ANN. HUM. GENET. 28* 201-249, 1965.

FRASER, G. R., MORGANS, M. E. AND TROTTER, W. R.* THE SYNDROME OF SPORADIC GOITRE AND CONGENITAL DEAFNESS. QUART. J. MED. 29* 279-295, 1960.

HOLLANDER, C. S., PROUT, T. E., RIENHOFF, M., RUBEN, R. J. AND ASPER, S. P., JR.* CONGENITAL DEAFNESS AND GOITER. STUDIES OF A PATIENT WITH A COCHLEAR DEFECT AND INADEQUATE FORMATION OF IODOTHYRONINES. AM. J. MED. 37* 630-637, 1964.

JOHNSEN, S.* FAMILIAL DEAFNESS AND GOITRE IN PERSONS WITH A LOW LEVEL OF PROTEIN-BOUND IODINE. ACTA OTOLARYNG. 140 (SUPPL.)* 168-177, 1958.

*26080 PENTOSURIA (L-XYLULOSURIA)

SUBJECTS EXCRETE 1-4 GMS. OF THE PENTOSE L-XYLULOSE IN THE URINE EACH DAY. IT IS A BENIGN DISTURBANCE WHICH OCCURS ALMOST EXCLUSIVELY IN ASHKENAZI JEWS OF POLISH-RUSSIAN EXTRACTION. HOWEVER, KHACHADURIAN (1962) AND POLITZER AND FLEISCHMANN

(1962) HAVE DESCRIBED IT IN LEBANESE FAMILIES. THE FREQUENCY IN ASHKENAZIM MAY BE AS HIGH AS ONE IN EACH 2500 BIRTHS. A LOADING METHOD FOR DEMONSTRATING THE HETEROZYGOTE IS AVAILABLE. BY DIRECT BIOCHEMICAL MEANS APPLIED TO ERYTHROCYTES WANG AND VAN EYS (1970) DEMONSTRATED THAT THE BASIC FAULT CONCERNS NADP-LINKED XYLITOL DEHYDROGENASE. HETEROZYGOTES COULD BE IDENTIFIED.

HIATT, H. H.* PENTOSURIA. IN, STANBURY, J. B., WYNGAARDEN, J. B. AND FREDRICK-SON, D. S. (EDS.)* THE METABOLIC BASIS OF INHERITED DISEASE. NEW YORK* MCGRAW-HILL, 1966 (2ND ED.). PP. 109-123.

KHACHADURIAN, A. K.* ESSENTIAL PENTOSURIA. AM. J. HUM. GENET. 14* 249-255, 1962.

POLITZER, W. M. AND FLEISCHMANN, H.* L-XYLULOSURIA IN A LEBANESE FAMILY. AM. J. HUM. GENET. 14* 256-260, 1962.

ROBERTS, P. D.* THE INHERITANCE OF ESSENTIAL PENTOSURIA. BRIT. MED. J. 1* 1478-1479, 1960.

WANG, Y. M. AND VAN EYS, J.* THE ENZYMATIC DEFECT IN ESSENTIAL PENTOSURIA. NEW ENG. J. MED. 282* 892-896, 1970.

26090 PERICARDIAL EFFUSION, CHRONIC

GENECIN (1959) DESCRIBED YOUNG ADULT BROTHERS WITH ASYMPTOMATIC CHRONIC PERICAR-DIAL EFFUSION. IN ONE THE PERICARDIAL FLUID CONTAINED ABUNDANT CHOLESTEROL CRYSTALS. THE OTHER BROTHER ALSO HAD MILD POLYCYTHEMIA, STRIKINGLY TORTUOUS RETINAL ARTERIOLES AND LOCALIZED AREAS OF CUTANEOUS FLUSHING.

GENECIN, A.* CHRONIC PERICARDIAL EFFUSION IN BROTHERS, WITH A NOTE ON *CHOLES-TEROL PERICARDITIS.* AM. J. MED. 26* 496-502, 1959.

*26100 PERNICIOUS ANEMIA, CONGENITAL, DUE TO FAILURE OF INTRINSIC FACTOR SECRETION

RECESSIVE

CONGENITAL PA HAS BEEN DESCRIBED IN 28 CASES ACCORDING TO MCNICHOLL AND EGAN (1968) WHO DESCRIBED AFFECTED BROTHER AND SISTER. THE DEFECT SEEMS TO BE ONE OF FAILURE OF INTRINSIC FACTOR SECRETION DESPITE NORMAL GASTRIC ACIDITY AND MUCOSAL MORPHOLOGY. THE DISORDER IS DISTINCT FROM SELECTIVE B12 MALABSORPTION AND FROM THE JUVENILE PA WITH GASTRIC ATROPHY, ACHLORHYDRIA, ENDOCRINE GLAND HYPOFUNCTION, CIRCULATING ANTIBODIES AND FREQUENT RETURN OF INTRINSIC FACTOR SECRETION WITH TREATMENT WITH CORTICOSTEROIDS AND THYROID HORMONE. IT IS ALSO PROBABLY DISTINCT FROM ADULT PA. THE CONGENITAL FORM WAS MANIFEST BY MEGALOBLASTIC ANEMIA PRESEN-TING AT ABOUT 1 YEAR OF AGE AND MENTAL RETARDATION.

MCNICHOLL, B. AND EGAN, B.* CONGENITAL PERNICIOUS ANEMIA* EFFECTS ON GROWTH, BRAIN, AND ABSORPTION OF B12. PEDIATRICS 42* 149-156, 1968.

*26110 PERNICIOUS ANEMIA, JUVENILE

WATERS AND MURPHY (1963) REPORTED THREE AFFECTED BROTHERS. BOTH PARENTS AND 5 OTHER SIBS HAD SUBNORMAL OR BORDERLINE VITAMIN B12 ABSORPTION. SEE ALSO LAMBERT, PRANKERD AND SMELLIE (1961). MOLLIN, BAKER AND DONIACH (1955) REPORTED JUVENILE PERNICIOUS ANEMIA IN THE OFFSPRING OF A FIRST COUSIN MARRIAGE. THE FATHER DEVELOPED CLASSIC PERNICIOUS ANEMIA IN MIDDLE AGE. GRASBECK (1960) DESCRIBED WHAT MAY BE A DISTINCT CONDITION. WHEREAS A DEFECT IN PRODUCTION OF INTRINSIC FACTOR WAS POSTULATED BY THE AUTHORS CITED ABOVE, GRASBECK FAVORED A SELECTIVE DEFECT IN INTESTINAL ABSORPTION OF VITAMIN B12 IN THIS DISORDER WHICH WAS UNINFLUENCED BY ADMINISTRATION OF INTRINSIC FACTOR. PROTEINURIA AND MALFORMATION OF THE URINARY TRACT WERE ALSO PRESENT. IMERSLUND AND BJORNSTAD (1963) AND LAMY ET AL. (1961) REPORTED ON THE SYNDROME OF CHRONIC RELAPSING MEGALOBLASTIC ANEMIA AND PERMANENT PROTEINURIA. CASES OF CHILDHOOD PERNICIOUS ANEMIA HAVE BEEN REPORTED IN WHICH, ALTHOUGH THE GASTRIC MUCOSA WAS HISTOLOGICALLY NORMAL INTRINSIC FACTOR WAS LACKING FROM THE ACID GASTRIC JUICE. NO ANTIBODIES TO INTRINSIC FACTOR OR TO GASTRIC PARIETAL CELLS WERE DETECTED IN THE PATIENT'S SERUM. STUDIES IN SIBS, PARENTS AND GRANDPARENTS SHOWED NO ABNORMALITY IN THE SECRETION OF GASTRIC ACID OR INTRINSIC FACTOR AND NORMAL VITAMIN B12 ABSORPTION (MCINTYRE ET AL., 1965).
IN ONE SUCH FAMILY (HERBERT, STREIFF AND SULLIVAN, 1964) TWO SIBS WERE AFFECTED. ADULT PERNICIOUS ANEMIA SHOWS GASTRIC ATROPHY, ANTIBODIES TO INTRINSIC FACTOR AND TO PARIETAL CELLS IN THE PLASMA AND A RELATIVELY HIGH FREQUENCY OF ASSOCIATED THYROIDITIS AND MYXEDEMA. SOME JUVENILE CASES ARE OF THIS TYPE. OTHER JUVENILE CASES (DESCRIBED ABOVE) SEEM TO SUFFER FROM A SELECTIVE FAILURE OF INTRINSIC FACTOR SECRETION. THIS MAY BE RECESSIVE. JUVENILE *CONGENITAL* PERNICIOUS ANEMIA WAS THE DESIGNATION SUGGESTED BY MILLER ET AL. (1966) FOR VITAMIN B12 DEFICIENCY DUE TO CONGENITAL LACK OF GASTRIC INTRINSIC FACTOR WITHOUT OTHER APPARENT ABNORMALITY OF THE STOMACH OR ITS SECRETIONS. FURTHERMORE, SERUM ANTIBODIES TO INTRINSIC FACTOR AND GASTRIC PARIETAL CELLS ARE CONSPICUOUSLY ABSENT. THE RELATION TO THE USUAL ADULT PERNICIOUS ANEMIA IS UNCLEAR. MOHAMED ET AL. (1966) REPORTED SISTERS WITH SELECTIVE MALABSORPTION OF VITAMIN B12 WITH ADEQUATE GASTRIC SECRETION OF FUNCTIONALLY COMPETENT INTRINSIC FACTOR AND HYDROCHLORIC ACID. PERSISTENT PROTEINURIA APPEARS TO BE AN INTEGRAL PART OF THE SYNDROME (MOHAMED ET AL., 1966). THE LATTER AUTHORS GAVE A GENETIC ANALYSIS OF PUBLISHED CASES. IN THE OLDEST KNOWN PATIENT, GOLDBERG AND FUDENBERG (1968) FOUND

NORMAL AMOUNTS OF BIOLOGICALLY ACTIVE INTRINSIC FACTOR IN THE GASTRIC JUICE AND
FOUND NEITHER ANTIBODIES TO INTRINSIC FACTOR NOR INHIBITORS OF INTRINSIC FACTORS.
THE MECHANISM OF DEFECTIVE ABSORPTION IS UNKNOWN.

FRANCOIS, R., REVOL, L., GERMAIN, D., BOURLIER, V., KARLIN, MME., COEUR, P.,
PELLET, H. AND MANUEL, Y.* LE SYNDROME D'IMERSLUND (A PROPOS DE TROIS CAS DANS UNE
MEME FRATRIE). ANN. PEDIAT. 43* 490-503, 1967.

GOLDBERG, L. S. AND FUDENBERG, H. H.* FAMILIAL SELECTIVE MALABSORPTION OF
VITAMIN B12. RE-EVALUATION OF AN IN VIVO INTRINSIC-FACTOR INHIBITOR. NEW ENG. J.
MED. 279* 405-407, 1968.

GRASBECK, R. AND KANTERO, I.* A CASE OF JUVENILE VITAMIN B12 DEFICIENCY.
(ABSTRACT) ACTA PAEDIAT. 47 (SUPPL. 118)* 140-141, 1959.

GRASBECK, R.* FAMILJAR SELEKTIV B12-MALABSORPTION WITH PROTEINURI ETT PERNICIO-
SALIKNANDE SYNDROME. NORD. MED. 63* 322-323, 1960.

HERBERT, V., STREIFF, R. R. AND SULLIVAN, L. W.* NOTES ON VITAMIN B12 ABSORP-
TION, AUTOIMMUNITY AND CHILDHOOD PERNICIOUS ANEMIA, RELATION OF INTRINSIC FACTOR
TO BLOOD GROUP SUBSTANCE. MEDICINE 43* 679-687, 1964.

IMERSLUND, O. AND BJORNSTAD, P.* FAMILIAL VITAMIN B12 MALABSORPTION. ACTA
HAEMAT. 30* 1-7, 1963.

LAMBERT, H. P., PRANKERD, T. A. J. AND SMELLIE, J. M.* PERNICIOUS ANAEMIA IN
CHILDHOOD. A REPORT OF TWO CASES IN ONE FAMILY AND THEIR RELATIONSHIPS TO THE
AETIOLOGY OF PERNICIOUS ANAEMIA. QUART. J. MED. 30* 71-90, 1961.

LAMY, M., BESANCON, F., LOVERDO, A. AND AFIFI, F.* SPECIFIC MALABSORPTION OF
VITAMIN B12 AND PROTEINURIA. MEGALOBLASTIC ANEMIA OF IMERSLUND-GRASBECK* STUDY OF
4 CASES. ARCH. FRANC. PEDIAT. 18* 1109-1120, 1961.

MCINTYRE, O. R., SULLIVAN, L. W., JEFFRIES, G. H. AND SILVER, R. H.* PERNICIOUS
ANEMIA IN CHILDHOOD. NEW ENG. J. MED. 272* 981-986, 1965.

MILLER, D. R., BLOOM, G. E., STREIFF, R. R., LO BUGLIO, A. F. AND DIAMOND, L.
K.* JUVENILE 'CONGENITAL' PERNICIOUS ANEMIA. CLINICAL AND IMMUNOLOGIC STUDIES.
NEW ENG. J. MED. 275* 978-983, 1966.

MOHAMED, S. D., MCKAY, E. AND GALLOWAY, W. H.* JUVENILE FAMILIAL MEGALOBLASTIC
ANAEMIA DUE TO SELECTIVE MALABSORPTION OF VITAMIN B(12). A FAMILY STUDY AND A
REVIEW OF THE LITERATURE. QUART J. MED. 35* 433-453, 1966.

MOLLIN, D. L., BAKER, S. J. AND DONIACH, I.* ADDISONIAN PERNICIOUS ANAEMIA
WITHOUT GASTRIC ATROPHY IN YOUNG MAN. BRIT. J. HAEMAT. 1* 278-290, 1955.

WATERS, A. H. AND MURPHY, M. E. B.* FAMILIAL JUVENILE PERNICIOUS ANAEMIA. A
STUDY OF THE HEREDITARY BASIS OF PERNICIOUS ANAEMIA. BRIT. J. HAEMAT. 9* 1-12,
1963.

R
E
C
E
S
S
I
V
E

*26120 PEROMELIA

IN A BRAZILIAN FAMILY OF PORTUGUESE ANCESTRY FREIRE-MAIA, QJELCE-SALGADO AND
KOEHLER (1959) FOUND AN APPARENT RECESSIVE TYPE OF PEROMELIA ('MAIMED LIMB').
ABNORMALITY WAS CONFINED TO THE UPPER LIMBS AND CONSISTED OF APLASIA OR HYPOPLASIA
OF MANY BONES. ONE AFFECTED MALE MARRIED TO THE DAUGHTER OF HIS HALF-SISTER HAD
TWO AFFECTED CHILDREN.

FREIRE-MAIA, N., QUELCE-SALGADO, A. AND KOEHLER, R. A.* HEREDITARY BONE
APLASIAS AND HYPOPLASIAS OF THE UPPER EXTREMITIES. ACTA GENET. STATIST. MED. 9*
33-40, 1959.

*26130 PEROMELIA WITH MICROGNATHISM

THIS SYNDROME IS PROBABLY DISTINCT FROM THE BRAZILIAN TYPE OF ACHEIROPODY (Q.V.)
AND FROM SIMPLE PEROMELIA (Q.V.). IN HANHART'S REPORT OF THREE CASES, TWO WERE
RELATED AND IN THE THIRD THE PARENTS WERE CONSANGUINEOUS.

HANHART, E.* UBER DIE KOMBINATION VON PEROMELIE MIT MIKROGNATHIE, EIN NEUER
SYNDROM BEIM MENSCHEN, ENTSPRECHEND DER AKROTERIASIS CONGENITA VON WRIEDT UND MOHR
BEIM RINDER. ARCH. KLAUS STIFT. VERERBUNGSFORSCH. 25* 531-543, 1950.

26140 PERONEUS TERTIUS MUSCLE, ABSENCE OF

FROM STUDIES IN THE NAVAJO, SPUHLER (1950) CONCLUDED THAT ABSENCE IS RECESSIVE.
THE MUSCLE IS A DORSIFLEXOR OF THE FOOT. WHEN THE SUBJECT STANDS WITH THE TOES IN
SHARP DORSIFLEXION, THE TENDONS OF THE PERONEUS TERTIUS BECOME PROMINENT OVER THE
CUBOID BONE JUST OUTSIDE THE MOST LATERAL TENDON OF THE EXTENSOR DIGITORUM LONGUS.

SPUHLER, J. N.* GENETICS OF THREE NORMAL MORPHOLOGICAL VARIATIONS* PATTERN OF
SUPERFICIAL VEINS OF THE ANTERIOR THORAX, PERONEUS TERTIUS MUSCLE, AND NUMBER OF

*26150 PEROXIDASE AND PHOSPHOLIPID DEFICIENCY IN EOSINOPHILES

IN YEMENITE JEWS IN ISRAEL, PRESENTEY (1969) AND PRESENTEY AND SZAPIRO (1969)
DESCRIBED A "NEW" ANOMALY OF EOSINOPHILES CHARACTERIZED BY NUCLEAR HYPERSIGMENTA-
TION, HYPOGRANULATION AND NEGATIVE PEROXIDASE AND PHOSPHOLIPID STAINING. NO
CONNECTION BETWEEN THE MORPHOLOGIC AND PRESUMED ENZYMATIC DEFECT AND ANY ILLNESS
HAS BEEN ESTABLISHED. RECESSIVE INHERITANCE SEEMS QUITE CLEAR.

PRESENTEY, B. Z. AND SZAPIRO, L.* HEREDITARY DEFICIENCY OF PEROXIDASE AND
PHOSPHOLIPIDS IN EOSINOPHILIC GRANULOCYTES. ACTA HAEMAT. 41* 359-362, 1969.

PRESENTEY, B. Z.* MORPHOLOGIC OBSERVATIONS AND GENETIC FOLLOW-UP OF A FAMILIAL
ANOMALY OF EOSINOPHILS. AM. J. CLIN. PATH. 51* 458-462, 1969.

*26160 PHENYLKETONURIA

THIS CAUSE OF MENTAL RETARDATION IS IMPORTANT BECAUSE IT IS TREATABLE BY DIETARY
MEANS. THE DEFECT CONCERNS PHENYLALANINE HYDROXYLASE. FEATURES OTHER THAN MENTAL
RETARDATION INCLUDE A "MOUSEY" ODOR, LIGHT PIGMENTATION, PECULIARITIES OF GAIT,
STANCE AND SITTING POSTURE, ECZEMA, AND EPILEPSY (PAINE, 1957). PECULIARITIES IN
THE DISTRIBUTION OF PHENYLKETONURIA HAVE BEEN NOTED. THE DISORDER IS RARE IN
ASHKENAZI JEWS (COHEN ET AL., 1961* CENTERWALL AND NEFF, 1961). CARTER AND WOOLF
(1961) NOTED THAT OF THE CASES SEEN IN LONDON AND PRESENTLY LIVING IN SOUTHEAST
ENGLAND, A DISPROPORTIONATELY LARGE NUMBER HAD PARENTS AND GRANDPARENTS BORN IN
IRELAND OR WEST SCOTLAND. THE FREQUENCY AT BIRTH IN NORTHERN EUROPEANS MAY BE
ABOUT 1 PER 10,000 (GUTHRIE AND SUSI, 1963). PKU IS ALSO RARE IN SOUTHERN
ITALIANS. WHEN IT DOES OCCUR IN THIS GROUP, IT SEEMS TO BE A DIFFERENT ENTITY,
NAMELY, THE FORM IN WHICH DEATH OCCURS ON LOW PHENYLALANINE DIET WITHOUT SUPERVI-
SION (EFRON, PERSONAL COMMUNICATION, NOV. 2, 1965). VICTOR H. AJERBACH (PHILADEL-
PHIA) ALSO CONCLUDED THERE IS A SECOND VARIETY OF PKU. EVIDENCE OF HETEROGENEITY
IN PHENYLKETONURIA WAS PRESENTED ALSO BY WOOLF ET AL. (1968). THE OCCURRENCE OF
MENTAL RETARDATION IN THE OFFSPRING OF HOMOZYGOUS MOTHERS IS AN EXAMPLE OF A
GENETIC DISEASE BASED ON THE GENOTYPE OF THE MOTHER. KERR ET AL. (1968) DEMONS-
TRATED "FETAL PKU" BY ADMINISTERING LARGE AMOUNTS OF PHENYLALANINE TO MOTHER
MONKEYS. THE OFFSPRING HAD REDUCED LEARNING ABILITY. THEY POINTED OUT THAT THE
DAMAGE IS AGGRAVATED BY THE NORMAL PLACENTAL PROCESS WHICH FUNCTIONS TO MAINTAIN
HIGHER LEVELS OF AMINO ACIDS IN THE FETUS THAN IN THE MOTHER. HUNTLEY AND
STEVENSON (1969) DESCRIBED TWO SISTERS WITH PKU WHO HAD IN ALL 28 PREGNANCIES. 16
ENDED IN SPONTANEOUS FIRST-TRIMESTER ABORTION. ALL CARRIED TO TERM HAD INTRAU-
TERINE GROWTH RETARDATION AND MICROCEPHALY. 9 OF THE 12 TERM INFANTS HAD CARDIAC
MALFORMATIONS. LEVY ET AL. (1970) SCREENED THE SERUM OF 280,919 "NORMAL"
TEENAGERS AND ADULTS WHOSE BLOOD HAD BEEN SUBMITTED FOR SYPHILIS TESTING. ONLY
THREE ADULTS WITH THE BIOCHEMICAL FINDINGS OF PKU WERE FOUND. EACH WAS MENTALLY
SUBNORMAL. NORMAL MENTALITY IS VERY RARE AMONG PATIENTS WITH PHENYLKETONURIA WHO
HAVE NOT RECEIVED DIETARY THERAPY.

R
E
C
E
S
S
I
V
E

AOKI, K. AND SIEGEL, F. L.* HYPERPHENYLALANINEMIA* DISAGGREGATION OF BRAIN
POLYRIBOSOMES IN YOUNG RATS. SCIENCE 168* 129-130, 1970.

ARTHUR, L. J. H. AND HULME, J. D.* INTELLIGENT, SMALL FOR DATES BABY BORN TO
OLIGOPHRENIC PHENYLKETONURIC MOTHER AFTER LOW PHENYLALANINE DIET DURING PREGNANCY.
PEDIATRICS 46* 235-239, 1970.

AUERBACH, V. H., DIGEORGE, A. M. AND CARPENTER, G. G.* PHENYLALINEMIA. A STUDY
OF THE DIVERSITY OF DISORDERS WHICH PRODUCE ELEVATION OF BLOOD CONCENTRATIONS OF
PHENYLALANINE. IN, NYHAN, W. L. (ED.)* AMINO ACID METABOLISM AND GENETIC
VARIATION. NEW YORK* MCGRAW-HILL, 1967. PP. 11-68.

CARTER, C. O. AND WOOLF, L. I.* THE BIRTHPLACES OF PARENTS AND GRANDPARENTS OF
A SERIES OF PATIENTS WITH PHENYLKETONURIA IN SOUTHEAST ENGLAND. ANN. HUM. GENET.
25* 57-64, 1961.

CENTERWALL, W. R. AND NEFF, C. A.* PHENYLKETONURIA* A CASE REPORT OF CHILDREN
OF JEWISH ANCESTRY. ARCH. PAEDIAT. 78* 379-384, 1961.

COHEN, B. E., BODONYI, E. AND SZEINBERG, A.* PHENYLKETONURIA IN JEWS. LANCET
1* 344-345, 1961.

CUNNINGHAM, G. C., DAY, R. W., BERMAN, J. L. AND HSIA, D. Y.-Y.* PHENYLALANINE
TOLERANCE TESTS IN FAMILIES WITH PHENYLKETONURIA AND HYPERPHENYLALANINEMIA. AM.
J. DIS. CHILD. 117* 626-635, 1969.

FRANKENBURG, W. K., DUNCAN, B. R., COFFELT, R. W., KOCH, R., COLDWELL, J. G.
AND SON, C. D.* MATERNAL PHENYLKETONURIA* IMPLICATIONS FOR GROWTH AND DEVELOPMENT.
J. PEDIAT. 73* 560-570, 1968.

GUTHRIE, R. AND SUSI, A.* A SIMPLE PHENYLALANINE METHOD FOR DETECTING PHENYLKE-
TONURIA IN LARGE POPULATIONS OF NEWBORN INFANTS. PEDIATRICS 32* 338-343, 1963.

HSIA, D. Y.-Y.* PHENYLKETONURIA AND ITS VARIANTS. PROG. MED. GENET. 7* 29-68,

HUNTLEY,   C. C. AND STEVENSON, R. E.* MATERNAL PHENYLKETONURIA. COURSE OF TWO
PREGNANCIES. OBSTET. GYNEC. 34* 694-700, 1969.

KERR, G. R., CHAMOVE, A. S., HARLOW, H. F. AND WAISMAN, H. A.* *FETAL PKU'* THE
EFFECT OF MATERNAL HYPERPHENYLALANINEMIA DURING PREGNANCY IN THE RHESUS MONKEY
(MACACA MULATTA). PEDIATRICS 42* 27-36, 1968.

KNOX, W. E.* PHENYLKETONURIA.   IN, STANBURY, J. B., WYNGAARDEN, J. B. AND
FREDRICKSON, D. S. (EDS.)* THE METABOLIC BASIS OF INHERITED DISEASE. NEW YORK*
MCGRAW-HILL, 1966 (2ND ED.). PP. 258-294.

LEVY, H. L., KAROLKEWICZ, V., HOUGHTON, S. A. AND MACCREADY, R. A.* SCREENING
THE 'NORMAL' POPULATION IN MASSACHUSETTS FOR PHENYLKETONURIA. NEW ENG. J. MED.
282* 1455-1458, 1970.

MENKES, J. H. AND AEBERHARD, E.* MATERNAL PHENYLKETONURIA. J. PEDIAT. 74* 924-
931, 1969.

O'FLYNN, M. E., TILLMAN, P. AND HSIA, D. Y.-Y.* HYPERPHENYLALANEMIA WITHOUT
PHENYLKETONURIA. AM. J. DIS. CHILD. 113* 22-30, 1967.

PAINE, R. S.* THE VARIABILITY IN MANIFESTATIONS OF UNTREATED PATIENTS WITH
PHENYLKETONURIA (PHENYLPYRUVIC ACIDURIA). PEDIATRICS 20* 290-302, 1957.

PERRY, T. L., HANSEN, S., TISCHLER, B., BUNTING, R. AND DIAMOND, S.* GLUTAMINE
DEPLETION IN PHENYLKETONURIA* POSSIBLE CAUSE OF THE MENTAL DEFECT. NEW ENG. J.
MED. 282* 761-766, 1970.

ROSENBLATT, D. AND SCRIVER, C. R.* HETEROGENEITY IN GENETIC CONTROL OF
PHENYLALANINE METABOLISM IN MAN. NATURE 218* 677-678, 1968.

WOOLF, L. I., CRANSTON, W. I. AND GOODWIN, B. L.* GENETICS OF PHENYLKETONURIA.
I. HETEROZYGOSITY FOR PHENYLKETONURIA. II. THIRD ALLELE AT THE PHENYLALANINE
HYDROXYLASE LOCUS IN MAN. NATURE 213* 882-885, 1967.

WOOLF, L. I., GOODWIN, B. L., CRANSTON, W. I., WADE, D. N., WOOLF, F., HUDSON,
F. P. AND MCBEAN, M. S.* A THIRD ALLELE AT THE PHENYLALANINE-HYDROXYLASE LOCUS IN
MILD PHENYLKETONURIA (HYPERPHENYLALANINAEMIA). LANCET 1* 114-117, 1968.

YU, J. S. AND O'HALLORAN, M. T.* ATYPICAL PHENYLKETONURIA IN A FAMILY WITH A
PHENYLKETONURIC MOTHER. PEDIATRICS 46* 707-711, 1970.

R
E
C
E
S
S
I
V
E

26170 PHOSPHOGLYCERATE KINASE DEFICIENCY OF ERYTHROCYTE

KRAUS (1968) ATTRIBUTED LIFE-LONG ANEMIA IN A 63 YEAR OLD CAUCASIAN WOMAN TO
DEFICIENCY OF RED CELL PHOSPHOGLYCERATE KINASE. NO RELATIVES WERE AVAILABLE FOR
STUDY, BUT A HISTORY OF ANEMIA IN THE PROBAND'S MOTHER AND TWO OF HER SIBS WAS
OBTAINED.   ONE WOULD EXPECT RECESSIVE INHERITANCE, HOWEVER. HEMOLYTIC ANEMIA DUE
TO DEFICIENCY OF PHOSPHOGLYCERATE KINASE APPEARED TO BE X-LINKED IN A KINDRED
STUDIED BY VALENTINE ET AL. (SEE X-LINKED CATALOG).

KRAUS, A. P., LANGSTON, M. F., JR. AND LYNCH, B. L.* RED CELL PHOSPHOGLYCERATE
KINASE DEFICIENCY.   A NEW CAUSE OF NON-SPHEROCYTIC HEMOLYTIC ANEMIA. BIOCHEM.
BIOPHYS. RES. COMMUN. 30* 173-177, 1968.

26180 PIERRE ROBIN SYNDROME (GLOSSOPTOSIS, MICROGNATHIA, CLEFT PALATE)

AFFECTED BROTHERS WERE REPORTED BY SMITH AND STOWE (1961) AND PICTURED BY MCKUSICK
ET AL. (1962).   SACHTLEBEN (1964) ALSO DESCRIBED 2 BROTHERS, WHO IN ADDITION TO
THE USUAL FEATURES HAD BILATERAL SYNDACTYLY OF THE SECOND AND THIRD TOES AND
EVIDENCE OF CARDIAC DISEASE. THE OLDER BROTHER HAD HYPOSPADIAS, BIPARTITE SCROTUM
AND MENTAL RETARDATION. SHAH ET AL. (1970) OBSERVED PIERRE ROBIN SYNDROME IN FOUR
SIBS INCLUDING A SET OF TWINS. BIXLER AND CHRISTIAN (1971) DESCRIBED THE FULL
ROBIN SYNDROME IN TWO SIBSHIPS RELATED TO EACH OTHER AS SECOND COUSINS. SINGH ET
AL. (1970) REPORTED A THIRD PAIR OF AFFECTED BROTHERS.

BIXLER, D. AND CHRISTIAN, J. C.* PIERRE ROBIN SYNDROME OCCURRING IN THREE
UNRELATED SIBSHIPS. THE CLINICAL DELINEATION OF BIRTH DEFECTS. X. THE ENDOCRINE
SYSTEM. BALTIMORE* WILLIAMS AND WILKINS, 1971.

MCKUSICK, V. A. AND COLLEAGUES* MEDICAL GENETICS 1961. J. CHRONIC DIS. 15*
417-572, 1962.

SACHTLEBEN, P.* ZUR PATHOGENESE UND THERAPIE DES PIERRE-ROBIN-SYNDROMS. ARCH.
KINDERHEILK. 171* 55-63, 1964.

SHAH, C. V., PRUZANSKY, S. AND HARRIS, W. S.* CARDIAC MALFORMATIONS WITH FACIAL
CLEFTS. AM. J. DIS. CHILD. 114* 238-244, 1970.

SINGH, R. P., JACO, N. T. AND VIGNA, V.* PIERRE ROBIN SYNDROME IN SIBLINGS.

AM. J. DIS. CHILD. 120* 560-561, 1970.

SMITH, J. L. AND STOWE, F. R.* THE PIERRE ROBIN SYNDROME (GLOSSOPTOSIS, MICROGNATHIA, CLEFT PALATE). A REVIEW OF 39 CASES WITH EMPHASIS ON ASSOCIATED OCULAR LESIONS. PEDIATRICS 27* 128-133, 1961.

26190 PILI TORTI (TWISTED HAIR)

THE SHAFTS OF THE HAIRS ARE FLATTENED AT IRREGULAR INTERVALS AND TWISTED THROUGH 180 DEGREES ABOUT THEIR AXES. THE HAIR IS COARSE, DRY AND LUSTERLESS. IT BREAKS OFF LEAVING A STUBBLE OF VARIABLE LENGTH. IN TWO OF SIX FAMILIES REPORTED BY GEDDA AND CAVALIERI (1963) THE PARENTS WERE RELATED AND IN TWO OTHERS OF THE SIX FAMILIES TWO SIBS WERE AFFECTED. BOTH PARENTS WERE UNAFFECTED IN ALL 5 FAMILIES. THE DENTAL ENAMEL HAS BEEN HYPOPLASTIC IN SOME OF THE CASES. USUALLY THE HAIR BECOMES NORMAL AT PUBERTY. THE CONDITION WAS FIRST DESCRIBED AND NAMED BY RONCHESE (1932) WHO OBSERVED 2 AFFECTED SISTERS. APPEL AND MESSINA (1942) DESCRIBED AN AFFECTED GIRL OF WHOM A BROTHER, A SISTER, A PATERNAL AUNT AND THE PATERNAL GRANDMOTHER WERE ALSO AFFECTED. A SIMILAR CONDITION OF THE HAIR OCCURRED IN THE PATIENTS WITH MENKES SYNDROME, AN X-LINKED RECESSIVE (Q.V.).

APPEL, B. AND MESSINA, S. J.* PILI TORTI HEREDITARIA. NEW ENG. J. MED. 226* 912-915, 1942.

GEDDA, L. AND CAVALIERI, R.* RILIEVI GENETICI DELLE DISTROFIE CONGENITE DEI CAPELLI. PROC. SEC. INTERN. CONG. HUM. GENET. (ROME, SEPT. 6-12, 1961.) 2* 1070-1077, 1963.

NICHAMIN, S. J.* TWISTED HAIRS (PILI TORTI). AM. J. DIS. CHILD. 95* 612-615, 1958.

RONCHESE, F.* TWISTED HAIRS (PILI TORTI). ARCH. DERM. SYPH. 26* 98-109, 1932.

26200 PILI TORTI AND NERVE DEAFNESS

BJORNSTAD (1965) FIRST COMMENTED ON THIS ASSOCIATION. AMONG 8 CASES OF PILI TORTI, FIVE HAD NERVE DEAFNESS. REED (1966) OBSERVED FOUR ADDITIONAL CASES AND ROBINSON AND JOHNSTON (1967) REPORTED A CASE. THE DEAFNESS IS EVIDENT IN THE FIRST YEAR OF LIFE. THE SYNDROME OCCURRED IN SIBS AMONG THE CASES OF BJORNSTAD AND REED.

BJORNSTAD, R.* PILI TORTI AND SENSORY-NEURAL LOSS OF HEARING. PROC. 17TH MEET. NTH. DERMAT. SOC. (COPENHAGEN, MAY 27-29, 1965).

REED, W. B.* BURBANK, CALIF.* PERSONAL COMMUNICATION, 1966.

ROBINSON, G. C. AND JOHNSTON, M. M.* PILI TORTI AND SENSORY NEURAL HEARING LOSS. J. PEDIAT. 70* 621-623, 1967.

26220 PINEALOMA WITH HYPERPINEALISM

AN INCREASING BODY OF EVIDENCE SUGGESTS AN ENDOCRINE FUNCTION OF THE PINEAL GLAND AND A ROLE IN REGULATION OF HYPOTHALAMIC RELEASING FACTORS, PARTICULARLY GONADO-TROPINS (REITER AND FRASCHINI, 1969). MENDENHALL (1950) DESCRIBED A FAMILY IN WHICH 3 OF 7 SIBS HAD HIRSUTISM, HYPERPIGMENTATION, PRECOCIOUS DENTITION, HYPERGLYCEMIA AND ENLARGED GENITALIA. TWO OF THE THREE ALSO HAD PITUITARY CYSTS.

MENDENHALL, E. M.* TUMOR OF THE PINEAL BODY WITH HIGH INSULIN RESISTANCE. J. INDIANA MED. ASS. 43* 32-36, 1950.

*26230 PINGELAPESE BLINDNESS

BRODY ET AL. (1970) DESCRIBED IN PINGELAPESE PEOPLE OF THE EASTERN CAROLINE ISLANDS IN THE PACIFIC, A SEVERE OCULAR ABNORMALITY MANIFESTED BY HORIZONTAL PENDULAR NYSTAGMUS, PHOTOPHOBIA, AMAUROSIS, COLOR BLINDNESS AND GRADUALLY DEVELOPING CATARACT. FROM 4 TO 10 PERCENT OF PINGELAPESE PEOPLE ARE BLIND FROM INFANCY. SEGREGATION ANALYSIS AND EQUAL SEX DISTRIBUTION SUPPORTED RECESSIVE INHERITANCE. THE HIGH GENE FREQUENCY WAS ATTRIBUTED TO REDUCTION IN THE POPULA-TION TO ABOUT 9 SURVIVING MALES BY A TYPHOON ABOUT 1780, COMBINED WITH SUBSEQUENT ISOLATION. WHETHER THE DISORDER IS A FORM OF CONGENITAL ACHROMATOPSIA OR A TAPETORETINAL DEGENERATION WITH PRIMARY INVOLVEMENT OF THE CONES WAS NOT CLEAR. CARR ET AL. (1970) STUDIED THE SAME GROUP AND CONCLUDED THAT IT IS INSTEAD CONGENITAL COMPLETE ACHROMATOPSIA. THE IMPRESSION OF TAPETORETINAL DEGENERATION WAS BASED, THEY THOUGHT, ON SEVERE MYOPIA WHICH WAS FOUND IN A MAJORITY OF THE AFFECTED PERSONS. THE DISORDER IS NONPROGRESSIVE.

BRODY, J. A., HUSSELS, I., BRINK, E. AND TORRES, J.* HEREDITARY BLINDNESS AMONG PINGELAPESE PEOPLE OF EASTERN CAROLINE ISLANDS. LANCET 1* 1253-1257, 1970.

CARR, R. E., MORTON, N. E. AND SIEGEL, I. M.* PINGELAP EYE DISEASE. (LETTER) LANCET 1* 667 ONLY, 1970.

*26240 PITUITARY DWARFISM I (PRIMORDIAL DWARFISM, SEXUAL ATELEIOTIC DWARFISM, ISOLATED

EARLY IN THIS CENTURY GILFORD CALLED DWARFS WITH NORMAL BODY PROPORTIONS ATELEIO-
TIC ('NOT ARRIVED AT PERFECTION') AND DISTINGUISHED SEXUAL AND ASEXUAL TYPES. THE
TWO TYPES CORRESPOND TO WHAT ARE REFERRED TO HERE AS PITUITARY DWARFISM I AND III.
THE FIRST HAS AN ISOLATED DEFICIENCY OF GROWTH HORMONE, WHEREAS THE SECOND HAS
DEFICIENCY OF ALL ANTERIOR PITUITARY HORMONES. THE EXISTANCE OF AN ISOLATED
GROWTH HORMONE DEFICIENCY IN RECESSIVELY INHERITED SEXUAL ATELEIOSIS WAS DEMONS-
TRATED BY RIMOIN, MERIMEE AND MCKUSICK (1966). FAMILIES OF THIS TYPE HAVE BEEN
REPORTED BY MCKUSICK (1955), VON VERSCHUER AND CONRADI (1938), DZIERZYNSKI (1938)
AND OTHERS. MOE (1968) REPORTED BROTHER AND SISTER WITH HYPOGLYCEMIA AND PRESUMED
ISOLATED SOMATOTROPIN DEFICIENCY. THE FATHER HAD DIABETES INSIPIDUS.

CARSNER, R. L. AND RENNELS, E. G.* PRIMARY SITE OF GENE ACTION IN ANTERIOR
PITUITARY DWARF MICE. SCIENCE 131* 829 ONLY, 1960.

DZIERZYNSKI, W.* NANOSOMIA PITUITARIA HYPOPLASTICA HEREDITARIA. ZBL. GES.
NEUROL. PSYCHIAT. 162* 411-421, 1938.

MCKUSICK, V. A.* PRIMORDIAL DWARFISM AND ECTOPIA LENTIS. AM. J. HUM. GENET. 7*
189-198, 1955.

MOE, P. J.* HYPOPITUITARY DWARFISM. THE IMPORTANCE OF EARLY THERAPY. ACTA
PAEDIAT. SCAND. 57* 300-304, 1968.

RIMOIN, D. L., MERIMEE, T. J. AND MCKUSICK, V. A.* GROWTH-HORMONE DEFICIENCY IN
MAN* AN ISOLATED, RECESSIVELY INHERITED DEFECT. SCIENCE 152* 1635-1637, 1966.

SEIP, M., VAN DER HAGEN, C. B. AND TRYGSTAD, O.* HEREDITARY PITUITARY DWARFISM
WITH SPONTANEOUS DWARFISM. ARCH. DIS. CHILD. 43* 47-52, 1968.

VON VERSCHUER, O. F. AND CONRADI, L.* EINE SIPPE MIT REZESSIV ERBLICHEM
PRIMORDIALEM ZWERGWUCHS. Z. MENSCHL. VERERB. KONSTITUTIONSL. 22* 261-267, 1938.

*26250 PITUITARY DWARFISM II

PERTZELAN ET AL. (1968) DESCRIBED A FORM OF DWARFISM IN WHICH THE ABNORMALITY OF
PITUITARY HORMONES IS LIMITED TO GROWTH HORMONE BUT THE LEVEL OF GROWTH HORMONE AS
MEASURED BY THE IMMUNO-ASSAY METHOD IS HIGH RATHER THAN LOW. IN ISRAEL ALL CASES
(13 FEMALES, 7 MALES) OF THIS TYPE WERE ORIENTAL JEWS. A FUNCTIONALLY ABNORMAL
ALTHOUGH IMMUNO-REACTIVE GROWTH HORMONE MOLECULE WAS POSTULATED. INHERITANCE WAS
CLEARLY RECESSIVE. BAILEY ET AL. (1967) OBSERVED TWO SIBS WITH SEVERE DWARFING,
RETARDED BONE AGE, HYPOGLYCEMIA AND EXCESSIVELY HIGH SERUM LEVELS OF GROWTH
HORMONE AS DETERMINED BY RADIO-IMMUNO-ASSAY. THE PARENTS WERE FIRST COUSINS.
THIS DISORDER COULD BE DETERMINED BY A GENE ALLELIC TO THAT PRODUCING LACK OF
GROWTH HORMONE. THE 30 YEAR OLD MAN REPORTED BY MERIMEE ET AL. (1968) HAD RAISED
LEVELS OF PLASMA HGH WHICH WAS NOT SUPPRESSED BY HYPERGLYCEMIA AND FURTHER
AUGMENTED BY INSULIN-INDUCED HYPOGLYCEMIA AND BY ARGININE INFUSION. WITH RESPECT
TO ALL METABOLIC INDICES EXAMINED HE SHOWED ATTENUATED RESPONSES TO EXOGENOUS
GROWTH HORMONE. SIMILARITIES TO ISOLATED GROWTH HORMONE DEFICIENCY CASES OF TYPE
I WERE EXAGGERATED HYPOGLYCEMIC RESPONSE TO EXOGENOUS INSULIN AND INSULINOPENIA
AFTER GLUCOSE OR ARGININE. A 'WARPED' HGH MOLECULE WHICH SATURATES RECEPTORS AND
PRIMARY END ORGANS UNRESPONSIVENESS ARE TWO ALTERNATIVE EXPLANATIONS.

BAILEY, J. D., BAIN, H. W., THOMPSON, M. W., GARGLIARDINO, J. J. AND MARTIN, J.
M.* ETIOLOGICAL FACTORS IN IDIOPATHIC HYPOPITUITARY DWARFISM. AM. PEDIAT. SOC.,
1967.

DAUGHADAY, W. W., LARON, Z., PERTZELAN, A. AND HEINS, J. N.* DEFECTIVE
SULFATION FACTOR GENERATION* A POSSIBLE ETIOLOGICAL LINK IN DWARFISM. TRANS. ASS.
AM. PHYSICIANS 82* 129-140, 1969.

LARON, Z., PERTZELAN, A. AND MANNHEIMER, S.* GENETIC PITUITARY DWARFISM WITH
HIGH SERUM CONCENTRATION OF GROWTH HORMONE. A NEW INBORN ERROR OF METABOLISM.Q
ISRAEL J. MED. SCI. 2* 152-155, 1966.

MERIMEE, T. J., HALL, J., RABINOWITZ, D., MCKUSICK, V. A. AND RIMOIN, D. L.* AN
UNUSUAL VARIETY OF ENDOCRINE DWARFISM* SUBRESPONSIVENESS TO GROWTH HORMONE IN A
SEXUALLY MATURE DWARF. LANCET 2* 191-193, 1968.

NAJJAR, S. S., KHACHADURIAN, A. K., ILBAWI, M. N. AND BLIZZARD, R. M.* DWARFISM
WITH ELEVATED LEVELS OF PLASMA GROWTH HORMONE. NEW ENG. J. MED. 284* 809-812,
1971.

PERTZELAN, A., ADAM, A. AND LARON, Z.* GENETIC ASPECTS OF PITUITARY DWARFISM
DUE TO ABSENCE OR BIOLOGICAL INACTIVITY OF GROWTH HORMONE. ISRAEL J. MED. SCI. 4*
895-900, 1968.

*26260 PITUITARY DWARFISM III (PANHYPOPITJITARISM)

PANHYPOPITUITARY DWARFISM IS NOT EXCESSIVELY RARE, THERE PROBABLY BEING 7 TO 10
THOUSAND CASES IN THE UNITED STATES. THE FORM INHERITED AS A SIMPLE RECESSIVE

PROBABLY IS RARE. MULTIPLE CASES IN MULTIPLE SIBSHIPS OBSERVED AMONG THE HUTTERITES, A RELIGIOUS ISOLATE IN THE UNITED STATES AND CANADA, INDICATE THE RECESSIVE INHERITANCE OF PANHYPOPITUITARISM. WE HAVE ALSO OBSERVED PANHYPOPITUI- TARISM IN A 50 YEAR OLD UNCLE AND 5 YEAR OLD NIECE. FURTHERMORE, THE FAMILIAL CASES IN THE INBRED POPULATION OF CERTAIN AREAS OF SWITZERLAND AND OF THE ISLAND OF VEGLIA (KRK) IN THE ADRIATIC, OBSERVED BY HANHART (1925, 1953), ARE PROBABLY EXAMPLES. THIS TYPE (ATELEIOTIC DWARFISM WITH HYPOGONADISM) IS SOMETIMES CALLED HANHART'S DWARFISM. THE NATURE OF MOST PANHYPOPITUITARISM AS A CONGENITAL MALFORMATION WITH LITTLE INDICATION OF A MENDELIAN BASIS IS SUPPORTED BY THE OBSERVATION BY ROSENFIELD ET AL. (1967) OF 16 YEAR OLD IDENTICAL TWINS, ONE NORMAL AND ONE WITH PANHYPOPITUITARISM. KIRCHHOFF (1954) DESCRIBED THREE AFFECTED SIBS WHO MAY HAVE HAD PANHYPOPITUITARISM, THE OLDEST BEING ALMOST 18 YEARS OLD. SELYE (1949) PICTURED THREE BROTHERS, AGES 25, 22, AND 11 WITH PANHYPOPITUITARISM. THE CASES DESCRIBED BY SCHMOLCK (1907) MAY HAVE BEEN OF THE PANHYPOPITUITARY TYPE. BAILEY ET AL. (1967) REPORTED TWO FAMILIES WITH A TOTAL OF 5 AFFECTED. IN ONE THE PARENTS WERE FIRST COUSINS. STEINER AND BOGGS (1965) DESCRIBED BROTHER AND SISTER, OFFSPRING OF FIRST COUSIN PARENTS, WITH CONGENITAL ABSENCE OF THE PITUITARY LEADING TO HYPOTHYROIDISM, HYPOADRENALISM AND HYPOGONADISM. A THIRD SIB WAS PROBABLY ALSO AFFECTED AND PROBABLY DIED OF HYPOGLYCEMIA IN THE NEWBORN PERIOD. THIS MAY BE A SEPARATE ENTITY FROM THE OTHER(S) DISCUSSED IN THIS LISTING. THE SELLA TURCICA WAS NORMAL IN SIZE IN THE CASES OF STEINER AND BOGGS (1965).

BAILEY, J. D., BAIN, H. W., THOMPSON, M. W., GAGLIARDINO, J. J. AND MARTIN, J. M.* ETIOLOGICAL FACTORS IN IDIOPATHIC HYPOPITUITARY DWARFISM. AM. PEDIAT. SOC., 1967.

FERRIER, P. E.* CONGENITAL ABSENCE OF HYPOPLASIA OF THE ENDOCRINE GLANDS. J. GENET. HUM. 17* 325-347, 1969.

FRASER, G. R.* STUDIES IN ISOLATES. J. GENET. HUM. 13* 32-46, 1964.

HANHART, E.* DIE ROLLE DER ERBFAKTOREN BEI DEN STORUNGEN DES WACHSTUMS. SCHWEIZ. MED. WSCHR. 83* 198-203, 1953.

HANHART, E.* UBER HEREDODEGENERATIVEN ZWERGWUCHS MIT DYSTROPHIA ADIPOSOGENITA- LIS. AN HAND VON UNTERSUCHUNGEN BEI DREI SIPPEN VON PROPORTIONIERTEN ZWERGEN. ARCH. KLAUS STIFT. VERERBUNGSFORSCH. 1* 181-257, 1925.

KIRCHHOFF, H. W., LEHMANN, W. AND SCHAEFER, U.* CLINICAL, HEREDITARY-BIOLOGIC AND CONSTITUTIONAL STUDIES OF PRIMORDIAL DWARFS. Z. KINDERHEILK. 75* 243-266, 1954.

ROSENFIELD, R. L., ROOT, A. W., BONGIOVANNI, A. M. AND EBERLEIN, W. R.* IDIOPATHIC ANTERIOR HYPOPITUITARISM IN ONE OF MONOZYGOTIC TWINS. J. PEDIAT. 70* 115-117, 1967.

SCHMOLCK, (NI)* MEHRFACHER ZWERGWUCHS IN VERWANDTEN FAMILIEN EINES HOCHGEBIRG- TALES. VIRCHOW ARCH. PATH. ANAT. 187* 105-111, 1907.

SELYE, H.* TEXTBOOKS OF ENDOCRINOLOGY. MONTREAL* U. MONTREAL, 1947. P. 268.

STEINER, M. M. AND BOGGS, J. D.* ABSENCE OF PITUITARY GLAND, HYPOTHYROIDISM HYPOADRENALISM AND HYPOGONADISM IN A 17-YEAR-OLD DWARF. J. CLIN. ENDOCR. 25* 1591-1598, 1965.

26270 PITUITARY DWARFISM WITH SMALL SELLA TURCICA

FERRIER AND STONE (1969) DESCRIBED AN APPARENTLY DISTINCT FORM OF FAMILIAL PITUITARY INSUFFICIENCY IN TWO SISTERS, AGED 10 AND 11 YEARS. THE FEATURES WERE SEVERE GROWTH RETARDATION FROM INFANCY, TENDENCY TO HYPOGLYCEMIA, DEFICIENT PRODUCTION OF GROWTH HORMONE, TSH AND ACTH, MARKED RETARDATION IN SKELETAL MATURATION, AND VERY SMALL SELLA TURCICA WITH ABNORMAL MORPHOLOGY OF THE PETROUS BONE.

FERRIER, P. E. AND STONE, E. F., JR.* FAMILIAL PITUITARY DWARFISM ASSOCIATED WITH AN ABNORMAL SELLA TURCICA. PEDIATRICS 43* 858-865, 1969.

26280 PLASMA CLOT RETRACTION FACTOR, DEFICIENCY OF

NEWCOMB ET AL. (1967) DESCRIBED AN APPARENTLY *NEW* BLEEDING SYNDROME CHARAC- TERIZED BY DEEP TISSUE BLEEDING, POOR WOUND HEALING, PSEUDOTUMOR FORMATION AND UMBILICAL CORD BLEEDING. A DEFECT IN CLOT RETRACTION WAS CORRECTABLE BY A PLASMA PROTEIN. FAMILY STUDIES SUPPORTED AUTOSOMAL RECESSIVE INHERITANCE.

NEWCOMB, T. F., KITCHENS, C. S. AND BERMAN, P. A.* A NEW BLEEDING SYNDROME WITH DEFECTIVE CLOT RETRACTION DUE TO DEFICIENCY OF A PLASMA PROTEIN. AM. SOC. HEMAT., TORONTO, 1967.

26290 PLEOCONIAL MYOPATHY

IN A CASE OF CHILDHOOD MYOPATHY, SHY ET AL. (1966) FOUND LARGE NUMBERS OF

R
E
C
E
S
S
I
V
E

MITOCHONDRIA. THE CLINICAL FEATURES WERE PROXIMAL WEAKNESS AND WASTING, PROLONGED
EPISODES OF FLACCID PARALYSIS AND SALT-CRAVING. TWO BROTHERS MAY HAVE BEEN
AFFECTED IN THIS SIBSHIP.

SHY, G. M., GONATAS, N. K. AND PEREZ, M.* TWO CHILDHOOD MYOPATHIES WITH
ABNORMAL MITOCHONDRIA* I. MEGACONIAL MYOPATHY. II. PLEOCONIAL MYOPATHY. BRAIN
89* 133-158, 1966.

26310 POLYCYSTIC KIDNEY, CATARACT AND CONGENITAL BLINDNESS

FAIRLEY, LEIGHTON AND KINCAID-SMITH (1963) OBSERVED THREE SIBS WITH SOME TYPE OF
EYE DEFECT CAUSING BLINDNESS AND SOME TYPE OF RENAL DEFECT. ONE DIED AT AGE 22
YEARS OF POLYCYSTIC KIDNEY, WAS BLIND FROM BIRTH AND SHOWED CENTRAL CATARACT. A
SECOND DIED AT 18 YEARS AND HAD THE SAME EYE DEFECT* ATROPHIC KIDNEYS WITH
PYRAMIDAL CYSTS WERE FOUND. THE THIRD SIB HAD RETINAL DYSTROPHY (OR DYSPLASIA)
AND LARGE KIDNEYS WITH MEDULLARY CYSTS. PIERSON ET AL. (1963) REPORTED TWO
SISTERS WHO DIED AT THE AGES OF 10 AND 15 DAYS. BOTH HAD A COMPLEX OCULAR
DYSPLASIA (MICROCORIA, HYPOPLASTIC RETINA, CATARACT, ABSENCE OF CILIARY BODY,
PERSISTENCE OF FETAL IRIDO-CORNEAL ANGLE) IN ASSOCIATION WITH MICROCYSTIC RENAL
DYSPLASIA. I HAVE HAD A MALE PATIENT (P 11614) WHO WAS BLIND FROM BIRTH, PROBABLY
AS A RESULT OF RETINAL APLASIA, AND DIED OF RENAL FAILURE AT AGE 12 YEARS.
AUTOPSY SHOWED CYSTIC DISEASE OF THE KIDNEYS.

FAIRLEY, K. F., LEIGHTON, P. W. AND KINCAID-SMITH, P.* FAMILIAL VISUAL DEFECTS
ASSOCIATED WITH POLYCYSTIC KIDNEY AND MEDULLARY SPONGE KIDNEY. BRIT. MED. J. 1*
1060-1063, 1963.

PIERSON, M., CORDIER, J., HERVOUET, F. AND RAUBER, G.* UNE CURIEUSE ASSOCIATION
MALFORMATIVE CONGENITALE ET FAMILIALE ATTEIGNANT L'OEIL ET LE REIN. J. GENET.
HUM. 12* 184-213, 1963.

*26320 POLYCYSTIC KIDNEY, INFANTILE, TYPE I

IT HAS LONG BEEN RECOGNIZED THAT THE AGE DISTRIBUTION OF CASES OF POLYCYSTIC
KIDNEYS HAS TWO PEAKS, ONE AT BIRTH AND ONE BETWEEN AGES 30-60 YEARS. FURTHER-
MORE, THE CASES WITH THE LATER PEAK SHOW THE FAMILIAL PATTERN OF AN AUTOSOMAL
DOMINANT. THREE TYPES OF CYSTIC KIDNEYS IN NEWBORNS, INFANTS AND CHILDREN WERE
DISTINGUISHED BY LUNDIN AND OLOW (1961). IN TYPE I THE KIDNEYS ARE OVERSIZED AND
SPONGY. THE LIVER AND PANCREAS MAY SHOW FIBROSIS AND-OR CYSTIC CHANGE. 'POTTER'S
FACE' (DEEP-SET EYES, MICROGNATHIA, LARGE, FLAPPY, LOW-SET EARS) IS PRESENT IN
MOST OR ALL. LUNDIN AND OLOW (1961) FOUND 9 CASES AMONG 21 SIBS. WHEN THESE
FIGURES WERE TREATED BY THE METHOD OF WEINBERG THE CORRECTED FIGURE OF 6 AFFECTED
IN 27 SIBS WAS ARRIVED AT (A SATISFACTORY AGREEMENT WITH THE RATIO EXPECTED OF A
RECESSIVE TRAIT).
(TYPE II ALSO HAS LARGE KIDNEYS BUT IS CHARACTERIZED BY MORE ABUNDANT
CONNECTIVE TISSUE THAN IN TYPE I. TYPE III HAS HYPOPLASTIC KIDNEYS. IN TYPE II
FAMILIAL AGGREGATION HAS BEEN OBSERVED, BUT THE EVIDENCE FOR RECESSIVE INHERITANCE
IS NOT COMPLETE.) CARTER (1970) SUMMARIZED A CLINICOPATHOLOGIC STUDY BY BLYTH AND
OCKENDEN (1969). CHILDHOOD POLYCYSTIC DISEASE FELL INTO FOUR CLASSES ACCORDING TO
AGE OF ONSET, CLINICAL COURSE, PROPORTION OF RENAL TUBULES INVOLVED AND DEGREE OF
HEPATIC FIBROSIS. ALL FOUR GROUPS, TERMED PERINATAL, NEONATAL, INFANTILE AND
JUVENILE, WERE THOUGHT TO BE RECESSIVE. THE TYPE WAS CONSISTENT WITHIN ANY ONE
FAMILY. OCCASIONALLY, THE 'ADULT' DOMINANT FORM PRESENTED IN CHILDHOOD.

BLYTH, H. M. AND OCKENDEN, B. G.* A CLINICO-PATHOLOGICAL AND FAMILY STUDY OF
POLYCYSTIC DISEASE OF THE KIDNEYS AND LIVER IN CHILDREN. (ABSTRACT) J. CLIN.
PATH. 22* 508 ONLY, 1969.

CARTER, C. O.* GENETICS OF POLYCYSTIC DISEASE OF KIDNEY. THE CLINICAL
DELINEATION OF BIRTH DEFECTS. BALTIMORE* WILLIAMS AND WILKINS, 1970.

LEE, K. H. AND CHANG, E.* DYSTOCIA DUE TO CONGENITAL POLYCYSTIC KIDNEYS. J.
OBSTET. GYNEC. 77* 1115-1116, 1970.

LUNDIN, P. M. AND OLOW, I.* POLYCYSTIC KIDNEYS IN NEWBORNS, INFANTS AND
CHILDREN. A CLINICAL AND PATHOLOGICAL STUDY. ACTA PAEDIAT. 50* 185-200, 1961.

26330 POLYCYTHEMIA RUBRA VERA

MODAN (1965) SUGGESTED THAT IN ONLY TWO REPORTS OF FAMILIAL PRV IS THE DIAGNOSIS
COMPLETELY DOCUMENTED (LAWRENCE AND GOETSCH, 1950* ERF, 1956). LAWRENCE AND
GOETSCH DESCRIBED 3 AFFECTED SIBS. TWO PATIENTS IN THE SERIES OF ERF WERE
BROTHERS AND THREE OTHERS HAD 'A DEFINITE FAMILY HISTORY.' LEVIN ET AL. (1967)
REPORTED A CURIOUS CASE OF TWO BROTHERS WITH POLYCYTHEMIA VERA AND THE PHILADEL-
PHIA CHROMOSOME. THE PRECISE MODE OF INHERITANCE IS UNKNOWN.

ERF, L. A.* RADIOACTIVE PHOSPHORUS IN THE TREATMENT OF PRIMARY POLYCYTHEMIA.
PROGR. HEMAT. 1* 153-165, 1956.

LAWRENCE, J. H. AND GOETSCH, A. T.* FAMILIAL OCCURRENCE OF POLYCYTHEMIA AND
LEUKEMIA. CALIF. MED. 73* 361-364, 1950.

LEVIN, W. C., HOUSTON, E. W. AND RITZMAN, S. E.* POLYCYTHEMIA VERA WITH PH-1 CHROMOSOMES IN TWO BROTHERS. BLOOD 30* 503-512, 1967.

MODAN, B.* POLYCYTHEMIA* A REVIEW OF EPIDEMOLOGICAL AND CLINICAL ASPECTS. J. CHRONIC DIS. 18* 605-645, 1965.

26340 POLYCYTHEMIA, BENIGN FAMILIAL, OF CHILDREN

AUERBACH, WOLFF AND METTIER (1958) REPORTED THREE FAMILIES. IN ONE, TWO BROTHERS AND A SISTER WERE AFFECTED AND IN THE SECOND THE PROBAND AND AN AUNT. THE PARENTS WERE NORMAL. UNLIKE POLYCYTHEMIA VERA, THE SUBJECTS DEMONSTRATED NO INCREASE IN WHITE COUNT, PLATELETS OR URIC ACID AND THE PROCESS WAS BENIGN. NADLER AND COHN (1939) DESCRIBED A FAMILY IN WHICH 4 OF 11 CHILDREN SHOWED POLYCYTHEMIA. THE MOTHER STATED THAT THESE FOUR CHILDREN HAD RED FACES FROM THE TIME OF BIRTH. THIS CONDITION WOULD MORE ACCURATELY BE CALLED BENIGN FAMILIAL ERYTHROCYTOSIS, SINCE ONLY THE ERYTHROID SERIES IS AFFECTED. SEE ERYTHROCYTOSIS, BENIGN FAMILIAL, IN DOMINANT CATALOG.

AUERBACH, M. L., WOLFF, J. A. AND METTIER, S. R.* BENIGN FAMILIAL POLYCYTHEMIA IN CHILDHOOD* REPORT OF TWO CASES. PEDIATRICS 21* 54-58, 1958.

NADLER, S. B. AND COHN, I.* FAMILIAL POLYCYTHEMIA. AM. J. MED. SCI. 198* 41-48, 1939.

26350 POLYDACTYLISM

THE ELLIS-VAN CREVELD AND LAWRENCE-MOON-BIEDL-BARDET SYNDROMES (Q.V.) ARE RECESSIVE DISORDERS WHICH HAVE POLYDACTYLISM AS FEATURES. SNYDER (1929) IN A STUDY OF NEGROES IN PAMLICO CO., N.C., ASSEMBLED EVIDENCE INTERPRETED AS INDICATING A RECESSIVE FORM OF SIMPLE POLYDACTYLY.

SNYDER, L. H.* A RECESSIVE FACTOR FOR POLYDACTYLISM IN MAN. STUDIES IN HUMAN INHERITANCE. J. HERED. 20* 73-77, 1929.

26360 POLYSACCHARIDE, STORAGE OF UNUSUAL

R
E
C
E
S
S
I
V
E

CRAIG AND UZMAN (1958) DESCRIBED TWO SIBS AFFECTED BY A METABOLIC DISORDER CHARACTERIZED PATHOLOGICALLY BY THE STORAGE OF AN UNUSUAL POLYSACCHARIDE.

CRAIG, J. M. AND UZMAN, L. L.* A FAMILIAL METABOLIC DISORDER WITH STORAGE OF AN UNUSUAL POLYSACCHARIDE COMPLEX. PEDIATRICS 22* 20-32, 1958.

*26370 PORPHYRIA, CONGENITAL ERYTHROPOIETIC (GUNTHER'S DISEASE)

FORMS OF HEREDITARY PORPHYRIA OTHER THAN THIS BEHAVE AS DOMINANT TRAITS. THE CONGENITAL ERYTHROPOIETIC FORM IS VERY RARE. DRABKIN (1963) REPORTED IN BRIEF A BRAZILIAN FAMILY IN WHICH 4 OF 9 SIBS WERE AFFECTED. MARKED SPLENOMEGALY AND CUTANEOUS MUTILATION WERE FEATURES. PORPHYRINS ARE DEMONSTRABLE IN THE ERYTHROPOIETIC CELLS, THUS PROVIDING DIFFERENTIATION FROM THE HEPATIC FORMS OF PORPHYRIA WHICH SHOW PORPHYRINS IN THE LIVER CELLS AND NOT IN THE RED BLOOD CELLS. HEMOLYTIC ANEMIA MAY BE HELPED BY SPLENECTOMY. GUNTHER CALLED THIS CONDITION CONGENITAL HAEMATOPORPHYRIA. WATSON RENAMED IT ERYTHROPOIETIC PORPHYRIA. ALTHOUGH RECESSIVE IN CATTLE AS WELL AS IN MAN, CONGENITAL ERYTHROPOIETIC PORPHYRIA IS SAID TO BE DOMINANT IN SWINE AND IN CATS (GLENN ET AL., 1968). ROMEO AND LEVIN (1969) CONCLUDED THAT THE PRIMARY ENZYME DEFECT CONCERNS UROPORPHYRINOGEN III COSYNTHETASE.

DRABKIN, D. L.* SOME HISTORICAL HIGHLIGHTS IN KNOWLEDGE OF PORPHYRINS AND PORPHYRIAS. ANN. N.Y. ACAD. SCI. 104* 658-665, 1963.

GLENN, B. L., GLENN, H. G. AND OMTVEDT, I. T.* CONGENITAL PORPHYRIA IN THE DOMESTIC CAT (FELIS CATUS)* PRELIMINARY INVESTIGATIONS ON INHERITANCE PATTERN. AM. J. VET. RES. 29* 1653-1657, 1968.

ROMEO, G. AND LEVIN, E. Y.* UROPORPHYRINOGEN III COSYNTHETASE IN HUMAN CONGENITAL ERYTHROPOIETIC PORPHYRIA. PROC. NAT. ACAD. SCI. 63* 856-863, 1969.

ROMEO, G., GLENN, B. L. AND LEVIN, E. Y.* UROPORPHYRINOGEN III COSYNTHETASE IN ASYMPTOMATIC CARRIERS OF CONGENITAL ERYTHROPOIETIC PORPHYRIA. BIOCHEM. GENET. 4* 719-726, 1970.

ROMEO, G., KABACK, M. M. AND LEVIN, E. Y.* UROPORPHYRINOGEN III COSYNTHETASE ACTIVITY IN FIBROBLASTS FROM PATIENTS WITH CONGENITAL ERYTHROPOIETIC PORPHYRIA. BIOCHEM. GENET. 4* 659-664, 1970.

SCHMID, R.* THE PORPHYRIAS. IN, STANBURY, J. B., WYNGAARDEN, J. B. AND FREDRICKSON, D. S. (EDS.)* THE METABOLIC BASIS OF INHERITED DISEASES. NEW YORK* MCGRAW-HILL, 1966 (2ND ED.). PP. 813-870.

WATSON, C. J.* THE PROBLEM OF PORPHYRIA - SOME FACTS AND QUESTIONS. NEW ENG. J. MED. 263* 1205-1215, 1960.

GITELMAN ET AL. (1966) REPORTED TWO AFFECTED SISTERS WHO WERE THE OFFSPRING OF PARENTS RELATED AS HALF-FIRST-COUSINS-ONCE-REMOVED. THEY HAD EXPERIENCED OCCASIONAL MILD EPISODES OF MUSCLE WEAKNESS AND HAD SUFFERED FOR MANY YEARS FROM A CHRONIC DERMATITIS CHARACTERIZED BY THICKENING WITH A PURPLE-RED HUE. ERYTHEMA OF THE SKIN IS A FEATURE OF EXPERIMENTAL MAGNESIUM DEPLETION IN THE RAT.

EARLE, D. P., SHERRY, S., EICHNA, L. W. AND CONAN, N. J.* LOW POTASSIUM SYNDROME DUE TO DEFECTIVE RENAL TUBULAR MECHANISMS FOR HANDLING POTASSIUM. AM. J. MED. 11* 283-301, 1951.

FRANCE, R. AND TOLLESON, W. J.* POTASSIUM DEPLETION OF UNDETERMINED ORIGIN IN TWO BROTHERS. TRANS. AM. CLIN. CLIMAT. ASS. 69* 106-112, 1958.

GITELMAN, H. J., GRAHAM, J. B. AND WELT, L. G.* A NEW FAMILIAL DISORDER CHARACTERIZED BY HYPOKALEMIA AND HYPOMAGNESEMIA. TRANS. ASS. AM. PHYSICIANS 79* 221-235, 1966.

26390 POTASSIUM-SODIUM DISORDER OF ERYTHROCYTE

SHEEP SHOW A POLYMORPHISM OF RED CELL POTASSIUM AND SODIUM CONCENTRATION. SO-CALLED LK SHEEP HAVE LOW POTASSIUM AND HIGH SODIUM WHEREAS HK SHEEP HAVE THE CONVERSE. LOW POTASSIUM IS DOMINANT TO HIGH POTASSIUM. A PRECISELY COMPARABLE SITUATION HAS NOT BEEN FOUND IN MAN. (SEE REVIEW BY LUSH (1966). IN A CHILD WITH HEMOLYTIC ANEMIA ZARKOWSKY ET AL. (1968) FOUND HIGH SODIUM (100 MEQ. PER LITER) AND LOW POTASSIUM (40 MEQ. PER LITER) IN THE RED CELLS. SPLENECTOMY WAS BENEFI-CIAL. BOTH PARENTS WERE OF HUNGARIAN DESCENT. THEY AND A FEMALE SIB HAD NORMAL BLOOD STUDIES. IN 3 MALES IN 3 SUCCESSIVE GENERATIONS, OSKI ET AL. (1969) FOUND HEMOLYTIC ANEMIA, STOMATOCYTIC RED CELLS, AND INCREASED RED CELL FRAGILITY. OLD CELLS WERE LESS DENSE THAN YOUNG CELLS AND HAD A HIGH-SODIUM, LOW-POTASSIUM CONTENT.

LUSH, I. E.* THE BIOCHEMICAL GENETICS OF VERTEBRATES EXCEPT MAN. PHILADELPHIA* W. B. SAUNDERS, 1966.

OSKI, F. A., NAIMAN, J. L., BLUM, S. F., ZARKOWSKY, H. S., WHAUN, J., SHOHET, S. B., GREEN, A. AND NATHAN, D. G.* CONGENITAL HEMOLYTIC ANEMIA WITH HIGH-SODIUM, LOW-POTASSIUM RED CELLS. NEW ENG. J. MED. 280* 909-916, 1969.

ZARKOWSKY, H. S., OSKI, F. A., SHA'AFI, R., SHOHET, S. B. AND NATHAN, D. G.* CONGENITAL HEMOLYTIC ANEMIA WITH HIGH-SODIUM, LOW-POTASSIUM RED CELLS. I. STUDIES OF MEMBRANE PERMEABILITY. NEW ENG. J. MED. 278* 573-581, 1968.

R
E
C
E
S
S
I
V
E

26400 PRADER-WILLI SYNDROME

JOHNSEN, CRAWFORD AND HAESSLER (1967) STUDIED 7 MENTALLY RETARDED CASES AGED 4 TO 19 YEARS. ALL SHOWED POVERTY OF FETAL MOVEMENTS AND EXTREME INFANTILE HYPOTONIA. WITH IMPROVEMENT IN MUSCLE TONE, FEEDING DIFFICULTIES ABATED BUT WERE REPLACED BY UNCONTROLLABLE HYPERPHAGIA. PLETHORIC OBESITY, RETARDED PSYCHOMOTOR DEVELOPMENT AND DIMINUTIVE HANDS AND FEET WERE NOTED. ALL TEENAGERS WERE LESS THAN 5 FEET TALL. STUDIES SHOWED THAT FAT SYNTHESIS FROM ACETATE DURING FASTING WAS 10 TIMES GREATER IN CASES THAN UNAFFECTED SIBS AND HORMONE STIMULATED LIPOLYSIS WAS DEPRESSED. THESE WORKERS SUGGESTED THAT THE CONDITION IS COMPARABLE TO THE GENETIC OBESE-HYPERGLYCEMIC MOUSE. SINCE DURING FASTING SUBSTRATE CONTINUES TO BE USED FOR NEW FAT AND LIPOLYSIS IS DEFICIENT, SURVIVAL DEPENDS ON A CONTINUOUS SUPPLY OF EXOGENOUS CALORIES. LANGDON-DOWN (1828-1896), WHO DESCRIBED MONGOLISM (DOWN'S SYNDROME), ALSO DESCRIBED THIS CONDITION IN 1887 (SEE ACCOUNT BY BRAIN, 1967). THE PATIENT WAS A MENTALLY SUBNORMAL GIRL WHO, WHEN 13 YEARS OLD, WAS 4 FEET 4 INCHES IN HEIGHT, AND WEIGHED 196 LBS. AT 25 YEARS OF AGE SHE WEIGHED 210 LBS. 'HER FEET AND HANDS REMAINED SMALL, AND CONTRASED REMARKABLY WITH THE APPENDAGES THEY TERMINATED. SHE HAD NO HAIR IN THE AXILLAE, AND SCARCELY ANY ON THE PUBIS. SHE HAD NEVER MENSTRUATED, NOR DID SHE EXHIBIT THE SLIGHTEST SEXUAL INSTINCT.' DOWN CALLED THE CONDITION POLYSARCIA. ZELLWEGER AND SCHNEIDER (1968) FOUND ONE INSTANCE OF AFFECTED SIBS, BROTHER AND SISTER (GABILAN AND ROYER, TO BE PUBLISHED* PROBABLY THE SAME AS GABILAN, 1962) AND ONE INSTANCE OF PARENTAL CONSANGUINITY IN THE SAME REPORT. I HAVE OBSERVED A SINGLE CASE IN AN INBRED AMISH COMMUNITY. THE FACT THAT ONLY ONE CASE IS PRESENT SPEAKS AGAINST RECESSIVE INHERITANCE. HOWEVER, PRADER AND WILLI (QUOTED BY HOEFNAGEL ET AL., 1967) FAVORED RECESSIVE INHERITANCE. GABILAN (1962) REPORTED ONE FAMILY WITH AFFECTED BROTHER AND SISTER, AS WELL AS A SECOND IN WHICH THE PARENTS OF THE PROBAND WERE FIRST COUSINS., BUT HIS PATIENTS WERE NOT ENTIRELY TYPICAL. THE ABUNDANT FAT, MUSCLE HYPOTONIA AND SMALL FEET AND HANDS ARE EXACTLY THE OPPOSITE OF THE SPARSE FAT, MUSCLE HYPERTROPHY AND LARGE HANDS AND FEET IN SEIP'S SYNDROME, A RECESSIVE. DUNN (1968) FOUND A HIGH PARENTAL AGE BUT OTHERS HAVE NOT. ONE OF THEIR PATIENTS HAD AN XYY KARYOTYPE. THE SUGGESTION OF A HYPOTHALAMIC DEFECT LOCATED IN THE VENTROMEDIAL OR VENTROLATERAL NUCLEUS IS PLAUSIBLE, BUT NO SUCH LESION HAS BEEN REPORTED, NOR WAS SUCH FOUND ON CAREFUL SEARCH IN A TYPICAL CASE (WARKANY, 1970).

BRAIN, R. T.* IN, WOLSTENHOLME, G. E. W. AND PORTER, R. (EDS.)* MONGOLISM. BOSTON* LITTLE BROWN AND CO., 1967. PP. 1-5.

DOWN, J. L.* MENTAL AFFECTIONS OF CHILDHOOD AND YOUTH. LONDON* CHURCHILL, 1887. P. 172.

DUNN, H. G.* THE PRADER-LABHART-WILLI SYNDROME* REVIEW OF THE LITERATURE AND REPORT OF NINE CASES. ACTA PAEDIAT. SCAND. 186 (SUPPL.)* 1-38, 1968.

GABILAN, J. C. AND ROYER, P.* LE SYNDROME DE PRADER, LABHART ET WILLI (ETUDE DE ONZE OBSERVATIONS). ARCH. FRANC. PEDIAT., TO BE PUBLISHED.

GABILAN, J. C.* SYNDROME DE PRADER, LABHART ET WILLI. J. PEDIAT. (PARIS) 1* 179-   , 1962.

HOEFNAGEL, D., COSTELLO, P. J. AND HATOUM, K.* PRADER-WILLI SYNDROME. J. MENT. DEFIC. RES. 11* 1-11, 1967.

JOHNSEN, S., CRAWFORD, J. D. AND HAESSLER, H. A.* FASTING HYPERLIPOGENESIS* AN INBORN ERROR OF ENERGY METABOLISM IN PRADER-WILLI SYNDROME. APS, 1967.

LAURANCE, B. M.* HYPOTONIA, MENTAL RETARDATION, OBESITY, AND CRYPTORCHIDISM ASSOCIATED WITH DWARFISM AND DIABETES IN CHILDREN. ARCH. DIS. CHILD. 42* 126-139, 1967.

WARKANY, J.* CINCINNATI, OHIO* PERSONAL COMMUNICATION, 1970.

ZELLWEGER, H. AND SCHNEIDER, H. J.* SYNDROME OF HYPOTONIA-HYPOMENTIA-HYPOGONA-DISM-OBESITY (HHHO) OR PRADER-WILLI SYNDROME. AM. J. DIS. CHILD. 115* 588-598, 1968.

26410 PROGERIA

PRECOCIOUS SENILITY OF STRIKING DEGREE IS CHARACTERISTIC OF THIS EXCEEDINGLY RARE DISORDER. DEATH FROM CORONARY ARTERY DISEASE IS FREQUENT AND MAY OCCUR BEFORE 10 YEARS OF AGE. SUGGESTION OF RECESSIVE INHERITANCE IS PROVIDED BY THE REPORT FROM EGYPT OF AFFECTED SISTERS, CHILDREN OF FIRST COUSINS (GABR ET AL., 1960). COCKAYNE'S SYNDROME (Q.V.) WHICH RESEMBLES PROGERIA IN SOME RESPECTS, IS CLEARLY AN AUTOSOMAL RECESSIVE. PATERSON (1922) RECORDED THE CASES OF TWO AFFECTED BROTHERS, OFFSPRING OF FIRST COUSIN PARENTS. PHOTOGRAPHS WERE NOT PUBLISHED, HOWEVER, AND THE DIAGNOSIS IS NOT COMPLETELY CERTAIN. THE FULL REPORT WAS SIMPLY THE FOLLOWING* 'A BOY, AGED 8 YEARS. CONDITION HAS BEEN PRESENT SINCE BIRTH. THE FATHER AND MOTHER ARE FIRST COUSINS. THERE ARE FOUR CHILDREN IN THE FAMILY* THE GIRLS ARE UNAFFECTED, BOTH BOYS ARE AFFECTED. THE SENILE CONDITION OF THE SKIN AND FACIES SHOULD BE NOTED. THE VESSELS SHOW ARTERIOSCLEROSIS. (THERE IS ALMOST COMPLETE ABSENCE OF SUBCUTANEOUS FAT.)' AMONG THE 9 OFFSPRING OF TWO SISTERS, RAVA (1967) FOUND 6 AFFECTED. ERECINSKI ET AL. (1961) DESCRIBED PHOTOGRAPHICALLY TYPICAL PROGERIA IN 2 BROTHERS.

ERECINSKI, K., BITTEL-DOBRZYNSKA, N. AND MOSTOWIEC, S.* ZESPOL PROGERII U DWOCH BRACI. POL. TYG. LEK. 16* 806-809, 1961.

GABR, M., HASHEM, N., HASHEM, M., FAHMI, A. AND SAFOUH, M.* PROGERIA, A PATHOLOGIC STUDY. J. PEDIAT. 57* 70-77, 1960.

PATERSON, D.* CASE OF PROGERIA. PROC. ROY. SOC. MED. 16* 42 ONLY, 1922.

RAVA, G.* SU UN NUCLEO FAMILIARE DI PROGERIA. MINERVA MED. 58* 1502-1509, 1967.

26420 PSEUDOGLIOMA

ALTHOUGH USUALLY INHERITED AS AN X-LINKED RECESSIVE, THE DISORDER WAS OBSERVED IN A BOY AND GIRL FROM A CONSANGUINEOUS MARRIAGE, BY MOUTINHO AND FRANCESCHETTI (1954).

MOUTINHO, H. AND FRANCESCHETTI, A.* PSEUDO-GLIOME FAMILIAL DU TYPE INFLAMMA-TOIRE AVEC CONSANGUINITE DES PARENTS. J. GENET. HUM. 3* 82-85, 1954.

26430 PSEUDOHERMAPHRODITISM, MALE, WITH GYNECOMASTIA

SAEZ ET AL. (1971) REPORTED TWO BROTHERS WITH MALE PSEUDOHERMAPHRODISM AND GYNECOMASTIA IN WHOM METABOLIC LED TO THE CONCLUSION THAT A DEFECT IN 17-KETOS-TEROID REDUCTASE LIMITED TO THE TESTIS WAS THE 'CAUSE.' THE PARENTS WERE APPARENTLY NON-CONSANGUINEOUS. SEVEN BROTHERS AND FIVE SISTERS WERE LIVING AND APPARENTLY WELL.

SAEZ, J. M., FREDERICH, A., DE PERETTI, E. AND BERTRAND, J.* CHILDREN WITH MALE PSEUDOHERMAPHRODITISM* ENDOCRINE AND METABOLIC STUDIES. THE CLINICAL DELINEATION OF BIRTH DEFECTS. X. THE ENDOCRINE SYSTEM. NEW YORK* NATIONAL FOUNDATION, 1971.

26440 PSEUDOHYPOPHOSPHATASIA

SCRIVER AND CAMERON (1969) DESCRIBED A FEMALE INFANT WITH CLASSIC CLINICAL FEATURES OF HYPOPHOSPHATASIA BUT CONSISTENTLY NORMAL LEVELS OF ALKALINE PHOSPHA-

R
E
C
E
S
S
I
V
E

TASE IN PLASMA BY THE USUAL TESTS WHICH USE HIGH SUBSTRATE CONCENTRATIONS. IT WAS FOUND THAT AT LOW SUBSTRATE CONCENTRATIONS THE PATIENT'S PLASMA HYDROLYZED PHOSPHOETHANOLAMINE MORE SLOWLY THAN DID NORMAL PLASMA.

SCRIVER, C. R. AND CAMERON, D.* PSEUDOHYPOPHOSPHATASIA. NEW ENG. J. MED. 281* 604-606, 1969.

26450 PSEUDOURIDINURIA AND MENTAL DEFECT

KIHARA (1967) DESCRIBED INCREASED URINARY EXCRETION OF PSEUDOURIDINE (5-RIBOSY-LURACIL) IN SIBS INSTITUTIONALIZED FOR MENTAL DEFICIENCY.

KIHARA, H.* PSEUDOURIDINURIA IN MENTALLY DEFECTIVE SIBLINGS. AM. J. MENT. DEFIC. 71* 593-596, 1967.

26460 PSEUDOVAGINAL PERINEOSCROTAL HYPOSPADIAS (PPSH)

SIMPSON ET AL. (1971) DESCRIBED A FAMILY WITH THREE AFFECTED BROTHERS WHOSE PARENTS WERE DOUBLE FIRST COUSINS. EACH OF THE AFFECTED SIBS HAD AN XY KARYOTYPE AND AMBIGUOUS GENITALIA LEADING TO REARING AS FEMALES. NO BREAST DEVELOPMENT OR MENSTRUATION OCCURRED AT PUBERTY, AND INSTEAD TYPICAL MASCULATION WAS OBSERVED. THE NAME OF THE DISORDER STEMS FROM THE FINDING OF A BLIND-ENDING PERINEAL OPENING RESEMBLING A VAGINA AND A SEVERELY HYPOSPADIAC PENIS WITH THE URETHRA OPENING ONTO THE PERINEUM. DE VAAL (1955) REPORTED THREE BROTHERS WHO WERE THOUGHT FOR A TIME TO BE GIRLS. THE PARENTS AND GRANDPARENTS ON ONE SIDE WERE FIRST COUSINS AND GREAT-GRANDPARENTS WERE ALSO RELATED.

DE VAAL, O. M.* GENITAL INTERSEXUALITY IN THREE BROTHERS, CONNECTED WITH CONSANGUINEOUS MARRIAGES IN THE THREE PREVIOUS GENERATIONS. ACTA PAEDIAT. 44* 35-39, 1955.

SIMPSON, J. L., NEW, M., PETERSON, R. E. AND GERMAN, J.* PSEUDOVAGINAL PERINEOSCROTAL HYPOSPADIAS (PPSH) IN SIBS. THE CLINICAL DELINEATION OF BIRTH DEFECTS. X. THE ENDOCRINE SYSTEM. BALTIMORE* WILLIAMS AND WILKINS, 1971.

*26470 PSEUDOVITAMIN D DEFICIENCY RICKETS

DENT ET AL. (1968) DESCRIBED A SEVERELY AFFECTED PATIENT. THE FINDINGS IN THIS DISORDER DIFFER FROM THOSE IN THE X-LINKED VITAMIN D RESISTANT RICKETS BY THE SEVERITY AND THE ACCOMPANYING MYOPATHY. THE RESPONSE TO VITAMIN D IS BETTER IN THIS DISORDER THAN IN THE X-LINKED CONDITION. THE SEVERE SKELETAL CHANGES SUGGEST THOSE OF MORQUIO SYNDROME OR SOME SIMILAR SKELETAL DYSPLASIA. THE BENEFICIAL EFFECTS OF THERAPY MAY BE OVERLOOKED. EARLIER ONSET AND DEPRESSION OF CALCIUM AS WELL AS PHOSPHORUS IN THE BLOOD HELP DISTINGUISH THIS DISORDER FROM THE X-LINKED CONDITION. PRADER ET AL. (1961) SUGGESTED DOMINANT INHERITANCE BUT LATER PRADER (CITED BY DENT ET AL., 1968) EXPRESSED DOUBTS. HE HAD A NEW FAMILY WITH FIRST COUSIN PARENTS WHO WERE HEALTHY WITH NORMAL PLASMA LEVELS OF CALCIUM AND PHOS-PHORUS. DENT ET AL. (1968) MADE BRIEF MENTION OF TWO OTHER PATIENTS KNOWN TO THEM, BOTH WITH NORMAL PARENTS WHO WERE, HOWEVER, RELATED AS FIRST COUSINS. WE HAVE OBSERVED AFFECTED BROTHER AND SISTER. VITAMIN-D-DEPENDENT RICKETS WAS THE TERM SUGGESTED BY FRASER AND SALTER (1958). SCRIVER (1970) SUPPORTED AUTOSOMAL RECESSIVE INHERITANCE AND SUGGESTED THAT THE CONDITION MAY BE MORE FREQUENT THAN PREVIOUSLY REALIZED. HAMILTON ET AL. (1970) DEMONSTRATED DEFECTIVE INTESTINAL ABSORPTION OF CALCIUM AS THE PRIMARY DEFECT.

FRASER, D. AND SALTER, R. B.* THE DIAGNOSIS AND MANAGEMENT OF THE VARIOUS TYPES OF RICKETS. PEDIAT. CLIN. N. AM. 417-441, 1958.

HAMILTON, R., HARRISON, J., FRASER, D., RADDLE, I., MORECKI, R. AND PAUNIER, L.* THE SMALL INTESTINE IN VITAMIN D DEPENDENT RICKETS. PEDIATRICS 45* 364-373, 1970.

DENT, C. E., FRIEDMAN, M. AND WATSON, L.* HEREDITARY PSEUDO-VITAMIN D DEFICIEN-CY RICKETS ('HEREDITARE PSEUDO-MANGELRACKITIS'). J. BONE JOINT SURG. 50B* 708-719, 1968.

PRADER, A., ILLIG, R. AND HEIERLI, E.* EINE BESONDERE FORM DER PRIMAREN VITAMIN-D-RESISTENTEN RACHITIS MIT HYPOCALCAMIE UND AUTOSOMAL-DOMINANT ERBGANG* DIE HEREDITARE PSEUDO-MANGELRACHITIS. HELV. PAEDIAT. ACTA 16* 452-468, 1961.

SCRIVER, C. R.* VITAMIN D DEPENDENCY. (EDITORIAL) PEDIATRICS 45* 361-363, 1970.

*26480 PSEUDOXANTHOMA ELASTICUM

THE FEATURES ARE CHARACTERISTIC CHANGES IN THE SKIN OF THE NECK, AXILLA AND OTHER FLEXURAL AREAS, IN BRUCH'S MEMBRANE RESULTING IN ANGIOID STREAKS ON FUNDUSCOPIC EXAMINATION AND IN ARTERIES PRODUCING GASTROINTESTINAL AND OTHER HEMORRHAGE, PRECOCIOUS CALCIFICATION AND OCCLUSIVE VASCULAR CHANGES. SERIES ASCERTAINED BECAUSE OF THE SKIN LESIONS SHOW A PREPONDERANCE OF FEMALES, WHEREAS SERIES OF CASES OF ANGIOID STREAKS SHOW A SEX RATIO OF ABOUT 1. THE POSSIBILITY OF AN AUTOSOMAL DOMINANT FORM OF PXE HAS BEEN RAISED BY THE RATHER NUMEROUS FAMILIES IN

WHICH SUCCESSIVE GENERATIONS ARE AFFECTED. WISE (1966) STATED THAT ABOUT A QUARTER OF ALL FAMILIES WITH TWO OR MORE AFFECTED HAVE CASES IN SUCCESSIVE GENERATIONS. THIS WOULD APPEAR TO BE TOO FREQUENT A FINDING TO BE EXPLICABLE IN ALL INSTANCES BY THE PHENOMENON OF QUASI-DOMINANCE. WISE (1966) COULD DISCERN NO QUANTITATIVE OR QUALITATIVE DIFFERENCE BETWEEN THE CASES IN FAMILIES WITH SUCCESSIVE GENERATIONS AFFECTED AND FAMILIES WITH UNAFFECTED BUT CONSANGUINEOUS PARENTS.

BERLYNE ET AL. (1961) SUGGESTED THAT PXE MAY BE INHERITED AS A PARTIAL X-LINKED RECESSIVE (I.E., THAT THE GENE MAY BE ON A PART OF THE X CHROMOSOME HOMOLOGOUS WITH PART OF THE Y CHROMOSOME). IF SUCH WERE THE CASE PATIENTS IN ANY ONE SIBSHIP WOULD TEND ALWAYS TO BE OF THE SAME SEX. THIS APPEARS NOT TO BE THE CASE. METACHROMASIA OF FIBROBLASTS WAS REPORTED BY CARTWRIGHT ET AL. (1969).

BERLYNE, G. M., BULMER, M. G. AND PLATT, R.* THE GENETICS OF PSEUDOXANTHOMA ELASTICUM. QUART. J. MED. 30* 201-212, 1961.

CARTWRIGHT, E., DANKS, D. M. AND JACK, I.* METACHROMATIC FIBROBLASTS IN PSEUDOXANTHOMA ELASTICUM AND MARFAN'S SYNDROME. (LETTER) LANCET 1* 533-534, 1969.

COFFMAN, J. D. AND SOMMERS, S. C.* FAMILIAL PSEUDOXANTHOMA ELASTICUM AND VALVULAR HEART DISEASE. CIRCULATION 19* 242-250, 1959.

GOODMAN, R. M., SMITH, E. W., PATON, D., BERGMAN, R. A., SIEGEL, C. L., OTTESEN, O. E., SHELLEY, W. M., PUSCH, A. L. AND MCKUSICK, V. A.* PSEUDOXANTHOMA ELASTICUM* A CLINICAL AND HISTOPATHOLOGICAL STUDY. MEDICINE 42* 297-334, 1963.

MESSIS, C. P. AND BUDZILOVICH, G. N.* PSEUDOXANTHOMA ELASTICUM* REPORT OF AN AUTOPSIED CASE WITH CEREBRAL INVOLVEMENT. NEUROLOGY 20* 703-709, 1970.

WISE, D.* IN, H. GOTTRON AND U. SCHNYDER (EDS.)* HEREDITARY DISORDERS OF CONNECTIVE TISSUES. VERERBUNG VON HAUTKRANKHEITEN. BERLIN* SPRINGER-VERLAG, 1966. P. 471.

*26490 PTA (PLASMA THROMBOPLASTIN ANTECEDENT, FACTOR XI) DEFICIENCY

THE DISORDER IS NOT COMPLETELY RECESSIVE BECAUSE THE HETEROZYGOTES HAVE A MILD BUT DEFINITE BLEEDING TENDENCY. ALMOST ALL PATIENTS HAVE BEEN OF JEWISH EXTRACTION (BIGGS AND MACFARLANE, 1962). ROSENTHAL (1964) COLLECTED 72 CASES FROM 46 JEWISH FAMILIES.

BIGGS, R. AND MACFARLANE, R. G.* HUMAN BLOOD COAGULATION AND ITS DISORDERS. OXFORD* BLACKWELL, 1962. (3RD ED.).

RAPAPORT, S. I., PROCTOR, R. R., PATCH, M. J. AND YETTRA, M.* THE MODE OF INHERITANCE OF PTA DEFICIENCY* EVIDENCE FOR THE EXISTENCE OF MAJOR PTA DEFICIENCY AND MINOR PTA DEFICIENCY. BLOOD 18* 149-165, 1961.

ROSENTHAL, R. L.* HAEMORRHAGE IN PTA (FACTOR XI) DEFICIENCY. (ABSTRACT) PROC. 10TH. INTERN. CONGR. SOC. HEMATOL., STOCKHOLM, 1964.

ROSENTHAL, R. L., DRESKIN, O. H. AND ROSENTHAL, N.* PLASMA THROMBOPLASTIN ANTECEDENT (PTA) DEFICIENCY* CLINICAL, COAGULATION, THERAPEUTIC AND HEREDITARY ASPECTS OF A NEW HEMOPHILIA-LIKE DISEASE. BLOOD 10* 120-131, 1955.

VINAZZER, H.* PARTIELLER FAMILIARER FAKTOR-XI-MANGEL. BLUT 15* 263-267, 1967.

26500 PTERYGIUM SYNDROME

WEBBING OF THE NECK, ANTECUBITAL FOSSAE AND POPLITEAL FOSSAE WITH STERNAL DEFORMITY AND MALE HYPOGONADISM MAY BEHAVE SOMETIMES AS A DOMINANT, BUT THERE APPEARS CLEARLY TO BE A RECESSIVE PTERYGIUM SYNDROME. I HAVE OBSERVED A FAMILY IN WHICH EACH OF TWO COUSIN SIBSHIPS CONTAINED TWO CASES (NORUM ET AL. 1969). OF THE 4, 3 WERE MALE AND ONE FEMALE. CURIOUS 'DENTS,' CUTANEOUS DEPRESSIONS, WERE PRESENT ON THE BACK OF THE ELBOWS AND FRONT OF THE KNEES.

NORUM, R. A., JAMES, V. L. AND MABRY, C. C.* PTERYGIUM SYNDROME IN THREE CHILDREN IN A RECESSIVE PEDIGREE PATTERN. THE CLINICAL DELINEATION OF BIRTH DEFECTS. II. MALFORMATION SYNDROMES. NEW YORK* NATIONAL FOUNDATION, 1969. PP. 233-235.

*26510 PULMONARY ALVEOLAR MICROLITHIASIS

THE CONDITION IS CHARACTERIZED BY MULTIPLE MINUTE CALCIFICATIONS LOCATED IN THE ALVEOLI AND PRODUCING A TYPICAL RADIOGRAPHIC APPEARANCE. SIBS HAVE BEEN AFFECTED IN A NUMBER OF CASES. INFORMATION ON CONSANGUINITY HAS APPARENTLY NOT BEEN COLLECTED IN A SYSTEMATIC MANNER* HOWEVER, IN SEVERAL OF THE REPORTED CASES NOTE WAS MADE OF THE FACT THAT THE PARENTS WERE RELATED. CAFFREY AND ALTMAN (1965) DESCRIBED THE DISORDER IN PREMATURE TWINS WHO DIED AT AGE 12 HOURS. THEY REVIEWED 66 CASES IN THE LITERATURE OF 68 CASES (INCLUDING THEIRS), 34 WERE FAMILIAL, OCCURRING IN 13 FAMILIES. A DISPROPORTIONATELY LARGE PROPORTION OF CASES MAY BE OF SPANISH EXTRACTION. IN SPAIN LOPEZ-AREAL ET AL. (1965) DESCRIBED 2 AFFECTED SISTERS IN ONE FAMILY AND A BOY AND HIS TWO SISTERS IN A SECOND FAMILY. O'NEILL

ET AL. (1967) OBSERVED THREE AFFECTED SIBS. AFFECTED BROTHER AND SISTER WITH FIRST COUSIN PARENTS WERE REPORTED BY BURGUET AND REGINSTER (1967). IN BEIRUT BALIKIAN ET AL. (1968) DESCRIBED THE DISORDER IN TWO PAIRS OF BROTHERS AND AN UNRELATED GIRL.

BALIKIAN, J. P., FULEIHAN, F. J. D. AND NUCHO, C. N.* PULMONARY ALVEOLAR MICROLITHIASIS. REPORT OF FIVE CASES WITH SPECIAL REFERENCE TO ROENTGEN MANIFES-TATIONS. AM. J. ROENTGEN. 103* 509-518, 1968.

BURGUET, W. AND REGINSTER, A.* L'HEREDITE DE LA MICROLITHIASE ALVEOLAIRE PULMONAIRE. A PROPOS D'UNE NOUVELLE OBSERVATION FAMILIALE. ANN. GENET. 10* 75-81, 1967.

CAFFREY, P. R. AND ALTMAN, R. S.* PULMONARY ALVEOLAR MICROLITHIASIS IN PREMATURE TWINS. J. PEDIAT. 66* 758-763, 1965.

GOMEZ, G., GOMEZ, G. E., LICHLEMBERGER, E., SANTAMARIA, A., CARVAJAL, L., JIMENEZ-PENULEA, B., SAAIBI, E., BARRERA, A. R., ORDUZ, E. AND CORREA-HENAO, A.* FAMILIAL PULMONARY ALVEOLAR MICROLITHIASIS* FOUR CASES FROM COLOMBIA, S. A.* IS MICROLITHIASIS ALSO AN ENVIRONMENTAL DISEASE.Q RADIOLOGY 72* 550-561, 1959.

LOPEZ-AREAL, L., ZUMARRAGA, R., TURNER, C. G., GRANIZO, I. F. M., VARA CUADRADO, F. AND DUQUE FRAILE, J.* MICROLITIASIS ALVEOLAR PULMONAR FAMILIAR E INFANTIL. (DESCRIPTION DE CINCO CASOS IN DOS FAMILIAS). REV. CLIN. ESP. 97* 389-395, 1965.

O'NEILL, R. P., COHN, J. E. AND PELLEGRINO, E. D.* PULMONARY ALVEOLAR MICROLI-THIASIS - A FAMILY STUDY. ANN. INTERN. MED. 67* 957-967, 1967.

SOSMAN, M. C., DODD, G. D., JONES, W. D. AND PILLMORE, G. U.* THE FAMILIAL OCCURRENCE OF PULMONARY ALVEOLAR MICROLITHIASIS. AM. J. ROENTGEN. 77* 947-1012, 1957.

VISWANATHAN, R.* PULMONARY ALVEOLAR MICROLITHIASIS. THORAX 17* 251-256, 1962.

26520 PULMONARY ARTERIAL STENOSES, CALCIFIED CARTILAGES, DEAFNESS, AND SHORT TERMINAL DIGITS

BEUREN (1970) TOLD ME OF AN APPARENTLY *NEW* SYNDROME OBSERVED IN HIS CLINIC IN THE SON AND DAUGHTER OF PARENTS RELATED AS FIRST COUSINS ONCE REMOVED. THE FEATURES WERE (1) SEVERE MULTIPLE PERIPHERAL PULMONARY ARTERIAL STENOSES, (2) CALCIFICATION OF THE CARTILAGES OF THE TRACHEA, BRONCHI, RIBS AND EARS, (3) DEAFNESS, AND (4) HYPOTELEPHALANGISM OF SOME FINGERS AND TOES. THE AFFECTED SIBS WERE SUCCESSIVELY BORN IN A SIBSHIP OF FIVE.

BEUREN, A. J.* GOTTINGEN, GERMANY* PERSONAL COMMUNICATION, 1970.

26530 PULMONARY CYSTIC LYMPHANGIECTASIS (LYMPHANGIOMATOSIS)

FRANK AND PIPER (1959) DESCRIBED TWO AFFECTED INFANTS WHO WERE NOT RELATED. ONE WAS STILLBORN AND THE OTHER LIVED ONLY ABOUT 2 HOURS. IN ONE CASE THERE WERE SIMILAR LESIONS IN THE HEART, PANCREAS, KIDNEYS AND MESENTERY. NOTHING IS KNOWN ABOUT POSSIBLE GENETIC BASIS.

FRANK, J. AND PIPER, P. G.* CONGENITAL PULMONARY CYSTIC LYMPHANGIECTASIS. J.A.M.A. 171* 1094-1098, 1959.

26540 PULMONARY HYPERTENSION, PRIMARY

IN TWO SISTERS AND A BROTHER COLEMAN, EDMUNDS AND TREGILLUS (1959) OBSERVED PRIMARY PULMONARY HYPERTENSION AND CONFIRMED THE DIAGNOSIS BY POST-MORTEM EXAMINATION. ALL THREE SIBS WERE AFFECTED IN THE FAMILY REPORTED BY TSAGARIS AND TIKOFF (1968). TWO WERE MALE AND ONE FEMALE. OTHER REPORTS HAVE SUGGESTED DOMINANT INHERITANCE (Q.V.). HOOD ET AL. (1968) REPORTED THE CONDITION IN THREE SISTERS. THEIR REVIEW OF THE LITERATURE LED THEM TO CONCLUDE THAT THE SINGLE GENERATION CASES TEND TO BE PREDOMINANTLY IN WOMEN AND TO HAVE LATER ONSET THAN THE MULTIPLE GENERATION CASES WHICH TEND TO SHOW MORE NEARLY EQUAL SEX DISTRIBU-TION.

COLEMAN, P. N., EDMUNDS, A. W. AND TREGILLUS, J.* PRIMARY PULMONARY HYPERTEN-SION IN THREE SIBS. BRIT. HEART J. 21* 81-88, 1959.

HOOD, W. B., JR., SPENCER, H., LASS, R. W. AND DALEY, R.* PRIMARY PULMONARY HYPERTENSION* FAMILIAL OCCURRENCE. BRIT. HEART J. 30* 336-343, 1968.

ROBERTSON, B., ROSENHAMER, G. AND LINDBERG, J.* IDIOPATHIC PULMONARY HYPERTEN-SION IN TWO SIBLINGS. CLINICAL, MICROANGIOGRAPHIC AND HISTOLOGIC OBSERVATIONS. ACTA MED. SCAND. 186* 569-577, 1969.

TSAGARIS, T. J. AND TIKOFF, G.* FAMILIAL PRIMARY PULMONARY HYPERTENSION. AM. REV. RESP. DIS. 97* 127-130, 1968.

R
E
C
E
S
S
I
V
E

COBLENTZ AND MATHIVAT (1952) DESCRIBED TWO SISTERS WITH PULMONIC STENOSIS. LAMY, DE GROUCHY AND SCHWEISGUTH (1957) FOUND INCREASED PARENTAL CONSANGUINITY IN PULMONIC STENOSIS AND DESCRIBED ONE INSTANCE OF TWO AFFECTED SIBS. CONSANGUINITY EFFECT IS TO BE EXPECTED OF A MULTIFACTORIAL TRAIT, SO THAT THIS LIKE THE OCCURRENCE OF AFFECTED SIBS IS NOT PROOF OF SIMPLE RECESSIVE INHERITANCE.

COBLENTZ, B. AND MATHIVAT, A.* STENOSE PULMONAIRE CONGENITALE CHEZ DEUX SOEURS. ARCH. MAL. COEUR. 45* 490-495, 1952.

LAMY, M., DE GROUCHY, J. AND SCHWEISGUTH, O.* GENETIC AND NON-GENTIC FACTORS IN THE ETIOLOGY OF CONGENITAL HEART DISEASE* A STUDY OF 1188 CASES. AM. J. HUM. GENET. 9* 17-41, 1957.

26560 PULMONIC STENOSIS AND CONGENITAL NEPHROSIS

FOURNIER AND COLLEAGUES (1963) OBSERVED A FAMILY IN WHICH 4 OF 5 CHILDREN HAD CLINICAL AND-OR AUTOPSY EVIDENCE OF PULMONARY STENOSIS AND CONGENITAL NEPHROTIC SYNDROME.

FOURNIER, A., PAGET, M., PAULI, A. AND DEVIN, P.* SYNDROMES NEPHROTIQUES FAMILIAUX. SYNDROME NEPHROTIQUE ASSOCIE A UNE CARDIOPATHIE CONGENITALE CHEZ QUATRE SOEURS. PEDIATRIE 18* 677-685, 1963.

*26570 PURETIC'S SYNDROME

PURETIC AND COLLEAGUES (1962) DESCRIBED A *NEW* FORM OF CONNECTIVE TISSUE DISORDER. IN ADDITION TO THE PROBAND, A BROTHER AND SISTER WERE APPARENTLY AFFECTED, HAVING DIED IN INFANCY WITH PAINFUL FLEXURAL CONTRACTURES OF THE ELBOWS, SHOULDER JOINTS AND KNEES WHICH DEVELOPED AT ABOUT 3 MONTHS OF AGE. IN ADDITION TO CONTRACTURES, THE PROBAND SHOWED (1) DEFORMITY OF THE FACE AND SKULL, (2) STUNTED GROWTH, (3) OSTEOLYSIS OF TERMINAL PHALANGES, (4) MULTIPLE LARGE SUBCU-TANEOUS NODES, SOME CALCIFIED, (5) DYSSEBORRHEIC, SCLERODERMIFORM AND ATROPHIC CHANGES OF THE SKIN, (6) RECURRENT SUPPURATIVE INFECTIONS OF THE SKIN, EYES, NOSE AND EARS. ISHIKAWA AND HORI (1964) DESCRIBED A TWO AND HALF YEAR OLD JAPANESE INFANT WHOSE SIBS HAD DIED AT 8 MONTHS PROBABLY OF THE SAME CONDITION. SYSTEMIC HYALINOSIS WAS SUGGESTED AS A DESIGNATION.

ISHIKAWA, H. AND HORI, Y.* SYSTEMATISIERTE HYALINOSE IN ZUSAMMENHANG MIT EPIDERMOLYSIS BULLOSA POLYDYSTROPHICA UND HYALINOSIS CUTIS ET MUCOSAE. ARCH. KLIN. EXP. DERM. 218* 30-51, 1964.

PURETIC, S., PURETIC, B., FISER-HERMAN, M. AND ADAMCIC, M.* A UNIQUE FORM OF MESENCHYMAL DYSPLASIA. BRIT. J. DERM. 74* 8-19, 1962.

*26580 PYCNODYSOSTOSIS (PYKNODYSOSTOSIS)

THE FEATURES ARE DEFORMITY OF THE SKULL (INCLUDING WIDE SUTURES), MAXILLA AND PHALANGES (ACRO-OSTEOLYSIS), OSTEOSCLEROSIS AND FRAGILITY OF BONE. THE DISORDER WAS FIRST DESCRIBED AND NAMED BY MAROTEAUX AND LAMY (1962). (ANDREN ET AL. (1962) SIMULTANEOUSLY AND INDEPENDENTLY DELINEATED THIS SYNDROME. THEY FOUND 11 PATIENTS REPORTED UNDER VARIOUS DESIGNATIONS AND ADDED THE CASES OF MONOZYGOTIC TWINS.) IN THE PAST A NUMBER OF THESE CASES HAVE PROBABLY BEEN DIAGNOSED AS OSTEOPETROSIS (E.G., SEIGMAN AND KILBY, 1950). THE PATIENT OF THE LATTER AUTHORS WAS A NEGRO FEMALE, THE OFFSPRING OF FIRST OR SECOND COUSINS. KAJII ET AL. (1966) DESCRIBED A JAPANESE CASE IN THE DAUGHTER OF A FIRST-COUSIN MARRIAGE. ALSO SEE CRANIOSTENO-SIS. FOR A SOMEWHAT SIMILAR THOUGH DISTINCT ENTITY SEE ACRO-OSTEOLYSIS WITH OSTEOPOROSIS AND CHANGES IN SKULL AND MANDIBLE (DOMINANT CATALOG). SEDANO ET AL. (1968) FOUND PARENTAL CONSANGUINITY IN ABOUT 30 PERCENT OF REPORTED CASES, REFLECTING THE RARITY OF THE PYCNODYSOSTOSIS GENE.

ANDREN, L., DYMLING, J.-F., HOGEMAN, K.-E. AND WENDEBERG, B.* OSTEOPETROSIS ACRO-OSTEOLYTICA. A SYNDROME OF OSTEOPETROSIS, ACRO-OSTEOLYSIS AND OPEN SUTURES OF THE SKULL. ACTA CHIR. SCAND. 124* 496-507, 1962.

ELMORE, S. M.* PYCNODYSOSTOSIS* A REVIEW. J. BONE JOINT SURG. 49A* 153-163, 1967.

ELMORE, S. M., NANCE, W. E., MCGEE, B. J., ENGEL-DE MONTMOLLIN, M. AND ENGEL, E.* PYCNODYSOSTOSIS, WITH A FAMILIAL CHROMOSOME ANOMALY. AM. J. MED. 40* 273-282, 1966.

KAJII, T., HOMMA, T. AND OHSAWA, T.* PYCNODYSOSTOSIS. J. PEDIAT. 69* 131-133, 1966.

MAROTEAUX, P. AND LAMY, M.* LA PYCNODYSOSTOSE. PRESSE MED. 70* 999-1002, 1962.

NANCE, W. E. AND ENGEL, E.* AUTOSOMAL DELETION MAPPING IN MAN. SCIENCE 155* 692-694, 1967.

SEDANO, H. D., GORLIN, R. J. AND ANDERSON, V. E.* PYCNODYSOSTOSIS. CLINICAL

R
E
C
E
S
S
I
V
E

SEIGMAN, E. L. AND KILBY, W. C.* OSTEOPETROSIS.   REPORT OF A CASE AND REVIEW OF RECENT LITERATURE.   AM. J. ROENTGEN. 63* 865-874, 1950.

*26590 PYLE'S DISEASE (METAPHYSEAL DYSPLASIA)

DESPITE THE BIZARRE ROENTOGENOGRAPHIC CHANGES, THERE ARE FEW CLINICAL FINDINGS OTHER THAN GENU VALGUM. THE SKULL IS ONLY MILDLY AFFECTED, THUS DISTINGUISHING THIS DISORDER FROM THE CRANIOMETAPHYSEAL DYSPLASIAS. THE FEMURS SHOW AN ERLEN-MEYER-FLASH CONFORMITY. THE HUMERUS IS ABNORMALLY BROAD AND *UNDERMODELED* IN ITS PROXIMAL TWO-THIRDS, THE RADIUS AND ULNA IN THEIR DISTAL TWO-THIRDS. AFFECTED SIBS WERE REPORTED BY BAKWIN AND KRIDA (1937), DANIEL (1960), PYLE (1931), FELD ET AL. (1955) AND HERMEL ET AL. (1953), AMONG OTHERS. PARENTAL CONSANGUINITY WAS PRESENT IN THE CASES OF DANIEL (1960). IT IS SUGGESTED BY GORLIN ET AL. (1969) THAT *PYLE'S DISEASE* BE RESERVED FOR THE FORM OF METAPHYSEAL DYSPLASIA WITH LITTLE INVOLVEMENT OF THE CRANIAL BONES. RESTUDY OF PYLE'S PATIENTS SHOWED LITTLE INVOLVEMENT OF THE SKULL (SILVERMAN, 1970). SEE CRANIOMETAPHYSEAL DYSPLASIA.

BAKWIN, H. AND KRIDA, A.* FAMILIAL METAPHYSEAL DYSPLASIA. AM. J. DIS. CHILD. 53* 1521-1527, 1937.

DANIEL, A.* PYLE'S DISEASE. INDIAN J. RADIOL. 14* 126-131, 1960.

FELD, H., SWITZER, R. A., DEXTER, M. W. AND LANGER, E. W.* FAMILIAL METAPHYSEAL DYSPLASIA. RADIOLOGY 65* 206-212, 1955.

GORLIN, R. J., SPRANGER, J. AND KOSZALKA, M. F.* GENETIC CRANIOTUBULAR BONE DYSPLASIAS AND HYPEROSTOSES. A CRITICAL ANALYSIS. THE CLINICAL DELINEATION OF BIRTH DEFECTS. IV. SKELETAL DYSPLASIAS. NEW YORK* NATIONAL FOUNDATION, 1969. PP. 79-95.

HERMEL, M. B., GERSHON-COHEN, J. AND JONES, D. T.* FAMILIAL METAPHYSEAL DYSPLASIA. AM. J. ROENTGENOL. 70* 413-421, 1953.

PYLE, E.* CASE OF UNUSUAL BONE DEVELOPMENT. J. BONE JOINT SURG. 13* 874-876, 1931.

SILVERMAN, F. N.* CINCINNATI, OHIO* PERSONAL COMMUNICATION, 1970.

26600 PYLORIC STENOSIS, CONGENITAL

MENDELIAN INHERITANCE OF PYLORIC STENOSIS CANNOT BE ESTABLISHED. CARTER (1961) ESTIMATED THAT THE RECURRENCE RISK WAS 10 PERCENT FOR MALES BORN AFTER AN AFFECTED CHILD AND 1.5 TO 2 PERCENT FOR FEMALES.

CARTER, C. O.* THE INHERITANCE OF CONGENITAL PYLORIC STENOSIS. BRIT. MED. BULL. 17* 251-254, 1961.

*26610 PYRIDOXINE DEPENDENCY

WALDINGER (1964) DESCRIBED THREE SIBS OF ITALIAN ANCESTRY IN WHOM PYRIDOXINE DEPENDENCY WAS MANIFEST AT BIRTH, BY CONVULSIONS. FOUR PREVIOUSLY REPORTED SIBSHIPS WITH MORE THAN ONE AFFECTED SIB WERE REFERRED TO. BEJSOVEC ET AL. (1967) DESCRIBED THREE SIBS WITH INTRAUTERINE CONVULSIONS. THE FIRST TWO (FEMALES) DIED IN STATUS EPILEPTICUS. THE THIRD WAS SHOWN TO HAVE PYRIDOXINE DEPENDENCY. THUS, THIS IS ONE FORM OF *CONVULSIVE DISORDER, FAMILIAL, WITH PRENATAL OR EARLY ONSET* (Q.V.). THE DISORDER WAS FIRST DESCRIBED BY HUNT (1954), BUT ONLY RECENTLY HAS THE DEFECT BEEN PROPOSED TO RESIDE IN GLUTAMIC ACID DECARBOXYLASE.

BEJSOVEC, M., KULENDA, Z. AND PONCA, E.* FAMILIAL INTRAUTERINE CONVULSIONS IN PYRIDOXINE DEPENDENCY. ARCH. DIS. CHILD. 42* 201-207, 1967.

HUNT, A. D., JR., STOKES, J., JR., MCCROY, W. W. AND STROUD, H. H.* PYRIDOXINE DEPENDENCY* REPORT OF A CASE OF INTRACTABLE CONVULSIONS IN AN INFANT CONTROLLED BY PYRIDOXINE. PEDIATRICS 13* 140-145, 1954.

SCRIVER, C. R.* VITAMIN B6 DEFICIENCY AND DEPENDENCY IN MAN. AM. J. DIS. CHILD. 113* 109-114, 1967.

SCRIVER, C. R. AND HUTCHISON, J. H.* THE VITAMIN B6 DEFICIENCY SYNDROME IN HUMAN INFANCY* BIOCHEMICAL AND CLINICAL OBSERVATIONS. PEDIATRICS 31* 240-250, 1963.

WALDINGER, C.* PYRIDOXINE DEFICIENCY AND PYRIDOXINE DEPENDENCY IN INFANTS AND CHILDREN. POSTGRAD. MED. 35* 415-422, 1964.

*26620 PYRUVATE KINASE (PK) DEFICIENCY OF ERYTHROCYTE (MORE THAN ONE TYPE)

THE DISEASE AS DESCRIBED BY BOWMAN AND PROCOPIO (1963) IS MUCH MORE SEVERE THAN THAT REPORTED BY TANAKA, VALENTINE AND MIWA (1962). BOWMAN AND PROCOPIO OBSERVED SEVERE HEMOLYTIC ANEMIA LEADING TO DEATH IN FIRST YEARS OF LIFE IF NOT TREATED BY

TRANSFUSIONS AND SPLENECTOMY. TANAKA, VALENTINE AND MIWA OBSERVED A COMPENSATED HEMOLYTIC ANEMIA IN YOUNG ADULTS WHO HAD BEEN RELATIVELY LITTLE INCAPACITATED. SEPARATE ALLELES OR EVEN GENES AT DIFFERENT LOCI MAY BE INVOLVED. NECHELES ET AL. (1966) ILLUSTRATED THE VARIABILITY WITH TWO UNRELATED PATIENTS. ONE HAD CHOLECYS-TITIS AND CHOLELITHIASIS FOR WHICH SURGERY WAS PERFORMED AT AGE 23. HE WAS WELL THEREAFTER UNTIL AGE 28 WHEN ANEMIA DEVELOPED, FOR WHICH SPLENECTOMY WAS PERFORMED WITH GOOD RESULTS. THE SECOND CASE WAS AN INFANT WHO REQUIRED EXCHANGE TRANSFU-SION IN THE NEONATAL PERIOD BECAUSE OF JAUNDICE AND ANEMIA. RESULTS OF SPLENEC-TOMY PERFORMED AT 14 MONTHS WERE EXCELLENT. FURTHER EVIDENCE OF HETEROGENEITY (POSSIBLY ALL ALLELIC) IN PYRUVATE KINASE DEFICIENCY WAS PRESENTED BY SACHS ET AL. (1967) AND BY PAGLIA ET AL. (1968), WHO FOUND A PK ENZYME OF ABNORMAL KINETICS IN PATIENTS WITH ANEMIA. LEUKOCYTES OF PATIENTS WITH RED CELL PK DEFICIENCY SHOW NORMAL ENZYME ACTIVITY. THE LIVER SHOWS, HOWEVER DEFICIENCY OF THE PK ISOZYME WHICH IS IDENTICAL TO THAT IN RED CELLS (BIGLEY AND KOLER, 1968). ZUELZER ET AL. (1968) POINTED OUT MARKED INTRAFAMILIAL VARIABILITY WHICH STUDIES SUGGESTED WAS DUE TO HETEROZYGOSITY FOR TWO DISTINCT INTERACTING MUTANTS IN MILDLY AFFECTED RELATIVES OF SEVERELY AFFECTED PROBANDS. PERSONS POSSIBLY HETEROZYGOUS FOR AN ANOMALOUS PYRUVATE KINASE HAD ANEMIA IN THE FAMILY REPORTED BY SACHS ET AL. (1968). THE EVIDENCE OF KOLER ET AL. (1964) INDICATE THE EXISTENCE OF AT LEAST TWO PK LOCI. SINCE PK IS AN ESSENTIAL ENZYME HOMOZYGOSITY FOR THE DEFICIENT STATE WOULD BE LETHAL OTHERWISE. ALTHOUGH NOT ALL PATIENTS WITH PK DEFICIENCY RES-PONDED, BLUME ET AL. (1970) REPORTED THAT INTRAVENOUS ADMINISTRATION OF INOSINE AND ADENINE WAS EFFECTIVE THERAPY, LEADING TO DECREASED HEMOLYSIS.

BIGLEY, R. H. AND KOLER, R. D.* LIVER PYRUVATE KINASE (PK) ISOZYMES IN A PK-DEFICIENT PATIENT. ANN. HUM. GENET. 31* 383-388, 1968.

BLUME, K. G., BUSCH, D., HOFFBAUER, R. W., ARNOLD, H. AND LOHR, G. W.* THE POLYMORPHISM OF NUCLEOSIDE EFFECT IN PYRUVATE KINASE DEFICIENCY. HUMANGENETIK 9* 257-259, 1970.

BOWMAN, H. S. AND PROCOPIO, F.* HEREDITARY NON-SPHEROCYTIC HEMOLYTIC ANEMIA OF THE PYRUVATE-KINASE DEFICIENT TYPE. ANN. INTERN. MED. 58* 567-591, 1963.

BOWMAN, H. S., MCKUSICK, V. A. AND DRONAMRAJU, K. R.* PYRUVATE KINASE DEFICIENT HEMOLYTIC ANEMIA IN AN AMISH ISOLATE. AM. J. HUM. GENET. 17* 1-8, 1965.

KEITT, A. S. AND BENNETT, D. C.* PYRUVATE KINASE DEFICIENCY AND RELATED DISORDERS OF RED CELL GLYCOLYSIS. AM. J. MED. 41* 762-785, 1966.

KOLER, R. D., BIGLEY, R. H., JONES, R. T., RIGAS, D. A., VANBELLINGHEN, P. AND THOMPSON, P.* PYRUVATE KINASE* MOLECULAR DIFFERENCES BETWEEN HUMAN RED CELL AND LEUKOCYTE ENZYMES. COLD SPRING HARBOR SYMP. QUANT. BIOL. 24* 213-221, 1964.

NECHELES, T. F., FINKEL, H. E., SHEEHAN, R. G. AND ALLEN, D. M.* RED CELL PYRUVATE KINASE DEFICIENCY. THE EFFECT OF SPLENECTOMY. ARCH. INTERN. MED. 118* 75-78, 1966.

OSKI, F. A. AND BOWMAN, H.* A LOW K(M) PHOSPHOENOLPYRUVATE MUTANT IN THE AMISH WITH RED CELL PYRUVATE KINASE DEFICIENCY. BRIT. J. HAEMAT. 17* 289-297, 1969.

PAGLIA, D. E., VALENTINE, W. N., BAUGHAN, M. A., MILLER, D. R., REED, C. F. AND MCINTYRE, O. R.* AN INHERITED MOLECULAR LESION OF ERYTHROCYTE PYRUVATE KINASE. IDENTIFICATION OF A KINETICALLY ABERRANT ISOZYME ASSOCIATED WITH PREMATURE HEMOLYSIS. J. CLIN. INVEST. 47* 1929-1946, 1968.

SACHS, J. R., WICKER, D. J., GILCHER, R. O., CONRAD, M. E. AND COHEN, R. J.* FAMILIAL HEMOLYTIC ANEMIA RESULTING FROM AN ABNORMAL RED BLOOD CELL PYRUVATE KINASE. J. LAB. CLIN. MED. 72* 359-362, 1968.

SEARCY, G. P., MILLER, D. R. AND TASKER, J. B.* CONGENITAL HEMOLYTIC ANEMIA IN THE BASENJI DOG DUE TO ERYTHROCYTE PYRUVATE KINASE DEFICIENCY. CANAD. J. COMP. MED. 35* 67-70, 1971.

TANAKA, K. R., VALENTINE, W. N. AND MIWA, S.* PYRUVATE KINASE (PK) DEFICIENCY HEREDITARY NONSPHEROCYTIC HEMOLYTIC ANEMIA. BLOOD 19* 267-295, 1962.

VALENTINE, W. N. AND TANAKA, K. R.* PYRUVATE KINASE DEFICIENCY HEREDITARY HEMOLYTIC ANEMIA. IN, STANBURY, J. B., WYNGAARDEN, J. B. AND FREDRICKSON, D. S. (EDS.)* THE METABOLIC BASIS OF INHERITED DISEASE. NEW YORK* MCGRAW-HILL, 1966 (2ND ED.). PP. 1051-1059.

ZUELZER, W. W., ROBINSON, A. R. AND HSU, T. H. J.* ERYTHROCYTE PYRUVATE KINASE DEFICIENCY IN NON-SPHEROCYTIC HEMOLYTIC ANEMIA* A SYSTEM OF MULTIPLE GENETIC MARKERS.Q BLOOD 32* 33-48, 1968.

26630 RED HAIR

IN COPENHAGEN, HAUGE AND HELWEG-LARSEN (1954) FOUND THE PREVALENCE OF *STRIKINGLY RED HAIR* TO BE 1.90 PERCENT. NEEL (1943) WAS OF THE OPINION THAT RED HAIR IS RECESSIVE WITH OCCASIONAL PENETRANCE IN HETEROZYGOTES AND HYPOSTASIS TO FACTORS DETERMINING BLACK OR BROWN HAIR COLOR. REED (1952) QUESTIONED WHETHER RED HAIR

R
E
C
E
S
S
I
V
E

'SEGREGATES' WHEN MACROSCOPIC METHODS FOR SCORING SUBJECTS ARE USED. RED HAIR HAS BEEN PRESENT IN PATIENTS WITH JOB'S SYNDROME (Q.V.). RIFE (1967) CONCLUDED THAT THE PROPORTION OF RED HAIRED OFFSPRING IN FAMILIES IN WHICH ONE OR BOTH PARENTS ARE RED HAIRED ARE TOO HIGH TO SUPPORT THE HYPOTHESIS THAT RED HAIR IS INHERITED AS A SIMPLE RECESSIVE. THE FAMILY DATA AND GENE FREQUENCY ANALYSIS SUGGESTED TO HIM THAT THE PRESENCE OF RED PIGMENT IN THE HAIR IS DOMINANT TO ITS ABSENCE AND IS HYPOSTATIC TO BROWN OR BLACK.

HAUGE, M. AND HELWEG-LARSEN, H. F.* STUDIES ON LINKAGE IN MAN* RED HAIR VERSUS BLOOD GROUPS, PTC AND EYE COLOUR. ANN. EUGEN. 18* 175-182, 1954.

NEEL, J. V.* CONCERNING INHERITANCE OF RED HAIR. J. HERED. 34* 93-96, 1943.

REED, T. E.* RED HAIR COLOUR AS A GENETICAL CHARACTER. ANN. EUGEN. 17* 115-139, 1952.

RIFE, D. C.* THE INHERITANCE OF RED HAIR. ACTA GENET. MED. GEM. 16* 342-349, 1967.

SINGLETON, W. R. AND ELLIS, B.* INHERITANCE OF RED HAIR FOR SIX GENERATIONS. J. HERED. 55* 261-266, 1964.

26640 REESE'S RETINAL DYSPLASIA

THIS DISORDER CONSISTS OF MALFORMATION OF THE RETINA AND PERSISTENCE OF THE PRIMARY VITREOUS. ABSENCE OF THE DEFINITIVE VITREOUS IS NOT SURPRISING SINCE ITS FORMATION IS DEPENDENT ON THE RETINA. THE ABNORMALITY MAY SIMULATE NORRIE'S DISEASE (SEE X-LINKED CATALOG). IT IS THE CHARACTERISTIC EYE CHANGE IN TRISOMY 13-15 (TRISOMY D-1, OR THE BARTHOLIN-PATAU SYNDROME), WHICH IS CHARACTERIZED BY DELAY IN THE DEVELOPMENT OF SEVERAL PROTEINS SUCH AS ADULT HEMOGLOBIN AND RED CELL CATALASE (LEE ET AL., 1966). MULTIPLE VISCERAL MANIFESTATIONS AND OTHERS SUCH AS POLYDACTYLY WERE KNOWN TO BE ASSOCIATED (HARRIS AND THOMSON, 1937* REESE AND BLODI, 1950* REESE AND STRAATSMA, 1958* YUDKIN, 1928) LONG BEFORE THE CHROMOSOMAL BASIS WAS ELUCIDATED. ASIDE FROM THE IMPORTANCE IN THE DIFFERENTIAL DIAGNOSIS OF MICROPHTHALMOS, ANOPHTHALMOS, NORRIE'S DISEASE, THE MAIN REASON FOR INCLUDING MENTION HERE OF REESE'S RETINAL DYSPLASIA IS THAT REESE AND STRAATSMA (1958) OBSERVED TWO SIBSHIPS WITH MULTIPLE AFFECTED MEMBERS - 2 OUT OF 3 IN ONE AND 3 OUT OF 4 IN A SECOND.

HARRIS, H. A. AND THOMSON, G. C.* PERSISTENT TRUNCUS ARTERIOSUS COMMUNIS WITH MICROPHTHALMOS, ORBITAL CYST AND POLYDACTYLY. ARCH. DIS. CHILD. 12* 59-66, 1937.

LEE, C. S. N., BOYER, S. H., BOWEN, P., WEATHERALL, D. J., ROSENBLUM, H., CLARK, D. B., DUKE, J. R., LIBORO, C., BIAS, W. AND BORGAONKAR, D. S.* THE D(1) TRISOMY SYNDROME* THREE SUBJECTS WITH UNEQUALLY ADVANCING DEVELOPMENT. BULL. JOHNS HOPKINS HOSP. 118* 374-394, 1966.

REESE, A. B. AND BLODI, F. C.* RETINAL DYSPLASIA. AM. J. OPHTHAL. 33* 23-32, 1950.

REESE, A. B. AND STRAATSMA, B. R.* RETINAL DYSPLASIA. AM. J. OPHTHAL. 45* 199-211, 1958.

YUDKIN, A. M.* CONGENITAL BILATERAL MICROPHTHALMOS ACCOMPANIED BY OTHER MALFORMATIONS OF THE BODY. AM. J. OPHTHAL. 11* 128-131, 1928.

*26650 REFSUM'S SYNDROME

RETINITIS PIGMENTOSA, CHRONIC POLYNEURITIS AND CEREBELLAR SIGNS ARE THE CARDINAL CLINICAL FEATURES. SOME CASES HAVE NERVE DEAFNESS AND MOST HAVE ELECTROCARDIOGRA-PHIC CHANGES. ICHTHYOSIS IS PRESENT IN SOME. HISTOLOGICALLY INTERSTITIAL HYPERTROPHIC POLYNEURITIS AND DEGENERATION OF NUCLEI AND FIBER TRACTS IN THE BRAIN STEM HAVE BEEN DESCRIBED. AN INSTRUCTIVE PEDIGREE IS THAT SHOWN BY BAKER (1962). THIS CONDITION HAS BEEN SHOWN TO BE A DISORDER OF LIPID METABOLISM. AN UNUSUAL FATTY ACID 3, 7, 11, 15- TETRAMETHYL-HEXADECANIC ACID HAS BEEN IDENTIFIED IN THE SERUM AND IN THE LIPID DEPOSITS OF THE LIVER, KIDNEY AND OTHER ORGANS. KLENK AND KAHLKE (1963) DISCOVERED THE ACCUMULATION OF THE BRANCHED CHAIN FATTY ACID, PHYTANIC ACID. ISOTOPIC STUDIES INDICATE THAT THERE IS LITTLE ENDOGENOUS SYNTHESIS OF PHYTANIC ACID AND THAT THE METABOLIC DEFECT INVOLVES DEGRADATION. IN THESE PATIENTS EXOGENOUS PHYTOL IS READILY CONVERTED TO PHYTANIC ACID. ELDJARN ET AL. (1966) SHOWED THAT A DIET FREE OF CHLOROPHYLL AND OF FOODS WHICH MIGHT CONTAIN PHYTOL, PHYTANIC ACID OR THEIR PRECURSORS, PHYTANIC ACID COULD BE REDUCED IN THE BLOOD AND CLINICAL IMPROVEMENT EFFECTED. PATIENTS AND CULTURED FIBROBLASTS FROM PATIENTS SHOW VERY LOW OXIDATION OF C14-LABELLED PHYTANIC ACID BUT NORMAL OXIDATION OF PRISTANIC ACID WHICH IS KNOWN TO BE THE FIRST PRODUCT OF PHYTANIC ACID DEGRADATION (STEINBERG ET AL., 1967). THE DEFECT THEN RESIDES IN THE ENZYME WHICH CATALYZES THE ALPHA-OXIDATIVE PROCESS BY WHICH PHYTANIC ACID IS SHORTENED BY ONE CARBON ATOM. STUDIES OF CULTURED FIBROBLASTS FROM PATIENTS WITH REFSUM'S DISEASE LED HERNDON ET AL. (1969) TO THE CONCLUSION THAT THE ENZYME INVOLVED IN ALPHA-HYDROXYLATION OF PHYTANATE IS DEFICIENT, WHILE ENZYMES INVOLVED IN LATER STEPS ARE NORMAL.

RECESSIVE

ASHENHURST, E. M., MILLAR, J. H. D. AND MILLIKEN, T. G.* REFSUM'S SYNDROME AFFECTING A BROTHER AND TWO SISTERS. BRIT. MED. J. 2* 415-417, 1958.

BAKER, A. B.* FAMILIAL PRIMARY AMYLOIDOSIS WITH POLYNEUROPATHY. CLINICAL NEUROLOGY. NEW YORK* HOEBER-HARPER, (2ND ED.) 4* 2287, 1962.

CLARK, D. B. AND CRITCHLEY, M.* HEREDOPATHIA ATACTICA POLYNEURITIFORMIS (REFSUM'S SYNDROME). PROC. ROY. SOC. MED. 44* 689-690, 1951.

ELDJARN, L., TRY, K., STOKKE, O., MUNTHE-KAAS, A. W., REFSUM, S., STEINBERG, D., AVIGAN, J. AND MIZE, C.* DIETARY EFFECTS ON SERUM-PHYTANIC-ACID LEVELS AND ON CLINICAL MANIFESTATIONS IN HEREDOPATHIA ATACTICA POLYNEURITIFORMS. LANCET 1* 691-693, 1966.

HERNDON, J. H., JR., STEINBERG, D. AND UHLENDORF, B. W.* REFSUM'S DISEASE* DEFECTIVE OXIDATION OF PHYTANIC ACID IN TISSUE CULTURES DERIVED FROM HOMOZYGOTES AND HETEROZYGOTES. NEW ENG. J. MED. 281* 1034-1038, 1969.

HERNDON, J. H., JR., STEINBERG, D., UHLENDORF, B. W. AND FALES, H. M.* REFSUM'S DISEASE* CHARACTERIZATION OF THE ENZYME DEFECT IN CELL CULTURE. J. CLIN. INVEST. 48* 1017-1032, 1969.

KAHLKE, W. AND WAGENER, H.* CONVERSION OF H3-PHYTOL TO PHYTANIC ACID AND ITS INCORPORATION INTO PLASMA LIPID FRACTIONS IN HEREDOPATHIA ATACTICA POLYNEURITIFORMIS. METABOLISM 15* 687-693, 1966.

KLENK, E. AND KAHLKE, W.* UBER DAS VORKOMMEN DER 3.7.11.15-TETRAMETHYL-HEXADECANSAURE (PHYTANSAURE) IN DER CHOLESTERINESTERN UND ANDERN LIPOIDFRAKTIONEN DER ORGANE BEI EINEM KRANKHEITSFALL UN BEKANNTER GENESE (VERDACHT AUF HEREDOPATHIA ATACTICA POLYNEURITIFORMIS REFSUM-SYNDROM). HOPPE SEYLER. Z. PHYSIOL. CHEM. 333* 133-142, 1963.

MIZE, C. E., HERNDON, J. H., JR., BLASS, J. P., MILNE, G. W. A., FOLLANSBEE, C., LAUDAT, P. AND STEINBERG, D. E.* LOCALIZATION OF THE OXIDATIVE DEFECT IN PHYTANIC ACID DEGRADATION IN PATIENTS WITH REFSUM'S DISEASE. J. CLIN. INVEST. 48* 1033-1040, 1969.

REFSUM, S.* HEREDOPATHIA ATACTICA POLYNEURITIFORMIS. J. NERV. MENT. DIS. 116* 1046-1050, 1952.

REFSUM, S., SALOMONSEN, L. AND SKATVEDT, M.* HEREDOPATHIA ATACTICA POLYNEURITIFORMIS IN CHILDREN. J. PEDIAT. 35* 335-343, 1949.

RICHTERICH, R., KAHLKE, W., VAN MECHELEN, P. AND ROSSI, E.* REFSUM'S SYNDROME (HEREDOPATHIA ATACTICA POLYNEURITIFORMIS)* EIN ANGEBORENER DEFEKT IM LIPID-STOFFWECHSEL MIT SPEICHERUNG VON 3,7,11,15-TETRAMETHYL-HEXADECANSAURE. KLIN. WSCHR. 41* 800-801, 1963.

RICHTERICH, R., VAN MECHELEN, P. AND ROSSI, E.* REFSUM'S DISEASE (HEREDOPATHIA ATACTICA POLYNEURITIFORMIS)* AN INBORN ERROR OF LIPID METABOLISM WITH STORAGE OF 3,7,11,15-TETRAMETHYL HEXADECANOIC ACID. I. REPORT OF A CASE. AM. J. MED. 39* 230-236, 1965.

STEINBERG, D., HERNDON, J. H., JR., UHLENDORF, B. W., MIZE, C. E., AVIGAN, J. AND MILNE, G. W. A.* REFSUM'S DISEASE* NATURE OF THE ENZYME DEFECT. SCIENCE 156* 1740-1742, 1967.

STEINBERG, D., MIZE, C. E., AVIGAN, J., FALES, H. M., ELDJARN, L., TRY, K., STOKKE, O. AND REFSUM, S.* STUDIES ON THE METABOLIC ERROR IN REFSUM'S DISEASE. J. CLIN. INVEST. 46* 313-322, 1967.

STEINBERG, D., MIZE, C. E., HERNDON, J. H., JR., FALES, H. M., ENGEL, W. K. AND VROOM, F. Q.* PHYTANIC ACID IN PATIENTS WITH REFSUM'S SYNDROME AND RESPONSE TO DIETARY TREATMENT. ARCH. INTERN. MED. 125* 75-87, 1970.

STEINBERG, D., VROOM, F. Q., ENGEL, W. K., CAMMERMEYER, J., MIZE, C. E. AND AVIGAN, J.* REFSUM'S DISEASE - A RECENTLY CHARACTERIZED LIPIDOSIS INVOLVING THE NERVOUS SYSTEM. ANN. INTERN. MED. 66* 365-395, 1967.

26660 REGIONAL ENTERITIS

ABOUT 10 PERCENT OF PERSONS WITH REGIONAL ENTERITIS HAVE ONE OR MORE CLOSE RELATIVES WITH GRANULOMATOUS DISEASE OF THE BOWEL. THE FAMILIAL PATTERN DOES NOT SUGGEST SIMPLE MENDELIAN INHERITANCE. IN 5 PERSONS OF ASHKENAZIC JEWISH ORIGIN (ANCESTORS FROM AREA OF RUSSIA-POLAND AROUND VILNA) SHEEHAN ET AL. (1967) FOUND RED CELL GLUCOSE-6-PHOSPHATE DEHYDROGENASE DEFICIENCY ASSOCIATED WITH REGIONAL ENTERITIS OR GRANULOMATOUS COLITIS. THE AFFECTED PERSONS WERE 2 MALES AND 3 FEMALES.

SHEEHAN, R. G., NECHELES, T. F., LINDEMAN, R. J., MEYER, H. J. AND PATTERSON, J. F.* REGIONAL ENTERITIS ASSOCIATED WITH ERYTHROCYTE G6PD-DEFICIENCY. NEW ENG. J. MED. 277* 1124-1126, 1967.

R
E
C
E
S
S
I
V
E

THERE ARE AT LEAST TWO REPORTS OF THE DEFECT IN SIBS. ON THE OTHER HAND, SIX CASES ARE KNOWN OF TWIN PAIRS OF WHICH ONLY ONE WAS AFFECTED (DAVIDSON AND ROSS, 1954). NO TWINS, BOTH AFFECTED, SEEM TO HAVE BEEN REPORTED. BILATERAL RENAL AGENESIS WAS REPORTED IN 2 MALE SIBS BY MADISSON (1934).

DAVIDSON, W. M. AND ROSS, G. I. M.* BILATERAL ABSENCE OF THE KIDNEYS AND RELATED CONGENITAL ANOMALIES. J. PATH. BACT. 68* 459-471, 1954.

MADISSON, H.* BILATERAL APLASIA* 4 CASES. CENTRABL. PATH. ANAT. 60* 1-8, 1934.

SCHMIDT, E. C. H., HARTLEY, A. A. AND BOWER, R.* RENAL APLASIA IN SISTERS. ARCH. PATH. 54* 403-406, 1952.

26680 RENAL AGENESIS, UNILATERAL

GORVOY, SMULEWICZ AND ROTHFELD (1962) DESCRIBED AFFECTED BROTHERS. THE DISORDER COULD, AS FAR AS THIS INFORMATION ALONE IS CONCERNED, BE X-LINKED. UNILATERAL ABSENCE OF THE KIDNEY WAS DESCRIBED IN A BOY AND HIS MATERNAL UNCLE BY BOUND (1943).

BOUND, J. P.* TWO CASES OF CONGENITAL ABSENCE OF ONE KIDNEY IN THE SAME FAMILY. BRIT. MED. J. 2* 747 ONLY, 1943.

GORVOY, J. D., SMULEWICZ, J. AND ROTHFELD, S. H.* UNILATERAL RENAL AGENESIS IN TWO SIBLINGS. CASE REPORT. PEDIATRICS 29* 270-273, 1962.

*26690 RENAL DYSPLASIA AND RETINAL APLASIA

LOKEN AND COLLEAGUES (1961) REPORTED BROTHER AND SISTER WITH THIS COMBINATION. IN THE SISTER RENAL DYSPLASIA WAS PROVED AT AUTOPSY. A SIMILAR SYNDROME IS SAID (WAARDENBURG, 1963) TO HAVE BEEN FOUND IN MICE BY KEELER. SENIOR, FRIEDMANN AND BRAUDO (1961) AND FAIRLEY, LEIGHTON AND KINCAID-SMITH (1963) HAVE ALSO REPORTED FAMILIES WITH AN OCULORENAL SYNDROME. IN THE FORMER FAMILY THE RENAL CHANGES RESEMBLED THOSE IN FANCONI'S FAMILIAL JUVENILE NEPHRONOPHTHIS (Q.V.). IN THE LATTER FAMILY THE RENAL CHANGE WAS LIKE POLYCYSTIC KIDNEY. IN AN AMISH ISOLATE, SCHIMKE (1969) FOUND TWO COUSINS WITH VASOPRESSIN-RESISTANT DIABETES INSIPIDUS, PROGRESSIVE AZOTEMIA, AND RETINITIS PIGMENTOSA. A MORE REMOTELY RELATED PERSON MAY ALSO HAVE BEEN AFFECTED. DESPITE SOME HISTOLOGIC SIMILARITIES TO JUVENILE NEPHRONOPHTHISIS AND TO MEDULLARY CYSTIC DISEASE, SCHIMKE CONCLUDED THAT THE TOTAL CLINICOGENETIC PICTURE SUPPORTED THE VIEW THAT THIS IS A DISTINCT ENTITY. DEKABAN (1969) DESCRIBED TWO BROTHERS WITH CONGENITAL RETINAL BLINDNESS AND A DEVELOPMEN-TAL RENAL ABNORMALITY LEADING TO UREMIA. AUTOPSY WAS PERFORMED IN ONE OF THE PATIENTS WHO DIED AT AGE 10 YEARS.

BIOS, E. AND ROYER, P.* ASSOCIATION DE NEPHROPATHIE TUBULO-INTERSTITIELLE CHRONIQUE ET DE DEGENERESCENCE TAPETO-RETINIENNE. ETUDE GENETIQUE. ARCH. FRANC. PEDIAT. 27* 471-481, 1970.

DEKABAN, A. S.* FAMILIAL OCCURRENCE OF CONGENITAL RETINAL BLINDNESS AND DEVELOPMENTAL RETINAL LESIONS. J. GENET. HUM. 17* 289-296, 1969.

FAIRLEY, K. F., LEIGHTON, P. W. AND KINCAID-SMITH, P.* FAMILIAL VISUAL DEFECTS ASSOCIATED WITH POLYCYSTIC KIDNEY AND MEDULLARY SPONGE KIDNEY. BRIT. MED. J. 1* 1060-1063, 1963.

FONTAINE, J.-L., BOULESTEIX, J., SARAUX, H., LASFARGUES, G., GRENET, P., GHIEM-MINH-DUNG, N., DHERMY, P., ROY, C. AND LAPLANE, R.* NEPHROPATHIE TUBULO-INTERSTI-TIELLE DE L'ENFANT AVEC DEGENERESCENCE TAPETO-RETINIENNE (SYNDROME DE SENIOR). A PROPOS D'UNE OBSERVATION. ARCH. FRANC. PEDIAT. 27* 459-470, 1970.

LOKEN, A. C., HANSSEN, O., HALVORSEN, S. AND JOLSTER, N. J.* HEREDITARY RENAL DYSPLASIA AND BLINDNESS. ACTA PAEDIAT. 50* 177-184, 1961.

SARAUX, H., DHERMY, P., FONTAINE, J.-L., BOULESTEIX, J., LASFARGUE, G., GRENET, P., N'GHEIM, M. AND LAPLANE, R.* SENIOR AND LOKEN'S TUBULAR DEGENERATION. ARCH. OPHTHAL. 30* 683-696, 1970.

SCHIMKE, R. N.* HEREDITARY RENAL-RETINAL DYSPLASIA. ANN. INTERN. MED. 70* 735-744, 1969.

SENIOR, B., FRIEDMANN, A. I. AND BRAUDO, J. L.* JUVENILE FAMILIAL NEPHROPATHY WITH TAPETORETINAL DEGENERATION* A NEW OCULORENAL DYSTROPHY. AM. J. OPHTHAL. 52* 625-633, 1961.

WAARDENBURG, P. J.* CONGENITAL AND EARLY INFANTILE RETINAL DYSFUNCTION (HIGH-GRADED AMBLYOPIA AND AMAUROSIS LEBER). IN, GENETICS AND OPHTHALMOLOGY. SPRING-FIELD, ILL.* CHARLES C THOMAS, VOL. 2, 1963. PP. 1567-1581.

26700 RENAL RETINAL DYSPLASIA

IN AN AMISH ISOLATE, SCHIMKE (1969) FOUND TWO COUSINS WITH VASOPRESSIN-RESISTANT DIABETES INSIPIDUS, PROGRESSIVE AZOTEMIA, AND RETINITIS PIGMENTOSA. A MORE REMOTELY RELATED PERSON MAY ALSO HAVE BEEN AFFECTED. DESPITE SOME HISTOLOGIC SIMILARITIES TO JUVENILE NEPHRONOPHTHISIS AND TO MEDULLARY CYSTIC DISEASE, SCHIMKE CONCLUDED THAT THE TOTAL CLINICOGENETIC PICTURE SUPPORTED THE VIEW THAT THIS IS A DISTINCT ENTITY.

SCHIMKE, R. N.* HEREDITARY RENAL-RETINAL DYSPLASIA. ANN. INTERN. MED. 70* 735-744, 1969.

26710 RENAL TUBULAR ACIDOSIS

HUTH, WEBSTER AND ELKINTON (1960) SEPARATED THE GROUP WITH ONSET IN INFANCY AND CHILDHOOD FROM THAT WITH ONSET IN LATER LIFE. THE FORMER SEEMS TO BE A GENETIC DISORDER TRANSMITTED AS AN AUTOSOMAL RECESSIVE, ALTHOUGH A PREDOMINANCE OF MALES HAS BEEN OBSERVED. WILSON ET AL. (1967) STUDIED TWO FAMILIES EACH WITH A CASE OF LATE ONSET RENAL TUBULAR ACIDOSIS AND FOUND ELEVATION OF SERUM IMMUNOGLOBULINS IN CLOSE RELATIVES BUT NO OTHER CASES OF RENAL TUBULAR ACIDOSIS. RENAL TUBULAR ACIDOSIS BECOMES APPARENT BECAUSE OF (1) PERIODIC PARALYSIS DUE TO HYPOKALEMIA, (2) RICKETS OR OSTEOMALACIA, (3) KIDNEY STONES, OR (4) NEPHROCALCINOSIS BY ABDOMINAL X-RAY.

HUTH, E. J., WEBSTER, G. D., JR. AND ELKINTON, J. R.* THE RENAL EXCRETION OF HYDROGEN ION IN RENAL TUBULAR ACIDOSIS. III. AN ATTEMPT TO DETECT LATENT CASES IN A FAMILY* COMMENTS ON NOSOLOGY, GENETICS AND ETIOLOGY OF THE PRIMARY DISEASE. AM. J. MED. 29* 586-598, 1960.

WILSON, I. D., WILLIAMS, R. C., JR. AND TOBIAN, L., JR.* RENAL TUBULAR ACIDOSIS* THREE CASES WITH IMMUNOGLOBULIN ABNORMALITIES IN THE PATIENTS AND THEIR KINDREDS. AM. J. MED. 43* 356-370, 1967.

26720 RENAL TUBULAR ACIDOSIS III (DISLOCATION OR BICARBONATE WASTING)

MORRIS ET AL. (1969) OBSERVED TWO UNRELATED INFANT GIRLS WITH A DISTINCT FORM OF BICARBONATE WASTING RTA WHICH THEY REFERRED TO AS DISLOCATION TYPE.

MORRIS, E., SEBASTIAN, A., KRANHOLD, J. AND MORRIS, R. C.* INFANTILE RENAL TUBULAR ACIDOSIS (RTA), A DISTINCT TYPE. (ABSTRACT) CLIN. RES. 17* 441 ONLY, 1969.

*26730 RENAL TUBULAR ACIDOSIS WITH PROGRESSIVE NERVE DEAFNESS

KONIGSMARK (1966) HAS OBSERVED A 17 YEAR OLD GIRL WHO HAD CALCULI REMOVED FROM BOTH KIDNEYS AT AGE 12. STUDIES AT THAT TIME SHOWED RENAL TUBULAR ACIDOSIS AND BILATERAL NEURAL DEAFNESS. ONE BROTHER, AGE 20, HAD SIMILAR RENAL DISEASE AND PROGRESSIVE NERVE DEAFNESS. THE PARENTS AND ANOTHER BROTHER WERE NORMAL AND THE PARENTS WERE UNRELATED. NANCE (1970) HAS OBSERVED SIBS WITH THIS COMBINATION OF ABNORMALITIES.

KONIGSMARK, B. W.* BALTIMORE, MD.* PERSONAL COMMUNICATION, 1966.

NANCE, W. E.* INDIANAPOLIS, IND.* PERSONAL COMMUNICATION, 1970.

NANCE, W. E., SWEENEY, A., MCLEOD, A. C. AND COOPER, M. C.* HEREDITARY DEAFNESS* A PRESENTATION OF SOME RECOGNIZED TYPES, MODES OF INHERITANCE, AND AIDS IN COUNSELING. STH. MED. BULL. 58* 41-57, 1970.

NANCE, W. E., UNGER, E. J. AND SWEENEY, A.* EVIDENCE FOR AUTOSOMAL RECESSIVE INHERITANCE OF THE SYNDROME OF RENAL TUBULAR ACIDOSIS WITH DEAFNESS. THE CLINICAL DELINEATION OF BIRTH DEFECTS. IX. EAR. BALTIMORE* WILLIAMS AND WILKINS, 1970.

WALKER, W. G.* RENAL TUBULAR ACIDOSIS AND DEAFNESS. THE CLINICAL DELINEATION OF BIRTH DEFECTS. IX. EAR. BALTIMORE* WILLIAMS AND WILKINS, 1970.

26740 RENAL, GENITAL AND MIDDLE EAR ANOMALIES

IN 4 FEMALE SIBS WINTER ET AL. (1968) OBSERVED RENAL HYPOPLASIA OR APLASIA, ANOMALIES OF THE INTERNAL GENITALIA ESPECIALLY VAGINAL ATRESIA AND IN THE TWO SURVIVING SISTERS, IN WHOM IT COULD BE INVESTIGATED, ANOMALY OF THE OSSICLES OF THE MIDDLE EAR. TURNER (1968) DESCRIBED A SIMILARLY AFFECTED PATIENT.

TURNER, G.* A SECOND FAMILY WITH RENAL, VAGINAL, AND MIDDLE EAR ANOMALIES. J. PEDIAT. 76* 641 ONLY, 1968.

WINTER, J. S. D., KOHN, G., MELLMAN, W. J. AND WAGNER, S.* A FAMILIAL SYNDROME OF RENAL, GENITAL, AND MIDDLE EAR ANOMALIES. J. PEDIAT. 72* 88-93, 1968.

26750 RETICULAR DYSGENESIA (CONGENITAL ALEUKIA)

IN 1959 DE VAAL AND SEYNHAEVE DESCRIBED NEWBORN MALE TWINS WHO HAD NORMAL NUMBERS OF ERYTHROCYTES AND PLATELETS BUT NO BLOOD LEUKOCYTES AT ALL. THEY DIED AT 5 AND 8 DAYS OF AGE OF SEPSIS. POSTMORTEM SHOWED ABSENT MYELOID ELEMENTS FROM THE BONE

R
E
C
E
S
S
I
V
E

MARROW AND ABSENT LYMPHOCYTES FROM THE THYMUS AND SPLEEN. SELIGMANN ET AL. (1968) SUGGESTED THAT THIS MAY BE GENERALIZED IMMUNOLOGIC DEFICIENCY DISORDER. THEY SUGGESTED THAT THE CASE OF GITLIN ET AL. (1964) MAY HAVE BEEN THE SAME DISORDER. IN THAT CASE THE THYMUS WAS HYPOPLASTIC WITHOUT HASSAL'S CORPUSCLES.

DE VAAL, O. M. AND SEYNHAEVE, V.* RETICULAR DYSGENESIA. LANCET 2* 1123-1125, 1959.

GITLIN, D., VAWTER, G. AND CRAIG, J. M.* THYMIC ALYMPHOPLASIA AND CONGENITAL ALEUKOCYTOSIS. PEDIATRICS 33* 184-192, 1964.

SELIGMANN, M., FUDENBERG, H. H. AND GOOD, R. A.* A PROPOSED CLASSIFICATION OF PRIMARY IMMUNOLOGIC DEFICIENCIES. AM. J. MED. 45* 817-825, 1968.

*26770 RETICULOSIS, FAMILIAL HISTIOCYTIC (OR HEMOPHAGOCYTIC)

ANEMIA, GRANULOCYTOPENIA AND THROMBOCYTOPENIA ARE PRODUCED IN PART BY PHAGOCYTOSIS OF BLOOD CELLS, IN PART BY REPLACEMENT OF THE MARROW BY HISTIOCYTIC INFILTRATION. FAMILIES HAVE BEEN REPORTED BY MARRIAN AND SANERKIN (1963) AND BY FARQUHAR AND COLLEAGUES (1952, 1958). IN THE LATTER FAMILY 4 SIBS WERE AFFECTED. THE FATHER SHOWED AUTOANTIBODY AND SHORTENED RED CELL LIFE-SPAN. FARQUHAR, MACGREGOR AND RICHMOND (1958) CONCLUDED THAT THE MINOR CHANGES OBSERVED IN THE FATHER AND ONE SIB REPRESENTED THE HETEROZYGOUS STATE. THEY WERE NOT CONCERNED ABOUT THE LACK OF CHANGES IN THE MOTHER SINCE EXPRESSION IN THE HETEROZYGOTE IS OFTEN VARIABLE. THE DISORDER DISCUSSED BY OMENN (1965) AND BY MILLER (1966) IS PROBABLY THIS. OMENN (1965) DESCRIBED AN INBRED AMERICAN FAMILY OF IRISH EXTRACTION WITH A LARGE NUMBER OF AFFECTED PERSONS IN MANY RELATED SIBSHIPS. MILLER (1966) DESCRIBED FIVE SISTERS - A COMPLETE SIBSHIP, INCLUDING A PAIR OF TWINS - WITH CLINICAL FEATURES OF FAILURE TO THRIVE, RECURRENT INFECTIONS, LYMPHADENOPATHY, HEPATOSPLENOMEGALY, PULMONARY INFILTRATION AND TERMINAL PANCYTOPENIA AND HYPERGAMMAGLOBULINEMIA. DEATH OCCURRED BETWEEN AGES 20 MONTHS AND 57 MONTHS. AUTOPSY SHOWED DIFFUSE RETICULUM CELL INFILTRATION OF MOST ORGANS INCLUDING THE CENTRAL NERVOUS SYSTEM, OBLITERATION OF ARCHITECTURE OF LYMPH GLANDS AND MARKED PLASMACYTOSIS.
THIS DISORDER, LYMPHOHISTIOCYTIC INFILTRATION (Q.V.), AND LETTERER-SIWE DISEASE (Q.V.) ARE NOT EASILY DISTINGUISHED AND MAY BE THE SAME ENTITY. THE FAMILY REPORTED BY FARQUHAR ET AL. (1952, 1958) WAS SCOTTISH. ANOTHER SCOTTISH FAMILY, WITH 3 AFFECTED SIBS, WAS REPORTED BY GOODALL, GUTHRIE AND BUIST (1965). BELL ET AL. (1968) DESCRIBED AFFECTED BROTHERS BORN 11 YEARS APART. MENINGOENCE-PHALITIS DURING INFANCY WAS A FEATURE IN EACH. HEMOPHAGOCYTOSIS IN BONE MARROW PREPARATIONS MADE THE DIAGNOSIS. DONAHUE (1968) HAS NARCOPSY INFORMATION ON 6 CASES WHICH OCCURRED IN AN INBRED MENNONITE GROUP IN ONTARIO.

BELL, R. J. M., BRAFIELD, A. J. E., BARNES, N. D. AND FRANCE, N. E.* FAMILIAL HAEMOPHAGOCYTIC RETICULOSIS. ARCH. DIS. CHILD. 43* 601-606, 1968.

DONAHUE, W. L.* TORONTO, CANADA* PERSONAL COMMUNICATION, 1968.

FARQUHAR, J. W. AND CLAIREAUX, A. E.* FAMILIAL HAEMOPHAGOCYTIC RETICULOSIS. ARCH. DIS. CHILD. 27* 519-525, 1952.

FARQUHAR, J. W., MACGREGOR, A. R. AND RICHMOND, J.* FAMILIAL HAEMOPHAGOCYTIC RETICULOSIS. BRIT. MED. J. 2* 1561-1564, 1958.

FRIEDMAN, R. M. AND STEIGBIGEL, N. H.* HISTIOCYTIC MEDULLARY RETICULOSIS. AM. J. MED. 38* 130-133, 1965.

GOODALL, H. B., GUTHRIE, W. AND BUIST, N. R. M.* FAMILIAL HAEMOPHAGOCYTIC RETICULOSIS. SCOT. MED. J. 10* 425-438, 1965.

MACMAHON, H. E., BEDIZEL, M. AND ELLIS, C. A.* FAMILIAL ERYTHROPHAGOCYTIC LYMPHOHISTIOCYTOSIS. PEDIATRICS 32* 868-879, 1963.

MARRIAN, V. J. AND SANERKIN, N. G.* FAMILIAL HISTIOCYTIC RETICULOSIS (FAMILIAL HAEMOPHAGOCYTIC RETICULOSIS). J. CLIN. PATH. 16* 65-69, 1963.

MILLER, D. R.* FAMILIAL RETICULOENDOTHELIOSIS* CONCURRENCE OF DISEASE IN FIVE SIBLINGS. PEDIATRICS 38* 986-995, 1966.

OMENN, G. S.* FAMILIAL RETICULOENDOTHELIOSIS WITH EOSINOPHILIA. NEW ENG. J. MED. 273* 427-432, 1965.

26780 RETINAL DYSTROPHY, RETICULAR PIGMENTARY, OF POSTERIOR POLE

THIS CONDITION, FIRST DESCRIBED BY SJOGREN IN 1950, IS CHARACTERIZED BY A PECULIAR NETWORK OF BLACK PIGMENTED LINES IN THE POSTERIOR POLE OF THE RETINA, RESEMBLING A FISHNET WITH ITS KNOTS. IN LATE STAGES THE NETWORK DISAPPEARS AND DRUSEN APPEAR. DEUTMAN AND RUMKE (1969) DESCRIBED THE DISORDER IN A DUTCH BROTHER AND SISTER WHOSE PARENTS WERE SECOND COUSINS. THE PARENTS OF SJOGREN'S FAMILY WERE ALSO RELATED. DEAFNESS AND SPHEROPHAKIA IN THAT FAMILY WERE PROBABLY INDEPENDENT RECESSIVE TRAITS.

DEUTMAN, A. F. AND RUMKE, A. M.* RETICULAR DYSTROPHY OF THE RETINAL PIGMENT

R
E
C
E
S
S
I
V
E

EPITHELIUM. DYSTROPHIA RETICULARIS LAMINAE PIGMENTOSA RETINAE OF H. SJOGREN.
ARCH. OPHTHAL. 82* 4-9, 1969.

SJOGREN, H.* DYSTROPHIA RETICULARIS LAMINAE PIGMENTOSAE RETINAE* EARLIER NOT
DESCRIBED HEREDITARY EYE DISEASE. ACTA OPHTHAL. 28* 279-295, 1950.

26790 RETINAL TELANGIECTASIA AND HYPOGAMMAGLOBULINEMIA

FRENKEL AND RUSSE (1967) DESCRIBED A 13 YEAR OLD BOY WITH THIS COMBINATION. HIS
10 YEAR OLD SISTER HAD LESS EXTENSIVE RETINAL TELANGIECTASES AND IMPAIRMENT OF
DELAYED HYPERSENSITIVITY BUT NO DEFICIENCY OF GAMMAGLOBULIN.

FRENKEL, M. AND RUSSE, H. P.* RETINAL TELANGIECTASIA ASSOCIATED WITH HYPOGAMMA-
GLOBULINEMIA. AM. J. OPHTHAL. 63* 215-220, 1967.

*26800 RETINITIS PIGMENTOSA

CHANGES WHICH MAY BE LABELLED RETINITIS PIGMENTOSA (OR ATYPICAL RETINITIS
PIGMENTOSA) ARE OBSERVED IN A NUMBER OF THE OTHER CONDITIONS LISTED HERE, E.G.,
ABETALIPOPROTEINEMIA, ALSTROM'S SYNDROME, REFSUM'S DISEASE, LAURENCE-MOON-BIEDL
SYNDROME, USHER'S SYNDROME, COCKAYNE'S SYNDROME, PALLIDAL DEGENERATION. IN A
SURVEY OF RETINITIS PIGMENTOSA IN FIVE SWISS CANTONS, AMMANN, KLEIN AND BOHRINGER
(1961) FOUND DEAF-MUTISM ASSOCIATED IN 16 OF 118 LIVING CASES (SEE USHER'S
SYNDROME).   FRANCESCHETTI'S STRIKING PEDIGREE (1953) IS REPRODUCED IN FRANCOIS'
BOOK (1961).

AMMANN, F., KLEIN, D. AND BOHRINGER, H. R.* RESULTATS PRELIMINAIRES D'UNE
ENQUETE SUR LA FREQUENCE ET LA DISTRIBUTION GEOGRAPHIQUE DES DEGENERESCENCES
TAPETO-RETINIENNES EN SUISSE (ETUDE DE CINQ CANTONS). J. GENET. HUM. 10* 99-127,
1961.

FRANCESCHETTI, A.* DEGENERESCENCE CHORIORETINIENNE FAMILIALE AVEC ANGIOSCLEROSE
CHOROIDIENNE, STADE TARDIF D'UNE RETINITIS PUNCTATA ALBESCENS, CONSTATEE 54 ANS
AUPARAVANT. OPHTHALMOLOGIA 125 (SUPPL. 37)* 340-347, 1953.

FRANCESCHETTI, A.* RETINITE PIGMENTAIRE RECESSIVE DANS DEUX GENERATIONS
CONSECUTIVE ('PSEUDO-DOMINANCE'). J. GENET. HUM. 2* 145-146, 1953.

FRANCOIS, J.* HEREDITY IN OPHTHALMOLOGY. ST. LOUIS* C. V. MOSBY CO., 1961. P.
444 FIG. 391.

KOBAYASHI, F.* GENETIC STUDY ON RETINITIS PIGMENTOSA. JAP. J. OPHTHAL. 4* 82-
91, 1960.

R
E
C
E
S
S
I
V
E

26810 RETINOSCHISIS WITH EARLY HEMERALOPIA

FAVRE (1958) DESCRIBED A BROTHER AND SISTER, AGE 16 AND 15 RESPECTIVELY, WITH
HEMERALOPIA, DEGENERATIVE NITREOUS CHANGES, PERIPHERAL AND CENTRAL RETINOSCHISIS,
ETC.   MACVICAR AND WILBRANDT (1970) DESCRIBED THE DISORDER IN TWO BROTHERS WHOSE
PARENTS WERE RELATED. NIGHT BLINDNESS HAD BEEN PRESENT SINCE CHILDHOOD.

FAVRE, M.* A PROPOS DE DEUX CAS DE DEGENERESCENCE HYALOIDEORETINIENNE. TWO
CASES OF HYALOID-RETINAL DEGENERATION. OPHTHALMOLOGICA 135* 604-609, 1958.

MACVICAR, J. E. AND WILBRANDT, H. R.* HEREDITARY RETINOSCHISIS AND EARLY
HEMERALOPIA. ARCH. OPHTHAL. 83* 629-636, 1970.

26820 RHABDOMYOLYSIS, ACUTE RECURRENT

ALTHOUGH THE GENETICS REMAINS UNCLEAR, RECESSIVE INHERITANCE IS PERHAPS MOST
LIKELY.   HED (1953) OBSERVED THREE AFFECTED BROTHERS. THREE OTHER BROTHERS AND
THE PARENTS WERE UNAFFECTED. THE SISTER OF A MALE PATIENT OF BOWDEN ET AL. (1956)
WAS ALSO AFFECTED.

BOWDEN, D. H., FRASER, D., SACKSON, S. H. AND WALKER, N. F.* ACUTE RECURRENT
RHABDOMYOLYSIS (PAROXYSMAL MYOHAEMOGLOBINURIA). MEDICINE 35* 335-353, 1956.

FARMER, T. A., HAMMACK, W. J. AND FROMMEYER, W. B.* IDIOPATHIC RECURRENT
RHABDOMYOLYSIS ASSOCIATED WITH MYOGLOBINURIA. REPORT OF A CASE. NEW ENG. J. MED.
264* 60-66, 1961.

HED, R.* MYOGLOBINURIA. ARCH. INTERN. MED. 92* 825-832, 1953.

KAHLER, H. J.* DIE MYOGLOBINURIEN. ERGEBN. INN. MED. KINDERHEILK. 11* 1-103,
1959.

*26830 ROBERT'S SYNDROME (SEVERE ABSENCE DEFORMITIES OF LONG BONES OF LIMBS ASSOCIATED
WITH CLEFT LIP-PALATE)

ROBERTS (1919) DESCRIBED THREE AFFECTED SIBS AND PICTURES WERE INCLUDED. THE
PARENTS WERE FIRST COUSINS OF ITALIAN EXTRACTION. THE BONES OF THE LEGS WERE
ALMOST ABSENT AND THOSE OF THE ARMS HYPOPLASTIC. THE SKULL LOOKED OXYCEPHALIC

(LIKE CROUZON'S) WITH PROMINENT EYES. STROER'S CASE (1939) MAY BE THE SAME ENTITY. AGAIN THE PARENTS WERE FIRST COUSINS. APPELT ET AL. (1966) ALSO DESCRIBED CASES AND POINTED OUT THAT CLITORAL OR PENILE ENLARGEMENT IS A FEATURE. THE SC PHOCOMELIA SYNDROME (Q.V.) IS A SIMILAR BUT DISTINCT DISORDER.

APPELT, J., GERKEN, H. AND LENZ, W.* TETRAPHOKOMELIE MIT LIPPEN-KIEFER-GAUMENSPALTE UND KLITORISHYPERTROPIE - EIN SYNDROM. PAEDIAT. PADOL. 2* 119-124, 1966.

HERRMANN, J., FEINGOLD, M., TUFFLI, G. A. AND OPITZ, J. M.* A FAMILIAL DYSMORPHOGENETIC SYNDROME OF LIMB DEFORMITIES, CHARACTERISTIC FACIAL APPEARANCE AND ASSOCIATED ANOMALIES* THE 'PSEUDOTHALIDOMIDE' OR 'SC-SYNDROME.' THE CLINICAL DELINEATION OF BIRTH DEFECTS. III. LIMB MALFORMATIONS. NEW YORK* NATIONAL FOUNDATION, 1969. PP. 81-89.

ROBERTS, J. B.* A CHILD WITH DOUBLE CLEFT OF LIP AND PALATE, PROTRUSION OF THE INTERMAXILLARY PORTION OF THE UPPER JAW AND IMPERFECT DEVELOPMENT OF THE BONES OF THE FOUR EXTREMITIES. ANN. SURG. 70* 252-254, 1919.

STROER, W. F. H.* UBER DER ZUSAMMENTREFFEN VON HASENSCHARTE MIT ERNSTEN EXTREMITATENMISSBILDUNGEN. ERBARZT 7* 101-104, 1939.

*26840 ROTHMUND-THOMSON SYNDROME (POIKILODERMA ATROPHICANS AND CATARACT)

THIS IS A HEREDITARY DERMATOSIS CHARACTERIZED BY ATROPHY, PIGMENTATION, AND TELANGIECTASIA AND FREQUENTLY ACCOMPANIED BY JUVENILE CATARACT, SADDLE NOSE, CONGENITAL BONE DEFECTS, DISTURBANCES OF HAIR GROWTH, AND HYPOGONADISM. PROGNOSIS FOR SURVIVAL IS FAIRLY GOOD. ROTHMUND'S FAMILY WAS FURTHER INVESTIGATED BY SIEMENS (CITED BY WAARDENBURG, 1961). IT IS POSSIBLE THAT THE CONDITION DESCRIBED BY THOMSON (1936) IS A DIFFERENT RECESSIVE DISORDER FROM THAT DESCRIBED BY ROTHMUND. SADDLE NOSE WAS NOT PRESENT AND CATARACT DID NOT OCCUR.

BLINSTRUB, R. S., LEHMAN, R. AND STEINBERG, T. H.* POIKILODERMA CONGENITALE. REPORT OF TWO CASES. ARCH. DERM. 89* 659-664, 1964.

BLOCK, B. AND STAUFFER, H.* SKIN DISEASES OF ENDOCRINE SYSTEM (DYSHORMONAL DERMATOSES). POIKILODERMA-LIKE CHANGES IN CONNECTION WITH UNDERDEVELOPMENT OF THE SEXUAL GLANDS AND DYSTROPHIA ADIPOSOGENITALIS. ARCH. DERM. SYPH. 19* 22-34, 1929.

COLE, H. N., GIFFEN, H. K., SIMMONS, J. T. AND STROUD, G. M., III* CONGENITAL CATARACTS IN SISTERS WITH CONGENITAL ECTODERMAL DYSPLASIA. J.A.M.A. 129* 723-728, 1945.

FRANCESCHETTI, A.* LES DYSPLASIES ECTODERMIQUES ET LES SYNDROMES HEREDITAIRES APPARENTES. DERMATOLOGICA 106* 129-156, 1953.

KRAUS, B. S., GOTTLIEB, M. A. AND MELITON, H. R.* THE DENTITION IN ROTHMUND'S SYNDROME. J. AM. DENT. ASS. 81* 894-915, 1970.

ROTHMUND, A.* UBER CATARACTEN IN VERBINDUNG MIT EINER EIGENTHUMLICHEN HAUTDE-GENERATION. GRAEFE. ARCH. OPHTHAL. 14* 159-182, 1868.

SEXTON, G. B.* THOMSON'S SYNDROME (POIKILODERMA CONGENITALE). CANAD. MED. ASS. J. 70* 662-665, 1954.

SIEMENS, H. W.* IN, WAARDENBURG, P. J., FRANCESCHETTI, A. AND KLEIN, D. (EDS.)* GENETICS AND OPHTHALMOLOGY. SPRINGFIELD, ILL.* CHARLES C THOMAS, 2* 896 ONLY, 1963.

TAYLOR, W. B.* ROTHMUND'S SYNDROME - THOMSON'S SYNDROME. ARCH. DERM. 75* 236-244, 1957.

THOMSON, M. S.* POIKILODERMA CONGENITALE. BRIT. J. DERM. 48* 221-234, 1936.

26850 ROWLEY-ROSENBERG SYNDROME (GROWTH RETARDATION, PULMONARY HYPERTENSION AND AMINOACIDURIA)

ROWLEY AND COLLEAGUES (1961) DESCRIBED A 'NEW' SYNDROME IN THREE OF SIX CHILDREN. FEATURES WERE GROWTH RETARDATION, POOR MUSCULAR DEVELOPMENT, SCANTY ADIPOSE TISSUE, RECURRENT PULMONARY INFECTION, ATELECTASIS, AND RIGHT VENTRICULAR HYPERTROPHY. ONE SURVIVOR HAD AMINOACIDURIA WITHOUT ELEVATION OF SERUM AMINO ACIDS AND INCREASED PLASMA UNESTERIFIED FATTY ACID CONCENTRATION (ROSENBERG ET AL., 1961).

ROSENBERG, L. E., MUELLER, P. S. AND WATKINS, D. M.* A NEW SYNDROME* FAMILIAL GROWTH RETARDATION, RENAL AMINOACIDURIA AND COR PULMONALE. II. INVESTIGATION OF RENAL FUNCTION, AMINO ACID METABOLISM, AND GENETIC TRANSMISSION. AM. J. MED. 31* 205-215, 1961.

ROWLEY, P. T., MUELLER, P. S., WATKINS, D. M. AND ROSENBERG, L. E.* FAMILIAL GROWTH RETARDATION, RENAL AMINOACIDURIA AND COR PULMONALE. I. DESCRIPTION OF A NEW SYNDROME, WITH CASE REPORTS. AM. J. MED. 31* 187-204, 1961.

ALTHOUGH MOST OF THE CASES HAVE BEEN SPORADIC, JOHNSON (1966) DESCRIBED AFFECTED SIBS. IN ADDITION TO THE ANOMALIES LISTED ABOVE, PULMONARY STENOSIS, KELOID FORMATION IN SURGICAL SCARS, LARGE FORAMEN MAGNUM, AND VERTEBRAL AND STERNAL ANOMALIES SHOULD BE MENTIONED. IN THE CASE REPORTED BY JELIU AND SAINT-ROME (1967), THE PARENTS WERE SECOND COUSINS. I FIND IT DIFFICULT TO ACCEPT THE SUGGESTION OF MULTIFACTORIAL INHERITANCE (ROY ET AL., 1968). I WOULD EXPECT A GRADED SEVERITY (FOR WHICH THERE IS NO EVIDENCE) AMONG CASES AND IN CLOSE RELATIVES, SINCE THERE IS NO OBVIOUS MECHANISM FOR A THRESHOLD EFFECT. THE LACK OF MUCH IF ANY FAMILIAL AGGREGATION IS AGAINST MULTIFACTORIAL INHERITANCE JUST AS IT IS AGAINST RECESSIVE INHERITANCE. MULTIFACTORIAL INHERITANCE IS UNLIKELY IN THE CASE OF SUCH RARE ENTITIES. THE DERMATOGLYPHIC CHANGES DESCRIBED BY GIROUX AND MILLER (1967) SUGGEST A CHROMOSOMAL ABNORMALITY. SUCH HAS NOT BEEN IDENTIFIED BUT A SMALL ABNORMALITY BEYOND THE LIMITS OF RESOLUTION OF EXISTING METHODS SEEMS THE MOST LIKELY CAUSE OF RUBINSTEIN'S SYNDROME. PADFIELD ET AL. (1968) STUDIED 17 CASES AND FOUND NO CASE AMONG 50 SIBS. THE FREQUENCY OF RUBINSTEIN'S SYNDROME IS ABOUT 1 PER 500 INSTITUTIONALIZED PERSON WITH MENTAL RETARDATION OVER AGE 5 YEARS. PFEIFFER (1968) DESCRIBED THE SYNDROME IN BOTH OF MONOZYGOTIC TWINS. FATHER-DAUGHTER INCEST PRODUCED ANOTHER CASE (PADFIELD ET AL., 1968). TAKEUCHI (1966) ALSO OBSERVED AFFECTED SIBS. RUBINSTEIN (1969) FOUND PARENTAL AGE TO BE ABOUT AVERAGE.

COFFIN, G. S.* BRACHYDACTYLY, PECULIAR FACIES AND MENTAL RETARDATION. AM. J. DIS. CHILD. 108* 351-359, 1964.

GIROUX, J. AND MILLER, J. R.* DERMATOGLYPHICS OF THE BROAD THUMB AND GREAT TOE SYNDROME. AM. J. DIS. CHILD. 113* 207-209, 1967.

JELIU, G. AND SAINT-ROME, G.* LE SYNDROME DE RUBINSTEIN-TAYBI. A PROPOS D'UNE OBSERVATION. UN. MED. CANADA 96* 22-29, 1967.

JOHNSON, C. F.* BROAD THUMBS AND BROAD GREAT TOES WITH FACIAL ABNORMALITIES AND MENTAL RETARDATION. J. PEDIAT. 68* 942-951, 1966.

PADFIELD, C. J., PARTINGTON, M. W. AND SIMPSON, N. E.* THE RUBINSTEIN-TAYBI SYNDROME. ARCH. DIS. CHILD. 43* 94-101, 1968.

PFEIFFER, R. A.* RUBINSTEIN-TAYBI-SYNDROM BEI WAHRSCHEINLICH EINEIIGEN ZWILLINGEN. HUMANGENETIK 6* 84-87, 1968.

ROY, F. H., SUMMITT, R. L., HIATT, R. L. AND HUGHES, J. G.* OCULAR MANIFESTATIONS OF THE RUBINSTEIN-TAYBI SYNDROME. CASE REPORT AND REVIEW OF THE LITERATURE. ARCH. OPHTHAL. 79* 272-278, 1968.

RUBINSTEIN, J. H. AND TAYBI, H.* BROAD THUMBS AND TOES AND FACIAL ABNORMALITIES. AM. J. DIS. CHILD. 105* 588-608, 1963.

RUBINSTEIN, J. H.* THE BROAD THUMB SYNDROME - PROGRESS REPORT 1968. THE CLINICAL DELINEATION OF BIRTH DEFECTS. II. MALFORMATION SYNDROMES. NEW YORK* NATIONAL FOUNDATION, 1969. PP. 25-41.

TAKEUCHI, M.* RUBINSTEIN'S SYNDROME IN TWO SIBLINGS. GUNMA J. MED. SCI. 15* 17-22, 1966.

26870 SACCHAROPINURIA

THIS CONDITION WAS OBSERVED BY CARSON ET AL. (1968) IN A 22 YEAR OLD, MODERATELY RETARDED, SOMEWHAT SHORT GIRL WITH EEG ABNORMALITIES BUT NO HISTORY OF FITS. NO OTHER FAMILY MEMBERS WERE AFFECTED. THE URINE CONTAINED LYSINE, CITRULLINE, AND HISTIDINE IN ADDITION SACCHAROPINE. THIS DISORDER IS PRESUMABLY DISTINCT FROM HYPERLYSINEMIA IN WHICH (IN ONE FORM AT LEAST) A DEFECT IN THE ENZYME WHICH CONVERTS LYSINE TO SACCHAROPINE IS PRESENT.

CARSON, N. A. J., SCALLY, B. G., NEILL, D. W. AND CARRE, I. J.* SACCHAROPINURIA* A NEW INBORN ERROR OF LYSINE METABOLISM. NATURE 218* 679 ONLY, 1968.

*26880 SANDHOFF'S DISEASE, OR GM(2) GANGLIOSIDOSIS TYPE II

THE INITIAL DESCRIPTION WAS MADE BY SANDHOFF ET AL. (1968). O'BRIEN (1971) STUDIED TWO MEXICAN-AMERICAN SISTERS AND A BOY OF ANGLO-SAXON EXTRACTION. ALL PATIENTS HAVE BEEN NON-JEWISH. HOWEVER, THE CLINICAL AND PATHOLOGIC PICTURE IS VERY SIMILAR TO TAY-SACHS DISEASE. WEAKNESS BEGINS IN THE FIRST SIX MONTHS OF LIFE. STARTLE REACTION, EARLY BLINDNESS, PROGRESSIVE MENTAL AND MOTOR DETERIORATION, DOLL-LIKE FACE, CHERRY RED SPOTS AND MACROCEPHALY ARE ALL PRESENT AS IN TAY-SACHS DISEASE. DEATH HAS OCCURRED BY AGE THREE. HEXOSAMINIDASES A AND B ARE BOTH DEFICIENT IN THIS DISORDER.

O'BRIEN, J. S.* GANGLIOSIDE STORAGE DISEASES. IN, HARRIS, H. AND HIRSCHHORN, K. (ED.)* ADVANCES IN HUMAN GENETICS, (VOL.3) 1971.

SANDHOFF, K., ANDREAE, U. AND JATZKEWITZ, H.* DEFICIENT HEXOSAMINIDASE ACTIVITY
IN AN EXCEPTIONAL CASE OF TAY-SACHS DISEASE WITH ADDITIONAL STORAGE OF KIDNEY
GLOBOSIDE IN VISCERAL ORGANS. LIFE SCI. 7* 283-288, 1968.

26890 SARCOSINEMIA

GERRITSEN AND WAISMAN (1966) FOUND HYPERSARCOSINEMIA AND SARCOSINURIA IN BROTHER
AND SISTER WITH MILD MENTAL RETARDATION AND FEW OTHER ABNORMALITIES. ABNORMAL
INCREASES IN BLOOD AND URINE SARCOSINE OCCURRED IN 2 OTHER SIBS, THE MOTHER, A
MATERNAL AUNT AND THE MATERNAL GRANDMOTHER (BUT NOT IN THE FATHER) WHEN SARCOSINE
OR ITS PRECURSOR DIMETHYLGLYCINE WAS ADMINISTERED. SARCOSINE DEHYDROGENASE MAY BE
DEFECTIVE. SCOTT ET AL. (1970) FOUND BY LOADING TESTS TO A DECREASED CAPACITY TO
CONVERT SARCOSINE TO GLYCINE, SUGGESTING A DEFICIENCY OF SARCOSINE DEHYDROGENASE
ACTIVITY, THE SUGGESTION CAN BE PROVEN ONLY BY LIVER BIOPSY. THEIR PATIENT HAD
MOTOR AND MENTAL RETARDATION.

GERRITSEN, T. AND WAISMAN, H. A.* HYPERSARCOSINEMIA* AN INBORN ERROR OF
METABOLISM. NEW ENG. J. MED. 275* 66-69, 1966.

SCOTT, C. R., CLARK, S. H., TENG, C. C. AND SWEDBERG, K. R.* CLINICAL AND
CELLULAR STUDIES OF SARCOSINEMIA. J. PEDIAT. 77* 805-811, 1970.

*26900 SC PHOCOMELIA SYNDROME

IN A FAMILY WITH SURNAME BEGINNING WITH S AND ANOTHER WITH SURNAME BEGINNING WITH
C, HERRMANN ET AL. (1969) DESCRIBED A SYNDROME CONSISTING OF THE FOLLOWING
FEATURES* (1) NEARLY SYMMETRICAL REDUCTIVE MALFORMATIONS OF THE LIMBS RESEMBLING
PHOCOMELIA* (2) FLEXION CONTRACTURES OF VARIOUS JOINTS* (3) MULTIPLE MINOR
ANOMALIES, INCLUDING CAPILLARY HEMANGIOMA OF THE FACE, FOREHEAD AND EARS,
HYPOPLASTIC CARTILAGES OF THE EARS AND NOSE, MICROGNATHIA, SCANTY, SILVERY-BLOND
HAIR, AND CLOUDY CORNEAS* (4) INTRAUTERINE AND EXTRAUTERINE GROWTH RETARDATION*
(5) POSSIBLY MENTAL RETARDATION* AND (6) AUTOSOMAL RECESSIVE INHERITANCE. THE
SAME SYNDROME WAS PROBABLY DESCRIBED BY O'BRIEN AND MUSTARD (1921) IN 3 OF 8
CHILDREN OF NORMAL PARENTS WHO WERE RELATED AS DOUBLE FIRST COUSINS.

HERRMANN, J., FEINGOLD, M., TUFFLI, G. A. AND OPITZ, J. M.* A FAMILIAL
DYSMORPHOGENETIC SYNDROME OF LIMB DEFORMITIES, CHARACTERISTIC FACIAL APPEARANCE
AND ASSOCIATED ANOMALIES* THE 'PSEUDOTHALIDOMIDE' OR 'SC-SYNDROME.' THE CLINICAL
DELINEATION OF BIRTH DEFECTS. III. LIMB MALFORMATIONS. NEW YORK* NATIONAL
FOUNDATION, 1969. PP. 81-89.

O'BRIEN, H. R. AND MUSTARD, H. S.* AN ADULT LIVING CASE OF TOTAL PHOCOMELIA.
J.A.M.A. 77* 1964-1967, 1921.

26910 SCHILDER'S DISEASE

ALL CASES REPORTED AS FAMILIAL SCHILDER'S DISEASE ARE PROBABLY IN FACT EITHER
KRABBE'S DISEASE, SUDANOPHILIC CEREBRAL SCLEROSIS, OR METACHROMATIC LEUKENCEPHALO-
PATHY (Q.V.). IF THE TERM IS TO BE PRESERVED AT ALL, ITS USE SHOULD BE CONFINED
TO SUDANOPHILIC CEREBRAL SCLEROSIS (Q.V.).

26920 SCHMIDT'S SYNDROME (DIABETES MELLITUS, ADDISON'S DISEASE, MYXEDEMA)

IT IS THOUGHT BY MANY THAT THIS SYNDROME HAS AN AUTOIMMUNE BASIS. OTHER POSSIBLE
AUTOIMMUNE CONDITIONS, E.G. HASHIMOTO'S STRUMA, SHOW FAMILIAL AGGREGATION.
WHETHER THE BASIS IS GENETIC CANNOT BE STATED WITH CERTAINTY, AND IF GENETIC IT IS
NOT CERTAIN THAT A SINGLE GENE CHANGE IS INVOLVED. PHAIR ET AL. (1965) REPORTED
BROTHER AND SISTER.

CARPENTER, C. C. J., SOLOMON, N., SILVERBERG, S. G., BLEDSOE, T., NORTHCUTT, R.
C., KLINENBERG, J. R., BENNETT, I. L. AND HARVEY, A. M.* SCHMIDT'S SYNDROME
(THYROID AND ADRENAL INSUFFICIENCY). A REVIEW OF THE LITERATURE AND A REPORT OF
FIFTEEN NEW CASES INCLUDING TEN INSTANCES OF COEXISTENT DIABETES MELLITUS.
MEDICINE 43* 153-180, 1964.

PHAIR, J. P., BONDY, P. K. AND ABELSON, D. M.* DIABETES MELLITUS, ADDISON'S
DISEASE AND MYXEDEMA REPORT OF TWO CASES. J. CLIN. ENDOCR. 25* 260-265, 1965.

SOLOMON, N., CARPENTER, C. J., BENNETT, I. L., JR. AND HARVEY, A. M.* SCHMIDT'S
SYNDROME (THYROID AND ADRENAL INSUFFICIENCY) AND COEXISTENT DIABETES MELLITUS.
DIABETES 14* 300-304, 1965.

26930 SCHWARTZ-LELAK SYNDROME

GORLIN ET AL. (1969) SUGGESTED THAT THE PATIENT DESCRIBED BY SCHWARTZ (1960) AS AN
EXAMPLE OF CRANIOMETAPHYSEAL DYSPLASIA AND THAT REPORTED BY LELEK (1961) AS AN
EXAMPLE OF CAMURATI-ENGELMANN'S DISEASE SUFFERED FROM A DISTINCT DISORDER.
ENLARGEMENT OF THE HEAD AND GENU VARUM OR GENU VALGUM WERE MAIN FEATURES. LONG
BONES WERE WIDENED WITH TRANSLUCENT FLARING OF THE METAPHYSES. SERUM ALKALINE
PHOSPHATASE LEVEL WAS ELEVATED IN BOTH CASES. BOTH PATIENTS WERE MALES. PARENTS
AND SIBS WERE UNAFFECTED AND NO MENTION WAS MADE OF PARENTAL CONSANGUINITY.

GORLIN, R. J., SPRANGER, J. AND KOSZALKA, M. F.* GENETIC CRANIOTUBULAR BONE DYSPLASIAS AND HYPEROSTOSES* A CRITICAL ANALYSIS. THE CLINICAL DELINEATION OF BIRTH DEFECTS. IV. SKELETAL DYSPLASIAS. NEW YORK* NATIONAL FOUNDATION, 1969.

LELEK, I.* CAMURATI-ENGELMANN DISEASE. FORTSCHR. ROENTGEN. 94* 702-712, 1961.

SCHWARTZ, E.* CRANIOMETAPHYSEAL DYSPLASIA. AM. J. ROENTGEN. 84* 461-466, 1960.

26940 SCLEROCORNEA

SCLEROCORNEA IS A CONGENITAL MALFORMATION OF THE CORNEA, SUCH THAT THE BOUNDARY BETWEEN THE CORNEA AND THE SCLERA IS OBSCURED. USUALLY THE INVOLVEMENT IS LIMITED TO THE PERIPHERAL PART OF THE CORNEA BUT IT MAY EXTEND TO THE ENTIRE CORNEA, SO-CALLED SCLEROCORNEA TOTALIS. THE MILD FORM IS INHERITED AS A DOMINANT, THE SEVERE FORM AS A RECESSIVE. THE PINNAE ARE MALFORMED IN SOME CASES. BLOCH (1965) REVIEWED THE FAMILIAL REPORTS. SEGREGATION ANALYSIS SHOWED SATISFACTORY AGREEMENT WITH THE RECESSIVE HYPOTHESIS. SEVERAL INSTANCES OF PARENTAL CONSANGUINITY ARE REPORTED. SCLEROCORNEA IS ALSO A FEATURE OF CORNEA PLANA (Q.V.).

BLOCH, N.* LES DIFFERENTS TYPES DE SCLEROCORNEE, LEURS MODES D'HEREDITE ET LES MALFORMATIONS CONGENITALES CONCOMITANTES. J. GENET. HUM. 14* 133-172, 1965.

*26950 SCLEROSTENOSIS (CORTICAL HYPEROSTOSIS WITH SYNDACTYLY)

SCLEROSTEOSIS IS A TERM APPLIED BY HAUSEN (1967) TO A DISORDER SIMILAR TO VAN BUCHEM'S HYPEROSTOSIS CORTICALIS GENERALISATA (Q.V.) BUT DIFFERING IN RADIOLOGIC APPEARANCE OF THE BONE CHANGES AND IN THE PRESENCE OF ASYMMETRIC CUTANEOUS SYNDACTYLY OF THE INDEX AND MIDDLE FINGERS IN MANY BUT NOT ALL CASES. THE JAW HAS AN UNUSUALLY SQUARE APPEARANCE IN THIS CONDITION. AFFECTED SIBS WERE OBSERVED BY HIRSCH (1929), FALCONER AND RYRIE (1937), HIGINBOTHAM AND ALEXANDER (1941), KELLEY AND LAWLAH (1946), TRUSWELL (1958) AND KLINTWORTH (1963). PARENTAL CONSANGUINITY WAS OBSERVED BY FALCONER AND RYRIE (1937) AND BY TRUSWELL (1958) AND THE CASES OF KELLEY AND LAWLAH (1946) AND OF WITKOP (1965) WERE FROM AN INBRED TRI-RACIAL GROUP OF SOUTHERN MARYLAND KNOWN AS THE "WE-SORTS."

FALCONER, A. W. AND RYRIE, B. J.* REPORT ON FAMILIAL TYPE OF GENERALIZED OSTEO-SCLEROSIS WITH REPORT ON PATHOLOGICAL CHANGES. MED. PRESS 195* 12-20, 1937.

HAUSEN, H. G.* SKLEROSTEOSE. IN, OPITZ, H. AND SCHMID, F. (EDS.)* HANDBUCH DER KINDERHEILKUNDE, 1967. PP. 351-355.

HIGINBOTHAM, N. L. AND ALEXANDER, S. F.* OSTEOPETROSIS. FOUR CASES IN ONE FAMILY. AM. J. SURG. 53* 444-454, 1941.

HIRSCH, I. S.* GENERALIZED OSTEITIS FIBROSA. RADIOLOGY 13* 44-84, 1929.

KELLEY, C. H. AND LAWLAH, J. W.* ALBERS-SCHONBERG DISEASE. A FAMILY SURVEY. RADIOLOGY 47* 507-513, 1946.

KLINTWORTH, G. K.* NEUROLOGIC MANIFESTATIONS OF OSTEOPETROSIS (ALBERS-SCHON-BERG'S DISEASE). NEUROLOGY 13* 512-519, 1963.

TRUSWELL, A. S.* OSTEOPETROSIS WITH SYNDACTYLY. A MORPHOLOGIC VARIANT OF ALBERS-SCHONBERG'S DISEASE. J. BONE JOINT SURG. 40B* 208-218, 1958.

WITKOP, C. J.* GENETIC DISEASE OF THE ORAL CAVITY. IN, TIECKE, R. W. (ED.)* ORAL PATHOLOGY. NEW YORK* MCGRAW-HILL CO., 1965.

26960 SEA-BLUE HISTOCYTE DISEASE

THIS DISORDER IS CHARACTERIZED BY SPLENOMEGALY, MILD THROMBOCYTOPENIA AND, IN THE BONE MARROW, NUMEROUS HISTOCYTES CONTAINING CYTOPLASMIC GRANULES WHICH STAIN BRIGHT BLUE WITH THE USUAL HEMATOLOGIC STAINS. THE NAME WAS COINED BY SILVERSTEIN ET AL. (1970). HOLLAND ET AL. (1965) SUGGESTED THAT THE SYNDROME IS THE CONSE-QUENCE OF AN INHERITED METABOLIC DEFECT ANALOGOUS TO GAUCHER'S DISEASE AND OTHER SPHINGOLIPOIDOSES. JONES ET AL. (1970) DESCRIBED AFFECTED BROTHER AND SISTER. PARENTAL CONSANGUINITY WAS POSSIBLE BECAUSE BOTH PARENTS CAME FROM THE SAME RESTRICTED AREA OF WEST VIRGINIA. LAKE ET AL. (1970) SUGGESTED THAT THE 'SEA-BLUE' DESIGNATION BE ABANDONED BECAUSE THE MARROW CONTAINS A SECOND VARIETY OF ABNORMAL CELL WHICH NEVER STAINS 'SEA-BLUE' AND BECAUSE THEY HAD OBSERVED A 'MALIGNANT' DISORDER WITH THE SAME TYPE OF CELLS AND PROGRESSIVE NEUROLOGIC DISEASE CHARACTERIZED BY ATAXIA, DEMENTIA AND SEIZURES. HETEROZYGOTES MAY HAVE SOME SEA-BLUE HISTIOCYTES IN THE BONE MARROW (ZLOTNICK, FRIED, 1970). WEWALKA (1970) GAVE A LONG-TERM FOLLOW-UP ON A CASE REPORTED IN 1950. HE COMMENTED ON EYE CHANGES* A WHITE RING SURROUNDING THE MACULA.

HOLLAND, P., HUG, G. AND SCHUBERT, W. K.* CHRONIC RETICULOENDOTHELIAL CELL STORAGE DISEASE. AM. J. DIS. CHILD. 110* 117-124, 1965.

JONES, B., GILBERT, E. F., ZUGIBE, F. T. AND THOMPSON, H.* SEA-BLUE HISTIOCYTE DISEASE IN SIBLINGS. LANCET 2* 73-75, 1970.

RECESSIVE

HISTIOCYTE. (LETTER) LANCET 2* 309 ONLY, 1970.

SILVERSTEIN, M. N., ELLEFSON, R. D. AND AHERN, E. J.* THE SYNDROME OF THE SEA-BLUE HISTIOCYTE. NEW ENG. J. MED. 282* 1-4, 1970.

WEWALKA, F. G.* SYNDROME OF THE SEA-BLUE HISTIOCYTE. (LETTER) LANCET 2* 1248 ONLY, 1970.

ZLOTNICK, A. AND FRIED, K.* SEA-BLUE-HISTIOCYTE SYNDROME. (LETTER) LANCET 2* 776 ONLY, 1970.

*26970 SEIP SYNDROME (BERARDINELLI SYNDROME, TOTAL LIPODYSTROPHY AND ACROMEGALOID GIGANTISM)

THE FEATURES ARE GENERALIZED LIPODYSTROPHY, HYPERLIPEMIA, HEPATOMEGALY, ACANTHOSIS NIGRICANS, ELEVATED BASAL METABOLIC RATE AND NON-KETONIC INSULIN-RESISTANT DIABETES MELLITUS. STUDIES OF PITUITARY AND ADRENAL FUNCTION INCLUDING GROWTH HORMONE ASSAYS HAVE BEEN NORMAL. POLYCYSTIC OVARIES, MUSCULAR HYPERTROPHY, AND MENTAL RETARDATION HAVE OCCURRED IN SOME CASES. TWO AFFECTED SIBS HAVE BEEN REPORTED IN EACH OF FIVE FAMILIES AND IN FOUR OTHER FAMILIES THE PARENTS WERE CONSANGUINEOUS (BRUNZELL ET AL., 1968). SEIP (1959) DESCRIBED AFFECTED BROTHER AND SISTER. LIPODYSTROPHIC MUSCULAR HYPERTROPHY (SENIOR, 1961) MAY BE THE SAME ENTITY. CONSANGUINITY AND MULTIPLE AFFECTED SIBS ARE KNOWN. SUBSTANCES WITH INSULIN-ANTAGONIZING AND FAT-MOBILIZING PROPERTIES HAVE BEEN FOUND IN THE URINE (HAMWI ET AL, 1966). LEPRECHAUNISM (Q.V.) HAS SOME SIMILAR FEATURES. SEE PRADER-WILLI SYNDROME FOR A CONDITION IN WHICH ABUNDANT FAT, MUSCLE HYPOTONIA AND SMALL HANDS AND FEET ARE EXACTLY THE OPPOSITE OF THE FINDINGS IN THIS SYNDROME. SEE SYSTEMIC CYSTIC ANGIOMATOSIS AND SEIP'S SYNDROME FOR DISCUSSION OF WHAT MAY BE THE SAME ENTITY.

BERARDINELLI, W.* A UNDIAGNOSED ENDOCRINOMETABOLIC SYNDROME* REPORT OF TWO CASES. J. CLIN. ENDOCR. 14* 193-204, 1954.

BRUNZELL, J. D., SHANKLE, S. W. AND BETHUNE, J. E.* CONGENITAL GENERALIZED LIPODYSTROPHY AND SYSTEMIC CYSTIC ANGIOMATOSIS* THE SIMULTANEOUS OCCURRENCE OF TWO UNUSUAL SYNDROMES IN A SINGLE FAMILY. ANN. INTERN. MED. 69* 501-516, 1968.

HAMWI, G. J., KRUGER, F. A., EYMONTT, M. J., SCARPELLI, D. G., GWINUP, G. AND BYRON, R.* LIPOATROPHIC DIABETES. DIABETES 15* 262-268, 1966.

LAWRENCE, R. D.* LIPODYSTROPHY AND HEPATOMEGALY WITH DIABETES, LIPAEMIA, AND OTHER METABOLIC DISTURBANCES. A CASE THROWING NEW LIGHT ON THE ACTION OF INSULIN. LANCET 1* 724-731, 773-775, 1946.

REED, W. B., DEXTER, R., CORLEY, C. AND FISH, C.* CONGENITAL LIPODYSTROPHIC DIABETES WITH ACANTHOSIS NIGRICANS. THE SEIP-LAURENCE SYNDROME. ARCH. DERM. 91* 326-334, 1965.

SEIP, M. AND TRYGSTAD, O.* GENERALIZED LIPODYSTROPHY. ARCH. DIS. CHILD. 38* 447-453, 1963.

SEIP, M.* LIPODYSTROPHY AND GIGANTISM WITH ASSOCIATED ENDOCRINE MANIFESTATION. A NEW DIENCEPHALIC SYNDROME.Q ACTA PAEDIAT. 48* 555-574, 1959.

SENIOR, B.* LIPODYSTROPHIC MUSCULAR HYPERTROPHY. ARCH. DIS. CHILD. 36* 426-431, 1961.

26980 SENILE PLAQUE FORMATION

CONSTANTINIDIS AND DE AJURIAGUERRA (1965) STUDIED THE BRAIN FROM 64 ELDERLY PERSONS, FROM 30 FAMILIES, WITH VARIOUS PSYCHIATRIC DIAGNOSES, FOR THE PRESENCE OF SENILE PLAQUES INDEPENDENT OF ASSOCIATED CEREBRAL LESIONS. OF 29 PAIRS OF SIBS, SENILE PLAQUES WERE FOUND IN BOTH IN 22, 4 WERE BOTH UNAFFECTED AND 3 HAD ONE AFFECTED. ALTHOUGH THE AUTHORS POSTULATED RECESSIVE INHERITANCE, IT SHOULD BE NOTED THAT OF 10 TWO GENERATION OBSERVATIONS, PARENT AND CHILD WERE AFFECTED IN 3 AND ONE GENERATION ONLY IN 7.

CONSTANTINIDIS, J. AND DE AJURIAGUERRA, J.* L'INCIDENCE FAMILIALE DES PLAQUES SENILES. CONFIN. PSYCHIAT. 8* 130-137, 1965.

26990 SIALURIA

MONTREUIL ET AL. (1967) DESCRIBED THE CHEMICAL ASPECTS OF A NEW FORM OF MELLITURIA CALLED SIALURIA. A 'YOUNG PATIENT' EXCRETED 5.8 TO 7.2 GM. OF N-ACETYL-NEURAMINIC ACID PER DAY. NO CLINICAL OR GENETIC INFORMATION WAS PROVIDED.

MONTREUIL, J., BISERTE, G., STRECKER, G., SPIK, G., FONTAINE, G. AND FARRIAUX, J.-P.* DESCRIPTION D'UN NOUVEAU TYPE DE MELITURIE* LA SIALURIE. C. R. ACAD. SCI. 265* 97-99, 1967.

27000 SIDBURY SYNDROME

SIDBURY, SMITH AND HARLAN (1967) OBSERVED THAT THREE OF FOUR CHILDREN OF A SECOND-COUSIN MARRIAGE DIED IN THE FIRST TWO WEEKS OF LIFE WITH THE FOLLOWING SYMPTOMS AFTER THE FIRST THREE DAYS* CONVULSIONS, LETHARGY, DEHYDRATION, MODERATE HEPATOMEGALY, DEPRESSED PLATELETS AND LEUCOCYTES AND AN UNUSUAL URINARY ODOR LIKE THAT OF SWEATY FEET. POSTMORTEM EXAMINATION SHOWED MAINLY CHANGES RELATED TO THE HEMATOLOGIC FINDINGS* HYPOPLASTIC MARROW, SCATTERED HEMORRHAGES OF VISCERA AND TERMINAL SEPTICEMIA. THE UNUSUAL ODOR IS THE RESULT OF BUTYRIC AND HEXANOIC ACIDS. THEY SUGGEST THAT THIS IS AN INBORN ERROR OF SHORT-CHAIN FATTY ACID METABOLISM AND MORE SPECIFICALLY THAT A DEFECT IN GREEN ACYL DEHYDROGENASE MAY BE INVOLVED. IN A SECOND FAMILY A BROTHER AND SISTER WITH UNRELATED PARENTS HAD A SIMILAR AILMENT. SEE ISOVALERICACIDEMIA.

SIDBURY, J. B., JR., SMITH, E. K. AND HARLAN, W.* AN INBORN ERROR OF SHORT-CHAIN FATTY ACID METABOLISM. THE ODOR-OF-SWEATY-FEET SYNDROME. J. PEDIAT. 70* 8-15, 1967.

27010 SITUS INVERSUS VISCERUM

FAMILIAL CONCENTRATION (LEININGER AND GIBSON, 1950) AND CONSANGUINEOUS PARENTS (COCKAYNE, 1938) HAVE BEEN OBSERVED.

COCKAYNE, E. A.* THE GENETICS OF TRANSPOSITION OF THE VISCERA. QUART. J. MED. 7* 479-493, 1938.

LEININGER, C. R. AND GIBSON, S.* TRANSPOSITION OF VISCERA IN SIBLINGS. J. PEDIAT. 37* 195-200, 1950.

*27020 SJOGREN-LARSSON SYNDROME (OLIGOPHRENIA, CONGENITAL ICHTHYOSIS, SPASTIC NEUROLOGIC DISORDER)

THE SKIN CHANGES ARE SIMILAR TO THOSE OF CONGENITAL ICHTHYOSIFORM ERYTHRODERMA (Q.V.). LINK AND ROLDAN (1958) REPORTED CASES. BLUMEL, WATKINS AND EGGERS (1958) REFERRED TO THE NEUROLOGIC DISORDER AS SPASTIC QUADRIPLEGIA. SJOGREN AND LARSSON (1956, 1957) SUGGESTED THAT ALL THEIR CASES (28 IN NUMBER) WERE DERIVED FROM THE SAME MUTATION, OCCURRING ABOUT 600 YEARS AGO AND THAT ABOUT 1.3 PERCENT OF THE POPULATION OF THE NORTH OF SWEDEN IS HETEROZYGOUS FOR THE GENE. ABOUT HALF THE CASES HAVE PIGMENTARY DEGENERATION OF THE RETINA. LESIONS OF THE OCULAR FUNDUS WERE DISCUSSED BY GILBERT ET AL. (1968).

BLUMEL, J., WATKINS, M. AND EGGERS, G. W. N.* SPASTIC QUADRIPLEGIA COMBINED WITH CONGENITAL ICHTHYOSIFORM ERYTHRODERMA AND OLIGOPHRENIA. AM. J. DIS. CHILD. 96* 724-726, 1958.

GILBERT, W. R., JR., SMITH, J. L. AND NYHAN, W. L.* THE SJOGREN-LARSSON SYNDROME. ARCH. OPHTHAL. 80* 308-316, 1968.

HEIJER, A. AND REED, W. B.* SJOGREN-LARSSON SYNDROME* CONGENITAL ICHTHYOSIS SPASTIC PARALYSIS, AND OLIGOPHRENIA. ARCH. DERM. 92* 545-552, 1965.

LINK, J. K. AND ROLDAN, E. C.* MENTAL DEFICIENCY, SPASTICITY, AND CONGENITAL ICHTHYOSIS. REPORT OF A CASE. J. PEDIAT. 52* 712-714, 1958.

RICHARDS, B. W.* CONGENITAL ICHTHYOSIS, SPASTIC DIPLEGIA AND MENTAL DEFICIENCY. (LETTER) BRIT. MED. J. 2* 714 ONLY, 1960.

SELMANOWITZ, V. J. AND PORTER, M. J.* THE SJOGREN-LARSSON SYNDROME. AM. J. MED. 42* 412-422, 1967.

SJOGREN, T. AND LARSSON, T.* OLIGOPHRENIA IN COMBINATION WITH CONGENITAL ICHTHYOSIS AND SPASTIC DISORDERS. A CLINICAL AND GENETIC STUDY. ACTA PSYCHIAT. NEUROL. SCAND. 32 (SUPPL. 113)* 1-112, 1957.

SJOGREN, T.* OLIGOPHRENIA COMBINED WITH CONGENITAL ICHTHYOSIFORM ERYTHRODERMIA, SPASTIC SYNDROME AND MACULARRETINAL DEGENERATION. A CLINICAL AND GENETIC STUDY. ACTA GENET. STATIST. MED. 6* 80-91, 1956.

ZALESKI, W. A.* CONGENITAL ICHTHYOSIS, MENTAL RETARDATION AND SPASTICITY (SJOGREN-LARSSON SYNDROME). CANAD. MED. ASS. J. 86* 951-954, 1962.

*27030 SKIN PEELING, FAMILIAL CONTINUOUS

KURBAN AND AZAR (1969) DESCRIBED 3 AFFECTED MALES AND AN AFFECTED FEMALE AMONG THE 9 OFFSPRING OF A FIRST COUSIN MARRIAGE. NO PREVIOUS INSTANCE OF FAMILIAL OCCURRENCE OF THIS CONDITION (OTHERWISE KNOWN AS DECIDUOUS SKIN, KERATOLYSIS EXFOLIATIVA CONGENITA, 'SKIN SHEDDING' ETC.) HAS BEEN DESCRIBED.

KURBAN, A. K. AND AZAR, H. A.* FAMILIAL CONTINUAL SKIN PEELING. BRIT. J. DERM. 81* 191-195, 1969.

*27040 SMITH-LEMLI-OPITZ SYNDROME

IN THREE UNRELATED MALES SMITH, LEMLI AND OPITZ (1964) FOUND A STRIKINGLY SIMILAR

R
E
C
E
S
S
I
V
E

COMBINATION OF CONGENITAL ANOMALIES* MICROCEPHALY, MENTAL RETARDATION, HYPOTONIA, INCOMPLETE DEVELOPMENT OF THE MALE GENITALIA, SHORT NOSE WITH ANTEVERTED NOSTRILS, AND, IN TWO, PYLORIC STENOSIS. A DECEASED MALE SIB OF ONE OF THESE WAS PROBABLY IDENTICALLY AFFECTED. NO PARENTAL CONSANGUINITY WAS DISCOVERED. PINSKY AND DIGEORGE (1965) REPORTED AFFECTED BROTHER AND SISTER. BLAIR AND MARTIN (1966) ALSO DESCRIBED THE CONDITION IN BROTHER AND SISTER. THE MALE HAD HYPOSPADIAS. DALLAIRE AND FRASER (1966) DESCRIBED AFFECTED BROTHERS. BLEPHAROPTOSIS HAS BEEN A FEATURE OF MANY CASES. LOWRY, MILLER AND MACLEAN (1968) DESCRIBED THE COMBINATION OF MICROGNATHIA, POLYDACTYLY AND CLEFT PALATE, RESEMBLING THE SYNDROME KNOWN IN THE GERMAN LITERATURE AS "TYPUS ROSTOCKIENSIS" OR "ULLRICH-FEICHTIGER SYNDROME" BUT SUGGESTING THE SMITH-LEMLI-OPITZ SYNDROME IN RESPECT TO DERMATOGLYPHICS.

BLAIR, H. R. AND MARTIN, J. K.* A SYNDROME CHARACTERIZED BY MENTAL RETARDATION, SHORT STATURE, CRANIOFACIAL DYSPLASIA, AND GENITAL ANOMALIES OCCURRING IN SIBLINGS. J. PEDIAT. 69* 457-459, 1966.

DALLAIRE, L. AND FRASER, F. C.* THE SYNDROME OF RETARDATION WITH UROGENITAL AND SKELETAL ANOMALIES IN SIBLINGS. J. PEDIAT. 69* 459-460, 1966.

DALLAIRE, L.* SYNDROME OF RETARDATION WITH UROGENITAL AND SKELETAL ANOMALIES (SMITH-LEMLI-OPITZ SYNDROME)* CLINICAL FEATURES AND MODE OF INHERITANCE. J. MED. GENET. 6* 113-120, 1969.

KENIS, H. AND HUSTINX, T. W.* A FAMILIAL SYNDROME OF MENTAL RETARDATION IN ASSOCIATION WITH MULTIPLE CONGENITAL ANOMALIES RESEMBLING THE SYNDROME OF SMITH-LEMLI-OPITZ. MAANDSCHR. KINDERGENEESK. 35* 37-48, 1967.

LOWRY, R. B., MILLER, J. R. AND MACLEAN, J. R.* MICROGNATHIA, POLYDACTYLY AND CLEFT PALATE. J. PEDIAT. 72* 859-861, 1968.

PINSKY, L. AND DIGEORGE, A. M.* A FAMILIAL SYNDROME OF FACIAL AND SKELETAL ANOMALIES ASSOCIATED WITH GENITAL ABNORMALITY IN THE MALE AND NORMAL GENITALS IN THE FEMALE. ANOTHER CAUSE OF MALE PSEUDOHERMAPHRODITISM. J. PEDIAT. 66* 1049-1054, 1965.

SMITH, D. W., LEMLI, L. AND OPITZ, J. M.* A NEWLY RECOGNIZED SYNDROME OF MULTIPLE CONGENITAL ANOMALIES. J. PEDIAT. 64* 210-217, 1964.

WEBER, J. W. AND SCHWARTZ, H.* DER TYPUS ROSTOCKIENSIS ULLRICH-FEICHTIGER DYSKRANIO-PYGO-PHALANGIE. HELV. PAEDIAT. ACTA. 15* 163-170, 1960.

27050 SMITH-STRANG DISEASE (OASTHOUSE URINE DISEASE)

THE URINE HAD A CHARACTERISTIC AND UNIQUE ODOR LIKE THAT OF AN OASTHOUSE. ALTHOUGH PHENYLPRUVIC ACID WAS FOUND IN THE URINE, THE ODOR WAS DIFFERENT FROM THAT OF PHENYLKETONURIA. THE DEFECT WAS THOUGHT TO CONCERN THE UTILIZATION OF THE ALPHA KETO ACIDS OF ALL ESSENTIAL AMINO ACIDS AS A RESULT OF WHICH ALPHA-KETO ACIDS, THEIR AMINO ACID PRECURSORS OR HYDROXY ACID DERIVATIVES ACCUMULATED IN THE BLOOD AND OVERFLOWED IN THE URINE. THE UNUSUAL ODOR WAS THOUGHT TO BE PRODUCED BY ALPHA HYDROXYBUTYRIC ACID BUT COULD BE SOME OTHER SUBSTANCE RATHER LIKE IT. NO FURTHER CASES HAVE BEEN DISCOVERED (STRANG, 1963). THE CASE OF HOOFT AND COLLEAGUES (1964) MAY BE OF THE SAME DISORDER. THE DISORDER SEEMS TO COMBINE THE FEATURES OF PHENYLKETONURIA AND OF METHIONINE MALABSORPTION. THE FERRIC CHLORIDE TEST IS POSITIVE. THE CASE OF HOOFT ET AL. (1965) WAS IN A GIRL WITH MENTAL RETARDATION, DIARRHEA, CONVULSIONS, POLYPNEA, BLUE EYES, STRIKINGLY WHITE HAIR.

HOOFT, C., TIMMERMANS, J., SNOECK, J., ANTENER, I., OYAERT, W. AND VAN DER - HENDE, C. H.* METHIONINE MALABSORPTION IN A MENTALLY DEFECTIVE CHILD. LANCET 2* 20 ONLY, 1964.

HOOFT, C., TIMMERMANS, J., SNOECK, J., ANTENER, I., OYAERT, W. AND VAN DER - HENDE, C. H.* METHIONINE MALABSORPTION SYNDROME. ANN. PAEDIAT. 205* 73-104, 1965.

JEPSON, J. B., SMITH, A. J. AND STRANG, L. B.* AN INBORN ERROR OF METABOLISM WITH URINARY EXCRETION OF HYDROXYACIDS, KETOACIDS AND AMINOACIDS. (LETTER) LANCET 2* 1334-1335, 1958.

SMITH, A. J. AND STRANG, L. B.* AN INBORN ERROR OF METABOLISM WITH THE URINARY EXCRETION OF ALPHA-HYDROXY-BUTYRIC ACID AND PHENYLPYRUVIC ACID. ARCH. DIS. CHILD. 33* 109-113, 1958.

STRANG, L. B.* LONDON, ENGLAND* PERSONAL COMMUNICATION, 1963.

*27060 SPASTIC DIPLEGIA, INFANTILE TYPE

HANHART (1936) DESCRIBED 7 CASES IN 4 RELATED SIBSHIPS. ALL EIGHT PARENTS COULD BE TRACED TO A COMMON ANCESTOR BORN IN THE 17TH CENTURY. PENROSE (1963) OBSERVED THE DISORDER WITH MENTAL DIFICIENCY IN TWO OFFSPRING OF A FIRST COUSIN MARRIAGE. THIS IS PROBABLY THE SAME DISORDER AS THAT REPORTED BY BOOK (1956) AND BOOK AND SJOGREN (1970) AS SPASTIC OLIGOPHRENIA.

BOOK, J. A. AND SJOGREN, T.* A PEDIGREE WITH ESSENTIAL MYOCLONUS AND GENETIC

SPASTIC OLIGOPHRENIA. CLIN. GENET. 1* 95-103, 1970.

BOOK, J. A.* GENETICAL INVESTIGATIONS IN A NORTH-SWEDISH POPULATION. POPULA-TION STRUCTURE, SPASTIC OLIGOPHRENIA, DEAF MUTISM. ANN. HUM. GENET. 20* 239-250, 1956.

HANHART, E.* EINE SIPPE MIT EINFACH-REZESSIVER DIPLEGIA SPASTICA INFANTILIS (LITTLESCHER KRANKHEIT) AUS, EINEM SCHWEIZER INSUCHTGEBIET. ERBARZT 11* 165-172, 1936. (SEE DE GENETICA MEDICA, L. GEDDA (ED.). 3* 68 ONLY, 1963.).

PENROSE, L. S.* THE BIOLOGY OF MENTAL DEFECT. NEW YORK* GRUNE AND STRATTON, (3RD ED.). 1963. P. 168.

27070 SPASTIC PARAPLEGIA AND RETINAL DEGENERATION

LOUIS-BAR AND PIROT (1945) DESCRIBED TWO BROTHERS WITH MACULAR DEGENERATION AND SPASTIC PARAPLEGIA REFERRED TO BY THE AUTHORS AS *STRUMPELL TYPE.* A THIRD BROTHER WAS SAID TO HAVE A FORME FRUSTE OF SPASTIC PARAPLEGIA. THEY COULD FIND NO REPORT OF SIMILAR CASES. FAMILY 1 OF LEDIC AND VAN BOGAERT (1960) MAY BE IDENTICAL. WE HAVE SEEN A FEMALE (S.S., 1217761) WITH LATE ONSET SPASTIC PARAPLEGIA AND RETINAL DEGENERATION MORE STRIKING PERIPHERALLY. A SISTER IS IDENTICALLY AFFECTED, AND ANOTHER SISTER HAD ONLY SPASTIC PARAPLEGIA (MAHLOUDJI AND CHUKE, 1968).

LEDIC, P. AND VAN BOGAERT, L.* CEREBELLAR AND SPASTIC HEREDO-DEGENERATION WITH MACULAR DEGENERATION. J. GENET. HUM. 9* 140-157, 1960.

LOUIS-BAR, D. AND PIROT, G.* SUR UNE PARAPLEGIE SPASMODIQUE AVEC DEGENERESCENCE MACULAIRE CHEZ DEUX FRERES. OPTHALMOLOGICA 109* 32-43, 1945.

MAHLOUDJI, M. AND CHUKE, P. O.* FAMILIAL SPASTIC PARAPLEGIA WITH RETINAL DEGENERATION. JOHNS HOPKINS MED. J. 123* 142-144, 1968.

*27080 SPASTIC PARAPLEGIA, HEREDITARY

R
E
C
E
S
S
I
V
E

BELL AND CARMICHAEL (1939) FOUND PROBABLE RECESSIVE INHERITANCE IN 49 OF 74 PEDIGREES. SPASTIC PARAPLEGIA, LIKE RETINITIS PIGMENTOSA AND OPTIC ATROPHY, IS A RELATIVELY NON-SPECIFIC MANIFESTATION. THE PYRAMIDAL TRACTS ARE HIGHLY VULNERABLE TO INSULT FROM MANY CAUSES BECAUSE OF THE LONG AXONE. THE PROTEIN-SYNTHESIZING MACHINERY IS IN THE CELL BODY AND MITROCHONDRIA ARE ALSO IN SHORT SUPPLY IN THE AXOPLASM SO THAT OXIDATIVE METABOLISM IS LIMITED. INTERFERENCE WITH AXOPLASMIC FLOW WHICH OCCURS FROM THE CELL BODY TO THE FARTHEST REACHES OF THE AXONE CAN EASILY OCCUR. RECESSIVE CASES WERE DESCRIBED BY FREUD (1893) AND BY JONES (1907).

AAGENAES, O.* HEREDITARY SPASTIC PARAPLEGIA* A FAMILY WITH TEN INJURED. ACTA PSYCHIAT. NEUROL. SCAND. 34* 489-494, 1959.

BELL, J. AND CARMICHAEL, E. A.* ON THE HEREDITY OF ATAXIA AND SPASTIC PARAPLE-GIA. IN, TREASURY OF HUMAN INHERITANCE. LONDON* CAMBRIDGE UNIV. PRESS, 4* (PART 3) 169-172, 1939.

FREUD, S.* UBER FAMILIARE FORMEN VON CEREBRALEN DIPLEGIEN. NEUROL. CENTRABLATT (MENDEL) 12* 512-515 AND 542-547, 1893.

JONES, E.* EIGHT CASES OF HEREDITARY SPASTIC PARAPLEGIA. REV. NEUROL. PSYCHIAT. 5* 98-106, 1907.

27090 SPASTIC PSEUDOSCLEROSIS (DISSEMINATED ENCEPHALOMYELOPATHY* CORTICOPALLIDODE-GENERATION)

DAVISON AND RABINER (1940) DESCRIBED TWO BROTHERS AND A SISTER WITH ONSET IN THE LATE 20'S. AUTOPSY WAS PERFORMED IN ONE. IT IS NOT CLEAR THAT A DISTINCT ENTITY IS INVOLVED.

DAVISON, C. AND RABINER, A. M.* SPASTIC PSEUDOSCLEROSIS (DISSEMINATED ENCEPHA-LOMYELOPATHY* CORTICOPALLIDOSPINAL DEGENERATION)* FAMILIAL AND NON-FAMILIAL INCIDENCE (CLINICOPATHOLOGIC STUDY). ARCH. NEUROL. PSYCHIAT. 44* 578-598, 1940.

27100 SPINA BIFIDA CYSTICA

LORBER (1965) SUGGESTED RECESSIVE INHERITANCE. HOWEVER, PENETRANCE MUST BE GREATLY REDUCED BECAUSE HE ESTIMATED THE RISK OF RECJRRENCE OF SPINA BIFIDA CYSTICA, ANENCEPHALY OR HYDROCEPHALUS IN SUBSEQUENTLY BORN OFFSPRING TO BE ABOUT 8 PERCENT. RECORD AND MCKEOWN (1950) HAD ESTIMATED THE RISK AT 4 PERCENT. TAKING SPINA BIFIDA AND ANENCEPHALY (Q.V.), CARTER AND ROBERTS (1967) ESTIMATED THE RISK IN ENGLAND OF A THIRD CHILD HAVING MAJOR CENTRAL NERVOUS SYSTEM MALFORMATION, TWO HAVING BEEN PREVIOUSLY AFFECTED, TO BE ABOUT 1 IN 10. LORBER AND LEVICK (1967) FOUND SPINA BIFIDA OCCULTA IN 14.3 PERCENT OF 188 MOTHERS AND 26.8 PERCENT OF 179 FATHERS OF CASES, AND IN 5 PERCENT OF 200 CONTROLS. SPINA BIFIDA OCCULTA WAS NOT COMMONER AMONG PARENTS WITH MORE THAN ONE AFFECTED CHILD AND IN A MAJORITY OF FAMILIES NEITHER PARENT HAD IT.

CARTER, C. O. AND ROBERTS, J. A. F.* THE RISK OF RECURRENCE AFTER TWO CHILDREN WITH CENTRAL-NERVOUS-SYSTEM MALFORMATIONS. LANCET 1* 306-308, 1967.

LORBER, J. AND LEVICK, K.* SPINA BIFIDA CYSTICA* INCIDENCE OF SPINA BIFIDA OCCULTA IN PARENTS AND IN CONTROLS. ARCH. DIS. CHILD. 42* 171-173, 1967.

LORBER, J.* THE FAMILY OF SPINA BIFIDA CYSTICA. PEDIATRICS 35* 589-595, 1965.

RECORD, R. G. AND MCKEOWN, T.* CONGENITAL MALFORMATION OF THE CENTRAL NERVOUS SYSTEM. III. RISK OF MALFORMATIONS IN SIBS OF MALFORMED INDIVIDUALS. BRIT. J. PREV. SOC. MED. 4* 217-220, 1950.

27110 SPINAL EXTRADURAL CYST

CHYNN (1967) DESCRIBED SPINAL EXTRADURAL CYST IN A NEGRO BROTHER AND SISTER, AGES 12 AND 10 AT THE TIME OF DIAGNOSIS. PROGRESSIVE WEAKNESS IN THE LEGS WAS THE MAIN SYMPTOM. ANOTHER SIB MAY ALSO HAVE BEEN AFFECTED. IN ALL THREE SIBS CONGENITAL LYMPHEDEMA OF THE LEG AND DOUBLE ROWS OF EYELASHES (DISTICHIASIS) WERE PRESENT. THE SYNDROME OF LYMPHEDEMA, DISTICHIASIS AND OTHER ANOMALIES HAS BEEN OBSERVED AS A DOMINANT (Q.V.). BERGLAND (1968) FOUND THREE SIBS OUT OF 4 AFFECTED BUT THIS APPEARS TO BE THE SAME FAMILY AS THAT DESCRIBED BY CHYNN (1967). SPINAL EXTRA-DURAL CYSTS ARE VERY RARE. SPINAL ANOMALIES OF THIS TYPE WERE PRESENT IN AFFECTED PERSONS WITH LYMPHEDEMA AND DISTICHIASIS REPORTED BY ROBINOW ET AL. (1970) BUT WERE ASYMPTOMATIC. IT IS LIKELY THAT *SPINAL EXTRADURAL CYST* IS NOT A SEPARATE GENETIC ENTITY BUT MERELY PART OF THE LYMPHEDEMA-DISTICHIASIS SYNDROME.

BERGLAND, R. M.* CONGENITAL INTRASPINAL EXTRADURAL CYST. REPORT OF THREE CASES IN ONE FAMILY. J. NEUROSURG. 28* 495-499, 1968.

CHYNN, K.-Y.* CONGENITAL SPINAL EXTRADURAL CYST IN TWO SIBLINGS. AM. J. ROENTGEN. 101* 204-215, 1967.

ROBINOW, M., JOHNSON, G. F. AND VERHAGEN, A. D.* DISTICHIASIS-LYMPHEDEMA. A HEREDITARY SYNDROME OF MULTIPLE CONGENITAL DEFECTS. AM. J. DIS. CHILD. 119* 343-347, 1970.

*27120 SPINAL MUSCULAR ATROPHY, RYUKYUAN TYPE

IN THE RYUKYU ISLANDS OF JAPAN, KONDO ET AL. (1970) DESCRIBED A FORM OF SPINAL MUSCULAR ATROPHY WHICH MAY BE DIFFERENT FROM ANY PREVIOUSLY DESCRIBED. THE DISEASE BEGAN IN EARLY INFANCY AND CAUSED SYMMETRIC PROXIMAL MUSCULAR ATROPHY, MORE SEVERE IN THE LOWER EXTREMITIES THAN IN THE UPPER. FASCICULATIONS, SLIGHT KYPHOSCOLIOSIS AND PES CAVUS WERE SEEN. THE EVIDENCE OF RECESSIVE INHERITANCE IS CONVINCING. A COMMON ANCESTOR OF ALL THE PATIENTS WAS THOUGHT TO BE A LORD WHO LIVED IN NORTHERN OKINAWA FROM 1314 TO 1429. THE MUTATION MUST HAVE OCCURRED BEFORE THE 14TH CENTURY. THE PRESENT DISTRIBUTION OF CASES COULD BE EXPLAINED BY THE ACTIVITIES OF ANCESTORS SEVERAL CENTURIES AGO. WHETHER THIS DISEASE IS SEPARATE FROM KUGELBERG-WELANDER DISEASE, A HETEROGENEOUS ENTITY, IS NOT CERTAIN, AND IT RESEMBLES LIMB-GIRDLE MUSCULAR DYSTROPHY (WHICH IS ALSO HETEROGENEOUS).

KONDO, K., TSUBAKI, T. AND SAKAMOTO, F.* THE RYUKYUAN MUSCULAR ATROPHY. AN OBSCURE HERITABLE NEUROMUSCULAR DISEASE FOUND IN THE ISLANDS OF SOUTHERN JAPAN. J. NEUROL. SCI. 11* 359-382, 1970.

27130 SPLEEN, ABSENCE OF (ASPLENIA SYNDROME)

CONGENITAL ABSENCE OF THE SPLEEN IS USUALLY ACCOMPANIED BY COMPLEX CARDIAC MALFORMATIONS, MALPOSITION AND MALDEVELOPMENT OF THE ABDOMINAL ORGANS, AND ABNORMAL LOBATION OF THE LUNGS. HEINZ AND HOWELL-JOLLY BODIES IN THE PERIPHERAL BLOOD ARE HEMATOLOGIC SIGNS OF ABSENT SPLEEN. A FEW CASES HAVE HAD MULTIPLE SPLEENS. MOST CASES ARE SPORADIC. HOWEVER, FAMILIAL INCIDENCE HAS BEEN OBSERVED TWICE. A PATIENT WITH THE TYPICAL ASPLENIA SYNDROME HAD A SIB WHO AT AUTOPSY SHOWED MULTIPLE ACCESSORY SPLEENS, PERSISTENT ATRIOVENTICULARIS COMMUNIS AND PARTIAL TRANSPOSITION OF THE ABDOMINAL VISCERA (POLHEMUS AND SCHAFER, 1952). IN A SECOND FAMILY 3 SIBS HAD ASPLENIA WITH CYANOTIC CONGENITAL HEART DISEASE (RUTTEN-BERG ET AL., 1964).

POLHEMUS, D. W. AND SCHAFER, W. B.* CONGENITAL ABSENCE OF SPLEEN. SYNDROME WITH ATRIOVENTRICULARIS AND SITUS INVERSUS. CASE REPORTS AND REVIEW OF LITERA-TURE. PEDIATRICS 9* 696-708, 1952.

RUTTENBERG, H. D., NEUFELD, H. N., LUCAS, R. V., JR., CAREY, L. S., ADAMS, P., JR., ANDERSON, R. C. AND EDWARDS, J. E.* SYNDROME OF CONGENITAL CARDIAC DISEASE WITH ASPLENIA. DISTINCTION FROM OTHER FORMS OF CONGENITAL CYANOTIC CARDIAC DISEASE. AM. J. CARDIOL. 13* 387-406, 1964.

*27140 SPLENIC HYPOPLASIA

KEVY ET AL. (1968) DESCRIBED A SIBSHIP WITH CONSANGUINEOUS PARENTS, IN WHICH ONE OF TWO BOYS AND TWO OF THREE GIRLS HAD SPLENIC HYPOPLASIA. ONE OF THE CHILDREN DIED AT 10 MONTHS OF OVERWHELMING HAEMOPHILUS INFLUENZAE SEPSIS. THE OTHER TWO HAD REPEATED EPISODES OF PNEUMOCOCCAL MENINGITIS AND H. INFLUENZAE SEPSIS.

ABSENCE OF THE SPLEEN WAS DEMONSTRATED BY RADIOACTIVE SCANNING AFTER INJECTION OF AU(198) COLLOID AND CHROMIUM-TAGGED, HEATED RED CELLS, BY THE PRESENCE OF HOWELL-JOLLY BODIES AND HEINZ BODIES IN THE PERIPHERAL BLOOD, AND BY FAILURE TO SYNTHE-SIZE ANTIBODY TO SHEEP RED BLOOD CELLS INJECTED INTRAVENOUSLY. THE SITUATION IS COMPARABLE TO THAT IN INFANTS IN WHOM THE SPLEEN IS REMOVED IN EARLY LIFE.

KEVY, S. V., TEFFT, M., VAWTER, G. F. AND ROSEN, F. S.* HEREDITARY SPLENIC HYPOPLASIA. PEDIATRICS 42* 752-758, 1968.

27150 SPLENOPORTAL VASCULAR ANOMALIES

BARBAGALLO SANGIORGI, PAGLIARO AND LA SETA (1965) DESCRIBED TWO FAMILIES. IN ONE, TWO OF 4 BROTHERS HAD SPLENOMEGALY, COMPENSATED CIRRHOSIS AND MILD DIABETES. SPLENIC VENOGRAPH SHOWED SPLENOCAVAL SHUNT AND ONE HAD CHRONIC HYPERAMMONIACAL ENCEPHALOPATHY. IN THE SECOND FAMILY A BROTHER AND TWO SISTERS HAD SPLENOMEGALY, ASCITES AND ANOMALOUS SPLENOPORTAL VENOUS SYSTEM. THE FATHER AND ANOTHER BROTHER WERE SYMPTOM FREE BUT HAD SPLENOMEGALY. THE VASCULAR ANOMALY MAY HAVE BEEN SECONDARY TO HEPATIC FIBROSIS AND THE DISORDER MAY BE EITHER IDENTICAL TO THAT DISCUSSED ELSEWHERE (SEE HEPATIC FIBROSIS) OR MAY HAVE BEEN NON-GENETIC.

BARBAGALLO SANGIORGI, G., PAGLIARO, L. AND LA SETA, A.* FAMILIAL OCCURRENCE OF CONGENITAL SPLENOPORTAL ANOMALIES. LANCET 1* 962-963, 1965.

*27160 SPONDYLOEPIPHYSEAL DYSPLASIA

GOLDING (1935) AND KLENERMAN (1961) DESCRIBED TWO SONS AND A DAUGHTER OF A FIRST COUSIN MARRIAGE SHOWING SHORT STATURE, FLAT VERTEBRAE AND SEVERE HIP DISEASE. IN THE PROBAND SYMPTOMS IN THE BACK BEGAN AT 15 YEARS FOLLOWED BY SYMPTOMS REFERABLE TO THE HIPS. MULTIPLE LOOSE BODIES WERE REMOVED FROM VARIOUS JOINTS OF ONE SIB - 18 FROM THE RIGHT HIP AT ABOUT AGE 26, SEVERAL FROM LEFT ELBOW AT AGE 28 AND 30 FROM THE LEFT HIP AT AGE 33. THE PROBAND WAS ABOUT 52 YEARS OLD AT THE TIME OF KLENERMAN'S REPORT. SEVERE OSTEOARTHRITIS OF THE HIPS WAS A FEATURE. THE AUTHORS SUGGESTED A RELATIONSHIP TO MORQUIO-BRAILSFORD'S CHONDRO-OSTEODYSTROPHY, BUT THIS SEEMS DOUBTFUL. MARTIN ET AL. (1970) DESCRIBED TWO BROTHERS, OFFSPRING OF A SECOND COUSIN MARRIAGE, WITH PLATYSPONDYLY, FLATTENING OF THE METATARSAL AND METACARPAL BEADS AND SYMMETRICAL POLYARTICULAR OSTEOARTHRITIS. NO BETA-2-GLOBULIN WAS DEMONSTRATED IN THEIR SERA. THE PATIENTS WERE NATIVES OF THE MAGDALEN ISLANDS IN THE GULF OF ST. LAWRENCE AND MANY OTHERS OF THAT POPULATION WERE FOUND TO HAVE EITHER ABSENCE OR RELATIVE DEFICIENCY OF BETA-2-GLOBULIN (MARTIN, 1970). HENCE, IT MAY REPRESENT A SEPARATE GENETIC TRAIT.

R
E
C
E
S
S
I
V
E

GOLDING, F. C.* CHONDRO-OSTEO DYSTROPHY. BRIT. J. RADIOL. 8* 457-465, 1935.

KLENERMAN, L.* AN ADULT CASE OF CHONDRO-OSTEODYSTROPHY. PROC. ROY. SOC. MED. 54* 71-73, 1961.

MARTIN, J. R.* MONTREAL, CANADA* PERSONAL COMMUNICATION, 1970.

MARTIN, J. R., MACEWAN, D. W., BLAIS, J. A., METRAKOS, J., GOLD, P., LANGER, F. AND HILL, R. O.* PLATYSPONDYLY, POLYARTICULAR OSTEOARTHRITIS, AND ABSENT BETA-2-GLOBULIN IN TWO BROTHERS. ARTH. RHEUM. 13* 53-67, 1970.

*27170 SPONDYLOEPIPHYSEAL DYSPLASIA, PSEUDO-ACHONDROPLASTIC TYPES

AS INDICATED UNDER THIS ENTRY IN THE DOMINANT CATALOG (Q.V.), HALL AND DORST (1969) SUGGESTED THE EXISTENCE OF AT LEAST FOUR TYPES OF PSEUDO-ACHONDROPLASTIC SED, TWO DOMINANT AND TWO RECESSIVE. SEE THEIR PUBLICATION FOR THE DIFFERENTIAL FEATURES AND FOR DESCRIPTION OF ILLUSTRATIVE CASES.

HALL, J. G. AND DORST, J. P.* PSEUDOACHONDROPLASTIC SED, RECESSIVE MAROTEAUX-LAMY TYPE. THE CLINICAL DELINEATION OF BIRTH DEFECTS. IV. SKELETAL DYSPLASIAS. NEW YORK* NATIONAL FOUNDATION, 1969. PP. 254-259.

27180 SPONDYLOMETAPHYSEAL DYSOSTOSIS

KOZLOWSKI ET AL. (1967) DELINEATED THIS ENTITY. THE CONDITION PROMPTS MEDICAL ATTENTION BECAUSE OF SHORT STATURE, USUALLY BETWEEN AGES 1 AND 4 YEARS. SHOR-TENING OF THE TRUNK IS THE MAIN FACTOR IN THE SHORT STATURE. UNUSUAL, PERHAPS UNIQUE, RADIOLOGIC CHANGES OCCUR IN THE DISTAL METAPHYSEAL OF THE FEMUR BEFORE AGE SIX. METAPHYSEAL CHANGES ARE STRIKING IN THE FEMORAL NECK AND TROCHANTERIC AREA. GENERALIZED PLATYSPONDYLY IS A STRIKING FEATURE. SIMILAR CASES OF THIS CONDITION, WHICH IS USUALLY TERMED MORQUIO'S SYNDROME, WERE FOUND IN THE LITERATURE. THE AUTHORS SUSPECTED AUTOSOMAL RECESSIVE INHERITANCE.

KOZLOWSKI, K., MAROTEAUX, P. AND SPRANGER, J.* LA DYSOSTOSE SPONDYLO-METAPHY-SAIRE. PRESSE MED. 75* 2769-2774, 1967.

MICHEL, J., GRENIER, B., CASTAING, J., AUGIER, J. L. AND DESBUQUOIS, G.* DEUX CASE FAMILIAUX DE DYSPLASIE SPONDYLO-METAPHYSAIRE. ANN. RADIOL. 13* 251-254, 1970.

PIFFARETTI, P. G., DELGADO, H. AND NUSSLE, D.* LA DYSOSTOSE SPONDYLO-METAPHY-

REMY, J., NUYTS, J. P., BOMBART, E. AND REMBERT, A.* LA DYSOSTOSE SPONDYLO-METAPHYSAIRE. A PROPOS DE DEUX OBSERVATIONS. ANN. RADIOL. 13* 419-425, 1970.

*27190 SPONGY DEGENERATION OF CENTRAL NERVOUS SYSTEM

SALIENT CLINICAL FEATURES ARE ONSET IN EARLY INFANCY, ATONIA OF NECK MUSCLES, HYPEREXTENSION OF LEGS AND FLEXION OF ARMS, BLINDNESS, SEVERE MENTAL DEFECT, MEGALOCEPHALY AND DEATH BY 18 MONTHS ON THE AVERAGE. PATHOLOGIC STUDIES SHOW SPONGY DEGENERATION OF THE WHITE MATTER. IN THIS COUNTRY THE DISORDER HAS BEEN OBSERVED IN INFANTS OF JEWISH EXTRACTION WHOSE ANCESTORS LIVED IN VILNA (BANKER ET AL., 1964). SPONGY DEGENERATION IS A NON-SPECIFIC MORPHOLOGIC CHANGE WHICH OCCURS IN A NUMBER OF SITUATIONS. SEE LACTIC ACIDOSIS WITH SPONGY DEGENERATION. SPONGY DEGENERATION RATHER CLOSELY RESEMBLING THAT OF VAN BOGAERT-BERTRAND'S DISEASE WAS OBSERVED IN A CASE OF HOMOCYSTINURIA (CHOU AND WAISMAN, 1965). THIS IS ALSO CALLED CANAVAN'S DISEASE. IN AN IRANIAN FAMILY WITH FIRST-COUSIN PARENTS, MAHLOUDJI ET AL. (1970) DESCRIBED FOUR AFFECTED SIBS OUT OF 9.

ADUCHI, M. AND ARONSON, S. M.* STUDIES ON SPONGY DEGENERATION OF THE CENTRAL NERVOUS SYSTEM (VAN BOGAERT-BERTRAND TYPE). IN, ARONSON, S. M. AND VOLK, B. W. (EDS.)* INBORN DISORDERS OF SPHINGOLIPID METABOLISM. OXFORD* PERGAMON PRESS, 1967. PP. 129-147.

BANKER, B. Q., ROBERTSON, J. T. AND VICTOR, M.* SPONGY DEGENERATION OF THE CENTRAL NERVOUS SYSTEM IN INFANCY. NEUROLOGY 14* 981-1001, 1964.

CHOU, S. M. AND WAISMAN, H. A.* SPONGY DEGENERATION OF THE CENTRAL NERVOUS SYSTEM. CASE OF HOMOCYSTINURIA. ARCH. PATH. 79* 357-363, 1965.

HOGAN, G. R. AND RICHARDSON, E. P., JR.* SPONGY DEGENERATION OF THE NERVOUS SYSTEM (CANAVAN'S DISEASE). REPORT OF A CASE IN AN IRISH-AMERICAN FAMILY. PEDIATRICS 35* 284-294, 1965.

MAHLOUDJI, M., DANESHBOD, K. AND KARJOO, M.* FAMILIAL SPONGY DEGENERATION OF THE BRAIN. ARCH. NEUROL. 22* 294-298, 1970.

MORCALDI, L., SALVATI, G., GIORDANO, G. G. AND GUAZZI, G. C.* CONGENITAL VAN BOGAERT-BERTRAND DISEASE IN A NON-JEWISH FAMILY. ACTA GENET. MED. GEM. 18* 142-157, 1969.

VAN BOGAERT, L.* FAMILIAL SPONGY DEGENERATION OF THE BRAIN. (COMPLEMENTARY STUDY OF THE FAMILY R). ACTA PSYCHIAT. NEUROL. SCAND. 39* 107-113, 1963.

ZU RHEIN, G. M., EICHMAN, P. L. AND PULETTI, F.* FAMILIAL IDIOCY WITH SPONGY DEGENERATION OF THE CENTRAL NERVOUS SYSTEM OF VAN BOGAERT-BERTRAND TYPE. NEUROLOGY 10* 998-1006, 1960.

27200 SUCROSURIA, HIATUS HERNIA AND MENTAL RETARDATION

SUCROSURIA HAS BEEN OBSERVED WITH MENTAL DEFICIENCY IN SEVERAL CASES. HOWEVER, PERRY ET AL. (1959) CONCLUDED THAT THE ASSOCIATION IS COINCIDENTAL. FURTHERMORE, SUCROSURIA HAS NOT BEEN PROVED TO REPRESENT AN INBORN ERROR. THIS IS PROBABLY NOT A SINGLE GENE DISORDER BUT RATHER A NON-SPECIFIC SYNDROME DUE TO ATONIC STATE OF SEVERELY MENTALLY RETARDED CHILDREN, WITH ABSORPTION OF UNDIGESTED SUCROSE FROM THE ATONIC BOWEL.

MONCRIEFF, A. A.* BIOCHEMISTRY OF MENTAL DEFECT. LANCET 2* 273-278, 1960.

PERRY, T. L., LIPPMAN, R. W., WALKER, D. AND SHAW, K. N. F.* SUCROSURIA AND MENTAL DEFICIENCY* A COINCIDENCE. PEDIATRICS 24* 774-779, 1959.

STERN, J. AND SYLVESTER, P. E.* SUCROSURIA, HIATUS HERNIA AND MENTAL RETARDA-TION. PROC. LONDON CONF. ON SCIENTIFIC STUDY OF MENTAL DEFICICIENCY. (1960), DAGENHAM* MAY AND BAKER LTD., 1962. PP. 153-159.

WOODRUFF, G. G., JR.* SUCROSURIA IN ASSOCIATION WITH MENTAL DEFICIENCY AND HIATAL HERNIA. J. PEDIAT. 52* 66-72, 1958.

27210 SUDANOPHILIC CEREBRAL SCLEROSIS

THE DISORDER SEEMS TO BEGIN RARELY IN EARLY INFANCY. HOWEVER, THE PAUCITY OF MYELIN IN THE CEREBRAL HEMISPHERES DURING THE FIRST 4-6 MONTHS OF LIFE WOULD MAKE HISTOPATHOLOGIC CLASSIFICATION ON THE BASIS OF MYELIN BREAKDOWN DIFFICULT AT THIS STAGE. PROGRESSION IS USUALLY SUBACUTE IN PACE. CORTICAL BLINDNESS IS OFTEN A CONSPICUOUS FEATURE. SIBS MAY SHOW GREAT DIFFERENCES IN THE SITE OF THE LESION, AGE OF ONSET AND RATE OF PROGRESSION (MEYER AND PILKINGTON, 1936).

GREENFIELD, J. G.* IN, NEUROPATHOLOGY. LONDON* EDWARD ARNOLD LTD., 1958. P. 460 FF.

MEYER, A. AND PILKINGTON, F.* SOME PROBLEMS OF PATHOGENESIS IN SCHILDER'S

R
E
C
E
S
S
I
V
E

DISEASE, WITH DESCRIPTION OF A NEW FAMILIAL CASE. J. MENT. SCI. 82* 812-826, 1936.

*27220 SULFATIDOSIS, JUVENILE, AUSTIN TYPE

AT LEAST THREE PATIENTS HAVE BEEN DESCRIBED (AUSTIN, 1965* THIEFFRY ET AL., 1967). THE DISORDER COMBINES FEATURES OF METACHROMATIC LEUKODYSTROPHY AND OF A MUCOPOLY-SACCHARIDOSIS. INCREASED AMOUNTS OF ACID MUCOPOLYSACCHARIDES ARE FOUND IN THE WINE AND SEVERAL TISSUES. WHEREAS IN THE CLASSIC FORM OF METACHROMATIC LEUKODYS-TROPHY ARYLSULFATASE A, B AND C ARE ABSENT IN THE AUSTIN TYPE OF JUVENILE SULFATIDOSIS. AUSTIN'S TWO PATIENTS WERE SIBS (IN THE M FAMILY). THE GARGOYLISM FEATURES ARE MILD. NEUROLOGIC DETERIORATION IS RAPID. BOTH MUCOPOLYSACCHARIDE AND SULFATIDE ARE FOUND IN THE URINE IN EXCESS. CEREBROSPINAL FLUID PROTEIN IS INCREASED. PERIPHERAL NERVES SHOW METACHROMATIC DEGENERATION OF MYELIN ON BIOPSY. RAMPINI ET AL. (1970) REPORTED THREE ADDITIONAL CASES.

AUSTIN, J. H.* METACHROMATIC LEUKODYSTROPHY. IN, CARTER, C. C. (ED.)* MEDICAL ASPECTS OF MENTAL RETARDATION. SPRINGFIELD, ILL.* CHARLES C THOMAS, 1965. P. 768.

RAMPINI, S., ISLER, W., BAERLOCHER, K., BISCHOFF, A., ULRICH, J. AND PLUSS, H. J.* DIE KOMBINATION VON METACHROMATISCHER LEUKODYSTROPHIE UND MUKOPOLYSACCHARIDOSE ALS SELBSTANDIGES KRANKHEITSBILD (MUKOSULFATIDOSE). HELV. PAEDIAT. ACTA 25* 436-461, 1970.

THIEFFRY, S., LYON, G. AND MAROTEAUX, P.* ENCEPHALOPATHIE METABOLIQUE ASSOCIANT UNE MUCOPOLYSACCHARIDOSE ET UNE SULFATIDOSE. ARCH. FRANC. PEDIAT. 24* 425-432, 1967.

*27230 SULFO-CYSTEINURIA (SULFITE OXIDASE DEFICIENCY)

IN AN INFANT WITH FATAL NEUROLOGIC DISEASE AND ECTOPIA LENTIS, MUDD ET AL. (1967) FOUND INCREASED S-SULFO-L-CYSTEINE, SULFITE AND THIOSULFITE IN THE URINE WITH MARKEDLY DECREASED INORGANIC SULFATE EXCRETION. A DEFICIENCY IN THE ACTIVITY OF SULFITE OXIDASE, AN ENZYME WHICH NORMALLY CATALYZES CONVERSION OF SULFITE TO SULFATE, WAS POSTULATED. SIBS HAD DIED, PROBABLY OF THE SAME DISORDER.

IRREVERRE, F., MUDD, S. H., HEIZER, W. D. AND LASTER, L.* SULFATE OXIDASE DEFICIENCY* STUDIES OF A PATIENT WITH MENTAL RETARDATION, DISLOCATED OCULAR LENSES, AND ABNORMAL URINARY EXCRETION OF S-SULFO-L-CYSTEINE, SULFITE AND THIOSULFATE. BIOCHEM. MED. 1* 187-199, 1967.

MUDD, S. H., IRREVERRE, F. AND LASTER, L.* SULFITE OXIDASE DEFICIENCY IN MAN* DEMONSTRATION OF THE ENZYMATIC DEFECT. SCIENCE 156* 1599-1602, 1967.

27240 SUXAMETHONIUM SENSITIVITY (PSEUDOCHOLINESTERASE DEFICIENCY)

HOMOZYGOUS PERSONS SUSTAINED PROLONGED APNEA AFTER ADMINISTRATION OF THE MUSCLE RELAXANT SUXAMETHONIUM IN CONNECTION WITH SURGICAL ANESTHESIS. PSEUDOCHOLINES-TERASE IN THE SERUM IS LOW IN ITS ACTIVITY AND IS FURTHERMORE ATYPICAL IN ITS SUBSTRATE BEHAVIOR. IN THE ABSENCE OF THE RELAXANT THE HOMOZYGOTE IS AT NO KNOWN DISADVANTAGE. THE DIBUCAINE NUMBER (PERCENTAGE INHIBITION BY DIBUCAINE) IDENTI-FIES THREE GENOTYPES. TWO FURTHER ALLELES ARE A SILENT GENE AND AN ALLELE IDENTIFIED BY FLUORIDE INHIBITION. A NON-ALLELE IS RESPONSIBLE FOR AN ELECTRO-PHORETIC VARIANT. DEFICIENCY OF PSEUDOCHOLINESTERASE IS UNUSUALLY FREQUENT AMONG ALASKAN ESKIMOS (GUTSCHE ET AL., 1967). HETEROGENEITY OF THE 'SILENT' CHOLINES-TERASE GENES WAS INDICATED BY THE STUDIES OF RUBINSTEIN ET AL. (1970). IN AN ESKIMO POPULATION WITH A GENE FREQUENCY FOR SERUM CHOLINESTERASE DEFICIENCY EXCEEDING 10 PERCENT, SCOTT ET AL. (1970) DETERMINED NORMAL ENZYME LEVELS AT VARIOUS AGES AND THE DEGREE OF OVERLAP OF HETEROZYGOUS AND HOMOZYGOUS CLASSES. (NO ASTERISK IS GIVEN IN THIS ENTRY, BECAUSE IN THE DOMINANT CATALOG THE TWO PSEUDOCHOLINESTERASE LOCI ARE LISTED.).

GOEDDE, H. W., DOENICKE, A. AND ALTLAND, K.* PSEUDOCHOLINESTERASEN* PHARMAKO-GENETIK, BIOCHEMIE, KLINIK. BERLIN* SPRINGER-VERLAG, 1967.

GUTSCHE, B. B., SCOTT, E. M. AND WRIGHT, R. C.* HEREDITARY DEFICIENCY OF PSEUDOCHOLINESTERASE IN ESKIMOS. NATURE 215* 322-323, 1967.

HODGKIN, W., GIBLETT, E. R., LEVINE, H., BAUER, W. AND MOTULSKY, A. G.* COMPLETE PSEUDOCHOLINESTERASE DEFICIENCY* GENETIC AND IMMUNOLOGIC CHARACTERIZA-TION. J. CLIN. INVEST. 44* 486-493, 1965.

LEHMANN, H. AND LIDDELL, J.* PSEUDOCHOLINESTERASE DEFICIENCY AND SOME OTHER PHARMACOGENETIC DISORDERS. IN, STANBURY, J. B., WYNGAARDEN, J. B. AND FREDRICK-SON, D. S. (EDS.)* THE METABOLIC BASIS OF INHERITED DISEASE. NEW YORK* MCGRAW-HILL, 1966 (2ND ED.). PP. 1356-1369.

LEHMANN, H. AND SILK, E.* FAMILIAL PSEUDOCHOLINESTERASE DEFICIENCY. BRIT. MED. J. 1* 128-129, 1961.

RUBINSTEIN, H. M., DIETZ, A. A., HODGES, L. K., LUBRANO, T. AND CZEBOTAR, V.*

R
E
C
E
S
S
I
V
E

SCOTT, E. M., WEAVER, D. D. AND WRIGHT, R. C.* DISCRIMINATION OF PHENOTYPES IN
HUMAN SERUM CHOLINESTERASE DEFICIENCY. AM. J. HUM. GENET. 22* 363-369, 1970.

27250 SYSTEMIC CYSTIC ANGIOMATOSIS AND SEIP SYNDROME

IN A NEGRO FAMILY BRUNZELL ET AL. (1968) OBSERVED A COMBINATION OF CONGENITAL
GENERALIZED LIPODYSTROPHY AND SYSTEMIC CYSTIC ANGIOMATOSIS IN 5 OF 12 SIBS. THE
AUTHORS FOUND PREVIOUS REPORTS OF ONLY 14 CASES OF CYSTIC ANGIOMATOSIS, NONE
FAMILIAL. PROGRESSIVE INCAPACITATING BONE INVOLVEMENT OCCURRED. TWO HAD SOFT
TISSUE (E.G., SUBCUTANEOUS) ANGIOMAS. THE LIPODYSTROPHY WAS ACCOMPANIED BY
ACANTHOSIS NIGRICANS, LARGE HANDS AND FEET, ACROMEGALOID FACIAL FEATURES, LIPENIA,
AND HEPATOSPLENOMEGALY AND WAS IN ALL WAYS IDENTICAL TO THAT OF SEIP'S SYNDROME
(Q.V.). THUS, ONE AND THE SAME GENE MAY BE RESPONSIBLE FOR THE SYNDROME IN
REPORTED CASES OF SEIP'S DISEASE AND IN THE AFFECTED PERSONS REPORTED BY BRUNZELL
ET AL. (1968). CYSTIC ANGIOMATOSIS MAY HAVE BEEN LATE IN DEVELOPING OR OVERLOOKED
IN REPORTED CASES.

BRUNZELL, J. D., SHANKLE, S. S. AND BETHUNE, J. E.* CONGENITAL GENERALIZED
LIPODYSTROPHY AND SYSTEMIC CYSTIC ANGIOMATOSIS* THE SIMULTANEOUS OCCURRENCE OF TWO
UNUSUAL SYNDROMES IN A SINGLE FAMILY. ANN. INTERN. MED. 69* 501-516, 1968.

27260 TAPETO-RETINAL DEGENERATION WITH ATAXIA

THERE APPEAR TO BE SEVERAL TYPES. IN ONE TYPE THE ATAXIA IS OF THE MARIE TYPE.
ALTHOUGH THE INHERITANCE IS USUALLY DOMINANT, RECESSIVE PEDIGREES HAVE BEEN
OBSERVED (WALSH, 1957). IN A SECOND FORM THE ATAXIA IS OF FRIEDREICH'S TYPE
(Q.V.). THE INHERITANCE IS RECESSIVE. MIXED OR MORE COMPLEX TYPES OF NEUROLOGIC
INVOLVEMENT WITH ATAXIA OCCUR IN A THIRD TYPE. AS ONE WOULD EXPECT, THIS IS A
HETEROGENEOUS CATEGORY. REFSUM'S DISEASE AND ABETALIPOPROTEINEMIA GIVE THIS
COMBINATION OF FINDINGS. SEE ALSO NERVOUS SYSTEM DISORDER RESEMBLING REFSUM'S
DISEASE AND HURLER'S DISEASE. SEE OLIVOPONTOCEREBELLAR ATAXIA WITH MACULAR
DYSTROPHY.

FRANCESCHETTI, A., FRANCOIS, J. AND BAHEL, J.* LES HEREDO-DEGENERESCENCES
CHOROIDO-RETINIENNES (DEGENERESCENCES TAPETO-RETINIENNES). PARIS* MASSON, 2*
1963.

WALSH, F. B.* CLINICAL NEURO-OPHTHALMOLOGY. BALTIMORE* WILLIAMS AND WILKINS,
1957 (2ND ED.). PP. 620.

27270 TAURODONTISM

THIS TRAIT IS CHARACTERIZED BY LARGE PULP CHAMBERS. THE CHANGES ARE USUALLY MOST
STRIKING IN THE MOLARS. SHAW (1928) CLAIMED THAT THE TRAIT IS INHERITED AS AN
AUTOSOMAL RECESSIVE BUT MUCH MORE EVIDENCE IS REQUIRED.

SHAW, J. C. M.* TAURODENT TEETH IN SOUTH AFRICAN RACES. J. ANAT. 62* 476-498,
1928.

*27280 TAY-SACHS DISEASE (AMAUROTIC FAMILY IDIOCY)

TAY-SACHS DISEASE IS CHARACTERIZED BY THE ONSET IN INFANCY OF DEVELOPMENTAL
RETARDATION, FOLLOWED BY PARALYSIS, DEMENTIA AND BLINDNESS, WITH DEATH IN THE
SECOND OR THIRD YEAR OF LIFE. A GRAY-WHITE AREA AROUND THE FOVEA CENTRALIS, DUE
TO LIPID-LADEN GANGLION CELLS, LEAVING A CENTRAL 'CHERRY-RED' SPOT IS A TYPICAL
FUNDOSCOPIC FINDING. PATHOLOGICAL VERIFICATION IS PROVIDED BY THE FINDING OF THE
TYPICALLY BALLOONED NEURONS IN THE CENTRAL NERVOUS SYSTEM. THE FREQUENCY OF THE
CONDITION IS MUCH HIGHER IN ASHKENAZI JEWS OF EASTERN EUROPEAN ORIGIN THAN IN
OTHERS. PARENTAL CONSANGUINITY IS FREQUENT IN NON-JEWISH CASES, RELATIVELY
INFREQUENT IN THE JEWISH CASES - FACTS WHICH ALSO EMPHASIZE THE DIFFERENCE IN GENE
FREQUENCY IN THE TWO GROUPS. THE GENE FREQUENCY IN NEW YORK CITY JEWS IS BETWEEN
0.013 AND 0.016 AND THAT IN NON-JEWS IS ONLY ABOUT ONE-HUNDREDTH OF THIS VALUE.
FRUCTOSE-1-PHOSPHATE ALDOLASE IS DEFICIENT IN THE SERUM AND GLUTAMIC OXALACETIC
TRANSAMINASE AND LACTIC DEHYDROGENASE ARE ELEVATED. AN EARLY AND PERSISTENT
EXTENSION RESPONSE TO SOUND ('STARTLE REACTION') IS USEFUL FOR RECOGNIZING THE
DISORDER. ZEMAN (1966) IS OF THE OPINION THAT ONLY THREE ENTITIES DESERVE BEING
CALLED AMAUROTIC IDIOCY, NAMELY, (1) CONGENITAL AMAUROTIC IDIOCY, (2) TAY-SACHS
DISEASE, AND (3) GENERALIZED GANGLIOSIDOSIS. IN ALL OF THESE EXCESSIVE ACCUMULA-
TION OF GANGLIOSIDES HAS BEEN DEMONSTRATED BY THIN-LAYER CHROMATOGRAPHY. IN THE
SO-CALLED JUVENILE AND ADULT FORMS OF AMAUROTIC IDIOCY NO ABNORMALITY OF GANGLIO-
SIDES OR OTHER LIPIDS HAS BEEN FOUND, THUS INDICATING THE TAXONOMIC INAPPROPRIA-
TENESS OF CLASSIFYING THESE WITH TAY-SACHS DISEASE. THE THREE TRUE GANGLIOSIDOSES
HAVE ONSET DURING INFANCY AND SHOW STRIKING MEGALENCEPHALY. BALINT ET AL. (1967)
FOUND THAT BOTH HOMOZYGOTES AND HETEROZYGOTES SHOW REDUCED SPHINGOMYELIN IN RED
BLOOD CELLS AND FOUND THIS REDUCTION USEFUL IN CARRIER IDENTIFICATION. ACCUMULA-
TION OF A GLYCOPROTEIN IN RED CELLS OF PATIENTS WITH TAY-SACHS DISEASE DEMONS-
TRATED BY BALINT AND KYRIAKIDES (1968) MAY HAVE BEARING ON THE NATURE OF THE
PRIMARY DEFECT. THE BASIC ENZYME DEFECT HAS BEEN SHOWN BY OKADA AND O'BRIEN
(1969) TO CONCERN ONE COMPONENT OF A HEXOSAMINIDASE. TOTAL HEXOSAMINIDASE

R
E
C
E
S
S
I
V
E

ACTIVITY WAS NORMAL BUT WHEN COMPONENTS A AND B WERE SEPARATED, COMPONENT A WAS FOUND TO BE ABSENT. HULTBERG (1969) CONFIRMED THE FINDINGS OF OKADA AND O'BRIEN (1969). OKADA ET AL. (1971) COMPARED THE FINDINGS IN REGARD TO HEXOSAMINIDASES A AND B IN THE THREE FORMS OF GANGLIOSIDE GM(2) STORAGE DISEASE (TAY-SACHS DISEASE, SANDHOFF'S DISEASE, AND JUVENILE GM(2) GANGLIOSIDOSIS).

ARONSON, S. M., VALSAMIS, M. P. AND VOLK, B. W.* INFANTILE AMAUROTIC FAMILY IDIOCY* OCCURRENCE, GENETIC CONSIDERATIONS AND PATHOPHYSIOLOGY IN THE NON-JEWISH INFANT. PEDIATRICS 26* 229-242, 1960.

BALINT, J. A. AND KYRIAKIDES, E. C.* STUDIES OF RED CELL STROMAL PROTEINS IN TAY-SACHS DISEASE. J. CLIN. INVEST. 47* 1858-1864, 1968.

BALINT, J. A., KYRIAKIDES, E. C. AND SPITZER, H. L.* ON THE CHEMICAL CHANGES IN THE RED CELL STROMA IN TAY-SACHS DISEASE* THEIR VALUE AS GENETIC TRACERS. IN, ARONSON, S. M. AND VOLK, B. W. (EDS.)* INBORN DISORDERS OF SPHINGOLIPID METABO-LISM. OXFORD* PERGAMON PRESS, 1967. PP. 423-430.

BRADY, R. O.* CEREBRAL LIPIDOSES. ANN. REV. MED. 21* 317-334, 1970.

FREDRICKSON, D. S. AND TRAMS, E. G.* GANGLIOSIDE LIPIDOSIS* TAY-SACHS DISEASE. IN, STANBURY, J. B., WYNGAARDEN, J. B. AND FREDRICKSON, D. S. (EDS.)* THE METABOLIC BASIS OF INHERITED DISEASE. NEW YORK* MCGRAW-HILL, 1966 (2ND ED.). PP. 523-538.

HANHART, E.* UBER 27 SIPPEN MIT INFANTILER AMAUROTISCHER IDIOTIE (TAY-SACHS). ACTA GENET. MED. GEM. 3* 331-364, 1954.

HULTBERG, B.* N-ACETYLHEXOSAMINIDASE ACTIVITIES IN TAY-SACHS DISEASE. (LETTER) LANCET 2* 1195 ONLY, 1969.

O'BRIEN, J. S., OKADA, S., CHEN, A. AND FILLERUP, D. L.* TAY-SACHS DISEASE* DETECTION OF HETEROZYGOTES AND HOMOZYGOTES BY SERUM HEXOSAMINIDASE ASSAY. NEW ENG. J. MED. 283* 15-20, 1970.

OKADA, S. AND O'BRIEN, J. S.* TAY-SACHS DISEASE* GENERALIZED ABSENCE OF A BETA-D-N-ACETYLHEXOSAMINIDASE COMPONENT. SCIENCE 165* 698-700, 1969.

OKADA, S., VEATH, M. L., LEROY, J. AND O'BRIEN, J. S.* GANGLIOSIDE GM(2) STORAGE DISEASES* HEXOSAMINIDASE DEFICIENCIES IN CULTURED FIBROBLASTS. AM. J. HUM. GENET. 23* 55-61, 1971.

SCHNECK, L., MAISEL, J. AND VOLK, B. W.* THE STARTLE RESPONSE AND SERUM ENZYME PROFILE IN EARLY DETECTION OF TAY-SACHS DISEASE. J. PEDIAT. 65* 749-756, 1964.

VOLK, B. W.* TAY-SACHS DISEASE. NEW YORK* GRUNE AND STRATTON, 1964.

ZEMAN, W.* INDIANAPOLIS, IND.* PERSONAL COMMUNICATION, 1966.

R
E
C
E
S
S
I
V
E

27290 TAY-SACHS DISEASE (JUVENILE TYPE)

COMPONENT A MAY BE A GROUP OF ENZYMES AND THE PARTIAL DEFICIENCY IN THE JUVENILE FORM MAY BE IN FACT TOTAL ABSENCE OF ONE OF THESE ENZYMES.

SUZUKI, Y. AND SUZUKI, K.* PARTIAL DEFICIENCY OF HEXOSAMINIDASE COMPONENT A IN JUVENILE G(M2)-GANGLIOSIDOSIS. NEUROLOGY 20* 848-851, 1970.

27300 TEETH, FUSED

DEPPENDORF (1912) DESCRIBED BILATERAL FUSION OF THE DECIDUOUS INCISORS IN SISTERS, AGED 4 AND 5 AND ONE HALF YEARS, AND ALSO A RARER CONDITION, BILATERAL FUSION OF A DECIDUOUS MANDIBULAR CANINE WITH THE SECOND INCISOR.

DEPPENDORF, (NI)* BEITRAGE ZUR VERSCHMELZUNG UND ZURLLINGSBILDUNG MENSCHLICHER ZAHNE IM MILCH- UND IM BLEIBENDEN GEBISS. DEUTSCH. MSCHR. ZAHNHEILK. 5* 427-432, 1912.

27310 TESTES, ABSENCE OF

ABEYARATNE ET AL. (1969) DESCRIBED 16 CASES OF APPARENT COMPLETE ABSENCE OF TESTES IN PHENOTYPIC MALES, INCLUDING ONE PAIR OF AFFECTED SIBS. BOBROW AND GOUGH (1970) ALSO DESCRIBED TWO AFFECTED BROTHERS. THIS FAMILIAL DISORDER MAY BE UNILATERAL IN A PORTION OF CASES. FAMILIAL OCCURRENCE WAS ALSO NOTED BY OVERZIER AND LINDEN (1956) AND BY KOOPMAN (1930), ACCORDING TO FERRIER (1969), WHO IN TWINS BLOOD SHOWED THEM PROBABLY TO BE MONOZYGOTIC DESCRIBED ANORCHIA IN ONLY ONE.

ABEYARATNE, M. R., AHERNE, W. A. AND SCOTT, J. E. S.* THE VANISHING TESTIS. LANCET 2* 822-824, 1969.

BOBROW, M. AND GOUGH, M. H.* BILATERAL ABSENCE OF TESTES. (LETTER) LANCET 1* 366 ONLY, 1970.

OVERZIER, C. AND LINDEN, H.* ECHTER AGONADISMUS (ANORCHISMUS) BEI GESCHWISTERN. GYNAECOLOGIA 142* 215-233, 1956.

27320 TESTICULAR FEMINIZATION, INCOMPLETE TYPE

THIS SYNDROME DIFFERS FROM COMPLETE TESTICULAR FEMINIZATION IN THE PRESENCE OF CLITORAL ENLARGEMENT AND SOMETIMES PARTIAL FUSION OF THE LABIA AT BIRTH AND VIRILIZATION AT PUBERTY. THE PEDIGREE PATTERN IS LIKE THAT OF AN X-LINKED RECESSIVE IN SEVERAL PUBLISHED FAMILIES, BUT PHILIP AND TROLLE (1965) DESCRIBED A FAMILY IN WHICH FOUR SIBS, THE PRODUCT OF A CONSANGUINEOUS MATING, AND THEIR PATERNAL COUSINS WERE AFFECTED.

PHILIP, J. AND TROLLE, D.* FAMILIAL MALE HERMAPHRODITISM WITH DELAYED AND PARTIAL MASCULINIZATION. AM. J. OBSTET. GYNEC. 93* 1076-1083, 1965.

27330 TESTICULAR TUMORS

HUTTER ET AL. (1967) REVIEWED THE REPORTS OF TESTICULAR TUMORS IN BROTHERS AND IN TWINS AND REPORTED AFFECTED BROTHERS.

HUTTER, A. M., LYNCH, J. J. AND SHNIDER, B. I.* MALIGNANT TESTICULAR TUMORS IN BROTHERS. A CASE REPORT. J.A.M.A. 199* 1009-1010, 1967.

27340 TETRAMELIC DEFICIENCIES, ECTODERMAL DYSPLASIA, DEFORMED EARS, AND OTHER ABNORMALITIES

FREIRE-MAIA (1970) DESCRIBED A BRAZILIAN FAMILY IN WHICH A BROTHER AND SISTER AND TWO DECEASED BROTHERS SHOWED SEVERE ABSENCE DEFORMITIES OF ALL FOUR LIMBS, HYPOTRICHOSIS, ABNORMAL TEETH, HYPOPLASTIC NIPPLES AND AREOLAE AND DEFORMED AURICLES. HIS CONSISTENT FEATURES INCLUDED HYPOPLASTIC NAILS, HYPOGONADISM, THYROID ENLARGEMENT, INCOMPLETE CLEFT LIP, MENTAL RETARDATION, AND ECG AND EEG ABNORMALITIES. BOTH LIVING SIBS SHOWED AN EXCESS OF TYROSINE AND-OR TRYPTOPHANE IN THE URINE. PARENTAL CONSANGUINITY WAS DENIED BUT THE PARENTS CAME FROM THE SAME FARM IN ONE OF THE MOST INBRED AREAS OF BRAZIL.

FREIRE-MAIA, N.* A NEWLY RECOGNIZED GENETIC SYNDROME OF TETRAMELIE DEFICIEN-CIES, ECTODERMAL DYSPLASIA, DEFORMED EARS, AND OTHER ABNORMALITIES. AM. J. HUM. GENET. 22* 370-377, 1970.

27350 THALASSEMIAS

IT SEEMS JUSTIFIED TO INCLUDE THALASSEMIA MAJOR IN A CATALOG OF RARE RECESSIVE PHENOTYPES. (NO ASTERISK IS USED BECAUSE IT IS NOT CERTAIN THAT MUTATION ELSEWHERE THAN AT THE ESTABLISHED STRUCTURAL LOCI FOR HEMOGLOBIN IS INVOLVED.) APPARENT HOMOZYGOTES HAVE BEEN OBSERVED IN THE OFFSPRING OF CONSANGUINEOUS MARRIAGES IN BIRMINGHAM, ENGLAND (LLOYD AND BROWN, 1962). THE GENE INVOLVED MAY HAVE ARISEN BY MUTATION AND NOT BEEN INTRODUCED BY EARLY TRAVELERS FROM THE MEDITERRANEAN. THE SAME ARGUMENT CAN BE PROPOSED FOR THE SICKLE HOMOZYGOTE (SEE SICKLE CELL ANEMIA). TWO VARIETIES OF THALASSEMIA HAVE BEEN RECOGNIZED ACCORDING TO THEIR BEHAVIOR IN THE HETEROZYGOUS STATE WITH ALPHA AND BETA CHAIN MUTANTS. THUS, BETA THALASSEMIA INTERACTS WITH HB S (A BETA CHAIN VARIANT) TO RESULT IN THE CLINICAL PICTURE CALLED SICKLE-THALASSEMIA AND ALPHA THALASSEMIA INTERACTS WITH HB I IN A COMPARABLE MANNER (ATWATER AND COLLEAGUES, 1960). A THIRD VARIETY IS CALLED DELTA THALASSEMIA BECAUSE THE DEFECT CONCERNS AN INABILITY TO MAKE DELTA CHAINS. THE HOMOZYGOTE HAS NO HB A2 (THOMPSON ET AL., 1965). HB LEPORE (SEE DOMINANT CATALOG) ALSO PRODUCES A THALASSEMIA PICTURE. A FOURTH VARIETY OF THALASSEMIA MAY BE CALLED BETA-DELTA TYPE AND MAY LIKE LEPORE HEMOGLOBIN REPRESENT THE RESULT OF FUSION OF THE GENES DETERMINING THE BETA AND DELTA HEMOGLOBIN CHAINS. (THESE GENES BY OTHER EVIDENCE APPEAR TO BE CONTIGUOUS.) COMINGS AND MOTULSKY (1966) SHOWED THAT CIS DELTA CHAINS ARE NOT SYNTHESIZED IN THIS CONDITION WHICH IS ALSO CALLED FETAL THALASSEMIA (BECAUSE OF HIGH HB F). IN THEIR PATIENT WITH THE ABNORMAL BETA-DELTA GENE (ACTUALLY PERHAPS A DELETION) ON ONE CHROMOSOME AND THE HB B(2) GENE IN THE OTHER, NO HB A2 WAS FORMED.

ATWATER, J., SCHWARTZ, I. R. AND TOCANTINS, L. M.* A VARIETY OF HUMAN HEMOGLO-BIN WITH 4 DISTINCT ELECTROPHORETIC COMPONENTS. BLOOD 15* 901-908, 1960.

BUTIKOFER, E., HOIGNE, R., MARTI, H. R. AND BETKE, K.* HAMOGLOBIN-H-THALASSA-MIE. MITTEILUNG EINES FALLES MIT FAMILIENUNTERSUCHUNG. SCHWEIZ. MED. WSCHR. 90* 1215-1217, 1960.

BANNERMAN, R. M. AND CALLENDER, S. T.* THALASSAEMIA IN BRITAIN. (LETTER) BRIT. MED. J. 2* 1288 ONLY, 1961.

CALLENDER, S. T., MALLETT, B. J. AND LEHMANN, H.* THALASSAEMIA IN BRITAIN. BRIT. J. HAEMAT. 7* 1-8, 1961.

COMINGS, D. E. AND MOTULSKY, A. G.* ABSENCE OF CIS DELTA CHAIN SYNTHESIS IN DELTA-BETA THALASSEMIA (F-THALASSEMIA). BLOOD 28* 54-69, 1966.

DITTMAN, W. A., HAUT, A., WINTROBE, M. M. AND CARTWRIGHT, G. E.* HEMOGLOBIN H ASSOCIATED WITH AN UNCOMMON VARIANT OF THALASSEMIA TRAIT. BLOOD 16* 975-983, 1960.

HAVARD, C. W. H., LEHMANN, H. AND SCOTT, R. B.* THALASSAEMIA MINOR IN AN ENGLISH WOMAN. BRIT. MED. J. 1* 304-305, 1958.

HELLER, P., YAKULIS, V. J., ROSENZWEIG, A. I., ABILDGAARD, C. F. AND RUCKNAGEL, D. L.* MILD HOMOZYGOUS BETA-THALASSEMIA* FURTHER EVIDENCE FOR THE HETEROGENEITY OF BETA-THALASSEMIA GENES. ANN. INTERN. MED. 64* 52-61, 1966.

HUISMAN, T. H., PUNT, K. AND SCHAAD, J. D.* THALASSEMIA MINOR ASSOCIATED WITH HEMOGLOBIN-B2 HETEROZYGOSITY* A FAMILY REPORT. BLOOD 17* 747-757, 1961.

ISRAELS, M. C. G. AND TURNER, R. L.* A BRITISH TARGET-CELL ANAEMIA. LANCET 2* 1363-1365, 1955.

LEHMANN, H.* THALASSAEMIA IN BRITAIN. (LETTER) BRIT. MED. J. 2* 1288-1289, 1961.

LLOYD, J. K. AND BROWN, G. A.* HOMOZYGOUS THALASSEMIA IN AN ENGLISH CHILD. (ABSTRACT) PROC. 10TH INTERN. CONGR. PEDIAT., LISBON, 1962. P. 23-24.

MOTULSKY, A. G.* CURRENT CONCEPTS OF THE GENETICS OF THE THALASSEMIAS. COLD SPRING HARBOR SYMPOS. QUANT. BIOL. 29* 399-413, 1964.

NECHELES, T. F., ALLEN, D. M. AND GERALD, P. S.* THE MANY FORMS OF THALASSEMIA* DEFINITION AND CLASSIFICATION OF THE THALASSEMIA SYNDROMES. ANN. N.Y. ACAD. SCI. 165* 5-12, 1969.

PEARSON, H. A. AND MOORE, M. M.* HUMAN HEMOGLOBIN GENE LINKAGE* REPORT OF A FAMILY WITH HEMOGLOBIN B(2), HEMOGLOBIN S, AND BETA-THALASSEMIA, INCLUDING A PROBABLE CROSSOVER BETWEEN THALASSEMIA AND DELTA LOCI. AM. J. HUM. GENET. 17* 125-132, 1965.

SCHWARTZ, E.* THE SILENT CARRIER OF BETA THALASSEMIA. NEW ENG. J. MED. 281* 1327-1333, 1969.

ANNOTATION* THALASSAEMIA IN BRITAIN. BRIT. MED. J. 2* 1139 ONLY, 1961.

THOMPSON, R. B., WARRINGTON, R., ODOM, J. AND BELL, W. N.* INTERACTION BETWEEN GENES FOR DELTA THALASSEMIA AND HEREDITARY PERSISTENCE OF FOETAL HEMOGLOBIN. ACTA GENET. STATIST. MED. 15* 190-200, 1965.

WEATHERALL, D. J.* THE BIOCHEMICAL LESION IN THALASSEMIA. BRIT. J. HAEMAT. 15* 1-5, 1968.

WEATHERALL, D. J.* THE THALASSAEMIA SYNDROME. PHILADELPHIA* F. A. DAVIS CO., 1965.

R
E
C
E
S
S
I
V
E

27360 THALIDOMIDE SUSCEPTIBILITY

KREMER AND FULLERTON (1961) DESCRIBED BROTHER AND SISTER WHO DEVELOPED NEUROPATHY AT THE SAME TIME INTERVAL AFTER STARTING THALIDOMIDE. GENETIC DIFFERENCES IN SUSCEPTIBILITY TO THE TERATOGENIC EFFECTS OF THALIDOMIDE ARE SUSPECTED BUT UNPROVED AND NOTHING IS KNOWN OF GENETIC DIFFERENCES IN THE METABOLISM OF THE DRUG.

KREMER, M. AND FULLERTON, P. M.* NEUROPATHY AFTER THALIDOMIDE ('DISTAVAL'). BRIT. MED. J. 2* 1498 ONLY, 1961.

27370 THIEMANN EPIPHYSEAL DISEASE

BOHME (1963), REPORTED TWO MALE SIBS WITH THIEMANN'S EPIPHYSEAL DISEASE, INVOLVING THE PROXIMAL INTERPHALANGEAL JOINTS OF THE FINGERS. THE METAPHYSES AND EPIPHYSES WERE BROAD AND SHORT. ONSET WAS AT 13 AND 17 YEARS RESPECTIVELY. THE PARENTS WERE NOT RELATED AND THEY AND OTHER FAMILY MEMBERS WERE NOT AFFECTED.

BOHME, A.* KASUISTISCHER BEITRAG ZUR THIEMANNSCHEN EPIPHYSENERKRANKUNG. Z. GES. INN. MED. 18* 491-495, 1963.

*27380 THROMBASTHENIA OF GLANZMANN AND NAEGELI

RECESSIVE INHERITANCE IS CLAIMED TO OBTAIN IN ALMOST ALL CASES (LELONG, 1960* MARX AND JEAN, 1962). A BLEEDING DIATHESIS WITH NORMAL BLEEDING TIME, PLATELET COUNT AND COAGULATION TIME BUT DEFICIENT CLOT RETRACTION AND ABNORMAL PLATELET MORPHOLO- GY IS FOUND. THERE PROBABLY IS MORE THAN ONE FORM OF THE DISEASE. GROSS ET AL. (1960) FOUND THAT THE PLATELETS OF ONE GROUP HAVE GREATLY REDUCED GLYCERALDEHYDE- PHOSPHATE DEHYDROGENASE (GAPDH) AND PYRUVATE KINASE (PK) ACTIVITY. THE PLATELETS SHOW REDUCED ADHESIVENESS, ON BLOOD SMEARS THERE IS NOTABLE ABSENCE OF PLATELET AGGREGATION AND BY ELECTRON MICROSCOPY THE 'ROUND' TYPE OF PLATELET PREDOMINATES. FRIEDMAN ET AL. (1964) DESCRIBED THE DISEASE IN A BOY AND GIRL WHO WERE DOUBLE

FIRST COUSINS (THE MOTHER OF ONE WAS A SISTER OF THE FATHER OF THE OTHER AND VICE VERSA). NO ABNORMALITY HAS BEEN DETECTED IN HETEROZYGOTES. FIVE FACTORS HAVE BEEN IDENTIFIED AS ESSENTIAL TO NORMAL PLATELET FUNCTION IN HEMOSTASIS* (1) A PLATELET PROPERTY, LACKING IN GLANZMANN'S THROMBASTHENIA, WHICH MAKES PLATELETS ADHERE AT THE SITE OF VESSEL INJURY, (2) A COLLAGENOUS AND ELASTIC FIBROUS SUBSTANCE FOR PLATELETS TO ADHERE TO, (3) A PLASMA FACTOR, LACKING IN VON WILLEBRAND'S DISEASE (A DOMINANT, Q.V.), (4) CALCIUM, AND (5) ADP WHICH IS RELEASED FROM DAMAGED RED CELLS AND TISSUE CELLS. THE DIFFICULT NOSOLOGY OF THIS UNDOUBTEDLY HETEROGENEOUS CATEGORY WAS DISCUSSED BY KANSKA ET AL. (1963) AND BY ALAGILLE ET AL. (1964). AN APPARENTLY UNIQUE CONGENITAL PLATELET DISORDER WAS DESCRIBED BY BOWIE, THOMPSON AND OWEN (1964). THERE IS SOME SUGGESTION OF A DOMINANT FORM (Q.V.) AS WELL AS THE BETTER ESTABLISHED RECESSIVE FORM (CAEN ET AL., 1966) AND THIS MAY BE A HETEROGENEOUS CATEGORY. ABSENT PLATELET AGGREGATION WAS EMPHASIZED BY CAEN ET AL. CRONBERG ET AL. (1967) DESCRIBED A KINDRED IN WHICH THREE PERSONS IN TWO SIBSHIP HAD A SEVERE CLOTTING DEFECT, WHEREAS OTHERS, INCLUDING ALL 4 PARENTS OF THE AFFECTED SIBSHIPS, HAD A MINOR DEFECT. THE MOST IMPRESSIVE ABNORMALITY IN VITRO WAS COMPLETE ABSENCE OF ABILITY OF THE PLATELETS TO AGGREGATE OR ADHERE TO GLASS. THE SAME WAS OBSERVED BY ZAIZOV ET AL. (1968) IN BROTHER AND SISTER WHOSE PARENTS WERE FIRST COUSINS ONCE REMOVED. PAPAYANNIS AND ISRAELS (1970) CONCLUDED THAT THE HETEROZYGOTE CAN BE IDENTIFIED BY THE CLOT RETRACTION TEST. SOME HETEROZYGOTES ARE MILD BLEEDERS.

ALAGILLE, D., JOSSO, F., BINET, J.-L. AND BLIN, M. L.* LA DYSTROPHIE THROMBOCY-TAIRE HEMORRAGIPARE. DISCUSSION NOSOLOGIQUE. NOUV. REV. FRANC. HEMAT. 4* 755-790, 1964.

BOWIE, E. J. W., THOMPSON, J. H., JR. AND OWEN, C. A., JR.* A NEW ABNORMALITY OF PLATELET FUNCTION. THROMB. DIATH. HAEMORRH. 11* 195-203, 1964.

CAEN, J. P., CASTALDI, P. A., LECLERC, J. C., INCEMAN, S., LARRIEU, M. J., PROBST, M. AND BERNARD, J.* CONGENITAL BLEEDING DISORDERS WITH LONG BLEEDING TIME AND NORMAL PLATELET COUNT. I. GLANZMAN'S THROMBASTHENIA (REPORT OF FIFTEEN PATIENTS). AM. J. MED. 41* 4-26, 1966.

CRONBERG, S., NILSSON, I. M. AND ZETTERQVIST, E.* INVESTIGATION OF A FAMILY WITH MEMBERS WITH BOTH SEVERE AND MILD DEGREE OF THROMBASTHENIA. ACTA PAEDIAT. SCAND. 56* 189-197, 1967.

FRIEDMAN, L. L., BOWIE, E. J. W., THOMPSON, J. H., JR., BROWN, A. L., JR. AND OWEN, C. A., JR.* FAMILIAL GLANZMANN'S THROMBASTHENIA. MAYO CLIN. PROC. 39* 908-918, 1964.

GROSS, R., GEROK, W., LOHR, G. W., VOGELL, W., WALLER, H. D. AND THEOPOLD, W.* UBER DIE NATUR DER THROMBASTHENIE. THROMBOPATHIE GLANZMANN-NAEGELI. KLIN. WSCHR. 38* 193-206, 1960.

KANSKA, B., NIEWIAROWSKI, S., OSTROWSKI, L., POPLAWSKI, A. AND PROKOPOWICZ, J.* MACROTHROMBOCYTIC THROMBOPATHIA. CLINICAL, COAGULATION AND HEREDITARY ASPECTS. THROMB. DIATH. HAEMORRH. 10* 88-100, 1963.

LELONG, J. C.* LA THROMBOPATHIE DE GLANZMANN-NAEGELI. PARIS* R. FOULON ET CIE., 1960.

MARX, R. AND JEAN, G.* STUDIEN ZUR PATHOGENESE DER THROMBASTHENIE GLANZMANN-NAEGELI. KLIN. WSCHR. 40* 942-953, 1962.

PAPAYANNIS, A. G. AND ISRAELS, M. C. G.* GLANZMANN'S DISEASE AND TRAIT. (LETTER) LANCET 2* 44 ONLY, 1970.

PITTMAN, M. A., JR. AND GRAHAM, J. B.* GLANZMANN'S THROMBOPATHY* AN AUTOSOMAL RECESSIVE TRAIT IN ONE FAMILY. AM. J. MED. SCI. 247* 293-303, 1964.

WALLER, H. D. AND GROSS, R.* GENETISCHE ENZYMDEFECTE ALS URSACHE VON THROMBOCY-TOPATHIEN. VERH. DEUTSCH. GES. INN. MED. 70* 476-494, 1964.

ZAIZOV, R., COHEN, I. AND MATOTH, Y.* THROMBASTHENIA* A STUDY OF TWO SIBLINGS. ACTA PAEDIAT. SCAND. 57* 522-526, 1968.

*27390 THROMBOCYTOPENIA

SCHAAR (1963) DESCRIBED FOUR AFFECTED BROTHERS. NO PLATELET-STIMULATING FACTOR OR ANTI-PLATELET ANTIBODY WAS PRESENT AND THERE WAS NO SKELETAL ANOMALY. BLOOM ET AL. (1966) DESCRIBED A FORM OF CONSTITUTIONAL APLASTIC ANEMIA (SEE ANEMIA, CONGENITAL HYPOPLASTIC) WITH 'AMEGAKARYOCYTIC THROMBOCYTOPENIA PRESENT AT BIRTH OR EARLY INFANCY, FOLLOWED LATER IN CHILDHOOD BY PANCYTOPENIA.' THEY CALLED IT TYPE II CONSTITUTIONAL APLASTIC ANEMIA. MATERNAL-FETAL INCOMPATIBILITY OF PLATELET ANTIGENS IS A CAUSE OF NEONATAL THROMBOCYTOPENIA IN MULTIPLE SIBS (PAGANELLI, 1969), SIMULATING RECESSIVE INHERITANCE. SEE PLATELET GROUPS IN DOMINANT CATALOG. THESE PATIENTS WERE CHRONICALLY THROMBOCYTOPENIC BUT RESPONDED TO THE TRANSFUSION OF NORMAL PLASMA. AUTOSOMAL RECESSIVE INHERITANCE HAS BEEN REPORTED BY ROBERTS AND SMITH (1950) AND BY WILSON ET AL. (1963).

BLOOM, G. E., WARNER, S., GERALD, P. S. AND DIAMOND, L. K.* CHROMOSOME ABNORMALITIES IN CONSTITUTIONAL APLASTIC ANEMIA. NEW ENG. J. MED. 274* 8-14, 1966.

PAGANELLI, V. H.* THROMBOCYTOPENIA IN NEWBORN SIBLINGS. (LETTER) J.A.M.A. 208* 1703 ONLY, 1969.

ROBERTS, M. H. AND SMITH, M. H.* THROMBOPENIC PURPURA. REPORT OF FOUR CASES IN ONE FAMILY. AM. J. DIS. CHILD. 79* 820-825, 1950.

SCHAAR, F. E.* FAMILIAL IDIOPATHIC THROMBOCYTOPENIC PURPURA. J. PEDIAT. 62* 546-551, 1963.

SHULMAN, I., PIERCE, M., LUKENS, A. AND CURRIMBHOY, Z.* A FACTOR IN NORMAL PLASMA REQUIRED FOR PLATELET PRODUCTION* CHRONIC THROMBOCYTOPENIA DUE TO ITS DEFICIENCY. BLOOD 16* 943-957, 1960.

VILDOSOLA, J. AND EMPARANZA, E.* HEREDITARY FAMILIAL THROMBOCYTOPENIA. (ABSTRACT) INTERN. CONG. PAEDIAT., LISBON, 1962. P. 36.

WILSON, S. J., LARSEN, W. E., SKILLMAN, R. S. AND WALTERS, T. R.* FAMILIAL THROMBOCYTOPENIC PURPURA. BLOOD 22* 827 ONLY, 1963.

*27400 THROMBOCYTOPENIA ABSENT RADIUS (TAR) SYNDROME

SHAW AND OLIVER (1959) DESCRIBED SIBS WITH ABSENT RADII AND THROMBOCYTOPENIA. THEY SUGGESTED THAT THIS DISORDER IS DISTINCT FROM FANCONI'S PANCYTOPENIC SYNDROME (Q.V.) BECAUSE THERE WAS NO HYPOPLASIA OF THE ERYTHRON AND THE BLOOD DISORDER WAS EVIDENT IN THE FIRST FEW MONTHS OF LIFE. THE RARE CONDITION HAD BEEN REPORTED IN SIBS BY GROSS, GROH AND WEIPPL (1956). IN OTHER REPORTED CASES CONGENITAL HEART DISEASE AND RENAL MALFORMATIONS WERE FOUND. THROMBOCYTOPENIA USUALLY GIVES RISE TO SYMPTOMS EARLY IN LIFE BUT IS TRANSIENT. THUS, THE PROCESS IS A MORE BENIGN ONE THAN IS FANCONI'S PANMYELOPATHY, IN WHICH LEUKEMIA IS A FURTHER COMPLICATION. OTHER DIFFERENCES FROM FANCONI'S DISEASE INCLUDE THE ABSENCE OF PARTICULAR CHANGE IN THE THUMB, OF PIGMENTARY ABNORMALITIES, AND OF CHROMOSOMAL BREAKS. IN A FAMILY STUDIED IN THIS DEPARTMENT (HALL ET AL., 1969) FOUR SISTERS WERE AFFECTED. ONE WITH TETRALOGY OF FALLOT HAD DIED. THE OLDEST WAS ALIVE AT AGE 27 AND HAD TWO NORMAL CHILDREN. THE OCCURRENCE OF HYPOPLASTIC RADIUS AND HYPOPLASTIC THROMBOCY-TOPENIA WITH TRISOMY 18 (RABINOWITZ ET AL., 1967) IS OF INTEREST ALTHOUGH ITS RELATIONSHIP TO THE MENDELIZING SYNDROME IS DOUBTFUL.

DIGNAN, P. S. J., MAUER, A. M. AND FRANTZ, C.* PHOCOMELIA WITH CONGENITAL HYPOPLASTIC THROMBOCYTOPENIA AND MYELOID LEUKEMOID REACTIONS. J. PEDIAT. 70* 561-573, 1967.

GROSS, H., GROH, C. AND WEIPPL, G.* KONGENITALE HYPOPLASTISCHE THROMBOPENIE MIT RADIUSAPLASIE, EIN SYNDROM MULTIPLER ABARTUNGEN. NEUE OEST. Z. KINDERHEILK. 1* 574, 1956.

HALL, J. G., LEVIN, J., KUHN, J. P., OTTENHEIMER, E. J., VAN BERKUM, K. A. P. AND MCKUSICK, V. A.* THROMBOCYTOPENIA WITH ABSENT RADIUS (TAR). MEDICINE 48* 411-439, 1969.

RABINOWITZ, J. G., MOSELEY, J. E., MITTY, H. A. AND HIRSCHORN, K.* TRISOMY 18, ESOPHAGEAL ATRESIA, ANOMALIES OF THE RADIUS, AND CONGENITAL HYPOPLASTIC THROMBOCY-TOPENIA. RADIOLOGY 89* 488-491, 1967.

SHAW, S. AND OLIVER, R. A. M.* CONGENITAL HYPOPLASTIC THROMBOCYTOPENIA WITH SKELETAL DEFORMITIES IN SIBLINGS. BLOOD 14* 374-377, 1959.

27410 THROMBOCYTOPENIC THROMBOPATHY

CULLUM, ET AL., (1967) DESCRIBED A FAMILY OF SICILIAN ORIGIN WITH A BLEEDING DISORDER CHARACTERIZED BY THROMBOCYTOPENIA, MORPHOLOGICALLY ABNORMAL PLATELETS, PROLONGED BLEEDING TIME, LOW PLATELET THROMBOPLASTIC ACTIVITY AND NORMAL CLOT RETRACTION. PHOSPHOLIPID CONTENT OF PLATELETS WAS INCREASED. THE AUTHORS SUGGESTED THAT ABNORMALLY RAPID REMOVAL OF THE BIZARRE PLATELETS MAY BE RESPON-SIBLE FOR THROMBOCYTOPENIA. THE MORPHOLOGIC ABNORMALITY OF THE PLATELET WAS THOUGHT TO BE DOMINANT. TWO MEMBERS OF THE FAMILY WERE JUDGED TO BE HOMOZYGOTES. THEIR PARENTS WERE FIRST COUSINS. ALL OF FIVE CHILDREN WERE APPARENT HETEROZY-GOTES. NONE OF THE HETEROZYGOTES HAD ABNORMAL BLEEDING.

CULLUM, C., COONEY, D. P. AND SCHRIER, S. L.* FAMILIAL THROMBOCYTOPENIC THROMBOCYTOPATHY. BRIT. J. HAEMAT. 13* 147-159, 1967.

27420 THUMB, DISTAL HYPEREXTENSIBILITY OF

ACCORDING TO GLASS AND KISTLER (1953), AMONG WHITES 24.7 PERCENT AND AMONG NEGROES 35.6 PERCENT SHOWED THE TRAIT. PENETRANCE WAS CALCULATED AS 96.5 PERCENT. HYPEREXTENSIBLE THUMB WAS JUDGED TO BE RECESSIVE, THE RESPONSIBLE GENE HAVING A FREQUENCY OF 0.496 IN U.S. WHITES.

27430 THYROID HORMONE UNRESPONSIVENESS

AMONG 2 OF 6 CHILDREN OF A CONSANGUINEOUS MARRIAGE, REFETOFF ET AL. (1967)
OBSERVED DEAF-MUTISM, STRIPPLED EPIPHYSES, GOITER AND ABNORMALLY HIGH PBI. THEY
POSTULATED END-ORGAN UNRESPONSIVENESS TO THYROID HORMONE. OTHER AUTOSOMAL END-
ORGAN UNRESPONSIVE STATES BEHAVE AS DOMINANTS. EXCEPTIONS TO THIS STATEMENT
INCLUDE UNRESPONSIVENESS TO THYROTROPIN AND ADRENAL UNRESPONSIVENESS TO ACTH.

   REFETOFF, S., DE WIND, L. T. AND DE GROOT, L. J.* FAMILIAL SYNDROME COMBINING
DEAF-MUTISM, STIPPLED EPIPHYSES, GOITER AND ABNORMALLY HIGH PBI* POSSIBLE TARGET
ORGAN REFRACTORINESS TO THYROID HORMONE. J. CLIN. ENDOCR. 27* 279-294, 1967.

*27440 THYROID HORMONOGENESIS, GENETIC DEFECT IN, I (ACCUMULATION, TRANSPORT OR
TRAPPING DEFECT)

THIS DEFECT IS CHARACTERIZED BY AN INABILITY OF THE THYROID TO MAINTAIN A
CONCENTRATION DIFFERENCE OF READILY EXCHANGEABLE IODINE BETWEEN THE PLASMA AND THE
THYROID GLAND. THE DEFECT IS ALSO FOUND IN THE SALIVARY GLAND AND GASTRIC MUCOSA.
IT IS PRESUMED TO ARISE EITHER BECAUSE OF A DEFICIENT SUPPLY OF ENERGY FOR THE
TRANSPORT SYSTEM OR BECAUSE OF ABNORMALITY OF A CARRIER OR RECEPTOR SUBSTANCE.
PARENTAL CONSANGUINITY WAS PRESENT IN THE CASE OF STANBURY AND CHAPMAN (1960).

   BEIERWALTES, W. H.* GENETICS OF THYROID DISEASE. IN, HAZARD, J. B. AND SMITH,
D. E. (EDS.)* THE THYROID. BALTIMORE* WILLIAMS AND WILKINS CO., 1964.

   STANBURY, J. B. AND CHAPMAN, E. M.* CONGENITAL HYPOTHYROIDISM WITH GOITER*
ABSENCE OF AN IODIDE-CONCENTRATING MECHANISM. LANCET 1* 1162-1165, 1960.

   STANBURY, J. B.* THE METABOLIC ERRORS IN CERTAIN TYPES OF FAMILIAL GOITER.
RECENT PROGR. HORMONE RES. 19* 547-577, 1963.

   STANBURY, J. B.* FAMILIAL GOITER. IN, STANBURY, J. B., WYNGAARDEN, J. B. AND
FREDRICKSON, D. S. (EDS.)* THE METABOLIC BASIS OF INHERITED DISEASE. NEW YORK*
MCGRAW-HILL, 1966 (2ND ED.). PP. 215-257.

*27450 THYROID HORMONOGENESIS, GENETIC DEFECT IN, IIA (ORGANIFICATION DEFECT I)

THIS DEFECT MAY INCLUDE TWO DISTINCT TYPES. IN BOTH, THE ABILITY TO IODINATE
TYROSYL RESIDUES WITH INTRATHYROIDAL IODINE IS IMPAIRED. A SEVERE TYPE MAY LACK
AN IODIDE PEROXIDASE. ACCUMULATED IODIDE IS PRECIPITOUSLY DISCHARGED FROM THE
GLAND ON ADMINISTRATION OF THIOCYANATE.

   LESZYNSKY, H. E.* GENETIC STUDIES IN FAMILIAL GOITROUS CRETINISM. (ABSTRACT)
ACTA ENDOCR. 46* 103-110, 1964.

   PARKER, R. H. AND BEIERWALTES, W. H.* INHERITANCE OF DEFECTIVE ORGANIFICATION
OF IODINE IN FAMILIAL GOITROUS CRETINISM. J. CLIN. ENDOCR. 21* 21-30, 1961.

*27460 THYROID HORMONOGENESIS, GENETIC DEFECT IN, IIB (ORGANIFICATION DEFECT II)

A MILDER TYPE OF ORGANIFICATION DEFECT IS ASSOCIATED WITH CONGENITAL DEAFNESS
(PENDRED'S SYNDROME) AND MAY BE THE RESULT OF LACK OF AN IODINASE. SEE PENDRED'S
SYNDROME. PATIENTS WITH THE MILDER DEFECT SHOW ONLY PARTIAL DISCHARGE OF IODINE
WHEN THIOCYANATE IS GIVEN. FRASER (1967) RAISES THE QUESTION OF WHETHER THE
ORGANIFICATION DEFECT WITHOUT DEAFNESS AS DESCRIBED BY STANBURY AND HEDGE (1950)
IS DIFFERENT FROM THE ORGANIFICATION DEFECT WITH DEAFNESS AS DESCRIBED BY PENDRED.
FRASER RAISES THE POSSIBILITY THAT VARIABILITY IN SEVERITY OF ONE AND THE SAME
DEFECT MAY BE INVOLVED. HE SUPPORTS THIS CONTENTION WITH THE DESCRIPTION OF A
PATIENT WITH UNILATERAL DEAFNESS WHOSE SISTER, ALSO WITH PENDRED'S SYNDROME, HAD
BILATERAL DEAFNESS. ALSO CASES OF THE FULL SYNDROME AND CASES WITH NEAR NORMAL
HEARING OCCURRED IN THE SAME FAMILY. A PARTIAL ORGANIFICATION DEFECT WITHOUT
DEAFNESS AND WITH GOITER AND EUTHYROID STATE WAS DESCRIBED IN 3 SIBS BY FURTH ET
AL. (1967).

   FRASER, G. R.* ADELAIDE, AUSTRALIA* PERSONAL COMMUNICATION, 1967.

   FURTH, E. D., CARVALHO, M. AND VIANNA, B.* FAMILIAL GOITER DUE TO AN ORGANIFI-
CATION DEFECT IN EUTHYROID SIBLINGS. J. CLIN. ENDOCR. 27* 1137-1140, 1967.

   STANBURY, J. B. AND HEDGE, A. N.* A STUDY OF A FAMILY OF GOITROUS CRETINS. J.
CLIN. ENDOCR. 10* 1471-1484, 1950.

*27470 THYROID HORMONOGENESIS, GENETIC DEFECT IN, III (COUPLING DEFECT)

PATIENTS WITH THE IODOTYROSYL COUPLING DEFECT FAIL TO COUPLE ENOUGH OF THESE
RESIDUES INTO IODOTHYRONINE HORMONES. THIS MAY BE THE RESULT OF ABSENCE OF A
HYPOTHETICAL 'COUPLING ENZYME' OR OF A STRUCTURAL ABNORMALITY IN THYROGLOBULIN
WHICH MAKES INTRAMOLECULAR COUPLING MORE DIFFICULT. THE DEFECT CAN BE DETECTED
WITH CERTAINTY ONLY BY SHOWING THAT IODOTHYRONINES FAIL TO APPEAR IN BIOPSY

R
E
C
E
S
S
I
V
E

ALEXANDER, N. M. AND BURROW, G. N.* THYROXINE BIOSYNTHESIS IN HUMAN GOITROUS CRETINISM. J. CLIN. ENDOCR. 30* 308-315, 1970.

MORRIS, J. H.* DEFECTIVE COUPLING OF IODOTYROSINE IN FAMILIAL GOITERS* REPORT OF TWO PATIENTS. ARCH. INTERN. MED. 114* 417-423, 1964.

*27480 THYROID HORMONOGENESIS, GENETIC DEFECT IN, IV (DEFECT OF IODOTYROSINE DEHALOGENASE, OR DEIODINASE)

THE IODOTYROSINE DEHALOGENASE DEFECT IS CHARACTERIZED BY AN INABILITY OF MANY TISSUES, INCLUDING THE THYROID, TO DEIODINATE MIT AND DIT. AS A RESULT INTRA-VENOUSLY ADMINISTERED LABELLED DIT APPEARS INTACT IN THE URINE. THIS IS THE ONLY THYROID DEFECT FOR WHICH THE SPECIFIC ENZYME INVOLVED HAS BEEN IDENTIFIED. HUTCHISON AND MCGIRR (1956) STUDIED THIS DISORDER IN AN INBRED GROUP OF ITINERANT TINKERS IN WESTERN SCOTLAND. WERDNIG-HOFFMANN PARALYSIS OCCURRED IN THE SAME GROUP. AMONG 7 SIBS FROM RELATED PARENTS, KUSAKABE AND MIYAKE (1964) FOUND THREE IN WHOM PERIPHERAL DEIODINATION OCCURRED BUT NONE WAS PRODUCED BY THYROID BIOPSY TISSUE. THUS, TWO ENTITIES MAY EXIST IN THIS CLASS.

HUTCHISON, J. H. AND MCGIRR, E. M.* SPORADIC NON-ENDEMIC GOITROUS CRETINISM. HEREDITARY TRANSMISSION. LANCET 1* 1035-1037, 1956.

KUSAKABE, T. AND MIYAKE, T.* THYROIDAL DEIODINATION DEFECT IN THREE SISTERS WITH SIMPLE GOITER. J. CLIN. ENDOCR. 24* 456-459, 1964.

*27490 THYROID HORMONOGENESIS, GENETIC DEFECT IN, V (PLASMA IODOPROTEIN DEFECT)

PATIENTS WITH THE SERUM IODOPROTEIN DISORDER HAVE LARGE AMOUNTS OF AN ALBUMIN-LIKE IODOPROTEIN IN THE PLASMA. THE SOURCE OF THIS COMPONENT COULD BE A NORMAL BUT MINOR PATHWAY OF IODINE METABOLISM IN THE THYROID WHICH EXPANDS BECAUSE OF A BLOCK IN THE NORMAL THYROGLOBULIN PATHWAY, OR IT MAY APPEAR SIMPLY AS A RESULT OF HYPERPLASIA OF THE GLAND FROM SOME UNDISCLOSED CAUSE, OR BECAUSE A STRUCTURAL ABNORMALITY OF THE CELL MEMBRANE PERMITS ALBUMIN TO ENTER AND LEAVE THE CELL, BEING IODINATED IN THE PROCESS. LISSITZKY ET AL. (1967) DESCRIBED A 12 YEAR OLD BOY WITH CONGENITAL GOITER AND HYPOTHYROIDISM. THE PARENTS WERE SECOND COUSINS. IN THE THYROID TISSUE THYROGLOBULIN WAS PRACTICALLY ABSENT AND WAS REPLACED BY IODINATED ALBUMIN-LIKE PROTEINS. ALTHOUGH THE SISTER WAS EUTHYROIDAL, SHE HAD GOITER WITH HIGH RAI UPTAKE BY THE THYROID AND LOW PBI AS IN HER BROTHER. COMPLICATING INTERPRETATION IS THE PRESENCE OF ASYMPTOMATIC GOITER IN THE MOTHER AND HER SISTER.

LISSITZKY, S., CODACCIONI, J.-L., BISMUTH, J. AND DEPIEDS, R.* CONGENITAL GOITER WITH HYPOTHYROIDISM AND IODO-SERUM ALBUMIN REPLACING THYROGLOBULIN. J. CLIN. ENDOCR. 27* 185-196, 1967.

27500 THYROTOXICOSIS (GRAVES' DISEASE)

BARTELS (1941) CLAIMED THAT THIS DISORDER IS INHERITED AS A SIMPLE AUTOSOMAL RECESSIVE WITH RELATIVE SEX LIMITATION TO FEMALES AND A REDUCED PENETRANCE (70-80 PERCENT) IN HOMOZYGOTES. MARTIN AND FISHER (1945) ALSO POSTULATED A RECESSIVE FACTOR PREDISPOSING TO EXOPHTHALMIC GOITER. IN CONTRAST, THESE WORKERS (1951) COULD FIND NO EVIDENCE OF HEREDITARY BASIS OF TOXIC NODULAR GOITER. INGBAR AND COLLEAGUES (1956) FOUND ABNORMALITIES OF THYROID METABOLISM IN EUTHYROID RELATIVES OF THYROTOXIC PATIENT. LEVIT IN EARLY STUDIES IN RUSSIA WAS MORE INCLINED TOWARD DOMINANT INHERITANCE (FRASER, 1967). NEITHER THE RECESSIVE NOR THE DOMINANT HYPOTHESIS HAS SATISFACTORY PROOF. IMPRESSIVELY EXTENSIVE INVOLVEMENT OCCURS IN SOME FAMILIES.

BARTELS, E. D.* HEREDITY IN GRAVES' DISEASE. COPENHAGEN* MUNKSGAARD, 1941.

FRASER, G. R.* ADELAIDE, AUSTRALIA* PERSONAL COMMUNICATION, 1967.

INGBAR, S. H., FREINKEL, N., DOWLING, J. T. AND KUMAGAI, L. F.* ABNORMALITIES OF IODINE METABOLISM IN EUTHYROID RELATIVES OF PATIENTS WITH GRAVES' DISEASE. (ABSTRACT) J. CLIN. INVEST. 35* 714 ONLY, 1956.

MARTIN, L. AND FISHER, R. A.* THE HEREDITARY AND FAMILIAL ASPECTS OF EXOPHTHAL-MIC GOITER AND NODULAR GOITRE. QUART. J. MED. 14* 207-219, 1945.

MARTIN, L. AND FISHER, R. A.* THE HEREDITARY AND FAMILIAL ASPECTS OF TOXIC NODULAR GOITRE (SECONDARY THYROTOXICOSIS). QUART. J. MED. 20* 293-297, 1951.

27510 THYROTROPIN DEFICIENCY, ISOLATED

ABOUT A DOZEN CASES HAVE BEEN REPORTED. APPARENTLY ALL WERE ISOLATED CASES. MOST PRESENTED WITH COMPLICATIONS OF ATHEROSCLEROSIS. THE PATIENT OF GRABOW AND CHOU (1968) HAD PERIPHERAL NEUROPATHY. ISOLATED TSH DEFICIENCY HAS BEEN DESCRIBED (ZISMAN ET AL., 1969) IN PATIENTS WITH PSEUDOHYPOPARATHYROIDISM (ALBRIGHT'S HEREDITARY OSTEODYSTROPHY, Q.V.).

R
E
C
E
S
S
I
V
E

NEUROPATHY. ARCH. NEUROL. 19* 284-291, 1968.

ODELL, W. D.* ISOLATED DEFICIENCIES OF ANTERIOR PITUITARY HORMONES* SYMPTOMS
AND DIAGNOSIS. J.A.M.A. 197* 1006-1016, 1966.

SAWIN, C. T. AND MCHUGH, J. E.* ISOLATED LACK OF THYROTROPIN IN MAN. J. CLIN.
ENDOCR. 26* 955-959, 1966.

ZISMAN, E., LOTZ, M., JENKINS, M. E. AND BARTTER, F. C.* STUDIES IN PSEUDOHYPO-
PARATHYROIDISM. TWO NEW CASES WITH A PROBABLE SELECTIVE DEFICIENCY OF THYROTRO-
PIN. AM. J. MED. 46* 464-471, 1969.

27520 THYROTROPIN, UNRESPONSIVENESS TO

STANBURY ET AL. (1968) DESCRIBED AN 8 YEAR OLD BOY WITH CONGENITAL HYPOTHYROIDISM
WHO WAS THE OFFSPRING OF PARENTS RELATED AS FIRST COUSINS ONCE REMOVED AND WHO
SHOWED HIGH SERUM LEVELS OF BIOLOGICALLY ACTIVE THYROTROPIN BUT NO RESPONSE TO
THYROTROPIN IN VIRO OR IN HIS THYROID TISSUE SLICES IN VITRO. END-ORGAN UNRESPON-
SIVENESS WAS SUGGESTED.

STANBURY, J. B., ROCMANS, P., BUHLER, U. K. AND OCHI, Y.* CONGENITAL HYPO-
THYROIDISM WITH IMPAIRED THYROID RESPONSE TO THYROTROPIN. NEW ENG. J. MED. 279*
1132-1136, 1968.

27530 TRACHEOBRONCHOMEGALY

JOHNSTON AND GREEN (1965) PRESENTED 5 CASES OF WHICH TWO WERE NEGRO BROTHER AND
SISTER. CHROMOSOME STUDIES WERE NORMAL. THE PARENTS AND FIVE OTHER SIBS APPEARED
TO BE UNAFFECTED. TWO SIBS DIED IN EARLY INFANCY. IN ONE MONGOLISM WAS DIAG-
NOSED. ALTHOUGH BRONCHOPULMONARY SUPPURATION LARGELY DETERMINES THE DEGREE OF
RESPIRATORY DISABILITY, INFECTION IS NOT RESPONSIBLE FOR THE UNDERLYING LESION OF
THE TRACHEOBRONCHIAL TREE. THE CHARACTERISTIC BRONCHOGRAPHIC PICTURE LED SEVERAL
WORKERS TO CALL IT TRACHIECTASIS WITH MULTIPLE DIVERTICULA. THE APPEARANCE IS
CREATED BY ENLARGEMENT OF THE AIRWAYS AND MUSCULO-MEMBRANOUS TISSUE PROJECTING
LIKE CORRUGATIONS BETWEEN THE CARTILAGINOUS RINGS. THE NEGRO PATIENT REPORTED BY
AABY AND BLAKE (1966) PROBABLY SUFFERED FROM EHLERS-DANLOS SYNDROME.

AABY, G. V. AND BLAKE, H. A.* TRACHEOBRONCHIOMEGALY. ANN. THORAC. SURG. 2* 64-
70, 1966.

JOHNSTON, R. F. AND GREEN, R. A.* TRACHEOBRONCHIOMEGALY* REPORT OF FIVE CASES
AND DEMONSTRATION OF FAMILIAL OCCURRENCE. AM. REV. RESP. DIS. 91* 35-50, 1965.

27540 TRICHOMEGALY (EXCESSIVE GROWTH OF EYELASHES AND BROW HAIR) WITH MENTAL
RETARDATION, DWARFISM AND PIGMENTARY DEGENERATION OF RETINA

EXCESSIVE GROWTH OF EYELASHES AND BROW HAIR IS PROBABLY A FAMILIAL TRAIT. OLIVER
AND MCFARLANE (1965) DESCRIBED AN ISOLATED CASE OF A MALE CHILD WITH LOW BIRTH
WEIGHT DWARFISM, VERY LONG EYELASHES AND EYEBROWS, MENTAL RETARDATION AND
PIGMENTARY DEGENERATION OF THE RETINA. THE KARYOTYPE WAS NORMAL AND THE PARENTS
WERE NOT CONSANGUINEOUS. I HAVE SEEN SIBS WITH LONG EYELASHES AND MENTAL
RETARDATION. CORBY ET AL. (1971) REPORTED A CASE OF THE FULL SYNDROME.

CANT, J. S.* ECTODERMAL DYSPLASIA. J. PEDIAT. OPHTHAL. 4 (NO. 4)* 13-17, 1967.

CORBY, D. G., LOWE, R. S., JR., HASKINS, R. C. AND HEBERTSON, L. M.* TRICHOME-
GALY, PIGMENTARY DEGENERATION OF THE RETINA, AND GROWTH RETARDATION. AM. J. DIS.
CHILD. 121* 344-345, 1971.

OLIVER, G. L. AND MCFARLANE, D. C.* CONGENITAL TRICHOMEGALY WITH ASSOCIATED
PIGMENTARY DEGENERATION OF THE RETINA, DWARFISM AND MENTAL RETARDATION. ARCH.
OPHTHAL. 74* 169-171, 1965.

*27550 TRICHO-RHINO-PHALANGEAL SYNDROME

GIEDION (1966) DELINEATED A NEW SYNDROME CONSISTING OF THIN AND SLOWLY GROWING
HAIR, PEAR-SHAPED NOSE WITH HIGH PHILTRUM, BRACHYPHALANGY WITH DEFORMATION OF THE
FINGERS AND WEDGE-SHAPED EPIPHYSES. GIEDION'S PATIENT, A GIRL, HAD 2 SUPERNU-
MERARY INCISORS. IN THE LITERATURE HE FOUND TWO PREVIOUS REPORTS EACH DESCRIBING
TWO AFFECTED SIBS. FURTHERMORE THE PARENTS WERE CONSANGUINEOUS IN ONE CASE. ONE
OF THE PAIRS OF AFFECTED SIBS WAS REPORTED AS PSEUDO-PSEUDOHYPOPARATHYROIDISM
(VAN DER WERFF TEN BOSCH, 1959). MURDOCH (1969) DESCRIBED THE CASE OF A MALE
WHOSE FATHER WHO DIED AT 43 YEARS OF A CEREBROVASCULAR ACCIDENT WAS PROBABLY ALSO
AFFECTED. THE PARENTS CAME FROM A SIMILAR ETHNIC BACKGROUND BUT WERE NOT KNOWN TO
BE RELATED. THE POSSIBILITY OF A DOMINANT FORM MUST BE KEPT IN MIND.

GIEDION, A.* DAS TRICHO-RHINO-PHALANGEAL SYNDROM. HELV. PAEDIAT. ACTA 21* 475-
482, 1966.

GIEDION, A.* ZAPFENEPIPHYSEN. NATURGESCHICHTE UND DIAGNOSTISCHE BEDEUTUNG
EINER STROUNG DES ENCHONDRALEN WACHSTUMS. ERGENB. MED. RADIOL. 8* 59-124, 1968.

RECESSIVE

MURDOCH, J. L.* TRICHO-RHINO-PHALANGEAL DYSPLASIA WITH POSSIBLE AUTOSOMAL DOMINANT TRANSMISSION. THE CLINICAL DELINEATION OF BIRTH DEFECTS. II. MALFORMA-TION SYNDROMES. NEW YORK* NATIONAL FOUNDATION, 1969. PP. 218-220.

VAN DER WERFF TEN BOSCH, J. J.* THE SYNDROME OF BRACHYMETACARPAL DWARFISM ('PSEUDO-PSEUDOHYPOPARATHYROIDISM') WITH AND WITHOUT GONADAL DYSGENESIS. LANCET 1* 69-71, 1959.

27560 TRIGONOCEPHALY

MULTIPLE AFFECTED SIBS HAVE BEEN OBSERVED BY DEMYER (1964). AGENESIS OF THE OLFACTORY BULBS AND TRACTS IS ASSOCIATED. IT IS AN ENTITY DISTINCT FROM HOLOPRO-SENCEPHALY (Q.V.) WITH WHICH IT, HOWEVER, SHARES SOME FEATURES.

DEMYER, W.* INDIANAPOLIS, IND.* PERSONAL COMMUNICATION, 1964.

27570 TRIMETHYLAMINURIA (FISH-ODOR SYNDROME)

HUMBERT ET AL. (1970) DESCRIBED A 6 YEAR OLD GIRL WITH MULTIPLE PULMONARY INFECTIONS BEGINNING IN THE NEONATAL PERIOD AND INTERMITTENTLY A FISHY ODOR. SPLENOMEGALY, ANEMIA AND NEUTROPENIA WERE ALSO PRESENT. THE URINE CONTAINED INCREASED AMOUNTS OF TRIMETHYLAMINE.

HUMBERT, J. R., HAMMOND, K. B., HATHAWAY, W. E., MARCOUX, J. G. AND O'BRIEN, D.* TRIMETHYLAMINURIA* THE FISH-ODOUR SYNDROME. (LETTER) LANCET 2* 770-771, 1970.

*27580 TRIOSEPHOSPHATE ISOMERASE (TPI) DEFICIENCY

A FORM OF NON-SPHEROCYTIC HEMOLYTIC ANEMIA OF DACIE'S TYPE II (IN VITRO AUTOHEMO-LYSIS IS NOT CORRECTED BY ADDED GLUCOSE) HAS BEEN FOUND TO HAVE A DEFICIENCY OF RED CELL TRIOSEPHOSPHATE ISOMERASE (SCHNEIDER ET AL., 1965). ASSOCIATION WITH RECURRENT INFECTION AND A PROGRESSIVE NEUROLOGIC DISORDER CHARACTERIZED BY SPASTICITY WAS NOTED. THE HOMOZYGOTES SHOW 6 PERCENT OF NORMAL TPI ACTIVITY IN RED CELLS AND 20 PERCENT IN WHITE CELLS. HETEROZYGOTES SHOW ABOUT 50 PERCENT.

RUDIGER, H. W., PASSARGE, E., HIRTH, L., GOEDDE, H. W., BLUME, K. G., LOHR, G. W., BENOHR, H. C. AND WALLER, H. D.* TRIOSEPHOSPHATE ISOMERASE GENE NOT LOCALIZED ON THE SHORT ARM OF CHROMOSOME 5 IN MAN. (LETTER) NATURE 228* 1320-1321, 1970.

SCHNEIDER, A. S., VALENTINE, W. N., HATTORI, M. AND HEINS, H. L., JR.* HEREDITARY HEMOLYTIC ANEMIA WITH TRIOSEPHOSPHATE ISOMERASE DEFICIENCY. NEW ENG. J. MED. 272* 229-235, 1965.

*27590 TROYER SYNDROME

IN AN AMISH GROUP IN OHIO, CROSS AND MCKUSICK (1967) OBSERVED 20 CASES OF SPASTIC PARAPLEGIA WITH DISTAL MUSCLE WASTING AND DESIGNATED IT TROYER SYNDROME FOR THE SURNAME OF MANY OF THE AFFECTED PERSONS. THE DISORDER HAS ITS ONSET IN EARLY CHILDHOOD WITH DYSARTHRIA, DISTAL MUSCLE WASTING AND DIFFICULTY IN LEARNING TO WALK. LOWER LIMB SPASTICITY AND CONTRACTURES USUALLY MAKE WALKING IMPOSSIBLE BY THE THIRD OR FOURTH DECADE. DROOLING AND MILD CEREBELLAR SIGNS OCCUR IN SOME. ALL HAVE WEAKNESS AND ATROPHY OF THENAR, HYPOTHENA AND DORSAL INTEROSSEOUS MUSCLES.

CROSS, H. E. AND MCKUSICK, V. A.* THE TROYER SYNDROME. A RECESSIVE FORM OF SPASTIC PARAPLEGIA WITH DISTAL MUSCLE WASTING. ARCH. NEUROL. 16* 473-485, 1967.

*27600 TRYPSINOGEN DEFICIENCY DISEASE

FAILURE TO THRIVE, NUTRITIONAL EDEMA, AND HYPOPROTEINEMIA WITH NORMAL SWEAT ELECTROLYTES WERE FEATURES OF AFFECTED INFANTS. A PROTEIN HYDROLYSATE DIET WAS BENEFICIAL. A MALE SIB OF TOWNES' FIRST PATIENT (1965) HAD DIED APPARENTLY OF THE SAME CONDITION. TOWNES' TWO PATIENTS WERE MALE (1965, 1967). MORRIS AND FISHER (1967) REPORTED A FEMALE WHO ALSO HAD IMPERFORATE ANUS. THE CLINICAL PICTURE IN ENTEROKINASE DEFICIENCY (Q.V.) IS CLOSELY SIMILAR BUT THE DEFECT IS NOT IN THE SYNTHESIS OF TRYPSINOGEN BUT IN THE SYNTHESIS OF THE ENTEROKINASE WHICH STIMULATES SECRETION OF PROTEOLYTIC ENZYMES BY THE PANCREAS.

MORRIS, M. D. AND FISHER, D. A.* TRYPSINOGEN DEFICIENCY DISEASE. AM. J. DIS. CHILD. 114* 203-208, 1967.

TOWNES, P. L., BRYSON, M. F. AND MILLER, G.* FURTHER OBSERVATIONS ON TRYPSINO-GEN DEFICIENCY DISEASE* REPORT OF A CASE. J. PEDIAT. 71* 220-224, 1967.

TOWNES, P. L.* TRYPSINOGEN DEFICIENCY DISEASE. J. PEDIAT. 66* 275-285, 1965.

*27610 TRYPTOPHANURIA WITH DWARFISM

TADA, ITO, WADA AND ARAKAWA (1963) DESCRIBED A 9 YEAR OLD GIRL WITH DWARFISM, MENTAL DEFECT, CUTANEOUS PHOTOSENSITIVITY AND GAIT DISTURBANCE RESEMBLING CEREBELLAR ATAXIA. THE CLINICAL FEATURES RESEMBLED HARTNUP'S DISEASE (Q.V.) BUT THE CHEMICAL FINDINGS WERE DIFFERENT. TRYPTOPHANE WAS EXCRETED IN THE URINE IN

R
E
C
E
S
S
I
V
E

EXCESS WITHOUT INCREASE IN INDICAN OR INDOLE ACETIC ACID EXCRETION. WITH TRYPTOPHANE LOADING THE PLASMA LEVEL OF TRYPTOPHANE INCREASED MARKEDLY AND REMAINED HIGHER LONGER THAN IN NORMALS AND TRYPTOPHANURIA WAS INCREASED WITH RELATIVELY LITTLE INCREASE IN KYNURENINE EXCRETION. THE DEFECT WAS THOUGHT TO CONCERN THE CONVERSION OF TRYPTOPHAN TO KYNURENINE. THE DISORDER WAS THOUGHT TO HAVE OCCURRED IN THREE CHILDREN (TWO MALES AND THE FEMALE PROBAND) IN THREE SIBSHIPS. ALL SIX PARENTS WERE TRACED TO A COMMON ANCESTRAL COUPLE. THE PROBAND SHOWED CONJUNCTIVAL TELANGIECTASIA WHICH TOGETHER WITH ATAXIA CREATES SIMILARITIES TO ATAXIA-TELANGIECTASIA (Q.V.).

TADA, K., ITO, H., WADA, Y. AND ARAKAWA, T.* CONGENITAL TRYPTOPHANURIA WITH DWARFISM ('H' DISEASE-LIKE CLINICAL FEATURES WITHOUT INDICANURIA AND GENERALIZED AMINOACIDURIA)* A PROBABLY NEW INBORN ERROR OF TRYPTOPHANE METABOLISM. TOHOKU J. EXP. MED. 80* 118-134, 1963.

27620 T-SUBSTANCE ANOMALY

SOME OF THE CHILDREN IN WHOM UNUSUAL, AS YET UNIDENTIFIED, T-SUBSTANCE HAS BEEN FOUND IN THE URINE BY PAPER CHROMATOGRAPHY HAVE HAD SEVERE MENTAL AND-OR PHYSICAL RETARDATION.

COLES, H. M.* T-SUBSTANCE ANOMALY WITH HORSESHOE KIDNEY. PROC. ROY. SOC. MED. 54* 330-331, 1961.

COLES, H. M., PRIESTMAN, A. AND WILKINSON, J. H.* T-SUBSTANCE ANOMALY. AN INBORN ERROR OF PURINE METABOLISM. LANCET 2* 1220-1223, 1960.

27630 TURCOT SYNDROME (MALIGNANT TUMORS OF THE CENTRAL NERVOUS SYSTEM ASSOCIATED WITH FAMILIAL POLYPOSIS OF THE COLON)

TURCOT, DEPRES AND ST. PIERRE (1959) DESCRIBED AFFECTED BROTHER AND SISTER. THE PARENTS WERE THIRD COUSINS (PERSONAL COMMUNICATION FROM TURCOT). BECAUSE OF THE ASSOCIATION OF COLONIC POLYPS WITH TUMORS OF MANY TYPES IN THE GARDNER'S SYNDROME, IT IS POSSIBLE THAT THE SIBS REPORTED BY TURCOT AND COLLEAGUES HAD THAT CONDITION, A DOMINANT (Q.V.). THE POSSIBILITY IS STRENGTHENED BY THE DESCRIPTION BY YAFFEE (1964) OF A CASE OF GARDNER'S SYNDROME WHOSE 'UNCLE DIED OF TURCOT'S SYNDROME.' THIS MIGHT SUGGEST THAT TURCOT SYNDROME IS MERELY AN UNUSUAL MODE OF PRESENTATION OF THE GARDNER SYNDROME, A DOMINANT. THE CONTRARY VIEW, THAT THERE EXISTS A GENUINE SYNDROME OF GLIOMA AND POLYPOSIS INHERITED AS A RECESSIVE, IS SUPPORTED BY THE FAMILY REPORTED BY BAUGHMAN ET AL. (1969). A BROTHER AND TWO SISTERS HAD THE FULL SYNDROME AND ANOTHER BROTHER MAY HAVE BEEN AFFECTED. THE PARENTS WERE HEALTHY AND UNRELATED.

BAUGHMAN, F. A., JR., LIST, C. F., WILLIAMS, J. R., MULDOON, J. P., SEGARRA, J. M. AND VOLKEL, J. S.* THE GLIOMA-POLYPOSIS SYNDROME. NEW ENG. J. MED. 281* 1345-1346, 1969.

TURCOT, J., DESPRES, J. P. AND ST. PIERRE, F.* MALIGNANT TUMORS OF THE CENTRAL NERVOUS SYSTEM ASSOCIATED WITH FAMILIAL POLYPOSIS OF THE COLON* REPORT OF TWO CASES. DIS. COLON RECTUM 2* 465-468, 1959.

YAFFEE, H. S.* GASTRIC POLYPOSIS AND SOFT TISSUE TUMORS. A VARIANT OF GARDNER'S SYNDROME. ARCH. DERM. 89* 806-808, 1964.

27640 TWINNING, DIZYGOTIC

WEINBERG (1909) SUGGESTED THAT HEREDITARY TWINNING IS TRANSMITTED ONLY THROUGH THE FEMALE LINE, APPLIES ONLY TO DIZYGOTIC TWINS, AND IS PROBABLY RECESSIVE. OBSERVATION OF MULTIPLE BIRTHS FOLLOWING USE OF PITUITARY GONADOTROPINS SUGGESTS A PITUITARY MECHANISM FOR GENE ACTION (MILHAM, 1964). WYSHAK AND WHITE (1965) PRESENTED EVIDENCE, BASED ON MORMON RECORDS, WHICH THEY INTERPRETED AS SUPPORTING RECESSIVE INHERITANCE. AMONG THE CHILDREN OF FEMALE MZ TWINS, 17.1 TWINS PER 1000 MATERNITIES OCCURRED AS COMPARED WITH 7.9 AMONG CHILDREN OF MALE MZ TWINS. FEMALE SIBS OF MZ TWINS HAD 17 PER 1000 TWINS, WHEREAS MALE SIBS HAD 13.1 PER 1000. SUPPOSEDLY THE GENE IS TOO FREQUENT FOR ONE TO EXPECT INCREASED CONSANGUINITY IN THE GRANDPARENTS OF DIZYGOTIC TWINS. TAYLOR (1931) REPORTED MULTIPLE SETS OF DIZYGOTIC TWINS IN FOUR GENERATIONS. IN THE SAME FAMILY MOTHER AND DAUGHTER DID NOT MENSTRUATE UNTIL AFTER THEIR FIRST PREGNANCIES, AT AGES 20 AND 22, RESPECTIVE-LY. THE DIFFERENTIATION OF MULTIFACTORIAL AND MONOFACTORIAL INHERITANCE OF TWINNING IS DIFFICULT. ETHNIC DIFFERENCES IN THE RATE OF DIZYGOTIC TWINNING IS EVIDENCE OF GENETIC FACTORS. IN INTERRACIAL MARRIAGES THE RATE FOLLOWS THAT OF THE MOTHER'S ETHNIC GROUP. FURTHERMORE, WHEN THE MOTHER IS A RACIAL HYBRID, THE DIZYGOTIC TWINNING FREQUENCY IS THAT OF THE RACE WITH THE LOWER FREQUENCY, INDICATING THE RECESSIVE NATURE OF THE GENETIC FACTORS (MORTON ET AL., 1967).

MILHAM, S., JR.* PITUITARY GONADOTROPIN AND DIZYGOTIC TWINNING. LANCET 2* 566 ONLY, 1964.

MORTON, N. E., CHUNG, C. S. AND MI, M.* GENETICS OF INTERRACIAL CROSSES IN HAWAII. MONOGRAPHS IN HUMAN GENETICS, VOL. 3. BASEL* S. KARGER, 1967.

TAYLOR, C. E.* FOUR GENERATIONS OF HETEROSEXUAL TWINS WITH PREPARTUM AMENORR-

HOEA IN TWO GENERATIONS. BRIT. MED. J. 2* 384 ONLY, 1931.

WEINBERG, W.* ZUR BEDEUTUNG DER MEHRLINGSGEBURTEN FUR DIE FRAGE DER BESTIMMUNG DES GESCHLECHTS. ARCH. RASS.-U. GES. BIOL. 6* 28-32, 1909.

WYSHAK, G. AND WHITE, C.* GENEALOGICAL STUDY OF HUMAN TWINNING. AM. J. PUBLIC HEALTH 55* 1586-1593, 1965.

27650 TYROSINE METABOLISM, DELAYED MATURATION IN

BLOXAM AND COLLEAGUES (1960) FOUND THAT 14 OF 1276 INFANTS TESTED HAD LARGE AMOUNTS OF P-HYDROXYPHENYL-PYRUVIC ACID, P-HYDROXYPHENYL-LACTIC ACID AND TYROSINE IN THE URINE. THE INFANTS WERE ON NORMAL DIET. A DELAY IN MATURATION OF AN ENZYME WAS POSTULATED. A GENETIC BASIS WAS PRESUMED AND IS INDEED PLAUSIBLE BUT NOT PROVED.

BLOXAM, H. R., DAY, M. G., GIBBS, N. K. AND WOOLF, L. I.* AN INBORN DEFECT IN THE METABOLISM OF TYROSINE IN INFANTS ON A NORMAL DIET. BIOCHEM. J. 77* 320-326, 1960.

27660 TYROSINE TRANSAMINASE DEFICIENCY

BUIST (1967) REFERRED TO STUDIES OF A CHILD WITH TYROSINEMIA AND TYROSINE TRANSAMINASE DEFICIENCY, BUT NORMAL P-HYDROXYPHENYLPYRUVIC ACID OXIDASE. PHENYLALANINE LEVEL WAS NORMAL. HYDROXYPHENYLPYRUVIC ACID WAS ELEVATED IN THE URINE.

BUIST, N.* IN, NYHAN, W. L. (ED.)* COMMENT* AMINO ACID METABOLISM AND GENETIC VARIATION. NEW YORK* MCGRAW-HILL, 1967. P. 117.

*27670 TYROSINEMIA

AMONG THE CHILDREN OF FIRST COUSIN PARENTS, LELONG ET AL. (1963) OBSERVED TWO SONS WITH CIRRHOSIS, FANCONI SYNDROME AND MARKED INCREASE IN PLASMA TYROSINE. IN THE SIB MOST EXTENSIVELY OBSERVED HEPATOSPLENOMEGALY WAS DISCOVERED AT 3 MONTHS OF AGE AND RICKETS AT 18 MONTHS. MALIGNANT CHANGES DEVELOPED IN THE LIVER AND DEATH FROM PULMONARY METASTASES OCCURRED SHORTLY BEFORE HIS 5TH BIRTHDAY. THE AUTHOR SUGGESTED THAT THE BASIC DEFECT CONCERNS AN ENZYME INVOLVED WITH TYROSINE METABOLISM. OTHER CASES ARE REPORTED IN THE EARLIER LITERATURE. HIMSWORTH HAS A SIMILAR CASE IN HIS BOOK ON THE LIVER. GENTZ, JAGENBURG AND ZETTERSTROM (1965) DESCRIBED 7 PATIENTS IN 4 FAMILIES WITH MULTIPLE RENAL TUBULAR DEFECTS LIKE THOSE OF THE DE TONI-DEBRE-FANCONI SYNDROME, NODULAR CIRRHOSIS OF THE LIVER AND IMPAIRED TYROSINE METABOLISM. P-HYDROXYPHENYLLACTIC ACID WAS EXCRETED IN UNUSUALLY LARGE AMOUNTS. A TOTAL LACK OF LIVER P-HYDROXYPHENYLPYRUVATE OXIDASE ACTIVITY WAS DEMONSTRATED. TYROSINE-ALPHA-KETOGLUTARATE TRANSAMINASE WAS NORMAL. SCRIVER, LAROCHELLE AND SILVERBERG (1967) IDENTIFIED THE DISEASE IN 35 FRENCH-CANADIAN INFANTS OF WHOM 16 WERE SIBS (I.E., TWO OR MORE IN EACH OF SEVERAL FAMILIES). MARKED TYROSINEMIA AND TYROSYLURIA WERE PRESENT. THE URINE CONTAINED PARA-HYDROXYPHENYLPYRUVIC ACID (PHPPA) AND LACTIC AND ACETIC DERIVATIVES. LOADING TEST WITH TYROSINE AND WITH PHPPA SUGGESTED DEFICIENT P-HYDROXYPHENYLPYRUVATE OXIDASE ACTIVITY, WHICH WAS CONFIRMED BY ASSAY OF LIVER BIOPSY SAMPLES. IN STAGE I INFANTS EXHIBIT HEPATIC NECROSIS AND HYPERMETHIONINEMIA. IN STAGE II NODULAR CIRRHOSIS AND CHRONIC HEPATIC INSUFFICIENCY WITHOUT HYPERMETHIONINEMIA ARE FOUND. IN STAGE III RENAL TUBULAR DAMAGE (BABER'S SYNDROME), OFTEN WITH HYPOPHOSPHATEMIC RICKETS, APPEARS. LOW TYROSINE DIET ARRESTED PROGRESSION OF THE DISEASE. ZETTERSTROM (1963) STUDIED 7 CASES COMING FROM AN ISOLATED AREA OF SOUTHWESTERN SWEDEN. HALVORSEN ET AL. (1966) GAVE DETAILS ON 6 CASES FROM NORWAY.

FRITZELL, S., JAGENBURG, O. R. AND SCHNURER, L. B.* FAMILIAL CIRRHOSIS OF THE LIVER, RENAL TUBULAR DEFECTS WITH RICKETS AND IMPAIRED TYROSINE METABOLISM. ACTA PAEDIAT. 53* 18-32, 1964.

GAULL, G. E., RASSIN, D. K., STURMAN, J. A.* SIGNIFICANCE OF HYPERMETHIONINAE-MIA IN ACUTE TYROSINOSIS. (LETTER) LANCET 1* 1318-1319, 1968.

GENTZ, J., JAGENBURG, R. AND ZETTERSTROM, R.* TYROSINEMIA. J. PEDIAT. 66* 670-696, 1965.

HALVORSEN, S. AND GJESSING, L. R.* STUDIES OF TYROSINOSIS. I. EFFECT OF LOW-TYROSINE AND LOW-PHENYLALANINE DIET. BRIT. MED. J. 2* 1171-1173, 1964.

HALVORSEN, S., PANDE, H., LOKEN, A. C. AND GJESSING, L. R.* TYROSINOSIS. A STUDY OF 6 CASES. ARCH. DIS. CHILD. 41* 238-249, 1966.

KANG, E. S. AND GERALD, P. S.* HEREDITARY TYROSINEMIA AND ABNORMAL PYRROLE METABOLISM. A PATIENT WITH HEREDITARY TYROSINEMIA IS DESCRIBED WHO DEVELOPED METABOLIC AND CLINICAL CHANGES COMPATIBLE WITH ACUTE INTERMITTENT PORPHYRIA. J. PEDIAT. 77* 397-406, 1970.

LA DU, B. N.* THE ENZYMATIC DEFICIENCY IN TYROSINEMIA. AM. J. DIS. CHILD. 113* 54-57, 1967.

RECESSIVE

LABERGE, C.* HEREDITARY TYROSINEMIA IN A FRENCH CANADIAN ISOLATE. AM. J. HUM. GENET. 21* 36-45, 1969.

LELONG, M., ALAGILLE, D., GENTIL, C. I., COLIN, J., LE TAN, V. AND GABILAN, J. C.* CIRRHOSE CONGENITALE ET FAMILIALE AVEC DIABETE PHOSPHO-GLUCO-AMINE, RACHITISME VITAMIN D-RESISTANT ET TYROSINURIE MASSIVE. REV. FRANC. ETUDE. CLIN. BIOL. 8* 37-50, 1963.

SCRIVER, C. R., LAROCHELLE, J. AND SILVERBERG, M.* HEREDITARY TYROSINEMIA AND TYROSYLURIA IN A FRENCH CANADIAN GEOGRAPHIC ISOLATE. AM. J. DIS. CHILD. 113* 41-46, 1967.

SCRIVER, C. R., PARTINGTON, M. AND SASS-KORTSAK, A.* CONFERENCE ON HEREDITARY TYROSINEMIA HELD AT THE HOSPITAL FOR SICK CHILDREN. CANAD. MED. ASS. J. 97* 1045-1100, 1967.

ZETTERSTROM, R.* TYROSINOSIS. ANN. N.Y. ACAD. SCI. 111* 220-226, 1963.

27680 TYROSINOSIS

CONFUSION EXISTS BETWEEN THE TERMS 'TYROSINEMIA' AND 'TYROSINOSIS.' LA DU (PERSONAL COMMUNICATION, 1966) SUGGESTS THAT THE PROBLEM IS BEST SOLVED BY RESERVING THE TERM 'TYROSINOSIS' FOR THE APPARENTLY UNIQUE CONDITION REPORTED BY MEDES (1932). THE DEFECT IN HER PATIENT MAY HAVE INVOLVED LIVER TYROSINE TRANSAMINASE, NOT P-HYDROXYPHENYLPYRUVIC ACID OXIDASE AS SHE POSTULATED. THE PATIENT WAS A 49 YEAR OLD MALE RUSSIAN JEW, DIAGNOSED AS HAVING MYASTHENIA GRAVIS.

MEDES, G.* A NEW ERROR OF TYROSINE METABOLISM* TYROSINOSIS. THE INTERMEDIARY METABOLISM OF TYROSINE AND PHENYLALANINE. BIOCHEM. J. 26* 917-940, 1932.

*27690 USHER SYNDROME (RETINITIS PIGMENTOSA AND CONGENITAL DEAFNESS)

LANG (1959) OBSERVED FIVE AFFECTED CHILDREN OUT OF TEN FROM A FIRST-COUSIN MARRIAGE. LINDENOV (1945) WROTE ON DEAF-MUTISM ASSOCIATED WITH RETINITIS PIGMENTOSA AND FEEBLEMINDEDNESS. KLOEPFER, LAGUAITE AND MCLAURIN (1966) IDENTI-FIED 537 PERSONS WITH HEARING LOSS IN A FRENCH 'CAJUN' GROUP IN LOUISIANA. OF THE 468 LIVING PERSONS WITH HEARING LOSS AT LEAST 158 OR ABOUT 30 PERCENT WERE KNOWN TO HAVE RETINITIS PIGMENTOSA AND CATARACT. THE FIRST DESCRIPTION OF THIS SYNDROME WAS BY LIEBREICH (1861) WHO COMMENTED ON A RELATIVELY HIGH FREQUENCY IN JEWS IN BERLIN. VON GRAEFE (1858) MAY HAVE GIVEN THE EARLIEST DESCRIPTION. HAMMERSCHLAG (1907) MADE A SIMILAR OBSERVATION IN VIENNA. HALLGREN (1959) FOUND 177 AFFECTED PERSONS IN 102 FAMILIES. IN ADDITION TO THE FEATURES NOTED IN THE TITLE OF HIS PAPER, CATARACT DEVELOPED BY AGE 40 IN MOST. MENTAL DEFICIENCY AND PSYCHOSIS OCCUR EACH IN ABOUT ONE-QUARTER OF CASES. A LARGE MAJORITY HAD A DISTURBANCE OF GAIT ATTRIBUTED TO A LESION OF THE LABYRINTH. IN FINLAND, NUUTILA (1970) FOUND 133 PERSONS WITH RETINITIS PIGMENTOSA AND CONGENITAL SENSORY DEAFNESS, 4 WITH RP AND PROGRESSIVE SENSORY DEAFNESS. ON THE BASIS OF 133 PATIENTS IN FINLAND, FORSIUS ET AL. (1971) CONCLUDED THAT THERE ARE TWO DISTINCT FORMS OF THE USHER SYNDROME* ONE CHARACTERIZED BY CONGENITAL DEAFNESS AND SEVERE RETINITIS PIGMENTO-SA, AND A SECOND LESS FREQUENT FORM IN WHICH THE INNER EAR AND RETINA ARE BOTH LESS SEVERELY AFFECTED. WHETHER THESE ARE ALLELIC FORMS OR NOT IS UNKNOWN.

DE HAAS, E. B. H., VAN LITH, G. H. M., RIJNDERS, J., RUMKE, A. M. L. AND VOLMER, C. H.* USHER'S SYNDROME, WITH SPECIAL REFERENCE TO HETEROZYGOUS MANIFESTA-TIONS. DOCUM. OPHTHAL. 28* 166-190, 1970.

FORSIUS, H., ERIKKSON, A., NUUTILA, A., VAINIO-MATTILA, B. AND KRAUSE, U.* A GENETIC STUDY OF THREE RARE RETINAL DISORDERS* DYSTROPHIA RETINAE DYSACUSIS SYNDROME, X-CHROMOSOMAL RETINOSCHISIS AND GROUPED PIGMENTS OF THE RETINA. THE CLINICAL DELINEATION OF BIRTH DEFECTS. VIII. EYE. BALTIMORE* WILLIAMS AND WILKINS, 1971.

HALLGREN, B.* RETINITIS PIGMENTOSA COMBINED WITH CONGENITAL DEAFNESS* WITH VESTIBULO-CEREBELLAR ATAXIA AND MENTAL ABNORMALITY IN A PROPORTION OF CASES. ACTA PSYCHIAT. NEUROL. SCAND. 34* (SUPPL. 138) 9-101, 1959.

HAMMERSCHLAG, V.* ZUR KENNTNIS DER HEREDITAR-DEGENERATIVEN TAUBSTUMMEN UND IHRE DIFFERENTIAL-DIAGNOSTISCHE BEDEUTUNG. Z. OHRENHEILK. 54* 18-36, 1907.

KLOEPFER, H. W., LAGUAITE, J. K. AND MCLAURIN, J. W.* THE HEREDITARY SYNDROME OF CONGENITAL DEAFNESS AND RETINITIS PIGMENTOSA* (USHER'S SYNDROME). LARYNGOSCOPE 76* 850-862, 1966.

LANG, H. A.* RETINAL DEGENERATION AND NERVE DEAFNESS. BRIT. MED. J. 2* 1096 ONLY, 1959.

LIEBREICH, R.* ABKUNFT AUS EHEN UNTER BLUTSVERWARDTEN ALS GRUND VON RETINITIS PIGMENTOSA. DTSCH. KLIN. 13* 53, 1861.

LINDENOV, H.* THE ETIOLOGY OF DEAF-MUTISM WITH SPECIAL REFERENCE TO HEREDITY. COPENHAGEN* E. MUNKSGAARD, 1945.

NUUTILA, A.* DYSTROPHIA RETINAE PIGMENTOSA-DYSACUSIS SYNDROME (DRD)* A STUDY OF THE USHER OR HALLGREN SYNDROME. J. GENET. HUM. 18* 57-88, 1970.

USHER, C. H.* BOWMAN'S LECTURE* ON A FEW HEREDITARY EYE AFFECTIONS. TRANS. OPHTHAL. SOC. U.K. 55* 164-245, 1935.

VON GRAEFE, A.* EXCEPTIONELLES VERHALTEN DES GESICHTSFELDES BEI PIGMENTENTAR-TUNG DER NERZHAUT. GRAEFES ARCH. OPHTHAL. 4 II* 250-253, 1858.

VERNON, M.* USHER'S SYNDROME-DEAFNESS AND PROGRESSIVE BLINDNESS. CLINICAL CASES, PREVENTION, THEORY AND LITERATURE SURVEY. J. CHRONIC DIS. 22* 133-151, 1969.

27700 VAGINA, ABSENCE OF (ROKITANSKY-KUSTER-HAUSER SYNDROME* UTERUS BIPARTITUS SOLIDUS RUDIMENTARIUS CUM VAGINA SOLIDA)

THE FEATURES, IN ADDITION TO CONGENITAL ABSENCE OF THE VAGINA, ARE NORMAL FEMALE SECONDARY SEXUAL CHARACTERISTICS, RUDIMENTARY UTERUS IN THE FORM OF BILATERAL AND NON-CANALICULATED MUSCULAR BUDS, NORMAL TUBES AND OVARIES AND NORMAL ENDOCRINE AND CYTOGENETIC EVALUATIONS. ANGER ET AL. (1966) REPORTED THREE AFFECTED SISTERS. PHANEUF (1947) DESCRIBED THE MALFORMATION IN TWO PAIRS OF SISTERS WHOSE MOTHERS WERE SISTERS. LAS CASAS DOS SANTOS (1888) REPORTED EARLY FAMILIAL CASES.

ANGER, D., HEMET, J. AND ENSEL, J.* FORME FAMILIALE DU SYNDROME DE ROKITANSKY-KUSTER-HAUSER. BULL. FED. GYNEC. OBSTET. FRANC. 18* 229-234, 1966.

LAS CASAS DOS SANTOS, (NI)* MISSBILDUNGEN DES UTERUS. Z. GEBURTSH. GYNAEK. 14* 140-184, 1888.

PHANEUF, L. E.* DISCUSSION (CONGENITAL MALFORMATIONS OF THE REPRODUCTIVE ORGANS). AM. J. OBSTET. GYNEC. 53* 48 ONLY, 1947.

*27710 VALINEMIA

URINARY AND SERUM VALINE WERE ELEVATED, WITHOUT ELEVATION OF LEUCINE AND ISOLEU-CINE, IN A CHILD WITH VOMITING, FAILURE TO THRIVE AND DROWSINESS (WADA ET AL., 1963). THE PARENTS, WHO WERE NOT KNOWN TO BE RELATED, BOTH SHOWED ABNORMALLY LARGE AMOUNTS OF VALINE IN THE URINE. THE DEFICIENT ENZYME IS VALINE TRANSA-MINASE. OBSERVATION OF THIS CONDITION AND SWEATY FEET DISEASE INDICATES THAT DIFFERENT ENZYMES ARE INVOLVED IN THE METABOLISM OF VALINE, LEUCINE AND ISOLEU-CINE. DANCIS ET AL. (1967) PRESENTED EVIDENCE THAT THE TRANSAMINATION OF VALINE IS DEPENDENT ON AN ENZYME SPECIFIC FOR VALINE. THEY SHOWED FURTHER THAT TRANSA-MINATION OF VALINE IS DEMONSTRABLE IN THE NORMAL PLACENTA. IT MIGHT BE POSSIBLE TO MAKE A PRENATAL DIAGNOSIS OF VALINEMIA BY NEEDLE BIOPSY OF THE PLACENTA, IN INSTANCES OF AN AFFECTED PREVIOUSLY BORN SIB.

DANCIS, J., HUTZLER, J., TADA, K., WADA, Y., MORIKAWA, T. AND ARAKAWA, T.* HYPERVALINEMIA* A DEFECT IN VALINE TRANSAMINATION. PEDIATRICS 39* 813-817, 1967.

TADA, K., WADA, Y. AND ARAKAWA, T.* HYPERVALINEMIA* ITS METABOLIC LESION AND THERAPEUTIC APPROACH. AM. J. DIS. CHILD. 113* 64-67, 1967.

WADA, Y., TADA, K., MINAGAWA, A., YOSHIDA, T., MORIKAWA, T. AND OKAMURA, T.* IDIOPATHIC HYPERVALINEMIA. PROBABLY A NEW ENTITY OF INBORN ERROR OF VALINE METABOLISM. TOHOKU J. EXP. MED. 81* 46-55, 1963.

27720 VENTRICLE, HYPOPLASIA OF RIGHT

HYPOPLASIA OF THE RIGHT VENTRICLE AND TRICUSPID VALVE WAS OBSERVED IN BROTHER AND SISTER BY DAVACHI ET AL. (1967), WHO POINTED OUT THAT AT LEAST TWO FAMILIES WITH MULTIPLE AFFECTED SIBS HAVE BEEN REPORTED (MEDD ET AL., 1961* SACKNER ET AL., 1961).

DAVACHI, F., MCLEAN, R. H., MOLLER, J. H. AND EDWARDS, J. E.* HYPOPLASIA OF THE RIGHT VENTRICLE AND TRICUSPID VALVE IN SIBLINGS. J. PEDIAT. 71* 869-874, 1967.

MEDD, W. E., NEUFELD, H. N., WEIDMAN, W. H. AND EDWARDS, J. E.* ISOLATED HYPOPLASIA OF THE RIGHT VENTRICLE AND TRICUSPID VALVE IN SIBLINGS. BRIT. HEART J. 23* 25-30, 1961.

SACKNER, M. A., ROBINSON, M. J., JAMISON, W. L. AND LEWIS, D. H.* ISOLATED RIGHT VENTRICULAR HYPOPLASIA WITH ATRIAL SEPTAL DEFECT OR PATENT FORAMEN OVALE. CIRCULATION 24* 1388-1402, 1961.

*27730 VERTEBRAL ANOMALIES

LAVY, PALMER AND MERRITT (1967) OBSERVED 4 OF 7 OFFSPRINGS OF A THIRD-COUSIN MARRIAGE HAVING CHARACTERISTIC VERTEBRAL ANOMALIES, INCLUDING HEMIVERTEBRAE AND BLOCK VERTEBRAE ACCOMPANIED BY DEFORMITY OF THE RIBS. ALL AFFECTED CHILDREN DIED OF RESPIRATORY INFECTION UNDER 1 YEAR OF AGE. MOSELEY AND BONFORTE (1969) DESCRIBED THE SAME DISORDER IN TWO APPARENTLY UNRELATED CHILDREN OF NON-CONSAN-GUINEOUS PUERTO RICAN PARENTS. CAFFEY (1967) DESCRIBED BROTHER AND SISTER WITH

R
E
C
E
S
S
I
V
E

SHORT NECK AND TRUNK IN CONTRAST TO EXTREMITIES OF NORMAL LENGTH. BOTH SHOWED 'HEMIVERTEBRAE AT PRACTICALLY ALL LEVELS IN THE SPINE.' THE SKELETONS WERE OTHERWISE NORMAL. WE (NORUM, 1969) HAVE OBSERVED 4 SIMILAR CASES IN TWO RELATED SIBSHIPS IN AN INBRED COMMUNITY IN EASTERN KENTUCKY. FUSED RIBS ALSO OCCURRED IN AFFECTED PERSONS. SEE COSTOVERTEBRAL SEGMENTATION ANOMALIES IN THE DOMINANT CATALOG. PHENOTYPICALLY THE DOMINANT AND RECESSIVE FORMS ARE VERY SIMILAR. ELLER AND MORTON (1970) DESCRIBED SIMILAR DEFORMITY OF THE CHEST AND SPINE, WITH ADDITIONAL CRANIOLACUNIA, RACHISCHISIS AND URINARY TRACT ANOMALIES, IN THE OFFSPRING OF A WOMAN WHO ADMITTED TO A SINGLE EXPOSURE TO LSD ABOUT THE TIME OF CONCEPTION. CANTU ET AL. (1971) DESCRIBED FIVE CASES IN AN INBRED KINDRED.

CAFFEY, J. P.* NORMAL VERTEBRAL COLUMN. PEDIATRIC X-RAY DIAGNOSIS. CHICAGO* YEAR BOOK MEDICAL PUBLISHERS, 1967. (5TH ED.) PP. 1101-1108.

CANTU, J. M., URRUSTI, J., ROSALES, G. AND ROJAS, A.* EVIDENCE FOR AUTOSOMAL RECESSIVE INHERITANCE OF COSTOVERTEBRAL DYSPLASIA. CLIN. GENET., IN PRESS, 1971.

ELLER, J. L. AND MORTON, J. M.* BIZARRE DEFORMITIES IN OFFSPRING OF USER OF LYSERGIC ACID DIETHYLAMIDE. NEW ENG. J. MED. 283* 395-397, 1970.

LAVY, N. W., PALMER, C. G. AND MERRITT, A. D.* A SYNDROME OF BIZARRE VERTEBRAL ANOMALIES. J. PEDIAT. 69* 1121-1125, 1967.

MOSELEY, J. E. AND BONFORTE, R. J.* SPONDYLOTHORACIC DYSPLASIA - A SYNDROME OF CONGENITAL ANOMALIES. AM. J. ROENTGEN. 106* 166-169, 1969.

NORUM, R. A.* COSTOVERTEBRAL ANOMALIES WITH APPARENT RECESSIVE INHERITANCE. THE CLINICAL DELINEATION OF BIRTH DEFECTS. IV. SKELETAL DYSPLASIAS. NEW YORK* NATIONAL FOUNDATION, 1969. PP. 326-329.

27740 VITAMIN B12 METABOLIC DEFECT

MUDD ET AL. (1969) DESCRIBED THE BIOCHEMICAL FINDINGS IN AN INFANT WHO DIED AT 7.5 WEEKS. THERE WAS A DEFECT IN THE TWO REACTIONS IN WHICH VITAMIN B12 DERIVATIVES ARE KNOWN TO FUNCTION AS COENZYMES* (1) METHIONINE FORMATION FROM 5-METHYLFOLATE-H(4) AND HOMOCYSTEINE, AND (2) ISOMERIZATION OF METHYLMALONYL-CO-A TO SUCCINYL-CO-A. THE INFANT SHOWED HOMOCYSTINEMIA, CYSTATHIONINEMIA AND CYSTATHIONINURIA, DECREASE IN METHIONINE, AND METHYLMALONIC ACIDURIA. DEFICIENT ACTIVITY WAS DEMONSTRATED IN THE TWO ENZYMES DEPENDENT ON B12 DERIVATIVES AS COENZYMES* METHYLFOLATE-H(4) METHYLTRANSFERASE AND METHYLMALONYL-CO-A ISOMERASE. SINCE VITAMIN B12 WAS PRESENT IN NORMAL CONCENTRATIONS IN THE LIVER, MUDD ET AL. CONCLUDED THAT THE GENE-DETERMINED DEFECT PROBABLY CONCERNED THE CONVERSION OF B12 TO COENZYMATICALLY ACTIVE DERIVATIVES. THIS MAY BE THE FIRST PROVEN INSTANCE OF DERANGED VITAMIN METABOLISM IN MAN.

R
E
C
E
S
S
I
V
E

MUDD, S. H., LEVY, H. L. AND ABELES, R. H.* A DERANGEMENT IN B12 METABOLISM LEADING TO HOMOCYSTINEMIA, CYSTATHIONINEMIA AND METHYLMALONIC ACIDURIA. BIOCHEM. BIOPHYS. RES. COMMUN. 35* 121-126, 1969.

27750 VITAMIN D DEPENDENT RICKETS

VITAMIN-D-DEPENDENT RICKETS WAS THE TERM SUGGESTED BY FRASER AND SALTER (1958). SCRIVER (1970) SUPPORTED AUTOSOMAL RECESSIVE INHERITANCE AND SUGGESTED THAT THE CONDITION MAY BE MORE FREQUENT THAN PREVIOUSLY REALIZED. HAMILTON ET AL. (1970) DEMONSTRATED DEFECTIVE INTESTINAL ABSORPTION OF CALCIUM AS THE PRIMARY DEFECT.

FRASER, D. AND SALTER, R. B.* THE DIAGNOSIS AND MANAGEMENT OF THE VARIOUS TYPES OF RICKETS. PEDIAT. CLIN. N. AM. 417-441, 1958.

HAMILTON, R., HARRISON, J., FRASER, D., RADDLE, I., MORECKI, R. AND PAUNIER, L.* THE SMALL INTESTINE IN VITAMIN D DEPENDENT RICKETS. PEDIATRICS 45* 364-373, 1970.

SCRIVER, C. R.* VITAMIN D DEPENDENCY. (EDITORIAL) PEDIATRICS 45* 361-363, 1970.

*27760 WEILL-MARCHESANI SYNDROME (SPHEROPHAKIA-BRACHYMORPHIA SYNDROME, CONGENITAL MESODERMAL DYSMORPHO-DYSTROPHY)

THE FEATURES ARE ECTOPIA LENTIS, SHORT STATURE AND BRACHYDACTYLY. THE LENS IS USUALLY ROUND AND ABNORMALLY SMALL, SO THAT THE SPHEROPHAKIA-BRACHYMORPHIA SYNDROME IS A SYNONYM. THE SYNDROME IS APPARENTLY NOT COMPLETELY RECESSIVE. PROBERT (1953) DESCRIBED A FAMILY IN WHICH FOUR SIBS (3 FEMALES, ONE MALE) HAD THE FULL SYNDROME, AND ONE OF THEIR PARENTS AND MANY RELATIVES IN A DOMINANT PEDIGREE PATTERN HAD BRACHYMORPHISM. MEYER AND HOLSTEIN (1941) DESCRIBED FOUR AFFECTED SIBS WHOSE PARENTS WERE RELATED. RENNERT (1969) DESCRIBED 'DIFFICULTY IN EXTENDING HIS ARMS OVER HIS HEAD' IN A 9 YEAR OLD BOY. THE SISTERS REPORTED BY FEINBERG (1960) CLEARLY DID NOT HAVE W-M. THEY ARE THE SAME CASES AS THOSE DESCRIBED BY GORLIN ET AL. (1960) AS A POSSIBLE NEW SYNDROME (SEE GORLIN'S SYNDROME).

FEINBERG, S. B.* CONGENITAL MESODERMAL DYSMORPHO-DYSTROPHY (BRACHYMORPHIC

TYPE). RADIOLOGY 74* 218-229, 1960.

GORLIN, R. J., CHAUDHRY, A. P. AND MOSS, M. L.* CRANIOFACIAL DYSOSTOSIS, PATENT DUCTUS ARTERIOSUS, HYPERTRICHOSIS, HYPOPLASIA OF LABIA MAJORA, DENTAL AND EYE ANOMALIES - A NEW SYNDROME.Q J. PEDIAT. 56* 778-785, 1960.

KLOEPFER, H. W. AND ROSENTHAL, J. W.* POSSIBLE GENETIC CARRIERS IN THE SPHEROPHAKIA-BRACHYMORPHIA SYNDROME. AM. J. HUM. GENET. 7* 398-424, 1955.

MEYER, S. J. AND HOLSTEIN, T.* SPHEROPHAKIA WITH GLAUCOMA AND BRACHYDACTYLY. AM. J. OPHTHAL. 24* 247-257, 1941.

PROBERT, L. A.* SPHEROPHAKIA WITH BRACHYDACTYLY. COMPARISON WITH MARFAN'S SYNDROME. AM. J. OPHTHAL. 36* 1571-1574, 1953.

RENNERT, O. M.* THE MARCHESANI SYNDROME. A BRIEF REVIEW. AM. J. DIS. CHILD. 117* 703-705, 1969.

STADLIN, W. AND KLEIN, D.* ECTOPIE CONGENITALE DU CRISTALLIN AVEC SPHEROPHAQUIE ET BRACHYMORPHIE ACCOMPANGEE DE PARESIS DU REGARD. (SYNDROME DE MARCHESANI). ANN. OCULIST. 181* 692-701, 1948.

*27770 WERNER SYNDROME

THE FEATURES ARE SCLERODERMA-LIKE SKIN CHANGES, ESPECIALLY IN THE EXTREMITIES, CATARACT, SUBCUTANEOUS CALCIFICATION, PREMATURE ARTERIOSCLEROSIS, DIABETES MELLITUS, AND A WIDENED AND PREMATURELY AGED FACIES. A PARTICULARLY INSTRUCTIVE PEDIGREE WAS REPORTED BY MCKUSICK ET AL. (1963).

BOYD, M. W. J. AND GRANT, A. P.* WERNER'S SYNDROME (PROGERIA OF THE ADULT)* FURTHER PATHOLOGICAL AND BIOCHEMICAL OBSERVATIONS. BRIT. MED. J. 2* 920-925, 1959.

EPSTEIN, C. J., MARTIN, G. M., SCHULTZ, A. L. AND MOTULSKY, A. G.* WERNER'S SYNDROME* A REVIEW OF ITS SYMPTOMATOLOGY, NATURAL HISTORY, PATHOLOGIC FEATURES, GENETICS AND RELATIONSHIP TO THE NATURAL AGING PROCESS. MEDICINE 45* 177-222, 1966.

MCKUSICK, V. A. AND COLLEAGUES* MEDICAL GENETICS 1962. J. CHRONIC DIS. 16* 457-634, 1963.

MOTULSKY, A. G., SCHULTZ, A. AND PRIEST, J.* WERNER'S SYNDROME* CHROMOSOMES, GENES, AND THE AGEING PROCESS. LANCET 1* 160-161, 1962.

27780 WILMS' TUMOR

RATHER NUMEROUS INSTANCES OF MULTIPLE AFFECTED SIBS HAVE BEEN DESCRIBED (FITZ-GERALD, HARDIN, 1955). STROM (1957) DESCRIBED A FAMILY WITH 5 CASES IN THREE GENERATIONS. A HEALTHY MALE HAD TWO AFFECTED CHILDREN (OUT OF 5) BY ONE WIFE AND ONE AFFECTED CHILD BY ANOTHER WIFE. A SISTER AND AN AUNT OF HIS HAD DIED IN INFANCY OR EARLY CHILDHOOD OF ABDOMINAL TUMOR. ANIRIDIA, HEMIHYPERTROPHY AND OTHER CONGENITAL ANOMALIES HAVE BEEN FOUND IN SOME CASES OF WILMS' TUMOR (MILLER, FRAUMENI AND MANNING, 1964).

FITZGERALD, W. L. AND HARDIN, H. C., JR.* BILATERAL WILMS' TUMOR IN A WILMS' TUMOR FAMILY* CASE REPORT. J. UROL. 73* 468-474, 1955.

MILLER, R. W., FRAUMENI, J. F., JR. AND MANNING, M. D.* ASSOCIATION OF WILMS' TUMOR WITH ANIRIDIA, HEMIHYPERTROPHY AND OTHER CONGENITAL MALFORMATIONS. NEW ENG. J. MED. 270* 922-927, 1964.

STROM, T.* A WILMS' TUMOR FAMILY. ACTA PAEDIAT. 46* 601-604, 1957.

*27790 WILSON'S DISEASE (HEPATOLENTICULAR DEGENERATION)

THE LIVER AND BASAL GANGLIA UNDERGO CHANGES WHICH EXPRESS THEMSELVES IN NEUROLOGIC MANIFESTATIONS AND SIGNS OF CIRRHOSIS. A DISTURBANCE IN COPPER METABOLISM IS SOMEHOW INVOLVED IN THE MECHANISM. LOW CERULOPLASMIN IS FOUND IN THE SERUM. SHOKEIR AND SHREFFLER (1969) ADVANCED THE HYPOTHESIS THAT CERULOPLASMIN FUNCTIONS IN ENZYMATIC TRANSFER OF COPPER TO COPPER-CONTAINING ENZYMES SUCH AS CYTOCHROME OXIDASE. SUPPORTING THE HYPOTHESIS WAS THE FINDING OF MARKEDLY REDUCED LEVELS OF ACTIVITY OF CYTOCHROME OXIDASE IN WILSON'S DISEASE AND MODERATE REDUCTIONS IN HETEROZYGOTES.

ANDERSON, P. J. AND POPPER, H.* CHANGES IN HEPATIC STRUCTURE IN WILSON'S DISEASE. AM. J. PATH. 36* 483-497, 1960.

BEARN, A. G. AND MCKUSICK, V. A.* AZURE LUNULAE. AN UNUSUAL CHANGE IN THE FINGERNAILS IN TWO PATIENTS WITH HEPATOLENTICULAR DEGENERATION (WILSON'S DISEASE). J.A.M.A. 166* 904-906, 1958.

BEARN, A. G.* A GENETICAL ANALYSIS OF THIRTY FAMILIES WITH WILSON'S DISEASE

BEARN, A. G.* WILSON'S DISEASE. IN, STANBURY, J. B., WYNGAARDEN, J. B. AND FREDRICKSON, D. S. (EDS.)* THE METABOLIC BASIS OF INHERITED DISEASE. NEW YORK* MCGRAW-HILL, 1966 (2ND ED.). PP. 761-779.

HOLTZMAN, N. A., NAUGHTON, M. A., IBER, F. L. AND GAUMNITZ, B. M.* CERULOPLAS-MIN IN WILSON'S DISEASE. J. CLIN. INVEST. 46* 993-1002, 1967.

LEVI, A. J., SHERLOCK, S., SCHEUER, P. J. AND CUMINGS, J. N.* PRESYMPTOMATIC WILSON'S DISEASE. LANCET 2* 575-579, 1967.

SHOKEIR, M. H. R. AND SHREFFLER, D. C.* CYTOCHROME OXIDASE DEFICIENCY IN WILSON'S DISEASE* A SUGGESTED CERULOPLASMIN FUNCTION. PROC. NAT. ACAD. SCI. 62* 867-872, 1969.

WALSHE, J. M. AND CUMINGS, J. N.* WILSON'S DISEASE. SOME CURRENT CONCEPTS. OXFORD* BLACKWELL, 1961. PP. 1-292.

*27800 WOLMAN'S DISEASE

WOLMAN AND COLLEAGUES (1961) DESCRIBED THREE SIBS IN WHOM INVOLVEMENT OF THE VISCERA WAS AN IMPORTANT FEATURE AND DEATH OCCURRED AT THE AGE OF ABOUT 3 MONTHS. XANTHOMATOUS CHANGES WERE OBSERVED IN THE LIVER, ADRENAL, SPLEEN, LYMPH NODES, BONE MARROW, SMALL INTESTINE, LUNGS AND THYMUS AND SLIGHT CHANGE IN THE SKIN, RETINA AND CENTRAL NERVOUS SYSTEM. THE ADRENALS WERE CALCIFIED. DEATH WAS THOUGHT TO BE DUE TO INTESTINAL MALABSORPTION RESULTING FROM INVOLVEMENT OF THE GUT. THE PARENTS, PERSIAN JEWS, WERE COUSINS. LIPIDS IN THE PLASMA WERE NORMAL OR MODERATELY ELEVATED. SEVERAL FEATURES SUGGESTED THAT THE ENTITY IS DISTINCT FROM HYPERCHOLESTEROLEMIA AND THE HYPERLIPIDEMIAS (Q.V.). THREE CASES, THE FIRST FROM THE U.S.A., WERE REPORTED BY CROCKER AND COLLEAGUES (1965) WHO GAVE NO INFORMATION ON ETHNICITY. THE RELATIVELY NON-SPECIFIC CLINICAL PICTURE INCLUDES POOR WEIGHT GAIN, VOMITING, DIARRHEA, INCREASING HEPATOSPLENOMEGALY WITH ABDOMINAL PROTRUBERANCE AND DEATH IN NUTRITIONAL FAILURE BY 2-4 MONTHS OF AGE. FOAM CELLS ARE FOUND IN BONE MARROW AND VACUOLATED LYMPHOCYTES IN PERIPHERAL BLOOD, AS IN NIEMANN-PICK DISEASE. DIFFUSE PUNCTATE CALCIFICATION OF THE ADRENALS IS TYPICAL. DISSEMINATED FOAM CELL INFILTRATION IS FOUND IN MANY ORGANS. GREAT INCREASES IN CHOLESTEROL ARE FOUND IN THE ORGANS. KONNO ET AL. (1966) REPORTED A JAPANESE FAMILY WITH THREE AFFECTED SIBS. SPIEGEL-ADOLF ET AL. (1966) REPORTED 3 AFFECTED SIBS IN AN AMERICAN FAMILY. PATRICK AND LAKE (1969) DEMONSTRATED DEFICIENCY OF AN ACID LIPASE WHICH APPARENTLY LEADS TO THE PROGRESSIVE ACCUMULATION OF TRIGLY-CERIDES AND CHOLESTEROL ESTERS IN LYSOSOMES IN THE TISSUES OF AFFECTED PERSONS. LOUGH ET AL. (1970) DESCRIBED AN AFFECTED INFANT OF GREEK ANCESTRY IN WHOM CALCIFIED ADRENALS WERE DEMONSTRATED ON THE 5TH DAY OF LIFE. YOUNG AND PATRICK (1970) COMMENTED ON THE EXISTENCE OF CASES WITH THE SAME BIOCHEMICAL AND HISTOLO-GIC CHANGES AS IN THE ACUTE INFANTILE FORM BUT WITH LATER ONSET AND A MUCH LESS FULMINANT COURSE. ONE OF THEIR CASES WAS ALIVE AND WELL AT AGE 8 YEARS, SHOWING NO CLINICAL ABNORMALITY OTHER THAN MODERATE HEPATOMEGALY. THE SAME ENZYME IS DEFICIENT IN ALL THESE CASES. HENCE, THEY SUGGESTED THE TERM *ACID LIPASE DEFICIENCY* FOR THE WHOLE GROUP WITH WOLMAN'S DISEASE AS THE DESIGNATION FOR THE ACUTE INFANTILE FORM.

CROCKER, A. C., VAWTER, G. F., NEUHAUSER, E. B. D., AND ROSOWSKY, A.* WOLMAN'S DISEASE* THREE NEW PATIENTS WITH A RECENTLY DESCRIBED LIPIDOSIS. PEDIATRICS 35* 627-640, 1965.

KAHANA, D., BERANT, M. AND WOLMAN, M.* PRIMARY FAMILIAL XANTHOMATOSIS WITH ADRENAL INVOLVEMENT (WOLMAN'S DISEASE). REPORT OF A FURTHER CASE WITH NERVOUS SYSTEM INVOLVEMENT AND PATHOGENETIC CONSIDERATIONS. PEDIATRICS 42* 70-76, 1968.

KONNO, T., FUJII, M., WATANUKI, T. AND KOIZUMI, K.* WOLMAN'S DISEASE* THE FIRST CASE IN JAPAN. TOHOKU J. EXP. MED. 90* 375-389, 1966.

LAKE, B. D. AND PATRICK, A. D.* WOLMAN'S DISEASE* DEFICIENCY OF E600-RESISTANT ACID ESTERASE ACTIVITY WITH STORAGE OF LIPIDS IN LYSOSOMES. J. PEDIAT. 76* 262-266, 1970.

LOUGH, J., FAWCETT, J. AND WIEGENSBERG, B.* WOLMAN'S DISEASE. AN ELECTRON MICROSCOPIC, HISTOCHEMICAL, AND BIOCHEMICAL STUDY. ARCH. PATH. 89* 103-110, 1970.

MARSHALL, W. C., OCKENDEN, B. G., FOSBROOKE, A. S. AND CUMINGS, J. N.* WOLMAN'S DISEASE. A RARE LIPIDOSIS WITH ADRENAL CALCIFICATION. ARCH. DIS. CHILD. 44* 331-341, 1969.

PATRICK, A. D. AND LAKE, B. D.* DEFICIENCY OF AN ACID LIPASE IN WOLMAN'S DISEASE. NATURE 222* 1067-1068, 1969.

SPIEGEL-ADOLF, M., BAIRD, H. W. AND MCCAFFERTY, M.* HEMATOLOGIC STUDIES IN NIEMANN-PICK AND WOLMAN'S DISEASE (CYTOLOGY AND ELECTROPHORESIS). CONFIN. NEUROL. 28* 399-406, 1966.

WOLMAN, M., STERK, V. V., GATT, S. AND FRENKEL, M.* PRIMARY FAMILY XANTHOMATO-

SIS WITH INVOLVEMENT AND CALCIFICATION OF THE ADRENALS. REPORT OF TWO MORE CASES IN SIBLINGS OF A PREVIOUSLY DESCRIBED INFANT. PEDIATRICS 28* 742-757, 1961.

YOUNG, E. P. AND PATRICK, A. D.* DEFICIENCY OF ACID ESTERASE ACTIVITY IN WOLMAN'S DISEASE. ARCH. DIS. CHILD. 45* 664-668, 1970.

27810 WOLMAN'S DISEASE WITH HYPOLIPOPROTEINEMIA AND ACANTHOCYTOSIS

ETO AND KITAGAWA (1970) DESCRIBED A DISORDER WHICH MAY BE A DISTINCT ENTITY. MALABSORPTION OF LIPID, VOMITING, GROWTH FAILURE, AND ADRENAL CALCIFICATION WERE PRESENT. HYPOLIPOPROTEINEMIA AND ACANTHOCYTOSIS SUGGEST THIS IS AN ENTITY DISTINCT FROM WOLMAN'S DISEASE.

ETO, Y. AND KITAGAWA, T.* WOLMAN'S DISEASE WITH HYPOLIPOPROTEINEMIA AND ACANTHOCYTOSIS* CLINICAL AND BIOCHEMICAL OBSERVATIONS. J. PEDIAT. 77* 862-867, 1970.

27820 WOOLLY HAIR, HYPOTRICHOSIS, EVERTED LOWER LIP, PSYCHOSIS, ETC.

SALAMON (1963) DESCRIBED THIS SYNDROME AS A RECESSIVE. THE PARENTS WERE CONSAN-GUINEOUS. WOOLLY HAIR, AS AN ISOLATED TRAIT, IS A DOMINANT (Q.V.).

SALAMON, T.* UBER EINE FAMILIE MIT RECESSIVER KRAUSHAARIGKEIT, HYPOTRICHOSE UND ANDEREN ANOMALIEN. HAUTARZT 14* 540-544, 1963.

*27830 XANTHINURIA

THE DISORDER IS CHARACTERIZED BY EXCRETION OF VERY LARGE AMOUNTS OF XANTHINE IN THE URINE AND A TENDENCY TO FORM XANTHINE STONES. URIC ACID IS STRIKINGLY DIMINISHED IN SERUM AND URINE. THE DEFECT IS THOUGHT TO INVOLVE XANTHINE OXIDASE AND A RENAL TUBULAR DEFECT IN REABSORPTION OF XANTHINE IS ALSO PRESENT. THE CONDITION MAY WELL BE INHERITED AS A RECESSIVE. HOWEVER, THE EVIDENCE IS MEAGER. DICKINSON AND SMELLIE (1959) DESCRIBED A WELL-STUDIED SINGLE CASE, A CHILD OF UNRELATED, UNAFFECTED PARENTS. WATTS ET AL. (1964) DESCRIBED A 23 YEAR OLD WOMAN IN WHOM THE DISORDER WAS SUSPECTED BECAUSE OF VERY LOW SERUM URIC ACID. THERE WERE NO URINARY CALCULI. ENZYME ASSAYS SHOWED VERY LITTLE OXIDATION OF BOTH HYPOXANTHINE AND XANTHINE PRESUMABLY DUE TO A DEFECT IN XANTHINE OXIDASE. AFFECTED BROTHERS HAVE BEEN OBSERVED (WYNGAARDEN, 1966). IN THE EIGHTH KNOWN PATIENT, STUDIED BY CHALMERS ET AL. (1969), A NEGRO MALE, CRYSTALLINE DEPOSITS OCCURRED IN SKELETAL MUSCLE.

CHALMERS, R. A., JOHNSON, M., PALLIS, C. AND WATTS, R. W. E.* XANTHINURIA WITH MYOPATHY. QUART. J. MED. 38* 493-512, 1969.

DICKINSON, C. J. AND SMELLIE, J. M.* XANTHINURIA. BRIT. MED. J. 2* 1217-1221, 1959.

ENGELMAN, K., WATTS, R. W. E., KLINENBERG, J. R., SJOERDSMA, A. AND SEEGMILLER, J. E.* CLINICAL, PHYSIOLOGICAL AND BIOCHEMICAL STUDIES OF A PATIENT WITH XAN-THINURIA AND PHEOCHROMOCYTOMA. AM. J. MED. 37* 839-861, 1964.

WATTS, R. W. E., ENGELMAN, K., KLINENBERG, J. R., SEEGMILLER, J. E. AND SJOERDSMA, A.* ENZYME DEFECT IN A CASE OF XANTHINURIA. NATURE 201* 395-396, 1964.

WYNGAARDEN, J. B.* XANTHINURIA. IN, STANBURY, J. B., WYNGAARDEN, J. B. AND FREDRICKSON, D. S. (EDS.)* THE METABOLIC BASIS OF INHERITED DISEASE. NEW YORK* MCGRAW-HILL, 1966 (2ND ED.). PP. 729-738.

27840 XANTHISM (RUFOUS ALBINISM)

THIS TRAIT OCCURS IN NEGROES AND IS CHARACTERIZED BY BRIGHT COPPER-RED COLORATION OF THE SKIN AND HAIR AND DILUTION OF THE COLOR OF THE IRIS. BARNICOT (1957) SUGGESTED THAT THIS IS A GENETIC TRAIT DISTINCT FROM ALBINISM. PEARSON, NETTLE-SHIP AND USHER (1911-1913) ARE SAID TO HAVE CITED A PEDIGREE IN WHICH BOTH XANTHISM AND ALBINISM OCCURRED. XANTHISM MAY BE THE SAME AS TYPE II ALBINISM (Q.V.), WHICH IN THE NEGRO SEEMS TO ANSWER THE DESCRIPTIONS CITED ABOVE.

BARNICOT, N. A.* HUMAN PIGMENTATION. MAN 57* 114-120, 1957.

PEARSON, K., NETTLESHIP, E. AND USHER, C. H.* A MONOGRAPH ON ALBINISM IN MAN. SERIES VI, VIII, IX, PARTS I, II AND IV. LONDON* CAMBRIDGE UNIV. PRESS, 6* 1911-1913.

27850 XANTHOMATOSIS, TENDINOUS AND TUBEROUS, WITHOUT HYPERLIPIDEMIA

HARLAN AND STILL (1968) DESCRIBED NEGRO BROTHER AND SISTER WITH MULTIPLE TENDINOUS AND TUBEROUS XANTHOMAS DESPITE PLASMA LIPIDS WHICH WERE QUANTITATIVELY AND QUALITATIVELY NORMAL. EVIDENCE OF XANTHOMATOUS INVOLVEMENT OF THE LUNGS WAS FOUND IN THE MALE. THE AUTHORS SUGGESTED THAT NORMOLIPEMIC XANTHOMATOSIS IS A DISTINCT ENTITY INHERITED AS AN AUTOSOMAL RECESSIVE AND THAT IT SHOULD BE CLASSIFIED AS A RETICULOENDOTHELIOSIS. SWANSON (1968) SUGGESTED THAT THIS MAY BE THE SAME ENTITY AS CEREBROTENDINOUS XANTHOMATOSIS. ALTHOUGH NEUROLOGICAL MANIFESTATIONS WERE NOT

R
E
C
E
S
S
I
V
E

EVIDENT, THESE MAY BE LATE IN APPEARING.

HARLAN, W. R., JR. AND STILL, W. J.* HEREDITARY TENDINOUS AND TUBEROUS XANTHOMATOSIS WITHOUT HYPERLIPIDEMIA. A NEW LIPID-STORAGE DISORDER. NEW ENG. J. MED. 278* 416-422, 1968.

SWANSON, P. D.* CEREBROTENDINOUS XANTHOMATOSIS. (LETTER) NEW ENG. J. MED. 278* 857 ONLY, 1968.

*27860 XANTHURENICACIDURIA

THIS DISORDER IS DUE TO A DEFECT IN KYNURENINASE, A VITAMIN B6 DEPENDENT ENZYME IN THE TRYPTOPHANE CATABOLIC PATHWAY. BOTH B6-RESPONSIVE AND B6-NONRESPONSIVE FORMS ARE KNOWN.

TADA, K., YOKOYAMA, Y., NAKAGAWA, H., YOSHIDA, T. AND ARAKAWA, T.* VITAMIN B6 DEPENDENT XANTHURENIC ACIDURIA. TOHOKU J. EXP. MED. 93* 115-124, 1967.

*27870 XERODERMA PIGMENTOSUM

SENSITIVITY TO SUNLIGHT WITH THE DEVELOPMENT OF CARCINOMATA AT AN EARLY AGE IS OBSERVED. ONSET, WITH FRECKLE-LIKE LESIONS IN EXPOSED AREAS, USUALLY OCCURS IN THE FIRST YEARS OF LIFE. THE POSSIBILITY OF PARTIAL SEX-LINKED RECESSIVE INHERITANCE WAS SUGGESTED BY HALDANE BUT IS NOW CONSIDERED UNLIKELY. PARENTAL CONSANGUINITY IS FREQUENT. THE SEX RATIO IS ABOUT 1. RUDER (CITED BY COCKAYNE) OBSERVED THE CONDITION IN 7 OUT OF 13 SIBS. IT IS NOT CLEAR WHETHER HETEROZYGOTES SHOW CHANGES. INCREASED FRECKLING HAS BEEN CLAIMED TO BE SUCH A MANIFESTATION. EL-HEFNAWI, SMITH AND PENROSE (1965) PRESENTED USEFUL PEDIGREES AND SUGGESTED LINKAGE WITH THE ABO BLOOD GROUP LOCUS. CLEAVER (1968) SHOWED THAT WHEREAS NORMAL SKIN FIBROBLASTS CAN REPAIR ULTRAVIOLET RADIATION DAMAGE TO DNA BY INSERTING NEW BASES INTO DNA, CELLS FROM PATIENTS WITH XERODERMA PIGMENTOSUM LACK THIS CAPACITY OR HAVE A MUCH REDUCED CAPACITY FOR REPAIR.

CLEAVER, J. E.* DEFECTIVE REPAIR REPLICATION OF DNA IN XERODERMA PIGMENTOSUM. NATURE 218* 652-656, 1968.

COCKAYNE, E. A.* INHERITED ABNORMALITIES OF THE SKIN AND ITS APPENDAGES. LONDON* OXFORD UNIV. PRESS, 1933.

DE GROUCHY, J., DE NAVA, C., FEINGOLD, J., FREZAL, J. AND LAMY, M.* ASYNCHRONIE CHROMOSOMIQUE DANS UN CAS DE XERODERMA PIGMENTOSUM. ANN. GENET. 10* 224-225, 1967.

EL-HEFNAWI, H., SMITH, S. M. AND PENROSE, L. S.* XERODERMA PIGMENTOSUM-ITS INHERITANCE AND RELATIONSHIP TO THE ABO BLOOD-GROUP SYSTEM. ANN. HUM. GENET. 28* 273-290, 1965.

MACKLIN, M. T.* XERODERMA PIGMENTOSUM* REPORT OF A CASE AND CONSIDERATION OF INCOMPLETE SEX LINKAGE IN INHERITANCE OF THE DISEASE. ARCH. DERM. SYPH. 49* 157-171, 1944.

*27880 XERODERMIC IDIOCY OF DE SANCTIS AND CACCHIONE

IN ADDITION TO XERODERMA PIGMENTOSUM THE FEATURES ARE MENTAL DEFICIENCY, DWARFISM AND GONADAL HYPOPLASIA. REED, MAY AND NICKEL (1965) DESCRIBED THE SYNDROME IN A CAUCASIAN BROTHER AND SISTER AND TWO 'JAPANESE' BROTHERS. ALTHOUGH THESE AUTHORS WERE OF THE VIEW THAT THIS IS FUNDAMENTALLY THE SAME ENTITY AS XERODERMA PIGMENTO-SUM WITHOUT ASSOCIATED ABNORMALITIES, IT SEEMS MORE LIKELY THAT IT IS DISTINCTIVE. CHOREO-ATHETOID NEUROLOGIC SIGNS OCCURRED IN THEIR CASES AND IN ONE SIB DEVELOPED LEUKEMIA (REED, 1967). YANO (1950) DESCRIBED THE AUTOPSY FINDINGS IN A JAPANESE CASE AND REED ET AL. (1969) REPORTED THE FINDINGS IN A JAPANESE-AMERICAN CASE. CEREBRAL AND OLIVOPONTOCEREBELLAR ATROPHY WAS FOUND. OF THE 5 PATIENTS DESCRIBED BY REED ET AL. (1969), 4 HAD ASSOCIATED NEUROLOGIC FEATURES (DESANCTIS-CACCHIONE SYNDROME). ONE OF THE PATIENTS WITH THE LATTER SYNDROME DEVELOPED ACUTE LYMPHATIC LEUKEMIA AT THE AGE OF 3 YEARS.

ELSASSER, G., FREUSBERG, O. AND THEML, F.* DAS XERODERMA PIGMENTOSUM UND DIE 'XERODERMISCHE IDIOTIE.' ARCH. DERM. 188* 651-655, 1950.

REED, W. B.* BURBANK, CALIF.* PERSONAL COMMUNICATION, 1967.

REED, W. B., LANDING, B., SUGARMAN, G., CLEAVER, J. E. AND MELNYK, J.* XERODERMA PIGMENTOSUM. CLINICAL AND LABORATORY INVESTIGATION OF ITS BASIC DEFECT. J.A.M.A. 207* 2073-2079, 1969.

REED, W. B., MAY, S. B. AND NICKEL, W. R.* XERODERMA PIGMENTOSUM WITH NEUROLO-GICAL COMPLICATIONS. ARCH. DERM. 91* 224-226, 1965.

YANO, K.* XERODERMA PIGMENTOSUM MIT STORUNGEN DES ZENTRALNERVENSYSTEMS* EINE HISTOPATHOLOGISCHE UNTERSUCHUNG. FOLIA PSYCHIAT. NEUROL. JAP. 4* 143-151, 1950.

27890 XYLOSIDASE DEFICIENCY

R
E
C
E
S
S
I
V
E

540 PAYLING-WRIGHT AND EVANS (1970) DESCRIBED A GIRL WHO HAD BEEN NORMAL UNTIL AGE 3 MONTHS WHEN THERE WAS ONSET OF SEIZURES. AT THE AGE OF NINE MONTHS, SHE WAS FLOPPY, MADE CHOREO-ATHETOTIC MOVEMENTS AND APPEARED TO LACK SIGHT OR HEARING. INVESTIGATIONS SHOWED SMALL HEAD, HYPSARRHYTHMIA BY EEG AND DILATED VENTRICLES BY AIR ENCEPHALOGRAPHY. LYMPHOCYTES GROWN IN SHORT-TERM CULTURE SHOWED VERY LOW BETA-XYLOSIDASE. THUS, THIS APPEARS TO BE A LYSOSOMAL DISORDER.

PAYLING-WRIGHT, C. R. AND EVANS, P. R.* A CASE OF BETA-XYLOSIDASE DEFICIENCY. (LETTER) LANCET 2* 43 ONLY, 1970.

RECESSIVE

X-LINKED PHENOTYPES

FANCONI, PRADER, ISLER, LUTHY AND SIEBENMANN (1964) SUGGESTED X-LINKED RECESSIVE INHERITANCE OF A SYNDROME OF ADDISON'S DISEASE AND CEREBRAL SCLEROSIS. ALL CASES HAVE BEEN MALE AND IN AT LEAST FIVE INSTANCES A BROTHER AND-OR A MATERNAL UNCLE OF THE PROBAND HAS BEEN SIMILARLY AFFECTED. HOEFNAGEL, VAN DEN NOORT AND INGBAR (1962) DESCRIBED THE HISTOLOGIC FINDINGS IN ENDOCRINE GLANDS, ESPECIALLY THE PITUITARY AND ADRENAL.

AGUILAR, M. J., O'BRIEN, J. S. AND TABER, P.* THE SYNDROME OF FAMILIAL LEUKODYSTROPHY, ADRENAL INSUFFICIENCY AND CUTANEOUS MELANOSIS. IN, ARONSON, S. M. AND VOLK, B. W. (EDS.)* INBORN DISORDERS OF SPHINGOLIPID METABOLISM. OXFORD* PERGAMON PRESS, 1967. PP. 149-166.

FANCONI, A., PRADER, A., ISLER, W., LUTHY, F. AND SIEBENMANN, R.* MORBUS ADDISON MIT HIRNSKLEROSE IM KINDESALTER. EIN HEREDITARES SYNDROM MIT X-CHROMO-SOMALER VERERBUNG.Q HELV. PAEDIAT. ACTA 18* 480-501, 1964.

HOEFNAGEL, D., BRUN, A., INGBAR, S. H. AND GOLDMAN, H.* ADDISON'S DISEASE AND DIFFUSE CEREBRAL SCLEROSIS. J. NEUROL. NEUROSURG. PSYCHIAT. 30* 56-60, 1967.

HOEFNAGEL, D., VAN DEN NOORT, S. AND INGBAR, S. H.* DIFFUSE CEREBRAL SCLEROSIS WITH ENDOCRINE ABNORMALITIES IN YOUNG MALES. BRAIN 85* 553-568, 1962.

TURKINGTON, R. W. AND STEMPFEL, R. S., JR.* ADRENOCORTICAL ATROPHY AND DIFFUSE CEREBRAL SCLEROSIS (ADDISON-SCHILDER'S DISEASE). J. PEDIAT. 69* 406-412, 1966.

*30020 ADRENAL HYPOPLASIA

THE ANATOMIC FEATURES WERE BOTH SEVERE HYPOPLASIA AND DISORGANIZATION. DEATH WITHOUT TREATMENT WAS EARLY IN LIFE. THERE ARE PROBABLY BOTH AUTOSOMAL RECESSIVE AND X-LINKED FORMS AND THERE MAY BE MORE THAN ONE OF EACH. WEISS AND MELLINGER (1970) REPORTED 3 AFFECTED BROTHERS OUT OF FOUR. A DIFFERENT MAN FATHERED EACH OF THE THREE AFFECTED SONS. HISTOLOGICALLY THERE WAS LACK OF ORGANIZATION OF THE CORTEX INTO CORDS. PRESENCE OF CLUMPS OF LARGE PALE STAINING CELLS IS ANOTHER FEATURE. SEVERAL OTHER FAMILIES CONSISTENT WITH X-LINKED INHERITANCE WERE FOUND (E.G., BOYD AND MACDONALD, 1960* UTTLEY, 1968* STEMPFEL AND ENGEL, 1960). BROCHNER-MORTENSEN (1956) DESCRIBED ADDISON'S DISEASE IN TWO BROTHERS AND TWO OF THEIR MATERNAL UNCLES. THREE OF THE PATIENTS HAD DIED AT AGES 19, 26 AND 33 YEARS. ADDISON'S DISEASE AND CEREBRAL SCLEROSIS (Q.V.) IS A WELL ESTABLISHED X-LINKED DISORDER. IN BROTHERS REPORTED BY MEAKIN ET AL. (1959), THE DIAGNOSIS WAS MADE IN THE ELDER AT 9 YEARS OF AGE AND IN THE SECOND AT 6 YEARS OF AGE. MARTIN (1971) DESCRIBED A PAIR OF BROTHERS IN WHOM THE SIGNS OF ADDISON'S DISEASE DEVELOPED AT AGE 5. IT SEEMS LIKELY THAT ADDISON'S DISEASE WITH THIS LATER ONSET IS DISTINCT FROM THAT DUE TO ADRENAL HYPOPLASIA AS DESCRIBED BY WEISS AND MELLINGER (1970) AND BY OTHERS.

BOYD, J. F. AND MACDONALD, A. M.* ADRENAL CORTICAL HYPOPLASIA IN SIBLINGS. ARCH. DIS. CHILD. 35* 561-568, 1960.

BROCHNER-MORTENSEN, K.* FAMILIAL OCCURRENCE OF ADDISON'S DISEASE. ACTA MED. SCAND. 155* 205-209, 1956.

MARTIN, M. M.* FAMILIAL ADDISON'S DISEASE. THE CLINICAL DELINEATION OF BIRTH DEFECTS. X. THE ENDOCRINE SYSTEM. BALTIMORE* WILLIAMS AND WILKINS, 1971.

STEMPFEL, R. S., JR. AND ENGEL, F. L.* A CONGENITAL, FAMILIAL SYNDROME OF ADRENOCORTICAL INSUFFICIENCY WITHOUT HYPOALDOSTERONISM. J. PEDIAT. 57* 443-451, 1960.

UTTLEY, W. S.* FAMILIAL CONGENITAL ADRENAL HYPOPLASIA. ARCH. DIS. CHILD. 43* 724-730, 1968.

WEISS, L. AND MELLINGER, R. C.* CONGENITAL ADRENAL HYPOPLASIA - AN X-LINKED DISEASE. J. MED. GENET. 7* 27-32, 1970.

*30030 AGAMMAGLOBULINEMIA (BRUTON TYPE)

PATIENTS ARE UNUSUALLY PRONE TO BACTERIAL INFECTION BUT NOT TO VIRAL INFECTION. A CLINICAL PICTURE RESEMBLING RHEUMATOID ARTHRITIS DEVELOPS IN MANY. BEFORE ANTIBIOTICS, DEATH OCCURRED IN THE FIRST DECADE. IN THE MORE USUAL X-LINKED FORM OF THE DISEASE PLASMA CELLS ARE LACKING. A RARER FORM OF AGAMMAGLOBULINEMIA (HITZIG AND WILLI, 1961), WHICH IS INHERITED AS AN AUTOSOMAL RECESSIVE (Q.V.), SHOWS MARKED DEPRESSION OF THE CIRCULATING LYMPHOCYTES AND LYMPHOCYTES ARE ABSENT FROM THE LYMPHOID TISSUE. THE ALYMPHOCYTOTIC TYPE IS EVEN MORE VIRULENT THAN THE X-LINKED FORM LEADING TO DEATH IN THE FIRST 18 MONTHS AFTER BIRTH, FROM SEVERE THRUSH, CHRONIC DIARRHEA, AND RECURRENT PULMONARY INFECTIONS. SELIGMAN ET AL. (1968) PROPOSED A CLASSIFICATION OF IMMUNOLOGIC DEFICIENCIES WHICH INCLUDED 11 ENTITIES OF WHICH A GENETIC BASIS HAS BEEN PROVED OR SUSPECTED IN ALL EXCEPT ONE - DIGEORGE'S THYMIC APLASIA. THE 10 OTHERS ARE BRUTON'S SEX-LINKED AGAMMAGLOBULINE-MIA, SELECTIVE INABILITY TO PRODUCE IGA (WHICH THEY STATE MAY BE AUTOSOMAL RECESSIVE IN SOME CASES), TRANSIENT HYPOGAMMAGLOBULINEMIA OF INFANCY, NON-SEX-

X
L
I
N
K
E
D

LINKED IMMUNOGLOBULIN DEFICIENCY, AGAMMAGLOBULINEMIA WITH THYMOMA, WISKOTT-ALDRICH SYNDROME, ATAXIA-TELANGIECTASIA, PRIMARY LYMPHOPENIC IMMUNOLOGIC DEFICIENCY OF THE TYPE FIRST REPORTED BY GITLIN AND CRAIG (1963), SWISS-TYPE AGAMMAGLOBULINEMIA, AND AUTOSOMAL RECESSIVE LYMPHOPENIA WITH NORMAL IMMUNOGLOBULINS (NEZELOF'S SYNDROME).

GARVIE, J. M. AND KENDALL, A. C.* CONGENITAL AGAMMAGLOBULINAEMIA. REPORT OF TWO FURTHER CASES. BRIT. MED. J. 1* 548-550, 1961.

GITLIN, D. AND CRAIG, J. M.* THE THYMUS AND OTHER LYMPHOID TISSUES IN CONGENI-TAL AGAMMAGLOBULINEMIA. I. THYMIC ALYMPHOPLASIA AND LYMPHOCYTIC HYPOPLASIA AND THEIR RELATION TO INFECTION. PEDIATRICS 32* 517-530, 1963.

HITZIG, W. H. AND WILLI, H.* HEREDITARY LYMPHOPLASMOCYTIC DYSGENESIS ('ALYMPHO-CYTOSE MIT AGAMMAGLOBULINAMIA'). SCHWEIZ. MED. WSCHR. 91* 1625-1633, 1961.

JANEWAY, C. A., APT, L. AND GITLIN, D.* AGAMMAGLOBULINEMIA. TRANS. ASS. AM. PHYSICIANS 66* 200-202, 1953.

SELIGMAN, M., FUDENBERG, H. H. AND GOOD, R. A.* A PROPOSED CLASSIFICATION OF PRIMARY IMMUNOLOGIC DEFICIENCIES. AM. J. MED. 45* 817-825, 1968.

*30040 AGAMMAGLOBULINEMIA, SWISS TYPE (THYMIC EPITHELIAL HYPOPLASIA)

THIS TYPE OF DISEASE DIFFERS FROM THE BRUTON TYPE BY THE PRESENCE OF LYMPHOCYTO-PENIA ('ALYMPHOCYTOSIS'), EARLIER AGE OF DEATH, VULNERABILITY TO VIRAL AND FUNGAL AS WELL AS BACTERIAL INFECTIONS, LACK OF DELAYED HYPERSENSITIVITY, ATROPHY OF THE THYMUS, AND LACK OF BENEFIT BY GAMMA GLOBULIN ADMINISTRATION. IT IS USUALLY INHERITED AS AN AUTOSOMAL RECESSIVE (Q.V.) BUT ALL CASES IN THREE FAMILIES STUDIED BY ROSEN ET AL. (1966) WERE MALE AND ONE KINDRED (FAMILY T) HAD 9 AFFECTED MALES IN 5 SIBSHIPS IN THREE GENERATIONS CONNECTED THROUGH FEMALES IN A TYPICAL X-LINKED RECESSIVE PEDIGREE PATTERN. MILLER AND SCHIEKEN (1967) SUGGESTED THAT ONE FORM OF THYMIC DYSPLASIA IS X-LINKED. AN IMPRESSIVE PEDIGREE WITH 6 AFFECTED MALES IN 3 GENERATIONS WAS PUBLISHED BY DOOREN ET AL. (1968), WHO FOLLOWING THE RECOMMENDA-TIONS OF A WORKSHOP ON IMMUNOLOGICAL DEFICIENCY DISEASES IN MAN (SANIBEL ISLAND, FORT MYERS, FLA., FEB. 1-5, 1967) CALLED THE CONDITION THYMIC EPITHELIAL HYPOPLA-SIA. IN THE SAME WORKSHOP ROSEN ET AL. (1968) POINTED OUT THAT A DIFFERENCE FROM THE AUTOSOMAL RECESSIVE IS LESS PROFOUND LYMPHOCYTOPENIA.

MILLER, M. E. AND SCHIEKEN, R. M.* THYMIC DYSPLASIA. A SEPARABLE ENTITY FROM 'SWISS AGAMMAGLOBULINEMIA.' AM. J. MED. SCI. 253* 741-750, 1967.

ROSEN, F. S. AND JANEWAY, C. A.* THE GAMMA GLOBULINS. III. THE ANTIBODY DEFICIENCY SYNDROMES. NEW ENG. J. MED. 275* 709-715 AND 769-775, 1966.

ROSEN, F. S., CRAIG, J. M., VAWTER, G. AND JANEWAY, C. A.* THE DYSGAMMAGLOBU-LINEMIAS AND X-LINKED THYMIC HYPOPLASIA. IN, GOOD, R. A. (ED.)* IMMUNOLOGIC DEFICIENCY DISEASES IN MAN. NEW YORK* NATIONAL FOUNDATION, 1968. PP. 67-70.

ROSEN, F. S., GOTOFF, S. P., CRAIG, J. M., RITCHIE, J. AND JANEWAY, C. A.* FURTHER OBSERVATIONS ON THE SWISS TYPE OF AGAMMAGLOBULINEMIA (ALYMPHOCYTOSIS). THE EFFECT OF SYNGENEIC BONE-MARROW CELLS. NEW ENG. J. MED. 274* 18-21, 1966.

*30050 ALBINISM, OCULAR

IN AFFECTED MEN THE PUPILLARY REFLEX IS CHARACTERISTIC OF ALBINISM. THE FUNDUS IS DEPIGMENTED AND THE CHOROIDAL VESSELS STAND OUT STRIKINGLY. NYSTAGMUS, HEAD NODDING, AND IMPAIRED VISION ALSO OCCUR. PIGMENTATION IS NORMAL ELSEWHERE THAN IN THE EYE. IN CARRIER FEMALES THE FUNDUS, ESPECIALLY IN THE PERIPHERY, SHOWS A MOSAIC OF PIGMENTATION, AS FIRST RECOGNIZED BY VOGT (1942). LYON (1962) POINTED OUT THAT THE FUNDUS FINDING IN HETEROZYGOUS FEMALES SUPPORTS HER THEORY. NYSTAGMUS IS FREQUENTLY AN ASSOCIATED FEATURE. IN FACT THE OCULAR ALBINISM HAS BEEN COMMENTED ON ONLY OBLIQUELY OR NOT AT ALL IN SOME REPORTS OF X-LINKED NYSTAGMUS IN FAMILIES WHICH ALMOST CERTAINLY HAD OCULAR ALBINISM. WAARDENBURG AND VAN DEN BOSCH'S FAMILY WAS EARLIER REPORTED BY ENGELHARD AS A FAMILY WITH HEREDITARY NYSTAGMUS. ONE FAMILY STUDIED BY FIALKOW ET AL. (1967) HAD BEEN REPORTED BY LEIN ET AL. (1956) AS SEX-LINKED NYSTAGMUS. FUNDUS DRAWINGS OF HETEROZYGOUS CARRIERS ARE PROVIDED BY FRANCOIS AND DEWEER, AND BY OTHERS. (SEE FRONTISPIECE, MCKUSICK, 1964.) THEORETICALLY ONE SHOULD BE ABLE TO COUNT THE NUMBER OF PIGMENTED SPOTS AND ARRIVE AT AN ESTIMATE OF THE NUMBER OF ANLAGE CELLS PRESENT AT THE TIME OF LYONIZATION. UNFORTUNATELY MOST OF THE AVAILABLE DRAWINGS ARE PROBABLY TOO CRUDE TO BE RELIED ON FOR THIS USE. FURTHERMORE, THE DRAWINGS SUGGEST APPRECIABLE VARIATION IN THE NUMBER AND SIZE OF PIGMENTED AREAS, A FINDING TO BE EXPECTED FROM THE CONSIDERATIONS OF THE LYON HYPOTHESIS. ISOLATED ALBINISM OF THE EYE IS INHERITED IN THE RABBIT AS AN AUTOSOMAL RECESSIVE (MAGNUSSEN, 1952). FIALKOW ET AL. (1967) ESTIMATED THAT THE RECOMBINATION FRACTION FOR OCULAR ALBINISM AND XG IS ABOUT 0.17. THIS WAS CONFIRMED BY PEARCE ET AL. (1968) IN AN ENGLISH KINDRED.

ENGELHARD, C. F.* EINE FAMILIE MIT HEREDITAREM NYSTAGMUS. ZBL. GES. NEUROL. PSYCHIAT. 28* 319-338, 1915.

FIALKOW, P. J., GIBLETT, E. R. AND MOTULSKY, A. G.* MEASURABLE LINKAGE BETWEEN

X
L
I
N
K
E
D

FRANCOIS, J. AND DEWEER, J. P.* ALBINISME OCULAIRE LIE AU SEXE ET ALTERATIONS CARACTERISTIQUES DU FOND D'OEIL CHEZ LES FEMMES HETEROZYGOTES. OPHTHALMOLOGIA 126* 209-221, 1953.

GILLESPIE, F. D.* OCULAR ALBINISM WITH REPORT OF A FAMILY WITH FEMALE CARRIERS. ARCH. OPHTHAL. 66* 774-777, 1961.

LEIN, J. N., STEWART, C. T. AND MOLL, F. C.* SEX-LINKED HEREDITARY NYSTAGMUS. PEDIATRICS 18* 214-217, 1956.

LYON, M. F.* SEX CHROMATIN AND GENE ACTION IN THE MAMMALIAN X-CHROMOSOME. AM. J. HUM. GENET. 14* 135-148, 1962.

MAGNUSSEN, K.* BEITRAG ZUR GENETIK UND HISTOLOGIE EINES ISOLIERTEN AUGENALBINI-SMUS BEIM KANINCHEN. Z. MORPH. ANTHROP. 44* 127-135, 1952.

MCKUSICK, V. A.* ON THE X CHROMOSOME OF MAN. WASHINGTON* AIBS, 1964.

NEGRELLI, B. C.* L'ALBINISME OCULAIRE LIE AU SEXE DANS LE CADRE DJ DEPISTAGE DES HETEROZYGOTES EN OPHTHALMOLOGIE. J. GENET. HUM. 8* 108 ONLY, 1959.

PEARCE, W. G., SANGER, R. AND RACE, R. R.* OCULAR ALBINISM AND XG. LANCET 1* 1282-1283, 1968.

VOGT, A.* DIE IRIS ALBINISMUS SOLUM BULBI. ATLAS SPALT-LAMPEN-MIKROSKOPIE 3* 846, 1942.

WAARDENBURG, P. J. AND VAN DEN BOSCH, J.* X-CHROMOSOMAL OCULAR ALBINISM IN DUTCH FAMILY. ANN. HUM. GENET. 21* 101-122, 1956.

30060 ALBINISM, OCULAR (FORSIUS-ERIKSSON TYPE)

FORSIUS AND ERIKSSON (1964) CONSIDERED THE OCULAR ALBINISM THEY DESCRIBED IN A FAMILY FROM THE ALAND ISLANDS IN THE SEA OF BOTHNIA TO BE A DISTINCT ENTITY. MALES IN 6 GENERATIONS WERE AFFECTED. IN ADDITION TO ALBINISM OF THE FUNDUS, THE FEATURES WERE HYPOPLASIA OF THE FOVEA, MARKED IMPAIRMENT OF VISION, NYSTAGMUS, MYOPIA, ASTIGMATISM AND PROTANOMALOUS COLOR BLINDNESS. FEMALE CARRIERS SHOWED SLIGHT DISTURBANCES OF COLOR DISCRIMINATION AND ELECTROMYOGRAPHICALLY DEMONSTRABLE NYSTAGMUS. WARBURG (1964) DESCRIBED OCULAR ALBINISM AND PROTANOPIA IN THE SAME FAMILY. ONLY TWO OF FOUR MALES WITH OCULAR ALBINISM SHOWED DYSCHROMATOPSIA. THE ABSENCE OF CHARACTERISTIC FUNDUS PIGMENTARY PATTERN IN FEMALE CARRIERS IN THE FAMILY OF FORSIUS AND ERIKSSCN MAY BE THE BEST INDICATION THAT THEY DEALT WITH A DISTINCT ENTITY. WAARDENBURG ET AL. (1969) CONCLUDED THAT THE DISORDER IS ENTIRELY DISTINCT FROM THE X-LINKED OCULAR ALBINISM. THE PIGMENT DEFICIENCY IS NOT COMPLETE AS IN OCULAR ALBINISM. THEY USE ALAND ISLAND DISEASE OR THE FORSIUS-ERIKSSON SYNDROME AS PREFERABLE DESIGNATIONS. LINKAGE STUDIES INDICATE A RECOMBINATION FRACTION OF ABOUT 0.12 (CONFIDENCE LIMITS WIDE) WITH THE XG BLOOD GROUP LOCUS (RACE AND SANGER, 1968), LEADING WAARDENBURG ET AL. (1969) TO THE SUGGESTION THAT ALAND ISLAND DISEASE AND OCULAR ALBINISM MAY BE ALLELIC, OR MAY BE PSEUDO-ALLELIC, I.E., DUE TO GENES AT ADJACENT LOCI. SCIALFA (1967) REPORTED A FAMILY WITH THIS DISORDER.

FORSIUS, H. AND ERIKSSON, A. W.* EIN NEUES AUGENSYNDROM MIT X-CHROMOSOMAL TRANSMISSION. EINE SIPPE MIT FUNDUSALBINISMUS, FOVEAHYPOPLASIE, NYSTAGMUS, MYOPIE, ASTIGMATISMUS UND DYSCHROMATOPSIE. KLIN. MBL. AUGENHEILK. 144* 447-457, 1964.

RACE, R. R. AND SANGER, R.* BLOOD GROUPS IN MAN. PHILADELPHIA* F. A. DAVIS CO., 1968 (5TH ED.). P. 549.

SCIALFA, A.* ALBINISME OCULAIRE ET DYSCHROMATOPSIE. ARCH. OPHTHAL. (PARIS) 27* 483-494, 1967.

WAARDENBURG, P. J., ERIKSSON, A. W. AND FORSIUS, H.* ALAND EYE DISEASE (SYNDROMA FORSIUS-ERIKSSON). PROG. NEURO-OPHTHAL. 2* 336-339, 1969.

WARBURG, M.* OCULAR ALBINISM AND PROTANOPIA IN THE SAME FAMILY. ACTA OPHTHAL. 42* 444-451, 1964.

*30070 ALBINISM-DEAFNESS SYNDROME

MARGOLIS (1962) DESCRIBED A 'NEW' X-LINKED SYNDROME - DEAF-MUTISM AND TOTAL ALBINISM. ALSO FROM ISRAEL, ZIPRKOWSKI AND HIS COLLEAGUES (1962) DESCRIBED AN X-LINKED SYNDROME CONSISTING OF DEAF-MUTISM AND PARTIAL ALBINISM (WITHOUT OCULAR ALBINISM). THEY WERE REPORTING ON THE SAME FAMILY. THE ALBINISM IS SHOWN BY THE PHOTOGRAPHS TO BE 'PARTIAL,' AS DESCRIBED BY ZIPRKOWSKI AND COLLEAGUES. INDEED, THE PIGMENTARY DISORDER MIGHT BE CALLED 'PIEBALD.' WOOLF (1965) OBSERVED THE SAME PHENOTYPE IN TWO HOPI AMERICAN INDIAN BROTHERS. WOOLF, DOLOWITZ AND ALDOUS (1965) DESCRIBED TWO HOPI BROTHERS WITH CONGENITAL DEAFNESS AND A REMARKABLY SIMILAR PATTERN OF PIGMENTARY VARIEGATION OF THE PIEBALD TYPE. ANOTHER BROTHER AND BOTH

PARENTS WERE NORMAL AND NO OTHER CASES ARE KNOWN IN SOUTHWEST INDIANS. THE DEAFNESS WAS SUBTOTAL NERVE TYPE. HEARING IMPAIRMENT IN HETEROZYGOTES WAS DEMONSTRATED BY FRIED ET AL. (1969).

FRIED, K., FEINMESSER, M. AND TSITSIANOV, J.* HEARING IMPAIRMENT IN FEMALE CARRIERS OF THE SEX-LINKED SYNDROME OF DEAFNESS WITH ALBINISM. J. MED. GENET. 6* 132-134, 1969.

MARGOLIS, E.* A NEW HEREDITARY SYNDROME - SEX-LINKED DEAF-MUTISM ASSOCIATED WITH TOTAL ALBINISM. ACTA GENET. STATIST. MED. 12* 12-19, 1962.

REED, W. B., STONE, V. M., BODER, E. AND ZIPRKOWSKI, L.* PIGMENTARY DISORDERS IN ASSOCIATION WITH CONGENITAL DEAFNESS. ARCH. DERM. 95* 176-186, 1967.

WOOLF, C. M.* ALBINISM AMONG INDIANS IN ARIZONA AND NEW MEXICO. AM. J. HUM. GENET. 17* 23-35, 1965.

WOOLF, C. M., DOLOWITZ, D. A. AND ALDOUS, H. E.* CONGENITAL DEAFNESS ASSOCIATED WITH PIEBALDNESS. ARCH. OTOLARYNG. 82* 244-250, 1965.

ZIPRKOWSKI, L., KRAKOWSKI, A., ADAM, A., COSTEFF, H. AND SADE, J.* PARTIAL ALBINISM AND DEAFMUTISM DUE TO A RECESSIVE SEX-LINKED GENE. ARCH. DERM. 86* 530-539, 1962.

*30080 ALBRIGHT'S HEREDITARY OSTEODYSTROPHY

THIS CONDITION COMPRISES BOTH PSEUDOHYPOPARATHYROIDISM AND PSEUDO-PSEUDOHYPOPARA-THYROIDISM, WHICH ARE PROBABLY ASPECTS OF A SINGLE ENTITY. THE FACTS (1) THAT NO INDUBITABLE INSTANCE OF MALE-TO-MALE TRANSMISSION HAS BEEN OBSERVED AND (2) THAT FEMALES ARE AFFECTED TWICE AS OFTEN AS MALES SUPPORT THE VIEW THAT THE DISORDER IS AN X-LINKED DOMINANT. ON THE OTHER HAND, HEMIZYGOUS MALES ARE NOT MORE SEVERELY AFFECTED THAN ARE HETEROZYGOUS FEMALES. IN FACT, THE TABULATION OF REPORTED PEDIGREES (MANN, ET AL., 1962) SHOWS THAT WHEREAS ONLY FOUR OF 36 FEMALE CASES WERE OF THE INCOMPLETE FORM, SIX OF 14 MALE CASES FAILED TO SHOW FULL EXPRESSION. THIS FINDING, CONTRARY TO THAT IN OTHER X-LINKED TRAITS AND CONTRARY TO PRESENT CONCEPTS OF THE X CHROMOSOME, MAKES IT POSSIBLE THAT THIS DISORDER IS IN FACT A SEX-INFLUENCED AUTOSOMAL DOMINANT. TYPE E BRACHYDACTYLY (MCKUSICK AND MILCH, 1964) RESEMBLES THIS ENTITY IN RESPECT TO SHORT STATURE, THE HAND ANOMALY AND ROUND FACE. MENTAL RETARDATION, CATARACT AND ECTOPIC CALCIFICATION ARE NOT PRESENT. IT IS CLEARLY AUTOSOMAL DOMINANT (Q.V.). MALE-TO-MALE TRANSMISSION WAS ALSO OBSERVED IN THE FAMILY REPORTED BY GOEMINNE (1965) BUT THE ABSENCE OF ECTOPIC CALCIFICATION, MENTAL RETARDATION AND CATARACT MAKES IT VIRTUALLY CERTAIN THAT THIS TOO WAS AN INSTANCE OF METACARPAL BRACHYDACTYLY AND NOT ALBRIGHT'S OSTEODYS-TROPHY. (GOEMINNE 1970) REMAINS OF THE OPINION THAT HIS *AUTOSOMAL* PEDIGREE REPRESENTS PPHP). HYPERPLASIA OF THE PARATHYROIDS IS THE ANATOMIC FINDING IN THESE CASES. TURNER'S SYNDROME, A CHROMOSOMAL ABERRATION, OFTEN SHOWS THE SAME HAND CHANGE. THIS ALBRIGHT'S SYNDROME IS NOT TO BE CONFUSED WITH POLYOSTOTIC FIBROUS DYSPLASIA (Q.V.) TO WHICH ALBRIGHT'S NAME IS ALSO ATTACHED EPONYMOUSLY. CASES IN WHICH THE PICTURE WAS PSEUDOHYPOPARATHYROIDISM AT ONE STAGE AND LATER PSEUDO-PSEUDOHYPOPARATHYROIDISM HAVE BEEN REPORTED BY PALUBINSKAS AND DAVIS (1959) AND OTHERS. LEE ET AL. (1968) FOUND HIGH PARATHORMONE AND THYROCALCITONIN IN A MOTHER AND HER AFFECTED SON AND DAUGHTER. THE AUTHORS STATED THAT THE ONLY OTHER FAMILY WITH FULL EXPRESSION IN TWO GENERATIONS WAS THAT OF MANN ET AL. (1962). WHEREAS NORMAL INDIVIDUALS SHOW AN INCREASE IN URINARY EXCRETION OF CYCLIC AMP (WHICH IS INVOLVED IN THE CELLULAR MECHANISMS OF RESPONSE TO SEVERAL HORMONES) ON ADMINISTRATION OF PARATHORMONE, CHASE ET AL. (1968) FOUND NO SUCH RESPONSE IN PATIENTS WITH PSEUDOHYPOPARATHYROIDISM. CHASE ET AL. (1969) FOUND THAT PARA-THYROID HORMONE CIRCULATES IN ABNORMALLY HIGH CONCENTRATION IN PSEUDOHYPOPARA-THYROIDISM AND SECRETION OF THE HORMONE RESPONDS NORMALLY TO PHYSIOLOGIC CONTROL BY CALCIUM. UNLIKE THE NORMAL, CYCLIC AMP DID NOT INCREASE IN THE URINE IN RESPONSE TO ADMINISTRATED PARATHORMONE. THEY SUGGESTED THAT THE BASIC DEFECT MAY BE DEFICIENT AMOUNT OR FUNCTION OF PARATHORMONE-SENSITIVE ADENYL CYCLASE IN BONE AND KIDNEY. LIKE OTHERS, CHASE ET AL. (1969) FOUND PSEUDOPSEUDOHYPOPARATHYROIDISM AND PSEUDOHYPOPARATHYROIDISM IN DIFFERENT MEMBERS OF THE SAME FAMILY, BUT SURPRISING FINDINGS WERE THAT PERSONS WITH PSEUDO-PSEUDOHYPOPARATHYROIDISM SHOWED (1) ABNORMALLY HIGH BASAL URINARY EXCRETION OF CYCLIC AMP, AND (2) NORMAL INCREASE IN URINARY AMP WITH PARATHORMONE INFUSION. POSSIBLY PATIENTS CHANGE IN REGARD TO THESE CHARACTERISTICS WHEN PASSING FROM THE PICTURE OF PSEUDO- TO PSEUDO-PSEUDOHY-POPARATHYROIDISM. CHASE AND AURBACH (1968) SHOWED THAT PARATHORMONE AND VASOPRES-SIN STIMULATES ADENYL CYCLASE IN ANATOMICALLY SEPARATE PART OF THE KIDNEY, CORTEX AND MEDULLA, RESPECTIVELY. TO MY KNOWLEDGE, THE CYCLIC AMP SYSTEM HAS NOT BEEN EXAMINED IN NEPHROGENIC DIABETES INSIPIDUS (Q.V.). INTELLIGENCE IS NORMAL IN SOME PATIENTS WITH PSEUDOHYPOPARATHYROIDISM.

CHASE, L. R. AND AURBACH, G. D.* RENAL ADENYL CYCLASE* ANATOMICALLY SEPARATE SITES FOR PARATHYROID HORMONE AND VASOPRESSIN. SCIENCE 159* 545-547, 1968.

CHASE, L. R., MELSON, G. L. AND AURBACH, G. D.* PSEUDOHYPOPARATHYROIDISM* DEFECTIVE EXCRETION OF 3 (PRIME)-5(PRIME)-AMP IN RESPONSE TO PARATHYROID HORMONE. J. CLIN. INVEST. 48* 1832-1844, 1969.

GOEMINNE, L.* ALBRIGHT'S HEREDITARY POLY-OSTEOCHONDRODYSTROPHY (PSEUDO-PSEUDO-

X
L
I
N
K
E
D

HYPOPARATHYROIDISM WITH DIABETES HYPERTENSION, ARTERITIS AND POLYARTHROSIS). ACTA GENET. MED. GEM. 14* 226-281, 1965.

GOEMINNE, L.* ZULTE, BELGIUM* PERSONAL COMMUNICATION, 1970.

HERMANS, P. E., GORMAN, C. A., MARTIN, W. J. AND KELLY, P. J.* PSEUDO-PSEUDOHY-POPOPARATHYROIDISM (ALBRIGHT'S HEREDITARY OSTEODYSTROPHY). A FAMILY STUDY. MAYO CLIN. PROC. 39* 81-91, 1964.

LEE, J. B., TASHJIAN, A. H., JR., STREETO, J. M. AND FRANTZ, A. G.* FAMILIAL PSEUDOHYPOPARATHYROIDISM. ROLE OF PARATHYROID HORMONE AND THYROCALCITONIN. NEW ENG. J. MED. 279* 1179-1184, 1968.

MANN, J. B., ALTERMAN, S. AND HILL, A. G.* ALBRIGHT'S HEREDITARY OSTEODYSTROPHY COMPRISING PSEUDOHYPOPARATHYROIDISM AND PSEUDO-PSEUDOHYPOPARATHYROIDISM, WITH A REPORT OF TWO CASES REPRESENTING THE COMPLETE SYNDROME OCCURRING IN SUCCESSIVE GENERATIONS. ANN. INTERN. MED. 56* 315-342, 1962.

MCKUSICK, V. A. AND MILCH, R. A.* THE CLINICAL BEHAVIOR OF GENETIC DISEASE* SELECTED ASPECTS. CLIN. ORTHOP. 33* 22-39, 1964.

PALUBINSKAS, A. J. AND DAVIES, H.* CALCIFICATION OF THE BASAL GANGLIA OF THE BRAIN. AM. J. ROENTGEN. 82* 806-822, 1959.

30090 ALCOHOLISM

CRUZ-COKE AND VARELA (1966) ADVANCED THE HYPOTHESIS THAT ALCOHOLISM IS DETERMINED BY AN X-LINKED RECESSIVE GENE. WINOKUR (1967) CONCLUDED FROM AN ANALYSIS OF DATA PUBLISHED BY AMARK (1951) THAT THE X-LINKED HYPOTHESIS IS UNTENABLE.

AMARK, C.* A STUDY IN ALCOHOLISM. CLINICAL, SOCIAL-PSYCHIATRIC AND GENETIC INVESTIGATIONS. ACTA PSYCHIAT. NEUROL. SCAND. 70 (SUPPL.)* 1-283, 1951.

CRUZ-COKE, R. AND VARELA, A.* INHERITANCE OF ALCOHOLISM. ITS ASSOCIATION WITH COLOUR-BLINDNESS. LANCET 2* 1282-1284, 1966.

WINOKUR, G.* X-BORNE RECESSIVE GENES IN ALCOHOLISM. (LETTER) LANCET 2* 466 ONLY, 1967.

*30100 ALDRICH SYNDROME

THE MANIFESTATIONS ARE ECZEMA, THROMBOCYTOPENIA, PRONENESS TO INFECTION, AND BLOODY DIARRHEA. DEATH OCCURS BEFORE AGE 10. ALDRICH'S ORIGINAL KINDRED WAS OF DUTCH EXTRACTION. VAN DEN BOSCH AND DRUKKER (1964) DESCRIBED SEVERAL FAMILIES IN THE NETHERLANDS. IN 3 OF 5 FEMALE CARRIERS THE PLATELET COUNT WAS BELOW THE LOWER LIMIT OF NORMAL. SEVERAL GROUPS (BLAESE ET AL., 1968* COOPER ET AL., 1968) HAVE PRESENTED EVIDENCE THAT THE IMMUNE DEFECT IS IN THE AFFERENT LIMB, I.E., IS ONE OF ANTIGEN PROCESSING OR RECOGNITION.

ALDRICH, R. A., STEINBERG, A. G. AND CAMPBELL, D. C.* PEDIGREE DEMONSTRATING A SEX-LINKED RECESSIVE CONDITION CHARACTERIZED BY DRAINING EARS, ECZEMATOID DERMATITIS AND BLOODY DIARRHEA. PEDIATRICS 13* 133-139, 1954.

BLAESE, R. M., STROBER, W., BROWN, R. S. AND WALDMANN, T. A.* THE WISKOTT-ALDRICH SYNDROME. A DISORDER WITH A POSSIBLE DEFECT IN ANTIGENS PROCESSING OR RECOGNITION. LANCET 1* 1056-1060, 1968.

COOPER, M. D., CHAE, H. P., LOWMAN, J. T., KRIVIT, W. AND GOOD, R. A.* WISKOTT-ALDRICH SYNDROME. AN IMMUNOLOGIC DEFICIENCY DISEASE INVOLVING THE AFFERENT LIMB OF IMMUNITY. AM. J. MED. 44* 499-513, 1968.

GELZER, J. AND GASSER, C.* WISKOTT-ALDRICH-SYNDROME. HELV. PAEDIAT. ACTA 16* 17-39, 1961.

KRIVIT, W. AND GOOD, R. A.* ALDRICH'S SYNDROME (THROMBOCYTOPENIA, ECZEMA AND INFECTION IN INFANTS). STUDIES OF THE DEFENSE MECHANISMS. AM. J. DIS. CHILD. 97* 137-153, 1959.

LEVIN, A. S., SPITLER, L. E., STILES, D. P. AND FUNDENBERG, H. H.* WISKOTT-ALDRICH SYNDROME, A GENETICALLY DETERMINED CELLULAR IMMUNOLOGIC DEFICIENCY* CLINICAL AND LABORATORY RESPONSES TO THERAPY WITH TRANSFER FACTOR. PROC. NAT. ACAD. SCI. 67* 821-828, 1970.

STEINBERG, A. G.* METHODOLOGY IN HUMAN GENETICS. J. MED. EDUC. 34* 315-334, 1959.

VAN DEN BOSCH, J. AND DRUKKER, J.* HET SYNDROOM VAN ALDRICH* EEN KLINISCH EN GENETISCH ONDERZOEK VAN ENIGE NEDERLANDSE FAMILIES. MAANDSCHR. KINDERGENEESK. 32* 359-373, 1964.

WOLFF, J. A.* WISKOTT-ALDRICH SYNDROME* CLINICAL, IMMUNOLOGIC, AND PATHOLOGIC OBSERVATIONS. J. PEDIAT. 70* 221-232, 1967.

X
L
I
N
K
E
D

THE ENAMEL IS OPAQUE WHITE, SOFT, AND EASILY ABRADED BUT APPEARS OF NORMAL THICKNESS IN UNERUPTED TEETH. THE CONDITION IS INHERITED AS AN X-LINKED RECESSIVE.

WITKOP, C. J.* HEREDITARY DEFECTS IN ENAMEL AND DENTIN. ACTA GENET. STATIST. MED. 7* 236-239, 1957.

*30120 AMELOGENESIS IMPERFECTA, HYPOPLASTIC TYPE (HEREDITARY ENAMEL HYPOPLASIA)

IN THIS CONDITION THE ENAMEL IS VERY HARD BUT IS ABNORMALLY THIN SO THAT THE TEETH APPEAR SMALL. THE SURFACE IS ROUGH. THIS TYPE IS INHERITED AS AN X-LINKED DOMINANT. POSSIBLE GENETIC RELATIONSHIP, E.G. ALLELISM, WITH THE FACTOR FOR THE HYPOMATURATION TYPE IS UNKNOWN. THEREFORE THE TWO HAVE BEEN LISTED AS SEPARATE LOCI. RUSHTON (1964) POINTED OUT DIFFERENCES IN MALES AND FEMALES WHICH MAY BE BASED ON THE LYON PHENOMENON. THE AFFECTED MALES HAVE ONLY A VERY THIN SMOOTH LAYER OF ENAMEL WHICH APPEARS NEARLY HOMOGENEOUS. THE FEMALES HAVE ENAMEL WHICH IN PARTS IS MUCH THICKER GIVING A VERTICALLY GROOVED APPEARANCE TO THE TEETH. WIDE VARIATION IN THE INVOLVEMENT IN FEMALES IS ALSO CONSISTENT WITH THE LYON HYPOTHESIS. THIS DISORDER, LIKE HYPOPHOSPHATEMIA, WAS CONSIDERED TO BE AUTOSOMAL DOMINANT BEFORE THE TRUE INHERITANCE WAS POINTED OUT BY SCHULZE (1952, 1957) AND OTHERS. THE HISTOLOGIC CHARACTERISTIC IS THE PRESENCE OF TWISTED ENAMEL RODS COURSING FROM THE DENTINO-ENAMEL JUNCTION TO THE ENAMEL SURFACE.

HALDANE, J. B. S.* A PROBABLE NEW SEX-LINKED DOMINANT IN MAN. J. HERED. 28* 58-60, 1937.

RUSHTON, M. A.* HEREDITARY ENAMEL DEFECTS. PROC. ROY. SOC. MED. 57* 53-58, 1964.

SCHULZE, C. AND LENZ, F. R.* UBER ZAHNSCHMELZHYPOPLASIE VON UNVOLLSTANDIG DOMINANTEM GESCHLECHTSGEBUNDENEN ERBGANG. Z. MENSCHL. VERERB. KONSTITUTIONSL. 31* 104-114, 1952.

SCHULZE, C.* ERBBEDINGTE STRUKTURANOMALIEN MENSCHLICHER ZAHNE. ACTA GENET. STATIST. MED. 7* 231-235, 1957.

WEINMANN, J. P., SVOBODA, J. F. AND WOODS, R. W.* HEREDITARY DISTURBANCES OF ENAMEL FORMATION AND CALCIFICATION. J. AM. DENT. ASS. 32* 397-418, 1945.

*30130 ANEMIA, HYPOCHROMIC

THIS CONDITION WAS FIRST DESCRIBED BY COOLEY (1945), WHO ALSO FIRST DESCRIBED THALASSEMIA. HE POINTED OUT POSSIBLE X-LINKAGE IN A FAMILY IN WHICH 19 MALES IN FIVE GENERATIONS WERE AFFECTED, WITH TRANSMISSION THROUGH UNAFFECTED FEMALES. RUNDLES AND FALLS REPORTED TWO FAMILIES, OF WHICH ONE WAS THE SAME AS THAT REPORTED BY COOLEY.
HYPOCHROMIC ANEMIA HAS, OF COURSE, OTHER CAUSES, NOTABLY IRON DEFICIENCY. WHAT IS REFERRED TO HERE ARE THE RARE CASES IN WHICH IT IS HEREDITARY. THE CONDITION IS ALSO KNOWN AS HEREDITARY IRON-LOADING ANEMIA (BYRD AND COOPER, 1961). THE FEATURES INCLUDE, (A) ANEMIA DETECTED FIRST IN CHILDHOOD IN SOME CASES, (B) DEATH FROM HEMOCHROMATOSIS AT A RELATIVELY YOUNG AGE, WITH THE NUMBER OF TRANSFUSIONS INADEQUATE TO ACCOUNT FOR THE HEMOCHROMATOSIS, (C) HYPERFERRICEMIA, AND (D) ABUNDANCE OF SIDEROCYTES IN PERIPHERAL BLOOD AFTER SPLENECTOMY. SOMEWHAT ENLARGED SPLEENS AND MINOR RED CELL ABNORMALITIES WITHOUT ANEMIA WERE OBSERVED IN FEMALE CARRIERS BY RUNDLES AND FALLS (1946).
BICKERS ET AL. (1962) DESCRIBED THE DISORDER IN A MAN WHOSE MOTHER, SISTER AND FIVE CHILDREN HAD HEMATOLOGIC INVOLVEMENT IN VARIOUS DEGREES. PYRIDOXINE RESPONSIVENESS WAS DEMONSTRATED IN AT LEAST TWO AFFECTED MEMBERS OF RUNDLES AND FALLS' FAMILY (BISHOP AND BETHEL, 1959* HORRIGAN AND HARRIS, 1964). CLOSE LINKAGE TO THE XG LOCUS WAS EXCLUDED BY ELVES, BOURNE AND ISRAELS (1966). ASSOCIATED HYPOLIPIDEMIA AND HYPOCHOLESTEROLEMIA WERE POINTED OUT BY SPITZER, NEWCOMB AND NOYES (1966). TWO POPULATIONS OF CELLS, AS TO MORPHOLOGY, IN HETEROZYGOTES WERE ILLUSTRATED BY PINKERTON (1967). PRASAD ET AL. (1968) STUDIED A NEGRO FAMILY IN WHICH BOTH SIDEROBLASTIC ANEMIA AND G6PD-DEFICIENCY WERE SEGREGATING. A MAXIMUM LIKELIHOOD ESTIMATE OF THE RECOMBINATION VALUE WAS 0.14. IN FEMALES DOUBLY HETEROZYGOUS IN COUPLING, A CORRELATION BETWEEN SMALL RED CELLS AND LOW G6PD WAS FOUND. IN A HETEROZYGOTE LEE ET AL. (1968) SEPARATED TWO POPULATIONS OF RED CELLS BY CENTRIFUGATION IN LAYERED GUM ACACIA SOLUTIONS OF DIFFERENT SPECIFIC GRAVITY. THE MICROCYTES HAD A LOWER LEVEL OF FREE PROTOPORPHYRIN THAN DID THE NORMAL CELLS BUT UNIMPAIRED CAPACITY TO CONVERT DELTA-AMINOLEVULINIC ACID TO PROTOPORPHYRIN, SUGGESTING A DEFECT AT OR BEFORE THE STEP IN WHICH DELTA-AMINOLEVULINIC ACID IS SYNTHESIZED. THE ENZYME DEFECT MAY CONCERN DELTA-AMINOLEVULINIC ACID SYNTHETASE, WHICH REQUIRES VITAMIN B6 AS A COFACTOR AND IS THE RATE-LIMITING STEP IN PORPHYRIN SYNTHESIS. IF SO, THIS ENZYME WOULD APPEAR TO BE DETERMINED BY A STRUCTURAL GENE ON THE X CHROMOSOME. THALASSEMIA MINOR IS THE OTHER CONDITION WHICH IN THIS COUNTRY PRODUCES HEREDITARY HYPOCHROMIC ANEMIA. WEATHERALL ET AL. (1970) WERE UNABLE TO DEMONSTRATE LYONIZATION OF THE XG LOCUS BY OBSERVING TWO POPULATIONS OF CELLS IN FEMALES HETEROZYGOUS FOR FAMILIAL SIDEROBLASTIC ANEMIA, CALLED HERE X-LINKED HYPOCHROMIC ANEMIA.

X
L
I
N
K
E
D

BICKERS, J. N., BROWN, C. L. AND SPRAGUE, C. C.* PYRIDOXINE RESPONSIVE ANEMIA. 549
BLOOD 19* 304-312, 1962.

BISHOP, R. C. AND BETHEL, F. H.* HEREDITARY HYPOCHROMIC ANEMIA WITH TRANSFUSION
HEMOSIDEROSIS TREATED WITH PYRIDOXIN. NEW ENG. J. MED. 261* 486-489, 1959.

BYRD, R. B. AND COOPER, T.* HEREDITARY IRON-LOADING ANEMIA WITH SECONDARY
HEMOCHROMATOSIS. ANN. INTERN. MED. 55* 103-123, 1961.

COOLEY, T. B.* A SEVERE TYPE OF HEREDITARY ANEMIA WITH ELLIPTOCYTOSIS*
INTERESTING SEQUENCE OF SPLENECTOMY. AM. J. MED. SCI. 209* 561-568, 1945.

ELVES, M. W., BOURNE, M. S. AND ISRAELS, M. C. G.* PYRIDOXINE-RESPONSIVE
ANAEMIA DETERMINED BY AN X-LINKED GENE. J. MED. GENET. 3* 1-4, 1966.

HARRIS, J. W. AND HORRIGAN, D. L.* PYRIDOXINE-RESPONSIVE ANEMIA-PROTOTYPE AND
VARIATIONS OF THE THEME. VITAMINS HORMONES 22* 721-753, 1964.

HORRIGAN, D. L. AND HARRIS, J. W.* PYRIDOXINE-RESPONSIVE ANEMIA* ANALYSIS OF 62
CASES. ADVANCES INTERN. MED. 12* 103-174, 1964.

LEE, G. R., MACDIARMID, W. D., CARTWRIGHT, G. E. AND WINTROBE, M. M.* HEREDI-
TARY, X-LINKED, SIDEROACHRESTIC ANEMIA. THE ISOLATION OF TWO ERYTHROCYTE
POPULATIONS DIFFERING IN XG(A) BLOOD TYPE AND PORPHYRIN CONTENT. BLOOD 32* 59-70,
1968.

PINKERTON, P. H.* X-LINKED HYPOCHROMIC ANEMIA. (LETTER) LANCET 1* 1106-1107,
1967.

PRASAD, A. S., TRANCHIDA, L., KONNO, E. T., BERMAN, L., ALBERT, S., SING, C. F.
AND BREWER, G. J.* HEREDITARY SIDEROBLASTIC ANEMIA AND GLUCOSE-6-PHOSPHATE
DEHYDROGENASE DEFICIENCY IN A NEGRO FAMILY. J. CLIN. INVEST. 47* 1415-1424, 1968.

RUNDLES, R. W. AND FALLS, H. F.* HEREDITARY (SEX-LINKED) ANEMIA. AM. J. MED.
SCI. 211* 641-658, 1946.

SPITZER, N., NEWCOMB, T. F. AND NOYES, W. D.* PYRIDOXINE-RESPONSIVE HYPOLIPIDE-
MIA AND HYPOCHOLESTEROLEMIA IN A PATIENT WITH PYRIDOXINE RESPONSIVE ANEMIA. NEW
ENG. J. MED. 274* 772-775, 1966.

WEATHERALL, D. J., PEMBERY, M. E., HALL, E. G., SANGER, R., TIPPETT, P. AND
GAVIN, J.* FAMILIAL SIDEROBLASTIC ANAEMIA* PROBLEM OF XG AND X CHROMOSOMES
INACTIVATION. LANCET 2* 744-748, 1970.

30140 ANEMIA, IRON DEFICIENCY

IN THE MOUSE AN X-BORNE LOCUS IS APPARENTLY CONCERNED WITH TRANSPORT OF IRON
ACROSS THE INTESTINAL MUCOSA, SPECIFICALLY FROM THE MUCOSAL CELL INTO THE BLOOD,
BECAUSE AN X-LINKED ANEMIA OF THE MOUSE HAS A DEFECT IN THIS TRANSPORT (PINKERTON
AND BANNERMAN, 1967). SO MUCH HOMOLOGY OF X CHROMOSOMAL CONSTITUTION EXISTS AMONG
MAMMALS THAT A SIMILAR DISORDER MAY TURN UP IN MAN.

EDWARDS, J. A. AND BANNERMAN, R. M.* HEREDITARY DEFECT OF INTESTINAL IRON
TRANSPORT IN MICE WITH SEX-LINKED ANEMIA. J. CLIN. INVEST. 49* 1869-1871, 1970.

PINKERTON, P. H. AND BANNERMAN, R. M.* HEREDITARY DEFECT OF IRON-ABSORPTION IN
MICE. NATURE 216* 482-483, 1967.

30150 ANGIOKERATOMA, DIFFUSE (FABRY'S DISEASE HEREDITARY DYSTOPIC LIPIDOSIS)

SKIN LESIONS OF VASCULAR NATURE ARE THE MAIN BASIS OF THE NAME. ATTACKS OF PAIN
IN THE ABDOMEN ARE OFTEN MISDIAGNOSED AS APPENDICITIS. SUCH PAINS AND THOSE
ELSEWHERE, SUCH AS IN THE EXTREMITIES, PROBABLY HAVE THEIR BASIS IN LIPID CHANGES
IN GANGLION CELLS OF THE AUTONOMIC NERVOUS SYSTEM. VASCULAR LESIONS OF LIPID
NATURE OCCUR AT OTHER SITES SUCH AS THE OCULAR FUNDI AND KIDNEY. RENAL FAILURE IS
THE USUAL CAUSE OF DEATH. HETEROZYGOUS FEMALES ALMOST NEVER HAVE SKIN LESIONS AND
SURVIVE LONGER DESPITE RENAL INVOLVEMENT. HAMBURGER AND COLLEAGUES (1964)
DESCRIBED A FAMILIAL NEPHROPATHY, MANIFESTED CLINICALLY BY PROTEINURIA AND RENAL
INSUFFICIENCY. RENAL BIOPSY SHOWED THAT THE EPITHELIAL CELLS OF THE GLOMERULAR
TUFTS AND TO A LESSER EXTENT THE TUBULAR EPITHELIAL CELLS, GLOMERULAR ENDOCAPIL-
LARY CELLS AND ARTERIOLAR MUSCULAR CELLS WERE SEVERELY DEFORMED WITH A LARGE
AMOUNT OF CYTOPLASMIC INCLUSION MATERIAL. THE INCLUSION MATERIAL WAS THOUGHT TO   X
BE LIPOID IN NATURE. THE FINDINGS RESEMBLE THOSE OF ANGIOKERATOMA CORPORIS
DIFFUSUM BUT THE ABSENCE OF OTHER SIGNS OF THIS DISEASE SUGGESTED THAT A NEW   L
ENTITY MAY BE INVOLVED. THE MOTHER'S FATHER DIED OF UREMIA. SKIN LESIONS ARE   I
EASILY OVERLOOKED. IT IS CLEAR, HOWEVER, THAT THEY MAY BE LACKING EVEN IN   N
PATIENTS WITH SEVERE VISCERAL MANIFESTATIONS (JOHNSTON, 1967). JOHNSTON ET AL.   K
(1969) ESTIMATED THE RECOMBINATION FRACTION OF ANGIOKERATOMA VERSUS XG TO BE 0.24   E
(95 PERCENT PROBABILITY LIMITS, 8-49.8 PERCENT) AND OF ANGIOKERATOMA VERSUS DEUTAN D
TO BE 0.17 (95 PERCENT PROBABILITY LIMITS, 1-50 PERCENT). FRANCESCHETTI ET AL.
(1969) REEXAMINED THE FAMILY WITH 'CORNEA VERTICILLATA' REPORTED BY GRUBER (1946)
AND SHOWED THAT FABRY'S DISEASE WAS THE 'CAUSE' OF THE CORNEAL CHANGE. THE EXTENT

OF INVOLVEMENT OF THE CORNEA IS ABOUT THE SAME IN MALES AND FEMALES. THUS, CARRIER FEMALES CAN BE IDENTIFIED. THE CORNEAL CONDITION WAS FORMERLY CALLED ALSO FLEISCHER'S VORTEX DYSTROPHY, OR WHORL-LIKE CORNEAL DYSTROPHY. ATABRINE PRODUCES AN INTERESTING PHENOCOPY. KINT (1970) SHOWED THAT THE ACTIVITY OF ALPHA-GALACTO-SIDASE IS DEFICIENT IN LEUKOCYTES OF MALE PATIENTS WITH FABRY'S DISEASE AND THAT CARRIER FEMALES CAN BE IDENTIFIED BY THIS METHOD. IN TWO PATIENTS MAPES ET AL. (1970) DEMONSTRATED A DECLINE IN THE PLASMA LEVEL OF GALACTOSYLGALACTOSYLGLUCOSYL-CERAMIDE WHEN NORMAL PLASMA WAS INFUSED TO PROVIDE ACTIVE ENZYME (CERAMIDE TRIHEXOSIDASE). THE FABRY LOCUS DOES 'LYONIZE' (ROMEO AND MIGEON, 1970). AT A MONTREAL HOSPITAL IN A PERIOD OF A FEW MONTHS CLARKE ET AL. (1971) SAW TWO MEN WITH FABRY'S DISEASE WITHOUT SKIN LESIONS, SUGGESTING THAT IT MAY BE A MORE FREQUENT CAUSE OF PROTEINURIA OR RENAL FAILURE THAN REALIZED. A DIFFERENCE FROM THE USUAL FORM OF FABRY'S DISEASE IS SUGGESTED BY THE FACT THAT LEUKOCYTE ALPHA-GALACTOSIDASE DEFICIENCY IN THE LEUKOCYTES WAS ONLY PARTIAL RATHER THAN BEING COMPLETE (KINT, 1970) AS IN THE USUAL CASES. THE RELATIONSHIP OF THE ALPHA-GALACTOSIDASE DEFICIENCY TO THE PRIMARY FAULT, DEFICIENCY OF CERAMIDE TRIHEXOSI-DASE, IS UNKNOWN.

BRADY, R. O., GAL, A. E., BRADLEY, R. M., MARTENSSON, E., WARSHAW, A. L. AND LASTER, L.* ENZYMATIC DEFECT IN FABRY'S DISEASE. CERAMIDETRIHEXOSIDASE DEFICIEN-CY. NEW ENG. J. MED. 276* 1163-1167, 1967.

CLARKE, J. T. R., KNAACK, J., CRAWHALL, J. C. AND WOLFE, L. S.* CERAMIDE TRIHEXOSIDOSIS (FABRY'S DISEASE) WITHOUT SKIN LESIONS. NEW ENG. J. MED. 284* 233-235, 1971.

FRANCESCHETTI, A. T., PHILIPPART, M. AND FRANCESCHETTI, A.* A STUDY OF FABRY'S DISEASE. I. CLINICAL EXAMINATION OF A FAMILY WITH CORNEA VERTICILLATA. DERMATOLOGICA 138* 209-221, 1969.

FROST, P., TANAKA, Y. AND SPAETH, G. L.* FABRY'S DISEASE - GLYCOLIPID LIPI-DOSES. HISTOCHEMICAL AND ELECTRON MICROSCOPIC STUDIES OF TWO CASES. AM. J. MED. 40* 618-627, 1966.

GRUBER, M.* CORNEA VERTICILLATA. (EINE EINFACH-DOMINANTE VARIANTE DER HORNHAUT DES MENSCHLICHEN AUGES). OPHTHALMOLOGICA 111* 120-129, 1946.

GRUBER, M.* CORNEA VERTICILLATA. II. MITTEILUNG. OPHTHALMOLOGICA 112* 88-91, 1946.

HAMBURGER, J., DORMONT, J., DE MONTERA, H. AND HINGLAIS, N.* SUR UNE SINGULIERE MALFORMATION FAMILIALE DE L'EPITHELIUM RENAL. SCHWEIZ. MED. WSCHR. 94* 871-876, 1964.

JOHNSTON, A. W.* FABRY'S DISEASE WITHOUT SKIN LESIONS. (LETTER) LANCET 1* 1277 ONLY, 1967.

JOHNSTON, A. W., FROST, P., SPAETH, G. L. AND RENWICK, J. H.* LINKAGE RELATION-SHIPS OF THE ANGIOKERATOMA (FABRY) LOCUS. ANN. HUM. GENET. 32* 369-374, 1969.

KINT, J. A.* FABRY'S DISEASE* ALPHA-GALACTOSIDASE DEFICIENCY. SCIENCE 167* 1268-1269, 1970.

MAPES, C. A., ANDERSON, R. L., SWEELEY, C. C., DESNICK, R. J. AND KRIVIT, W.* ENZYME REPLACEMENT IN FABRY'S DISEASE, AN INBORN ERROR OF METABOLISM. SCIENCE 169* 987-989, 1970.

OPITZ, J. M., STILES, F. C., WISE, D., RACE, R. R., SANGER, R., VON GEMMINGEN, G. R., KIERLAND, R. R., CROSS, E. G. AND DEGROOT, W. P.* THE GENETICS OF ANGIO-KERATOMA CORPORIS DIFFUSUM (FABRY'S DISEASE) AND ITS LINKAGE RELATIONS WITH THE XG LOCUS. AM. J. HUM. GENET. 17* 325-342, 1965.

PHILIPPART, M., SARLIEVE, L. AND MANACORDA, A.* URINARY GLYCOLIPIDS IN FABRY'S DISEASE. THEIR EXAMINATION IN THE DETECTION OF ATYPICAL VARIANTS AND THE PRE-SYMPTOMATIC STATE. PEDIATRICS 43* 201-206, 1969.

RAHMAN, A. N., SIMEONE, F. A., HACKEL, D. B., HALL, P. W., III, HIRSCH, E. Z. AND HARRIS, J. W.* ANGIOKERATOMA CORPORIS DIFFUSUM UNIVERSALE (HEREDITARY DYSTOPIC LIPIDOSIS). TRANS. ASS. AM. PHYSICIANS 74* 366-377, 1961.

ROMEO, G. AND MIGEON, B. R.* GENETIC INACTIVATION OF THE ALPHA-GALACTOSIDASE LOCUS IN CARRIERS OF FABRY'S DISEASE. SCIENCE 170* 180-181, 1970.

SWEELEY, C. C. AND KLIONSKY, B.* FABRY'S DISEASE* CLASSIFICATION AS A SPHINGO-LIPIDOSIS AND PARTIAL CHARACTERIZATION OF A NOVEL GLYCOLIPID. J. BIOL. CHEM. 238* 3148-3150, 1963.

WISE, D., WALLACE, H. J. AND JELLINEK, E. H.* ANGIOKERATOMA CORPORIS DIFFUSUM* A CLINICAL STUDY OF EIGHT AFFECTED FAMILIES. QUART. J. MED. 31* 177-206, 1962.

X
L
I
N
K
E
D

30160 ANGIOMATOSIS, DIFFUSE CORTICO-MENINGEAL, OF DIVRY AND VAN BOGAERT

FEATURES IN ADDITION TO THE CORTICO-MENINGEAL ANGIOMATOSIS WERE DEMYELINATION OF
THE WHITE SUBSTANCE OF THE CENTRUM OVALE WITH HEMIANOPSIA, AND 'MARBLED SKIN'
RESULTING FROM A TELANGIECTATIC NETWORK. THREE AFFECTED BROTHERS WERE DESCRIBED.

DIVRY, P. AND VAN BOGAERT, L.* UNE MALADIE FAMILIALE CARACTERISEE PAR UNE
ANGIOMATOSE DIFFUSE CORTICO-MENINGEE NON CALCIFIANTE ET UNE DEMYELINISATION
PROGRESSIVE DE LA SUBSTANCE BLANCHE. J. NEUROL. NEUROSURG. PSYCHIAT. 9* 41-54,
1946.

30170 ANOSMIA

ANOSMIA MAY BE AN X-LINKED DOMINANT TRAIT* NO MALE-TO-MALE TRANSMISSION HAS BEEN
OBSERVED, ALTHOUGH ONLY A FEW AFFECTED MALES HAVE HAD CHILDREN (GLASER, 1918).
THE MAIN REASON FOR CONSIDERING ANOSMIA SEPARATELY IS THAT IT IS NOT CLEAR WHETHER
IT IS ALWAYS MERELY PART OF THE KALLMANN SYNDROME (Q.V.) OR MAY BE A DISTINCT
MUTATION. AFFECTED MALES IN GLASER'S FAMILY IN WHICH X-LINKED INHERITANCE WAS
SUGGESTED HAD 'EXCESSIVE SEX INTEREST.' IT WAS A RUSSIAN JEWISH FAMILY LIKE THOSE
OF KALLMANN AND COLLEAGUES.
     THE ANATOMIC BASIS OF ANOSMIA IS AGENESIS OF THE OLFACTORY LOBES. DE MORSIER
COLLECTED 28 REPORTED CASES OF AGENESIS OF THE OLFACTORY LOBES IN WHICH COMPLETE
AUTOPSY WAS PERFORMED AND FOUND THAT ABNORMALITIES OF THE SEXUAL ORGANS, MAINLY
CRYPTORCHIDISM AND TESTICULAR ATROPHY, HAD BEEN NOTED IN 14. HE SUGGESTED THAT
THE GENITAL ATROPHY IS SECONDARY TO INVOLVEMENT OF THE HYPOTHALAMUS AS WELL AS THE
OLFACTORY LOBES.

DE MORSIER, G.* ETUDES SUR LES DYSTROPHIES CRANIO-ENCEPHALIQUES. I. AGENESIE
DES LOBES OLFACTIFS (TELENCEPHALOSCHIZIS LATERAL) ET DES COMMISSURES CALLEUSE ET
ANTERIEURE (TELENCEPHALOSCHIZIS MEDIAN)* LA DYSPLASIE OLFACTO-GENITALE. SCHWEIZ.
ARCH. NEUROL. PSYCHIAT. 74* 309-361, 1954.

GLASER, O.* HEREDITARY DEFICIENCIES IN THE SENSE OF SMELL. SCIENCE 48* 647-
648, 1918.

30180 ANUS, IMPERFORATE

WEINSTEIN (1965) REPORTED THREE FAMILIES WITH MULTIPLE AFFECTED MALES IN A PATTERN
STRONGLY SUGGESTING X-LINKED RECESSIVE INHERITANCE. IN A LATER PAPER, WINKLER AND
WEINSTEIN (1970) DESCRIBED TWO FAMILIES, EACH WITH TWO SISTERS WITH IMPERFORATE
ANUS AND-OR ECTOPIC ANUS (RECTOVAGINAL FISTULA). THEY THEN PROPOSED AUTOSOMAL
RECESSIVE INHERITANCE FOR SOME CASES.

WEINSTEIN, E. D.* SEX-LINKED IMPERFORATE ANUS. PEDIATRICS 35* 715-717, 1965.

WINKLER, J. M. AND WEINSTEIN, E. D.* IMPERFORATE ANUS AND HEREDITY. J. PEDIAT.
SURG. 5* 555-558, 1970.

*30190 BORJESON SYNDROME (MENTAL DEFICIENCY, EPILEPSY, ENDOCRINE DISORDERS)

FEATURES WERE SEVERE MENTAL DEFECT, EPILEPSY, HYPOGONADISM, HYPOMETABOLISM, MARKED
OBESITY, SWELLING OF SUBCUTANEOUS TISSUE OF FACE, NARROW PALPEBRAL FISSURE, LARGE
BUT NOT DEFORMED EARS. THREE FEMALES WHO MIGHT BE CARRIERS HAD MODERATE MENTAL
RETARDATION. THIS IS A 'NEW' SYNDROME DESCRIBED IN A SINGLE KINDRED. BAAR AND
GALINDO (1965) DESCRIBED A SINGLE CASE THEY THOUGHT REPRESENTED THE SAME ENTITY.

BAAR, H. S. AND GALINDO, J.* THE BORJESON-FORSSMAN-LEHMANN SYNDROME. J. MENT.
DEFIC. RES. 9* 125-130, 1965.

BORJESON, M., FORSSMAN, H. AND LEHMANN, O.* AN X-LINKED, RECESSIVELY INHERITED
SYNDROME CHARACTERIZED BY GRAVE MENTAL DEFICIENCY, EPILEPSY, AND ENDOCRINE
DISORDER. ACTA MED. SCAND. 171* 13-21, 1962.

*30200 BULLOUS DYSTROPHY, HEREDITARY MACULAR TYPE

THE FEATURES ARE FORMATION OF BULLAE WITHOUT EVIDENT TRAUMA, ABSENCE OF ALL HAIR,
HYPERPIGMENTATION, DEPIGMENTATION, ACROCYANOSIS, DWARFISM, MICROCEPHALY, MENTAL
INFERIORITY, SHORT TAPERING FINGERS, SOMETIMES ANOMALIES OF THE NAILS. MOST
PATIENTS DIE BEFORE ATTAINING ADULTHOOD. THIS DISORDER HAS BEEN RECOGNIZED ONLY
IN A SINGLE KINDRED LIVING IN THE NETHERLANDS AND DESCRIBED IN THREE PUBLICATIONS
AS LISTED BELOW.

CAROL, W. L. L. AND KOOIJ, R.* MACULAR TYPE OF HEREDITARY BULLOUS DYSTROPHY.   X
MAANDSCHR. KINDERGENEESK. 6* 39-51, 1936.

MENDES DA COSTA, S. AND VAN DER VALK, J. W.* TYPUS MACULATUS DER BULLOSEN   L
HEREDITAREN DYSTOPHIE. ARCH. DERM. SYPH. 91* 1-8, 1908.   I
                                                                              N
WOERDEMAN, M. J.* DYSTROPHIA BULLOSA HEREDITARIA, TYPUS MACULATUS. NEDERL. T.   K
GENEESK. 102* 111-116, 1958.   E
                                                                              D
30210 CARPAL SUBLUXATION

SO MUCH HOMOLOGY OF X CHROMOSOME EXISTS AMONG MAMMALS THAT THE DESCRIPTION OF

SUBLUXATION OF THE CARPUS AS AN X-LINKED TRAIT IN DOGS IS OF GREAT INTEREST. THE HOMOLOGOUS CONDITION IN MAN IS NOT KNOWN. THE TRAIT IN DOGS IS VERY CLOSELY LINKED TO THE LOCUS FOR HEMOPHILIA A. THE TWO MUTANT GENES WERE IN REPULSION AND NO RECOMBINATION WAS OBSERVED IN 49 OPPORTUNITIES (PICK ET AL., 1967). INTER-SPECIES X-CHROMOSOME HOMOLOGIES ARE DISCUSSED BY MCKUSICK (1964) AND BY OHNO (1967). X-LINKED TRAITS IN THE MOUSE ARE CATALOGED BY GREEN (1966).

GREEN, E. L.* BIOLOGY OF THE LABORATORY MOUSE. NEW YORK* MCGRAW-HILL, 1966 (2ND ED.).

MCKUSICK, V. A.* ON THE X CHROMOSOM OF MAN. WASHINGTON* AM. INST. BIOL. SCI., 1964.

OHNO, S.* SEX CHROMOSOMES AND SEX-LINKED GENES. BERLIN* SPRINGER-VERLAG, 1967.

PICK, J. R., GOYER, R. A., GRAHAM, J. B. AND RENWICK, J. H.* SUBLUXATION OF THE CARPUS IN DOGS. AN X CHROMOSOMAL DEFECT CLOSELY LINKED WITH THE LOCUS FOR HEMOPHILIA A. LAB. INVEST. 17* 243-248, 1967.

*30220 CATARACT, CONGENITAL TOTAL, WITH POSTERIOR SUTURAL OPACITIES IN HETEROZYGOTES

WALSH AND WEGMAN (1937) DESCRIBED POSSIBLE X-LINKED CATARACT IN THE *WE-SORTS,* A TRI-RACIAL GROUP OF SOUTHERN MARYLAND. THE AFFECTED MALES HAD NUCLEAR CATARACTS WITH SEVERE VISUAL IMPAIRMENT. HETEROZYGOUS FEMALES HAD SUTURE CATARACTS WITH ONLY SLIGHT REDUCTION IN VISION. FRACCARO ET AL. (1967) FOUND THE SAME TYPE OF EXPRESSION IN MALES AND FEMALES. LINKAGE STUDIES INDICATED THAT THE XG LOCUS AND THE CATARACT LOCUS MAY BE WITHIN MEASURABLE DISTANCE. THESE AUTHORS POINTED OUT THAT THE PEDIGREES OF STIEREN (1907) AND OF HALBERTSMA (1934), WHICH HAVE BEEN FREQUENTLY CITED AS EXAMPLES OF X-LINKED CATARACT, ARE NOT ACCEPTABLE. IN STIEREN'S PEDIGREE 7 OF 17 AFFECTED MALES HAD CONGENITAL HYDROCEPHALUS AND ALL AFFECTED MALES WERE BORN BLIND AND DIED IN CONVULSIONS. THUS, THEY MAY HAVE SUFFERED FROM A COMPLEX SYNDROME OF WHICH CATARACT WAS ONLY ONE FEATURE. FURTHERMORE, TWO UNAFFECTED MALES HAD DAUGHTERS WHO GAVE BIRTH TO AFFECTED SONS. IN HALBERTSMA'S FAMILY, BESIDE 10 AFFECTED MALES, 3 FEMALES HAD CONGENITAL CATARACT AND ONE HAD SENILE CATARACT. FRASER AND FRIEDMANN (1967) OBSERVED A FAMILY WITH POSSIBLE X-LINKED CATARACT. KRILL ET AL. (1969) DESCRIBED A CONVIN-CINGLY X-LINKED PEDIGREE. SUTURE CATARACT WAS FOUND AS AN EARLY MANIFESTATION IN HEMIZYGOUS MALES. CATARACT IS A FEATURE OF NEARLY ALL CASES OF LOWE'S SYNDROME (Q.V.).

FRACCARO, M., MORONE, G., MANFREDINI, U. AND SANGER, R.* X-LINKED CATARACT. ANN. HUM. GENET. 31* 45-50, 1967.

FRASER, G. R. AND FRIEDMANN, A. I.* THE CAUSES OF BLINDNESS IN CHILDHOOD. A STUDY OF 776 CHILDREN WITH SEVERE VISUAL HANDICAPS. BALTIMORE* JOHNS HOPKINS PRESS, 1967. P. 59.

HALBERTSMA, K. T. A.* FAMILIARE AANGEBOREN CATARACT. NEDERL. T. GENEESK. 78* 1705-1709, 1934.

KRILL, A. E., WOODBURY, G. AND BOWMAN, J. E.* X-CHROMOSOMAL-LINKED SUTURAL CATARACTS. AM. J. OPHTHAL. 68* 867-872, 1969.

STIEREN, E.* A STUDY IN ATAVISTIC DESCENT OF CONGENITAL CATARACT THROUGH FOUR GENERATIONS. OPHTHAL. REC. 16* 234-238, 1907.

WALSH, F. B. AND WEGMAN, M. E.* PEDIGREE OF HEREDITARY CATARACT, ILLUSTRATING SEX-LIMITED TYPE. BULL. HOPKINS HOSP. 61* 125-135, 1937.

30230 CATARACT, CONGENITAL WITH MICROCORNEA OR SLIGHT MICROPHTHALMIA

WAARDENBURG (LOC. CIT. P. 880) OBSERVED A FAMILY WITH CLEAR X-LINKED RECESSIVE INHERITANCE. WITKOP-OOSTENRIJK (1956) DESCRIBED A FAMILY IN WHICH X-LINKED DOMINANCE (POSSIBLY WITH LETHALITY IN THE AFFECTED HEMIZYGOTE) MIGHT BE THE GENETIC MECHANISM. AUTOSOMAL DOMINANT AND AUTOSOMAL RECESSIVE FORMS ALSO EXIST. CAPELLA ET AL. (1963) ALSO OBSERVED PROBABLE X-LINKED CATARACT. NINE MEN HAD CATARACT, FOUR ALSO HAD MICROCORNEA IN ONE OR BOTH EYES AND ONE HAD SMALL PHTHISICAL EYES. IT IS UNCERTAIN THAT CATARACT WITH MICROCORNEA IS AN ENTITY SEPARATE FROM *CATARACT, CONGENITAL TOTAL, WITH POSTERIOR SUTURAL OPACITIES IN HETEROZYGOTES,* BECAUSE SOME PATIENTS OF WALSH AND WEGMAN AND ONE OF KRILL ET AL. SHOWED MICROCORNEA.

CAPELLA, J. A., KAUFMAN, H. E., LILL, F. J. AND COOPER, G.* HEREDITARY CATARACTS AND MICROPHTHALMIA. AM. J. OPHTHAL. 56* 454-458, 1963.

WITKOP-OOSTENRIJK, G. A.* MICROPHTHALMUS, MICROCORNEA EN AANGEBOREN CATARACT. NEDERL. T. GENEESK. 100* 2910-2913, 1956.

WAARDENBURG, P. J., FRANCESCHETTI, A. AND KLEIN, D. (EDS.)* GENETICS AND OPHTHALMOLOGY. SPRINGFIELD, ILL.* CHARLES C THOMAS, 1* 851-888, 1961.

30240 CENTRAL INCISORS, ABSENCE OF

X
L
I
N
K
E
D

HUSKINS DESCRIBED AN ENGLISH FAMILY WITH AFFECTED MEMBERS OF AT LEAST THREE GENERATIONS. HE SPECIFICALLY STATED THAT THERE WAS "NO EVIDENCE OF ANY OTHER DEFECTIVE CONDITION BEING ASSOCIATED WITH THIS DENTAL ANOMALY." THERE WAS ONE AFFECTED FEMALE IN THE FAMILY. WE KNOW OF NO OTHER REPORT OF X-LINKAGE.

HUSKINS, C. L.* ON THE INHERITANCE OF AN ANOMALY OF HUMAN DENTITION. J. HERED. 21* 279-282, 1930.

*30250 CEREBELLAR ATAXIA

SHOKEIR (1970) DESCRIBED 3 KINDREDS WITH A TOTAL OF 16 AFFECTED PERSONS IN AN X-LINKED RECESSIVE PEDIGREE PATTERN. ONE OF THE AFFECTED PERSONS WAS A FEMALE WITH THE XO TURNER SYNDROME. ABSENCE OF EXTRAPYRAMIDAL SIGNS DISTINGUISHED THE DISORDER FROM THAT DESCRIBED BY MALAMUD. THE ABSENCE OF KYPHOSCOLIOSIS AND PES CAVUS AND PRESERVATION OF POSTERIOR COLUMN FUNCTION WERE FEATURES DISTINGUISHING THE DISORDER FROM FRIEDREICH'S ATAXIA. THE DISEASE DID NOT SEEM TO AFFECT LIFE-SPAN AND INTELLIGENCE WAS UNIMPAIRED. ONSET WAS IN THE LATE TEENS OR EARLY TWENTIES. THERE WAS NO VISUAL DIFFICULTY EXCEPT THAT ATTRIBUTABLE TO NYSTAGMUS.

SHOKEIR, M. H. K.* X-LINKED CEREBELLAR ATAXIA. (ABSTRACT) AM. J. HUM. GENET. 22* 37A-38A, 1970.

SHOKEIR, M. H. K.* X-LINKED CEREBELLAR ATAXIA. CLIN. GENET. 1* 225-231, 1970.

*30260 CEREBELLAR ATAXIA WITH EXTRAPYRAMIDAL INVOLVEMENT

MALAMUD'S FAMILY HAD AN UNUSUAL FORM OF NEUROLOGIC DISEASE IN THAT THE CLINICAL PICTURE DOMINATED AT THE OUTSET BY CEREBELLAR SIGNS WAS LATER CHARACTERIZED BY EXTRAPYRAMIDAL SIGNS. ANATOMICAL CHANGES INVOLVED BOTH THE CEREBELLAR AND THE EXTRAPYRAMIDAL SYSTEMS.

MALAMUD, N. AND COHEN, P.* UNUSUAL FORM OF CEREBELLAR ATAXIA WITH SEX-LINKED INHERITANCE. NEUROLOGY 8* 261-266, 1958.

*30270 CEREBRAL SCLEROSIS, DIFFUSE, SCHOLZ TYPE

FORD REFERS TO THIS FORM AS THE SUBACUTE CHILDHOOD TYPE. IT BEGINS AT AGE 8-10 YEARS AND IS CHARACTERIZED BY DEAFNESS, BLINDNESS, WEAKNESS AND SPASTICITY OF THE LEGS, AND DEMENTIA. SURVIVAL IS SHORTER AFTER ONSET OF SYMPTOMS. HOWEVER, IN SCHOLZ' FAMILY, ALTHOUGH THE AFFECTED MALES IN THE YOUNGEST GENERATION SHOWED THIS PICTURE, THEIR MATERNAL GRANDFATHERS, AGE 65 AND 60, HAD THE PICTURE OF SPASTIC PARAPLEGIA.
    WALSH (1957) DESCRIBED UNDER THE HEADING OF SCHILDER'S DISEASE, OR ENCEPHALI-TIS PERIAXIALIS DIFFUSA, A KINDRED IN WHICH FOUR MALES, OFFSPRING OF SISTERS, SUCCUMBED TO AN ILLNESS POSSIBLY OF THE TYPE SHOWN BY SCHOLZ' YOUNGEST PATIENTS. SEE ALSO ADDISON'S DISEASE AND CEREBRAL SCLEROSIS. SCHOLZ (1925) USED HISTOLOGIC TECHNIQUES WHICH WOULD HAVE REMOVED METACHROMATIC MATERIAL. THE CASES OF SCHOLZ WERE RESTUDIED BY PEIFFER (1959) USING FROZEN SECTIONS AND STRIKING METACHROMASIA WAS DEMONSTRATED.

BECKER, P. E.* ANDERE NEUROLOGISCHE ERBKRANKHEITEN. HANDBUCH DER INNEREN MEDIZIN, SPRINGER, BERLIN-GOTTINGEN-HEIDELBERG. 4. AUFL. V-III* 1003, 1953.

PEIFFER, J.* UBER DIE METACHROMATISCHEN LEUKODYSTROPHIEN (TYP SCHOLZ). ARCH. PSYCHIAT. NERVENKR. 199* 386-416, 1959.

SCHOLZ, W.* KLINISCHE, PATHOLOGISCH-ANATOMISCHE UND ERBBIOLOGISCHE UNTERSUCHUN-GEN BEI FAMILIARER, DIFFUSER HIRNSKLEROSE IM KINDESALTER. ZBL. GES. PSYCHIAT. 9* 651-717, 1925.

WALSH, F. B.* CLINICAL NEURO-OPHTHALMOLOGY. BALTIMORE* WILLIAMS AND WILKINS, 1957 (2ND ED.). P. 664 ONLY.

*30280 CHARCOT-MARIE-TOOTH PERONEAL MUSCULAR ATROPHY

THIS CONDITION IS ESSENTIALLY A DEGENERATION OF SPINAL NERVE ROOTS, ESPECIALLY THE MOTOR ROOTS TO THE DISTAL PARTS OF THE EXTREMITIES. AUTOSOMAL DOMINANT AND RECESSIVE FORMS ALSO EXIST. WORATZ (CITED BY BECKER, 1966) STUDIED A FAMILY IN WHICH X-LINKED DOMINANT INHERITANCE WAS PRESENT. A VERY LARGE NUMBER OF PERSONS IN 6 GENERATIONS WERE AFFECTED. TEN AFFECTED FATHERS HAD ONLY AFFECTED DAUGHTERS (15) AND ONLY NORMAL SONS (8), WHEREAS AFFECTED MOTHERS (26) HAD AFFECTED SONS (23) AND AFFECTED DAUGHTERS (21) AS WELL AS UNAFFECTED OFFSPRING. MALES WERE MORE SEVERELY AFFECTED THAN FEMALES. HERRINGHAM (1889) REPORTED A FAMILY WITH 20 AFFECTED MALES IN 4 GENERATIONS. ERWIN (1944) OBSERVED 7 CASES IN 5 GENERATIONS.

ALLAN, W.* RELATION OF HEREDITARY PATTERN TO CLINICAL SEVERITY AS ILLUSTRATED BY PERONEAL ATROPHY. ARCH. INTERN. MED. 63* 1123-1131, 1939.

ERWIN, W. G.* A PEDIGREE OF SEX-LINKED RECESSIVE PERONEAL ATROPHY. J. HERED. 35* 24-26, 1944.

HERRINGHAM, W. P.* MUSCULAR ATROPHY OF THE PERONEAL TYPE AFFECTING MANY MEMBERS

X
L
I
N
K
E
D

WORATZ, G.* CITED BY BECKER, P. E.* HUMANGENETIK 5* 427 ONLY, 1966.

30290 CHARCOT-MARIE-TOOTH PERONEAL MUSCULAR ATROPHY AND FRIEDREICH'S ATAXIA, COMBINED

IN THE FAMILIES REPORTED BY VAN BOGAERT AND MOREAU (1939, 1941), CHARCOT-MARIE-TOOTH DISEASE AND FRIEDREICH'S ATAXIA OCCURRED IN THE SAME INDIVIDUALS IN A PATTERN OF SEX-LINKED RECESSIVE INHERITANCE. POSSIBLY THIS IS A MUTATION DISTINCT FROM THAT RESPONSIBLE FOR THE TWO DISORDERS SEPARATELY. IF THE GENES FOR PERONEAL MUSCULAR ATROPHY AND FRIEDREICH'S ATAXIA ARE CLOSELY SITUATED ON THE X CHROMOSOME, DELETION IS ANOTHER POSSIBLE EXPLANATION FOR THE FINDING IN THIS FAMILY. IN BIEMOND'S KINDRED SOME INDIVIDUALS HAD CHARCOT-MARIE-TOOTH DISEASE (IN A PEDIGREE PATTERN CONSISTENT WITH X-LINKED INHERITANCE), WHEREAS TWO FEMALES OF ONE SIBSHIP HAD FRIEDREICH'S ATAXIA. IN ADDITION MANY MEMBERS OF THE KINDRED HAD DEAF-MUTISM (IN A PATTERN CONSISTENT WITH AUTOSOMAL RECESSIVE INHERITANCE). THUS, THREE SEEMINGLY INDEPENDENT HEREDITARY TRAITS WERE OBSERVED IN THE SAME FAMILY. VAN BOGAERT'S FAMILY IS PROBABLY THE ONLY ONE IN WHICH THE TWO NEUROLOGIC DISEASES OCCURRED ALWAYS TOGETHER IN AN X-LINKED PATTERN.

BIEMOND, A.* NEUROTISCHE MUSKELATROPHIE UND FRIEDREICHSCHE TABES IN DERSELBEN FAMILIE. DEUTSCH. Z. NERVENHEILK. 104* 113-145, 1928.

VAN BOGAERT, L. AND MOREAU, M.* COMBINAISON DE L'AMYOTROPHIE DE CHARCOT-MARIE-TOOTH ET DE LA MALADIE DE FRIEDREICH, CHEZ PLUSIEURS MEMBRES D'UNE MEME FAMILLE. ENCEPHALE 34* 312-320, 1939-1941.

30300 CHOROIDAL SCLEROSIS

IN HIS ATLAS OF THE FUNDUS OCULI (1934), WILMER SHOWED (PLATE 82) THE FUNDUS OF A 35 YEAR OLD AFFECTED MAN WHOSE MATERNAL GRANDFATHER WAS ALSO AFFECTED. FURTHER-MORE TWO BROTHERS AND THE MATERNAL GRANDFATHER OF THE PROBAND'S MATERNAL GRANDFA-THER WERE ALSO AFFECTED, I.E., THE PROBAND HAD INHERITED THE DISORDER FROM HIS GREAT-GREAT-GRANDFATHER THROUGH THE INTERMEDIACY OF A CARRIER MOTHER AND GREAT-GRANDMOTHER. FOLLOW-UP BY LETTER IN 1962 PROVIDED NO FURTHER INFORMATION.
STANKOVIC (1958) REPORTED A SIMILAR FAMILY, WHICH IS OF FURTHER INTEREST BECAUSE FEMALE CARRIERS SHOWED PARTIAL EXPRESSION.
A DIFFICULTY IN INTERPRETATION OF THESE REPORTS IS THE UNCERTAINTY THAT THE DISORDER IS DISTINCT FROM RETINITIS PIGMENTOSA (Q.V.) AND PERHAPS CHOROIDEREMIA (Q.V.). IN RETINITIS PIGMENTOSA (SEE JACOBSON AND STEPHENS, 1962) THE FUNDI ARE SOMETIMES REPORTED AS SHOWING 'SEVERE CHOROIDAL SCLEROSIS.' SORSBY (1963) IS OF THE OPINION THAT THE CASES REPORTED BY SORSBY AND SAVORY (1956) AS X-LINKED CHOROIDAL SCLEROSIS WERE INSTANCES OF CHOROIDEREMIA.

JACOBSON, J. H. AND STEPHENS, G.* HEREDITARY CHOROIDORETINAL DEGENERATION. STUDY OF A FAMILY INCLUDING ELECTRORETINOGRAPHY AND ADAPTOMETRY. ARCH. OPHTHAL. 67* 321-335, 1962.

SORSBY, A. AND SAVORY, M.* CHOROIDAL SCLEROSIS. A POSSIBLE INTERMEDIATE SEX-LINKED FORM. BRIT. J. OPHTHAL. 40* 90-95, 1956.

SORSBY, A.* QUOTED BY FRANCESCHETTI, A., FRANCOIS, J. AND BABEL, J.* LES HEREDO-DEGENERESCENCES CHORIO-RETINIENNES (DEGENERESCENCES TAPETO RETINIENNES). PARIS* MASSON, 2* 1963. P. 777.

STANKOVIC, I.* L'ANGIOSCLEROSE CHOROIDIENNE FAMILIALE LIEE AU SEXE. BULL. SOC. FRANC. OPHTAL. 71* 411-417, 1958.

*30310 CHOROIDEREMIA (PROGRESSIVE TAPETO-CHOROIDAL DYSTROPHY)

AFFECTED MALES SUFFER PROGRESSIVE LOSS OF VISION (REDUCTION OF CENTRAL VISION, CONSTRICTION OF VISUAL FIELDS, NIGHT BLINDNESS) BEGINNING AT AN EARLY AGE, AND THE CHOROID AND RETINA UNDERGO COMPLETE ATROPHY. HETEROZYGOUS FEMALES SHOW NO VISUAL DEFECT BUT OFTEN SHOW STRIKING FUNDOSCOPIC CHANGES SUCH AS IRREGULAR PIGMENTATION AND ATROPHY AROUND THE OPTIC DISC. FULLY AFFECTED FEMALES HAVE BEEN REPORTED (FRASER AND FRIEDMANN, 1967* SHAPIRA AND SITNEY, 1943). THESE RAISE THE USUAL QUESTIONS OF X-CHROMOSOMAL ABERRATION, UNFORTUNATE LYONIZATION IN A HETEROZYGOTE, HOMOZYGOSITY, ETC. AN EXTENSIVE STUDY IN HOLLAND WAS CONDUCTED BY KURSTJENS (1965).
THE TERM CHOROIDEREMIA, WHICH IS COMPARABLE TO IRIDEREMIA AND MEANS ABSENCE OF CHOROID, IS INAPPROPRIATE, SINCE THERE IS NO CONGENITAL ABSENCE OF THE CHOROID. THE CONDITION IS AN ABIOTROPHY BEGINNING SHORTLY AFTER BIRTH AND PROGRESSING GRADUALLY. WAARDENBURG FAVORED AN ALTERNATIVE DESIGNATION 'TAPETOCHOROIDAL DYSTROPHY' (PAMEYER, ET AL., 1960). HARRIS AND MILLER (1968) OBSERVED VISUAL IMPAIRMENT IN A HETEROZYGOTE IN THE FAMILY REPORTED EARLIER BY MCCULLOCH AND MCCULLOCH (1948).

FRASER, G. R. AND FRIEDMANN, A. I.* THE CAUSES OF BLINDNESS IN CHILDHOOD. A STUDY OF 776 CHILDREN WITH SEVERE VISUAL HANDICAPS. BALTIMORE* JOHNS HOPKINS PRESS, 1967.

HARRIS, G. S. AND MILLER, J. R.* CHOROIDEREMIA* VISUAL DEFECTS IN A HETEROZY-

X
L
I
N
K
E
D

GOTE. ARCH. OPHTHAL. 80* 423-429, 1968.

KURSTJENS, J. H.* CHOROIDEREMIA AND GYRATE ATROPHY OF THE CHOROID AND RETINA. DOCUM. OPHTHAL. 19* 1-122, 1965.

MCCULLOCH, C. AND MCCULLOCH, R. J. P.* A HEREDITARY AND CLINICAL STUDY OF CHOROIDEREMIA. TRANS. AM. ACAD. OPHTHAL. OTOLARYNG. 52* 160-190, 1948.

SHAPIRA, T. M. AND SITNEY, J. A.* CHOROIDEREMIA. AM. J. OPHTHAL. 26* 182-183, 1943.

SORSBY, A., FRANCESCHETTI, A., JOSEPH, R. AND DAVEY, J. B.* CHOROIDEREMIA. CLINICAL AND GENETIC ASPECTS. BRIT. J. OPHTHAL. 36* 547-581, 1952.

PAMEYER, J. K., WAARDENBURG, P. J. AND HENKES, H. E.* CHOROIDEREMIA. BRIT. J. OPHTHAL. 44* 724-738, 1960.

*30320 CHOROIDO-RETINAL DEGENERATION WITH RETINAL REFLEX IN HETEROZYGOUS WOMEN

FALLS AND COTTERMAN (1948) DESCRIBED AN X-LINKED FORM OF CHOROIDO-RETINAL DEGENERATION WHICH IS DISTINGUISHED FROM OTHER TYPES BY THE PRESENCE IN HETEROZY-GOUS WOMEN OF A TAPETAL-LIKE RETINAL REFLEX. SEE RETINITIS PIGMENTATION AND CHOROIDO-RETINAL DYSTROPHY FOR PHENOTYPICALLY RELATED ENTITIES.

FALLS, H. F. AND COTTERMAN, C. W.* CHOROIDORETINAL DEGENERATION. A SEX-LINKED FORM IN WHICH HETEROZYGOUS WOMEN EXHIBIT A TAPETAL-LIKE RETINAL REFLEX. ARCH. OPHTHAL. 40* 685-703, 1948.

30330 CHOROIDO-RETINAL DYSTROPHY

HOARE (1965) DESCRIBED A CHORIORETINAL DISORDER IN 10 MALES IN SEVEN SIBSHIPS WHICH WERE OFFSPRING OF SISTERS. THE MATERNAL GRANDFATHER OF THE AFFECTED MALES WAS PROBABLY ALSO AFFECTED. THE CONDITION WAS DETECTED IN CHILDHOOD. SOME CARRIER WOMEN SHOWED FUNDUS ABNORMALITIES WITH VISUAL IMPAIRMENT BEGINNING IN MIDDLE AGE AND PROBABLY SHOWING PROGRESSION. THE CONDITION IN MALES RESEMBLED RETINITIS PIGMENTOSA IN FUNDUS PICTURE AND NIGHT BLINDNESS BUT DIFFERED BY THE ABSENCE OF ANNULAR SCOTOMA, BY EARLY INVOLVEMENT OF CENTRAL VISION, AND BY RELATIVELY LITTLE VASCULAR CHANGE.

HOARE, G. W.* CHOROIDO-RETINAL DYSTROPHY. BRIT. J. OPHTHAL. 49* 449-459, 1965.

*30340 CLEFT PALATE

IN A BRITISH COLUMBIA INDIAN FAMILY, LOWRY (1970) FOUND 12 MALES WITH INCOMPLETE CLEFT OF THE SECONDARY PALATE. IN SOME THE CLEFT WAS SUBMUCOUS. PALATOPHARYNGEAL INCOMPETENCE WAS A LEADING FEATURE. THE PEDIGREE PATTERN SUGGESTED X-LINKED RECESSIVE INHERITANCE. THE HIGH SEX RATIO FOR CLEFT PALATE IN BRITISH COLUMBIA INDIANS COULD BE DUE TO THE EXISTENCE OF AN X-LINKED FORM OF SUBMUCOUS CLEFT PALATE (LOWRY AND RENWICK, 1969).

LOWRY, R. B. AND RENWICK, D. H.* INCIDENCE OF CLEFT LIP AND PALATE IN BRITISH COLUMBIA INDIANS. J. MED. GENET. 6* 67-69, 1969.

LOWRY, R. B.* SEX LINKED CLEFT PALATE IN A BRITISH COLUMBIA INDIAN FAMILY. PEDIATRICS 46* 123-128, 1970.

30350 CLEFT PALATE WITH HYPERTELORISM AND MEDIAN FRONTAL PROMINENCE

WEINSTEIN AND COHEN (1966) SUGGESTED THAT AN X-LINKED FORM EXISTS. AFFECTED MALES AND CARRIER FEMALES SHOWED HYPERTELORISM AND MEDIAN FRONTAL PROMINENCE. FOUR MALES IN THREE SIBSHIPS CONNECTED THROUGH 5 PRESUMABLY HETEROZYGOUS FEMALES WERE AFFECTED. GORLIN (1967) SUGGESTS THAT THE CONDITION IN THIS FAMILY MAY HAVE BEEN WHAT HE TERMED THE OTO-PALATO-DIGITAL SYNDROME.

GORLIN, R. J.* MINNEAPOLIS, MINN.* PERSONAL COMMUNICATION, 1967.

WEINSTEIN, E. D. AND COHEN, M. M.* SEX-LINKED CLEFT PALATE. REPORT OF A FAMILY AND REVIEW OF 77 KINDREDS. J. MED. GENET. 3* 17-22, 1966.

30360 COFFIN SYNDROME

THE FEATURES ARE MENTAL RETARDATION WITH PECULIAR PUGILISTIC NOSE, LARGE EARS, TAPERED FINGERS, DRUMSTICK TERMINAL PHALANGES BY X-RAY, PECTUS CARINATUM.

*30370 COLOR BLINDNESS, BLUE-MONO-CONE-MONO-CHROMATIC TYPE

THIS DISORDER WAS PREVIOUSLY INTERPRETED AS TOTAL COLOR BLINDNESS. PRESENT INFORMATION (SPIVEY, 1965) INDICATES THAT AFFECTED PERSONS CAN SEE SMALL BLUE OBJECTS ON A LARGE YELLOW FIELD AND VICE VERSA. THESE CASES HAVE BEEN VARIOUSLY CALLED PARTIAL COMPLETE COLOR BLINDNESS, OR INCOMPLETE ACHROMATOPSIA. BLACKWELL AND BLACKWELL (1961) HAVE DESCRIBED ACHROMATOPTIC FAMILIES IN WHICH A FEW BLUE CONES SEEMED TO BE PRESENT. SEE COMMENTS OF ALPERN, FALLS AND LEE (1960). SLOAN

X
L
I
N
K
E
D

(1964) HAS EVIDENCE OF THE PRESENCE OF A FEW RED CONES IN CASES OF OTHERWISE COMPLETE ACHROMATOPSIA. ALTHOUGH THIS IS LISTED AS A SEPARATE MUTATION ITS GENETIC RELATIONSHIP (E.G., ALLELISM) TO THE TWO PARTIAL COLOR BLINDNESS LOCI IS UNKNOWN.

ALPERN, M., FALLS, H. F. AND LEE, G. B.* THE ENIGMA OF TYPICAL TOTAL MONOCHROMACY. AM. J. OPHTHAL. 50* 996-1012, 1960.

BLACKWELL, H. R. AND BLACKWELL, O. M.* ROD AND CONE RECEPTOR MECHANISMS IN TYPICAL AND ATYPICAL CONGENITAL ACHROMATOPSIA. VISION RES. 1* 62-107, 1961.

SLOAN, L. L.* BALTIMORE, MD.* PERSONAL COMMUNICATION, 1964.

SLOAN, L. L.* CONGENITAL ACHROMATOPSIA* A REPORT OF 19 CASES. J. OPT. SOC. AM. 44* 117-128, 1954.

SPIVEY, B. E.* THE X-LINKED RECESSIVE INHERITANCE OF ATYPICAL MONOCHROMATISM. ARCH. OPHTHAL. 74* 327-333, 1965.

*30380 COLOR BLINDNESS, PARTIAL, DEUTAN SERIES

IN WESTERN EUROPEANS ABOUT 8 PER CENT OF MALES ARE COLOR BLIND. OF THESE ABOUT 75 PERCENT HAVE A DEFECT IN THE DEUTAN SERIES AND ABOUT 25 PERCENT HAVE A DEFECT IN THE PROTAN SERIES. WAALER (1968) DISTINGUISHED TWO TYPES OF NORMAL COLOR VISION ACCORDING TO 'GREENPOINT,' I.E., THE POINT AT WHICH THE SUBJECT SEES PURE GREEN, AND TWO TYPES ACCORDING TO 'BLUEPOINT.' HE PRESENTED THE FOLLOWING GENETIC HYPOTHESIS* MALES CAN BE OF EITHER G(1)B(1), G(1)B(2) OR G(2)B(2). FEMALES CAN BE OF SIX GENOTYPES. AMONG 59 CHILDREN OF DOUBLY HETEROZYGOUS MOTHERS ONE POSSIBLE CROSS-OVER WAS FOUND. HE SUGGESTED THE USE OF THIS POLYMORPHISM IN LINKAGE STUDIES.

ADAM, A. AND FRASER, G. R.* THE LINKAGE BETWEEN PROTAN AND DEUTAN LOCI. (LETTER) AM. J. HUM. GENET. 22* 691-693, 1970.

WAALER, G. H.* HEREDITY OF TWO NORMAL TYPES OF COLOUR VISION. NATURE 218* 688-689, 1968.

*30390 COLOR BLINDNESS, PARTIAL, PROTAN SERIES

THE TWO-LOCUS HYPOTHESIS FOR COLOR BLINDNESS IS SUPPORTED BY THREE SETS OF OBSERVATIONS.
A. THE RELATIVE FREQUENCY OF COLOR BLINDNESS IN MALES AND FEMALES IS MOST CONSISTENT WITH THE EXISTENCE OF TWO LOCI. GIVEN A FREQUENCY OF COLOR-BLIND MALES OF .08 AND A TOTAL GENE FREQUENCY FOR COLOR BLINDNESS ALSO OF .08, THEN ON A ONE-LOCUS HYPOTHESIS THE FREQUENCY OF COLOR-BLIND FEMALES SHOULD BE .08 X .08, OR .64 PERCENT. ON A TWO-LOCUS HYPOTHESIS, WITH THE PROTAN AND DEUTAN SERIES REPRESENTING 25 AND 75 PERCENT, RESPECTIVELY, THEN THE FREQUENCY OF COLOR-BLIND FEMALES SHOULD BE LESS, ASSUMING THAT DOUBLY HETEROZYGOUS FEMALES ARE NORMAL*
FEMALES COLOR-BLIND FOR PROTAN
SERIES - .02 X .02 = .04 PERCENT
FEMALES COLOR-BLIND FOR DEUTAN
SERIES - .06 X .06 = .36 PERCENT
.40 PERCENT
(THE EXPECTED FREQUENCY OF DOUBLY HETEROZYGOUS FEMALES IS THE PRODUCT OF THE FREQUENCIES OF SINGLY HETEROZYGOUS FEMALES - (2 X .02 X .98) (2 X .06 X .94), OR 0.0044.) IN FACT, THE DATA ON RELATIVE FREQUENCY OF COLOR BLINDNESS IN MALES AND FEMALES COLLECTED IN NORWAY BY WAALER (1927) AND IN SWITZERLAND BY VON PLANTA (1928) AGREE WITH THE VALUES PREDICTED BY A TWO-LOCUS THEORY.
B. THE TWO-LOCUS THEORY IS ALSO SUPPORTED BY THE FACT THAT FEMALES WHO BY THE NATURE OF THE COLOR VISION DEFECT IN THEIR SONS ARE KNOWN TO CARRY GENES FOR BOTH TYPES OF COLOR BLINDNESS USUALLY DO NOT SHOW A DEFECT IN COLOR VISION. THIS IS ESSENTIALLY THE COMPLEMENTARITY TEST OF ALLELISM. (THE DOUBLE HETEROZYGOTES IN THE PEDIGREES OF KONDO AND BRUNNER HAD NORMAL COLOR VISION.)
COMPLEMENTARITY IS ALSO INDICATED BY THE FINDINGS IN THE FAMILIES BY FRANCESCHETTI AND KLEIN (1957). IT IS POSSIBLE, OF COURSE, THAT THE MOTHER IN EACH FAMILY WAS A MANIFESTING HETEROZYGOTE. IT IS TO BE HOPED THAT THE PRESUMABLY DOUBLY HETEROZYGOUS DAUGHTERS HAVE A LARGE NUMBER OF SONS AND THAT THE COLOR VISION OF THESE SONS IS TESTED IN THE FUTURE.
C. THE PEDIGREE OF VANDERDONCK AND VERRIEST (1960) AND THAT OF SINISCALCO ET AL., (1964) INDICATES INDEPENDENT ASSORTMENT OF DEUTAN AND PROTAN GENES AMONG THE OFFSPRING OF A DOUBLY HETEROZYGOUS FEMALE.
THE NAGEL ANOMALOSCOPE, USED IN DETERMINATION OF THE TYPE OF COLOR BLINDNESS, CONSISTS OF A VIEWING TUBE WITH A CIRCULAR BIPARTITE FIELD, ONE HALF ILLUMINATED WITH YELLOW AND THE OTHER HALF WITH A MIXTURE OF GREEN AND RED. THE YELLOW HALF IS NOT VARIABLE EXCEPT IN BRIGHTNESS. THE OTHER HALF CAN BE VARIED CONTINUOUSLY FROM RED TO GREEN. THE SUBJECT'S COLOR SENSE IS TESTED BY HAVING HIM MIX COLORS IN THE VARIABLE HALF-FIELD UNTIL HE ACHIEVES A SUBJECTIVE MATCH TO THE YELLOW FIELD. CERTAIN COLOR COMBINATIONS ARE CONSIDERED NORMAL WHEREAS SPECIFIC DIFFERENCES FROM THE NORMAL INDICATE THE TYPE AND DEGREE OF ANOMALOUS COLOR VISION.
ISHIHARA PLATES ALONE ARE UNRELIABLE IN DISTINGUISHING DEUTAN AND PROTAN TYPES. ALTHOUGH THE NAGEL ANOMALOSCOPE IS THE 'LAST COURT OF APPEAL' IN MAKING

X
L
I
N
K
E
D

THE DIFFERENTIATION, IT IS EXPENSIVE, TIME-CONSUMING, DIFFICULT FOR UNSOPHISTI-
CATED SUBJECTS, AND, OF COURSE, NOT USABLE *IN THE FIELD.* TWO *BOOK* TESTS, THE
TOKYO MEDICAL COLLEGE TEST AND THE AO-HRR (HARDY-RAND-RITTLER) PSEUDOISOCHROMATIC
PLATES, ESPECIALLY WHEN TOGETHER, REPRESENT PROBABLY THE METHODS WHICH ARE BOTH
THE EASIEST AND THE MOST RELIABLE NOW AVAILABLE (SLOAN, 1961).

IDENTIFICATION OF A SMALL PROPORTION OF DEUTEROHETEROZYGOTES IS POSSIBLE BY
MEANS OF THE LUMINOSITY QUOTIENT, DETERMINED BY A MODIFICATION OF THE NAGEL
ANOMALOSCOPE DESIGNED BY CRONE. MOST CASES OF PROTO-HETEROZYGOTES CAN BE
IDENTIFIED AS SUCH WITH A HIGH DEGREE OF CERTAINTY USING THIS METHOD.

IT APPEARS (NEMOTO AND MURAO, 1961) THAT THE ORDER OF DOMINANCE IN COLOR
BLINDNESS IS NORMAL - ANOMALY - ANOPIA (FRANCESCHETTI*S HYPOTHESIS).

CRONE, R. A.* SPECTRAL SENSITIVITY IN COLOR-DEFECTIVE SUBJECTS AND HETEROZYGOUS
CARRIERS. AM. J. OPHTHAL. 48* 231-238, 1959.

FRANCESCHETTI, A. AND KLEIN, D.* TWO FAMILIES WITH PARENTS OF DIFFERENT TYPES
OF RED-GREEN BLINDNESS. ACTA GENET. STATIST. MED. 7* 255-259, 1957.

FRASER, G. R.* ESTIMATION OF THE RECOMBINATION FRACTION BETWEEN THE PROTAN AND
DEUTAN LOCI. AM. J. HUM. GENET. 21* 593-599, 1969.

KALMUS, H.* DIAGNOSIS AND GENETICS OF DEFECTIVE COLOUR VISION. OXFORD*
PERGAMON PRESS, 1965. P. 59.

NEMOTO, H. AND MURAO, M.* A GENETIC STUDY OF COLOR BLINDNESS. JAP. J. HUM.
GENET. 6* 165-173, 1961.

SCHMIDT, I.* A SIGN OF MANIFEST HETEROZYGOSITY IN CARRIERS OF COLOR DEFICIENCY.
AM. J. OPTOM. 32* 404-408, 1955.

SINISCALCO, M., FILIPPI, G. AND LATTE, B.* RECOMBINATION BETWEEN PROTAN AND
DEUTAN GENES* DATA ON THEIR RELATIVE POSITIONS IN RESPECT OF THE G6PD LOCUS.
NATURE 204* 1062-1064, 1964.

SLOAN, L. L.* EVALUATION OF THE TOKYO MEDICAL COLLEGE COLOR VISION TEST. AM.
J. OPHTHAL. 52* 650-659, 1961.

THULINE, H. C., HODGKIN, W. E., FRASER, G. R. AND MOTULSKY, A. G.* GENETICS OF
PROTAN AND DEUTAN COLOR-VISION ANOMALIES* AN INSTRUCTIVE FAMILY. AM. J. HUM.
GENET. 21* 581-592, 1969.

VANDERDONCK, R. AND VERRIEST, G.* FEMME PROTANOMALE ET HETEROZYGOTE MIXTE
(GENES DE LA PROTANOMALIE ET DE LA DEUTERANOPIE EN POSITION DE REPULSION) AYANT
DEUX FILS DEUTERANOPES, UN FILS PROTANOMAL ET DEUX FILS NORMAUX. BIOTYPOLOGIE 21*
110-120, 1960.

VON PLANTA, P.* DIE HAUFIGKEIT DER ANGEBORENEN FARBENSINNSTORUNGEN BEI KNABEN
UND MADCHEN UND IHRE FESTSTELLUNG DURCH DIE UBLICHEN KLINISCHEN PROBEN. GRAEFE.
ARCH. OPHTHAL. 120* 253-281, 1928.

WAALER, G. H. M.* UBER DIE ERBLICHKEITSVERHALTNISSE DER VERSCHIEDENEN ARTEN VON
ANGEBORENER ROTGRUNBLINDHEIT. ZTSCH. F. INDUKT. ABSTAMMUNGS- U. VERERBUNGSL. 45*
279-333, 1927.

*30400 COLOR BLINDNESS, PARTIAL, TRITANOMALY

THE DEFECT IN *BLUE SENSE* IS LESS SEVERE THAN IN TRITANOPIA, AN AUTOSOMAL
DOMINANT (Q.V.). THIS CONDITION IS CONSIDERABLY RARER THAN PROTAN AND DEUTAN
COLOR BLINDNESS. THE FREQUENCY OF TRITAN DEFECTS IS IMPERFECTLY KNOWN BECAUSE OF
LACK OF DIAGNOSTIC TOOLS AND LESSER PRACTICAL IMPORTANCE IN SIGNALING AND TRAFFIC
CONTROL.

KALMUS, H.* DIAGNOSIS AND GENETICS OF DEFECTIVE COLOUR VISION. OXFORD*
PERGAMON PRESS, 1965. P. 59.

*30410 CORPUS CALLOSUM, PARTIAL AGENESIS OF

MENKES, PHILIPPART AND CLARK (1964) DESCRIBED A FAMILY WITH FIVE MALES (IN FOUR
SIBSHIPS OF TWO GENERATIONS CONNECTED THROUGH FEMALES) WITH PARTIAL AGENESIS OF
THE CORPUS CALLOSUM. CLINICAL FEATURES INCLUDED SEVERE INTELLECTUAL RETARDATION
AND INTRACTABLE SEIZURES. POSTMORTEM STUDIES OF ONE PATIENT SHOWED A COMBINATION
OF ANATOMIC AND CHEMICAL ABNORMALITIES.

MENKES, J. H., PHILIPPART, M. AND CLARK, D. B.* HEREDITARY PARTIAL AGENESIS OF
CORPUS CALLOSUM. ARCH. NEUROL. 11* 198-208, 1964.

30420 CUTIS VERTICIS GYRATA, THYROID APLASIA AND MENTAL RETARDATION

AKESSON (1965) DESCRIBED FIVE MALES IN THREE SIBSHIPS OF TWO GENERATIONS WHO MAY
HAVE HAD THIS COMBINATION OF MANIFESTATIONS. ONLY THE PROBAND WAS EXAMINED IN
FULL. HE POINTED OUT THAT ALTHOUGH X-LINKED INHERITANCE SEEMED LIKELY MOST OTHER
CASES OF CUTIS VERTICIS GYRATA AND MENTAL RETARDATION SEEM TO HAVE AUTOSOMAL

AKESSON, H. O.* CUTIS VERTICIS GYRATA, THYROAPLASIA AND MENTAL DEFICIENCY. ACTA GENET. MED. GEM. 14* 200-204, 1965.

30430 CYANIDE, INABILITY TO SMELL

INITIAL STUDIES (REVIEWED BY STERN) SHOWED MALE-FEMALE FREQUENCIES AND FAMILY DATA CONSISTENT WITH X-LINKED RECESSIVE INHERITANCE OF INABILITY TO SMELL CYANIDE. FURTHER STUDIES SEEM TO INDICATE THAT THE SITUATION IS MORE COMPLEX (KIRK, 1953). THE SAME CONCLUSION WAS REACHED BY BROWN AND ROBINETTE (1967) AND BY GILES ET AL. (1968). THE WORK OF THE LAST GROUP OF WORKERS EXCLUDES X-LINKAGE.

ALLISON, A. C.* CYANIDE SMELLING DEFICIENCY AMONG AFRICANS. MAN 53* 176-177, 1953.

BROWN, K. S. AND ROBINETTE, R. R.* NO SIMPLE PATTERN OF INHERITANCE IN ABILITY TO SMELL SOLUTIONS OF CYANIDE. NATURE 215* 406-408, 1967.

BROWN, K. S., MACLEAN, C. M. AND ROBINETTE, R. R.* THE DISTRIBUTION OF THE SENSITIVITY TO CHEMICAL ODORS IN MAN. HUM. BIOL. 40* 456-472, 1968.

FUKUMOTO, Y., NAKAJIMA, H., UETAKE, M., MATSUYAMA, A. AND YOSHIDA, T.* SMELL ABILITY TO SOLUTION OF POTASSIUM CYANIDE AND ITS INHERITANCE. JAP. J. HUM. GENET. 2* 7-16, 1957.

GILES, E., HANSEN, A. T., MCCULLOUGH, J. M., METZGER, D. G. AND WOLPOFF, M. H.* HYDROGEN CYANIDE AND PHENYLTHIOCARBAMIDE SENSITIVITY, MID-PHALANGEAL HAIR AND COLOR BLINDNESS IN YUCATAN, MEXICO. AM. J. PHYS. ANTHROP. 28* 203-212, 1968.

KIRK, R. L. AND STENHOUSE, N. S.* ABILITY TO SMELL SOLUTIONS OF POTASSIUM CYANIDE. NATURE 171* 698-699, 1953.

SRIVASTAVA, R. P.* ABILITY TO SMELL SOLUTIONS OF SODIUM CYANIDE. EASTERN ANTHROPOLOGIST (LUCKNOW) 14* 189-191, 1961.

STERN, C.* IN, FREEMAN, W. H. (ED.)* PRINCIPLES OF HUMAN GENETICS. SAN FRANCISCO* (2ND. ED.) 1960. P. 232, TABLE 35.

*30440 DEAFNESS, CONDUCTIVE TYPE, WITH STAPES FIXATION

SHINE AND WATSON (1967) DESCRIBED A HAWAIIAN-CHINESE FAMILY WITH 9 MALES IN TWO GENERATIONS AFFECTED WITH CONDUCTIVE HEARING LOSS AND VESTIBULAR DISTURBANCE. AT OPERATION THE FOOTPLATE OF THE STAPES WAS FOUND TO BE FIXED. WHEN IT WAS MOBILIZED, PROFUSE DRAINAGE OF PERILYMPH AND CEREBROSPINAL FLUID OCCURRED INDICATING ABNORMAL PATENCY OF THE COCHLEAR AQUEDUCT. NANCE ET AL. (1970, 1971) HAVE OBSERVED A SIMILAR FAMILY OF EUROPEAN EXTRACTION, INDICATING THAT THIS IS A BONA FIDE SYNDROME.

SHINE, I. AND WATSON, J. R.* A NEW SYNDROME OF SEX-LINKED CONGENITAL CONDUCTIVE DEAFNESS. TO BE PUBLISHED, 1967.

MCRAE, K. N., UCHIDA, I. A. AND LEWIS, M.* SEX-LINKED CONGENITAL DEAFNESS. AM. J. HUM. GENET. 21* 415-419, 1969.

NANCE, W. E., SETLEFF, R., MCLEOD, A. C., SWEENEY, A., COOPER, M. C. AND MCCONNELL, F.* X-LINKED MIXED DEAFNESS WITH CONGENITAL FIXATION OF THE STAPEDIAL FOOTPLATE AND PERILYMPHATIC GUSHER. THE CLINICAL DELINEATION OF BIRTH DEFECTS. IX. EAR. BALTIMORE* WILLIAMS AND WILKINS, 1970.

NANCE, W. E., SWEENEY, A., MCLEOD, A. C. AND COOPER, M. C.* HEREDITARY DEAFNESS* A PRESENTATION OF SOME RECOGNIZED TYPES, MODES OF INHERITANCE, AND AIDS IN COUNSELING. STH. MED. BULL. 58* 41-57, 1970.

*30450 DEAFNESS, CONGENITAL, PERCEPTIVE TYPE

PROBABLY ABOUT 1.5 PERCENT OF GENETIC DEAFNESS IS DETERMINED BY AN X-BORNE GENE. THE X-LINKED FORM OF CONGENITAL DEAFNESS HAS BEEN DESCRIBED FROM MISSOURI (DOW, POYNTER, 1930), JAPAN (MITSUDA ET AL., 1952), BELFAST (STEVENSON, CITED BY DERAEMAEKER), BELGIUM (DERAEMAEKER, 1958), PHILADELPHIA (SATALOFF ET AL. 1955) AND AUSTRALIA (PARKER, 1958). FRASER (1965) FOUND SEVERAL FAMILIES IN ENGLAND. IN THE FAMILY REPORTED BY DOW AND POYNTER FOUR AFFECTED MALES MARRIED DEAF-MUTE WOMEN WHO PROBABLY HAD THE AUTOSOMAL RECESSIVE FORM OF THE DISEASE BECAUSE NO CHILDREN WERE AFFECTED. THE DEAFNESS IS OF PERCEPTIVE TYPE.

DERAEMAEKER, R.* SEX-LINKED CONGENITAL DEAFNESS. ACTA GENET. STATIST. MED. 8* 228-231, 1958.

DOW, G. S. AND POYNTER, C. I.* THE DAR FAMILY. EUGEN. NEWS 15* 128-130, 1930.

FRASER, G. R.* SEX-LINKED RECESSIVE CONGENITAL DEAFNESS AND THE EXCESS OF MALES IN PROFOUND CHILDHOOD DEAFNESS. ANN. HUM. GENET. 29* 171-196, 1965.

X
L
I
N
K
E
D

MITSUDA, H., INOUE, S. AND KAZAMA, Y.* EINE FAMILIE MIT REZESSIV GESCHLECHTSGE-BUNDENER TAUBSTUMMHEIT. JAP. J. HUM. GENET. 27* 142, 1952.

PARKER, N.* CONGENITAL DEAFNESS DUE TO A SEX-LINKED RECESSIVE GENE. AM. J. HUM. GENET. 10* 196-200, 1958.

RICHARDS, B. W.* SEX-LINKED DEAF-MUTISM. ANN. HUM. GENET. 26* 195-199, 1963.

SATALOFF, J., PASTORE, P. N. AND BLOOM, E.* SEX-LINKED HEREDITARY DEAFNESS. AM. J. HUM. GENET. 7* 201-203, 1955.

30460 DEAFNESS, HIGH TONE NEURAL

LIVAN (1961) DESCRIBED AN X-LINKED VARIETY OF NERVE DEAFNESS CHARACTERIZED BY HIGHTONE LOSS WHICH MAY BE DISTINCT FROM THE OTHER FORMS OF X-LINKED DEAFNESS LISTED HERE.

LIVAN, M.* CONTRIBUTE ALLA CONSCENZA DELLA SORBITA EREDITARIE. ARCH. ITAL. OTOL. 72* 331-339, 1961.

*30470 DEAFNESS, PROGRESSIVE

SUFFICIENT HEARING IS PRESENT AT FIRST THAT SPEECH DEVELOPS NORMALLY, THEN DETERIORATES.

MOHR, J. AND MAGEROY, K.* SEX-LINKED DEAFNESS OF A POSSIBLY NEW TYPE. ACTA GENET. STATIST. MED. 10* 54-62, 1960.

*30480 DIABETES INSIPIDUS, NEPHROGENIC

THE DEFECT CONCERNS THE ABILITY OF THE RENAL TUBULE TO RESPOND TO ANTIDIURETIC HORMONE. A PARTIAL DEFECT IS DEMONSTRABLE IN FEMALES. NAKANO (1969) DESCRIBED THE DISORDER IN FOUR GENERATIONS OF A SAMOAN FAMILY. TEN BENSEL AND PETERS (1970) DESCRIBED HYDRONEPHROSIS IN AFFECTED MALE SIBS OF THE FAMILY REPORTED BY CANNON (1955). THE PEDIGREE THEY PRESENTED COVERING 5 GENERATIONS WITH 12 AFFECTED MALES IS TYPICALLY OF X-LINKAGE. CANNON HAD CLAIMED MALE-TO-MALE TRANSMISSION IN 3 INSTANCES AND AUTOSOMAL DOMINANT INHERITANCE. HIS INFORMATION MUST HAVE BEEN IN ERROR.

ABELSON, H.* NEPHROGENIC DIABETES INSIPIDUS. PEDIAT. RES. 2* 271-282, 1968.

BODE, H. H. AND MIETTINEN, O. S.* NEPHROGENIC DIABETES INSIPIDUS* ABSENCE OF CLOSE LINKAGE WITH XG. AM. J. HUM. GENET. 22* 221-227, 1970.

CANNON, J. F.* DIABETES INSIPIDUS. CLINICAL AND EXPERIMENTAL STUDIES WITH CONSIDERATION OF GENETIC RELATIONSHIPS. ARCH. INTERN. MED. 96* 215-272, 1955.

CARTER, C. AND SIMPKISS, M.* THE CARRIER STATE IN NEPHROGENIC DIABETES INSIPIDUS. LANCET 2* 1069-1073, 1956.

NAKANO, K. K.* FAMILIAL NEPHROGENIC DIABETES INSIPIDUS. HAWAII MED. J. 28* 205-208, 1969.

ORLOFF, J. AND BURG, M. B.* VASOPRESSIN-RESISTANT DIABETES INSIPIDUS. IN, STANBURY, J. B., WYNGAARDEN, J. B. AND FREDRICKSON, D. S. (EDS.)* THE METABOLIC BASIS OF INHERITED DISEASES. NEW YORK* MCGRAW-HILL, 1966 (2ND ED.). PP. 1247-1261.

TEN BENSEL, R. W. AND PETERS, E. R.* PROGRESSIVE HYDRONEPHROSIS, HYDROURETER, AND DILATATION OF THE BLADDER IN SIBLINGS WITH CONGENITAL NEPHROGENIC DIABETES INSIPIDUS. J. PEDIAT. 77* 439-443, 1970.

*30490 DIABETES INSIPIDUS, NEUROHYPOPHYSEAL TYPE

IN ADDITION TO THE X-LINKED FORMS OF DIABETES INSIPIDUS, AUTOSOMAL DOMINANT FORMS ALSO EXIST. FORSSMAN HAD FIVE FAMILIES* TWO PROBABLY AUTOSOMAL AND THREE X-LINKED. OF THE THREE X-LINKED FAMILIES, ONE WAS OF THE PITRESSIN-RESISTANT TYPE, WHEREAS THE OTHER TWO FAMILIES WERE SUSCEPTIBLE. THE LATTER TWO FAMILIES PRESUMABLY REPRESENT THE NEUROHYPOPHYSEAL TYPE. GREEN ET AL. (1967) REPORTED A FAMILY WITH DIABETES INSIPIDUS IN DOMINANT PATTERN, EITHER X-LINKED OR AUTOSOMAL. AUTOPSY IN ONE OF THE AFFECTED MEMBERS SHOWED MARKED REDUCTION OF NEURONES IN THE SUPRAOPTIC AND PARAVENTRICULAR NUCLEI OF THE HYPOTHALAMUS. BREAST FEEDING WAS NORMAL IN ONE OF THESE PATIENTS, DESPITE THE VIRTUAL ABSENCE OF HYPOTHALAMIC NUCLEI THOUGHT TO BE RESPONSIBLE FOR PRODUCTION OF OXYTOCIN WHICH IS CONSIDERED ESSENTIAL FOR BREAST FEEDING.

FORSSMAN, H.* ON HEREDITARY DIABETES INSIPIDUS WITH SPECIAL REGARD TO A SEX-LINKED FORM. ACTA MED. SCAND. 159 (SUPPL.)* 1945.

FORSSMAN, H.* TWO DIFFERENT MUTATIONS OF THE X-CHROMOSOME CAUSING DIABETES INSIPIDUS. AM. J. HUM. GENET. 7* 21-27, 1955.

GREEN, J. R., BUCHAN, G. C., ALVORD, E. C., JR. AND SWANSON, A. G.* HEREDITARY AND IDIOPATHIC TYPES OF DIABETES INSIPIDUS. BRAIN 90* 707-714, 1967.

*30500 DYSKERATOSIS, CONGENITAL (ZINSSER-COLE-ENGMAN SYNDROME)

THE FEATURES ARE CUTANEOUS PIGMENTATION, DYSTROPHY OF THE NAILS, LEUCOPLAKIA OF THE ORAL MUCOSA, CONTINUOUS LACRIMATION DUE TO ATRESIA OF THE LACRIMAL DUCTS, OFTEN THROMBOCYTOPENIA, ANEMIA, AND IN MOST CASES TESTICULAR ATROPHY. ONLY MALES ARE AFFECTED IN A PATTERN CONSISTENT WITH X-LINKED RECESSIVE INHERITANCE. MILGROM ET AL. (1964) DESCRIBED THE CONDITION IN A NEGRO MALE. THEY POINTED OUT THAT THE TWO SERIOUS COMPLICATIONS ARE ANEMIA AND CANCER, WHICH DEVELOPS IN THE LEUKOPLAKIA OF THE ANUS OR MOUTH, OR MAY DEVELOP IN THE SKIN. BRYAN AND NIXON (1965) DESCRIBED A PEDIGREE WITH FOUR AND POSSIBLY FIVE AFFECTED MALES IN A RELATIONSHIP NICELY CONSISTENT WITH X-LINKED RECESSIVE INHERITANCE. THE PATIENTS HAD PANCYTO-PENIA WHICH LED THE AUTHORS (INCORRECTLY, I THINK) TO THE CONCLUSION THAT FANCONI'S PANMYELOPATHY AND DYSKERATOSIS CONGENITA ARE ONE AND THE SAME ENTITY. ADDISON AND RICE (1965) DESCRIBED A MALE WITH SEEMINGLY TYPICAL SKIN AND MUCOSAL CHANGES, AS WELL AS PANCYTOPENIA. HIS SISTER HAD POIKILODERMA AND ORAL LEUKOPLA-KIA, PROGRESSING TO SQUAMOUS CARCINOMA FATAL AT AGE 24 YEARS. SORROW AND HITCH (1963) DESCRIBED A FEMALE PATIENT WHO HAD FATAL CERVICAL AND VAGINAL SQUAMOUS CARCINOMA. THE RELATION OF THE DISORDER IN THESE FEMALE PATIENTS TO THE CONDITION WHICH IS CLEARLY X-LINKED IS NOT CLEAR.

ADDISON, M. AND RICE, M. S.* THE ASSOCIATION OF DYSKERATOSIS CONGENITA AND FANCONI'S ANAEMIA. MED. J. AUST. 1* 797-799, 1965.

BRYAN, H. G. AND NIXON, R. K.* DYSKERATOSIS CONGENITA AND FAMILIAL PANCYTO-PENIA. J.A.M.A. 192* 203-208, 1965.

GARB, J.* DYSKERATOSIS CONGENITA WITH PIGMENTATION, DYSTROPHIA UNGUIUM AND LEUKOPLAKIA ORIS. ARCH. DERM. 77* 704-712, 1958.

MILGROM, H., STOLL, H. L., JR. AND CRISSEY, J. T.* DYSKERATOSIS CONGENITA. A CASE WITH NEW FEATURES. ARCH. DERM. 89* 345-349, 1964.

KOSZEWSKI, B. J. AND HUBBARD, T. F.* CONGENITAL ANEMIA IN HEREDITARY ECTODERMAL DYSPLASIA. ARCH. DERM. 74* 159-166, 1956.

SORROW, J. M., JR. AND HITCH, J. M.* DYSKERATOSIS CONGENITA. FIRST REPORT OF ITS OCCURRENCE IN A FEMALE AND A REVIEW OF THE LITERATURE. ARCH. DERM. 88* 340-347, 1963.

*30510 ECTODERMAL DYSPLASIA, ANHIDROTIC

THE AFFECTED MALES SHOW ABSENCE OF TEETH, HYPOTRICHOSIS, AND ABSENCE OF SWEAT GLANDS. HETEROZYGOUS WOMEN MAY SHOW REDUCTION OR MALFORMATION OF TEETH AND MILD ABNORMALITIES OF SWEAT GLANDS AND BREASTS. IN ROBERT'S FAMILY 1929, SKIN INVOLVEMENT IN HETEROZYGOUS FEMALES WAS PATCHY. HALPERIN AND CURTIS' CASE 1942 SHOWED MENTAL DEFECT ALSO, BUT THIS IS NOT AN INVARIABLE FEATURE OF CASES, EVEN IN THEIR FAMILY. THIS WAS THE CONDITION AFFECTING THE 'TOOTHLESS MEN OF SIND,' MEMBERS OF A HINDU KINDRED WHICH RESIDES IN THE VICINITY OF HYDERABAD AND WAS DESCRIBED BY DARWIN (1875) AND BY THADANI (1934). DARWIN (1875) WROTE AS FOLLOWS* 'I MAY GIVE AN ANALOGOUS CASE, COMMUNICATED TO ME BY MR. W. WEDDERBURN, OF A HINDOO FAMILY IN SCINDE, IN WHICH TEN MEN, IN THE COURSE OF FOUR GENERATIONS, WERE FURNISHED, IN BOTH JAWS TAKEN TOGETHER, WITH ONLY FOUR SMALL AND WEAK INCISOR TEETH AND WITH EIGHT POSTERIOR MOLARS. THE MEN THUS AFFECTED HAVE VERY LITTLE HAIR ON THE BODY, AND BECOME BALD EARLY IN LIFE. THEY ALSO SUFFER MUCH DURING HOT WEATHER FROM EXCESSIVE DRYNESS OF THE SKIN. IT IS REMARKABLE THAT NO INSTANCE HAS OCCURRED OF A DAUGHTER BEING AFFECTED...THOUGH THE DAUGHTERS IN THE ABOVE FAMILY ARE NEVER AFFECTED, THEY TRANSMIT THE TENDENCY TO THEIR SONS* AND NO CASE HAS OCCURRED OF A SON TRANSMITTING IT TO HIS SONS. THE AFFECTION THUS APPEARS ONLY IN ALTERNATE GENERATIONS, OR AFTER LONG INTERVALS.' HUTT (1935) CALLED ATTENTION TO DARWIN'S DESCRIPTION. SINGH, JOLLY, AND KAUR (1962) DESCRIBED A SEVERE CASE IN A 27 YEAR OLD SIKH WOMAN IN INDIA. TWO BROTHERS HAD DIED OF THE DISEASE. WHETHER THIS WAS A HOMOZYGOUS AFFECTED OR A HETEROZYGOUS MANIFESTING FEMALE IS UNCERTAIN, ESPECIALLY SINCE NO INFORMATION WAS PROVIDED ON WHETHER THE FATHER WAS AFFECTED. CONSANGUINEOUS MATINGS OF THE TYPES WHICH ARE EXPECTED TO RESULT IN HOMOZYGOUS AFFECTED FEMALES ARE FREQUENT IN SOME INDIAN GROUPS. OTHER DEFECTS INCLUDE SADDLE-NOSE AND THOSE INVOLVING THE LACRIMAL GLANDS, BREASTS AND CORNEA. MOST PATIENTS ARE SHORT OF STATURE AND SHOW HYPERPIGMENTATION AROUND THE EYES. AUTOPSY IN ONE PATIENT (REED ET AL., 1970) SHOWED ABSENCE OF MUCOUS GLANDS IN THE PHARYNX, LARYNX, TRACHEA, AND LARGE AND SMALL BRONCHI. THE FINDING WAS THOUGHT TO BE THE BASIS FOR INCREASED SUSCEPTIBILITY TO RESPIRATORY INFECTIONS OBSERVED IN LIFE. MUCOUS GLANDS WERE ALSO ABSENT IN THE UPPER ESOPHAGUS AND HYPOPLASTIC IN THE COLON.

BOWEN, R.* HEREDITARY ECTODERMAL DYSPLASIA OF THE ANHIDROTIC TYPE. STH. MED. J. 50* 1018-1021, 1957.

DARWIN, C.* THE VARIATION OF ANIMALS AND PLANTS UNDER DOMESTICATION. LONDON* JOHN MURRAY, 1875. (2ND ED.) P. 319.

X
L
I
N
K
E
D

GRANT, R. AND FALLS, H. F.* ANODONTIA* REPORT OF A CASE ASSOCIATED WITH ECTODERMAL DYSPLASIA OF THE ANHIDROTIC TYPE. AM. J. ORTHODONT. 30* 661-672, 1944.

HALPERIN, S. L. AND CURTIS, G. M.* ANHIDROTIC ECTODERMAL DYSPLASIA ASSOCIATED WITH MENTAL DEFICIENCY. AM. J. MENT. DEFIC. 46* 459-463, 1942.

HUTT, F. B.* AN EARLIER RECORD OF THE TOOTHLESS MEN OF SIND. J. HERED. 26* 65-66, 1935.

JESPERSON, H. G.* HEREDITARY ECTODERMAL DYSPLASIA OF ANHIDROTIC TYPE. ACTA PAEDIAT. 51* 712-720, 1962.

KLINE, A. H., SIDBURY, J. B., JR. AND RICHTER, C. P.* THE OCCURRENCE OF ECTODERMAL DYSPLASIA AND CORNEAL DYSPLASIA IN ONE FAMILY. J. PEDIAT. 55* 355-366, 1959.

MALAGON, V. AND TAVERAS, J. E.* CONGENITAL ANHIDROTIC ECTODERMAL AND MESODERMAL DYSPLASIA. ARCH. DERM. 74* 253-258, 1956.

REED, W. B., LOPEZ, D. A. AND LANDING, B.* CLINICAL SPECTRUM OF ANHIDROTIC ECTODERMAL DYSPLASIA. ARCH. DERM. 102* 134-143, 1970.

ROBERTS, E.* THE INHERITANCE OF ANHIDROSIS ASSOCIATED WITH ANODONTIA. J.A.M.A. 93* 277-279, 1929.

SIMPSON, J. L., ALLEN, F. H., JR., NEW, M. AND GERMAN, J.* ABSENCE OF CLOSE LINKAGE BETWEEN THE LOCUS FOR XG AND THE LOCUS FOR ANHIDROTIC ECTODERMAL DYSPLASIA. VOX SANG. 17* 465-467, 1969.

SINGH, A., JOLLY, S. S. AND KAUR, S.* HEREDITARY ECTODERMAL DYSPLASIA. BRIT. J. DERM. 74* 34-37, 1962.

THADANI, K. I.* THE TOOTHLESS MEN OF SIND. J. HERED. 25* 483-484, 1934.

*30520 EHLERS-DANLOS SYNDROME

AS ONE PART OF THE GENETIC HETEROGENEITY OF THIS SYNDROME, BEIGHTON (1968) DESCRIBED TWO FAMILIES IN WHICH X-LINKED INHERITANCE IS PROBABLE. CLOSE LINKAGE WITH XG BLOOD GROUPS AND COLOR-BLINDNESS WAS EXCLUDED. THE CLINICAL FEATURES INCLUDED HYPEREXTENSIBLE SKIN AND BRUISING TENDENCY. FRAGILITY OF SKIN WAS UNIMPRESSIVE.

BEIGHTON, P.* X-LINKED RECESSIVE INHERITANCE IN THE EHLERS-DANLOS SYNDROME. BRIT. MED. J. 2* 409-411, 1968.

*30530 ENDOCARDIAL FIBROELASTOSIS

FIXLER ET AL. (1970) DESCRIBED FOUR MALES IN THREE SIBSHIPS, RELATED THROUGH FEMALES, WITH THE CONTRACTED FORM OF ENDOCARDIAL FIBROELASTOSIS. THE AFFECTED MALES DIED OF HEART FAILURE IN THE FIRST YEARS OF LIFE. AN AUTOSOMAL RECESSIVE FORM OF ENDOCARDIAL FIBROELASTOSIS APPEARS TO BE WELL ESTABLISHED AND FIBROELASTO-SIS IS FREQUENTLY FOUND ASSOCIATED WITH MALFORMATIONS OF THE HEART. DILATED AND CONTRACTED FORMS OF FIBROELASTOSIS ARE RECOGNIZED ON THE BASIS OF THE STATE OF THE LEFT VENTRICLE AT AUTOPSY. THE CLINICAL PICTURE OF THE TWO TYPES DIFFER. IT IS NOT CERTAIN THAT THE GENETICS IS DIFFERENT FOR THE TWO TYPES. FEMALE CASES OF THE CONTRACTED FORM HAVE BEEN DESCRIBED.

FIXLER, D. E., COLE, R. B., PAUL, M. H., LEV, M. AND GIROD, D. A.* FAMILIAL OCCURRENCE OF THE CONTRACTED FORM OF ENDOCARDIAL FIBROELASTOSIS. AM. J. CARDIOL. 26* 208-213, 1970.

*30540 FACIOGENITAL DYSPLASIA

AARSKOG (1970) HAS DESCRIBED AN X-LINKED DISORDER CHARACTERIZED BY OCULAR HYPERTELORISM, ANTIVERTED NOSTRILS, BROAD UPPER LIP, AND PECULIAR PENOSCROTAL RELATIONS ('SADDLE-BAG SCROTUM'). AFFECTED MALES CAN REPRODUCE. SCOTT (1971) EMPHASIZED THE OCCURRENCE OF LIGAMENTOUS LAXITY MANIFEST BY HYPEREXTENSIBILITY OF THE FINGERS, GENU RECURVATUM AND FLAT FEET. FURTHERMORE, HYPERMOBILITY IN THE CERVICAL SPINE WITH ANOMALY OF THE ODONTOID RESULTED IN NEUROLOGIC DEFICIT. IN HIS FAMILY, 9 MALES IN 5 SIBSHIPS WERE AFFECTED.

AARSKOG, D.* A FAMILIAL SYNDROME OF SHORT STATURE ASSOCIATED WITH FACIAL DYSPLASIA AND GENITAL ANOMALIES. J. PEDIAT. 77* 856-861, 1970.

SCOTT, C. I., JR.* UNUSUAL FACIES, JOINT HYPERMOBILITY, GENITAL ANOMALY AND SHORT STATURE* A NEW DYSMORPHIC SYNDROME. THE CLINICAL DELINEATION OF BIRTH DEFECTS. X. THE ENDOCRINE SYSTEM. BALTIMORE* WILLIAMS AND WILKINS, 1971.

*30550 FIBRIN-STABILIZING FACTOR (FACTOR XIII) DEFICIENCY

FIBRIN-STABILIZING FACTOR (FACTOR XIII) IS A CONSTITUENT OF HUMAN PLASMA WHICH, WHEN ACTIVATED, LINKS ADJACENT MOLECULES OF FIBRIN TO FORM A STABLE CLOT,

CHARACTERIZED BY INSOLUBILITY IN 5M UREA OR 1 PERCENT MONOCHLOROACETIC ACID.
RATNOFF AND STEINBERG (1968) POINTED OUT THAT ALTHOUGH IN SOME FAMILIES DEFICIENCY
IS UNQUESTIONABLY INHERITED AS AN AUTOSOMAL RECESSIVE, X-LINKED INHERITANCE IS
LIKELY IN OTHER FAMILIES. IF TRUE, THE CONCLUSION SUGGESTS THAT EITHER (1) FACTOR
XIII IS COMPOSED OF TWO POLYPEPTIDE CHAINS, OR (2) TWO OR MORE ENZYMES OR CLOTTING
FACTORS ARE INVOLVED IN FIBRIN-STABILIZATION. STEINBERG AND RATNOFF (1970) FOUND
A HIGHLY SIGNIFICANT DIFFERENCE IN THE FREQUENCY OF PARENTAL CONSANGUINITY BETWEEN
FAMILIES WITH ONLY MALES AFFECTED AND FAMILIES WITH AFFECTED FEMALES. THEY
ADVANCED THIS AS EVIDENCE FOR THE EXISTENCE OF BOTH X-LINKED AND AUTOSOMAL FORMS.

RATNOFF, O. D. AND STEINBERG, A. G.* INHERITANCE OF FIBRIN-STABILIZING-FACTOR
DEFICIENCY. LANCET 1* 25-26, 1968.

STEINBERG, A. G. AND RATNOFF, O. D.* INHERITANCE OF FACTOR XIII. (LETTER) AM.
J. HUM. GENET. 22* 597-598, 1970.

*30560 FOCAL DERMAL HYPOPLASIA (FDH)

FDH APPEARS TO BE AN X-LINKED DOMINANT WITH LETHALITY IN MALES. THE FEATURES
INCLUDE ATROPHY AND LINEAR PIGMENTATION OF THE SKIN, HERNIATION OF FAT THROUGH THE
DERMAL DEFECTS AND MULTIPLE PAPILLOMAS OF THE MUCOUS MEMBRANES OR SKIN. IN
ADDITION, DIGITAL ANOMALIES CONSIST OF SYNDACTYLY, POLYDACTYLY, CAMPTODACTYLY AND
ABSENCE DEFORMITIES. ORAL ANOMALIES, IN ADDITION TO LIP PAPILLOMAS, INCLUDE
HYPOPLASTIC TEETH. OCULAR ANOMALIES (COLOBOMA OF IRIS AND CHOROID, STRABISMUS,
MICROPHTHALMIA) HAVE ALSO BEEN PRESENT IN SOME CASES. GOLTZ ET AL. (1962) NOTED
THAT ALL FIVE OF THEIR CASES WERE FEMALE, THAT THE DISORDER OCCURRED ONLY IN
FEMALE ANTECEDENTS AND OTHER RELATIVES AND THAT MISCARRIAGES ARE FREQUENT IN THESE
FAMILIES. THEY HAD AFFECTED FEMALES IN FOUR SUCCESSIVE GENERATIONS IN ONE FAMILY
AND IN TWO GENERATIONS OF ANOTHER. THE MOTHER OF WODNIANSKY'S FEMALE PATIENT
(1957) HAD SKIN CHANGES AND A SISTER HAD SYNDACTYLY OF THE 3RD AND 4TH FINGERS AND
TOES BILATERALLY. WARBURG (1970) OBSERVED MICROPHTHALMOS WITH BILATERAL COLOBOMA
OF THE IRIS AND ECTOPIA LENTIS. KISTENMACHER ET AL. (1970) DESCRIBED AN AFFECTED
MALE AND RAISED THE QUESTION OF 'DURCHBRENNER' OF HADORN, I.E., THE OCCASIONAL
SURVIVAL OF A LETHAL.

GOLTZ, R. W., HENDERSON, R. R., HITCH, J. M. AND OTT, J. E.* FOCAL DERMAL
HYPOPLASIA SYNDROME. A REVIEW OF THE LITERATURE AND REPORT OF TWO CASES. ARCH.
DERM. 101* 1-11, 1970.

GOLTZ, R. W., PETERSON, W. C., JR., GORLIN, R. J. AND RAVITS, H. G.* FOCAL
DERMAL HYPOPLASIA. ARCH. DERM. 86* 708-717, 1962.

GORLIN, R. J., MESKIN, L. H., PETERSON, W. C., JR. AND GOLTZ, R. W.* FOCAL
DERMAL HYPOPLASIA SYNDROME. ACTA DERMATOVENER. 43* 421-440, 1963.

HOLDEN, J. D. AND AKERS, W. A.* GOLTZ'S SYNDROME* FOCAL DERMAL HYPOPLASIA. AM.
J. DIS. CHILD. 114* 292-300, 1967.

KISTENMACHER, M. L., TOROSOLO, M. A., PUNNETT, H. H. AND DIGEORGE, A. M.* FOCAL
DERMAL HYPOPLASIA IN A MALE. (ABSTRACT) AM. J. HUM. GENET. 22* 19A ONLY, 1970.

WARBURG, M.* FOCAL DERMAL HYPOPLASIA. OCULAR AND GENERAL MANIFESTATIONS WITH A
SURVEY OF THE LITERATURE. ACTA OPHTHAL. 48* 525-536, 1970.

WODNIANSKY, P.* UBER DIE FORMEN DER CONGENITALEN POIKILODERMIE. ARCH. KLIN.
EXP. DERM. 205* 331-342, 1957.

30570 GERMINAL CELL APLASIA (SERTOLI-CELL-ONLY SYNDROME* DEL CASTILLO SYNDROME)

EDWARDS AND BANNERMAN (1971) OBSERVED TWO BROTHERS, AGES 14 AND 12, WITH GYNECOMA-
STIA AND OBESITY. THEIR DISORDER MIGHT HAVE BEEN CLASSIFIED SIMPLY AS ADOLESCENT
OR PUBERTAL GYNECOMASTIA WERE IT NOT FOR THE EXISTENCE OF TWO MATERNAL UNCLES WITH
A HISTORY OF PUBERTAL GYNECOMASTIA AND IN THE ONE OF THEM AVAILABLE FOR STUDY
CLINICAL FEATURES AND TESTICULAR BIOPSY CONSISTENT WITH THE DEL CASTILLO SYNDROME.
BY THE AGE OF 26, HE SHOWED NO GYNECOMASTIA. IN THE 14 YEAR OLD NEPHEW THE SPERM
COUNT WAS PROBABLY LOW BUT SPERM WAS PRESENT. THE AUTHORS SUGGESTED THAT IN THIS
BOY THEY HAD AN OPPORTUNITY TO OBSERVE THE DEL CASTILLO SYNDROME AT AN EARLIER
STAGE THAN HAD PREVIOUSLY BEEN POSSIBLE. THEY SUGGESTED THAT, AS IN OTHER SIMILAR
CONDITIONS SUCH AS THE TESTICULAR FEMINIZATION SYNDROME AND AND REIFENSTEIN
SYNDROME, THE INHERITANCE IS EITHER X-LINKED OR AUTOSOMAL DOMINANT MALE-LIMITED.
SEVERAL KINDREDS WITH MULTIPLE AFFECTED MALES ARE KNOWN.

EDWARDS, J. A. AND BANNERMAN, R. M.* FAMILIAL GYNECOMASTIA. THE CLINICAL
DELINEATION OF BIRTH DEFECTS. X. THE ENDOCRINE SYSTEM. BALTIMORE* WILLIAMS AND
WILKINS, 1971.

WEYENETH, R.* ETIOPATHOGENIE ET DIAGNOSTIC DE LA STERILITE MASCULINE. PRAXIS
45* 21-34, 1956.

30580 GERODERMIA OSTEODYSPLASTICA

BOREUX (1969) DESCRIBED A DISORDER WHICH THEY CONCLUDED IS INHERITED AS AN X-

X
L
I
N
K
E
D

LINKED RECESSIVE WITH OCCASIONAL MANIFESTATION IN FEMALES. AS THE NAME INDICATES THE FEATURES INCLUDE CHANGES IN THE SKIN SUGGESTING PRECOCIOUS AGING AND OSSEOUS CHANGES INCLUDING OSTEOPOROSIS AND MULTIPLE LINES LIKE GROWTH RINGS OF A TREE. BOREUX SUGGESTED THAT THE PHYSIOGNOMY RESEMBLES THAT OF WALT DISNEY'S DWARFS (FROM 'SNOW WHITE').

BOREUX, G.* LA GERODERMIE OSTEODYSPLASIQUE A HEREDITE LIEE AU SEXE, NOUVELLE ENTITE CLINIQUE ET GENETIQUE. J. GENET. HUM. 17* 137-178, 1969.

BROCHER, J. E. W., KLEIN, D., BAMATTER, F., FRANCESCHETTI, A. AND BOREUX, G.* RONTGENOLOGISCHE BEFUNDE BEI GERODERMA OSTEODYSPLASTICA HEREDITARIA. FORTSCHR. ROENTGENSTR. 109* 185-198, 1968.

*30590 GLUCOSE-6-PHOSPHATE DEHYDROGENASE VARIANTS

SINCE IDENTIFICATION OF DEFICIENCY OF G6PD AND OF ITS X-CHROMOSOMAL DETERMINATION IN THE 1950'S AND DEMONSTRATION OF ELECTROPHORETIC VARIANTS OF THIS ENZYME IN THE EARLY 1960'S (BOYER ET AL., 1962), THE GENETIC, CLINICAL AND BIOCHEMICAL SIGNIFICANCE OF THIS POLYMORPHISM HAS BEEN FOUND TO BE VERY GREAT. DEFICIENCY OF THE RED CELL ENZYME, IN VARIOUS FORMS, IS THE BASIS OF FAVISM, PRIMAQUINE SENSITIVITY AND OTHER DRUG-SENSITIVE HEMOLYTIC ANEMIA, ANEMIA AND JAUNDICE IN THE NEWBORN, AND CHRONIC NONSPHEROCYTIC HEMOLYTIC ANEMIA (BEUTLER ET AL., 1968). DIFFERENT VARIANTS OF THE ENZYME ARE FOUND IN HIGH FREQUENCY IN AFRICAN, MEDITERRANEAN AND ASIATIC POPULATIONS (PORTER ET AL., 1964) AND HETEROZYGOTE ADVANTAGE VIZ-A-VIZ MALARIA (LUZZATTO ET AL., 1969) HAS BEEN INVOKED TO ACCOUNT FOR THE HIGH FREQUENCY OF THE PARTICULAR ALLELES IN PARTICULAR POPULATION.

THE VARIETY OF FORMS OF THE ENZYME IS NUMEROUS, AS ILLUSTRATED BY THE TABLES OF YOSHIDA, BEUTLER AND MOTULSKY (SEE LATER). THE WORLD HEALTH ORGANIZATION (1967) GAVE ITS ATTENTION TO PROBLEMS OF NOMENCLATURE AND STANDARD PROCEDURES FOR STUDY. THEY DEMONSTRATED POLYMORPHISM AT THIS X-LINKED LOCUS RIVALS THAT OF THE AUTOSOMAL LOCI FOR THE POLYPEPTIDE CHAINS OF HEMOGLOBIN. AS IN THE LATTER INSTANCE, SINGLE AMINO ACID SUBSTITUTION HAS BEEN DEMONSTRATED AS THE BASIS OF THE CHANGE IN THE G6PD MOLECULE RESULTING FROM MUTATION (YOSHIDA ET AL., 1967).

POLYMORPHISM AT THE G6PD LOCUS HAS MADE IT A USEFUL X-CHROMOSOME MARKER, LIKE COLORBLINDNESS AND THE XG BLOOD GROUP LOCUS, AND CLOSE LINKAGE OF THE COLORBLINDNESS LOCI, THE G6PD LOCUS AND THE LOCUS FOR HEMOPHILIA A (ADAM ET AL., 1966* BOYER AND GRAHAM, 1965) HAS BEEN DEMONSTRATED. AS A BIOCHEMICAL PHENOTYPE IDENTIFIABLE AT THE CELLULAR LEVEL, G6PD VARIANTS HAVE BEEN USEFUL IN SOMATIC CELL GENETICS, PERMITTING, FOR EXAMPLE, ONE OF THE CRITICAL PROOFS IN MAN OF THE LYON HYPOTHESIS (DAVIDSON ET AL., 1963).

THE RELATIVE STABILITY OF THE X CHROMOSOME DURING EVOLUTION HAS BEEN SHOWN BY THE FACT THAT THE G6PD LOCUS IS X-BORNE ALSO IN A NUMBER OF OTHER SPECIES (OHNO, 1967).

ADAM, A., TIPPETT, P., GAVIN, J., NOADES, J., SANGER, R. AND RACE, R. R.* THE LINKAGE RELATION OF XG TO G-6-PD IN ISRAELIS* THE EVIDENCE OF A SECOND SERIES OF FAMILIES. AM. J. HUM. GENET. 30* 211-218, 1966.

AZEVEDO, E. AND YOSHIDA, A.* BRAZILIAN VARIANT OF GLUCOSE-6-PHOSPHATE DEHYDROGENASE (GD MINAS GERAIS). NATURE 222* 380-382, 1969.

AZEVEDO, E., KIRKMAN, H. N., MORROW, A. C. AND MOTULSKY, A. G.* VARIANTS OF RED CELL GLUCOSE-6-PHOSPHATE DEHYDROGENASE AMONG ASIATIC INDIANS. ANN. HUM. GENET. 31* 373-380, 1968.

BEACONSFIELD, P., RAINSBURY, R. AND KALTON, G.* GLUCOSE-6-PHOSPHATE DEHYDROGENASE DEFICIENCY AND THE INCIDENCE OF CANCER. ONCOLOGIA 19* 11-19, 1965.

BEUTLER, E. AND ROSEN, R.* NONSPHEROCYTIC CONGENITAL HEMOLYTIC ANEMIA DUE TO A NEW G-6-PD VARIANT* G-6-PD ALHAMBRA. PEDIATRICS 45* 230-235, 1970.

BEUTLER, E., MATHAI, C. K. AND SMITH, J. E.* BIOCHEMICAL VARIANTS OF GLUCOSE-6-PHOSPHATE DEHYDROGENASE GIVING RISE TO CONGENITAL NONSPHEROCYTIC HEMOLYTIC DISEASE. BLOOD 31* 131-150, 1968.

BOYER, S. H. AND GRAHAM, J. B.* LINKAGE BETWEEN THE X CHROMOSOME LOCI FOR GLUCOSE-6-PHOSPHATE DEHYDROGENASE ELECTROPHORETIC VARIATION AND HEMOPHILIA A. AM. J. HUM. GENET. 17* 320-324, 1965.

BOYER, S. H., PORTER, I. H. AND WEILBAECHER, R. G.* ELECTROPHORETIC HETEROGENEITY OF GLUCOSE-6-PHOSPHATE DEHYDROGENASE AND ITS RELATIONSHIP TO ENZYME DEFICIENCY IN MAN. PROC. NAT. ACAD. SCI. 48* 1868-1876, 1962.

DAVIDSON, R. G., NITOWSKY, H. M. AND CHILDS, B.* DEMONSTRATION OF TWO POPULATIONS OF CELLS IN THE HUMAN FEMALE HETEROZYGOUS FOR GLUCOSE-6-PHOSPHATE DEHYDROGENASE VARIANTS. PROC. NAT. ACAD. SCI. 50* 481-485, 1963.

OHNO, S.* SEX CHROMOSOMES AND SEX-LINKED GENES. BERLIN, NEW YORK* SPRINGER, 1967.

LUZZATTO, L., USANGA, E. A. AND REDDY, S.* GLUCOSE-6-PHOSPHATE DEHYDROGENASE DEFICIENT RED CELLS* RESISTANCE TO INFECTION BY MALARIAL PARASITES. SCIENCE 164* 839-842, 1969.

PORTER, I. H., BOYER, S. H., WATSON-WILLIAMS, E. J., ADAM, A., SZEINBERG, A. AND SINISCALCO, M.* VARIATION OF GLUCOSE-6-PHOSPHATE DEHYDROGENASE IN DIFFERENT POPULATIONS. LANCET 1* 895-899, 1964.

WHO* NOMENCLATURE OF GLUCOSE-6-PHOSPHATE DEHYDROGENASE IN MAN. BULL. WHO 36* 319-322, 1967. ALSO CANAD. MED. ASS. J. 97* 422-424, 1967.

WHO* SCIENTIFIC GROUP ON THE STANDARDIZATION OF PROCEDURES FOR THE STUDY OF GLUCOSE-6-PHOSPHATE DEHYDROGENASE. WHO TECHN. REP. SER., NO. 366, 1967.

X
L
I
N
K
E
D

YOSHIDA, A.* A SINGLE AMINO ACID SUBSTITUTION (ASPARAGINE TO ASPARTIC ACID)   565
BETWEEN NORMAL (B PLUS) AND THE COMMON NEGRO VARIANT (A PLUS) OF HUMAN GLUCOSE-6-
PHOSPHATE DEHYDROGENASE.   PROC. NAT. ACAD. SCI. 57* 835-840, 1967.

YOSHIDA, A., BAUR, E. W. AND MOTULSKY, A. G.* A PHILIPPINO GLUCOSE-6-PHOSPHATE
DEHYDROGENASE VARIANT (G6PD UNION) WITH ENZYME DEFICIENCY AND ALTERED SUBSTRATE
SPECIFICITY.   BLOOD 35* 506-513, 1970.

YOSHIDA, A., STAMATOYANNOPOULOS, G. AND MOTULSKY, A. G.* NEGRO VARIANT OF
GLUCOSE-6-PHOSPHATE DEHYDROGENASE DEFICIENCY (A-) IN MAN.   SCIENCE 155* 97-99,
1967.

TABLE OF HUMAN GLUCOSE–6–PHOSPHATE DEHYDROGENASE VARIANTS[1,5]

by

AKIRA YOSHIDA,[2] ERNEST BEUTLER,[3] AND ARNO G. MOTULSKY[4]

So many G6PD variants have been described that it has become very difficult to determine whether or not a newly discovered variant is distinct from any other. This difficulty can be partially overcome by performing a number of physicochemical tests and comparing the results with those already reported for the known variants. The purpose here is to provide an up-to-date table summarizing the currently available data on G6PD variants. For convenience, the variants described in the table are somewhat arbitrarily divided into five groups, in accord with their activity in red cells and their associated clinical manifestations:

Class 1: Severe enzyme deficiency with chronic non-spherocytic hemolytic anemia.

Class 2: Severe enzyme deficiency (less than 10% of normal)

Class 3: Moderate to mild enzyme deficiency (10-60% of normal)

Class 4: Very mild or no enzyme deficiency (60-100% of normal)

Class 5: Increased enzyme activity (more than twice normal)

Distinction between these classes is not always clear. For example, G-6-PD Mediterranean has been placed in class 2, but has been reported to be associated with non-spherocytic congenital hemolytic anemia. Furthermore, some of the variants listed in class 1 because of the severe functional lesion which they cause actually have higher enzyme activities in vitro than some of the variants with "moderate to mild enzyme deficiency" (class 3).

Within the classes, the variant enzymes are arranged in order of their electrophoretic mobility: i.e., the faster one is first.

The variants of each class are also subdivided into four groups according to the state of their characterization, as designated by the WHO Technical Report, No. 366, 1967:

Group I: Variants have been fairly completely characterized, and appear to be distinctive.

Group II: Insufficient information is available to ascertain that it is unique. These variants are shown with quotation marks.

Group III: Variants have been described, but insufficient data have been given to warrant their inclusion in the tabulation.

Group IV: Variants have been characterized, but seem to be identical to one of the variants given in the table.

The data in the table are the raw values which were described in the reports; no critical judgment of the dependability and accuracy of these reported values was made. In general, Km for NADP alone should not be considered a prime criterion for distinguishing a variant.

In order to distinguish closely similar variants, it is necessary to examine their properties in side-by-side comparison under the same conditions. Unfortunately, many variant blood samples are no longer available or are difficult to obtain. Another difficulty involved in distinguishing G6PD variants is that several, particularly those which were reported earlier than 1967, were

1.   This work is supported by a grant from the World Health Organization International Reference Center for G6PD Variants and by U.S. Public Health Service grants GM15253 and HE07449 from the National Institutes of Health.
2.   Department of Medicine (Division of Medical Genetics), University of Washington, Seattle, Washington 98105.
3.   Division of Medicine, City of Hope National Medical Center, Duarte, California 91010.
4.   Departments of Medicine (Division of Medical Genetics) and Genetics, University of Washington, Seattle, Washington 98105.
5.   Acknowledgments: We are grateful to Dr. P. McCurdy and Dr. G. Stamatoyannopoulos for making their results known to us before publication. This table is to be published also in the Bulletin of the World Health Organization. It is included here with the permission of WHO.

not characterized by the standard method recommended by the WHO Technical Report. We believe that all characterization should be performed by the methods recommended in the WHO Technical Report. In addition, more extensive characterization by improved methods is in each case desirable. Comparison of the utilization of deamino NADP was very useful in distinguishing G6PD variants which were not distinguished by other criteria. Study of exact amino acid substitutions of these variants could distinguish the variants from each other without ambiguity. Thus far, amino acid substitutions have been elucidated in only two G6PD variants (G6PD A+ and G6PD Hektoen) but technical improvements will facilitate such structural study in the future. Until such studies can be carried out on all variants, a descriptive register of variants should be maintained. The compilation which follows includes all of the published and unpublished variants known to the authors through August 1970. We propose to prepare supplemental tables as further variants are described. In compiling the type and quantity of data included in the present tabulation we have undoubtedly made errors both in interpretation and in transcription. We will welcome having such errors called to our attention, so that they may be corrected in subsequent tabulations.

CLASS AND GROUP	VARIANT (REFERENCES)	POPULATION ORIGIN	RED CELL ENZYME ACTIVITY (% OF NORMAL)	ELECTRO-PHORETIC MOBILITY (% OF NORMAL)	K_m G6P (µM)	K_m NADP (µM)	2-d G6P UTILIZATION (% of G6P)	DEAMINO NADP UTILIZATION (% of NADP)	HEAT STABILITY	pH OPTIMA	POPULATION FREQUENCY OR COMMENT
NORMAL	B (1-3)	Various	100	100	50-70	2.9-4.4	<4	55-60	Normal	Normal (Truncate)	Usual
SEVERE ENZYME DEFICIENCY ASSOCIATED WITH CHRONIC NON-SPHEROCYTIC HEMOLYTIC ANEMIA											
I.	Ohio (4)	Italian	2-16	110 (Tris-glycine)	Slightly increased	Slightly increased	<4		Very low		Rare
	Torrance (5)	U. S.	2.4	103 (Ph)	48-60	2.4			Very low	8.0-8.5	Reversibly inactivated at pH 8
	Bat-Yam (6)	Iraqui Jew	0	100 (TEB)	27		40-45		Very low	Biphasic	Rare
	Albuquerque (7)	U.S. White	1	100 (TEB, Tris, Ph)	115	11	0		Very low	Sharp peak at 8.5	Rare
	Bangkok (8)	Thai	5	100(TEB, Tris, Ph)	60	5.3	8.4		Very low	8-8.5	
	Oklahoma (9,10)	West Europe	4-10	100 (Tris)	127-200	20	<4		Low	Narrow peak at 8.2	Rare
	Duarte (7)	U. S. White	8.5	100 (TEB, Tris, Ph)	58	5	5.4		Very low	7.0	Rare
	Hong Kong (11)	Chinese	0-15	100(TEB, pH 8.0)	½ normal	Normal	Slightly increased		Normal	Normal	
	Chicago (12)	West Europe	9-26	100 (Tris)	58-76	3.1-3.7	<4		Very low	Normal	Rare

SEVERE ENZYME DEFICIENCY ASSOCIATED WITH CHRONIC NON-SPHEROCYTIC HEMOLYTIC ANEMIA (Continued)

CLASS AND GROUP	VARIANT (REFERENCES)	POPULATION ORIGIN	RED CELL ENZYME ACTIVITY (% of NORMAL)	ELECTRO-PHORETIC MOBILITY (% of NORMAL)	K_m G6P (μM)	K_m NADP (μM)	2-d G6P UTILIZATION (% of G6P)	DEAMINO NADP UTILIZATION (% of NADP)	HEAT STABILITY	pH OPTIMA	POPULATION FREQUENCY OR COMMENT
I. (Cont.)	Tripler (13)	U.S. White	35	97 (TEB) 97 (Tris) 90 (Ph)	30		3.7	62.4	Very low	Slightly biphasic	
	Alhambra (14)	Finnish Swedish	9-20	96 (TEB) 95 (Tris) 85 (Ph)	55	2.6	2		Low	Rare	
	Milwaukee (15)	Puerto Rican White	0.5	92 (Tris)	224		3.7			8.0	Rare
	Ramat-Gan (6)	Iraqui Jew	0	90-92 (TEB)	35		40		Very low	Biphasic	Rare
	Ashdod (6)	Jew N. Africa	10	90-92 (TEB)	100		40		Slightly low	Biphasic	Rare
	Freiburg (16, 16a)	German	10-20	85 (TEB) 90 (Ph)	87-118	4				Biphasic	Rare
	Worcester (17)	U.S. White	0	86 (TEB, pH 7.6) 70 (TEB, pH 9.1 Cellulose acetate)	11.2	61	<2	21	Very low	Sharp peak at 8.0	
II	"Beaujon" (18)	French	0	Fast (Acrylamide-Tris-glycine, pH 8.6)	182					Peak at 9.5	Rare
	"Clichy" (18)	Greek	2	100 (Acrylamide-Tris-glycine, pH 8.6)	178					Abnormal plateau 9-10	Rare

CLASS AND GROUP	VARIANT (REFERENCES)	POPULATION ORIGIN	RED CELL ENZYME ACTIVITY (% of NORMAL)	ELECTRO-PHORETIC MOBILITY (% of NORMAL)	K_m G6P (μM)	K_m NADP (μM)	2-d G6P UTILIZATION (% of G6P)	DEAMINO NADP UTILIZATION (% of NADP)	HEAT STABILITY	pH OPTIMA	POPULATION FREQUENCY OR COMMENT
				SEVERE ENZYME DEFICIENCY ASSOCIATED WITH CHRONIC NON-SPHEROCYTIC HEMOLYTIC ANEMIA (Continued)							
II. (Cont.)	"Strasbourg" (19)	French	6	100 (Cellulose acetate pH 8.6)	96	13			Low	Peak at pH 9.0	
	"Paris" (18)	West Europe	4	?	280				Very low	Sharp at 9.5	Rare

III. The following G6PD variants of this group have been described, but insufficient data have been given to warrant their inclusion in the tabulation: Eyssen (2), Fulham (20), Nashville 1 (21), Berlin (22).

IV. The following G6PD variants of this group have been characterized, but they seem to be identical to one of the variants given in the table: Nashville 2 (21), similar to Chicago

SEVERE ENZYME DEFICIENCY

	VARIANT	POPULATION ORIGIN	RED CELL ENZYME ACTIVITY	ELECTRO-PHORETIC MOBILITY	K_m G6P	K_m NADP	2-d G6P UTILIZATION	DEAMINO NADP UTILIZATION	HEAT STABILITY	pH OPTIMA	POPULATION FREQUENCY OR COMMENT
I.	Hualien-Chi (23)	Taiwan	1	110 (Tris) 120 (Ph)	10.1	42			Normal	Biphasic (6.28-10.0)	
	San Juan (24)	Puerto Rican	10	110 (Tris) 105 (Ph)	16.2 ± 0.7		21.6		Very low	Biphasic (7.0 & 9.5)	Rare
	Markham (25)	New Guinea	1.5-10	105-108 (Tris)	4.4-6.3		162-222		Low	Biphasic	Common. Uses NAD as cofactor
	Taiwan-Hakka (26)	Hakka-Chinese	2-9	110 (Ph) 105 (Tris)	10.7-12.2		9.8-21.1		Normal to sl. low	Biphasic (7.0 & 9.5-10.0)	Common. Uses NAD as cofactor
	Union (27)	Philippino	<3	107 (TEB, Ph)	8-12	3.6-5.2	180	400	Low	Very biphasic (5.5 & 9.0)	Common. Does not use NAD as cofactor

SEVERE ENZYME DEFICIENCY (Continued)

CLASS AND GROUP	VARIANT (REFERENCES)	POPULATION ORIGIN	RED CELL ENZYME ACTIVITY (% of NORMAL)	ELECTRO-PHORETIC MOBILITY (% of NORMAL)	K_m G6P (µM)	K_m NADP (µM)	2-d G6P UTILIZATION (% of G6P)	DEAMINO NADP UTILIZATION (% of NADP)	HEAT STABILITY	pH OPTIMA	POPULATION FREQUENCY OR COMMENT
I. (Cont.)	Teheran (23)	Iran	<1	100 (Tris) 110 (Ph)	46.8		<4		Normal	Biphasic (5.5 & 10.0)	
	Hualien (23)	Taiwan	0	105 (Tris)	8.7		72.2		Very low	Biphasic (6.5 & 9.75)	
	Indonesia (28)	Indonesia	<5	100 (Tris)	25-52	4-9			Normal to slightly low	Slightly biphasic	
	Camplellpur (29)	Pakistani	2-7	100 (Tris) 100 (Ph)	11.4-13.9		5.6-16.4		Very low	Biphasic (7.5 & 9.5)	Common, 2% in this population
	Mediterranean (30-34)	Greeks Sardinians Sephardic Jews Asiatic Indians Asian, N.W. Ind.	0-7	100 (TEB, Tris, Ph)	19-26	1.2-1.6	23-27	350	Low	Biphasic	Common; sometimes assoc. with Favism or NSHA; may be heterogenous (see below)
	Corinth (35)	Greeks Mediterraneans S.E. Asia	0-7	100 (TEB, Tris, Ph)	19-26	1.2-1.6	23-27	55-60	Low	Biphasic	May be common
	Panay (36)	Philippino	5	96 (Tris, Ph)	30	4.7	Normal		Slightly low	Biphasic	May be common
	Orchomenos (37)	Greeks	0-7	92-94 (Ph) 100 (TEB Tris)	11	2.1	105	350		Biphasic	

SEVERE ENZYME DEFICIENCY (Continued)

CLASS AND GROUP	VARIANT (REFERENCES)	POPULATION ORIGIN	RED CELL ENZYME ACTIVITY (% of NORMAL)	ELECTRO-PHORETIC MOBILITY (% of NORMAL)	K_m G6P (μM)	K_m NADP (μM)	2-d G6P UTILIZATION (% of G6P)	DEAMINO NADP UTILIZATION (% of NADP)	HEAT STABILITY	pH OPTIMA	POPULATION FREQUENCY OR COMMENT
I. (Cont.)	Lifta (6)	Iraqui Jew	0	87-90 (TEB)	25		60		Very low	No clear optimum	Rare
	Carswell (38)	Irish	10	78 (TEB) 92 (Tris) 78 (Ph)	44	6.4	3.5		Normal	Normal or slightly displaced	Rare
II.	"Taiwan-Ami 6" (23)	Taiwanese	1	105 (Tris) 110 (Ph)	30.2		29.0		Very low	Biphasic (6.5 & 10.0)	
	"Taiwan-Ami 5" (23)	Taiwanese	0	105 (Tris)	35.3		52.8			Biphasic (7.0 & 9.5)	
	"Zahringen" (39)	German	1 - 4	105 (Ph)	28	4.7	30		Low	7.5 & 8.5	Rare. Assoc. with Favism. Similar to San Juan

III. The following G6PD variants of this group have been described, but insufficient data have been given to warrant their inclusion in the tabulation: Sao Paulo 3 (21); Joliet 3 (40).

IV. The following G6PD variants of this group have been characterized, but they seem to be identical to one of the variants given in the table: Athens-like (37, similar to Athens; "U-M" (37), similar to Markham or Union; Taiwan-Ami 1 (23), similar to Markham or Union; Taiwan-Ami 2 (23), similar to Taiwan-Hakka; Johnstown (41), similar to A-; Panay like (26), similar to Panay; El Morro (24), similar to Mediterranean; New Guinea II (25), similar to Mediterranean; Hong Kong 2 (11), similar to Canton; Singapore (42), similar to Canton; Joliet 1 (40), similar to Columbus.

MODERATE TO MILD ENZYME DEFICIENCY

CLASS AND GROUP	VARIANT (REFERENCES)	POPULATION ORIGIN	RED CELL ENZYME ACTIVITY (% of NORMAL)	ELECTROPHORETIC MOBILITY (% of NORMAL)	K_m G6P (μM)	K_m NADP (μM)	2-d G6P UTILIZATION (% of G6P)	DEAMINO NADP UTILIZATION (% of NADP)	HEAT STABILITY	pH OPTIMA	POPULATION FREQUENCY OR COMMENT
I. (Cont.)	Barbieri (31)	Italian	24-40	135 (Tris, pH 7.6)	Increased	Increased			Normal		Rare
	Puerto Rico (43)	Puerto Rican	38	112 (Tris)	18.6		2.7		Slightly low	Normal	Rare
	A- (2,10,44,45)	Negro	8-20	110 (TEB, Tris) 115 (Ph)	Normal	Normal	<4	50-60	Normal	Normal	Common
	Debrousse (formerly Constantine) (46)	Arab	20	113 (Ph) 110 (Tris)	19-29	1.9-3.3	4-11		Normal	Normal	Common
	Taipei-Hakka (26)	Chinese	6-9	105 (Tris) 110 (Ph)	27.7-43.4	3.3-5.4			Slightly low	Truncate (9.75-10.0)	
	Kabyle (47)	Algerian	14-36	104 (TEB) 110 (Ph)	68		Normal		Normal	Normal	
	Chibuto (48)	Negro Bantu	20	108 (TEB) 109 (Ph)	30	8.2	<4		Slightly low	Normal	Rare
	Melissa (37)	Greeks	25	107 (TEB) 105 (Tris) 105 (Ph)	18.1 22.0	3.1-3.7	3.7	59-65	Truncate		
	Canton (49)	South Chinese	4-24	105 (Tris) 105 (Ph)	17.7-38.3		1.2-20.8		Low	Biphasic (6.5-7.0 & 9.0-9.5)	May be heterogenous

MODERATE TO MILD ENZYME DEFICIENCY (Continued)

CLASS AND GROUP	VARIANT (REFERENCES)	POPULATION ORIGIN	RED CELL ENZYME ACTIVITY (% of NORMAL)	ELECTRO-PHORETIC MOBILITY (% of NORMAL)	K_m G6P (μM)	K_m NADP (μM)	2-d G6P UTILIZATION (% of G6P)	DEAMINO NADP UTILIZATION (% of NADP)	HEAT STABILITY	pH OPTIMA	POPULATION FREQUENCY OR COMMENT
I. (Cont.)	Columbus (4)	Negro	36	100 (Tris)	Normal	Normal	Normal				Rare
	Athens (50)	Greeks	20-25	98 (TEB)	16-19	2.5-6.5	10-15	126	Slightly low	Slightly biphasic	Common
	Washington (43)	Negro	16-33	95 (Tris)	49-57.4		1.6		Normal	Normal	
	Benevento (41)	Italian	13	93 (Tris)	4.6		245		Low	Biphasic (5.5 & 9.75)	
	West Bengal (51)	Asiatic Indian	9	90 (TEB) 82 (Tris)	31	6.6	4		Normal	Normal	Rare
	Mexico (52)	Mexican	10-22	85-88 (TEB) 91 (Tris) 90 (Ph)	32-40	2-3	26-33	130-160		Truncate	
	Seattle (53,54)	Welsh Scottish	8-21	80 (TEB) 90 (Tris)	15-25	2.4-2.8	7-11		Normal	Slightly biphasic	Rare
	Kerala (51)	Asiatic, S.E. Indian	50	75 (TEB) 90 (Tris)	23	1.5	7.4		Normal	Biphasic	Rare
	Tel Hashomer (55,56)	Tunisian Jew	25-40	60-70 (TEB)	30-40		Normal		Normal	Slightly biphasic	Rare

CLASS AND GROUP	VARIANT (REFERENCES)	POPULATION ORIGIN	RED CELL ENZYME ACTIVITY (% of NORMAL)	ELECTRO-PHORETIC MOBILITY (% of NORMAL)	K_m G6P (μM)	K_m NADP (μM)	2-d G6P UTILIZATION (% of G6P)	DEAMINO NADP UTILIZATION (% of NADP)	HEAT STABILITY	pH OPTIMA	POPULATION FREQUENCY OR COMMENT
				MODERATE TO MILD ENZYME DEFICIENCY (Continued)							
I. (Cont.)	Capetown (57)	Cape Colored Norwegian	53-80	55-65 (TEB) 76-88 (Tris) 35-48 (Ph)	11-14	0.2-1	7-16		Normal	Biphasic	
	Port-Royal (58)	Sicilian	50-75	85 (TEB)	20		7.5	10	Low		Probably rare
II.	"Attica" (59)	Greece	50	105 (Cellogel, pH 7.5)	40.7	4.7	1.8		Normal	Normal	

III. The following G6PD variants of this group have been described, but insufficient data have been given to warrant their inclusion in the tabulation: Madison (60); Andra Pradesh (61); Sao Paulo (21); Joliet 2 (40).

IV. The following G6PD variants of this group have been characterized, but seem to be identical to one of the variants given in the table: Loyola (D-) (53,62), identical to Seattle; and Seattle-like (59,63).

CLASS AND GROUP	VARIANT (REFERENCES)	POPULATION ORIGIN	RED CELL ENZYME ACTIVITY (% of NORMAL)	ELECTRO-PHORETIC MOBILITY (% of NORMAL)	K_m G6P (μM)	K_m NADP (μM)	2-d G6P UTILIZATION (% of G6P)	DEAMINO NADP UTILIZATION (% of NADP)	HEAT STABILITY	pH OPTIMA	POPULATION FREQUENCY OR COMMENT
				VERY MILD OR NO ENZYME DEFICIENCY							
I.	Inhambane (48)	African Bantu	100	112 (TEB) 115 (Ph)	38	4.7	<4		Normal	Slightly biphasic	Rare
	Steilacoom (64)	Negro	100	>110 (TEB) 107 (Ph)	62	3	<4		Normal	Normal	
	A+ (2,10,65)	Negro	80-100	110 (TEB, Tris) 115 (Ph)	Normal	Normal	<4	50-60	Normal	Normal	Common

VERY MILD OR NO ENZYME DEFICIENCY (continued)

CLASS AND GROUP	VARIANT (REFERENCES)	POPULATION ORIGIN	RED CELL ENZYME ACTIVITY (% of NORMAL)	ELECTRO-PHORETIC MOBILITY (% of NORMAL)	K_m G6P (µM)	K_m NADP (µM)	2-d G6P UTILIZATION (% of G6P)	DEAMINO NADP UTILIZATION (% of NADP)	HEAT STABILITY	pH OPTIMA	POPULATION FREQUENCY OR COMMENT
I. (Cont.)	Levadia (66)	Greeks	100	107 (TEB) 104 (Tris) 108 (Ph)	40.6	3.5	2.6	60		Normal	
	Lourenzo Marques (48)	African Bantu	100	106 (TEB) 106 (Ph)	66	4.3	<4		Normal	Normal	Rare
	King County (35)	Negro	100	105 (TEB)	61	4	6			Normal	Rare
	Thessaly (67)	Greeks	100-110	98 (TEB) 104-105 (Tris) 98 (Ph)	28.5	12.3	9.7	70		Normal	
	Karditsa (37)	Greeks	85	95 (TEB, Tris) 91-92 (Ph)	24.7	6.5	6.5	52.4		Normal	
	Western (68)	Greeks	60	95 (TEB, Ph)	38	2.2	3.6	42		Normal	
	Manjacaze (48)	African Bantu	100	90 (TEB) 90 (Ph)	141	3.8	<4		Normal	Normal	Rare
	Baltimore Austin (69,73)	Negro	75	90 (Tris)	65	3.1	<4		Normal	Normal	Rare
	Ijebu-Ode (70)	Negro	100	85 (TEB)	60	24			Low	Biphasic	Rare
	Minas Gerais (71)	Brazilian	>70	82 (Ph)	41	4	9			Normal	Rare

CLASS AND GROUP	VARIANT (REFERENCES)	POPULATION ORIGIN	RED CELL ENZYME ACTIVITY (% of NORMAL)	ELECTRO-PHORETIC MOBILITY (% of NORMAL)	K_m G6P (μM)	K_m NADP (μM)	2-d G6P UTILIZATION (% of G6P)	DEAMINO NADP UTILIZATION (% of NADP)	HEAT STABILITY	pH OPTIMA	POPULATION FREQUENCY OR COMMENT
I. (Cont.)						VERY MILD OR NO ENZYME DEFICIENCY (Continued)					
	Tacoma (68)	Negro	100	94 (TEB) 80-82 (Ph)	66	4	2.6	69		Normal	Can be distinguished from Ibadan Austin, Madrona & Minas Gerais by side-by-side comparison.
	Madrona (72)	Negro	70-80	80 (Ph)	32	3.5	Normal			Normal	Rare
	Ibadan-Austin (69,73)	Negro	72	80 (Tris)	62-72	3.3	<4		Normal	Normal	Rare
	Ita-Bala (69)	Negro	100	65 (TEB)	91	11			Slightly low	Normal	Rare
I.						INCREASED ENZYME ACTIVITY					
	Hektoen (74-77)	U.S. White	400	100 (TEB, Tris) 120 (Ph, pH 6.5)	51	3.0	3	44	Normal	Normal	Rare
III.	The following G6PD variants of this group have been described, but insufficient data have been given to warrant their inclusion in the tabulation: Hartford (78).										

REFERENCES IN TABLES OF G6PD VARIANTS

1. Yoshida, A.: Glucose-6-phosphate dehydrogenase of human erythrocytes. I. Purification and characterization of normal (B+) enzyme. J. Biol. Chem. 241:4966-4976, 1966.

2. Boyer, S.H., Porter, I.H., and Weilbaecher, R.G.: Electrophoretic heterogeneity of glucose-6-phosphate dehydrogenase and its relationship to enzyme deficiency in man. Proc. Nat. Acad. Sci. 48:1868-1876, 1962.

3. Kirkman, H.N. and Hendrickson, E.M.: Glucose-6-phosphate dehydrogenase from human erythrocytes. II. Subactive states of the enzyme from normal persons. J. Biol. Chem. 237:2371-2376, 1962.

4. Pinto, P.V.C., Newton, W.A., Jr., and Richardson, K.E.: Evidence for four types of erythrocyte glucose-6-phosphate dehydrogenase from G-6-PD-deficient human subjects. J. Clin. Invest. 45:823-831, 1966.

5. Tanaka, K.R., and Beutler, E.: Hereditary hemolytic anemia due to glucose-6-phosphate dehydrogenase Torrance: A new variant. J. Lab. Clin. Med. 73:657-667, 1969.

6. Ramot, B., Ben-Bassat, I., and Shchory, M.: New glucose-6-phosphate dehydrogenase variants observed in Israel. Association with congenital non-spherocytic hemolytic disease. J. Lab. Clin. Med. 74:895-901, 1969.

7. Beutler, E., Mathai, C.K., and Smith, J. E.: Biochemical variants of glucose-6-phosphate dehydrogenase giving rise to congenital nonspherocytic hemolytic disease. Blood 31:131-150, 1968.

8. Talalak, P., and Beutler, E.: G-6-PD Bangkok: A new variant found in congenital nonspherocytic hemolytic disease (CNHD). Blood 33:772-776, 1969.

9. Kirkman, H.N., and Riley, H.D., Jr.: Congenital nonspherocytic hemolytic anemia. Am. J. Dis. Child. 102:313-320, 1961.

10. Kirkman, H.N., McCurdy, P.R., and Naiman, J. L.: Functionally abnormal glucose-6-phosphate dehydrogenases. Cold Spring Harbor Symposia Quantit. Biol. 29:391-398, 1964.

11. Wong, P.W.K., Shih, L.-Y., and Hsia, D. Y.-Y.: Characterization of glucose-6-phosphate dehydrogenase among Chinese. Nature 208:1323-1324, 1965.

12. Kirkman, H.N., Rosenthal, I.M., Simon, E.R., Carson, P.E., and Brinson, A.G.: "Chicago I" variant of glucose-6-phosphate dehydrogenase in congenital hemolytic disease. J. Lab. Clin. Med. 63:715-725, 1964.

13. Engstrom, P.F., and Beutler, E.: G-6-PD Tripler: A unique variant associated with chronic hemolytic disease. Blood 36:10-13, 1970.

14. Beutler, E., and Rosen, R.: Nonspherocytic congenital hemolytic anemia due to a new G-6-PD variant: G-6-PD Alhambra. Pediatrics 45:230-235, 1970.

15. Westring, D.W., and Pisciotta, A.V.: Anemia, cataracts, and seizures in patient with glucose-6-phosphate dehydrogenase deficiency. Arch. Intern. Med. 118:385-390, 1966.

16. Weinreich, J., Busch, D., Gottstein, U., Schaefer, J., and Rohr, J.: Uber zwei neue Falle von hereditarer nichtspharozytarer hamolytischer Anamie bein Glucose-6-phosphat-dehydrogenase-defekt in einer nord Deutschen Familie. Klin. Wschr. 46:146-149, 1968.

16a. Busch, D. and Boie, K.: Glucose-6-phosphat-dehydrogenase-defekt in Deutschland II. Eigenschaften des Enzyms (Typ Freiburg). Klin. Wschr. 48:74-78, 1970.

17. Snyder, L.M., Necheles, T.F., and Roddy, W.J.: G6PD Worcester, a new variant, associated with X-linked optic atrophy. Am. J. Med. 49:125-132, 1970.

18. Boivin, P., and Galand, C.: Nouvelles variantes de la glucose-6-phosphate dehydrogenase erythrocytaire. Rev. Franc. Etud. Clin. Biol. 13:30-39, 1968.

19. Waitz, R., Boivin, P., Oberling, F., Casenave, J.P., North, M.L., and Mayer, S.: Variante Gd (-) Strasbourg de la glucose-6-phosphate-dehydrogenase. Nouv. rev. franc. hemat. 10:312-314, 1970.

20. Huskisson, E.C., Murphy, B., and West, C.: Glucose-6-phosphate dehydrogenase deficiency and chronic haemolysis in an English family. J. Clin. Path. 23:135-139, 1970.

21. Nance, W.E.: Ph.D. thesis, University of Wisconsin, Madison, Dept. of Med. Genet., 1967.

22. Helge, H., and Börner, K.: Kongenitale nichtspharozytare hamolytische Anamie, Katarakt und Glucose-6-phosphat-dehydrogenase-mangel. Deutsch. Med. Wschr. 91:1584-1589, 1966.

23. McCurdy, P.R.: Personal communication.

24. McCurdy, P.R., and Maldonado, N.: Personal communication.

25. Kirkman, H.N., Kidson, C., and Kennedy M.: Variants of human glucose-6-phosphate dehydrogenase. Studies of samples from New Guinea. Pp. 126-145 in E. Beutler (ed.) Hereditary Disorders of Erythrocyte Metabolism. New York: Grune & Stratton, 1968.

26. McCurdy, P.R., Blackwell, R.Q., Todd, D., Tso, S.C., and Tuchinda, S.: Further studies on glucose-6-phosphate dehydrogenase deficiency in Chinese subjects. J. Lab. Clin. Med. 75:788-797, 1970.

27. Yoshida, A., Baur, E.W., and Motulsky, A.G.: A Philippino glucose-6-phosphate dehydrogenase variant (G6PD Union) with enzyme deficiency and altered substrate specificity. Blood 35:506-513, 1970.

28. Kirkman, H.N., and Luan Eng, L.I.: Variants of glucose-6-phosphate dehydrogenase in Indonesia. Nature 221:959, 1969.

29. McCurdy, P.R., and Mahmood, L.: Personal communication.

30. Kirkman, H.N., Schettini, F., and Pickard, B.M.: Mediterranean variant of glucose-6-phosphate dehydrogenase. J. Lab. Clin. Med. 63:726-735, 1964.

31. Marks, P.A., Banks, J., and Gross, R.T.: Genetic heterogeneity of glucose-6-phosphate dehydrogenase deficiency. Nature 194:454-456, 1962.

32. Ramot, B., Bauminger, S., Brok, F., Gafni, D., and Schwartz, J.: Characterization of glucose-6-phosphate dehydrogenase in Jewish mutants. J. Lab. Clin. Med. 64:895-904, 1964.

33. Benöhr, H.D., and Waller, H.D.: Eigenschaften der Glucose-6-P Dehydrogenase, Tubingen. Klin. Wschr. 48:71-74, 1970.

34. Ben-Bassat, J., and Ben-Ishay, D.: Hereditary hemolytic anemia associated with glucose-6-phosphate dehydrogenase deficiency (Mediterranean type). Israel J. Med. Sci. 5:1053-1059, 1969.

35. Yoshida, A.: Unpublished observations.

36. Fernandez, M.N., and Fairbanks, V.F.: Glucose-6-phosphate dehydrogenase deficiency in the Philippines: Report of a new variant-G6PD Panay. Mayo Clin. Proc. 43:645-660, 1968.

37. Stamatoyannopoulos, G.: Unpublished observations.

38. Siegel, N.H., and Beutler, E.: Unpublished observations.

39. Johannsen, L.P., Witt, I., and Kunzer, W.: Favismus bei einer Deutschen Familie. Deutsch. Med. Wschr. 93:2463-2470, 1968.

40. Carson, P.E., and Frischer, H.: Glucose-6-phosphate dehydrogenase deficiency and related disorders of the pentose phosphate pathway. Am. J. Med. 41:744-761, 1966.

41. McCurdy, P.R., Dillon, D., and Conrad, M.: Personal communication.

42. Motulsky, A.G.: Unpublished observations.

43. McCurdy, P.R.: Personal communication.

44. Yoshida, A., Stamatoyannopoulos, G., and Motulsky, A.: Negro variant of glucose-6-phosphate dehydrogenase deficiency (A-) in man. Science 155:97-99, 1967.

45. Kirkman, H.N., and Hendrickson, E.M.: Sex-linked electrophoretic difference in glucose-6-phosphate dehydrogenase. Am. J. Hum. Genet. 15:241-258, 1963.

46. Kissin, C., and Cotte, J.: Etude d'un variant de glucose-6-phosphate dehydrogenase: le type Constantine. Enzym. biol. clin. 11:277-284, 1970.

47. Kaplan, J.C., Rosa, R., Seringe, P., and Hoeffel, J.C.: Le polymorphisme genetique de la glucose-6-phosphate deshydrogenase erythrocytaire chez l'homme. II. Etude d'une nouvelle variete a activite diminuee: le type "Kabyle." Enzym. biol. clin. 8:332-340, 1967.

48. Reys, L., Manso, C., and Stamatoyannopoulos, G.: Genetic studies on Southeastern Bantu of Mozambique. I. Variants of glucose-6-phosphate dehydrogenase. Am. J. Hum. Genet. 22:203-215, 1970.

49. McCurdy, P. R., Kirkman, H.N., Naiman, J.L., Jim, R.T.S., and Pickard, B.M.: A Chinese variant of glucose-6-phosphate dehydrogenase. J. Lab. Clin. Med. 67:374-385, 1966.

50. Stamatoyannopoulos, G., Yoshida, A., Bacopoulos, C., and Motulsky, A.G.: Athens variant of glucose-6-phosphate dehydrogenase. Science 157: 831-833, 1967.

51. Azevedo, E., Kirkman, H.N., Morrow, A.C., and Motulsky, A.G.: Variants of red cell glucose-6-phosphate dehydrogenase among Asiatic Indians. Ann. Hum. Genet. 31:373-379, 1968.

52. Motulsky, A., et al.: Unpublished observations.

53. Shows, T.B., Jr., Tashian, R.E., Brewer, G.J., and Dern, R.J.: Erythrocyte glucose-6-phosphate dehydrogenase in Caucasians: new inherited variant. Science 145:1056-1057, 1964.

54. Kirkman, H.N., Simon, E.R., and Pickard, B.M.: Seattle variant of glucose-6-phosphate dehydrogenase. J. Lab. Clin. Med. 66: 834-840, 1965.

55. Kirkman, H.N., Ramot, B., and Lee, J.T.: Altered aggregational properties in a genetic variant of human glucose-6-phosphate dehydrogenase. Biochem. Genet. 3:137-150, 1969.

56. Ramot, B., and Brok, F.: A new glucose-6-phosphate dehydrogenase mutant (Tel-Hashomer mutant). Ann. Hum. Genet. 28:167-172, 1964.

57. Botha, M.C., Dern, R.J., Mitchell, M., West, C., and Beutler, E.: G6PD Capetown, a variant of glucose-6-phosphate dehydrogenase. Am. J. Hum. Genet. 21:547-551, 1969.

58. Kaplan, J. C., Hanzlickova-Leroux, A., Nicholas, A.M., Rosa, R., Weiler, C., and Lepercq, G.: A new glucose-6-phosphate dehydrogenase variant (G6PD Port-Royal). Enzym. biol. clin. 12:15-32, 1971.

59. Rattazzi, M.C., Lenzerini, L., Khan, P.M., and Luzzatto, L.: Characterization of glucose-6-phosphate dehydrogenase variants. II. G6PD Kephalonia, G6PD Attica, and G6PD "Seattle-like" found in Greece. Am. J. Hum. Genet. 21:154-167, 1969.

60. Nance, W.E., and Uchida, I.: Turner's syndrome, twinning, and an unusual variant of glucose-6-phosphate dehydrogenase. Am. J. Hum. Genet. 16:380-392, 1964.

61. Rattazzi, M.C., and Lenzerini, L.: Preliminary studies on the characterization of some glucose-6-phosphate dehydrogenase variants. Atti. Ass. Genet. Ital. 12:158-160, 1967.

62. Beutler, E., and Dern, R.J.: Unpublished observations.

63. Lenzerini, L., Khan, M.P., Filippi, G., Rattazzi, M.C., and Ray, A.K.: Characterization of glucose-6-phosphate dehydrogenase variants. I. Occurrence of a G6PD Seattle-like variant in Sardinia and its interaction with G6PD Mediterranean variant. Am. J. Hum. Genet. 21:142-153, 1969.

64. Yoshida, A., Baur, E., and Voigtlander, G.: Unpublished observations.

65. Yoshida, A.: Human glucose-6-phosphate dehydrogenase: Purification and characterization of Negro type variant (A+) and comparison with normal enzyme (B+). Biochem. Genet. 1:81-99, 1967.

66. Stamatoyannopoulos, G., Kotsakis, P., Voigtlander, V., Akrivakis, A., and Motulsky, A. G.: Electrophoretic diversity of glucose-6-phosphate dehydrogenase among Greeks. Am. J. Hum. Genet. 22:587-596, 1970.

67. Stamatoyannopoulos, G., Voigtlander, V., and Akrivakis, A.: Thessaly variant of glucose-6-phosphate dehydrogenase. Humangenetik 9:23-25, 1970.

68. Yoshida, A., and Baur, E.: Unpublished observations.

69. Long, W.K., Kirkman, H.N., and Sutton, H.E.: Electrophoretically slow variants of glucose-6-phosphate dehydrogenase from red cells of Negroes. J. Lab. Clin. Med. 65:81-87, 1965.

70. Luzzatto, L., and Afolayan, A.: Enzymic properties of different types of human erythrocyte glucose-6-phosphate dehydrogenase, with characterization of two new genetic variants. J. Clin. Invest. 47: 1833-1842, 1968.

71. Azevedo, E.S., and Yoshida, A.: Brazilian variant of glucose-6-phosphate dehydrogenase (Gd Minas Gerais). Nature 222: 380-382, 1969.

72 Hook, E.B., Stamatoyannopoulos, G., Yoshida, A. and Motulsky, A.G.: Glucose-6-phosphate dehydrogenase Madrona: A slow electrophoretic glucose-6-phosphate dehydrogenase variant with kinetic characteristics similar to those of normal type. J. Lab. Clin. Med. 72:404-409, 1968.

73. Porter, I.H., Boyer, S.H., Watson-Williams, E.J., Adam, A., Szeinberg, A., and Siniscalco, M.: Variation of glucose-6-phosphate dehydrogenase in different populations. Lancet 1:895-899, 1964.

74. Dern, R.J.: A new hereditary quantitative variant of G-6-PD characterized by a marked increase in enzyme activity. J. Lab. Clin. Med. 68: 560-565, 1966.

75. Yoshida, A.: Genetic variants of human glucose-6-phosphate dehydrogenas. Jap. J. Genet. 44:258-265, 1969.

76. Dern, R.J., McCurdy, P.R., and Yoshida, A.: A new structural variant of glucose-6-phosphate dehydrogenase with a high production rate (G6PD Hektoen). J. Lab. Clin. Med. 73:283-290, 1969.

77. Yoshida, A.: Amino acid substitution (histidine to tyrosine) in a glucose-6-phosphate dehydrogenase variant (G6PD Hektoen) associated with over-production. (Abstract) Sci. Prog., Am. Soc. Hum. Genet., San Francisco, p. 49, Oct. 1-4, 1969.

78. Brewer, G.J., Gall, J.C., Honeyman, M.S., Gershowitz, H., Dern, R.J., and Hames, C.G.: Inheritance of quantitative expression of G-6-PD deficiency in heterozygous Negro females—a twin study. (Abstract) Clin. Res. 13:165, 1965.

*30600 GLYCOGEN STORAGE DISEASE VIII (DEFICIENCY OF PHOSPHORYLASE KINASE)

WILLIAMS AND FIELD (1961) FOUND LOW LEUKOCYTE PHOSPHORYLASE ACTIVITY IN TWO AFFECTED BROTHERS AND NORMAL IN AN UNAFFECTED BROTHER AND IN THE FATHER. AN INTERMEDIATELY LOW LEVEL IN THE MOTHER, TOGETHER WITH AFFECTED MALES, SUGGESTED X-LINKED INHERITANCE. WALLIS ET AL. (1966) RESTUDIED THE FAMILY AND WITH NEW METHODS FOUND SUPPORT FOR X-LINKAGE. HUIJING (1967) SHOWED THAT THERE ARE TWO FORMS OF THE TYPE VI (SEE RECESSIVE CATALOG). BOTH HAVE LOW PHOSPHORYLASE ACTIVITY IN THE ABSENCE OF ADENOSINE MONOPHOSPHATE (AMP), BUT ONE (WHICH IS AUTOSOMAL RECESSIVE) HAS NORMAL PHOSPHORYLASE KINASE ACTIVITY, WHILE THE OTHER (WHICH IS X-LINKED RECESSIVE) HAS LOW PHOSPHORYLASE KINASE ACTIVITY. HUIJING AND FERNANDEZ (1969) STUDIED TWO KINDREDS, ONE OF WHICH HAD 6 AFFECTED PLUS TWO POSSIBLY AFFECTED MALES. THE OTHER HAD 20 AFFECTED MALES, TWO AFFECTED FEMALES AND 7 PROBABLY AFFECTED MALES. SINCE PHOSPHORYLASE KINASE IS KNOWN TO BE ENZYMICALLY ACTIVATED (KREBS ET AL. 1964), IT IS POSSIBLE THAT IT IS AN ACTIVATING ENZYME THAT IS CONTROLLED BY THE X-CHROMOSOME. IT MAY BE SIGNIFICANT, HOWEVER, THAT PHOSPHORYLASE B KINASE DEFICIENCY OF SKELETAL MUSCLE IS X-LINKED IN MICE (LYON ET AL. 1967). HUG ET AL. (1969) STUDIED FEMALE PATIENTS WITH GLYCOGENOSIS DUE TO DEFICIENCY OF PHOSPHORYLASE KINASE. HUIJING AND FERNANDEZ (1970) SUGGESTED THAT THESE PATIENTS WERE HETEROZYGOTES. HUIJING (1970) POINTED OUT SIMILARITIES AND DIFFERENCES OF THE HUMAN AND MURINE DEFECTS. PHOSPHORYLASE KINASE DEFICIENCY PRODUCES THE MILDEST OF THE GLYCOGENOSES OF MAN. ALTHOUGH HUIJING (1970) REFERRED TO IT AS GLYCOGEN STORAGE DISEASE TYPE VIA, IT SEEMS BEST FOR REASONS STATED ELSEWHERE TO GIVE IT A DIFFERENT NUMBER* HENCE VIII IS USED HERE.

HERS, H. G.* ETUDES ENZYMATIQUES SUR FRAGMENTS HEPATIQUES* APPLICATION A LA CLASSIFICATION DES GLYCOGENOSES. REV. INT. HEPAT. 9* 35-55, 1959.

HUG, G., SCHUBERT, W. K. AND CHUCK, G.* DEFICIENT ACTIVITY OF DEPHOSPHOPHOS-PHORYLASE KINASE AND ACCUMULATION OF GLYCOGEN IN THE LIVER. J. CLIN. INVEST. 48* 704-715, 1969.

HUIJING, F. AND FERNANDEZ, J.* LIVER GLYCOGENOSIS AND PHOSPHORYLASE KINASE DEFICIENCY. (LETTER) AM. J. HUM. GENET. 22* 484-485, 1970.

HUIJING, F. AND FERNANDEZ, J.* X-CHROMOSOMAL INHERITANCE OF LIVER GLYCOGENOSIS WITH PHOSPHORYLASE KINASE DEFICIENCY. AM. J. HUM. GENET. 21* 275-284, 1969.

HUIJING, F.* GLYCOGEN-STORAGE DISEASE TYPE VIA* LOW PHOSPHORYLASE KINASE ACTIVITY CAUSED BY A LOW ENZYME-SUBSTRATE AFFINITY. BIOCHIM. BIOPHYS. ACTA 206* 199-201, 1970.

HUIJING, F.* PHOSPHORYLASE KINASE DEFICIENCY. BIOCHEM. GENET. 4* 187-194, 1970.

HUIJING, F.* PHOSPHORYLASE KINASE IN LEUCOCYTES OF NORMAL SUBJECTS AND OF PATIENTS WITH GLYCOGEN-STORAGE DISEASE. BIOCHIM. BIOPHYS. ACTA 148* 601-603, 1967.

KREBS, E. G., LOVE, D. S., BRATVOLD, G. E., TRAYSER, K. A., MEYER, W. L. AND FISCHER, E. H.* PURIFICATION AND PROPERTIES OF RABBIT SKELETAL MUSCLE PHOSPHORY-LASE B KINASE. BIOCHEMISTRY 3* 1022-1033, 1964.

LYON, J. B., JR., PORTER, J. AND ROBERTSON, M.* PHOSPHORYLASE B KINASE INHERITANCE IN MICE. SCIENCE 155* 1550-1551, 1967.

WALLIS, P. G., SIDBURY, J. B., JR. AND HARRIS, R. C.* HEPATIC PHOSPHORYLASE DEFECT. STUDIES ON PERIPHERAL BLOOD. AM. J. DIS. CHILD. 111* 278-282, 1966.

WILLIAMS, H. E. AND FIELD, J. B.* LOW LEUKOCYTE PHOSPHORYLASE IN HEPATIC PHOSPHORYLASE DEFICIENT GLYCOGEN STORAGE DISEASE. J. CLIN. INVEST. 40* 1841-1845, 1961.

30610 GONADAL DYSGENESIS, XY FEMALE TYPE

THE PATIENTS APPEAR TO BE NORMAL FEMALES, WHO DO NOT, HOWEVER, DEVELOP SECONDARY SEXUAL CHARACTERISTICS AT PUBERTY, DO NOT MENSTRUATE AND HAVE 'STREAK GONADS.' THEY ARE CHROMATIN NEGATIVE AND HAVE A 44 + XY KARYOTYPE. AFFECTED SISTERS WERE REPORTED BY COHEN AND SHAW (1965) AND TWINS BY FRASIER ET AL. (1964). STERNBERG AND BARCLAY (1967) OBSERVED THREE CASES, EACH IN A DIFFERENT SIBSHIP OF A FAMILY, CONNECTED THROUGH NORMAL FEMALES (PROPOSITA, MATERNAL COUSIN AND MATERNAL AUNT). A HIGH INCIDENCE OF NEOPLASIA (GONADOBLASTOMAS AND GERMINOMAS) IN STREAK GONADS OF PATIENTS WITH THE XY KARYOTYPE WAS CLAIMED BY TAYLOR ET AL. (1966). THE PATIENTS ARE OF ESSENTIALLY NORMAL STATURE AND HAVE NO SOMATIC STIGMATA OF TURNER'S SYNDROME EXCEPT, OF COURSE, THE LACK OF SECONDARY SEXUAL CHARACTERISTICS. IN THIS CONDITION, AS IN THE TESTICULAR FEMINIZATION SYNDROME, IT IS UNCLEAR WHETHER THE GENE WHICH MAY BE RESPONSIBLE IS ON THE X CHROMOSOME OR ON AN AUTOSOME AND EXPRESSED ONLY IN CHROMOSOMAL MALES. WHETHER THE ABNORMAL GENE DIRECTLY SUP-PRESSES TESTIS-DETERMINING LOCI ON THE CHROMOSOME OR BLOCKS SOME EARLY STAGE OF TESTICULAR MORPHOGENESIS IS ALSO UNKNOWN. THE POSSIBILITY OF A CHROMOSOMAL BASIS HAS NOT BEEN EXCLUDED IN THESE CASES. THE SISTERS REPORTED BY COHEN AND SHAW

X
L
I
N
K
E
D

(1965) HAD A MARKER AUTOSOME, WHICH WAS PRESENT ALSO IN THE MOTHER. THEY REFERRED TO ANOTHER INSTANCE OF XY 'SISTERS' WITH AN ABNORMAL AUTOSOME. ONE OF THEIR 2 PATIENTS HAD GONADOBLASTOMA. TWO SISTERS REPORTED BY FINE, MELLINGER AND CANTON (1962) WERE OF NORMAL STATURE BUT WERE CHROMATIN NEGATIVE. ONE OF THESE CASES AND ONE OF THOSE REPORTED BY BARON, RUCKI AND SIMM (1962) HAD GONADOBLASTOMA. IN THE LAST FAMILY, TWO 'FEMALES' AND A MALE WERE AFFECTED, THE MALE SHOWING NO TESTES. ALL THREE SIBS WERE SEX CHROMATIN NEGATIVE. BARR ET AL. (1967) REPORTED ON A SIBSHIP IN WHICH (1) A GENETIC MALE HAD MALE PSEUDOHERMAPHRODITISM, WAS REARED AS A FEMALE BUT DEVELOPED SIGNS OF MASCULINIZATION AT PUBERTY AND HAD UNDESCENDED BUT OTHERWISE NORMAL, TESTES AND SMALL FALLOPIAN TUBES, AND (2) A SECOND GENETIC MALE (180 CM. TALL) HAD PURE GONADAL DYSGENESIS WITH SMALL UTERUS AND STREAK GONADS. THE SECOND PATIENT WAS AT FIRST THOUGHT TO HAVE THE TESTICULAR FEMINIZATION SYNDROME. A SISTER HAD A SON WITH HYPOSPADIAS (URETHRAL ORIFICE AT THE BASE OF THE PENIS). ESPINER ET AL. (1970) DESCRIBED FIVE XY FEMALES IN THREE SIBSHIPS OF TWO GENERATIONS. THEY EMPHASIZED THAT THE AFFECTED PERSONS WERE UNUSUALLY TALL.

BARON, J., RUCKI, T. AND SIMM, S.* FAMILIAL GONADAL MALFORMATIONS. GYNAECOLO-GIA 153* 298-308, 1962.

BARR, M. L., CARR, D. H., PLUNKETT, E. R., SOLTAN, H. C. AND WIENS, R. G.* MALE PSEUDOHERMAPHRODITISM AND PURE GONADAL DYSGENESIS IN SISTERS. AM. J. OBSTET. GYNEC. 99* 1047-1055, 1967.

COHEN, M. M. AND SHAW, M. W.* TWO XY SIBLINGS WITH GONADAL DYSGENESIS AND A FEMALE PHENOTYPE. NEW ENG. J. MED. 272* 1083-1088, 1965.

ESPINER, E. A., VEALE, A. M. O., SANDS, V. E. AND FITZGERALD, P. H.* FAMILIAL SYNDROME OF STREAK GONADS AND NORMAL MALE KARYOTYPE IN FIVE PHENOTYPIC FEMALES. NEW ENG. J. MED. 283* 6-11, 1970.

FINE, G., MELLINGER, R. C. AND CANTON, J. N.* GONADOBLASTOMA OCCURRING IN A PATIENT WITH FAMILIAL GONADAL DYSGENESIS. AM. J. CLIN. PATH. 38* 615-629, 1962.

FRASIER, S. D., BASHORE, R. A. AND MOSIER, H. D.* GONADOBLASTOMA ASSOCIATED WITH PURE GONADAL DYSGENESIS IN MONOZYGOUS TWINS. J. PEDIAT. 64* 740-745, 1964.

JUDD, H. L., SCULLY, R. E., ATKINS, L., NEER, R. M. AND KLIMAN, B.* PURE GONADAL DYSGENESIS WITH PROGRESSIVE HIRSUTISM. DEMONSTRATION OF TESTOSTERONE PRODUCTION BY GONADAL STREAKS. NEW ENG. J. MED. 282* 881-885, 1970.

STERNBERG, W. H., BARCLAY, D. L. AND KLOEPFER, H. W.* FAMILIAL XY GONADAL DYSGENESIS. NEW ENG. J. MED. 278* 695-700, 1968.

STERNBERG, W. H. AND BARCLAY, D. L.* FAMILIAL XY GONADAL DYSGENESIS. (LETTER) LANCET 2* 946 ONLY, 1967.

TAYLOR, H., BARTER, R. H. AND JACOBSON, C. B.* NEOPLASMS OF DYSGENETIC GONADS. AM. J. OBSTET. GYNEC. 96* 816-823, 1966.

30620 GOUT

SOME CASES OF GOUT HAVE BEEN FOUND TO HAVE A PARTIAL DEFICIENCY OF HYPOXANTHINE-GUANINE PHOSPHORIBOSYL TRANSFERASE, THE ENZYME WHICH IS COMPLETELY ABSENT IN THE LESCH-NYHAN SYNDROME (Q.V.). CHARACTERISTICS OF THE ENZYME IN THESE CASES SUGGESTS THAT A STRUCTURAL MUTATION IS INVOLVED AND SOME OF THE PEDIGREES ARE CONSISTENT WITH X-LINKED RECESSIVE INHERITANCE. THUS, THE SAME LOCUS AS THE LESCH-NYHAN LOCUS MAY BE INVOLVED AND SEPARATE LISTING IS NOT WARRANTED. THE GOUT IS EARLY IN ONSET IN THESE PATIENTS AND SOME HAVE MEGALOBLASTIC BONE MARROW CHANGES AND-OR NEUROLOGIC ABNORMALITIES. THAT GOUT IS A HIGHLY HETEROGENEOUS CATEGORY OF DISEASE IS SUGGESTED BY THE STUDIES OF KELLEY ET AL. (1967). IN FIVE PATIENTS THESE WORKERS SHOWED A PARTIAL DEFICIENCY OF HYPOXANTHINE-GUANINE PHOSPHORIBOSYL-TRANSFERASE, THE ENZYME DEFICIENT IN LESCH-NYHAN SYNDROME (AN X-LINKED CONDITION). ALL 5 WERE MALE. TWO BROTHERS IN ONE FAMILY WERE 24 AND 11 YEARS OLD. THREE BROTHERS IN A SECOND FAMILY WERE 42, 49 AND 55 YEARS OLD. IN THE FIRST FAMILY NEPHROLITHIASIS BEGAN AT AGE 6 OR 7 FOLLOWED IN ONE BY GOUTY ARTHRITIS AT AGE 13. IN THE THREE BROTHERS ACUTE GOUTY ARTHRITIS BEGAN BETWEEN AGES 20 AND 31 AND TWO HAD HAD RECURRENT NEPHROLITHIASIS. THE TWO BROTHERS OF THE FIRST FAMILY HAD SPINOCEREBELLAR DERANGEMENT DISTINCT FROM THE NEUROLOGIC DISORDER OF THE LESCH-NYHAN SYNDROME. THE CHARACTERISTICS OF THE ENZYME WERE THE SAME IN EACH FAMILY BUT DIFFERENT BETWEEN FAMILIES. THE DIFFERENCES CONCERNED RELATIVE ACTIVITIES FOR GUANINE AND HYPOXANTHINE AND HEAT STABILITY.

KELLEY, W. N., GREENE, M. L., ROSENBLOOM, F. M., HENDERSON, J. F. AND SEEGMIL-LER, J. E.* HYPOXANTHINE-GUANINE PHOSPHORIBOSYLTRANSFERASE DEFICIENCY IN GOUT. ANN. INTERN. MED. 70* 155-206, 1969.

KELLEY, W. N., ROSENBLOOM, F. M., HENDERSON, J. F. AND SEEGMILLER, J. E.* A SPECIFIC ENZYME DEFECT IN GOUT ASSOCIATED WITH OVERPRODUCTION OF URIC ACID. PROC. NAT. ACAD. SCI. 57* 1735-1739, 1967.

X
L
I
N
K
E
D

30630 GRANULOMAS, CONGENITAL CEREBRAL

STURGILL AND BROWN (1966) DESCRIBED 4 BROTHERS WHO DIED IN THE FIRST 24 HOURS OF LIFE OF CONGENITAL CEREBRAL GRANULOMAS. THE LESIONS SUGGESTED TOXOPLASMOSIS OR SALIVARY GLAND VIRUS DISEASE. HOWEVER, NO ORGANISMS OR INCLUSIONS WERE DEMONSTRATED. TWO SISTERS WERE HEALTHY. CONSANGUINITY WAS NOT COMMENTED UPON.

STURGILL, B. C. AND BROWN, A. K.* CONGENITAL CEREBRAL GRANULOMAS. REPORT OF FOUR CASES IN MALE SIBLINGS. PEDIATRICS 37* 769-775, 1966.

*30640 GRANULOMATOUS DISEASE DUE TO LEUKOCYTE MALFUNCTION

QUIE, WHITE, HOLMES AND GOOD (1967) HAVE OBSERVED A FORM OF FATAL GRANULOMATOUS DISEASE IN MALES IN AN X-LINKED PEDIGREE PATTERN. THE LEUKOCYTES PHAGOCYTIZE STAPHYLOCCI NORMALLY BUT ARE DEFECTIVE IN THEIR ABILITY TO DIGEST THE ORGANISM. THE AUTHORS THOUGHT THAT THE CONDITION WAS X-LINKED. WINDHORST ET AL. (1967) DID FAMILY STUDIES ESTABLISHING X-LINKED RECESSIVE INHERITANCE AND DEMONSTRATING TWO POPULATIONS OF LEUKOCYTES IN HETEROZYGOUS FEMALES. BAEHNER AND NATHAN (1967) DEMONSTRATED A DEFECT IN A LEUKOCYTE OXIDASE. THE INTACT LEUKOCYTES FAILED TO REDUCE NITROBLUE TETRAZOLIUM OR TO SHOW INCREASED OXYGEN CONSUMPTION DURING PHAGOCYTOSIS. CARSON AND COLLEAGUES (1965) REPORTED 16 MALES IN 8 FAMILIES WITH A SYNDROME OF CHRONIC SUPPURATIVE LYMPHADENITIS, CHRONIC DERMATITIS, CHRONIC PULMONARY DISEASE AND HEPATOSPLENOMEGALY WITH SUBSEQUENT FATAL OUTCOME. HYPERGAMMAGLOBINEMIA WAS OFTEN PRESENT. THE MOTHER OF THE AFFECTED BOY DESCRIBED BY MACFARLANE ET AL. (1967) HAD A CHRONIC DERMATITIS OF THE NECK (JESSNER'S BENIGN LYMPHOCYTIC INFILTRATION) AND PARTIAL DEFECT DEMONSTRABLE IN VITRO QUALITATIVELY IDENTICAL TO THAT IN HER SON. REDUCED NICOTINAMIDE-ADENINE DINUCLEOTIDE OXIDASE OF NORMAL HUMAN POLYMORPHONUCLEAR LEUKOCYTES HAS PROPERTIES THAT QUALIFY IT AS THE ENZYME RESPONSIBLE FOR THE RESPIRATORY BURST DURING PHAGOCYTOSIS. BAEHNER AND KARNOVSKY (1968) FOUND DEFICIENCY OF THE ENZYME IN FIVE PATIENTS WITH CHRONIC GRANULOMATOUS DISEASE. THOMPSON ET AL. (1969) FOUND LEUKOCYTE ABNORMALITY IN BOTH PARENTS OF A PATIENT WITH CHRONIC GRANULOMATOUS DISEASE, SUGGESTING THAT THIS WAS AN AUTOSOMAL RECESSIVE FORM OR REQUIRING SOME MORE COMPLEX EXPLANATION. CONTROVERSY OVER THE INHERITANCE, X-LINKED OR AUTOSOMAL, IS ILLUSTRATED BY THE LETTER OF WINDHORST (1969) AND ACCOMPANYING REPLY.

BAEHNER, R. L. AND KARNOVSKY, M. L.* DEFICIENCY OF REDUCED NICOTINAMIDE-ADENINE DINUCLEOTIDE OXIDASE IN CHRONIC GRANULOMATOUS DISEASE. SCIENCE 162* 1277-1279, 1968.

BAEHNER, R. L. AND NATHAN, D. G.* LEUKOCYTE OXIDASE* DEFECTIVE ACTIVITY IN CHRONIC GRANULOMATOUS DISEASE. SCIENCE 155* 835-836, 1967.

CARSON, M. J., CHADWICK, D. L., BRUBAKER, C. A., CLELAND, R. S. AND LANDING, B. H.* THIRTEEN BOYS WITH PROGRESSIVE SEPTIC GRANULOMATOSIS. PEDIATRICS 35* 405-412, 1965.

EDWARDS, J. H.* INHERITANCE OF CHRONIC GRANULOMATOUS DISEASE. (LETTER) LANCET 2* 850-851, 1969.

HOLMES, B., PAGE, A. R. AND GOOD, R. A.* STUDIES OF THE METABOLIC ACTIVITY OF LEUKOCYTES FROM PATIENTS WITH A GENETIC ABNORMALITY OF PHAGOCYTIC FUNCTION. J. CLIN. INVEST. 46* 1422-1432, 1967.

MACFARLANE, P. S., SPEIRS, A. L. AND SOMMERVILLE, R. G.* FATAL GRANULOMATOUS DISEASE OF CHILDHOOD AND BENIGN LYMPHOCYTIC INFILTRATION OF THE SKIN (CONGENITAL DYSPHAGECYTOSIS). LANCET 1* 408-410, 1967.

NATHAN, D. G., BAEHNER, R. L. AND WEAVER, D. K.* FAILURE OF NITRO BLUE TETRAZOLIUM REDUCTION IN THE PHAGOCYTIC VACUOLES OF LEUKOCYTES IN CHRONIC GRANULOMATOUS DISEASE. J. CLIN. INVEST. 48* 1895-1904, 1969.

QUIE, P. G., WHITE, J. G., HOLMES, B. AND GOOD, R. A.* IN VITRO BACTERICIDAL CAPACITY OF HUMAN POLYMORPHONUCLEAR LEUKOCYTES* DIMINISHED ACTIVITY IN CHRONIC GRANULOMATOUS DISEASE OF CHILDHOOD. J. CLIN. INVEST. 46* 668-679, 1967.

THOMPSON, E. N., CHANDRA, R. K., COPE, W. A. AND SOOTHILL, J. F.* LEUCOCYTE ABNORMALITY IN BOTH PARENTS OF A PATIENT WITH CHRONIC GRANULOMATOUS DISEASE. LANCET 1* 799-800, 1969.

WINDHORST, D., HOLMES, B. AND GOOD, R. A.* A NEWLY DEFINED X-LINKED TRAIT IN MAN WITH DEMONSTRATION OF THE LYON EFFECT IN CARRIER FEMALES. LANCET 1* 737-739, 1967.

WINDHORST, D. B.* INHERITANCE OF CHRONIC GRANULOMATOUS DISEASE. (LETTER) LANCET 2* 543-544, 1969.

30650 GYNECOMASTIA, FAMILIAL

IN SOME FAMILIES MALE-TO-MALE TRANSMISSION BESPEAKS AUTOSOMAL DOMINANT INHERITANCE. IN THE FAMILY DESCRIBED BY ROSEWATER, GWINUP AND HAMWI (1965), GYNECOMASTIA WITH HYPOGONADISM OCCURRED IN FOUR MALES OF THREE SIBSHIPS IN TWO GENERATIONS CONNECTED THROUGH FEMALES IN A PATTERN CONSISTENT WITH X-LINKED OR AUTOSOMAL DOMINANT INHERITANCE. THEIR CASES DIFFER FROM THE REIFENSTEIN SYNDROME BY THE

ROSEWATER, S., GWINUP, G. AND HAMWI, G. J.* FAMILIAL GYNECOMASTIA. ANN. INTERN. MED. 63* 377-385, 1965.

*30660 HEMOLYSIS OF TRYPSIN-TREATED RED CELLS

HEISTO ET AL. (1964) FOUND THAT FRESHLY TAKEN SERUM OF ABOUT 12 PERCENT OF MALE DONORS AND ABOUT 23 PERCENT OF FEMALE DONORS WOULD HEMOLYZE TRYPSIN-TREATED RED CELLS IRRESPECTIVE OF THE ABO OR RH GROUPS. THE MALE AND FEMALE FREQUENCIES AND FAMILY STUDIES VIRTUALLY PROVED X-LINKAGE. FURTHER INVESTIGATIONS SHOULD BE MADE.

HEISTO, H., HARBOE, M. AND GODAL, H. C.* WORM HAEMOLYSINS ACTIVE AGAINST TRYPSINIZED RED CELLS* OCCURRENCE, INHERITANCE AND CLINICAL SIGNIFICANCE. PROC. 10TH CONGR. INTERN. SOC. BLOOD TRANSF. (STOCKHOLM). PP. 787-789, 1964.

*30670 HEMOPHILIA A (CLASSICAL HEMOPHILIA)

CLASSICAL HEMOPHILIA IS THE RESULT OF A HEREDITARY DEFECT IN ANTIHEMOPHILIC GLOBULIN (FACTOR VIII). A PARTIAL DEFICIENCY IN HETEROZYGOUS CARRIERS HAS BEEN DEMONSTRATED BY RAPAPORT ET AL. (1960), AMONG SEVERAL.
ALEXANDER AND GOLDSTEIN (1953) FIRST NOTED LOW LEVELS OF FACTOR VIII IN CASES OF VON WILLEBRAND'S DISEASE ("VASCULAR HEMOPHILIA"), AN AUTOSOMALLY INHERITED DISORDER. THIS WAS CONFIRMED BY OTHER WORKERS INCLUDING NILSSON AND COLLEAGUES (1957), WHO STUDIED VON WILLEBRAND'S ORIGINAL FAMILY IN THE ALAND ISLANDS. THUS, AN AUTOSOMAL LOCUS SEEMS ALSO INVOLVED IN SOME WAY IN FACTOR VIII FORMATION. THE POSSIBLE ALLELIC RELATIONSHIP OF MILD FACTOR VIII DEFICIENCY IS SUGGESTED BY FAMILIES SUCH AS THAT OF GRAHAM AND COLLEAGUES (1953) AND THAT OF BOND AND COLLEAGUES (1962) IN WHICH THE CARRIER FEMALES AS WELL AS HEMIZYGOUS MALES SHOWED DEPRESSION OF FACTOR VIII LEVELS AND SOMETIMES CLINICAL HEMOPHILIA, ALTHOUGH THE LEVELS OF FACTOR VIII WERE NOT AS LOW AS IN HEMIZYGOUS AFFECTED MALES. SUTTON (IN METABOLIC BASIS OF INHERITED DISEASE, STANBURY, ET AL., EDITORS, 1960) AND WOOLF (1962) HAVE MADE THE INTERESTING SUGGESTION THAT IN MAN AS IN BACTERIA FEEDBACK REPRESSION, OPERATING AT THE LEVEL OF THE GENE OR AT THE LEVEL OF RNA, MAY BE INVOLVED IN SETTING THE RATE OF PROTEIN SYNTHESIS. SPECIFICALLY, IF A MUTATION IS OF A TYPE IN WHICH NO PROTEIN OF A PARTICULAR TYPE IS FORMED, THEN NO ABNORMALITY IN LEVEL WOULD BE EXPECTED IN HETEROZYGOTES. ON THE OTHER HAND, IF A "WARPED MOLECULE" IS SYNTHESIZED AS A RESULT OF THE MUTATION, THEN FEEDBACK REPRESSION MIGHT OCCUR EVEN THOUGH THE MOLECULE WAS DEFECTIVE IN THE PERFORMANCE OF ITS PHYSIOLOGIC FUNCTION. SUTTON AND WOOLF SUGGESTED THAT THE FINDINGS IN THE HETEROZYGOTE FOR MILD HEMOPHILIA FIT THE LATTER MODEL, WHEREAS THOSE OF SEVERE HEMOPHILIA MAY FIT THE FIRST MODEL. THE CONCEPT IS COMPATIBLE WITH THE LYON HYPOTHESIS AND QUITE INDEPENDENT OF IT. FROM STUDY OF A FAMILY IN WHICH BOTH HEMOPHILIA A AND HEMOPHILIA B WERE SEGREGATING WOODLIFF AND JACKSON (1966) CONCLUDED THAT THE TWO LOCI ARE FAR APART, AS IS ALSO SUGGESTED BY LINKAGE STUDIES OF THE INDIVIDUAL DISORDERS WITH MARKER TRAITS. SPLENIC TRANSPLANTATION TO DOGS WITH HEMOPHILIA A CORRECTS THE COAGULATION DEFECT (NORMAN ET AL., 1968).
ZACHARSKI ET AL. (1968) SHOWED THAT LEUKOCYTES (PROBABLY LYMPHOCYTES) IN VITRO SYNTHESIZE FACTOR VIII. AS OF THIS WRITING THE BEST OPINION SEEMS TO BE THAT FACTOR VIII LIKE MANY OTHER PROTEINS IS SYNTHESIZED IN THE LIVER AND THAT ITS PRESENCE IN THE SPLEEN IS ONLY A TEMPORARY, PERHAPS STORAGE PHENOMENON. RISE IN FACTOR VIII LEVEL IS INDUCED, FOR EXAMPLE, BY ADMINISTRATION OF EPINEPHRINE. AMONG 54 PATIENTS WITH HEMOPHILIA A, FEINSTEIN ET AL. (1969) FOUND THAT THE PLASMA OF 52 SHOWED NO NEUTRALIZING ACTIVITY WITH A HUMAN ANTIBODY TO FACTOR VIII. THE PLASMA FROM THE OTHER TWO HAD NEUTRALIZING ACTIVITY COMPARABLE TO THAT OF NORMAL PLASMA. USING NEUTRALIZATION OF A FACTOR-VIII INHIBITOR AS A MEASURE OF CROSS-REACTING MATERIAL IN THE PLASMA OF HEMOPHILICS, DENSON (1968) FOUND THAT 33 HEMOPHILIC PLASMAS (PRESUMABLY FROM SEPARATE PATIENTS) SHOWED LITTLE NEUTRALIZA-TION WHEREAS 3 HEMOPHILIC PLASMAS SHOWED ABOUT THE SAME NEUTRALIZATION AS NORMAL PLASMA. THE FINDING SEEMS TO INDICATE THE PRESENCE OF CRM-POSITIVE AND CRM-NEGATIVE FORMS OF HEMOPHILIA. HOYER AND BRECKENRIDGE (1968) ALSO FOUND HETERO-GENEITY IN HEMOPHILIA A. FOR BOTH HEMOPHILIA A AND HEMOPHILIA B TWO SUBTYPES EXIST - ONE WITHOUT ANY PROTEIN IMMUNOLOGICALLY DEMONSTRABLE AND ONE WITH IMMUNOLOGICALLY NORMAL BUT HEMOSTATICALLY DEFECTIVE PROTEIN (DENSON ET AL., 1969). IN BOTH HEMOPHILIA A AND B, THE CRM-POSITIVE FORM IS THE RARER. WHETHER HEMOPHI-LIA A IS CRM-POSITIVE OR CRM-NEGATIVE MAY BE A FUNCTION OF THE SENSITIVITY OF THE TECHNIQUE USED TO TEST IMMUNOLOGICALLY FOR THE PRESENCE OF CROSS-REACTING MATERIAL. STITES ET AL. (1970) DEMONSTRATED CRM IN ALL HEMOPHILIA A PATIENTS AND IN NO PATIENT WITH VON WILLEBRAND'S DISEASE. LINKAGE STUDIES INDICATE THAT HEMOPHILIA A AND B ARE NOT ALLELIC. THE INDEPENDENCE OF THEIR LOCI WAS NICELY CONFIRMED WHEN ROBERTSON AND TRUEMAN (1964) FOUND A FAMILY WITH BOTH HEMOPHILIA A AND HEMOPHILIA B AND IN IT A MALE DEFICIENT IN BOTH FACTORS. EARLY REPORTS OF HEMOPHILIA FAMILIES EMANATED FROM THIS COUNTRY BEGINNING WITH A NEWSPAPER ACCOUNT IN 1792 (MCKUSICK, 1962) AND CONTINUING WITH REPORTS BY OTTO IN 1803 AND HAY IN 1813 (MCKUSICK, 1962).
STITES ET AL. (1971) WERE ABLE TO DETECT FACTOR VIII IMMUNOLOGICALLY IN ALL OF 14 PATIENTS WITH HEMOPHILIA A THEY STUDIED. LITTLE OR NO FACTOR VIII WAS IDENTIFIED IN PATIENTS WITH VON WILLEBRAND'S DISEASE. THEY WERE USING AN UNUSUALLY SENSITIVE METHOD. ZIMMERMAN ET AL. (1971) FOUND IMMUNOREACTIVE MATERIAL IN ALL OF 22 PATIENTS WITH HEMOPHILIA A. VON WILLEBRAND'S DISEASE, ON THE OTHER HAND, APPEARS TO BE TRUE FACTOR VIII DEFICIENCY.

X
L
I
N
K
E
D

570

ALEXANDER, B. AND GOLDSTEIN, R.* DUAL HEMOSTATIC DEFECT IN PSEUDOHEMOPHILIA. (ABSTRACT) J. CLIN. INVEST. 32* 551 ONLY, 1953.

ARRANTS, J. E., JORDAN, P. H., JR. AND NEWCOMB, T. F.* VON WILLEBRAND'S DISEASE* A CAUSE FOR MASSIVE POSTOPERATIVE BLEEDING - REPORT OF A CASE. ANN. SURG. 156* 845-851, 1962.

BENNETT, E. AND HUEHNS, E. R.* IMMUNOLOGICAL DIFFERENTIATION OF THREE TYPES OF HEMOPHILIA AND IDENTIFICATION OF SOME FEMALE CARRIERS. LANCET 2* 956-958, 1970.

BOND, T. P., LEVIN, W. C., CELANDER, D. R. AND GUEST, M. M.* 'MILD HEMOPHILIA' AFFECTING BOTH MALES AND FEMALES. NEW ENG. J. MED. 266* 220-223, 1962.

DENSON, K. W. E.* TWO FORMS OF HAEMOPHILIA.Q (LETTER) LANCET 2* 222-223, 1968.

DENSON, K. W. E., BIGGS, R., HADDON, M. E., BORRETT, R. AND COBB, K.* TWO TYPES OF HAEMOPHILIA (A+ AND A-)* A STUDY OF 48 CASES. BRIT. J. HAEMAT. 17* 163-171, 1969.

FEINSTEIN, D., CHONG, M. N. Y., KASPER, C. K. AND RAPAPORT, S. I.* HEMOPHILIA A* POLYMORPHISM DETECTABLE BY A FACTOR VIII ANTIBODY. SCIENCE 163* 1071-1072, 1969.

GRAHAM, J. B., MCLENDON, W. W. AND BRINKHOUS, K. M.* MILD HEMOPHILIA* AN ALLELIC FORM OF THE DISEASE. AM. J. MED. SCI. 225* 46-53, 1953.

GROZDEA, J., COLOMBIES, P., BIERME, R. AND DUCOS, J.* MYELOPEROXIDASIS AND GENETICS OF HAEMOPHILIA A. (LETTER) LANCET 2* 220 ONLY, 1969.

HOYER, L. W. AND BRECKENRIDGE, R. T.* TWO FORMS OF HAEMOPHILIA.Q (LETTER) LANCET 2* 457 ONLY, 1968.

MCKUSICK, V. A.* HEMOPHILIA IN EARLY NEW ENGLAND. A FOLLOW-UP OF FOUR KINDREDS IN WHICH HEMOPHILIA OCCURRED IN PRE-REVOLUTIONARY PERIOD. J. HIST. MED. 17* 342-365, 1962.

MCKUSICK, V. A.* THE EARLIEST RECORD OF HEMOPHILIA IN AMERICA.Q BLOOD 19* 243-244, 1962.

NILSSON, I. M., BLOMBACK, M. AND RAMGREN, O.* INVESTIGATIONS ON HEMOPHILIA A AND B CARRIERS. BIBL. HAEMAT. 26* 26-29, 1966.

NILSSON, I. M., BLOMBACK, M. AND VON FRANCKEN, I.* ON AN INHERITED AUTOSOMAL HEMORRHAGIC DIATHESIS WITH ANTIHEMOPHILIC GLOBULIN (AHG) DEFICIENCY AND PROLONGED BLEEDING TIME. ACTA MED. SCAND. 159* 35-57, 1957.

NILSSON, I. M., BLOMBACK, M., RAMGREN, O. AND VON FRANCKEN, I.* HAEMOPHILIA IN SWEDEN. II. CARRIERS OF HAEMOPHILIA A AND B. ACTA MED. SCAND. 171* 223-235, 1962.

NORMAN, J. C., COVELLI, V. H. AND SISE, H. S.* TRANSPLANTATION OF THE SPLEEN. (EDITORIAL) ANN. INTERN. MED. 78* 700-704, 1968.

RAPAPORT, S. I., PATCH, M. J. AND MOORE, F. J.* ANTI-HEMOPHILIC GLOBULIN LEVELS IN CARRIERS OF HEMOPHILIA A. J. CLIN. INVEST. 39* 1619-1625, 1960.

ROBERTSON, J. H. AND TRUEMAN, R. G.* COMBINED HEMOPHILIA AND CHRISTMAS DISEASE. BLOOD 24* 281-288, 1964.

SCHIFFMAN, S. AND RAPAPORT, S. I.* INCREASED FACTOR VIII LEVELS IN SUSPECTED CARRIERS OF HEMOPHILIA A* TAKING CONTRACEPTIVES BY MOUTH. NEW ENG. J. MED. 275* 599 ONLY, 1966.

STITES, D. P., HERSHGOLD, E. J., PERLMAN, J. D. AND FUDENBERG, H. H.* FACTOR VIII DETECTION BY HEMAGGLUTINATION INHIBITION* HEMOPHILIA A AND VON WILLEBRAND'S DISEASE. SCIENCE 171* 196-197, 1971.

STITES, D. P., HERSHGOLD, E. J., PERLMAN, J. D. AND FUDENBERG, H. H.* PRESENCE OF THE PRODUCT OF A 'SILENT GENE' IN HEMOPHILIA A. (ABSTRACT) AM. J. HUM. GENET. 22* 16A ONLY, 1970.

X

L
I
N
K
E
D

WOODLIFF, H. J. AND JACKSON, J. M.* COMBINED HAEMOPHILIA AND CHRISTMAS DISEASE. A GENETIC STUDY OF A PATIENT AND HIS RELATIVES. MED. J. AUST. 53* 658-661, 1966.

WOOLF, L. I.* GENE EXPRESSION IN HETEROZYGOTES. NATURE 194* 609-610, 1962.

ZACHARSKI, L. R., BOWIE, E. J. W., TITUS, J. L. AND OWEN, C. A., JR.* SYNTHESIS OF ANTIHEMOPHILIC FACTOR (FACTOR VIII) BY LEUKOCYTES* PRELIMINARY REPORT. MAYO CLIN. PROC. 43* 617-619, 1968.

ZIMMERMAN, T. S., RATNOFF, O. D. AND LITTELL, A. S.* DETECTION OF CARRIERS OF CLASSIC HEMOPHILIA USING AN IMMUNOLOGIC ASSAY FOR ANTIHEMOPHILIC FACTOR (FACTOR

VIII). J. CLIN. INVEST. 50* 255-258, 1971.

ZIMMERMAN, T. S., RATNOFF, O. D. AND POWELL, A. E.* IMMUNOLOGIC DIFFERENTIATION OF CLASSIC HEMOPHILIA (FACTOR VIII DEFICIENCY) AND VON WILLEBRAND'S DISEASE, WITH OBSERVATIONS ON COMBINED DEFICIENCIES OF ANTIHEMOPHILIC FACTOR AND PROACCELERIN (FACTOR V) AND ON AN ACQUIRED CIRCULATING ANTICOAGULANT AGAINST ANTIHEMOPHILIC FACTOR. J. CLIN. INVEST. 50* 244-245, 1971.

30680 HEMOPHILIA A WITH VASCULAR ABNORMALITY

EGEBERG (1965) STUDIED A NORWEGIAN FAMILY IN WHICH AT LEAST 7 PERSONS HAD A DISORDER COMBINING FEATURES OF HEMOPHILIA A AND OF VON WILLEBRAND'S DISEASE. THE AFFECTED MALES SHOWED MILD TO MODERATELY SEVERE BLEEDING TENDENCY AND THE FEMALES A LESS SEVERE TENDENCY. FACTOR VIII WAS DECREASED, MORE IN MALES THAN IN FEMALES. BLEEDING TIME WAS PROLONGED AND CAPILLARY FRAGILITY DEMONSTRATED IN BOTH SEXES. THE PEDIGREE WAS COMPATIBLE WITH X-LINKED TRANSMISSION.

EGEBERG, O.* AN INHERITED HEMORRHAGIC TRAIT WITH CHARACTERISTICS RESEMBLING BOTH MILD HEMOPHILIA OF TYPE A AND VON WILLEBRAND'S DISEASE. SCAND. J. CLIN. LAB. INVEST. 17* (SUPPL. 84) 25-32, 1965.

*30690 HEMOPHILIA B (CHRISTMAS DISEASE)

CHRISTMAS DISEASE IS THE RESULT OF A HEREDITARY DEFECT IN FACTOR IX (PTC* PLASMA THROMBOPLASTIC COMPONENT). LINKAGE STUDIES SUGGEST THAT THE GENES RESPONSIBLE FOR HEMOPHILIAS A AND B ARE NOT ALLELIC. BLACKBURN AND COLLEAGUES (1962) DESCRIBED TWO UNRELATED GIRLS WITH CHRISTMAS DISEASE (PTC DEFICIENCY) AND A 'PRIMARY' VASCULAR ABNORMALITY. IN BOTH INSTANCES ALL OTHER MEMBERS OF THE FAMILY WERE NORMAL. THIS MAY BE A SITUATION COMPARABLE TO THE COMBINATION OF AHG AND VASCULAR DEFECTS IN WILLEBRAND'S DISEASE. THE COMBINATION OF FACTOR IX WITH FACTOR VII DEFICIENCY IN AN X-LINKED PATTERN OF INHERITANCE WAS DESCRIBED BY SEVERAL WORKERS (E.G., NOUR-ELDIN AND WILKINSON, 1959). HOWEVER, VERSTRAETE, VERMYLEN AND VANDENBROUCKE (1962) FOUND FACTOR VII DEFICIENCY IN ALL AFFECTED MALES OF FOUR FAMILIES WITH CHRISTMAS DISEASE AND SUGGESTED THAT IT IS A CONSISTENT SECONDARY PHENOMENON. BY THE LATTER VIEW NO SEPARATE MUTATION FOR THE COMBINED DEFECT NEED BE POSTULATED. TWOMEY AND HOUGIE (1967) DEFINED A VARIANT OF HEMOPHILIA B WHICH DIFFERS FROM THE USUAL FORM IN THE PRESENCE OF A PROLONGED PROTHROMBIN TIME. THEY PRESENTED EVIDENCE THAT A STRUCTURALLY ABNORMAL AND INACTIVE FORM OF FACTOR IX, FORMED IN THESE CASES, ACTS AS AN INHIBITOR OF THE NORMAL REACTION BETWEEN FACTOR VII AND ANIMAL BRAIN. THEY CALLED THE VARIANT HEMOPHILIA B(M), AFTER THE INITIAL OF THE FAMILY SURNAME. ONLY A MINORITY OF HEMOPHILIA B CASES ARE OF THIS TYPE. EVIDENCE FOR MORE THAN ONE FORM OF HEMOPHILIA B WAS PRESENTED BY HOUGIE AND TWOMEY (1967) WHO FOUND THAT IN SOME FAMILIES AFFECTED PERSONS HAVE PROLONGED PROTHROMBIN TIMES THOUGHT TO BE DUE TO INHIBITION BY AN ABNORMAL AND DEFECTIVE FACTOR IX MOLECULE. HETEROZYGOUS FEMALES SHOW PROLONGED PROTHROMBIN TIMES. THEY DESIGNATED THE VARIANT HEMOPHILIA B(M). ROBERTS ET AL. (1968) ALSO DEMONSTRATED HETEROGENEITY IN HEMOPHILIA B. ABOUT 90 PERCENT OF PATIENTS SHOWED REDUCED PTC-INHIBITOR-NEUTRALIZING ACTIVITY PROPORTIONAL TO THE REDUCTION IN PTC CLOTTING ACTIVITY. THESE WERE INTERPRETED AS CRM-NEGATIVE MUTANTS. ABOUT 10 PERCENT OF PATIENTS SHOWED FULLY EFFECTIVE PTC-INHIBITOR-NEUTRALIZING ACTIVITY. THESE WERE INTERPRETED AS CRM-POSITIVE MUTANTS. LASCARI ET AL. (1969) DESCRIBED A DAUGHTER OF AN AFFECTED MALE WHO HAD AN XX KARYOTYPE, FACTOR IX LEVEL OF 5 PERCENT AND HEMARTHROSIS. THE FACTOR IX LEVEL IN THE MOTHER WAS 100 PERCENT. THE GIRL WAS THOUGHT TO BE A MANIFESTING HETEROZYGOTE. TWOMEY ET AL. (1969) DESCRIBED A VARIANT OF HEMOPHILIA B IN WHICH AN 'EARLY ONE-STAGE INHIBITOR' BELIEVED TO BE AN ALTERED FACTOR IX MOLECULE IS PRESENT. THE INHIBITOR WAS FOUND IN ABOUT 14 PERCENT OF CHRISTMAS DISEASE PATIENTS. THEY CALLED THIS FORM HEMOPHILIA B(M) FOR THE FAMILY SURNAME WHICH BEGAN WITH M. DENSON ET AL. (1968) DEMONSTRATED WHAT WAS PROBABLY THE SAME BIOLOGICALLY INEFFECTIVE MOLECULE BY IMMUNOLOGIC MEANS. UNFORTUNATE LYONIZATION WAS POSTULATED IN AN AFFECTED GIRL PROBABLY HETEROZYGOUS FOR THE CHRISTMAS DISEASE GENE. VELTKAMP ET AL. (1970) DESCRIBED A VARIANT CALLED HEMOPHILIA B LEYDEN WHICH IS CHARACTERIZED BY DISAPPEARANCE OF THE BLEEDING DIATHESIS AS THE PATIENT AGES. CORRELATED WITH THE CLINICAL IMPROVEMENT IS A RISE IN FACTOR IX FROM ABOUT 1 PERCENT TO 20 TO 60 PERCENT OF NORMAL. THE TENNA KINDRED MAY HAVE THE SAME DISORDER.

BLACKBURN, E. K., MONAGHAN, J. H., LEDERER, H. AND MACFIE, J. M.* CHRISTMAS DISEASE ASSOCIATED WITH PRIMARY CAPILLARY ABNORMALITIES. BRIT. MED. J. 1* 154-156, 1962.

BROWN, P. E., HOUGIE, C. AND ROBERTS, H. R.* THE GENETIC HETEROGENEITY OF HEMOPHILIA B. NEW ENG. J. MED. 283* 61-64, 1970.

DENSON, K. W., BIGGS, P. AND MANNUCCI, P. M.* AN INVESTIGATION OF THREE PATIENTS WITH CHRISTMAS DISEASE DUE TO AN ABNORMAL TYPE OF FACTOR IX. J. CLIN. PATH. 21* 160-165, 1968.

DIDISHEIM, P. AND VANDERVOORT, R. L. E.* DETECTION OF CARRIERS FOR FACTOR IX (PTC) DEFICIENCY. BLOOD 20* 150-155, 1962.

HOUGIE, C. AND TWOMEY, J. J.* HEMOPHILIA B(M)* A NEW TYPE OF FACTOR-IX DEFICIENCY. LANCET 1* 698-700, 1967.

X

L
I
N
K
E
D

LASCARI, A. D., HOAK, J. C. AND TAYLOR, J. C.* CHRISTMAS DISEASE IN A GIRL. AM. J. DIS. CHILD. 117* 585-588, 1969.

NOUR-ELDIN, F. AND WILKINSON, J. F.* FACTOR-VII DEFICIENCY WITH CHRISTMAS DISEASE IN ONE FAMILY. LANCET 1* 1173-1176, 1959.

ROBERTS, H. R., GRIZZLE, J. E., MCLESTER, W. D. AND PENICK, G. D.* GENETIC VARIANTS OF HEMOPHILIA B* DETECTION BY MEANS OF A SPECIFIC PTC INHIBITOR. J. CLIN. INVEST. 47* 360-365, 1968.

VELTKAMP, J. J., MEILOF, J., REMMELTS, H. G., VAN DER VLERK, D. AND LOELIGER, E. A.* ANOTHER GENETIC VARIANT OF HAEMOPHILIA B* HAEMOPHILIA B LEYDEN. SCAND. J. HAEMAT. 7* 82-90, 1970.

VERSTRAETE, M., VERMYLEN, C. AND VANDENBROUCKE, J.* HEMOPHILIA B ASSOCIATED WITH A DECREASED FACTOR VII ACTIVITY. AM. J. MED. SCI. 243* 20-26, 1962.

WHITTAKER, D. L., COPELAND, D. L. AND GRAHAM, J. B.* LINKAGE OF COLOR BLINDNESS WITH HEMOPHILIAS A AND B. AM. J. HUM. GENET. 14* 149-158, 1962.

*30700 HYDROCEPHALUS DUE TO CONGENITAL STENOSIS OF AQUEDUCT OF SYLVIUS

THE HYDROCEPHALUS MAY BECOME ARRESTED AND THE PRINCIPAL MANIFESTATIONS MAY BE MENTAL DEFICIENCY AND SPASTIC PARAPLEGIA. HYPOPLASIA AND CONTRACTURE OF THE THUMB ARE CHARACTERISTIC (EDWARDS 1961) BUT WERE NOT PRESENT IN ANY OF THE 7 AFFECTED MALES IN THE FAMILY STUDIED BY BICKERS AND ADAMS (1949) AND LATER BY HOLMES AND NASH (1967). SEE CATARACT, CONGENITAL TOTAL, FOR DESCRIPTION OF CONGENITAL HYDROCEPHALUS WITH CATARACT. SAJID AND COPPLE (1968) FOUND BASILAR IMPRESSIONS AS AN ASSOCIATED FEATURE IN TWO BROTHERS AND SUGGESTED ITS USEFULNESS IN DIAGNOSIS.

BICKERS, D. S. AND ADAMS, R. D.* HEREDITARY STENOSIS OF THE AQUEDUCT OF SYLVIUS AS A CAUSE OF CONGENITAL HYDROCEPHALUS. BRAIN 72* 246-262, 1949.

EDWARDS, J. H.* THE SYNDROME OF SEX-LINKED HYDROCEPHALUS. ARCH. DIS. CHILD. 36* 486-493, 1961.

EDWARDS, J. H., NORMAN, R. M. AND ROBERTS, J. M.* SEX-LINKED HYDROCEPHALUS. REPORT OF A FAMILY WITH 15 AFFECTED MEMBERS. ARCH. DIS. CHILD. 36* 481-485, 1961.

FANCONI, G.* ZUR DIAGNOSE UND THERAPIE HYDROCEPHALISCHER UND VERWANDTER ZUSTANDE. SCHWEIZ. MED. WSCHR. 64* 214-223, 1934.

HOLMES, L. B. AND NASH, A.* X-LINKED HYDROCEPHALUS, COMPARISON OF PATHOLOGY IN TWO GENERATIONS. MEETING, AM. SOC. HUM. GENET., TORONTO, DEC. 13, 1967.

RIBIERRE, M., COUVREUR, J. AND CANETTI, J.* LES HYDROCEPHALIES PAR STENOSE DE L'AQUEDUC DE SYLVIUS DANS LA TOXOPLASMOSE CONGENITALE. ARCH. FRANC. PEDIAT. 27* 501-510, 1970.

SAJID, M. H. AND COPPLE, P. J.* FAMILIAL AQUEDUCTAL STENOSIS AND BASILAR IMPRESSION. NEUROLOGY 18* 260-262, 1968.

SHANNON, M. W. AND NADLER, H. L.* X-LINKED HYDROCEPHALUS. J. MED. GENET. 5* 326-328, 1968.

30710 HYPERTELORISM WITH ESOPHAGEAL ABNORMALITY AND HYPOSPADIAS (G SYNDROME)

OPITZ ET AL. (1969) DESCRIBED FOUR BROTHERS WITH HYPERTELORISM, A NEUROMUSCULAR DEFECT OF THE ESOPHAGUS AND SWALLOWING MECHANISM, HOARSE CRY, HYPOSPADIAS, CRYPTORCHIDISM, BIFID SCROTUM, AND, IN ONE, IMPERFORATE ANUS. TWO OTHER BROTHERS HAD DIED OF ASPIRATION. THE PARENTS WERE NOT RELATED. THE MOTHER WAS THOUGHT TO HAVE MINOR STIGMATA SUCH AS HYPERTELORISM, HAD DIFFICULTY SWALLOWING FLUIDS UNTIL AGE 11 MONTHS WHEN A LINGUAL FRENULUM (ALSO PRESENT IN AT LEAST ONE OF THE AFFECTED SONS) WAS RESECTED. FOUR LIVING SISTERS WERE WELL EXCEPT FOR ONE WITH USHER'S SYNDROME (CONGENITAL DEAFNESS AND RETINITIS PIGMENTOSA) AND ONE WITH SWALLOWING DIFFICULTIES LIKE THE MOTHER. AS IS HIS PRACTICE, OPITZ (1969) DESIGNATED THE CONDITION, 'G SYNDROME' AFTER THE FAMILY IN WHICH HE OBSERVED IT. COBURN (1970) DESCRIBED AN ISOLATED CASE IN A MALE INFANT.

COBURN, T. P.* G SYNDROME. AM. J. DIS. CHILD. 120* 466 ONLY, 1970.

OPITZ, J. M., FRIAS, J. L., GUTENBERGER, J. E. AND PELLETT, J. R.* THE G SYNDROME OF MULTIPLE CONGENITAL ANOMALIES. THE CLINICAL DELINEATION OF BIRTH DEFECTS. II. MALFORMATION SYNDROMES. NEW YORK* NATIONAL FOUNDATION, 1969. PP. 95-101.

30720 HYPERURICEMIA, ATAXIA, DEAFNESS

ROSENBERG ET AL. (1970) DESCRIBED A KINDRED IN WHICH FIVE PERSONS HAD HYPERURICE- MIA, RENAL INSUFFICIENCY, ATAXIA AND DEAFNESS. SERUM URATE LEVELS WERE ELEVATED IN OTHER MEMBERS OF THE KINDRED WHO DID NOT HAVE RENAL INSUFFICIENCY, INDICATING THAT THE HYPERURICEMIA WAS NOT SECONDARY TO RENAL DISEASE. RED CELL HYPOXANTHINE-

X
L
I
N
K
E
D

WITH X-LINKED INHERITANCE WITH FULL EXPRESSION IN SOME FEMALES, INCOMPLETE
EXPRESSION IN OTHERS.

ROSENBERG, A. L., BERGSTROM, L., TROOST, B. T. AND BARTHOLOMEW, B. A.*
HYPERURICEMIA AND NEUROLOGIC DEFICITS* A FAMILY STUDY. NEW ENG. J. MED. 282* 992-
997, 1970.

30730 HYPOGONADISM, MALE

VARIOUSLY TERMED IN THE LITERATURE ARE SEVERAL CONDITIONS WHICH AFFECT ONLY
PERSONS WITH THE USUAL MALE KARYOTYPE AND WHICH ARE FAMILIAL WITH A PATTERN OFTEN
SUGGESTING X-LINKED INHERITANCE. AT LEAST FIVE DISTINCT ENTITIES ARE PROBABLY
INVOLVED* (1) MALE HYPOGONADISM WITH OR WITHOUT GYNECOMASTIA, (2) MALE PSEUDOHER-
MAPHRODITISM (Q.V.), (3) THE TESTICULAR FEMINIZATION SYNDROME (Q.V.), (4)
GYNECOMASTIA (Q.V.), AND (5) THE KALLMANN SYNDROME (Q.V.). AS SEEN LATER, THERE
MAY BE AT LEAST TWO DISTINCT FORMS OF THE TESTICULAR FEMINIZATION SYNDROME. MALE
PSEUDOHERMAPHRODITISM IS ALSO PROBABLY A HETEROGENEOUS CATEGORY. AUTOSOMAL
DOMINANT (MALE-LIMITED), AUTOSOMAL RECESSIVE (MALE-LIMITED) OR X-LINKED INHERI-
TANCE ARE ALL POSSIBLE IN THIS GROUP OF ENTITIES. WHEN HYPOSPADIAS AND GYNECOMAS-
TIA ARE ASSOCIATED WITH HYPOGONADISM, THE DESIGNATION OF REIFENSTEIN SYNDROME IS
OFTEN ATTACHED. GYNECOMASTIA MAY OCCUR ALONE AS A FAMILIAL ANOMALY OR BE A
FEATURE OF ONE OF THE OTHER THREE CLASSES. THE NECESSITY FOR STUDIES, GENETIC AND
PHYSIOLOGIC, TO BRING ORDER OUT OF THIS NOSOLOGIC CHAOS IS EVIDENT. YET OTHER
FORMS OF MALE HYPOGONADISM - THAT ASSOCIATED WITH ICHTHYOSIS (Q.V.) AND THAT
ASSOCIATED WITH ATAXIA (Q.V.) - WILL BE SEPARATELY DISCUSSED.
PETERS AND COLLEAGUES (1955) DESCRIBED GYNECOMASTIA, INGUINAL TESTES, AND
SLIGHT HYPOGONADAL TRAITS IN TWO HALF-BROTHERS (SONS OF THE SAME MOTHER) AND IN A
COUSIN, THE SON OF THE MOTHER'S SISTER. ONE AFFECTED MALE HAD INTERCOURSE AND
EJACULATION. THE FAMILY OF GILBERT-DREYFUS AND COLLEAGUES (1957) IS YET ANOTHER
EXAMPLE* MATERNAL UNCLES WERE AFFECTED. REIFENSTEIN (1947) RESTUDIED THE FAMILY
REPORTED BY YOUNG (1937). THE ANOMALY IS CLEARLY IDENTICAL TO THAT IN REIFENS-
TEIN'S FAMILY WHICH WE HAVE ALSO RESTUDIED. SINCE A SEPARATE, RATHER CLEAR-CUT
ENTITY SEEMS TO BE REPRESENTED IN THESE CASES, I PROPOSED TO REFER TO IT AS
REIFENSTEIN'S SYNDROME (Q.V.).
THERE IS LIKELY TO BE HETEROGENEITY LEFT WITHIN THE GROUP OF MALE HYPOGONA-
DISM EVEN AFTER THE TYPES DISCUSSED SEPARATELY HEREAFTER ARE REMOVED. SOME CASES
MAY BE PRIMARY AS INDICATED BY HIGH LEVELS OF URINARY GONADOTROPINS WHEREAS OTHERS
ARE CASES OF SECONDARY HYPOGONADISM WITH LOW GONADOTROPINS. THE CASES OF SOHVAL
AND SOFFER AND THOSE OF REIFENSTEIN WERE OF THE PRIMARY TYPE. ROTH (1947)
DESCRIBED FOUR BROTHERS OF CZECHOSLOVAKIAN EXTRACTION, WITH UNRELATED PARENTS, WHO
HAD INFANTILE EXTERNAL GENITALIA, HYPOGONADOTROPIC HYPOGONADISM, GYNECOMASTIA, AND
RETINAL DEGENERATION. ONE WAS NOTABLY OBESE. THUS SOME ASPECTS OF THE BIEDL-
BARDET SYNDROME WERE PRESENT.

BIBEN, R. L. AND GORDAN, G. S.* FAMILIAL HYPOGONADOTROPIC EUNUCHOIDISM. J.
CLIN. ENDOCR. 15* 931-942, 1955.

BRIMBLECOMBE, S. L.* BILATERAL CRYPTORCHIDISM IN THREE BROTHERS. BRIT. MED. J.
1* 526 ONLY, 1946.

GILBERT-DREYFUS., SAVOIE., SEBAOUN., ALEXANDRE, C. AND BELAISCH, J.* ETUDE D'UN
CAS FAMILIAL D'ANDROGYNOIDISME AVEC HYPOSPADIAS GRAVE, GYNECOMASTIE ET HYPEROES-
TROGENIE. ANN. ENDOCR. 18* 93-101, 1957.

HURXTHAL, L. M.* SUBLINGUAL USE OF TESTOSTERONE IN 7 CASES OF HYPOGONADISM*
REPORT OF 3 CONGENITAL EUNUCHOIDS OCCURRING IN ONE FAMILY. J. CLIN. ENDOCR. 3*
551-556, 1943.

PETERS, J. H., SIEBER, W. K. AND DAVIS, N.* FAMILIAL GYNECOMASTIA ASSOCIATED
WITH GENITAL ABNORMALITIES* REPORT OF A FAMILY. J. CLIN. ENDOCR. 15* 182-198,
1955.

REIFENSTEIN, E. C., JR.* HEREDITARY FAMILIAL HYPOGONADISM. PROC. AM. FED.
CLIN. RES. 3* 86 ONLY, 1947. RECENT PROGR. HORMONE RES. 3* 224-225, 1947.

ROTH, A. A.* FAMILIAL EUNUCHOIDISM. THE LAURENCE-MOON-BIEDL SYNDROME. J.
UROL. 57* 427-442, 1947.

SIMPSON, S. L.* TWO BROTHERS, WITH INFANTILISM OR EUNUCHOIDISM. PROC. ROY.
SOC. MED. 39* 512-513, 1946.

SOHVAL, A. R. AND SOFFER, L. J.* CONGENITAL FAMILIAL TESTICULAR DEFICIENCY.
AM. J. MENT. DEFIC. 14* 328-348, 1953.

YOUNG, H. H.* GENITAL ABNORMALITIES, HERMAPHRODITISM AND RELATED ADRENAL
DISEASES. BALTIMORE* WILLIAMS AND WILKINS, 1937. PP. 405-409.

30740 HYPOGONADISM, MALE, AND ATAXIA

VOLPE'S CASES HAD EUNUCHOID SKELETAL FEATURES AND LOW URINARY GONADOTROPINS, AND
IN ADDITION THERE WAS CEREBELLAR ATAXIA. MATHEWS (1964) DESCRIBED TWO BROTHERS

WITH PURE CEREBELLAR ATAXIA BEGINNING AT ABOUT AGE 20 AND ASSOCIATED WITH MARKED HYPOGONADISM DUE APPARENTLY TO LOW GONADOTROPIN EXCRETION.

MATHEWS, W. B. AND RUNDLE, A. T.* FAMILIAL CEREBELLAR ATAXIA AND HYPOGONADISM. BRAIN 87* 463-468, 1964.

VOLPE, R., METZLER, W. S. AND JOHNSTON, M. W.* FAMILIAL HYPOGONADOTROPHIC EUNUCHOIDISM WITH CEREBELLAR ATAXIA. J. CLIN. ENDOCR. 23* 107-115, 1963.

30750 HYPOGONADISM, MALE, WITH MENTAL RETARDATION AND SKELETAL ANOMALIES

SOHVAL AND SOFFER (1953) DESCRIBED TWO BROTHERS WHO WERE IDENTICALLY AFFECTED WITH MENTAL RETARDATION, MULTIPLE SKELETAL ANOMALIES AND HYPOGONADISM. THE TESTICULAR HISTOPATHOLOGY WAS DISTINCTIVE. ALL THE SEMINIFEROUS TUBULES WERE INVOLVED BY ONE OF TWO DISTINCT PROCESSES* TRUE GERMINAL APLASIA OR COMPLETE FIBROSIS, WITH NO GRADATIONS BETWEEN THEM. BOTH BROTHERS HAD FASTING HYPERGLYCEMIA AND GLUCOSE INTOLERANCE. SKELETAL ANOMALIES WERE RESTRICTED TO THE CERVICAL SPINE AND SUPERIOR RIBS.

SOHVAL, A. R. AND SOFFER, L. J.* CONGENITAL FAMILIAL TESTICULAR DEFICIENCY. AM. J. MED. DEFIC. 14* 328-348, 1953.

*30760 HYPOMAGNESEMIC TETANY

VAINSEL ET AL. (1970) DESCRIBED A 5 MONTH OLD BOY WHO HAD CONVULSIONS AND PERSISTENT TETANY, ASSOCIATED WITH HYPOMAGNESEMIA AND HYPOCALCEMIA. VITAMIN D THERAPY CORRECTED THE HYPOCALCEMIA WITHOUT IMPROVING THE CLINICAL STATUS. AUTOPSY SHOWED CALCINOSIS OF THE MYOCARDIUM, KIDNEYS AND A CEREBRAL ARTERY. TWO BROTHERS OF THE PROBAND HAD DIED OF A CLINICALLY SIMILAR DISORDER AND THREE OF FOUR SURVIVING BROTHERS HAD CONVULSIONS. OTHERS, E.G. SKYBERG ET AL. (1967, 1969), HAVE REPORTED CASES, ALL IN MALES, AND X-LINKED RECESSIVE INHERITANCE SEEMS LIKELY.

SKYBERG, D., STROMME, J. H., NESBAKKEN, R. AND HARNAES, K.* CONGENITAL PRIMARY HYPOMAGNESEMIA, AN INBORN ERROR OF METABOLISM. ACTA PAEDIAT. SCAND. (SUPPL. 177)* 26-27, 1967.

SKYBERG, D., STROMME, J. H., NORMANN, T., JOHANNESSEN, B. K. AND SEIP, M.* SELECTIVE MALABSORPTION OF MAGNESIUM. AN INBORN ERROR OF METABOLISM. IN, ALLAN, J. D. AND OTHERS (EDS.)* ENZYMOPENIC ANEMIAS, LYSOSOMES, AND OTHER PAPERS* PROC. 6TH SYMPOSIUM OF SOCIETY FOR STUDY OF INBORN ERRORS OF METABOLISM. EDINBURGH AND LONDON* E. AND S. LIVINGSTON, 1969.

VAINSEL, M., VANDEVELDE, G., SMULDERS, J., VOSTERS, M., HUBAIN, P. AND LOEB, H.* TETANY DUE TO HYPOMAGNESAEMIA WITH SECONDARY HYPOCALCEMIA. ARCH. DIS. CHILD. 45* 254-258, 1970.

*30770 HYPOPARATHYROIDISM

PENDEN'S FAMILY SHOWED NEONATAL TRUE IDIOPATHIC HYPOPARATHYROIDISM. SHE SUGGESTED THAT MOST FAMILIAL CASES OF EARLY ONSET ARE OF THE X-LINKED TYPE. THE AUTOSOMAL VARIETY HAS A LATER ONSET. NO AFFECTED MALES REPRODUCED IN PENDEN'S FAMILY AND PROBABLY NOT IN OTHERS OF THE X-LINKED TYPE. BUCHS (1957) REPORTED THREE AFFECTED BROTHERS WHO PRESENTED WITH NEONATAL TETANY. ALTHOUGH MATERNAL HYPERPARATHYROI-DISM WITH FETAL PARATHYROID SUPPRESSION WAS NOT EXCLUDED, IT IS UNLIKELY BECAUSE SUBSEQUENT CHILDREN WERE NORMAL.

BUCHS, S.* FAMILIARER HYPOPARATHYREOIDISMUS. ANN. PAEDIAT. 188* 124-127, 1957.

PENDEN, V. H.* TRUE IDIOPATHIC HYPOPARATHYROIDISM AS A SEX-LINKED RECESSIVE TRAIT. AM. J. HUM. GENET. 12* 323-337, 1960.

*30780 HYPOPHOSPHATEMIA (VITAMIN-D-RESISTANT RICKETS)

LOW SERUM PHOSPHORUS WITH VITAMIN-D-RESISTANT RICKETS BEHAVES AS A SEX-LINKED DOMINANT TRAIT. HETEROZYGOUS FEMALES HAVE ON THE AVERAGE LESS PRONOUNCED DEPRESSION OF SERUM PHOSPHATE AND LESS SEVERE SKELETAL CHANGE. AFFECTED PERSONS SHOW A REDUCTION IN RENAL PHOSPHATE TM TO ABOUT 50 PERCENT OF NORMAL. MALES AND FEMALES ARE NOT SIGNIFICANTLY DIFFERENT IN THIS RESPECT. IT IS UNSETTLED WHETHER THE BASIC DEFECT CONCERNS (1) RENAL RESORPTION OF PHOSPHATE, OR (2) INTESTINAL ABSORPTION OF CALCIUM WITH SECONDARY HYPERPARATHYROIDISM. AVIOLI ET AL. (1967) OBSERVED A DEFECT IN METABOLISM OF VITAMIN D TO A BIOLOGICALLY ACTIVE SUBSTANCE AND SUGGESTED THAT THIS IS THE BASIC DEFECT. FALLS ET AL. (1968) PRESENTED DATA THEY INTERPRETED AS INDICATING THAT HYPERPHOSPHATURIA IS DUE TO SECONDARY HYPERPARATHYROIDISM. SEE WILLIAMS' (1968) DISCUSSION OF THE NATURE OF THE DEFECT. STICKLER (1969) CONCLUDED THAT HYPOPHOSPHATEMIA IS PRESENT ALREADY IN THE NEONATAL PERIOD, THAT ALKALINE PHOSPHATASE IS ELEVATED AT ONE MONTH OF AGE AND THAT EARLY TREATMENT WITH HIGH DOSES OF VITAMIN D DOES NOT PREVENT GROWTH FAILURE. THE CONCEPT OF VITAMIN D RESISTANCE HAS SHORTCOMINGS BECAUSE THE MIMICRY OF NUTRI-TIONAL RICKETS IS NOT CLOSE. THE X-LINKED DISORDER NEVER SHOWS MYOPATHY, TETANY OR HYPOCALCEMIA. FURTHERMORE, COMPLETE HEALING WITH VITAMIN D IN HIGH DOSAGE AND RESTORATION OF NORMAL GROWTH IS DIFFICULT OR IMPOSSIBLE. PONCHON ET AL. (1969)

X
L
I
N
K
E
D

CONCLUDED THAT THE LIVER IS THE MAJOR IF NOT THE ONLY PHYSIOLOGIC SITE OF HYDROXYLATION OF VITAMIN D3 (CHOLECALCIFEROL) TO ITS BIOLOGICALLY ACTIVE METABO- LITE 25-HYDROXYCHOLECALCIFEROL. THE POSSIBILITY OF A DEFECT IN THIS SYSTEM IN HYPOPHOSPHATEMIC RICKETS IS BEING INVESTIGATED. ON THE BASIS OF A FOLLOW-UP STUDY MCNAIR AND STICKLER (1969) QUESTIONED WHETHER VITAMIN D THERAPY HAS ANY BENEFICIAL EFFECT ON GROWTH. SURPRISINGLY THEY FURTHER CONCLUDED THAT MALES AND FEMALES ARE AFFECTED TO AN EQUAL DEGREE. BY AN ORAL PHOSPHATE TOLERANCE TEST, CONDON ET AL. (1970) DEMONSTRATED DEFECTIVE INTESTINAL ABSORPTION OF PHOSPHATE. EARP ET AL. (1970) FOUND 25-HCC INEFFECTIVE IN FIVE PATIENTS. BASED ON EXPERIENCE WITH A WELL-STUDIED CASE, SCHOEN AND REYNOLDS (1970) ARE OF THE OPINION THAT TREATMENT INSTITUTED THE FIRST DAY OF LIFE, OR AT LEAST WELL BEFORE WEIGHT BEARING, CAN RESULT IN NORMAL GROWTH. IF TRUE, THIS PLACES GREAT IMPORTANCE ON THE FAMILY HISTORY IN IDENTIFYING INFANTS WHO NEED SUCH THERAPY. THOMAS AND FRY (1970) DESCRIBED THE DEVELOPMENT OF PARATHYROID ADENOMA, HYPERPARATHYROIDISM AND OSTEITIS FIBROSA CYSTICA AS COMPLICATIONS OF VITAMIN D-RESISTANT RICKETS.

ARCHARD, H. O. AND WITKOP, C. J., JR.* HEREDITARY HYPOPHOSPHATEMIA (VITAMIN D-RESISTANT RICKETS) PRESENTING PRIMARY DENTAL MANIFESTATIONS. ORAL SURG. 22* 184-193, 1966.

AVIOLI, L. V., WILLIAMS, T. F., LUND, J. AND DELUCA, H. F.* METABOLISM OF VITAMIN D(3) - (3)H IN VITAMIN D-RESISTANT RICKETS AND FAMILIAL HYPOPHOSPHATEMIA. J. CLIN. INVEST. 46* 1907-1915, 1967.

BLACKARD, W. G., ROBINSON, R. R. AND WHITE, J. E.* FAMILIAL HYPOPHOSPHATEMIA* REPORT OF A CASE, WITH OBSERVATIONS REGARDING PATHOGENESIS. NEW ENG. J. MED. 266* 899-905, 1962.

BURNETT, C. H., DENT, C. E., HARPER, C. AND WARLAND, B. J.* VITAMIN D-RESISTANT RICKETS. ANALYSIS OF TWENTY-FOUR PEDIGREES WITH HEREDITARY AND SPORADIC CASES. AM. J. MED. 36* 222-232, 1964.

CONDON, J. R., NASSIM, J. R. AND RUTTER, A.* DEFECTIVE INTESTINAL PHOSPHATE ABSORPTION IN FAMILIAL AND NON-FAMILIAL HYPOPHOSPHATEMIA. BRIT. MED. J. 3* 138-141, 1970.

EARP, H. S., NEY, R. L., GITELMAN, H. J., RICHMAN, R. AND DELUCA, H. F.* EFFECTS OF 25-HYDROXYCHOLECALCIFEROL IN PATIENTS WITH FAMILIAL HYPOPHOSPHATEMIA AND VITAMIN-D-RESISTANT RICKETS. NEW ENG. J. MED. 283* 627-630, 1970.

FALLS, W. F., JR., CARTER, N. W., RECTOR, F. C., JR. AND SELDIN, D. W.* FAMILIAL VITAMIN D-RESISTANT RICKETS* STUDY OF SIX CASES WITH EVALUATION OF THE PATHOGENETIC ROLE OF SECONDARY HYPERPARATHYROIDISM. ANN. INTERN. MED. 68* 553-560, 1968.

MCNAIR, S. L. AND STICKLER, G. B.* GROWTH IN FAMILIAL HYPOPHOSPHATEMIC VITAMIN-D-RESISTANT RICKETS. NEW ENG. J. MED. 281* 511-516, 1969.

PONCHON, G., KENNAN, A. L. AND DELUCA, H. F.* *ACTIVATION* OF VITAMIN D BY THE LIVER. J. CLIN. INVEST. 48* 2032-2037, 1969.

SCHOEN, E. J. AND REYNOLDS, J. B.* SEVERE FAMILIAL HYPOPHOSPHATEMIC RICKETS. NORMAL GROWTH FOLLOWING EARLY TREATMENT. AM. J. DIS. CHILD. 120* 58-61, 1970.

STICKLER, G. B.* FAMILIAL HYPOPHOSPHATEMIC VITAMIN D RESISTANT RICKETS. THE NEONATAL PERIOD AND INFANCY. ACTA PAEDIAT. SCAND. 58* 213-219, 1969.

THOMAS, W. C., JR. AND FRY, R. M.* PARATHYROID ADENOMAS IN CHRONIC RICKETS. AM. J. MED. 49* 404-407, 1970.

WILLIAMS, T. F.* PATHOGENESIS OF FAMILIAL VITAMIN D-RESISTANT RICKETS. (EDITORIAL) ANN. INTERN. MED. 68* 706-707, 1968.

WINTERS, R. W., GRAHAM, J. B., WILLIAMS, T. F., MCFALLS, V. W. AND BURNETT, C. H.* A GENETIC STUDY OF FAMILIAL HYPOPHOSPHATEMIA AND VITAMIN D RESISTANT RICKETS WITH A REVIEW OF THE LITERATURE. MEDICINE 37* 97-142, 1958.

30790 HYPOSPADIAS-HYPERTELORISM SYNDROME

IN ADDITION TO HYPOSPADIAS AND HYPERTELORISM, THE FEATURES IN SOME CASES ARE MILD TO MODERATELY SEVERE MENTAL RETARDATION, CLEFT LIP AND CLEFT PALATE. ONLY MALES ARE AFFECTED AND THE DISORDER IS TRANSMITTED THROUGH FEMALES WHO SHOW HYPERTE- LORISM (OPITZ ET AL. 1965). AFFECTED MALES HAVE NOT REPRODUCED. THUS MALE- LIMITED AUTOSOMAL DOMINANT INHERITANCE CANNOT BE EXCLUDED. HYPOSPADIAS AND HYPERTELORISM WERE FEATURES OF TWO BROTHERS WHO ALSO HAD OSTEOCHONDRITIS DISSECANS AT MULTIPLE SITES AS DESCRIBED IN THE RECESSIVE CATALOG (SEE HYPERTELORISM, CRYPTORCHIDISM, ETC.).

OPITZ, J. M. AND SMITH, D. W.* NEW SYNDROME OF HYPOSPADIAS AND HYPERTELORISM, OCCASIONALLY ASSOCIATED WITH CLEFT LIP AND CLEFT PALATE AND MENTAL RETARDATION, AFFECTING MALES AND TRANSMITTED BY FEMALES WITH HYPERTELORISM. TO BE PUBLISHED.

X
L
I
N
K
E
D

STUDIES USING HUMAN-MOUSE SOMATIC CELL HYBRIDS INDICATE, BY REASONING SIMILAR TO THAT USED FOR LOCATING THE THYMIDINE KINASE LOCUS TO CHROMOSOME 17, THAT THE HGPRT LOCUS IS ON THE X CHROMOSOME (NABHOLZ ET AL., 1969). THE FEATURES OF THE LESCH-NYHAN SYNDROME. ARE MENTAL RETARDATION, SPASTIC CEREBRAL PALSY, CHOREOATHETOSIS, URIC ACID URINARY STONES AND SELF-DESTRUCTIVE BITING OF FINGERS AND LIPS. A 200 FOLD INCREASE IN THE CONVERSION OF C(14)-LABELLED GLYCINE TO URIC ACID WAS OBSERVED BY NYHAN, OLIVIER AND LESCH (1965). X-LINKAGE WAS FIRST SUGGESTED BY HOEFNAGEL ET AL. (1965) AND IS SUPPORTED BY A RAPIDLY ACCUMULATING NUMBER OF FAMILIES. SEEGMILLER ET AL. (1967) DEMONSTRATED DEFICIENCY IN THE ENZYME HYPOXANTHINE-GUANINE PHOSPHORIBOSYLTRANSFERASE. THAT THE ENZYME DEFICIENCY RESULTED IN EXCESSIVE PURINE SYNTHESIS SUGGESTS THAT THE ENZYME (OR THE PRODUCT OF ITS FUNCTION) NORMALLY PLAYS A CONTROLLING ROLE IN PURINE METABOLISM. ROSENBLOOM ET AL. (1967) AND MIGEON ET AL. (1968) DEMONSTRATED TWO POPULATIONS OF FIBROB-LASTS, AS REGARDS THE RELEVANT ENZYME ACTIVITY, IN HETEROZYGOUS FEMALES, THUS PROVIDING SUPPORT BOTH FOR X-LINKAGE AND FOR THE LYON HYPOTHESIS. MEGALOBLASTIC ANEMIA HAS BEEN FOUND BY SOME (VAN DER ZEE ET AL., 1968). FUJIMOTO ET AL. (1968) PRESENTED EVIDENCE THAT THE DISEASE CAN BE RECOGNIZED IN THE FETUS WELL BEFORE THE 20 WEEKS WHICH IS CONSIDERED A LIMIT ON THERAPEUTIC ABORTION. THE METHOD USED WAS AN AUTORADIOGRAPHIC TEST FOR HGPRT ACTIVITY, APPLIED TO CELLS OBTAINED BY AMNIOCENTESIS. BOYLE ET AL. (1970) MADE THE PRENATAL DIAGNOSIS AND PERFORMED THERAPEUTIC ABORTION. HENDERSON ET AL. (1969) FOUND THAT THE LOCUS FOR HGPRT IS CLOSELY LINKED TO THE XG LOCUS. SEE *HYPERURICEMIA, ATAXIA, DEAFNESS* FOR A SYNDROME WITH SOME SIMILARITIES TO THE LESCH-NYHAN SYNDROME BUT NORMAL RED CELL HGPRT LEVELS. MCDONALD AND KELLEY (1971) PRESENTED EVIDENCE OF GENETIC HETERO-GENEITY IN THE LESCH-NYHAN SYNDROME. IN THE PATIENT THEY REPORTED, HGPRT SHOWED ALTERED KINETICS.

BLAND, J. H.* (GENERAL CHAIRMAN) SEMINARS ON THE LESCH-NYHAN SYNDROME. FED. PROC. 27* 1017-1112, 1968.

BOYLE, J. A., RAIVIO, K. O., ASTRIN, K. H., SHULMAN, J. D., GRAF, M. L., SEEGMILLER, J. E. AND JACOBSON, C. B.* LESCH-NYHAN SYNDROME* PREVENTIVE CONTROL BY PRENATAL DIAGNOSIS. SCIENCE 169* 688-689, 1970.

COX, R. P., KRAUSS, M. R., BALIS, M. E. AND DANCIS, J.* EVIDENCE FOR TRANSFER OF ENZYME PRODUCT AS THE BASIS OF METABOLIC COOPERATION BETWEEN TISSUE CULTURE FIBROBLASTS OF LESCH-NYHAN DISEASE AND NORMAL CELLS. PROC. NAT. ACAD. SCI. 67* 1573-1579, 1970.

DEMARS, R., SARTO, G., FELIX, J. S. AND BENKE, P.* LESCH-NYHAN MUTATION* PRENATAL DETECTION WITH AMNIOTIC FLUID CELLS. SCIENCE 164* 1303-1305, 1969.

FUJIMOTO, W. Y., SEEGMILLER, J. E., UHLENDORF, B. W. AND JACOBSON, C. B.* BIOCHEMICAL DIAGNOSIS OF X-LINKED DISEASE IN UTERO. (LETTER) LANCET 2* 511-512, 1968.

HENDERSON, J. F., KELLEY, W. N., ROSENBLOOM, F. M. AND SEEGMILLER, J. E.* INHERITANCE OF PURINE PHOSPHORIBOSYLTRANSFERASES IN MAN. AM. J. HUM. GENET. 21* 61-70, 1969.

HOEFNAGEL, D., ANDREW, E. D., MIREAULT, N. G. AND BERNDT, W. O.* HEREDITARY CHOREOATHETOSIS, SELF-MUTILATION AND HYPERURICEMIA IN YOUNG MALES. NEW ENG. J. MED. 273* 130-135, 1965.

KOGUT, M. D., DONNELL, G. N., NYHAN, W. L. AND SWEETMAN, L.* DISORDER OF PURINE METABOLISM DUE TO PARTIAL DEFICIENCY OF HYPOXANTHINE-GUANINE PHOSPHORIBOSYLTRANS-FERASE. AM. J. MED. 48* 148-161, 1970.

MCDONALD, J. A. AND KELLEY, W. N.* LESCH-NYHAN SYNDROME* ALTERED KINETIC PROPERTIES OF MUTANT ENZYMES. SCIENCE 171* 689-691, 1971.

MIGEON, B. R.* X-LINKED HYPOXANTHINE-GUANINE PHOSPHORIBOSYL TRANSFERASE DEFICIENCY* DETECTION OF HETEROZYGOTES BY SELECTIVE MEDIUM. BIOCHEM. GENET. 4* 377-384, 1970.

MIGEON, B. R., DER KALOUSTIAN, V. M., NYHAN, W. L., YOUNG, W. J. AND CHILDS, B.* X-LINKED HYPOXANTHINE-GUANINE PHOSPHORIBOSYL TRANSFERASE DEFICIENCY* HETEROZY-GOTE HAS TWO CLONAL POPULATIONS. SCIENCE 160* 425-427, 1968.

NABHOLZ, M., MIGGIANO, V. AND BODMER, W.* GENETIC ANALYSIS WITH HUMAN-MOUSE SOMATIC CELL HYBRIDS. NATURE 223* 358-363, 1969.

NEWCOMBE, D. S., SHAPIRO, S. L., SHEPPARD, G. L. AND DREIFUSS, F. E.* TREATMENT OF X-LINKED PRIMARY HYPERURICEMIA WITH ALLOPURINOL. J.A.M.A. 198* 315-317, 1966.

NYHAN, W. L., OLIVIER, W. J. AND LESCH, M.* A FAMILIAL DISORDER OF URIC ACID METABOLISM AND CENTRAL NERVOUS SYSTEM FUNCTION. J. PEDIAT. 67* 257-263, 1965.

NYHAN, W. L., RESEK, J., SWEETMAN, L., CARPENTER, D. G. AND CARTER, C. H.* GENETICS OF AN X-LINKED DISORDER OF URIC ACID METABOLISM AND CEREBRAL FUNCTION.

X
L
I
N
K
E
D

PEDIAT. RES. 1* 5-13, 1967.

ROSENBLOOM, F. M., KELLEY, W. N., HENDERSON, J. F. AND SEEGMILLER, J. E.* LYON HYPOTHESIS AND X-LINKED DISEASE. (LETTER) LANCET 2* 305-306, 1967.

ROSENBLOOM, F. M., KELLEY, W. N., MILLER, J., HENDERSON, J. F. AND SEEGMILLER, J. E.* INHERITED DISORDER OF PURINE METABOLISM. CORRELATION BETWEEN CENTRAL NERVOUS SYSTEM DYSFUNCTION AND BIOCHEMICAL DEFECTS. J.A.M.A. 202* 175-177, 1967.

SASS, J. K., ITABASHI, H. H. AND DEXTER, R. A.* JUVENILE GOUT WITH BRAIN INVOLVEMENT. ARCH. NEUROL. 13* 639-655, 1965.

SEEGMILLER, J. E., ROSENBLOOM, F. M. AND KELLEY, W. N.* ENZYME DEFECT ASSO-CIATED WITH A SEX-LINKED HUMAN NEUROLOGICAL DISORDER AND EXCESSIVE PURINE SYNTHESIS. SCIENCE 155* 1682-1684, 1967.

SHAPIRO, S. L., SHEPPARD, G. L., JR., DREIFUSS, F. E. AND NEWCOMBE, D. S.* X-LINKED RECESSIVE INHERITANCE OF A SYNDROME OF MENTAL RETARDATION WITH HYPERURICE-MIA. PROC. SOC. EXP. BIOL. MED. 122* 609-611, 1966.

SPERLING, O., FRANK, M., OPHIR, R. LIBERMAN, U. A., ADAM, A. AND DE VRIES, A.* PARTIAL DEFICIENCY OF HYPOXANTHINE-GUANINE PHOSPHORIBOSYLTRANSFERASE ASSOCIATED WITH GOUT AND URIC ACID LITHIASIS. EUROP. J. CLIN. BIOL. RES. 15* 942-947, 1970.

VAN DER ZEE, S. P. M., SCHRETLEN, E. D. A. M. AND MONNENS, L. A. H.* MEGALOBLA-STIC ANAEMIA IN THE LESCH-NYHAN SYNDROME. (LETTER) LANCET 1* 1427 ONLY, 1968.

*30810 ICHTHYOSIS

CZORSZ (1928) DESCRIBED A PRESUMED HOMOZYGOUS, AFFECTED FEMALE. IN 1929 OREL FOUND IN THE LITERATURE 10 FAMILIES WITH THE X-LINKED FORM. TURPIN AND HIS COLLEAGUES (1945) DESCRIBED ASSOCIATED CHANGES IN THE FUNDUS OCULI OF AFFECTED MALES. KERR, WELLS AND SANGER (1964) PRESENTED EVIDENCE SUGGESTING THAT THE X-LINKED ICHTHYOSIS LOCUS MAY BE WITHIN 'MAPPABLE' DISTANCE OF THE XG LOCUS. IN ADDITION TO THE GENETIC DIFFERENCE BETWEEN X-LINKED ICHTHYOSIS AND ICHTHYOSIS VULGARIS, CLINICAL AND HISTOLOGIC DIFFERENCES EXIST (WELLS AND JENNINGS, 1967). IN THE X-LINKED FORM ONSET IS AT BIRTH AND SCALP, EARS, NECK AND ONE OR MORE FLEXURES ARE INVOLVED, WITH MORE STRIKING SCALING ON THE ABDOMEN THAN THE BACK AND EXTENSION OF THE SCALING DOWN THE FRONT OF THE LEG ONTO THE DORSUM OF THE FOOT. HISTOLOGICALLY THE EPIDERMIS IS ATROPHIC IN ICHTHYOSIS VULGARIS AND HYPERTROPHIC IN THE X-LINKED VARIETY. CLOSER SITUATION OF THE XG AND ICHTHYOSIS LOCI WAS INDICATED BY STUDIES OF ADAM ET AL. (1969) WHO ESTIMATED THE RECOMBINATION FRACTION AS 0.105 AND OF WENT ET AL. (1969) WHO FOUND A VALUE OF 0.115. CLOSE LINKAGE WITH THE DEUTAN, PROTAN AND G6PD LOCI WAS EXCLUDED (ADAM ET AL., 1969). WENT ET AL. (1969) FOUND MILD ABNORMALITY OF THE SKIN IN ABOUT ONE FOURTH OF HETEROZYGOTES. SCHNYDER (1970) GAVE A USEFUL CLASSIFICATION OF THE INHERITED ICHTHYOSES.

ADAM, A., ZIPRKOWSKI, L., FEINSTEIN, A., SANGER, R., TIPPETT, P., GAVIN, J. AND RACE, R. R.* LINKAGE RELATIONS OF X-BORNE ICHTHYOSIS TO THE XG BLOOD GROUPS AND TO OTHER MARKERS OF THE X IN ISRAELIS. ANN. HUM. GENET. 32* 323-332, 1969.

COCKAYNE, E. A.* INHERITED ABNORMALITIES OF THE SKIN AND ITS APPENDAGES. LONDON* OXFORD U. PRESS, 1933. P. 213.

CZORSZ, B.* MSCHR. UNFALHEILK. MEDIZIN. 2* 180. ALSO Z. HAUT. GESCHLECHTSKR. 26* 463, 1928.

HARRIS, H.* A PEDIGREE OF SEX-LINKED ICHTHYOSIS VULGARIS. ANN. EUGEN. 14* 9 ONLY, 1947.

KERR, C. B. AND WELLS, R. S.* SEX-LINKED ICHTHYOSIS. ANN. HUM. GENET. 29* 33-50, 1965.

KERR, C. B., WELLS, R. S. AND SANGER, R.* X-LINKED ICHTHYOSIS AND THE XG GROUPS. LANCET 2* 1369-1370, 1964.

OREL, H.* DIE VERERBUNG DER ICHTHYOSIS CONGENITA UND DER ICHTHYOSIS VULGARIS. Z. KINDERHEILK. 47* 312-340, 1929.

SCHNYDER, U. W.* INHERITED ICHTHYOSES. ARCH. DERM. 102* 240-252, 1970.

TURPIN, R., DESVIGNES, (NI). AND DEMASSIEUX, (NI)* SEM. HOP. PARIS 21* 343, 1945.

WELLS, R. S. AND JENNINGS, M. C.* X-LINKED ICHTHYOSIS AND ICHTHYOSIS VULGARIS. CLINICAL AND GENETIC DISTINCTIONS IN A SECOND SERIES OF FAMILIES. J.A.M.A. 202* 485-488, 1967.

WENT, L. N., DEGROOT, W. P., SANGER, R., TIPPETT, P. AND GAVIN, J.* X-LINKED ICHTHYOSIS* LINKAGE RELATIONSHIP WITH THE XG BLOOD GROUPS AND OTHER STUDIES IN A LARGE DUTCH KINDRED. ANN. HUM. GENET. 32* 333-346, 1969.

IN THE APPARENTLY UNIQUE FAMILY REPORTED BY LYNCH AND HIS COLLEAGUES FIVE MALES IN THREE GENERATIONS SHOWED BOTH SECONDARY HYPOGONADISM (ASSOCIATED WITH LOW TITERS OF PITUITARY GONADOTROPHIC HORMONES) AND CONGENITAL ICHTHYOSIS. THIS IS CLASSED AS A DEFINITE X-LINKED RECESSIVE TRAIT BECAUSE IF THE SYNDROME WERE INHERITED AS AN AUTOSOMAL DOMINANT, THE ICHTHYOSIS COMPONENT WOULD BE EXPECTED TO HAVE BEEN DISPLAYED BY FEMALES. THE AUTHORS SUGGESTED THAT CLOSE LINKAGE MAY BE RESPONSIBLE FOR THE OCCURRENCE OF HYPOGONADISM WITH ICHTHYOSIS, A WELL-KNOWN X-LINKED TRAIT. HOWEVER, ICHTHYOSIS AND HYPOGONADISM IS LISTED AS A SEPARATE MUTATION SINCE LINKAGE CAN ONLY BE POSTULATED. IF INDEED THE TWO TRAITS ARE DUE TO TWO LINKED GENES ONE CAN SAY WITH 95 PERCENT CONFIDENCE THAT THE RECOMBINATION VALUE IS NOT GREATER THAN 20 PERCENT. THE DISORDER WAS TRANSMITTED BY SIX FEMALES IN WHOM THERE WAS OPPORTUNITY FOR CROSS-OVER.

LYNCH, H. T., OZER, F., MCNUTT, C. W., JOHNSON, J. E. AND JAMPOLSKY, N. A.* SECONDARY MALE HYPOGONADISM AND CONGENITAL ICHTHYOSIS. ASSOCIATION OF TWO RARE GENETIC DISEASES. AM. J. HUM. GENET. 12* 440-447, 1960.

*30830 INCONTINENTIA PIGMENTI

INCONTINENTIA PIGMENTI IS A DISTURBANCE OF SKIN PIGMENTATION INCONSTANTLY ASSOCIATED WITH A VARIETY OF MALFORMATIONS OF THE EYE, TEETH, SKELETON, HEART, ETC. THE PIGMENTARY DISTURBANCE, AN AUTOCHTHONOUS TATTOOING, IS EVIDENT AT OR SOON AFTER BIRTH AND MAY BE PRECEDED BY A PHASE SUGGESTING INFLAMMATION IN THE SKIN. IN THE FULLY DEVELOPED DISEASE, THE SKIN SHOWS SWIRLING PATTERNS OF MELANIN PIGMENTATION, ESPECIALLY ON THE TRUNK, SUGGESTING THE APPEARANCE OF 'MARBLE CAKE.' HISTOLOGICALLY, DEPOSITS OF MELANIN PIGMENT ARE SEEN IN THE CORIUM* THE DESIGNATION WAS BASED ON THE IDEA THAT THE BASAL LAYER OF THE EPIDERMIS IS 'INCONTINENT' OF MELANIN. PEDIGREE PATTERNS SUGGEST X-LINKED DOMINANCE WITH LETHALITY IN THE MALE. THE PHENOTYPE IN THE AFFECTED FEMALES MIGHT BE CONSISTENT WITH RANDOM X CHROMOSOME INACTIVATION AS IN THE LYON HYPOTHESIS.
THE CUTANEOUS PHENOTYPE HAS OTHER INTERESTING FEATURES, NAMELY, THAT IN THE FIRST MONTHS OF LIFE IT HAS SOME CHARACTERISTICS OF AN INFLAMMATORY PROCESS AND THAT THE PIGMENTARY CHANGES HAVE USUALLY DISAPPEARED COMPLETELY BY THE AGE OF 20 YEARS. CAFFEY'S DISEASE (INFANTILE HYPEROSTOSIS), WHICH IS FAMILIAL AND POSSIBLY GENETIC, DISPLAYS A SIMILAR BEHAVIOR, WITH PRONOUNCED SIGNS SUGGESTING AN INFLAMMATORY PROCESS IN MANY BONES WITH SUBSEQUENT QUIESCENCE AND IN MANY CASES DISAPPEARANCE OF ALL EVIDENCE OF PREVIOUS DISEASE. KUSTER AND OLBING (1964) REPORTED A MENTALLY RETARDED WOMAN WITH INCOMPLETE DENTITION AND A HISTORY OF SKIN LESIONS AT BIRTH. SHE HAD ONE SON AND 11 DAUGHTERS. SIX OF THE GIRLS SHOWED INCOMPLETE DENTITION AND INCONTINENTIA PIGMENTI.
CYTOPLASMIC (OR OTHER NONCHROMOSOMAL) INHERITANCE WITH LETHALITY IN THE MALE COULD ALSO ACCOUNT FOR THE PEDIGREE PATTERN. FEATURES OF THE HISTOLOGIC AND CLINICAL PICTURE HAVE SUGGESTED VIRAL ETIOLOGY TO SEVERAL WORKERS (E.G., HABER, 1952). CYTOPLASMIC INCLUSIONS LIKE THOSE OF MOLLUSCUM CONTAGIOSUM HAVE BEEN IDENTIFIED (THOMAS W. MURRELL, JR.* RICHMOND* PERSONAL COMMUNICATION).
AS A THIRD POSSIBILITY, THE PEDIGREE PATTERN IS PROBABLY CONSISTENT ALSO WITH AN AUTOSOME X CHROMOSOME TRANSLOCATION. NO CHROMOSOMAL ABNORMALITY WAS FOUND IN TWO CASES OF INCONTINENTIA PIGMENTI STUDIED BY BENIRSCHKE (PERSONAL COMMUNICATION). IN THE FAMILY STUDIED, THE MOTHER AND TWO DAUGHTERS WERE AFFECTED* THERE HAD BEEN ONE MALE ABORTION. GARROD (1906) MAY HAVE DESCRIBED THE FIRST CASE, A GIRL WITH TYPICAL PIGMENTARY CHANGES TOGETHER WITH MENTAL DEFICIENCY AND TETRAPLEGIA.

CARNEY, R. G. AND CARNEY, R. G., JR.* INCONTINENTIA PIGMENTI. ARCH. DERM. 102* 157-162, 1970.

GARROD, A. E.* PECULIAR PIGMENTATION OF THE SKIN IN AN INFANT. TRANS. CLIN. SOC. LOND. 39* 216 ONLY, 1906.

HABER, H.* THE BLOCH-SULZBERGER SYNDROME (INCONTINENTIA PIGMENTI). BRIT. J. DERM. 64* 129-140, 1952.

KUSTER, F. AND OLBING, H.* INCONTINENTIA PIGMENTI. BERICHT UBER NEUN ERKRANKUNGER IN EINER FAMILIE UND EINEM OBDUKTIONSBEFUND. ANN. PAEDIAT. 202* 92-100, 1964.

LENZ, W.* MEDIZINISCHE GENETIK. EINE EINFUHRUNG IN IHRE GRUNDLAGEN UND PROBLEME. STUTTGART* GEORG THIEME VERLAG, 1961. P. 89.

PFEIFFER, R. A.* ZUR FRAGE DER VERERBUNG DER INCONTINENTIA PIGMENTI BLOCH-SIEMENS. Z. MENSCHL. VERERB. KONSTITUTIONSL. 35* 469-493, 1960.

REED, W. B., CARTER, C. AND COHEN, T. M.* INCONTINENTIA PIGMENTI. DERMATOLOGICA 134* 243-250, 1967.

30840 INTRAUTERINE GROWTH RETARDATION, MICROCEPHALY, AND MENTAL RETARDATION

IN THEIR REPORT ON INTRAUTERINE GROWTH RETARDATION, WARKANY, MONROE AND SUTHERLAND (1961) DESCRIBED A FAMILY IN WHICH FOUR MALES IN THREE GENERATIONS IN A PATTERN CONSISTENT WITH X-LINKED RECESSIVE INHERITANCE SHOWED LOW-BIRTH WEIGHT DESPITE

X
L
I
N
K
E
D

TERM GESTATION AND WERE EITHER STILLBORN OR SHOWED SLOW PHYSICAL AND MENTAL DEVELOPMENT. THREE PRESUMED HETEROZYGOUS FEMALES HAD LOW BIRTH WEIGHT BUT BECAME NORMAL ADULTS CAPABLE OF REPRODUCTION. MICROCEPHALY WAS PRESENT IN THE AFFECTED MALES AND MENTAL RETARDATION REQUIRED INSTITUTIONALIZATION. THIS MAY BE THE SAME CONDITION AS THAT DESCRIBED SIMPLY AS MENTAL RETARDATION IN THIS X-LINKED CATALOG.

WARKANY, J., MONROE, B. B. AND SUTHERLAND, B. S.* INTRAUTERINE GROWTH RETARDA-TION. AM. J. DIS. CHILD. 102* 249-279, 1961.

*30850 IRIS, HYPOPLASIA OF, WITH GLAUCOMA

FRANK-KAMENETZKI (1925) DESCRIBED THIS DISORDER IN TWO RUSSIAN KINDREDS. THE ATROPHY OR HYPOPLASIA OF THE IRIS SEEMED, FROM THE FINDINGS IN YOUNG FAMILY MEMBERS, TO BE PRIMARY AND GLAUCOMA SECONDARY. MAKAROW (CITED BY WAARDENBURG, FRANCESCHETTI, KLEIN, TEXTBOOK, 1961, P. 609) PROBABLY DESCRIBED THE SAME DISORDER, ALSO IN RUSSIA. NO OTHER FAMILIES ARE KNOWN. THE SIMILARITY TO RIEGER'S ANOMALY (SEE DOMINANT CATALOG) IS NOTEWORTHY.

FRANK-KAMENETZKI, S. G.* EINE EIGENARTIGE HEREDITARE GLAUKOMFORM MIT MANGEL DES IRISSTROMAS UND GESCHLECHTSGEBUNDENER VERERBUNG. KLIN. MBL. AUGENHEILK. 74* 133-150, 1925.

30860 JAUNDICE, FAMILIAL OBSTRUCTIVE, OF INFANCY

MCELFRESH (1962) DESCRIBED A FORM OF NEO-NATAL HYPERBILIRUBINEMIA IN SIX MALES OF TWO GENERATIONS IN A PATTERN CONSISTENT WITH X-LINKED RECESSIVE INHERITANCE. ONE AFFECTED MEMBER OF THE EARLIER GENERATION WAS JAUNDICED WITH LIGHT STOOLS FOR THE FIRST FIVE MONTHS OF LIFE. HE WAS 31 AND WELL, WITH TWO NORMAL CHILDREN, AT THE TIME OF REPORT.

MCELFRESH, A. E.* FAMILIAL OBSTRUCTIVE JAUNDICE DURING INFANCY. (ABSTRACT) AM. J. DIS. CHILD. 104* 531-532, 1962.

30870 KALLMANN SYNDROME (SECONDARY, HYPOGONADOTROPIC, HYPOGONADISM WITH ANOSMIA* DYSPLASIA OLFACTOGENITALIS OF DE MORSIER)

AFFECTED MALES SHOW ANOSMIA AND HYPOGONADISM SECONDARY TO LOW GONADOTROPIN PRODUCTION. TRANSMITTING FEMALES HAVE PARTIAL OR COMPLETE ANOSMIA. GONADOTROPINS HAVE TO OUR KNOWLEDGE NOT BEEN STUDIED IN THE CARRIER FEMALES. AFFECTED MALES AT TIMES HAVE CHILDREN. UNILATERAL RENAL AGENESIS HAS OCCURRED IN SOME AFFECTED MALES. ANOSMIA IS DUE TO AGENESIS OF THE OLFACTORY LOBES. WHETHER A MUTATION RESULTING IN ANOSMIA IS SEPARATE FROM THAT FOR THE KALLMANN SYNDROME IS DISCUSSED ELSEWHERE. COLOR BLINDNESS WAS ALSO SEGREGATING IN KALLMANN'S FAMILIES. HOWEVER, THE INFORMATION WAS TOO LIMITED TO GIVE CONCLUSIVE EVIDENCE ON POSSIBLE X-LINKAGE OF THIS SYNDROME. HOCKADAY (1966) DESCRIBED TWO CASES. IN THE SECOND THE FATHER WAS FOUND TO HAVE *COMPLETE ANOSMIA ON TESTING.* ANOSMIA MUST BE INQUIRED ABOUT IN CASES OF HYPOGONADISM SINCE PATIENTS RARELY VOLUNTEER THE INFORMATION. INDEED, THE PATIENT IS SOMETIMES UNAWARE OF ANOSMIA SO THAT TESTS ARE NECESSARY. PITTMAN (1966) FOUND ANOSMIA IN 16 OF 28 CASES OF HYPOGONADOTROPHIC HYPOGONADISM. WITH TREATMENT FERTILITY MAY BE RESTORED IN THESE CASES AND OBSERVATIONS DIFFERENTIA-TING X-LINKED FROM AUTOSOMAL INHERITANCE MAY BE FORTHCOMING. SEE THE AUTOSOMAL RECESSIVE CATALOG FOR POSSIBLE AUTOSOMAL RECESSIVE INHERITANCE OF KALLMANN SYNDROME. BARDIN ET AL. (1969) CONCLUDED THAT THESE PATIENTS HAVE A DEFECT IN BOTH PITUITARY AND LEYDIG CELL FUNCTION. THEY DEMONSTRATED IMPAIRED SECRETION OF FSH AND LH AND LEYDIG CELL INSENSITIVITY TO GONADOTROPIN. SPARKES ET AL. (1968) DESCRIBED HYPOGONADOTROPIC HYPOGONADISM WITH ANOSMIA IN TWO BROTHERS AND IN A HALF-SISTER OF THEIRS. THE THREE AFFECTED SIBS HAD THE SAME MOTHER WHO ALTHOUGH OBVIOUSLY NOT FULLY AFFECTED HAD MINOR SIGNS (LATE MENARCHE AND IRREGULAR MENSES) DESPITE WHICH SHE MANAGED TO HAVE 9 LIVEBORN CHILDREN. THE AFFECTED GIRL HAD NO MENSES OR BREAST DEVELOPMENT AT AGE 18 AND OVARIES WHICH WERE HISTOLOGICALLY EXACTLY LIKE THOSE OF THE FETUS. ANOSMIA WAS PRESENT. THE AUTHORS SUGGESTED X-LINKED INHERITANCE. SCHROFFNER AND FURTH (1970) FOUND FAILURE OF RESPONSE TO CLOMIPHENE, AS MEASURED BY PLASMA LEVELS OF GONADOTROPINS. THE FATHER HAD ANOSMIA. THE FATHER OF ONE OF HOCKADAY'S PATIENT'S ALSO HAD ANOSMIA (1966).

BARDIN, C. W., ROSS, G. T., RIFKIND, A. B., CARGILLE, C. M. AND LIPSETT, M. B.* STUDIES OF THE PITUITARY-LEYDIG CELL AXIS IN YOUNG MEN WITH HYPOGONADOTROPIC HYPOGONADISM AND HYPOSMIA* COMPARISON WITH NORMAL MEN, PREPUBERAL BOYS, AND HYPOPITUITARY PATIENTS. J. CLIN. INVEST. 48* 2046-2056, 1969.

HENKIN, R. I.* ABNORMALITIES OF TASTE AND OLFACTION IN PATIENTS WITH CHROMATIN NEGATIVE GONADAL DYSGENESIS. J. CLIN. ENDOCR. 27* 1436-1440, 1967.

HOCKADAY, T. D. R.* HYPOGONADISM AND LIFE-LONG ANOSMIA. POSTGRAD. MED. J. 42* 572-574, 1966.

KALLMANN, F. J., SCHOENFELD, W. A. AND BARRERA, S. E.* THE GENETIC ASPECTS OF PRIMARY EUNUCHOIDISM. AM. J. MENT. DEFIC. 48* 203-236, 1944.

NOWAKOWSKI, H. AND LENZ, W.* GENETIC ASPECTS IN MALE HYPOGONADISM. RECENT PROGR. HORMONE RES. 17* 53-95, 1961.

PAULSEN, C. A.* FAMILIAL HYPOGONADOTROPIC HYPOGONADISM WITH ANOSMIA. ARCH. INTERN. MED. 121* 534-538, 1968.

PITTMAN, J.* BOSTON, MASS.* PERSONAL COMMUNICATION, 1966.

SCHROFFNER, W. G. AND FURTH, E. D.* HYPOGONADOTROPIC HYPOGONADISM WITH ANOSMIA (KALLMANN'S SYNDROME) UNRESPONSIVE TO CLOMIPHENE CITRATE. J. CLIN. ENDOCR. 31* 267-270, 1970.

SPARKES, R. S., SIMPSON, R. W. AND PAULSEN, C. A.* FAMILIAL HYPOGONADOTROPIC HYPOGONADISM WITH ANOSMIA. ARCH. INTERN. MED. 121* 534-538, 1968.

*30880 KERATOSIS FOLLICULARIS SPINULOSA DECALVANS CUM OPHIASI

AFFECTED MEN SHOW THICKENING OF THE SKIN OF THE NECK, EARS, AND EXTREMITIES, ESPECIALLY THE PALMS AND SOLES, LOSS OF EYEBROWS, EYELASHES AND BEARD, THICKENING OF THE EYELIDS WITH BLEPHARITIS AND ECTROPION, AND CORNEAL DEGENERATION. THE TERM 'CUM OPHIASI' MEANS 'WITH OPHIASIS,' I.E., BALDNESS IN ONE OR MORE WINDING STREAKS ABOUT THE HEAD. THE TERM COMES FROM THE GREEK FOR SNAKE. DECALVANS REFERS TO THE LOSS OF HAIR. AUTOSOMAL DOMINANT INHERITANCE HAS ALSO BEEN DESCRIBED (THELEN 1940).

IN SIEMENS' PUBLICATION POINTING OUT X-LINKED INHERITANCE, TWO FAMILIES WERE DESCRIBED. IN THE ONE NOT OBSERVED PERSONALLY BY SIEMENS (DESCRIBED BY LAMERIS, 1905, AND BY ROCHAT, 1906) THE INHERITANCE APPEARED TO BE X-LINKED RECESSIVE, WHEREAS THE OTHER WAS AN EXAMPLE OF X-LINKED DOMINANT (OR INTERMEDIATE) INHERI- TANCE. THE LAMERIS KINDRED WAS STUDIED FURTHER BY JONKERS (1950) AND THE PEDIGREE WAS REPRODUCED BY WAARDENBURG, FRANCESCHETTI, AND KLEIN (GENETICS AND OPHTHALMOLO- GY, VOL. I, 1961). RESTUDY INDICATED THAT THE INHERITANCE IS THE SAME AS IN SIEMENS' PEDIGREE.

JONKERS, G. H.* HYPERKERATOSIS FOLLICULARIS AND CORNEA DEGENERATION. OPHTHAL- MOLOGICA 120* 365-367, 1950.

LAMERIS, (NI)* ICHTHYOSIS FOLLICULARIA. NEDERL. T. GENEESK. P. 1524, 1905.

ROCHAT, (NI)* LA PARALIPIE DE L'OCULOMATOEUR EXTERNE D'ORIGINE AURICULAIRE. ARCH. INTERNAT. LARYNG. 21* 125-131, 1906.

SENDI, H.* QUELQUES CAS DE KERATOSIS FOLLICULARIS SPINULOSA DECALVANS (SIE- MENS). M.D. THESIS, GENEVA, 1957.

SIEMENS, H. W.* UEBER EINEN IN DER MENSCHLICHEN PATHOLOGIE NOCH NICHT BEOBACH- TETEN VERERBUNGSMODUS* DOMINANTGE-SCHLECHTSGEBUNDENE VERERBUNG. ARCH. RASS.-U. GES. BIOL. 17* 47-61, 1925.

30890 LEBER'S OPTIC ATROPHY

PART OF THE DIFFICULTY IN STUDYING THE GENETICS OF THIS DISORDER ARISES FROM DIAGNOSTIC CONFUSION IN A DISEASE CATEGORY WHICH IS ALMOST CERTAINLY HETERO- GENEOUS. THERE ARE MANY PECULIARITIES TO THE FAMILIAL DISTRIBUTION OF LEBER'S OPTIC ATROPHY. IN EUROPEANS 84.8 PERCENT OF CASES ARE MALE BUT IN JAPANESE ONLY 59.1 PERCENT. IN EUROPEANS THE PEAK AGE OF ONSET SEEMS TO BE ABOUT AGE 20 YEARS. THE DISORDER IS USUALLY TRANSMITTED THROUGH THE MOTHER. NINETY-FIVE PER CENT OF AFFECTED MALES APPARENTLY GET THEIR DISEASE FROM THE MOTHER, SOME OF WHOM (ABOUT A SEVENTH) ARE AFFECTED WHEREAS THE REMAINDER HAVE AFFECTED RELATIVES. EIGHTY-FOUR PERCENT OF AFFECTED FEMALES GET THEIR DISEASE FROM THE MOTHER AND ABOUT HALF OF THEIR MOTHERS ARE AFFECTED.

RECENT STUDIES RAISE DOUBTS ABOUT WHETHER MALES EVER TRANSMIT THE CONDITION. FURTHERMORE, THE INTERRELATIONSHIP OF A GENETIC FACTOR WITH AN ENVIRONMENTAL FACTOR (PERHAPS TOBACCO) HAS BEEN RAISED (WILSON, 1963, 1965). THE GENETIC COMPONENT MAY WELL PROVE TO BE AUTOSOMAL. IMAI AND MORIWAKI SUGGEST CYTOPLASMIC INHERITANCE. WILSON (1965) HAS SUGGESTED THAT THIS GENERALIZED NEUROLOGIC DISEASE RESULTS FROM CYANIDE INTOXICATION BECAUSE CYANIDE IN THE DIET AND IN TOBACCO SMOKE IS FOR GENETIC REASONS NOT ADEQUATELY DETOXIFIED TO THIOCYANATE.

BELL, J.* HEREDITARY OPTIC ATROPHY (LEBER'S DISEASE). IN, TREASURY OF HUMAN INHERITANCE. LONDON* CAMBRIDGE UNIV. PRESS, 2* 325-423, 1933.

IMAI, Y. AND MORIWAKI, D.* A PROBABLE CASE OF CYTOPLASMIC INHERITANCE IN MAN* A CRITIQUE OF LEBER'S DISEASE. J. GENET. HUM. 33* 163-167, 1936.

WAARDENBURG, P. J.* BEITRAG ZUR VERERBUNG DER FAMILIAREN SEHNERVENATROPHIE (LEBERSCHEN KRANKHEIT). KLIN. MBL. AUGENHEILK. 73* 619-652, 1924.

WILSON, J.* LEBER'S HEREDITARY OPTIC ATROPHY* A POSSIBLE DEFECT OF CYANIDE METABOLISM. CLIN. SCI. 29* 505-515, 1965.

WILSON, J.* LEBER'S HEREDITARY OPTIC ATROPHY* SOME CLINICAL AND AETIOLOGICAL CONSIDERATIONS. BRAIN 86* 347-362, 1963.

*30900 LOWE'S OCULOCEREBRORENAL SYNDROME

X
L
I
N
K
E
D

THE FEATURES ARE HYDROPHTHALMIA, CATARACT, MENTAL RETARDATION, VITAMIN D RESISTANT RICKETS, AMINOACIDURIA, AND REDUCED AMMONIA PRODUCTION BY THE KIDNEY. STREIFF AND COLLEAGUES (1958) SUGGESTED X-LINKAGE BECAUSE ALL CASES ARE MALE AND AFFECTED BROTHERS HAVE BEEN DESCRIBED. IN ONE CASE TWO BROTHERS AND A COUSIN (THE MOTHERS WERE SISTERS) WERE AFFECTED. BY SLIT LAMP RICHARDS AND COLLEAGUES (1965) FOUND LENS OPACITIES IN HETEROZYGOTES. AMINOACIDURIA IN THE MOTHER OF A PATIENT, AFTER LOADING WITH ORNITHINE, WAS REPORTED AS A HETEROZYGOTE MANIFESTATION BY CHUTORIAN AND ROWLAND (1966) AND A HIGH INCIDENCE OF MATERNAL CATARACT HAS BEEN NOTED. MCCANCE, MATHESON, GRESHAM AND ELKINTON (1960) DESCRIBED A CONDITION WHICH IS PROBABLY QUITE DISTINCT BUT WHICH MAY ALSO BE X-LINKED, THEIR SUBJECTS HAVING BEEN TWO BROTHERS WITH UNRELATED UNAFFECTED PARENTS. FEATURES WERE POOR APPETITE, FAILURE TO GROW, CORNEAL OPACITIES, PARTIAL BLINDNESS, NYSTAGMUS, MENTAL RETARDA- TION, INTENTION TREMOR, HYPERCHLOREMIC ACIDOSIS, VERY ACID URINE, DEFECT IN URINARY PRODUCTION OF AMMONIUM ION, DEATH FROM PROGRESSIVE RENAL FAILURE, UNDERDEVELOPED GLOMERULI, STRUCTURAL ABNORMALITIES IN THE BRAIN, AND ABSENCE OF TESTES. SVORC ET AL. (1967) DESCRIBED AN AFFECTED FEMALE CHILD AND REFERRED TO TWO OTHERS IN THE LITERATURE. SUCH CASES MAY HAVE A DIFFERENT GENETIC MECHANISM THAN X-LINKAGE OR MAY REPRESENT INFELICITOUS LYONIZATION IN HETEROZYGOUS FEMALES. MATSUDA ET AL. (1969) DESCRIBED A JAPANESE BOY WITH TYPICAL CLINICAL FEATURES OF LOWE'S SYNDROME, BUT THE METABOLIC ACIDOSIS WAS SHOWN TO BE DUE TO FAILURE NOT OF URINARY ACIDIFICATION BUT OF BICARBONATE REABSORPTION. MATSUDA ET AL. (1970) SUGGESTED THAT THIS IS A SPECIAL TYPE OF LOWE'S SYNDROME AND THAT IT MAY HAVE AUTOSOMAL RECESSIVE INHERITANCE. HE SUGGESTED THAT THE CASES DESCRIBED BY OETLIKER AND ROSSI (1969) WERE OF THIS TYPE. IN MATSUDA'S STUDY THE FATHER SHOWED AMINOACIDURIA AFTER ORNITHINE LOADING. MILD 'SNOWFLAKE' LENTICULAR OPACITIES IN CARRIER FEMALES WERE DESCRIBED BY MARTIN AND CARSON (1967).

ACKER, K. J., ROELS, H., BEELAERTS, W., PASTERNACK, A. AND VALCKE, R.* THE HISTOLOGIC LESIONS OF THE KIDNEY IN THE OCULO-CEREBRO-RENAL SYNDROME OF LOWE. NEPHRON 4* 193-214, 1967.

AURICCHIO, S., FRISCHKNECHT, W. AND SHMERLING, D.* PRIMARE TUBULOPATHIEN. III. EIN FALL VON OCULO-CEREBRO-RENALEM SYNDROM (LOWE-SYNDROME). HELV. PAEDIAT. ACTA 16* 647-655, 1961.

CHUTORIAN, A. AND ROWLAND, L. P.* LOWE'S SYNDROME. NEUROLOGY 16* 115-122, 1966.

HARRIS, L. S., GITTER, K. A., GALIN, M. A. AND PLECHATY, G. P.* OCULO-CEREBRO- RENAL SYNDROME. REPORT OF A CASE IN A BABY GIRL. BRIT. J. OPHTHAL. 54* 278-280, 1970.

LOWE, C. U.* OCULO-CEREBRAL-RENAL SYNDROME. MAANDSCHR. KINDERGENESK. 28* 77- 80, 1960.

LOWE, C. U., TERREY, M. AND MACLACHLAN, E. A.* ORGANIC-ACIDURIA, DECREASED RENAL AMMONIA PRODUCTION, HYDROPHTHALMOS, AND MENTAL RETARDATION. AM. J. DIS. CHILD. 83* 164-184, 1952.

MATSUDA, I., SUGAI, M. AND KAJII, T.* ORNITHINE LOADING TEST IN LOWE'S SYNDROME. J. PEDIAT. 77* 127-129, 1970.

MATSUDA, I., TAKEDA, T., SUGAI, M. AND MATSUURA, N.* OCULOCEREBRORENAL SYNDROME. AM. J. DIS. CHILD. 117* 205-212, 1969.

MARTIN, V. A. F. AND CARSON, N. A. J.* INBORN METABOLIC DISORDERS WITH ASSOCIATED OCULAR LESIONS IN NORTHERN IRELAND. TRANS. OPHTHAL. SOC. U.K. 87* 847- 870, 1967.

MCCANCE, R. A., MATHESON, W. J., GRESHAM, G. A. AND ELKINTON, J. R.* THE CEREBRO-OCULAR-RENAL DYSTROPHIES* A NEW VARIANT. ARCH. DIS. CHILD. 35* 240-249, 1960.

OETLIKER, O. AND ROSSI, E.* THE INFLUENCE OF EXTRACELLULAR FLUID VOLUME ON THE RENAL BICARBONATE THRESHOLD* A STUDY OF TWO CHILDREN WITH LOWE'S SYNDROME. PEDIAT. RES. 3* 140-148, 1969.

PALLISGAARD, G. AND GOLDSCHMIDT, E.* THE OCULO-CEREBRO-RENAL SYNDROME OF LOWE IN FOUR GENERATIONS OF ONE FAMILY. ACTA PAEDIAT. SCAND. 60* 146-148, 1971.

RICHARDS, W., DONNELL, G. N., WILSON, W. A., STOWENS, D. AND PERRY, T.* THE OCULO-CEREBRO-RENAL SYNDROME OF LOWE. AM. J. DIS. CHILD. 109* 185-203, 1965.

STREIFF, E. B., STRAUB, W. AND GOLAY, L.* LES MANIFESTATIONS OCULAIRES DU SYNDROME DE LOWE. OPHTHALMOLOGICA 135* 632-639, 1958.

SVORC, J., MASOPUST, J., KOMARKOVA, A., MACEK, M. AND HYANEK, J.* OCULOCERE- BRORENAL SYNDROME IN A FEMALE CHILD. AM. J. DIS. CHILD. 114* 186-190, 1967.

WILSON, W. A., RICHARDS, W. AND DONNELL, G. N.* OCULO-CEREBRAL-RENAL SYNDROME OF LOWE* A REVIEW OF EIGHT CASES NOTING THE GENETIC INHERITANCE. ARCH. OPHTHAL. 70* 5-11, 1963.

X
L
I
N
K
E
D

WITZLEBEN, C. L., SCHOEN, E. J., TU, W. H. AND MCDONALD, L. W.* PROGRESSIVE MORPHOLOGIC RENAL CHANGES IN THE OCULO-CEREBRO-RENAL SYNDROME OF LOWE. AM. J. MED. 44* 319-324, 1968.

*30910 MACULAR DYSTROPHY

HALBERTSMA'S PEDIGREE IS CONSISTENT WITH X-LINKED INHERITANCE EXCEPT FOR AN INSTANCE OF APPARENT FATHER-TO-SON TRANSMISSION IN THE FIRST GENERATION. COLOR BLINDNESS ALSO WAS SEGREGATING IN HALBERTSMA'S FAMILY, BUT ANALYSIS IN TERMS OF LINKAGE IS IMPOSSIBLE BECAUSE IN THOSE MALES WITH MACULAR DYSTROPHY THE RETINAL DISEASE MAY HAVE BEEN RESPONSIBLE FOR THE COLOR BLINDNESS. FALLS (1952) STUDIED A FAMILY OF X-LINKED MACULAR DYSTROPHY WITH AFFECTED IDENTICAL MALE TWINS. A CYSTIC MACULOPATHY MAY BE THE ONLY FINDING IN X-LINKED RETINOSCHISIS (Q.V.).

FALLS, H. F.* THE ROLE OF THE SEX CHROMOSOME IN HEREDITARY OCULAR PATHOLOGY. TRANS. AM. OPHTHAL. SOC. 50* 421-467, 1952.

HALBERTSMA, K. T. A.* UEBER EINIGE ERBLICHE FAMILIARE AUGENERKRANKUNGEN. I. ERBLICHE FAMILIARE ENTARTUNG DES GELBEN FLECKES (ZUSAMMEN MIT FARBENBLINDHEIT). KLIN. MBL. AUGENHEILK. 80* 794-812, 1928.

30920 MANIC-DEPRESSIVE PSYCHOSIS

WINOKUR AND TANNA (1969) SUGGESTED X-LINKED DOMINANT INHERITANCE. THE EVIDENCE IS WEAK, AT THE BEST.

WINOKUR, G. AND TANNA, V. L.* POSSIBLE ROLE OF X-LINKED DOMINANT FACTOR IN MANIC DEPRESSIVE DISEASE. DIS. NERV. SYST. 30* 89-94, 1969.

*30930 MEGALOCORNEA

AFFECTED MALES SHOW LARGE CORNEA AS AN ISOLATED DEFECT. HETEROZYGOUS WOMEN MAY SHOW SLIGHT INCREASE IN CORNEAL DIAMETER (RIDDELL, 1941). AUTOSOMAL DOMINANT INHERITANCE IS PROBABLY MUCH RARER. MEGALOCORNEA OCCURS AT TIMES AS PART OF THE MARFAN SYNDROME (INHERITED AS AN AUTOSOMAL DOMINANT).

GRONHOLM, V.* UEBER DIE VERERBUNG DER MEGALOKORNEA NEBST EINEM BEITRAG ZUR FRAGE DES GENETISCHEN ZUSAMMENHANGES ZWISCHEN MEGALOKORNEA UND HYDROPHTHALMUS. (TWO PRESUMED HOMOZYGOUS FEMALES OCCURRED IN THIS FAMILY). KLIN. MBL. AUGENHEILK. 67* 1-15, 1921.

RIDDELL, W. J. B.* UNCOMPLICATED HEREDITARY MEGALOCORNEA. ANN. EUGEN. 11* 102-107, 1941.

*30940 MENKES SYNDROME (KINKY HAIR DISEASE)

IN A FAMILY OF ENGLISH-IRISH DESCENT LIVING IN NEW YORK, MENKES AND COLLEAGUES (1962) DESCRIBED AN X-LINKED RECESSIVE DISORDER CHARACTERIZED BY EARLY RETARDATION IN GROWTH, PECULIAR HAIR AND FOCAL CEREBRAL AND CEREBELLAR DEGENERATION. SEVERE NEUROLOGIC IMPAIRMENT BEGAN WITHIN A MONTH OR TWO OF BIRTH AND PROGRESSED RAPIDLY TO DECEREBRATION. FIVE MALES WERE AFFECTED BUT THE GENE COULD BY INFERENCE BE IDENTIFIED IN FOUR GENERATIONS. THE FAILURE TO GROW BROUGHT THE AFFECTED INFANTS TO MEDICAL ATTENTION AT THE AGE OF A FEW WEEKS AND DEATH OCCURRED IN THE FIRST OR SECOND YEAR OF LIFE. THE HAIR WAS STUBBY AND WHITE. MICROSCOPICALLY IT SHOWED TWISTING, VARYING DIAMETER ALONG THE LENGTH OF THE SHAFT AND OFTEN FRACTURES OF THE SHAFT AT REGULAR INTERVALS. RATHER EXTENSIVE BIOCHEMICAL INVESTIGATIONS SHOWED ELEVATED PLASMA GLUTAMIC ACID AS THE ONLY CONSISTENT ABNORMALITY. THE ANATOMIC CHANGE IN THE CENTRAL NERVOUS SYSTEM WAS DESCRIBED ON THE BASIS OF TWO AUTOPSIES. BRAY (1965) OBSERVED TWO BROTHERS WHO DIED AS INFANTS WITH SPASTIC DEMENTIA, SEIZURES AND DEFECTIVE HAIR. BLOOD AND URINE AMINO ACIDS WERE NORMAL. WHETHER THIS IS THE SAME DISORDER AS THAT IN MENKES' FAMILY IS UNCLEAR. THE CONDITION DESCRIBED BY YOSHIDA ET AL. (1964) MAY BE THE SAME. FRENCH AND SHERARD (1967) PRESENTED EVIDENCE THAT THIS DISORDER MAY REPRESENT AN ABNORMALITY OF LIPID METABOLISM. THEIR 16 MONTH OLD PATIENT SHOWED (1) SCANT, WHITISH, LACKLUSTER, KINKY HAIR WHICH MICROSCOPICALLY SHOWED PILI TORTI, MONILETHRIX AND TRICHORRHEXIS NODOSA, (2) RETARDED GROWTH, (3) MICROGNATHIA AND HIGHLY ARCHED PALATE, (4) DECLINE IN MENTAL DEVELOPMENT, (5) ONSET OF FOCAL AND GENERALIZED SEIZURES, (6) SPASTIC QUADRIPARESIS WITH CLENCHED FISTS, OPISTHOTONOS AND SCISSORING. BIOCHEMICAL STUDIES SHOWED DEPRESSED SERUM TOCOPHEROL AND NORMAL AMINO ACID CONTENT OF HAIR SERUM AND URINE. AN ABNORMAL AUTOFLUORESCENCE IS DISPLAYED BY HAIR AND BY PURKINJE CELLS AXONS. 'KINKY HAIR DISEASE' HAS PROVED A DESIGNATION USEFUL IN DETECTION OF NEW CASES, SINCE THE HAIR CHANGE IS AN EASILY REMEMBERED FEATURE BY WHICH PHYSICIANS CAN BE ALERTED TO THE CONDITION (O'BRIEN, 1968).

BRAY, P. F.* SEX-LINKED NEURODEGENERATIVE DISEASE ASSOCIATED WITH MONILETHRIX. PEDIATRICS 36* 417-420, 1965.

FRENCH, J. H. AND SHERARD, E. S.* STUDIES OF THE BIOCHEMICAL BASIS OF KINKY HAIR DISEASE. PRS, 1967.

MENKES, J. H., ALTER, M., STEIGLEDER, G. K., WEAKLEY, D. R. AND SUNG, J. H.* A SEX-LINKED RECESSIVE DISORDER WITH RETARDATION OF GROWTH, PECULIAR HAIR AND FOCAL

X
L
I
N
K
E
D

O'BRIEN, J. S.* LOS ANGELES, CALIF.* PERSONAL COMMUNICATION, 1968.

YOSHIDA, T., TADA, K., MIZUNO, T., WADA, Y., AKABANE, J., OGASAWARA, J., MINAGAWA, A., MORIKAWA, T. AND OKAMURA, T.* A SEX-LINKED DISORDER WITH MENTAL AND PHYSICAL RETARDATION CHARACTERIZED BY CEREBROCORTICAL ATROPHY AND INCREASE OF GLUTAMIC ACID IN THE CEREBROSPINAL FLUID. TOHOKU J. MED. SCI. 83* 261-269, 1964.

*30950 MENTAL DEFICIENCY

AMONG THE NUMEROUS TYPES OF MENTAL DEFICIENCY AN HEREDITARY X-LINKED FORM EXISTS. AN APPARENTLY X-LINKED NON-PROGRESSIVE FORM OF MENTAL DEFICIENCY WITHOUT EVIDENT SOMATIC MALFORMATION AND WITHOUT MOTOR OR SENSORY DYSFUNCTION WAS DESCRIBED BY MARTIN AND BELL (1943) AND POSSIBLY THE SAME MUTATION WAS DESCRIBED BY ALLAN AND HERNDON (1944). PRIEST AND COLLEAGUES (1961), AS WELL AS OTHERS, FOUND MORE MALES IN STATE INSTITUTIONS FOR MENTAL DEFECTIVES AND FOUND THAT AFFECTED SIBS WERE MORE OFTEN MALE. HOWEVER, MALES ARE PROBABLY MORE LIKELY TO BE INSTITUTIONALIZED. FURTHERMORE, SEVERAL AUTOSOMAL CONDITIONS SHOW A MALE PREPONDERANCE WHICH ALMOST CERTAINLY HAS A BASIS OTHER THAN X-LINKAGE IN A PROPORTION OF CASES. ANOTHER KINDRED WITH CONVINCINGLY X-LINKED MENTAL RETARDATION WAS REPORTED BY RENPENNING AND HIS COLLEAGUES (1962). LUBS (1969) FOUND A MARKER X CHROMOSOME CONSISTING OF A SECONDARY CONSTRICTION NEAR THE END OF THE LONG ARM GIVING THE APPEARANCE OF LARGE SATELLITES. THE ANOMALOUS CHROMOSOME WAS NOT PERFERENTIALLY LYONIZED AS OCCURS WITH AN ISOCHROMOSOME X FOR EXAMPLE. THE HEMIZYGOUS MALES HAD MENTAL RETARDATION. THE AUTHOR THOUGHT THAT EITHER THE ANOMALOUS REGION ITSELF OR A CLOSELY LINKED RECESSIVE GENE MIGHT ACCOUNT FOR THE X-LINKED INHERITANCE OF MENTAL DEFICIENCY IN THIS FAMILY. TURNER ET AL. (1970) EMPHASIZED THE LACK OF PHYSICAL ABNORMALITY IN THIS DISORDER.

ALLAN, W. AND HERNDON, C. N.* RETINITIS PIGMENTOSA AND APPARENTLY SEX-LINKED IDIOCY IN A SINGLE SIBSHIP. J. HERED. 35* 41-43, 1944.

ALLAN, W., HERNDON, C. N. AND DUDLEY, F. C.* SOME EXAMPLES OF THE INHERITANCE OF MENTAL DEFICIENCY* APPARENTLY SEX-LINKED IDIOCY AND MICROCEPHALY. AM. J. MENT. DEFIC. 48* 325-334, 1944.

LOSOWSKI, M. S.* HEREDITARY MENTAL DEFECT SHOWING THE PATTERN OF SEX INFLUENCE. J. MENT. DEFIC. RES. 5* 60-62, 1961.

LUBS, H. A.* A MARKER X CHROMOSOME. AM. J. HUM. GENET. 21* 231-244, 1969.

MARTIN, J. P. AND BELL, J.* A PEDIGREE OF MENTAL DEFECT SHOWING SEX-LINKAGE. J. NEUROL. PSYCHIAT. 6* 154-157, 1943.

PRIEST, J. H., THULINE, H. C., LAVECK, G. D. AND JARVIS, D. B.* AN APPROACH TO GENETIC FACTORS IN MENTAL RETARDATION. STUDIES OF FAMILIES CONTAINING AT LEAST TWO SIBLINGS ADMITTED TO A STATE INSTITUTION FOR THE RETARDED. AM. J. MENT. DEFIC. 66* 42-50, 1961.

RENPENNING, H., GERRARD, J. W., ZALESKI, W. A. AND TABATA, T.* FAMILIAL SEX-LINKED MENTAL RETARDATION. CANAD. MED. ASS. J. 87* 954-956, 1962.

ROSANOFF, A. J.* SEX-LINKED INHERITANCE IN MENTAL DEFICIENCY. AM. J. PSYCHIAT. 11* 289-297, 1931.

SNYDER, R. D. AND ROBINSON, A.* RECESSIVE SEX-LINKED MENTAL RETARDATION IN THE ABSENCE OF OTHER RECOGNIZABLE ABNORMALITIES. REPORT OF A FAMILY. CLIN. PEDIAT. 8* 669-674, 1969.

TURNER, G., TURNER, B. AND COLLINS, E.* RENPENNING'S SYNDROME - X-LINKED RETARDATION. J. DEVEL. MED. CHILD. NEUROL., IN PRESS, 1970.

WORTIS, H., POLLACK, M. AND WORTIS, J.* FAMILIES WITH TWO OR MORE MENTALLY RETARDED OR MENTALLY DISTURBED SIBLINGS* THE PREPONDERANCE OF MALES. AM. J. MENT. DEFIC. 70* 745-752, 1966.

30960 MENTAL RETARDATION AND MUSCULAR ATROPHY

ALLAN, HERNDON AND DUDLEY (1943-44) DESCRIBED A PHENOMENAL FAMILY IN WHICH MANY AFFECTED MALES HAD, IN ADDITION TO MENTAL RETARDATION, MUSCULAR WEAKNESS FIRST NOTED AT ABOUT SIX MONTHS BY INABILITY TO HOLD UP THE HEAD (GIVING THE FAMILY'S DESIGNATION OF 'LIMBER-NECK'). WALKING WAS DELAYED OR NEVER ACHIEVED. SPEECH WAS ALMOST UNINTELLIGIBLE. MUSCULAR ATROPHY AND WEAKNESS WAS GENERALIZED. CONTRACTURES OF THE HAMSTRING RESULTED IN PECULIAR STANCE.

ALLAN, W., HERNDON, C. N. AND DUDLEY, F. C.* SOME EXAMPLES OF THE INHERITANCE OF MENTAL DEFICIENCY* APPARENTLY SEX-LINKED IDIOCY AND MICROCEPHALY. AM. J. MENT. DEFIC. 48* 325-334, 1943-44.

30970 MICROPHTHALMIA

X
L
I
N
K
E
D

IN STEPHEN'S CASES WHITE OPACIFICATION OF THE CORNEA (POSSIBLY THIS SHOULD BE TERMED SCLEROCORNEA) AND BLINDNESS WERE PRESENT. ROBERTS' CASES ALSO HAD CORNEAL CHANGE. MENTAL DEFICIENCY WAS PRESENT IN SOME IN ROBERTS' FAMILY, BUT INTELLIGENCE WAS NORMAL IN AT LEAST TWO OF SIX CASES OF MICROPHTHALMIA EXAMINED. NO MENTAL DEFECT WAS PRESENT EXCEPT IN MICROPHTHALMIA CASES. ON THE OTHER HAND, STEPHENS' CASES WERE OF UNIVERSITY LEVEL OF INTELLIGENCE. SJOGREN AND LARSSON (1949) DESCRIBED MICROPHTHALMIA AND OLIGOPHRENIA BEHAVING AS AN AUTOSOMAL RECESSIVE SYNDROME.

ANOPHTHALMIA AND MICROPHTHALMIA ARE TERMS USED INTERCHANGEABLY. THE FAMILY REPORTED BY HOEFNAGEL, KEENAN, AND ALLEN (1963) WAS PROBABLY ONE OF X-LINKED MICROPHTHALMIA. MOST CASES OF TRUE ANOPHTHALMOS HAVE BEEN RECESSIVE (Q.V.). PSEUDOGLIOMA, MICROPHTHALMIA AND NORRIE'S DISEASE ARE CONFUSED IN THE LITERATURE (WARBURG, 1966). THE AFFECTED PERSONS IN ROBERTS' PEDIGREE (ORIGINALLY REPORTED BY ASH IN 1922) WERE CLEARLY INSTANCES OF NORRIE'S DISEASE. IN ONLY ABOUT HALF OF THE CASES WAS THE EYE MICROPHTHALMIC OR MORE PRECISELY PHTHISICAL. HISTOLOGIC STUDY OF THE EYE IN ONE MENTALLY RETARDED BLIND BOY FROM THIS FAMILY (WHITNALL AND NORMAN, 1940) SHOWED CHANGES LIKE THOSE OBSERVED BY WARBURG IN NORRIE'S DISEASE (Q.V.). STEPHENS' PATIENTS ARE MORE DIFFICULT TO EVALUATE, MAINLY BECAUSE THEY WERE RATHER OLD AT THE TIME OF FIRST EXAMINATION AND INFORMATION IS LIMITED TO THE FACTS THAT THE EYES WERE SMALL AND CORNEAS CLOUDY. WARBURG (1966) THINKS THESE ALSO MAY HAVE BEEN INSTANCES OF NORRIE'S DISEASE. CONGENITAL CATARACT WAS ALSO PRESENT IN SOME OF THE PATIENTS IN A FAMILY REPORTED BY CAPELLA ET AL. (1963). CATARACTS AND MICROPHTHALMIA WAS DOMINANT (Q.V.) IN A SECOND FAMILY THEY REPORTED.

CAPELLA, J. A., KAUFMAN, H. E., LILL, F. J. AND COOPER, G.* HEREDITARY CATARACTS AND MICROPHTHALMIA. AM. J. OPHTHAL. 56* 454-458, 1963.

HOEFNAGEL, D., KEENAN, M. E. AND ALLEN, F. H.* HEREDOFAMILIAL BILATERAL ANOPHTHALMIA. ARCH. OPHTHAL. 69* 760-764, 1963.

ROBERTS, J. A. F.* SEX-LINKED MICROPHTHALMIA SOMETIMES ASSOCIATED WITH MENTAL DEFECT. BRIT. MED. J. 2* 1213-1216, 1937. (IN, WAARDENBURG, P. J., FRANCESCHETTI, A. AND KLEIN, D. (EDS.)* GENETICS AND OPHTHALMOLOGY. SPRINGFIELD, ILL.* CHARLES C THOMAS, 2* 768-770, 1961. THEY THINK THIS WAS AN INSTANCE OF PSEUDOGLIOMA OR OF RETINAL DYSPLASIA.

SJOGREN, T. AND LARSSON, T.* MICROPHTHALMOS AND ANOPHTHALMOS WITH OR WITHOUT COINCIDENT OLIGOPHRENIA. ACTA PSYCHIAT. NEUROL. 56 (SUPPL.)* 1-103, 1949.

STEPHENS, F. E.* A CASE OF SEX-LINKED MICROPHTHALMIA. J. HERED. 38* 307-310, 1947.

WARBURG, M.* COPENHAGEN, DENMARK* PERSONAL COMMUNICATION, 1966.

WHITNALL, S. E. AND NORMAN, R. M.* MICROPHTHALMIA AND VISUAL PATHWAYS, CASE ASSOCIATED WITH BLINDNESS AND IMBECILITY, AND SEX-LINKED. BRIT. J. OPHTHAL. 24* 229-244, 1940.

*30980 MICROPHTHALMIA OR ANOPHTHALMOS, WITH DIGITAL ANOMALIES

THE EYE ANOMALY WAS UNILATERAL IN SOME OF THE AFFECTED PERSONS IN LENZ' REMARKABLE PEDIGREE. NARROW SHOULDERS, DOUBLE THUMBS, OTHER SKELETAL ANOMALIES, AND DENTAL, UROGENITAL AND CARDIOVASCULAR MALFORMATIONS WERE OBSERVED. THE MOTHER OF THE PROBAND, A 13 YEAR OLD BOY BORN BLIND, HAD A DEFORMITY OF THE FIFTH FINGER, SUGGESTING MILD EXPRESSION.

HOEFNAGEL, D., KEENAN, M. E. AND ALLEN, F. H.* HEREDOFAMILIAL BILATERAL ANOPHTHALMIA. ARCH. OPHTHAL. 69* 760-764, 1963.

LENZ, W.* RECESSIV-GESCHLECHTSGEBUNDENE MIKROPHTHALMIE MIT MULTIPLEN MISSBILDUNGEN. ZTSCHR. KINDERHEILK. 77* 384-390, 1955.

*30990 MUCOPOLYSACCHARIDOSIS TYPE II (HUNTER SYNDROME)

THE FORM OF THE HURLER SYNDROME (GARGOYLISM) WHICH IS SEX-LINKED DIFFERS FROM THE AUTOSOMAL TYPE IN BEING ON THE AVERAGE LESS SEVERE AND IN NOT SHOWING CLOUDING OF THE CORNEA. FEATURES ARE DYSOSTOSIS WITH DWARFISM, GROTESQUE FACIES, HEPATOSPLENOMEGALY FROM MUCOPOLYSACCHARIDE DEPOSITS, CARDIOVASCULAR DISORDERS FROM MUCOPOLYSACCHARIDE DEPOSITS IN THE INTIMA, MENTAL RETARDATION, DEAFNESS, EXCRETION OF LARGE AMOUNTS OF CHONDROITIN SULFATE B AND HEPARITIN SULFATE IN THE URINE. DANES AND BEARN (1965) FIND THAT FIBROBLASTS FROM PATIENTS WITH THIS DISORDER SHOW METACHROMATIC CYTOPLASMIC INCLUSIONS AND THAT ABOUT HALF THE FIBROBLASTS OF HETEROZYGOTES SHOW SUCH INCLUSIONS. BERG ET AL. (1968) CONCLUDED THAT THE HUNTER LOCUS AND THE XM LOCUS ARE WITHIN MEASURABLE DISTANCE OF EACH OTHER, THE BEST ESTIMATE OF THE RECOMBINATION FRACTION BEING 0.09.

BERG, K., DANES, B. S. AND BEARN, A. G.* THE LINKAGE RELATION OF THE LOCI FOR THE XM SERUM SYSTEM AND THE X-LINKED FORM OF HURLER'S SYNDROME (HUNTER'S SYNDROME). AM. J. HUM. GENET. 20* 398-401, 1968.

CANTZ, M., CHRAMBACH, A. AND NEUFELD, E. F.* CHARACTERIZATION OF THE FACTOR DEFICIENT IN THE HUNTER SYNDROME BY POLYACRYLAMIDE GEL ELECTROPHORESIS. BIOCHEM.

DANES, B. S. AND BEARN, A. G.* HURLER'S SYNDROME* A GENETIC STUDY OF CLONES IN
CELL CULTURE WITH PARTICULAR REFERENCE TO THE LYON HYPOTHESIS. J. EXP. MED. 126*
509-522, 1967.

DANES, B. S. AND BEARN, A. G.* HURLER'S SYNDROME* DEMONSTRATION OF AN INHERITED
DISORDER OF CONNECTIVE TISSUE IN CELL CULTURE. SCIENCE 149* 987-989, 1965.

GERICH, J. E.* HUNTER'S SYNDROME* BETA-GALACTOSIDASE DEFICIENCY IN SKIN. NEW
ENG. J. MED. 280* 799-802, 1969.

MCKUSICK, V. A.* HERITABLE DISORDERS OF CONNECTIVE TISSUE. ST. LOUIS* C. V.
MOSBY CO., 1966 (3RD ED.).

OCKERMANN, P. A. AND KOHLIN, P.* GLYCOSIDASES IN SKIN AND PLASMA IN HUNTER'S
SYNDROME. ABNORMALITY OF A BETA-GALACTOSIDASE IN SKIN. ACTA PAEDIAT. SCAND. 57*
281-284, 1968.

VAN PELT, J. F.* GARGOYLISM. THESIS, NIJMEGEN, 1960.

31000 MUSCULAR DYSTROPHY, MABRY TYPE

MABRY ET AL. (1965) DESCRIBED A KINDRED WITH 9 MALES AFFECTED BY A LATE-ONSET FORM
OF MUSCULAR DYSTROPHY. THESE AUTHORS THOUGHT IT TO BE DIFFERENT FROM THE TYPES OF
DUCHENNE, BECKER AND DREIFUSS. THEY SUGGESTED THAT IT DIFFERED FROM THE BECKER
TYPE, WHICH IT RESEMBLED MOST CLOSELY, BY EARLIER ONSET (ABOUT PUBERTY) AND SOME
HISTOLOGICAL FEATURES.

MABRY, C. C., ROECKEL, I. E., MUNICH, R. L. AND ROBERTSON, D.* X-LINKED
PSEUDOHYPERTROPHIC MUSCULAR DYSTROPHY WITH A LATE ONSET AND SLOW PROGRESSION. NEW
ENG. J. MED. 273* 1062-1070, 1965.

*31010 MUSCULAR DYSTROPHY, PROGRESSIVE, TARDIVE TYPE OF BECKER

THE ONSET IS OFTEN IN THE 20'S AND 30'S AND SURVIVAL TO A RELATIVELY ADVANCED AGE
IS FREQUENT. SEVERAL AFFECTED MALES IN BECKER'S LARGE KINDRED HAD PRODUCED
CHILDREN AND THE RESULTING PEDIGREE PATTERN WAS CONSISTENT WITH X-LINKED INHERI-
TANCE. OTHERS HAVE DESCRIBED SUCH FAMILIES. ALLELISM WITH THE DUCHENNE TYPE IS
POSSIBLE. LINKAGE STUDIES MIGHT ESTABLISH NON-ALLELISM AS IN THE CASE OF
HEMOPHILIAS A AND B. THERE MAY BE MORE THAN ONE FORM OF X-LINKED LATE FORM OF
MUSCULAR DYSTROPHY. EMERY (1962) HAS RESTUDIED THE FAMILY OF DREIFUSS AND HOGAN
(1961) AND FOUND FEATURES DIFFERENT FROM THOSE IN THE FAMILIES REPORTED BY BECKER.
A REVIEW OF REPORTS WAS GIVEN BY ZELLWEGER AND HANSON (1967), WHO ALSO REPORTED A
FAMILY WITH MANY MALES AFFECTED. EMERY ET AL. (1969) PRESENTED EVIDENCE SUGGES-
TING LINKAGE OF THE BECKER MUSCULAR DYSTROPHY LOCUS AND THE DEUTAN COLOR-BLINDNESS
LOCUS. THIS SHOULD BE CHECKED IN OTHER FAMILIES, USING ALSO G6PD AS A MARKER.
THAT DUCHENNE AND BECKER TYPES ARE AT DIFFERENT LOCI WOULD BE INDICATED BY SUCH A
FINDING, SINCE THE DUCHENNE TYPE IS NOT LINKED TO COLOR-BLINDNESS.

BECKER, P. E.* EINE NEUE X-CHROMOSOMALE MUSKELDYSTROPHIE. ACTA PSYCHIAT.
NEUROL. SCAND. 193* 427 ONLY, 1955.

BECKER, P. E.* NEUE ERGEBNISSE DER GENETIK DER MUSKELDYSTROPHIEN. ACTA GENET.
STATIST. MED. 7* 303-310, 1957.

BECKER, P. E.* TWO NEW FAMILIES OF BENIGN SEX-LINKED RECESSIVE MUSCULAR
DYSTROPHY. REV. CANAD. BIOL. 21* 551-566, 1962.

BLYTH, H. AND PUGH, R. J.* MUSCULAR DYSTROPHY IN CHILDHOOD* THE GENETICAL
ASPECT* A FIELD STUDY IN THE LEEDS REGION OF CLINICAL TYPES AND THEIR INHERITANCE.
ANN. HUM. GENET. 23* 127-163, 1959.

DREIFUSS, F. E. AND HOGAN, G. R.* SURVIVAL IN X-CHROMOSOMAL MUSCULAR DYSTROPHY.
NEUROLOGY 11* 734-737, 1961.

EMERY, A. E. H.* BALTIMORE, MD.* PERSONAL COMMUNICATION, 1962.

EMERY, A. E. H., CLACK, E. R., SIMON, S. AND TAYLOR, J. L.* DETECTION OF
CARRIERS OF BENIGN X-LINKED MUSCULAR DYSTROPHY. BRIT. MED. J. 4* 522-523, 1967.

EMERY, A. E. H., SMITH, C. A. B. AND SANGER, R.* THE LINKAGE RELATIONS OF THE
LOCI FOR BENIGN (BECKER TYPE) X-BORNE MUSCULAR DYSTROPHY, COLOUR BLINDNESS AND THE
XG BLOOD GROUPS. ANN. HUM. GENET. 32* 261-269, 1969.

SHAW, R. F. AND DREIFUSS, F. E.* MILD AND SEVERE FORMS OF X-LINKED MUSCULAR
DYSTROPHY. ARCH. NEUROL. 20* 451-460, 1969.

ZELLWEGER, H. AND HANSON, J. W.* SLOWLY PROGRESSIVE X-LINKED RECESSIVE MUSCULAR
DYSTROPHY (TYPE IIIB). REPORT OF CASES AND REVIEW OF THE LITERATURE. ARCH.
INTERN. MED. 120* 525-535, 1967.

X
L
I
N
K
E
D

USUALLY THE ONSET IS BEFORE AGE SIX AND THE VICTIM IS CHAIR-RIDDEN BY AGE 12 AND DEAD BY AGE 20. THE MYOCARDIUM IS AFFECTED. AN AUTOSOMAL RECESSIVE FORM OF MUSCULAR DYSTROPHY CAN CLOSELY SIMULATE THE SEX-LINKED FORM BUT THE MYOCARDIUM IS PROBABLY NOT AFFECTED.

CHUNG, MORTON, AND PETERS (1960), AMONG OTHERS, HAVE CONCLUDED THAT A MINORITY OF HETEROZYGOUS FEMALE CARRIERS HAVE AN INCREASE IN SERUM ALDOLASE AND EVEN FEWER HAVE PHYSICAL DISABILITY AND CREATINURIA. LEYBJRN, THOMSON AND WALTON (1961), ON THE OTHER HAND, COULD DEMONSTRATE NO ABNORMALITY OF CREATINE AND CREATININE EXCRETION OR OF SERUM LEVELS OF ALDOLASE AND TRANSAMINASES IN CARRIER FEMALES. SERUM PHOSPHOCREATINE KINASE (CREATINE PHOSPHOKINASE) IS ELEVATED BEYOND THE NORMAL RANGE IN MANY FEMALE CARRIERS, ACCORDING TO SCHAPIRA AND COLLEAGUES (1960) AND AEBI AND COLLEAGUES (1961-62). MIYOSHI ET AL. (1968) FOUND FOUR ELECTROPHORETICALLY SEPARABLE MYOGLOBIN SUBFRACTIONS IN NORMAL MUSCLE AND FOUND IN DUCHENNE'S MUSCULAR DYSTROPHY BUT NOT OTHER TYPES A STRIKING CHANGE IN THE QUANTITIES OF THE TYPES. DECREASED BODY POTASSIUM CONCENTRATIONS WERE REPORTED BY BLAHD ET AL. (1967) IN PATIENTS WITH MUSCULAR DYSTROPHY AND PARTICULARLY INTERESTINGLY IN RELATIVES WHO MAY HAVE BEEN HETEROZYGOTES. BOTH THE DUCHENNE AND THE LIMB-GIRDLE TYPES OF MUSCULAR DYSTROPHY WERE REPRESENTED IN THEIR SERIES. MENTAL RETARDATION OF MILD DEGREE IS A PLEIOTROPIC EFFECT OF THE DUCHENNE GENE, (ZELLWEGER AND NIEDERMEYER, 1965), ALTHOUGH THE MECHANICS IS UNKNOWN. ROY AND DUBOWITZ (1970) SUGGESTED THAT ELECTRONMICROSCOPY MAY BE USEFUL IN IDENTIFYING CARRIERS.

AEBI, U., RICHTERICH, R., STILLHART, H., COLOMBO, J. P. AND ROSSI, E.* PROGRESSIVE MUSCULAR DYSTROPHY. II. BIOCHEMICAL IDENTIFICATION OF THE CARRIER STATE IN THE RECESSIVE SEX-LINKED JUVENILE (DUCHENNE) TYPE BY SERUM CREATINE-PHOSPHOKINASE DETERMINATIONS. ENZYM. BIOL. CLIN. 1* 61-74* HELV. PAEDIAT. ACTA 16* 543-564, 1961-62.

BLAHD, W. H., LEDERER, M. AND CASSEN, B.* THE SIGNIFICANCE OF DECREASED BODY POTASSIUM CONCENTRATIONS IN PATIENTS WITH MUSCULAR DYSTROPHY AND NONDYSTROPHIC RELATIVES. NEW ENG. J. MED. 276* 1349-1352, 1967.

CHUNG, C. S., MORTON, N. E. AND PETERS, H. A.* SERUM ENZYMES AND GENETIC CARRIERS IN MUSCULAR DYSTROPHY. AM. J. HUM. GENET. 12* 52-66, 1960.

GARDNER-MEDWIN, D.* MUTATION RATE IN THE DUCHENNE TYPE OF MUSCULAR DYSTROPHY. J. MED. GENET. 7* 334-337, 1970.

LEYBURN, P., THOMSON, W. H. S. AND WALTON, J. N.* AN INVESTIGATION OF THE CARRIER STATE IN THE DUCHENNE TYPE MUSCULAR DYSTROPHY. ANN. HUM. GENET. 25* 41-49, 1961.

MIYOSHI, K., SAIJO, K., KURYU, Y., OSHIMA, Y., NAKANO, M. AND KAWAI, H.* MYOGLOBIN SUBFRACTIONS* ABNORMALITY IN DUCHENNE TYPE OF PROGRESSIVE MUSCULAR DYSTROPHY. SCIENCE 159* 736-737, 1968.

MORTON, N. E. AND CHUNG, C. S.* FORMAL GENETICS OF MUSCULAR DYSTROPHY. AM. J. HUM. GENET. 11* 360-379, 1959.

PROSSER, E. J., MURPHY, E. G. AND THOMPSON, M. W.* INTELLIGENCE AND THE GENE FOR DUCHENNE MUSCULAR DYSTROPHY. ARCH. DIS. CHILD. 44* 221-230, 1969.

ROSMAN, N. P. AND KAKULAS, B. A.* MENTAL DEFICIENCY ASSOCIATED WITH MUSCULAR DYSTROPHY-A NEUROLOGICAL STUDY. BRAIN 89* 769-788, 1966.

ROSMAN, N. P.* THE CEREBRAL DEFECT AND MYOPATHY IN DUCHENNE MUSCULAR DYSTROPHY. A COMPARATIVE CLINICOPATHOLOGICAL STUDY. NEUROLOGY 20* 329-335, 1970.

ROY, S. AND DUBOWITZ, V.* CARRIER DETECTION IN DUCHENNE MUSCULAR DYSTROPHY. A COMPARATIVE STUDY OF ELECTRON MICROSCOPY, LIGHT MICROSCOPY, AND SERUM ENZYMES. J. NEUROL. SCI. 11* 65-80, 1970.

SCHAPIRA, F., DREYFUS, J.-C., SCHAPIRA, G. AND DEMOS, J.* ETUDE DE L'ALDOLASE ET DE LA CREATINE KINASE DU SERUM CHEZ LES MERES DE MYOPATHIES. REV. FRANC. ETUD. CLIN. BIOL. 5* 990-994, 1960.

SKYRING, A. P. AND MCKUSICK, V. A.* CLINICAL, GENETIC AND ELECTROCARDIOGRAPHIC STUDIES OF CHILDHOOD MUSCULAR DYSTROPHY. AM. J. MED. SCI. 242* 534-547, 1961.

ZELLWEGER, H. AND NIEDERMEYER, E.* CENTRAL NERVOUS SYSTEM MANIFESTATIONS IN CHILDHOOD MUSCULAR DYSTROPHY (CMD) I. ANN. PAEDIAT. 205* 25-42, 1965.

X
L
I   *31030 MUSCULAR DYSTROPHY, TARDIVE TYPE OF DREIFUSS, WITH CONTRACTURES
N
K   DREIFUSS AND HOGAN (1961) AND EMERY (1964) STUDIED A VIRGINIAN KINDRED IN WHICH
E   THERE WERE EIGHT AFFECTED MALES IN THREE GENERATIONS IN TYPICAL X-LINKED PEDIGREE
D   PATTERN. ONSET OF MUSCLE WEAKNESS WAS NOTED AROUND THE AGE OF FOUR OR FIVE, FIRST
AFFECTING THE LOWER EXTREMITIES WITH A TENDENCY TO WALK ON THE TOES. BY THE EARLY
TEENS WADDLING GAIT WITH INCREASED LUMBAR LORDOSIS WAS MARKED AND WEAKNESS OF THE
SHOULDER GIRDLE MUSCULATURE APPEARED LATER. SLOW PROGRESSION WITH CONTINUED

GAINFUL EMPLOYMENT IS THE RULE. FLEXION DEFORMITIES OF THE ELBOWS DATING FROM EARLY CHILDHOOD, MILD PECTUS EXCAVATUM, SIGNS OF CARDIAC INVOLVEMENT AND ABSENCE OF MUSCLE PSEUDOHYPERTROPHY, INVOLVEMENT OF THE FOREARM MUSCLES AND MENTAL RETARDATION DISTINGUISHED THE DREIFUSS FORM FROM THE BECKER FORM. PEARSON, KAR, PETER AND MUNSAT (1965) FOUND A DIFFERENCE OF MUSCLE LDH ELECTROPHORETIC PATTERN IN THIS TYPE AS COMPARED WITH THE DUCHENNE TYPE.

DREIFUSS, F. E. AND HOGAN, G. R.* SURVIVAL IN X-CHROMOSOMAL MUSCULAR DYSTROPHY. NEUROLOGY 11* 734-737, 1961.

EMERY, A. E. H. AND DREIFUSS, F. E.* UNUSUAL TYPE OF BENIGN X-LINKED MUSCULAR DYSTROPHY. J. NEUROL. NEUROSURG. PSYCHIAT. 29* 338-342, 1966.

EMERY, A. E. H.* THE CARRIER IN X-LINKED MUSCULAR DYSTROPHY. PH.D THESIS, JOHNS HOPKINS UNIVERSITY, 1964.

PEARSON, C. M., KAR, N. C., PETER, J. B. AND MUNSAT, T. L.* MUSCLE LACTATE DEHYDROGENASE PATTERNS IN TWO TYPES OF X-LINKED MUSCULAR DYSTROPHY. AM. J. MED. 39* 91-97, 1965.

31040 MYOPATHY, CENTRONUCLEAR (MYOTUBULAR MYOPATHY)

VAN WIJNGAARDEN ET AL. (1969) DESCRIBED THIS DISORDER IN FIVE AFFECTED MALES IN FOUR SIBSHIPS CONNECTED THROUGH FEMALES WHO IN TWO INSTANCES SHOWED PARTIAL MANIFESTATIONS ON MUSCLE BIOPSY. THE PATIENTS WERE BORN AS FLOPPY INFANTS AND HAD SERIOUS RESPIRATORY PROBLEMS EARLY IN LIFE, EXTRAOCULAR, FACIAL AND NECK MUSCLES WERE ALWAYS AFFECTED.

VAN WIJNGAARDEN, G. K., FLEURY, P., BETHLEM, J. AND MEIJER, H.* FAMILIAL 'MYOTUBULAR' MYOPATHY. NEUROLOGY 19* 901-908, 1969.

*31050 NIGHT BLINDNESS, CONGENITAL STATIONARY, WITH MYOPIA

NIGHT BLINDNESS (NYCTALOPIA) IS A SYMPTOM OF SEVERAL CHORIORETINAL DEGENERATIONS. THE DISTINCTIVE FEATURE OF THE MUTATION LISTED HERE IS THE STATIONARY NATURE OF THE NIGHT BLINDNESS. THERE IS AN AUTOSOMAL DOMINANT VARIETY REPORTED IN MANY FAMILIES OF WHICH THE MOST FAMOUS IS THAT DESCENDANT FROM JEAN NOUGARET, BORN IN PROVENCE IN 1637, AND STUDIED BY CUNIER (1838), NETTLESHIP (1909, 1912) AND OTHERS. (AN ABNORMAL SEGREGATION RATIO WITH FEWER AFFECTED PERSONS THAN ANTICI-PATED HAS BEEN SUGGESTED IN THIS FAMILY, BUT OTHER LARGE PEDIGREES DO NOT SHOW THIS.) THE X-LINKED FORM IS DISTINGUISHED FROM THE AUTOSOMAL FORM BY THE ASSOCIATION OF MYOPIA. MORTON (1893) DESCRIBED A FAMILY WITH X-LINKED MYOPIA AND NIGHT BLINDNESS. FRASER AND FRIEDMANN (1967) DESCRIBED A FAMILY FROM THE SAME AREA NEAR CARDIFF, WALES.
MYOPIA HAS NOT BEEN LISTED AS A SEPARATE X-LINKED MUTATION BECAUSE IT IS NOT COMPLETELY CERTAIN THAT IT INDEED OCCURS WITH THIS MODE OF INHERITANCE AND INDEPENDENT OF NIGHT BLINDNESS OR OPHTHALMOPLEGIA. WORTH (1906) REPORTED FOUR FAMILIES WITH MYOPIA WHICH APPARENTLY WAS X-LINKED. AT NETTLESHIP'S SUGGESTION HE LOOKED FOR ASSOCIATED NIGHT BLINDNESS AND FOUND IT IN THE AFFECTED MEMBERS OF ONLY ONE OF THE FAMILIES. IN OSWALD'S FAMILY WITH MYOPIA TRANSMITTED IN A PATTERN OTHERWISE CONSISTENT WITH X-LINKED INHERITANCE APPARENT MALE-TO-MALE TRANSMISSION OCCURRED IN THE FIRST GENERATION. FRANCOIS AND DE ROUCK (1965) DESCRIBED TWO FAMILIES WITH 'DEGENERATIVE' MYOPIA TRANSMITTED AS AN X-LINKED RECESSIVE. IN ONE OF THE FAMILIES CONGENITAL HEMERALOPIA WAS ASSOCIATED.

CUNIER, F.* OBSERVATIONS CURIEUSE D'UNE ACHROMATOPSIE HEREDITAIRE DEPUIS 5 GENERATIONS. ANN. OCULIST. 1* 488-489, 1838.

FRANCOIS, J. AND DE ROUCK, A.* SEX-LINKED MYOPIC CHORIORETINAL HEREDODEGENERA-TION. AM. J. OPHTHAL. 60* 670-678, 1965.

FRASER, G. R. AND FRIEDMANN, A. I.* THE CAUSES OF BLINDNESS IN CHILDHOOD. A STUDY OF 776 CHILDREN WITH SEVERE VISUAL HANDICAPS. BALTIMORE* JOHNS HOPKINS PRESS, 1967. P. 72.

KLEINER, W.* UBER DEN GROSSEN SCHWEIZERISCHEN STAMMBAUM, IN DEM MIT KURZSICHTI-GKEIT KOMBINIERTE NACHTBLINDHEIT SICH FORTERBT. ARCH. RASS.-U. GES. BIOL. 15* 1-17, 1923.

MORTON, A. S.* TWO CASES OF HEREDITARY CONGENITAL NIGHT-BLINDNESS WITHOUT VISIBLE FUNDUS CHANGE. TRANS. OPTHAL. SOC. U.K. 13* 147-150, 1893.

NETTLESHIP, E.* ON SOME HEREDITARY DISEASES OF THE EYE (BOWMAN LECTURE). RETINITIS PIGMENTOSA, NIGHT BLINDNESS WITH MYOPIA, OCULAR ALBINISM. TRANS. OPHTHAL. SOC. U.K. 29* 57-148, 1909. A PEDIGREE OF CONGENITAL NIGHT BLINDNESS WITH MYOPIA. TRANS. OPHTHAL. SOC. U.K. 32* 21-45, 1912.

WHITE, T.* LINKAGE AND CROSSING-OVER IN THE HUMAN SEX CHROMOSOMES. J. GENET. 40* 403-437, 1940.

WORTH, C.* HEREDITARY INFLUENCE IN MYOPIA. TRANS. OPHTHAL. SOC. U.K. 26* 141-144, 1906.

WARBURG (1961) REPORTED SEVEN CASES OF A HEREDITARY DEGENERATIVE DISEASE IN SEVEN
GENERATIONS OF A DANISH FAMILY. THE PROBAND WAS A 12 MONTH OLD BOY. HE WAS
NORMAL EXCEPT FOR LENS OPACITIES FOUND AT INITIAL EXAMINATION AT THREE MONTHS OF
AGE. BOTH IRISES WERE ATROPHIC. THE FUNDUS WAS FILLED WITH A PROLIFERATING
RETROLENTAL YELLOWISH MASS. AT EIGHT MONTHS OF AGE THE LEFT EYE WAS ENUCLEATED ON
SUSPICION OF RETINOBLASTOMA. HISTOLOGICAL EXAMINATION SHOWED A HEMORRHAGIC
NECROTIC MASS IN THE POSTERIOR CHAMBER SURROUNDED BY UNDIFFERENTIATED GLIAL
TISSUE. HISTOLOGIC DIAGNOSIS WAS PSEUDOTUMOR OF THE RETINA, RETINAL HYPERPLASIA,
HYPERPLASIA OF RETINAL, CILIARY, AND IRIS PIGMENT EPITHELIUM, HYPOPLASIA AND
NECROSIS OF THE INNER LAYER OF THE RETINA, CATARACT, PHTHISIS BULBI. SIX
RELATIVES HAD A SIMILAR OCULAR DISEASE. IN FIVE OF THESE SEVEN CASES DEAFNESS
DEVELOPED IN LATER YEARS, AND IN FOUR OF THE SEVEN CASES THE MENTAL CAPACITY WAS
LOW. WARBURG FOUND 48 SIMILAR CASES IN NINE FAMILIES DESCRIBED IN THE LITERATURE
UNDER DIFFERENT CATEGORIES WHICH SHE BELIEVES BELONG TO THIS DISEASE.
WARBURG (1963) PRESENTED TWO NEW FAMILIES WITH 11 PATIENTS SUFFERING FROM
THIS DISEASE. PATIENTS EXAMINED VARIED FROM 2 MONTHS TO 58 YEARS OF AGE. AT
EARLIEST EXAMINATION PSEUDOGLIOMA, SYNECHIAE AND ATROPHY OF THE IRIS WERE
OBSERVED. BLINDNESS WAS FOUND DURING INFANTS' FIRST MONTH OF LIFE. BY EIGHT
MONTHS CATARACT WAS OBSERVED AND AT 10 YEARS THE EYES WERE ATROPHIC WITH BAND-
SHAPED CORNEAL DEGENERATION AND DENSE CATARACT. BY THE AGE OF 50 YEARS THE
ATROPHY HAD ADVANCED TO OPAQUE WHITE CORNEA, OBLITERATED ANTERIOR CHAMBER,
ATROPHIC WHITE IRIS, AND CATARACTOUS LENS. THOUGH SOME AFFLICTED HAD NORMAL
INTELLIGENCE, MANY WERE MENTALLY DEFICIENT. FIVE OF NINE IN ONE FAMILY WERE HARD
OF HEARING AND TWO OF THESE FIVE HAD DIABETES. THE MODE OF INHERITANCE IN BOTH
FAMILIES WAS X-CHROMOSOMAL RECESSIVE.
WHITNALL AND NORMAN (1940) REPORTED THE NEUROPATHOLOGY OF A CASE. THE OPTIC
NERVES AND LATERAL GENICULATE BODIES WERE SMALL. WARBURG, HAUGE AND SANGER (1965)
DEMONSTRATED NO LINKAGE WITH THE XG BLOOD GROUPS. FAMILIES WITH NORRIE'S DISEASE
HAVE OFTEN BEEN REPORTED AS PSEUDOGLIOMA OR AS MICROPHTHALMIA IN THE LITERATURE.
THE MENTAL RETARDATION IS A DETERIORIATION INASMUCH AS THE AFFECTED INFANTS SEEM
TO BE NORMAL FOR THE FIRST 1-2 YEARS. IN 1959 TAYLOR ET AL. REPORTED A GREEK
FAMILY WITH THIS CONDITION LIVING IN EPISKOPI IN CYPRUS. THE CONDITION WAS
POPULARLY KNOWN AS EPISKOPI BLINDNESS. THE PUBLISHED PEDIGREE SHOWED 16 AFFECTED
MALES IN 5 GENERATIONS. ALL AFFECTED MALES WERE RETARDED. MISTAKENLY DUKE-ELDER
IN HIS SYSTEM OF OPHTHALMOLOGY CLASSIFIED THE DISORDER AS BAND-SHAPED KERATOPATHY.
IN THE FAMILY REPORTED BY FORSSMAN, 'PSEUDOGLIOMA' WAS COMBINED WITH MENTAL
DEFICIENCY PRESENT FROM INFANCY AND APPARENTLY OF PROGRESSIVE NATURE. FORSSMAN'S
PATIENTS (1960) WERE FIRST DESCRIBED BY DAHLBERG-PARROW (1956). THREE OF THE
BLIND BOYS WERE RE-EXAMINED BY WARBURG (1966) WHO CONCLUDED THAT THE HISTORIES AND
OCULAR FINDINGS WERE TYPICAL OF NORRIE'S DISEASE. IN THE EXTENSIVE PEDIGREE FROM
A CANADIAN INDIAN GROUP REPORTED BY WILSON (1949), HISTOLOGIC CHANGES MAY HAVE
BEEN LIKE THOSE OF NORRIE'S DISEASE. ZIMMERMAN (1964) FOUND RETINAL DYSPLASIA IN
ONE OF THESE CASES.
CLARKE (1898) DESCRIBED POSSIBLE HOMOZYGOUS AFFECTED FEMALES. A MAN BLIND
FROM PROBABLE BILATERAL 'PSEUDOGLIOMA' MARRIED HIS FIRST COUSIN. OF THEIR SIX
CHILDREN, 2 GIRLS AND 1 BOY HAD UNILATERAL OR BILATERAL 'PSEUDOGLIOMA.' AS
DISCUSSED UNDER MICROPHTHALMIA (Q.V.), 'PSEUDOGLIOMA,' MICROPHTHALMOS AND NORRIE'S
DISEASE ARE CONFUSED IN THE LITERATURE.
PSEUDOGLIOMA IS A NON-SPECIFIC TERM FOR ANY CONDITION MORE OR LESS MIMICKING
RETINOBLASTOMA. THUS PSEUDOGLIOMA CAN HAVE AS DIVERSE CAUSES AS INFLAMMATION,
HEMORRHAGE, TRAUMA, NEOPLASIA OR CONGENITAL MALFORMATION. MANY OF THE CAUSES LEAD
ONLY TO UNILATERAL INVOLVEMENT. NORRIE'S DISEASE IS A FORM OF BILATERAL AND
CONGENITAL PSEUDOGLIOMA. IT SHOULD BE EVIDENT FROM THE ABOVE DISCUSSION THAT
PSEUDOGLIOMA IS MERELY ANY CONDITION OF THE EYE LIABLE TO BE MISTAKEN FOR TRUE
GLIOMA AND THEREFORE NOT AN ACCEPTABLE DIAGNOSIS EITHER CLINICALLY OR PATHOLOGI-
CALLY (DUKE-ELDER, 1958).

ANDERSON, S. R. AND WARBURG, M.* NORRIE'S DISEASE. ARCH. OPHTHAL. 66* 614-618,
1961.

CLARKE, E.* 'PSEUDO-GLIOMA' IN BOTH EYES. TRANS. OPHTHAL. SOC. U.K. 18* 136-
138, 1898.

DAHLBERG-PARROW, R.* CONGENITAL SEX-LINKED PSEUDOGLIOMA AND GRAVE MENTAL
DEFICIENCY. ACTA OPHTHAL. 34* 250-254, 1956.

DUKE-ELDER, J. R.* PSEUDOGLIOMA IN CHILDREN* ASPECTS OF CLINICAL AND PATHOLOGI-
CAL DIAGNOSIS. STH. MED. J. 51* 754-759, 1958.

FORSSMAN, H.* MENTAL DEFICIENCY AND PSEUDOGLIOMA, A SYNDROME INHERITED AS AN X-
LINKED RECESSIVE. AM. J. MENT. DEFIC. 64* 984-987, 1960.

HOLMES, L. B.* NORRIE'S DISEASE - AN X-LINKED SYNDROME OF RETINAL MALFORMATION,
MENTAL RETARDATION AND DEAFNESS. NEW ENG. J. MED. 284* 367-368, 1971.

NANCE, W. E., HARA, S., HANSEN, A., ELLIOTT, J., LEWIS, M. AND CHOWN, B.*
GENETIC LINKAGE STUDIES IN A NEGRO KINDRED WITH NORRIE'S DISEASE. AM. J. HUM.
GENET. 21* 423-429, 1969.

TAYLOR, P. J., COATES, T. AND NEWHOUSE, M. L.* EPISKOPI BLINDNESS* HEREDITARY

X
L
I
N
K
E
D

WARBURG, M.* COPENHAGEN, DENMARK* PERSONAL COMMUNICATION, 1966.

WARBURG, M.* NORRIE'S DISEASE (ATROFIA BULBORUM HEREDITARIA). ACTA OPHTHAL. 41* 134-146, 1963.

WARBURG, M.* NORRIE'S DISEASE, A CONGENITAL PROGRESSIVE OCULO-ACOUSTICO-CEREBRAL DEGENERATION. ACTA OPHTHAL. 89 (SUPPL.)* 1-147, 1966.

WARBURG, M., HAUGE, M. AND SANGER, R.* NORRIE'S DISEASE AND THE XG BLOOD GROUP SYSTEM* LINKAGE DATA. ACTA GENET. 15* 103-115, 1965.

WHITNALL, S. E. AND NORMAN, R. M.* MICROPHTHALMIA AND THE VISUAL PATHWAYS. A CASE ASSOCIATED WITH BLINDNESS AND IMBECILITY, AND SEX-LINKED. BRIT. J. OPHTHAL. 24* 229-244, 1940.

WILSON, W. M. G.* CONGENITAL BLINDNESS (PSEUDOGLIOMA) OCCURRING AS A SEX-LINKED DEVELOPMENTAL ANOMALY. CANAD. MED. ASS. J. 60* 580-584, 1949.

*31070 NYSTAGMUS

NYSTAGMUS IS, OF COURSE, ONLY A SYMPTOM AND HAS MANY CAUSES. IN FACT IT OCCURS AS PART OF THE SYMPTOM COMPLEX IN CERTAIN OTHER SEX-LINKED TRAITS (E.G., PELIZAEUS-MERZBACHER, SPASTIC PARAPLEGIA, OCULAR ALBINISM, ETC.). WHAT IS REFERRED TO HERE IS A HEREDITARY FORM WHICH OCCURS ALONE AND OF WHICH THE NEUROANATOMICAL BASIS IS STILL UNKNOWN.
AUTOSOMAL DOMINANT AND RECESSIVE FORMS ARE LESS FREQUENT THAN THE X-LINKED FORM. WAARDENBURG (PERSONAL COMMUNICATION) FEELS THERE IS NO REASON TO SEPARATE AN X-LINKED RECESSIVE FROM AN X-LINKED DOMINANT FORM AS SOME HAVE ATTEMPTED. IN SOME FAMILIES THE DISORDER IS RECESSIVE IN ONE LINE AND DOMINANT IN ANOTHER (HEMMES, 1924* WAARDENBURG, FRANCESCHETTI AND KLEIN, TEXTBOOK, 1961). THE EXPLANATION COULD BE THAT THE MUTATION IS IDENTICAL BUT THAT THERE IS A SERIES OF 'WILDTYPE' ISOALLELES WHICH HAVE DIFFERENT EFFECTS ON PENETRANCE OF THE MUTATION IN THE HETEROZYGOUS FEMALE.

BILLINGS, M. L.* NYSTAGMUS THROUGH FOUR GENERATIONS. J. HERED. 33* 457 ONLY, 1942.

COX, R. A.* CONGENITAL HEAD-NODDING AND NYSTAGMUS* REPORT OF A CASE. ARCH. OPHTHAL. 15* 1032-1036, 1936.

CUENDET, J. F. AND DELLA PORTA, V.* UNE FAMILLE DE NYSTAGMIQUES. OPHTHALMOLO-GICA 117* 199-201, 1949.

HEMMES, G. C.* OVER HEREDITAIREN NYSTAGMUS. THESIS, UTRECHT, 1924.

RUCKER, C. W.* SEX-LINKED NYSTAGMUS ASSOCIATED WITH RED-GREEN COLOR-BLINDNESS. AM. J. HUM. GENET. 1* 52-54, 1949.

WAARDENBURG, P. J.* ZUM KAPITEL DES AUSSEROKULAREN ERBLICHEN NYSTAGMUS. ACTA GENET. STATIST. MED. 4* 298-312, 1953.

31080 NYSTAGMUS, MYOCLONIC

THIS CONDITION MAY BE AN X-LINKED DOMINANT AND DISTINCT FROM SIMPLE NYSTAGMUS (Q.V.).

IN THE FAMILY DESCRIBED BY VAN BOGAERT AND DE SAVITSCH (1937), TEN SONS OF FOUR AFFECTED MEN WERE ALL NORMAL WITH THE EXCEPTION OF ONE INSTANCE OF AN AFFECTED SON OF AN AFFECTED MAN WHO WAS MARRIED TO A RELATIVE* TEN OF THE SONS OF 13 DAUGHTERS OF AFFECTED MEN WERE AFFECTED.

VAN BOGAERT, L. AND DE SAVITSCH, E.* SUR UNE MALADIE CONGENITALE ET HEREDOFAMI-LIALE COMPORTANT UN TREMBLEMENT RYTHMIQUE DE LA TETE DES GLOBES OCULAIRES ET DES MEMBRES SUPERIEURS. (SES RELATIONS AVEC LE NYSTAGMUS-MYOCLONIE ET LE NYSTAGMUS CONGENITAL HEREDITAIRE.) ENCEPHALE 32* 113-139, 1937.

31090 OCCIPITAL HAIR, WHITE LOCK OF

ONLY A SINGLE PEDIGREE SHOWING X-LINKED INHERITANCE IS KNOWN TO US, THAT OF KARL PEARSON, WHO STATED THAT THE PEDIGREE WAS THAT 'OF A WELL-KNOWN FAMILY.' THE FOLLOWING IS A QUOTATION FROM PEARSON (1909).
A CASE OF SOME INTEREST, THE PARTIAL ALBINISM, CONSISTING OF A WHITE LOCK, APPEARS TO BE INHERITED ONLY THROUGH THE FEMALE AND TO OCCUR ONLY IN THE MALES. II.3 (REPORTED BY IV.7), IV.7 AND VI.1 HAD PATCHES OF WHITE HAIR ON THE BACK OF THE HEAD. THE PATCH ON VI.1 IS ABOUT THE SIZE OF A SHILLING, IT IS SLIGHTLY TO THE RIGHT OF THE MEDIAN PLANE AND ABOVE THE OCCIPUT* THE SKIN FROM WHICH IT SPRINGS DOES NOT APPEAR LESS PIGMENTED OR OTHERWISE DIFFERENTIATED FROM THE ADJACENT SKIN. OFFSPRING OF V.3 ARE KNOWN TO EXIST AND ARE SAID NOT TO BE AFFECTED, BUT DETAILS COULD NOT BE ASCERTAINED.

X
L
I
N
K
E
D

PEARSON, K., NETTLESHIP, E. AND USHER, C. H.* A MONOGRAPH ON ALBINISM IN MAN. CAMBRIDGE* DRAPERS COMPANY RESEARCH MEMOIRS, 1911-1913, 1* 255, FIG. 638, PLATE 53.

*31100 OPHTHALMOPLEGIA, EXTERNAL, AND MYOPIA

IN THE PROBABLY UNIQUE FAMILY OF SALLERAS AND ORTIZ DE ZARATE (1950), AFFECTED MEN SHOWED BILATERAL PTOSIS, COMPLETE OR PARTIAL OPHTHALMOPLEGIA, ABNORMAL SHAPE OR FUNCTION OF THE PUPIL, MYOPIA, AND PROGRESSIVE DEGENERATION OF THE RETINA AND CHOROID. OFTEN THERE WAS ALSO ABSENCE OF PATELLAR AND ACHILLES REFLEXES, SPINA BIFIDA, AND CARDIAC AND OTHER CONGENITAL MALFORMATIONS. SOME CARRIER WOMEN SHOWED ABSENT DEEP TENDON REFLEXES ONLY. HEREDITARY OPHTHALMOPLEGIA WITHOUT MYOPIA IS FREQUENTLY AN AUTOSOMAL DOMINANT OR RECESSIVE. THE PEDIGREE WAS BROUGHT UP TO DATE IN 1966.

ORTIZ DE ZARATE, J. C.* RECESSIVE SEX-LINKED INHERITANCE OF CONGENITAL EXTERNAL OPHTHALMOPLEGIA AND MYOPIA COINCIDENT WITH OTHER DYSPLASIAS. BRIT. J. OPHTHAL. 50* 606-607, 1966.

SALLERAS, A. AND ORTIZ DE ZARATE, J. C.* RECESSIVE SEX-LINKED INHERITANCE OF EXTERNAL OPHTHALMOPLEGIA AND MYOPIA COINCIDENT WITH OTHER DYSPLASIAS. BRIT. J. OPHTHAL. 34* 662-667, 1950.

SOLOMON, L. M., FRETZIN, D. AND PRUZANSKY, S.* PILOSEBACEOUS DYSPLASIA IN THE ORAL-FACIAL-DIGITAL SYNDROME. ARCH. DERM. 102* 598-602, 1970.

31110 OPTIC ATROPHY - SPASTIC PARAPLEGIA SYNDROME

BRUYN AND WENT (1964) DESCRIBED A DEGENERATIVE DISORDER OF THE CENTRAL NERVOUS SYSTEM ASSOCIATED WITH OPTIC ATROPHY IN AT LEAST 18 MEMBERS OF A FAMILY. ONE OF THESE WAS FEMALE BUT THE DIAGNOSIS WAS IN SOME DOUBT IN THIS CASE. THE NEUROLOGIC DISORDER SHOWED FEATURES INTERMEDIATE BETWEEN THOSE OF HEREDITARY SPASTIC PARAPLEGIA (STRUMPELL-LORRAIN) AND HALLERVORDEN-SPATZ DISEASE. THE LABORATORY STUDIES (WENT, 1964) SHOWED SOME PECULIARITIES, E.G., ABNORMAL ORAL GLUCOSE TOLERANCE TESTS AND MILD RED CELL MACROCYTOSIS, BUT HAVE THUS FAR NOT CONTRIBUTED PARTICULARLY TO AN UNDERSTANDING OF THE DISORDER.

BRUYN, G. W. AND WENT, L. N.* A SEX-LINKED HEREDO-DEGENERATIVE NEUROLOGICAL DISORDER, ASSOCIATED WITH LEBER'S OPTIC ATROPHY. I. CLINICAL STUDIES. J. NEUROL. SCI. 1* 59-80, 1964.

WENT, L. N.* A SEX-LINKED HEREDO-DEGENERATIVE NEUROLOGICAL DISORDER ASSOCIATED WITH LEBER'S OPTIC ATROPHY. GENETIC ASPECTS. ACTA GENET. STATIST. MED. 14* 220-239, 1964.

WENT, L. N.* A SEX-LINKED HEREDO-DEGENERATIVE NEUROLOGICAL DISORDER, ASSOCIATED WITH LEBER'S OPTIC ATROPHY. II. LABORATORY INVESTIGATIONS. J. NEUROL. SCI. 1* 81-87, 1964.

*31120 ORAL-FACIAL-DIGITAL (OFD) SYNDROME

GORLIN AND COLLEAGUES (1961) FIRST REPORTED THIS CONDITION IN THE ENGLISH LITERATURE. CLEFTS OF THE JAW AND TONGUE IN THE AREA OF THE LATERAL INCISORS AND CANINES, OTHER MALFORMATIONS OF THE FACE AND SKULL, MALFORMATION OF THE HANDS, SPECIFICALLY SYNDACTYLY, FAMILIAL TREMBLING, AND MENTAL RETARDATION ARE FEATURES. OTHERS INCLUDE SMALL NOSTRILS, LATERAL DISPLACEMENT OF THE INNER CANTHI, LOBULATE TONGUE, PECULIARLY IRREGULAR AND ASYMMETRICAL CLEFTS OF THE PALATE, MULTIPLE MILIA ON PINNAE, ALOPECIA. ABNORMAL FRENULAE IN THE MOUTH APPEAR TO LEAD TO THE CLEFTING OF JAW, TONGUE AND UPPER LIP. ALL CASES (WITH EXCEPTION MENTIONED BELOW) ARE FEMALE. RUESS AND COLLEAGUES (1962) STATE THAT THE SEX RATIO IN AFFECTED SIBSHIPS DIFFERS SIGNIFICANTLY FROM 1*1 IN THE DIRECTION OF 2*1 (F*M). FURTHERMORE, AN EXCESSIVE NUMBER OF ABORTIONS IN AFFECTED SIBSHIPS IS REPORTED. X-LINKED DOMINANT INHERITANCE IS SUGGESTED, WITH THE TRAIT LETHAL IN THE HEMIZYGOUS MALE. HOWEVER, PATAU AND COLLEAGUES (1961) INTERPRET THIS SYNDROME AS A PARTIAL AUTOSOMAL TRISOMY WHICH IS LETHAL IN THE MALE. THE EXISTENCE OF AN AUTOSOMAL ABERRATION HAS BEEN CLAIMED IN SEVERAL OF THE CASES STUDIED BY THIS GROUP. THE POSSIBILITY THAT THE CHROMOSOMAL SEGMENT INSERTED INTO A LARGE AUTOSOME WAS DERIVED FROM AN X CHROMOSOME AND THAT THE PHENOTYPIC CHANGES WERE THE RESULT OF POSITION EFFECTS WAS CONSIDERED UNLIKELY BY PATAU (PERSONAL COMMUNICATION). THE ONLY MALE REPORTED AS PRESUMED OFD SYNDROME (KUSHNICK, MASSA, BAUKEMA, 1963) PROBABLY HAD MOHR'S SYNDROME (Q.V.). DOEGE ET AL. (1964) REPORTED A KINDRED WITH 15 AFFECTED FEMALES. CHROMOSOME STUDIES OF 8 OF THEM DID NOT UNCOVER ANY ABNORMALITY. WAHRMAN, BERANT, JACOBS, AVIAD AND BEN-HJR (1966) DESCRIBED THE CONDITION IN AN XXY MALE. THIS GREATLY STRENGTHENS THE IDEA THAT INHERITANCE IS MALE-LETHAL X-LINKED DOMINANT. INCONTINENTIA PIGMENTI (Q.V.) MAY HAVE THE SAME INHERITANCE. SEE TREMBLING CHIN IN THE DOMINANT CATALOG. SEE MOHR SYNDROME IN RECESSIVE CATALOG FOR INFORMATION BEARING ON THE DIFFERENTIAL DIAGNOSIS. IN 1960 FUHRMANN AND VOGEL DESCRIBED CLEFT LIP-PALATE AND SYNDACTYLY IN A FEMALE INFANT AND PARTIAL MANIFESTATION (SYNDACTYLY, FINGER DEFORMITY AND SPLIT IN TIP OF TONGUE) IN THE MOTHER. THE LIP CLEFT WAS MEDIAN. THEY CITED OTHER CASES OF THIS SYNDROME AND SUGGESTED AUTOSOMAL DOMINANT INHERITANCE. SUBSEQUENTLY FUHRMANN ET AL. (1966) CONCLUDED THAT THIS WAS A CASE OF OFD SYNDROME AND THAT INHERITANCE IS

X
L
I
N
K
E
D

X-LINKED DOMINANT WITH LETHALITY IN MALE. VAILLAUD ET AL. (1968) DESCRIBED A REMARKABLE PEDIGREE IN WHICH 10 FEMALES HAD OFD. THE GRANDMOTHER AND 9 OF HER GRANDDAUGHTERS THROUGH THREE UNAFFECTED SONS HAD OFD. THE 9 AFFECTED INCLUDED ALL DAUGHTERS OF THE THREE CARRIER MALES. THE AUTHORS ACCEPTED THE INTERPRETATION OF X-LINKED DOMINANCE WITH LETHALITY IN THE HEMIZYGOUS MALES, WHICH HAS BEEN APPLIED TO PREVIOUSLY PUBLISHED PEDIGREES. IN ADDITION, HOWEVER, TO EXPLAIN THE FINDINGS IN THIS SPECIFIC FAMILY THEY POSTULATED THAT THE OFD GENE IS ON A TERMINAL SEGMENT OF THE X CHROMOSOME HOMOLOGOUS WITH A SEGMENT OF THE Y CHROMOSOME AND THAT THE THREE CARRIER MALES HAD INHERITED A Y CHROMOSOME WHICH IN SOME WAY MASKED EXPRESSION OF THE OFD GENE. GORLIN (1970) SUGGESTS THAT THE TWO SISTERS WITH 'SEVERE ACHONDROPLASIA' DESCRIBED BY WALLACE ET AL. (1970) HAD THIS CONDITION. CERTAINLY THE APPEARANCE OF THE UPPER LIP WAS TYPICAL OF OFD IN BOTH.

DODGE, J. A. AND KERNOHAN, D. C.* ORAL-FACIAL-DIGITAL SYNDROME. ARCH. DIS. CHILD. 42* 214-219, 1967.

DOEGE, T. C., CAMPBELL, M. M., BRYANT, J. S. AND THULINE, H. C.* MENTAL RETARDATION AND DERMATOGLYPHICS IN A FAMILY WITH THE ORAL-FACIAL-DIGITAL SYNDROME. AM. J. DIS. CHILD. 116* 615-622, 1968.

DOEGE, T. C., THULINE, H. C., PRIEST, J. H., NORBY, D. E. AND BRYANT, J. S.* STUDIES OF A FAMILY WITH THE ORAL-FACIAL-DIGITAL SYNDROME. NEW ENG. J. MED. 271* 1073-1080, 1964.

FUHRMANN, W., STAHL, A. AND SCHROEDER, T. M.* DAS ORO-FACIO-DIGITALE SYNDROME, ZUGLEICH EINE DISKUSSION DER ERBGANGE MIT GESCHLECHTSBEGRENZTEM LETALEFFEKT. HUMANGENETIK 2* 133-164, 1966.

GORLIN, R. J. AND PSAUME, J.* ORODIGITOFACIAL DYSOSTOSIS - A NEW SYNDROME. J. PEDIAT. 61* 520-530, 1962.

GORLIN, R. J.* MINNEAPOLIS, MINN.* PERSONAL COMMUNICATION, 1970.

GORLIN, R. J., ANDERSON, V. E. AND SCOTT, C. R.* HYPERTROPHIED FRENULI, OLIGOPHRENIA, FAMILIAL TREMBLING AND ANOMALIES OF THE HAND. REPORT OF FOUR CASES IN ONE FAMILY AND A FORME FRUSTE IN ANOTHER. NEW ENG. J. MED. 264* 486-489, 1961.

KUSHNICK, T., MASSA, T. P. AND BAUKEMA, R.* OROFACIODIGITAL SYNDROME IN MALE* CASE REPORT. J. PEDIAT. 63* 1130-1134, 1963.

PATAU, K., THERMAN, E., INHORN, S. L., SMITH, D. W. AND RUESS, A. L.* PARTIAL TRISOMY SYNDROMES. II. AN INSERTION AS CAUSE OF THE OFD SYNDROME IN MOTHER AND DAUGHTER. CHROMOSOMA 12* 573-584, 1961.

REINWEIN, H., SCHILLI, W., RITTER, H., BREHME, H. AND WOLF, V.* UNTERSUCHUNGEN AN EINER FAMILIE MIT ORAL-FACIAL-DIGITAL-SYNDROM. HUMANGENETIK 2* 165-177, 1966.

RUESS, A. L., PRUZANSKY, S., LIS, E. F. AND PATAU, K.* THE ORAL-FACIAL-DIGITAL SYNDROME* A MULTIPLE CONGENITAL CONDITION OF FEMALES WITH ASSOCIATED CHROMOSOMAL ABNORMALITIES. PEDIATRICS 29* 985-995, 1962.

VAILLAUD, J. C., MARTIN, J., SZEPETOWSKI, G. AND ROBERT, J. M.* LE SYNDROME ORO-FACIO-DIGITAL. ETUDE CLINIQUE ET GENETIQUE A PROPOS DE 10 CAS OBSERVES DANS UNE MEME FAMILLE. REV. PEDIAT. 4* 383-392, 1968.

WAHRMAN, J., BERANT, M., JACOBS, J., AVIAD, I. AND BEN-HUR, N.* THE ORAL-FACIAL-DIGITAL SYNDROME* A MALE-LETHAL CONDITION IN A BOY WITH 47-XXY CHROMOSOMES. PEDIATRICS 37* 812-821, 1966.

WALLACE, D. C., EXTON, L. A., PRITCHARD, D. A., LEUNG, Y. AND COOKE, R. A.* SEVERE ACHONDROPLASIA. DEMONSTRATION OF PROBABLE HETEROGENEITY WITHIN THIS CLINICAL SYNDROME. J. MED. GENET. 7* 22-26, 1970.

31130 OTO-PALATO-DIGITAL (OPD) SYNDROME

DUDDING ET AL. (1967) DESCRIBED THREE MALE SIBS WITH CONDUCTION DEAFNESS, CLEFT PALATE, CHARACTERISTIC FACIES AND A GENERALIZED BONE DYSPLASIA. A BROAD NASAL ROOT GIVES THE PATIENT A PUGILISTIC APPEARANCE. WIDE-SPACING OF THE TOES CREATES A RESEMBLANCE TO THE FOOT OF A TREE FROG. X-LINKAGE AND AUTOSOMAL INHERITANCE COULD NOT BE DISTINGUISHED. ROENTGENOLOGIC FEATURES WERE REVIEWED IN THE SAME PATIENTS BY LANGER (1967). (THE MALE PATIENT REPORTED BY TAYBI (1962) MAY HAVE HAD THIS CONDITION). CONDUCTIVE HEARING LOSS, SOMEWHAT BROAD THUMBS AND GREAT TOES, SHORT FINGERNAILS, FIFTH FINGER CLINODACTYLY, DISLOCATION OF THE HEAD OF THE RADIUS, PECTUS EXCAVATUM, MILD DWARFISM WERE ALSO FEATURES. A SECONDARY OSSIFICA-TION CENTER AT THE BASE OF THE SECOND METACARPAL AND METATARSAL IS CHARACTERISTIC. TURNER (1970) HAS OBSERVED AFFECTED HALF-BROTHERS WHO HAD DIFFERENT FATHERS, THUS SUPPORTING X-LINKED INHERITANCE.

DUDDING, B. A., GORLIN, R. J. AND LANGER, L. O.* THE OTO-PALATO-DIGITAL SYNDROME. A NEW SYMPTOM-COMPLEX CONSISTING OF DEAFNESS, DWARFISM, CLEFT PALATE, CHARACTERISTIC FACIES, AND A GENERALIZED BONE DYSPLASIA. AM. J. DIS. CHILD. 113* 214-221, 1967.

X
L
I
N
K
E
D

LANGER, L. O., JR.* THE ROENTGENOGRAPHIC FEATURES OF THE OTO-PALATO-DIGITAL (OPD) SYNDROME. AM. J. ROENTGEN. 100* 63-70, 1967.

TAYBI, H.* GENERALIZED SKELETAL DYSPLASIA WITH MULTIPLE ANOMALIES. A NOTE ON PYLE'S DISEASE. AM. J. ROENTGEN. 88* 450-457, 1962.

TURNER, G.* SYDNEY, AUSTRALIA* PERSONAL COMMUNICATION, 1970.

31140 PAINE'S SYNDROME (MICROCEPHALY WITH SPASTIC DIPLEGIA)

IN THE FRENCH-CANADIAN FAMILY DESCRIBED BY PAINE (1960) THE PATTERN OF INHERITANCE WAS QUITE CONSISTENT WITH X-LINKAGE. MYOCLONIC FITS WERE ONE FEATURE AND ANOTHER WAS ELEVATED LEVEL OF AMINO ACIDS IN THE SPINAL FLUID WITH INVERSION OF THE USUAL RATIO OF PLASMA LEVEL TO SPINAL FLUID LEVEL. AUTOPSY IN ONE CASE SHOWED AN APPARENT DEVELOPMENTAL MALFORMATION (HYPOPLASIA OF THE CEREBELLUM, INFERIOR OLIVES AND PONS), SUPPORTING THE VIEW THAT THIS ENTITY IS DISTINCT FROM THE TWO FORMS OF DIFFUSE SCLEROSIS (Q.V.) AND FROM HYDROCEPHALUS DUE TO STENOSIS OF THE AQUEDUCT OF SYLVIUS (Q.V.) WHICH IS SOMETIMES ACCOMPANIED BY SPASTIC PARAPLEGIA AND MICROCE-PHALY AFTER ARREST OF THE HYDROCEPHALUS. SUBSEQUENT STUDIES FAILED TO SUBSTAN-TIATE THE AMINO ACID CHANGES (EFRON, 1966).

EFRON, M. S.* BOSTON, MASS.* PERSONAL COMMUNICATION, 1966.

PAINE, R. S.* EVALUATION OF FAMILIAL BIOCHEMICALLY DETERMINED MENTAL RETARDA-TION IN CHILDREN, WITH SPECIAL REFERENCE TO AMINOACIDURIA. NEW ENG. J. MED. 262* 658-665, 1960.

PAINE, R. S.* WASHINGTON, D.C.* PERSONAL COMMUNICATION, 1963.

*31150 PARKINSONISM

LIKE SOME OTHER TRAITS LISTED HERE, PARKINSONISM IS ONLY A SYMPTOM AND HAS MANY CAUSES. CASES OF IDIOPATHIC PARALYSIS AGITANS (THAT IS, CASES IN WHICH ARTERIOSC-LEROSIS AND ENCEPHALITIS ARE CONSIDERED UNLIKELY CAUSES) HAVE BEEN FOUND TO HAVE FAMILY HISTORIES CONSISTENT WITH AUTOSOMAL DOMINANT INHERITANCE. THE FILIPINO KINDRED SHOWING X-LINKED RECESSIVE INHERITANCE (OBSERVED BY MCKUSICK AND COLLEA-GUES) APPEARS TO BE UNIQUE. ONSET OF SYMPTOMS OCCURS AT THE AGE OF ABOUT 40 YEARS.

JOHNSTON, A. W. AND MCKUSICK, V. A.* SEX-LINKED RECESSIVE INHERITANCE IN SPASTIC PARAPLEGIA AND PARKINSONISM. PROC. SEC. INTERN. CONG. HUM. GENET., (ROME, SEPT. 6-12, 1961.) 3* 1652-1654, 1961.

*31160 PELIZAEUS-MERZBACHER DISEASE

THE DIFFUSE CEREBRAL SCLEROSIS GROUP RIVALS THE SPINOCEREBELLAR DEGENERATION GROUP IN CLINICAL, PATHOLOGIC, AND GENETIC CONFUSION. IT IS CURRENTLY UNDER INTENSE INVESTIGATION AND IS GRADUALLY BEING ELUCIDATED THROUGH BIOCHEMICAL CHARACTERIS-TICS. SOME, E.G., FORD (1960), REFER TO THE PELIZAEUS-MERZBACHER FORM AS THE CHRONIC INFANTILE TYPE. IT BEGINS IN INFANCY AS EARLY AS THE EIGHTH DAY AND USUALLY NO LATER THAN THE THIRD MONTH AND IS VERY SLOWLY PROGRESSIVE SO THAT THE VICTIM MAY SURVIVE TO MIDDLE AGE. ONE OF PELIZAEUS' PATIENTS LIVED TO 52 YEARS OF AGE AND IN TYLER'S NEGRO FAMILY AN AFFECTED MALE WAS STILL LIVING AT AGE 51. AT FIRST, ROTARY MOVEMENTS OF THE HEAD AND EYES DEVELOP BUT CURIOUSLY MAY LATER DISAPPEAR. AFFECTED CHILDREN ARE KNOWN IN THESE FAMILIES AS 'HEAD NODDERS' AND 'EYE WAGGERS.' SPASTICITY OF THE LEGS AND LATER THE ARMS, CEREBELLAR ATAXIA, DEMENTIA, AND PARKINSONIAN SYMPTOMS ARE OTHER FEATURES DEVELOPING OVER THE FIRST DECADE OR TWO OF LIFE. SOME HETEROZYGOUS FEMALES SHOW THE DISORDER. THE BRAIN OF SUCH A FEMALE IN MERZBACHER'S FAMILY WAS STUDIED BY SPIELMEYER (CITED BY TYLER, 1958) WITH DEMONSTRATION OF CHANGES. SIDMAN, DICKIE AND APPEL (1964) DESCRIBED AN X-LINKED DEMYELINATION DISORDER IN MICE WHICH IS SIMILAR TO PELIZAEUS-MERZBACHER DISEASE IN MAN.

FORD, F. R.* DISEASES OF THE NERVOUS SYSTEM IN INFANCY, CHILDHOOD AND ADOLES-CENCE. SPRINGFIELD, ILL.* CHARLES C THOMAS, 1960. (4TH ED.). PP. 831-833.

GERTNER, M., ZALAY, E. AND HIRSCHHORN, K.* CELLULAR METACHROMASIA IN POMPE'S DISEASE AND PELIZAEUS-MERZBACHER DISEASE. CLIN. GENET. 1* 28-29, 1970.

MERZBACHER, L.* GESETZMASSIGKEITEN IN DER VERERBUNG UND VERBREITUNG VERSCHIE-DENER HEREDITAR-FAMILIAREN ERKRANKUNGEN. ARCH. RASS.-U. GES. BIOL. 6* 172-198, 1909.

NISENBAUM, C., SANDBANK, U. AND KOHN, R.* PELIZAEUS-MERZBACHER DISEASE 'INFANTILE ACUTE TYPE.' REPORT OF A FAMILY. ANN. PAEDIAT. 204* 365-376, 1965.

PENROSE, L. S.* BIOLOGY OF MENTAL DEFECT. LONDON* SIDGWICK AND JACKSON LTD., (2ND ED.) 1954.

SIDMAN, R. L., DICKIE, M. M. AND APPEL, S. H.* MUTANT MICE (QUAKING AND JIMPY) WITH DEFICIENT MYELINATION IN THE CENTRAL NERVOUS SYSTEM. SCIENCE 144* 309-311, 1964.

X
L
I
N
K
E
D

TYLER, H. R.* PELIZAEUS-MERZBACHER DISEASE* A CLINICAL STUDY. ARCH. NEUROL. PSYCHIAT. 80* 162-169, 1958.

ZEMAN, W., DEMYER, W. AND FALLS, H. F.* PELIZAEUS-MERZBACHER DISEASE. A STUDY IN NOSOLOGY. J. NEUROPATH. EXP. NEUROL. 23* 334-354, 1964.

31170 PERIODIC PARALYSIS, FAMILIAL

KHAN (1935) DESCRIBED A LARGE FAMILY IN WHICH 8 MALES WERE AFFECTED WITH FAMILIAL PERIODIC PARALYSIS IN A PATTERN CONSISTENT WITH X-LINKED RECESSIVE INHERITANCE. BY THIS HYPOTHESIS, AT LEAST 4 FEMALES WERE HETEROZYGOUS CARRIERS. THE X-LINKED RECESSIVE PATTERN OF INHERITANCE IN KHAN'S FAMILY WAS PROBABLY ONLY FORTUITOUS BASED ON THE DISEASE'S PREDILECTION FOR MALES. OF 627 REPORTED CASES REVIEWED BY SAGILD, 411 WERE MEN. FURTHERMORE 99 OF 109 PROBANDS WERE MEN. AMONG 52 CASES OF THE DISEASE IN DENMARK ONLY 4 WERE FEMALE, A SEX-RATIO OF 12*1. WHEN AFFECTED, WOMEN SHOW A LESS SEVERE CLINICAL PICTURE. SOME OF SAGILD'S FAMILIES, ESPECIALLY WHEN ONLY PART IS CONSIDERED, HAVE A PEDIGREE PATTERN CONSISTENT WITH X-LINKED RECESSIVE INHERITANCE. HOWEVER, NUMEROUS INSTANCES OF MALE-TO-MALE TRANSMISSION HAVE BEEN OBSERVED. SAGILD'S CONCLUSION WAS THAT THE HYPOKALEMIC VARIETY OF FAMILIAL PERIODIC PARALYSIS IS INHERITED AS AN AUTOSOMAL DOMINANT WITH MARKED REDUCTION IN PENETRANCE IN THE FEMALE. THE HYPERKALEMIC FORM OF THE DISEASE AFFECTS MALES AND FEMALES EQUALLY.

KHAN, M. Y.* FAMILIAL PERIODIC PARALYSIS. INDIAN MED. GAZ. 70* 28-29, 1935.

SAGILD, U.* HEREDITARY TRANSIENT PARALYSIS. COPENHAGEN, MUNKSGARRD, 1959.

*31180 PHOSPHOGLYCERATE KINASE (PGK) DEFICIENCY HEMOLYTIC ANEMIA

VALENTINE ET AL. (1969) FOUND HEMOLYTIC ANEMIA WITH DEFICIENT RED AND WHITE CELL PHOSPHOGLYCERATE KINASE, IN A LARGE CHINESE KINDRED. MILD HEMOLYSIS WAS PRESENT IN PRESUMED HETEROZYGOTES. CHEN ET AL. (1971) DESCRIBED AN ELECTROPHORETIC VARIANT OF PGK WITH ENZYME ACTIVITY IN THE NORMAL RANGE. PGK AND G6PD ARE PROBABLY NOT CLOSELY LINKED.

CHEN, S.-H., MALCOLM, L. A., YOSHIDA, A. AND GIBLETT, E. R.* PHOSPHOGLYCERATE KINASE* AN X-LINKED POLYMORPHISM IN MAN. AM. J. HUM. GENET. 23* 87-91, 1971.

VALENTINE, W. N., HSIEH, H.-S., PAGLIA, D. E., ANDERSON, H. M., BAUGHAN, M. A., JAFFE, E. R. AND GARSON, O. M.* HEREDITARY HEMOLYTIC ANEMIA ASSOCIATED WITH PHOSPHOGLYCERATE KINASE DEFICIENCY IN ERYTHROCYTES AND LEUKOCYTES. A PROBABLE X-CHROMOSOME-LINKED SYNDROME. NEW ENG. J. MED. 280* 528-534, 1969.

31190 PIERRE ROBIN SYNDROME WITH CONGENITAL HEART MALFORMATION AND CLUBFOOT

GORLIN ET AL. (1970) DESCRIBED A KINDRED IN WHICH MULTIPLE MALES, RELATED THROUGH NORMAL FEMALES HAD THIS COMBINATION. OTHER POSSIBLE REPORTS OF THE SYNDROME WERE NOTED, E.G., SACHTLEBEN (1964) HAD TWO BROTHERS WITH CLEFT PALATE, CONGENITAL HEART DISEASE AND CLUBFOOT.

GORLIN, R. J., CERVENKA, J., ANDERSON, R. C., SAUK, J. J. AND BEVIS, W. D.* ROBIN'S SYNDROME. A PROBABLY X-LINKED RECESSIVE SUBVARIETY EXHIBITING PERSISTENCE OF LEFT SUPERIOR VENA CAVA AND ATRIAL SEPTAL DEFECT. AM. J. DIS. CHILD. 119* 176-178, 1970.

SACHTLEBEN, P.* ZUR PATHOGENESE UND THERAPIE DES PIERRE-ROBIN-SYNDROMES. ARCH. KINDERHEILK. 171* 55-63, 1964.

*31200 PITUITARY DWARFISM IV (X-LINKED PANHYPOPITUITARISM)

PHELAN ET AL. (1971) REPORTED FOUR CASES IN THREE SIBSHIPS CONNECTED THROUGH FEMALES AND SCHIMKE ET AL. (1971) DESCRIBED PANHYPOPITUITARISM IN TWO HALF-BROTHERS WITH THE SAME MOTHER.

PHELAN, P. D., CONNELLY, J., MARTIN, F. I. R. AND WETTENHALL, H. N. B.* X-LINKED RECESSIVE HYPOPITUITARISM. THE CLINICAL DELINEATION OF BIRTH DEFECTS. X. THE ENDOCRINE SYSTEM. BALTIMORE* WILLIAMS AND WILKINS, 1971.

SCHIMKE, R. N., SPAULDING, J. J. AND HOLLOWELL, J. G.* X-LINKED CONGENITAL PANHYPOPITUITARISM. THE CLINICAL DELINEATION OF BIRTH DEFECTS. X. THE ENDOCRINE SYSTEM. BALTIMORE* WILLIAMS AND WILKINS, 1971.

31210 PSEUDOHERMAPHRODITISM, MALE

THE TESTICULAR FEMINIZATION SYNDROME (Q.V.) IS ONE TYPE OF MALE PSEUDOHERMAPHRODI-TISM AND IN ITSELF MAY COMPRISE, AS NOTED ABOVE, AT LEAST TWO DISTINCT ENTITIES. THE REIFENSTEIN SYNDROME (Q.V.) IS ANOTHER. IN ADDITION THERE IS AT LEAST ONE OTHER FORM IN WHICH THE EXTERNAL GENITALIA ARE AMBIGUOUS AND MASCULINIZATION IS RELATIVELY STRIKING. TESTES ARE THE ONLY GONADS PRESENT. SOME CASES (FOR EXAMPLE SIX OF THE NINE CASES IN THE SERIES OF ALEXANDER AND FERGUSON-SMITH, 1961) HAVE A RUDIMENTARY UTERUS AND FALLOPIAN TUBES. THE SEX CHROMOSOME CONSTITUTION IS XY (ALEXANDER AND FERGUSON-SMITH, 1961). IT WILL BE EVIDENT THAT IT IS OFTEN

DIFFICULT TO KNOW WHETHER CASES BELONG IN THE GENERAL CATEGORY DISCUSSED HERE OR IN THAT OF HYPOGONADISM. WHEREAS THE HISTOLOGIC FINDINGS IN THE TESTIS OF TESTICULAR FEMINIZATION SYNDROME IS CHARACTERISTIC, THOSE IN THE FORM OF MALE PSEUDOHERMAPHRODITISM DISCUSSED HERE ARE ONLY THE NON-SPECIFIC ONES FOUND IN ANY CRYPTORCHID TESTIS. THE DEFECT IN MALE PSEUDOHERMAPHRODITISM MAY INVOLVE THE MALE MORPHOGENETIC HORMONE NORMALLY PRODUCED BY THE FETAL TESTIS.

MALE PSEUDOHERMAPHRODITISM IS FAMILIAL IN MANY INSTANCES, ALTHOUGH THE NOW AVAILABLE INFORMATION ON THIS POINT IS LESS EXTENSIVE THAN FOR TESTICULAR FEMINIZATION. MULTIPLE AFFECTED SIBS HAVE BEEN REPORTED BY SEVERAL AUTHORS (E.G., ALEXANDER AND FERGUSON-SMITH, 1961* EVANS AND RILEY, 1953* AND WITSCHI AND MENGERT, 1942). MALE-LIMITED AUTOSOMAL RECESSIVE INHERITANCE IS NOT EXCLUDED FOR AT LEAST SOME OF THE CASES, AND OF COURSE AUTOSOMAL DOMINANT INHERITANCE IS POSSIBLE IF MATERNAL UNCLES ARE AFFECTED. ASSEMBLY OF MORE PEDIGREE DATA, INFORMATION ON THE FREQUENCY OF CONSANGUINITY, AND LINKAGE STUDIES MAY BE OF VALUE.

IN TWO SIBS (L. L. A. 921527 AND M. A. 920004) WITH AMBIGUOUS GENITALIA, TESTES, AND XY KARYOTYPE, RECENTLY STUDIED IN THIS HOSPITAL, WE HAVE FOUND THAT ONE WAS XG(A+) AND THE OTHER XG(A-), SUGGESTING NO CLOSE LINKAGE. THE FINDING MAY INDICATE AUTOSOMAL INHERITANCE.

ALEXANDER, D. S. AND FERGUSON-SMITH, M. A.* CHROMOSOMAL STUDIES IN SOME VARIANTS OF MALE PSEUDOHERMAPHRODITISM. PEDIATRICS 28* 758-763, 1961.

BERGADA, C., CLEVELAND, W. W., JONES, H. W., JR. AND WILKINS, L.* GONADAL HISTOLOGY IN PATIENTS WITH MALE PSEUDOHERMAPHRODITISM AND ATYPICAL GONADAL DYSGENESIS. RELATION TO THEORIES OF SEX DIFFERENTIATION. ACTA ENDOCR. 40* 493-520, 1962.

EVANS, T. N. AND RILEY, G. M.* PSEUDOHERMAPHRODITISM. A CLINICAL PROBLEM. OBSTET. GYNEC. 2* 363-378, 1953.

WITSCHI, E. AND MENGERT, W. F.* ENDOCRINE STUDIES ON HUMAN HERMAPHRODITES AND THEIR BEARING ON THE INTERPRETATION OF HOMOSEXUALITY. J. CLIN. ENDOCR. 2* 279-286, 1942.

31220 RADIAL LOOP, PLAIN, ON RIGHT INDEX FINGER

WALKER (1941) SUGGESTED THAT THIS PATTERN IS SEX LINKED. HOLT (1962) COULD NOT CONFIRM THE SUGGESTION OF X-LINKAGE.

HOLT, S. B.* LONDON, ENGLAND* PERSONAL COMMUNICATION, 1962.

WALKER, J. F.* A SEX LINKED RECESSIVE FINGERPRINT PATTERN. J. HERED. 32* 279-280, 1941.

31230 REIFENSTEIN SYNDROME

THE FEATURES OF THIS FORM OF MALE PSEUDOHERMAPHRODITISM ARE HYPOSPADIAS, HYPOGONA-DISM, GYNECOMASTIA, NORMAL XY KARYOTYPE AND A PEDIGREE PATTERN CONSISTENT WITH X-LINKED RECESSIVE INHERITANCE. ALTHOUGH THE AFFECTED MALES ARE INFERTILE, GERM CELLS WITH MITOTIC (AND PERHAPS MEIOTIC) ACTIVITY ARE DEMONSTRATED BY TESTICULAR BIOPSY. NO SPERMATOZOA ARE FOUND. SOME OF THE HISTOLOGIC FEATURES SUCH AS LEYDIG CELL HYPERPLASIA AND HYALINE TUBULAR GHOSTS RESEMBLE THOSE OF THE XXY KLINEFELTER SYNDROME. HOWEVER, THE PRESENCE OF GERM CELLS, THE HYPOSPADIAS AND THE FAMILIAL NATURE ARE DISTINGUISHING FEATURES. A DEFECT IN PRODUCTION OF FETAL ANDROGEN IS THOUGHT TO BE RESPONSIBLE FOR THE HYPOSPADIAS. SOME OF THE PATHOLOGIC CHANGES IN THE TESTIS MAY RESULT FROM HIGH FSH SECONDARY TO ANDROGEN DEFICIENCY. TREATMENT WITH TESTOSTERONE FROM AN EARLY AGE MIGHT RESTORE FERTILITY.

BOCZKOWSKI, K. AND TETER, J.* FAMILIAL MALE PSEUDOHERMAPHRODITISM. ACTA ENDOCR. 49* 497-509, 1965.

BOWEN, P., LEE, C. N. S., MIGEON, C. J., KAPLAN, N. M., WHALLEY, P. J., MCKUSICK, V. A. AND REIFENSTEIN, E. C.* HEREDITARY MALE PSEUDOHERMAPHRODITISM WITH HYPOGONADISM, HYPOSPADIAS AND GYNECOMASTIA (REIFENSTEIN*S SYNDROME). ANN. INTERN. MED. 62* 252-270, 1965.

31240 RENAL TUBULAR ACIDOSIS II (PROXIMAL, RATE, OR BICARBONATE WASTING TYPE)

THIS VARIETY IS APPARENTLY DISTINCT FROM CLASSIC RTA I, WHICH IS INHERITED AS A DOMINANT. MOST, OR PERHAPS ALL, THE CASES HAVE BEEN MALES. HENCE, X-LINKED RECESSIVE INHERITANCE IS POSSIBLE.

X
L
I
N
K
E
D

EDELMANN, C. M., JR.* BRONX, N. Y.* PERSO5AL COMMUNICATION, 1970.

SEBASTIAN, A., MCSHERRY, E. AND MORRIS, R. C., JR.* ON THE MECHANISM OF RENAL POTASSIUM WASTING IN RENAL TUBULAR ACIDOSIS ASSOCITED WITH THE FANCONI SYNDROME (TYPE 2 RTA). J. CLIN. INVEST. 50* 231-243, 1971.

SORIANO, J. R., BOICHIS, H., STARK, H. AND EDELMANN, C. M., JR.* PROXIMAL RENAL TUBULAR ACIDOSIS. A DEFECT IN BICARBONATE REABSORPTION WITH NORMAL URINARY ACIDIFICATION. PEDIAT. RES. 1* 81-98, 1967.

*31250 RETICULOENDOTHELIOSIS

FALLETTA ET AL. (1970) DESCRIBED A LATIN AMERICAN FAMILY IN WHICH 17 MALES IN TWO GENERATIONS DIED UNDER THE AGE OF 6 YEARS, FOLLOWING AN ILLNESS CHARACTERIZED BY FEVER, PALLOR, JAUNDICE, HEPATOSPLENOMEGALY, AND LYMPHADENOPATHY. MEDIAN AGE OF ONSET WAS 14 MONTHS (4-62 MONTHS) AND MEDIAN DURATION OF ILLNESS WAS 22 DAYS (1-50 DAYS). HISTOLOGIC CHANGES WERE CONSISTENT WITH MALIGNANT RETICJLOENDOTHELIOSIS. ALL AFFECTED MALES WERE RELATED THROUGH THEIR MOTHERS.

FALLETTA, J. M., FERNBACH, D. J., SINGER, D. B., SHORE, N. A., LANDING, B. AND HEATH, C. W., JR.* AN X-LINKED RECESSIVE *MALIGNANT* RETICULOENDOTHELIOSIS. (ABSTRACT) SOCIETY FOR PEDIATRIC RESEARCH, ATLANTIC CITY, 1970.

*31260 RETINITIS PIGMENTOSA

THE X-LINKED FORM IS ALSO CALLED CHOROIDORETINAL DEGENERATION, OR PIGMENTARY RETINOPATHY. AFFECTED MALES SHOW TYPICAL *BONE CORPUSCLE* CLUMPS OF PIGMENT ON FUNDOSCOPIC EXAMINATION AND PROGRESSIVE CHOROIDAL SCLEROSIS LEADING TO COMPLETE BLINDNESS. HETEROZYGOUS WOMEN MAY SHOW A TAPETORETINAL REFLEX (BRILLIANT, SCINTILLATING, GOLDEN HUED, PATCHY APPEARANCE MOST STRIKING AROUND THE MACULA) BUT NO VISUAL DEFECT. RETINITIS PIGMENTOSA IS SOMETIMES AUTOSOMAL DOMINANT, SOMETIMES AUTOSOMAL RECESSIVE. IN ADDITION TO THESE HEREDITARY FORMS WITHOUT ASSOCIATED MANIFESTATIONS, RETINITIS PIGMENTOSA IS ONE COMPONENT OF CERTAIN HEREDITARY SYNDROMES, NOTABLY THE LAURENCE-MOON-BARDET-BIEDL SYNDROME. THUS THERE MAY BE AT LEAST SEVEN OR EIGHT DISTINCT GENETIC VARIETIES OF THE PHENOTYPE. THE X-LINKED FORM IS ONE OF THE RARER. ALL FAMILIES DO NOT SHOW THE EXPRESSION IN FEMALE CARRIERS DESCRIBED ABOVE. THUS, THERE SEEMS TO BE A FULLY RECESSIVE AND AN INTERMEDIATE X-LINKED FORM* THEIR RELATION TO EACH OTHER IS UNKNOWN. THE GYRATE CHOROIDAL ATROPHY DESCRIBED BY WAARDENBURG (1932) AS X-LINKED WAS FOUND ON FURTHER STUDY TO BE RETINITIS PIGMENTOSA (WAARDENBURG, FRANCESCHETTI AND KLEIN, TEXTBOOK, 1961, P. 799). AS IS REVIEWED BY JACOBSON AND STEPHENS (1962), THERE ARE SOME PHENOTYPIC DIFFERENCES BETWEEN FAMILIES REPORTED. THE GENETIC SIGNIFICANCE OF THESE DIFFERENCES IS UNKNOWN. IN THE FAMILY REPORTED BY HECK (1963), HETEROZYGOUS FEMALES SOMETIMES WERE FULLY AFFECTED AND SOMETIMES SHOWED ONLY A BLUE-YELLOW COLOR DEFECT (A RARE ANOMALY). *TAPETAL REFLEX* WAS NOT PRESENT, AS IN THE HETEROZYGOTES REPORTED BY FALLS AND COTTERMAN. THE DEGENERATION OF THE RETINA WAS VARIABLE IN TYPE, BEING PIGMENTARY DEGENERATION, NON-PIGMENTARY DEGENERATION AND MACULAR DEGENERATION IN DIFFERENT AFFECTED MALES. CATARACT WAS PRESENT IN TWO WITH PIGMENTARY DEGENERATION. THE MOST FREQUENT FORM OF RETINITIS PIGMENTOSA IS THE RECESSIVELY INHERITED FORM(S), THE DOMINANT FORMS ARE NEXT IN FREQUENCY AND THE X-LINKED FORM IS RAREST, BEING LESS THAN 5 PERCENT IN MOST SERIES.

ALLAN, W.* EUGENIC SIGNIFICANCE OF RETINITIS PIGMENTOSA. ARCH. OPHTHAL. 18* 938-947, 1937.

FALLS, H. F.* THE ROLE OF THE SEX CHROMOSOME IN HEREDITARY OCULAR PATHOLOGY. TRANS. AM. OPHTHAL. SOC. 50* 421-467, 1952.

HECK, A. F.* PRESUMPTIVE X-LINKED INTERMEDIATE TRANSMISSION OF RETINAL DEGENERATIONS. VARIATIONS AND COINCIDENTAL OCCURRENCE WITH ATAXIA IN A LARGE FAMILY. ARCH. OPHTHAL. 70* 143-149, 1963.

JACOBSON, J. H. AND STEPHENS, G.* HEREDITARY CHOROIDORETINAL DEGENERATION. STUDY OF A FAMILY INCLUDING ELECTRORETINOGRAPHY AND ADAPTOMETRY. ARCH. OPHTHAL. 67* 321-335, 1962.

KLEIN, D., FRANCESCHETTI, A., HUSSELS, I., RACE, R. R. AND SANGER, R.* X-LINKED RETINITIS PIGMENTOSA AND LINKAGE STUDIES WITH THE XG BLOOD-GROUPS. LANCET 1* 974-975, 1967.

MCQUARRIE, M. D.* TWO PEDIGREES OF HEREDITARY BLINDNESS IN MAN. J. GENET. 30* 147-153, 1935.

USHER, C. H.* BOWMAN LECTURE ON A FEW HEREDITARY EYE AFFECTIONS. TRANS. OPHTHAL. SOC. U.K. 55* 164-245, 1935.

WAARDENBURG, P. J.* DAS MENSCHLICHE AUGE UND SEINE ERBANLAGAN. MARTINUS NIJHOFF, *S-GRAVENHAGE, 1932.

WARBURG, M. AND SIMONSEN, S. E.* SEX-LINKED RECESSIVE RETINITIS PIGMENTOSA. A PRELIMINARY STUDY OF THE CARRIERS. ACTA OPHTHAL. 46* 494-499, 1968.

*31270 RETINOSCHISIS

RETINOSCHISIS IS INTRARETINAL SPLITTING DUE TO DEGENERATION. THE ABNORMALITY MAY NOT BE CLINICALLY MANIFEST UNTIL MIDDLE LIFE. THE AFFECTED MALES SHOW CYSTIC DEGENERATION LEADING TO SPLIT IN THE RETINA, DETACHMENT OF THE RETINA, AND FINALLY COMPLETE RETINAL ATROPHY WITH SCLEROSIS OF THE CHOROID. GIESER AND FALLS (1961) OBSERVED A MACULAR CYST IN ONE EYE OF A POSSIBLE FEMALE CARRIER IN A KINDRED WITH NINE AFFECTED MALES AND SUGGESTED THAT IT MIGHT REPRESENT AN EXPRESSION OF THE CARRIER STATE.
RETINOSCHISIS IS, IN THE OPINION OF GIESER AND FALLS (1961), THE SAME

CONDITION AS THAT DESCRIBED BY MANN AND MACRAE (1938) AS CONGENITAL VASCULAR VEIL IN THE VITREOUS AND ALSO THE SAME AS THE X-LINKED RETINAL DETACHMENT DESCRIBED BY SORSBY AND COLLEAGUES (1951). RETINOSCHISIS IS PROBABLY DISTINCT FROM PSEUDOGLIOMA, ALTHOUGH POSSIBLY EVEN THIS CANNOT BE CONSIDERED SETTLED. SO-CALLED CONGENITAL FALCIFORM FOLD OF THE RETINA (ABLATIO FALCIFORMIS RETINAE CONGENITA) IS PROBABLY YET ANOTHER EXPRESSION OF THE SAME GENE AS THAT FOR RETINOSCHISIS. WEVE (1938) OBSERVED FALCIFORM FOLD AND PSEUDOGLIOMA IN THE SAME FAMILY. FORSIUS AND COLLEAGUES (1963) DESCRIBED A FAMILY WITH A HOMOZYGOUS AFFECTED FEMALE WHO WAS THE DAUGHTER OF AN AFFECTED MALE AND HIS SECOND COUSIN. ALL THREE OF THE HOMOZYGOTE'S SONS, BY TWO DIFFERENT HUSBANDS, WERE AFFECTED. YANOFF ET AL. (1968) REPORTED THE HISTOLOGIC APPEARANCE IN THE EYE OF A 50 MONTH OLD BOY WHOSE BROTHER WAS ALSO AFFECTED. THE SPLITTING OCCURRED IN THE SENSORY RETINA, PREDOMINANTLY IN THE NERVE FIBER LAYER. CYSTIC MACULOPATHY IS SOMETIMES THE ONLY FINDING IN THESE PATIENTS. THE BASIC LESION IS CYSTIC DEGENERATION IN THE DEEP NERVE LAYER. IVES ET AL. (1970) FOUND LOOSE LINKAGE WITH THE XG LOCUS.

FORSIUS, H., ERIKSSON, A. AND VAINIO-MATTILA, B.* GESCHLECHTSGEBUNDENE ERBLICHE RETINOSCHISIS IN ZWEI FAMILIEN IN FINNLAND. KLIN. MBL. AUGENHEILK. 143* 806-816, 1963.

FORSIUS, H., ERIKKSON, A., NUUTILA, A., VAINIO-MATTILA, B. AND KRAUSE, U.* A GENETIC STUDY OF THREE RARE RETINAL DISORDERS* DYSTROPHIA RETINAE DYSACUSIS SYNDROME, X-CHROMOSOMAL RETINOSCHISIS AND GROUPED PIGMENTS OF THE RETINA. THE CLINICAL DELINEATION OF BIRTH DEFECTS. VIII. EYE. BALTIMORE* WILLIAMS AND WILKINS, 1971.

FORSIUS, H., VAINIO-MATTILA, B. AND ERIKSSON, A.* X-LINKED HEREDITARY RETINOSCHISIS. BRIT. J. OPHTHAL. 46* 678-681, 1962.

GIESER, E. P. AND FALLS, H. F.* HEREDITARY RETINOSCHISIS. AM. J. OPHTHAL. 51* 1193-1200, 1961.

IVES, E. J., EWING, C. C. AND INNES, R.* X-LINKED JUVENILE RETINOSCHISIS AND XG LINKAGE IN FIVE FAMILIES. (ABSTRACT) AM. J. HUM. GENET. 22* 17A-18A, 1970.

KLEINERT, H.* EINE RECESSIV-GESCHLECHTSGEBUNDENE FORM DER IDIOPATHISCHEN NETZHAUTSPALTUNG BEI NICHTMYOPEN JUGENDLICHEN. GRAEFE. ARCH. OPHTHAL. 154* 295-305, 1953.

MANN, I. AND MACRAE, A.* CONGENITAL VASCULAR VEILS IN THE VITREOUS. BRIT. J. OPHTHAL. 22* 1-10, 1938.

SORSBY, A., KLEIN, M., GANN, J. H. AND SIGGINS, G.* UNUSUAL RETINAL DETACHMENT, POSSIBLY SEX LINKED. BRIT. J. OPHTHAL. 35* 1-10, 1951.

VAINIO-MATTILA, B., ERIKSSON, A. W. AND FORSIUS, H.* X-CHROMOSOMAL RECESSIVE RETINOSCHISIS IN THE REGION OF PORI. AN OPHTHALMO-GENETICAL ANALYSIS OF 103 CASES. ACTA OPHTHAL. 47* 1135-1148, 1969.

WEVE, H.* ABLATIO FALCIFORMIS CONGENITA (RETINAL FOLD). BRIT. J. OPHTHAL. 22* 456-470, 1938.

YANOFF, M., KERTESZ RAHN, E. AND ZIMMERMAN, L. E.* HISTOPATHOLOGY OF JUVENILE RETINOSCHISIS. ARCH. OPHTHAL. 79* 49-53, 1968.

31280 SACRAL DEFECT WITH ANTERIOR SACRAL MENINGOCELE

COHN AND BAY-NIELSEN (1969) DESCRIBED SEVEN CASES OF ANTERIOR SACRAL MENINGOCELE WITH PARTIAL ABSENCE OF THE SACRUM AND COCCYX. SYMPTOMS INCLUDED CONSTIPATION AND URINARY INCONTINENCE. ALL THE AFFECTED PERSONS WERE FEMALE. ONE UNAFFECTED FEMALE APPEARS TO HAVE TRANSMITTED THE DISORDER. A MAJORITY OF REPORTED CASES ARE FEMALE. THE AUTHORS SUGGESTED X-LINKED DOMINANT INHERITANCE. ABORTIONS DO NOT SEEM TO HAVE BEEN INCREASED IN THE FAMILY.

COHN, J. AND BAY-NIELSEN, E.* HEREDITARY DEFECTS OF THE SACRUM AND COCCYX WITH ANTERIOR SACRAL MENINGOCELE. ACTA PAEDIAT. SCAND. 58* 268-274, 1969.

*31290 SPASTIC PARAPLEGIA

SPASTIC PARAPLEGIA IS AN AUTOSOMAL DOMINANT IN MANY FAMILIES, AN AUTOSOMAL RECESSIVE IN MANY OTHERS. THE FAMILY OF JOHNSTON AND MCKUSICK (1962) SHOWED X-LINKED RECESSIVE INHERITANCE. WOLFSLAST'S FAMILY (1943), WITH WHAT HE TERMED SPASTIC DIPLEGIA, IS ANOTHER POSSIBLE EXAMPLE. ONE AFFECTED MALE WAS LIVING AT AGE 50 AND A SECOND AT AGE 20. NYSTAGMUS WAS DESCRIBED IN A FEMALE CARRIER. PROF. P. E. BECKER OF GOTTINGEN IS OF THE OPINION, HOWEVER, THAT WOLFSLAST'S FAMILY SUFFERED FROM THE PELIZAEUS-MERZBACHER SYNDROME, AND VERSCHUER IN HIS TEXTBOOK STATES THE SAME OPINION. A MORE LIKELY CASE OF X-LINKED SPASTIC PARAPLEGIA IS THAT OF BLUMEL ET AL. (1957). EARLY ONSET, SLOW PROGRESSION, AND LONG SURVIVAL WITH EVENTUAL INVOLVEMENT OF THE CEREBELLUM, CEREBRAL CORTEX AND OPTIC NERVES ARE FEATURES OF THE X-LINKED FORM AS OBSERVED BY JOHNSTON AND MCKUSICK. THURMON (1971) HAS STUDIED TWO KINDREDS RATHER EXTENSIVELY AFFECTED WITH PROBABLE X-LINKED SPASTIC PARAPLEGIA.

X
L
I
N
K
E
D

BLUMEL, J., EVANS, E. B. AND EGGERS, G. W. N.* HEREDITARY CEREBRAL PALSY. A PRELIMINARY REPORT. J. PEDIAT. 50* 454-458, 1957.

JOHNSTON, A. W. AND MCKUSICK, V. A.* A SEX-LINKED RECESSIVE INHERITANCE OF SPASTIC PARAPLEGIA. AM. J. HUM. GENET. 14* 83-94, 1962.

THURMON, T. F.* NEW ORLEANS, LA.* PERSONAL COMMUNICATION, 1971.

WOLFSLAST, W.* EINE SIPPE MIT RECESSIVER GESCHLECHTSGEBUNDENER SPASTISCHER DIPLEGIE. Z. MENSCHL. VERERB. KONSTITUTIONSL. 27* 189-198, 1943.

31300 SPATIAL VISUALIZATION, APTITUDE FOR

STAFFORD (1961), USING THE IDENTICAL BLOCKS TEST AS A MEASURE OF SPATIAL VISUALI-ZATION, STUDIED 104 FATHERS AND MOTHERS AND THEIR 58 TEEN-AGE SONS AND 70 DAUGHTERS. MALES SHOWED HIGHER AVERAGE SCORES THAN FEMALES IN BOTH THE PATERNAL AND OFFSPRING GROUP. NO CORRELATION OF SCORES EXISTED BETWEEN FATHERS AND MOTHERS AND NONE BETWEEN FATHERS AND SONS. THE CORRELATIONS BETWEEN FATHERS AND DAUGH-TERS, BETWEEN MOTHERS AND SONS AND BETWEEN MOTHERS AND DAUGHTERS WAS WHAT WOULD BE EXPECTED ON THE ASSUMPTION THAT THE APTITUDE FOR VISUALIZING SPACE IS AN X-LINKED RECESSIVE TRAIT. GARRON (1970) POINTED OUT THAT IF SPATIAL AND NUMERICAL ABILITIES ARE DETERMINED BY AN X-LINKED RECESSIVE GENE PATIENTS WITH TURNER SYNDROME SHOULD SHOW SUPERIOR NOT INFERIOR PERFORMANCE.

GARRON, D. C.* SEX-LINKED, RECESSIVE INHERITANCE OF SPATIAL AND NUMERICAL ABILITIES, AND TURNER'S SYNDROME. PSYCHOL. REV. 77* 147-152, 1970.

STAFFORD, R. E.* SEX DIFFERENCES IN SPATIAL VISUALIZATION AS EVIDENCE OF SEX-LINKED INHERITANCE. PERCEPT. MOTOR SKILLS 13* 428 ONLY, 1961.

31310 SPIEGLER-BROOKE'S TUMORS

THE DEMONSTRATION, IN THE SAME PATIENTS AND SAME FAMILIES, OF CYLINDROMA AS DESCRIBED BY SPIEGLER AND OF EPITHELIOMA ADENOIDES CYSTICUM AS DESCRIBED BY BROOKE SUPPORTS THEIR GENETIC IDENTITY (GUGGENHEIM AND SCHNYDER, 1961). (SEE EPITHE-LIOMA, HEREDITARY BENIGN CYSTIC, IN DOMINANT CATALOG FOR FURTHER DISCUSSION OF NOSOLOGY.) SCHMIDT-BAUMLER (1931) RAISED THE QUESTION OF X-LINKED DOMINANT INHERITANCE. THE PEDIGREE OF BLANDY AND COLLEAGUES (1961) SHOWED AN AFFECTED MALE WHO HAD ALL DAUGHTERS AFFECTED AND ALL SONS UNAFFECTED. UP TO THE END OF 1954, EVANS FOUND 47 REPORTED CASES, OF WHICH 30 WERE FEMALE. GUGGENHEIM AND SCHNYDER FOUND THAT 132 OF 212 REPORTED CASES WERE IN FEMALES. HOWEVER, AGAINST X-LINKAGE IS THE FACT THAT MALE-TO-MALE TRANSMISSION HAS BEEN FREQUENTLY OBSERVED. WE HAVE ONE PEDIGREE WITH AT LEAST NINE AFFECTED PERSONS AND AT LEAST ONE INSTANCE OF MALE-TO-MALE TRANSMISSION. THE DISORDER IS PROBABLY AN AUTOSOMAL DOMINANT WITH STRONGER EXPRESSION IN THE FEMALE. STRONGER EXPRESSION IN PRESUMED HETEROZYGOUS FEMALES THAN IN HEMIZYGOUS MALES IS CONTRARY TO WHAT IS EXPECTED IN X-LINKED DOMINANT INHERITANCE. THE POSSIBILITY OF X-LINKAGE IN A SMALL PROPORTION OF FAMILIES IS NOT COMPLETELY EXCLUDED, HOWEVER.

BLANDY, J. P., GAMMIE, W. F. P., STOVIN, P. G. I. AND SWETTENHAM, K.* TURBAN TUMOURS IN BROTHER AND SISTER. BRIT. J. SURG. 49* 136-140, 1961.

CHALSTREY, L. J.* TURBAN TUMORS. ST. BART'S HOSP. J. 59* 378-383, 1955.

EVANS, C. D.* TURBAN TUMOUR. BRIT. J. DERM. 66* 434-443, 1954.

GUGGENHEIM, W. AND SCHNYDER, U. W.* ZUR NOSOLOGIE DER SPIEGLER-BROOKE SCHEN TUMOREN. DERMATOLOGICA 122* 274-278, 1961.

REGAN, W. J.* TURBAN TUMOURS. PROC. ROY. SOC. MED. 49* 337-339, 1956.

SCHMIDT-BAUMLER, H.* FAMILIARES CYLINDROME. EIN BEITRAG ZUR FRAGE DER GESCHLECHTSBEGRENZTEN VERERBUNG. ARCH. DERM. SYPH. 163* 114-125, 1931.

WIEDMANN, A.* WEITERE BEITRAGE ZUR KENNTNIS DER SOGENANNTEN ZYLINDROME DER KOPFHAUT. ARCH. DERM. SYPH. 159* 180-187, 1929.

*31320 SPINAL AND BULBAR MUSCULAR ATROPHY

KENNEDY, ALTER AND SUNG (1968) DESCRIBED 9 MALES IN TWO UNRELATED KINDREDS. ONSET OF FASCICULATIONS FOLLOWED BY MUSCLE WEAKNESS AND WASTING OCCURRED AT APPROXIMATE-LY 40 YEARS OF AGE. BULBAR SIGNS AND FACIAL FASCICULATIONS WERE CHARACTERISTIC. DYSPHAGIA PERSISTED MORE THAN 10 YEARS IN ONE MAN OF EACH FAMILY. BABINSKI SIGN WAS NEGATIVE IN ALL. THE DISORDER IS COMPATIBLE WITH LONG LIFE. PYRAMIDAL, SENSORY AND CEREBELLAR SIGNS WERE ABSENT. THREE OF THEIR PATIENTS HAD GYNECOMAS-TIA. JAPANESE FAMILIES REPORTED BY TSUKAGOSHI ET AL. (1965) AND SOME OTHER ISOLATED CASES (SMITH AND PATEL, 1965) MAY HAVE HAD THE SAME DISORDER. INFANTILE MUSCULAR ATROPHY (WERDING-HOFFMAN DISEASE) IS AN AUTOSOMAL RECESSIVE. JUVENILE HEREDITARY PROXIMAL SPINAL MUSCULAR ATROPHY BEGINS IN CHILDHOOD OR ADOLESCENCE AND IS SLOWLY PROGRESSIVE USUALLY WITHOUT BULBAR INVOLVEMENT. INHERITANCE IS EITHER AUTOSOMAL RECESSIVE OR AUTOSOMAL DOMINANT. THE PROBAND IN MURAKAMI'S FAMILY (1957) WAS A 55-YEAR-OLD JAPANESE FARMER. KURLAND (1957) MENTIONED TWO FAMILIES

X
L
I
N
K
E
D

598

SEEN BY HIM IN JAPAN. QUARFORDT ET AL. (1970) DESCRIBED FOUR BROTHERS WITH ADULT-ONSET PROXIMAL SPINAL MUSCULAR ATROPHY. TYPE II HYPERLIPOPROTEINEMIA WAS PRESENT IN ALL FOUR AND WAS ABSENT FROM THEIR ONE UNAFFECTED SIB, A SISTER. SOME CHILDREN OF AFFECTED MALES, TOO YOUNG TO SHOW THE NEUROLOGIC ABNORMALITY, ALSO SHOWED HYPERLIPOPROTEINEMIA.

KENNEDY, W. R., ALTER, M. AND SUNG, J. H.* PROGRESSIVE PROXIMAL SPINAL AND BULBAR MUSCULAR ATROPHY OF LATE ONSET* A SEX-LINKED RECESSIVE TRAIT. NEUROLOGY 18* 671-680, 1968.

KURLAND, L. T.* EPIDEMIOLOGIC INVESTIGATIONS OF AMYOTROPHIC LATERAL SCLEROSIS. III. A GENETIC INTERPRETATION OF INCIDENCE AND GEOGRAPHIC DISTRIBUTION. MAYO CLIN. PROC. 32* 449-462, 1957.

LEE, G. R., MACDIARMID, W. D., CARTWRIGHT, G. E. AND WINTROBE, M. M.* HEREDI-TARY, X-LINKED, SIDEROACHRESTIC ANEMIA. THE ISOLATION OF TWO ERYTHROCYTE POPULATIONS DIFFERING IN XG(A) BLOOD TYPE AND PORPHYRIN CONTENT. BLOOD 32* 59-70, 1968.

MURAKAMI, U.* CLINICO-GENETIC STUDY OF HEREDITARY DISORDERS OF THE NERVOUS SYSTEM, ESPECIALLY ON PROBLEMS OF PATHOGENESIS. FOLIA PSYCHIAT. NEUROL. JAP. 1 (SUPPL.)* 1-209, 1957.

QUARFORDT, S. H., DEVIVO, D. C., ENGEL, W. K., LEVY, R. I. AND FREDRICKSON, D. S.* FAMILIAL ADULT-ONSET PROXIMAL SPINAL MUSCULAR ATROPHY. ARCH. NEUROL. 22* 541-549, 1970.

SMITH, J. B. AND PATEL, A.* THE WOHLFART-KUGELBERG-WELANDER DISEASE* REVIEW OF THE LITERATURE AND REPORT OF A CASE. NEUROLOGY 15* 469-473, 1965.

TAKIKAWA, K.* A PEDIGREE OF PROGRESSIVE BULBAR PARALYSIS APPEARING IN SEX-LINKED RECESSIVE INHERITANCE. JAP. J. HUM. GENET. 28* 116 ONLY, 1953.

TSUKAGOSHI, H., NAKANISHI, T., KONDO, K. AND TSUBAKI, T.* HEREDITARY, PROXIMAL, NEUROGENIC MUSCULAR ATROPHY IN ADULT. ARCH. NEUROL. 12* 597-603, 1965.

*31330 SPINAL ATAXIA

A KINDRED WITH X-LINKED INHERITANCE OF WHAT THE AUTHORS THOUGHT WAS PROBABLY FRIEDREICH'S ATAXIA WAS REPORTED BY TURNER AND ROBERTS (1938). ONSET WAS AT ABOUT FIVE YEARS AND THE VICTIM WAS BEDFAST BY ABOUT 20 YEARS. THE FIRST CARRIER FEMALE IN THE KINDRED WAS OF ENGLISH EXTRACTION. IN 1910 BRANDENBERG DESCRIBED FOUR MALES WITH FRIEDREICH'S ATAXIA IN THREE GENERATIONS OF A FAMILY, RELATED THROUGH FEMALES IN A PATTERN CONSISTENT WITH X-LINKAGE.

BRANDENBERG, F.* KASUISTISCHE BEITRAGE ZUR GLEICHGESCHLECHTLICHEN VERERBUNG. ARCH. RASS.-U. GES. BIOL. 7* 290-305, 1910.

TURNER, E. V. AND ROBERTS, E.* A FAMILY WITH A SEX-LINKED HEREDITARY ATAXIA. J. NERV. MENT. DIS. 87* 74-80, 1938.

*31340 SPONDYLO-EPIPHYSEAL DYSPLASIA, LATE

THE TRUNK IS PARTICULARLY SHORT AND THE HIPS SHOW DEGENERATIVE DISEASE. CHANGES IN THE SPINE AND HIPS BECOME EVIDENT BETWEEN 10 AND 14 YEARS OF AGE. IN ADULTS VERTEBRAL CHANGES, ESPECIALLY IN THE LUMBAR REGION, ARE DIAGNOSTIC. OCHRONOSIS IS SUGGESTED BY APPARENT INTERVERTEBRAL DISK CALCIFICATION. IN FACT, THE VERTEBRAL BODIES ARE MALFORMED AND FLATTENED AND MOST OF THE DENSE AREA IS PART OF THE VERTEBRAL PLATE.

BARBER, H. S.* AN UNUSUAL FORM OF FAMILIAL OSTEODYSTROPHY. LANCET 1* 1220-1221* AND 2* 154-155, 1960.

BANNERMAN, R. M.* X-LINKED SPONDYLOEPIPHYSEAL DYSPLASIA TARDA (SDT). THE CLINICAL DELINEATION OF BIRTH DEFECTS. IV. SKELETAL DYSPLASIAS. NEW YORK* NATIONAL FOUNDATION, 1969. PP. 48-51.

HOBAEK, A.* PROBLEMS OF HEREDITARY CHONDRODYSPLASIA. OSLO, NORWAY* OSLO U. PRESS, 1961.

JACOBSEN, A. W.* HEREDITARY OSTEOCHONDRO-DYSTROPHIA DEFORMANS. A FAMILY WITH TWENTY MEMBERS AFFECTED IN FIVE GENERATIONS. J.A.M.A. 113* 121-124, 1939.

LAMY, M. AND MAROTEAUX, P.* LES CHONDRODYSTROPHIES GENOTYPIQUES. PARIS* L'EXPANSION, 1960. PP. 67FF.

LANGER, L. O., JR.* SPONDYLOEPIPHYSEAL DYSPLASIA TARDA. HEREDITARY CHONDRODYS-PLASIA WITH CHARACTERISTIC VERTEBRAL CONFIGURATION IN THE ADULT. RADIOLOGY 82* 833-839, 1964.

MAROTEAUX, P., LAMY, M. AND BERNARD, J.* LA DYSPLASIE SPONDYLO-EPIPHYSAIRE TARDIVE. PRESSE MED. 65* 1205-1208, 1957.

X
L
I
N
K
E
D

ERPENSTEIN AND PFEIFFER (1967) DESCRIBED TRANSMISSION OF OLIGODONTIA OR HYPODONTIA THROUGH FOUR GENERATIONS OF A FAMILY. MALES HAD OLIGODONTIA, FEMALES HAD HYPODONTIA. NO MALE-TO-MALE TRANSMISSION WAS OBSERVED. HOWEVER, ONLY TWO AFFECTED MALES HAD CHILDREN (4 UNAFFECTED SONS, 1 DAUGHTER WITH HYPODONTIA). X-LINKAGE IS LIKELY. IN AT LEAST 18 PERSONS IN 4 GENERATIONS DAHLBERG (1937) NOTED ABSENCE OF AT LEAST SIX ANTERIOR TEETH IN BOTH DENTITIONS. HE SUGGESTED X-LINKED DOMINANT INHERITANCE, BUT AGAINST THIS IS ONE UNAFFECTED DAUGHTER OF THE ONE AFFECTED MALE WITH CHILDREN IN THE KINDRED.

DAHLBERG, A. A.* INHERITED CONGENITAL ABSENCE OF SIX INCISORS, DECIDUOUS AND PERMANENT. J. DENT. RES. 16* 59-62, 1937.

ERPENSTEIN, H. AND PFEIFFER, R. A.* GESCHLECHSGEBUNDEN-DOMINANT ERBLICHE ZAHNUNTERZAHL. HUMANGENETIK 4* 280-293, 1967.

31360 TELECANTHUS WITH ASSOCIATED ABNORMALITIES

OCULAR HYPERTELORISM IS OFTEN INCORRECTLY DIAGNOSED WHEN A FLAT NASAL BRIDGE, EPICANTHAL FOLDS, EXTERNAL STRABISMUS, WIDELY SPACED EYEBROWS, BLEPHAROPHIMOSIS OR SOME COMBINATION OF THESE IS PRESENT. TELECANTHUS IS A PREFERABLE TERM WHEN INCREASED DISTANCE SEPARATES THE INNER CANTHI. DYSTOPIA CANTHORUM IS A SYNONYM. CHRISTIAN ET AL. (1969) AND OPITZ ET AL. (1969) REPORTED, IN ALL, FOUR FAMILIES IN WHICH TELECANTHUS WITH OR WITHOUT HYPERTELORISM WAS ASSOCIATED IN MALES WITH HYPOSPADIAS, CRYPTORCHIDISM, CLEFT LIP AND PALATE, URINARY MALFORMATIONS, AND IN SOME MENTAL RETARDATION. FEMALE CARRIERS HAVE LESS SEVERE TELECANTHUS AND ESCAPED CONGENITAL MALFORMATION. EXCEPT FOR ONE ALLEGED AND UNCONFIRMED INSTANCE IN A REMOTE BRANCH OF ONE OF THE FAMILIES OF OPITZ ET AL., NO MALE-TO-MALE TRANSMISSION WAS OBSERVED. THUS X-LINKED INHERITANCE IS POSSIBLE.

CHRISTIAN, J. C., BIXLER, D., BLYTHE, S. C. AND MERRITT, A. D.* FAMILIAL TELECANTHUS WITH ASSOCIATED CONGENITAL ANOMALIES. THE CLINICAL DELINEATION OF BIRTH DEFECTS. II. MALFORMATION SYNDROMES. NEW YORK* NATIONAL FOUNDATION, 1969. PP. 82-85.

OPITZ, J. M., SUMMITT, R. L. AND SMITH, D. W.* THE BBB SYNDROME. FAMILIAL TELECANTHUS WITH ASSOCIATED CONGENITAL ANOMALIES. THE CLINICAL DELINEATION OF BIRTH DEFECTS. II. MALFORMATION SYNDROMES. NEW YORK* NATIONAL FOUNDATION, 1969. PP. 86-94.

*31370 TESTICULAR FEMINIZATION SYNDROME

THIS VARIETY OF SEX ANOMALY HAS BEEN OF RELATIVELY LONG INTEREST TO GENETICISTS LARGELY THROUGH THE PUBLICATIONS OF PETTERSSON AND BONNIER (1937). BOTH THE NATURE OF THE BASIC DEFECT AND THE MODE OF INHERITANCE ARE IN QUESTION. THE AFFECTED MALES HAVE FEMALE EXTERNAL GENITALIA, FEMALE BREAST DEVELOPMENT, BLIND VAGINA, ABSENT UTERUS AND FEMALE ADNEXA, ABDOMINAL OR INGUINAL TESTES, AND A NORMAL MALE (2A + XY) KARYOTYPE. THE PATIENTS OFTEN COME TO MEDICAL ATTENTION BECAUSE OF A PRESUMED INGUINAL HERNIA. MANY HAVE ABSENT PUBIC AND AXILLARY HAIR ('HAIRLESS PSEUDOFEMALE'). THE HAIR OF THE HEAD IS LUXURIANT, WITHOUT TEMPORAL BALDING. THE PHENOTYPE IS OFTEN VOLUPTUOUSLY FEMININE* NETTER (1958) REPORTED THIS DISORDER IN A FAMOUS PHOTOGRAPHIC MODEL, MARSHALL AND HARDER (1958) REPORTED AFFECTED MONOZYGOTIC TWINS WHO WORKED AS AIRLINE STEWARDESSES, AND POLAILLON (1891) DESCRIBED PROSTITUTION IN AN AFFECTED PERSON.
      IN ONE SUCH PATIENT STUDIED BY WILKINS (1957) THE HAIR FOLLICLES OF THE AXILLARY AND PUBIC AREAS, ALTHOUGH ANATOMICALLY NORMAL, WERE UNRESPONSIVE TO LOCAL OR PARENTERAL ADMINISTRATION OF ANDROGENS AND THE BEARD, VOICE, AND CLITORIS WERE SIMILARLY UNRESPONSIVE. FEMALE CARRIERS, PRESUMED HETEROZYGOTES, MAY SHOW NO, OR ALMOST NO, SECONDARY SEX HAIR BUT HAVE NORMAL MENSTRUATION, CONCEPTION AND PREGNANCIES. THE BASIC DEFECT IN CASES OF THE HAIRLESS PSEUDOFEMALE TYPE MIGHT BE END-ORGAN UNRESPONSIVENESS TO ANDROGEN, A SITUATION COMPARABLE TO NEPHROGENIC DIABETES INSIPIDUS, AND PSEUDOHYPOPARATHYROIDISM (INHERITED AS AN AUTOSOMAL DOMINANT). (THESE CONDITIONS ARE ANALOGOUS TO THE SITUATION IN THE SEABRIGHT BANTAM COCK WHICH HAS A FEMALE COMB STRUCTURE DESPITE OBVIOUS DEMONSTRATIONS OF VIRILITY.) IT IS LIKELY THAT MORE THAN ONE DISTINCT ENTITY IS INCLUDED IN THE TESTICULAR FEMINIZATION SYNDROME. WILKINS STATES* 'IN ABOUT ONE-THIRD OF THE CASES OF MALE PSEUDOHERMAPHRODITISM 'OF FEMININE TYPE' SEXUAL HAIR HAS BEEN ENTIRELY LACKING.' MILLER CONSIDERS 'FEMINIZING LABIAL TESTES' OF THE TYPE DESCRIBED BY LUBS, VILAR AND BERGENSTAL (1959) TO BE A SEPARATE FORM OF MALE PSEUDOHERMAPHRODITISM.
      THE HISTOLOGICAL CHANGES IN THE TESTIS IN THIS SYNDROME TEND TO BE CHARAC-TERISTIC AND NOT THE NON-SPECIFIC ONES OF CRYPTORCHIDISM. FURTHERMORE, THE DEGREE OF FEMINIZATION APPEARS TO BE CORRELATED WITH THE DEGREE OF CHANGE IN THE TESTIS.
      WHETHER THE TRAIT IS X-LINKED OR AUTOSOMAL IS UNCERTAIN. THE EVIDENCE FROM LINKAGE STUDIES IS INCONCLUSIVE.
      MAINLY USING DATA ON THE FREQUENCY OF INGUINAL HERNIA IN FEMALES, JAGIELLO AND ATWELL (1962) ESTIMATED THE FREQUENCY OF TESTICULAR FEMINIZATION AS BEING OF THE ORDER OF ONE IN 65,000 MALES. THIS VALUE IMPLIES A MUTATION RATE OF 0.5-0.4X10-5 GENES PER GENERATION (DEPENDING ON WHETHER THE DISORDER IS AUTOSOMAL DOMINANT OR X-LINKED RECESSIVE).
      PROFESSOR J. MCL. MORRIS, YALE UNIVERSITY, CALLED MY ATTENTION TO THE

X
L
I
N
K
E
D

FOLLOWING CASE OF GAYRAL AND COLLEAGUES (1960)* A WOMAN, WHO WAS SISTER, MOTHER, AND GRANDMOTHER OF AFFECTED MALES, SHOWED ASYMMETRY IN THE DEVELOPMENT OF THE BREASTS, BODY HAIR, AND VULVA. THE RIGHT BREAST WAS SMALLER THAN THE LEFT AND THERE WAS NO PUBIC HAIR TO THE RIGHT OF THE MID-LINE. SHE HAD ALWAYS HAD MENSTRUAL IRREGULARITY BUT HAD THREE CHILDREN, AN AFFECTED MALE, A CARRIER DAUGHTER, AND A DAUGHTER WHO WAS THE MOTHER OF THREE UNAFFECTED SONS. THE FINDINGS MAY BE BEST EXPLAINED BY AN X-LINKED RECESSIVE (OR INCOMPLETELY RECESSIVE) GENE WHOSE EFFECTS ARE TO RENDER TISSUES RESISTANT TO MALE HORMONE. THE PATCHY CHANGES IN THE HETEROZYGOUS FEMALE SUGGEST, FURTHERMORE, THAT THE CAUSATIVE GENE IS X-LINKED WITH LYONIZATION PHENOMENON.

FRENCH ET AL. (1966) FOUND THAT TESTOSTERONE FAILED TO AFFECT THE URINARY EXCRETION OF NITROGEN, PHOSPHORUS AND CITRIC ACID WHEN GIVEN IN A DOSAGE MUCH GREATER THAN THAT WHICH IN CONTROLS DECREASED EXCRETION OF ALL THREE. CONVERSION OF TESTOSTERONE TO ESTROGEN DOES NOT OCCUR, IT SEEMS. PLASMA ESTROGEN LEVELS WERE THOSE OBSERVED IN THE NORMAL FEMALE. LEYDIG CELL STIMULATION TO ESTROGEN PRODUCTION OCCURS PROBABLY BECAUSE OF FAILURE OF THE FEED-BACK REPRESSION OF THE PITUITARY WHICH SHARES THE UNRESPONSIVENESS TO TESTOSTERONE. SOUTHERN ET AL. (1961) SHOWED NORMAL TESTOSTERONE LEVELS. THE MEANS FOR ESTABLISHING X-LINKED INHERITANCE INCLUDED DEMONSTRATION OF LINKAGE WITH AN X CHROMOSOME MARKER, DEMONSTRATION OF LYONIZATION IN HETEROZYGOUS FEMALES AND DEMONSTRATION THAT THE PROPORTION OF NEW MUTATION CASES IS ONE THIRD RATHER THAN ONE-HALF (EXPECTED OF AN AUTOSOMAL DOMINANT). POSSIBLY BY ARTIFICIAL INSEMINATION METHODS, X-LINKED INHERITANCE COULD BE TESTED IN THE TESTICULAR FEMINIZATION OF CATTLE (NES, 1966). LYON AND HAWKES (1970) DESCRIBED A HOMOLOGOUS PHENOTYPE IN THE MOUSE AND SHOWED THAT IT IS GENETIC, THE TFM LOCUS BEING SITUATED IN THE MIDDLE OF THE X CHROMOSOME. OHNO AND LYON (1970) SHOWED THAT IN THESE MICE CERTAIN ENZYMES OF THE MOUSE KIDNEY, E.G., ALCOHOL DEHYDROGENASE, ARE NOT INDUCIBLE AS IS USUALLY POSSIBLE. THEY POSTULATED THAT THE TFM LOCUS IS A REPRESSIVE REGULATORY LOCUS CONTROLLING MANY TESTOSTERONE INDUCIBLE ENZYMES. IN AFFECTED HEMIZYGOTES ALL THESE ENZYMES BECOME NON-INDUCIBLE. ACCORDING TO THEIR SUGGESTION, THIS IS A REGULATOR MUTATION LIKE THE NON-INDUCIBLE MUTATION IN THE LAC-REPRESSOR LOCUS OF E. COLI AS ELUCIDATED BY JACOB AND MONOD (1963). BARDIN ET AL. (1970) DESCRIBED STUDIES OF THE PSEUDOHERMAPHRODITIC RAT WHICH SEEMS TO HAVE A DISORDER ANALOGOUS TO TESTICULAR FEMINIZATION. ANDROGEN-DEPENDENT DIFFERENTIATION IS ABSENT. DEFECTIVE FORMATION OF DIHYDROTESTOSTERONE WAS APPARENTLY NOT THE EXPLANATION.

CLINICALLY CASES OF INCOMPLETE, OR PARTIAL, TESTICULAR FEMINIZATION ARE RECOGNIZED. THESE DIFFER FROM THE CLASSIC "COMPLETE" FORM IN THE PRESENCE OF ENLARGED CLITORIS AT BIRTH AND VIRILIZATION AT PUBERTY. FAMILIAL OCCURRENCE HAS BEEN

ADACHI, K. AND KANO, M.* ADENYL CYCLASE IN HUMAN HAIR FOLLICLES* ITS INHIBITION BY DIHYDROTESTOSTERONE. BIOCHEM. BIOPHYS. RES. COMMUN. 41* 884-890, 1970.

ALBRIGHT, F., BURNETT, C. H., SMITH, P. H. AND PARSON, W.* PSEUDO-HYPOPARA-THYROIDISM, AN EXAMPLE OF "SEABRIGHT-BANTAM SYNDROME." REPORT OF 3 CASES. ENDOCRINOLOGY 30* 922-932, 1942.

BARDIN, C. W., BULLOCK, L., SCHNEIDER, G., ALLISON, J. E. AND STANLEY, A. J.* PSEUDOHERMAPHRODITE RAT* END ORGAN INSENSITIVITY TO TESTOSTERONE. SCIENCE 167* 1136-1137, 1970.

BURGERMEISTER, J. J.* CONTRIBUTION A L'ETUDE D'UN TYPE FAMILIAL D'INTERSEXUA-LITE. J. GENET. HUM. 2* 51-82, 1953.

FRENCH, F. S., BAGGETT, B., VAN WYK, J. J., TALBERT, L. M., HUBBARD, W. R., JOHNSTON, F. R., WEAVER, R. P., FORCHIELLI, E., RAO, G. S. AND SARDA, I. R.* TESTICULAR FEMINIZATION* CLINICAL, MORPHOLOGICAL AND BIOCHEMICAL STUDIES. J. CLIN. ENDOCR. 25* 661-677, 1965.

FRENCH, F. S., VAN WYK, J. J., BAGGETT, B., EASTERLING, W. E., TALBERT, L. M., JOHNSTON, F. R. AND FORCHIELLI, E.* FURTHER EVIDENCE OF A TARGET ORGAN DEFECT IN THE SYNDROME OF TESTICULAR FEMINIZATION. J. CLIN. ENDOCR. 26* 493-503, 1966.

GAYRAL, L., BARRAUD, M., CARRIE, J. AND CANDEBAT, L.* PSEUDO-HERMAPHRODISME A TYPE DE "TESTICULE FEMINISANT"* 11 CAS. ETUDE HORMONALE ET ETUDE PSYCHOLOGIQUE. TOULOUSE MED. 61* 637-647, 1960.

GRUMBACH, M. M. AND BARR, M. L.* CYTOLOGIC TESTS OF CHROMOSOMAL SEX IN RELATION TO SEXUAL ANOMALIES IN MAN. RECENT PROGR. HORMONE RES. 14* 255-334, 1958.

HAUSER, G. A.* TESTIKULARE FEMINISIERUNG. IN* DIE INTERSEXUALITAT. OVERZIER, C. (ED.)* STUTTGART* GEORG THIEME VERLAG, 1961. PP. 261-282.

JACOB, F. AND MONOD, J.* GENERAL REPRESSION, ALLOSTERIC INHIBITION, AND CELLULAR DIFFERENTIATION. IN, LOCKE, M. (ED.)* CYTODIFFERENTIATION AND MACROMOLE-CULAR SYNTHESIS. LONDON* ACADEMIC PRESS, 1963. PP. 30-64.

JAGIELLO, G., AND ATWELL, J. D.* PREVALENCE OF TESTICULAR FEMINISATION. LANCET 1* 329 ONLY, 1962.

LUBS, H. A., JR., VILAR, O. AND BERGENSTAL, D. M.* FAMILIAL MALE PSEUDOHERMAPH-RODITISM WITH LABIAL TESTES AND PARTIAL FEMINIZATION* ENDOCRINE STUDIES AND

X
L
I
N
K
E
D

GENETIC ASPECTS. J. CLIN. ENDOCR. 19* 1110-1120, 1959.

LYON, M. F. AND HAWKES, S. G.* X-LINKED GENE FOR TESTICULAR FEMINIZATION IN THE MOUSE. NATURE 225* 1217-1219, 1970.

MARSHALL, H. K. AND HARDER, H. I.* TESTICULAR FEMINIZING SYNDROME IN MALE PSEUDOHERMAPHRODE* REPORT OF TWO CASES IN IDENTICAL TWINS. OBSTET. GYNEC. 12* 284-293, 1958.

MAUVAIS-JARVIS, P., BERCOVICI, J. P., CREPY, O. AND GAUTHIER, F.* STUDIES ON TESTOSTERONE METABOLISM IN SUBJECTS WITH TESTICULAR FEMINIZATION SYNDROME. J. CLIN. INVEST. 49* 31-40, 1970.

MILLER, O. J.* DEVELOPMENTAL SEX ABNORMALITIES. IN, PENROSE, L. S. (ED.)* RECENT ADVANCES IN HUMAN GENETICS. LONDON* J. AND A. CHURCHILL LTD., 1961. PP. 39-55.

NES, N.* TESTIKULAER FEMINISERING HOS STORFE. NORD. MED. 18* 19-29, 1966.

NORTHCUTT, R. C., ISLAND, D. P. AND LIDDLE, G. W.* AN EXPLANATION FOR THE TARGET ORGAN UNRESPONSIVENESS TO TESTOSTERONE IN THE TESTICULAR FEMINIZATION SYNDROME. J. CLIN. ENDOCR. 29* 422-425, 1969.

OHNO, S. AND LYON, M. F.* X-LINKED TESTICULAR FEMINIZATION IN THE MOUSE AS A NON-INDUCIBLE REGULATORY MUTATION OF THE JACOB-MONOD TYPE. CLIN. GENET. 1* 121-127, 1970.

PETTERSSON, G. AND BONNIER, G.* INHERITED SEX-MOSAIC IN MAN. HEREDITAS 23* 49-69, 1937.

PUCK, T. T., ROBINSON, A. AND TJIO, J. H.* FAMILIAL PRIMARY AMENHORRHEA DUE TO TESTICULAR FEMINIZATION* A HUMAN GENE AFFECTING SEX DIFFERENTIATION. PROC. SOC. EXP. BIOL. MED. 103* 192-196, 1960.

SCHREINER, W. E.* UBER EINE HEREDITARE FORM VON PSEUDOHERMAPHRODISMUS MASCU-LINUS (TESTICULARE FEMINISIERUNG). GYNAECOLOGIA 148* 355-357, 1959.

SOUTHERN, A. L. AND SAITO, A.* THE SYNDROME OF TESTICULAR FEMINIZATION. A REPORT OF THREE CASES WITH CHROMATOGRAPHIC ANALYSIS OF THE URINARY NEUTRAL 17-KETOSTEROIDS. ANN. INTERN. MED. 55* 925-931, 1961.

SOUTHERN, A. L.* THE SYNDROME OF TESTICULAR FEMINIZATION. IN, LEVINE, R. AND LUFT, R. (EDS.)* ADVANCES IN METABOLIC DISEASES. NEW YORK* ACADEMIC PRESS, 1965. PP. 227-256.

STENCHEVER, M. A., NG, A. B. P., JONES, G. K. AND JARVIS, J. A.* TESTICULAR FEMINIZATION SYNDROME. CHROMOSOMAL, HISTOLOGIC, AND GENETIC STUDIES IN A LARGE KINDRED. OBSTET. GYNEC. 33* 649-657, 1969.

STRICKLAND, A. L. AND FRENCH, F. S.* ABSENCE OF RESPONSE TO DIHYDROTESTOSTERONE IN THE SYNDROME OF TESTICULAR FEMINIZATION. J. CLIN. ENDOCR. 29* 1284-1286, 1969.

WILKINS, L.* THE DIAGNOSIS AND TREATMENT OF ENDOCRINE DISORDERS IN CHILDHOOD AND ADOLESCENCE. SPRINGFIELD, ILL.* CHARLES C THOMAS, 1957 (2ND ED.).

31380 TESTICULAR FEMINIZATION, INCOMPLETE TYPE

THIS SYNDROME RESEMBLES THE COMPLETE FORM IN RESPECT TO FEMALE PHENOTYPE, BILATERAL TESTES AND 46,XY KARYOTYPE, BUT DIFFERS BY CLITORAL ENLARGEMENT FROM BIRTH AND VIRILIZATION AT PUBERTY. THE LABIA MAY BE PARTIALLY FUSED. ALTHOUGH THE DEGREE OF MASCULINIZATION OF THE EXTERNAL GENITALIA IS VARIABLE, MOST PATIENTS ARE RAISED AS FEMALES. THE TESTES RESEMBLES THOSE OF COMPLETE TESTICULAR FEMINIZATION. IN THE FAMILY DESCRIBED BY LUBS ET AL. (1959) SOME SPERMATOGENESIS WAS FOUND. THERE IS PARTIAL RESPONSIVENESS TO ANDROGEN (WINTERBORN ET AL. (1970). ALTHOUGH X-LINKED RECESSIVE OR MALE-LIMITED AUTOSOMAL DOMINANT INHERITANCE IS SUGGESTED BY SOME PEDIGREES SUCH AS THAT OF LUBS ET AL. (1959), AN AUTOSOMAL RECESSIVE FORM (Q.V.) SEEMS TO EXIST ALSO.

LUBS, H. A., JR., VILAR, O. AND BERGENSTAL, D. M.* FAMILIAL MALE PSEUDOHERMAPH-RODITISM WITH LABIAL TESTES AND PARTIAL FEMINIZATION* ENDOCRINE STUDIES AND GENETIC ASPECTS. J. CLIN. ENDOCR. 19* 1110-1120, 1959.

WINTERBORN, M. H., FRANCE, N. E. AND RAITI, S.* INCOMPLETE TESTICULAR FEMINIZA-TION. ARCH. DIS. CHILD. 45* 811-812, 1970.

*31390 THROMBOCYTOPENIA

VESTERMARK AND VESTERMARK (1964) FOUND X-LINKED 'ESSENTIAL' THROMBOCYTOPENIA IN TWO GENERATIONS OF A FAMILY. ONE AFFECTED MALE BECAME SYMPTOM-FREE SPONTANEOUSLY AFTER PUBERTY AND ONE BECAME SYMPTOM-FREE AFTER SPLENECTOMY AT THE AGE OF 18 YEARS BUT DIED LATER OF ADRENAL HEMORRHAGE. THREE OTHER PATIENTS HAD, IN ADDITION TO HEMORRHAGIC DIATHESIS, A MILD TENDENCY TO INFECTION AND ECZEMA. THIS CONDITION

X
L
I
N
K
E
D

MAY BE DISTINCT FROM ALDRICH'S SYNDROME (Q.V.). IN ADDITION TO ALDRICH SYNDROME AND SEPARATE FROM IT, A PROBABLE X-LINKED THROMBOCYTOPENIA HAS BEEN DESCRIBED BY ATA, FISHER, AND HOLMAN (1965) IN 9 MALES IN 6 SIBSHIPS IN 4 GENERATIONS OF A KINDRED, CONNECTED BY FEMALES. IN ADDITION ONE FEMALE WAS AFFECTED. SHE WAS KARYOLOGICALLY NORMAL AND THE FATHER HAD NO HISTORY OF BLEEDING. THEREFORE, SHE PROBABLY REPRESENTS UNFORTUNATE LYONIZATION. SHE DIFFERED FROM THE AFFECTED MALES IN RECOVERING SPONTANEOUSLY. CANALES AND MAUER (1967) STUDIED A FAMILY CONTAINING 7 THROMBOCYTOPENIC MALES IN AN X-LINKED RECESSIVE PEDIGREE PATTERN. ALTHOUGH NO ECZEMA OR UNDUE SUSCEPTIBILITY TO INFECTION WAS NOTED AND BLEEDING SYMPTOMS WERE MILD, 5 OF THE 7 SHOWED REDUCED OR ABSENT ISOHEMAGGLUTININS AND INCREASED GAMMA-A GLOBULIN.

ATA, M., FISHER, O. D. AND HOLMAN, C. A.* INHERITED THROMBOCYTOPENIA. LANCET 1* 119-123, 1965.

CANALES, L. AND MAUER, A. M.* SEX-LINKED HEREDITARY THROMBOCYTOPENIA AS A VARIANT OF WISKOTT-ALDRICH SYNDROME. NEW ENG. J. MED. 277* 899-901, 1967.

VESTERMARK, B. AND VESTERMARK, S.* FAMILIAL SEX-LINKED THROMBOCYTOPENIA. ACTA PEDIAT. 53* 365-370, 1964.

31400 THROMBOCYTOPENIA WITH ELEVATED SERUM IGA AND RENAL DISEASE

GUTENBERGER ET AL. (1970) DESCRIBED A KINDRED IN WHICH 10 MALES AND TWO FEMALES HAD THROMBOCYTOPENIA APPARENTLY AS A RESULT OF REDUCED PLATELET PRODUCTION. EIGHT OF THE THROMBOCYTOPENIC PERSONS HAD ELEVATED IGA LEVELS IN THE SERUM. RENAL BIOPSY IN THREE THROMBOCYTOPENIC BROTHERS WITH HEMATURIA SHOWED VARYING DEGREES OF GLOMERULONEPHRITIS. THE TWO THROMBOCYTOPENIC WOMEN WERE MOTHERS OF AFFECTED SONS. ONE OF THESE TWO WOMEN ALSO HAD ELEVATED IGA. THE AUTHORS CONCLUDED THAT THE DISORDER IS X-LINKED AND PROBABLY DISTINCT FROM THE WISKOTT-ALDRICH SYNDROME AND FROM 'SIMPLE' X-LINKED THROMBOCYTOPENIA.

GUTENBERGER, J., TRYGSTAD, C. W., STIEHN, E. R., OPITZ, J. M., THATCHER, L. G. AND BLOODWORTH, J. M. B., JR.* FAMILIAL THROMBOCYTOPENIA, ELEVATED SERUM IGA LEVELS AND RENAL DISEASE. AM. J. MED. 49* 729-741, 1970.

31410 THUMB, CONGENITAL CLASPED

IN THIS DISORDER THE THUMB IS ADDUCTED AND FLEXED ACROSS THE PALM DUE TO A DEFECT IN THE EXTENSORS OF THE THUMB. WECKESSER ET AL. (1968) DESCRIBED AN INTERESTING NEGRO FAMILY IN WHICH 7 MALES IN 4 SIBSHIPS WERE AFFECTED. THE PATTERN WAS ENTIRELY CONSISTENT WITH X-LINKED RECESSIVE INHERITANCE. FINDINGS IN CHILDREN AND GRANDCHILDREN OF AFFECTED MALES WERE NOT DESCRIBED. WHITE AND JENSEN (1952) OBSERVED THE ANOMALY IN MOTHER AND TWO CHILDREN AND NAMBA ET AL. (1965) DESCRIBED IT IN BROTHER AND SISTER. A PREPONDERANCE OF AFFECTED MALES (27 OUT OF 42) IS CONSISTENT WITH X-LINKAGE, ESPECIALLY WHEN THE LIKELY HETEROGENEITY OF CONGENITAL CLASPED THUMB IS TAKEN INTO ACCOUNT. (WECKESSER ET AL. (1968) CLASSIFIED THEIR CASES IN 4 GROUPS.) CLASPED THUMB OCCURS IN SOME FAMILIES WITH X-LINKED HYDROCE-PHALUS DUE TO STENOSIS OF THE AQUEDUCT OF SYLVIUS (Q.V.).

NAMBA, K., MUDA, Y. AND HACHIGUCHI, T.* CONGENITAL CLASPED THUMB. ORTHOP. SURG. 16* 1031-1035, 1965.

WECKESSER, E. C., REED, J. R. AND HEIPLE, K. G.* CONGENITAL CLASPED THUMB (CONGENITAL FLEXION-ADDUCTION DEFORMITY OF THE THUMB). A SYNDROME, NOT A SPECIFIC ENTITY. J. BONE JOINT SURG. 50A* 1417-1428, 1968.

WHITE, J. W. AND JENSEN, W. E.* THE INFANT'S PERSISTENT THUMB-CLUTCHED HAND. J. BONE JOINT SURG. 34A* 680-688, 1952.

*31420 THYROXINE-BINDING GLOBULIN (TBG) OF SERUM, VARIANTS OF

THYROXINE-BINDING GLOBULIN IS REDUCED SO THAT PATIENTS SHOW REDUCED PROTEIN BOUND IODINE (PBI) BUT ARE EUTHYROID. NICOLOFF, DOWLING AND PATTON (1964) OBSERVED 6 CASES (3 MALES, 3 FEMALES) IN 3 SIBSHIPS OF TWO GENERATIONS OF A FAMILY. NO MALE-TO-MALE TRANSMISSION WAS OBSERVED. NIKOLAI AND SEAL (1966) STUDIED TWO FAMILIES IN WHICH X-LINKAGE IS POSSIBLE. MARSHALL, LEVY AND STEINBERG (1966) DESCRIBED AN EXTENSIVELY STUDIED FAMILY IN WHICH THE FINDINGS WERE MOST CONSISTENT WITH X-LINKAGE. FEMALE CARRIERS SHOWED AN INTERMEDIATE LEVEL OF TBG. WITH A MUTATION, PRESUMABLY AT THE SAME LOCUS, AN INCREASE IN TBG CAN OCCUR. BECAUSE OF INCREASE IN TOTAL BINDING GLOBULIN PROTEIN-BOUND IODINE IS INCREASED IN FOUR PERSONS IN THREE GENERATIONS. THE PEDIGREE PATTERN WAS EQUALLY CONSISTENT WITH AUTOSOMAL AND X-LINKED DOMINANCE. BEIERWALTES AND ROBBINS (1959) FOUND HIGH TBG IN A FATHER AND HIS ONLY DAUGHTER. BOTH HIS SONS HAD NORMAL TBG LEVELS. THE DAUGHTER'S LEVEL WAS NOT AS HIGH AS THE FATHER'S. THUS IN THIS FAMILY ALSO X-LINKED DOMINANCE WAS SUGGESTED. JONES AND SEAL (1967) REPORTED A FAMILY WITH ELEVATED TBG IN 9 PERSONS IN 3 GENERATIONS, AGAIN IN A PATTERN SUGGESTING X-LINKAGE. THEY SUGGESTED GENE DUPLICATION AS THE MECHANISM OF THE ELEVATION. X-LINKED INHERITANCE WAS STRONGLY SUPPORTED BY THE FINDINGS OF DEFICIENCY OF TBG IN A PATIENT WITH THE XO TURNER SYNDROME (REFETOFF AND SELENKOW, 1968). THE MATERNAL GRANDFATHER AND A HALF BROTHER WERE ALSO TBG-DEFICIENT AND AT LEAST 3 FEMALES, INCLUDING THE MOTHER, HAD INTERMEDIATE LEVELS. KRAEMER AND WISWELL (1968) PRESENTED SUGGESTIVE BUT NOT

X
L
I
N
K
E
D

CONCLUSIVE EVIDENCE OF AUTOSOMAL TRANSMISSION AND SOME OTHER PUBLISHED PEDIGREES ARE CONSISTENT WITH THIS MODE. THORSON ET AL. (1966) PRESENTED EVIDENCE FOR TWO THYROID-BINDING GLOBULINS, THUS CREATING THE POSSIBILITY OF APPRECIABLE GENETIC HETEROGENEITY IN BOTH HIGH AND LOW TBG. FOR A REVIEW, SEE RIVAS ET AL. (1971).

BEIERWALTES, W. H. AND ROBBINS, J.* FAMILIAL INCREASE IN THYROXINE BINDING SITES IN SERUM ALPHA GLOBULIN. J. CLIN. INVEST. 38* 1683-1688, 1959.

FIALKOW, P. J., GIBLETT, E. R. AND MUSA, B.* INCREASED SERUM THYROXINE-BINDING GLOBULIN CAPACITY* INHERITANCE AND LINKAGE RELATIONSHIPS. J. CLIN. ENDOCR. 30* 66-70, 1970.

FLORSHEIM, W. H., DOWLING, J. T., MEISTER, L. AND BODFISH, R. E.* FAMILIAL ELEVATION OF SERUM THYROXINE-BINDING CAPACITY. J. CLIN. ENOCR. 22* 735-740, 1962.

JONES, J. E. AND SEAL, U. S.* X-CHROMOSOME LINKED INHERITANCE OF ELEVATED THYROXINE-BINDING GLOBULIN. J. CLIN. ENDOCR. 27* 1521-1528, 1967.

KRAEMER, E. AND WISWELL, J. G.* FAMILIAL THYROXINE-BINDING GLOBULIN DEFICIENCY. METABOLISM 17* 260-262, 1968.

MARSHALL, J. S., LEVY, R. P. AND STEINBERG, A. G.* HUMAN THYROXINE-BINDING GLOBULIN DEFICIENCY. A GENETIC STUDY. NEW ENG. J. MED. 274* 1469-1473, 1966.

NICOLOFF, J. T., DOWLING, J. T. AND PATTON, D. D.* INHERITANCE OF DECREASED THYROXINE-BINDING BY THE THYROXINE-BINDING GLOBULIN. J. CLIN. ENDOCR. 24* 294-298, 1964.

NIKOLAI, T. F. AND SEAL, U. S.* X-CHROMOSOME LINKED FAMILIAL DECREASE IN THYROXINE-BINDING GLOBULIN ACTIVITY. J. CLIN. ENDOCR. 26* 835-841, 1966.

NIKOLAI, T. F. AND SEAL, U. S.* X-CHROMOSOME LINKED INHERITANCE OF THYROXINE-BINDING GLOBULIN DEFICIENCY. J. CLIN. ENDOCR. 27* 1515-1520, 1967.

REFETOFF, S. AND SELENKOW, H. A.* FAMILIAL THYROXINE-BINDING GLOBULIN DEFICIEN-CY IN A PATIENT WITH TURNER'S SYNDROME (XO). GENETIC STUDY OF A KINDRED. NEW ENG. J. MED. 278* 1081-1087, 1968.

RIVAS, M. L., MERRITT, A. D. AND OLIVER, L.* GENETIC VARIANTS OF THYROXINE BINDING GLOBULIN (TBG). THE CLINICAL DELINEATION OF BIRTH DEFECTS. X. THE ENDOCRINE SYSTEM. BALTIMORE* WILLIAMS AND WILKINS, 1971.

THORSON, S. C., TAUXE, W. N. AND TASWELL, H. F.* EVIDENCE FOR THE EXISTENCE OF TWO THYROXINE-BINDING GLOBULIN MOIETIES* CORRELATION BETWEEN PAPER AND STARCH-GEL ELECTROPHORETIC PATTERNS UTILIZING THYROXINE-BINDING GLOBULIN-DEFICIENT SERA. J. CLIN. ENDOCR. 26* 181-188, 1966.

31430 TORTICOLLIS, KELOIDS, CRYPTORCHIDISM, AND RENAL DYSPLASIA

GOEMINNE (1968) DESCRIBED A SYNDROME HE CONCLUDED IS INHERITED AS AN X-LINKED TRAIT WITH INCOMPLETE DOMINANCE. NONE OF THE AFFECTED MALES REPRODUCED. AFFECTED PERSONS INCLUDED (1) A MALE WITH CONGENITAL MUSCULAR TORTICOLLIS, (2) A MALE WITH TORTICOLLIS, CRYPTORCHIDISM AND VARICOSE VEINS, (3) A MALE WITH TORTICOLLIS, MANY SPONTANEOUS KELOIDS, UNILATERAL CRYPTORCHIDISM, OLIGOSPERMIA, CHRONIC PYELONEPHRI-TIS WITH UNILATERAL RENAL ATROPHY, MULTIPLE CUTANEOUS NEVI, A BASAL CELL EPITHE-LIOMA, AND VARICOSE VEINS, (4) A MALE WITH TORTICOLLIS, KELOIDS AND CRYPTORCHI-DISM, (5) A FEMALE WITH TORTICOLLIS AND PIGMENTED NEVI, AND (6) A FEMALE WITH FACIAL ASYMMETRY, CHRONIC PYCLONEPHRITIS AND NEVI. THE PEDIGREE WAS CONSISTENT WITH THE POSTULATED MODE OF INHERITANCE BUT NO AFFECTED MALE REPRODUCED.

GOEMINNE, L.* A NEW PROBABLY X-LINKED INHERITED SYNDROME* CONGENITAL TORTICOL-LIS, MULTIPLE KELOIDS, CRYPTORCHIDISM AND RENAL DYSPLASIA. ACTA GENET. MED. GEM. 17* 439-467, 1968.

31440 VALVULAR HEART DISEASE, CONGENITAL

MONTELEONE AND FAGAN (1969) DESCRIBED 6 DEFINITE AND 1 PROBABLE CASE OF CONGENITAL HEART DISEASE IN MALES IN FOUR SIBSHIPS OF THREE GENERATIONS OF A NEGRO KINDRED IN A PATTERN SUGGESTING X-LINKED RECESSIVE INHERITANCE. FOUR HAD MITRAL AND AORTIC REGURGITATION, OF WHOM TWO ALSO HAD TRICUSPID REGURGITATION. THE FIFTH DEFINITE CASE HAD ONLY MITRAL REGURGITATION. HISTOLOGICALLY CHANGES IN THE MITRAL VALVE OF ONE CASE RESEMBLED THOSE SEEN IN THE *FLOPPY VALVE SYNDROME* (READ ET AL., 1965) OR IN MARFAN SYNDROME (WHICH WAS SUGGESTED BY NO OTHER FEATURE OF THE CASES).

MONTELEONE, P. L. AND FAGAN, L. F.* POSSIBLE X-LINKED CONGENITAL HEART DISEASE. CIRCULATION 39* 611-614, 1969.

READ, R. C., THAL, A. P. AND WENDT, V. E.* SYMPTOMATIC VALVULAR MYXOMATOUS TRANSFORMATION (THE FLOPPY VALVE SYNDROME). A POSSIBLE FORME FRUSTE OF THE MARFAN SYNDROME. CIRCULATION 32* 897-910, 1965.

*31450 VAN DEN BOSCH SYNDROME

X
L
I
N
K
E
D

THE COMPONENTS OF THIS SYNDROME TRANSMITTED AS AN X-LINKED RECESSIVE ARE (1) MENTAL DEFICIENCY, (2) CHOROIDEREMIA, (3) ACROKERATOSIS VERRUCIFORMIS, (4) ANHIDROSIS, AND (5) SKELETAL DEFORMITY. AN INTERESTING AND POSSIBLY IMPORTANT POINT IS THAT AT LEAST 3 OF THESE FIVE COMPONENTS HAVE BEEN DESCRIBED AS ISOLATED X-LINKED TRAITS. THE SYNDROME HAS BEEN OBSERVED IN A SINGLE KINDRED.

VAN DEN BOSCH, J.* A NEW SYNDROME IN THREE GENERATIONS OF A DUTCH FAMILY. OPHTHALMOLOGICA 137* 422-423, 1959.

31460 WILDERVANCK SYNDROME (CERVICO-OCULO-ACOUSTIC SYNDROME)

THE WILDERVANCK SYNDROME CONSISTS OF CONGENITAL PERCEPTIVE DEAFNESS, KLIPPEL-FEIL ANOMALY (FUSED CERVICAL VERTEBRAE), AND ABDUCENS PALSY WITH RETRACTIO BULBI (DUANE SYNDROME). THE DISORDER IS LIMITED, OR ALMOST COMPLETELY LIMITED, TO FEMALES, RAISING THE QUESTION OF SEX-LINKED DOMINANCE WITH LETHALITY IN THE HEMIZYGOUS MALE. THIS SYNDROME (AT LEAST PROFOUND CHILDHOOD DEAFNESS AND KLIPPEL-FEIL MALFORMATION) MAY BE RESPONSIBLE FOR AT LEAST 1 PERCENT OF DEAFNESS AMONG GIRLS. THE DEAFNESS IS PERCEPTIVE IN TYPE AND HAS BEEN SHOWN BY RADIOLOGIC STUDIES TO BE DUE TO A BONY MALFORMATION OF THE INNER EAR. KIRKHAM (1969) DESCRIBED A FAMILY WHICH WAS AFFECTED THROUGH 5 GENERATIONS WITH PERCEPTIVE DEAFNESS AND IN WHICH TWO MEMBERS HAD DUANE'S SYNDROME.

FRASER, W. I. AND MACGILLIVRAY, R. C.* CERVICO-OCULO-ACOUSTIC DYSPLASIA ('THE SYNDROME OF WILDERVANCK'). J. MENT. DEFIC. RES. 12* 322-329, 1968.

KIRKHAM, T. H.* CERVICO-OCULO-ACUSTICUS SYNDROME WITH PSEUDOPAPILLOEDEMA. ARCH. DIS. CHILD. 44* 504-508, 1969.

KIRKHAM, T. H.* DUANE'S SYNDROME AND FAMILIAL PERCEPTIVE DEAFNESS. BRIT. J. OPHTHAL. 53* 335-339, 1969.

MCLAY, K. AND MARAN, A. G. D.* DEAFNESS AND THE KLIPPEL-FEIL SYNDROME. J. LARYNG. 83* 175-184, 1969.

WILDERVANCK, L. S.* A CERVICO-OCULO-ACUSTICUS SYNDROME BELONGING TO THE STATUS DYSRAPHICUS. PROC. SEC. INTERN. CONG. HUM. GENET., (ROME, SEPT. 6-12, 1961.) 3* 1409-1412, 1961.

WILDERVANCK, L. S.* EEN CERVICO-OCULO-ACUSTICUSSYNDROOM. NEDERL. T. GENEESK. 104* 2600-2605, 1960.

WILDERVANCK, L. S., HOEKSEMA, P. E. AND PENNING, L.* RADIOLOGICAL EXAMINATION OF THE INNER EAR OF DEAF-MUTES PRESENTING THE CERVICO-OCULO-ACUSTICUS SYNDROME. ACTA OTOLARYNG. 61* 445-453, 1966.

*31470 XG BLOOD GROUP SYSTEM

THE ANTIGEN CALLED XG(A) BEHAVES AS AN X-LINKED DOMINANT. IT WAS FOUND IN 89 PERCENT OF 188 CAUCASIAN FEMALES AND IN 62 PERCENT OF 154 MALES. THE ANTISERUM WAS DERIVED FROM A PATIENT WITH HEREDITARY HEMORRHAGIC TELANGIECTASIA WHO HAD RECEIVED MANY TRANSFUSIONS. THE ANTIGEN IS WELL DEVELOPED AT BIRTH. IN THE FEW NEGROES TESTED THE PHENOTYPE FREQUENCIES SEEM TO BE ABOUT THE SAME AS IN CAUCA-SIANS. 'EVIDENCE IS ACCUMULATING THAT HOMOZYGOTES REACT AS STRONGLY AS HEMIZY-GOTES AND MORE STRONGLY THAN HETEROZYGOTES.' THE EFFICIENT ESTIMATE OF THE FREQUENCY OF THE XG(A) ALLELE IN CAUCASIANS, MAKING USE OF THE DATA ON FEMALES AS WELL AS MALES, IS 0.651 (SANGER ET AL., 1962).
THE XG(A) BLOOD GROUP IS OF GREAT USE TO GENETICS ESPECIALLY FOR STUDY OF LINKAGE AND DETERMINATION WHERE NON-DISJUNCTION OCCURS LEADING TO X CHROMOSOME ANEUPLOIDY. EVIDENCE ON LYONIZATION OF THE XG LOCUS IS CONFLICTING. EVIDENCE FOR LYONIZATION CAME FROM A STUDY OF X-LINKED HYPOCHROMIC ANEMIA (Q.V.) BY LEE AND COLLEAGUES (1968). LAWLER AND SANGER (1970) FOUND THAT A GROUP OF FEMALES WITH PHILADELPHIA-CHROMOSOME-POSITIVE MYELOID LEUKEMIA CASES HAD THE FREQUENCY OF XG TYPES EXPECTED OF FEMALES. THIS COULD MEAN EITHER THAT THE XG LOCUS IS NOT SUBJECT TO INACTIVATION OR THAT ALL PH-POSITIVE CELLS ARE NOT MONOCLONAL. ALSO ASSUMED, OF COURSE, IS THAT THE ERYTHROID CELLS IN THE PATIENTS STUDIED ARE DERIVED FROM A PH-POSITIVE CELL AND THAT NO RED CELLS DERIVED FROM PH-NEGATIVE PRECURSORS PERSIST.

COOK, I. A., POLLEY, M. J. AND MOLLISON, P. L.* A SECOND EXAMPLE OF ANTI-XG(A). LANCET 1* 857-859, 1963.

LEE, G. R., MACDIARMID, W. D. AND CARTWRIGHT, G. E.* HEREDITARY, X-LINKED, SIDEROACHRESTIC ANEMIA. THE ISOLATION OF TWO ERYTHROCYTE POPULATIONS DIFFERING IN XG BLOOD TYPE AND PORPHYRIN CONTENT. BLOOD 32* 59-70, 1968.

MANN, J. D., CAHAN, A., GELB, A. G., FISHER, N., HAMPER, J., TIPPETT, P., SANGER, R. AND RACE, R. R.* A SEX-LINKED BLOOD GROUP. LANCET 1* 8-10, 1962.

SANGER, R., RACE, R. R., TIPPETT, P., HAMPER, J., GAVIN, J. AND CLEGHORN, T. E.* THE X-LINKED BLOOD GROUP SYSTEM XG* MORE TESTS ON UNRELATED PEOPLE AND ON FAMILIES. VOX SANG. 7* 571-578, 1962.

X
L
I
N
K
E
D

THE XH ANTIGEN WAS FIRST DESCRIBED BY BUNDSCHUH (1966), WHO SUGGESTED X-LINKAGE BECAUSE THE ANTIGEN IS MORE FREQUENT IN WOMEN (97 PERCENT) THAN IN MEN (88 PERCENT). THE ANTIGEN IS DEMONSTRATED WITH ANTISERUM PRODUCED BY INJECTING RABBITS WITH POOL SERUM FROM HEALTHY WOMEN AND ABSORPTION OF THE IMMUNE SERUM WITH SELECTED MALE SERA. GENETIC ANALYSIS IS COMPLICATED BY THE FACT THAT BOTH GENETIC AND NON-GENETIC FACTORS SEEM TO INFLUENCE THE QUANTITY OF THE ANTIGEN PRESENT.

KUEPPERS, F.* STUDIES ON THE XH ANTIGEN IN HUMAN SERUM. HUMANGENETIK 7* 98-103, 1969.

*31490 XM SYSTEM

BERG AND BEARN (1966) DISCOVERED AN X-LINKED SERUM PROTEIN TYPE BY MEANS OF HETEROANTISERUM MADE SPECIFIC BY ABSORPTION. SINCE THE GROUP SPECIFIC ANTIGEN APPEARS TO BE LOCATED IN THE ALPHA-2-MACROGLOBULIN OF SERUM, THE NAME XM WAS ASSIGNED TO THE SYSTEM. THE DISTRIBUTION OF PHENOTYPES IN FAMILIES AND IN POPULATIONS WAS CONSISTENT WITH X-LINKAGE. BERG ET AL. (1968) CONCLUDED THAT THE HUNTER LOCUS AND THE XM LOCUS ARE WITHIN MEASURABLE DISTANCE OF EACH OTHER, THE BEST ESTIMATE OF THE RECOMBINATION FRACTION BEING 0.09.

BERG, K. AND BEARN, A. G.* A COMMON X-LINKED SERUM MARKER AND ITS RELATION TO OTHER LOCI ON THE X CHROMOSOME. TRANS. ASS. AM. PHYSICIANS 79* 165-176, 1966.

BERG, K. AND BEARN, A. G.* AN INHERITED X-LINKED SERUM SYSTEM IN MAN. THE XM SYSTEM. J. EXP. MED. 123* 379-397, 1966.

BERG, K., DANES, B. S. AND BEARN, A. G.* THE LINKAGE RELATION OF THE LOCI FOR THE XM SERUM SYSTEM AND THE X-LINKED FORM OF HURLER'S SYNDROME (HUNTER'S SYN-DROME). AM. J. HUM. GENET. 20* 398-401, 1968.

31500 ZONULAR CATARACT AND NYSTAGMUS

FALLS (1952) REPORTED A FAMILY IN WHICH THIS COMBINATION OF TRAITS APPEARED TO BE X-LINKED. HE POINTED OUT THAT THE FAMILY WAS 'INCOMPLETELY STUDIED.'

FALLS, H. F.* THE ROLE OF THE SEX CHROMOSOME IN HEREDITARY OCULAR PATHOLOGY. TRANS. AM. OPHTHAL. SOC. 50* 421-467, 1952.

X
L
I
N
K
E
D

Author Index

The names are those of authors referred to in the catalogs. The numbers after the names are those of the entries in which the author is mentioned. Entries beginning with the digit ''1'' are in the dominant catalog. Entries beginning with the digit ''2'' are in the recessive catalog. Entries beginning with the digit ''3'' are in the X-linkage catalog.

BUDD, M. A...............24350
BUDZILOVICH, G............22390
BUDZILOVICH, G. N.........20810, 26480
BUENO, M.................23410
BUERK, E.................12520
BUERMANN, A..............19040
BUHLER, U. K.............27520
BUIST, N.................27660
BUIST, N. R. M...........26770
BULL, J..................18430
BULL, J. C...............21910
BULL, J. M. C............17400
BULL, J. W. D............10950
BULLOCK, L...............31370
BULMER, M. G.............21970, 26480
BUNCH, L. D..............10540
BUNDEY, S................16090
BUNIM, J. J..............18030
BUNTIN, P. T.............16220
BUNTING, R...............21220, 26160
BURCH, T. A..............18030
BURCHELL, H. B...........18730
BURG, M. B...............30480
BURGER, R. A.............24180
BURGERMEISTER, J. J......31370
BURGERT, E. O., JR.......14170, 20590,
    21230
BURGESS, E. A............22300, 22960,
    23250, 23720, 25100
BURGI, W.................24790
BURGOON, C. F., JR.......15480
BURGUET, W...............26510
BURIAN, F................19370
BURKE, B. S..............15720
BURKE, E. C..............10010, 14110,
    15650, 19300, 22680, 23540
BURKE, J.................10420, 23950
BURKE, V.................21230, 22390,
    26040
BURKET, R. L.............21870
BURKHOLDER, G. V.........10010
BURKHOLDER, P............10420, 23950
BURKI, E.................22000
BURKLAND, C. E...........19160
BURKS, J.................15080, 24610
BURLAND, J. G............11840
BURMAN, D................16910
BURNETT, C. H............25890, 30780,
    31370
BURNETT, J. W............24710
BURNETT, L...............15240
BURNEY, D. W.............14630
BURNIE, K. L.............10560
BURNS, R. A..............16960
BURNS, S. L..............24030
BURNSIDE, R. M...........19330
BURROW, G. N.............27470
BURSTON, D...............18860
BURTON, C................24320
BUSCH, D.................26620, 30590
BUSCH, G.................19050
BUSCH, K. F. B...........16670
BUSCH, K.-T..............18050
BUSINCO, L...............13470
BUSSE, R. J., JR.........23400
BUSSEY, H. J. R..........17490
BUSTAMENTE, W............24250
BUTIKOFER, E.............27350
BUTLER, A. M.............10420, 17480
BUTLER, E. A.............14170
BUTLER, H. G.............24580
BUTLER, R................15200, 15220,
    20020, 20740
BUTT, H. R...............14350, 23750
BUTTEN, A. F. H..........22850
BUTTERWORTH, T...........12560, 18200
BUTTIMER, R. J...........11080
BUXTON, P. H.............20370
BYERLY, B. H.............12760
BYERS, R. K..............14310
BYRD, J. R...............23330, 23340
BYRD, R. B...............30130

BYRON, R.................26970
BYRON, R. L., JR.........17500
BYWATERS, E. G. L........14790

CABANNES, R..............14170
CACCAMISE, W. C..........25810
CADWALADER, W. B.........21810
CADY, B..................21200
CAEN, J..................19340
CAEN, J. P...............18780, 27380
CAESAR, R................25240
CAFFEY, J................12700, 15060,
    15650, 16630, 23050, 23900
CAFFEY, J. P.............27730
CAFFREY, P. R............26510
CAFLISCH, A..............17810
CAGIANUT, B..............18000
CAHAN, A.................31470
CAHANE, D................20160
CAHILL, G. F., JR........22210
CAHILL, K. M.............24330
CAIN, W. A...............20890
CALDERON, A..............23750
CALDWELL, J. B. H........16550
CALDWELL, J. R...........22310
CALHOUN, F. P............14250, 14300
CALLAGHAN, P.............24350
CALLAHAN, J..............23060
CALLAHAN, J. A...........10890
CALLAWAY, J. L...........12420
CALLENDER, S. T..........17090, 27350
CALVELLI, G. J., JR......20650
CALVERT, H. T............20120
CAMACHO, A. M............20200
CAMBIER, J...............11820
CAMERON, A. H............20010
CAMERON, D...............23170, 26440
CAMERON, J. M............13240
CAMERON, K. M............14500
CAMERON, O...............25440
CAMERON, S. J............19330
CAMIEL, M. R.............17530
CAMMERMEYER, J...........26650
CAMP, C. D...............16950
CAMP, M. B...............16240
CAMPBELL, A. M. G........14310, 16240
CAMPBELL, C. J...........12780
CAMPBELL, D. C...........30100
CAMPBELL, M..............11520
CAMPBELL, M. M...........31120
CAMPBELL, P. E...........13260
CAMPBELL, R. A...........23540, 24120
CAMPBELL, S..............23540, 25610
CANADA, W. J.............17550
CANALES, L...............31390
CANBY, J. P..............23580
CANDEBAT, L..............31370
CANETTI, J...............30700
CANIJO, M................10480
CANN, H. M...............23670
CANNON, F. E.............12870
CANNON, J. F.............12580, 14340,
    30480
CANNON, P. J.............24120
CANT, J. S...............27540
CANTOLINO, S. J..........13680, 18510
CANTON, J. N.............30610
CANTOR, H. E.............20460
CANTU, J. M..............27730
CANTWELL, A. R., JR......13260
CANTZ, M.................30990
CAPELLA, J. A............30230, 30970
CAPLAN, D. B.............12160
CAPLAN, R. M.............24710
CAPOTORTI, L.............24380
CAPP, G. I...............14170
CAPUTE, A. J.............15110
CARATZALI, A.............13740
CARAVATI, C. M...........17370
CARBONELL JUANICO, M.....16600
CARDINALE, G. J..........25100
CARESANO, A..............25140

HEINENBERG, S..............14170
HEINER, D. C..............10610
HEINRICHSBAUER, F..........22660
HEINS, H. L., JR..........27580
HEINS, J. N..............26250
HEIPLE, K. G..............31410
HEISTO, H..............30660
HEIZER, W. D..............27230
HELGE, H..............30590
HELLER, H..............10480, 24910
HELLER, I. H..............16240
HELLER, J..............24910
HELLER, P..............14170, 27350
HELLIER, F. F..............13900, 14930
HELLRIEGEL, K..............17840
HELLSING, G..............13430
HELLYER, D. T..............11400
HELMEN, C..............19260
HELWEG-LARSEN, H. F........12520, 26630
HELWIG, E. B..............10590
HELWIG, F. C..............13290
HELWIG, H..............24620
HEMET, J..............27700
HEMINGWAY, E..............14350
HEMMES, G. C..............31070
HEMMES, G. D..............18020
HEMSTED, E. H..............14070
HENDERSON, A. S..............21870
HENDERSON, J. F..............10260, 30620, 30800
HENDERSON, J. L..............21810
HENDERSON, N. S..............14770, 15420
HENDERSON, R. R..............21660, 30560
HENDRICKS, C. A..............24710
HENDRICKSON, E. M..............30590
HENDRIKX, A..............12250
HENI, F..............14400
HENKES, H. E..............15390, 20400, 30310
HENKIN, R. I..............25680, 30870
HENLEY, K. S..............21160
HENLEY, W. L..............24750
HENLY, W. S..............15560
HENNEMAN, P. H..............19170
HENNESSY, T. G..............19330
HENNINGSEN, K..............17210
HENSEN, A..............13450
HENSON, J. B..............13000
HENSON, T. E..............16060
HEPPER, N. G..............20740
HERBER, R..............22290
HERBERT, V..............21170, 26110
HERBICH, J..............17150
HERBST, E..............18340
HERDMAN, R. C..............12730, 20060, 20850, 25610
HERLANT, M..............10460
HERMAN, E..............25730
HERMAN, G..............17520
HERMAN, R. H..............17050, 22840
HERMANN, H..............10060, 22640
HERMANN, P..............15710
HERMANS, P. E..............30080
HERMANSKY, F..............20330, 21450
HERMEL, M. B..............26590
HERNANDEZ, F. A..............22470
HERNDON, C. N..............18010, 18640, 23520, 30950, 30960
HERNDON, J. H., JR........10190, 26650
HERPOL, J..............23630
HERRAULT, A..............24670
HERRELL, W. E..............25450
HERRICK, S. E..............19330
HERRIN, J. T..............23720
HERRINGHAM, W. P..............30280
HERRLIN, K.-M..............23080
HERRMANN, C., JR..........15930, 17250
HERRMANN, J..............26830, 26900
HERRON, M. A..............20210
HERS, H. G..............23000, 23270, 30600
HERSH, A. H..............11270

HERSHGOLD, E. J..............30670
HERSHKO, C..............22010
HERTZOG, K. P..............11270, 11330
HERVOUET, F..............26310
HERZBERG, J. J..............10940
HESLIN, D. J..............17680
HESS, C. E..............23190
HESS, J. W..............25610
HESSELBERG, C..............20690
HESSEN, I..............18730
HESTON, L. L..............10430, 18150
HETZAR, W..............16590
HEUPKE, G..............14170
HEUSCHER-ISLER, R..............18010
HEWER, R. L..............22930
HEWITT, L. F..............16390
HEWSON, S. E..............24710
HEY, M..............18730
HEYL, T..............24710
HEYN, R. M..............25890
HEYNS, W..............12250
HIATT, H. H..............26080
HIATT, R. L..............26860
HIBBS, R. E..............17480
HICKEN, N. F..............17520
HICKEY, M. E..............22740
HICKMAN, G. C..............14010
HICKMAN, R. O..............21980, 23040
HICKMANS, E. M..............21280
HICKS, E. P..............16240
HICKS, P..............13460, 22780
HIEKKALA, H..............24030
HIEN-VOLPEL, K. F..............13210
HIGASHI, O..............22910
HIGGINS, F..............22740
HIGINBOTHAM, N. L..............26950
HILBERT, R..............11680
HILBISH, T. F..............13370
HILD, J. R..............13130
HILGARTNER, M..............21950
HILGERS, J. H. C..............17800
HILL, A. G..............30080
HILL, B. J..............17140
HILL, E..............13760, 13770
HILL, E. M..............24710
HILL, J. E..............23510
HILL, L. L..............15650
HILL, R. J..............14170
HILL, R. L..............14170, 14710
HILL, R. O..............27160
HILL, T. R..............17650
HILL, W..............10850, 11730
HILLBORG, P. O..............23080
HILLMAN, D. A..............23920
HILLMAN, J. W..............15790
HILLMAN, R. E..............23160, 23310
HINDS, J. R..............21960
HINGLAIS, N..............30150
HINTERBUCHNER, L. P..............25580
HINTON, G. G..............23940
HINTZ, R. L..............23370, 23610, 24430
HINZ, J. E..............14170
HIRAKO, T..............16100
HIRANO, A..............10540, 16870, 20430
HIRD, F. J. R..............23720
HIROHATA, R..............20350
HIROKAWA, K..............22550
HIRONO, H..............23620
HIROOKA, M..............21160
HIRSCH, E. Z..............30150
HIRSCH, I. S..............26950
HIRSCH, M..............22470
HIRSCH, M. S..............20760
HIRSCHBERG, E..............20010
HIRSCHFELD, J..............13920
HIRSCHHORN, H. H..............18930
HIRSCHHORN, K..............15240, 20770, 21650, 22790, 23230, 25730, 31160
HIRSCHHORN, R..............23230
HIRSCHMAN, R. J..............20590

VALTIN, H.................12570, 22200
VAMOS-HURWITZ, E..........23000
VAN BOGAERT, L............27190
VAN BUSKIRK, F. W.........11400
VAN DER WERFF TEN BOSCH, J.27550
VAN LEEUWEN, A............14280
VAN ROOD, J. J...........14280
VAN SCOTT, E. J..........20320
VAN ALLEN, M. W..........10510
VAN ASSEN, J.............19290
VAN BALEN, A. T. M.......12210, 13970,
    14320, 14330
VAN BERKUM, K. A. P......27400
VAN BLOMMESTEIN, A.......15390
VAN BOGAERT, L...........16730, 18260,
       20130, 21000, 21370, 27070, 30160,
       30290, 31080
VAN BOGAERT, L. V........25000
VAN BOLHUIS, A. H........12460
VAN BUCHEM, F. S. P......23910
VAN CREVELD, S...........17070
VAN DE KAMER, J. H.......22300
VAN DE SAR, A............12260
VAN DEN BOSCH, J.........20400, 25120,
       30050, 30100, 31450
VAN DEN NOORT, S.........30010
VAN DER HAGEN, C. B......26240
VAN DER WIEL , H. J......15790
VAN DER HAGEN, C. B......13410
VAN DER HENDE, C.........25090
VAN DER HENDE, C. H......27050
VAN DER HOEVE, J.........24450
VAN DER VALK, J. W.......30200
VAN DER VLERK, D.........30690
VAN DER WEERDT, C. M.....17350
VAN DER WOUDE, A.........11930
VAN DER ZEE, S. P. M.....30800
VAN DYKE, R. A...........14590
VAN EPPS, C..............18670
VAN EPPS, E. F...........10940
VAN EYES, J..............22880
VAN EYS, J...............25080
VAN GEHUCHTEN, P.........24520
VAN GELDER, D. W.........10710, 20750
VAN GEMUND, J. J.........22350
VAN GOOL, J..............11700
VAN HOOF, F..............23000, 23270
VAN HOOVER, G............21380
VAN LEEUWEN, A...........14280
VAN LITH, G. H. M........27690
VAN LOGHEM, E............14700
VAN LOGHEM, J. L.........17350
VAN MECHELEN, P..........23650
VAN ORDSTRAND, H. S......13500, 17850
VAN PELT, J. F...........30990
VAN ROOD, J. J...........14280
VAN ROOYEN, R. J.........17040
VAN ROS, G...............14170
VAN ROSSUM, A............20910
VAN SANDE, M.............20780
VAN SCOTT, E.............20320
VAN SCOTT, E. J..........10940
VAN SPRANG, F. J.........23580
VAN STEKELENBURG, G. K...23580
VAN WIJNGAARDEN, G. K....25190, 31040
VAN WYK, J. J............20170, 31370
VAN'T HOFF, W............17050
VANBELLINGHEN, P.........26620
VANCE, J. E..............13110
VANDENBROUCKE, J.........30690
VANDENSCHRIECK, H. G.....12250
VANDEPITTE, J............14170
VANDERDONCK, R...........30390
VANDERHAEGHEN, J.-J......14650
VANDERVOORT, R. L. E.....30690
VANDEVELDE, G............31760
VANGELDEREN, H. H........22390
VANHEULE, R..............23800
VANHOUTTE, J. J..........17530
VANN, R. L...............20240
VANNOTTI, A..............15360
VARA CUADRADO, F.........26510

VARADI, D. P.............13000
VARCO, R. L..............20250
VARDAS, E................17230
VARELA, A................30090
VARGHESE, P. J...........23800
VASSAR, P. S.............23590
VASSELLA, F..............24730, 25680
VAUGHN, J. G.............23620
VAUZELLE, J. L...........12300
VAWTER, G................26750, 30040
VAWTER, G. F.............27140, 27800
VEALE, A. M..............17510
VEALE, A. M. O...........17490, 30610
VEATH, M. L..............27280
VEEGER, W................22230
VEENHOVEN-VON RIESZ, L. E.17350
VELDEN, W. H.............13120
VELEZ, A. H..............23450
VELLA, F.................14170
VELLIOS, F...............16660
VELTKAMP, J. J...........13450, 30690
VENKATACHALAM, P. S......23450
VENNING, P...............18900
VENTER, J................20970
VENTRUTO, V..............14170
VENTURA, G...............24480
VERBEECK, J..............23630
VEREL, D.................17860
VERGOS, D................14170
VERGOZ, D................14170
VERHAEGEN, H.............22410
VERHAGEN, A. D...........15340, 27110
VERLOOP, M. C............20330
VERMA, B. S..............19390
VERMASSEN, A.............23800
VERMEULEN, A.............17030
VERMYLEN, C..............30690
VERNANT, C...............16220
VERNANT, P...............14290, 25310
VERNIER, R. L............14120, 25610,
    25630
VERNON, M................27690
VERRET, S................25690
VERRIEST, G..............16350, 25810,
    30390
VERSTRAETE, M............30690
VERWILGHEN, R............22410
VESA, L..................16120
VESELL, E. S.............15000, 18580,
    20990
VESSIE, P. R.............14310
VESTERMARK, B............31390
VESTERMARK, S............22600, 31390
VETTER, K. K.............20340
VIALATTE, J..............26040
VIAMONTE, M., JR.........22870
VIANNA, B................27460
VICK, N. A...............25510
VICK, R. L...............19250
VICKERS, R. A............16230
VICTOR, M................16430, 25390,
    27190
VIDAL, F.................12180
VIERUCCI, A..............15200
VIETOR, W. P. J..........17050
VIETTI, T. J.............20990
VIGNA, V.................26180
VIGNES....................11010
VIGO, (NI)...............12160
VILANOVA, X..............16100
VILAR, O.................31370, 31380
VILDOSOLA, J.............27390
VILJOEN, E...............18290
VILLARET, M..............10170
VILLIERS, J. D...........14560
VINAZZER, H..............26490
VINETA TEIXIDO, J........16600
VINEYARD, W. R...........10760, 18460
VINH, L. T...............10670
VINOGRAD, J. R...........14170
VIPARELLI, V.............13510
VIRCHOW, H...............13380

Subject Index

In addition to the preferred title of each entry, alternative designations and individual phenotypic features are indexed. The numbers refer to individual entries, each of which presumably represents a separate locus. Entries beginning with the digit ''1'' are in the dominant catalog. Those beginning with the digit ''2'' are in the recessive catalog. Those beginning with the digit ''3'' are in the X-linkage catalog.

ABDOMINAL MUSCLES, ABSENCE OF, WITH URINARY TRACT ABNORMALITY AND CRYPTOR-
 CHIDISM.. 10010
ABDUCENS PALSY.. 10020
*ABETALIPOPROTEINEMIA (ACANTHOCYTOSIS)... 20010
ABO BLOOD GROUP SEE BLOOD GROUP-ABO SYSTEM (11030)
ABSENCE DEFECT OF LIMBS, SCALP AND SKULL.. 10030
ABSENCE DEFORMITIES OF EXTREMITIES SEE PEROMELIA (26120), ACHONDROGENE-
 SIS (20060, 20070)
ABSENCE OF RODS AND CONES, CONGENITAL SEE AMAUROSIS CONGENITA (20400),
 RETINAL APLASIA (17990)
ABSENCE OF SKIN SEE EPIDERMOLYSIS BULLOSA WITH ABSENCE OF SKIN (13200)
ABSENCE OF SKIN, BLISTERING, ABNORMALITY OF NAILS................................. 10040
*ACANTHOCYTOSIS.. 10050
ACANTHOCYTOSIS SEE ABETALIPOPROTEINEMIA
ACANTHOCYTOSIS SEE WOLMAN'S DISEASE WITH HYPOBETALIPOPROTEINEMIA AND
 ACANTHOCYTOSIS (27810), ABETALIPOPROTEINEMIA (20010)
ACANTHOSIS NIGRICANS.. 10060
ACANTHOSIS NIGRICANS SEE SEIP SYNDROME (26970)
*ACATALASEMIA (TWO OR MORE TYPES)... 20020
ACATALASIA SEE ACATALASEMIA (20020)
ACCESSORY BONES IN FEET SEE SYMPHALANGISM, PROXIMAL (18580)
*ACETOPHENETIDIN SENSITIVITY.. 20030
ACETYLATION, POLYMORPHISM OF SEE ISONIAZID (INH) INACTIVATION (24340)
ACETYLTRANSFERASE DEFICIENCY SEE ISONIAZID (INH) INACTIVATION (24340)
ACHALASIA, FAMILIAL ESOPHAGEAL.. 20040
ACHARD SYNDROME... 10070
ACHEIROPODY SEE PEROMELIA (26120)
*ACHEIROPODY (BRAZILIAN TYPE)... 20050
*ACHONDROGENESIS, TYPE I (PARENTI-FRACCARO OR LETHAL TYPE)........................ 20060
*ACHONDROGENESIS, TYPE II (GREBE OR BRAZILIAN TYPE).............................. 20070
ACHONDROPLASIA.. 20080
*'ACHONDROPLASIA' AND SWISS-TYPE AGAMMAGLOBULINEMIA............................... 20090
*ACHONDROPLASIA, CLASSICAL.. 10080
*ACHROMATIC REGIONS OF TETRAZOLIUM STAINED STARCH GELS............................ 10090
ACHROMATOPSIA SEE COLOR BLINDNESS, TOTAL (21690)
ACHROMATOPSIA, CONGENITAL COMPLETE SEE PINGELAPESE BLINDNESS (26230)
*ACID PHOSPHATASE DEFICIENCY.. 20095
ACID PHOSPHATASE OF RED CELLS SEE FAVISM (13470)
ACID PHOSPHATASE, ERYTHROCYTE, ELECTROPHORETIC VARIANTS OF SEE PHOSPHA-
 TASE, ACID, OF ERYTHROCYTE (17150)
ACIDOSIS SEE AMINOACIDURIA WITH OTHER FEATURES (20480), LACTIC ACIDOSIS
 (14980, 24540)
ACOMPLEMENTEMIA SEE COMPLEMENT COMPONENT C-PRIME-2, DEFICIENCY OF
 (21700)
*ACOUSTIC NEUROMA, BILATERAL.. 10100
ACROCEPHALOPOLYSYNDACTYLY TYPE I (ACPS I, OR NOACK'S SYNDROME).................... 10110
*ACROCEPHALOPOLYSYNDACTYLY TYPE II (ACPS II, CARPENTER'S SYNDROME)............... 20100
*ACROCEPHALOSYNDACTYLY TYPE I (TYPICAL APERT'S SYNDROME).......................... 10120
ACROCEPHALOSYNDACTYLY TYPE II (APERT-CROUZON DISEASE, OR VOGT'S CEPHALODA-
 CTYLY)... 10130
*ACROCEPHALOSYNDACTYLY TYPE III (ACROCEPHALY, SKULL ASYMMETRY AND MILD
 SYNDACTYLY).. 10140
*ACROCEPHALOSYNDACTYLY TYPE IV (WAARDENBURG TYPE)................................. 10150
*ACROCEPHALOSYNDACTYLY TYPE V (PFEIFFER TYPE)..................................... 10160
ACROCEPHOSYNDACTYLY OF MOHR SEE OCULODENTODIGITAL DYSPLASIA SYNDROME
 (16420)
ACROCYANOSIS.. 10170
ACROCYANOSIS SEE HEMANGIOMATOSIS, CUTANEOUS, WITH ASSOCIATED FEATURES
 (23480), ALBUMIN, VARIANTS OF SERUM (10360)
*ACRODERMATITIS ENTEROPATHICA... 20110
ACRODYSOSTOSIS.. 10180
ACROFACIAL DYSOSTOSIS OF NAGER SEE MANDIBULO-FACIAL DYSOSTOSIS WITH
 LIMB ANOMALIES (15440)
ACROGERIA... 20120
*ACROKERATOSIS VERRUCIFORMIS (HOPF).. 10190
ACROKERATOSIS VERRUCIFORMIS SEE VAN DEN BOSCH SYNDROME (31450)
ACROLEUKOPATHY, SYMMETRIC... 10200
*ACROMEGALOID CHANGES, CUTIS VERTICIS GYRATA AND CORNEAL LEUKOMA................. 10210
ACROMEGALY.. 10220
ACROMELALGIA, HEREDITARY ('RESTLESS LEGS').. 10230
ACRO-OSTEOLYSIS... 10240
ACRO-OSTEOLYSIS SEE OCULO-AURICULO-VERTEBRAL DYSPLASIA (25770), PURE-
 TIC'S SYNDROME (26570), PYCNODYSOSTOSIS (26580), NEUROPATHY, HEREDITARY
 SENSORY RADICULAR (16240)
*ACRO-OSTEOLYSIS WITH OSTEOPOROSIS AND CHANGES IN SKULL AND MANDIBLE
 (CHENEY SYNDROME).. 10250
ACRO-OSTEOLYSIS, NEUROGENIC... 20130
ACROPACHY SEE CLUBBING OF DIGITS (11990), PACHYDERMOPERIOSTOSIS (16710)
ACROPATHIE ULCERO-MUTILANTE SEE NEUROPATHY, HEREDITARY SENSORY RADICU-
 LAR (16240)
ACTH DEFICIENCY... 20140
ACTH, ADRENAL UNRESPONSIVENESS TO SEE ADRENAL UNRESPONSIVENESS TO ACTH

          (20220)
    ADDISON'S DISEASE   SEE HYPOADRENOCORTICISM (24020, 24030), ADRENAL
        UNRESPONSIVENESS TO ACTH (20220), SCHMIDT'S SYNDROME (26920)
*ADDISON'S DISEASE AND CEREBRAL SCLEROSIS................................. 30010
    ADDISON'S DISEASE AND SPASTIC PARAPLEGIA............................... 20150
*ADENINE PHOSPHORIBOSYLTRANSFERASE VARIANT................................ 10260
    ADENOCARCINOMA OF KIDNEY   SEE HYPERNEPHROMA (14470)
    ADENOMA SEBACEUM   SEE TUBEROUS SCLEROSIS (19110)
    ADENOMATOSIS, MULTIPLE ENDOCRINE   SEE ENDOCRINE ADENOMATOSIS, MULTIPLE
        (13110)
*ADENOSINE DEAMINASE POLYMORPHISM.. 10270
    ADENOSINE TRIPHOSPHATASE DEFICIENCY, ANEMIA DUE TO..................... 10280
*ADENOSINE TRIPHOSPHATE, ELEVATED, OF ERYTHROCYTES....................... 10290
*ADENYLATE KINASE DEFICIENCY, ANEMIA DUE TO.............................. 20160
*ADENYLATE KINASE ELECTROPHORETIC VARIANTS............................... 10300
    ADIE SYNDROME... 10310
    ADIPOSIS DOLOROSA (DERCUM'S DISEASE).................................. 10320
    ADRENAL ADENOMA   SEE MACROSOMIA ADIPOSA CONGENITA (24810)
    ADRENAL AND OVARY 17-HYDROXYLATION, DEFICIENCY IN   SEE ADRENAL HYPERPLA-
        SIA V (WITH DEFECT IN 17-HYDROXYLASE) (20210)
    ADRENAL CALCIFICATION   SEE WOLMAN'S DISEASE (27800)
*ADRENAL HYPERPLASIA I (WITH DEFECT IN 21-HYDROXYLASE)................... 20170
*ADRENAL HYPERPLASIA II (WITH DEFECT IN 11-BETA-HYDROXYLASE)............. 20180
*ADRENAL HYPERPLASIA III (WITH DEFECT IN 3-BETA-HYDROXYSTEROID DEHYDROGENASE).. 20190
*ADRENAL HYPERPLASIA IV (WITH DEFECT IN ENZYME PRIOR TO DELTA 5-PREGNENO-
        LONE)* LIPOID HYPERPLASIA OF ADRENAL CORTEX WITH MALE PSEUDOHERMAPHRO-
        DITISM.. 20200
    ADRENAL HYPERPLASIA V (WITH DEFECT IN 17-HYDROXYLASE).................. 20210
*ADRENAL HYPOPLASIA.. 30020
*ADRENAL UNRESPONSIVENESS TO ACTH.. 20220
    ADRENOCORTICAL ADENOMA   SEE MACROSOMIA ADIPOSA CONGENITA (24810)
    ADRENOCORTICAL CARCINOMA.. 20230
    ADRENOCORTICAL CARCINOMA   SEE GARNER'S SYNDROME (17530)
    ADRENOCORTICAL HYPOPLASIA   SEE HYPOADRENOCORTICISM (24020, 24030)
    ADRENOCORTICAL INSUFFICIENCY   SEE HYPOADRENOCORTICISM (24020, 24030),
        ALDOSTERONE DEFICIENCY (20340)
    ADRENOGENITAL SYNDROME   SEE ADRENAL HYPERPLASIA (20170, 20210)
    ADYNAMIA EPISODICA HEREDITARIA   SEE PERIODIC PARALYSIS II (HYPERKALEMIC
        TYPE) (17050)
*AFIBRINOGENEMIA, CONGENITAL... 20240
    AG SYSTEM   SEE LIPOPROTEIN TYPES - AG SYSTEM (15200)
*AGAMMAGLOBULINEMIA (BRUTON TYPE).. 30030
*AGAMMAGLOBULINEMIA, SWISS OR ALYMPHOCYTOTIC TYPE........................ 20250
*AGAMMAGLOBULINEMIA, SWISS TYPE (THYMIC EPITHELIAL HYPOPLASIA)........... 30040
    AGAMMAGLOBULINEMIA, SWISS TYPE, AND ACHONDROPLASIA   SEE ACHONDROPLASIA
        AND SWISS TYPE AGAMMAGLOBULINEMIA (20090)
    AGANGLIOSIS   SEE NEUROBLASTOMA (25670), MEGACOLON, AGANGLIONIC (24920)
    AGENESIS OF CEREBELLAR VERMIS   SEE CEREBELLO-PARENCHYMAL DISORDER IV
        (21330)
    AGENESIS OF CEREBRAL WHITE MATTER..................................... 20260
    AGENESIS OF OLFACTORY LOBES   SEE KALLMANN SYNDROME (24420, 24430, 30870)
    AGENESIS, BILATERAL RENAL   SEE RENAL AGENESIS, BILATERAL (26670)
    AGLOSSIA-ADACTYLIA.. 10330
    AGLYCOGENOSIS   SEE HYPOGLYCEMIA DUE TO DEFICIENCY OF GLYCOGEN SYNTHETASE
        IN THE LIVER (24060)
*AGRANULOCYTOSIS, INFANTILE GENETIC, OF KOSTMANN........................ 20270
    AINHUM.. 10340
    ALACRIMA   SEE ECTODERMAL DYSPLASIA, ANHIDROTIC (12930, 12940, 22490,
        30510)
    ALACRIMIA CONGENITA.. 20280
    ALACRIMIA CONGENITA   SEE DYSAUTONOMIA
    ALACTASIA, INTESTINAL   SEE DISACCHARIDE INTOLERANCE III (22310)
    ALAND ISLAND DISEASE   SEE ALBINISM, OCULAR (FORSIUS-ERIKSSON TYPE)
        (30060)
    ALANINEMIA   SEE HYPER-BETA-ALANINEMIA (23740)
    ALANINURIA WITH MICROCEPHALY, DWARFISM, ENAMEL HYPOPLASIA, DIABETES MELLITUS.. 20290
    ALAR-NASAL CARTILAGES, COLOBOMA OF, WITH TELECANTHUS.................. 20300
    ALBERS-SCHONBERG'S DISEASE   SEE OSTEOPETROSIS (25970)
    ALBINISM   SEE OCULOCEREBRAL SYNDROME WITH HYPOPIGMENTATION (25780)
*ALBINISM I... 20310
*ALBINISM II.. 20320
    ALBINISM II   SEE XANTHISM (27840)
    ALBINISM III   SEE CHEDIAK-HIGASHI SYNDROME (21450)
    ALBINISM IV   SEE DEAFMUTISM WITH TOTAL ALBINISM (22090)
*ALBINISM WITH HEMORRHAGIC DIATHESIS AND PIGMENTED RETICULOENDOTHELIAL CELLS... 20330
*ALBINISM, OCULAR... 30050
    ALBINISM, OCULAR (FORSIUS-ERIKSSON TYPE).............................. 30060
    ALBINISM, PARTIAL   SEE PIEBALD TRAIT (17280)
    ALBINISM-DEAFNESS.. 10350
*ALBINISM-DEAFNESS SYNDROME... 30070
    ALBINISM-LIKE DISEASE   SEE OCULOCEREBRAL SYNDROME WITH HYPOPIGMENTATION
        (25780)

ALBINOIDISM   SEE ALBINISM II (20320)
ALBRIGHT'S HEREDITARY OSTEODYSTROPHY   SEE THYROTROPIN DEFICIENCY, ISO-
    LATED (27510)
*ALBRIGHT'S HEREDITARY OSTEODYSTROPHY... 30080
ALBUMIN NASKAPI   SEE ALBUMIN, VARIANTS OF SERUM (10360)
*ALBUMIN, VARIANTS OF SERUM... 10360
ALCOHOL DEHYDROGENASE.. 10370
ALCOHOLISM.. 30090
*ALDER ANOMALY.. 10380
ALDER ANOMALY   SEE FUCHS' ATROPHIA GYRATA CHOROIDEAE ET RETINAE (22990)
ALDOLASE DEFICIENCY OF LIVER   SEE FRUCTOSE INTOLERANCE, HEREDITARY
    (22960)
*ALDOSTERONE DEFICIENCY, DUE TO, DEFECT IN 18-HYDROXYLASE OR 18-DEHYDROGENASE.. 20340
ALDOSTERONISM, SENSITIVE TO DEXAMETHASONE... 10390
ALDRICH SYNDROME   SEE THROMBOCYTOPENIA (18800, 27390, 31390)
*ALDRICH SYNDROME.. 30100
ALEUKIA CONGENITA   SEE RETICULAR DYSGENESIS (26750)
ALKALINE PHOSPHATASE   SEE PHOSPHATASE, ALKALINE (17170, 17180)
ALKALI-RESISTANT ADULT HEMOGLOBIN   SEE HEMOGLOBIN RAINIER (14170)
ALKALOSIS, CONGENITAL, WITH DIARRHEA   SEE CHLORIDE DIARRHEA, FAMILIAL
    (21470)
*ALKAPTONURIA... 20350
ALLOALBUMINEMIA   SEE ALBUMIN, VARIANTS OF SERUM (10360)
ALOPECIA   SEE BULLOUS DYSTROPHY, HEREDITARY MACULAR TYPE (30200), KERA-
    TOSIS FOLLICULARIS SPINULOSA DECALVANS CUM OPHIASI (30800), ECTODERMAL
    DYSPLASIA, ANHIDROTIC (30510), MONILETHRIX (15800), HYPOTRICHOSIS,
    SYNDACTYLY AND RETINITIS PIGMENTOSA (24200), ATRICHIA WITH PAPULAR
    LESIONS (20950), CARTILAGE-HAIR HYPOPLASIA (21230), BALDNESS (10920)
ALOPECIA AREATA.. 10400
ALOPECIA CONGENITA WITH KERATOSIS PALMO-PLANTARIS................................. 10410
ALOPECIA-EPILEPSY-OLIGOPHRENIA SYNDROME OF MOYNAHAN (FAMILIAL CONGENITAL
    ALOPECIA, EPILEPSY, MENTAL RETARDATION AND UNUSUAL EEG)........................ 20360
*ALPERS' DIFFUSE DEGENERATION OF CEREBRAL GRAY MATTER (POLIODYSTROPHIA
    CEREBRI PROGRESSIVA) WITH HEPATIC CIRRHOSIS................................... 20370
ALPHA(1)-ACID GLYCOPROTEIN VARIANTS   SEE GLYCOPROTEIN ALPHA-1-ACID, OF
    SERUM (13860)
ALPHA-1-ANTITRYPSIN VARIANTS   SEE ANTITRYPSIN, ELECTROPHORETIC VARIANT
    OF SERUM (10740)
ALPHA-2-GLOBULINS, POLYMORPHISM OF   SEE HAPTOGLOBIN (14010), GROUP-
    SPECIFIC COMPONENT (GC) (13920), PA POLYMORPHISM OF ALPHA-2-GLOBULIN
    (26010)
*ALPORT SYNDROME (HEREDITARY NEPHROPATHY AND DEAFNESS)........................... 10420
ALSTROM SYNDROME... 20380
*ALYMPHOCYTOSIS, PURE (THYMIC DYSPLASIA WITH NORMAL IMMUNOGLOBINS AND
    IMMUNOLOGIC DEFICIENCY)... 20390
*ALZHEIMER'S DISEASE OF BRAIN.. 10430
AMAUROSIS CONGENITA   SEE RETINAL APLASIA (17990)
*AMAUROSIS CONGENITA OF LEBER I.. 20400
*AMAUROSIS CONGENITA OF LEBER II... 20410
*AMAUROTIC FAMILY IDIOCY, JUVENILE TYPE (BATTEN'S DISEASE IN ENGLAND, VOGT-
    SPIELMEYER'S DISEASE ON THE CONTINENT)....................................... 20420
AMAUROTIC FAMILY IDIOCY, INFANTILE   SEE TAY-SACHS DISEASE (27280)
AMAUROTIC IDIOCY AND METACHROMATIC LEUKODYSTROPHY, COMBINED FEATURES OF
    SEE METACHROMATIC LEUKODYSTROPHY AND AMAUROTIC IDIOCY (24980)
AMAUROTIC IDIOCY, ADULT TYPE.. 20430
*AMAUROTIC IDIOCY, CONGENITAL FORM... 20440
AMAUROTIC IDIOCY, LATE INFANTILE TYPE (JANSKY-BIELSCHOWSKY)...................... 20450
*AMAUROTIC IDIOCY, LATE INFANTILE, WITH MULTILAMELLAR CYTOSOMES................. 20460
AMELIA AND TERMINAL TRANSVERSE HEMIMELIA.. 10440
*AMELOGENESIS IMPERFECTA, HYPOCALCIFICATION TYPE............................... 10450
*AMELOGENESIS IMPERFECTA, PIGMENTED HYPOMATURATION TYPE........................ 20470
*AMELOGENESIS IMPERFECTA, HYPOMATURATION TYPE.................................. 30110
*AMELOGENESIS IMPERFECTA, HYPOPLASTIC TYPE (HEREDITARY ENAMEL HYPOPLASIA)...... 30120
AMENORRHEA, HYPERTENSION AND HYPOKALEMIC ALKALOSIS   SEE ADRENAL HYPERP-
    LASIA V (20210)
AMENORRHEA-GALACTORRHEA SYNDROME.. 10460
AMINOACIDURIA WITH MENTAL DEFICIENCY, DWARFISM, MUSCULAR DYSTROPHY, OSTEO-
    POROSIS AND ACIDOSIS... 20480
AMMONEMIA, AMMONIA INTOXICATION   SEE HYPERAMMONIA (23720, 23730), LYSINE
    INTOLERANCE (24790), CITRULLINEMIA (21570)
AMMONIA INTOXICATION   SEE LYSINE INTOLERANCE (24790)
AMNIOTIC BANDS   SEE CONSTRICTING BANDS, CONGENITAL (21710)
*AMYLASE, SERUM (TWO LOCI)... 10470
AMYLOIDOSIS   SEE MEDITERRANEAN FEVER, FAMILIAL (24910), URTICARIA,
    DEAFNESS AND AMYLOIDOSIS (19190)
AMYLOIDOSIS   SEE URTICARIA, DEAFNESS AND AMYLOIDOSIS (19190)
*AMYLOIDOSIS I (ANDRADE OR PORTUGUESE TYPE).................................... 10480
*AMYLOIDOSIS II (INDIANA OR RUKAVINA TYPE)..................................... 10490
AMYLOIDOSIS III (CARDIAC FORM)... 10500
*AMYLOIDOSIS IV (IOWA OR VAN ALLEN TYPE)....................................... 10510
AMYLOIDOSIS, CORNEAL   SEE CORNEAL DYSTROPHY, LATTICE TYPE (12220)
AMYLOIDOSIS, CUTANEOUS BULLOUS... 20490

*AMYLOIDOSIS, FAMILIAL VISCERAL.. 10520
AMYLOID-PRODUCING MEDULLARY THYRIOD CANCER   SEE PHEOCHROMOCYTOMA AND
   AMYLOID PRODUCING MEDULLARY THYROID CARCINOMA (17140), NEUROMATA,
   MUCOSAL, WITH ENDOCRINE TUMORS (16230)
AMYOTONIA CONGENITA (OPPENHEIM'S DISEASE) 20500
*AMYOTROPHIC DYSTONIC PARAPLEGIA... 10530
*AMYOTROPHIC LATERAL SCLEROSIS... 10540
AMYOTROPHIC LATERAL SCLEROSIS-PARKINSONISM DEMENTIA COMPLEX OF GUAM (ALS-PD).. 10550
*AMYOTROPHIC LATERAL SCLEROSIS, JUVENILE... 20510
AMYOTROPHIC LATERAL SCLEROSIS, JUVENILE, WITH DEMENTIA............................ 20520
AMYOTROPHIC LATERAL SCLEROSIS   SEE MUSCULAR ATROPHY, PROGRESSIVE (15870,
   25350)
AMYOTROPHY OF HANDS   SEE SPASTIC PARAPLEGIA WITH AMYOTROPHY OF HANDS
   (18270)
ANAL STENOSIS   SEE RIEGER'S SYNDROME (18050)
*ANALBUMINEMIA... 20530
ANALGESIA   SEE BIEMOND'S CONGENITAL AND FAMILIAL ANALGESIA (21030),
   INSENSITIVITY TO PAIN (24300)
*ANALPHALIPOPROTEINEMIA (TANGIER DISEASE).. 20540
ANAL-SACRAL ANOMALIES... 20550
ANDERSON'S DISEASE   SEE GLYCOGEN STORAGE DISEASE IV (23250)
ANDROGEN-RESISTANT MALE PSEUDOHERMAPHRODITISM   SEE TESTICULAR FEMINIZA-
   TION SYNDROME (31370)
ANEMIA   SEE SPHEROCYTOSIS, HEREDITARY (18290), VARIOUS HEMOGLOBINOPA-
   THIES LISTED UNDER HEMOGLOBIN (14170), PERNICIOUS ANEMIA (17090),
   STOMATOCYTOSIS (18500)
ANEMIA AND TRIPHALANGEAL THUMBS... 20560
ANEMIA WITH MULTINUCLEATED ERYTHROBLASTS.. 10560
ANEMIA, AUTOIMMUNE HEMOLYTIC.. 20570
ANEMIA, CHLORAMPHENICOL-INDUCED... 20580
ANEMIA, CONGENITAL   SEE ANEMIA AND TRIPHALANGEAL THUMBS (20560)
ANEMIA, CONGENITAL HYFOPLASTIC, OF BLACKFAN AND DIAMOND (CHRONIC CONGENI-
   TAL AREGENERATIVE ANEMIA, ERYTHROGENESIS IMPERFECTA, 'PURE RED CELL
   ANEMIA').. 20590
ANEMIA, CONSTITUTIONAL APLASTIC OR CONSTITUTIONAL INFANTILE PANMYELOPATHY
   SEE FANCONI'S PANCYTOPENIA (22790)
*ANEMIA, FAMILIAL PYRIDOXINE-RESPONSIVE.. 20600
ANEMIA, FAMILIAL SIDEROBLASTIC   SEE ANEMIA, HYPOCHROMIC (30130)
ANEMIA, HEMOLYTIC   SEE PHOSPHOHEXOSE ISOMERASE, VARIANTS OF (17240),
   GLUTATHIONE PEROXIDASE DEFICIENCY, HEMOLYTIC ANEMIA DUE TO (23170)
*ANEMIA, HYPOCHROMIC... 30130
ANEMIA, HYPOCHROMIC MICROCYTIC.. 20610
ANEMIA, IRON DEFICIENCY... 30140
*ANEMIA, NON-HEMOLYTIC NORMOCHROMIC.. 10570
ANEMIA, NONSPHEROCYTIC HEMOLYTIC.. 20620
ANEMIA, NONSPHEROCYTIC HEMOLYTIC, ASSOCIATED WITH ABNORMALITY OF RED-CELL
   MEMBRANE.. 20630
ANEMIA, NONSPHEROCYTIC HEMOLYTIC, POSSIBLY DUE TO DEFECT IN PORPHYRIN
   METABOLISM.. 20640
ANEMIA, NONSPHEROCYTIC HEMOLYTIC   SEE PYRUVATE KINASE DEFICIENCY OF
   ERYTHROCYTE (26620), GLUTATHIONE REDUCTASE HEMOLYTIC ANEMIA DUE TO
   DEFICIENCY OF (23180), GLUTATHIONE PEROXIDASE DEFICIENCY, HEMOLYTIC
   ANEMIA DUE TO (23170), TRIOSEPHOSPHATE ISOMERASE DEFICIENCY (27580),
   DIPHOSPHOGLYCERATE MUTASE DEFICIENCY (22280)
ANEMIA, NONSPHEROCYTIC HEMOLYTIC, ASSOCIATED WITH ABNORMALITY OF RED-CELL
   MEMBRANE   SEE RED CELL PHOSPHOLIPID DEFECT WITH HEMOLYSIS (17970)
ANENCEPHALY... 20650
ANESTHESIA, HYPERTHERMIA AFTER   SEE HYPERTHERMIA OF ANESTHESIA (14560)
ANEURYSM OF AORTA   SEE ERDHEIM'S CYSTIC MEDIAL NECROSIS OF AORTA (13290)
ANEURYSM, INTRACRANIAL 'BERRY'.. 10580
ANEURYSMS, MULTIPLE ARTERIAL   SEE EHLERS-DANLOS SYNDROME (13000, 22540,
   30520)
ANGIOID STREAKS   SEE PSEUDOXANTHOMA ELASTICUM (26480), CALCINOSIS,
   TUMORAL (21190), HYPEROSTOSIS CORTICALIS DEFORMANS JUVENILIS (23900)
ANGIOKERATOMA, DIFFUSE (FABRY'S DISEASE HEREDITARY DYSTOPIC LIPIDOSIS)....... 30150
ANGIOLIPOMAS, MULTIPLE.. 10590
ANGIOMA RACEMOSUM VENOSUM... 10600
ANGIOMATA   SEE BLUE RUBBER BLEB NEVUS (11220)
ANGIOMATOSIS   SEE HEMANGIOMATOSIS, CUTANEOUS, WITH ASSOCIATED FEATURES
   (23480)
ANGIOMATOSIS, CYSTIC, WITH LIPODYSTROPHY   SEE LIPODYSTROPHY AND CYSTIC
   ANGIOMATOSIS (24700)
ANGIOMATOSIS, DIFFUSE CORTICO-MENINGEAL, OF DIVRY AND VAN BOGAERT............. 30160
ANGIOMATOSIS, SYSTEMIC CYSTIC   SEE SYSTEMIC CYSTIC ANGIOMATOSIS AND SEIP
   SYNDROME (27250)
*ANGIONEUROTIC EDEMA (TWO TYPES)... 10610
ANGIO-OSTEO-HYPERTROPHY SYNDROME   SEE KLIPPEL-TRENAUNAY-WEBER SYNDROME
   (14900)
*ANHIDROSIS... 20660
ANHIDROSIS   SEE NEUROPATHY, CONGENITAL SENSORY, WITH ANHIDROSIS (25680)
ANHIDROTIC ECTODERMAL DYSPLASIA   SEE ECTODERMAL DYSPLASIA, ANHIDROTIC
   (12930, 12940, 22490, 30510)

*ANIRIDIA.. 10620
 ANIRIDIA   SEE WILMS' TUMOR (27780)
 ANIRIDIA, CEREBELLAR ATAXIA AND MENTAL DEFICIENCY......................... 20670
 ANKYLOBLEPHARON FILIFORME   SEE CLEFT LIP-PALATE, MUCOUS CYSTS OF LOWER
    LIP, POPLITEAL PTERYGIUM, DIGITAL AND GENITAL ANOMALIES (11950)
 ANKYLOSING SPONDYLITIS... 10630
 ANKYLOSING VERTEBRAL HYPEROSTOSIS WITH TYLOSIS........................... 10640
 ANKYLOSIS OF INTERPHALANGEAL JOINTS   SEE SYMPHALANGISM (18560, 18570)
 ANNULAR ERYTHEMA... 10650
 ANODONTIA   SEE TEETH, ABSENCE OF (31350)
*ANODONTIA, PARTIAL.. 10660
 ANODONTIA, PARTIAL   SEE TEETH, ABSENCE OF (31350)
 ANOMALOUS PULMONARY VENOUS RETURN....................................... 10670
 ANONYCHIA... 10680
 ANONYCHIA... 20680
*ANONYCHIA-ECTRODACTYLY.. 10690
 ANONYCHIA-ONYCHODYSTROPHY... 10700
 ANOPHTHALMOS   SEE MICROPHTHALMIA OR ANOPHTHALMOS, WITH DIGITAL ANOMALIES
    (30980)
*ANOPHTHALMOS, TRUE OR PRIMARY... 20690
 ANORCHIA   SEE LOWE'S OCULO-CEREBRO-RENAL SYNDROME (30900), TESTES,
    ABSENCE OF (27310)
 ANORECTAL ANOMALIES... 10710
 ANORECTAL ANOMALIES   SEE ANUS, IMPERFORAT (20750, 30180)
 ANOSMIA... 30170
 ANOSMIA   SEE CYANIDE, INABILITY TO SMELL (30430), KALLMANN SYNDROME
    (24420, 30870)
 ANOSMIA FOR ISOBUTYRIC ACID... 20700
 ANOSMIA, CONGENITAL... 20720
 ANOTIA AND MEATAL ATRESIA... 20710
 ANTICOAGULANT RESISTANCE   SEE COUMARIN RESISTANCE (12270)
 ANTIMONGOLOID SLANT OF EYES   SEE MANDIBULOFACIAL-DYSOSTOSIS (15450),
    RUBINSTEIN'S SYNDROME (26860)
 ANTITHROMBIN DEFICIENCY... 10730
 ANTITHROMBIN III DEFICIENCY... 20720
 ANTITHROMBIN, FAMILIAL HEMORRHAGIC DIATHESIS DUE TO..................... 20730
*ANTITRYPSIN DEFICIENCY OF PLASMA.. 20740
*ANTITRYPSIN, ELECTROPHORETIC VARIANT OF SERUM.......................... 10740
 ANUS, IMPERFORATE.. 20750
 ANUS, IMPERFORATE.. 30180
 ANUS, IMPERFORATE   SEE TRYPSINOGEN DEFICIENCY DISEASE (27600)
 AORTIC ARCH ANOMALY WITH PECULIAR FACIES AND MENTAL RETARDATION......... 10750
 AORTIC ARCH SYNDROME ('YOUNG FEMALE ARTERITIS,' 'PULSELESS DISEASE,' OR
    TAKAYASU'S ARTERITIS)... 20760
 AORTIC STENOSIS   SEE SUPRAVALVAR AORTIC STENOSIS (18550)
 APERT-CROUZON DISEASE (VOGT'S CEPHALODACTYLY)   SEE ACROCEPHALOSYNDACTYLY
    TYPE II (10130)
 APERT'S SYNDROME   SEE ACROCEPHALOSYNDACTYLY TYPE I (10120)
 APICAL DYSTROPHY   SEE BRACHYDACTYLY, TYPE B (11300)
*APLASIA CUTIS CONGENITA... 10760
*APLASIA CUTIS CONGENITA (CONGENITAL DEFECT OF SKIN, CONGENITAL DEFECT OF
    SKULL AND SCALP)... 20770
 APLASIA CUTIS CONGENITA   SEE ABSENCE DEFECT OF LIMBS, SCALP AND SKULL
    (10030), EPIDERMOLYSIS BULLOSA WITH CONGENITAL LOCALIZED ABSENCE OF
    SKIN AND DEFORMITY OF NAILS (13200)
 APPENDICITIS, PRONENESS TO.. 10770
 APPLE PEEL SYNDROME   SEE JEJUNAL ATRESIA (24360)
 ARACHNODACTYLY   SEE MARFAN SYNDROME (15470), ACHARD SYNDROME (10070)
 ARCUS CORNEAE (ARCUS SENILIS).. 10780
 AREFLEXIC DYSTASIA   SEE ROUSSY-LEVY HEREDITARY AREFLEXIC DYSTASIA (18080)
*ARGININEMIA... 20780
 ARGININOSUCCINIC ACID SYNTHETASE DEFICIENCY   SEE CITRULLINEMIA (21570)
*ARGININOSUCCINICACIDURIA... 20790
 ARHINENCEPHALY   SEE HOLOPROSENCEPHALY, FAMILIAL ALOBAR (23610)
 ARMS, MALFORMATION OF... 10790
*ARTERIAL CALCIFICATION, GENERALIZED, OF INFANCY........................ 20800
 ARTERIES, ANOMALIES OF... 10800
 ARTERIES, HYPOPLASIA OF   SEE INTERNAL CAROTID ARTERIES, HYPOPLASIA OF
    (24310)
 ARTERIOPATHY, FAMILIAL   SEE SUPRAVALVULAR AORTIC STENOSIS (18550)
 ARTERIOVENOUS FISTULA, PULMONARY   SEE TELANGIECTASIA, HEREDITARY HEMORR-
    HAGIC (18730)
 ARTHRITIS, SACRO-ILIAC.. 10810
 ARTHROCHALASIS MULTIPLEX CONGENITA   SEE JOINT LAXITY (24380)
 ARTHROGRYPOSIS   SEE PSEUDO-ARTHROGRYPOSIS (17730)
 ARTHROGRYPOSIS MULTIPLEX CONGENITA..................................... 20810
 ARTHROGRYPOSIS MULTIPLEX CONGENITA   SEE MUSCULAR DYSTROPHY, CONGENITAL
    PRODUCING ARTHROGRYPOSIS (25390)
*ARTHROGRYPOSIS-LIKE DISORDER... 20820
 ARTHROGRYPOSIS-LIKE DISORDER   SEE PSEUDO-ARTHROGRYPOSIS (17730)
 ARTHROGRYPOSIS-LIKE HAND ANOMALY AND SENSORI-NEURAL DEAFNESS............ 10820
*ARTHRO-OPHTHALMOPATHY, HEREDITARY PROGRESSIVE.......................... 10830

REGURGITATION (15770)
CERVICO-OCULO-ACUSTIC SYNDROME   SEE WILDERVANCK SYNDROME (31460)
*CHARCOT-MARIE-TOOTH DISEASE... 11820
CHARCOT-MARIE-TOOTH DISEASE AND NEPHRITIS... 11830
*CHARCOT-MARIE-TOOTH PERONEAL MUSCULAR ATROPHY...................................... 21440
CHARCOT-MARIE-TOOTH PERONEAL MUSCULAR ATROPHY   SEE GAMSTORP-WOHLFART
    SYNDROME (13720)
*CHARCOT-MARIE-TOOTH PERONEAL MUSCULAR ATROPHY...................................... 30280
CHARCOT-MARIE-TOOTH PERONEAL MUSCULAR ATROPHY AND FRIEDREICH'S ATAXIA,
    COMBINED.. 30290
*CHEDIAK-HIGASHI SYNDROME... 21450
CHEDIAK-HIGASHI SYNDROME   SEE LYMPHOHISTIOCYTIC INFILTRATION, GENERA-
    LIZED (24750)
CHEILOSIS-SEBORRHEA-AMINOACIDURIA... 21460
CHEMODECTOMA   SEE PARAGANGLIOMATA (16800)
CHENEY SYNDROME   SEE ACRO-OSTEOLYSIS WITH OSTEOPOROSIS, ETC. (10250)
*CHERUBISM (FAMILIAL FIBROUS DYSPLASIA OF THE JAWS)................................. 11840
CHIARI-FROMMEL SYNDROME   SEE AMENORRHEA-GALACTORRHEA SYNDROME (10460)
CHIEF CELL HYPERPLASIA   SEE HYPERPARATHYROIDISM (14500)
CHILBLAINS   SEE ACROCYANOSIS (10170)
CHIN REFLEX   SEE PALMO-MENTAL REFLEX (16770)
CHIN, CLEFT   SEE CLEFT CHIN (11900)
CHIN, QUIVERING OF   SEE TREMBLING CHIN (19010), SPINAL AND BULBAR MUSCU-
    LAR ATROPHY (31320)
*CHLORIDE DIARRHEA, FAMILIAL.. 21470
CHOANAL ATRESIA, POSTERIOR... 21480
'CHOCOLATE CYST' OF OVARY   SEE ENDOMETRIOSIS (13120)
CHOLANGITIS, SCLEROSING   SEE FIBROSCLEROSIS, MULTIFOCAL (22880)
*CHOLESTASIS AND LYMPHEDEMA... 21490
CHOLESTASIS, INTRAHEPATIC   SEE INTRAHEPATIC CHOLESTASIS (24330), BYLER'S
    DISEASE (21160)
CHOLESTERINOSIS   SEE CEREBRAL CHOLESTERINOSIS (21370)
CHOLESTEROL ESTER STORAGE DISEASE OF LIVER... 21500
CHOLESTEROL-ESTERIFICATION DEFECT   SEE LECITHIN* CHOLESTEROL ACETYLTRAN-
    SFERASE (LCAT) DEFICIENCY (24590)
CHOLINESTERASE   SEE PSEUDOCHOLINESTERASE (17740-17760)
CHOLINESTERASE DEFICIENCY   SEE SUXAMETHONIUM SENSITIVITY (27240)
CHOLINESTERASE, REDUCTION IN RED CELL.. 11850
CHOLINESTERASE, REDUCTION IN RED CELL   SEE PSEUDOCHOLINESTERASE VARIANTS
    (17740, 17750)
CHONDROCALCINOSIS ('CALCIUM GOUT')... 11860
*CHONDRODYSPLASIA PUNCTATA (CHONDRODYSTROPHIA CALCIFICANS CONGENITA)............. 11865
*CHONDRODYSPLASIA PUNCTATA (CHONDRODYSTROPHIA CALCIFICANS CONGENITA, CHON-
    DRODYSTROPHIA CALCIFICANS PUNCTATA, CONRADI'S DISEASE)......................... 21510
CHONDRODYSTROPHIA CALCIFICANS CONGENITA   SEE CHONDRODYSPLASIA PUNCTATA
    (21510)
CHONDRODYSTROPHY   SEE CARTILAGE-HAIR HYPOPLASIA (21230), ELLIS-VAN
    CREVELD SYNDROME (22550)
CHONDRODYSTROPHY, JOINT DISLOCATION, GLAUCOMA, AND MENTAL RETARDATION.......... 21520
CHONDROSARCOMA... 21530
CHONDRO-TRICHO-HYPOPLASIA   SEE CARTILAGE-HAIR HYPOPLASIA (21230)
CHORDOMA... 21540
*CHOREA, HEREDITARY BENIGN... 11870
*CHOREOATHETOSIS, FAMILIAL PAROXYSMAL.. 11880
CHOREOATHETOSIS, PAROXYSMAL MOVEMENT-INDUCED (KINETOGENIC)   SEE DYS-
    TONIA, FAMILIAL PAROXYSMAL (12820)
CHORIORETINOPATHY   SEE MICROCEPHALY (25120)
CHOROID PLEXUS, INTRAVENTRICULAR PAPILLOMA OF   SEE PAPILLOMA, OF CHOROID
    PLEXUS (26050)
CHOROID PLEXUS, PAPILLOMA OF   SEE PAPILLOMA OF CHOROID PLEXUS (26050)
CHOROIDAL ATROPHY, OR SCLEROSIS   SEE FUNDUS DYSTROPHY (13690)
CHOROIDAL SCLEROSIS.. 21550
CHOROIDAL SCLEROSIS.. 30300
CHOROIDEREMIA   SEE VAN DEN BOSCH SYNDROME (31450)
*CHOROIDEREMIA (PROGRESSIVE TAPETO-CHOROIDAL DYSTROPHY)............................ 30310
*CHOROIDO-RETINAL DEGENERATION WITH RETINAL REFLEX IN HETEROZYGOUS WOMEN....... 30320
CHOROIDO-RETINAL DYSTROPHY... 30330
CHRISTMAS DISEASE   SEE HEMOPHILIA B (30690)
CHROMOSOMAL ABERRATIONS   SEE NON-DISJUNCTION (25730), SATELLITE ASSOCIA-
    TION (18110)
CHYLOUS ASCITES   SEE ASCITES, CHYLOUS (20830)
'CIGARETTE-PAPER SCARS'   SEE NECROBIOSIS LIPOIDICA AND PERIODONTOSIS
    (16170), EHLERS-DANLOS SYNDROME (13000, 22540, 30520)
CIRRHOSIS OF LIVER   SEE ALPERS' DEGENERATION OF CEREBRAL GRAY MATTER
    WITH HEPATIC CIRRHOSIS (20370), ANTITRYPSIN DEFICIENCY OF PLASMA (207
CIRRHOSIS WITH POLIODYSTROPHY   SEE POLIODYSTROPHY WITH CIRRHOSIS (26300)
CIRRHOSIS, FAMILIAL.. 11890
CIRRHOSIS, FAMILIAL.. 21560
CIRRHOSIS, FAMILIAL CONGENITAL, WITH PHOSPHOGLUCOAMINOACIDURIA, VITAMIN
    RESISTANT RICKETS AND TYROSINURIA   SEE TYROSINEMIA (27670)
*CITRULLINURIA... 21570
CLAW-FOOT, FAMILIAL, WITH ABSENT TENDON JERKS   SEE ROUSSY-LEVY HEREDI-

```
      DIAPHYSEAL ACLASIS    SEE EXOSTOSES, MULTIPLE (13370)
     *DIASTEMA, DENTAL MEDIAL.....................................................  12590
      DIASTEMATOMYELIA............................................................  22250
     *DIASTROPHIC DWARFISM.......................................................  22260
      DIBASICAMINOACIDURIA I......................................................  12600
     *DIBASICAMINOACIDURIA II....................................................  22270
      DIEGO BLOOD GROUP    SEE BLOOD GROUP-DIEGO SYSTEM (11050)
      DIGEORGE'S SYNDROME    SEE THYMUS AND PARATHYROIDS, ABSENCE OF (18840)
      DIGITAL CONTRACTURES    SEE HYPERTELORISM, ETC. (23970)
      DILANTIN-LIKE SYNDROME    SEE FIBROMATOSIS, GINGIVAL, WITH HYPERTRICHOSIS
         (13540)
      DIMPLES, FACIAL.............................................................  12610
     *DIPHOSPHOGLYCERATE MUTASE DEFICIENCY OF ERYTHROCYTE, ANEMIA DUE TO..........  22280
     *DISACCHARIDE INTOLERANCE I (CONGENITAL SUCROSE-ISOMALTOSE MALABSORPTION*
         CONGENITAL SUCROSE INTOLERANCE).........................................  22290
     *DISACCHARIDE INTOLERANCE II (CONGENITAL LACTOSE INTOLERANCE)...............  22300
     *DISACCHARIDE INTOLERANCE III (ADULT LACTASE DEFICIENCY)....................  22310
      DISAPPEARING CARPAL BONES    SEE OSTEOLYSIS, HEREDITARY, OF CARPAL BONES
         WITH NEPHROPATHY (16630)
      DISLOCATION OF HEAD OF FIBULA    SEE FIBULA, RECURRENT DISLOCATION OF HEAD
         OF (13580)
      DISLOCATION OF JOINTS    SEE CHONDRODYSTROPHY, JOINT DISLOCATION, GLAUCOMA
         AND MENTAL RETARDATION (21520), LARSEN'S SYNDROME (24560)
      DISLOCATION OF JOINTS, RECURRENT FAMILIAL    SEE JOINT LAXITY (14790,
         24380)
      DISLOCATION OF KNEES, CONGENITAL    SEE LARSEN'S SYNDROME (24560)
      DISLOCATION OF RADIUS    SEE PTERYGIUM, ANTECUBITAL (17820)
      DISSECTING ANEURYSM OF AORTA    SEE ERDHEIM'S CYSTIC MEDIAL NECROSIS OF
         AORTA (13290), MARFAN SYNDROME (15470)
      DISSEMINATED SCLEROSIS (MULTIPLE SCLEROSIS).................................  12620
      DISSEMINATED SCLEROSIS (MULTIPLE SCLEROSIS).................................  22320
      DISSEMINATED SCLEROSIS WITH NARCOLEPSY......................................  22330
      DISSEMINATED SCLEROSIS-LIKE DISORDER    SEE ATAXIA, SPASTIC (10860),
         PELIZAEUS-MERZBACHER DISEASE (16940, 16950, 26060), MULTIPLE SCLEROSIS-
         LIKE DISEASE (15840)
      DISTAL MYOPATHY    SEE MYOPATHY, LATE DISTAL HEREDITARY (16050)
      DISTICHIASIS    SEE ALACRIMIA CONGENITA (20280), SPINAL EXTRADURAL CYST
         (27110), LYMPHEDEMA, WITH DISTICHIASIS (15340)
     *DISTICHIASIS (TWO ROWS OF EYELASHES).......................................  12630
      DIVERTICULA, SMALL BOWEL    SEE DEAFNESS, NERVE TYPE, MESENTERIC DIVERTI-
         CULA, ETC. (22140)
      DIVERTICULOSIS OF TRACHEA    SEE TRACHEOBRONCHOMEGALY (27530)
      DIZYGOTIC TWINNING    SEE TWINNING, DIZYGOTIC (27640)
      DOHLE BODIES    SEE MAY-HEGGLIN ANOMALY (15510)
      DOMBROCK BLOOD GROUP    SEE BLOOD GROUP-DOMBROCK SYSTEM (11060)
      DOUBLE ATHETOSIS (STATUS MARMORATUS, OR 'LITTLE'S DISEASE WITH INVOLUNTARY
         MOVEMENTS').............................................................  12640
      DOUBLE LIP    SEE BLEPHAROCHALASIS AND 'DOUBLE LIP' (10990)
      DOUBLE NAIL FOR FIFTH TOE...................................................  12650
     *DOYNE'S HONEYCOMB DEGENERATION OF RETINA....................................  12660
      DPNH - DIAPHORASE DEFICIENCY    SEE METHEMOGLOBINEMIA (25080)
      DRUSEN OF BRUCH'S MEMBRANE..................................................  12670
      DRUSEN OF OPTIC DISKS    SEE PSEUDOPAPILLEDEMA (17780)
      DUANE SYNDROME    SEE WILDERVANCK SYNDROME (31460)
     *DUANE SYNDROME (RETRACTION SYNDROME)........................................  12680
      DUARTE VARIANT    SEE GALACTOSEMIA (23040)
      DUBIN-JOHNSON DISEASE    SEE HYPERBILIRUBINEMIA II (14360, 23750)
      DUCHENNE MUSCULAR DYSTROPHY    SEE MUSCULAR DYSTROPHY, PSEUDOHYPERTROPHIC
         PROGRESSIVE, DUCHENNE TYPE (31020)
      DUFFY BLOOD GROUP    SEE BLOOD GROUP-DUFFY SYSTEM (11070)
      DUODENAL ATRESIA............................................................  22340
      DUPUYTREN'S CONTRACTURE.....................................................  12690
      DUPUYTREN'S CONTRACTURE    SEE FIBROSCLEROSIS, MULTIFOCAL (22880)
      DWARFISM    SEE AMINOACIDURIA WITH OTHER FEATURES (20480), CARTILAGE-HAIR
         HYPOPLASIA (21230), TRYPTOPHANURIA WITH DWARFISM (27610), SILVER-RUS-
         SELL DWARFISM (18240)
      DWARFISM AND SKIN CHANGES    SEE BLOOM'S SYNDROME (21090)
      DWARFISM OF HANHART    SEE PITUITARY DWARFISM II (26250)
     *DWARFISM, ATELEIOTIC (PRIMORDIAL DWARFISM)    SEE PITUITARY DWARFISM I
         (26240)
      DWARFISM, BIRD-HEADED, OF SECKEL    SEE BIRD-HEADED DWARF (21060)
     *DWARFISM, CORTICAL THICKENING OF TUBULAR BONES, AND TRANSIENT HYPOCALCEMIA....  12700
      DWARFISM, LEVI OR 'SNUB-NOSED' TYPE.........................................  12710
      DWARFISM, LOW BIRTH-WEIGHT TYPE, WITH UNRESPONSIVENESS TO GROWTH HORMONE.....  22350
      DWARFISM, PITUITARY    SEE PITUITARY DWARFISM (26240-26270, 31200)
      DWARFISM, SHORT SPINE    SEE MORQUIO SYNDROME (25230), BRACHYRAPHIA
         (11350), SPONDYLOEPIPHYSEAL DYSPLASIA TARDA TYPE (18410)
      DWARFISM, 'SNUB-NOSED' TYPE.................................................  22360
      DWARFISM, TYPE UNCLEAR......................................................  22370
      DWARFISM, WITH STIFF-JOINTS AND OCULAR ABNORMALITIES........................  12720
      DYGGVE-MELCHIOR-CLAUSEN DISEASE.............................................  22380
      DYSAUTONOMIA    SEE NEUROPATHY, CONGENITAL SENSORY, WITH ANHIDROSIS (25680)
```

EXOSTOSES OF HEEL.. 13360
*EXOSTOSES, MULTIPLE... 13370
EXTRASYSTOLES   SEE CARDIAC ARRHYTHMIA (11500)
EXTREMITIES, ABSENCE DEFORMITIES OF   SEE ROBERT'S SYNDROME (26830),
    ECTRODACTYLY (12980)
EYE AND KIDNEY ABNORMALITIES, ASSOCIATED   SEE RENAL DYSPLASIA AND RE-
    TINAL APLASIA (26690), ALPORT SYNDROME (10420), POLYCYSTIC KIDNEY,
    CATARACT AND CONGENITAL BLINDNESS (26310)
EYEBROW, WHORL IN... 13380
EYELASHES   SEE DISTICHIASIS (12630), TRISTICHIASIS (19080)
EYELASHES, LONG   SEE TRICHOMEGALY (27540)
EYELID FOLD, NORDIC TYPE   SEE BLEPHAROCHALASIS OF UPPER LID (11000)
EYELIDS, 'BAGGY'   SEE BLEPHAROCHALASIS (10990, 11000)
EYELIDS, HYPERPIGMENTATION OF   SEE HYPERPIGMENTATION OF EYELIDS (14510)
FABRY'S DISEASE   SEE ANGIOKERATOMA, DIFFUSE (30150)
FACIAL ASYMMETRY, EAR ANOMALY, SIMIAN CREASE.................................... 13390
FACIAL DIPLEGIA OF LATE ONSET   SEE FACIAL PARALYSIS (13420)
FACIAL DIPLEGIA, CONGENITAL   SEE MOEBIUS SYNDROME (15790)
FACIAL HYPERTRICHOSIS.. 13400
FACIAL PALSY, CONGENITAL UNILATERAL.. 13410
FACIAL PARALYSIS.. 13420
FACIAL PARALYSIS   SEE CRANIAL NERVES, PARESIS OF (21810, 21820)
FACIAL SPASM.. 13430
FACIES, PECULIAR   SEE RUBINSTEIN SYNDROME (26860)
*FACIOGENITAL DYSPLASIA.. 30540
FACIO-SCAPULO-HUMERAL MUSCULAR DYSTROPHY   SEE MUSCULAR DYSTROPHY, FACIO-
    SCAPULO-HUMERAL (15890)
FACTOR I DEFICIENCY   SEE AFIBRINOGENEMIA, CONGENITAL (20240)
FACTOR II DEFICIENCY   SEE HYPOPROTHROMBINEMIA (24170)
FACTOR V (PROACCELERIN) EXCESS WITH SPONTANEOUS THROMBOSIS..................... 13440
FACTOR V AND FACTOR VIII, COMBINED DEFICIENCY OF.............................. 22730
*FACTOR V DEFICIENCY (OWREN'S PARAHEMOPHILIA' LABILE FACTOR DEFICIENCY)....... 22740
*FACTOR VII DEFICIENCY (HYPOPROCONVERTINEMIA)................................. 22750
*FACTOR VIII DEFICIENCY.. 13450
FACTOR VIII DEFICIENCY   SEE HEMOPHILIA A (30670), VON WILLEBRAND'S
    DISEASE (19340)
FACTOR IX DEFICIENCY   SEE HEMOPHILIA B (30690)
*FACTOR X DEFICIENCY (DEFICIENCY OF STUART-PROWER FACTOR).................... 22760
FACTOR XI DEFICIENCY   SEE PTA DEFICIENCY (26490)
FACTOR XII DEFICIENCY   SEE HAGEMAN FACTOR DEFICIENCY (23400)
FACTOR XIII DEFICIENCY   SEE FIBRIN-STABILIZING FACTOR DEFICIENCY (30550)
FAHR'S DISEASE   SEE CEREBRAL CALCIFICATION, NON-ARTERIOSCLEROTIC
    (21360), ARTERIAL CALCIFICATION, GENERALIZED, OF INFANCY (20800)
FAIRBANK'S DISEASE   SEE EPIPHYSEAL DYSPLASIA, MULTIPLE (13240)
FAMILIAL MEDITERRANEAN FEVER   SEE MEDITERRANEAN FEVER, FAMILIAL (24910)
FANCONI RENOTUBULAR SYNDROME.. 13460
*FANCONI SYNDROME I (CHILDHOOD AND INFANTILE FORM WITHOUT CYSTINOSIS)........ 22770
*FANCONI SYNDROME II ('ADULT' FORM WITHOUT CYSTINOSIS)...................... 22780
FANCONI'S NEPHRONOPHTHISIS   SEE NEPHRONOPHTHISIS, FAMILIAL JUVENILE
    (25610)
*FANCONI'S PANCYTOPENIA (CONSTITUTIONAL INFANTILE PANMYELOPATHY)............. 22790
*FARBER'S LIPOGRANULOMATOSIS.. 22800
FASCICULATION, MUSCULAR   SEE ATAXIA WITH FASCICULATIONS (10870)
FASCICULATIONS   SEE SPINAL AND BULBAR MUSCULAR ATROPHY (31320)
FASCICULATIONS, BENIGN   SEE MYOKYMIA (16010)
FAT-INDUCED HYPERLIPEMIA   SEE HYPERLIPOPROTEINEMIA I (23860)
FATTY METAMORPHOSIS OF VISCERA... 22810
FAVISM.. 13470
FAZIO-LONDE'S DISEASE   SEE BULBAR PARALYSIS, PROGRESSIVE, OF CHILDHOOD
    (21150)
FDH SYNDROME   SEE FOCAL DERMAL HYPOPLASIA (30560)
FEMALE PSEUDO-TURNER SYNDROME   SEE PTERYGIUM COLLI SYNDROME (17810)
FEMUR-FIBULA-ULNA (FFU) SYNDROME... 22820
FERTILE EUNUCH.. 22830
FETAL HEMOGLOBIN, HEREDITARY PERSISTENCE OF   SEE HEMOGLOBIN F (14170)
FEVER OF UNKNOWN ORIGIN   SEE MEDITERRANEAN FEVER, FAMILIAL (24910),
    PERIODIC FEVER (17030)
FEVER, FAMILIAL LIFELONG PERSISTENT... 22840
FFU SYNDROME   SEE FEMUR-FIBULA-ULNA SYNDROME (22820)
FIBRIN MONOMER AGGREGATION PRODUCING CLOTTING DISTURBANCE   SEE FIBRINO-
    GEN VARIANTS (13480)
FIBRINOGEN BALTIMORE   SEE FIBRINOGEN, VARIANTS (13480)
FIBRINOGEN DEFICIENCY   SEE AFIBRINOGENEMIA, CONGENITAL (20240)
*FIBRINOGEN VARIANTS.. 13480
FIBRINOGENOPATHIES   SEE FIBRINOGEN VARIANTS (13480)
FIBRINOLYTIC DEFECT... 13490
*FIBRIN-STABILIZING FACTOR (FIBRINASE, OR FACTOR XIII) DEFICIENCY........... 22850
*FIBRIN-STABILIZING FACTOR (FACTOR XIII) DEFICIENCY........................ 30550
*FIBROCYSTIC PULMONARY DYSPLASIA... 13500
*FIBRODYSPLASIA OSSIFICANS PROGRESSIVA..................................... 13510
FIBROMATOSIS OF SMALL INTESTINE   SEE NEUROFIBROMATOSIS (16220)
FIBROMATOSIS, CONGENITAL GENERALIZED....................................... 13520

FIBROMATOSIS, GINGIVAL.. 13530
*FIBROMATOSIS, GINGIVAL, WITH HYPERTRICHOSIS............................. 13540
*FIBROMATOSIS, GINGIVAL, WITH ABNORMAL FINGERS, FINGERNAILS, NOSE AND EARS
    AND SPLENOMEGALY... 13550
FIBROMATOSIS, JUVENILE... 22860
FIBROMUSCULAR HYPERPLASIA OF THE RENAL ARTERIES........................ 22870
FIBRO-OSSEOUS DYSPLASIA OF THE JAWS.................................... 13560
FIBROSCLEROSIS, MULTIFOCAL... 22880
FIBROSIS OF EXTRAOCULAR MUSCLE... 13570
FIBROSIS, PULMONARY   SEE PULMONARY FIBROSIS, IDIOPATHIC (17850)
FIBROUS DYSPLASIA OF JAW   SEE CHERUBISM (11840)
FIBULA AND ULNA, HYPOPLASIA OF   SEE ULNA AND FIBULA, HYPOPLASIA OF
    (19140), NIEVERGELT SYNDROME (16340), MESOMELIC DWARFISM (24970)
FIBULA AND ULNA, PARTIAL ABSENCE OF   SEE ACHONDROGENESIS (20060, 20070)
FIBULA APLASIA AND COMPLEX BRACHYDACTYLY............................... 22890
FIBULA, RECURRENT DISLOCATION OF HEAD OF.............................. 13580
FIBULA, SHORT   SEE MENTAL RETARDATION SYNDROME (24960)
FIFTH FINGER SYNDROME.. 13590
FINGER, ABSENT TERMINAL PHALANX OF FIFTH FINGERS   SEE FIFTH FINGER
    SYNDROME (13590)
FINGER, RADIALLY CURVED FIFTH   SEE CAMPTODACTYLY (11420)
FINGERPRINTS   SEE RADIAL LOOP, PLAIN, ON RIGHT INDEX FINGER (31220)
*FINGERPRINTS, ABSENCE OF.. 13600
FINGERPRINTS, ABSENCE OF   SEE ECTODERMAL DYSPLASIA, ABSENT DERMATOGLY-
    PHIC PATTERN, ETC. (12920)
FINGERS, CURVED   SEE BRACHYDACTYLY, TYPE A2 (11260)
FINGERS, RELATIVE LENGTH OF.. 13610
FISH-ODOR SYNDROME   SEE TRIMETHYLAMINURIA (27570)
FISSURED TONGUE   SEE GEOGRAPHIC TONGUE AND FISSURED TONGUE (13740)
FISTULA AURIS CONGENITA   SEE DEAFNESS, WITH EAR PITS (12510), BRANCHIAL
    CLEFT ANOMALIES (11360), EARPITS (12870)
FLEISCHER'S VORTEX DYSTROPHY OF CORNEA   SEE ANGIOKERATOMA, DIFFUSE
    (30150)
FLETCHER FACTOR DEFICIENCY... 22900
FLEXION CONTRACTURE OF FINGERS   SEE FINGERPRINTS, ABSENCE OF (13600)
FLEXION CONTRACTURES OF FINGERS, CONGENITAL   SEE WHISTLING FACE-WINDMILL
    VANE HAND SYNDROME (19370)
FLOPPY MITRAL VALVE SYNDROME   SEE MITRAL REGURGITATION (15770)
FLUSHING OF EARS AND SOMNOLENCE....................................... 13620
FLUSHING OF SKIN   SEE PAIN, SUBMANDIBULAR, OCULAR AND RECTAL, WITH
    FLUSHING (16740)
*FLYNN-AIRD SYNDROME... 13630
*FOCAL DERMAL HYPOPLASIA (FDH).. 30560
FOCAL EPITHELIAL HYPERPLASIA OF THE ORAL MUCOSA....................... 13640
*FOCAL FACIAL DERMAL DYSPLASIA (HEREDITARY SYMMETRICAL APLASTIC NEVI OF
    TEMPLES).. 13650
FOERSTER'S ATONIC-ASTATIC SYNDROME   SEE ATONIC-ASTATIC SYNDROME OF
    FOERSTER (20910)
FOLIC ACID, SELECTIVE DEFECT IN ABSORPTION OF   SEE MEGALOBLASTIC ANEMIA,
    ETC. (24930)
FOLLICULITIS ULERYTHEMATOSUS RETICULATA   SEE ATROPHODERMIA VERMICULATA
    (20970)
FOOT BLISTERING   SEE EPIDERMOLYSIS BULLOSA OF HANDS AND FEET (13180)
FORAMINA PARIETALIA PERMAGNA   SEE PARIETAL FORAMINA, SYMMETRICAL (16850)
FORBES' DISEASE   SEE GLYCOGEN STORAGE DISEASE III (23240)
FORBES-ALBRIGHT SYNDROME   SEE AMENORRHEA-GALACTORRHEA SYNDROME (10460)
FOREFINGERS, CURVED   SEE BRACHYDACTYLY, TYPE A2 (11260)
FORELOCK, WHITE   SEE PIEBALD TRAIT (17280)
*FORMIMINOTRANSFERASE DEFICIENCY...................................... 22910
FORSIUS-ERIKSSON SYNDROME   SEE ALBINISM, OCULAR (FORSIUS-ERIKSSON TYPE)
    (30060)
FOVEAL DYSTROPHY   SEE MACULAR DEGENERATION OF THE RETINA (24820)
*FRAGILITAS OCULI (CORNEAL FRAGILITY, KERATOGLOBUS, BLUE SCLERAE) WITH
    JOINT HYPEREXTENSIBILITY... 22920
FRANCESCHETTI SYNDROME   SEE MANDIBULO-FACIAL DYSOSTOSIS (15440, 15450,
    24840)
FRANCOIS' SYNDROME   SEE DERMO-CHONDRO-CORNEAL DYSTROPHY OF FRANCOIS
    (22180)
FRASER SYNDROME OF MULTIPLE MALFORMATIONS   SEE CRYPTOPHTHALMOS WITH OTHER
    MALFORMATIONS (21900)
FRECKLES   SEE LENTIGINES (15090)
FREEMAN-SHELDON SYNDROME   SEE WHISTLING FACE-WINDMILL VANE HAND SYNDROME
    (19370)
FRENULI, HYPERTROPHIED   SEE ORAL-FACIAL-DIGITAL (OFD) SYNDROME (31120)
FRIEDREICH'S ATAXIA... 13660
*FRIEDREICH'S ATAXIA.. 22930
FRONTODIGITAL SYNDROME.. 13670
FRONTOMETAPHYSEAL DYSPLASIA... 22940
FRUCTOKINASE DEFICIENCY   SEE FRUCTOSURIA (22980)
FRUCTOSE AND GALACTOSE INTOLERANCE.................................... 22950
*FRUCTOSE INTOLERANCE, HEREDITARY (FRUCTOSEMIA)....................... 22960
FRUCTOSEMIA   SEE FRUCTOSE INTOLERANCE, HEREDITARY (22960)

GLUCOSEPHOSPHATE ISOMERASE (GPI) DEFICIENCY   SEE PHOSPHOHEXOSE
    ISOMERASE, VARIANTS OF (17240)
GLUCOSEPHOSPHATE ISOMERASE DEFICIENCY HEMOLYTIC ANEMIA   SEE PHOSPHOHE-
    XOSE ISOMERASE, VARIANTS OF (17240)
*GLUCOSE-6-PHOSPHATE DEHYDROGENASE VARIANTS............................... 30590
GLUCOSE-6-PHOSPHATE DEHYDROGENASE   SEE FAVISM (13470)
GLUCOSE-6-PHOSPHATE DEHYDROGENASE, INSTABILITY OF, IN LEUKOCYTES   SEE
    CHRONIC GRANULOMATOUS DISEASE DUE TO LEUKOCYTE MALFUNCTION (23370,
    30640)
*GLUTAMIC OXALOACETIC TRANSAMINASE OF MITOCHONDRIA, ELECTROPHORETIC VARIANT
    OF... 13820
GLUTAMICACIDEMIA   SEE MENKES SYNDROME (30940)
*GLUTATHIONE PEROXIDASE DEFICIENCY, HEMOLYTIC ANEMIA DUE TO................. 23170
GLUTATHIONE PEROXIDASE DEFICIENCY OF LEUKOCYTES   SEE GRANULOMATOUS
    DISEASE DUE TO LEUKOCYTE MALFUNCTION (23370, 30640)
*GLUTATHIONE REDUCTASE ELECTROPHORETIC VARIANTS........................... 13830
*GLUTATHIONE REDUCTASE, HEMOLYTIC ANEMIA DUE TO DEFICIENCY OF, IN RED CELLS.... 23180
*GLUTATHIONE SYNTHETASE DEFICIENCY OF ERYTHROCYTES, HEMOLYTIC ANEMIA DUE TO.... 23190
GLUTEN-INDUCED ENTEROPATHY   SEE CELIAC SPRUE (11690)
GLYCERALDEHYDE-3-PHOSPHATE DEHYDROGENASE VARIANTS......................... 13840
GLYCERIC ACIDURIA   SEE OXALOSIS II (26000)
GLYCINEMIA (HYPERGLYCINEMIA WITH KETOACIDOSIS AND LEUKOPENIA) PROPIONICA-
    CIDEMIA.. 23200
GLYCINURIA   SEE GLUCOGLYCINURIA (13810), IMINO GLYCINURIA (24260)
GLYCINURIA WITH OR WITHOUT OXALATE UROLITHIASIS........................... 13850
GLYCOGEN DEFICIENCY   SEE HYPOGLYCEMIA DUE TO DEFICIENCY OF GLYCOGEN
    SYNTHETASE IN THE LIVER (24060)
GLYCOGEN STORAGE DISEASE LIMITED TO HEART (ANTOPOL'S DISEASE).............. 23210
GLYCOGEN STORAGE DISEASE I (VON GIERKE'S DISEASE HEPATORENAL FORM OF
    GLYCOGEN STORAGE DISEASE* GLUCOSE-6-PHOSPHATASE DEFICIENCY* HEPATORENAL
    GLYCOGENOSIS).. 23220
GLYCOGEN STORAGE DISEASE II (POMPE'S DISEASE CARDIAC FORM OF GENERALIZED
    GLYCOGENOSIS* CARDIOMEGALIA GLYCOGENICA DIFFUSA* ETC.)................. 23230
GLYCOGEN STORAGE DISEASE III (FORBES' DISEASE CORI'S DISEASE* LIMIT
    DEXTRINOSIS)... 23240
GLYCOGEN STORAGE DISEASE IV (ANDERSEN'S DISEASE BRANCHER DEFICIENCY*
    AMYLOPECTINOSIS* FAMILIAL CIRRHOSIS WITH DEPOSITION OF ABNORMAL GLYCO-
    GEN).. 23250
GLYCOGEN STORAGE DISEASE V (MCARDLE'S DISEASE MYOPHOSPHORYLASE DEFICIENCY
    GLYCOGENOSIS).. 23260
GLYCOGEN STORAGE DISEASE VI (HERS' DISEASE PHOSPHORYLASE DEFICIENCY
    GLYCOGEN-STORAGE DISEASE OF LIVER)..................................... 23270
*GLYCOGEN STORAGE DISEASE VII (PHOSPHOFRUCTOKINASE DEFICIENCY GLYCOGEN
    DISEASE OF MUSCLE)... 23280
*GLYCOGEN STORAGE DISEASE VIII (DEFICIENCY OF PHOSPHORYLASE KINASE).......... 30600
GLYCOGEN SYNTHETASE DEFICIENCY   SEE HYPOGLYCEMIA DUE TO OF GLYCOGEN
    SYNTHETASE IN THE LIVER DEFICIENCY (24060)
GLYCOLIC ACIDURIA   SEE OXALOSIS I (25990)
GLYCOLIPIDOSIS   SEE ANGIOKERATOMA DIFFUSE (30150)
GLYCOPROTEIN STORAGE DISEASE... 23290
GLYCOPROTEIN* LACK OF BETA(2)-GLYCOPROTEIN I.............................. 23300
*GLYCOPROTEIN, ALPHA-1-ACID, OF SERUM..................................... 13860
GLYCOPROTEIN, CONCENTRATION OF BETA-2-GLYCOPROTEIN I IN SERUM............. 13870
*GLYCOSURIA, RENAL (ALSO SEE FANCONI SYNDROME)........................... 23310
GLYOXALASE II (HYDROXYACYL-GLUTATHIONE HYDROLASE) DEFICIENCY............. 23320
GM TYPES   SEE IMMUNOGLOBULIN TYPES* GM (14710)
GOITER   SEE BLEPHAROCHALASIS (10990, 11000)
GOITER WITH IODO-ALBUMIN REPLACING THYROGLOBULIN   SEE THYROID HORMONO-
    GENESIS, GENETIC DEFECT IN, V (27490)
GOITER, FAMILIAL   SEE THYROID HORMONOGENESIS, GENETIC DEFECTS IN (27440-
    27490)
GOITER, NON-TOXIC, WITH INTRATHYROIDAL CALCIFICATION..................... 13880
GOLDENHAR'S SYNDROME   SEE OCULO-AURICULO-VERTEBRAL DYSPLASIA (25770)
GOLTZ SYNDROME   SEE FOCAL DERMAL HYPOPLASIA (30560)
*GONADAL DYSGENESIS, XX TYPE.. 23330
GONADAL DYSGENESIS, XX TYPE, WITH DEAFNESS............................... 23340
GONADAL DYSGENESIS, XY FEMALE TYPE....................................... 30610
GONADOTROPIN DEFICIENCY, ISOLATED   SEE EUNUCHOIDISM, FAMILIAL HYPOPO-
    GONADOTROPHIC (22720)
GORLIN'S SYNDROME (CRANIOFACIAL DYSOSTOSIS, HYPERTRICHOSIS, HYPOPLASIA OF
    LABIA MAJORA, DENTAL AND EYE ANOMALIES, PATENT DUCTUS ARTERIOSUS,
    NORMAL INTELLIGENCE)... 23350
GOUT.. 13890
GOUT.. 30620
GOUT   SEE NEPHROPATHY, FAMILIAL, WITH GOUT (16200), HYPOXANTHINE GUANINE
    PHOSPHORIBOSYL TRANSFERASE DEFICIENCY (30800)
GPI DEFICIENCY   SEE PHOSPHOHEXOSE ISOMERASE, VARIANTS OF (17240)
GRANULE CELL HYPERTROPHY   SEE CEREBELLO-PARENCHYMAL DISORDER VI (11750)
GRANULOCYTOPENIA WITH IMMUNOGLOBULIN ABNORMALITY......................... 23360
GRANULOMAS, CONGENITAL CEREBRAL.. 30630
*GRANULOMATOUS DISEASE DUE TO LEUKOCYTE MALFUNCTION....................... 23370
*GRANULOMATOUS DISEASE DUE TO LEUKOCYTE MALFUNCTION....................... 30640

GRANULOMATOUS DISEASE OF BOWEL   SEE REGIONAL ENTERITIS (26660)
GRANULOSA CELL TUMOR OF OVARY   SEE POLYPOSIS, INTESTINAL II (PEUTZ-
    JEGHERS) (17520)
GRANULOSIS RUBRA NASI.. 13900
GRAVES' DISEASE   SEE THYROTOXICOSIS (27500)
GRAYING OF HAIR, EARLY... 13910
GRAYING, PREMATURE   SEE WAARDENBURG'S SYNDROME (19350), BOOK'S SYNDROME,
    OR PHC SYNDROME (11230)
GREIG'S SYNDROME   SEE HYPERTELORISM (14540)
GROUPED PIGMENTATION OF THE MACULA... 23380
*GROUP-SPECIFIC COMPONENT (GC)... 13920
GROWTH HORMONE DEFICIENCY   SEE PITUITARY DWARFISM I AND II (26240, 26250)
GROWTH HORMONE EXCESS WITH DWARFISM   SEE PITUITARY DWARFISM II (26080)
GRUBER'S SYNDROME   SEE MECKEL SYNDROME (24900)
GUMS, HYPERPLASIA OF   SEE FIBROMATOSIS, GINGIVAL (13530), RUTHERFURD'S
    SYNDROME (18090)
GYNECOMASTIA   SEE SPINAL AND BULBAR MUSCULAR ATROPHY (31320)
GYNECOMASTIA, FAMILIAL   SEE REIFENSTEIN SYNDROME (31230)
GYNECOMASTIA, FAMILIAL... 30650
GYNECOMASTIA, HEREDITARY... 13930
GYNECOMASTIA, HEREDITARY... 23390
G6PD DEFICIENCY   SEE GLUCOSE-6-PHOSPHATE DEHYDROGENASE VARIANTS (30590),
    REGIONAL ENTERITIS (26660)
G6PD WORCESTER UNDER G6PD VARIANTS   SEE BEHR'S SYNDROME (21000)
*HAGEMAN FACTOR DEFICIENCY... 23400
HAILEY-HAILEY DISEASE   SEE PEMPHIGUS, BENIGN FAMILIAL (16960)
HAIR WHORL ('COW-LICK,' 'CROWN').. 13940
HAIR, ABNORMALITY OF   SEE CARTILAGE-HAIR HYPOPLASIA (21230), NETHERTON'S
    DISEASE (25650), MENKES SYNDROME (30940)
HAIR, ANOMALIES OF   SEE MONILETHRIX (15800, 25220)
HAIR, EARLY GRAYING OF   SEE GRAYING OF HAIR, EARLY (13910)
HAIR, MIDPHALANGEAL   SEE MIDPHALANGEAL HAIR (15720)
HAIR, WHITE LOCK OF OCCIPITAL   SEE OCCIPITAL HAIR, WHITE LOCK OF (31090)
HAIRLESSNESS   SEE HYPOTRICHOSIS (24190)
HAIRY EARS (HYPERTRICHOSIS PINNAE AURIS)...................................... 13950
HAIRY ELBOWS.. 13960
HALLERMANN-STREIFF SYNDROME... 13970
HALLERMANN-STREIFF SYNDROME... 23410
*HALLERVORDEN AND SPATZ, SYNDROME OF.. 23420
HALO NEVI (LEUKODERMA ACQUISITUM CENTRIFUGUM OF SUTTON)....................... 23430
HAMMAN-RICH SYNDROME   SEE PULMONARY FIBROSIS, IDIOPATHIC (17850)
HAND CLASPING PATTERN... 13980
HANDEDNESS.. 13990
HAND-FOOT-UTERUS (HFU) SYNDROME... 14000
HANHART'S ABSENCE DEFORMITY OF LIMBS WITH MICROGNATION   SEE PEROMELIA
    WITH MICROGNATHISM (26130)
HANHART'S DWARFISM (ATELEIOTIC DWARFISM WITH HYPOGONADISM)   SEE PITUI-
    TARY DWARFISM II (26250)
HAPSBURG JAW   SEE PROGNATHISM, MANDIBULAR (17670)
*HAPTOGLOBIN, ALPHA LOCUS (HP).. 14010
*HAPTOGLOBIN, BETA LOCUS (BP)... 14020
HARLEQUIN FETUS   SEE ICHTHYOSIS, CONGENITAL, 'HARLEQUIN FETUS' TYPE
    (24250)
*HARTNUP'S DISEASE.. 23450
HASHIMOTO'S STRUMA.. 14030
HAY FEVER   SEE ATOPIC HYPERSENSITIVITY (20920)
HEART AND HAND SYNDROME I   SEE HOLT-ORAM SYNDROME (14290)
HEART AND HAND SYNDROME   SEE TABATZNIK HEART-HAND SYNDROME (18680),
    HOLT-ORAM SYNDROME (14290)
HEART ANOMALY   SEE ELLIS-VAN CREVELD SYNDROME (22550), ATROPHODERMIA
    VERMICULATA (20970)
*HEART BLOCK.. 14040
HEART BLOCK   SEE ATRIOVENTRICULAR DISSOCIATION (20960), ATRIAL SEPTAL
    DEFECT WITH ATRIO-VENTRICULAR CONDUCTION DEFECT (10890)
HEART BLOCK AND OPHTHALMOPLEGIA... 23460
*HEART BLOCK, CONGENITAL.. 23470
HEART MALFORMATION   SEE ATRIAL SEPTAL DEFECT (10880)
HEART MALFORMATION, CONGENITAL   SEE VALVULAR HEART DISEASE, CONGENITAL
    (27710)
HEART, MALFORMATION OF.. 14050
HEBERDEN'S NODES.. 14060
HEINZ BODY ANEMIA... 14070
HEINZ BODY ANEMIA   SEE HEMOGLOBIN UBE AND HEMOGLOBIN ZURICH (14170)
HEMANGIOBLASTOMA, CEREBELLAR AND SPINAL   SEE VON HIPPEL-LINDAU SYNDROME
    (19330)
HEMANGIOMA, CAVERNOUS   SEE GLOMUS TUMORS, MULTIPLE (13800)
HEMANGIOMAS.. 14080
HEMANGIOMAS   SEE GLOMUS TUMOR, MULTIPLE (13800), BLUE RUBBER BLEB NEVUS
    (11220)
HEMANGIOMAS OF SMALL INTESTINE.. 14090
HEMANGIOMATA   SEE MACROCEPHALY (24800), KLIPPEL-TRENAUNAY-WEBER SYNDROME
    (14900), VON HIPPEL-LINDAU SYNDROME (19330), STURGE-WEBER SYNDROME

          (18530)
HEMANGIOMA-THROMBOCYTOPENIA SYNDROME (KASSABACH-MERRITT SYNDROME).............. 14100
HEMANGIOMATOSIS, CUTANEOUS, WITH ASSOCIATED FEATURES........................... 23480
HEMANGIOMATOSIS, DISSEMINATED... 14110
HEMATURIA   SEE HYDROXYPROLINEMIA (23700)
HEMATURIA, BENIGN FAMILIAL.. 14120
HEMERALOPIA   SEE NIGHT BLINDNESS, HEMERALOPIA MEANS DAY BLINDNESS BUT IS
     OFTEN CONFUSED WITH NIGHT BLINDNESS FOR WHICH THE ACCURATE TERM IS
     NYCTALOPIA (16350), OGUCHI'S DISEASE (25810)
*HEMERALOPIA, ESSENTIAL, WITH HIGH GRADE MYOPIA............................... 23490
HEMIFACIAL ATROPHY, PROGRESSIVE (PARRY-ROMBERG SYNDROME)...................... 14130
HEMIFACIAL MICROSOMIA... 14140
HEMIHYPERTROPHY.. 23500
HEMIHYPERTROPHY   SEE SILVER-RUSSELL DWARFISM (18240)
HEMIMELIC EPIPHYSIAL DYSPLASIA   SEE DYSPLASIA EPIPHYSEALIS HEMIMELICA
     (12780)
HEMIPLEGIC MIGRAINE, FAMILIAL.. 14150
HEMIVERTEBRAE   SEE COSTOVERTEBRAL SEGMENTATION ANOMALIES (12260)
HEMIVERTEBRAE, MULTIPLE   SEE VERTEBRAL ANOMALIES (27730)
*HEMOCHROMATOSIS.. 14160
HEMOCHROMATOSIS   SEE SPHEROCYTOSIS, HEREDITARY (18290)
HEMOCHROMATOSIS, IDIOPATHIC NEONATAL (OR PERINATAL) GIANT CELL HEPATITIS..... 23510
*HEMOCHROMATOSIS, JUVENILE.. 23520
HEMOGLOBIN (5 LOCI - ALPHA, BETA, GAMMA, DELTA, EPSILON)...................... 14170
HEMOGLOBIN A2, COMPLETE ABSENCE OF... 23530
*HEMOLYSIS OF TRYPSIN-TREATED RED CELLS....................................... 30660
HEMOLYTIC ANEMIA   SEE GLUCOSE-6-PHOSPHATE DEHYDROGENASE VARIANTS
     (30590), PHOSPHOGLYCERATE KINASE DEFICIENCY HEMOLYTIC ANEMIC (31180)
HEMOLYTIC-UREMIC SYNDROME... 23540
HEMOPHAGOCYTIC RETICULOSIS   SEE RETICULOSIS, FAMILIAL HISTIOCYTIC (26770)
HEMOPHILIA A   SEE FACTOR VIII DEFICIENCY (13450)
*HEMOPHILIA A (CLASSICAL HEMOPHILIA).. 30670
HEMOPHILIA A WITH VASCULAR ABNORMALITY....................................... 30680
*HEMOPHILIA B (CHRISTMAS DISEASE)... 30690
HEMOSIDEROSIS, CONGENITAL   SEE CEREBRO-HEPATO-RENAL SYNDROME (21410)
HEMOSIDEROSIS, PULMONARY, WITH DEFICIENCY OF GAMMA-A GLOBULIN................. 23550
'HEPARIN EXCESS'   SEE HYPERHEPARINEMIA (14400)
HEPATIC DISEASE WITH CYANOSIS   SEE CYANOSIS AND HEPATIC DISEASE (21940)
HEPATIC FIBROSIS   SEE SPLENOPORTAL VASCULAR ANOMALIES (27150)
HEPATIC FIBROSIS, CONGENITAL   SEE POLYCYSTIC KIDNEY, INFANTILE, TYPE I
     (26320)
HEPATITIS, GIANT CELL   SEE GIANT CELL HEPATITIS, NEONATAL (23110)
HEPATITIS, NEONATAL   SEE HEMOCHROMATOSIS, IDIOPATHIC NEONATAL (23510)
HEPATOLENTICULAR DEGENERATION   SEE WILSON'S DISEASE (27790)
HEPATOMA   SEE CIRRHOSIS, FAMILIAL (11890, 21560)
HEREDOPATHIA ATACTICA POLYNEURITIFORMIS   SEE REFSUM'S SYNDROME (26650)
HEREDO-RETINOPATHIA CONGENITALIS MONOLHBRIDA RECESSIVA AUTOSOMALIS   SEE
     AMAUROSIS CONGENITA OF LEBER I (20400)
HERLITZ FORM OF EPIDERMOLYSIS BULLOSA   SEE EPIDERMOLYSIS BULLOSA LETALIS
     (22670)
HERMAPHRODITISM, MALE PSEUDO   SEE PSEUDO-HERMAPHRODITISM, MALE (26430,
     31210)
*HERMAPHRODITISM, TRUE... 23560
HERNIA, DOUBLE INGUINAL.. 14230
HERNIA, HIATUS.. 14240
HERNIA, UMBILICAL   SEE EMG SYNDROME (22560)
HERS' DISEASE   SEE GLYCOGEN STORAGE DISEASE VI (23270)
HETEROCHROMIA IRIDIS   SEE PIEBALD TRAIT (17280), WAARDENBURG'S SYNDROME
     (19350), MEGACOLON, AGANGLIONIC (24920), HORNER'S SYNDROME (22560)
HETEROCHROMIA IRIDIS.. 14250
HEXOKINASE.. 14260
*HEXOKINASE DEFICIENCY HEMOLYTIC ANEMIA...................................... 23570
*HEXOSEPHOSPHATE ISOMERASE DEFICIENCY HEMOLYTIC ANEMIA....................... 23575
HEXOSEPHOSPHATE ISOMERASE DEFICIENCY   SEE PHOSPHOHEXOSE ISOMERASE,
     VARIANTS OF (17240)
HHHO SYNDROME   SEE PRADER-WILLI SYNDROME (26400)
HIATUS HERNIA   SEE MICROCEPHALY, HIATUS HERNIA AND NEPHROTIC SYNDROME
     (25130)
HIDROTIC ECTODERMAL DYSPLASIA   SEE ECTODERMAL DYSPLASIA, HIDROTIC (12950)
HIGH DENSITY LIPOPROTEIN DEFICIENCY   SEE ANALPHALIPOPROTEINEMIA (20540)
HIP, DISLOCATION OF, CONGENITAL.. 14270
HIPPEL-LINDAU SYNDROME   SEE VON HIPPEL-LINDAU SYNDROME (19330)
HIRSCHSPRUNG'S DISEASE   SEE MEGACOLON, AGANGLIONIC (24920), MEGACOLON,
     AGANGLIONIC (24920)
HIRSUTISM   SEE FIBROMATOSIS, GINGIVAL (13530)
HISTAMINE TEST, POSTIVE (NO AXONE FLARE)   SEE DYSAUTONOMIA (22390),
     NEUROPATHY, CONGENITAL SENSORY WITH ANHIDROSIS (25680)
*HISTIDINEMIA... 23580
HISTIOCYTOSIS X   SEE LETTERER-SIWE DISEASE (24640)
*HISTIOCYTOSIS, FAMILIAL LIPOCHROME... 23590
HISTOPHAGOCYTIC RETICULOSIS   SEE RETICULOSIS, HISTOCYTIC (26770)
*HL-A HISTOCOMPATIBILITY TYPE... 14280

HYPERLIPIDEMIA VI (FAMILIAL HYPERCHYLOM ICRONEMIA WITH HYPERPREBETALIPOPRO-
    TEINEMIA, MIXED HYPERLIPEMIA, COMBINED FAT AND CARBOHYDRATE-INDUCED
    HYPERLIPEMIA)... 23850
HYPERLIPOGENESIS   SEE PRADER-WILLI SYNDROME (26400)
HYPERLIPOPROTEINEMIA (TYPE II) AND DEAFNESS................................... 14430
HYPERLIPOPROTEINEMIA I (FAMILIAL HYPERCHYLOMICRONEMIA, IDIOPATHIC HYPERLI-
    PERMIA OF BURGER-GRUTZ TYPE, ESSENTIAL FAMILIAL HYPERLIPEMIA)............... 23860
*HYPERLIPOPROTEINEMIA II (HYPERBETALIPOPROTEINEMIA, HYPER-LOW-DENSITY-
    LIPOPROTEINEMIA, ESSENTIAL FAMILIAL HYPERCHOLESTEROLEMIA, FAMILIAL
    HYPERCHOLESTEROLEMIC XANTHOMATOSIS, XANTHOMA TUBEROSUM MULTIPLEX,
    FAMILIAL XANTHOMA)... 14440
HYPERLIPOPROTEINEMIA III (FAMILIAL HYPERBETA AND PREBETALIPOPROTEINEMIA,
    FAMILIAL HYPERCHOLESTEROLEMIA WITH HYPERLIPEMIA, HYPERLIPEMIA WITH
    FAMILIAL HYPERCHOLESTEROLEMIC XANTHOMATOSIS, CARBOHYDRATE-INDUCED
    HYPERLIPEMIA)... 14450
HYPERLIPOPROTEINEMIA IV (CARBOHYDRATES INDUCED HYPERLIPEMIA)................. 14460
*HYPERLYSINEMIA.. 23870
HYPERLYSINEMIA   SEE LYSINE INTOLERANCE (24790)
HYPERMETABOLISM DUE TO DEFECT IN MITOCHONDRIA............................... 23880
HYPERMETABOLISM DUE TO DEFECT IN MITOCHONDRIA   SEE MYOPATHY WITH GIANT
    ABNORMAL MITOCHONDRIA (25540)
HYPERMETHIONINEMIA... 23890
HYPERMETHIONINEMIA   SEE HOMOCYSTINURIA (23620)
HYPERNEPHROMA (ADENOCARCINOMA OF KIDNEY)................................... 14470
*HYPEROSTOSIS CORTICALIS DEFORMANS JUVENILIS (JUVENILE PAGET'S DISEASE,
    CHRONIC CONGENITAL IDIOPATHIC HYPERPHOSPHATASEMIA)....................... 23900
HYPEROSTOSIS CORTICALIS GENERALISATA (VAN BUCHEM'S DISEASE HYPERPHOSPHA-
    TASEMIA TARDA)... 23910
HYPEROSTOSIS FRONTALIS INTERNA (MORGAGNI-STEWART-MOREL SYNDROME).......... 14480
HYPEROSTOSIS GENERALISATA WITH STRIATIONS   SEE OSTEOPATHIA STRIATA
    (16650)
HYPEROXALURIA... 14490
HYPERPARATHYROIDISM... 14500
HYPERPARATHYROIDISM, NEONATAL FAMILIAL PRIMARY............................ 23920
HYPERPHOSPHATASEMIA   SEE HYPEROSTOSIS CORTICALIS DEFORMANS JUVENILIS
    (23900)
HYPERPHOSPHATASEMIA TARDA   SEE HYPEROSTOSIS CORTICALIS GENERALISTA
    (23910)
*HYPERPHOSPHATASIA WITH MENTAL RETARDATION................................ 23930
HYPERPHOSPHATASIA, CONGENITA   SEE HYPEROSTOSIS CORTICALIS DEFORMANS
    JUVENILIS (23900)
HYPERPHOSPHATEMIA   SEE CALCINOSIS, TUMORAL (21190)
*HYPERPIGMENTATION OF EYELIDS... 14510
HYPERPIGMENTATION OF FULDAUER AND KUIJPERS............................... 14520
HYPERPIGMENTATION OF FULDAUER AND KUIJPERS   SEE NAEGELI'S SYNDROME
    (16100), INCONTINENTIA PIGMENTI (30830), ACANTHOSIS NIGRICANS (10060)
HYPERPIGMENTATION, GENERALIZED   SEE MELANOSIS, UNIVERSAL (15580)
HYPERPIPECOLATEMIA... 23940
HYPERPLASIA, GINGIVAL   SEE FIBROMATOSIS, GINGIVAL (13530, 13540), FACIAL
    HYPERTRICHOSIS (13400)
*HYPERPROLINEMIA, TYPE I... 23950
*HYPERPROLINEMIA, TYPE II... 23961
HYPERPYREXIA IN ANESTHESIA   SEE HYPERTHERMIA OF ANESTHESIA (14560),
    SUXAMETHONIUM SENSITIVITY (27240)
HYPERPYREXIA, MALIGNANT, OF ANESTHESIA   SEE HYPERTHERMIA OF ANESTHESIA
    (14560)
HYPER-REFLEXIA, HEREDITARY.. 14530
HYPERSEGMENTATION OF THE NUCLEI OF THE POLYMORPHONUCLEAR LEUKOCYTES   SEE
    UNDRITZ ANOMALY (19150)
HYPERSEROTONEMIA... 23960
HYPERTELORISM   SEE TELECANTHUS WITH ASSOCIATED ABNORMALITIES (31360),
    FACIOGENITAL DYSPLASIA (30540), LISSENCEPHALY SYNDROME (24720)
*HYPERTELORISM (GREIG'S SYNDROME)...................................... 14540
HYPERTELORISM WITH ESOPHAGEAL ABNORMALITY AND HYPOSPADIAS (G SYNDROME)..... 30710
HYPERTELORISM, CRYPTORCHIDISM, DIGITAL CONTRACTURES, STERNAL DEFORMITY,
    AND OSTEOCHONDRITIS DISSECANS... 23970
HYPERTELORISM, MICROTIA, FACIAL CLEFTIN((HMC) SYNDROME................ 23980
HYPERTENSION   SEE FIBROMUSCULAR HYPERPLASIA OF RENAL ARTERIES (22870),
    PSEUDO-ALDOSTERONISM (17720)
HYPERTENSION, ESSENTIAL... 14550
HYPERTENSION, PULMONARY   SEE PULMONARY HYPERTENSION, PRIMARY (17860,
    26540)
HYPERTHELIA   SEE NIPPLES, SUPERNUMERARY (16370)
*HYPERTHERMIA OF ANESTHESIA... 14560
HYPERTHYROIDISM   SEE THYROTOXICOSIS (27500)
HYPERTONIA   SEE KOK'S DISEASE (14940)
HYPERTRICHOSIS   SEE FIBROMATOSIS, GINGIVAL (13530, 13540), HAIRY EARS
    (13950), HAIRY ELBOWS (13960)
HYPERTRICHOSIS CUBITI   SEE HAIRY ELBOWS (13960)
*HYPERTRICHOSIS, UNIVERSALIS.. 14570
*HYPERTROPHIA MUSCULORUM VERA... 14580
*HYPERTROPHIC NEUROPATHY OF DEJERINE-SOTTAS........................... 14590

```
      (26400)
 HYPOTRICHOSIS          SEE WOOLLY HAIR, HYPOTRICHOSIS EVERTED LOWER LIP, ETC.
      (27820)
*HYPOTRICHOSIS ('HAIRLESSNESS')............................................... 24190
 HYPOTRICHOSIS, SYNDACTYLY AND RETINITIS PIGMENTOSA........................... 24200
*HYPOXANTHINE GUANINE PHOSPHORIBOSYL TRANSFERASE DEFICIENCY................... 30800
 ICHTHYOSIFORM ERYTHRODERMA, BULLOUS FORM      SEE BULLOUS ERYTHRODERMA
      ICHTHYOSIFORMIS CONGENITA (BROCQ) (11380)
*ICHTHYOSIFORM ERYTHRODERMA, BROCQ'S CONGENITAL, NON-BULLOUS FORM............. 24210
*ICHTHYOSIFORM ERYTHRODERMA, UNILATERAL, WITH EPSILATERAL MALFORMATIONS
      ESPECIAL ABSENCE DEFORMITY OF LIMBS..................................... 24220
*ICHTHYOSIS.................................................................. 30810
 ICHTHYOSIS AND MALE HYPOGONADISM............................................ 30820
 ICHTHYOSIS CONGENITA     SEE HARLEQUIN FETUS (23440)
*ICHTHYOSIS CONGENITA (LAMELLAR EXFOLIATION, OR DESQUAMATION OF THE NEW-
      BORN, COLLODION FETUS, ETC.)........................................... 24230
 ICHTHYOSIS CONGENITA AND CATARACT     SEE CATARACT AND CONGENITAL ICHTHYO-
      SIS (21240)
 ICHTHYOSIS CONGENITA WITH BILIARY ATRESIA.................................. 24240
*ICHTHYOSIS HYSTRIX GRAVIOR (LAMBERT TYPE ICHTHYOSIS, 'PORCUPINE MAN')....... 14660
*ICHTHYOSIS VULGARIS (ICHTHYOSIS SIMPLEX)................................... 14670
 ICHTHYOSIS, BULLOUS TYPE.................................................. 14680
 ICHTHYOSIS, CONGENITAL, 'HARLEQUIN FETUS' TYPE............................ 24250
 ICSH DEFICIENCY     SEE FERTILE EUNUCH (22830)
 IMERSLUND SYNDROME     SEE PERNICIOUS ANEMIA, JUVENILE (26110)
 IMIDAZOLE AMINOACIDURIA          SEE AMAUROTIC FAMILY IDIOCY, JUVENILE TYPE
      (20420)
*IMINOGLYCINURIA........................................................... 24260
 IMMUNE DEFECT DUE TO ABSENCE OF THYMUS.................................... 24270
*IMMUNE DEFECT WITH LYMPHOTOXIC FACTOR.................................... 24280
*IMMUNOGLOBULIN TYPES* AM(1).............................................. 14690
*IMMUNOGLOBULIN TYPES* AM(2).............................................. 14700
*IMMUNOGLOBULIN TYPES* GM................................................. 14710
*IMMUNOGLOBULIN TYPES* INV................................................ 14720
 IMPERFORATE ANUS        SEE ANORECTAL ANOMALIES (10710), ANUS, IMPERFORATE
      (20750, 30180)
 INCISORS, ABSENCE OF     SEE CENTRAL INCISORS, ABSENCE OF (30240)
 INCISORS, ABSENCE OF LATERAL     SEE LATERAL INCISORS, ABSENCE OF (15040)
 INCISORS, CENTRAL       SEE DIASTEMA, DENTAL MEDIAL (12590), CENTRAL INCI-
      SORS, ABSENCE OF (30240)
 INCISORS, LONG UPPER CENTRAL............................................. 14730
 INCISORS, PROTRUBERANT UPPER     SEE MALOCCLUSION DUE TO PROTRUBERANT UPPER
      FRONT TEETH (15430)
 INCISORS, 'SHOVEL-SHAPED'................................................ 14740
 INCONTINENTIA PIGMENTI     SEE NAEGELI'S SYNDROME (16100)
*INCONTINENTIA PIGMENTI.................................................... 30830
 INCUS, MALFORMATION OF    SEE MOHR SYNDROME (25210), ORAL-FACIAL-DIGITAL
      SYNDROME (31120)
 INDIANA AMYLOIDOSIS     SEE AMYLOIDOSIS II (10490)
 INDICANURIA, FAMILIAL    SEE 'BLUE DIAPER SYNDROME' (21100)
 INDIFFERENCE TO PAIN    SEE INSENSITIVITY TO PAIN (24300)
 INDOLYLACROYL GLYCINURIA WITH MENTAL RETARDATION......................... 24290
 INFANTILE CORTICAL HYPEROSTOSIS     SEE CAFFEY'S DISEASE (11400)
 INFANTILE MUSCULAR ATROPHY     SEE MUSCULAR ATROPHY, INFANTILE (25330)
 INFANTILE NEUROAXONAL DYSTROPHY     SEE NEUROAXONAL DYSTROPHY, INFANTILE
      (25660)
 INFANTILE SPINAL AMYOTROPHY     SEE MUSCULAR ATROPHY, INFANTILE (25330)
 INH INACTIVATION     SEE ISONIAZID INACTIVATION (24340)
 INNERVATION OF INTESTINE, CONGENITAL ABNORMALITY OF    SEE MEGACOLON,
      AGANGLIONIC (24920)
*INSENSITIVITY TO PAIN (INDIFFERENCE TO PAIN* CONGENITAL ANALGIA) (ALSO
      SEE NEUROPATHY, SENSORY.  ALSO SEE BIEMOND'S CONGENITAL AND FAMILIAL
      ANALGESIA)............................................................ 24300
 INTERNAL CAROTID ARTERIES, HYPOPLASIA OF................................. 24310
 INTERSTITIAL CELL STIMULATING HORMONE DEFICIENCY     SEE FERTILE EUNUCH
      (22830)
 INTESTINAL DISACCHARIDASE DEFICIENCY         SEE DISACCHARIDE INTOLERANC
      (22290-22310)E
 INTESTINAL MONOSACCHARIDASE DEFICIENCY     SEE GLUCOSE-GALACTOSE MALABSORP-
      TION (23160)
 INTRACRANIAL HYPERTENSION, IDIOPATHIC.................................... 24320
 INTRAHEPATIC CHOLESTASIS................................................. 24330
 INTRAHEPATIC CHOLESTASIS    SEE BYLER'S DISEASE (21160)
 INTRAUTERINE GROWTH RETARDATION, MICROCEPHALY, AND MENTAL RETARDATION..... 30840
 INTRINSIC FACTOR, LACK OF    SEE PERNICIOUS ANEMIA, CONGENITAL, DUE TO
      FAILURE OF INTRINSIC FACTOR SECRETION (26100)
 INTRINSIC FACTOR, SPECIFIC DEFICIENCY OF    SEE PERNICIOUS ANEMIA, JU-
      VENILE (26110)
 INV     SEE IMMUNOGLOBIN TYPES* INV (14720)
 IRIS COLOBOMA     SEE BIEMOND SYNDROME II (10970)
 IRIS DYSGENESIS     SEE RIEGER'S SYNDROME (18050)
*IRIS HYPOPLASIA WITH GLAUCOMA........................................... 14760
```

712   IRIS, HYPOPLASIA OF   SEE MICROCORIA, CONGENITAL (15660), TEETH, ABSENCE
          OF (31350), RIEGER'S SYNDROME (18050), MYOTONIC DYSTROPHY (16090)
    *IRIS, HYPOPLASIA OF, WITH GLAUCOMA.. 30850
     IRON-DEFICIENCY ANEMIA   SEE ANEMIA, HYPOCHROMIC MICROCYTIC (20610)
     ISOCITRATE DEHYDROGENASE POLYMORPHISM...................................... 14770
    *ISONIAZID (INH) INACTIVATION.. 24340
    *ISOVALERICACIDEMIA... 24350
     JAUNDICE, CONGENITAL, FAMILIAL NONHEMOLYTIC, WITH KERNICTERUS   SEE
          CRIGLER-NAJJAR SYNDROME (21880)
     JAUNDICE, FAMILIAL OBSTRUCTIVE, OF INFANCY................................ 30860
     JAUNDICE, FAMILIAL, DUE TO INTRAHEPATIC CHOLESTASIS   SEE INTRAHEPATIC
          CHOLESTASIS (24330)
     JAUNDICE, NEONATAL OBSTRUCTIVE   SEE GIANT CELL HEPATITIS, NEONATAL
          (23110)
     JAVRE'S HYALOIDO-TAPETORETINAL DEGENERATION   SEE HYALOIDO-TAPETORETINAL
          DEGENERATION OF FAVRE (23650)
     JAW, CYSTS OF   SEE CHERUBISM (11840), BASAL CELL NEVUS SYNDROME (10940),
          CYSTS OF JAW (12390)
     JAW, OSTEOMA OF   SEE POLYPOSIS, INTESTINAL III (17530), OSTEOMA OF
          MANDIBLE (16640), TORUS PALATINUS AND TORUS MANDIBULARIS (18970)
     JAW, WINKING   SEE MARCUS GUNN PHENOMENON (15460)
     JAW-JERKING   SEE EPILEPSY, PRIMARY READING (13220)
    *JEJUNAL ATRESIA ('APPLE PEEL' SYNDROME)................................... 24360
     JERVELL AND LANGE-NIELSEN SYNDROME   SEE DEAFMUTISM AND FUNCTIONAL HEART
          DISEASE (22040)
     JEUNE'S SYNDROME   SEE ASPHYXIATING THORACIC DYSTROPHY OF THE NEWBORN
          (20850)
    *JOB'S SYNDROME... 24370
     JOINT CONTRACTURES   SEE PSEUDO-ARTHROGRYPOSIS (17720)
     JOINT CONTRACTURES WITH OTHER ABNORMALITIES.............................. 14780
     JOINT HYPERFLEXIBILITY   SEE HEMANGIOMATOSIS, CUTANEOUS, WITH ASSOCIATED
          FEATURES (23480)
     JOINT LAXITY (ARTHROCHALASIS MULTIPLEX CONGENITA)........................ 24380
    *JOINT LAXITY, FAMILIAL.. 14790
     JORDANS' ANOMALY OF LEUKOCYTES... 24390
     JOSEPH'S SYNDROME.. 24400
     JUMPING FRENCHMAN OF MAINE (SEE ALSO HYPER-REFLEXIA, HEREDITARY).......... 24410
     KALLMANN SYNDROME (HYPOGONADOTROPIC HYPOGONADISM AND ANOSMIA)............. 24420
     KALLMANN SYNDROME (SECONDARY, HYPOGONADOTROPIC, HYPOGONADISM WITH ANOSMIA*
          DYSPLASIA OLFACTOGENITALIS OF DE MORSIER)............................ 30870
     KALLMANN SYNDROME WITH FACIAL CLEFTING................................... 24430
     KAPOSI'S SARCOMA... 14800
    *KARTAGENER'S SYNDROME (DEXTROCARDIA, BRONCHIECTASIS AND SINUSITIS)........ 24440
     KELL BLOOD GROUP   SEE BLOOD GROUP KELL-CELLANO SYSTEM (11090)
     KELOIDS.. 14810
     KELOIDS   SEE TORTICOLLIS, KELOIDS, CRYPTORCHIDISM, AND RENAL DYSPLASIA
          (31430)
     KENNY SYNDROME   SEE DWARFISM, CORTICAL THICKENING OF TUBULAR BONES, AND
          TRANSIENT HYPOCALCEMIA (12700)
    *KERATITIS FUGAX HEREDITARIA.. 14820
     KERATOACANTHOMA   SEE EPITHELIOMA, SELF-HEALING SQUAMOUS (FERGUSON-SMITH
          TYPE) (13280)
     KERATOCONUS.. 14830
     KERATOCONUS.. 24450
     KERATOCONUS POSTICUS CIRCUMSCRIPTUS...................................... 24460
     KERATOPACHYDERMIA   SEE DEAFNESS, CONGENITAL WITH KERATOPACHYDERMIA AND
          CONSTRICTIONS OF FINGERS AND TOES (12450)
     KERATOPATHY, BAND-SHAPED   SEE CORNEAL DYSTROPHY, BAND-SHAPED (21750)
     KERATOSES, SEBORRHEIC   SEE SEBORRHEIC KERATOSES (18200)
     KERATOSIS   SEE PORKERATOSIS OF MIBELLI (17580)
     KERATOSIS FOLLICULARIS   SEE DARIER-WHITE DISEASE (12420)
    *KERATOSIS FOLLICULARIS SPINULOSA DECALVANS CUM OPHIASI................... 30880
    *KERATOSIS PALMARIS ET PLANTARIS FAMILIARIS (TYLOSIS)..................... 14840
    *KERATOSIS PALMARIS ET PLANTARIS WITH ESOPHAGEAL CANCER................... 14850
     KERATOSIS PALMARIS ET PLANTARIS   SEE KNUCKLE PADS LEUKONYCHIA AND SEN-
          SINEURAL DEAFNESS (14920)
     KERATOSIS PALMO-PLANTARIS PAPULOSA....................................... 14860
     KERATOSIS PALMO-PLANTARIS STRIATA.. 14870
     KERATOSIS PALMO-PLANTARIS TRANSGRADIENS OF SIEMENS   SEE MAL DE MELEDA
          (24830)
    *KERATOSIS PALMO-PLANTARIS WITH CORNEAL DYSTROPHY......................... 24480
    *KERATOSIS PALMO-PLANTARIS WITH PERIODONTOPATHIA (PAPILLON-LEFEVRE SYNDROME)... 24500
     KERATOSIS PALMO-PLANTARIS   SEE SCLERO-ATROPHIC AND KERATOTIC DERMATOSIS
          OF LIMBS (18160), ALOPECIA CONGENITA WITH KERATOSIS PALMO-PLANTARIS
          (10410)
     KETOACIDURIA WITH MENTAL DEFICIENCY AND OTHER FEATURES (RICHARDS-RUNDLE
          SYNDROME)... 24510
     KIDD BLOOD GROUP   SEE BLOOD GROUP-KIDD SYSTEM (11100)
     KIDNEY, ADENOCARCINOMA OF   SEE HYPERNEPHROMA (14470)
     KINESOGENIC CHOREOATHETOSIS   SEE DYSTONIA, FAMILIAL PAROXYSMAL (12820)
     KINKY HAIR DISEASE   SEE MENKES SYNDROME (30940)
     KIRNER'S DEFORMITY   SEE DYSTELEPHALANGY (12800)

KLEEBLATTSCHADEL (CLOVERLEAF SKULL) SYNDROME.................................... 14880   713
KLIPPEL-FEIL SYNDROME.. 14890
KLIPPEL-FEIL SYNDROME   SEE VERTEBRAL ANOMALIES (27730), WILDERVANCK
    SYNDROME (31460), CERVICAL VERTEBRAL FUSION (11810, 21430)
KLIPPEL-TRENAUNAY-WEBER SYNDROME... 14900
KNEE JOINT, DISLOCATION OF   SEE CAMPTODACTYLY (11420)
KNUCKLE PADS... 14910
*KNUCKLE PADS, LEUKONYCHIA AND SENSINEURAL DEAFNESS............................ 14920
KOCHER-DEBRE-SEMELAIGNE SYNDROME (CHILDHOOD HYPOTHYROIDISM WITH MUSCULAR
    'HYPERTROPHY')   SEE CRETINISM, ATHYREOTIC (21870)
*KOILONYCHIA, HEREDITARY... 14930
*KOK'S DISEASE... 14940
KOSTMANN'S AGRANULOCYTOSIS   SEE AGRANULOCYTOSIS, INFANTILE GENETIC, OF
    KOSTMANN'S (20270)
*KRABBE'S DISEASE (GLOBOID CELL SCLEROSIS)..................................... 24520
KRAMER SYNDROME   SEE OCULOCEREBRAL SYNDROME WITH HYPOPIGMENTATION (25780)
KRAUSE-REESE SYNDROME   SEE ENCEPHALO-RETINAL DYSPLASIA (13100)
KUGELBERG-WELANDER DISEASE   SEE MUSCULAR ATROPHY, JUVENILE (15860, 25340)
KURU.. 24530
KUSKOKWIN DISEASE   SEE ARTHROGRYPOSIS-LIKE DISORDER (20820)
*KYPHOSCOLIOSIS, OSTEOPENIA, CONGENITAL CONTRACTURES.......................... 14950
KYPHOSIS, LUMBAR   SEE VERTEBRAL HYPOPLASIA WITH LUMBAR KYPHOSIS (19290)
LABIA MINORA, INCOMPLETE ADHESION OF.. 14960
*LACRIMAL DUCT DEFECT.. 14970
LACRIMAL DUCT DEFECT   SEE CLEFT LIP-PALATE WITH SPLIT HAND AND FOOT
    (11940)
LACRIMAL DUCTS, ANOMALY OF   SEE ORBITAL MARGIN, HYPOPLASIA O (16560)F
LACTASE DEFICIENCY, INTESTINAL, IN ADULT   SEE DISACCHARIDE INTOLERANCE
    III (22310)
LACTASE, DEFECT IN INTESTINAL   SEE DISACCHARIDE INTOLERANCE III (22310)
LACTIC ACIDOSIS   SEE FRUCTOSE-1, 6-DIPHOSPHATASE, HEPATIC, DEFICIENCY
    OF, ALANINURIA, ETC. (20290)
LACTIC ACIDOSIS, CHRONIC ADULT FORM... 14980
*LACTIC ACIDOSIS, FAMILIAL INFANTILE.. 24540
*LACTIC DEHYDROGENASE VARIANT X OF TESTIS..................................... 14990
LACTIC DEHYDROGENASE VARIANTS IN SERUM VARIANTS OF SUBUNIT A................ 15000
LACTIC DEHYDROGENASE VARIANTS IN SERUM VARIANTS OF SUBUNIT B................ 15010
LACTOSE INTOLERANCE   SEE DISACCHARIDE INTOLERANCE II AND III (22300,
    22310)
LACTOSYL CERAMIDOSIS.. 24550
LACUNAE, SYMMETRICAL PARIETAL   SEE PARIETAL FORAMINA, SYMMETRICAL
    (16850), CRANIUM BIFIDUM OCCULTUM (12320)
LAFORA'S DISEASE   SEE MYOCLONIC EPILEPSY (25480)
LAMINA DURA, ABSENCE OF... 15020
LANDING'S DISEASE   SEE GANGLIOSIDOSIS, GENERALIZED (23050, 23060)
LANDOUZY-DEJERINE MUSCULAR DYSTROPHY   SEE MUSCULAR DYSTROPHY FACIO-
    SCAPULO-HUMERAL (15890)
*LARSEN'S SYNDROME... 24560
LARYNGEAL ABDUCTOR PARALYSIS.. 24570
LARYNX, CONGENITAL PARTIAL ATRESIA OF... 15030
LARYNX, POSTERIOR CLEFT OF   SEE CLEFT LARYNX, POSTERIOR (21580)
*LATERAL INCISORS, ABSENCE OF... 15040
LATTICE DEGENERATION OF RETINA LEADING TO RETINAL DETACHMENT................... 15050
*LAURENCE-MOON SYNDROME.. 24580
LAWRENCE-SEIP SYNDROME   SEE SEIP SYNDROME (26970)
LCAT DEFICIENCY   SEE LECITHIN* CHOLESTEROL ACETYLTRANSFERASE (LCAT)
    DEFICIENCY (24590)
LD SYSTEM   SEE LIPOPROTEIN TYPES - LD SYSTEM (15210)
LDH VARIANTS   SEE LACTIC DEHYDROGENASE VARIANTS (14990-15010)
LEBER'S CONGENITAL AMAUROSIS   SEE AMAUROSIS CONGENITA (NOT TO BE CON-
    FUSED WITH LEBER'S OPTIC ATROPHY) (20400)
LEBER'S DISEASE   SEE LEBER'S OPTIC ATROPHY (30890)
LEBER'S OPTIC ATROPHY   SEE OPTIC ATROPHY - SPASTIC PARAPLEGIA SYNDROME
    (31110)
LEBER'S OPTIC ATROPHY... 30890
LECITHIN CHOLESTEROL ACETYLTRANSFERASE (LCAT) DEFICIENCY (NORUM'S DISEASE)... 24590
*LEG, ABSENCE DEFORMITY OF, WITH CONGENITAL CATARACT.......................... 24600
LEGG-CALVE-PERTHES DISEASE.. 15060
LEIGH'S ENCEPHALOMYELOPATHY   SEE NECROTIZING ENCEPHALOPATHY INFANTILE
    SUBACUTE (25600)
LEIOMYOMA OF VULVA AND ESOPHAGUS.. 15070
LEIOMYOMATA OF SKIN... 24610
*LEIOMYOMATA, HEREDITARY MULTIPLE, OF SKIN.................................... 15080
LENTIGINES... 15090
LENTIGINES   SEE MITRAL REGURGITATION, CONDUCTIVE DEAFNESS, ETC. (15870),
    LEOPARD SYNDROME (15110)
LENTIGINOSIS, CENTROFACIAL NEURO-DYSRAPHIC.................................... 15100
LENZ SYNDROME   SEE MICROPHTHALMIA OR ANOPHTHALMOS, WITH DIGITAL ANOMA-
    LIES (30980)
LEONTIASIS OSSEA   SEE HYPEROSTOSIS CORTICALIS GENERALISATA (23910),
    CRANIODIAPHYSEAL DYSPLASIA (21830)
*LEOPARD SYNDROME... 15110

*LIPOPROTEIN TYPES - AG SYSTEM.. 15200
*LIPOPROTEIN TYPES - LD SYSTEM.. 15210
*LIPOPROTEIN TYPES - LP SYSTEM.. 15220
 LIPOPROTEIN TYPES - LT SYSTEM.. 15230
 LIPOPROTEIN, VARIANT OF BETA ('DOUBLE BETA-LIPOPROTEIN')..................... 15240
*LISSENCEPHALY SYNDROME... 24720
 LIVER CANCER... 24730
 LOBSTER-CLAW DEFORMITY   SEE SPLIT-HAND DEFORMITY (18360)
 LOOSEJOINTEDNESS   SEE EHLERS-DANLOS SYNDROME (13000, 22540, 30520),
    JOINT LAXITY (14790, 24380), EPIPHYSEAL DYSPLASIA, MULTIPLE (13240),
    HEMANGIOMATOSIS (14110, 23480)
 'LOP EARS' OR 'BAT EARS'   SEE EARS WITHOUT HELIX (12880)
 LOW BIRTH WEIGHT DWARFISM WITH SKELETAL DYSPLASIA............................ 24740
 LOW BIRTH WEIGHT DWARFISM   SEE BIRD-HEADED DWARF (21060)
*LOWE'S OCULOCEREBRORENAL SYNDROME.. 30900
 LP SYSTEM   SEE LIPOPROTEIN TYPES - LP SYSTEM (15220)
 LT SYSTEM   SEE LIPOPROTEIN TYPES-LT (15230)
 LUDER-SHELDON SYNDROME... 15250
 LUFT'S DISEASE   SEE HYPERMETABOLISM DUE TO DEFECT IN MITOCHONDRIA (23880)
 LUMBOSACRAL VERTEBRAL FUSION AND BLEPHAROPTOSIS   SEE VERTEBRAL FUSION,
    POSTERIOR LUMBOSACRAL, WITH BLEPHAROPTOSIS (19280)
 LUNG   SEE FIBROCYSTIC PULMONARY DYSPLASIA (13500)
 LUNG DEGENERATION   SEE ANTITRYPSIN DEFICIENCY OF PLASMA (20740)
 LUNULAE OF FINGERNAILS... 15260
 LUPUS ERYTHEMATOSUS, SYSTEMIC (SLE).. 15270
 LUTEINIZING HORMONE DEFICIENCY, ISOLATED   SEE FERTILE EUNUCH (22830)
 LUTHERAN BLOOD GROUP   SEE BLOOD GROUP-LUTHERAN SYSTEM (11120)
 L-XYLULOSURIA   SEE PENTOSURIA (26080)
 LYMPHANGIECTASIA, INTESTINAL... 15280
 LYMPHANGIECTASIS OF BOWEL   SEE ENTEROPATHY, PROTEIN-LOSING (22630)
 LYMPHANGIECTASIS, PULMONARY CYSTIC   SEE PULMONARY CYSTIC LYMPHANGIECTA-
    SIS (26530)
 LYMPHATIC LEUKEMIA   SEE LEUKEMIA, CHRONIC LYMPHATIC (15140)
 LYMPHEDEMA   SEE SPINAL EXTRADURAL CYST, ASCITES, CHYLOUS (20830)
 LYMPHEDEMA AND CEREBRAL ARTERIOVENOUS ANOMALY................................ 15290
 LYMPHEDEMA AND PTOSIS.. 15300
*LYMPHEDEMA, HEREDITARY I (NONNE-MILROY, OR EARLY-ONSET TYPE)................. 15310
 LYMPHEDEMA, HEREDITARY II (MEIGE, OR LATE-ONSET TYPE)........................ 15320
 LYMPHEDEMA, WITH ADULT ONSET AND YELLOW NAILS................................ 15330
*LYMPHEDEMA, WITH DISTICHIASIS.. 15340
 LYMPHOCYTES, ABSENCE OF   SEE ALYMPHOCYTOSIS, PURE (20390)
 LYMPHOHISTIOCYTIC INFILTRATION, GENERALIZED.................................. 24750
 LYMPHOHISTIOCYTOSIS OF NERVOUS SYSTEM.. 24760
 LYMPHOID SYSTEM DETERIORATION, PROGRESSIVE................................... 24770
 LYMPHOPENIA   SEE LYMPHOID SYSTEM DETERIORATION, PROGRESSIVE (24770),
    AGAMMAGLOBULINEMIA, SWISS OR ALYMPHOCYTOTIC TYPE (20250)
*LYMPHOPENIC HYPERGAMMAGLOBULINEMIA, ANTIBODY DEFICIENCY, AUTO-IMMUNE
    HEMOLYTIC ANEMIA AND GLOMERULONEPHRITIS.................................... 24780
*LYSINE INTOLERANCE... 24790
 LYSINEMIA   SEE HYPERLYSINEMIA (23870)
 LYSINURIA   SEE DIBASICAMINOACIDURIA I AND II (12600, 22270)
 MACROCEPHALY... 24800
 MACROCEPHALY, PSEUDOPAPILLEDEMA AND MULTIPLE HEMANGIOMATA.................... 15350
 MACRODACTYLY   SEE MEGALODACTYLY (15550)
 MACROGLOBULINEMIA, WALDENSTROM'S... 15360
 MACROGLOSSIA   SEE EMG SYNDROME (22560)
 MACROGNATHIA   SEE PROGNATHISM, MANDIBULAR (17670)
 MACROSOMIA ADIPOSA CONGENITA... 24810
 MACULAR COLOBOMA   SEE COLOBOMA OF MACULA (12030)
 MACULAR DEGENERATION   SEE SPASTIC PARAPLEGIA AND RETINAL DEGENERATION
    (27070), OLIVOPONTOCEREBELLAR ATROPHY (16450)
*MACULAR DEGENERATION OF THE RETINA... 24820
 MACULAR DEGENERATION OF THE RETINA   SEE TAPETO-RETINAL DEGENERATION WITH
    ATAXIA (27260)
*MACULAR DEGENERATION, POLYMORPHIC.. 15370
 MACULAR DEGENERATION, SENILE... 15380
*MACULAR DYSTROPHY.. 30910
 MACULAR DYSTROPHY OF CORNEA   SEE CORNEAL DYSTROPHIES (12150-12230,
    21740-21780)
 MACULAR DYSTROPHY* BUTTERFLY-SHAPED PIGMENT DYSTROPHY OF FOVEA............... 15390
 MADELUNG DEFORMITY... 15400
 MADELUNG'S DEFORMITY   SEE DYSCHONDROSTEOSIS (12730), EXOSTOSES, MULTIPLE
    (13370)
 MAFFUCCI'S SYNDROME   SEE OSTEOCHONDROMATOSIS (16600)
 MAGNESIUM AND POTASSIUM DEPLETION   SEE POTASSIUM AND MAGNESIUM DEPLETION
    (26380)
 MAGNESIUM, LOW LEVELS OF   SEE HYPOMAGNESEMIC TETANY (30760)
*MAL DE MELEDA (KERATOSIS PALMO-PLANTARIS TRANSGRADIENS OF SIEMENS).......... 24830
*MALATE DEHYDROGENASE, ELECTROPHORETIC VARIANTS OF MITOCHONDRIAL BOUND....... 15410
*MALATE DEHYDROGENASE, ELECTROPHORETIC VARIANT OF SOLUBLE CYTOPLASMIC........ 15420
 MALE TURNER SYNDROME   SEE PTERYGIUM COLLI SYNDROME (17810)
 MALHERBE CALCIFYING EPITHELIOMA   SEE EPITHELIOMA, CALCIFICANS OF MAL-

MIGRAINE, FAMILIAL HEMIPLEGIC   SEE HEMIPLEGIC MIGRAINE, FAMILIAL (14150)
MILIA   SEE FINGERPRINTS, ABSENCE OF (13600)
*MILIA, MULTIPLE ERUPTIVE... 15740
MILK PROTEINS, VARIANTS OF... 15750
MILROY'S DISEASE   SEE LYMPHEDEMA, HEREDITARY I (15310)
MIRROR MOVEMENTS, HEREDITARY... 15760
MITOCHONDRIA   SEE HYPERMETABOLISM DUE TO DEFECT IN MITOCHONDRIA (23880),
    MYOPATHY WITH GIANT ABNORMAL MITOCHONDRIA (25540), PLEOCONIAL MYOPATHY
    (26290)
MITOCHONDRIAL ABNORMALITIES WITH MYOPATHY.................................. 25190
MITOCHONDRIAL MYOPATHY WITH SALT CRAVING................................... 25200
*MITRAL REGURGITATION.. 15770
MITRAL REGURGITATION   SEE VALVULAR HEART DISEASE, CONGENITAL (31440)
MITRAL REGURGITATION, CONDUCTIVE DEAFNESS, AND FUSION OF CERVICAL VERTE-
    BRAE AND OF CARPAL AND TARSAL BONES.................................... 15780
MITRAL VALVE, 'FLOPPY'   SEE MITRAL REGURGITATION (15770)
MOEBIUS SYNDROME   SEE FACIAL PALSY, CONGENITAL UNILATERAL (13410)
*MOEBIUS SYNDROME (CONGENITAL FACIAL DIPLEGIA)............................. 15790
*MOHR SYNDROME... 25210
MOLES   SEE NEVI (16290)
MONGOLISM   SEE NON-DISJUNCTION
MONGOLOID FACIES   SEE LERI'S PLEONOSTEOSIS (15120)
*MONILETHRIX.. 15800
MONILETHRIX... 25220
MONILETHRIX   SEE MENKES SYNDROME (30940)
MONILIASIS   SEE HYPOADRENOCORTICISM, ETC. (24030)
MONONEURITIS   SEE NEURITIS WITH BRACHIAL PREDILECTION (16210)
MONOPHALANGY OF GREAT TOE.. 15810
MONOPHALANGY OF GREAT TOE   SEE FIERODYSPLASIA OSSIFICANS PROGRESSIVA
    (13510)
MONOSACCHARIDE MALABSORPTION   SEE GLUCOSE-GALACTOSE MALABSORPTION (23160)
MORGAGNI-STEWART-MOREL SYNDROME   SEE HYPEROSTOSIS FRONTALIS INTERNA
    (14480)
MORPHOLOGIC TRAITS (SOMETIMES CALLED ANTHROPOLOGIC TRAITS)................. 15820
*MORQUIO SYNDROME, NON-KERATOSULFATE-EXCRETING TYPE....................... 25230
MORQUIO-LIKE DISEASE   SEE BRACHYRAPHIA (11350), SPONDYLOEPIPHYSEAL
    DYSPLASIAS (27160)
MORQUIO'S DISEASE, OR BRAILSFORD-MORQUIO SYNDROME   SEE MUCOPOLYSACCHARI-
    DOSIS IV (25300)
MORQUIO-ULLRICH SYNDROME   SEE MUCOPOLYSACCHARIDOSIS IV (25300)
MORVAN'S SYNDROME   SEE NEUROPATHY, HEREDITARY SENSORY RADICULAR (16240)
MOSAICISM   SEE NON-DISJUNCTION (25730), SATELLITE ASSOCIATION, ETC.
    (18110)
MOSAICISM, CHROMOSOMAL   SEE SATELLITE ASSOCIATION RESULTING IN FAMILIAL
    CHROMOSOMAL MOSAICISM (18110)
MOSAICISM, FAMILIAL CHROMOSOMAL   SEE SATELLITE ASSOCIATION RESULTING IN
    CHROMOSOMAL MOSAICISM (18110)
*MOUTH, INABILITY TO OPEN COMPLETELY, AND SHORT FINGER-FLEXOR TENDONS...... 15830
MOYNIHAN SYNDROME   SEE ALOPECIA-EPILEPSY-OLIGOPHRENIA SYNDROME (20360)
MSUD   SEE MAPLE SYRUP URINE DISEASE (24860)
*MUCOLIPIDOSIS I (LIPOMUCOPOLYSACCHARIDOSIS).............................. 25240
*MUCOLIPIDOSIS II (I-CELL DISEASE).. 25250
*MUCOLIPIDOSIS III (PSEUDO-HURLER POLYDYSTROPHY).......................... 25260
MUCOPOLYSACCHARIDOSES, OTHER POSSIBLE   SEE OSTEOARTHROPATHY OF SCHINZ
    AND FURTWAENGLER (25900), FARBER'S LIPOGRANULOMATOSIS (22800)
MUCOPOLYSACCHARIDOSES, UNCLASSIFIED TYPES................................. 25270
MUCOPOLYSACCHARIDOSIS   SEE FUCOSIDOSIS (23000), DYGGVE-MELCHIOR-CLAUSEN
    DISEASE (22380)
MUCOPOLYSACCHARIDOSIS TYPE I (HURLER SYNDROME GARGOYLISM)............... 25280
*MUCOPOLYSACCHARIDOSIS TYPE III (SANFILIPPO SYNDROME)..................... 25290
*MUCOPOLYSACCHARIDOSIS TYPE IV (MORQUIO SYNDROME)......................... 25300
*MUCOPOLYSACCHARIDOSIS TYPE V (SCHEIE'S SYNDROME, LATE HURLER'S SYNDROME,
    ETC.)... 25310
*MUCOPOLYSACCHARIDOSIS TYPE VI (MAROTEAUX-LAMY SYNDROME).................. 25320
*MUCOPOLYSACCHARIDOSIS TYPE II (HUNTER SYNDROME).......................... 30990
MUCOPOLYSACCHARIDOSIS-LIKE CONDITION   SEE MUCOLIPIDOSIS III (25260)
MUCOUS CYSTS OF LOWER LIP   SEE CLEFT LIP AND-OR PALATE WITH MUCOUS CYSTS
    OF LOWER LIP (11930)
MUCOVISCIDOSIS   SEE CYSTIC FIBROSIS (21970)
MULTILOCULAR ENCEPHALOMALACIA   SEE ENCEPHALOMALACIA, MULTILOCULAR (22570)
MULTINUCLEARITY OF ERYTHROBLASTS   SEE ANEMIA WITH MULTINUCLEATED ERYTH-
    ROBLASTS (10560)
MULTIPLE EXOSTOSES   SEE EXOSTOSES, MULTIPLE (13370)
MULTIPLE SCLEROSIS   SEE DISSEMINATED SCLEROSIS (12620, 22320), PELI-
    ZAEUS-MERZBACHER DISEASE (16950, 26060, 31160)
MULTIPLE SCLEROSIS-LIKE DISEASE (SEE ATAXIA, SPASTIC)..................... 15840
MUSCLE CRAMPS   SEE MYOKYMIA (16010), GLYCOGEN STORAGE DISEASE V
    (MCARDLE'S DISEASE (23260), CENTRAL CORE DISEASE OF MUSCLE (11700)
MUSCLE, ANOMALIES OF   SEE POLAND SYNDROME (17380), PALMARIS LONGUS
    MUSCLE, ABSENCE OF (16760), MUSCULAR DYSTROPHY, FACIO-SCAPUTO-HUMERAL
    (15890), PERONEUS TERTIUS MUSCLE, ABSENCE OF (26140)
MUSCLE, TWITCHES   SEE MYOKYMIA (16010)

MUSCLES, ABSENCE OF   SEE MUSCULAR DYSTROPHY, FACIO-SCAPULO-HUMERAL
    (15890)
*MUSCULAR ATROPHY, ATAXIA, RETINITIS PIGMENTOSA, DIABETES INSIPIDUS............ 15850
*MUSCULAR ATROPHY, INFANTILE (WERDNIG-HOFFMANN)............................... 25330
 MUSCULAR ATROPHY, JUVENILE (KUGELBERG-WELANDER SYNDROME).................... 15860
*MUSCULAR ATROPHY, JUVENILE (KUGELBERG-WELANDER)............................. 25340
 MUSCULAR ATROPHY, PROGRESSIVE... 15870
 MUSCULAR ATROPHY, PROGRESSIVE... 25350
 MUSCULAR ATROPHY, PROGRESSIVE   SEE AMYOTROPHIC LATERAL SCLEROSIS (10540,
    20510)
 MUSCULAR ATROPHY, PROXIMAL SPINAL, OF LATE ONSET   SEE SPINAL AND BULBAR
    MUSCULAR ATROPHY (31320)
 MUSCULAR DYSTROPHY   SEE MUSCULAR DYSTROPHY FACIO-SCAPULO-HUMERAL
    (15890), MYOPATHY, LATE DISTAL HEREDITARY (16050), MYOTONIC DYSTROPHY
    (16090), OCULOPHARYNGEAL MUSCULAR DYSTROPHY (16430), AMINOACIDURIA WITH
    OTHER FEATURES (20480)
*MUSCULAR DYSTROPHY I (LIMB-GIRDLE, PELVO-FEMORAL OR LEYDEN-MOEBIUS TYPE)...... 25360
*MUSCULAR DYSTROPHY II (RESEMBLING X-LINKED DUCHENNE MUSCULAR DYSTROPHY)....... 25370
 MUSCULAR DYSTROPHY LIMITED TO FEMALES   SEE MYOPATHY, LIMITED TO FEMALES
    (16060)
 MUSCULAR DYSTROPHY, BARNES TYPE... 15880
 MUSCULAR DYSTROPHY, CONGENITAL PROGRESSIVE, WITH MENTAL RETARDATION.......... 25380
*MUSCULAR DYSTROPHY, CONGENITAL, PRODUCING ARTHROGRYPOSIS..................... 25390
 MUSCULAR DYSTROPHY, CONGENITAL, WITH INFANTILE CATARACT AND HYPOGONADISM..... 25400
 MUSCULAR DYSTROPHY, CONGENITAL, WITH RAPID PROGRESSION...................... 25410
*MUSCULAR DYSTROPHY, FACIO-SCAPULO-HUMERAL................................... 15890
 MUSCULAR DYSTROPHY, MABRY TYPE... 31000
*MUSCULAR DYSTROPHY, PROGRESSIVE, TARDIVE TYPE OF BECKER..................... 31010
 MUSCULAR DYSTROPHY, PROXIMAL... 15900
*MUSCULAR DYSTROPHY, PSEUDOHYPERTROPHIC PROGRESSIVE, DUCHENNE TYPE........... 31020
 MUSCULAR DYSTROPHY, SIMULATION OF   SEE ENGELMANN'S DISEASE (13130)
*MUSCULAR DYSTROPHY, TARDIVE TYPE OF DREIFUSS, WITH CONTRACTURES.............. 31030
 MUSCULAR HYPOPLASIA, CONGENITAL UNIVERSAL, OF KRABBE....................... 15910
 MUSCULAR SHORTENING AND DYSTROPHY.. 15920
 MYASTHENIA GRAVIS.. 15930
 MYASTHENIA GRAVIS.. 25420
 MYASTHENIA GRAVIS   SEE AUTOIMMUNE DISEASES (10910)
 MYASTHENIA, FAMILIAL LIMB-GIRDLE... 15940
 MYASTHENIC MYOPATHY... 25430
 MYCOSIS FUNGOIDES... 25440
 MYELINATED OPTIC NERVE FIBERS... 15950
 MYELOMA, MULTIPLE... 25450
*MYELOPEROXIDASE DEFICIENCY.. 25460
 MYELOPROLIFERATIVE DISEASE.. 25470
 MYOCARDIOPATHY   SEE CARDIOMYOPATHY, FAMILIAL IDIOPATHIC (11520)
 MYOCLONIC EPILEPSY   SEE PHOTOMYOCLONUS, ETC. (17250)
*MYOCLONIC EPILEPSY OF UNVERRICHT AND LUNDBORG............................. 25480
*MYOCLONIC EPILEPSY, HARTUNG TYPE... 15960
 MYOCLONIC VARIANT OF CEREBRAL LIPIDOSIS   SEE AMAUROTIC FAMILY IDIOCY,
    JUVENILE TYPE (20420)
 MYOCLONUS AND ATAXIA.. 15970
 MYOCLONUS EPILEPSY   SEE ATAXIA WITH MYOCLONUS EPILEPSY AND PRESENILE
    DEMENTIA (20870)
 MYOCLONUS, CEREBELLAR ATAXIA AND DEAFNESS................................. 15980
*MYOCLONUS, HEREDITARY ESSENTIAL.. 15990
*MYOGLOBIN MUTANTS.. 16000
 MYOGLOBINURIA   SEE RHABDOMYOLYSIS, ACUTE RECURRENT (26820), GLYCOGEN
    STORAGE DISEASE V (23260)
 MYOKINASE   SEE ADENYLATE KINASE (10300)
*MYOKYMIA... 16010
 MYOKYMIA   SEE GAMSTORP-WOHLFART SYNDROME (13720)
 MYOMATA UTERI   SEE LEIOMYOMATA, HEREDITARY MULTIPLE, OF SKIN (15080)
 MYOPATHY PRODUCING CONGENITAL OPHTHALMOPLEGIA AND "FLOPPY BABY" SYNDROME...... 25500
 MYOPATHY WITH ABNORMAL LIPID METABOLISM................................... 25510
 MYOPATHY WITH ABNORMALLY LARGE NUMBER OF MITOCHONDRIA   SEE PLEOCONIAL
    MYOPATHY (26290)
 MYOPATHY, CENTRONUCLEAR (MYOTUBULAR MYOPATHY)............................. 25520
 MYOPATHY, CENTRONUCLEAR (MYOTUBULAR MYOPATHY)............................. 31040
*MYOPATHY, CONGENITAL (BATTEN-TURNER TYPE)................................ 25530
 MYOPATHY, CONGENITAL, WITH CRYSTALLINE INTRANUCLEAR INCLUSIONS............ 16020
*MYOPATHY, DISTAL, WITH ONSET IN INFANCY................................. 16030
 MYOPATHY, DUE TO GLYCOLYTIC ABNORMALITY................................. 16040
*MYOPATHY, LATE DISTAL HEREDITARY....................................... 16050
 MYOPATHY, LIMITED TO FEMALES... 16060
 MYOPATHY, MITOCHONDRIAL, WITH SALT CRAVING   SEE MITOCHONDRIAL MYOPATHY
    WITH SALT CRAVING (25200)
 MYOPATHY, MYOTUBULAR   SEE MYOPATHY, CENTRONUCLEAR MYOTUBULAR MYOPATHY
    (25520, 31040)
 MYOPATHY, NEMALINE   SEE NEMALINE MYOPATHY (16180)
 MYOPATHY, WITH GIANT ABNORMAL MITOCHONDRIA............................. 25540
*MYOPIA... 16070
 MYOPIA   SEE OPHTHALMOPLEGIA, EXTERNAL, AND MYOPIA (31100), SPONDYLOEPI-

PHYSEAL DYSPLASIA, CONGENITAL TYPE (18390), ALPORT SYNDROME (10420),
ARTHRO-OPHTHALMOPATHY, HEREDITARY PROGRESSIVE (10830), DEAFNESS, COCH-
LEAR, ETC. (22120)
MYOPIA, HIGH GRADE, WITH ESSENTIAL HEMERALOPIA   ,SEE HEMERALOPIA, ESSEN-
TIAL, WITH HIGH GRADEMYOPIA (23490)
MYOPIA, INFANTILE SEVERE... 25550
MYOSCLEROSIS, CONGENITAL, OF LOWENTHAL................................... 25560
MYOSITIS OSSIFICANS PROGRESSIVA   SEE FIBRODYSPLASIA OSSIFICANS PROGRES-
SIVA (13510)
MYOTONIA   SEE KOK'S DISEASE (14940), GAMSTORP-WOHLFART SYNDROME (13720)
*MYOTONIA CONGENITA (ALSO SEE PARAMYOTONIA CONGENITA)..................... 16080
*MYOTONIA, GENERALIZED... 25570
MYOTONIC DYSTROPHY   SEE EPITHELIOMA, CALCIFICANS OF MALHERBE (13260),
RIEGER'S SYNDROME (18050), PARAMYOTONIA CONGENITA OF EULENBURG (16830),
PERIODIC PARALYSIS II, (HYPERKALEMIC TYPE (17060)
*MYOTONIC DYSTROPHY (STEINERT'S DISEASE)................................. 16090
*MYOTONIC MYOPATHY, DWARFISM, CHONDRODYSTROPHY, AND OCULAR AND FACIAL
ABNORMALITIES... 25580
MYOTUBULAR MYOPATHY   SEE MYOPATHY, CENTRONUCLEAR (25520, 31040)
MYSTAGMUS   SEE ALBINISM OCULAR (30050, 30060)
MYXEDEMA.. 25590
MYXEDEMA   SEE SCHMIDT'S SYNDROME (26920)
*NAEGELI'S SYNDROME... 16100
NAGER'S ACROFACIAL DYSOSTOSIS   SEE MANDIBULO-FACIAL DYSOSTOSIS WITH LIMB
ANOMALIES (15440)
NAIL DYSPLASIA   SEE DEAFNESS, ECTODERMAL DYSPLASIA, POLYDACTYLISM AND
SYNDACTYLISM (12460), FIBROMATOSIS, GINGIVAL (13530)
NAIL, ABNORMALITIES OF   SEE LYMPHEDEMA OF ADULT ONSET AND YELLOW NAILS
(15330)
NAILBEDS, PIGMENTATION OF... 16110
*NAIL-PATELLA SYNDROME.. 16120
NAILS   SEE PACHYONYCHIA CONGENITAL (16720)
NAILS, ABNORMALITIES OF   SEE ANONYCHIA-ECTRODACTYLY (10690), ECTODERMAL
DYSPLASIA (30510), EPIDERMOLYSIS BULLOSA WITH CONGENITAL LOCALIZED
ABSENCE OF SKIN (13200), NAIL-PATELLA SYNDROME (16120), BRACHYDACTYLY
(TYPE A5) (11290)
NAILS, SPOON   SEE KOILONYCHIA, HEREDITARY (14930)
NAILS, THICKENING OF   SEE ONYCHOLYSIS, PARTIAL, WITH SCLERONYCHIA (16480)
NANOCEPHALY   SEE BIRD-HEADED DWARF (21060)
NANOPHTHALMOS (PURE MICROPHTHALMOS)..................................... 16130
NARCOLEPSY... 16140
*NASAL GROOVE, FAMILIAL TRANSVERSE...................................... 16150
NAVICULAR BONE, ACCESSORY.. 16160
NECROBIOSIS LIPOIDICA AND PERIODONTOSIS................................ 16170
NECROTIZING ENCEPHALOPATHY   SEE LACTIC ACIDOSIS (24540)
*NECROTIZING ENCEPHALOPATHY, INFANTILE SUBACUTE........................ 25600
*NEMALINE MYOPATHY.. 16180
NEONATAL OBSTRUCTIVE JAUNDICE   SEE GIANT CELL HEPATITIS, NEONATAL (23110)
NEPHRITIS, FAMILIAL, WITHOUT DEAFNESS OR OCULAR DEFECT................. 16190
NEPHRITIS-DEAFNESS SYNDROME   SEE ALPORT SYNDROME (10420)
NEPHROBLASTOMA   SEE WILMS' TUMOR (27780)
NEPHROCALCINOSIS   SEE RENAL TUBULAR ACIDOSIS (17980, 26720, 31240)
*NEPHRONOPHTHISIS, FAMILIAL JUVENILE................................... 25610
NEPHROPATHY   SEE PHOTOMYOCLONUS (17250), NAIL PATELLA SYNDROME (16120),
OSTEOLYSIS, HEREDITARY, OF CARPAL BONES WITH NEPHROPATHY (16630),
ASPHYXIATING THORACIC DYSTROPHY OF THE NEWBORN (20850)
NEPHROPATHY, BALKAN OR DANUBIAN   SEE DANUBIAN ENDEMIC FAMILIAL NEPHROPA-
THY (12410)
NEPHROPATHY, FAMILIAL, WITH GOUT...................................... 16200
NEPHROSIS WITH DEAFNESS AND URINARY TRACT AND OTHER MALFORMATIONS...... 25620
*NEPHROSIS, CONGENITAL.. 25630
NEPHROSIS, CONGENITAL   SEE PULMONIC STENOSIS (26550)
NEPHROTIC SYNDROME   SEE MICROCEPHALY, ETC. (25130)
NERVE COMPRESSION SYNDROME   SEE NEUROPATHY, HEREDITARY, WITH LIABILITY
TO PRESSURE PALSIES (16250)
NERVOUS SYSTEM DISORDER RESEMBLING REFSUM'S DISEASE AND HURLER'S DISEASE...... 25640
*NETHERTON'S DISEASE.. 25650
NEURAMINICACIDURIA   SEE SIALURIA (26990)
*NEURITIS WITH BRACHIAL PREDILECTION.................................. 16210
NEUROARTHROMYODYSPLASIA (NEURAL TYPE OF ARTHROGRYPOSIS)   SEE ARTHROGRY-
POSIS MULTIPLEX CONGENITA (20810)
*NEUROAXONAL DYSTROPHY, INFANTILE (SEITELBERGER)...................... 25660
NEUROBLASTOMA.. 25670
*NEUROFIBROMATOSIS... 16220
NEUROFIBROMATOSIS   SEE ACOUSTIC NEUROMA, BILATERAL (10100)
*NEUROMATA, MUCOSAL, WITH ENDOCRINE TUMORS........................... 16230
NEUROPATHY   SEE AMYLOIDOSIS (10480, 10490)
*NEUROPATHY, CONGENITAL SENSORY, WITH ANHIDROSIS..................... 25680
*NEUROPATHY, HEREDITARY SENSORY RADICULAR........................... 16240
*NEUROPATHY, HEREDITARY, WITH LIABILITY TO PRESSURE PALSIES......... 16250
NEUROPATHY, HYPERTROPHIC OF DEJERINE-SOTTAS   SEE HYPERTROPHIC NEUROPATHY
OF DEJERINE-SOTTAS (14590)

*NEUROPATHY, PROGRESSIVE SENSORY, OF CHILDREN.................................. 25690
  NEUROPATHY, SENSORY   SEE DEAFNESS, NERVE TYPE, MESENTRIC DIVERTICULA,
    ETC. (22140)
  NEUROPATHY, WITH PARAPROTEIN IN SERUM, CEREBROSPINAL FLUID AND URINE.......... 16260
  NEURO-VISCERAL LIPIDOSIS   SEE GANGLIOSIDOSIS, GENERALIZED (23050, 23060)
  NEUROVISCERAL STORAGE DISEASE WITH CURVILINEAR BODIES......................... 25700
  NEUTROPENIA   SEE NEUTROPENIA, LETHAL CONGENITAL WITH EOSINOPHILIA
    (25710), AGRANULOCYTOSIS, INFANTILE GENETIC, OF KOSTMANN (20270),
    CHEDIAK-HIGASHI SYNDROME (21450), FANCONI'S PANCYTOPENIA (22790),
    GLYCINEMIA (23200)
*NEUTROPENIA, CHRONIC FAMILIAL... 16270
  NEUTROPENIA, CYCLIC... 16280
  NEUTROPENIA, LETHAL CONGENITAL, WITH EOSINOPHILIA........................... 25710
  NEVI   SEE MELANOSIS, NEUROCUTANEOUS (24940)
*NEVI (PIGMENTED MOLES)... 16290
*NEVI FLAMMEI, FAMILIAL MULTIPLE.. 16300
  NEVI HALO   SEE HALO NEVI (23430)
  NEVI, MULTIPLE   SEE MELANOMA, MALIGNANT (15560)
  NEVOID BASAL CELL SYNDROME   SEE BASAL CELL NEVUS SYNDROME (10940)
*NEVUS FLAMMEUS OF THE NAPE OF THE NECK....................................... 16310
  NEVUS SEBACEUS OF JADASSOHN... 16320
  NEVUS SEBACEUS, LINEAR, WITH CONVULSIONS AND MENTAL RETARDATION............. 16330
  NIELSON SYNDROME   SEE PTERYGIUM COLLI SYNDROME (17810)
*NIEMANN-PICK DISEASE (SPHINGOMYELIN LIPIDOSIS)............................... 25720
*NIEVERGELT SYNDROME... 16340
*NIGHT BLINDNESS, CONGENITAL STATIONARY (HEMERALOPIA)........................ 16350
*NIGHT BLINDNESS, CONGENITAL STATIONARY, WITH MYOPIA......................... 31050
  NIGHTBLINDNESS   SEE HEMERALOPIA, ESSENTIAL (23490)
*NIPPLES INVERTED (MAMMILLAE INVERTITA)...................................... 16360
  NIPPLES, ABSENCE OF   SEE BREASTS AND NIPPLES, ABSENCE OF (11370)
  NIPPLES, SUPERNUMERARY... 16370
  NOACK'S SYNDROME   SEE ACROCEPHALOPOLYSYNDACTYLY I (10120)
*NODAL RHYTHM... 16380
  NON-DISJUNCTION... 25730
  NON-HEME PROTEIN OF ERYTHROCYTE... 16390
  NONNE-MILROY DISEASE   SEE LYMPHEDEMA (15310)
  NON-SPHEROCYTIC HEMELYTIC ANEMIA   SEE ANEMIA, NONSPHEROCYTIC HEMOLYTIC
    (20620)
  NOONAN SYNDROME   SEE TURNER PHENOTYPE (19130)
NORRIE'S DISEASE (ATROPHIA BULBORUM HEREDITARIA PSEUDOGLIOMA)............... 31060
  NORUM'S DISEASE   SEE LECITHIN* CHOLESTEROL ACETYLTRANSFERASE (LCAT)
    DEFICIENCY (24590)
  NOSE, ANOMALOUS SHAPE OF ('POTATO NOSE').................................. 16400
  NOSE, ANOMALY OF   SEE ALAR-NASAL CARTILAGES, COLOBOMA OF, WITH TELECAN-
    THUS (20300)
  NOSE, BIFID   SEE BIFID NOSE (21040)
  NOSE, HYPOPLASIA OF   SEE ACRODYSOSTOSIS (10180)
  NOSEBLEEDS   SEE EPISTAXIS, HEREDITARY (13250), TELANGIECTASIA (18730)
  NYCTALOPIA   SEE NIGHT BLINDNESS (16350, 31050), HEMERALOPIA (23490)
  NYHAN SYNDROME   SEE HYPOXANTHINE GUANINE PHOSPHORIBOSYL TRANSFERASE
    DEFICIENCY (30800)
  NYSTAGMUS... 25740
*NYSTAGMUS... 31070
  NYSTAGMUS   SEE ZONULAR CATARACT AND NYSTAGMUS (31500), PHOTOMYOCLONUS
    (17250), ALBINISM, OCULAR (30050, 30060), LENTIGINES (15090), SPLIT-
    HAND WITH CONGENITAL NYSTAGMUS, ETC. (18380)
*NYSTAGMUS, CONGENITAL... 16410
  NYSTAGMUS, MYOCLONIC... 31080
  OASTHOUSE URINE DISEASE   SEE SMITH AND STRANG DISEASE (27050)
  OAV SYNDROME   SEE OCULO-AURICULO-VERTEBRAL DYSPLASIA (25770)
  OBESITY   SEE MACROSOMIA ADIPOSA CONGENITA (24810), PRADER-WILLI SYNDROME
    (26400)
  OBESITY-HYPOVENTILATION SYNDROME (PICKWICKIAN SYNDROME)................... 25750
  OCCIPITAL HAIR, WHITE LOCK OF... 31090
  OCHRONOSIS   SEE ALKAPTONURIA (20350)
  OCKERMAN'S DISORDER   SEE MANNOSIDOSIS
  OCULAR ALBINISM   SEE ALBINISM, OCULAR (30050, 30060)
*OCULAR MYOPATHY WITH CURARE SENSITIVITY.................................. 25760
  OCULAR PAIN   SEE PAIN SUBMANDIBULAR OCULAR AND RECTAL, WITH FLUSHING
    (16740)
  OCULO-AURICULO-VERTEBRAL DYSPLASIA (OAV SYNDROME* GOLDENHAR SYNDROME)..... 25770
*OCULOCEREBRAL SYNDROME WITH HYPOPIGMENTATION............................. 25780
  OCULO-CEREBRO-RENAL SYNDROME OF LOWE   SEE LOWE'S OCULO-CEREBRO-RENAL
    SYNDROME (30900)
OCULODENTODIGITAL DYSPLASIA (ODD SYNDROME) OCULO-DENTO-OSSEOUS SYNDROME... 16420
  OCULOMOTOR PALSY   SEE CRANIAL NERVES, RECURRENT PARESIS OF (21820)
  OCULO-OSTEO-CUTANEOUS SYNDROME.. 25790
*OCULOPHARYNGEAL MUSCULAR DYSTROPHY..................................... 16430
  ODD SYNDROME   SEE OCULODENTODIGITAL DYSPLASIA (16420)
  ODONTOGENIC KERATOCYSTS   SEE BASAL CELL NEVUS SYNDROME (10940)
  ODOR   SEE SMITH AND STRANG DISEASE (27050)
  ODOR, PECULIAR... 25800

SYNDROME (26570)
*OSTEOLYSIS, HEREDITARY MULTICENTRIC.. 25960
*OSTEOLYSIS, HEREDITARY, OF CARPAL BONES WITH NEPHROPATHY........................... 16630
OSTEOMAS OF MANDIBLE.. 16640
OSTEO-ONYCHO-DYSPLASIA HEREDITARIA (ALBUMINURICA)   SEE NAIL-PATELLA
   SYNDROME (16120)
OSTEOPATHIA STRIATA... 16650
OSTEOPENIA   SEE KYPHOSCOLIOSIS, OSTEOPENIA, CONGENITAL CONTRACTURES
   (14950)
*OSTEOPETROSIS ('MARBLE BONES,' OSTEOSCLEROSIS FRAGILIS GENERALISATA,
   ALBERS-SCHONBERG'S DISEASE)... 16660
*OSTEOPETROSIS ('MARBLE BONES,' ALBERS-SCHONBERG DISEASE)........................... 25970
*OSTEOPOIKILOSIS.. 16670
OSTEOPOROSIS   SEE HOMOCYSTINURIA (23620), AMINOACIDURIA WITH OTHER
   FEATURES (20480), FANCONI SYNDROME I (22770)
OSTEOPOROSIS, JUVENILE.. 25980
OSTEOSCLEROSIS   SEE OSTEOPATHIA STRIATA (16650), DWARFISM, CORTICAL
   THICKENING OF BONE AND TRANSIENT HYPOCALCEMIA (12700)
OTO-PALATO-DIGITAL (OPD) SYNDROME... 31130
OTO-RENO-GENITAL SYNDROME   SEE RENAL, GENITAL AND MIDDLE EAR ANOMALIES
   (26740)
OTOSCLEROSIS.. 16680
OVALOCYTOSIS, HEREDITARY HEMOLYTIC.. 16690
OVARIAN TUMOR... 16700
OVARIAN TUMOR   SEE ELLIS-VAN CREVELD SYNDROME (22550)
OVARY AND ADRENAL, 17-HYDROXYLATION DEFICIENCY IN   SEE ADRENAL HYPERPLA-
   SIA V (20210)
OWREN'S PARAHEMOPHILIA   SEE FACTOR V DEFICIENCY (22740)
OXALATE URINARY CALCULI   SEE HYPEROXALURIA (14490)
OXALOSIS   SEE HYPEROXALURIA (14490)
*OXALOSIS I... 25990
*OXALOSIS II.. 26000
OXYCEPHALY   SEE CROUZON'S CRANIOFACIAL DYSOSTOSIS (12350), ACROCEPHALO-
   SYNDACTYLY (10130), CRANIOSTENOSIS
OXYDASE VARIANTS   SEE ACHROMATIC REGIONS OF TETRAZOLIUM STAINED STARCH
   GELS (10090)
P BLOOD GROUP   SEE BLOOD GROUP-P SYSTEM (11140)
PA POLYMORPHISM OF ALPHA-2-GLOBULIN... 26010
PACHYDERMOPERIOSTOSIS (PRIMARY OR IDIOPATHIC HYPERTROPHIC OSTEOARTHROPATHY).. 16710
*PACHYONYCHIA CONGENITA... 16720
PACHYONYCHIA CONGENITA   SEE STEATOCYSTOMA MULTIPLE (18460)
PAGET'S DISEASE OF BONE... 16730
PAGET'S DISEASE, JUVENILE   SEE HYPEROSTOSIS CORTICALIS DEFORMANS JUVENI-
   LIS (23900)
PAIN, INSENSITIVITY TO   SEE INSENSITIVITY TO PAIN (24300)
PAIN, SUBMANDIBULAR, OCULAR AND RECTAL, WITH FLUSHING.............................. 16740
PAINE'S SYNDROME (MICROCEPHALY WITH SPASTIC DIPLEGIA).............................. 31140
PALATAL INVAGINATIONS   SEE DENS IN DENTE AND PALATAL INVAGINATIONS
   (12530)
PALATOPHARYNGEAL INCOMPETENCE... 16750
PALLIDAL DEGENERATION, PROGRESSIVE, WITH RETINITIS PIGMENTOSA...................... 26020
*PALLIDO-PYRAMIDAL SYNDROME... 26030
PALLIDUM ATROPHY, FAMILIAL PROGRESSIVE   SEE PALLIDO-PYRAMIDAL SYNDROME
   (26030)
PALMARIS LONGUS MUSCLE, ABSENCE OF.. 16760
PALMO-MENTAL REFLEX... 16770
*PANCREATIC INSUFFICIENCY AND BONE MARROW DYSFUNCTION (SHWACHMAN SYNDROME)..... 26040
PANCREATIC LIPASE, CONGENITAL ABSENCE OF   SEE LIPASE, CONGENITAL ABSENCE
   OF PANCREATIC (24660)
*PANCREATITIS, HEREDITARY... 16780
PANCYTOPENIA   SEE PANCREATIC INSUFFICIENCY AND BONE MARROW DYSFUNCTION
   (26040)
PANCYTOPENIA, FANCONI'S   SEE FANCONI'S PANCYTOPENIA (22790)
PAPILLAE, ABSENT FUNGIFORM   SEE DYSAUTONOMIA (22390)
PAPILLAE, PIGMENTED FUNGIFORM   SEE TONGUE, PIGMENTED FUNGIFORM PAPILLAE
   OF (18940)
PAPILLEDEMA   SEE INTRACRANIAL HYPERTENSION, IDIOPATHIC (24320), MACROCE-
   PHALY, PSEUDOPAPILLEDEMA (15350)
PAPILLOMA OF CHOROID PLEXUS... 26050
PAPILLOMATOSIS, FAMILIAL CUTANEOUS... 16790
PAPILLON-LEFEVRE SYNDROME   SEE KERATOSIS PALMO-PLANTARIS WITH PERIODON-
   TOPATHIA (24500)
*PARAGANGLIOMATA.. 16800
PARAHEMOPHILIA   SEE FACTOR V DEFICIENCY (22740)
PARALYSIS AGITANS   SEE PALLIDO-PYRAMIDAL SYNDROME (26030), PARKINSONISM
   (16860, 31150)
PARALYSIS AGITANS, JUVENILE, OF HUNT... 16810
PARALYSIS OF CRANIAL NERVES, CONGENITAL   SEE CRANIAL NERVES, CONGENITAL
   PARESIS OF (21810)
PARAMOLAR TUBERCLE OF BOLK.. 16820
PARAMYLOIDOSIS   SEE AMYLOIDOSIS I (10480)
PARAMYOCLONUS MULTIPLEX   SEE MYOCLONUS, HEREDITARY ESSENTIAL (15990),

PLATELET ABNORMALITIES, QUALITATIVE.. 17340
*PLATELET GROUPS.. 17350
PLATELETS, DEFECTS IN   SEE THROMBASTHENIA OF GLANZMANN AND NAEGELI
     (18780, 27380), SIDBURY SYNDROME (27000)
PLATELETS, DISORDERS OF   SEE THROMBASTHENIA THROMBOCYTOPENIA, HEREDITARY
     (18790), THROMBOCYTOPENIA (18800, 27390, 31390), HB KOLN (14170),
     VON WILLEBRAND'S DISEASE (19340), ALDRICH'S SYNDROME (30100), FANCONI'S
     PANCYTOPENIA (22790)
PLATYBASIA   SEE BASILAR IMPRESSION, PRIMARY (10950)
PLEOCONIAL MYOPATHY.. 26290
PNEUMOTHORAX, SPONTANEOUS.. 17360
POIKILODERMA CONGENITA   SEE ROTHMUND-THOMSON SYNDROME (26840)
POIKILODERMA, HEREDITARY SCLEROSING.. 17370
POLAND SYNDROME (OR POLAND'S SYNDACTYLY)... 17380
POLYCYSTIC KIDNEY   SEE CEREBRO-HEPATO-RENAL SYNDROME (21410)
POLYCYSTIC KIDNEY, CATARACT AND CONGENITAL BLINDNESS............................... 26310
POLYCYSTIC KIDNEY, CATARACT AND CONGENITAL BLINDNESS   SEE RENAL DYSPLA-
     SIA AND RETINAL APLASIA (26690)
*POLYCYSTIC KIDNEY, INFANTILE, TYPE I.. 26320
*POLYCYSTIC KIDNEYS.. 17390
POLYCYSTIC KIDNEYS   SEE MECKEL SYNDROME (24900)
*POLYCYSTIC KIDNEYS, MEDULLARY TYPE.. 17400
POLYCYSTIC LIVER   SEE POLYCYSTIC KIDNEYS (17390, 26320)
POLYCYTHEMIA   SEE HEMOGLOBIN CHESAPEAKE, HEMOGLOBIN YPSI (14170)
POLYCYTHEMIA RUBRA VERA.. 26330
POLYCYTHEMIA, BENIGN FAMILIAL, OF CHILDREN... 26340
POLYCYTHEMIA, BENIGN FAMILIAL   SEE ERYTHROCYTOSIS, BENIGN FAMILIAL
     (13310)
POLYDACTYLISM.. 26350
POLYDACTYLY   SEE ELLIS-VAN-CREVELD SYNDROME (22550), LAURENCE-MOON
     SYNDROME (24580), BIEMOND SYNDROME II (10970), ACROCEPHALOPOLYSYNDACTY-
     LY (10110, 20100)
POLYDACTYLY WITHOUT THUMB   SEE POLYDACTYLY, PREAXIAL III (17460)
POLYDACTYLY, IMPERFORATE ANUS, VERTEBRAL ANOMALIES................................. 17410
POLYDACTYLY, POSTAXIAL   SEE ELLIS-VAN CREVELD SYNDROME (22550),
     LAURENCE-MOON SYNDROME (24580), BIEMOND SYNDROME II (21030)
POLYDACTYLY, POSTAXIAL   SEE MECKEL SYNDROME (24900)
*POLYDACTYLY, POSTAXIAL (PROBABLY AT LEAST TWO TYPES)............................. 17420
POLYDACTYLY, POSTAXIAL, WITH MEDIAN CLEFT OF UPPER LIP............................ 17430
POLYDACTYLY, PREAXIAL   SEE TRIPHALANGEAL THUMB, OPPOSABLE (19070)
POLYDACTYLY, PREAXIAL I ('THUMB POLYDACTYLY')..................................... 17440
*POLYDACTYLY, PREAXIAL II (POLYDACTYLY OF TRIPHALANGEAL THUMB).................... 17450
*POLYDACTYLY, PREAXIAL III ('INDEX FINGER POLYDACTYLY')........................... 17460
*POLYDACTYLY, PREAXIAL IV (POLYSYNDACTYLY).. 17470
POLYDYSSPONDYLY   SEE COSTOVERTEBRAL SEGMENTATION ANOMALIES (12260)
POLYDYSTROPHIC OLIGOPHRENIA   SEE MUCOPOLYSACCHARIDOSIS TYPE III (25290)
POLYMASTIA   SEE NIPPLES, SUPERNUMERARY (16370)
POLYNEUROPATHY, HEREDITARY   SEE CHARCOT-MARIE-TOOTH DISEASE (11820)
POLYONCOSIS, HEREDITARY CUTANEOMANDIBULAR   SEE BASAL CELL NEVUS SYNDROME
     (10940)
POLYOSTOTIC FIBROUS DYSPLASIA.. 17480
*POLYPOSIS COLI, JUVENILE TYPE.. 17490
POLYPOSIS OF INTESTINE   SEE TURCOT SYNDROME (27630)
POLYPOSIS, FAMILIAL, OF ENTIRE GASTROINTESTINAL TRACT............................. 17500
*POLYPOSIS, INTESTINAL I (FAMILIAL POLYPOSIS OF THE COLON)........................ 17510
*POLYPOSIS, INTESTINAL II (PEUTZ-JEGHERS SYNDROME)............................... 17520
*POLYPOSIS, INTESTINAL III (GARDNER'S SYNDROME).................................. 17530
POLYPOSIS, INTESTINAL IV (SCATTERED, DISCRETE POLYPS)............................ 17540
POLYPOSIS, SKIN PIGMENTATION, ALOPECIA AND FINGERNAIL CHANGES (CRONKITE-
     CANADA SYNDROME)... 17550
POLYSACCHARIDE, STORAGE OF UNUSUAL... 26360
POLYSEROSITIS   SEE MEDITERRANEAN FEVER, FAMILIAL (24910)
*POLYSYNDACTYLY... 17560
*POLYSYNDACTYLY WITH PECULIAR SKULL SHAPE... 17570
POMPE'S DISEASE   SEE GLYCOGEN STORAGE DISEASE II (23230)
POPLITEAL PTERYGIUM SYNDROME   SEE PTERYGIUM COLLI SYNDROME (17810),
     CLEFT LIP-PALATE, MUCOUS CYSTS OF THE LOWER LIP, POPLITEAL PTERYGIUM,
     ETC. (11950)
POPLITEAL WEBBING   SEE CLEFT LIP AND-OR PALATE WITH MUCOUS CYSTS OF THE
     LOWER LIP (11930)
*POROKERATOSIS OF MIBELLI... 17580
*POROKERATOSIS, DISSEMINATED SUPERFICIAL ACTINIC (DSAP)........................... 17590
PORPHYRIA   SEE PROTOPORPHYRIA (17700), COPROPORPHYRIA (12130)
*PORPHYRIA, ACUTE INTERMITTENT (SWEDISH TYPE OF PORPHYRIA)....................... 17600
*PORPHYRIA, CONGENITAL ERYTHROPOIETIC (GUNTHER'S DISEASE)........................ 26370
PORPHYRIA, HEPATIC-CUTANEOUS TYPE (PORPHYRIA CUTANEA TARDA)...................... 17610
*PORPHYRIA, VARIEGATA (SOUTH AFRICAN TYPE OF PORPHYRIA).......................... 17620
PORTUGUESE AMYLOIDOSIS   SEE AMYLOIDOSIS I (10480)
PORT-WINE STAIN   SEE NEVUS FLAMMEUS OF THE NAPE OF THE NECK (16310)
POSTERIOR CLEFT OF LARYNX   SEE CLEFT LARYNX, POSTERIOR (21580)
POSTERIOR POLYMORPHOUS CORNEAL DYSTROPHY OF SCHLICHTING   SEE CORNEAL
     DYSTROPHY, HEREDITARY POLYMORPHOUS POSTERIOR (12200)

POSTMINIMI, PEDUNCULATED   SEE POLYDACTYLY, POSTAXIAL (17420)
*POTASSIUM AND MAGNESIUM DEPLETION (SEE ALSO PSEUDO-ALDOSTERONISM).............. 26380
POTASSIUM-SODIUM DISORDER OF ERYTHROCYTE.................................... 26390
PRADER-WILLI SYNDROME.. 26400
PREALBUMIN   SEE ANTITRYPSIN, ELECTROPHORETIC VARIANT OF SERUM (10740)
PREALBUMIN, POLYMORPHISM OF SERUM.. 17630
PRE-AURICULAR PITS   SEE BRANCHIAL CLEFT ANOMALIES, INCLUDING BRANCHIAL
    CYSTS (11360)
*PRECOCIOUS PUBERTY.. 17640
PRECOCITY, SEXUAL   SEE PINEALOMA WITH HYPERPINEALISM (26220)
PREGNANCY-ASSOCIATED GLOBULIN   SEE PA POLYMORPHISM (26010)
PREMOLAR HYPODONTIA   SEE BOOK'S SYNDROME, OR PHC SYNDROME (11230)
PRESENILE DEMENTIA   SEE ATAXIA WITH MYOCLONUS EPILEPSY AND PRESENILE
    DEMENTIA (20870), ALZHEIMER'S DISEASE OF BRAIN (10430), PICK'S DISEASE
    OF BRAIN (17270)
PRESENILE DEMENTIA WITH SPASTIC PARALYSIS.................................. 17650
PRESENILE DEMENTIA, KRAEPELIA TYPE... 17660
PRESSURE PALSIES   SEE NEUROPATHY, HEREDITARY, WITH LIABILITY TO PRESSURE
    PALSIES (16250)
PRIMORDIAL DWARFISM   SEE PITUITARY DWARFISM I (26240)
PROACCELERIN DEFICIENCY   SEE FACTOR V DEFICIENCY (22740)
PROACCELERIN EXCESS   SEE FACTOR V EXCESS WITH SPONTANEOUS THROMBOSIS
    (13440)
PROCTALGIA FUGAX   SEE PAIN, SUBMANDIBULAR OCULAR AND RECTAL WITH FLU-
    SHING (16740)
PROGERIA... 26410
*PROGNATHISM, MANDIBULAR... 17670
PROGRESSIVE BULBAR ATROPHY   SEE AMYOTROPHIC LATERAL SCLEROSIS (10540,
    20510)
PROGRESSIVE INFANTILE SPINAL MUSCULAR ATROPHY (WERDNIG-HOFFMANN)   SEE
    MUSCULAR ATROPHY, INFANTILE (25330)
PROGRESSIVE SPINAL MUSCULAR ATROPHY, JUVENILE   SEE MUSCULAR ATROPHY,
    JUVENILE (15860, 25340)
PROLIDASE VARIANTS   SEE PEPTIDASE VARIANTS (16970-17020)
PROLINEMIA   SEE HYPERPROLINEMIA TYPES I AND II (23950)
PROLINURIA   SEE IMINOGLYCINURIA (24260)
PRONATION-SUPINATION OF THE FOREARM, IMPAIRMENT OF......................... 17680
PROPIONICACIDEMIA   SEE GLYCINEMIA (HYPERGLYCINEMIA WITH KETOACIDOSIS AND
    LEUKOPENIA (23200)
PROPORTIONATE DWARFISM   SEE PITUITARY DWARFISM I (26240)
PRO-SPCA DEFICIENCY   SEE FACTOR VII DEFICIENCY (22750)
PROTANOPIA   SEE COLOR BLINDNESS, PARTIAL (30390)
PROTEIN INTOLERANCE   SEE DIBASICAMINOACIDURIA (12600, 22270)
PROTEIN, SERUM TYPES   SEE SERUM PROTEIN TYPES (18230)
PROTEIN-LOSING ENTEROPATHY   SEE LYMPHANGIECTASIA, INTESTINAL (15280)
PROTEINOSIS, LIPOID   SEE LIPOID PROTEINOSIS OF URBACH AND WIETHE (24710)
PROTEINURIA   SEE PERNICIOUS ANEMIA, JUVENILE (26110)
PROTEOLYTIC CAPACITY OF PLASMA... 17690
PROTHROMBIN CARDEZA   SEE DYSPROTHROMBINEMIA (12970)
PROTHROMBIN DEFICIENCY   SEE HYPOPROTHROMBINEMIA (24170)
PROTHROMBIN, DEFECT OF   SEE DYSPROTHROMBINEMIA (12790)
*PROTOPORPHYRIA, ERYTHROPOIETIC.. 17700
PROXIMAL FOCAL FEMORAL DEFICIENCY (PFFD)   SEE FEMUR-FIBULA-ULNA (FFU)
    SYNDROME (22820)
PRUNE BELLY SYNDROME   SEE ABDOMINAL MUSCLES, ABSENCE OF, WITH URINARY
    TRACT ABNORMALITY (10010)
PRURIGO BESNIER   SEE ATOPIC HYPERSENSITIVITY (20920)
PRURITUS, HEREDITARY LOCALIZED... 17710
PSEUDO-ACHONDROPLASTIC TYPE OF SPONDYLOEPIPHYSEAL DYSPLASIA   SEE SPONDY-
    LOEPIPHYSEAL DYSPLASIA (27170)
PSEUDO-ALDOSTERONISM (LIDDLE SYNDROME).................................... 17720
PSEUDO-ARTHROGRYPOSIS (HEREDITARY CONGENITAL RIGIDITY OF ELBOWS AND KNEES).... 17730
PSEUDOCHOLINESTERASE DEFICIENCY   SEE SUXAMETHONIUM SENSITIVITY (27240)
*PSEUDOCHOLINESTERASE TYPES, E(1) VARIANTS................................. 17740
*PSEUDOCHOLINESTERASE TYPES, E(2) VARIANTS................................. 17750
PSEUDOCHOLINESTERASE TYPES   SEE CHOLINESTERASE, REDUCTION IN RED CELL
    (11850)
PSEUDOCHOLINESTERASE, INCREASE IN PLASMA LEVEL OF......................... 17760
PSEUDO-CROUZON'S DISEASE   SEE CRANIAL DYSOSTOSIS WITH PRONOUNCED DIGITAL
    IMPRESSIONS (12280)
PSEUDOGLAUCOMA... 17770
PSEUDOGLIOMA.. 26420
PSEUDOGOUT   SEE CHONDROCALCINOSIS (11860)
PSEUDOHERMAPHRODITISM, MALE, WITH GYNECOMASTIA............................ 26430
PSEUDOHERMAPHRODITISM, MALE   SEE PSEUDOVAGINAL PERINEOSCROTAL HYPOSPA-
    DIAS (26460), HYPOGONADISM, MALE (24110, 30730)
PSEUDOHERMAPHRODITISM, MALE... 31210
PSEUDO-HURLER POLYDYSTROPHY   SEE MUCOLIPIDOSIS III (25260)
PSEUDOHYPOPARATHYROIDISM AND PSEUDO-PSEUDOHYPOPARATHYROIDISM   SEE AL-
    BRIGHT'S HEREDITARY OSTEODYSTROPHY (30080)
PSEUDOHYPOPHOSPHATASIA.. 26440
PSEUDOPAPILLEDEMA... 17780

RETINAL DYSPLASIA OF REESE   SEE REESE'S RETINAL DYSPLASIA (26640)
RETINAL DYSTROPHY   SEE CHOROIDEREMIA (30310), MACULAR DYSTROPHY (30910)
RETINAL DYSTROPHY, RETICULAR PIGMENTARY, OF POSTERIOR POLE................... 26780
RETINAL TELANGIECTASIA AND HYPOGAMMAGLOBULINEMIA............................. 26790
*RETINITIS PIGMENTOSA.. 26800
*RETINITIS PIGMENTOSA.. 31260
*RETINITIS PIGMENTOSA (RP)... 18010
RETINITIS PIGMENTOSA AND CONGENITAL DEAFNESS   SEE USHER SYNDROME (27690)
*RETINOBLASTOMA... 18020
*RETINOSCHISIS... 31270
RETINOSCHISIS WITH EARLY HEMERALOPIA.. 26810
RETRACTION SYNDROME   SEE DUANE SYNDROME (12680)
RHABDOMYOLYSIS, ACUTE RECURRENT... 26820
RHABDOMYOMA, CARDIAC   SEE TUBEROUS SCLEROSIS (19110)
RHEUMATOID ARTHRITIS.. 18030
RIBBING'S DISEASE (HEREDITARY MULTIPLE DIAPHYSEAL SCLEROSIS)................. 18040
RIBS, BIFID   SEE BASAL CELL NEVUS SYNDROME (10940)
RICHARD-RUNDLE SYNDROME   SEE KETOACIDURIA, ETC. (24510)
RICKETS   SEE HYPOPHOSPHATEMIA (30780), VITAMIN-D-RESISTANT RICKETS
    (19310)
RIEDEL'S SCLEROSING THYROIDITIS   SEE FIBROSCLEROSIS, MULTIFOCAL (22880)
*RIEGER'S SYNDROME (HYPODONTIA, MESOECTODERMAL DYSGENESIS OF IRIS AND
    CORNEA, AND MYOTONIC DYSTROPHY)... 18050
RILEY-DAY SYNDROME   SEE DYSAUTONOMIA, FAMILIAL (22390)
*RINGED HAIR (PILI ANNULATI).. 18060
*ROBERT'S SYNDROME (SEVERE ABSENCE DEFORMITIES OF LONG BONES OF LIMBS
    ASSOCIATED WITH CLEFT LIP-PALATE)...................................... 26830
ROBIN SYNDROME   SEE PIERRE ROBIN SYNDROME (26180, 31190)
ROBINOW DWARFISM... 18070
ROKITANSKY-KUSTER-HAUSER SYNDROME   SEE VAGINA, ABSENCE OF (27700)
ROMBERG SYNDROME   SEE HEMIFACIAL ATROPHY, PROGRESSIVE (14130)
'ROOTLESS TEETH'   SEE DENTINE DYSPLASIA (12540)
*ROTHMUND-THOMSON SYNDROME (POIKILODERMA ATROPHICANS AND CATARACT).......... 26840
ROTOR DISEASE   SEE HYPERBILIRUBINEMIA III (14370)
*ROUSSY-LEVY HEREDITARY AREFLEXIC DYSTASIA.................................. 18080
ROWLEY-ROSENBERG SYNDROME (GROWTH RETARDATION, PULMONARY HYPERTENSION AND
    AMINOACIDURIA)... 26850
RUBINSTEIN SYNDROME (BROAD THUMBS AND GREAT TOES, CHARACTERISTIC FACIES,
    MENTAL RETARDATION).. 26860
RUSSELL DWARFISM   SEE SILVER-RUSSELL DWARFISM (18240)
*RUTHERFURD'S SYNDROME... 18090
SABRE SHINS   SEE BOWING OF LEGS, ANTERIOR, WITH DWARFISM (21130)
SACCHAROPINURIA... 26870
SACRAL DEFECT WITH ANTERIOR SACRAL MENINGOCELE............................. 31280
SADDLE NOSE   SEE DEAFNESS WITH ECTODERMAL DYSPLASIA (12520), ROTHMUND-
    THOMSON SYNDROME (26840), ECTODERMAL DYSPLASIA ANHIDROTIC (30510)
SALT CRAVING   SEE MITOCHONDRIAL MYOPATHY WITH SALT CRAVING (25200)
SALT-LOSING SYNDROME   SEE ADRENAL HYPERPLASIA, HYPOADRENOCORTICISM
    (24020), HYPOALDOSTERONISM (20340)
*SANDHOFF'S DISEASE, OR GM(2) GANGLIOSIDOSIS TYPE II....................... 26880
SANFILIPPO SYNDROME   SEE MUCOPOLYSACCHARIDOSIS III (25290)
SARCOIDOSIS... 18100
SARCOMA   SEE CHONDROSARCOMA (21530)
SARCOMA, OSTEOGENIC   SEE OSTEOGENIC SARCOMA (25950)
SARCOSINEMIA.. 26890
SATELLITE ASSOCIATION RESULTING IN FAMILIAL CHROMOSOMAL MOSAICISM.......... 18110
*SC PHOCOMELIA SYNDROME.. 26900
SC(1) TRAIT OF SALIVA... 18120
SCALP AND SKULL, DEFECT OF   SEE APLASIA CUTIS CONGENITA (10760)
SCALP, ABSENCE DEFORMITY OF   SEE ABSENCE DEFECT OF LIMBS, SCALP AND
    SKULL (10030)
SCAPHOCEPHALY   SEE CRANIOSTENOSIS OR CRANIOSYNOSTOSIS (12310, 21850,
    21860)
SCAPULA, CONTOUR OF VERTEBRAL BORDER OF.................................... 18130
SCAPULA, HIGH   SEE SPRENGEL'S DEFORMITY (18440)
SCAPULOPERONEAL AMYOTROPHY.. 18140
SCHAMBERG'S DISEASE   SEE PIGMENTED PURPURIC ERUPTION (17290)
SCHEIE'S SYNDROME   SEE MUCOPOLYSACCHARIDOSIS V (25310)
SCHEUERMANN'S DISEASE   SEE OSTEODYSTROPHY AND MENTAL RETARDATION
SCHILDER'S DISEASE.. 26910
SCHIMKE SYNDROME (PTC SYNDROME)   SEE PHEOCHROMOCYTOMA AND AMYLOID PRODU-
    CING MEDULLARY THYROID CARCINOMA (17140)
SCHIZOPHRENIA... 18150
SCHMIDT'S SYNDROME (DIABETES MELLITUS, ADDISON'S DISEASE, MYXEDEMA)........ 26920
SCHOLZ' CEREBRAL SCLEROSIS   SEE CEREBRAL SCLEROSIS, DIFFUSE, SCHOLZ TYPE
    (30270)
SCHWARTZ-LELAK SYNDROME.. 26930
SCIMITAR SYNDROME   SEE ANOMALOUS PULMONARY VENOUS RETURN (10670)
*SCLERO-ATROPHIC AND KERATOTIC DERMATOSIS OF LIMBS......................... 18160
SCLEROCORNEA.. 18170
SCLEROCORNEA.. 26940
SCLERONYCHIA   SEE ONYCHOLYSIS, PARTIAL, WITH SCLERONYCHIA (16480)

(31110), HYDROCEPHALUS DUE TO CONGENITAL STENOSIS OF AQUEDUCT OF SYL-
VIUS (30700)
SPASTIC PARAPLEGIA AND RETINAL DEGENERATION...................................... 27070
SPASTIC PARAPLEGIA WITH AMYOTROPHY OF HANDS....................................... 18270
SPASTIC PARAPLEGIA WITH ASSOCIATED EXTRAPYRAMIDAL SIGNS......................... 18280
*SPASTIC PARAPLEGIA, HEREDITARY.. 27080
SPASTIC PARAPLEGIA, HEREDITARY   SEE LISSENCEPHALY SYNDROME (24720),
PALLIDO-PYRAMIDAL SYNDROME (26030)
SPASTIC PSEUDOSCLEROSIS (DISSEMINATED ENCEPHALOMYELOPATHY* CORTICOPALLIDO-
DEGENERATION).. 27090
SPATIAL VISUALIZATION, APTITUDE FOR.. 31300
SPATZ-HALLERVORDEN SYNDROME   SEE HALLERVORDEN AND SPATZ, SYNDROME OF
(23420)
*SPHEROCYTOSIS, HEREDITARY.. 18290
SPHEROPHAKIA   SEE WEILL-MARCHESANI SYNDROME (27760)
SPHEROPHAKIA-BRACHYMORPHIA SYNDROME   SEE WEILL-MARCHESANI SYNDROME
(27760)
SPHINGOMYELIN LIPIDOSIS   SEE NIEMANN-PICK DISEASE (25720)
SPIEGLER-BROOKE'S TUMORS   SEE EPITHELIOMA, HEREDITARY MULTIPLE BENIGN
CYSTIC (13270)
SPIEGLER-BROOKE'S TUMORS.. 31310
SPIELMEYER-VOGT DISEASE   SEE AMAUROTIC FAMILY IDIOCY, JUVENILE TYPE
(20420), SANDHOFF'S DISEASE (26880)
SPINA BIFIDA CYSTICA.. 27100
*SPINAL AND BULBAR MUSCULAR ATROPHY.. 31320
SPINAL ATAXIA   SEE HYPOGONADISM MALE, WITH ATAXIA (30740)
*SPINAL ATAXIA.. 31330
SPINAL EXTRADURAL CYST.. 27110
*SPINAL MUSCULAR ATROPHY, RYUKYUAN TYPE.. 27120
SPINOCEREBELLAR ATAXIA   SEE FRIEDREICH'S ATAXIA (13660, 22930), CEREBEL-
LAR ATAXIA (11720, 11730, 21290, 30250, 30260)
*SPINOCEREBELLAR ATAXIA AND PLAQUE-LIKE DEPOSITS................................... 18300
SPINOCEREBELLAR ATAXIA WITH EXTERNAL OPHTHALMOPLEGIA AND RETINAL DEGENERA-
TION   SEE OLIVOPONTOCEREBELLAR ATROPHY III (16450)
SPINOCEREBELLAR ATROPHY WITH PUPILLARY PARALYSIS.................................. 18310
*SPINO-PONTINE ATROPHY.. 18320
SPLEEN, ABSENCE OF (ASPLENIA SYNDROME).. 27130
*SPLENIC HYPOPLASIA... 27140
SPLENO-GONADAL FUSION WITH LIMB DEFECTS AND MICROGNATHIA.......................... 18330
SPLENOPORTAL VASCULAR ANOMALIES... 27150
SPLIT HAND WITH CLEFT PALATE AND LIP   SEE CLEFT LIP-PALATE WITH SPLIT
HAND AND FOOT (11940)
SPLIT HANDS AND FEET WITH PERCEPTIVE HEARING LOSS   SEE DEAFMUTISM AND
SPLIT HANDS AND FEET (22060)
SPLIT LOWER LIP.. 18340
SPLIT-HAND AND FOOT WITH HYPODONTIA... 18350
*SPLIT-HAND DEFORMITY... 18360
SPLIT-HAND DEFORMITY   SEE CLEFT HAND AND ABSENT TIBIA (11910)
SPLIT-HAND DEFORMITY WITH MANDIBULOFACIAL DYSOSTOSIS.............................. 18370
SPLIT-HAND WITH CONGENITAL NYSTAGMUS, FUNDAL CHANGES, CATARACTS.................. 18380
SPONDYLOCOSTAL DYSPLASIA   SEE COSTOVERTEBRAL SEGMENTATION ANOMALIES
(12260)
*SPONDYLO-EPIPHYSEAL DYSPLASIA, LATE.. 31340
*SPONDYLOEPIPHYSEAL DYSPLASIA, CONGENITAL TYPE.................................... 18390
*SPONDYLOEPIPHYSEAL DYSPLASIA, PSEUDO-ACHONDROPLASTIC TYPES....................... 18400
SPONDYLOEPIPHYSEAL DYSPLASIA, TARDA TYPE.. 18410
*SPONDYLOEPIPHYSEAL DYSPLASIA, TARDA TYPE... 27160
*SPONDYLOEPIPHYSEAL DYSPLASIA, PSEUDO-ACHONDROPLASTIC TYPES....................... 27170
SPONDYLOLISTHESIS AND SPINA BIFIDA OCCULTA.. 18420
SPONDYLOMETAPHYSEAL DYSOSTOSIS.. 27180
SPONDYLOSIS, CERVICAL.. 18430
SPONDYLOTHORACIC DYSPLASIA   SEE VERTEBRAL ANOMALIES (27730)
SPONGE KIDNEY   SEE POLYCYSTIC KIDNEYS, MEDULLARY TYPE (17400)
*SPONGY DEGENERATION OF CENTRAL NERVOUS SYSTEM.................................... 27190
SPOON NAILS   SEE KOILONYCHIA, HEREDITARY (14930)
SPRENGEL'S DEFORMITY ('HIGH SCAPULA')... 18440
SPRUE   SEE CELIAC SPRUE (11690)
STAPES FOOTPALATE FIXATION   SEE MITRAL REGURGITATION, CONDUCTIVE DEAF-
NESS, AND FUSION OF CERVICAL VERTEBRAE AND OF CARPAL AND TARSAL BONES
(15780)
STAPES FOOTPLATE FIXATION   SEE CLEFT PALATE, DEAFNESS, OLIGODONTIA
(21630)
STARTLE SYNDROME   SEE HYPER-REFLEXIA, HEREDITARY (14530)
*STEATOCYSTOMA MULTIPLEX (SEBACEOUS CYSTS, MULTIPLE).............................. 18450
*STEATOCYSTOMA MULTIPLEX WITH PACHYONYCHIA CONGENITA.............................. 18460
STEATORRHEA, IDIOPATHIC   SEE CELIAC SPRUE (11690), CYSTIC FIBROSIS
(21970)
STEATOSIS, FATAL NEONATAL HEPATIC   SEE FATTY METAMORPHOSIS OF VISCERA
(22810)
STEINERT'S DISEASE   SEE MYOTONIC DYSTROPHY (16090)
STEIN-LEVENTHAL SYNDROME.. 18470
STELLATE CATARACT   SEE CATARACT, OPACITY OF THE SUTURES (11650)

STENOSIS OF AQUEDUCT OF SYLVIUS   SEE HYDROCEPHALUS (23660)
STERNAL DEFORMITY   SEE HYPERTELORISM, ETC. (23970)
STERNUM, PREMATURE OBLITERATION OF SUTURES OF................................ 18480
STIFF FINGERS   SEE SYMPHALANGISM DISTAL (18570)
STIFF JOINTS   SEE OSTEOARTHROPATHY OF SCHINZ AND FURTWAENGLER (25900),
    MUCOPOLYSACCHARIDOSIS I, II, III, V AND VI (25280, 30990, 25290, 25310,
    25320)
STIFF SKIN SYNDROME.. 18490
STILLING-TURK-DUANE SYNDROME   SEE DUANE SYNDROME (12680)
STIPPLED EPIPHYSES   SEE CHONDRODYSPLASIA PUNCTATA (21510), THYROID
    HORMONE UNRESPONSIVENESS (27430)
STOLTZFUS BLOOD GROUP   SEE BLOOD GROUP-STOLTZFUS SYSTEM (11180)
STOMATOCYTOSIS.. 18500
STORAGE DISEASE LIKE HURLER'S   SEE MANNOSIDOSIS (24850)
STRABISMUS.. 18510
STRABISMUS   SEE DUANE SYNDROME, ALSO ABDUCENS PALSY (10020)
STREBLODACTYLY   SEE CAMPTODACTYLY (11420)
STREBLOMICRODACTYLY   SEE CAMPTODACTYLY (11420), CLINODACTYLY (11970)
*STRIAE DISTENSAE.. 18520
STRIATION OF BONE   SEE OSTEOPATHIA STRIATA (16650)
STUART FACTOR DEFICIENCY   SEE FACTOR X DEFICIENCY (22760)
STUB THUMB   SEE BRACHYDACTYLY, TYPE D (11320)
STURGE-WEBER SYNDROME.. 18530
SUBAORTIC STENOSIS, MUSCULAR   SEE VENTRICULAR HYPERTROPHY, HEREDITARY
    (19620)
SUBGLOTTIC BAR.. 18540
SUBLUXATION OF KNEE JOINT   SEE CAMPTODACTYLY (11420)
SUBMANDIBULAR PAIN   SEE PAIN, SUBMANDIBULAR, OCULAR AND RECTAL, WITH
    FLUSHING (16740)
SUCROSE INTOLERANCE   SEE DISACCHARIDE INTOLERANCE I (22290)
SUCROSE ISOMALTOSE MALABSORPTION   SEE DISACCHARIDE INTOLERANCE I (22290)
SUCROSURIA, HIATUS HERNIA AND MENTAL RETARDATION.......................... 27200
SUDANOPHILIC CEREBRAL SCLEROSIS.. 27210
SUDDEN DEATH   SEE CARDIAC CONDUCTION SYSTEM, DEFECT IN (11510), DEAFMU-
    TISM AND FUNCTIONAL HEART DISEASE (22030), VENTRICULAR FIBRILLATION
    WITH PROLONGED Q-T INTERVAL (19250)
SULFATIDE LIPIDOSIS   SEE METACHROMATIC LEUKODYSTROPHY, INFANTILE (25010)
*SULFATIDOSIS, JUVENILE, AUSTIN TYPE..................................... 27220
SULFITE OXIDASE DEFICIENCY   SEE SULFO-CYSTEINURIA (27230)
*SULFO-CYSTEINURIA (SULFITE OXIDASE DEFICIENCY).......................... 27230
*SUPRAVALVAR AORTIC STENOSIS... 18550
SUXAMETHONIUM RESISTANCE   SEE PSEUDOCHOLINESTERASE, INCREASE IN PLASMA
    LEVEL OF (17760)
SUXAMETHONIUM SENSITIVITY (PSEUDOCHOLINESTERASE DEFICIENCY)............... 27240
SWEAT GLAND TUMORS OF SKIN   SEE SYRINGOMAS, MULTIPLE (18660)
SWEATING EXCESSIVE   SEE HYPERHIDROSIS, GUSTATORY (14410)
SWEATY FEET DISEASE   SEE ISOVALERICACIDEMIA (24350), SIDBURY SYNDROME
    (27000)
SWEATY FEET, ODOR LIKE   SEE ISOVALERICACIDEMIA (24350), SIDBURY SYNDROME
    (27000)
SWEDISH TYPE PORPHYRIA   SEE PORPHYRIA, ACUTE INTERMITTENT (17600)
SWYER SYNDROME   SEE GONADAL DYSGENESIS XY FEMALE TYPE (30610)
SYMONDS-SHAW 'FAMILIAL CLAW FOOT WITH ABSENT DEEP TENDON REFLEXES'   SEE
    ROUSSY-LEVY HEREDITARY AREFLEXIC DYSTASIA (18080)
SYMPHALANGISM   SEE DIASTROPHIC DWARFISM (22260)
SYMPHALANGISM OF TOES.. 18560
*SYMPHALANGISM, DISTAL.. 18570
*SYMPHALANGISM, PROXIMAL (HEREDITARY ABSENCE OF THE PROXIMAL INTERPHALAN-
    GEAL JOINTS).. 18580
SYMPHYSIS PUBIS, WIDE SEPARATION OF   SEE CLEIDOCRANIAL DYSOSTOSIS (11970)
SYNDACTYLISM   SEE DEAFNESS, ECTODERMAL DYSPLASIA, POLYDACTYLISM AND
    SYNDACTYLISM (12460), LEUKONYCHIA TOTALIS (15160), ACROCEPHALOSYNDACTY-
    LY (10120-10160), HYPEROSTOSIS CORTICALIS GENERALISATA (23910)
SYNDACTYLY   SEE ECTODERMAL DYSPLASIA, ANHIDROTIC, WITH CLEFT LIP AND
    CLEFT PALATE (12940), HYPOTRICHOSIS, SYNDACTYLY AND RETINITIS PIGMENTO-
    SA (24200), OCULODENTODIGITAL DYSPLASIA (16420), POLAND SYNDROME
    (17380), SCLEROSTENOSIS (26950)
*SYNDACTYLY, TYPE I (ZYGODACTYLY)....................................... 18590
*SYNDACTYLY, TYPE II (SYNPOLYDACTYLY)................................... 18600
*SYNDACTYLY, TYPE III (RING AND LITTLE FINGER SYNDACTYLY)............... 18610
SYNDACTYLY, TYPE IV (HASS TYPE)... 18620
*SYNDACTYLY, TYPE V (SYNDACTYLY WITH METACARPAL AND METATARSAL FUSION)... 18630
SYNOSTOSES (TARSAL, CARPAL AND DIGITAL)................................. 18640
SYNOSTOSES, MULTIPLE, WITH BRACHYDACTYLY................................ 18650
SYNOSTOSIS   SEE HUMERORADIAL SYNOSTOSIS (23640)
SYNPOLYDACTYLY   SEE SYNDACTYLY, TYPE II (18600)
SYRINGOMAS, MULTIPLE.. 18660
SYRINGOMYELIA, LUMBOSACRAL.. 18670
SYSTEMIC CYSTIC ANGIOMATOSIS AND SEIP SYNDROME.......................... 27250
TABATZNIK HEART-HAND SYNDROME.. 18680
TALIPES EQUINOVARUS   SEE CLUB FOOT (11980)
TANGIER DISEASE   SEE ANALPHALIPOPROTEINEMIA (20540)

UTERINE MYOMATA   SEE LEIOMYOMATA, HEREDITARY MULTIPLE, OF SKIN (15080)
UVULA, BIFID (SPLIT UVULA, CLEFT UVULA)... 19210
VAGINA, ABSENCE OF (ROKITANSKY-KUSTER-HAUSER SYNDROME* UTERUS BIPARTITUS
    SOLIDUS RUDIMENTARIUS CUM VAGINA SOLIDA)................................... 27700
VAGINAL ATRESIA   SEE RENAL, GENITAL AND MIDDLE EAR ANOMALIES (26740)
VAGINAL SEPTUM   SEE HYDROMETROCOLPOS (23670)
VAGINAL SEPTUM, LONGITUDINAL   SEE BRACHYCAMPTODACTYLY (11240)
*VALINEMIA.. 27710
VALVULAR HEART DISEASE, CONGENITAL.. 31440
VAN BUCHEM'S DISEASE   SEE HYPEROSTOSIS CORTICALIS GENERALISATA (23910)
*VAN DEN BOSCH SYNDROME... 31450
VAN DER WOUDE SYNDROME   SEE CLEFT LIP AND-OR PALATE WITH MUCOUS CYSTS OF
    LOWER LIP (11930)
VARICOSE VEINS... 19220
VARICOSE VEINS   SEE VENULAR INSUFFICIENCY, SYSTEMIC (19270)
VASCULAR HELIX OF UMBILICAL CORD... 19230
VASOPRESSIN-RESISTANT DIABETES INSIPIDUS   SEE DIABETES INSIPIDUS, NEPH-
    ROGENIC (30480)
VEINS, PATTERN OF, ON ANTERIOR THORAX.. 19240
VENTRICLE, HYPOPLASIA OF RIGHT... 27720
*VENTRICULAR FIBRILLATION WITH PROLONGED Q-T INTERVAL............................. 19250
*VENTRICULAR HYPERTROPHY, HEREDITARY.. 19260
VENULAR INSUFFICIENCY, SYSTEMIC.. 19270
VERMIS OF CEREBELLUM, AGENESIS OF   SEE CEREBELLO-PARENCHYMAL DISORDER IV
    (21330)
VERTEBRAE   SEE CERVICAL VERTEBRAL BRIDGE (11800), KLIPPEL-FEILL SYNDROME
    (14890), CERVICAL VERTEBRAL FUSIONS (11810, 21430)
VERTEBRAE   SEE COSTOVERTEBRAL SEGMENTATION ANOMALIES (12260)
*VERTEBRAL ANOMALIES... 27730
VERTEBRAL ANOMALIES   SEE COSTOVERTEBRAL SEGMENTATION ANOMALIES (12260)
VERTEBRAL FUSION, POSTERIOR LUMBOSACRAL, WITH BLEPHAROPTOSIS...................... 19280
VERTEBRAL HYPOPLASIA WITH LUMBAR KYPHOSIS.. 19290
VERTIGO   SEE ATAXIA, PERIODIC VESTIBULO-CEREBELLAR (10850)
VERTIGO, EPISODIC   SEE MENIERE'S DISEASE (15600)
VESICOURETERAL REFLUX.. 19300
VESICOURETERAL REFLUX, NONOBSTRUCTIVE ("MEGACYSTIC SYNDROME")   SEE
    MEGADUODENUM AND-OR MEGACYSTIS (15530)
VESTIBULO-CEREBELLAR ATAXIA   SEE ATAXIA, PERIODIC VESTIBULO-CEREBELLAR
    (10850)
VISCEROMEGALY   SEE EMG SYNDROME (22560)
VISCEROMEGALY WITH UMBILICAL HERNIA AND MICROGLOSSIA   SEE EMG SYNDROME
    (22560)
VITAMIN B12 METABOLIC DEFECT... 27740
VITAMIN B6 DEPENDENCY   SEE PYRIDOXINE DEPENDENCY (26610)
VITAMIN D DEPENDENT RICKETS.. 27750
VITAMIN D DEPENDENT RICKETS   SEE PSEUDOVITAMIN D DEFICIENCY RICKETS
    (26470)
VITAMIN-B12, SELECTIVE MALABSORPTION OF   SEE PERNICIOUS ANEMIA, JUVENILE
    (26110)
*VITAMIN-D-RESISTANT RICKETS... 19310
VITAMIN-D-RESISTANT RICKETS   SEE HYPOPHOSPHATEMIA (30780)
VITELLIFORM DYSTROPHY   SEE MACULAR DEGENERATION, POLYMORPHIC (15370)
VITELLINE DEGENERATION OF MACULA   SEE MACULAR DEGENERATION, POLYMORPHIC
    (15370)
VITELLIRUPTIVE DYSTROPHY   SEE MACULAR DEGENERATION, POLYMORPHIC (15370)
VITILIGO.. 19320
VITREO-RETINAL DEGENERATION   SEE HYALOIDEO-RETINAL DEGENERATION OF
    WAGNER (14320)
VITREOUS DEGENERATION   SEE HYALOIDEO-RETINAL DEGENERATION OF WAGNER
    (14320)
VOGT'S CEPHALODACTYLY (APERT-CROUZON DISEASE)   SEE ACROCEPHALOSYNDACTYLY
    TYPE II (10130)
VON GIERKE'S DISEASE   SEE GLYCOGEN STORAGE DISEASE I (23220)
VON EULENBERG'S PARAMYOTONIA   SEE PARAMYOTONIA CONGENITA OF EULENBURG
    (16830)
*VON HIPPEL-LINDAU SYNDROME.. 19330
VON RECKLINGHAUSEN'S DISEASE   SEE NEUROFIBROMATOSIS (16220)
VON RECKLINGHAUSEN'S NEUROFIBROMATOSIS   SEE NEUROFIBROMATOSIS (16220)
*VON WILLEBRAND'S DISEASE.. 19340
VORTEX DYSTROPHY OF THE CORNEA   SEE ANGIOKERATOMA, DIFFUSE (30150)
VORTEX PILORUM   SEE HAIR WHORL (13940)
VROLIK TYPE OF OSTEOGENESIS IMPERFECTA   SEE OSTEOGENESIS IMPERFECTA
    CONGENITA (25940)
VROLIK TYPE OSTEOGENESIS IMPERFECTA   SEE OSTEOGENESIS IMPERFECTA CON-
    GENITA (25940)
*WAARDENBURG'S SYNDROME.. 19350
WAGNER'S DISEASE   SEE HYALOIDEO-RETINAL DEGENERATION OF WAGNER (14320)
WALDENSTROM'S MACROGLOBULINEMIA   SEE MACROGLOBULINEMIA, WALDENSTROM'S
    (15360)
WEB, ANTECUBITAL   SEE PTERYGIUM, ANTECUBITAL (17820)
WEBER-COCKAYNE TYPE OF EPIDERMOLYSIS BULLOSA   SEE EPIDERMOLYSIS BULLOSA
    OF HANDS AND FEET (13130)